Matteson & McConnell's
Gerontological Nursing
Concepts *and* Practice

THIRD EDITION

Adrianne Dill Linton, PhD, RN
Associate Professor and Chair
Department of Chronic Nursing Care
University of Texas Health Science Center at San Antonio
School of Nursing
San Antonio, Texas

Helen W. Lach, PhD, RN, CS
Assistant Professor
School of Nursing, College of Health Sciences
Saint Louis University
St. Louis, Missouri

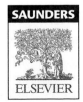

SAUNDERS

ELSEVIER

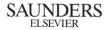

SAUNDERS
ELSEVIER

11830 Westline Industrial Drive
St. Louis, MO 63146

MATTESON & MCCONNELL'S GERONTOLOGICAL
NURSING: CONCEPTS AND PRACTICE, THIRD EDITION

ISBN-13: 978-1-4160-0166-9
ISBN-10: 1-4160-0166-2

Previous editions copyrighted 1997 and 1988.

ISBN-13: 978-1-4160-0166-9
ISBN-10: 1-4160-0166-2

Acquisitions Editor: Catherine Jackson
Developmental Editor: Amanda Sunderman Politte
Publishing Services Manager: Jeff Patterson
Senior Project Manager: Clay S. Broeker
Design Direction: Jyotika Shroff

Printed in the United States of America

Last digit is the print number: 9 8 7 6 5 4 3 2 1

To our families

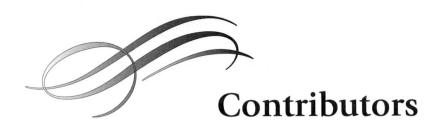

Contributors

Candace M. Ball, MS
PhD Candidate
Southern Illinois University Carbondale
Carbondale, Illinois

Anna J. Biggs, PhD, RN
Assistant Professor of Nursing
Saint Louis University
Doisy College of Health Sciences
School of Nursing
St. Louis, Missouri

Pamela Z. Cacchione, PhD, RN, BCGNP
Associate Professor
Saint Louis University School of Nursing
Gerontological Nurse Practitioner
Barnes-Jewish Extended Care
St. Louis, Missouri

Patrick J. Cacchione, MPA
President
Advocacy Strategies, Inc.
Co-founder and former Chair
Supportive Care of the Dying: A Coalition for
    Compassionate Care
St. Louis, Missouri

Elizabeth A. Capezuti, PhD, RN, FAAN
Associate Professor & Co-Director, The John A.
    Hartford Foundation Institute for Geriatric Nursing
Division of Nursing, The Steinhardt School of
    Education
New York University
New York, New York

David W. Carroll, MSN, RN
Clinical Instructor
University of Texas Health Science Center at San
    Antonio
San Antonio, Texas

Maria B. Carroll, MSN, RN, BC, GCNS
Gerontological Clinical Nurse Specialist
Barnes-Jewish Hospital
St. Louis, Missouri

James H. Cook, Jr., PhD, NCC, LPC
Behavioral Therapist
Saint Louis University
St. Louis, Missouri

Mary Z. Dunn, PhD, APRN, BC
University of Texas Health Science Center at San
    Antonio
School of Nursing
San Antonio, Texas

Coleen R. Elmers, RN, MSN
Leadership Educator
Baptist Health System
San Antonio, Texas

Julie K. Gammack MD
Assistant Professor, Division of Geriatric Medicine
Saint Louis University Health Science Center
St. Louis, Missouri

Lisa J. Hooter, RN, MSN, CDE
Staff Development Educator
St. Luke's Hospital
Baptist Health System
San Antonio, Texas

**Mary Ann House-Fancher ACNP, MSN,
    CCRN**
Acute Care Nurse Practitioner
Division of Cardiothoracic Surgery
University of Florida
Gainesville, Florida

Kathleen T. Lucke, PhD, RN
Assistant Professor
Department of Acute Nursing
University of Texas Health Science Center at San
    Antonio
San Antonio, Texas

Ronald J. Lynch, ARMP, MSN
Nurse Practitioner
Orlando Heart Center
Orlando, Florida

Pamela Millsap, MSN, RN
Research Instructor
Department of Neurology, Alzheimer's Disease
    Research Center
Washington University School of Medicine
St. Louis, Missouri

John E. Morley, MB, BCh
Dammert Professor of Gerontology
Director, Division of Geriatric Medicine
Saint Louis University Health Sciences Center
Director, GRECC
St. Louis VA Medical Center
St. Louis, Missouri

Carolyn D. Philpot, MSN(R), RN, GNP-BC
Clinical Assistant Professor
Geriatric Nurse Practitioner
Division of Geriatric Medicine
Saint Louis University Health Science Center
St. Louis, Missouri

Todd M. Ruppar, MSN(R), APRN, BC
Graduate Research Assistant
MU Sinclair School of Nursing
University of Missouri-Columbia
Columbia, Missouri

Susan A. Ruzicka, RN, PhD
Assistant Professor
University of Texas Health Science Center at San
    Antonio
School of Nursing
San Antonio, Texas

**Carrie M. Smith, MSN, RN, APRN, BC, ANP,
GNP**
Research Assistant
Saint Louis University
School of Nursing
St. Louis, Missouri

Jane Hsiao-Chen Tang, MSN, RN, PhD(c)
Project Director, Research Translation and
    Dissemination Core
Gerontological Nursing Interventions Research Center
Doctoral Candidate
University of Iowa College of Nursing
Iowa City, Iowa

Susan A. Taylor, BS, NHA
Nursing Home Administrator
National Health Care
Maryland Heights, Missouri

Marita G. Titler, PhD, RN, FAAN
Director, Research, Quality, and Outcomes
    Management
Department of Nursing Services and Patient Care
University of Iowa Hospitals and Clinics
Director, Research Translation and Dissemination Core
Gerontological Nursing Interventions Research Center
University of Iowa College of Nursing
Iowa City, Iowa

Nina Tumosa, PhD
Health Education Officer
St. Louis Veterans Affairs Medical Center
Professor
Internal Medicine/Geriatrics
Saint Louis University
St. Louis, Missouri

**Cheryl Lyn Zukerberg PhD, RN,C, PHN,
MSN, GNP**
Associate Professor
Gerontological Nursing Coordinator
Department of Baccalaureate Nursing
Biola University
La Mirada, California

Reflections Box Writers

Mary M. Austin, MSN, RN, NHA
President of Senior Pathways
Phoenixville, Pennsylvania

Elizabeth R.A. Beattie, PhD, RN, FGSA
Research Compliance Associate
Office of Human Research Compliance Review Office
    of the Vice President for Research
University of Michigan
Ann Arbor, Michigan
Adjunct Associate Professor
Adult and Gerontological Nursing
College of Nursing
University of Iowa
Iowa City, Iowa

Kathleen C. Buckwalter, PhD, RN, FAAN
Sally Mathis Hartwig Distinguished Professor of
    Nursing
Director, The University of Iowa John A. Hartford
    Center of Geriatric Nursing Excellence
University of Iowa
Iowa City, Iowa

Sandy C. Burgener, PhD, APRN-BC, FAAN
Associate Professor
College of Nursing
University of Illinois at Urbana-Champaign
Chicago, Illinois

Pamela Z. Cacchione, PhD, RN, BCGNP
Associate Professor
Saint Louis University School of Nursing;
Gerontological Nurse Practitioner
Barnes-Jewish Extended Care
St. Louis, Missouri

Yu-Ping Chang, PhD(c), MSN, RN
Nursing Instructor
Taiwan

**Deborah Marks Conley, MSN, APRN,BC, CS,
    FNGNA**
Certified Gerontological Clinical Nurse Specialist
Assistant Professor of Nursing
Nebraska Methodist Hospital & College
Omaha, Nebraska

Susan M. Davies, PhD MSc BSc RGN RHV
Senior Lecturer in Gerontological Nursing School of
    Nursing and Midwifery
Sheffield, United Kingdom

Karen S. Feldt, PhD, RN, GNP
Chief of Community Health
ERA Care Communities
Seattle, Washington

Geri R. Hall, PhD, ARNP, CNS, FAAN
Clinical Professor and Advanced Practice Nurse
University of Iowa College of Nursing
Iowa City, Iowa

J Taylor Harden, RN, PhD, FAAN
Assistant to the Director for Special Populations
National Institute on Aging National Institutes of
    Health
Bethesda, Maryland

Sheila Hoffmeister
St. Louis, Missouri

Kathryn A. Houston, GNP
Private Practice
St. Louis, Missouri

Rebecca A. Lorenz, RN, MHS, PhD(c)
Saint Louis University
St. Louis, Missouri
Funded by the National Institute of Nursing Research

Sithokozile Maposa, RN, BA, MSN
Community Health Nurse
Zimbabwe

Mary Ann Matteson, PhD, RN
Professor Emerita
School of Nursing
University of Texas Health Science Center
San Antonio, Texas

Eleanor S. McConnell, RN, PhD, APRN, BC
Associate Professor
Duke University School of Nursing
Clinical Nurse Specialist
Geriatric Research, Education and Clinical Center
Department of Veterans Affairs Medical Center
Durham, North Carolina

Marsha McGuire, RN, BC, GCNS, CWOCN
Geriatric Clinical Nurse Specialist
Wound, Ostomy, Continence Nurse
Saint Louis University Hospital
St. Louis, Missouri

Deanna Gray Miceli, DNSc, APRN, FAANP
Adjunct Assistant Professor
University of Pennsylvania
Philadelphia, Pennsylvania

Marilyn Pattillo, PhD, RN, APRN
Gerontological Nurse Practitioner
University of Texas at Austin
School of Nursing
Austin, Texas

Catherine C. Powers, MSN, APRN, BC
Clinical Nurse Specialist
Barnes-Jewish Hospital
One Barnes-Jewish Hospital Plaza
St. Louis, Missouri

Debra L. Schutte, PhD RN
Assistant Professor
Adult & Gerontology Area of Study
The University of Iowa College of Nursing
Iowa City, Iowa

May L. Wykle, PhD, RN, FAAN, FGSA
Dean and Florence Cellar Professor of Gerontological
    Nursing Frances
Payne Bolton School of Nursing
Case Western Reserve University
Cleveland, Ohio

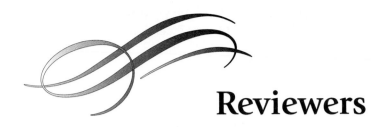

Reviewers

Margaret T. Bowers, RN, MSN, APRN, BC
Assistant Clinical Professor
School of Nursing and Division of Cardiovascular
 Medicine
Duke University Health System
Durham, North Carolina

Charles E. Brady III, MD
Associate Professor of Medicine
Internal Medicine
University of Texas Health Science Center at San
 Antonio
San Antonio, Texas

Tracy Brady, RN, BSN
Nurse Consultant
San Antonio, Texas

Joan K. Carter, PhD, RN
Professor Emeritus
Saint Louis University School of Nursing
St. Louis, Missouri

Kathleen B. Colling, PhD, RN
Assistant Research Scientist and Faculty
University of Michigan School of Nursing
Ann Arbor, Michigan

Laurie Flint Dodge, MSN, APRN, ANP, GNP
Gerontologic Nurse Practitioner Program Coordinator
Department of Family Nursing Care
University of Texas Health Science Center at San
 Antonio
San Antonio, Texas

Lois Kazmier Halstead PhD, RN
Associate Dean, College of Nursing
Rush University
Chicago, IL

Kris L'Ecuyer, RN, MSN, CCNS
Associate Professor of Nursing
Saint Louis University School of Nursing
St. Louis, Missouri

Geralyn Meyer, PhD, RN
Assistant Professor
Saint Louis University School of Nursing
St. Louis, Missouri

Jessica Pitts, RN, MSN, CS
Post-Master's Student, Nursing
University of North Carolina at Chapel Hill
Chapel Hill, North Carolina

Janet Specht, PhD, RN
Associate Professor
University of Iowa
Iowa City, Iowa

Marilyn Sullivan, RN, DSN
MSN Program Director
Graduate School of Nursing
Our Lady of the Lake College
Baton Rouge, Louisiana

**Carol Ann Hricz Townsend, RN, BSN, MSN,
 GNP, BC**
Geriatric Nurse Practitioner
VA Gainesville
Gainesville, Florida

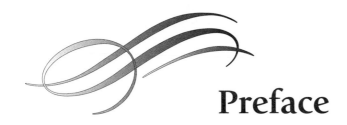

Preface

The first edition of *Gerontological Nursing: Concepts and Practice* was published in 1988. It was written to provide a comprehensive, research-based reference for nurses who cared for and about older adults. Almost 20 years later, the need for such a text is greater than ever. The aging population continues to grow, creating challenges, opportunities, and a demand for more nurses prepared in this specialty. In addition, generalist nurses continue to seek sources of information to guide their practice because the populations being served in all settings of care reflect our changing demographics.

Since the inception of this book, the base of research in gerontological nursing and care of older adults has dramatically increased. A primary goal of this text is to provide a comprehensive survey of the literature both from nursing as well as our colleagues in psychology, sociology, public health and medicine to build a holistic view of aging and health. This book describes the aging process across the health care continuum from wellness to illness. Physiological, sociological, and psychological aspects of aging are described in detail, as well as assessment and practice in all settings using the nursing process.

This book is organized into six sections. Section 1 provides an introduction to practice in gerontological nursing, describing issues and trends in the field, assessment of the older adult, and the use of nursing research and theory in practice. Section 2 is an exploration of the foundations of gerontological nursing practice from other fields including gerontology, ethics, nutrition, and pharmacology. Section 3 addresses physiological changes and needs of older persons. A systems approach is used to describe physiological aging changes,

health maintenance and promotion, common conditions in the older adult, and relevant nursing care. Special attention is given to research, differentiating between changes related to age and those related to lifestyle or pathology. The nursing process is applied as detailed nursing assessment is presented, followed by common nursing diagnoses, related interventions, and evaluation criteria. Sample care plans using NANDA, NOC, and NIC classifications are included. Section 4 covers key aspects of aging from the psychological and social perspectives as well as issues at the end of life. Section 5 addresses important competencies nurses need to fulfill clinical and leadership roles in gerontological nursing practice. Section 6 explores gerontological nursing across the continuum of care settings, including the community, assisted living, acute care, subacute care, and long-term care.

At the outset, we viewed this third edition as an update of the second edition. However, we quickly found that the incredible advances in our understanding of aging and health care merited a much more complete revision. Therefore, this edition contains a completely new literature review, updated references, and new content areas. Extensive reference lists reflect a thorough review of the recent literature in nursing, medicine, and social science. We have reorganized the presentation of aging changes and nursing care by system or domain to minimize repetition and ensure better readability for both students and busy practitioners. Throughout the book, tables are used to summarize theoretical and practice concepts for easy accessibility, and numerous assessment forms are reproduced to provide a comprehensive reference.

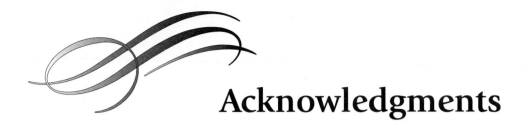

Acknowledgments

We would like to thank our families, friends, and colleagues who have supported us during the revision process. We especially thank our contributors who have shared their expertise with us and those who contributed to earlier versions of this text. We are also grateful to Amanda Politte, developmental editor, for her professional editorial guidance, support, and patience; Catherine Jackson, acquisitions editor; Heather Bays, editorial assistant; and Clay Broeker, project manager. Tracy Brady provided important technical assistance. Last, but certainly not least, we express appreciation to Drs Mary Ann Matteson and Eleanor McConnell whose vision and hard work made the first edition a reality and paved the way for subsequent editions.

Adrianne Dill Linton
Helen W. Lach

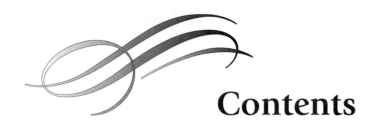

Contents

Section Two Foundations of Gerontological Nursing Practice, 123

Chapter 13 Respiratory System, 353
Adrianne Dill Linton

Chapter 14 Neurological System, 406
Pamela Millsap

Chapter 19 Age-Related Changes in the Special Senses, 600
Adrianne Dill Linton

Section Four Psychosocial Aging, 629

Chapter 20 Age-Related Psychological Changes, 631
David W. Carroll & Adrianne Dill Linton

Chapter 22 End of Life Care of the Older Adult, 712
Pamela Z. Cacchione & Patrick J. Cacchione

Section Five Competencies and Roles in Gerontological Nursing, 737

Chapter 23 Leadership Skills, 739
Nina Tumosa & Helen W. Lach

Chapter 26 Case Management, 777
Todd M. Ruppar

Chapter 27 Health Promotion and Health Education for Older Adults, 785
Helen W. Lach

Chapter 28 Quality Improvement, 810

Carolyn D. Philpot, Julie K. Gammack, Susan J. Taylor, & John E. Morley

Section Six Gerontological Nursing in the Context of Care, 825

Chapter 29 The Geriatric Continuum of Care, 827

Susan A. Ruzicka

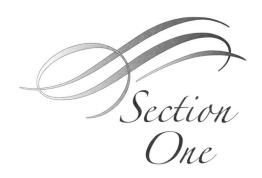

Section One

Introduction to Practice in Gerontological Nursing

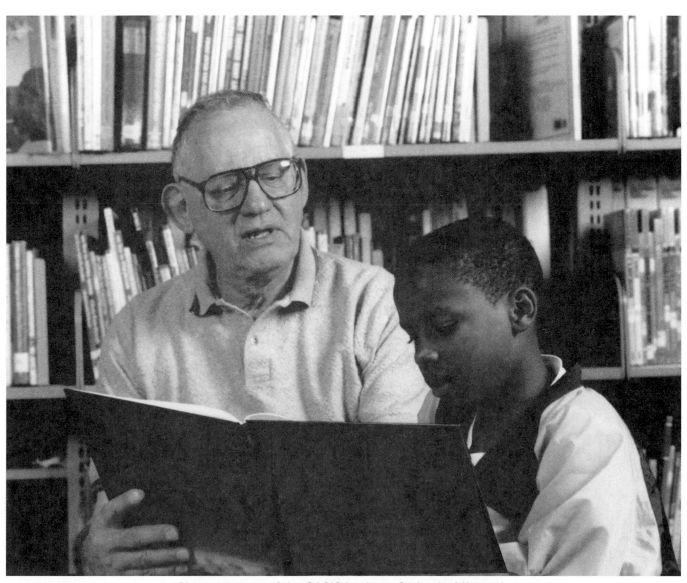

Chapter 1

Gerontological Nursing: Issues and Trends in Practice

Helen W. Lach

Objectives

Define gerontological nursing and place in the context of practice.
Trace the history of gerontological nursing and its influence on health care of the older adult.
Examine the roles and competencies for gerontological nurses.
Explore trends in gerontological nursing.

There has never been a more exciting time in gerontological nursing. We stand at the beginning of a century that will see huge growth in the number of older adults. Figure 1-1 illustrates the projected growth of the older adult population through the first half of the twenty-first century, as baby boomers reach later adulthood. Already the majority of patients in the hospital and nursing homes, as well as a good portion of home care patients, are age 65 and older. Those of us committed to providing quality health care to this burgeoning population are bracing ourselves for the onslaught and hoping for increasing support for our knowledge and skills.

The possibilities are great, with increasing opportunities for practice in a variety of roles and settings. Advanced practice nurses with geriatric and gerontological expertise will be especially poised to provide consultation and care in a variety of settings. Faculty with expertise in aging will be in great demand. As gerontological nurses, we will be limited only by our own creativity as we move forward to face the future. We are challenged to spread our expertise to all nurses. This chapter defines and explores the scope of gerontological nursing, as well as its possibilities, by examining its past, present, and future.

DEFINING GERONTOLOGICAL NURSING

Older adults are an extremely diverse group of individuals who possess a broad range of abilities and needs in all domains of function. This reality, along with the varied lifestyles, environmental conditions, and life histories characteristic of older adults, creates the need for highly individualized nursing care. Nursing of the elderly is thus a complex specialty—one that must allow for many different perspectives and accommodate diverse research findings and theoretical approaches.

Gunter and Estes in 1979 provided a definition of gerontological nursing that is still salient today: "a health service that incorporates generic nursing methods and specialized knowledge about the aged to establish conditions within the [patient] and within the environment that will do the following:

1. Increase health-promoting behaviors in the aged
2. Minimize and compensate for health-related losses and impairments related to aging
3. Provide comfort and sustenance through the distressing and debilitating events of aging, including dying and death
4. Facilitate the diagnosis, palliation, and treatment of disease in the aged" (pp. 91-92)

To devise a complete definition of gerontological nursing practice, the various environments in which gerontological nursing is practiced must be considered, along with how they influence the process and outcomes of gerontological nursing. Additionally, the following factors affect the practice of gerontological nursing:

1. Characteristics of the recipients of gerontological nursing

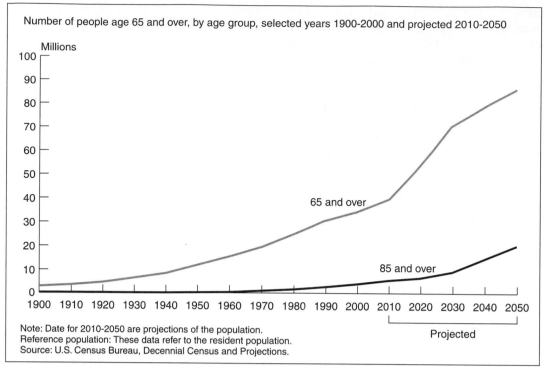

Number of people age 65 and over, by age group, selected years 1900-2000 and projected 2010-2050

Note: Date for 2010-2050 are projections of the population.
Reference population: These data refer to the resident population.
Source: U.S. Census Bureau, Decennial Census and Projections.

Figure 1-1   Changing demographics in the United States. Number of people ages 65 and older, by age group, 1900 to 2000 and projected 2010 to 2050. (Reprinted from Federal Interagency Forum on Aging-Related Statistics. [2004]. *Older Americans 2004: Key indicators of well-being.* Washington, DC: Federal Interagency Forum.)

2. The environment in which health care is delivered
3. Essential knowledge and competencies of gerontological nurses
4. Roles and standards for care
5. Application of the nursing process to care of the older adult: assessment, nursing diagnosis, nursing interventions, and nursing-sensitive outcomes

This section provides an overview of the first two factors; later in this chapter, roles and foundations for gerontological nursing are explored. It is beyond the scope of this chapter to address all of the issues in gerontological nursing. However, later sections address specific nursing issues related to aging changes, health problems, roles and competencies, and specific settings.

The Aging Population

During the last century, declines in mortality rates from medical and public health efforts have resulted in increased life expectancy and a growing older population. Today, one in eight Americans is over age 65, and those who reach that age can expect to live an additional 18.1 years (Administration on Aging [AOA], 2004). Women outnumber men, and women are more likely to be single and live alone. Aging is thus considered an important women's health issue.

The older population is expected to more than double over the next two decades as the baby boomer cohort contributes a bulge in population growth that will begin in 2012 and reach its peak in 2029 (Manton, 2003). The fastest growing group is the oldest of the old, those over 85, who will increase to 9.6 million by 2030. Minority populations are projected to grow at faster rates than the white population, which will increase the cultural diversity among older people. Life expectancy is not likely to increase further; however, some believe that advances in medicine may continue this trend (Merck Institute, 2002).

Patterns of Health and Disease among Older Adults

The older population continues to experience greater health problems and use more of the health care budget than other age-groups. Although the mortality rates for the leading causes of death have decreased, they continue to remain the major killers of older adults. Heart disease, cancer, and stroke accounted for 60% of deaths among older Americans in 2000 (Merck Institute, 2002). The hospitalization rate for older adults is more than three times the comparable rate for younger adults, and they average more doctor visits (AOA, 2004). Although only about 4.5% of older people live in nursing homes, the rate increases with advancing age so that 18.2% of adults age 85 and older live in nursing homes. A recent study of noninstitutionalized people found higher medication rates for older adults. The highest rate was among women over 65, with 57% taking 5 or more medications and 12% taking 10 or more medications (Kaufman, Kelly, Rosenberg, Anderson, & Mitchell, 2002).

Chronic versus acute disease is an important way to characterize disease patterns in the elderly (Figure 1-2). The majority of older adults have at least one chronic condition, and most suffer from more than one. Of the population approaching older age, 89% have risk factors for developing chronic conditions such as being overweight, smoking, getting little exercise, and having high cholesterol (National Academy on an Aging Society, 2000). The impact of chronic diseases is related to the severity of the disease, the treatment options available, and the support for self-management of disease symptoms (Bennett & Flaherty-Robb, 2003). Because of the growing impact of chronic illness, health care will need to move increasingly toward community-based care and away from institutional care (Quinn et al., 2004).

Along with chronic disease, older adults suffer disproportionately from functional disability, with over half (52.5%) of individuals over 85 limited in their activity because of chronic conditions (AOA, 2004). Despite the high number of older people with disabilities, the rates have actually declined, as shown in Figure 1-3 (Merck Institute, 2002), suggesting that management of disease and underlying health of the aged may be improving.

With the growing population, appropriate resources could help minimize the impact of chronic disease (Bennett & Flaherty-Robb, 2003). On the other hand, the growing population may mean significant increases in the numbers of people with chronic disease and resulting disabilities.

Mental health problems in older adults have always been underrecognized and undertreated. The older patient is less likely to receive treatment for mental health problems from either inpatient or community-based mental health providers (Merck Institute, 2002). At the same time, the mortality rate attributed to suicide for men over age 65 remains the highest of any age-group. It is anticipated that in the coming decades the number of older adults with major psychiatric disorders will increase to 15 million individuals (Merck Institute, 2002).

Minority elders tend to have increased risk of illness and disability across the later years. Non-Hispanic blacks and Hispanics are less likely to report having good health than whites, but they are more likely to experience the top chronic health conditions and to have difficulty performing activities of daily living than their white counterparts (Federal Interagency Forum, 2000). In addition, minorities are less likely to have insurance or access to care. Reducing health disparities among all age-groups, including older adults, will increasingly become a national priority (Office of Minority Health, 2002).

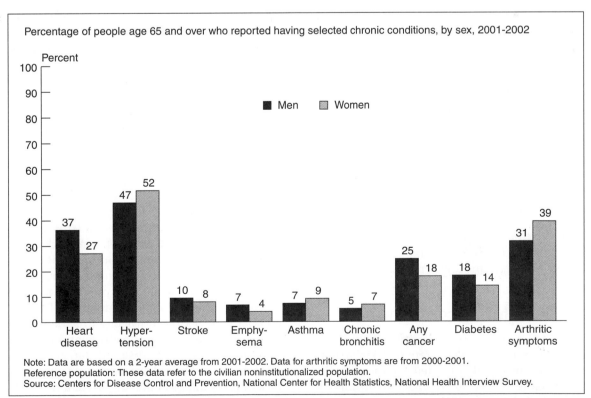

Percentage of people age 65 and over who reported having selected chronic conditions, by sex, 2001-2002

Note: Data are based on a 2-year average from 2001-2002. Data for arthritic symptoms are from 2000-2001.
Reference population: These data refer to the civilian noninstitutionalized population.
Source: Centers for Disease Control and Prevention, National Center for Health Statistics, National Health Interview Survey.

Figure 1-2 High prevalence of chronic disease. (Reprinted from Federal Interagency Forum on Aging-Related Statistics. [2004]. *Older Americans 2004: Key indicators of well-being.* Washington, DC: Federal Interagency Forum.)

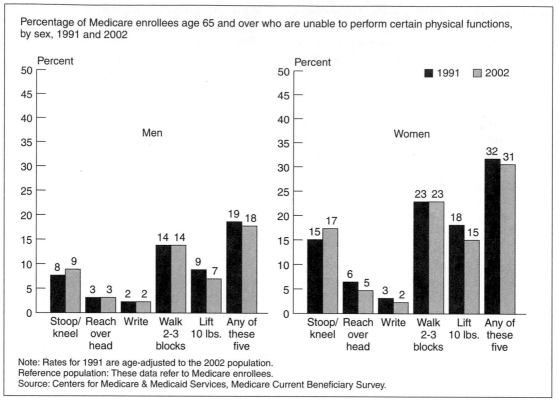

Percentage of Medicare enrollees age 65 and over who are unable to perform certain physical functions, by sex, 1991 and 2002

Note: Rates for 1991 are age-adjusted to the 2002 population.
Reference population: These data refer to Medicare enrollees.
Source: Centers for Medicare & Medicaid Services, Medicare Current Beneficiary Survey.

Figure 1-3 Indicators of disability in the older population. (Reprinted from Federal Interagency Forum on Aging-Related Statistics. [2004]. *Older Americans 2004: Key indicators of well-being.* Washington, DC: Federal Interagency Forum.)

A Healthier View of Aging

Although the statistics often present a dim view of aging, the reality is that a large percentage of older adults live active and productive later years. Only 4.5% of people over 65 live in nursing homes; an additional 5% report living in some kind of senior housing, which may have supportive services (AOA, 2004). Nearly three quarters (72%) report their health to be good, very good, or excellent (Federal Interagency Forum, 2000), despite the presence of chronic conditions. For the older population, 4 of the 10 *Healthy People 2000* targets were met: increased mammography, colorectal screening, flu vaccinations, and smoking cessation (AOA, 2004). If health trends continue to improve, future cohorts may experience healthier old age, increasing the demand for preventive and health promotion services.

Context of Health Services to the Aged

Nursing care of the older adult takes place within the environment of a complex health care delivery system. A fragmented and medically oriented system of health care has predictable effects on the practice of nursing, such as demands for greater clinical nursing sophistication and an ability to see the nursing role broadly, including providing advocacy for older patients.

Tremendous tension exists between the health system problems and the fact that many nurses caring for older adults have little formalized training in care of the aged. The result of poor preparation in nursing care of the elderly is nurses who are frustrated when the care provided fails to solve patient problems and is perceived by patients and families as inadequate.

The specialized knowledge required to assess and treat the older adult has been developing through research and care over the past few decades, and continues to build as new geriatric nursing scientists are trained. Unfortunately, health professionals inaccurately assume that they already know how to care for the elderly because they have older patients in their practice or setting (Drinka, 2002). This provides a barrier to increasing content on gerontological nursing into broader education and training for nurses at all levels. In addition, few faculty are prepared to develop and teach gerontology content (Burggraf & Barry, 1998). To combat this lack of knowledge in geriatric care, efforts are needed at all levels of nursing and in all settings to develop and share expertise.

Numerous studies have documented and decried the lack of gerontological nursing content in nursing curricula at both the baccalaureate and associate degree levels that persists into the twenty-first century. Although most schools now report some gerontological content in their curriculum, few offer stand-alone courses (Grocki & Fox, 2004). Curricula integrating gerontology may not provide adequate content. The inclusion of required stand-alone courses in gerontological nursing may increase students' interest in the specialty by increasing its visibility (Lindeman, 2000). One champion for increasing visibility and education in gerontological nursing has been the John A. Hartford Foundation, investing $35 million to support academic preparation, practice, and research capacity (Mezey & Fulmer, 2002).

Another area of conflict in nursing care for the older population is nursing's well-conceived and long-standing commitment to considering both the wellness and illness needs of patients. Despite this, nurses are frequently in the position of having to focus on only a narrow portion of an individual patient's problems because of the goals of the systems in which they work. This adds to the frustration of working with older people, because there is a gap between what should be and what is feasible in many practice settings.

For example, in the acute care setting, the major focus is on diagnosis and treatment of acute medical problems, with little attention to the impact of testing and treatment on the older patient. Nurses who work with older patients in the hospital need time and expertise to assess the patient's responses and prevent functional losses. The nurse in the hospital setting is in the best position to assess and monitor changes in a patient's function and to intervene to promote maintenance of functional independence. Once function is lost in the acute care setting, there is little opportunity to assist patients to regain self-care abilities before the patient is discharged (Mahoney, Sager, & Jalaluddin, 1998). Function lost in the hospital may never be regained, resulting in the older adult requiring a higher level of care than might have been necessary.

Some hospitals have developed special units and innovative ideas in acute care for the older patient (Flaherty et al., 2003; Miller, 2002). Many of these units have reinstituted the role of the clinical nurse specialist to educate the staff, lead an interdisciplinary team, and assist with discharge planning. However, only a small number of older hospitalized patients have access to this kind of care. Examples of long-term care programs that provide good care and improve quality of life are the exception rather than the norm. Community health nurses struggle to find adequate resources to support older adults at home. Unfortunately, although many effective models of care for older patients have been developed through demonstration projects, few have been incorporated into the health care system (Barker, 2003).

Additional effort is needed to effect real change in the health care system so that nurses have the resources to provide quality care to our older patients. Belza and Baker (2000) provide a blueprint for improving care for older adults that is described in Box 1-1. Although their recommendations address improving care for the well elderly, achievement of these goals would improve care for all older adults.

Advanced Practice

Research has shown the benefits of advanced practice nurses (APNs) with specialized gerontological nursing training in improving care of the older adult. APNs have been part of interdisciplinary models of care that have been developed and evaluated. For example, the Program of All-inclusive Care of the Elderly (PACE) has reduced nursing home admission among frail elderly (Eng, 2002). Other settings have included day hospitals and geriatric assessment programs that have shown reduced costs and improved function for patients (Rubenstein, 2004; Sochalski, 2001).

The impact of APNs on nursing practice was demonstrated in a study showing that restraint use could be reduced without adding cost or causing injury (Evans, Strumpf, & Allen-Taylor, 1997). The cost-effectiveness of using APNs in discharge planning for the frail elderly has also been established (Naylor, Brooten, & Campbell, 1999). A recent study showed decreased hospitalization rates for nursing home residents cared for by nurse practitioners (Kane, Flood, Bershadsky, & Keckhafer, 2004.) APNs have also been shown to improve health outcomes in nursing home residents, including health trajectory, incontinence, pressure ulcers, and aggressive behavior (Ryden et al., 2000).

Gerontological nurses take a holistic approach to the person rather than focusing on individual diseases, addressing the broad range of health and quality-of-life issues affecting this population. Gerontological APNs can affect the direct care of the older population, as well as the health care delivery system and health policy, to ensure that models of care and nursing interventions are designed that are appropriate for the needs of this population. There is great need for additional APNs who can serve as clinical leaders and change agents to improve care of older patients.

Before discussing further the roles and competencies for gerontological nursing practice, it is worthwhile to reflect on the history of the specialty of gerontological nursing and on emerging trends in clinical practice.

HISTORY OF GERONTOLOGICAL NURSING

Although the need for a gerontological nursing specialty was identified as early as 1900, it was not until 1966 that the specialty was formally recognized, as other specialties in nursing were being formed. The growth of the specialty has been slow but steady, as new roles are developed and incorporated into the health care system.

BOX 1-1 Recommendations for Improving Care for Older Adults

Reconceptualizing Ways of Thinking about Well Older Adults
■ Consider person-environment fit when conceptualizing well older adults.

Practice Initiatives
■ Develop community-based wellness centers staffed by multidisciplinary teams to provide primary care, skill training, and services such as memory training, falls prevention, nutritional assessment and counseling, consulting with families, counseling for transitions and lifestyle change, strength training, and home safety appraisals.
■ Identify evidence-based best practices for the care of well older adults.

Building the Science of Nursing Research in Geriatrics
■ Fund consensus conferences on topics related to well older adults, followed by a call for proposals and allocation of funds based on decisions made at the consensus conferences.
■ Increase predoctoral and postdoctoral training opportunities for nurse researchers in geriatrics.
■ Increase traineeships and fellowships to attract doctoral-prepared nurses to geriatrics.

Education and Training Opportunities
■ Integrate gerontology and geriatric content in curricula: team teach, provide a variety of clinical experiences, and work with state boards to increase the number of state board questions related to geriatrics and gerontology.
■ Offer stipends for undergraduate and graduate students, coupled with a service payback.
■ Offer 10-week summer training institutes for undergraduate students interested in geriatrics and gerontology. Recruit from health sciences, humanities, and arts and sciences.
■ Offer a well older adults subspecialty track in adult, geriatric, women's health, and family nurse practitioner programs.
■ Provide additional gerontological training for midcareer faculty and clinicians not prepared in gerontology.
■ Establish training grants for predoctoral nursing students in geriatrics.
■ Create professorships in aging with a focus on well older adults in schools of nursing.
■ Lobby for continuing nursing education in gerontology to be required for relicensure.
■ Create gerontological and geriatric nursing institutes in schools of nursing with a focus on well older adults.

Autonomy and Safety
■ Organize a consensus-building conference in which experts in the field of bioethics and aging and representatives from older adult advocacy groups draft and disseminate a position paper to address autonomy and safety.
■ Capitalize on the Joint Commission on Accreditation of Healthcare Organizations system of examination of sentinel events in which undesirable events for well older adults would be identified and refined along with effective therapeutic options.

From Belza, B., & Baker, M. W. (2000). Maintaining health in well older adults: Initiatives for schools of nursing and the John A. Hartford Foundation for the 21st century. *Journal of Gerontological Nursing*, 26(7), 8-17.

A number of nursing pioneers dedicated to improving care for older adults shaped the specialty to what it is today. Some of these pioneers are well known, and we will discuss the contributions of some of them. Many others have been the dedicated nurse clinicians at the bedside and researchers who have worked to learn more about the special needs of older patients, sought certification and specialized training, and helped grow the specialty (Box 1-2).

The first article on nursing care of the aged was published in 1904 (Bishop, 1904), the same year as the World's fair in St. Louis where the ice cream cone and hot dog were introduced. During the early part of the century, care for the infirm aged was provided in almshouses, along with orphans, people with mental illness, and other indigents. Nurses wrote about the plight of the elderly in these settings (e.g., Dock, 1908), but little changed until the 1930s. Gradually, board and care

homes were formed that led to the development of today's nursing homes (Ebersole, Hess, & Luggen, 2004).

It was not until 1950 that Newton published a gerontological nursing text. Like many nursing texts of the day, the material was short on scientific rationale and long on practical experience of the times. During the following years, interest in nursing research developed, and some of the earliest studies concerned older adults with chronic disease (e.g., Mack, 1952). Norton, McLaren, and Exton-Smith (1962) conducted a landmark study describing the problems of hospitalized older adults and the conditions under which nurses cared for them in the United Kingdom. At about the same time, Doris Schwartz and her colleagues (Schwartz, Henley, & Zeitz, 1964) published their study of the psychosocial needs of elderly ambulatory patients.

The budding research efforts, along with political action geared toward establishing health insurance for

BOX 1-2 Gerontological Nursing Time Line

1904 *American Journal of Nursing* publishes an article on care of the aged.

1920s Many older individuals live on "poor farms."

1935 Social Security Act is passed; federal monies are made available to older individuals who are needy or who have limited financial resources.

1940s Older adults are cared for in hospitals; no focused plans are made for discharging older adults home.

1950 First geriatric nursing text by Newton is published.

1950s Population of older adults gradually increases; increased emphasis on wellness activities; nursing education programs are moved into institutions of higher education.

1960s Nursing process is defined; theoretical frameworks of nursing are developed; gerontological nurses begin to identify frameworks and theories that would be effective for the older individual's care; educational grants and funding for professional nurses become available, including grants for graduate nursing students to specialize in older adult care.

1961 American Nurses Association (ANA) recommends the formation of a special interest group for geriatric nurses.

1962 Seventy nurses attend the first national ANA meeting of the Conference Group on Geriatric Nursing Practice in Detroit, Michigan; the main item on the agenda is their name, indicating the "identity crisis" they are experiencing at this early stage.

1966 ANA Conference Group on Geriatric Nursing Practice is recognized.

1970 ANA develops standards of geriatric nursing practice; first publication of standards for geriatric nursing practice.

1973 The North American Nursing Diagnosis Association (NANDA) publishes the first list of nursing diagnoses; ANA certification in geriatric nursing practice is offered.

1975 The *Journal of Gerontological Nursing* becomes the first professional nursing journal for gerontological nurses.

1976 The Geriatric Nursing Division changes its name to the Gerontological Nursing Division; the first gerontological nursing textbook is published: *Nursing and the Aged,* by Irene Burnside; the First National Conference of Gerontological Nurse Practitioners is held.

1979 The First National Conference on Gerontological Nursing is sponsored by the *Journal of Gerontological Nursing;* certification for gerontological nursing is first offered.

1980 The *Geriatric Nursing Journal* is first published; nursing is defined in a social policy statement.

1981 ANA publishes a statement on the scope of gerontological nursing practice; National Conference of Gerontological Nurse Practitioners founded.

1984 The Council of Gerontological Nursing is formed (ANA); the National Gerontological Nursing Association is formed.

1986 The first conference of the National Association of Directors of Nursing Administration in Long-Term Care (NADONA) is held.

1989 ANA certification is established for gerontological clinical nurse specialist.

Continued

BOX 1-2 Gerontological Nursing Time Line—cont'd	
1990s	Establishment of the National Institute of Nursing Research promotes the expansion of gerontological nursing knowledge base.
1991	Educators are still having difficulty ensuring gerontological content in basic nursing curricula.
1993	Approximately 12,000 nurses are certified in gerontological nursing specialties.
1996	Many older adults become part of managed care systems; the John A. Hartford Foundation funds the Institute for Geriatric Nursing (IGN) at New York University, leading to the larger Hartford Geriatric Nursing Initiative.
1998	Advanced practice nurse certification is made available for nurse practitioners and clinical nurse specialists in gerontology.
2000	The *Curriculum Guidelines for Geriatric Nursing Care* are published by the American Association of Colleges of Nursing (AACN) in conjunction with the IGN for baccalaureate programs.
2001	ANA publishes an updated *Scope and Standards of Gerontological Nursing.*
2003	Funded by Atlantic Philanthropies, Inc., the Nurse Competencies in Aging program is developed to increase knowledge of gerontology for nurses outside of the specialty.
2004	Terry T. Fulmer becomes the first nursing president of the Gerontological Society of America; competencies for nurse practitioners and clinical nurse specialists are published by AACN and IGN.

Data from Miller, C. A. (1993). Nursing care of older adults (2nd ed.). Philadelphia: Lippincott; ANA, 1995; Eliopoulos, C. (1997). Gerontological nursing (4th ed.). Philadelphia: Lippincott; and Ebersole, P., & Hess, P. (1998). Gerontological nursing (5th ed.). St. Louis: Mosby.

seniors, set the stage for the establishment of gerontological nursing as a specialty. In 1962 the American Nurses Association (ANA) convened the first meeting of the Conference Group on Geriatric Nursing Practice. Four years later the Division of Geriatric Nursing Practice was established, giving nursing of the aged specialty status along with maternal-child health, medical-surgical nursing, psychiatric nursing, and community health nursing.

1965 to 1980

The period following the enactment of Medicare and Medicaid was one of rapid growth in the health care industry. Federal funding was allocated for training nurses, which stimulated growth in nursing practice and education that led to expanded roles for nurses. As more nurses were prepared at the master's and doctoral levels, interest in theory to build nursing as a science grew. This time saw the establishment of the *Journal of Gerontological Nursing,* the first conference on gerontological nursing, and the first gerontological master's program at Duke University (Burnside, 1988). ANA published the first *Standards of Geriatric Nursing Practice* (1970) and offered the first specialty certification.

Medicare and Medicaid spawned tremendous growth in both the hospital and nursing home industries. Medicare legislation provided payment for medical care for older persons with physicians as gatekeepers of the system, but excluded most preventive and long-term care services. Reimbursement was based on provider charges plus incentives for expansion of services. Tremendous problems were encountered in obtaining reasonable standards of care in nursing homes. Lax regulations and liberal funding levels led to flagrant abuses of infirm older people. Medicare reimbursement regulations were slow to keep pace with the increasing support in health policy research for preventive care, community-based long-term care, and expanded nursing roles.

Large-scale longitudinal studies of the aging process began to mature during the 1960s and 1970s, providing the scientific basis for much of the modern perspectives on aging (see Chapter 6 for background and examples). In the 1970s the Veteran's Administration (VA) funded a number of Geriatric Research and Education Clinical Centers (GRECCs) at VA medical centers across the country. These "centers of excellence" focused on improving care for the aging veteran population, with a mission of increasing knowledge of aging, advancing research education and care for aging veterans, and transmitting knowledge to health care providers. The centers resulted in a large number of aging research studies and model programs (VA, 2004). Nurses working in the VA system had significant educational opportunities to learn about care of the older adult as a result of GRECC programs, at times more than nurses in other settings.

1981 to 1990

This decade was a watershed period in gerontological nursing during which the ANA published the first statement on the scope of gerontological nursing practice and the National Gerontological Nurses Association was formed. Several foundation program initiatives also helped shape the future of gerontological nursing. The W. K. Kellogg Foundation supported development of geriatric nurse practitioners in Western states to care for rural elderly (Ebersole, 2001). Further support for nurse practitioners was provided by Ross Laboratories, which sponsored the first national conference for these specialists. Specialty master's programs increased graduating, primarily clinical nurse specialists. The Robert Wood Johnson Foundation supported collaboration between nursing schools and nursing homes through the Teaching Nursing Home Program (Mezey & Fulmer, 2002). This program focused on maintaining patient function; outcomes showed reduced hospitalization and health care costs for teaching nursing home residents, and the program helped support Medicare coverage for gerontological nurse practitioners in nursing homes (Hutchins, 2002).

In health care, public policy began to shift away from federal involvement in social programs of all types, including health care financing. The Omnibus Budget Reconciliation Act (OBRA) of 1981 liberalized Medicare home health benefits by removing the limit on the number of visits allowed and the requirements for prior hospitalization. This led to rapid growth in home health and dramatically increased the acuity of patients being cared for in the home.

The Tax Equity and Fiscal Responsibility Act of 1983 changed Medicare reimbursement for hospitals, from a cost-based system to a prospective payment system, creating (for the first time since 1965) an incentive for hospitals to contain costs rather than expand services and costs. Concern about the high cost of health care resulted in more widespread implementation of new models for care provision, such as reimbursement for care coordination (or "case-management" services), increased use of nonphysicians as gatekeepers for care, increased centralization of diverse community-based services, and prepaid care.

The 1980s were characterized by an increased interest in health promotion and fitness and a slowly growing understanding of the limitations of technology to cure all ills. The recognition that people were living longer led to increased interest in preventing or reducing the effects of chronic disease. The goal became to increase "active life expectancy" and reduce the period of disability to a short time at the end of life rather than the duration of later life (Fries & Crapo, 1986). During this same period, increased interest in the ethical aspects of long-term care was evident, fueled by clinical dilemmas such as economic concerns that the elderly were consuming more than their fair share of health care resources (Callahan, 1987) and legal cases about the right to die. A focus on advance directives resulted in legislation supporting self-determination.

Fundamental changes also occurred during this period in delivery of health care services. The number of hospital beds decreased, and new institutions for the delivery of medical care emerged, including "urgent care" centers, ambulatory surgery facilities, and outpatient rehabilitation centers. These innovations helped contain costs through decreased overhead and hospitalization and by fostering the development of new care models. They also tended to further fragment care, increasing the potential for difficulties among those with complex care needs. For example, ambulatory surgery for cataract removal became a common outpatient procedure for older people. Some older adults undergoing this procedure are at high risk for developing acute delirium as a result of exposure to the sedative medications used intraoperatively, and they may have difficulty learning new skills required during the recovery phase, such as eyedrop instillation. These innovations in technology and health service delivery called for increased vigilance on the part of nurses to ensure that patients have adequate monitoring, information, and skill to perform self-care.

1991 to the Present

From the 1990s and into the present, we are experiencing some of the benefits of gerontological education and research initiatives. Increased numbers of nurses obtained advanced practice degrees, and the focus shifted to nurse practitioner roles and away from the clinical nurse specialist. A growing emphasis on primary care and position cutbacks caused by financial concerns of many health care settings contributed to this trend. With attention to health care reform, there is ongoing interest in exploring the roles of APNs in care of the aged. They may substitute for more costly services, such as physician or hospital services, or provide care to those who are underserved, such as older adults in rural areas. Both APN roles developed methods for reimbursement by Medicare for approved services.

It is no longer a rarity to find health care providers from many disciplines with specialized training in gerontology and geriatrics. The growth in programs such as PACE is a testament to the success of prior work. This program has built from a demonstration project in the 1970s to over 40 programs nationwide that are recognized Medicare/Medicaid providers. Although further work on the specific effects of APNs in care of the elderly is needed, evidence for their effectiveness is beginning to build (Bourbonniere & Evans, 2002).

This time saw a great deal of growth in managed care as a means to control spiraling health care costs. Managed care programs include health maintenance organizations (HMOs) and other prospective payment insurance systems designed to provide health care services at a fixed rate for the consumer. The managed care program controls costs by managing service utilization and contracting with providers such as hospitals for group discounts on services. Managed care is available to older Medicare and Medicaid patients, although only about 13% of seniors have enrolled in managed care options (Anderson & Robinson, 2001). As we move forward, workers who are in managed care plans now may elect to stay with those plans as they retire, gradually increasing the numbers of older adults in these plans (Jensen & Morrissey, 2004).

In health care, increased interest in complementary and alternative approaches to management of disease and even prevention of aging has fostered a multibillion-dollar industry in herbal treatments, nutritional supplements, and antiaging products. Regulatory oversight is often inadequate because the products fit under loopholes in the law; for example, many herbal and chemical preparations can qualify as "dietary supplements," which require minimal proof of safety or efficacy. Health professionals need to be proactive to protect and educate patients and consumers about these alternative treatments (Mehlman et al., 2004).

In research, several developments have fostered improved care for older adults, including increased emphasis on the outcomes of health care and the maturation of the National Institute on Aging (NIA) and the National Institute of Nursing Research (NINR). The medical outcomes movement fostered increased attention on whether the care received by older adults and others was appropriate and effective. Outcomes research was spearheaded in the 1990s by the U.S. Agency for Health Care Policy and Research (AHCPR; now the Agency for Healthcare Research and Quality [AHRQ]) under the Medical Treatment Effectiveness Program. One of the goals of this program was to examine various treatment approaches for common conditions and determine if a suitable scientific basis existed to make recommendations for treatment. This led to the development of several clinical guidelines, including pain, incontinence, and pressure sores. Since then, a growing emphasis on evidence-based practice has developed, so that practitioners can access the best available evidence in providing patient care in many areas (Conn, Burks, Rantz, & Knudsen, 2002). The need for further research is supported through identified gaps in knowledge.

Maturation of the extramural research program of the NIA provides a growing scientific basis for clinical care of the elderly. Large-scale epidemiological studies of the aged have matured and have provided increased understanding of the aging process and common health issues. Some of the important research programs include the following:

- Established Populations for Study of the Elderly
- Alzheimer's Disease Research Centers
- Claude D. Pepper Older Americans Independence Centers, named in honor of the late senator, a long-time political advocate for the needs of the elderly

The National Institute of Nursing Research has supported expansion of the knowledge base for gerontological nursing practice. In addition to funding individual and cooperative studies of common clinical problems affecting the elderly, the NINR funds original research projects and provides support for nurse scientist training. Thus a cadre of well-prepared nurse scientists to study nursing care problems of the aged has been emerging.

The John A. Hartford Foundation has provided a major initiative to support gerontological nursing across the spectrum (Mezey & Fulmer, 2002). This initiative included the development of the Institute for Geriatric Nursing at New York University and Centers of Geriatric Nursing Excellence at the University of Iowa, University of Arkansas, University of Pennsylvania, University of California at San Francisco, and Oregon Health Sciences University. In addition, the Foundation has provided support for enhancing gerontological curricula at the undergraduate level, continuing education for nurses, preparation of advanced practice nurses, and predoctoral and postdoctoral training. Several initiatives have been conducted in partnership with the American Association of Colleges of Nursing. All of these programs seek to enhance competency in care of the older patient throughout the educational and health care systems.

Pioneers in Gerontological Nursing

Many nurses influenced the development of gerontological nursing, attended the first conventions and meetings, and published their work. Four nurses with exceptional careers are highlighted here: Virginia Stone, Mary Opal Wolanin, Irene Mortenson Burnside, and Doris Schwartz. All had long and varied careers, and their contributions continue to influence nursing care for older people today. Of note, comments and tributes to each of these important women describe them as nurses who were highly caring, not only for their patients, but for students and others. Each faced an uphill climb attempting to focus attention on the problems and needs of the vulnerable older adult.

Virginia Stone (1912-1993). Virginia Stone obtained her doctorate in 1959 with one of the few dissertations focusing on gerontology, "Personal Adjustments by the Aged to Their Living Environments" (Wilson, 1994). Stone attended the first meeting convened by the ANA on gerontological nursing and started the first graduate program at Duke University in 1965. Her contributions to care of the elderly were recognized from the local to international levels. She helped lead the ANA to develop standards of practice in gerontological nursing, as well as specialty certification. Her advice was sought by other schools, the VA, and even the World Health Organization. A key focus of her career was identifying and meeting the educational needs of nurses on care of the older adult.

Mary Opal Wolanin (1920-1997). Mary Opal Wolanin was a nurse for many years before gradually developing her interest in gerontological nursing while taking care of stroke patients (Thames, 1997). She examined the benefits of rehabilitation, which later formed the subject of her writings. She served as faculty at the University of Arizona and supported inclusion of gerontological nursing content in the nursing curriculum. She became an expert on long-term care nursing and administration. Wolanin and Phillips' book on caring for cognitively impaired older adults, *Confusion:*

Prevention and Care (1981), was an important first guide to help nurses caring for patients with dementia or acute confusion.

Doris Schwartz (1917-1999). Doris Schwartz had a wide career in nursing and public health education. She started one of the first geriatric nurse practitioner programs at Cornell Medical College and published some of the first gerontological nursing research (Schwartz et al., 1964). She was the first gerontological nurse to receive funding from the National Institutes of Health. Doris Schwartz fought for improved care for the elderly. She challenged nurses to curb the use of restraints in the care of older people, leading to the seminal work in this area by her colleagues Lois Evans and Neville Strumpf (1989). Author of books and articles, her writings on her career, *My 50 Years in Nursing; Give Us to Go Blithely* (Schwartz, 1995) is an inspiring description of her experiences.

Irene Burnside (1924-2003). Irene Burnside started her career in psychiatric nursing and focused on the psychosocial needs of older adults. Her teaching spanned decades and included work with the Ethel Percy Andrus Gerontology Center at the University of

---

Box 1-3 *Reflections on the Development of Gerontological Nursing*

I received a diploma in nursing from the Hospital of the University of Pennsylvania in 1962. I spent about 10 years after graduation primarily raising a family and working part time in hospitals. I developed an affinity for the older people I met along the way, so when I went back to school in 1975 to earn a BSN at the University of North Carolina, I decided that I wanted to focus on nursing care of the aged. I looked for articles and textbooks on the subject and found very few. The only textbook that I found at that time was written by Irene Burnside. The book was readable, informative, and inspiring—inspiring because it demonstrated a deep understanding and compassion for both the older patients and the nurses who cared for them. Irene Burnside is a role model for nursing and for aging, a person who is rightfully included in this chapter as one of the founders of the art and science of gerontological nursing.

Toward the end of my undergraduate work, I found out that Duke University had a master's program in gerontological nursing, in which I enrolled immediately after graduation. There I had a great opportunity to have Virginia Stone as a teacher and mentor. Her positive view of aging and her enthusiasm for advanced practice nursing gave me the courage to create a clinical specialist position at the Duke Center on Aging Older Americans Resources and Services center. At the time, these positions were few and far between.

During my career, I was able to meet, work with, and be inspired by many gerontological nursing leaders in the late 1970s and early 1980s when the field was in its relative infancy. Thelma Wells, Terry Fulmer, Priscilla Ebersole, Cornelia Beck, and Mary Opal Wolanin generously shared their wisdom, experience, and friendship, each contributing her special skills and knowledge. In the late 1980s, Mary Opal Wolanin moved to San Antonio, Texas, about the same time that I did, so I was fortunate to be with her as she aged. She was in a retirement center and had difficulty getting around, eventually wheelchair bound. But, she continued writing grants, carrying out research, providing geriatric clinical experiences for students, and acting as an outspoken advocate for residents who were infirm.

Gerontological nursing has come a long way in the past 25 years. It is because of these leaders with their vision and passion that we have progressed as far as we have. I am grateful to have been a small part of that and know that the future is in good hands.

Mary Ann Matteson
Mary Ann Matteson, PhD, RN
Professor Emerita
School of Nursing
University of Texas Health Sciences Center
San Antonio, Texas

Southern California. She published many articles and books advocating for psychosocial care of older adults at vulnerable times in their lives (Buckwalter & Hertz, 2003). She advocated an approach to care of the elderly focusing on what is left, not what is gone (Ebersole, 2003). In addition, she pioneered therapeutic group work recognizing the value of reminiscence and life review for older adults (Burnside & Schmidt, 1994).

Many other nurses have contributed to the growth of gerontological nursing and will be recognized in future texts. Reflections on gerontological nursing are provided in Box 1-3 by Mary Ann Matteson, who helped pioneer the first edition of this textbook, showing the personal experiences of another influential gerontological nurse.

Looking to the Future

The history of gerontological nursing and current trends in the specialty underscore the importance of maintaining an approach to practice based on a strong nursing tradition influenced by knowledge from gerontology and geriatrics. While the need for nurses with this preparation expands, the picture is clouded. There is an anticipated shortage of nurses prepared for advanced practice positions, and a shortage of nursing faculty to prepare the future generations of gerontological nurses. The specialty continues to attract fewer nurses than the more generalist specialties. Some advocate working to improve the competencies of all nurses and APNs as a method of improving care for older patients, because we can never attract and train enough specialty nurses to meet the demand. It will be up to the current generation of gerontological nurses to create and research interventions to improve the health and well-being of future generations of older adults.

THE PRACTICE OF GERONTOLOGICAL NURSING
Opportunities for Gerontological Nurses

Opportunities for gerontological nurses are better than ever because of growing demand for services, better preparation of practitioners, and an enhanced research base. The tremendous variety of human situations and needs that confront the gerontological nurse is striking. There is ample opportunity for direct care, counseling, teaching, and advocacy in most positions. Research and policy contributions of gerontological nurses continue to receive recognition. Box 1-4 provides a list of roles that builds on the original work of Futrell and associates (1980) describing possible roles for gerontological nurses. The frontiers of gerontological nursing lie in *how* these roles are enacted, in what settings of care, with what creativity, and with what rewards or sacrifices.

BOX 1-4 Potential Roles for Gerontological Nurses

Direct care provider

Independent practitioner

Health educator

Researcher

Nursing faculty

Consultant to community agencies and long-term care facilities

Collaborator with other disciplines

Provider of direct care and interventions

Quality assurance coordinator

Clinical research coordinator

Advocate

Continuing education provider

Care manager/case manager

Health planner

Health and social policy maker

Administrator

Counselor

Program evaluator

Leader

The ongoing transition from institution-based care to community-based care will continue through this century. Gerontological nurses are therefore likely to be found in greater numbers in home health agencies, day hospitals or day care programs, hospices, primary care settings, and wellness programs than ever before. Gerontological nurses can expect to practice with relative autonomy in these settings, assuming ever-increasing responsibility for independent nursing assessment and initiating referrals to other disciplines as indicated by the patient's functional status. A smaller proportion of the care of the aged will be given in nursing homes and hospitals, although there is likely to be a demand for increased sophistication of nursing care for the aged in these settings. As pressures continue to mount for cost containment in health care generally, nurses will be forced to think critically about how to achieve therapeutic end points efficiently.

For example, the University of Pennsylvania School of Nursing has been a leader in development of model nursing care programs, such as nurse-run clinics for assessment and treatment of urinary incontinence, that have spawned similar models of care in non-university-affiliated private practice settings (Bourbonniere & Evans, 2002). More recently, this school has established additional gerontological nursing demonstration programs, including a geriatric day hospital, a hospital-based geropsychiatric nursing consultation liaison service, and a PACE program.

Elements of Gerontological Nursing Practice

Recipients of Gerontological Nursing. Recipients of gerontological nursing include those who seek assistance for themselves or a loved one in adjusting to age-related changes or health conditions in later life, or any individual over 65 years of age who receives nursing care from a professional nurse who practices according to the definition listed earlier. According to Orem (1991), any aged individual whose self-care demands exceed the ability to meet those demands is an appropriate recipient of gerontological nursing care.

Although chronological age is a poor indicator of the impact of aging on an individual, and an even poorer indicator of needs, it is used to mark the target population in this text for two reasons. First, there are no universally accepted markers of an individual's place on the continuum of aging. Second, aging is a social phenomenon as well as a physiological and psychological one, and the chronological age of 65 years has significant meaning in our society. It is the usual age of retirement, when society begins to allow individuals, as a normal course of events, to begin to relinquish their adult roles. It is also the age at which most Americans become eligible to benefit from the major health care financing system for the elderly, Medicare. Some states define the scope of practice for gerontological nurses as including adults who are age 60 and older.

Although a marker for gerontological nursing patients does not exist, the frail elderly have emerged as a target population that could benefit from specialized care. Frail older adults have been considered at high risk for disability, hospitalization, nursing home placement, and death (Fried et al., 2001). The term *frailty* has long been used in geriatrics and gerontology to identify the most vulnerable elders, but until recently, no standardized method for screening has existed to identify those who need this care. Researchers are now exploring methods to screen for frailty in order to target services to those most in need. Ideally, nurses will be able to identify those at risk for frailty and provide interventions to prevent development of decline and adverse health outcomes.

Essential Foundations for the Practice of Gerontological Nursing. Specific competencies are needed by the clinical gerontological nurse in addition to generic professional nursing preparation. These competencies are influenced by the level at which the nurse will function and the role expectations of the nurse. For example, APNs have expanded expertise and skills to fulfill specialized roles. Also, gerontological nurses in a clinical role require an expertise different from that of a gerontological nurse scientist. However, a common body of assumptions, knowledge, skills, and attitudes that are essential for good clinical nursing practice with the aged has been developed and provides the basic foundation for all levels of practice. This knowledge and its relationship to other related fields are depicted in Figure 1-4. The following describes the key assumptions, attitudes, knowledge, skills, and competencies that make up the foundation of gerontological nursing practice.

ASSUMPTIONS. The elderly have specific, although diverse, responses reflecting the interplay among age-related biological changes, illness, developmental tasks, and the social environment. They are capable of attaining the full range of the health-illness continuum, despite the increased incidence of chronic disease in later life and the increased vulnerability to illness. The context in which older persons currently receive health care is disease oriented, fragmented, and institutionally based. However, nurses take a holistic approach to the older adult and are concerned with preserving health and function, as well as preventing and curing disease. For these reasons, nurses are key health care providers for the elderly and need to consider the assumptions that guide their care for older adults. Important assumptions for gerontological nurses to consider are noted in Box 1-5.

KNOWLEDGE, SKILLS, AND COMPETENCIES. Science has provided a growing body of knowledge regarding health and illness in older adults. The gerontological nurse should be knowledgeable about basic professional and nursing practice, theories, and research, as well as specific information needed to care for the older adult. In addition, gerontological nurses should be skillful in applying generic nursing methods to care of the older adult, as well as adapting those methods based on the individual's age-related changes, health conditions, and psychosocial environment. Boxes 1-6 and 1-7 describe the essential knowledge, skills, and competencies that the gerontological nurse should strive to develop.

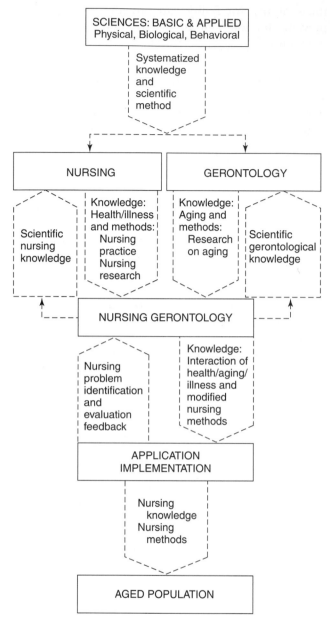

Figure 1-4 Knowledge base of gerontological nursing. (Adapted from Gunter, L., & Estes, C. [1979]. *Education for gerontologic nursing.* New York: Springer Publishing Company. Copyright 1979, p. 38. Used by permission.)

ATTITUDES. Most gerontological experts and clinicians would agree that nurses need to be able to recognize their biases toward aging and older people, but specifying the attitudes desirable for the gerontological nurse is considerably more difficult. The predominant culture in our society worships youth and productivity. McBride (2000) identifies the potential consequences of negative attitudes toward and stereotypes of aging:

- The needs of older adults are invisible.
- Older people are presumed to be the opposite of lively and fun.
- Morbidity is treated as morbidly dull.

BOX 1-5 Assumptions to Guide Gerontological Nursing Practice

- Older individuals and their families can be viewed as open systems, capable of change, growth, and mutual interaction.

- Human beings have the potential to develop their intellectual and practical skills and the motivation essential for self-care and care of dependent family members.

- Human development requires the formation and maintenance of specific environmental conditions that promote known developmental processes at each period of the life cycle.

- Older individuals are affected in unique ways by the combined effects of the aging process, disease processes, lifestyle, and the environment.

- Older people are capable of making independent decisions, unless some well-documented pathological process interferes with this ability. This capability is presumed to be intact unless demonstrated otherwise.

- Older adults are interested in learning more about health and aging, with a primary motivation of maintaining their independence. Health teaching can help older people maintain or improve their health; manage disease, complications, or disabilities; and improve health habits.

- Health status and developmental status are two separate but related concepts. Health is a multidimensional concept that allows for the presence of well-being despite the presence of pathological processes in body subsystems.

- Older people have the potential to benefit from a wide variety of health services, if appropriately targeted. Nurses are not and should not be the sole providers of care but should function within an interdisciplinary team context.

- Given the necessary information, older people can reduce their dependence on medical and institutional services.

- Gerontological nursing is practiced within the framework of professional nursing and therefore is subject to professional norms and the code of ethics.

- The focus is on forestalling wrinkles (that is, on surface issues) rather than tackling problems/possibilities.
- People involved in facilitating elderly individuals are regarded as being at the low end of the career pecking order.

BOX 1-6 Knowledge Base for Gerontological Nursing

- Physical, psychological, and social aspects of aging throughout the life span; the resulting impact on the individual and family

- Pathophysiology, epidemiology, treatment of chronic diseases, and the impact of disease processes and therapeutic regimens

- Health services and resources available to the elderly in the community, and how that relates to the national spectrum of health services

- Signs and symptoms of atypical manifestation of disease in older individuals, as well as common geriatric syndromes

- Altered pharmacology of drugs in the older adult

- The influence of environmental factors on human performance and health status in the aged

- The impact of ethnicity on age-related changes, disease, and developmental events

- Approaches to health promotion, disease prevention, and risk reduction in later life

- Ethical reasoning and problem solving

- Key issues for older patients relevant to the various settings of care

- Current theory, research, and evidence for nursing interventions, and standards of care for the older adult

---

- There is relatively little interest in understanding the strengths or advantages of later years.

Anecdotal data suggest that negative attitudes toward the elderly, based on stereotypical thinking, have negative effects on health outcomes. Gerontological nursing has been noted to be one of the profession's most challenging practice areas (ANA, 2001).

Obtaining the necessary attitudes, knowledge, skills, and competencies for the successful practice of gerontological nursing is not a simple process. Ideally, generic nursing programs should provide adequate preparation for professional nurses in gerontological nursing; however, the curricula of most schools of nursing historically have lacked adequate gerontological nursing content. Practice settings with advance practice gerontological nurses have a built-in resource for providing in-service education for staff.

Other avenues for developing the needed competencies are provided by a range of continuing education programs. These vary in depth of content and in

opportunities for precepted clinical practice. The federally funded, multidisciplinary Geriatric Education Centers provide high-quality continuing education in gerontology and nursing. The Internet now offers online options ranging from self-study programs to live interactive hosted discussions. In addition, journals, textbooks, and audiovisual aids may be used by nurses for self-study. It is the responsibility of the gerontological nurse to develop her or his foundational base and stay abreast of current knowledge in the field.

STANDARDS. Gerontological nursing should be practiced in accordance with standards developed by the nursing profession. The ANA's Division of Gerontological Nursing Practice has developed and refined standards for practice, most recently revised in 2001, which provide an excellent guide for evaluation of nursing practice. Standards are provided both for clinical care and for the professional role (Box 1-8). Clinical competence is demonstrated through appropriate utilization of the nursing process. Professional competence is derived from behaviors appropriate to the professional role. Each standard is described in detail, including rationale and measurement criteria, available from ANA (2001).

SCOPE OF PRACTICE. Although the scope of nursing practice is defined by state regulation, nursing practice is also influenced by the *needs of the patients* in a given *setting*. The range of health and illness needs that older adults experience is extremely broad. There is a place for nursing action at nearly every point along the health-illness continuum. Likewise, there is potential for nursing practice in every location in which older people are found.

The *focus* of nursing care in the many settings where gerontological nursing is practiced may be as broad as the range of needs encountered. For example, in a senior congregate housing project, nurses may be responsible for organizing and teaching an exercise class, and, on the same day, be responsible for initiating advanced emergency care to a person who has suffered a cardiopulmonary arrest. The nurse caring for an older patient in an intensive care unit is responsible for administering highly technological interventions to patients with multiple organ system dysfunctions. That nurse is also responsible for monitoring the patient's psychoemotional response to illness and the intensive care environment, because failure to do so may result in a technical success in controlling organ system pathology without concomitant restoration of the individual's functional ability.

PROCESS. Figure 1-5 diagrams the elements of gerontological nursing practice. The goal of each gerontological nurse-patient interaction is to establish conditions within patient and environment that will promote

---

BOX 1-7 Skills and Competencies for Gerontological Nursing

- Use research findings from gerontology, as well as nursing and the biomedical and behavioral sciences, to develop evidence-based practices.

- Interact effectively with individuals who have sensory and cognitive loss.

- Perform comprehensive assessment of the older person using standardized tools and individualized approaches based on level of nursing practice.

- Identify the theoretical underpinnings for practice .

- Serve as a collaborative partner in interdisciplinary teamwork.

- Implement rehabilitative and restorative nursing techniques.

- Help patients integrate past needs and meet developmental needs.

- Develop caring, collaborative relationships with the older person and family members in developing goals for nursing care, even if the individual has significant communication or cognitive impairments.

- Modify the environment to maximize the older person's ability to function independently.

- Provide case management services to support the patient and family.

- Provide excellent palliative, supportive, and spiritual care for those who are dying.

- Counsel the grieving.

- Consider ethical dilemmas encountered by older people, their kin, and their health care providers.

- Establish developmentally appropriate criteria for evaluation of nursing care.

- Participate in professional quality improvement activities designed to improve health care for older adults.

- Manage the group process for educational and therapeutic groups of older adults, professionals, or others.

- Teach professional caregivers, paraprofessional and lay caregivers, and older adults about the aging process, disease management, and health promotion.

- Provide leadership by modeling appropriate care for older patients.

- Supervise the efforts of professional, paraprofessional, and lay caregivers in providing nursing care to the aged.

- Advocate for older adults in the health care setting, in the community, and in the public policy arena.

- Engage in lifelong learning activities to maintain up-to-date knowledge.

---

healthy behaviors; compensate for disease-related losses and impairments; prevent further disease-related losses; promote comfort; and facilitate the diagnosis, palliation, and treatment of disease. These goals are achieved through interactions between patient and nurse, which are guided by the nursing process activities of assessment, diagnosis, planning, intervention, and evaluation. Discussion of the nursing process with older patients, as well as comprehensive assessment methods, is provided in Chapter 2.

Organization of Nursing for Older Adults

The organization of nursing personnel to care for older persons is also complex and may be confusing to non-nurses. A diverse group provides nursing care to older adults in America. At least 11 different levels of preparation exist for those providing gerontological nursing (see Table 1-1), and the only consistent credentialing mechanism throughout the United States for these various providers of nursing care is the state licensing mechanism

BOX 1-8   Standards of Clinical Gerontological Nursing Care with Rationales

Standard I. Assessment
The gerontological nurse collects patient health data.
Rationale: Information obtained from older adults, families, significant others, and the interdisciplinary team and nursing knowledge is used to develop the comprehensive plan of care. These assessments must always be culturally and ethnically appropriate.

Standard II. Diagnosis
The gerontological nurse analyzes the assessment data in determining diagnoses.
Rationale: The gerontological nurse, either independently or in collaboration with interdisciplinary care providers, evaluates health assessment data to develop comprehensive diagnoses that guide interventions.

Standard III. Outcome Identification
The gerontological nurse identifies expected outcomes individualized to the older adult.
Rationale: The ultimate goals of providing gerontological nursing care are to influence health outcomes and improve or maintain the health status of the older adult. Outcomes often focus on maximizing the state of well-being, functional status, and quality of life.

Standard IV. Planning
The gerontological nurse develops a plan of care that prescribes interventions to attain expected outcomes.
Rationale: A plan of care is used to structure and guide therapeutic interventions and achieve expected outcomes. It is developed in conjunction with the older adult, significant others, and interdisciplinary team members.

Standard V. Implementation
The gerontological nurse implements the interventions identified in the plan of care.
Rationale: The gerontological nurse uses a wide range of culturally competent interventions, including health promotion, health maintenance, prevention of illness, health restoration, rehabilitation, and palliation. The gerontological nurse implements the plan of care in collaboration with the older adult and others.

Standard VI. Evaluation
The gerontological nurse evaluates the older adult's progress toward attainment of expected outcomes.
Rationale: Nursing practice is dynamic and evolving. The gerontological nurse continually evaluates the older adult's responses to treatment and interventions. Collection of new data, revision of the database, alteration of diagnoses, and modification of the plan of care are essential.

Standards of Professional Gerontological Nursing Performance

Standard I. Quality of Care
The gerontological nurse systematically evaluates the quality of care and effectiveness of nursing practice.
Rationale: The dynamic nature and growing body of gerontological knowledge and research provide both the impetus and the means for gerontological nurses to improve the quality of patient care.

Standard II. Performance Appraisal
The gerontological nurse evaluates his or her own nursing practice in relation to professional practice standards and relevant statutes and regulations.
Rationale: The gerontological nurse is accountable to the public for providing competent clinical care and has an inherent responsibility to practice according to standards established by the professional and regulatory bodies.

Standard III. Education
The gerontological nurse acquires and maintains current knowledge applicable to nursing practice.
Rationale: Scientific, cultural, societal, and political changes require a continuing commitment from the gerontological nurse to pursue knowledge to maintain competency, enhance nursing expertise, and advance the profession. Formal education, continuing education, certification, and experiential learning are some of the means for professional growth.

Standard IV. Collegiality
The gerontological nurse contributes to the professional development of peers, colleagues, and others.
Rationale: The gerontological nurse is responsible for sharing knowledge, research, and clinical information with colleagues and others through formal and informal teaching methods and collaborative educational programs.

Standard V. Ethics
The gerontological nurse's decisions and actions on behalf of older adults are determined in an ethical manor.
Rationale: The gerontological nurse is responsible for providing nursing services and health care that are responsive to the public's trust and the older adult's rights. Formal and informal care providers must also be prepared to provide the care needed and desired by the older adult to render services in an appropriate setting.

Continued

BOX 1-8 Standards of Clinical Gerontological Nursing Care with Rationales—cont'd

Standard VI. Collaboration

The gerontological nurse collaborates with the older adult, the older adult's caregivers, and all members of the interdisciplinary team to provide comprehensive care.

Rationale: The complex nature of comprehensive care for older adults and their caregivers requires expertise from all members of the interdisciplinary team. Collaboration between health care consumers and providers is optimal for planning, implementing, and evaluating care. Communication among members of the interdisciplinary team provides a forum to evaluate the effectiveness of the plan of care and to use appropriate resources to achieve identified goals.

Standard VII. Research

The gerontological nurse interprets, applies, and evaluates research findings to inform and improve gerontological nursing practice.

Rationale: Gerontological nurses are responsible for improving current nursing practice and future health care for older adults by participating in the generation, testing, utilization, and evaluation of research findings. At the basic level of practice, the gerontological nurse participates in research studies, identifies clinical problems, and interprets and uses research findings to improve clinical care to older adults. At the advanced practice level, the gerontological nurse may be a full research participant in the generation, testing, utilization, critical evaluation, and dissemination of knowledge related to gerontological health care research.

Standard VIII. Resource Utilization

The gerontological nurse considers factors related to safety, effectiveness, and cost in planning and delivering patient care.

Rationale: The older adult is entitled to health care that is safe, ethical, effective, acceptable, and affordable. Treatment decisions consider quality of care and appropriate utilization of resources.

Modified from American Nurses Association. (2001). *Scope and standards of gerontological nursing practice* (2nd ed.). Washington, DC: American Nurses Publishing.

NOTE: Advanced practice nurses have a broader scope of practice, which is described in detail in *Nursing: Scope and Standards of Practice* (American Nurses Association, 2004).

for registered nurses and licensed practical nurses. Additional credentialing mechanisms that help differentiate gerontological nurses of different levels are earned degrees and the certification program sponsored by the ANA for specialist practitioners.

Additionally, nurses may function in a variety of capacities, such as direct caregivers, physician extenders, managers, teachers, consultants, and researchers; they may practice in many different settings, including hospitals, rehabilitation centers, ambulatory care clinics, mental health centers, long-stay institutions, and the home. The varied roles result in confusion as to precisely what nurses are prepared to do in health care, and at what level. This situation is particularly difficult for consumers of nursing services who reached maturity in the era before the proliferation of roles and responsibilities that characterize modern nursing.

Five levels of nursing personnel are involved in care of the elderly:

Level I: nursing assistants
Level II: licensed practical nurses
Level III: professional nurses
Level IV: advanced practice nurses (clinical specialists, nurse practitioners, nursing administrators)
Level V: nursing/gerontological scientists

Although the need for the involvement of diverse levels of caregivers in the care of older adults is recognized, under the definition of gerontological nursing used in this text, only level III to level V practitioners qualify for definition as gerontological nurses. The other two levels of providers assist professional nurses in the conduct of gerontological nursing but are not gerontological nurses. Practitioners at the first two levels carry out selected aspects of care under the supervision of the professional nurse. There are positions in gerontology for nurses at all levels of practice, as well as a great need.

Certification as a "gerontological nurse" is available for both the associate and bachelor's level professional nurse, recognizing expertise in assessing, managing, and evaluating clinical care for the older adult. Nurses will have worked at least 2 years full time, have 2000 hours of clinical practice, and have 30 hours of education contact hours in the specialty to sit for the examination. The gerontological nurse will provide direct care, as well as management and development of other nurses, and evaluation of services (ANA, 2001), making certified nurses valuable in almost any medical setting. Nurses with this certification would be excellent candidates to fill roles such as the "geriatric resource nurse," a unit-based nurse who serves as a consultant to other staff

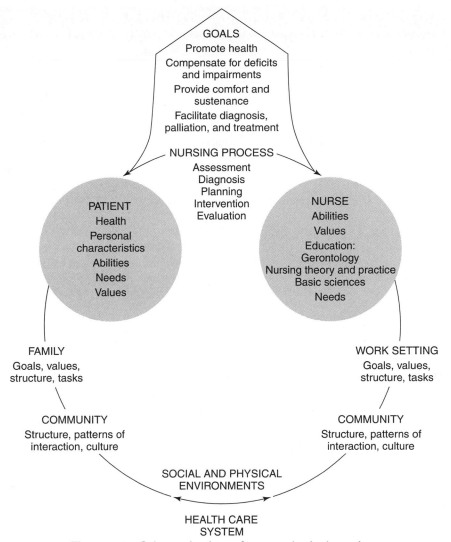

Figure 1-5 Schematic view of gerontological nursing.

regarding older patients (Lopez et al., 2002), or staffing specialty geriatric units or subacute units.

Advanced practice nurses (APNs) can be either gerontological nurse practitioners or gerontological clinical nurse specialists. Both roles encompass advanced practice, education, consultation, research, case management, administration, and advocacy for older adults. In addition, they develop advanced knowledge of theory, research, and practice. Depending on state regulations and preparation of the APN, the APN may order and interpret laboratory tests and prescribe pharmacological and nonpharmacological therapies, but these are most often performed by nurse practitioners.

The APN has a master's degree in nursing, which includes over 500 hours of precepted clinical practice, and the APN must pass a certification examination. In addition to the skills and knowledge listed previously, Bourbonniere and Evans (2002) reviewed studies that

used APNs and reported positive patient outcomes. They identified additional skills that seem to facilitate good APN practice, including communication, interpersonal relations, contextual thinking; clinical skills in assessment and monitoring, intervention, problem solving, and evaluation. The APN is an expert in providing care for older adults, families, and groups in a variety of settings.

Nurse practitioners (NPs) often provide direct care for older patients, focusing on assessment, differential diagnosis, and management of acute episodic and chronic illness, as well as emphasizing health promotion and disease prevention (American Academy of Nurse Practitioners, 2002). Gerontological NPs work in many types of settings, such as primary care practices and clinics, hospitals, and nursing home practices, often in collaboration with physicians. The NP role was developed to provide increased access to care for underserved

Table 1-1 *Levels of Nursing Practitioners Involved in Care of the Aged*

Practitioner	Functions	Educational Preparation
Nursing assistant (NA), also known as nurse's aid (NA), patient care aid (PCA) or patient care technician, direct care workers, unlicensed assistive personnel	Assists professional nurse in patient care tasks	Certified through short courses or technical colleges or through in-service training; competency-based evaluation must be passed
Licensed practical nurse (LPN) or licensed vocational nurse (LVN)	Assists professional nurse in patient care tasks	Technical college or vocational preparation; must pass licensure examination and maintain licensure to practice
Registered nurse (RN)	Practices professional nursing with patients in any health care setting Responsibilities include direct care, management and development of professional and other nursing personnel, and evaluation of care and services for the older adult (ANA, 2001)	Multiple levels of entry, including the following: ■ Diploma (hospital-based program) ■ Associate nursing degree (AND) in 2-year program ■ Baccalaureate degree (bachelor of science in nursing [BSN]) in 4-year university-based program Must pass examination and maintain licensure to practice
Advanced practice nurse ■ Nurse practitioner ■ Clinical nurse specialist	Performs basic nursing, but in addition has knowledge of theory, research, and practice to serve as one or more of the following: clinician, independent practitioner, educator, consultant, researcher, manager, or administrator (ANA, 2001)	Master's degree with supervised practicum hours required for certification of either type Provided by American Nurses Credentialling Center Licensure varies by state; may require certification
Nursing scientist	Advanced practice of nursing Educator Researcher	Doctor of nursing science (DNS) or doctor of philosophy (PhD) in nursing or other related field (e.g., psychology, public health)

populations, and it has grown as health insurance plans have included NPs as primary care providers (Keane & Becker, 2001).

The clinical nurse specialist (CNS) is prepared with expertise in a defined area such as gerontological nursing, and has *clinical* expertise in the assessment, diagnosis, and treatment of illness and the prevention or remediation of risk behaviors through nursing interventions (Fulton, 2004). The CNS often works through other nurses, focusing on educating nurses and improving nursing care, and influencing care related to staff, patients, families, and communities. The CNS most often works for health care agencies such as hospitals, home care providers, or nursing homes.

Overlap exists between the two advanced roles, and the profession has discussed combining the two, but at this time they continue as separate entities. Health care financing issues may play a part in determining the outcome of this discussion. NPs are often hired under the same medical model paradigm as physicians, with an expectation of reimbursement for their services. Because

they are required to see a certain number of patients to meet this expectation, their time to consult with nursing staff and health care agencies may be limited. The CNS is usually hired under a more traditional nursing model, so that the CNS's workload is negotiated with the agency administration. As a result, the CNS is more likely to fulfill the consultative role and less likely to be involved in direct patient care.

To meet the growing population demands, opportunities are expected to grow for gerontological nurses at all the levels discussed and in both advanced practice roles. Increasing awareness of the contributions of nursing to the care of this population will enhance the public and professional images of gerontological nursing.

SUMMARY

Gerontological nursing practice builds on the theories and methods of nursing practice generally. The nurse must consider the developmental issues unique to those of advanced years and be particularly astute in addressing environmental demands in providing care. These traits, in addition to skillful assessment and use of nursing interventions, are likely to result in enhanced health outcomes for the older person and more rewarding practice for the nurse.

Strumpf (2000) summarized the following problems that need to be addressed to advance gerontological nursing: a modest science, inadequate delivery systems, limited availability of information, and insufficient expertise. Nurses of this century need to develop and test interventions and models of care that will improve the health and well-being of older adults along the health-illness continuum. This knowledge then must be disseminated to a wide range of nurses and health professionals to improve health care.

Gerontological nursing remains at a crossroads. As the older population grows, increased public awareness of and interest in their problems should place gerontological nursing in the spotlight. Nurses have the knowledge and skills to improve the health care for this most vulnerable population. The challenge put to us by McConnell (1997) from the last edition of this text remains:

Can we lead health care of the aged into a more enlightened era, where well-prepared, rehabilitation-oriented teams of motivated professionals provide individualized, goal-oriented, cost-effective care for older people? Or will gerontological nurses become guardians of the status quo—where need for care is equated with the potential for reimbursement, where custodial care predominates in the name of cost containment, where nurses base their practice on myth and custom rather than on scientific reasoning and ethical principles—and follow the medical profession's lead into a fragmented system of care? The choice is ours to make.

REFERENCES

Administration on Aging. (2004). A profile of older Americans: 2004. Retrieved September 1, 2004, from www.aoa.gov/prof/Statistics/profile/2004/6.asp.

American Academy of Nurse Practitioners. (2002). *Scope of practice for nurse practitioners*. Washington, DC: American Academy of Nurse Practitioners.

American Nurses Association. (1970). *Standards of geriatric nursing practice*. Kansas City, MO: Division of Geriatric Nursing Practice, American Nurses Association.

American Nurses Association. (2001). *Scope and standards of gerontological nursing practice* (2nd ed.). Washington, DC: American Nurses Publishing.

Anderson, M. M., & Robinson, D. (2001). The role of managed care in health care delivery. In D. Robinson & C. P. Kish (Eds.), *Core concepts in advanced practice nursing*. St. Louis: Mosby.

Barker, W. H. (2003). Geriatrics in North America. In R. C. Tallis & H. M. Fillit (Eds.), *Brocklehurst's textbook of geriatric medicine and gerontology* (6th ed.). London: Churchill Livingstone.

Belza, B., & Baker, M. W. (2000). Maintaining health in well older adults: Initiatives for schools of nursing and the John A. Hartford Foundation for the 21st century. *Journal of Gerontological Nursing, 26*(7), 8-17.

Bennett, J. A., & Flaherty-Robb, M. K. (2003). Issues affecting the health of older citizens: Meeting the challenge. *Online Journal of Nursing Issues*, May 31.

Bishop, L. (1904). The relations of old age to disease with illustrative cases. *American Journal of Nursing, 4*, 679.

Bourbonniere, M., & Evans, L. K. (2002). Advanced practice nursing in the care of frail older adults. *Journal of the American Geriatrics Society, 50*, 2062-2076.

Buckwalter, K. C., & Hertz, J. E. (2003). Irene R. Mortenson Burnside: Tribute to a gerontological pioneer, colleague, friend and teacher. *Journal of Gerontological Nursing, 29*(11), 3-5.

Burggraf, V., & Barry, R. (1998). Gerontological nursing in the 21st century. *Journal of Gerontological Nursing, 24*(6), 29-35.

Burnside, I. M. (1988). *Nursing and the aged*. New York: McGraw-Hill.

Burnside, I. M., & Schmidt, M. G. (1994). *Working with older adults: Group process and technique*. Boston: Jones & Bartlett.

Callahan, D. (1987). *Setting limits: Medical goals for an aging society*. New York: Simon & Schuster.

Conn V. S., Burks, K. O., Rantz, M., & Knudsen, K. S. (2002). Evidence-based practice for gerontological nursing. *Journal of Gerontological Nursing, 28*(2), 45-52.

Dock, L. (1908). Alsmhouse nursing. *American Journal of Nursing, 8*(5), 361-363.

Drinka, T. K. (2002). From double jeopardy to double indemnity: Subtleties of teaching interdisciplinary geriatrics. *Educational Gerontology, 28*, 433-449.

Ebersole, P. (2001). Behind the scenes: Visionary foundations. *Geriatric Nursing, 22*(4), 210.

Ebersole, P. (2003). Irene Mortenson Burnside: Her light shines on. *Geriatric Nursing, 24*(4), 232-235.

Ebersole, P., & Hess, P. (1998). *Gerontological nursing* (5th ed.). St. Louis: Mosby.

Ebersole, P., Hess, P., & Luggen, A. S. (2004). *Toward healthy aging: Human needs and nursing response* (6th ed.). St. Louis: Mosby.

Eliopoulos, C. (1997). *Gerontological nursing* (4th ed.). Philadelphia: Lippincott.

Eng, C. (2002). Future consideration for improving end-of-life care for older persons: Program of All-inclusive Care of the Elderly (PACE). *Palliative Medicine, 5*(2), 903-910.

Evans, L., & Strumpf, N. E. (1989). Tying down the elderly: A review of the literature on physical restraint. *Journal of the American Geriatrics Society, 37*, 65-74.

Evans, L. K., Strumpf, N. E., & Allen-Taylor, S. L. (1997). A clinical trial to reduce restraints in nursing homes. *Journal of the American Geriatrics Society, 45*, 675-681.

Federal Interagency Forum on Aging-Related Statistics. (2000). *Older Americans 2000: Key indicators of well-being*. Washington, DC: Federal Interagency Forum.

Flaherty J. H., Tariq, S. H., Raghavan, S., Bakshi, S., Moinuddin, A., & Morley, J. E. (2003). A model for managing delirious older inpatients. *Journal of the American Geriatrics Society, 51*(7), 1031-1035.

Fried, L. P., Tangen, C. M., Walston, J, Newman, A. B., Hirsch, C., Gottdiener, J., et al. (2001). Frailty in older adults: Evidence for a phenotype. *Journal of Gerontology, Medical Sciences, 56A*(3), M146-M156.

Fries, J. F., & Crapo, L. M. (1986). The elimination of premature disease. In K. Dychtwald (Ed.), *Wellness and health promotion for the elderly*. Rockville, MD: Aspen.

Fulton, J. S. (2004). Just the facts. *Clinical Nurse Specialist, 18*(5), 219-221.

Futrell, M., Brovender, S., McKinnon-Mullett, E., & Brower, H.T. (1980). *Primary health care of the older adult*. North Scituate, MA: Duxbury Press.

Grocki, J. H., & Fox, G. E., Jr. (2004). Gerontology coursework in undergraduate nursing programs in the United States: A regional study. *Journal of Gerontological Nursing, 30*(3), 46-51.

Gunter, L., & Estes, C. (1979). *Education for gerontic nursing*. New York: Springer.

Hutchins, D. (2002). Evaluating Robert Wood Johnson's teaching nursing home program. Retrieved September 1, 2004, from www.rwjf.org/reports/grr/026434.

Jensen, G. A., & Morrisey, M. A. (2004). Are healthier older adults choosing managed care? *Gerontologist, 44*(10), 85-94.

Kane, R. L., Flood, S., Bershadsky, B., & Keckhafer, G. (2004). Effect of an innovative Medicare managed care program on the quality of care for nursing home residents. *Gerontologist, 44*(1), 95-103.

Kaufman, D. W., Kelly, J. P., Rosenberg, L., Anderson, T. E., & Mitchell, A. A. (2002). Recent patterns of medication use in the ambulatory adult population of the United States: The Slone survey. *Journal of the American Medical Association, 287*(3), 337-344.

Keane, A., & Becker, D. (2001). Emerging roles of the advanced practice nurse. In L. A. Joel (Ed.), *Advanced practice nursing: Essentials for role development*. Philadelphia: F. A. Davis.

Lindeman, C. A. (2000). The future of nursing education. *Journal of Nursing Education, 39*(1), 5-12.

Lopez, M., Delmore, B., Ake, J. M., Kim, Y. R., Golden, P., Bier, J., & Fulmer, T. (2002). Implementing a geriatric resource nurse model. *Journal of Nursing Administration, 32*(11), 577-585.

Mack, M. (1952). Personal adjustment of chronically ill people under home care. *Nursing Research, 1*, 9-30.

Mahoney, J. E., Sager, M. A., & Jalaluddin, M. (1998). New walking dependence associated with hospitalization for acute medical illness: Incidence and significance. *Journal of Gerontology, Medical Sciences, 53A*, M307-312.

Manton, K. G. (2003). The future of old age. In R.C. Tallis & H. M. Fillit (Eds.), *Brocklehurst's textbook of geriatric medicine and gerontology* (6th ed.). London: Churchill Livingstone.

McBride, A. B. (2000). Nursing and gerontology. *Journal of Gerontological Nursing, 26*(7), 18-27.

McConnell, E. S. (1997). Conceptual bases for gerontological nursing practice: Models, trends, and issues. In M. A. Matteson, E. S. McConnell, & A. D. Linton (Eds.), *Gerontological nursing: Concepts and practice* (2nd ed.). Philadelphia: Saunders.

Mehlman, M. J., Binstock, R. H., Juengst, E. T., Ponsaran, R. S., & Whitehouse, P. J. (2004). Anti-aging medicine: Can consumers be better protected? *Gerontologist, 44*(3), 304-310.

Merck Institute of Aging and Health & Gerontological Society of America. (2002). The state of aging and health in America. Retrieved September 1, 2004, from www.agingsociety.org/agingsociety/publications/state/index.html.

Mezey, T., & Fulmer, T. (2002). The future history of gerontological nursing. *Journal of Gerontology, Medical Sciences, 57A*(7), M438-M441.

Miller, C. A. (1993). *Nursing care of older adults* (2nd ed.). Philadelphia: Lippincott.

Miller, S. K. (2002). Acute care of the elderly units: A positive outcomes case study. *AACN Clinical Issues, 13*(1), 34-42.

National Academy on an Aging Society. (1999). *Chronic conditions: A challenge for the 21st century*. Washington, DC: National Academy on an Aging Society.

National Academy on an Aging Society. (2000). *At risk: Developing chronic conditions later in life*. Washington, DC: National Academy on an Aging Society.

Naylor, M. D., Brooten, D., & Campbell, R. (1999). Comprehensive discharge planning and home follow-up of hospitalized elders: A randomized clinical trial. *Journal of the American Medical Association, 281*, 613-620.

Newton, K. (1950). *Geriatric nursing*. St. Louis: Mosby.

Norton, D., McLaren, R., & Exton-Smith, N. (1962; reprinted 1975). *An investigation of geriatric nursing problems in hospital*. National Corporation for the Care of Old People. Edinburgh: Churchill Livingstone.

Office of Minority Health. (2002). Protecting the health of minority communities. Retrieved September 1, 2004, from www.omhrc.gov/rah/indexNew.htm.

Orem, D. (1991). *Nursing: Concepts of practice* (4th ed.). St. Louis: Mosby.

Quinn, M. E., Berding, C., Daniels, E., Gerlach, M. J., Harris, K., Nugent, K., et al. (2004). Shifting paradigms: Teaching gerontological nursing from a new perspective. *Journal of Gerontological Nursing, 30*(1), 21-27.

Rubenstein, L. Z. (2004). Comprehensive geriatric assessment: From miracle to reality. *Journal of Gerontology, Medical Sciences, 50A*, 473-477.

Ryden, M. B., Snyder, M., Gross, C. R., Savik, K., Pearson, V., Krichbaum, K., Mueller, C. (2000). Value-added outcomes: The use of advanced practice nurses in long term care facilities. *Gerontologist, 40*(6), 654-662.

Schwartz, D. (1995). *My 50 years in nursing; give us to go blithely*. New York: Springer.

Schwartz, D., Henley, B., & Zeitz, L. (1964). *The elderly ambulatory patient: Nursing and psychosocial needs*. New York: Macmillan.

Sochalski, J. A. (2001). Outcomes of a nurse-managed geriatric day hospital. *Gerontologist, 41*(special issue), 51.

Strumpf, N. E. (2000). Improving care for the frail elderly: The challenge for nursing, *Journal of Gerontological Nursing, 26*(7), 36-44.

Thames, D. (1997). Mary Opal Wolanin: A life worth living . . . a life of giving. *Geriatric Nursing, 18*(5), 229-231.

Veterans Administration. (2004). Retrieved September 1, 2004, from www1.va.gov/geriatricsshg/docs.GRECC/doc.

Wilson, R. L.(1994). Tribute to Virginia Stone. *Geriatric Nursing, 15*(4), 180-181.

Wolanin, M. O., & Phillips, L. R. (1981). *Confusion: Prevention and care*. St. Louis: Mosby.

Chapter 2

Assessment: Focus on Function

Helen W. Lach & Carrie M. Smith

Objectives

Discuss the rationale for functional assessment of the older adult.

Describe special considerations in assessment of the older adult.

Distinguish three different types of assessment: initial, functional, and ongoing.

Outline the elements of a comprehensive nursing assessment focused on function using Gordon's functional domains.

BACKGROUND

Assessment of function in the older adult has become the hallmark of gerontological care. Some have called functional decline the final common pathway of chronic disease in aging. Although the significance of function in health and illness has long been appreciated, its importance was not recognized until the 1950s, as the numbers of older and disabled persons grew and the prevalence of chronic disease increased. Historically, the importance of function was affirmed by the U.S. Commission on Chronic Illness and the World Health Organization (WHO) (2002), which fostered the development of a scientific base for measurement over the past few decades. Further theoretical research and instrument development examined key constructs of functional health: activities of daily living (ADLs) and instrumental activities of daily living (IADLs), as well as psychological and social variables. Today much research focuses on the prevention and treatment of functional decline and frailty, rehabilitation, and the prevention of disability. Assessment with a focus on function builds on this tradition to improve the care of colder adults.

DEFINITION

Functional status is defined as a person's ability to perform the activities necessary to ensure well-being, and is conceptualized as the integration of three domains of function: biological, psychological (cognitive and affective), and social. Functional assessment is derived from a systems model, which recognizes the interrelationships of these domains and their interaction with the environment. In the older adult, adaptive responses to stressors in any of these domains can contribute to behavior and well-being. Although individual health and developmental processes can cause wide variation in the clinical profiles of older adults, broadening traditional assessment to include all three of these domains gives a comprehensive picture of the adaptation of the older adult. Each domain provides a critical component of the person's overall health, need for care, and prognosis.

The interrelationships of the biopsychosocial domains are mediated by chronic disease burden and functional status as illustrated in Figure 2-1. Quality of life is influenced by each of these factors when deficits exist. As the chronic disease burden increases, the risk for functional impairment rises and the quality of life is threatened. With functional decline, the risks for increased health care utilization, nursing home placement, and death increase (Fried, Ferrucci, Darer, Williamson, & Anderson, 2004).

Nursing assessment has traditionally been holistic, grounded in addressing the wholeness of the individual and the interrelationships of the biopsychosocial domains. Nursing and other disciplines have also addressed measurement issues for screening and comprehensive assessment, program development, service delivery, and evaluation in older populations. Because

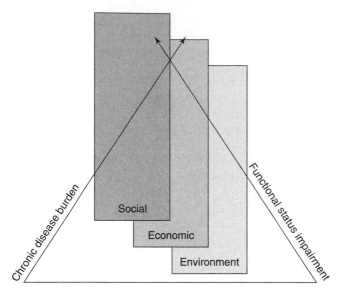

Figure 2-1 Interrelationships of chronic disease burden and functional impairment.

nurses are often the primary contact with older adults throughout the health care system, they are especially poised to assess the older adult, identify unmet needs, and make referrals to maintain or improve function.

Comprehensive assessment is often provided for older adults with complex problems through geriatric assessment programs that are made up of interdisciplinary teams of geriatric professionals offered through acute care, academic geriatric centers, or community programs. This form of care is discussed further in Chapter 25. Although interdisciplinary assessment and care are ideal for people with multiple diagnoses and complex situations, the roles of various professionals overlap and nurses should be able to independently perform a comprehensive assessment of older adults that has a focus on function.

The purpose of nursing assessment of the older adult is to identify patterns of functioning that deviate from baseline or from accepted standards (norms). Additionally, it is an opportunity to identify health promotion and disease prevention activities that may enhance the overall well-being of the older adult. A systematic approach is advocated to ensure comprehensiveness and efficiency. Nurses should develop an approach that accommodates their nursing framework, the objectives of the work setting, and the needs of the patients being served. Approaches to comprehensive assessment may vary depending on the practice setting.

First, this chapter describes special considerations for the older adult throughout the nursing process. Examples using standardized nursing diagnoses, nursing outcomes, and nursing interventions are provided. Next, approaches to assessment are outlined according to the older adult's entry into the health care system. A model for conducting a comprehensive nursing assessment

focused on the individual's function is presented. Specific measures and tools that may be used during the assessment process are discussed in depth in Chapter 3.

THE NURSING PROCESS: SPECIAL CONSIDERATIONS FOR THE OLDER ADULT

Knowledge of age-related changes and the societal responses to the aging population that are described throughout this text lead to modifications in generic nursing approaches when working with older adults. Older adults are a heterogeneous group, and providing individualized care to each person should be the norm. Much of gerontological nursing consists of the application of nursing processes and methods with special attention to the unique influences of the aging process on health and illness. It is important to keep in mind the similarities and differences between gerontological nursing practice and generalist nursing practice. Typically, the following elements of nursing practice remain the same, regardless of age:

- Goals of nursing
- Generic nursing process and methods
- Professional practice norms, including basic standards of practice, code of ethics, and accountability

The modifications in practice presented in Box 2-1 are commonly required when working with older adults, based on age-related changes and common health conditions, the location of care, and developmental issues.

Although the nursing process is divided into discrete, linear steps for the purposes of discussion, in practice these steps are more of a cyclical process carried on many, many times in each encounter. Assessment can enhance later nursing interventions, so it is important for the nurse to evaluate the impact of the assessment on the individual. For example, when the nurse assesses activity patterns in the older person, the very act of inquiring about this domain of function may "raise their consciousness" that activity is important regardless of age. This small step may enhance the effectiveness of subsequent health teaching about the need to exercise, for the person's "teachable moment" may occur earlier in the process of care than would have been the case if the topic had not come up in the assessment. The following sections review the various components of the nursing process and modifications that are helpful with the older adult.

Assessment

Assessment of an older person is a complex, time-consuming process, and it is usually impossible to perform a comprehensive assessment of an older person in one encounter. The older adult has a wealth of information to be gathered, and it may take time to establish

BOX 2-1 Modifications in Nursing Process with Older Adults		
MODIFICATIONS NECESSARY BECAUSE OF AGE-RELATED CHANGES AND HEALTH CONDITIONS	**MODIFICATIONS NECESSARY BECAUSE OF LOCATION OF CARE**	**MODIFICATIONS NECESSARY BECAUSE OF DEVELOPMENTAL LEVEL**
Slower pace of the nursing process	Financial resources available to implement a plan of care	Goals and priority setting
Emphasis on functional abilities	Health care professionals available to implement a plan of care	Attention to competency levels in those with cognitive impairment
Attention to the effects of the aging process on disease presentation and responses to disease and treatments	Priority setting	Awareness of losses and impact on the older adult
Emphasis on nursing diagnoses and geriatric syndromes common to older adults	The older adult's goals	Emphasis on coping and self-management of chronic diseases
Attention to the social, economic, and political influences on health care for this age-group	Increased attention to environmental modifications as an intervention or as a source of problems for the older adult	Increased attention to concerns about the dying process and end-of-life care
Increased alertness for signs of an intensified stress state, and iatrogenic responses to interventions		
Multidimensional effects of problems		

his or her trust. In addition, older adults may enjoy talking or reminiscing during the encounter, and the nurse may need to refocus the conversation in order to obtain the necessary information. Enough time should be planned to attain the nurse's goals, while matching the pace of the older person. Several encounters may be needed to accomplish this. Although the depth of the assessment may vary depending on the level of the nurse and the nurse's scope of practice, the topics and issues are the same.

Knowledge of normal age-related changes is essential for successful care of the older adult. Health providers often have the misconception that common conditions and symptoms are part of normal aging rather than disease processes, which may result in underdiagnosis and undertreatment of problems. Older adults also have these misconceptions and may not report symptoms, assuming they just have to live with them. The nurse should be able to accurately distinguish between normal aging changes and pathological findings.

The older adult also frequently has atypical symptoms of disease, making assessment challenging. The classic issues related to altered presentation include polypharmacy, the presence of multiple chronic conditions, and varied significance of symptoms (Henderson, 2001). Table 2-1 provides examples of some common variations in symptoms seen in the older patient compared with younger patients. Because of the wide range of symptoms possible in the older adult, it is important to consider all the possible causes of symptoms, and performing a comprehensive assessment may be indicated. It is important to get to know the individual patient in order to plan appropriate care, as illustrated by the experiences of Dr. Geri Hall (Box 2-2). When we know the patient, we can identify which symptoms are normal for her or him and which signal a change in health.

Before the Assessment. Before the actual encounter, the nurse can begin the process of assessment and planning. A review of the older adult's medical record or chart is always recommended before the encounter, when possible, and may help provide direction for the assessment. The medical record provides information about the past medical, personal, and social history; management plan for current health problems; medications; immunization history; and laboratory and diagnostic test results. Past screening and health promotion activities may also be listed in the chart, allowing the

Table 2-1 *How Illness Changes with Age*

Problem	Classic Presentation in Young Patient	Presentation in Elderly
Urinary tract infection	Dysuria, frequency, urgency	Incontinence, confusion, anorexia; dysuria often absent; frequency, urgency, nocturia may be present
Myocardial infarction	Severe substernal chest pain, diaphoresis, nausea, shortness of breath	Sometimes no chest pain or an atypical pain location such as the jaw, neck, or shoulder; shortness of breath, tachypnea, arrhythmia, hypotension, restlessness, syncope, confusion
Pneumonia	Cough, productive purulent sputum, chills and fever, pleuritis, chest pain, elevated white blood cell (WBC) count	Cough may be productive, dry, or absent; chills, fever, and elevated WBC count may be absent; tachypnea, slight cyanosis, confusion, anorexia, nausea and vomiting, tachycardia may be present
Congestive heart failure	Increased dyspnea, orthopnea, paroxysmal nocturnal dyspnea, fatigue, weight gain, pedal edema, night cough, nocturia, bibasilar rales	May have classic presentation plus anorexia, restlessness, cyanosis, falls
Hyperthyroidism	Heat intolerance, fast pace, exopthalmos, increased pulse, hyperreflexia, tremor	Slowing down, lethargy, weakness, depression, atrial fibrillation, congestive heart failure
Depression	Sad mood and thoughts, withdrawal, crying, weight loss, insomnia	Classic signs may or may not be present, apathy, memory and concentration problems, psychomotor retardation, increased somatic symptoms, increased sleep

Adapted from Henderson, M. L. (1985). Altered presentations. *American Journal of Nursing, 85*(10), 1103-1106.

nurse to identify if the health prevention standards have been met and determine health maintenance and preventive measures that need to be performed. In addition, the nurse should gather information from other health care providers who are familiar with the person, including staff from residential settings, home health or other community agency staff, or other allied health professionals.

The Assessment Encounter. With this knowledge, a tentative plan for the focus of the assessment, what will be covered, and how the assessment will be conducted can be formulated. For example, if the person has a history of congestive heart failure, the nurse should plan to perform a pertinent history and physical examination to assess the management of this chronic health problem. This is in addition to assessment of any current concerns the individual may have, which the nurse may not be knowledgeable about until the encounter. The nurse should plan to screen for problems

that have a high prevalence in the aged with an impact on functional ability (e.g., dysmobility, vision changes, urinary incontinence, falls, polypharmacy, acute confusion). It is important for the nurse to prepare for the visit to the extent possible while realizing that flexibility in the plan is essential.

Unless there is an emergency, the nurse should begin with the person's concerns. A plan for conducting the assessment in a way that flows smoothly, results in the least number of position changes for the older adult, and allows for adequate rest periods when needed yet remains comprehensive should also be developed. Box 2-3 provides key points to keep in mind for the assessment.

Several processes occur simultaneously during an assessment encounter. For example, while discussing with the older person the reason for seeking care, the nurse will use all of his or her senses to evaluate the older person's response to the questions, the ability to articulate concerns, mood, sensory function, comfort

---

Box 2-2   *Reflections on Nursing Assessment*

Comprehensive nursing assessment has been an integral part of my career for at least 30 years. It is, without any doubt, the most exciting, challenging, and interesting part of every position I've held.

In nursing school (1964–1967), assessment meant taking vital signs, knowing the medical history and progress notes, following the dialogue on the nursing notes, and understanding the orders in the kardex. All patients received basic daily care, while special needs were listed as treatments on a clipboard and checked off as tasks were completed. Social histories were limited to whether the patient smoked or consumed alcohol. We got to know our patients as "patients;" people who existed for us solely in the context of when they were in the hospital. To be fair, some patients were in the hospital for lengthy stays, so we got to meet families. We would see that patients have lives outside of the hospital, but we rarely were concerned about it. Discharge planning meant referring a visiting nurse and making sure the patient could take medications and change dressings per our schedule. Spending time talking with a patient was viewed as "idle chatter," and to be avoided at all times in the pursuit of "doing important nursing work."

That form of practice is not very satisfying because it failed to tap into the qualities that brought us into nursing: our interest in people and desire to help them. How could we help people if we had no idea of how their illnesses impacted on their lives? We might as well have been practicing on "Mrs. Chase!" (The Chase Family were manikins in the Nursing Arts lab.)

As I developed in my career I found it increasingly important to know the context of people's lives in order to help them adapt to the changes needed to manage their illnesses. One physician I knew from rehabilitation used to say "All diabetics are cheaters and liars." He wanted us to see that we needed to know more about people in order to help them manage their disease. Such a comment is unthinkable today.

In 1978, I took a position developing a comprehensive multidisciplinary assessment for case management of frail elders. We were able to relate to our patients as people who were as real as ourselves. We performed assessments on 900 subjects over the next few years. The work was fascinating as we began to learn the patient's stories. We not only knew that someone was a retired factory worker, we knew why they retired, what their family thought about it, and how that impacted on health and day-to-day function.

The instrument we used was lengthy (about 50 pages) and we were required to ask and record data that did not have meaning to our work because the researchers were afraid we would miss something. The instrument was cumbersome and unnecessarily invaded patients' privacy. From that I learned that the professional should only gather information that is important for planning care.

Developing assessment skills takes time, yet few skills are more professionally satisfying. The key to excellence is keeping assessment in the context of conversation so the patients are encouraged and able to share their most pressing concerns. If, after the information needs are satisfied, we can tell the patient's story, then we have completed an excellent assessment.

Geri R. Hall

Geri R. Hall, PhD, ARNP, CNS, FAAN
Clinical Professor and Advanced Practice Nurse
University of Iowa
Iowa City, Iowa

---

level, overall body integrity, and grooming. At the same time the nurse will modify the interaction style to accommodate sensory deficits (through voice modulation and attention to seating arrangements), provide support and instill confidence and trust, provide information about health concerns, and provide reinforcement for positive health behaviors.

Early in the assessment it is helpful to be aware of any special communication barriers (visual problems, hearing loss, aphasia, impaired cognition) so that adjustments in communication techniques can be made. Modify the environment to match the older person's needs by reducing noise levels (especially "white noise" generated from activity in hallways, other people in the room, television, radio, outdoor noise, intercoms). Ensure a comfortable temperature, adequate space and lighting, and privacy. Avoid glare from windows or shiny surfaces that can interfere with vision. Assist the person to sit in an upright position if in bed, to promote vision and eye contact, hearing, and alertness. Face the person to allow for lip reading. Make sure assistive devices, including hearing aids and glasses, are on and in good working order. Hand-held voice amplifiers can be valuable equipment for the nurse to use with hearing-impaired persons. They are easily obtained and are relatively inexpensive.

To enhance the person's ability to engage fully in the encounter, consider personal factors involved, such as comfort, by positioning the older person comfortably. Inquire about pain, thirst, and the need to use the toilet (and intervene beforehand or reschedule the interview if possible). Proceed in a relaxed pace, and do not rush the interaction. Maximize the use of silence to allow the person to collect his or her thoughts in order to formulate

---

BOX 2-3 10 Key Points in Older Adult Assessment

1. Identify personal biases/stereotypes about older adults so they can be avoided
2. Be aware of age-related changes in each body system
3. Distinguish between normal and pathological changes
4. Know the atypical presentations of illness
5. Allow time for trust to develop and to gather assessment information
6. Make accommodations for any impairments to promote comfort
7. Screen for conditions common in the older adult population
8. Be alert to signs and symptoms of elder abuse and neglect
9. Always consider medications and their effects as a cause/contributor to a problem
10. Use collateral sources to validate the patient's report

Adapted from Hall, G. R., & Smith, M. (2001). Life on the front lines: The clinical assessment of elderly patients. In G. R. Hall, M. L. Henderson, & M. Smith (Eds.), *Assessing the elderly.* New York: Lippincott Williams & Wilkins.

---

and answer questions or verbalize concerns. Be relaxed and patient. It is important to remember, however, that the nurse is responsible for maintaining the focus of the conversation, and may have to redirect the older adult.

Additionally, the nurse should be aware that assessments can produce anxiety in the older adult, and because examinations are often conducted in unfamiliar environments, the situation can even be threatening. To compensate for anxiety that may interfere with formal testing (for example, during mental status testing), the nurse should take a matter-of-fact approach to asking questions, and identify and respond to any concerns expressed. Introduce testing techniques as part of the normal examination for all older adults and explain how the information will help individualize the person's care.

The assessment encounter also provides the opportunity for the nurse and older person to identify or establish mutual expectations. The nurse can clarify his or her role and responsibilities with regard to the older person's care. The individual can be encouraged to discuss his or her needs and concerns and help identify strategies for meeting needs. The mutual interaction and collaboration between the nurse and the older adult fosters the expectation that they both will participate in decision making and care. The older adult will be in control to the greatest extent possible, with the nurse serving a supportive role. For those who are not able to articulate their needs or concerns, the nurse serves a supportive and advocacy role, compensating for limitations and, whenever possible, engaging family and friends to assist

in assessment. This approach sets up a relationship with the older adult in which his or her needs are central.

For the nurse providing care, there can be many opportunities, often over a period of days, to learn more about the older adult, especially in institutional settings. Much assessment information is directly accessible to the nurse during patient care encounters. Whenever possible, the nurse should take advantage of natural opportunities for gathering data (during the bath, at meals, during transfers), because actual performance is an important assessment finding. Direct observation of activities of daily living such as getting dressed, drinking fluids, eating a meal, and ambulating is the most reliable method of data collection. Observing communication patterns with others allows the nurse to assess the individual's socialization ability.

Assessing the individual at more than one encounter and at different times of the day may be advantageous to the nurse assessing functional status. Older adults have "good" days and "bad" days, and in some cases assessing at different times of the day can yield different results. For example, early morning stiffness or pain or late afternoon and evening fatigue can negatively affect performance so that the assessment is not characteristic of the person's usual functioning. Also, the older person may not feel wholly cooperative in the assessment encounter if not feeling at his or her best.

Following the assessment, it is important to confirm findings with family members, caregivers, nursing staff (including nursing assistants), or other health professionals, to elicit their perception of the older person's health problems, concerns, and functional status. These collateral sources can help the nurse form a clear picture of the patient's health and environment. The nurse will want to consider the individual's confidentiality during such discussions. When the person has cognitive impairment, information regarding his or her cognitive and functional abilities should be elicited from a knowledgeable informant. A knowledgeable informant is someone close to the person who can provide information about the person's capabilities, usually a significant other, a child, some other family member, or a friend. Also, validation of important information such as medications with an objective data source such as the medical record or list from the pharmacy is desirable. This helps increase the accuracy of the data.

Health conditions in the older adult can have many contributing factors and in turn, affect many other components of the person's life. For example, urinary incontinence may be related to hormonal changes, pathogens, pharmacological agents, neurological dysfunction, structural anomalies, pelvic musculature, functional problems, or psychological factors. The incontinence may cause accidents and embarrassment for the older individual, who begins to limit his or her social activities. The incontinence increases the individual's risk for skin problems, falls, and social isolation. Comprehensive assessment will allow the nurse to identify all of the contributing factors and outcomes related to the individual's health conditions.

Cultural patterns and beliefs have a significant impact on individual behaviors. An understanding of these behaviors will assist the nurse in identifying realistic goals for care. The nurse will need to ask questions to assess cultural factors during the assessment as an essential part of providing comprehensive and holistic care. Before asking questions, the nurse should consider his or her own personal cultural biases or beliefs that may affect health care practice. Ideally, awareness of these beliefs helps the nurse overcome negative stereotypes and be more objective in communicating with patients. Cultural and racial disparities exist, and the nurse must be proactive in promoting cultural competence.

In summary, gerontological nurses should consider the many potential contributors to a problem and the multiple ramifications of a problem on the individual's life. This is most readily accomplished by using a multi-dimensional framework for assessment such as the example presented later in this chapter.

Diagnosis

The act of *diagnosing*, or specifying the problems or needs for nursing intervention from assessment data, is the next step in the nursing process. A nursing diagnosis was originally defined by the North American Nursing Diagnosis Association (NANDA) as "a clinical judgment about individual, family or community responses to actual and potential health problems/life processes. Nursing diagnoses provide the basis for selection of nursing interventions to achieve outcomes for which the nurse is accountable" (NANDA International, 2003, p. 263). The standard format for communicating nursing diagnoses includes a diagnostic label, followed by risk factors or contributing factors, or signs and symptoms. For example, a hospitalized older woman might have the diagnosis "risk for impaired skin integrity related to immobility secondary to hip fracture." A list of key NANDA-approved nursing diagnoses common in the older adult is presented in Box 2-4. In this box, the diagnoses are grouped by the functional health patterns that correspond to the later assessment format.

Nurses have diagnosed patient problems since the time of Nightingale, but now nursing diagnosis terminology provides a way to consistently document problems. NANDA was first convened in 1973 as a broad constituency of practicing nurses and nursing theorists who believed in the importance of classifying the phenomena that nurses assess and treat. NANDA remains the driving force behind establishing a broadly accepted classification of nursing diagnoses that can be used to

---

BOX 2-4 Common Nursing Diagnoses for Older Adults by Health Patterns

Health Perception-Health Management
Altered health maintenance
Risk for injury: fall
Risk for poisoning: drug toxicity
Risk for infection
Impaired home maintenance
Health-seeking behaviors
Ineffective management of therapeutic regimen
Elder mistreatment

Nutritional-Metabolic Pattern
Impaired skin integrity: pressure ulcer
Impaired skin integrity: dry skin
Altered nutrition: less than body requirements
Impaired swallowing
Altered oral mucous membrane
Fluid volume deficit: dehydration
Risk for altered body temperature

Elimination Pattern
Constipation
Diarrhea
Bowel incontinence
Urinary incontinence

Activity-Exercise Pattern
Decreased cardiac output
Altered tissue perfusion
Ineffective breathing pattern
Activity intolerance
Impaired physical mobility
Self-care deficit
Diversional activity deficit

Sleep-Rest Pattern
Sleep pattern disturbance
Cognitive-Perceptual Pattern
Chronic confusion
Acute confusion
Pain
Sensory/perceptual alterations
Unilateral neglect
Knowledge deficit

Self-Perception–Self-Concept Pattern
Depression
Body image disturbance
Powerlessness
Anxiety and fear
Self-esteem disturbance
Hopelessness

Role-Relationship Pattern
Relocation stress syndrome
Grieving
Social isolation
Impaired communication
Caregiver role strain

Continued

BOX 2-4 Common Nursing Diagnoses for Older Adults by Health Patterns—cont'd

Role-Relationship Pattern—cont'd
Risk for violence: directed at self or others
Self-determination
Altered family processes

Sexuality-Reproductive Pattern
Sexual dysfunction
Altered sexuality patterns

Coping-Stress Tolerance Pattern
Ineffective coping

Value-Belief Pattern
Spiritual distress

---

support a variety of key clinical, administrative, and research activities.

Use of NANDA labels contributes to increased consistency in use of language, facilitating communication between nurses across the functional areas of practice, administration, teaching, and research. Second, using a nursing diagnosis taxonomy facilitates the statistical reporting of patient problems in various settings of care. Without a systematic means of classifying nursing phenomena, it is impossible to develop general information about the frequency with which these problems are encountered.

Building on the work of NANDA, the University of Iowa's Center for Nursing Classification has developed taxonomies for nursing interventions and outcomes (Nursing Interventions Classification [NIC] and Nursing Outcomes Classification [NOC]) that are discussed in further detail later. Use of these three taxonomies in clinical and research programs allows the identification of the work of nursing, which has been hard to define and quantify in the past. It is hoped that in the future these labels will be included in computerized systems in various health care settings, so that nurses can easily pick from a computer screen the diagnoses, outcomes, and interventions appropriate for patients. When this becomes available, nursing will be able to identify the frequency of various patient problems and nursing inventions that will help define nursing. For now, the use of references is needed to accurately use the methodology.

Medical diagnoses may be used by the advanced practice nurse (APN) in classifying problems in addition to the NANDA nursing diagnoses. The *International Classification of Diseases, 9th Revision* (ICD-9) contains the list of codes that are assigned to particular diagnoses and is the current standard for recognized medical diagnoses (Hart & Hopkins, 2003). It was developed by the World Health Organization in order to have an international standard for collecting mortality data. In addition to its original purpose, the ICD-9 codes are used extensively to determine reimbursement for health services. As a result, APNs may need to document diagnoses using ICD-9 codes in order to receive payment for their services and should be familiar with this process.

Planning

The nurse planning care for the older person should be aware of environmental influences on the individual's life situation and on the nurse's practice world. Two important types of environmental influences are the health care system and the social system. These may affect the nurse's priorities, or focus, in caring for a patient; the resources available to the patient and nurse for goal attainment; and the time available for goal achievement. An example is individuals cared for by the Department of Veterans Affairs. Patients in this health care system may have resources available to them that are not available to indigent patients in a free health clinic. The nurse working with either type of individual must consider what goals are appropriate for that person, given the options and resources available. Healthful outcomes are possible in both situations, but the specific goals and strategies are likely to be quite different.

Differences in social systems can also affect care. Individuals from large, healthy families in which the long-standing cultural norm is to "take care of your own" may have a wider range of options for assistance than individuals with limited family or friends or limited finances. These influences may dramatically affect judgments about what goals are attainable, which in turn help to shape nursing activities with that person.

Mutual goal setting is emphasized in working with older adults. Even if the individual requires much assistance, he or she remains entitled to the privileges accorded adults. Basic civil rights are sometimes abridged by well-meaning helpers, who assume that disability renders the older person incapable of setting goals or making decisions. It is vital to respect the adult status of the older person, and mutual goal setting is a fundamental way to accomplish this. The nurse should assume the older adult is responsible for providing assessment information and making decisions unless otherwise determined.

Involvement of family members in the planning of nursing care is important for older people with self-care deficits or who require assistance, because the majority of long-term care is provided in the home by family members. It is not always a simple matter to determine which family members are appropriate to include, but defining the functional family unit is essential in assessment of those in need of long-term care. Consideration should be given to family members' goals and needs also, such as socialization and respite.

Nursing care for older adults is likely to include interdisciplinary team involvement. Greater numbers of health care providers increase the complexity of the planning process but result in the expertise of a wide variety of specialists. There is a risk that without careful joint planning of care, disciplines may work at cross-purposes, resulting in suboptimal care. Nurses should be knowledgeable about behaviors that facilitate positive team interaction and be prepared to support the patient or family member in establishing goals for health care. Chapter 25 provides an overview of interdisciplinary teamwork, addressing issues in communication and collaboration.

Once goals have been established for the individual, the nurse should identify the desired outcomes related to the goals using the Nursing Outcomes Classification (NOC; Iowa Outcomes Project, 2003). Similar to nursing diagnoses, the NOC provides a standardized language that describes what the patient is experiencing, and the outcomes are developed in such a way that changes can be measured. The outcomes are also designed to be sensitive to nursing interventions, helping to define the contribution of nursing to patient care. The language and definitions were developed from extensive expert review and research.

NOC outcomes are categorized similarly to nursing diagnoses and include a definition and indicators that can be used to track the outcome. For example, a hip fracture patient has a risk for impaired skin integrity.

The goal for this patient is to prevent pressure sores, so the NOC outcome would be *tissue integrity: skin* (see Box 2-4). The indicator would be whether the skin remains lesion free, and the rating scale for this outcome is 1 to 5 (with 1 identifying that the skin is extremely compromised and 5 identifying that the skin is not compromised). The nurse can track the patient's progress using the rating scale over time, and use the information to document that the goal was met.

Intervention

The range of interventions available to nurses who work with older adults is as broad as with any other age-group. However, interventions may need to be modified to adapt to the special needs of older people. The Nursing Interventions Classification (NIC) provides a broad standardized list of interventions that make up the final step in the documentation of nursing actions. In addition, common interventions for specific outcomes are linked or grouped together for ease of use. NIC interventions are described with a definition and list of nursing activities. If we use our prior example, interventions are used that maintain skin integrity, and NIC provides a number of activities that may be appropriate to our patient. Box 2-5 shows how the patient

---

BOX 2-5 Sample of Nursing Process Using NANDA Nursing Diagnoses, NOC Outcomes, and NIC Interventions

NURSING PROCESS	EXAMPLE
Patient assessment	Mrs. P. is an 84-year-old woman in the hospital following a hip fracture repair.
Nursing diagnosis	Risk for impaired skin integrity related to immobility secondary to hip fracture
Nursing outcome	Tissue integrity: skin
Indicators	Tissue is lesion free.
Measurement	1 — Extremely 2 — Substantially 3 — Moderately 4 — Mildly 5 — Not compromised
Nursing interventions	Pressure Management
Activities	Assess risk with Braden scale
	Turning schedule every 2 hours
	Apply therapeutic mattress
	Use devices to keep heels and bony prominences off the bed
	Monitor for sources of pressure and friction
	Monitor skin for areas of redness and breakdown

care plan can be put together with the assessment, diagnosis, outcome, and intervention using NANDA, NIC, and NOC. These basic nursing activities should be familiar to all nurses. Using the standardized language allows the information to be computerized and coded.

The APN has more autonomy in prescribing interventions than does the registered nurse. State law dictates specific prescriptive privileges for APNs, and controlled substance dispensing is also regulated by the federal Drug Enforcement Agency. Pharmacological, diagnostic (laboratory and diagnostic tests), and other therapeutic interventions (ordering durable medical equipment, home oxygen, etc.) can be prescribed by the APN in addition to traditional nursing interventions.

Implementation of interventions with the older individual is affected by the aging process: some interventions are used more frequently, others are used less frequently, and sometimes the manner of implementing a given activity may need to be modified. For example, the increased need for services and the fragmented nature of the health care system for older adults requires nurses to be involved in coordination of services more often than with younger adults. Case management has helped decrease care fragmentation and is a service often provided by nurses to special populations, including the elderly. The high prevalence of functional disability in the aged also results in more use of rehabilitative and restorative nursing techniques and assistance with self-care activities than in younger adult groups.

A situation where interventions may be used less is related to dietary restrictions in adults of advanced age. Typically, adults in their sixties and seventies who have cardiac disease or high cholesterol may be strongly encouraged to monitor and control their dietary intake of fats, particularly saturated fats. This may also be recommended for them into their eighties and nineties, but this group is also at high risk for weight loss and poor nutritional intake. Despite this, they may continue to be careful about their diet and restrict their intake. Health care providers will want to encourage older adults who have lost weight or who are frail to liberalize their diets so that they have more choices of foods they enjoy, and will eat well and prevent undernutrition.

A good example of the need to modify nursing interventions is health teaching, an intervention commonly used with patients of all ages. Many health education materials have been developed with a younger population in mind (or likely without the older adult in mind) such as information on exercise. The pictures in the material may show young people participating in extremely vigorous activities that are not appealing to older adults. The print may be small and colors used in such a way that blue and green cannot be distinguished. For an older population, educational materials need to use a large font, provide contrast in colors, and include age-appropriate interventions. More details on health education are presented in Chapter 27.

Evaluation

Evaluation of nursing practice includes setting criteria and measuring progress using those criteria. If outcomes are measured (e.g., using NOC), the nurse will have documentation of the patient's progress. The evaluation process is the same in gerontological nursing; however, the generally accepted criteria for "success" and the time frame in which progress is measured may vary. Also, setting priorities and goals may be different with the older individual as compared with the young. For example, in the younger adult the goals of health promotion are often to improve health and fitness, whereas in the older adult the goals may be to maintain health and prevent decline.

Expectations for meeting evaluation criteria may also vary with the older person. Health conditions in younger people may improve in a relatively short period of time. However, in the older adult with chronic illness, the time needed to see improvement may be greatly extended. Even in acute illness, the time period for evaluation of results may need to be prolonged. For example, a 35-year-old who sustains a hip fracture in an automobile accident is likely to be able to regain independent functional ability sooner than an 80-year-old with the same type of fracture. The older person is apt to have complicating medical problems, which will prolong the recovery process. It is self-defeating for both patient and nurse to use the same standards for all patients.

COMPREHENSIVE NURSING ASSESSMENT: FOCUS ON FUNCTION

Typically, older adults seen in a health care setting for the first time will have a comprehensive assessment that includes a history and physical examination. Often a physician will do it, but this varies depending on the setting; at times a nurse will complete part of the history and assessment, and the physician will perform the physical examination. APNs may conduct the complete assessment independently. In an interdisciplinary setting, the assessment may be divided between multiple health professionals. Competent care of the older adult also includes a complete functional assessment (Kane, Ouslander, & Abrass, 2004).

This chapter describes a comprehensive nursing functional assessment of the older adult, based on Gordon's functional health patterns (2002). This differs from the typical history and physical examination commonly used under the traditional medical model, but there is significant overlap between the two assessments. The functional assessment can be performed independently by nurses. As this assessment focuses on function and problems that are common in older adults, the items are complementary to the traditional history and physical.

In older adults, especially those with complex medical, psychological, and social problems, this information is essential to provide a baseline for ongoing care addressing the biological, psychological (cognitive and affective), and social domains of function described earlier.

The following discussion of assessment reviews the typical history and physical examination, and then moves into details of the comprehensive nursing functional assessment. Each of the topics and items in the comprehensive functional assessment could be included in a traditional encounter or used in a separate nursing assessment. It is important for the nurse to be cognizant of the various methods and determine how best to obtain functional assessment data depending on the setting and situation.

The Initial History and Physical Examination

During the initial history, a wealth of information is gathered from the older adult and other sources. Specifically, identifying data such as age, gender, occupation, and marital status are obtained. Current medications, food and drug allergies, and type of reactions to the offending agent(s) are identified. Medication review includes a list of: prescription medications, over-the-counter medications, vitamin and mineral supplements, and additional complementary and alternative medications. The past medical, family, personal, and social histories are reviewed and recorded.

The past medical history includes a discussion of the person's health promotion and health maintenance practices. A detailed evaluation of these areas is also warranted in the older adult. Immunization utilization, safety practices (use of seat belts and smoke detectors), and screening tests (mammogram, Mantoux) received are assessed (Bickley & Szilagyi, 2003). In addition, lifestyle practices such as alcohol, tobacco, and drug use need to be explored, as well as exercise participation. Educational history, literacy, and health literacy, as well as preferred ways of learning for teaching purposes (reading, attending a class, watching a video), should be documented.

The data elicited from the initial history are standardized across health care settings even though the specific documentation of the data may vary. A few common terms are used to organize data from the history that all nurses should be aware of. The descriptions of these terms are listed in the order in which they are usually gathered during the history and documented in the medical record. The *chief complaint* is a brief statement in the person's own words describing the main reason health care is being sought at this time. The individual generally expresses this in the first few minutes of the interview. The *history of present illness* is a narrative written by the health care professional from the individual's perspective, which details the problems that have led to seeking health care. Each key problem should be characterized by the onset, location, duration, associated symptoms, and aggravating and alleviating factors of the problem, and the effect of any self-treatments for the problem.

The *review of systems* documents the presence or absence of common signs and symptoms that can occur within each body system. This information helps the health professional develop a mental list of plausible causes of the problem. This list is referred to as the *differential diagnosis* and should include any physical or mental disorders that could reasonably explain the patient's signs and symptoms.

It is important to note that when taking the history of present illness, a pertinent review of systems related to the problem should be elicited. The responses are recorded in the history of present illness section and, depending on whether they help "rule in" or "rule out" a medical diagnosis, are termed *pertinent positives* or *pertinent negatives*, respectively. Specific information to consider regarding common geriatric problems that aid in diagnosis is described later in this chapter.

The initial physical examination is a thorough, systematic assessment of the body systems to determine overall health and functioning. This initial examination is extremely important because it provides a baseline for comparison of all subsequent physical examinations. Unusual findings on physical examination may lead to the early diagnosis and treatment of disorders that may not be otherwise identified if the person is asymptomatic.

The first portion of the assessment is the introductory, or "first impression," phase of the encounter. The nurse observes the older person's overall appearance and physical function, sensory function, and ability to communicate. During these first moments, a substantial amount of information can be gathered, including: general state of health, level of consciousness, facial expressions, height, weight, body build, skin color, personal hygiene, dress, posture, gait, and motor coordination. Signs of distress or unusual body odors should also be noted. Altogether, this initial assessment and data collection is termed the *general survey* (Bickley & Szilagyi, 2003).

Key issues and concerns should be identified early in the encounter, and mutual expectations concerning the assessment should be discussed. As a result, the assessment may become targeted in certain areas, stemming from the chief complaint. Furthermore, problem areas for which careful attention is warranted may become evident, serving as a focal point in future assessment. This introductory encounter provides cues about potential sensory and cognitive deficits, general health status and concerns or problems, social support, and expectations for care.

A Functional Nursing Framework

Assessment data can be organized in different ways. A comprehensive framework helps the nurse collect data systematically so that all components of the biological, social, and psychological domains are included to provide a holistic assessment. This text uses Gordon's framework (2002) as a model, which organizes the assessment into 11 categories of functional health patterns: health perception–health management pattern, nutritional-metabolic pattern, elimination pattern, activity-exercise pattern, sleep-rest pattern, cognitive-perceptual pattern, self-perception-self–concept pattern, role-relationship pattern, sexuality-reproductive pattern, coping–stress tolerance pattern, and value-belief pattern.

During the assessment, data are collected to validate the objective (signs) and subjective (symptoms) findings from the initial encounter to form diagnoses. For example, the cue (the objective or subjective finding or observation) collected about functional ability, such as not being able to bend down to take off shoes, leads to the inference (the nurse's interpretation of the meaning of the cue) that activities of daily living and self-care may be impaired. Inferences and cues are validated through the history and physical examination performed during the assessment to determine the causes of and contributing factors to functional impairment.

The history or interview is extremely important in helping to determine diagnoses. Sometimes, the history alone can establish the etiology of the problem, and it is confirmed by the physical examination and laboratory and diagnostic tests. Interviewing styles among health care providers are varied, and specific techniques will help elicit the most pertinent information. First, active listening by the nurse is essential. Other techniques that should be employed include the following: starting with open-ended questions and following with directed questions for clarification, offering multiple choice answers to minimize bias, providing reassurance, and summarizing the information gathered (Bickley & Szilagyi, 2003). Interviewing and history taking is a skill, and it requires practice.

Gordon's (2002) 11 categories of functional health patterns are reviewed next, with specific questions for the history, physical examination, and laboratory and diagnostic test components that may be assessed in that domain. These items are to be used as guidelines, and clinical judgment of the nurse must be used in deciding which portions to include in a particular encounter. However, it is important to document a comprehensive assessment of the older individual at least periodically in order to provide a baseline profile. Changes can be more easily identified later that will alert the health provider of early decline when interventions are likely to be more successful. Additionally, the comprehensive assessment does not have to follow the exact order outlined in this book. For example, if someone has a chief complaint that fits into one of the domains, that domain should be the first one assessed, with the others assessed at a later time.

The Assessment

Health Perception–Health Management Pattern

HISTORY/INTERVIEW/SUBJECTIVE ASSESSMENT

1. **General.** "How would you describe your health?"
2. **Health maintenance/promotion practices.** What are older adults' perceptions of their own aging, health issues, and self-care requirements for health promotion? "What do you do to take care of yourself?" Ask about exercise, diet, rest, stress management, and seat belt use. Some of these items are addressed more fully under later patterns. Do they use tobacco, alcohol, or drugs? If so, quantify the amount and frequency. Are they up to date on their immunizations (influenza, tetanus, and pneumonia)? Do they see the dentist, eye doctor, and primary care provider (PCP) on a regular basis?
3. **Current health problems/management.** "Describe the health problems you are having now and how they are being managed (diet, medications, exercise or activity limitations, therapy, and so on)." Consider the overall degree of disability observed, relative to the health problems and medical diagnoses identified. Elicit understanding of health problems and rationale for management. Ask about management of health problems and any difficulty carrying out regimen. If treatment plan is not consistently carried out, do they understand the risks? Has a new health problem evolved requiring new information for self-care?
4. **Medications.** Elicit information about medication usage, rationale for use, and side effects. Do they perform monitoring activities such as obtaining blood pressure measurements or blood glucose readings?
5. **Limitations.** "Are there things you would like to do but can't because of your health or medical problems?" Elicit the impact of health problems and treatment modalities on functioning. Are they satisfied with health outcomes?
6. **Self-care.** If the individual lives at home, is he or she able to maintain the home and perform activities of daily living and maintain a suitable home environment? Is assistance available to perform those things the individual is unable to accomplish?
7. **Advanced care planning.** "Have you thought about what health care services you would want if you were severely injured or had a terminal illness in which you could not communicate?" "Have you discussed

these wishes with your family?" "Do you have an advance directive, durable power of attorney, or living will?" If so, "Does your PCP have a copy?"

PHYSICAL EXAMINATION/OBJECTIVE ASSESSMENT. The goal of the health perception–health management domain is to gain a broad overview of individuals' perceptions of themselves on the health and illness continuums and their ability to function within their environment. Assessment of health promotion practices, disease prevention strategies, and lifestyle habits helps achieve this goal. Because of the broad nature of this domain and the fact that assessments of many of the specific issues that may come up during the interview are discussed in more depth in one of the other domains, the following provides examples of objective assessments that may result from the patient history for this section:

- Observe for indicators of effective health care management related to special care measures (e.g., skin care, smoking cessation, weight control, glucose monitoring). Observe the overall appearance. Examine the face, hair, nails, and other areas of exposed skin for cleanliness. Note if clothes appear clean or contain soiled areas; note odors such as smoke.
- Check weight and compare with last documented weight and goal weight.

LABORATORY ASSESSMENT. Monitor health conditions as appropriate. For example, evaluate hemoglobin A_{1c} to assess blood glucose control over the last 3 months for those with diabetes. Evaluate performance of ADLs that may be of concern.

Observe the individual walking into the examination room, as well as across the room and back. For example, you could use the timed "up and go" test (Podsiadlo & Richardson, 1991) to document mobility. Other standardized assessment tools are discussed in Chapter 3.

Nutritional-Metabolic Pattern

HISTORY/ INTERVIEW/SUBJECTIVE ASSESSMENT

1. **General.** "How is your appetite? Has it recently changed?"
2. **Dietary habits.** Obtain food intake profile: 24-hour recall or 3-day diary to determine recommended dietary allowance (RDA) equivalents. Determine food preferences, cultural traditions, and knowledge of dietary needs. Are there any foods they are unable to eat (dairy products, food allergies) or has any special diet been recommended (potassium or calcium rich, low sodium, low calorie or high calorie)?
3. **Difficulties.** Do they have difficulty ingesting food: chewing, salivating, altered taste sensation, swallowing, nausea, regurgitation, stomach fullness, bloating,

impaired manual dexterity (paresis, weakness, joint pain or deformity, tremors), impaired cognition, or fatigue?
4. **Weight.** Have they experienced a recent (past 6 months) weight gain or loss? If so, was it intentional? Elicit their perception of current weight.
5. **Hydration.** Assess fluid intake, including fluids with meals, between-meal beverages, and foods with high water content.
6. **Other factors influencing intake.** Ask about underlying illnesses (special diets, dexterity problems limiting ability to feed oneself), medical treatment (medications), environmental factors (lack of assistance needed to shop for food or prepare food), or economic factors (lack of financial resources to purchase adequate food).
7. **Nutritional supplements.** Do they take any nutritional supplements (e.g., vitamins, vitamin B_{12} shots monthly, minerals, herbs, shakes, power bars, other foods)? Were these recommended by a health professional?

PHYSICAL EXAMINATION/OBJECTIVE ASSESSMENT

1. **General appearance.** Observe for dry skin, alopecia, muscle weakness, pale conjunctiva, agitation or confusion, lethargy.
2. **Anthropometric measurements.** Obtain height and weight and calculate body mass index (BMI) (Table 2-2 and Box 2-6). Abnormal range includes either above 25 or below 18.5 (U.S. Department of Health and Human Services, 2000). This value is not absolute in the older population, because of the decreased muscle mass that occurs with aging that may underestimate the amount of body fat present. Evidence suggests that older adults who are mild-to-moderately overweight do not have the same cardiovascular and additional risk factors of younger adults (Heiat, Vaccarino, & Krumholz, 2001). Additionally, because of the high risk of malnutrition and weight loss in frail older adults, a mild elevation in BMI may be advantageous in this population and is supported by many geriatric professionals. Generally, caloric and dietary restriction should be carefully considered because they may result in inadequate intake in older persons, which may be a greater risk to their long-term health. Consider their responses to your questions regarding weight. Are their caloric demands being met or exceeded? Patients with healing wounds or febrile illnesses will have increased caloric requirements. It may be helpful in these cases to calculate their requirements and adjust intake appropriately (see Chapter 8).
3. **Hydration/mucous membranes.** Assess oral cavity and hydration status, an important issue because thirst sensation is often diminished with age. Observe

Table 2-2 Body Mass Index (BMI) Chart

BMI	19	20	21	22	23	24	25	26	27	28	29	30	31	32	33	34	35
Height (Inches)								Body Weight (Pounds)									
58	91	96	100	105	110	115	119	124	129	134	138	143	148	153	158	162	167
59	94	99	104	109	114	119	124	128	133	138	143	148	153	158	163	168	173
60	97	102	107	112	118	123	128	133	138	143	148	153	158	163	168	174	179
61	100	106	111	116	122	127	132	137	143	148	153	158	164	169	174	180	185
62	104	109	115	120	126	131	136	142	147	153	158	164	169	175	180	186	191
63	107	113	118	124	130	135	141	146	152	158	163	169	175	180	186	191	197
64	110	116	122	128	134	140	145	151	157	163	169	174	180	186	192	197	204
65	114	120	126	132	138	144	150	156	162	168	174	180	186	192	198	204	210
66	118	124	130	136	142	148	155	161	167	173	179	186	192	198	204	210	216
67	121	127	134	140	146	153	159	166	172	178	185	191	198	204	211	217	223
68	125	131	138	144	151	158	164	171	177	184	190	197	203	210	216	223	230
69	128	135	142	149	155	162	169	176	182	189	196	203	209	216	223	230	236
70	132	139	146	153	160	167	174	181	188	195	202	209	216	222	229	236	243
71	136	143	150	157	165	172	179	186	193	200	208	215	222	229	236	243	250
72	140	147	154	162	169	177	184	191	199	206	213	221	228	235	242	250	258
73	144	151	159	166	174	182	189	197	204	212	219	227	235	242	250	257	265
74	148	155	163	171	179	186	194	202	210	218	225	233	241	249	256	264	272
75	152	160	168	176	184	192	200	208	216	224	232	240	248	256	264	272	279
76	156	164	172	180	189	197	205	213	221	230	238	246	254	263	271	279	287

From National Institutes of Health & National Heart, Lung, and Blood Institute. (1998). *Clinical guidelines on the identification, evaluation, and treatment, of overweight and obesity in adults: The evidence report.* National Institutes of Health.

To use this table, find the appropriate height in the left-hand column. Move across to a given weight. The number at the top of the column is the BMI at that height and weight. Pounds have been rounded off.

oral mucous membranes for dryness, cracking, bleeding, ulcers, and signs of infection. Specifically, note condition of mouth, tongue, mucous membranes, gums, and teeth. Remove dentures and assess denture fit, paying particular attention to the underlying gums. Is fluid intake adequate? Are mucous membranes moist? Geriatric sources report 30 ml/kg of body weight as a formula for determining fluid standards for older people (Jensen & Powers, 2003; Reuben et al., 2003). Chidester and Spangler (1997) found that a different formula, 100 ml/kg for the first 10 kg of body weight, 50 ml/kg for the next 10 kg, and 15 ml for all remaining kg, appeared to be superior to the 30 ml/kg formula because of its ability to remain accurate in older adults with low body weight or high body weight.

4. **Integumentary.** Assess the skin. Observe the skin color, and assess the temperature and sensation (paresthesias can be indicative of vitamin B_{12} deficiency). Note skin turgor, dryness or excessive oiliness, flaking, bruises, lacerations, moles, lesions, rashes, or discolorations. Additionally, if there is a skin alteration such as a stoma, incision, fistula, skin graft, or pressure sore, note evidence of poor healing or infection, tissue granulation, circulation, odor, and skin integrity of the surrounding area.

5. **Cardiovascular.** Assess specific areas of the cardiovascular and musculoskeletal system related to nutrition, including blood pressure and pulse. Assess for edema.

6. **Musculoskeletal.** Evaluate general muscle bulk and strength. Check grip strength with consideration of handedness. Observe for deformities or difficulties of the upper extremities and hands that might affect feeding ability.

7. **Observation.** If possible, observe eating behaviors. Note actual intake, food preferences, ability to feed self and swallow food, enjoyment in eating, position and comfort, time needed to finish the meal, and any encouragement needed.

LABORATORY ASSESSMENT. Initial evaluation should include a complete blood count (CBC), serum albumin level, and cholesterol level (Jensen & Powers, 2003; Sheiman, 2002). The CBC helps screen for a nutritional anemia such as an iron deficiency, vitamin B_{12} deficiency, or folate deficiency. Low serum albumin (hypoalbuminemia) typically reflects decreased protein stores, inflammation, or body injury (Jensen & Powers, 2003; Sheiman, 2002). Low cholesterol (hypocholesterolemia) reflects decreased intake of dietary cholesterol, found in animal products. Both are markers of poor nutritional status associated with increased morbidity and mortality risk (Jensen & Powers, 2003). Prealbumin can also be measured and reflects more recent changes in protein status. Additional laboratory

---

BOX 2-6 Calculation of Body Mass Index (BMI)

Calculation Using Kilograms and Meters

$$BMI = \frac{Weight\ (kg)}{Height\ (m^2)}$$

Calculation Using Pounds and Inches

$$BMI = \frac{Weight\ (lb) \times 705}{Height\ (in)^2}$$

Example: A woman is 65 inches tall and weighs 156 pounds.

$$\frac{156 \times 705}{65^2} = \frac{109980}{4225} = BMI\ 26.03$$

---

tests that may be helpful include a metabolic panel, thyroid-stimulating hormone (TSH), vitamin B_{12}, folate, and hepatic profile. The metabolic panel will include electrolytes, a serum glucose level, and kidney function tests that help determine hydration status. A TSH is a screen for thyroid dysfunction that is related to a person's metabolic rate. Screen for vitamin B_{12} and folate deficiencies. Finally, a hepatic profile, sometimes included as part of the metabolic panel, assesses the liver, which plays a large role in carbohydrate and fat metabolism.

Elimination Pattern

HISTORY/INTERVIEW (URINARY, SUBJECTIVE ASSESSMENT)

1. **General.** "Have you noticed any recent changes or problems with urination?" Inquire about recent pattern of urinary elimination, including frequency, amount, dysuria, urgency, losing urine, and nocturia. Ask if they have noticed blood in the urine, cloudy urine, difficulty starting the urine stream (straining) or a decrease in the force of the stream with dribbling at the end of the stream, feelings of urinary retention, malodorous urine, or suprapubic or flank pain. Approximately how many times do they void during the day and at night?
2. **Hydration considerations.** Estimate output, keeping in mind hydration status and fluid intake. Be alert to older adults who have a significant deviation from the norm. Identify perceptions about how fluid intake affects urination, and any self-restriction of intake to treat incontinence.
3. **Urinary incontinence.** "Have you had any difficulty losing your urine or making it to the bathroom on time?" If so, inquire about urgency, amount, and frequency. What causes the leakage? Is it associated with

coughing, lifting, or not getting to the bathroom in time? If they have had difficulty with incontinence, how are they managing the problem and what products are they currently using or have they used in the past? When incontinence is present, ask them to keep a voiding record for several days, documenting voiding times, amounts, whether continent or incontinent, and assistance or equipment (or both) needed when using the toilet to help identify the type of incontinence. Has urinary dysfunction affected daily activities, socialization, and quality of life?
4. **Urinary alterations.** Do they have an indwelling catheter or perform self-catheterization to empty their bladder? Do they have an ileal conduit? Can they manage these independently?

PHYSICAL EXAMINATION/OBJECTIVE ASSESSMENT

1. **Genitourinary assessment for older adults without symptoms.** Observe, percuss, and palpate for a distended bladder. Palpate the abdomen to assess for pain.
2. **In-depth genitourinary assessment for older adults with urinary symptoms:**
   Men and women. Note evidence of renal or urinary tract problem: check for fever, chills, fecal impaction (rectal examination) if history of constipation or incontinence; check costovertebral angle tenderness if suspected kidney infection.
   Women. Examine external genitalia, and perform a pelvic examination. Assess for vaginal discharge, atrophic vaginitis, vaginal and bladder prolapse (cystocele), and pelvic muscle strength; note rectal tone.
   Men. Examine external genitalia. Perform a rectal examination to palpate for enlarged prostate; check rectal tone.
3. **Incontinence.** Identify contributing factors: medications, impaired mobility, fecal impaction, dehydration, urinary tract infection, unfamiliar environment, cognitive impairment, lack of timely assistance, pain, depression, psychological reaction, or a new medical problem resulting in weakness.
4. **Urinary alterations.** When there is a catheter or an ileal conduit, note the color and clarity of the urine. Assess the stoma (color, shape, size) and the skin surrounding the stoma for excoriation, and determine if the appliance is secure.

LABORATORY AND DIAGNOSTIC TESTS. *Urine Tests.* A postvoid residual should be checked when retention is suspected or incontinence is present. Obtain a urine specimen, and a urine dipstick or urinalysis (UA) should be performed to help narrow the differential diagnosis list (most common are urinary tract infection [UTI], incontinence, and benign prostatic hyperplasia [BPH] and prostate cancer in men) and guide treatment. A dipstick or UA result with positive nitrites and elevated leukocytes accompanied by a typical presentation is highly suggestive of a UTI. Hematuria may be present in complicated UTIs but can be indicative of a more serious problem, and further workup should be performed. If a complicated UTI is suspected, a culture and sensitivity should be done, but this is not routinely done for uncomplicated UTIs.

Serum Tests. Depending on the history and physical examination, renal function tests may be ordered (creatinine and blood urea nitrogen) and a prostate-specific antigen (PSA) test may be ordered for men. Monitoring PSA levels in older men with less than a 10-year life expectancy remains controversial.

HISTORY/INTERVIEW/SUBJECTIVE ASSESSMENT (BOWEL)

1. **General.** "Has there been a recent change in bowel habits?"
2. **Usual bowel function.** Frequency, amount, color, consistency, diameter and size of bowel movements, fecal incontinence, and any pain or discomfort when passing stools or in abdomen. Do they strain with defecation, notice blood in stool or on toilet paper, or have feelings of incomplete evacuation? Ask about their last bowel movement.
3. **Bowel alterations.** Do they have an ileostomy or colostomy? Can they manage it independently? Is fluid and dietary fiber intake adequate? Inquire about past and current bowel problems and previous treatments (especially laxatives, enema use): constipation, impaction, hemorrhoids, anal fissures, diarrhea, fecal incontinence (see incontinence under urinary elimination for factors to consider), or excessive flatus. What are their expectations for bowel habits?

PHYSICAL EXAMINATION/OBJECTIVE ASSESSMENT

1. **Abdominal examination.** Observe for distention, percuss and palpate for masses, stool in colon, tenderness; auscultate for bowel sounds; percuss for dullness or tympany.
2. **Rectal examination.** Presence/absence of stool, consistency, presence of hemorrhoids, fissures, sphincter tone, fecal incontinence.
3. **Bowel alterations.** Assess the stoma and skin of a colostomy, similar to an ileal conduit described previously. Additional issues to consider include the odor, color, and consistency of the stool. Consider hydration issues in cases of constipation, diarrhea, and ileostomies.
4. **Medication review.** Review all medications to identify possible contributing factors to bowel problems.

LABORATORY AND DIAGNOSTIC TESTS. Guaiac testing is done to identify occult blood in the stool to screen for cancer and gastrointestinal bleeding and is typically done whenever a rectal examination is performed. In addition, the American Cancer Society (2005) recommends flexible sigmoidoscopy or colonoscopy along with fecal occult blood testing for older adults to routinely screen for colon and rectal cancer. In the case of intractable diarrhea, collect a stool specimen to check for *Clostridium difficile* (common in institutional settings), ova and parasites, and other organisms.

Activity-Exercise Pattern

HISTORY/INTERVIEW/SUBJECTIVE ASSESSMENT

1. **General.** "How often do you participate in regular physical activity?" Elicit beliefs about value of activity/exercise; note presence of any limitations.
2. **Typical day.** Ask the individual to recall a "typical" day's activities and a recent day's activities within the past week to determine alterations in habits or activities. Ask about activity patterns, meals, out-of-house activities, sleep adequacy and rest periods (discussed more under the sleep-rest pattern domain), and socialization. Does pain limit daily activities? "Does fatigue limit your activity?" Are they currently employed? Are they able to perform their job responsibilities adequately? Do they spend large amounts of time in bed or in a chair or wheelchair?
3. **Physical activity.** Inquire about usual exercise/activity pattern and any limitations or changes. "Do you currently participate in routine physical activity? What types of exercise have you done in the past that you enjoyed?" Assess frequency, duration, and intensity of activity. Does the activity meet the minimum recommendations of at least 30 minutes of physical activity most days of the week (Christmas & Andersen, 2000)? Are there barriers to participating in physical activity? Assess whether the activities include fitness elements of aerobic exercise for endurance, stretching for flexibility, strength training for muscle strength, and balance exercises.
4. **Assessment of ADLs/IADLs.** Can they perform activities independently (bathing, dressing, toileting, transferring, feeding)? Are they able to function independently at home (telephone use, transportation, grocery shopping, preparing meals, housework/cleaning, medication administration, manage finances)? If they have difficulty or need help with any activities, how are the activities managed? Why do they need help? Who provides assistance and how often? Is the assistance adequate to meet needs?
5. **Limitations.** Do they have any medical or physical problems that interfere with participation in

physical activities, personal care, home maintenance, or other activities? Are precautions taken for those who have a high degree of immobility, such as turning, moving, and skin care?

6. **Driving assessment.** Do they currently drive? Do they have an active driver's license? If so, have they had any accidents in the last 5 years? If any accidents occurred, obtain a detailed history regarding the accident(s). Was alcohol involved? Did it occur at night? Have they ever received minor traffic violations or had their license revoked? Have they had a driving test performed recently? Have they made adjustments to their driving (avoid driving at night, only drive when traffic is light, only drive to familiar locations)? Do they have a health condition that may affect their ability to drive, such as osteoarthritis (difficulty with movement because of pain), seizure disorder or other neurological disorder(s), diabetes (possible hypoglycemia), or sleep apnea? Are medications a potential problem, such as antihypertensives, hypoglycemic agents, pain medications, or other medications that cause drowsiness (Messinger-Rapport, 2002)? Has anyone ever suggested they should no longer drive? Was it a health care professional? Do they feel safe driving? Are they the primary driver in the family? Do they have a reliable vehicle that is well maintained? Do they wear their seat belt while in the car? Who else drives in the family? How are transportation needs managed within the family?

7. **Cardiovascular/altered tissue perfusion.** Ask about high blood pressure, heart trouble, angina, dizziness, edema, numbness or tingling in extremities, coldness in extremities, or claudication.

8. **Respiratory.** Do they have shortness of breath, cough, dyspnea, increased sputum production, orthopnea, or previous infection? Do the signs/symptoms occur at rest or with activity, or both? Do they have a history of any lung or breathing problems? Do they smoke or live with someone who smokes? Do they have allergies or environmental pollution that interferes with breathing?

9. **Musculoskeletal.** Is there a history of joint pain or swelling, stiffness, injuries, or other musculoskeletal problems that could affect activity?

10. **Falls.** Have they fallen in the past year? How did it occur? Did injury result? "Do you have any concerns about falling (falling again)?" "Do you limit your activities because you are concerned about falling? Describe any changes you have made. Do you use any assistive devices?" Are there other risk factors present such as muscle weakness, fatigue, balance or gait problems, visual or hearing impairments, cognitive impairment, or use of medications resulting in symptoms of dizziness, urinary urgency or

frequency, or sedation? Ask about environmental hazards at the home, including stairs, throw rugs, poor lighting, clutter, or uneven pavement of driveway or sidewalk. Have they made any modifications such as grab rails in the bathroom? Has a bone density test (dual energy X-ray absorptiometry [DEXA]) been done? Have they been diagnosed with osteopenia or osteoporosis, putting them at high risk for injury from falls? If so, are they being treated for their condition?

11. **Social/recreational activities.** Do they have outside interests or hobbies that provide enjoyment and diversion? Have they made recent changes in diversional activities? Do health problems limit participation in hobbies or recreational activities? If they have given up activities, have they identified other areas of interest to pursue?

PHYSICAL EXAMINATION/OBJECTIVE ASSESSMENT

1. **Vital signs.** Check vital signs at rest, after moderate activity (such as dressing or bathing), and vigorous activity (such as walking a long distance or after exercising). Check orthostatic vital signs, including blood pressure (BP) and heart rate (HR) in the supine and standing positions. A greater than 20 mm Hg drop in systolic BP or a diastolic BP drop of 10 mm Hg within 3 minutes of standing defines orthostatic hypotension (Consensus Committee of the American Autonomic Society and the American Academy of Neurology, 1996). An increase in HR of greater than 15 to 20 beats per minute may also be considered significant for orthostasis (Carlson, 1999; Engstrom & Aminoff, 1997). Based on a recent review of the literature, Irvin and White (2004) recommend having the person lie supine for 10 minutes before checking the initial BP and HR; assessing BP and HR and subjective symptoms of dizziness immediately on standing; and last, rechecking the BP and HR after the person has remained standing for 3 minutes.

2. **Cardiovascular.** A comprehensive cardiovascular assessment should be performed. Particular attention should be given to assessment of capillary refill; apical, radial, and peripheral pulses; and edema.

3. **Respiratory.** A complete examination is important. Observe respiratory pattern (rate, depth, rhythm, and type), nasal flaring, cyanosis, asymmetrical chest expansion, and use of accessory muscles. Note body positions such as sitting up and leaning forward in order to breathe easier. Auscultate lungs and note crackles, wheezes, or diminished sounds. Assess coughing pattern and sputum. If possible, obtain a pulse oximetry reading.

4. **Musculoskeletal.** Inspect muscles for symmetry, mass, tremor, or spasms. Assess range of motion:

active or passive, in all joints. Note stiffness, pain, limited range, contractures, and kyphosis or other deformities. Assess muscle strength and tone.

5. **Balance/coordination/gait.** Assess balance while sitting and standing. Also assess ability to stand, transfer, and ambulate, paying attention to gait while walking and turning around. Look at the step height, length, and symmetry, as well as sway or hesitancy. Do they use an assistive device? Is the device appropriate, of the correct height and setting, and do they know how to use it properly? Coordination can be assessed through the performance of neurological examination techniques, including rapidly alternating movements, point-to-point movements, and specific gait and stance testing (Bickley & Szilagyi, 2003, pp. 578-582).

6. **Assessment of ADLs/IADLs.** Have them demonstrate activities if this is a potential area of concern (see standardized measures in Chapter 3). Determine level of independence and if assistance is needed. Are there mechanical restrictions of movement such as casts or splints? In the acute care setting, are traction, incisions, restraints, intravenous lines, catheters, or ventilators significantly impairing mobility? Can they maneuver safely within the confines of the mechanical restriction?

7. **Driving assessment.** Focus on identifying deficits in visual acuity, hearing, cognitive/neurological, and musculoskeletal systems (Messinger-Rapport, 2002) that may predispose the older adult to driving difficulties and subsequent hazards.

8. **Fall assessment.** If the person has a history of falling; a specific fall assessment should be performed, including evaluation of gait, balance, muscle strength, medications, vision, and cardiovascular status. Falls are associated with significant morbidity and mortality rates in older adults and warrant further investigation. In the institutional setting, use a fall risk assessment to document individuals who have a high risk of falling.

LABORATORY AND DIAGNOSTIC TESTS. If there are new signs or symptoms of activity intolerance, further investigation is warranted. A CBC should be drawn to assess for anemia, and the white blood cell count should be evaluated to determine if an infectious process is occurring. With complaints of shortness of breath, check oxygenation status by pulse oximetry if available. Keep in mind that pulse oximetry readings may not be accurate when there are significant fluid volume changes or anemia. More advanced tests including a chest x-ray or electrocardiography can be used to help establish a diagnosis.

Screening tests related to the activity-exercise domain also need to be considered. A cardiac exercise stress test should be performed for individuals who want to start an exercise program, particularly those with cardiac risk factors or who were previously sedentary (Kennedy-Malone, Fletcher, & Plank, 2004, p. 4). The U.S. Preventive Services Task Force (2002) recommends routine osteoporosis screening via bone density testing in women over age 65, and beginning at age 60 for high-risk women. Women with osteopenia and osteoporosis are at an increased risk for injury from falls and should be identified so treatment can be offered and preventive measures instituted.

Sleep-Rest Pattern

HISTORY/INTERVIEW/SUBJECTIVE ASSESSMENT

1. **General.** "Do you typically feel rested after sleeping? Do you have the energy to get through your day?" Inquire about expectations regarding sleep and understanding about altered sleep patterns with aging.

2. **Current patterns.** Ask about usual bedtime, arousal time, and nap frequency and duration. Ask about any difficulty getting to sleep, staying asleep, waking up too early, nocturia, nightmares, fear of oversleeping (will not wake up at night if need to, such as caregiver for someone who has frequent needs), and quality of sleep. Ask about pain as an inhibitor of restful sleep.

3. **Changes.** Any recent change in sleep pattern? If recent difficulty getting to sleep, could anxiety or stress be contributing? Do they drink caffeinated beverages? Do they eat or exercise less than 2 hours before going to bed? Do certain medications keep them awake (theophylline, albuterol)? Do they nap during the day? Do certain medications make them drowsy (pain medications)? Do they drink alcohol? Are they depressed? Do they have a history of sleep apnea?

4. **Sleep routines.** Ask about sleeping aids (prescription, over-the-counter, alternative medications) and bedtime rituals: television, music, warm bath, food, drugs, alcohol, and so on. Inquire about the qualities of the environment (noise, temperature, pets, etc.).

5. **For sleep difficulties:**
   - Have them keep a sleep/wake diary to record naps, bedtime, nighttime sleeping duration, how they feel when awakening, daytime lethargy, dreams or nightmares, nighttime awakenings (nocturia, pain, dreams, worries, and noise), effectiveness of bedtime aids. Does environment (noise, lights, restraints, roommate, and so on) affect sleep?
   - Ask a family member or other individual (if available) to observe sleeping, noting positioning, movement, restlessness, periods of wakefulness, snoring, apnea, talking, and efforts to get out of bed.

PHYSICAL EXAMINATION/OBJECTIVE ASSESSMENT

1. Observe for adverse impact of sleeping patterns or sleep medication functioning (daytime naps, lethargy, irritability).
2. Review medications to help identify potential causes or contributing factors.

DIAGNOSTIC TESTING. A sleep study may be indicated for the rare older adult with a significant sleeping disturbance that does not respond to more conservative measures to aid in diagnosis.

Cognitive-Perceptual Pattern

HISTORY/INTERVIEW/SUBJECTIVE ASSESSMENT

1. **Cognition.** "Have there been any noticeable changes in your memory or thinking?"
   A. **Memory.** Have they been forgetful? "Have friends or families expressed concerns regarding your memory or ability to function? Have the changes been sudden or gradual?" Have the changes followed a stepwise pattern? "How long have the changes been going on?" Do they forget recent events or minor details? Do they forget major events or important information they would be expected to know? If the changes have been sudden, ask about recent medication changes, signs/symptoms of urinary or respiratory infection, and other reversible causes of delirium. The differential diagnosis for acute confusion of older adults is extensive, and a partial list may include transient ischemic attack, stroke, the postictal state after a seizure, hypoxia, and electrolyte disturbances, so probe for details to assist in identifying the cause.
   B. **Communication.** Inquire about any difficulties with communication: articulating words, forming ideas, sensory deficits, language barriers, memory impairment, or information processing and comprehension. Have they made any changes in activities as a result of communication issues such as hearing or vision?
   C. **Orientation.** Ask questions to determine orientation to time, including day, time of day, year, season, and so on. Do they recognize familiar people and acquaintances? Are they oriented to place? Do they recognize familiar streets? Could they find places outside their neighborhood? Do they get lost at home or elsewhere?
   D. **Functional considerations.** Does cognitive impairment affect their ability to manage daily activities and obligations such as appointments, managing money, or keeping track of personal belongings (executive functioning)? Note changes in activities in both the activity-exercise and role-relationship sections that might be related to cognitive decline. Do they understand situations and explanations? Have there been changes in personality or behavior? Would the individual be able to handle a home emergency? Is there risk for injury when left alone (fire, wandering)?

2. **Perception:**
   A. **Sensory systems.** "Have you noticed any recent changes in your vision or hearing? Ask about problems arising from changes in sensory function: vision, hearing, tactile, smell, or taste.
      - **Vision.** When was their last eye examination? Did it include pupil dilation? Do they wear corrective lenses or contacts? If so, how long ago did they receive a new prescription? Have they noticed any change in central or peripheral vision, decreased clarity of vision, or poor night vision? Have they experienced double vision or intolerance to light? Do they drive?
      - **Olfaction.** Are there changes in sense of smell that are problematic (e.g., food unappetizing)?
      - **Auditory.** Do they have difficulty understanding conversations, television, or radio? Have hearing changes impaired ability to participate in activities? Do they wear a hearing aid? If so, does it work properly? When was their last hearing test? Any ringing in the ears?
      - **Tactile.** Have they noticed any numbness or tingling sensations? If so, are they constant or intermittent?
      - **Gustatory.** Have food preferences changed related to changes in taste? Do they need to season food liberally? Can they distinguish between salty, sweet, and bitter flavors?
   B. **Pain assessment.** "Do you have any pain?"
      - Perform a history of present illness with the symptom of pain as with the assessment of any other symptom. Pain is acknowledged as "whatever the patient says it is." Include questions addressing: onset (acute or chronic), location (localized, referred, subcutaneous, and visceral), duration (constant, intermittent), intensity (have rate on standardized scale), characteristics (stabbing, shooting, sore, grinding, gnawing, ache, etc.), aggravating and alleviating factors, and self-treatments (heat, cold, immobilize, elevate, medication). How do they cope with the pain (distraction)? Does the pain have a pattern (same time each day, after certain activities)? What do they believe is the cause of their pain?
      - Inquire about previous experiences with pain and perceptions of effectiveness of treatments. Elicit beliefs about pain, and perceptions of it as a normal part of aging, a common

misperception held by many older adults. How does pain affect their mood, activities, self-care abilities, or other areas of their life? Are they able to obtain adequate rest?

PHYSICAL EXAMINATION/OBJECTIVE ASSESSMENT

1. **Cognitive assessment.** Assess level of consciousness. Conduct a standardized mental status examination with a standardized tool such as the Mini-Mental State Examination (MMSE) (Folstein, Folstein, & McHugh, 1975). Testing should be administered to all older adults to provide a baseline for future cognitive assessments, as well as to screen for cognitive dysfunction. Assess for apraxia and agnosia as potential signs of dementia. When there is a sudden change in cognition, evaluation for delirium, or acute confusion should be considered. Further discussion of specific screening tools is included in Chapter 3.

   - Further assessment of communication style is advised beyond the administration of mental status tests. Note the usual pattern of communication: verbosity, content, quality of speech (tone, pitch, pace, dialect, slurring, stuttering), language barrier, and eye contact. Be alert to signs of aphasia. Assess for situational factors that affect communication and cognition: pain, environment (sensory deprivation or overload, relocation), acute illness, impaired mobility, metabolic alterations (fluid and electrolyte imbalance), surgery, medications, sensory deficits, drugs, anxiety and fear, sleep deprivation, grief, or a psychological disorder (depression, anxiety).

2. **Sensory examination:**
   - **Vision.** Assess visual fields by confrontation to identify hemianopia or other visual field defects. Assess pupils for size, shape, symmetry, and reactivity to light. Use a Snellen chart (wall or handheld) to assess bilateral visual acuity. If using a wall chart, have patients read from a newspaper or magazine to assess close vision. If using the handheld chart, ask them to read a clock from 20 feet away to assess distance vision. Remember to have them use corrective lenses if needed. If they have trouble differentiating colors, assess for colorblindness.
   - **Olfaction.** Test olfaction by having them close their eyes, and occlude one nostril at a time while placing familiar scents under their nose such as coffee, vanilla, cloves, or soap to detect any difficulty identifying distinct scents (Bickley & Szilagyi, 2003).
   - **Auditory.** Test for auditory acuity using a whisper test. Cover one of the patient's ears with your finger and whisper a word with two equal syllables such as "baseball" into the opposite ear while

standing 1 to 2 feet away (Bickley & Szilagyi, 2003). The Weber and Rinne tests, which both can easily be performed with a tuning fork, can also be used to help distinguish between conductive and sensorineural hearing loss (Bickley & Szilagyi, 2003). For any older adult with hearing difficulties, check the auditory canals with an otoscope to look for cerumen buildup. This is a common occurrence in older adults and easily treatable. Presbycusis is the normal bilateral hearing loss resulting in a diminished ability to hear high-frequency sounds that occurs in older adults as they age; it should be considered in the diagnosis of hearing impairments (Boltz, 2002). Tinnitus can be caused by certain medications (aspirin in high doses, aminoglycosides), and medications should be reviewed when this complaint is voiced.

   - **Tactile.** Assess the sensory system as indicated, including pain and temperature sensation, light touch, vibratory and position sense, and discriminative sensations (Bickley & Szilagyi, 2003).
   - **Gustatory.** For complaints of changes in taste consider medications, smoking, radiation, or specific neurological problems as an etiology or contributing factor (Yen, 2004), while remembering that diminished taste accompanies normal aging. Decreased salivation may also be a contributing factor to taste alterations in those who are dehydrated, on anticholinergic medications, or with disorders of salivary function such as Sjögren's syndrome.
   - **Kinesthetic.** Observe for one-sided neglect in those with hemiparesis. Have them close their eyes, place their extremities in different positions, and describe the location and position of the extremity.

3. **Pain assessment.** Perform a pertinent physical examination based on the site of the pain. From the history and physical examination, attempt to determine the type of pain (somatic, visceral, and neuropathic) experienced and the possible etiologies. Acute pain (chest pain, severe abdominal pain) indicating a pathological process should be promptly and thoroughly investigated. Observe effectiveness of pain-coping measures on behavior, verbalization of comfort, participation in self-care and activities, and social interaction pattern.

Self-Perception–Self-Concept Pattern

HISTORY/INTERVIEW/SUBJECTIVE ASSESSMENT

1. **General.** "How do you feel about yourself as a person? Are you happy with the person you are right now? How would you describe yourself?" Ask how

have they adjusted to the effects of aging (structural and functional changes)? Has their body image been altered? Have the effects of aging and illness affected the individual's self-concept?

2. **Self-perception.** Have they achieved self-acceptance and recognition of self-worth? Ask the individual: "Are you satisfied with your life? Would you change any part of your life? Live any part over? Do you have any regrets? Can you describe what your life has meant to you?"

3. **Affective/psychological assessment.** "How have you been feeling lately?"
   A. **Symptoms.** Do they experience: feelings of prolonged sadness, decreased pleasure in activities, feelings of worthlessness, sense of loss, inability to cope, or feelings of guilt? Have they noticed an inability to concentrate, forgetfulness, irritability, lack of motivation, worrying about the past, rumination, apprehension, nervousness, or a lack of self-confidence? Have they had a recent loss (relationship, health, status, role, financial) that has been traumatic? Are these symptoms interfering with their ability to function on a daily basis? How have they been coping with or treating these symptoms (alcohol, drug use)? Do they feel they need professional help?
   B. **History.** Do they have a history of depression, anxiety, or another psychological disorder that was treated, or are they currently undergoing treatment? If so, elicit information about past and current treatments, perceptions of the effectiveness of those treatments, and current beliefs regarding the disorder and its effect on their lifestyle and quality of life.
   C. **Goals.** What are their goals for the future? Do they have plans in place to achieve those goals?

OBJECTIVE ASSESSMENT

1. **Psychosocial development.** Identify their stage of development. Typically, most people over age 65 are reflective about their life and are in the stage of "ego integrity versus despair," according to Erikson (1950). Determine if they are adjusting to this stage (feel fulfillment in life, do not fear death). When there are difficulties (feels regretful, fears death), the nurse should identify barriers that may be preventing the individual from achieving mastery of this stage and distinguish which barriers may be responsive to intervention (untreated depression, functional deficits that can be compensated for).

2. **Affective/psychological assessment.** Pay attention to affect during the history. Is their affect appropriate to the situation? Do they display a range of emotional behaviors? Do facial expressions and nonver-

bal cues coincide with verbal content? When possible, verify their perception of their social and emotional status with other sources.
   A. **Screening.** All older adults should be screened at least annually for depression, which is often underdiagnosed and undertreated in this group. Most geriatric experts agree that the Geriatric Depression Scale (Yesavage et al., 1983) is the preferred screening tool for use with older adults, including those with cognitive impairment. In addition to the recommended annual screening, any older adult with the aforementioned symptoms in the interview should be screened for depression at that time. Furthermore, those with symptoms of depression should be assessed for suicidal ideation, including any plans for carrying out the act. "Have you had any thoughts of harming yourself or anyone else?" If so, "Have you thought about how you are going to carry out the act? Do you have a plan?" If the major symptoms are nervousness, irritability, worrying about the past, rumination, or apprehension, the nurse should consider the possibility of an anxiety disorder.
   B. **Goals.** The goal-related questions explore the individual's adjustment to later life and may also help identify those at risk for depression or suicide. Those who are depressed may be simply "surviving" and may not have future goals, and suicidal individuals may not see a future for themselves. It is important for the nurse to maintain a high index of suspicion for both depression and suicide risk in individuals who cannot identify goals for themselves.

Role-Relationship Pattern

HISTORY/INTERVIEW/SUBJECTIVE ASSESSMENT

1. **General.** "How would you describe your role within your family and community? What do you consider to be your most important role?"

2. **Roles.** What are the formal and informal roles for this individual? Formal roles include familial roles such as child, parent, spouse, sibling, grandparent, and godparent. Informal roles include caregiver, cook, family decision maker, and driver. Each person may have multiple formal and informal roles that may need to be considered. Have there been role losses or changes related to health or other functional issues? Are they satisfied with their current roles? Obtain information about educational level, parenting history, and work history that may be pertinent to their current and previous roles. Are they recently retired? Do they provide care for an ill

spouse or other family member? Or do they receive assistance from a caregiver (spouse, child, or other family member) or from a formal support service (home health service)?

A. **Family roles.** Elicit information about marital status, family situation, and living arrangements. Who lives in their household, and what is their age, sex, and health status? Identify other family members who have contact with them, their roles, and where they live. Who manages the money in the household, and are they aware of their financial situation? Are they having any difficulties? Do they have sufficient funds to meet financial obligations?

B. **Friends/community roles.** Ask about involvement with friends and neighbors. Identify involvement in church, community groups, senior centers, or other social activities. How active are they and what roles do they play? Are they able to function independently in these roles?

3. **Relationships/socialization.** "Do you consider yourself a social person? Are you around others most of the time or are you alone a lot?" How do they describe their level of socialization? Are they satisfied with this amount of contact and socialization? Do they feel isolated or lonely? Obtain information about the number of persons seen in the past week. Do they have a confidant (either family or friends)? How often do they have contact? What is the quality of various relationships? Are there any conflicts? Who helps in times of need or when things become difficult (hospitalization, illness, crisis)? Have they had a temporary or permanent relocation? If so, what impact has relocation had on social interaction patterns or activity participation?

A. **Family.** "How are family decisions made? Describe how family members relate to one another." Would they like family relationships to be different? Is there a family crisis or stressor that is currently taxing the family? Do they have sufficient funds to meet financial obligations?

B. **Environmental factors.** Environmental factors such as distance from friends and financial resources can have a significant impact on their ability to participate in social activities. Do they have a telephone? Can the individual dial the appropriate telephone numbers to obtain assistance when needed (neighbor, relative, emergency 911, personal response system)? Do they have adequate transportation to attend desired social activities? Is it difficult to attend social activities because of the time required and the distance from home? Do they have adequate financial resources to participate in social activities?

4. **Destructive relationships/elder mistreatment.** During the relationship assessment, the nurse should screen for potentially harmful relationships. The older adult population is a vulnerable group, and therefore screening for elder abuse and neglect is an essential component of a comprehensive assessment. Elder mistreatment can be difficult to detect at times, and the gerontological nurse needs to maintain a high index of suspicion for elder abuse or neglect in those with risk factors. Identified risk factors for elder abuse and neglect in community-dwelling elders include female gender, advanced age (80 or older), nonwhite race, low income, living alone, functional deficits, and cognitive impairment (Administration for Children and Families, 1998; Lachs, Williams, O'Brien, Hurst, & Horwitz, 1997). Specific predictors of self-neglect for elders living in the community are depressive symptoms and cognitive impairment (Abrams, Lachs, McAvay, Keohane, & Bruce, 2002; Dyer, Pavlik, Murphy, & Hyman, 2000). Elder mistreatment is independently associated with a shortened life span (Lachs, Williams, O'Brien, Pillemer, & Charlson, 1998) and therefore early detection and intervention is paramount. Nevertheless, mistreatment must never be assumed by the nurse (Marshall, Benton, & Brazier, 2000; Wagner, Greenberg, & Capezuti, 2002). The patient and alleged abuser should be interviewed separately, using a nonjudgmental, nonconfrontational approach, beginning with general questions (Wagner et al., 2002; Wieland, 2000). This discussion may be difficult for the older adult, and the nurse should conduct the interview in a supportive environment at a pace that is comfortable for the patient.

A. **Abuse.** "Do you feel safe in your home (where you live)? Are you afraid of anyone? Has anyone tried to hurt you in any way? Have you ever been a victim of abuse? What were the circumstances? How was it resolved? How did you cope? Do you still feel vulnerable? Have you ever talked to someone about this before?" Do they express fear or ambivalent feelings about any family members or friends?

B. **Violence.** Has the individual ever been a victim of a crime or interpersonal violence? If the answer is yes, a detailed history will need to be completed similar to the questions listed previously for an older adult with a history of abuse.

C. **Neglect.** If they are receiving care from someone because of functional limitations, screening for caregiver neglect is important. "Are you alone a lot? Do you feel your needs are being met? Do you have a good relationship with your caregiver? Are you eating three meals a day? How often do you bathe?"

D. **Self-neglect.** "Do you feel you are able to take care of yourself adequately (ADLs, IADLs, especially hygiene)? Do you live in a safe environment? Are you able to keep your home (where you live) clean?"

PHYSICAL EXAMINATION/OBJECTIVE ASSESSMENT

1. **Observation of social patterns/relationships.** If possible, observe the frequency and patterns of interaction with family and friends, and identify the type of assistance provided (psychological support and visits, financial assistance, direct care, telephone calls, transportation, gifts). Observe how decision making proceeds, if conflicts arise, and how conflict is dealt with.

2. **Role assessment.** If the patient is a caregiver or a person who is routinely receiving physical assistance from another person (care recipient), the caregiver should be assessed.
   A. **Caregiver.** If they are a caregiver for another person it is essential to assess for caregiver burden, because the caregiver's capabilities and coping abilities can have a direct impact on the care received by the recipient. Briefly, this includes identification of the care recipient's need for assistance, the effect of caregiving on the caregiver (limited social/leisure activities), and the coping styles of the caregiver (Gallo, Fulmer, Paveza, & Reichel, 2000, p. 167).
   B. **Care recipient.** Alternatively, if they are the care recipient, their current caregiver should be assessed for burden. When possible, observe interaction patterns to assess for possible mistreatment. The nurse has a duty to report suspected elder mistreatment to the proper authorities in each state (Adult Protective Services, usually) (Gallo et al., 2000, p. 169).

3. **Elder mistreatment examination.** An examination focused on elder mistreatment is particularly indicated in three situations: an older adult with unusual injuries, an older adult with multiple risk factors for elder abuse or neglect (described previously), or any situation in which the nurse has a high index of suspicion for elder mistreatment. A review of the important elements of the examination follows:
   A. **General survey.** Observe personal hygiene. Are their clothes disheveled or soiled? Are they dressed appropriately for the weather? Do they have a strong body odor? Are their fingernails clean and trim? Is their hair clean? Do they have poor oral hygiene?
   B. **Screening.** Screening for cognitive impairment will help the nurse determine if the history is reliable. Functional deficits can be discovered through screening in order to detect if assistance needs are being met.
   C. **Physical examination.** A complete physical examination to assess for bodily injury is warranted.

The nurse should look for suspicious bruises, fractures, lacerations, or burns, and inquire about the surrounding circumstances.

Sexuality-Reproductive Pattern

HISTORY/INTERVIEW/SUBJECTIVE ASSESSMENT. Obtaining the sexual history may be challenging for the nurse because of the potential discomfort that occurs when discussing this topic. Nevertheless, the information gathered from this interview is needed and the topic should not be omitted. Personal biases and discomfort of the nurse in discussing sexuality should be identified and managed before conducting the history and physical examination, because an objective view is necessary.

1. **Introduction.** The topic may be introduced as follows to help alleviate any fears or discomfort: "As part of the health history for all adults, we routinely ask questions about sexual history and function." Then the nurse can begin the interview by asking, "Are you sexually active?" At times it may be better to ask more specific questions in case the term *sexually active* is not completely understood (Bickley & Szilagyi, 2003, p. 45). For example, "Have you recently been physically intimate with someone?" If so, "Has that included sexual intercourse?"

2. **Males and females.** Elicit beliefs and expectations about sexual activity in later life and about personal desires. Does the individual recognize intimacy (warm, close, nonsexual relationships) as a form of sensuality? Ask about previous negative sexual experiences such as rape, child abuse, or domestic violence that may affect current perceptions of sexuality (Gentili & Kuno, 2003). For those who are currently sexually active, who are previously sexually active, or who were involved in a negative sexual experience, inquire about sexually transmitted disease (STD) history and treatment. Do they report any sexual difficulties or changes (new partner, no longer sexually active)? Are they interested in improving sexual relationships through counseling, gynecological or urological evaluation, or medication? Does illness (cardiovascular disease, diabetes, human immunodeficiency virus) or medications (antidepressants, antihypertensives, chemotherapeutic agents) affect sexual activity? Have they had prior surgeries that may affect sexual functioning (radical prostatectomy in men) or feelings about sexuality (mastectomy or hysterectomy in women)? Have there been changes in their sexual abilities or their partner's abilities (e.g., started medication so that they are now sexually active)?

3. **Sexually active.** Inquire about: gender and number of current and past partners, type of intercourse (oral, vaginal, anal), patterns and frequency of sexual

activity, recent changes in patterns of sexual activity, satisfaction with activity (including decreased opportunity), and any current problems or concerns about intimacy needs. Are intimacy needs being fulfilled? Are their problems related to a partner's health or sexual difficulty? Are they protecting themselves from STDs (condoms) if they have multiple partners or are they in a mutually monogamous relationship?

A. **Women.** Ask about discomfort or painful intercourse (dyspareunia), insufficient vaginal lubrication, itching or burning in the genital area, and decreased desire. If they have experienced any of these problems, what treatments (abstinence, lubricants, medications, sexual counseling) have they tried, and did they have any effect? Inquire about signs/symptoms of STDs, including itching, burning, redness, or rash in genital area; change in or malodor of vaginal discharge; or pain in genital area.

B. **Men.** Ask about painful intercourse, impotence (erectile dysfunction), decreased desire, and premature ejaculation. If they have experienced any of these problems, what treatments (medications, sexual counseling) have they tried, and did they have any effect? Inquire about signs/symptoms of STDs, including itching, burning, redness, or rash in genital area; burning with urination; or penile discharge.

PHYSICAL EXAMINATION/OBJECTIVE ASSESSMENT

1. **Pay attention to verbal and nonverbal congruency.** Does the verbal content and enthusiasm with which they describe sexuality and intimacy indicate satisfaction? Do they articulate wishes that things could be different and therefore better? The fear of embarrassment may prevent them from honestly disclosing their true feelings regarding personal sexuality. If incongruency exists between verbal and nonverbal responses, the nurse should attempt to probe for concerns through a more detailed history, if necessary.

2. **Problem-focused physical examination.** For many, a physical examination of the genitalia is not necessary, unless a screening examination is indicated at this time (testicular for males, pelvic examinations for females). However, when there are signs/symptoms of an STD or physical sexual complaints, a pertinent physical examination should be performed.

Coping-Stress Tolerance Pattern

HISTORY/INTERVIEW/SUBJECTIVE ASSESSMENT

1. **General.** "How would you currently describe your overall stress level? Is it at a low, moderate, or high level?"

2. **Stress assessment.** "What are the current causes of and contributors to your stress? Are these stressors temporary or permanent? Are they worsening, improving, or stable? Have you been going through a lot of recent changes?"

3. **Stress management/coping.** "What are you currently doing to manage your stress? Do you feel it is manageable on your own? Do you feel you are coping effectively?" Ask for examples of effective and ineffective ways of coping (confrontation, avoidance, discussion, praying, meditation, humor, activity increase or decrease, seek presence of others, crying; indulgence in food, cigarettes, alcohol, drugs, etc.). "How have you managed similar stresses/crises in the past? Are those same skills helpful now?"

4. **Loss.** Have there been recent losses (actual or perceived): status, prestige, valued possessions, divorce, independence, death of loved one, change in environment, financial, health status/disease or effects of aging, peer relationship, lack of recognition from others? "How has your life changed since the loss? Are you able to function in your daily life?"

OBJECTIVE ASSESSMENT. Assess the range of coping skills being employed and their effectiveness. How do they perceive their stress level and their ability to manage the stress? Do they feel able to ask for professional help if it becomes necessary (counseling)? Have they successfully managed stress or have they used poor coping strategies (using food, drugs, or alcohol, or suicide attempts) in the past? Do they engage in healthy stress-reducing activities such as socializing, keeping a journal, gardening, listening to music, crafts, cooking, hobbies, caring for a pet, or exercising?

Certain adults possess specific characteristics that are associated with the use of positive coping methods in managing stress. Some of these personal characteristics are resilience, perceived self-efficacy, internal motivation, learned resourcefulness, and hardiness. These characteristics can be uncovered during the interview and can potentially be used to distinguish those persons who may be coping effectively from others who are at risk for ineffective coping.

Value-Belief Pattern

HISTORY/INTERVIEW/SUBJECTIVE ASSESSMENT. Initiating a discussion about spiritual beliefs can be challenging. The difficulties that are present when performing a sexual history (discussed previously) are comparable in certain ways to conducting a spiritual assessment. In both cases the topic is one that is a sensitive subject that must be broached delicately, and one in which the providers must be knowledgeable and comfortable with their own beliefs before an effective interview can occur. However, both areas are important for the nurse to assess because of each area's effect on health and well-being.

1. **Introduction.** Starting with an explanatory statement is an appropriate way to start. "As your health care provider I need to ask you some questions about your spiritual beliefs so I can learn more about you and care for you better. Each person has unique beliefs and it is important that I understand what things are important to you." Ideally, this will allow them to feel at ease and comfortable with the assessment. However, not all adults desire to discuss their religious and spiritual beliefs with their health care providers (McCord et al., 2004) and a few may resist.

2. **Values/beliefs.** "What are your values and beliefs about spirituality? Do you actively practice a religious faith? Do you consider yourself a spiritual person? Does spirituality play a role in your everyday life? Do you identify with a particular religion? Are you involved with others in the community with similar beliefs? Do you seek religious guidance?"

3. **Barriers.** Ask about barriers to participation in religious rituals, such as lack of transportation, lack of appropriate attire, impaired mobility, poor hearing and vision, urinary incontinence, pain, feelings of hopelessness, or depression. Are there referrals to community groups or religious opportunities that would help them be involved with others with similar beliefs?

4. **Internal conflict.** Do they verbalize doubts or inner conflicts about religion and their own faith?
   - At the end of life, or when these issues may play a role in decision making such as discussions of advance directives, a more in-depth spiritual assessment of this area is warranted.

5. **Open-ended question.** "Are there specific things you feel are important for us (health care providers) to know about your beliefs in order to take care of you better that we haven't talked about?"

OBJECTIVE ASSESSMENT

1. **Documentation.** Document important spiritual concepts that are expressed. This includes important beliefs that have the potential to affect the administration of health care. Note content of speech such as references to religious affiliation or relationship with a spiritual being. Does it appear that their spiritual needs are being met? Are they involved in a spiritual group on a regular basis, or are they comfortable expressing their faith alone? Follow up on references to death and dying.

2. **Spiritual distress.** Assess responses to internal conflict questioning. Do they feel despair or loss of faith or lack of meaning in their lives? Consider referral to a spiritual counselor or clergy for spiritual distress.

Concluding the Assessment Encounter

Overall, the comprehensive nursing assessment focused on function will provide the nurse with essential information in order to determine appropriate diagnoses and develop an individualized treatment plan for each patient as discussed under the nursing process. Additionally, the nurse must consider the far-reaching, multidimensional effects of problems occurring in the older adult and methods to manage these problems. Gordon's model provides a holistic approach to assessment that incorporates aspects of the biological, psychological, and social domains that can assist the nurse in performing a comprehensive functional assessment.

The procedures of the setting will determine how and when the plan is discussed and further developed with the patient, family, or other health care providers who may be involved with the individual's care. Additional diagnostic or laboratory tests may need to be performed before making any final decisions. The comprehensive assessment should provide the basis for a good working relationship with the older patient, with a goal of providing care that will maximize his or her function and potential.

ONGOING ASSESSMENT AND CARE OF THE OLDER ADULT

Older adults often have multiple health problems and should be seen by a primary care provider (PCP) at regular intervals. A PCP can be a physician, a physician's assistant, or an advanced practice nurse. Ideally, the PCP will be consistent, because continuity of care is essential for effective health care management in the geriatric population. Many elders see a variety of health care specialists in addition to their PCP, possibly including a podiatrist, an ophthalmologist, and a cardiologist, among other providers who contribute to their care. It is critical to have the PCP be the one consistent provider who is knowledgeable about the older adult and knows him or her well. Ideally, the PCP will have advanced training in geriatric care, but this is usually the exception instead of the norm. Although more professionals are choosing to specialize in this area, with the older adult population increasing at a rapid rate and with the limited supply of current professionals in this specialty, many older adults do not have access to a PCP with geriatric expertise.

The PCP typically provides most of the older adult's health care needs, including health promotion and disease prevention counseling, disease screening, and many treatments. Secondary prevention measures such as screening for breast cancer, colorectal cancer, sensory and memory impairments, prostate cancer, depression, and other conditions constitute a significant portion of the routine health care services that should be assessed at least annually in many older adults. Detailed recommendations for health maintenance and health screening for older adults are provided in later discussions on health maintenance. The PCP may not provide all of these services independently and often delegates specific tasks to nurses and other qualified health care personnel, but ultimately, the responsibility for the coordination and management of health care services rests with the PCP.

After the initial history and physical and the comprehensive assessment are completed on the new older adult, most subsequent encounters will consist of a problem-focused assessment. When new complaints are identified, problem-focused assessment elicits more detailed, in-depth information in a diagnostic category to rule in or rule out a diagnosis. Medical diagnosis will usually require further diagnostic and laboratory testing, in addition to the history and physical examination, to establish the diagnosis. In addition, for complex cases, referral to other health professionals may be necessary. Often, a problem-focused assessment is performed during follow-up visits for established diagnoses such as congestive heart failure or chronic obstructive pulmonary disorder to determine if it is being managed effectively or if the treatment plan needs adjustment.

The geriatric syndromes prompt a unique subset of problem-focused assessments. These syndromes, such as urinary incontinence, falls, cognitive impairment, malnutrition, and pressure ulcers, are encountered frequently by the gerontological nurse. Because they are common, the nurse should be familiar with broad preventive measures, risk factors for development, and common presentations of these problems, as well as appropriate assessment and intervention strategies to use in the diagnosis and management of these syndromes. Research-based quality indicators for several geriatric syndromes and other issues pertinent to older adults have been developed and may help guide primary care practice (Shekelle, MacLean, Morton, & Wenger, 2001). Gerontological APNs may develop roles in which they provide consultation for complex patients with particular geriatric syndromes. For example, nurses may develop specialized knowledge and develop roles such as incontinence or skin care nurses.

As a final component of ongoing care, the primary care provider will also want to address health care directives. The PCP should encourage all individuals to complete a durable power of attorney for health care decisions and a living will, and give a copy to the PCP so it can be discussed. This will enable the PCP to address emergency or catastrophic events should they arise. This information will also help inform discussions about screening options, treatment choices, and long-term care plans.

SUMMARY

Comprehensive assessment of the older adult should have a focus on function and is an essential part of the role of the gerontological nurse. The older adult population is unique, and adjustments to the traditional assessment of the adult are required. This chapter described the adaptations in the nursing process that will assist the nurse in addressing the special needs of older adults. Furthermore, a framework for a comprehensive nursing assessment has been provided. The numerous topics that should be included in the assessment have been described and can be easily adapted for use in a variety of health care settings. Nurses can improve their detection of common health problems using a standardized approach. Chapter 3 continues with a discussion of specific screening tools and assessment techniques that will further assist the nurse in performing a comprehensive assessment.

REFERENCES

Abrams, R. C., Lachs, M., McAvay, G., Keohane, D. J., & Bruce, M. L. (2002). Predictors of self-neglect in community-dwelling elders. *American Journal of Psychiatry, 159*(10), 1724-1730.

Administration for Children and Families, Administration on Aging, U.S. Department of Health and Human Services. (1998). *The national elder abuse incidence study.* Rockville, MD: Author.

American Cancer Society. (2005). *Cancer facts and figures 2005.* Atlanta, GA: Author.

Bickley, L. S., & Szilagyi, P. G. (2003). *Bates' guide to physical examination and history taking* (8th ed.). Philadelphia: Lippincott Williams & Wilkins.

Boltz, M. (2002). Sensory impairment. In V. T. Cotter & N. E. Strumpf (Eds.), *Advanced practice nursing with older adults: Clinical guidelines.* New York: McGraw-Hill.

Carlson, J. E. (1999). Assessment of orthostatic blood pressure: Measurement technique and clinical applications. *Southern Medical Journal, 92*(2), 167-173.

Chidester, J. C., & Spangler, A. A. (1997). Fluid intake in the institutionalized elderly. *Journal of the American Dietetic Association, 97*(1), 23-28.

Christmas, C., & Andersen, R. A. (2000). Exercise and older patients: Guidelines for the clinician. *Journal of the American Geriatrics Society, 48*(3), 318-324.

Consensus Committee of the American Autonomic Society and the American Academy of Neurology. (1996). Consensus statement on the definition of orthostatic hypotension, pure autonomic failure, and multiple system atrophy. *Neurology, 46*(5), 1470.

Dyer, C. B., Pavlik, V. N., Murphy, K. P., & Hyman, D. J. (2000). The high prevalence of depression and dementia in elder abuse or neglect. *Journal of the American Geriatrics Society, 48*(2), 205-208.

Engstrom, J. W., & Aminoff, M. J. (1997). Evaluation and treatment of orthostatic hypotension. *American Family Physician, 56*(5), 1378-1385.

Erikson, E. H. (1950). *Childhood and society.* New York: W. W. Norton.

Folstein, M. F., Folstein, S. E., & McHugh, P. R. (1975). "Mini-mental state." A practical guide for grading the cognitive state of patients for the clinician. *Journal of Psychiatric Research, 12*(3), 189-198.

Fried, L. P., Ferrucci, L., Darer, J., Williamson, J. D., & Anderson, G. (2004). Untangling the concepts of disability, frailty, and comorbidity: Implications for improved targeting and care. *Journal of Gerontology Medical Sciences, 59*(3), 255-263.

Gallo, J. J., Fulmer, T., Paveza, G. J., & Reichel, W. (2000). *Handbook of geriatric assessment* (3rd ed.). Gaithersburg, MD: Aspen.

Gentili, A., & Kuno, H. (2003). Disorders of sexual function. In E. Flaherty, T. T. Fulmer, & M. Mezey (Eds.), *Geriatric nursing review syllabus: A core curriculum in advanced practice geriatric nursing.* New York: American Geriatrics Society.

Gordon, M. (2002). *Manual of nursing diagnosis* (10th ed.). St. Louis: Mosby.

Hart, A. C., & Hopkins, C. A. (Eds.). (2003). *International classification of diseases, 9th revision: Expert for hospitals, volumes 1, 2, and 3* (6th ed.). Salt Lake City: Ingenix.

Heiat, A., Vaccarino, V., & Krumholz, H. (2001). An evidence-based assessment of federal guidelines for overweight and obesity as they apply to elderly persons. *Archives of Internal Medicine, 161*(9), 1194-1203.

Henderson, M. L. (2001). Assessing the elderly: Altered presentations. Reprinted in G. R. Hall, M. L. Henderson, & M. Smith (Eds), *Assessing the elderly.* Philadelphia: Lippincott Williams & Wilkins.

Iowa Outcomes Project. (2003). *Nursing outcomes classification (NOC)* (3rd ed.) (S. Moorhead, M. Johnson, & M. Maas, Eds.). St. Louis: Mosby.

Irvin, D. J., & White, M. (2004). The importance of accurately assessing orthostatic hypotension. *Geriatric Nursing, 25*(2), 99-101.

Jensen, G. L., & Powers, J. S. (2003). Malnutrition. In E. F. Flaherty, T. T. Fulmer, & M. Mezey (Eds.), *Geriatric nursing review syllabus: A core curriculum in advanced practice geriatric nursing.* New York: American Geriatrics Society.

Kane, R. L., Ouslander, J. G., & Abrass, I. B. (2004). *Essentials of clinical geriatrics.* New York: McGraw-Hill.

Kennedy-Malone, L., Fletcher, K. R., & Plank, L. M. (2004). *Management guidelines for nurse practitioners working with older adults* (2nd ed.). Philadelphia: F. A. Davis.

Lachs, M. S., Williams, C., O'Brien, S., Hurst, L., & Horwitz, R. (1997). Risk factors for reported elder abuse and neglect: A nine-year observational cohort study. *Gerontologist, 37*(4), 469-474.

Lachs, M. S., Williams, C. S., O'Brien, S., Pillemer, K. A., & Charlson, M. E. (1998). The mortality of elder mistreatment. *Journal of the American Medical Association, 280*(5), 428-432.

Marshall, C. E., Benton, D., & Brazier, J. M. (2000). Elder abuse: Using clinical tools to identify clues of mistreatment. *Geriatrics, 55*(2), 42-53.

McCord, G., Gilchrist, V. L., Grossman, S. D., King, B. D., McCormick, K. F., Oprandi, A. M., et al. (2004). Discussing spirituality with patients: A rational and ethical approach. *Annals of Family Medicine, 2*(4), 356-361.

Messinger-Rapport, B. J. (2002). How to assess and counsel the older driver. *Cleveland Clinic Journal of Medicine, 69*(3), 184-185, 189-190, 192.

NANDA International. (2003). *NANDA nursing diagnoses: Definitions and classification 2003–2004.* Philadelphia: NANDA.

National Heart, Lung, and Blood Institute. (2000). The practical guide: Identification, evaluation, and treatment of obesity in adults. Retrieved September 24, 2005, from www.nhlbi.nih.gov/guidelines/obesity/prctgd_c.pdf.

Podsiadlo, D., & Richardson, S. (1991). The timed "up and go": A test of basic functional mobility for frail elderly persons. *Journal of the American Geriatrics Society, 39,* 142-148.

Reuben, D. B., Herr, K. A., Pacala, J.T., Pollock, B.G., Potter, J.F., & Semla, T. P. (2003). *Geriatrics at your fingertips: 2003* (5th ed.). Malden, MA: American Geriatrics Society.

Sheiman, S. L. (2002). Nutritional problems. In V. T. Cotter & N. E. Strumpf (Eds.), *Advanced practice nursing with older adults: Clinical guidelines.* New York: McGraw-Hill.

Shekelle, P. G., MacLean, C. H., Morton, S. C., & Wenger, N. S. (2001). ACOVE quality indicators. *Annals of Internal Medicine, 135*(8 pt 2), 653-667.

U.S. Department of Health and Human Services. (2000). *The practical guide: Identification, evaluation, and treatment of overweight and obesity in adults* (NIH publication no. 00-4084). Rockville, MD: Author.

U.S. Preventive Services Task Force. (2002). Screening for osteoporosis in postmenopausal women: Recommendations and rationale. *Annals of Internal Medicine, 137*(6), 526-528.

Wagner, L., Greenberg, S., & Capezuti, E. (2002). Elder abuse and neglect. In V. T. Cotter & N. E. Strumpf (Eds.), *Advanced practice nursing with older adults: Clinical guidelines.* New York: McGraw-Hill.

Wieland, D. (2000). Abuse of older persons: An overview. *Holistic Nursing Practice, 14*(4), 40-50.

World Health Organization. (2002). *Towards a common language for functioning, disability and health: ICF the International classification of functioning, disability and health.* Geneva, Switzerland: Author.

Yen, P. K. (2004). Nutrition and sensory loss. *Geriatric Nursing, 25*(2), 118-119.

Yesavage, J. A., Brink, T. L , Rose, T. L, Lum, O., Huang, V, Adey, M., & Leirer, V. O. (1983). Development and validation of a geriatric depression screening scale: A preliminary report. *Journal of Psychiatric Research, 17,* 37-49.

Chapter 3

Tools for Screening and Assessment

Helen W. Lach & Carrie M. Smith

Objectives

Identify the purpose and four domains for screening in the older adult.

Describe considerations for choosing screening instruments for various clinical settings.

Review selected screening instruments from each of the four domains.

A variety of screening tools can be used during assessment to assist the nurse in detecting functional impairments or other conditions that may be amenable to intervention. They are added to the basic history and physical examination components described in the previous chapter. Screening methods serve to uncover problems that are not yet diagnosed and that place an individual at high risk because of the high prevalence and morbidity associated with the problem. After detection, early diagnosis and treatment can occur. The importance of screening tools is described by a nurse practitioner in Box 3-1.

Early detection is assumed to be advantageous to the older adult who, without screening, may not be identified until overt signs or symptoms occur, often indicating advanced disease with a worse prognosis. Screening measures tend to be brief, containing only essential diagnostic information. A positive result on a screening instrument indicates that the older adult has some of the characteristics of the disorder that the tool seeks to detect (e.g., depression) or that impairment exists in specific areas examined by the tool. For example, a person's inability to dress himself or herself would reflect impairment in activities of daily living. In either case, a more detailed evaluation is necessary to confirm the problem and etiology. This evaluation may include gathering additional physical examination data, laboratory and diagnostic test results, a more extensive history, or some combination of the three, to validate the screening results.

Older adults should be routinely screened for common physical, psychological, and cognitive impairments such as depression, dementia, or deficits in activities of daily living. In addition, screening for pain is essential in this age-group for two reasons: many comorbid conditions are often present in older adults that predispose them to pain, and pain is often underreported because of the misperception that pain is a normal part of aging. Even if the older adult does not have these conditions at the time of screening, it is useful to have systematic documentation of his or her symptoms and function as a baseline for future comparison.

The older adult's ability to participate in meaningful social interactions is another crucial area to consider. Impairment in socialization can have far-reaching effects on the older adult's physical, psychological, and functional well-being, leading to poor outcomes. Therefore identifying risk factors for social isolation such as bereavement, living alone, absence of a confidant or someone to turn to in an emergency, substance abuse, or caregiver stress should be followed by an indepth assessment. Finally, it is important to remember that terminally ill elders with a limited life span may continue to have screening needs and that enhanced quality of life is the ultimate aim.

CHOOSING A SCREENING TOOL

Several standardized measures exist for assessment and screening purposes that can be used with older adults. Some have been used as standards for assessment for many years, and others are newer, assessing additional or more specific domains of function. With multiple tools to choose from, selecting a screening instrument and deciphering the results can be a challenge. The nurse must consider many factors when selecting a screening

---

Box 3-1 *Reflections on Using Assessment Tools in Practice*

Older adults and their families transition through states of health and illness in their life cycle where they are often cared for by nurses. In the encounter with an aging population, gerontological nurses aid older adults and families to optimum states of wellness by not only treating their illnesses, but managing their outcomes as they affect daily living. It is in this context that assessment tools are vitally important in clinical practice.

Older adults collectively experience a wide array of health care issues, and individually experience a myriad of health concerns. As such, gerontological nurses must be prepared to effectively and efficiently assess and manage a host of problems in a timely fashion. One encounter with an older adult may require assessment and management of up to 10 or more chronic health problems per patient. Typically, the scope of problems encountered by the older adult extends to families, caregiving situations, and other dynamic interactions, such as qualification for available services, all of equal value in the geriatric assessment. Use of assessment tools helps to streamline important lines of inquiry about diseases and conditions.

Considering that a typical review of systems for the many chronic illnesses, not including assessment of the family and caregiving situation, is exhausting for the patient and even the experienced provider, use of assessment tools provides a helpful solution as an indicator of a health concern or disease progression, stability, or resolution. Consider the value of assessment tools in the overall management of this older adult. In this case, assessment tools helped hone in on the stability of this gentleman's multiple health problems:

An 86-year-old man visits the gerontological nurse practitioner for assessment of his progressive memory deterioration, isolated systolic hypertension, coronary artery disease, diabetes mellitus, spinal degenerative joint disease, peptic ulcer disease, and peripheral neuropathy. Unable to offer any reliable symptoms for which the nurse can judge the medical stability of these illnesses, attention is devoted to questions about daily living, including activities of daily living. What is learned through the functional assessment tools are the new onset of deficits of shortness of breath with walking, forgetting to use the toilet, and an increase in nocturia. These symptoms translate to a new onset of congestive heart failure confirmed by physical examination and diagnostic studies.

Further, administration of cognitive assessment tools found a clear deterioration by review of the summed score, which showed worsening memory. A drop in scores indicated a significant cognitive decline not usual in such a short period of time. This information translated to worsening cognition and the need for acute treatment. It was evident that the hypoxia occurring from the new congestive heart failure contributed to greater cognitive difficulties.

Another asset of assessment tools is the content, which may be significant itself, in addition to the summed rating of the score indicating presence or absence of a condition. Although assessment tools focus on one measurable construct, they may also explore a number of symptoms that may warrant further attention. These symptoms can signal an impending or looming problem. An example is the use of the Geriatric Depression Scale (GDS; Yesavage et al., 1983), which can lead to a diagnosis of depression when it is coupled with other pertinent clinical findings. But when the GDS score is marginally or borderline significant (in the case of a high but not positive score), the presence of pertinent symptoms on the GDS is relevant in clinical practice because they can be monitored for progression or isolated as evidence of other disease phenomena.

Although standards of care and clinical practice guidelines determine successful treatment intervention for defined diseases at any age, it is the assessment tool that enables the gerontological nurse to help the patient the most. Findings from assessment tools allow for important decisions to be made that ultimately guide interventions geared toward maintenance of independence and autonomy. Gerontological nurses recognize the importance of assessment tools in practice by reliance on findings revealed from and within assessment tools.

Deanna Gray Miceli

Deanna Gray Miceli, DNSc, APRN, FAANP
Adjunct Assistant Professor
University of Pennsylvania
Philadelphia, Pennsylvania
Nurse Practitioner/Research Scientist, Office of Planning and Development
New Jersey Department of Health and Senior Services
Trenton, New Jersey

---

instrument (Schretzman & Strumpf, 2002), including, but not limited to, the following:

- The purpose of the instrument
- Limitations of the setting
- Clinical relevance
- Ease of use
- Amount of training required
- Equipment needs and costs
- Appropriateness for use with older adults
- Special patient characteristics that may prevent obtaining accurate results

Furthermore, the measure must have demonstrated reliability and validity, and it must have appropriate sensitivity and specificity for the condition being screened. These terms are described in detail later. These factors can be grouped into three categories: general considerations, nurse or administrator considerations, and patient considerations.

General Considerations

General considerations when selecting a screening instrument include identification of the tool's purpose, clinical relevance of the information gathered from the tool, appropriateness for use with an older adult population, cost of equipment needed, and evidence from research studies performed to test the instrument. The nurse must determine the specific purpose for which the tool was designed and the population it was designed to assess. Discovering if the tool has been tested in an older population with characteristics of the target population is important. The information elicited from the tool should be useful and provide additional data not obtained during other parts of the patient assessment.

Some instruments require the purchase of specific equipment in order to gather the data needed. The cost of or difficulty in obtaining materials may be a deterrent to using the tool, and should be considered. Finally, studies describing the properties of the instrument and how it has been used need to be examined to assess the quality of the instrument. See Box 3-2 for a list of important factors to consider when choosing an instrument.

The terms *reliability, validity, sensitivity,* and *specificity* are frequently used to describe the screening characteristics of an instrument. When choosing a screening instrument, the nurse should review the research studies that have been performed to test the instrument to determine if it is an appropriate assessment tool. Examining the reliability, validity, sensitivity, and specificity of the tool is a good starting point to determine if the tool is suitable for use in a particular situation.

Reliability, sometimes called *accuracy* or *precision,* refers to the ability of the tool to provide a consistent and dependable measurement (Polit & Beck, 2004). *Intrarater reliability* refers to a nurse's ability to use a tool with consistent results. If patients with depression are assessed, the nurse should find scores that show they are depressed. In addition, if several different nurses assess the same patients using the same tool, they should find the same results. This is known as *interrater reliability* (Bickley & Szilagyi, 2003). For many instruments,

training is needed to use them reliably. The training may include reviewing guidelines, watching a tape of someone administering the tool, learning how to work equipment, or tips on how to ask questions. For example, nurses may feel uncomfortable asking some of the questions that test memory or depression. However, to reliably administer tests for these conditions, the interviewer must ask the questions in a consistent, matter-of-fact way and not provide clues regarding the answers, or respond to inappropriate answers.

Validity, on the other hand, assesses a tool's ability to measure the phenomena it is supposed to measure. It is more difficult to measure than reliability, yet it remains an important consideration when choosing an instrument. Validity is tested by comparing the tool with the best possible measure of reality (Bickley & Szilagyi, 2003; Polit & Beck, 2004). For example, a depression scale is tested by comparing it with a clinician's diagnosis of depression. If the tool is valid, the results using the tool will be consistent with the diagnosis. A few correlations exist between the reliability and validity of instruments, with low reliability being indicative of low validity; however, high reliability has no bearing on an instrument's validity (Polit & Beck, 2004). Research studies consider reliability and validity as the "psychometric properties" of a tool.

Additional quality indicators of an assessment instrument include sensitivity and specificity. These are criteria used primarily to evaluate screening and diagnostic instruments (Polit & Beck, 2004). The *sensitivity* of a tool refers to how well the tool identifies those who have the condition (Stommel & Wills, 2004). These are designated as "true positives." "False positives" are persons incorrectly identified by a tool as having the condition. The specificity of a tool refers to how well the tool identifies those who do not have the condition. These are designated "true negatives." "False negatives," the opposite of false positives, are persons who are not identified by the tool as having the condition, yet they are truly positive.

Ideally, a screening test correctly identifies most of the patients who have the condition (high sensitivity) with a minimum of false positives (high specificity). A tool with high sensitivity (90%) helps rule out disease and is most helpful in screening. On the other hand, a tool with high specificity (90%) helps rule in disease and may be more helpful in diagnosis (Bickley & Szilagyi, 2003). However, in general, as the sensitivity of an instrument increases (fewer false negatives), the specificity decreases (more false positives), making it a challenge to develop a tool that is both highly sensitive and highly specific (Polit & Beck, 2004).

Determining what levels of sensitivity and specificity are needed depends on the screening topic. If you are screening for breast cancer, a high sensitivity is needed. You want to identify as many women who may have the

---

BOX 3-2 Considerations in Selecting Screening Tools

- The purpose of the instrument
- Time limitations of the setting
- Ease of administration and scoring
- Amount of training required
- Equipment needs and costs
- Appropriateness for use with older adults
- Clinical relevance
- Reliability
- Validity
- Sensitivity and specificity

disease as possible. A diagnosis is confirmed later with more definitive tests. For other conditions, less screening accuracy may be acceptable. It is important to note that the sensitivity and specificity of a screening test may vary according to the conditions under which the test is administered.

Nursing Considerations

The time limitations of the setting, the ease of use of the tool, and the amount of training required to administer and score the tool (if applicable) are the main considerations for choosing a tool for clinical practice. First, the time it takes to administer the instrument must fit into the time designated for patient visits. The time needed to complete a lengthy screening instrument may not fit into a 15-minute office visit. The utility of most screening tools is that they allow the clinician to assess the patient for more problems in a shorter period of time. Either they are quicker than a more formal evaluation, or they can be completed before the examination, thus saving time. For example, patients may be able to complete forms at home and bring them to the office visit or complete them in the waiting room.

The tool's usability is another essential factor to consider. The ability of the nurse to obtain highly accurate results from a tool that is self-explanatory, even if used infrequently, is most desirable. Often, the amount of education and training required to correctly use a tool significantly affects whether it is chosen for clinical use. Unfortunately, because of the combination of scarce health care resources and time limitations experienced by many employers, the necessary time and effort needed to train staff to use more complex tools is lacking. However, with most tools, some minimal training should be performed.

Patient Considerations

Several patient characteristics can affect the validity of assessment results or the patient's ability to fully participate in the assessment, or both of these areas. The characteristics that may affect validity include cognitive impairment and educational level. For example, patients with severe cognitive decline may not understand questions in order to respond appropriately. Some cognitive screening tools require tasks that are based on a minimal educational level, so the results for less educated patients may be lower. Language and cultural differences can also confound the results if the individual has different meanings for words used in the instrument. Some may be unable to fully participate in the assessment process because of language barriers, illiteracy, or physical handicaps. The ability to complete the instrument or assessment without fatigue is another important consideration with older adults (VanSwearingen & Brach,

2001). Some of these barriers may be able to be overcome, and that should be the goal.

Nevertheless, the nurse needs to be alert to these characteristics before using an assessment instrument, while remembering that these characteristics do not always preclude an individual from being screened. For example, a translator may be able to administer a tool to a non–English-speaking patient, or versions in other languages may be available that have been tested and validated. Instead, the characteristics of the individual assessment tool will assist the nurse in deciding if screening is appropriate and if the results would be valid. It is preferable to use a screening tool only if it appears the results will be valid. If the nurse has questions about the potential validity of the results based on some of the described characteristics, the screening should be omitted and a clinical assessment should be performed if indicated.

Overall, choosing an instrument can be difficult but is made easier when keeping in mind the considerations described. With practice, the important questions covered will become second nature and limited time will be needed to evaluate or choose an appropriate tool. By using correct screening and assessment techniques, the nurse can make a significant impact on the individual's life through early intervention and treatment.

REVIEW OF SCREENING AND ASSESSMENT INSTRUMENTS

Selected screening instruments for use with older adults are briefly reviewed to provide an overview for the gerontological nurse. The tools are broadly categorized into the three domains discussed in the preceding chapter: biological (physical and functional), psychological (cognitive and affective), and social. A description of each tool is given, along with practical information regarding use of the tool. Some of the tools described are primarily used for research purposes. Familiarity with these instruments is important because of the frequency with which the nurse will see these tools referenced in the literature.

As discussed previously, before choosing an instrument, a review of relevant research findings is recommended to ensure that the instrument is psychometrically sound and is appropriate for the nurse's patient population and clinical setting. Of note, some of the basic instruments have been used for many years and continue to be common in practice and research; however, the basic research on the instruments was done some years ago.

For the purposes of this chapter we describe a few examples of instruments for each assessment domain. Nurses should be aware that many other excellent screening tools exist, and we encourage the reader to become familiar with many of the tools, especially for those conditions that are commonly seen in the nurse's clinical practice or area of research. The most commonly used tools are provided in this chapter to serve as a resource, and others are available in the literature and assessment texts (e.g., Gallo, Fulmer, Paveza, & Reichel, 2003).

Instruments for Functional Assessment

Instruments and scales have been developed for specific domains of function. Use of standardized measures can improve clinical decision making, because important aspects of that domain are less likely to be missed. Additionally, communication can be facilitated among disciplines when summary scores of recognized and accepted measures give brief, meaningful information about an older adult's functioning.

Assessment of Physical (General) Health.

Measures of physical health attempt to provide a global determination of overall health, and some are considered measures of quality of life. Resnick and Parker (2001) note that health status has been used to (1) describe recovery after acute events, (2) explore the trajectory of chronic diseases, (3) explore outcomes of aging, and (4) evaluate health promotion interventions. Some measures inquire about the presence of illness or disease, whereas others may cover items related to activities of daily living and instrumental activities of daily living.

Commonly used indicators of health include diagnoses and conditions present, symptoms, disabilities, categories or numbers of drugs taken, severity of illness indicators, and quantification of health care utilization (e.g., number of hospital days per year). Self-ratings of health and disability may also be included in such measures. Included here are a few examples of measures of general physical health. Three scales of health status are reviewed: the Cumulative Illness Rating Scale, Sickness Impact Profiles, and Short-Form 36. Pain assessment tools are also addressed here under physical health.

CUMULATIVE ILLNESS RATING SCALE. The Cumulative Illness Rating Scale (CIRS) is a research-oriented instrument designed to measure overall health through assessment of medical comorbidities to describe the burden of disease. The CIRS is a rating of the degree of impairment (5-point scale from none to extremely severe) in 12 organ systems (cardiac; vascular; respiratory; eyes, ears, nose, and throat; upper gastrointestinal; lower gastrointestinal; hepatic; renal; other genitourinary; musculoskeletal-integumentary; neurological; and endocrine-metabolic) and includes a psychiatric/behavioral category (Linn, Linn, & Gurel, 1968; Parmelee, Thuras, Katz, & Lawton, 1995). The CIRS is completed by a trained health professional following a complete history and physical examination.

The total CIRS score reflects the cumulative medical burden of the individual and has potential use in determining medical prognosis (Linn, 1967). The reliability and validity of the CIRS has been established, with the validity specifically being tested in both community-dwelling older adults and older adults residing in a long term-care setting (Miller et al., 1992; Parmelee et al., 1995). Miller and colleagues (1992) developed a modified CIRS for Geriatrics (CIRS-G) that yielded positive psychometric properties in assessment of older adults suffering from bereavement and depression. The CIRS is often used in geropsychiatric studies (e.g., Mistry et al., 2004; Taylor, McQuoid, & Krishnan, 2004) and other studies to describe the medical health status of the participants.

SICKNESS IMPACT PROFILE. The Sickness Impact Profile (SIP) was developed to assess health status as a measure of health care outcomes (Bergner, Bobbitt, Carter, & Gilson, 1981; Bergner, Bobbitt, Pollard, Martin, & Gilson, 1976; Gilson et al., 1975). It was designed to be used generically in different populations (such as hip fracture patients), in individuals and in groups of patients, and across geographical and cultural groups. The SIP contains 136 items, can be administered by an interviewer or can be self-administered, and is reported to take between 15 and 45 minutes to complete (Andresen, 1997). The statements describe health-related dysfunction in 12 categories: sleep and rest, eating, work, home management, recreation and pastimes, ambulation, mobility, body care and movement, social interaction, alertness behavior, emotional behavior, and communication. For example, the social interaction section includes such statements as, "I make many demands, for example, insist that people do things for me, tell them how to do things" and "I am going out less to visit people."

Reliability and validity of the SIP have been established (Bergner et al., 1981; Bergner et al., 1976; de Bruin, Buys, de Witte, & Diederiks, 1994). The tool has been used with a variety of populations and as an outcome measure in studies of the effects of interventions to reduce frailty, in a variety of settings (Cress et al., 1995; Shannon, Yip, & Wilber, 2004). Many different versions have been derived since the SIP's original development in 1975 (e.g., de Bruin et al., 1994; van Straten et al., 1997), including a nursing home version (Gerety et al., 1994). The SIP is being used to examine the impact of chronic disease and whether a profile exists unique to populations with different chronic diseases, and to evaluate the efficacy of treatment programs. Overall, the SIP is a research and clinical tool that has been used in a variety of health care settings as an outcome measure and a generic quality-of-life indicator, and in functional assessment.

**SHORT-FORM 36 GENERAL HEALTH QUES-
TIONNAIRE.** The Short-Form 36 (SF-36) is a popular
instrument that resulted from the Medical Outcomes
Study (MOS), a study performed to help determine how
patient outcomes are affected by specific health care system components, examining the structure, process, and
outcomes of care (Tarlov et al., 1989). Health services
researchers identified a need to develop a measure of
the individual's perspective of her or his health status
that was easy to administer, took only a brief time to
complete, and had acceptable psychometric properties.
Perceptions of health are related to severity of illness
and symptoms, as well as quality of life.

Earlier health status measures such as the SIP are
lengthy and impractical for clinical use. Therefore a 20-
item Short-Form 20 (SF-20) was originally developed
and incorporated into the screening process for the
MOS, but following further research the 36-item SF-36
has proved to be a better instrument and has replaced
the SF-20. More recently, the 12-item Short-Form 12
(SF-12) was constructed, which focuses primarily on the
physical and mental health components of the SF-36
(Ware, Kosinski, & Keller, 1996). Both the SF-36 and the
SF-12 yield valuable information when used in large
population studies (Jenkinson et al., 1997; Walters,
Munro, & Brazier, 2001). This measure is now widely
used in research and health care settings to measure
population health.

Eight health concepts are assessed by the SF-36: physical functioning, bodily pain, social functioning, general
mental health, vitality, general health perceptions, role
limitations due to physical functioning, and role limitations due to emotional problems (Ware & Sherbourne,
1992). The test can be administered by an interviewer in
person or over the telephone, or it can be self-administered. It takes between 5 and 10 minutes to complete or
administer (Ware & Sherbourne, 1992). Some differences have been found in the SF-36 results depending
on the method of administration; one study found that
self-assessment scores were significantly lower (indicating poorer perceived health) than interviewer-
administered scores performed in the clinic setting
(Lyons et al., 1999). Instruction for scoring the SF-36
is required, may take practice, and is ideally done by
computer.

Many studies have found the SF-36 to be a reliable
and valid tool in measuring health status of older adults
(Bayliss, Bayliss, Ware, & Steiner, 2004), the outcomes
of medical procedures (Lawrence et al., 2004), and interventions (Jensen, Roy, Buchanan, & Berg, 2004). Early
problems were identified for older adults completing
the SF-36, including missing data and difficulty completing independently (Hayes, Morris, Wolfe, & Morgan,
1995), both of which can be corrected by interviewer
administration. The SF-12 is an acceptable alternative in
many cases to the SF-36 (Ware, Kosinski, & Keller, 1996),

although it is still easier to score on the computer. The
SF-12 provides a mental health and physical health subscale and can be completed in 5 minutes or less. Resnick
and Parker (2001) proposed a simplified scoring system
for the SF-12 that involves summing the scores rather
than computing weights, as well as changes in the subscale items. The gerontological nurse should remember
that these tools are predominantly used in the study of
population characteristics, and despite yielding individual health perceptions, the SF tool's significance on an
individual basis is somewhat limited.

PAIN ASSESSMENT. Pain is common among older
patients as a result of chronic conditions, as well as
acute illness (Potter & Biswas, 2002), and is often called
the sixth vital sign. Despite the frequency of this symptom, pain is often missed or ignored, resulting in
unnecessary discomfort. The problem is especially difficult when patients have dementia and have difficulty
communicating their symptoms. However, even most
nursing home patients with cognitive impairment can
use a scale or answer questions about their pain
(Wynne, Ling, & Remsburg, 2000). Pain assessment
scales provide a quick way of rating the intensity of pain
that can be used to evaluate treatment outcomes. Nurses
often use the simple method of asking patients to rate
their pain on a scale of 1 to 10. Two visual scales for
documenting pain intensity that can be used for nursing
assessment to supplement the history and physical
examination are reviewed.

Faces Pain Scale. The Faces Pain Scale (FPS) (Bieri,
Reeve, & Champion, 1990) was developed to assess
pain in children and showed good reliability and validity (Figure 3-1). The FPS depicts a series of facial pictures that change with the intensity of pain level,
particularly the brow, mouth, and eyes. They are not
children's faces. The tool was tested with older adults by
Herr, Mobily, Kohout, and Wagenaar (1998) and showed
good reliability and validity in a sample of community
older adults. The tool provides a consistent method for
assessing and monitoring changes in pain.

Visual Analog Scale. The Visual Analog Scale (VAS)
(Jacox et al., 1994) provides a numerical rating of pain,
usually on a scale from 0 to 10, with 10 being the worst
possible pain and 0 representing no pain at all (Figure 3-2). The VAS provides a pictorial representation of
the rating scale that may help patients choose the best
rating of the severity of their pain.

Functional Status. Measures of functional status
are a key component of assessment for the older adult
and reveal the individual's physical abilities and the
impact of disease on self-care (Grundy, 2003). In addition, these measures identify the type and amount of
assistance the individual needs and can help inform
decisions about services and living situation. Activities

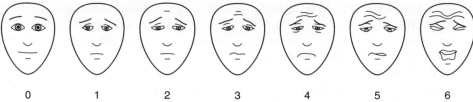

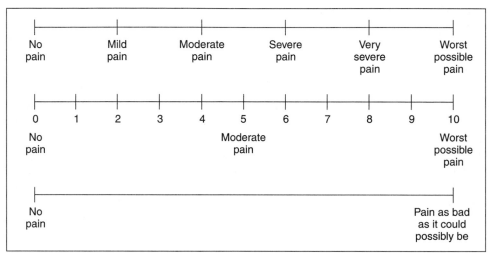

Figure 3-1 Faces Pain Scale. (From Bieri, D., Reeve, R., & Champion, G. (1990). The Faces Pain Scale for the self-assessment of severity of pain experienced by children: Development, initial validation, and preliminary investigation for ratio scale properties. *Pain, 41,* 139.)

Figure 3-2 Visual Analog Scale. (From Jacox, A., Carr, D. B., Payne, R., Berde, C. B., Breitbart, W., & Caine, J. M. (1994). *Management of cancer pain: Clinical practice guideline no. 9.* Rockville, MD: Agency for Health Care Policy and Research, pp. 139-150.)

of daily living (ADLs) include bathing, dressing, feeding, transfers, continence, and ambulation. These basic activities are important for the individual to manage his or her own personal care and independent living. The instrumental activities of daily living (IADLs) include activities that are usually necessary for maintaining a household, such as housekeeping, shopping, taking medicines, using transportation, using the telephone, cooking, and managing money. More advanced measures of functional status examine broader engagement in society by exploring participation in social and productive activities.

Functional decline has long been associated with aging and chronic disease, and is predictive of nursing home placement and mortality risk (Ostir et al., 1999). The utility of measuring functional status is to identify early decline and intervene before disability is severe and interventions are less likely to be successful. In addition, it is important to track changes in function related to disease and treatments, and should be considered in making medical decisions. There are numerous tools to examine functional status. Some of the most common tools are presented here, but many more are available in the literature.

Measures often rely on self-report, but direct observation is considered more reliable and sensitive to change because it is freer from bias, although it can be time consuming. It is important to confirm the self-report of the individual with a family member or caregiver when possible. "Environmental artifacts" may influence performance of ADLs (Katz et al., 1963). For example, in the hospital or nursing home, nurses may supervise or assist patients during bathing (getting into showers or tubs) and transfers. Care may be provided by the nurse for the sake of safety and convenience and to economize on time, instead of encouraging the individual to do as much as possible. This can result in learned helplessness and functional status ratings that are lower than they might be in the absence of such restrictions (Katz et al., 1963). The nurse administering the tools should be aware of the impact of the environment on the ratings of the individual and consider the actual abilities of the individual and not just her or his current performance.

KATZ INDEX OF ACTIVITIES OF DAILY LIVING. The Katz Index of ADLs (Katz et al., 1963) is a well-known, widely used clinical and research instrument used to assess ability to perform self-care (Figure 3-3). It

Independent means without supervision, direction, or active personal assistance, except as specifically noted below. This is based on actual status and not ability. A patient who refuses to perform a function is considered as not performing the function, even though he or she is deemed able.

Bathing (Sponge, Shower, or Tub)
Independent: Assistance only in bathing a single part (back or disabled extremity) or bathes self completely
Dependent: Assistance in bathing more than one part of body; assistance in getting in or out of tub; does not bathe self

Dressing
Independent: Gets clothes from closets and drawers; puts on clothes, outer garments, braces; manages fasteners; act of tieing shoes is excluded
Dependent: Does not dress self or remains partly underdressed

Going to Toilet
Independent: Gets to toilet; gets on and off toilet; arranges clothes; cleans organs of excretion (may manage own bedpan used at night only and may or may not be using mechanical supports)
Dependent: Uses bedpan or commode or receives assistance in getting to and using toilet

Transfer
Independent: Moves in and out of bed and in and out of chair independently (may or may not be using mechanical supports)
Dependent: Assistance in moving in or out of bed and/or chair; does not perform one or more transfers

Continence
Independent: Urination and defecation entirely self-controlled
Dependent: Partial or total incontinence in urination or defecation; partial or total control by enemas, catheters, or regulated use of urinals and/or bedpans

Feeding
Independent: Gets food from plate or its equivalent

Evaluation Form		
Name	Date of Evaluation	
For each area of functioning listed below, circle description that applies (the word "assistance" means supervision, directions, or personal assistance).		
Bathing – either sponge bath, tub bath, or shower		
Receives no assistance (gets in and out of tub by self if tub is usual means of bathing)	Receives assistance in bathing only one part of body (such as back or a leg)	Receives assistance in bathing more than one part of body (or does not bathe self)
Toileting – going to the "toilet room" for bowel and urine elimination; cleaning self after elimination and arranging clothes		
Goes to "toilet room," cleans self, and arranges clothes without assistance (may use object for support such as cane, walker, or wheelchair and may manage night bedpan or commode, emptying same in morning)	Receives assistance in going to "toilet room" or in cleansing self or in arranging clothes after elimination or in use of night bedpan or commode	Does not go to room termed "toilet" for the elimination process
Transfer		
Moves in and out of bed and in and out of chair without assistance (may use object for support such as cane or walker)	Moves in or out of bed with assistance	Does not get out of bed
Continence		
Controls urination and bowel movement completely by self	Has occasional "accidents"	Supervision helps keep urine or bowel control; catheter is used or is incontinent
Feeding		
Feeds self without assistance	Feeds self except for getting assistance in cutting meat or buttering bread	Receives assistance in feeding or is fed partly or completely by tubes or intravenous fluids

Figure 3-3 Katz Index of ADLs. (From Katz, S., Ford, A. B., Moskowitz, R. W., Jackson, B. A., & Jaffe, M. W. [1963]. Studies of illness in the aged. The index of ADL: A standardized measure of biological and psychosocial functioning. *Journal of the American Medical Association, 185,* 94-98.)

was originally developed to study treatment outcomes and the prognosis of older adults and the chronically ill. The six different functions measured are bathing, dressing, toileting, transfer ability, continence, and feeding ability. Each function is rated according to the level of assistance required to complete the task, with the choices being independent, assistance required, or completely dependent. A health professional or caregiver familiar with the individual's functional ability rates the items, and the scale takes less than 5 minutes to complete.

The six functions are conceived as being hierarchically ordered, with loss of function beginning with more complex activities, and ending with the most basic activities being retained. A combined measure of all six functions can be used to monitor change over time. A recent study of over 1000 older adult patients (age 70 or older) found that self-reported results from the Katz Index of ADLs (all areas except continence were assessed) are strongly related to patient hospital costs (Chuang et al., 2003). Patients who were dependent in ADLs had significantly higher hospital costs than patients who were independent in ADLs, even after adjusting for the Diagnosis-Related Group and length of stay of the patient.

BARTHEL INDEX. The Barthel Index (Figure 3-4) (Fortinsky, Granger, & Seltzer, 1981) is similar to the Katz Index and evaluates self-care abilities. It also includes items related to mobility functions (such as walking 50 yards, using stairs) and was originally developed for assessment of persons with neuromuscular or musculoskeletal disorders in an inpatient rehabilitation

setting (Mahoney & Barthel, 1965). The tool is scored by the health professional on performance of 10 activities as either being independent or needing assistance. The modified Barthel Index contains 15 specific items, with the scores graded for four different degrees of independence, and items are individually weighted. The maximum score of 100 indicates independence (lowest score is 0) in all items but may not reflect the individual's ability to live alone because of a lack of assessment of more complex functions such as housekeeping and preparing meals (Mahoney & Barthel, 1965). The modified Barthel Index is primarily used as a clinical tool and is a useful complement to clinical judgment when predicting rehabilitation potential and outcomes, disposition, and care requirements for older adult inpatients.

LAWTON INSTRUMENTAL ACTIVITIES OF DAILY LIVING SCALE. The Lawton Instrumental Activities of Daily Living (IADLs) Scale (Lawton & Brody, 1969) constitutes a range of activities more complex than those needed for personal self-care and aims to assess a person's ability to function in his or her environment (Figure 3-5). Eight areas are evaluated: the individual's ability to cook; shop; use the telephone; and manage medications, finances, transportation needs, laundry, and housework. The Lawton IADLs Scale tends to emphasize tasks commonly performed by women and may put men at a disadvantage because of social roles. For example, men may have been excluded during married life from food preparation or doing laundry, tasks considered essential daily functions. Items that tap

Barthel Index with Corresponding Values for Independent Performance of Tasks

INDEX	"CAN DO BY MYSELF"	"CAN DO WITH HELP OF SOMEONE ELSE"	"CANNOT DO AT ALL"
SELF-CARE INDEX			
1. Drinking from a cup	4	0	0
2. Eating	6	0	0
3. Dressing upper body	5	3	0
4. Dressing lower body	7	4	0
5. Putting on brace or artificial limb	0	−2	0 (not applicable)
6. Grooming	5	0	0
7. Washing or bathing	6	0	0
8. Controlling urination	10	5 (accidents)	0 (incontinent)
9. Controlling bowel movements	10	5 (accidents)	0 (incontinent)
MOBILITY INDEX			
10. Getting in and out of chair	15	7	0
11. Getting on and off toilet	6	3	0
12. Getting in and out of tub or shower	1	0	0
13. Walking 50 yards on the level	15	10	0
14. Walking up/down one flight of stairs	10	5	0 (not applicable)
15. IF NOT WALKING: Propelling or pushing wheelchair	5	0	0

Figure 3-4 Barthel Index. (From Granger, C. V., Albrecht, G. L., & Hamilton, B. B. [1979]. Outcome of comprehensive medical rehab: Measures of PULSES profile and the Barthel Index. *Archives of Physical Medicine and Rehabilitation, 60,* 145-154.)

Male Score		Female Score
	A. Ability to use telephone	
1	1. Operates telephone on own initiative; looks up and dials numbers, etc.	1
1	2. Dials a few well-known numbers	1
1	3. Answers telephone but does not dial	1
0	4. Does not use telephone at all	0
	B. Shopping	
1	1. Takes care of all shopping needs independently	1
0	2. Shops independently for small purchases	0
0	3. Needs to be accompanied on any shopping trip	0
0	4. Completely unable to shop	0
	C. Food preparation	
	1. Plans, prepares, and serves adequate meals independently	1
	2. Prepares adequate meals if supplied with ingredients	0
	3. Heats and serves prepared meals, or prepares meals but does not maintain adequate diet	0
	4. Need to have meals prepared and served	0
	D. Housekeeping	
	1. Maintains house alone or with occasional assistance (e.g., heavy-work domestic help)	1
	2. Performs light daily tasks such as dish washing and bed making	1
	3. Performs light daily tasks but cannot maintain acceptable level of cleanliness	1
	4. Needs help with all home maintenance tasks	1
	5. Does not participate in any housekeeping tasks	0
	E. Laundry	
	1. Does personal laundry completely	1
	2. Launders small items; rinses socks, stockings, etc.	1
	3. All laundry must be done by others	0
	F. Mode of transportation	
1	1. Travels independently on public transportation or drives own car	1
1	2. Arranges own travel via taxi, but does not otherwise use public transportation	1
0	3. Travels on public transportation when assisted or accompanied by another	1
0	4. Travel limited to taxi or automobile, with assistance of another	0
0	5. Does not travel at all	0
	G. Responsibility for own medication	
1	1. Is responsible for taking medication in correct dosages at correct time	1
0	2. Takes responsibility if medication is prepared in advance in separate dosages	0
0	3. Is not capable of dispensing own medication	0
	H. Ability to handle finances	
1	1. Manages financial matters independently (budgets, writes checks, pays rent and bills, goes to bank); collects and keeps track of income	1
1	2. Manages day-to-day purchases, but needs help with bank for major purchases, etc.	1
0	3. Incapable of handling money	0

Figure 3-5 Lawton IADLs Scale. (From Lawton, M. P., & Brody, E. M. [1969]. Assessment of older people: Self-maintaining and instrumental activities of daily living. *Gerontologist, 9,* 179. Copyright Gerontological Society of America. Reproduced by permission of the publisher.)

social role performance in older men (such as "fixing things around the house" or gardening) have not been included in the Lawton IADLs Scale.

The Lawton IADLs Scale is scored by a health professional according to self-reported level of independence during an interview or following completion of a self-administered questionnaire (Lawton, 1988). Validation from knowledgeable informants should be obtained when possible. Fillenbaum (1985) introduced a shorter five-item IADLs scale that is valid and reliable. Measuring IADLs in community-dwelling older adults is particularly important because impairments in ability to perform IADLs often precede other functional impairments and may indicate worsening of chronic illness and lead to a loss of independence. Identifying needs allows for the appropriate matching of services and family support to enable the individual to live independently for as long as possible.

OLDER AMERICANS RESOURCES AND SERVICES. The need to study functional assessment led to the development of a comprehensive measure of ADLs and IADLs. The Older Americans Resources and Services (OARS) questionnaire is divided into two sections: the Multidimensional Functional Assessment Questionnaire (MFAQ) and the Services Assessment Questionnaire (SAQ) (George & Fillenbaum, 1985). The addition of the second component establishes links between health care service use and functional status, making it a valuable research tool. The MFAQ is designed to assess the community-dwelling older adult's functional ability using five subscales (social resources, economic resources, mental health, physical health, and ADLs), and the SAQ assesses need and utilization of 24 generic health services.

The ADLs section of the MFAQ can be used by itself as a self-reported or interviewer-administered questionnaire and provides information about perceived ability to perform both basic ADLs and IADLs. One important limitation of the tool is its length, and the 105 questions in the full questionnaire take about 1 hour to complete (van Hook & Berkman, 1996). Most questions are answered by the patient, but a few questions are supposed to be completed by a knowledgeable informant, and a few should be answered by the interviewer. However, when specific sections of the tool (such as the 26-item ADL and IADL scales) are used independently, the time factor is significantly diminished. The interviewer scores each of the five areas (domains) on a 6-point scale along a continuum from excellent functioning to total impairment. This comprehensive tool was an important contribution to the study of function in older adults, but it is not widely used today, except for the social resources subscale, which is discussed later in this chapter under social assessment.

ADVANCED ACTIVITIES OF DAILY LIVING. Reuben and Solomon (1989) introduced the idea of advanced activities of daily living (AADLs), more complex tasks than IADLs that are not functionally essential, yet contribute to strong mental health, productive activity, and an enhanced quality of life. Healthy, active older adults living in the community score very well on the usual scales measuring ADLs and IADLs, because they are independent. Yet with advancing age and chronic disease, they may cut back on more advanced activities. Measuring high-level activities may be valuable in

assessing early levels of functional decline that are not identified with the usual scales.

AADLs are not routinely measured in many settings, but the gerontological nurse should be familiar with this term and its meaning. AADLs are described as voluntary physical, occupational, recreational, and social activities, which are highly individualized. Because of this, development of a general scale similar to those measuring ADLs or IADLs is difficult. Many instruments explore specific domains of AADLs, such as physical activity and exercise (e.g., the Physical Activity Scale for the Elderly; Washburn, Smith, Jette, & Janney, 1993). However, a few scales have been developed for research studies that attempt to examine more general AADLs, and two are reviewed here.

Functional Performance Inventory. Leidy (1999) developed the Functional Performance Inventory (FPI) for use in studies of people with pulmonary disease to evaluate the impact of disease on higher-level activity. The goal was to incorporate the social, spiritual, and recreational domains identified by individuals with pulmonary disease as common activities, in addition to the ADLs and IADLs. The FPI is self-administered in 15 minutes and has 65 items and 6 subscales: body care, household maintenance, physical exercise, recreation, spiritual activities, and social activities. Items are rated from 1 to 4 based on how easily they can be performed. The tool has good internal consistency, with a Cronbach's alpha of .96 and demonstrated significant correlation with related functional measures indicating good construct validity. Although the FPI has not been widely tested with other groups, it provides a tested tool of advanced activities in people with pulmonary disease.

Activity Checklist. The Activity Checklist has been used in a study of community-dwelling older adults (Everard, Lach, Fisher, & Baum, 2000) and was developed from the Activity Card Sort, a tool used by occupational therapists to evaluate activity engagement (Baum, 1993, 1995). Individuals describe their activity participation in a wide list of 55 options, and note if they do the activity, do it less than previously, do it more than previously, or if they never did the activity. The checklist takes 15 to 20 minutes to complete. Four categories of activities are included that make up the four subscales: instrumental activities such as housework, social activities such as attending parties, low-demand leisure activities such as reading or watching television, and high-demand leisure activities such as swimming or hiking. An individual's score is calculated based on what the individual does now, compared with what he or she has done in the past. As a result the score is individualized, and a person is not penalized for not participating in activities he or she never did. The checklist showed concurrent validity with the Activity Card Sort, with internal consistency of .72 to .90 for the subscales, and test-retest reliability ranged from .83 to .95.

The checklist was used in a cross-sectional study of community-dwelling older adults participating in an older adult organization (Everard et al., 2000). The results showed that maintenance of instrumental, social, and high-demand leisure activities was associated with better self-reported physical health, and maintenance of low-demand leisure activities was associated with worse physical health. The instrument may be useful in determining participation or changes in a wide range of activities over time.

PHYSICAL PERFORMANCE TEST. The Physical Performance Test (PPT) is a good example of a measure that tests actual physical performance. The PPT combines validated items from several scales that evaluate multiple dimensions of physical function at various levels of difficulty (Reuben & Siu, 1990). The test has nine items requiring direct observation and timed measurement of performance of various ADLs and IADLs, and takes about 10 to 15 minutes (highly impaired individuals may take longer). The variables assessed include fine motor function, upper coarse motor function, balance, mobility, coordination, and endurance. Specific observed ADLs include eating, transferring, dressing, and locomotion.

PPT items range from minimal difficulty, such as eating or writing a sentence, to moderate difficulty, such as lifting a book, to very difficult, such as climbing stairs. Items are scored on a 5-point scale based on the time it takes the individual to complete the task (climbing stairs also includes ability to climb up and down up to four flights of stairs). The scale has a maximum score of 36 points; a seven-item version omits the stair-climbing task and has a maximum score of 28 points. Reliability and validity tests were satisfactory, and there is high agreement between self-reported ability and the patient's actual ability as observed by the tester (Reuben & Siu, 1990).

The PPT is a brief and easily administered and scored test for screening for functional impairments. It holds practical appeal because it addresses a wide range of function, but is not cumbersome, as are some more detailed comprehensive evaluations. A modified version has been developed to measure function in nursing home residents with items that are more appropriate for a frail population (Binder, Miller, & Ball, 2001). The nursing home version takes 5 to 10 minutes to complete.

Tinetti Balance and Gait Evaluation. The Tinetti test is an example of a more specific performance and mobility evaluation (Tinetti, 1986; Tinetti, Williams, & Mayewski, 1986). The tool is completed in about 5 minutes while observing the individual perform a series of maneuvers such as sitting in a chair, getting up, standing, walking, and turning (Tables 3-1 and 3-2). The clinician rates each component of balance and gait from 0 to 2, with more points assigned for better performance.

Widely used as a clinical tool, it was recently used in a small study evaluating a walking program in an assisted living facility (Taylor et al., 2003). Individuals in the walking program improved their scores on the Tinetti measure after 9 weeks of participating in a walking club.

Get Up and Go Test. A simpler measure of gait and balance is the "get up and go" test (Mathias, Nayak, & Isaacs, 1986), which can be completed in a couple of minutes. The individual begins seated in a chair, gets up and walks 3 meters, turns around, returns to the chair, and sits down. The original scoring used a 5-point rating scale, with 1 being a normal score and 5 abnormal. A variety of versions of the test have been used. Later versions are timed rather than scored to provide a more accurate and continuous score and may use different distances (Podsiadlo & Richardson, 1991; Rikli & Jones, 1999). The get up and go test has been used to identify individuals at risk of falling (Huang, Gau, Lin, & George, 2003) and to measure changes in exercise trials in a long-term care facility (Baum, Jarjoura, Polen, Faur, & Rutecki, 2003).

Psychological Function: Cognitive and Affective Assessment. Psychological impairment, most notably depression and dementia, is strongly correlated with decreased quality of life and functional deficits. Impairments of this nature may go unnoticed by those who see the person infrequently, and the patient may be able to perform well in a social situation. Older adults may not report symptoms even if they are aware of them and may consider them a normal part of the aging process. Concerns about stigma of mental health problems may also inhibit the older adult from admitting that a psychological problem exists.

It is recommended that cognitive and affective functions be measured independently of one another, because impairments in both areas may coexist in the same individual and may be difficult to differentiate. The social environment may adversely affect the emotional state, leading to symptoms such as sadness, loneliness, anxiety, and "paranoia," which may result in poor performance on tests of cognitive function although no organic dementing process may exist. Therefore screening for cognitive and affective function should be a part of any geriatric assessment, keeping in mind that screening alone is insufficient to confirm a diagnosis.

Instruments for assessment of cognitive functioning are discussed first. This is because during a functional assessment, determining the reliability of the individual early on is important, in order to evaluate whether the individual's responses can be accepted and if a knowledgeable informant will be needed. Many tools have been developed to assess cognition. There is variation in the cognitive functions evaluated and the questions included in different mental status examinations, and

Table 3-1 _Assessment of Gait in the Elderly*_

Components[†]	Observation		Scoring
	Normal	**Abnormal**	
Initiation of gait (patient asked to begin walking down hallway)	Begins walking immediately without observable hesitation; initiation of gait is single, smooth motion	Hesitates; multiple attempts; initiation of gait not a smooth motion	0 = Any hesitancy or multiple attempts to start 1 = No hesitancy
Step height (begin observing after first few steps: observe one foot, then the other; observe from side)	Swing foot completely clears floor but by no more than 1-2 in	Swing foot is not completely raised off floor (may hear scraping) or is raised too high (>1-2 in)[‡]	0 = Right foot does not clear floor completely with step 1 = Right foot completely clears floor 0 = Left foot does not clear floor completely with step 1 = Left foot completely clears floor
Step length (observe distance between toe of stance foot and heel of swing foot; observe from side; do not judge first few or last few steps; observe one side at a time)	At least the length of individual's foot between the stance toe and swing heel (step length usually longer but foot length provides basis for observation)	Step length less than described under normal[‡]	0 = Right swing foot does not pass left stance 1 = Right foot passes left stance foot 0 = Left swing foot does not pass right stance 1 = Left foot passes right stance foot
Step symmetry (observe the middle part of the patch, not the first or last steps; observe from side, observe distance between heel of each swing foot and toe of each stance foot)	Step length same or nearly same on both sides for most step cycles	Step length varies between sides or patient advances with same foot with every step	0 = Right and left step length not equal (estimate) 1 = Right and left step appear equal
Step continuity	Begins raising heel of one foot (toe off) as heel of other foot touches the floor (heel strike); no breaks or stops in stride; step lengths equal over most cycles	Places entire foot (heel and toe) on floor before beginning to raise other foot; or stops completely between steps; or step length varies over cycles[‡]	0 = Stopping or discontinuity between steps 1 = Steps appear continuous

these may include the following: attention, memory, orientation, calculation, language, visual-spatial ability, concentration, and abstraction and judgment. Samples of common screening instruments for cognitive impairment are described next. However, the nurse should be aware that additional tools may be available, and some are more sensitive and diagnostic.

COGNITION

**Mini-Mental State Examination.** The Mini-Mental State Examination (MMSE) (Figure 3-6) is the most widely used brief screening instrument to detect cognitive impairment. It is interviewer administered and tests orientation, registration, attention and calculation,

recall, language, and ability to follow a three-part command (Folstein, Folstein, & McHugh, 1975). The test contains reading and writing portions that may be difficult for those with visual impairment or physical limitations such as arthritis or hemiplegia (Tombaugh & McIntyre, 1992).

The MMSE takes approximately 7 minutes to complete (Borson, Scanlan, Brush, Vitaliano, & Dokmak, 2000) and contains 17 items resulting in a maximum score of 30. A score of 23 or less may be found in individuals with dementia, schizophrenia, delirium, or an affective disorder. The severity of cognitive impairment can be classified into three levels, with scores between 24 and 30 indicating no cognitive impairment, scores between 18 and 23 indicating mild cognitive impairment, and

Table 3-1 *Assessment of Gait in the Elderly*—cont'd

Components[†]	Observation		Scoring
	Normal	**Abnormal**	
Path deviation (observe from behind; observe one foot over several strides; observe in relation to line on floor [e.g., tiles] if possible; difficult to assess if patient uses a walker)	Foot follows close to straight line as patient advances	Foot deviations from side to side or toward one direction[§]	0 = Marked deviation 1 = Mild or moderate deviation or uses walking aid 2 = Straight without walking aid
Trunk stability (observe from behind; side-to-side motion of trunk may be a normal gait pattern, need to differentiate this from instability)	Trunk does not sway; knees or back is not flexed; arms are not abducted in effort to maintain stability	Any of the preceding features present[§]	0 = Marked sway or used walking aid 1 = No sway, but flexion of the knees or back, or spreads arms out while walking 2 = No sway, no flexion, no use of arms, and no use of walking aid
Walk stance (observe from behind)	Feet should almost touch as one passes other	Feet apart with stepping[∥]	0 = Heels apart 1 = Heels almost touching while walking
Turning while walking	No staggering; turning continuous with walking; and steps are continuous while turning	Staggers; stops before initiating turn; or steps are discontinuous	

From Tinetti, M. (1986). Performance-oriented assessment of mobility problems in elderly patients. *Journal of the American Geriatrics Society, 34,* 119-126; and Tinetti, M. E., Williams, T. F., & Mayewski, R. (1986). Fall risk index for elderly patients based on number of chronic disabilities. *American Journal of Medicine, 80,* 429-434.

SCORING: Less than 9 on gait assessment = High fall risk.

*The patient stands with the examiner at end of obstacle-free hallway, using usual walking aid. Examiner asks patient to walk down hallway at his or her usual pace. Examiner observes one component of gait at a time. For some components the examiner walks behind the patient; for other components, the examiner walks next to patient. May require several trips to complete.

[†]Also ask patient to talk at a "more rapid than usual" pace and observe whether any walking aid is used correctly.

[‡]Abnormal gait finding may reflect a primary neurological or musculoskeletal problem directly related to the finding or reflect a compensatory maneuver for other, more remote problem.

[§]Abnormality may be corrected by walking aid such as cane; observe with and without walking aid if possible.

[∥]Abnormal finding is usually a compensatory maneuver rather than a primary problem.

scores between 0 and 17 indicating severe cognitive impairment. One study has suggested increasing the cognitively intact cutoff score to 26 or 27 in those with symptoms of cognitive impairment to increase the sensitivity of the MMSE (Kukull et al., 1994). The MMSE has been extensively studied and has been determined to have satisfactory reliability and validity (Tombaugh & McIntyre, 1992). Versions of the MMSE for telephone use have been validated (Newkirk et al., 2004; Roccaforte, Burke, Bayer, & Wengel, 1992).

MMSE scores may be significantly affected by social and demographic variables such as age, education, reading level, and ethnicity, which potentially contribute to false-positive results (Baker et al., 2002; Crum, Anthony, Bassett, & Folstein, 1993; Mayeaux et al., 1995; Tombaugh & McIntyre, 1992). As a result, the administrator should consider these factors in interpreting the results in those with low levels of education and literacy, or with advanced age. Overall, the MMSE is a highly useful clinical and research tool to assess several domains of cognition.

Short Blessed Orientation-Memory-Concentration Test. The Blessed information-memory-concentration test was a measure developed in England that resulted from attempting to determine the relationship between the neurophysiology of the brain and cognitive impairment as individuals age (Blessed, Tomlinson, & Roth, 1968). A positive correlation was found with participant scores on the Blessed information-memory-concentration test and the number of senile plaques found later in the postmortem cortex of the participant's brain. The original test had 29 items that were

Table 3-2 *Assessment of Balance in the Elderly*

Maneuver	Response			Scoring
	Normal	**Adaptive**	**Abnormal**	
Sitting balance	Steady, stable	Holds onto chair to keep upright	Leans, slides down in chair	0 = Leans or slides in chair 1 = Steady and safe
Arising from chair	Able to arise in a single movement without using arms	Uses arms (on chair or walking aid) to pull or push up; and/or moves forward in chair before attempting to arise	Multiple attempts required or unable without human assistance	0 = Unable without help 1 = Able, using arms to help 2 = Able without using arms
Immediate standing balance (first 3-5 sec)	Steady without holding onto walking aid or other object for support	Steady, but uses walking aid or other object for support	Any sign of unsteadiness[†]	0 = Unable without help 1 = Able with more than one attempt 2 = Able to rise in one attempt
Standing balance	Steady, able to stand with feet together without holding object for support	Steady, but cannot put feet together	Any sign of unsteadiness regardless of stance or holds onto object	0 = Unsteady (swaggers, moves feet, trunk sway) 1 = Steady, but uses walker or other support 2 = Steady without walker or other support
Balance with eyes closed (with feet as close together as possible)	Steady without holding onto any object with feet together	Steady with feet apart	Any sign of unsteadiness or needs to hold onto an object	0 = Unsteady 1 = Steady
Turning balance (360 degrees)	No grabbing or staggering; no need to hold onto any objects; steps are continuous (turn is a flowing movement)	Steps are discontinuous (patient puts one foot completely on floor before raising other foot)	Any sign of unsteadiness or holds onto an object	0 = Discontinuous steps 1 = Continuous steps 0 = Unsteady (grabs, swaggers) 1 = Steady
Nudge on sternum (patient standing with feet as close together as possible, examiner pushes with light even pressure over sternum three times; reflects ability to withstand displacement)	Steady, able to withstand pressure	Needs to move feet, but able to maintain balance	Begins to fall, or examiner has to help maintain balance	0 = Begins to fall 1 = Staggers, grabs, and catches self 2 = Steady

Table 3-2 *Assessment of Balance in the Elderly*—cont'd

Maneuver	Normal	Adaptive	Abnormal	Scoring
		Response		
Neck turning (patient asked to turn head side to side and look up while standing with feet as close together as possible)	Able to turn head at least halfway side to side and able to bend head back to look at ceiling; no staggering, grabbing, or symptoms of light-headedness, unsteadiness, or pain	Decreased ability to turn side to side to extend neck, but no staggering, grabbing, or symptoms of light-headedness, unsteadiness, or pain	Any sign of unsteadiness or symptoms when turning head or extending neck	Not scored
One-leg standing balance	Able to stand on one leg for 5 sec without holding object for support	Not applicable	Unable	Not scored
Back extension (ask patient to lean back as far as possible, without holding onto object if possible)	Good extension without holding object or staggering	Tries to extend, but decreased range of motion (compared with other patients of same age) or needs to hold object to attempt extension	Will not attempt or no extension seen or staggers	Not scored
Reaching up (have patient attempt to remove an object from a shelf high enough to require stretching or standing on toes)	Able to take down object without needing to hold onto other object for support and without becoming unsteady	Able to get object but needs to steady self by holding onto something for support	Unable or unsteady	Not scored
Bending down (patient is asked to pick up small object, such as pen, from the floor)	Able to bend down and pick up object and is able to get up easily in single attempt without needing to pull self up with arms	Able to get object and get upright in single attempt but needs to pull self up with arms or hold onto something for support	Unable to bend down or unable to get upright after bending down or takes multiple attempts to upright self	Not scored
Sitting down	Able to sit down in one smooth movement	Needs to use arms to guide self into chair or not a smooth movement	Falls into chair, misjudges distances (lands off center)	0 = Unsafe (misjudged distance, falls into chair) 1 = Uses arms or not a smooth motion 2 = Safe, smooth motion

From Tinetti, M. (1986). Performance-oriented assessment of mobility problems in elderly patients. *Journal of the American Geriatrics Society, 34*, 119-126; and Tinetti, M. E., Williams, T. F., & Mayewski, R. (1986). Fall risk index for elderly patients based on number of chronic disabilities. *American Journal of Medicine, 80*, 429-434.
SCORING: Less than 10 on balance assessment = High fall risk.
*The patient begins this assessment seated in a hard, straight-backed, armless chair.
†*Unsteadiness* is defined as grabbing at objects for support, staggering, moving feet, or more than minimal trunk sway.

Mini-Mental State Examination Sample Items

Orientation to Time
"What is the date?"

Registration
"Listen carefully. I am going to say three words. You say them back after I stop. Ready? Here they are. . .
HOUSE [pause], CAR [pause], LAKE [pause]. Now repeat those words back to me."
[Repeat up to five times, but score only the first trial.]

Naming
"What is this?" [Point to a pencil or pen.]

Reading
"Please read this and do what it says." [Show examinee the words on the stimulus form.]
CLOSE YOUR EYES

Figure 3-6 Sample items from the Mini-Mental State Examination. (Reproduced by special permission of the publisher, Psychological Assessment Resources, Inc., 16204 North Florida Avenue, Lutz, FL 33549, from *The Mini-Mental State Examination* by Marshall Folstein and Susan Folstein, copyright 1975, 1998, 2001 by Mini Mental LLC, Inc. Published 2001 by Psychological Assessment Resources, Inc. Further reproduction is prohibited without permission of PAR, Inc. The MMSE can be purchased from PAR, Inc. by calling [813] 968-3003.)

individually scored, with higher scores indicative of worsening cognitive functioning.

A U.S. study by Katzman and colleagues (1983) was able to validate a much shorter version called the short Blessed orientation-memory-concentration test, or short Blessed test (SBT), that is often used today. The SBT is interviewer administered in about 5 minutes, and has only six items with scores ranging from a perfect score of 0 to the worst possible score of 28 (Lorentz, Scanlan, & Borson, 2002). The test differentiates between those with normal cognitive functioning or minimal impairment (score of 8 or less), moderate impairment (score of 9 to 19), and severe impairment (score of 20 or more). Correct scoring of the SBT requires some instruction, with errors multiplied by a weighted score to determine the final score.

The SBT is highly correlated with the MMSE, and both tools have established reliability in dementia screening (Fillenbaum, Heyman, Wilkinson, & Haynes, 1987; Stuss, Meiran, Guzman, Lafleche, & Willmer, 1996). One item on the SBT, the time to recite the months of the year in reverse order, has also been found to be a reliable and valid measure of central processing speed in older women (Ball, Bisher, & Birge, 1999). Distinct advantages of the SBT over the MMSE include brevity (fewer items), objectiveness (scoring the interlocking pentagons on the MMSE is subjective), and generalizability (questions applicable in all settings, persons unable to read or write can participate) (Fillenbaum et al., 1987). However, the SBT may be affected by demographic variables, including gender and educational level (Stuss et al., 1996). The SBT is frequently administered clinically

and in research settings to assess older adults' cognitive abilities.

Mini-Cog. The Mini-Cog was developed in an effort to meet the need for a very brief dementia screening tool that is practical for use in the primary care setting with diverse patient populations (Borson et al., 2000). The two-item test can be interviewer administered in an average of 3 minutes. The first part includes the clock-drawing test, which has been studied independently as a screening test for dementia (Royall, Cordes, & Polk, 1998; Watson, Arfken, & Birge, 1993). The clock-drawing test shows good correlation to the MMSE and other tests, as well as good sensitivity, specificity, and test-retest reliability (Shulman, 2000). The second component is a three-item recall test. A study with 249 culturally, linguistically, and educationally diverse older adults found that Mini-Cog results were not significantly influenced by the participant's education or primary language (Borson et al., 2000). When directly compared with the MMSE, the Mini-Cog yielded higher sensitivity and greater diagnostic value while maintaining adequate specificity in both a community and a random sample of older adults (Borson et al., 2000; Borson, Scanlan, Chen, & Ganguli, 2003).

In addition to its excellent clinical properties, the Mini-Cog can be used realistically as a first-line screening tool in primary care. It can be administered and scored by individuals with little or no training, does not require special equipment, is brief, and is acceptable to a heterogeneous older adult population (Borson et al., 2000; Scanlan & Borson, 2001). This tool shows great promise for widespread clinical use in dementia screening, and it provides evidence of the ability of short screening tests to be as effective as, if not more effective than, longer ones.

ASSESSMENT OF ACUTE CONFUSION OR DELIRIUM. Screening instruments used in mental status assessment were originally developed to aid in the diagnosis of dementia, but very few are able to distinguish delirium, sometimes called acute confusion. Delirium can be superimposed on an individual with preexisting dementia, making the diagnosis even more challenging. Older adults with acute medical conditions, especially those who are hospitalized, are at high risk for delirium, which has been shown to lead to poor outcomes (e.g., increased use of health care resources, morbidity, and death) (Cacchione, 2002). Screening instruments to differentiate delirium and dementia have been developed and tested to aid the clinician in evaluating the patient who develops a sudden change in mental status. These changes may be the first sign of a significant medical condition, so identifying delirium is helpful to trigger a medical evaluation. Two instruments are reviewed here: the NEECHAM Confusion Scale and the Confusion Assessment Method.

NEECHAM

Confusion Scale. The NEECHAM Confusion Scale (Champagne, Neelon, McConnell, & Funk, 1987) was developed as an observational tool for assessing delirium and takes 10 minutes to complete if the components are not already completed as part of a clinical assessment. The tool has nine items and is calculated by adding scores from three subscales that look at behavior, processing, and physiological control. The range of scores is from 0 (minimal responsiveness) to 30 (normal function). Scores of 0 to 19 indicate moderate to severe confusion, scores of 20 to 24 indicate mild or early development of confusion, and scores above 24 are classified as "not confused." Sensitivity is reported to be 95%, specificity 78%, and predictive value 57%. In another study, sensitivity and specificity were reported at 30% and 92%, and the predictive value was 81% (Siemsen, Miller, Newman, & Lucas, 1992), and good internal consistency has been reported in a sample from acute care (Neelon, Champagne, Carlson, & Funk, 1996). The overall reliability of the NEECHAM Confusion Scale for determining level of delirium is good. The NEECHAM Confusion Scale is both feasible and clinically useful for assessing delirium.

Confusion Assessment Method. The Confusion Assessment Method (CAM) was designed to assist in the detection of delirium in hospitalized elderly (Inouye et al., 1990). The clinician identifies four features of delirium after patient assessment: acute onset and fluctuating course, inattention, disorganized thinking, and

altered level of consciousness (Box 3-3). The diagnosis of delirium requires the presence of either the first two or the last two features. The CAM has a sensitivity of 94% to 100% and a specificity of 90% to 95% when compared with geropsychiatric diagnosis and takes about 5 minutes to complete. The CAM has been used in clinical and research settings, and it has been translated into several languages. An alternate version has been developed for use in intensive care unit (ICU) patients (Ely et al., 2001), and a chart-based version has been developed for use in research or quality improvement programs (Inouye et al., 2005).

One study showed that hospital nurses had low reliability when using the CAM when a formal cognitive assessment was not performed (Inouye et al., 2001). The nurses were less likely to identify the features of delirium in patients who had hypoactive delirium, vision

---

BOX 3-3 Confusion Assessment Method (CAM)

Feature 1: Acute Onset and Fluctuating Course
This feature is usually obtained from a family member or nurse and is shown by positive responses to the following questions: Is there evidence of an acute change in mental status? Did the abnormal behavior fluctuate, or increase and decrease, in severity?

Feature 2: Inattention
This feature is shown by a positive response to the following question: Did the patient have difficulty focusing attention (e.g., being easily distractible, having difficulty keeping track of what was being said)?

Feature 3: Disorganized Thinking
This feature is shown by a positive response to the following question: Was the patient's thinking disorganized or incoherent, such as rambling or irrelevant conversation, unclear or illogical flow of ideas, or unpredictable switching from subject to subject?

Feature 4: Altered Level of Consciousness
This feature is shown by any answer other than alert to the following question: Overall, how would you rate this patient's level of consciousness? Answers: alert (normal), vigilant (hyperalert), lethargic (drowsy, easily aroused), stupor (difficult to arouse), or coma (not able to be aroused).

Diagnosis of delirium by the CAM requires the presence of features 1 and 2, and either 3 or 4.

From Inouye, S. K., van Dyck, C. H., Alessi, C. A., Balkin, S., Siegal, A. P., & Horwitz, R. I. (1990). Clarifying confusion: The confusion assessment method. A new method for detection of delirium. *Annals of Internal Medicine, 113*(12), 941-948.

impairment, or cognitive impairment, or who were over age 80. Use of the CAM would be improved with training of nurses on symptoms and assessment of cognitive impairment and delirium.

Affective (Mood) Assessment. A number of screening tools for depression have been validated in older persons. When older people have multiple chronic illnesses and functional impairments, the meaning of poor scores can be uncertain. Nonetheless, depression is common and screening tools can be helpful to detect major depression in older persons, thus opening opportunity for treatment. Three common tools in practice and the literature are reviewed here.

GERIATRIC DEPRESSION SCALE. The Geriatric Depression Scale (GDS) is a widely used self-rated scale that was developed specifically for use with older adults (Yesavage et al., 1983). The original GDS consists of 30 yes-or-no items that take approximately 5 minutes to complete (Box 3-4). The questions on the GDS were designed to focus on the psychological aspects of depression, in contrast to other tools that include somatic variables that are also associated with common chronic medical conditions. The original questionnaire has been studied extensively against other measures and in various settings, including community and inpatient populations (Koenig et al., 1993; Yesavage et al., 1983).

The GDS has been found to be feasible, accurate, and acceptable for use in clinical practice. At a cutoff score of 11, the 95% confidence intervals for sensitivity and specificity were high (84% to 93%). The tool is filled out by the individual, so it might be necessary in some cases to provide further explanations about instructions or to read items from the test.

BOX 3-4 Geriatric Depression Scale

Instructions to patient: Choose the best answer (YES or NO) to each question about how you felt the past week:

1. Are you basically satisfied with your life?*†	YES	NO
2. Have you dropped many of your activities and interests?*	YES	NO
3. Do you feel that your life is empty?*	YES	NO
4. Do you often get bored?*†	YES	NO
5. Are you hopeful about the future?	YES	NO
6. Are you bothered by thoughts you can't get out of your head?	YES	NO
7. Are you in good spirits most of the time?*	YES	NO
8. Are you afraid that something bad is going to happen to you?*	YES	NO
9. Do you feel happy most of the time?*	YES	NO
10. Do you often feel helpless?*†	YES	NO
11. Do you often get restless and fidgety?	YES	NO
12. Do you prefer to stay at home, rather than going out and doing new things?*†	YES	NO
13. Do you frequently worry about the future?	YES	NO
14. Do you feel you have more problems with memory than most?*	YES	NO
15. Do you think it is wonderful to be alive now?*	YES	NO
16. Do you often feel downhearted and blue?	YES	NO
17. Do you feel pretty worthless the way you are now?*†	YES	NO
18. Do you worry a lot about the past?	YES	NO
19. Do you find life very exciting?	YES	NO
20. Is it hard for you to get started on new projects?	YES	NO
21. Do you feel full of energy?*	YES	NO
22. Do you feel that your situation is hopeless?*	YES	NO
23. Do you think that most people are better off than you are?*	YES	NO
24. Do you frequently get upset over little things?	YES	NO
25. Do you frequently feel like crying?	YES	NO
26. Do you have trouble concentrating?	YES	NO
27. Do you enjoy getting up in the morning?	YES	NO
28. Do you prefer to avoid social gatherings?	YES	NO
29. Is it easy for you to make decisions?	YES	NO
30. Is your mind as clear as it used to be?	YES	NO

Scoring: Score 0 for each item that is "nondepressive" and 1 point for each "depressive" answer ("depressive" answers are NO for questions 1, 5, 7, 9, 15, 19, 21, 27, 29, and 30 and YES for all others). Normal score for the aged is 0 to 10.

From Yesavage, J. A., Brink, T. L., Rose, T. L., Lum, O., Huang, V., Adey, M., & Leirer, V. O. (1983). Development and validation of a geriatric depression screening scale. *Journal of Psychiatric Research, 17,* 37-49.

*Item on short form.

†Item on five-item form.

Shorter versions of the GDS have been developed and tested and show acceptable properties for screening. They provide the advantage of taking less time to complete and score, which can increase their use in the clinical setting. A 15-item version was developed that takes about 3 minutes to complete that also provides good accuracy (Sheikh & Yesavage, 1986). The 15-item GDS, with a cutoff score of 5, takes 3 to 5 minutes and showed 94% sensitivity and 83% specificity in 74 geriatric outpatients (Hoyl et al., 1999). A 5-item version that takes less than 1 minute to complete showed 97% sensitivity and 85% specificity with a cutoff score of 2 in the same population (Hoyl et al., 1999). In a large study, Weeks, McGann, Michaels, and Penninx (2003) compared the 15- and 5-item versions of the GDS in 816 inpatients. They found that the 5-item version had 97% sensitivity, but a high number of false positives. As a result, the authors recommend using the 5-item version, but for those who screen positive, the additional questions for the 15-item version should be asked to further screen out those who do not have depression.

The overlap among the symptoms of dementia and depression, as well as the concern that demented patients may be unable to answer the questions reliably, has been of concern to researchers and clinicians alike. Studies have yielded mixed results (Snow et al., 2005), with some showing poor predictive ability of the GDS when used in patients with dementia, and others showing acceptable properties. To overcome this problem, an alternative instrument was developed that includes both patient and collateral input, the Cornell Scale for Depression in Dementia (CSDD) (Alexopoulos, Robert, Robert, & Shamoian, 1988). In addition, a collateral version of the GDS was developed by Nitcher, Burke, Roccaforte, and Wingel (1993). The same GDS items are reworded to be answered by another person, for example, "Are *they* basically satisfied with their life?"

A recent study has indicated that those with dementia can provide accurate self-report of depression (Snow et al., 2005). Another study found acceptable levels of sensitivity and specificity for subjects with and without dementia in a sample that included normal controls and people with up to moderate levels of dementia (Lach, Chang, & Edwards, 2005). Scores on the three individual and collateral versions were compared with physician diagnosis of depression. Individuals were able to accurately report symptoms using the screening tools; however, a higher cutoff score is recommended for collateral sources, because they tend to report more symptoms.

BECK DEPRESSION INVENTORY. The Beck Depression Inventory (BDI) consists of 13 items related to mood, self-image, and somatic complaints that are scored on a 4-point scale according to the degree of severity for each item (Beck & Beck, 1972). The questionnaire is shortened from the original 21-item form (Beck, Ward, Medelson, Mock, & Erbaugh, 1961) and can be self-administered or administered by the clinician in about 5 minutes. A score of greater than 16 indicates severe depression, whereas a score of less than 4 represents minimal or no depression. The BDI has been shown to permit effective discrimination among groups of patients with varying degrees of depression with good reliability and validity (Gallagher, 1986). It also reflects changes in the intensity of depression over time (Beck & Beck, 1972). The BDI is somewhat more complex to complete than the GDS, but has been widely used.

CENTER FOR EPIDEMIOLOGICAL STUDIES DEPRESSION SCALE. The Center for Epidemiological Studies Depression Scale (CES-D) was developed as a tool for screening community-dwelling older adults for depression (Radloff, 1977). The 20 items ask about depressive symptoms and are rated by the individual on a 4-point scale (0 to 3), based on how the individual has felt over the past week. A score greater than 16 suggests depression and warrants further evaluation. The tool also includes four items evaluating positive affect so that a continuous score of affect can be obtained. The CES-D takes about 5 minutes to complete.

The CES-D was used extensively in a large population-based study of community-dwelling older adults, the Established Population for the Epidemiological Studies of the Elderly (EPESE) (Ossip-Klein, Rothenberg, & Andresen, 1997), and shorter versions have been developed. The CES-D has been widely used to identify depression in research with older adults (e.g., Berkman et al., 1986; Blazer, Burchett, Service, & George, 1991; Sinclair, Lyness, King, Cox, & Caine, 2001); however, the length and complexity of scoring make it less practical for the clinical setting.

Social Function. Measures of social functioning have historically taken into consideration two distinctly different dimensions: the social network and social support. Berkman (1983) described the *social network* as the web of social relationships that surrounds a person, including the number and frequency of contacts, the presence of a confidant, the durability of the network, geographical proximity, and reciprocity (mutual helping). *Social support* is defined as the emotional, instrumental, or financial aid that is obtained from the social network. All social networks do not provide the same degree of support and assistance, and the individual's objective perception may not relate to the quantity of help; therefore some measurement of perceived support is needed in social functioning instruments (Kane, 2003).

Social networks tend to be dynamic, especially so in the elderly, who confront many significant life changes. Therefore repeated assessment is necessary, particularly during stressful circumstances. Adequate social resources have long been considered to act as a "buffer" against adverse effects and facilitate independence and functional ability, whereas their absence may play a role in mental and physical decline. Maintaining social engagement seems to be an important determinant of health and successful aging (Rowe & Kahn, 1997). Two measures of social support are reviewed here, and clinical assessment of social support should be part of any good geriatric assessment.

OLDER AMERICANS RESOURCES AND SERVICES SOCIAL RESOURCES SCALE. The Social Resources Scale (Figure 3-7) is a well-known measure of social function (George & Fillenbaum, 1985). This scale is a subscale of the OARS Multidimensional Functional Assessment noted earlier in the chapter and takes 5 to 10 minutes to complete. It obtains information about family structure (marital status, living-in companions, frequency of family visits), contact with friends, availability of a confidant, satisfaction with the social interaction pattern, and availability of someone to help if the individual becomes sick or disabled.

In a study in which data from the OARS survey were used to control for variables, Blazer (1982) found that three parameters in the Social Resources Scale predicted mortality rate in an elderly community population 30 months after the initial assessment: perceived support, frequency of social contact, and available attachments. Ten potentially confounding variables that influence mortality risk, such as physical health status, cognitive functioning, cigarette smoking, stressful life events, and so forth, were controlled in the analysis. By accounting for variables within the physical and social context, possible causes of death were statistically controlled. Blazer notes that the influence of emotional status at the time of measurement may contribute to the perception of social support.

NORBECK SOCIAL SUPPORT QUESTIONNAIRE. The Norbeck Social Support Questionnaire identifies an individual's social support network and his or her perceptions about that support (Norbeck, Lindsey, & Carrieri, 1981, 1983). The questionnaire asks about specific people within the social network and the amount of tangible and emotional support they provide. It can be self-administered in 10 to 20 minutes or completed during an interview. A social network score is determined through adding the number of people listed in the individual's social network and the duration and frequency of contact. Changes in social network are also identified. The questionnaire has demonstrated good reliability and concurrent and predictive validity (Gigliotti, 2002).

CAREGIVER BURDEN. Another common social issue the nurse will encounter in practice has to do with caregivers and how they are coping with helping an older adult who may be a spouse, family member, or other. Although there are clearly positive aspects to caregiving, the purpose of using a measure of burden is to identify the caregiver's problems so that support and resources can be provided. One measure is reviewed here.

The Caregiver Burden Inventory (CBI) (Novak & Guest, 1989) purports to be a diagnostic tool to measure the many dimensions of caregiver burden. The CBI has 24 items and takes about 5 minutes to fill out. The instrument measures five factors: (1) *time dependence,* or burden related to restrictions on the caregiver's time; (2) *developmental burden,* or the caregiver's feelings of being unable to carry out her or his own developmental tasks; (3) *physical burden,* or the caregiver's feelings of fatigue or damage to physical health; (4) *social burden,* or feelings of role conflict; and (5) *emotional burden,* or negative feelings about caregiving. The instrument may be useful for identifying different patterns of burden, as well as social and psychological needs of caregivers, and has been used clinically and for research.

Other Assessment Tools

A wide variety of excellent screening and assessment tools are available to assist the gerontological nurse in screening for various problems and conditions. It is beyond the scope of this chapter to provide an exhaustive review of all of them, so we have focused on common measures for the key assessment domains. Table 3-3 provides a brief selection of additional assessment tools to address specific topics, as well as many previously described. Nurses will want to consider the important health problems for the patients in their practice in order to choose screening instruments that will help them provide quality care for that population.

SUMMARY

Standardized assessment tools should be used with a specific goal in mind and in accordance with their guidelines for use. Before using instruments, permission from the author may be necessary. Many instruments have detailed instructions available to assist practitioners in their use, and some have videotapes or training options. The strengths, weaknesses, and accuracy of the test being used should be considered, and its use should complement clinical practice (Kane, Ouslander, & Abrass, 2004). Results should be interpreted within the context of other information about the individual. Although much remains to be learned, careful use of instruments that are appropriate to the setting and population being served can result in improved clinical decision making, outcomes, and service delivery.

Now I'd like to ask you some questions about your family and friends.

Are you single, married, widowed, divorced, or separated?
1 Single   3 Widowed   5 Separated
2 Married   4 Divorced   – Not answered

If "2," ask following:

Does your spouse live here also?
          1 Yes
          2 No
          – Not answered

Who lives with you?
(Check "yes" or "no" for each of the following.)

Yes   No
_____   _____   No one
_____   _____   Husband or wife
_____   _____   Children
_____   _____   Grandchildren
_____   _____   Parents
_____   _____   Grandparents
_____   _____   Brothers and sisters
_____   _____   Other relatives (does not include in-laws covered in the above categories)
_____   _____   Friends
_____   _____   Nonrelated paid help (includes free room)
_____   _____   Others (specify) _____
                          _____

In the past year how often did you leave here to visit your family and/or friends for weekends or holidays or to go on shopping trips or outings?
          1 Once a week or more
          2 1-3 times a month
          3 Less than once a month or only on holidays
          4 Never
          – Not answered

How many people do you know well enough to visit with in their homes?
          3 Five or more
          2 Three to four
          1 One to two
          0 None
          – Not answered

About how many times did you talk to someone—friends, relatives or others—on the telephone in the past week (either you called them or they called you)? (If subject has no phone, question still applies.)
          3 Once a day or more
          2 Twice
          1 Once
          0 Not at all
          – Not answered

How many times during the past week did you spend some time with someone who does not live with you, that is, you went to see them, or they came to visit you, or you went out to do things together?

How many times in the past week did you visit with someone, either with people who live here or people who visited you here?
          3 Once a day or more
          2 Two to six
          1 Once
          0 Not at all
          – Not answered

Do you have someone you can trust and confide in?
          2 Yes
          0 No
          – Not answered

Figure 3-7   Social Resources Scale. (From Duke University Center for the Study of Aging and Human Development. [1978]. *Multidimensional functional assessment: The OARS methodology.* Durham, NC: Duke University Press.)   *Continued*

Do you find yourself feeling lonely quite often, sometimes, or almost never?
    0 Quite often
    1 Sometimes
    2 Almost never
    – Not answered

Do you see your relatives and friends as often as you want to, or are you somewhat unhappy about how little you see them?
    1 As often as wants to
    2 Somewhat unhappy about how little
    – Not answered

Is there someone *(outside this place)* who would give you any help at all if you were sick or disabled, for example, your husband/wife, a member of your family, or a friend?
    1 Yes
    0 No one willing and able to help
    – Not answered

        If "yes" ask a and b.

a. Is there someone (outside this place) who would take care of you as long as needed, or only for a short time, or only someone who would help you now and then (for example, taking you to the doctor, or fixing lunch occasionally, etc.)?

    1 Someone who would take care of subject indefinitely (as long as needed)
    2 Someone who would take care of subject for a short time (a few weeks to 6 months)
    3 Someone who would help subject now and then (taking to the doctor, or fixing lunch, etc.)
    – Not answered

b. Who is this person?
        Name _____
        Relationship _____

RATING SCALE
        Rate the current social resources of the person being evaluated along the 6-point scale presented below. Circle the *one* number that best describes the person's present circumstances.

1. Excellent Social Resources: Social relationships are very satisfying and extensive; at least one person would take care of him (her) indefinitely.

2. Good Social Resources: Social relationships are fairly satisfying and adequate and at least one person would take care of him (her) indefinitely, *or*
Social relationships are very satisfying and extensive, and only short-term help is available.

3. Mildly Socially Impaired: Social relationships are unsatisfactory (of poor quality and/or few) but at least one person would take care of him [her] indefinitely, *or*
Social relationships are fairly satisfactory and adequate, and only short-term help is available.

4. Moderately Socially Impaired: Social relationships are unsatisfactory (of poor quality and/or few) and only short-term care is available, *or*
Social relationships are at least adequate or satisfactory, but help would only be available now and then.

5. Severely Socially Impaired: Social relationships are unsatisfactory (of poor quality and/or few) and help would be available only now and then, *or*
Social relationships are at least satisfactory or adequate, but help is not available even now and then.

6. Totally Socially Impaired: Social relationships are unsatisfactory (of poor quality and/or few) and help is not available even now and then.

Note: Italicized questions apply to those living in institutions.

Figure 3-7, cont'd.

Table 3-3 *Assessment Instruments*

Content Area	Instrument	Comment
Advance directives	Values History (Doukas & McCullough, 1991)	Interview to identify values and beliefs about terminal care, as well as the individual's specific directives
Alcohol abuse	CAGE (Ewing, 1984)	Brief four-item screening for alcohol abuse
	Michigan Alcohol Screening Test—Geriatric (MAST-G) (Blow et al., 1992)	Screening tool for identifying alcohol abuse with 24 items
Caregiver burden	Caregiver Burden Inventory (Novak & Guest, 1989)	Evaluates caregiver burden in five areas: time dependence, developmental, physical, social, and emotional burden
	Zarit Burden Interview (Zarit, Orr, & Zarit, 1985)	A 29-item questionnaire to determine caregiver burden
Cognitive assessments	Clock Completion Test (Royall, Cordes, & Polk, 1998; Watson, Arfken, & Birge, 1993)	Single-item cognitive screening test
	Mini-Cog (Borson et al., 2000)	Two-item test to screen for cognitive impairment
	Mini-Mental State Examination (MMSE) (Folstein, Folstein, & McHugh, 1975)	Screen for cognitive impairment evaluating orientation, registration, attention, calculation, and recall
	Short Blessed test (Katzman et al., 1983)	Six-item screening test for cognitive impairment examining orientation, memory, and concentration
	Saint Louis University Mental Status Examination (SLUMS) (Division of Geriatric Medicine, 2005)	Cognitive screening test; identifies early cognitive impairment
Delirium assessment tools	Confusion Assessment Method (CAM) (Inouye et al., 1990)	Delirium screening tool identifies features of delirium
	NEECHAM Confusion Scale (Champagne et al., 1987)	Observational screening tool for delirium
Dementia-related tools	Alzheimer's Disease Assessment Scale (ADAS) (Rosen, Mohs, & Davis, 1984)	Assessment of clinical symptoms of Alzheimer's disease; widely used in clinical trials
	Clinical Dementia Rating Scale (CDR) (Morris, 1993)	For use by a trained clinician to determine severity of dementia. Used by National Institutes of Health (NIH)–funded Alzheimer's Disease Research Centers
	Global Deterioration Scale (Reisberg, Ferris, De Leon, & Crook, 1982)	A rating scale for severity of dementia based on amount of memory loss, used to determine prognosis
	Memory and Behavior Problems Checklist (Teri et al., 1992)	Identifies problem behavior frequency and impact
	Home Safety Inventory (Lach, Reed, Smith, & Carr, 1995)	Checklist to help identify dementia-related safety problems in home setting
	Hachinski Ischemic Score (Hachinski, Lliff, & Zilkha, 1975)	Scale to identify risk factors for vascular dementia to assist in diagnosis
Depression	Cornell Scale for Depression in Dementia (Alexopoulos et al., 1988)	Depression screening tool for use with a caregiver or proxy
	Geriatric Depression Scale (Yesavage et al., 1983)	Depression screening tool specific to older adults with 30-item, 15-item, and 5-item versions
	Beck Depression Inventory (Beck et al., 1961)	Depression screening tool
	Center for Epidemiological Studies Depression Scale (CES-D) (Radloff, 1977)	Screening tool for depression developed for community-dwelling older adults

Continued

Table 3-3 *Assessment Instruments—cont'd*

Content Area	Instrument	Comment
Fall risk	Morse Fall Scale (Morse, Morse, & Tylko, 1989)	Widely used fall risk assessment tool for the institutional setting
	Hendrich II Fall Risk Model (Hendrich, Bender, & Nyhuis, 2003)	Fall risk assessment for acute care
Fear of falling/falls efficacy	Falls Efficacy Scale (FES) (Tinetti, Richman, & Powell, 1990)	Measure of self-confidence at avoiding falling during usual daily activities
	Activities-specific Balance Confidence (ABC) scale (Powell & Myers, 1995)	Measure of falls efficacy with broader number of activity items
	Survey of Activities and Fear of Falling in the Elderly (SAFFE) (Lachman et al., 1998)	Measure of fear of falling and activity restriction
Functional assessment	Barthel Index (Fortinsky, Granger, & Seltzer, 1981)	Assessment of independence in activities of daily living
	Katz Index of ADLs (Katz et al., 1963)	Assessment of independence in activities of daily living
	Older Adult Resources and Services (OARS) ADLs and IADLs Scale (George & Fillenbaum, 1985)	Combined tool for assessment of independence in activities of daily living and instrumental activities of daily living
	Lawton Instrumental Activities of Daily Living Scale (Lawton & Brody, 1969)	Assessment of independence in instrumental activities of daily living
	Functional Fitness Test (Rikli & Jones, 1999)	Performance test of fitness in key areas that affect function, such as 6-minute walk, get up and go test, and chair stand for older adults with normative scores by age
General assessment	Fulmer SPICES (Fulmer, 1991)	A general assessment of common problems in the older adult: **S**leep disorders **P**roblems with eating or feeding **I**ncontinence **C**onfusion **E**vidence of falls **S**kin breakdown
Health care outcome measures	Charleson Comorbidity Index (Charlson, Pompei, Ales, & MacKenzie, 1987)	Developed to assess comorbidity and predict mortality risk
	Cumulative Illness Rating Scale (Linn, Linn, & Gurel, 1968)	Measures burden of illness; completed after history and physical examination
	Functional Independence Measure (FIM) (Laughlin, Granger, & Hamilton, 1992)	Functional status measure for the rehabilitation setting
	Minimum Data Set (MDS) (Morris et al., 1990)	Required resident assessment tool used in long-term care facilities
	Outcome and Assessment Information Set (OASIS) (Center for Health Policy Research, University of Colorado Health Sciences Center, 1994)	Required patient assessment measure for home health care
	Short-Form 36 (SF-36) (Ware, Kosinski, & Keller, 1996)	Outcome measure of health- and function-related quality of life, widely used in health care research
	Sickness Impact Profile (SIP) (Bergner et al., 1981)	General measure of health status
Hearing	Hearing Handicap Inventory for the Elderly (HHIE) (Lichtenstein, Bess, & Logan, 1988)	Questionnaire to identify impact of hearing loss on older adults

Table 3-3 *Assessment Instruments—cont'd*

Content Area	Instrument	Comment
Home safety assessment	*Check for Safety: A Home Fall Prevention Checklist for Older Adults* (Stephens & Olson, 2004)	Comprehensive brochure developed for the Centers for Disease Control and Prevention for public education
Medications	Medication Appropriateness Index (MAI) (Hanlon et al., 1992)	Tool to identify 10 problems in medication prescribing (e.g., indication, dosage accuracy, duplication with other drugs, etc.)
Nutritional status	Determine Your Nutritional Health Checklist (Gallaher-Allred, 1993)	Basic screening tool for frail elderly; can be completed by individual; more advanced screening tools also developed as part of the Nutrition Screening Initiative
	Mini-Nutritional Assessment (Guigoz, Vellas, & Garry, 1994)	A clinical assessment tool for evaluating nutritional status in older adults
Skin assessment	Braden Scale (Bergstrom, Braden, Laguzza, & Holman, 1988)	Widely used in hospital and long-term care settings to predict risk for skin breakdown
Social assessment	Norbeck Social Support Scale (Norbeck, Lindsey, & Carrieri, 1981)	Scale to assess individual's social network and perceptions of social support
	OARS Social Resources Scale (George & Fillenbaum, 1985)	Assessment of support network (amount of contact and help available)
Vision	Snellen chart	Test of far vision using standard wall chart at 20 feet developed in 1862

REFERENCES

Alexopoulos, G. S., Robert, C. A., Robert, C. Y., & Shamoain, C. A. (1988). Cornell Scale for Depression in Dementia. *Biological Psychiatry, 23,* 271-284.

Andresen, E. M. (1997). Measures of general health status. In E. Andresen, B. Rothenberg, & J. G. Zimmer (Eds.), *Assessing the health status of older adults.* New York: Springer.

Baker, D. W., Gazmararian, J. A., Sudano, J., Patterson, M., Parker, R. M., & Williams, M. V. (2002). Health literacy and performance on the Mini-Mental State Examination. *Aging and Mental Health, 6*(1), 22-29.

Ball, L. J., Bisher, G. B., & Birge, S. F. (1999). A simple test of central processing speed: An extension of the short Blessed test. *Journal of the American Geriatrics Society, 47*(1), 1359-1363.

Baum, C. M. (1993). *The effects of occupation on behaviors of persons with senile dementia of the Alzheimer's type and their carers.* Doctoral dissertation, George Warren Brown School of Social Work, Washington University, St. Louis.

Baum, C. M. (1995). The contribution of occupation to function in persons with Alzheimer's disease. *Journal of Occupation Science: Australia, 2*(2), 59-67.

Baum, E. E., Jarjoura, D., Polen, A. E., Faur, D., & Rutecki, G. (2003). Effectiveness of a group exercise program in a long-term care facility: A randomized pilot trial. *Journal of the American Medical Directors Association, 4*(2), 74-80.

Bayliss, E. A., Bayliss, M. S., Ware, J. E., & Steiner, J. F. (2004). Predicting declines in physical function in persons with multiple medical conditions: What can we learn from the medical problem list? *Health and Quality of Life Outcomes, 2*(1), 47-49.

Beck, A. T., & Beck, R. W. (1972). Screening depressed patients in family practice: A rapid technique. *Postgraduate Medicine, 52,* 81-85.

Beck, A. T., Ward, C. H., Medelson, M., Mock, J., & Erbaugh, J. (1961). An inventory for measuring depression. *Archives of General Psychiatry, 4,* 561-571.

Bergner, M., Bobbitt, R. A., Carter, W. B., & Gilson, B. S. (1981). The sickness impact profile: Development and final revision of a health status measure. *Medical Care, 19*(8), 787-805.

Bergner, M., Bobbitt, R. A., Pollard, W. E., Martin, D. P., & Gilson, B. S. (1976). The sickness impact profile: Validation of a health status measure. *Medical Care, 14*(1), 57-67.

Bergstrom, N., Braden, B. J., Laguzza, A., & Holman, V. (1988). The Braden scale for predicting pressure sore risk. *Nursing Research, 36,* 205-210.

Berkman, L. F. (1983). The assessment of social networks and social support in the elderly. *Journal of the American Geriatrics Society, 31*(12), 743-749.

Berkman, L. F., Berkman, C. S., Kasl, S., Freeman, D. H., Leo, L., Ostfeld, A. M., et al. (1986). Depressive symptoms in relation to physical health and functioning in the elderly. *American Journal of Epidemiology, 124,* 327-388.

Bickley, L. S., & Szilagyi, P. G. (2003). *Bates' guide to physical examination and history taking* (8th ed.). Philadelphia: Lippincott Williams & Wilkins.

Bieri, D., Reeve, R., & Champion, G. (1990). The Faces Pain Scale for the self-assessment of severity of pain experienced by children: Development, initial validation, and preliminary investigation for ratio scale properties. *Pain, 41,* 139-150.

Binder, E. F., Miller, J. P., & Ball, L. J. (2001). Development of a test of physical performance for the nursing home setting. *Gerontologist, 41*(5), 671-679.

Blazer, D., Burchett, B., Service, C., & George, L. K. (1991). The association of age and depression among the elderly: An epidemiological exploration. *Journal of Gerontology, 46,* M210-M215.

Blazer, D. G. (1982). Social support and mortality in an elderly community sample. *American Journal of Epidemiology, 115*(5), 684-693.

Blessed, G., Tomlinson, B. E., & Roth, M. (1968). The association between quantitative measures of dementia and of senile change in the cerebral gray matter of elderly subjects. *British Journal of Psychiatry, 114,* 797-811.

Blow, F. C., Brower, K. J., Schulenberg, J. E., Demo-Danaberg, L. M., Young, J. S., & Beresford, T. P. (1992). The Michigan Alcoholism Screening Test—Geriatric Version (MAST-G): A new elderly-specific screening instrument. *Alcohol Clinical and Experimental Research, 16,* 372.

Borson, S., Scanlan, J., Brush, M., Vitaliano, P., & Dokmak, A. (2000). The mini-cog: A cognitive "vital signs" measure for dementia screening in multi-lingual elderly. *International Journal of Geriatric Psychiatry, 15*(11), 1021-1027.

Borson, S., Scanlan, J. M., Chen, P., & Ganguli, M. (2003). The mini-cog as a screen for dementia: Validation in a population-based sample. *Journal of the American Geriatrics Society, 51*(10), 1451-1454.

Cacchione, P. Z. (2002). Four acute confusion assessment instruments: Reliability and validity for use in long-term care facilities. *Journal of Gerontological Nursing, 28*(1), 12-19.

Center for Health Policy Research, University of Colorado Health Sciences Center. (1994). *A study to develop outcome-based quality measures for home care.* Denver, CO: Author.

Champagne, M., Neelon, V., McConnell, E., & Funk, S. (1987). The NEECHAM Confusion Scale: Assessing acute confusion in the hospitalized and nursing home elderly. *Gerontologist, 27*(October special), 4A.

Charlson, M. E., Pompei, P., Ales, K. L., & MacKenzie, C. R. (1987). A new method of classifying prognostic comorbidity in longitudinal studies: Development and validation. *Journal of Chronic Diseases, 40,* 373-383.

Chuang, K. H., Covinsky, K. E., Sands, L. P., Fortinsky, R. H., Palmer, R. M., & Landefeld, C. S. (2003). Diagnosis-related group-adjusted hospital costs are higher in older medical patients with lower functional status. *Journal of the American Geriatrics Society, 51*(12), 1729-1734.

Cress, M. E., Schechtman, K. B., Mulrow, C. D., Fiatarone, M. A., Gerety, M. B., & Buchner, D. M. (1995). Relationship between physical performance and self-perceived physical function. *Journal of the American Geriatrics Society, 43*(2), 93-101.

Crum, R. M., Anthony, J. C., Bassett, S. S., & Folstein, M. F. (1993). Population-based norms for the Mini-Mental State Examination by age and educational level. *Journal of the American Medical Association, 269*(18), 2386-2391.

de Bruin, A. F., Buys, M., de Witte, L. P., & Diederiks, J. P. (1994). The sickness impact profile: SIP68, a short generic version. First evaluation of the reliability and reproducibility. *Journal of Clinical Epidemiology, 47*(8), 863-871.

Division of Geriatric Medicine. (2005). Saint Louis University Mental Status (SLUMS) examination. Retrieved June 10, 2005, from http://medschool.slu.edu/agingsuccessfully/pdfsurveys/slumsexam_05.pdf.

Doukas, D., & McCullough, L. (1991). The Values History: The evaluation of the patient's values and advance directives. *Journal of Family Practice, 31*(1), 145-153.

Ely, E. W., Margolin, R., Francis, J., May, L., Truman, B., Dittus, R., et al. (2001). Evaluation of delirium in critically ill patients: Validation of the Confusion Assessment Method for the Intensive Care Unit (CAM-ICU). *Critical Care Medicine, 29*(7), 1370-1379.

Everard, K. M., Lach, H. W., Fisher, E. B., & Baum, M. C. (2000). Relationship of activity and social support to the functional health of older adults. *Journals of Gerontology, Psychological Sciences and Social Sciences, 55*(4):S208-S212.

Ewing, J. (1984). Detecting alcoholism: The CAGE questionnaire. *Journal of the American Medical Association, 252,* 1905-1907.

Fillenbaum, G. G. (1985). Screening the elderly. A brief instrumental activities of daily living measure. *Journal of the American Geriatrics Society, 33*(10), 698-706.

Fillenbaum, G. G., Heyman, A., Wilkinson, W. E., & Haynes, C. S. (1987). Comparison of two screening tests in Alzheimer's disease. The correlation and reliability of the Mini-Mental State Examination and the modified Blessed test. *Archives of Neurology, 44*(9), 924-927.

Folstein, M. F., Folstein, S. E., & McHugh, P. R. (1975). "Mini-Mental State": A practical method for grading the cognitive state of patients for the clinician. *Journal of Psychiatric Research, 12,* 189-198.

Fortinsky, R. H., Granger, C. V., & Seltzer, G. B. (1981). The use of functional assessment in understanding home care needs. *Medical Care, 19*(5), 489-497.

Fulmer, T. (1991). The geriatric nurse specialist role: A new model. *Nursing Management, 22*(3), 91-93.

Gallagher, D. (1986). The Beck Depression Inventory and older adults: Review of its development and utility. *Clinics in Gerontology, 5,* 149-163.

Gallaher-Allred, C. R. (1993). *Implementing nutrition screening and intervention strategies.* Washington, DC: Nutrition Screening Initiative.

Gallo, J. J., Fulmer, T., Paveza, G. J., & Reichel, W. (2003). *Handbook of geriatric assessment* (3rd ed.). Boston: Jones & Bartlett.

George, L. K., & Fillenbaum, G. G. (1985). OARS methodology: A decade of experience in geriatric assessment. *Journal of the American Geriatrics Society, 33*(9), 607-615.

Gerety, M. B., Cornell, J. E., Mulrow, C. D., Tuley, M., Hazuda, H. P., Lichtenstein, M., et al. (1994). The Sickness Impact Profile for Nursing Homes (SIP-NH). *Journal of Gerontology, 49*(1), M2-M8.

Gigliotti, E. (2002). A confirmation of the factor structure of the Norbeck Social Support Questionnaire. *Nursing Research, 51*(5), 276-284.

Gilson, B. S., Gilson, J. S., Bergner, M., Bobbitt, R. A., Kressel, S., Pollard, W. E., et al. (1975). The Sickness Impact Profile: Development of an outcome measure of health care. *American Journal of Public Health, 65*(12), 1304-1310.

Grundy, E. M. (2003). The epidemiology of aging. In R. C. Tallis & H. M. Fillit (Eds.), *Brocklehurst's textbook of geriatric medicine and gerontology* (6th ed.). London: Churchill Livingstone.

Guigoz, V., Vellas, B., & Garry, P. J. (1994). A practical assessment tool for grading the nutritional state of elderly patients. *Facts and Research in Gerontology, Supplement #2,* 15-59.

Hachinski, V., Lliff, L., & Zilkha, E. (1975). Cerebral blood flow in dementia. *Archives of Neurology, 32,* 632-637.

Hanlon, J. T., Schmader, K. E., Samsa, G. P., Weinberger, M., Uttech, K. M., Lewis, I. K., Cohen, H. J., Feussner, J. R. (1992). A method for assessing drug therapy appropriateness. *Journal of Clinical Epidemiology, 45*(10), 1045-1051.

Hayes, V., Morris, J., Wolfe, C., & Morgan, M. (1995). The SF-36 health survey questionnaire: Is it suitable for use with older adults? *Age and Aging, 24,* 120-125.

Hendrich, A. L., Bender, P. S., & Nyhuis, A. (2003). Validation of the Hendrich II Fall Risk Model: A large concurrent case/control study of hospitalized patients, *Applied Nursing Research, 16*(1), 9-21.

Herr, K. A., Mobily, P. R., Kohout, F. J., & Wagenaar, D. (1998). Evaluation of the Faces Pain Scale for use with elderly. *Clinical Journal of Pain, 14,* 29-38.

Hoyl, M. T., Alessi, C. A., Harker, J. O., Josephson, K. R., Pietruszka, F. M., Koelfgen, M., et al. (1999). Development and testing of a five-item version of the Geriatric Depression Scale. *Journal of the American Geriatrics Society, 47,* 873-878.

Huang, H. C., Gau, M. L., Lin, W. C., & George, K. (2003). Assessing risk of falling in older adults. *Public Health Nursing, 20*(5), 399-411.

Inouye, S. K., Foreman, M. D., Mion, L. C., Katz, K. H., & Cooney, L. M. (2001). Nurses' recognition of delirium and its symptoms: Comparison of nurse and researcher ratings. *Archives of Internal Medicine, 161*(20), 2467-2473.

Inouye, S. K., Leo-Summers, L., Zhang, Y., Bogardus, S. T., Leslie, D. L., & Agostini, J. V. (2005). A chart-based method for identification of delirium: Validation compared with interviewer ratings using the Confusion Assessment Method. *Journal of the American Geriatrics Society, 53*(2), 312-318.

Inouye, S. K., van Dyck, C. H., Alessi, C. A., Balkin, S., Siegal, A. P., & Horwitz, R. I. (1990). Clarifying confusion: The Confusion Assessment Method. A new method for detection of delirium. *Annals of Internal Medicine, 113*(12), 941-948.

Jacox, A., Carr, D. B., Payne, R., Berde, C. B., Breitbart, W., & Caine, J. M. (1994). *Management of cancer pain: Clinical practice guideline no. 9.* Rockville, MD: Agency for Health Care Policy and Research.

Jenkinson, C., Layte, R., Jenkinson, D., Lawrence, K., Peterson, S., Paice, C., et al. (1997). A shorter form health survey: Can the SF-12 replicate results from the SF-36 in longitudinal studies? *Journal of Public Health Medicine, 19*(2), 179-186.

Jensen, G. L., Roy, M. A., Buchanan, A. E., & Berg, M. B. (2004). Weight loss interventions for obese older women: Improvements in performance and function. *Obesity Research, 12*(11), 1814-1820.

Kane, R. A. (2003). Social assessment of geriatric patients. In R. C. Tallis & H. M. Fillit (Eds.), *Brocklehurst's textbook of geriatric medicine and gerontology* (6th ed.). London: Churchill Livingstone.

Kane, R. L., Ouslander, J. G., & Abrass, I. B. (2004). *Essentials of clinical geriatrics.* New York: McGraw-Hill.

Katz, S., Ford, A. B., Moskowitz, R. W., Jackson, B. A., & Jaffe, M. W. (1963). Studies of illness in the aged. The index of ADL: A standardized measure of biological and psychosocial functioning. *Journal of the American Medical Association, 185,* 94-98.

Katzman, R., Brown, T., Fuld, P., Peck, A., Schechter, R., & Schimmel, H. (1983). Validation of a short orientation-memory-concentration test of cognitive impairment. *American Journal of Psychiatry, 140*(6), 734-738.

Koenig, H. G., Cohen, H. J., Blazer, D. G., Krishnan, K. R. R., & Sibert, T. E. (1993). Profile of depressive symptoms in younger and older medical inpatients with major depression. *Journal of the American Geriatrics Society, 41,* 1169-1700S.

Kukull, W. A., Larson, E. B., Teri, L., Bowen, J., McCormick, W., & Pfanschmidt, M. L. (1994). The Mini-Mental State Examination score and the clinical diagnosis of dementia. *Journal of Clinical Epidemiology, 47*(9), 1061-1067.

Lach, H. W., Chang, Y. P., & Edwards, D. F. (2005). Validity of the geriatric depression scales for dementia patients. *Gerontologist, 45*(special issue 11), 246.

Lach, H. W., Reed, A. T., Smith, L. J., & Carr, D. B. (1995). Alzheimer's disease: Assessing safety problems in the home. *Geriatric Nursing, 16*(4), 160-164.

Lachman, M. E., Howland, J., Tennstedt, S., Jette, A., Assman, S., & Peterson, E. W. (1998). Fear of falling and activity restriction: The Survey of Activities and Fear of Falling in the Elderly (SAFFE). *Journal of Gerontology, 53B,* P43-P50.

Laughlin, J. A., Granger, C. V., & Hamilton, B. B. (1992). Outcomes measurement in medical rehabilitation. *Rehab Management, 5*(1) 57-58.

Lawrence, V. A., Hazuda, H. P., Cornell, J. E., Pederson, T., Bradshaw, P. T., Mulrow, C. D., & Page, C. P. (2004). Functional independence after major abdominal surgery in the elderly. *Journal of the American College of Surgeons, 199*(5), 762-772.

Lawton, M. P. (1988). Scales to measure competence in everyday activities. *Psychopharmacology Bulletin, 24*(4), 609-613, 789-791.

Lawton, M. P., & Brody, E. M. (1969). Assessment of older people: Self-maintaining and instrumental activities of daily living. *Gerontologist, 9,* 179-186.

Leidy, N. K. (1999). Psychometric properties of the Functional Performance Inventory in patients with chronic obstructive pulmonary disease. *Nursing Research, 48*(1), 20-28.

Lichtenstein, M. J., Bess, F. H., & Logan, S. A. (1988). Validation of screening tools for identifying hearing-impaired elderly in primary care. *Journal of the American Medical Association, 259*(19), 2875-2878.

Linn, B. S., Linn, M. W., & Gurel, L. (1968). Cumulative Illness Rating Scale. *Journal of the American Geriatrics Society, 16*(9), 622-626.

Linn, M. W. (1967). A rapid disability rating scale. *Journal of the American Geriatrics Society, 15*(2), 211-214.

Lorentz, W. J., Scanlan, J. M., & Borson, S. (2002). Brief screening tests for dementia. *Canadian Journal of Psychiatry, 47*(8), 723-733.

Lyons, R. A., Wareham, K., Lucas, M. Price, D., Williams, J., & Hutchings, H. A. (1999). SF-36 scores vary by method of administration: Implications for study design. *Journal of Public Health Medicine, 21*(1), 41-45.

Mahoney, F. I., & Barthel, D. W. (1965). Functional evaluation: The Barthel Index. *Maryland State Medical Journal, 14,* 61-65.

Mathias, S., Nayak, U. S. L., & Isaacs, B. (1986). Balance in the elderly: The "get up and go test." *Archives of Physical Medicine and Rehabilitation, 67,* 387-389.

Mayeaux, E. J., Jr., Davis, T. C., Jackson, R. H., Henry, D., Patton, P., Slay, L., et al. (1995). Literacy and self-reported educational levels in relation to Mini-Mental State Examination scores. *Family Medicine, 27*(10), 658-662.

Mayfield, D. G., McLeod, G., & Hall, P. (1974). The CAGE questionnaire: Validation of a new alcoholism screening instrument. *American Journal of Psychiatry, 131,* 1121-1123.

Miller, M. D., Paradis, C. F., Houck, P. R., Mazumdar, S., Stack, J. A., Rifai, A. H., et al. (1992). Rating chronic medical illness burden in geropsychiatric practice and research: Application of the Cumulative Illness Rating Scale. *Psychiatry Research, 41*(3), 237-248.

Mistry, R., Gokhman, I., Bastani, R., Gould, R., Jimenez, E., Maxwell, A., et al. (2004). Measuring medical burden using CIRS in older veterans enrolled in UPBEAT, a psychogeriatric treatment program: A pilot study. *Journal of Gerontology Medical Sciences, 59*(10), 1068-1075.

Morris, J. C. (1993). The Clinical Dementia Rating (CDR): Current version and scoring rules. *Neurology, 43,* 2412-2414.

Morris, J. N., Hawes, C., Fries, B. E., Phillips, C. D., Mor, V., Katz, S., Murphy, K., et al. (1990). Designing the national resident assessment instrument for nursing homes. *Gerontologist, 30*(3), 293-307.

Morse, J. M., Morse, R., & Tylko, S. (1989). Development of a scale to identify the fall-prone patient. *Canadian Journal of Aging, 8,* 366-377.

Neelon, V. J., Champagne, M. T., Carlson, J. R., & Funk, S. G. (1996). The NEECHAM Confusion Scale: Construction, validation, and clinical testing. *Nursing Research, 45*(6), 324-330.

Newkirk, L. A., Kim, J. M., Thompson, J. M., Tinklenberg, J. R., Yesavage, J. A., & Taylor, J. L. (2004). Validation of a 26-point telephone version of the Mini-Mental State Examination. *Journal of Geriatric Psychiatry and Neurology, 17*(2), 81-87.

Nitcher, R. L., Burke, W. J., Roccaforte, W. H., & Wingel, S. P. (1993). A collateral source version of the geriatric depression rating scale. *American Journal of Geriatric Psychiatry, 1*(2), 143-152.

Norbeck, J. S., Lindsey, A. M., & Carrieri, V. L. (1981). The development of an instrument to measure social support. *Nursing Research, 30,* 264-269.

Norbeck, J. S., Lindsey, A. M., & Carrieri, V. L. (1983). Further development of the Norbeck Social Support Questionnaire. *Nursing Research, 32,* 4-9.

Novak, M., & Guest, C. (1989). Application of a multidimensional caregiver burden inventory. *Gerontologist, 29,* 798-803.

Ossip-Klein, D., Rothenberg, B. M., & Andresen, E. M. (1997). Screening for depression. In E. Andresen, B. Rothenberg, & J. G. Zimmer (Eds.), *Assessing the health status of older adults.* New York: Springer.

Ostir, G. V., Calson, J. E., Black, S. A., Rudkin, L., Goodwin, J. S., & Markides, K. S. (1999). Disability in older adults. 1: Prevalence, causes, and consequences. *Behavioral Medicine, 24*(4), 147-156.

Parmelee, P. A., Thuras, P. D., Katz, I. R., & Lawton, M. P. (1995). Validation of the Cumulative Illness Rating Scale in a geriatric residential population. *Journal of the American Geriatrics Society, 43*(2), 130-137.

Podsiadlo, D., & Richardson, S. (1991). The timed "up and go;" a test of basic functional mobility of frail elderly persons. *Journal of the American Geriatrics Society, 39,* 142-148.

Polit, D. F., & Beck, C. T. (2004). *Nursing research: Principles and methods* (7th Ed.). Philadelphia: Lippincott Williams & Wilkins.

Potter, J. F., & Biswas, N. (2002). Chronic pain. In R. J. Ham, P. D. Sloane, & G. A. Warshaw (Eds.), *Primary care geriatrics: A case-based approach.* St. Louis: Mosby.

Powell, L. E., & Myers, A. M. (1995). The Activities-specific Balance Confidence (ABC) scale. *Journal of Gerontology, 50A,* S28-S34.

Radloff, L. S. (1977). The CES-D scale: A self-report depression scale for research in the general population. *Applied Psychological Measurement, 1,* 385-401.

Reisberg, B., Ferris, S. H., De Leon, M. J., & Crook, T. (1982). The Global Deterioration Scale for the assessment of primary degenerative dementia. *American Journal of Psychiatry, 139,* 1136-1139.

Resnick, B., & Parker, R. (2001). Simplified scoring and psychometrics of the revised 12-item short form health survey. *Outcomes Management for Nursing Practice, 5*(4), 161-166.

Reuben, D. B., & Siu, A. L. (1990). An objective measure of physical function of elderly outpatients: The Physical Performance Test. *Journal of the American Geriatrics Society, 38,* 1105-1112.

Reuben, D. B., & Solomon, D. H. (1989). Assessment in geriatrics: Of caveats and names. *Journal of the American Geriatric Society, 37*(6), 570-572.

Rikli, R. E., & Jones, C. J. (1999). Development and validation of a functional fitness test for community-residing older adults. *Journal of Aging and Physical Activity, 7*(2), 129-161.

Roccaforte, W. H., Burke, W. J., Bayer, B. L., & Wengel, S. P. (1992). Validation of a telephone version of the Mini-Mental State Examination. *Journal of the American Geriatrics Society, 40*(7), 697-702.

Rosen, W. G., Mohs, R. C., & Davis, K. L. (1984). A new rating scale for Alzheimer's disease. *American Journal of Psychiatry, 141,* 1356-1364.

Rowe, J. W., & Kahn, R. L. (1997). Successful aging. *Gerontologist, 37,* 433-440.

Royall, D. R., Cordes, J. A., & Polk, M. (1998). CLOX: An executive clock drawing task. *Journal of Neurology, Neurosurgery and Psychiatry, 64,* 588-594.

Scanlan, J., & Borson, S. (2001). The mini-cog: Receiver operating characteristics with expert and naïve raters. *International Journal of Geriatric Psychiatry, 16*(2), 216-222.

Schretzman, D., & Strumpf, N. E. (2002). Principles guiding care of older adults. In V. T. Cotter & N. E. Strumpf (Eds.), *Advanced practice nursing with older adults: Clinical guidelines.* New York: McGraw-Hill.

Shannon, G. R., Yip, J. Y., & Wilber, K. H. (2004). Does payment structure influence change in physical functioning after rehabilitation therapy? *Home Health Services Quarterly, 23*(1), 63-78.

Sheikh, V. I., & Yesavage, V. A. (1986). Geriatric Depression Scale (GDS): Recent evidence and development of a shorter version. In T. L. Brink (Ed.), *Clinical gerontology: A guide to assessment and intervention.* New York: Haworth.

Shulman, K. I. (2000). Clock-drawing: Is it the ideal cognitive screening test? *International Journal of Geriatric Psychiatry, 15,* 548-561.

Siemsen, G. C., Miller, J., Newman, A. H., & Lucas, C. M. (1992). The predictive value of the NEECHAM scale. In S. G. Funk, E. M. Tournquist, M. T. Champagne, & R. A. Weise (Eds.), *Key aspects of managing eldercare: Managing falls, incontinence, and cognitive impairment.* New York: Springer.

Sinclair, P. A., Lyness, J. M., King, D. A., Cox, C., & Caine, E. D. (2001). Depression and self-reported functional status in older primary care patients. *American Journal of Psychiatry, 158*(3), 416-419.

Snow, A. L., Kunik, M. E., Molinari, V. A., Orengo, C. A., Doody, R., Graham, D. P., & Norris, M. P. (2005). Accuracy of self-reported depression in persons with dementia. *Journal of the American Geriatrics Society, 53,* 389-396.

Stephens, J. A., & Olson, S. J. (2004). Check for safety: A home fall prevention checklist for older adults. Retrieved July 10, 2005, from www.cdc.gov/ncipc/pub-res/toolkit/Check%20for%20Safety COLOR.pdf.

Stommel, M., & Wills, C. E. (2004). *Clinical research: Concepts and principles for advanced practice nurses.* Philadelphia: Lippincott Williams & Wilkins.

Stuss, D. T., Meiran, N., Guzman, D. A., Lafleche, G., & Willmer, J. (1996). Do long tests yield a more accurate diagnosis of dementia than short tests? A comparison of 5 neuropsychological tests. *Archives of Neurology, 53*(10), 1033-1039.

Tarlov, A. R., Ware, J. E., Jr., Greenfield, S., Nelson, E. C., Perrin, E., & Zubkoff, M. (1989). The Medical Outcomes Study: An application of methods for monitoring the results of medical care. *Journal of the American Medical Association, 262*(7), 925-930.

Taylor, L., Whittington, F., Hollingsworth, C., Ball, M., King, S., Patterson, V., et al. (2003). Assessing the effectiveness of a walking program on physical function of residents living in an assisted living facility. *Journal of Community Health Nursing, 20*(1), 15-26.

Taylor, W., D., McQuoid, D. R., & Krishnan, K. R. (2004). Medical comorbidity in late-life depression. *International Journal of Geriatric Psychiatry, 19*(10), 935-943.

Teri, L., Traus, P., Logsdon, R., Uomoto, J., Zarit, S., & Vitaliano, P. P. (1992). Assessment of behavioral problems in dementia: The revised memory and behavior problems checklist. *Psychology and Aging, 7*(4), 622-623.

Tinetti, M. (1986). Performance-oriented assessment of mobility problems in elderly patients. *Journal of the American Geriatrics Society, 34,* 119-126.

Tinetti, M. E., Richman, D., & Powell, L. (1990). Falls efficacy as a measure of fear of falling. *Journal of Gerontology, 45B,* P239-P243.

Tinetti, M. E., Williams, T. F., & Mayewski, R. (1986). Fall risk index for elderly patients based on number of chronic disabilities. *American Journal of Medicine, 80,* 429-434.

Tombaugh, T. N., & McIntyre, N. J. (1992). The Mini-Mental State Examination: A comprehensive review. *Journal of the American Geriatrics Society, 40*(9), 922-935.

van Hook, M. P., & Berkman, B. (1996). Assessment tools for general health care settings: PRIME-MD, OARS, and SF-36. *Health and Social Work, 21*(3), 230-234.

van Straten, A., de Haan, R. J., Limburg, M., Schuling, J., Bossuyt, P. M., & van den Bos, G. A. M. (1997). A stroke-adapted 30-item version of the Sickness Impact Profile to assess quality of life (SA-SIP30). *Stroke, 28*(1), 2155-2161.

VanSwearingen, J. M., & Brach, J. S. (2001). Making geriatric assessment work: Selecting useful measures. *Physical Therapy, 81*(6), 1233-1252.

Walters, S. J., Munro, J. F., & Brazier, J. E. (2001). Using the SF-36 with older adults: A cross-sectional community-based survey. *Age and Ageing, 30,* 337-343.

Ware, J. E., Jr., Kosinski, M., & Keller, S. D. (1996). A 12-item short-form health survey: Construction of scales and preliminary tests of reliability and validity. *Medical Care, 34*(3), 220-233.

Ware, J. E., Jr., & Sherbourne, C. D. (1992). The MOS 36-item short-form health survey (SF-36): Conceptual framework and item selection. *Medical Care, 30*(6), 473-483.

Washburn, R. A., Smith, K. W., Jette, A. M., & Janney, C. A. (1993). The Physical Activity Scale for the Elderly (PASE): Development and evaluation. *Journal of Clinical Epidemiology, 46,* 153-162.

Watson, Y. I., Arfken, C. L., & Birge, S. J. (1993). Clock completion: An objective screening test for dementia. *Journal of the American Geriatrics Society, 41*(11), 1235-1240.

Weeks, S. K., McGann, P. E., Michaels, T. K., & Penninx, B. W. (2003). Comparing various short-form Geriatric Depression Scale leads to the GDS-5/15. *Journal of Nursing Scholarship, 35*(2), 133-137.

Wynne, C. F., Ling, S. M., & Remsburg, R. (2000). Comparison of pain assessment instruments in cognitively intact and cognitively impaired nursing home residents. *Geriatric Nursing, 21*(1), 20-23.

Yesavage, J. A., Brink, T. L., Rose, T. L., Lum, O., Huang, V., Adey, M., & Leirer, V. O. (1983). Development and validation of a geriatric depression screening scale. *Journal of Psychiatric Research, 17,* 37-49.

Zarit, S. H., Orr, N. K., & Zarit, J. M. (1985). *The hidden victims of Alzheimer's disease: Families under stress.* New York: New York University Press.

Application of Nursing Theory

Helen W. Lach

Define theory *and discuss its relevance to gerontological nursing practice.*

Discuss the progress in knowledge development in nursing.

Provide an overview of conceptual models and grand theories of nursing.

Discuss middle-range theories relevant to gerontological nursing.

OVERVIEW OF NURSING THEORY

The importance of theory to nursing is often misunderstood as a purely academic endeavor with little relevance to practice. In some cases, we have adopted theoretical concepts to such a degree that they are now invisible. An example is systems theory, which identifies that individuals are in interaction with their environment, each affecting the other. This concept is so well integrated into most of our thinking that we forget that this concept was developed and described in nursing theory. Some other theories are not well understood and are thought to be inaccessible to the practicing nurse. Ideally, theory can help inform practice by shaping how the nurse goes about nursing. For example, nursing theory encourages a holistic view of the patient rather than a disease- or symptom-oriented view that is often the approach of medicine (Fawcett, Newman, & McAllister, 2004). As a result, the nurse and advanced practice nurse take a broader view of the patient than someone following the medical model, considering all the psychological, social, and environmental factors contributing to the patient's health situation.

It is critical to the gerontological nurse to gain a good understanding of nursing theory and to use a tested theoretical base to guide nursing practice. For example, a nurse may be caring for an older patient who lives alone and who is experiencing functional decline. Because the

nurse uses Orem's Self-Care Deficit Theory (Orem, Taylor, & Renpenning, 2001) to guide her or his practice, the nurse identifies the patient's self-care deficits and designs nursing interventions and evaluates them in relationship to how well they help the individual maintain independence in self-care. The theory in this case provides a systematic framework for practice. Theory allows nurses to "understand why they are doing what they are doing and be able to explain it to other health professionals" (Tomey & Alligood, 2002, p. 11). The many goals of nursing theory are listed in Box 4-1.

Bernick (2004) provides another example in a recent article describing her use of Watson's Caring-Healing Model in practice. She notes that this theory helps shape the way she provides care that is "concerned with the individual/family/group's human responses to their health and illness situation, with the goal of allowing for caring and healing" (p. 134). Although individual nurses could develop their own theoretical framework, the use of developed, discussed, and tested theory creates the science of nursing. Once a framework is developed, it can be debated and tested through research. The theory can be refined, and ultimately we develop evidence for how to deliver nursing care so that our patients obtain the best outcomes possible. This scholarly work is what makes nursing a discipline and a professional endeavor.

Several definitions provided by Alligood and Tomey (2002) help us to understand nursing theory and its relationship to practice: conceptual model, theory, grand theory, and middle-range theory (Box 4-2). A *conceptual model* is "a broad frame of reference for systematic approaches to the phenomena with which the discipline is concerned" (p. 223). A *theory* is "a group of related concepts that propose actions that guide practice" (p. 225). Theory provides a systematic way of viewing phenomena in order to describe, predict, explain, or prescribe (Dollins & Niemer, 2001). As such, theory can be tested through research. Some theories are nearly as

BOX 4-1 Goals of Nursing Theory

- Identify the domain and goals of nursing
- Provide knowledge to improve nursing practice, education, research, and administration
- Guide research to establish evidence base for nursing
- Identify areas to be studied
- Identify research techniques and tools that will be tested to validate nursing interventions
- Identify nature of contribution that research will make to the advancement of knowledge
- Establish criteria for measuring quality of nursing care, education, and research
- Guide development of nursing care delivery systems
- Provide systematic structure and rationale for nursing activities
- Develop curriculum plans for nursing education

From Perry, A. G. (2005). Theoretical foundations of nursing practice. In *Fundamentals of nursing* (6th ed.). St. Louis: Mosby.

broad as conceptual models, such as the *grand theories* of nursing, but other theories are specific to certain aspects of practice or specific care situations.

Not all authors seem to agree on which theories should be called "grand theories" and which should be called "conceptual frameworks." For the purposes of

this text, the major theories are summarized in one section. Theories with a more narrow scope are called *middle-range theories*. Middle-range theories are related to specific situations or contexts and can guide gerontological nursing practice. Several are described later in the chapter.

Theory has helped nursing identify the four major concepts of importance for practice, sometimes called the *nursing metaparadigm* (McEwen, 2002) or key concepts for nursing knowledge: person, environment, health, and nursing. *Person* identifies the individuals who are recipients of care. Many nursing theories suggest a respect for the individual, as well as self-determination for the individual, and the holistic view of the individual as more than the sum of his or her parts. External factors surrounding or interacting with the patient make up the *environment*. Even Florence Nightingale was concerned with broad environmental factors affecting people, both sick and well, from food and water to societal factors (Pfettscher, 2002).

Health is the desired outcome of nursing. Conceptualizations of health in nursing often view health as a continuum, as more than just the absence of disease, with a wellness component that can be achieved or strived for (e.g., Pender, in Pender, Murdaugh, & Parsons, 2001). *Nursing* is a science and an art. Hauner and Henderson (1955) defined *nursing* as follows: "to assist the individual, sick or well, in the performance of those activities contributing to health or its recovery (or

Box 4-2 Terms Used in Nursing Theory

Term	Definition
Conceptual model	"A broad frame of reference" (Alligood & Tomey, 2002) or perspective for considering a phenomenon such as the discipline of nursing.
Theory	Describes more specific relationships among concepts that can guide and predict actions. Has been described as "the knowledge that explains things" (Keller, 2001), and can be tested through research.
Grand theory	Many nursing theorists have developed what have been called *grand theories*. They are broad in scope and "define general parameters on which nursing function is based" (Beery et al., 2001).
Middle-range theory	Theory that is narrow in scope, addressing a specific problem or situation. Middle-range theories have been further described, based on how specific they are, as high middle-range, middle middle-range, and low middle-range theories (Liehr & Smith, 1999).
Nursing metaparadigm	The four components that are important for understanding and researching nursing: person, environment, health, and nursing (McEwen, 2002).
Ways of knowing in nursing	The four types of knowledge that help to describe and study nursing: empirics, ethics, personal knowing, and aesthetics (Chinn & Kramer, 2004).

Box 4-3 *Reflections on Using Nursing Theory*

In the last edition of this book I stated that "gerontological nursing practice builds upon the theories and methods of nursing practice generally." I have found general nursing theory, particularly the work of Dorothea Orem, to be a great framework for nursing practice. First, Orem's theory helps focus attention on the areas of health that only nurses address, such as self-care. Orem demonstrates that nursing care results from interactions between a patient who has a deficit in the need for self-care and the ability to provide it independently, and a nurse trained to compensate for deficits. Orem's theory also helps identify strategies for providing nursing assistance to patients, from counseling to providing complete care for someone who is ill.

Other theories are helpful in nursing practice. The Transtheoretical Model developed by Prochaska and colleagues provides interventions to help patients make behavior changes, and identify those who are likely to benefit from an intervention. The theory of trajectory in illness focuses attention on identifying the various points along a health or illness course and how these may affect the patient. Uncertainty theory helps identify the concept that people will work to move out of a state of uncertainty. The Nagi Disablement Model (see Box 4-4) provides an important way to think about the common path of older adults on a downward spiral toward disability, and helps predict the impact of disease. This text provides more detail about these theories, and I encourage nurses to explore them in order to discover the ways they can help guide nursing practice. Good theory can help the nurse think about nursing assessment and interventions in new ways that can enrich nursing practice.

Eleanor S. McConnell

Eleanor S. McConnell, RN, PhD APRN, BC
Associate Professor
Duke University
School of Nursing
Durham, North Carolina

to a peaceful death), that he would perform unaided if he had the necessary strength, will, or knowledge and to do this in such a way as to help him gain independence as rapidly as possible."

Definitions of advanced practice nursing explicitly identify advanced knowledge of theory as a core competency (e.g., American Nurses Association, 2001), and theory can help nurses understand the relationship of research findings to practice (Brown, 2000). Box 4-3 describes the use of theory in practice for one of this text's founding authors, and Box 4-4 describes a key theory that is relevant to geriatrics: the Nagi Disablement Model (Verbrugge & Jette, 1994). To help apply nursing theory to gerontological nursing, this chapter first provides some background on the development of nursing theory over the past 50 years and how thinking about nursing theory has changed. Some of the major nursing theories are reviewed, with implications for practice. Finally, several key middle-range theories with particular relevance to gerontological nursing practice are presented. Later chapters discuss theories from nursing and other disciplines that are related to the content. For example, theories of health behavior change are discussed in Chapter 27.

DEVELOPMENT OF NURSING THEORY AND NURSING KNOWLEDGE

Nurses became interested in theory that would guide nursing practice beginning in the 1950s, as the discipline strived to be recognized as a discipline. Budding nursing scientists understood that research needed to be based in theory that would help explain their findings and put them into a framework that would enable them to communicate their findings to other disciplines. Many early nurse scientists obtained their doctoral degrees in other disciplines with their own theoretical bases. Although concepts from fields such as psychology, education, and sociology have informed nursing practice and research, they do not fully explain nursing. These pioneers recognized that nursing was different, and therefore the discipline of nursing needed to develop its own theoretical bases to support our practice and research.

For the next 30 years, discussion and debate centered on the need for nursing theory and the development of numerous conceptual models and grand theories of nursing. These theories have led to a sound scientific basis for many aspects of practice, education, and curricula. Several of these major theories are described in the next section of this chapter. In addition, nursing has identified the kinds of knowledge we need to improve our understanding of nursing practice.

Four fundamental ways of understanding or "knowing" in nursing were first identified by Carper in 1978, and have been expanded on by Chinn and Kramer (2004), as framing nursing theory and science: empirics, ethics, personal knowing, and aesthetics. Chinn and Kramer describe these ways of knowing: "Each kind of knowledge is important for practice, and the best practices depend on integrating all together to form a whole" (p. 1).

- Empirical knowledge is considered the science of nursing, the traditional use of the scientific method,

Box 4-4 Nagi Disablement Model

The Nagi Disablement Model (Verbrugge & Jette, 1994) provides yet another theory that can be used to guide clinical practice and research, and is especially useful for gerontological nurses. One dilemma confronted by nurses and other clinicians is predicting which patients with a specific chronic disease are likely to have problems carrying out daily activities, such as work, or being independent in their self-care. Another dilemma is how to intervene to prevent disablement. Disablement is the inability to carry out customary or desired roles. The Nagi Disablement Model was developed to describe the process of developing disability and to identify factors that affect the development of disablement (Figure 4-1). This would ultimately help identify promising interventions to prevent or alleviate disability.

The Nagi Disablement Model proposes that development of disability is governed not simply by whether or not a disease exists, but on the extent to which the pathological processes that underlie the disease have resulted in impairments in organ system function or limitations in the abilities to carry out basic tasks such as reaching, lifting, moving from one position to another, or walking. Imagine being responsible for caring for someone with diabetes mellitus (DM). Some people with DM become unable to dress themselves, owing to peripheral neuropathy, blindness, or both. In order to know which patients will need assistance to prevent lost function, nurses need to examine peripheral sensation and test visual acuity. Disability in self-care resulting from peripheral neuropathy or blindness can be treated through modifications to the older adult's physical environment and through patient and family education. Patients with peripheral neuropathy can be independent in dressing if clothing fasteners are adapted so that fine motor control is not needed; patients with blindness can regain independence in dressing if their environment is structured so that clothing is stored in consistent places, with labels affixed to denote different colors.

The Nagi Disablement Model also suggests that intermediate steps along the pathway to disability can be identified before the onset of dependence in self-care. Longitudinal studies have been conducted to test this hypothesis, helping us to learn if intervening to preserve function before disability develops is an effective strategy (Leveille, Fried, McMullen, & Guralnik, 2004). Studies such as these will help refine our ability to predict who will have problems carrying out customary roles, as well as enhance our ability to treat and prevent disability.

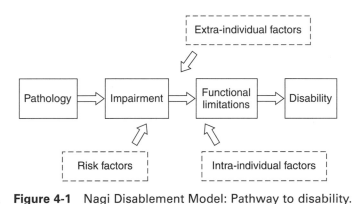

Figure 4-1   Nagi Disablement Model: Pathway to disability.

Box and figure from Verbrugge, L. M., & Jette, A. M. (1994). The disablement process. *Social Science & Medicine, 38*(1), 1-14.

using problem solving and logical reasoning. Through traditional science, nurses test hypotheses that are derived from theory, with a goal of explanation and prediction. In addition, descriptive and inductive methods of research are used to develop theory.

- Ethics in nursing is understood as guiding our work, directing what should be done in various situations and defining nursing obligations. Ethical knowledge is developed through consideration of morality, values and beliefs, and moral reasoning.

- Personal knowing in nursing comes from experiencing the provision of care, the relationships and transactions, and considering the personal role of the self in care situations. It explores the personal meaning of caring, and the discovery of the self through experience of being a nurse. Personal knowing is expressed in the passion, commitment, and integrity of the nurse.

- The last form of nursing, aesthetic knowing, helps describe the art of nursing, the way that the nurse performs actions that shape the experience in a unique way, depending on the individual nurse. Aesthetic knowing can also be expressed in regular art forms.

The model of Chinn and Kramer (2004) depicted in Figure 4-2 shows the questions, actions, and outcomes of these four ways of knowing in nursing, and how they fit together to form the whole of nursing practice.

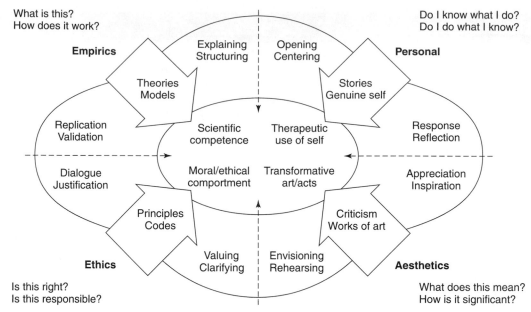

Figure 4-2 Processes for developing nursing knowledge. (From Chinn, P. L., & Kramer, M. K. [2004]. *Integrated knowledge development in nursing* [6th ed.]. St. Louis: Mosby, p. 9.)

Together they support the science of nursing and continued development of knowledge to guide practice.

This rich background of nursing knowledge development has led the profession to a new era, a "theory utilization phase," in which the confirmation of theory in practice is being explored (Tomey & Alligood, 2002). Research into the effectiveness of interventions, to identify new interventions, and to encourage implementation of effective interventions is well underway. In addition, much work now focuses on the development of middle-range theories that will support specific nursing practices. As background to our discussion of more specific theories, we first explore some of the major nursing theories and their application in nursing practice.

CONCEPTUAL MODELS AND GRAND THEORIES OF NURSING

Conceptual models and grand theories of nursing have been developed by a number of nursing scholars and theorists to help describe the practice and realm of nursing. It is beyond the scope of this chapter to give great detail about all the individual nursing theories. However, the key concepts of a sample of theories are presented here, as well as some comments on how they have been incorporated into practice (Box 4-5). Readers are encouraged to learn more about these and other nursing theories through texts designed to provide more detailed information (e.g., Fawcett, 2000; Tomey & Alligood, 2002). The following theorists are included here:

- Dorothea Orem: Self-Care Deficit Theory of Nursing
- Sister Callista Roy: Adaptation Model

- Dorothy Johnson: Behavioral System Model
- Martha Rogers: Unitary Human Being
- Myra Levine: Conservation Model
- Imogene King: Goal Attainment

Dorothea Orem: Self-Care Deficit Theory of Nursing

Orem's Self-Care Deficit Theory is a broad model describing nursing practice. The key concept of Orem's work is self-care, defined as "the practice of activities that maturing and mature persons initiate and perform, within time frames, on their own behalf in the interests of maintaining life and healthful functioning and continuing personal development" (Orem et al., 2001, p. 521). Self-care requisites are the things individuals need to accomplish in order to meet this goal, for example, obtaining food and water. Self-care deficits occur when the individual is unable to meet his or her self-care needs, and this deficit gives rise to the need for nursing. The practice of nursing focuses on identifying the patient's self-care deficits and providing education or assistance as needed to promote healing or health. Orem, Taylor, and Renpenning's book *Nursing: Concepts of Practice* (2001) describes a model for nursing practice through Orem's theory. Self-care deficit has been integrated into nursing diagnoses (NANDA International, 2003). Self-care is also a key concept in gerontological nursing because of the importance of maintaining independence for older adults and the focus of gerontological nursing on helping the patient regain or improve functional abilities, achieving self-care.

Box 4-5 Nursing Theorists	
AUTHOR	TITLE
Grand Theories and Conceptual Models	
Orem, D. (Orem, Taylor, & Renpenning, 2001)	Self-Care Deficit Theory of Nursing
Roy, C. (Roy & Andrews, 1999)	Adaptation Model
Johnson, D. (1980)	Behavioral System Model
Rogers, M. (1983)	Unitary Human Beings
Levine, M. (1990)	Conservation Model
King, I. (1981)	Goal Attainment
Middle-Range Theories	
Leininger, M., & McFarland, M. R. (2002)	Culture Care
Kolcaba, K. (1994)	Theory of Comfort
Corbin, J., & Strauss, A. (1992)	Chronic Illness Trajectory Framework
Norbeck, J, Lindsey, A., & Carrierei, V. (1981)	Model of Social Support
Mishel, M. (1988)	Theory of Uncertainty in Illness
Phillips, L., & Rempusheski, V. (1986)	Family Caregiving Dynamics Model
Schumacher, K. L., Stewart, B. J., & Archbold, P. (1998)	Doing Family Caregiving Well
Hall, G., & Buckwalter, K. (1987)	Progressively Lowered Stress Threshold Model
Matteson, M., Linton, A., & Barnes, S. (1996)	Cognitive Development Model
Algase, D., Beck, C., Kolanowski, A., Whall, A., Berent, S., Richards, K., & Beattie, E. (1996)	Need-Driven Dementia-Compromised Behavior Model
Dunn, K. (2004)	Adaptation to Chronic Pain

Sister Callista Roy: Adaptation Model

The process of adaptation is the major concept in Roy's work, defined as an ongoing life process. Humans are an adaptive system, a whole with parts that function together, interdependent and with a purpose (Roy & Andrews, 1999). Adaptation occurs in four modes: physiological, self-concept (psychological and spiritual), role functioning (social), and interdependence. Nursing is focused on promoting adaptation for the individual in these four areas to promote health, quality of life, or death with dignity. Roy describes how to apply her concepts through the nursing process. The concept of adaptation has provided a goal for nursing practice that has been widely applied in practice, education, and research (Beery et al., 2001). In gerontological nursing, we recognize that for the older patient, adaptation may be more difficult or slower because of the loss of reserves to deal with illness or injury, so that, for example, recovery may be slower than for the younger patient.

Dorothy Johnson: Behavioral System Model

Johnson describes individuals as whole behavioral systems with interdependent parts (Johnson, 1980), a different perspective than the medical approach of looking at the biological systems. Each individual or behavior system has a patterned, repetitive, purposeful way of behaving. There are several behavioral subsystems to accomplish the various tasks needed by the individual. The goal is to perform activities that promote equilibrium or a stabilized state, or state of harmony, or health. Health is an expanded consciousness or evolution that is not exclusive of disease. The goal of nursing is to support equilibrium, or balance within the individual, through nurturing, protection, or stimulation. Johnson's model has been helpful in developing and testing behavioral nursing interventions. Herbert (1989) describes how the model was used with an older woman who had suffered a stroke, showing application of the model to nursing practice with older adults.

Martha Rogers: Unitary Human Being

Rogers describes human beings as unitary energy fields that are irreducible, indivisible wholes, promoting a holistic approach to the individual. Individuals are open systems with interaction between individuals and the environment, which are integral to one another (Rogers, 1983). Human energy fields are constantly changing and evolving toward more complex patterns. There is a totality of experience and existence. Energy fields have patterns that are unique and revealed through manifestations such as behaviors and characteristics. Nursing promotes health through promoting integrity of the human field, directing or redirecting patterning of energy fields. This theory provides a way to consider how nursing interventions such as music, humor, touch, and meditation can positively influence health (Rogers, 2002), and encourages avoidance of a reductionist approach to the care of individuals. Gerontological nurses particularly use a holistic approach to patients that encompasses mind, body, spirit, and the environment.

Myra Levine: Conservation Model

Levine described three concepts in her Conservation Model: wholeness, adaptation, and conservation (Levine, 1990). She identified the individual as a whole with integrity and individual response. Adaptation is retaining the integrity of the whole within the realities of the internal and external environment. The individual can generate four types of responses: fight or flight, inflammatory response, stress response, and perceptual awareness. Conservation describes the way complex organisms or systems continue to function even when challenged. Four principles guide this model: conservation of energy, conservation of structural integrity, conservation of personal integrity, and conservation of social integrity. Nursing uses these principles to promote the wholeness of the individual, and these principles have application to older adults. For example, the older adult with chronic obstructive pulmonary disease may be taught methods to conserve energy while completing activities of daily living, which often leave them exhausted. By conserving energy doing these necessary tasks, the person may then have energy left to participate in other enjoyable activities during the day, enhancing the person's quality of life.

Imogene King: Goal Attainment

King (1981) described health as a dynamic life experience, "requiring continuous adjustments through the use of one's resources to achieve the maximum potential for daily living" (p. 5). Nursing is an interaction and interpersonal relationship between the nurse and patient within health care as an organization. This interaction occurs either with an individual or groups and encourages the active participation of the individual in determining his or her own health. Together, the nurse and patient make transactions toward goal setting and goal attainment to improve health, which includes effective care, satisfaction, and enhanced growth and development (Chinn & Kramer, 2004). This theory supports the need to develop a relationship with the patient so that care can be individualized, an important concept in gerontological nursing given the wide range of health and disease states among this population.

There are other major nursing theorists, and the authors encourage nurses to learn more about the many conceptual models. The following section provides more specific guidance for gerontological nursing practice through the discussion of a sample of middle-range theories.

MIDDLE-RANGE THEORIES

Middle-range nursing theories, as noted earlier, are more specific and are usually related to concepts and situations specific to nursing practice; therefore they are less abstract than the grand theories and conceptual models. They provide guidance for assessment, planning, intervention, and evaluation of nursing care. However, middle-range theories vary in scope, and three levels of middle-range theories have been proposed (Liehr & Smith, 1999). The high middle-range theories are the most broad, with application to almost any nursing situation; middle middle-range theories narrow the scope to more limited situations; and low middle-range theories are very specific. The theories that follow include representations of each of these levels of middle-range theory.

Gerontological nurses have been active in developing middle-range theories to understand some of our important practice problems, for example, care of people with dementia (Whall & Colling, 2005). Several middle-range theories that are important and helpful in gerontological nursing practice are reviewed here, and their application is discussed. Again, nurses are encouraged to read about concepts and nursing theory related to problems and issues in their own practice. The first middle-range theories are general, but important in gerontological nursing. The latter theories are more specific to gerontological practice settings.

- Culture Care
- Theory of Comfort
- Chronic Illness Trajectory Framework
- Model of Social Support
- Theory of Uncertainty in Illness
- Family Caregiving Dynamics Model
- Doing Family Caregiving Well
- Progressively Lowered Stress Threshold Model
- Cognitive Development Model
- Need-Driven Compromised Behavior Model
- Theory of Adaptation to Chronic Pain

Culture Care Diversity and Universality

Leininger started the specialty of transcultural nursing through her writings on the concepts of culture and health (Leininger & McFarland, 2002). The goal is to provide care that is congruent to the individual's culture and beliefs, which determines how the nurse will work with the individual patient and what kind of care is called for. Nurses are challenged to be open to the myriad of cultures they may encounter because of the increasing mobility of people worldwide. Leininger sees care as a universal need that nursing can meet. Developing cultural competence is a theme in practice, education, and research today as nurses attempt to provide appropriate care to patients from all over the globe and from all walks of life.

From this theory, the nurse encountering an older Korean woman who has recently immigrated to the United States would work to understand how this patient's culture shapes her choices in health practices. For example, she may be shy and unwilling to visit a male gynecologist for an examination, yet that is the only physician available at the local clinic. Because she cannot afford to go elsewhere, she does not receive an annual Papanicolaou (Pap) test that the nurse has recommended.

Theory of Comfort

Kolcaba's (1994) Theory of Comfort is a theory supporting basic nursing care. The need for comfort arises from a variety of health care situations. Comfort needs can come from many sources, including physical needs, psychosocial needs, spiritual needs, or environmental needs. A primary function of nursing is to assess and provide comfort measures, which are interventions designed to address the comfort needs of the individual. This theory can be applied in any setting and with any type of patient, and has been tested in a variety of studies and practice settings. Because the chronic diseases that result in pain and discomfort are common among older patients, identifying and addressing comfort needs is often an important component of care.

Chronic Illness Trajectory Framework

Chronic disease is extremely common among older adults, so that understanding how people cope with illness throughout its course is important for gerontological nursing. The trajectory framework of Corbin and Strauss (1992) describes common phases that occur as people experience the ups and downs of chronic illness over time, as well as common responses to these phases. The framework provides a guide for nursing assessment and interventions to assist patients in adapting to and coping with the challenges that occur. The trajectory onset begins when symptoms of disease appear, leading to a crisis phase. The course of chronic illness then continues with periods of exacerbation and remission resulting in acute, stable, unstable, and downward phases. Illness affects the various components of life, and people attempt to adapt and manage their disease. The downward spiral can result in a terminal or dying phase, although the phases are not necessarily linear or moving in the same direction at all times.

Nursing researchers have used this theory to explore ways to help patients with chronic diseases such as multiple sclerosis (Gullick, 1998). An update of the model has included a greater emphasis on chronic disease prevention in the pretrajectory phase and increased prominence of the nurse in chronic disease management (Corbin, 1998). Again, because chronic disease is more prevalent with age, older patients can be placed along this trajectory framework, and this information can help guide nursing interventions.

Model of Social Support

Norbeck's theory focuses on the importance of social support as a buffer for life stresses, and a force for promoting positive mental and physical health (Norbeck, Lindsey, & Carrierei, 1981). The dimensions of social support include the individual's characteristics, the situational demands, the needs of the individual for social support, and the availability of social support to meet the individual's needs. Norbeck studied the needs of several populations for social support in a variety of health situations and proposed that social support is a universal need (Norbeck & Tilden, 1988). This model encourages nurses to promote an environment to provide social support and assist individuals in developing broader networks if needed. Social support is a particularly important factor for older adults, who often suffer the losses of many members of their network, including family members, friends, and acquaintances.

Theory of Uncertainty in Illness

Merle Mishel (1988, 1990) developed the Theory of Uncertainty in Illness through her work with cancer patients to help explain how people cope with chronic and life-threatening illness (Bailey & Stewart, 2002). Again it would commonly apply to older adults who are at higher risk for chronic disease. The theory has assumptions about how people respond cognitively to illness, especially when they are unable to determine the meaning of illness-related events. Uncertainty is neutral, but the individual appraises the information and gives meaning as either positive or negative. Originally Mishel thought people would adapt and return to their preillness state. However, her research supported the idea that most people adopt a new view of life in the face of the experiences of illness. Illness acts as a catalyst for change.

Family Caregiving Dynamics Model

This theory was originally developed to help understand the dynamics of the caregiving situation so nurses could intervene to meet the needs of both elderly patients and their family caregivers (Phillips & Rempusheski, 1986). Phillips and colleagues further refined the model and have tested it through research (Phillips et al., 1995; Phillips, Brewer, & Torres de Ardon, 2001). The concepts of the model include first the structure, or background, of the individuals and their prior relationship. Second are context factors, which are important to the current situation. These include both interactional context factors, such as the caregiver's role expectations and expectations of the care recipient, and situational context factors, such as the care recipient's abilities. Third are perceptions that the caregiver and care recipient have about the situation, such as caregiving burden. This model provides a framework for understanding poor caregiving, with attention to many factors, including the prior relationship history of the caregiver and the care recipient.

Doing Family Caregiving Well

Another conceptualization of caregiving is provided by Schumacher, Stewart, and Archbold (1998) in their work on Doing Family Caregiving Well. They identified concepts in two groups, with the first group including four concepts related to how well the caregiver perceives she or he is providing care. Caregiving mastery and caregiver competence are broad concepts that describe caregivers' overall perceptions of their abilities. Caregiver preparedness and caregiver self-efficacy are concepts more specific to the tasks of caregiving. The second group of concepts related to how professionals would evaluate the caregiving situation. These include competence, or

having the knowledge and skills to provide care; providing care with predictability or routines; and finding enrichment from the caregiving experience in meaning or pleasure. These concepts can change over time as caregiving situations change, and are amenable to intervention. As this work develops, it will provide nurses with a framework to identify caregiver perspectives, as well as methods of improving caregiving that will assist older patients.

Progressively Lowered Stress Threshold Model

One of the first middle-range theories to help guide care of people with dementia is the Progressively Lowered Stress Threshold Model (Hall & Buckwalter, 1987). This model focuses on the effects of stress on the individual with dementia, who has diminished capacity to process stimuli and a reduced threshold for coping with stress. Stressors can be noise, illness, hunger, grief, change in caregivers, bathing, or any demand beyond the individual's ability to cope. Stressors accumulate, and when the individual's threshold is met, anxiety and dysfunctional behavior such as catastrophic reactions occur. This is often seen in the individual with "sundowning," in which the individual has reached his or her limit by late afternoon and acts out because of inability to continue to cope with the stressors accumulated over the course of the day. Severe reactions can be extreme and violent in some cases, and dysfunctional behaviors produce very difficult situations for caregivers to manage.

The ability to cope with stress in the environment declines with increasing cognitive impairment. Caregivers can help individuals with dementia to improve their quality of life and avoid undue stress much of the time. The caregiver can assess the level of stress that the individual patient can tolerate and identify situations that produce stress. Interventions include providing periods of decreased stress during the day, avoiding stressful situations when possible, and finding ways to help the individual cope when stressful situations cannot be avoided. This model has provided great insight into understanding behavior in individuals with dementia and has been used to develop interventions and educational programs (Smith, Gerdner, Hall, & Buckwalter, 2004).

Cognitive Development Model

The Cognitive Development Model (Matteson, Linton, & Barnes, 1996) explores the loss of abilities in people with Alzheimer's disease and other dementias. The theory proposes that intellectual losses occur in approximately the opposite order to that in which they are attained, based on Piaget's theory of intellectual development. These stages include (1) sensorimotor,

(2) preoperational, (3) concrete operations, and (4) formal operations. This information can help guide nursing assessment, and interventions are based on the patient's current level of intellect. Caregivers can anticipate that intellectual losses will continue throughout the disease.

Need-Driven Dementia-Compromised Behavior Model

The Need-Driven Dementia-Compromised Behavior Model provides additional important insights for caring for patients with dementia. This model developed out of work with dementia patients as a means to understand disruptive and disturbing behaviors such as vocalizations and wandering, particularly in the long-term care setting (Kolanowski, 1999). Rather than viewing these behaviors as a problem, this model conceptualizes them as "potentially understandable needs, that if responded to, will enhance quality of life" (Algase et al., 1996). Background factors such as the individual's personality and past experiences interact with proximal factors in the environment, resulting in the individual's response. Demographic characteristics, psychosocial variables, and the function that is compromised by the dementia are all background factors. Proximal factors include the individual's physical and social environment, as well as her or his psychological and physiological need state. Because of cognitive impairment, the individual's response may not be effective, as in the case of vocalizations or extreme passivity, but is the individual's best effort to respond to the situation. Behaviors can best be managed by trying to understand what the patient is trying to tell you through his or her behavior. The caregiver can explore the individual's background for clues about the behavior, in addition to factors in the current environment.

Theory of Adaptation to Chronic Pain

Dunn (2004) developed the Theory of Adaptation to Chronic Pain because of the prevalence of chronic disease resulting in unmanaged pain in this population, with consequences including depression and loss of function. The management of pain is based on the magnitude of the pain stimulus, the autonomic physiological response, and the adaptive ability of the coping strategies used by the individual. Religious and nonreligious coping strategies are used. Spiritual aspects are emphasized because this dimension is often neglected in practice. A positive outcome results in physical and spiritual well-being. Dunn's model supports the work of others, such as Ramsey and Bleiszner (1999), who explored how women's faith helped them through their lives in coping with a variety of issues through the development of what they called "spiritual resiliency."

SUMMARY

Theory should provide a means to understand various phenomena in gerontological nursing and guide practice, which can then be validated through nursing research. The outcome of this scholarly work is to determine the best practices for caring for our patients. Each of the major theorists explored concepts important to gerontological nursing practice: self-care, adaptation, holism, conservation, systems theory, and goal attainment. The middle-range theories guide us in managing more specific issues, such as caring for people from different cultures, comfort needs, managing chronic and life-threatening illnesses, and providing social support. Gerontological nurses have more specific direction from the theories on family caregiving, managing patients with dementia, and chronic pain. Gerontological nurses may apply these concepts without being aware of the theoretical influences on their practice. However, professional nursing practice should be guided by thoughtful application of theory, based on an understanding of nursing concepts and their historical development. We hope that this chapter will encourage nurses to explore the literature about issues in their practice and encourage theory development and research into areas that remain challenging.

REFERENCES

Algase, D., Beck, C., Kolanowski, A., Whall, A., Berent, S., Richards, K., & Beattie, E. (1996). Need-driven dementia-compromised behavior: An alternative view of disruptive behavior. *American Journal of Alzheimer's Disease, 11*(6), 10-19.

Alligood, M. R., & Tomey, A. M. (Eds.). (2002). *Nursing theory: Utilization and application* (2nd ed.). St. Louis: Mosby.

American Nurses Association. (2001). *Scope and standards of gerontological nursing practice* (2nd ed.). Washington, DC: American Nurses Publishing.

Bailey, D. E., & Stewart, J. L. (2002). Uncertainty in illness. In A. M. Tomey & M. R. Alligood (Eds.), *Nursing theorists and their work* (5th ed.). St. Louis: Mosby.

Beery, T., Dolline, A. M, Gers, M., LaCharity, L, Robinson, D., & Torok, L. S. (2001). Grand nursing theories and conceptual models. In D. Robinson & C. P. Kish (Eds.), *Core concepts in advanced practice nursing*. St. Louis: Mosby.

Bernick, L. (2004). Caring for older adults: Practice guided by Watson's Caring-Healing Model. *Nursing Science Quarterly, 17*(2), 128-134.

Brown, S. J. (2000). Direct clinical practice. In A. B. Hamric, J. A. Spross, & C. M. Hanson (Eds.), *Advanced practice nursing: An integrative approach* (3rd ed.). St. Louis: Elsevier.

Carper, B. A. (1978). Fundamental patterns of knowing in nursing. *Advances in Nursing Science, 1*(1), 13-24.

Chinn, P. L., & Kramer, M. K. (2004). *Integrated knowledge development in nursing* (6th ed.). St. Louis: Mosby.

Corbin, J. M. (1998). The Corbin and Strauss chronic illness trajectory model: An update. *Scholarly Inquiry for Nursing Practice, 12*(1), 33-41.

Corbin, J. M., & Strauss, A. (1992). A nursing model for chronic illness management based upon the trajectory framework. In P. Woog (Ed.), *The chronic illness trajectory framework: The Corbin and Strauss nursing model*. New York: Springer.

Dollins, A. M., & Niemer, L. M. (2001). Nursing theory and advanced practice. In D. Robinson & C. P. Kish (Eds.), *Core concepts in advanced practice nursing*. St. Louis: Mosby.

Dunn, K. S. (2004). Toward a middle-range theory of adaptation to chronic pain. *Nursing Science Quarterly, 17*(1), 78-84.

Fawcett, J. (2000). *Analysis and evaluation of contemporary nursing knowledge: Nursing models and theories*. Philadelphia: F. A. Davis.

Fawcett, J., Newman, D. M., & McAllister, M. (2004). Advanced practice nursing and conceptual models of nursing. *Nursing Science Quarterly, 17*(2), 135-138.

Gullick, E. E. (1998). Symptom and activities of daily living trajectory in multiple sclerosis: A 10-year study. *Nursing Research, 47*(3), 137-146.

Hall, G. R., & Buckwalter, K. C. (1987). Progressively lowered stress threshold: A conceptual model for care of adults with Alzheimer's disease. *Archives of Psychiatric Nursing, 1*(6), 399-406.

Hauner, B., & Henderson, V. (1955). *Textbook of the principles and practice of nursing*. New York: Macmillan.

Herbert, J. (1989). A model for Anna: Using the Johnson model of nursing in the care of one 75-year-old stroke patient. *Journal of Clinical Practice, Education and Management, 3*(42), 30-34.

Johnson, D. E. (1980). The behavioral system model for nursing. In J. P. Riehl & C. Roy (Eds.), *Conceptual models for nursing practice* (2nd ed.). New York: Appleton-Century-Crofts.

Keller, A. W. (2001). Nursing's utilization of theory. In D. Robinson & C. P. Kish (Eds.), *Core concepts in advanced practice nursing*. St. Louis: Mosby.

King, I. (1981). *A theory for nursing: Systems, concepts, process*. New York: John Wiley & Sons.

Kolcaba, K. (1994). A theory of holistic comfort for nursing. *Journal of Advanced Nursing, 19*, 1178-1184.

Kolanowski, A. M. (1999). An overview of the need-driven dementia-compromised behavior model. *Journal of Gerontological Nursing, 25*(9), 7-9.

Leininger, M., & McFarland, M. R. (2002). *Transcultural nursing: Concepts, theories, research and practice*. New York: McGraw-Hill.

Leveille, S. G., Fried, L. P., McMullen, W., & Guralnik, J. M. (2004). Advancing the taxonomy of disability in older adults. *Journal of Gerontology, 59A*, 86-93.

Levine, M. E. (1990). Conservation and integrity . . . Levine's conservation model. In M. E. Parker (Ed.), *Nursing theories in practice*. New York: National League for Nursing.

Liehr, P., & Smith, M. J. (1999). Middle range theory: Spinning research and practice to create knowledge for the new millennium. *Advances in Nursing Science, 21*(4), 81-91.

Matteson, M. A., Linton, A. D., & Barnes, S. J. (1996). Cognitive developmental approach to dementia. *Journal of Nursing Scholarship, 28*(3), 233-240.

McEwen, M. (2002). Overview of theory in nursing. In M. McEwen & E. M. Willis, *Theoretical Basis for Nursing*. Philadelphia: Lippincott.

Mishel, M. H. (1988). Uncertainty in illness. *Image: Journal of Nursing Scholarship, 22*, 225-231.

Mishel, M. H. (1990). Reconceptualization of the uncertainty in illness theory. *Image: Journal of Nursing Scholarship, 24*, 256-262.

NANDA International. (2003). *NANDA nursing diagnoses: Definitions and classification 2003-2004*. Philadelphia: NANDA.

Norbeck, J. S., Lindsey, A. M., & Carrierei, V. L. (1981). The development of an instrument to measure social support. *Nursing Research, 9*, 30264-30269.

Norbeck, J. S., & Tilden, V. P. (1988). International nursing research in social support: Theoretical and methodological issues. *Journal of Advanced Nursing, 13*(2), 173-178.

Orem, D., Taylor, S. G., & Renpenning, K. M. (2001). *Nursing: Concepts of practice* (6th ed.). St. Louis: Mosby.

Pender, N. J., Murdaugh, C. L., & Parsons, M. A. (2001). *Health promotion in nursing practice* (4th ed.). New York: Appleton & Lange.

Perry, A. G. (2005). Theoretical foundations of nursing practice. In *Fundamentals of nursing* (6th ed.). St. Louis: Mosby.

Pfettscher, S. A. (2002). Florence Nightengale: Modern nursing. In A. M. Tomey & M. R. Alligood (Eds.), *Nursing theorists and their work* (5th ed.). St. Louis: Mosby.

Phillips, L. R., Brewer, B. B., & Torres de Ardon, E. (2001). The elder image scale: A method for indexing history and emotion in family caregiving. *Journal of Nursing Measurement, 9*(1), 23-47.

Phillips, L. R., Morrison, E., Steffl, B., Chae, Y. M., Cromwell, S. L., & Russell, C. K. (1995). Effects of the situational context and interactional process on the quality of family caregiving. *Research in Nursing and Health, 18*, 205-216.

Phillips, L. R., & Rempusheski, V. F. (1986). Caring for the frail elderly at home: Toward a theoretical explanation of the dynamics of poor quality family caregiving. *Advances in Nursing Science, 8*(4), 62-84.

Prochaska, J. O., Redding, C. A., & Evers, K. E. (2002). The Transtheoretical Model and stages of change. In K. Glanz, B. K. Rimer, & B. M. Lewis (Eds.), *Health behavior and health education: Theory, research, and practice*. San Francisco: Jossey-Bass.

Ramsey, J. L., & Bleiszner, R. (1999). *Spiritual resiliency in older women: Models of strength for challenges through the life span*. Thousand Oaks, CA: Sage.

Rogers, M. E. (1983). Science of unitary human being: A paradigm for nursing. In I. W. Clements & F. B. Roberts (Eds.), *Family health: A theoretical approach to nursing care*. New York: John Wiley & Sons.

Rogers, M. E. (2002). Unitary health care: Martha Rogers science of unitary human beings. Retrieved October 15, 2004, from www.medweb.uwcm.ac.uk/martha.

Roy, C., & Andrews, H. A. (1999). *The Roy adaptation model* (2nd ed.). Stamford, CT: Appleton & Lange.

Schumacher, K. L., Stewart, B. J., & Archbold, P. G. (1998). Conceptualization and measurement of doing family caregiving well. *Image: Journal of Nursing Scholarship, 30*(1), 63-69.

Smith, M., Gerdner, L. A., Hall, G. R., & Buckwalter, K. C. (2004). History, development, and future of the Progressively Lowered Stress Threshold: A conceptual model for dementia care. *Journal of the American Geriatrics Society, 52*(10), 1755-1760.

Tomey, A. M., & Alligood, M. R. (2002). *Nursing theorists and their work* (5th ed.). St. Louis: Mosby.

Verbrugge, L. M., & Jette, A. M. (1994). The disablement process. *Social Science & Medicine, 38*(1), 1-14.

Whall, A. L., & Colling, K. B. (2005). Middle range theories of dementia care. In Fitzpatrick, J. J., & Wallace, M. (Eds.), *Encyclopedia of nursing research* (2nd ed.). New York: Springer.

Chapter 5

Evidence-Based Practice

Marita G. Titler & Jane Hsiao-Chen Tang

Objectives

Differentiate among research utilization, evidence-based practice, and conduct of research.

Define key terms in evidence-based practice.

Describe the steps of evidence-based practice.

Identify clinical topics of evidence-based practice for care of older adults.

Describe strategies for implementation of evidence-based practices.

Describe sites of care delivery for older adults and the potential influence on adoption of evidence-based practices.

Identify resources for evidence-based practice.

Describe the role of nurses in promoting use of evidence in care of older adults.

Identify future trends in evidence-based practice and translation science.

One in eight Americans (12.4%) is age 65 years or older (U.S. Census Bureau, 2000a), and by the year 2020, this is predicted to be 53.7 million (16.5% of the population) (U.S. Census Bureau, 2000a, 2000b). Approximately 50% of all hospital beds are occupied by patients older than 65 years of age, and about 25% of all inpatient hospital days are used by people older than 75 years of age (Eliopoulos, 1997). Evidence-based practice (EBP) has the potential to significantly reduce morbidity in older adults because of the sound scientific base for practice in a number of areas (e.g., treatment of hypertension; pain management). The Agency for Healthcare Research and Quality (AHRQ) (Farquhar, Stryer, & Slutsky, 2002; McCormick, Cummings, & Kovner, 1997) and others (Bottrell, Abraham, Fulmer, & Mezey, 1999; Mion, 1998; Rochon, Dikinson, & Gordon, 1997; Titler & Mentes, 1999) are responsive to the needs of this vulnerable population by funding synthesis reports and studies on prevention and treatment

of illnesses prevalent in older adults. Despite the availability of the evidence on health care interventions whose efficacy has been documented, EBPs are not consistently implemented by providers (Baker & Feder, 1997; Burns, Pahor, & Shorr, 1997; Kirchhoff, 2004; Schnelle, Cruise, Rahman, & Ouslander, 1998; Titler & Mentes, 1999).

"The stark reality [is] that we invest billions in research to find appropriate treatments, we spend more than $1 trillion on healthcare annually, we have extraordinary capacity to deliver the best care in the world, but we repeatedly fail to translate that knowledge and capacity into clinical practice" (Institute of Medicine, 2003, p. 2). For example, failure to rescue, decubitus ulcers, and postoperative sepsis accounted for 60% of all patient safety incidents among Medicare patients hospitalized from 2000 through 2002; decubitus ulcers accounted for $2.57 billion in excess inpatient costs to Medicare over 3 years (2000-2002); and postoperative pulmonary embolism or deep vein thrombosis accounted for $1.4 billion in excess inpatient costs to Medicare over 3 years (2000-2002) (Health Grades, Inc., 2004). It is all nurses' responsibility to use the current best research evidence in care of older adults. This chapter discusses the process of EBP in relation to care of older adults.

OVERVIEW OF EVIDENCE-BASED PRACTICE

The relationships among conduct, dissemination, and use of research findings in practice are illustrated in Figure 5-1. Conduct of research is the analysis of data collected from a homogeneous group of subjects who meet study inclusion and exclusion criteria for the purpose of answering specific research questions or testing specified hypotheses. Research design, methods, and statistical analyses are guided by the state of the science in the area of investigation. Traditionally, conduct of

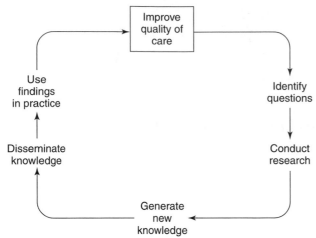

Figure 5-1 The model of the relationship among conduct, dissemination, and use of research. (Redrawn from Weiler, K., Buckwalter, K., & Titler, M. [1994]. Debate: Is nursing research used in practice? In J. McCloskey & H. Grace [Eds.], *Current issues in nursing* [4th ed.]. St. Louis: Mosby. For permission to use or reproduce, please contact Dr. Titler.)

research has included dissemination of findings via research reports in journals and at scientific conferences. In comparison, research utilization is the process of using research findings to improve patient care. It encompasses dissemination of scientific knowledge; critique of studies; synthesis of research findings; determining applicability of findings for practice; developing an evidence-based standard or guideline; implementing the standard; and evaluating the practice change with respect to staff, patients, and cost/resource utilization (Titler et al., 2001).

Evidence-based practice (EBP) has been defined by some experts as the synthesis and use of scientific findings from randomized clinical trials only (Dickersin & Manheimer, 1998; Estabrooks, 1998, 2004; Geyman, 1998; Mion, 1998), whereas others define EBP more broadly to include use of empirical evidence from other scientific methods (e.g., descriptive studies) and use of information from case reports and expert opinion (Cook, 1998; Sackett, Straus, Richardson, Rosenberg, & Haynes, 2000). Sackett and colleagues (2000) define evidence-based practice as "the integration of best research evidence with clinical expertise and patient values." Evidence-based practice encompasses use of research findings in clinical and operational decision making, as well as use of case reports and expert opinion in deciding the practices to be used in health care. When enough research evidence is available, it is recommended that the evidence base for practice be based on the research. Box 5-1 describes the efforts of the National Institute on Aging in developing a research base for practice, written from the perspective of a nurse researcher.

In some cases, a sufficient research base may not be available, and health care providers may supplement research findings with other types of evidence such as expert opinion and case reports when developing an EBP guideline. As more research is done in a specific area, the research evidence can be used to update and refine the guideline. When EBPs are effectively implemented, patient outcomes improve and resource use declines (Lubarsky et al., 1997; McCormick et al., 1997; Newman, Pyne, Leigh, Rounce, & Cowling, 2000; Schneider & Eisenberg, 1998; Titler, 1998). There is no guarantee, however, that the evidence is used in practice (Berg, Atkins, & Tierney, 1997; Dickersin & Manheimer, 1998; Kamerow, 1997), and use of evidence by nurses and physicians is sporadic at best (Atkins, Kamerow, & Eisenberg, 1998; Bostrom & Suter, 1993; Carroll et al., 1997; Cronenwett, 1995; Herr et al., 2004; Kirchhoff, 2004; McCurren, 1995; Pettengill, Gilles, & Clar, 1994; Rutledge, Greene, Mooney, Nail, & Ropka, 1996; Schneider & Eisenberg, 1998; Titler et al., 2003). Selected key terms used in evidence-based practice are defined in Box 5-2.

Multifaceted active dissemination strategies are needed to promote use of evidence in health care decision making and must address both the individual practitioner and organizational perspective. When nurses decide individually what evidence to use in practice, considerable variability in practice patterns results, potentially resulting in adverse patient outcomes. For example, a solely "individual" perspective of evidence-based practice would leave the decision about use of evidence-based pressure ulcer prevention techniques to each nurse. Some nurses may be familiar with the research findings for preventing pressure ulcers whereas others may not. This is likely to result in different and conflicting practices being used as nurses change shifts every 8 to 12 hours. From an organizational perspective, policies and procedures on prevention of pressure ulcers are written, based on evidence, and then adoption of these practices by nurses is systematically promoted in the organization.

MODELS OF EVIDENCE-BASED PRACTICE

Multiple models of EBP are available (Barnsteiner, Ford, & Howe, 1995; Berwick, 2003; Dufault, 2001; Goode & Piedalue, 1999; Logan, Harrison, Graham, Dunn, & Bissonnette, 1999; Olade, 2004; Rosswurm & Larrabee, 1999; Rycroft-Malone et al., 2002; Soukup, 2000; Stetler, 2003; Titler & Everett, 2001; Titler et al., 2001; Wagner et al., 2001). Common elements of these models are syntheses of evidence, implementation, evaluation of the impact on patient care, and consideration of the context/setting in which the evidence is implemented.

Box 5-1 *Reflections on Gerontological Research Supporting Evidence-Based Practice*

"The remarkable growth of the older population worldwide poses both opportunities and challenges. Notable progress in several areas of research—biomedical, social, and behavioral—have improved health and function and contributed to reduced rates of disability for older people. At the same time, unprecedented numbers of elders in the coming decades will face the risks of disease, frailty, and dependence. The need to understand the factors that promote health and independence and those that lead to disease and disability has never been more urgent" (Hodes, 2005).

It is in this context that the mission of the National Institute on Aging (NIA), part of the National Institutes of Health (NIH), takes on increasing urgency and relevance for supporting research in aging. It is also in this context that commitments to aging research and the translation of research into evidence-based practice takes on urgent importance. The NIA, by congressional authorization, has primary responsibility for research into Alzheimer's disease, and a substantial part of this research provides the foundation for practice in this area today. I have been fortunate to work with the NIA over the past 8 years in research and training endeavors.

The NIA's mission is to improve the health and well-being of older Americans through research, and specifically to do the following:

- Support and conduct high-quality research on
  - Aging processes
  - Age-related diseases, such as Alzheimer's disease
  - Special problems and needs of the aged
- Train and develop highly skilled research scientists from all population groups
- Develop and maintain state-of-the-art resources to accelerate research progress
- Disseminate information and communicate with the public and interested groups on health and research advances and on new directions for research

Since the NIA's founding, we have learned much about the biological, behavioral, and social changes that occur with advancing age. We now know that aging itself is not the cause of disease, disability, and frailty. Rather, disease and disabling processes influenced by age-related changes in the body and by unhealthy choices and sedentary lifestyles are the most important factors in compromising the quality of life for older people. NIA research has benefited older adults across ages, diseases, and conditions.

The eruption of knowledge that has occurred in the past 25 years and that continues today as the foundation for evidence-based practice has set the course for a hopeful roadmap to tomorrow. NIA-funded researchers are making a difference! The evidence base supporting advances in Alzheimer's disease reveals that 15 years ago, we did not know any of the genes that could cause Alzheimer's disease. Less than 3 years ago, we did not understand how plaques and tangles related to each other. Just over 5 years ago, the NIA did not fund prevention clinical trials and we had no way to identify people at risk for Alzheimer's disease. Today we know the three major genes for early-onset Alzheimer's disease and we know one of the major risk factor genes for late-onset disease.

Nurses such as Dr. Cornelia Beck at the University of Arkansas, Dr. Ruth Mulnard at the University of California–Irvine, Dr. Olivia Washington at Wayne State University, and Dr. May Wykle at Case Western Reserve University are just a few examples of nurses funded by the NIA and contributing to research evidence benefiting practice and older adults. We have come a long way to the evidence that what is good for the heart is probably good for the brain. For example, three institutes, the NIA, the National Institute of Mental Health (NIMH), and the National Institute of Neurological Disorders and Stroke (NINDS), have joined efforts to launch the evidence-based Cognitive and Emotional Health Project (CEHP). Current evidence indicates that a large number of older adults are at substantial risk for cognitive impairment from many causes as they age. The same is true for emotional disorders. Although research into biological mechanisms and environmental and social effects is yielding promising results in both animal and human studies, much remains to be discovered. Advances in understanding the positive and negative changes in cognition and emotion in adulthood, and what can be done to preserve and enhance positive outcomes, is at the core of the missions of the participating institutes. The overall goal of the CEHP is to assess the state of longitudinal and epidemiological research on demographic, social, and biological determinants of cognitive and emotional health in aging adults and the pathways by which cognitive and emotional health may reciprocally influence each other.

Despite these and other efforts, more can be done to assist nurses and other health care providers to use substantiated evidence from clinical trials and other empirical evidence from various research designs and studies. The NIA Web site at www.nia.nih.gov and the publications Web site at www.nia.nih.gov/HealthInformation/Publications are useful sites for dissemination of aging research results that should assist practitioners and others to build a strong evidenced base for practice.

J Taylor Harden

J Taylor Harden, RN, PhD, FAAN
Assistant to the Director for Special Populations
National Institute on Aging
National Institutes of Health
Bethesda, Maryland

BOX 5-2 Selected Key Terms Used in Evidence-Based Practice

TERM	DEFINITION
Audit and feedback	Audit and feedback is monitoring of critical indicators of practice (e.g., meperidine use) and providing the data/information back to those responsible for patient care (Davis et al., 1995; Oxman et al., 1995; Schoenbaum et al., 1995). Audit and feedback is an ongoing process that is done periodically (e.g., every 3 months) during the implementation, evaluation, and sustainability phases of translating evidence into practice. Feedback reports can use data aggregated at different levels such as the individual provider, patient care unit, service line, organization, or health system. It is helpful to provide data that compares indicators over time to demonstrate improvements (or lack thereof) in the evidence-based practices (Jamtvedt et al., 2004).
"Best" practice	A term that has many meanings, including use of the best scientific evidence, use of best empirical evidence (case reports), use of evidence-based findings, use of institutional data (e.g., fall rates), and use of evidence from another institution that has been able to achieve outcomes (e.g., length of stay) that your institution is striving for. Because of the overwhelming diversity of meaning, we recommend avoiding use of this term.
Change champion	Change champions are practitioners from the local peer group who continually promote the evidence-based practice. He or she imparts information about the evidence-based practice, encourages peers to align their practice with the evidence, demonstrates skills and knowledge necessary to carry out the evidence-based practice, and teaches new and existing personnel about the evidence-based practice (Titler & Everett, 2001).
Clinical practice guideline	A systematically developed statement designed to help practitioner and patient make decisions about appropriate health care for specific clinical circumstances (NHS Research and Development: Centre for Evidence Based Medicine, 2001).
Clinical significance	A judgment about the interpretation of the statistical results (that the difference or relationship has meaning for patient care) (Mateo & Kirchhoff, 1999).
Conduct of research	The scientific process of investigating a phenomenon (e.g., acute pain management in older adults) that begins with a problem statement, the current state of the science in the identified area, and a series of research questions or hypotheses to address the problem and advance the science of the phenomenon under study. The research questions are followed by a description of the study design (randomized clinical trial, experimental, quasi-experimental, exploratory, cross-sectional correlational design, etc.), specification of subject inclusion criteria, and study methods that include subject recruitment, instrumentation (e.g., questionnaires, bioinstruments), data collection, and delivery of the study intervention. Data analysis procedures, explication of findings to address each research question, and implications for future research and for practice conclude the scientific process. Many investigators believe that research unpublished is research undone, and thus include publication of the study as the final step in the conduct of research.
Confidence interval (CI)	Quantifies the uncertainty in measurement. It is usually reported as a 95% CI, which is the range of values within which we can be 95% sure that the true value for the whole population lies. For example, for an NNT (see definition later in this box) of 10 with a 95% CI of 5 to 15, we would have 95% confidence that the true NNT value lies between 5 and 15 (Mount Sinai Hospital–University Health Network: Centre for Evidence-Based Medicine, 2001).

BOX 5-2 Selected Key Terms Used in Evidence-Based Practice—cont'd

Control group

Research participants who do not receive experimental treatment and whose data are used for comparison with the experimental group (Mateo & Kirchhoff, 1999).

Cost-effectiveness analysis

Converts effects into health terms and describes the costs for some additional health gain (e.g., cost of preventing each additional myocardial infarction) (NHS Research and Development: Centre for Evidence Based Medicine, 2001).

Cross-sectional study

The observation of a defined population at a single point in time or time interval. Exposure and outcome are determined simultaneously. See also glossary of study designs (NHS Research and Development: Centre for Evidence Based Medicine, 2001).

Demographics

Background variables (age, sex, education, etc.) that define the sample or participants (Mateo & Kirchhoff, 1999).

Effectiveness

Effectiveness is determining if an intervention or treatment works in the real world without controls of an efficacy study.

Efficacy

Efficacy describes research that is designed to test interventions under tightly controlled conditions (e.g., dedicated person to deliver the intervention in a controlled clinical setting) with a homogeneous patient population (e.g., women 65 to 80 years of age with osteoporosis). Efficacy studies are done before application of the intervention in the real world (Brown, 2002).

Evidence-based guideline

A written guide of evidence-based health care practices/actions. The recommendations for practice should be referenced and identify the strength of the evidence for each of the practice recommendations. Component parts of evidence-based guidelines vary but usually include a brief description of the practice topic (e.g., acute pain), the types of patients that the guideline can be used for (e.g., elders, hospitalized elders, children, adults), the assessment and interventions used to carry out the EBPs, and the risk/benefits of the EBPs.

Experimental group

Research participants who receive experimental treatment (Mateo & Kirchhoff, 1999).

Focus groups

Focus groups are discussions and group interviews with six to eight people to elicit information about a specific topic. This methodology can be used as a type of qualitative evaluation following implementation of an EBP guideline. It can also be employed as a strategy for implementing an EBP guideline. For example, focus groups might be used to elicit information from potential users of the EBP regarding components they view as potentially problematic to implement, barriers to and facilitators of use of the EBP, and system changes (e.g., documentation systems) necessary for implementing the EBP.

Macrosystem

This term is used interchangeably with *organizational context* to convey the organization or health system "at large" in which the EBP is being implemented. Macrosystems are composed of multiple microsystems.

Meta-analysis

An overview that uses quantitative methods to summarize results.

OR

Mathematical summary of results of several studies.

(Mateo & Kirchhoff, 1999; NHS Research and Development: Centre for Evidence Based Medicine, 2001)

Continued

BOX 5-2 Selected Key Terms Used in Evidence-Based Practice—cont'd

Microsystem	The patient care unit(s), ambulatory clinic(s), or other specific patient care areas within the macrosystem in which the EBP is implemented. For example, an EBP on acute pain management may be first implemented in two or three patient care units or microsystems before being "rolled out" across the entire organization or macrosystem. Microsystems are composed of the unit culture, leadership, nature of the personnel, and manner in which people in the unit relate to one another in delivery of services/patient care, and routine monitoring of performance within the specified patient care unit.
Number needed to treat (NNT)	The number of patients who need to be treated to prevent one bad outcome. It is the inverse of the absolute relative risk (ARR): NNT = 1/ARR (NHS Research and Development: Centre for Evidence Based Medicine, 2001).
Opinion leaders	Opinion leaders are informal leaders from the local health care setting who are viewed as important and respected sources of influence among their peer group (e.g., nurses, physicians). A key characteristic of opinion leaders is that they are trusted to evaluate new information in the context of group norms. Opinion leaders are evaluators who are trusted to judge the fit between a technology or new practice and the local situation (Titler & Everett, 2001).
Organizational context	The organizational context is the health system environment in which the proposed EBP is to be implemented. This may be an acute care, home health care, or long-term care system. The core elements that help describe the organizational context include the prevailing culture of the system (e.g., patient centered); the nature of human relationships in the system, including the leadership styles that are operational (e.g., teamwork, clear role delineation); and the organization's approach to routine monitoring of performance of systems and services within the organization (e.g., routine use of audit and feedback) (Kitson, Harvey, & McCormack, 1998).
Outcome effectiveness	The ability of an intervention or care process to produce (or fail to produce) desired outcomes (e.g., decreased pain intensity, decreased length of stay) in the typical practice environment with a variety of patients, many of whom have other factors that may affect the amount of benefit or outcome of the intervention (Brown, 2002). This is often used to denote the application of an intervention in the "real world" of practice. Evaluation of an EBP project is a type of outcome effectiveness. Evaluation of an EBP is important to determine (1) if the intervention can be used successfully in day-to-day practice and (2) if application of interventions in the real world of practice results in similar outcomes as those achieved in efficacy studies of the intervention.
Outcome evaluation	A quality improvement technique that monitors outcomes, usually of patients, to determine if the outcomes from application of the EBP are similar to those intended, such as a decrease in pain intensity scores. Staff and fiscal outcomes might also be used in outcome evaluation.
Outreach/academic detailing	*Outreach* and *academic detailing* are terms often used synonymously to convey the use of a trained individual who meets one-on-one with practitioners in their setting to provide information about the EBP. Information conveyed during outreach may include data on provider performance, information about the EBP, or consultation regarding specific issues in use of the EBP. Studies have demonstrated that outreach visits alone or used in combination with other translation interventions result in positive changes in practice behaviors of nurses and physicians (Titler, 2005).

Although review of these models is beyond the scope of this chapter, implementing evidence in practice must be guided by a conceptual model to organize the strategies being used and to elucidate the extraneous variables (e.g., behaviors and facilitators) that may influence adoption of EBPs (e.g., organizational size, characteristics of users). Conceptual models used in translating research into practice studies, funded by AHRQ, include adult learning, health education, social influence, marketing, organizational, and behavior theories (Farquhar

BOX 5-2 Selected Key Terms Used in Evidence-Based Practice—cont'd	
Performance gap assessment	Performance gap assessment is baseline evaluation of practice performance that informs members of an organization about a particular practice, and opportunities for improving performance related to a specific indicator (e.g., frequency of acute pain assessment) or set of indicators (e.g., acute pain management of hospitalized elders) (Oxman et al., 1995; Schoenbaum et al., 1995). This is a data-driven strategy/intervention used early in the implementation phase of translating evidence into practice to convey to individuals the congruency or incongruency between their current clinical practice and recommended practices from evidence-based guidelines, EBP reports, or systematic reviews.
Process evaluation	Process evaluation is a quality improvement technique that monitors specific indicators directly related to the EBP. Monitoring nurses' use of a standard pain intensity scale for pain assessment is a type of process monitor to determine if nurses' processes of acute pain management are aligned with the evidence on this topic. Process evaluation is usually undertaken to determine if the EBP is being used/implemented consistently by care providers.
Randomized controlled clinical trial	A group of patients is randomized into an experimental group and a control group. These groups are followed-up for the variables or outcomes of interest (NHS Research and Development: Centre for Evidence Based Medicine, 2001).
Strength of evidence	This is an overall grade of the strength of evidence on a specific topic. Although various grading schemas are used, practice recommendations are usually graded using A, B, C, and so forth, with A being consistent findings from several randomized clinical trials and D or E grades used to convey conflicting research results, and/or use of expert opinion, case reports, or consensus (AHRQ, 2002).
Sustainability	The ability of an organization or individual to continue use of the EBP in routine clinical care following initial implementation.
Systematic reviews	Systematic reviews are a summary of past research on a topic of interest. The summary is arrived at through a rigorous scientific process similar to methods used in primary research. The scientific process used in systematic reviews includes the following: the review question(s), how studies will be located, methods used for critical appraisal of the primary studies, criteria for inclusion and exclusion of studies, synthesis methods (e.g., meta-analysis, narrative summary across studies), and summary recommendations for practice and future research. The final product is a summary of the best available scientific evidence following application of the aforementioned process (AHRQ, 2002; Joanna Briggs Institute, 2000, 2001).
Translation research	Translation research is the scientific investigation of methods and variables that influence rate and extent of adoption of evidence-based practices by individuals and organizations to improve clinical and operational decision making in the delivery of health care services. This includes testing the effect of strategies/interventions for promoting the adoption of EBPs, with the outcomes being the rate and extent of health care provider use of these practices (Titler & Everett, 2001).

et al., 2002). Translation science investigators (Doebbeling et al., 2002; Jones, 2000; Titler & Everett, 2001; Titler et al., 2003) have used E. Rogers' Diffusion of Innovation Model (Rogers, 1995, 2003), the Promoting Action on Research Implementation in Health Services Model (Rycroft-Malone et al., 2002), the "push/pull" framework (Lavis et al., 2003; Nutley & Davies, 2000; Nutley, Davies, & Walter, 2003), the decision-making framework (Lomas et al., 1991), and the Institute for Health Improvement (IHI) model (Berwick, 2003) in translation science and EBP.

Iowa Model of Evidence-Based Practice

The Iowa Model of Evidence-Based Practice is overviewed here as an example of an EBP model (Figure 5-2). This model has been widely disseminated and adopted in academic and clinical settings (Estabrooks, Winther,

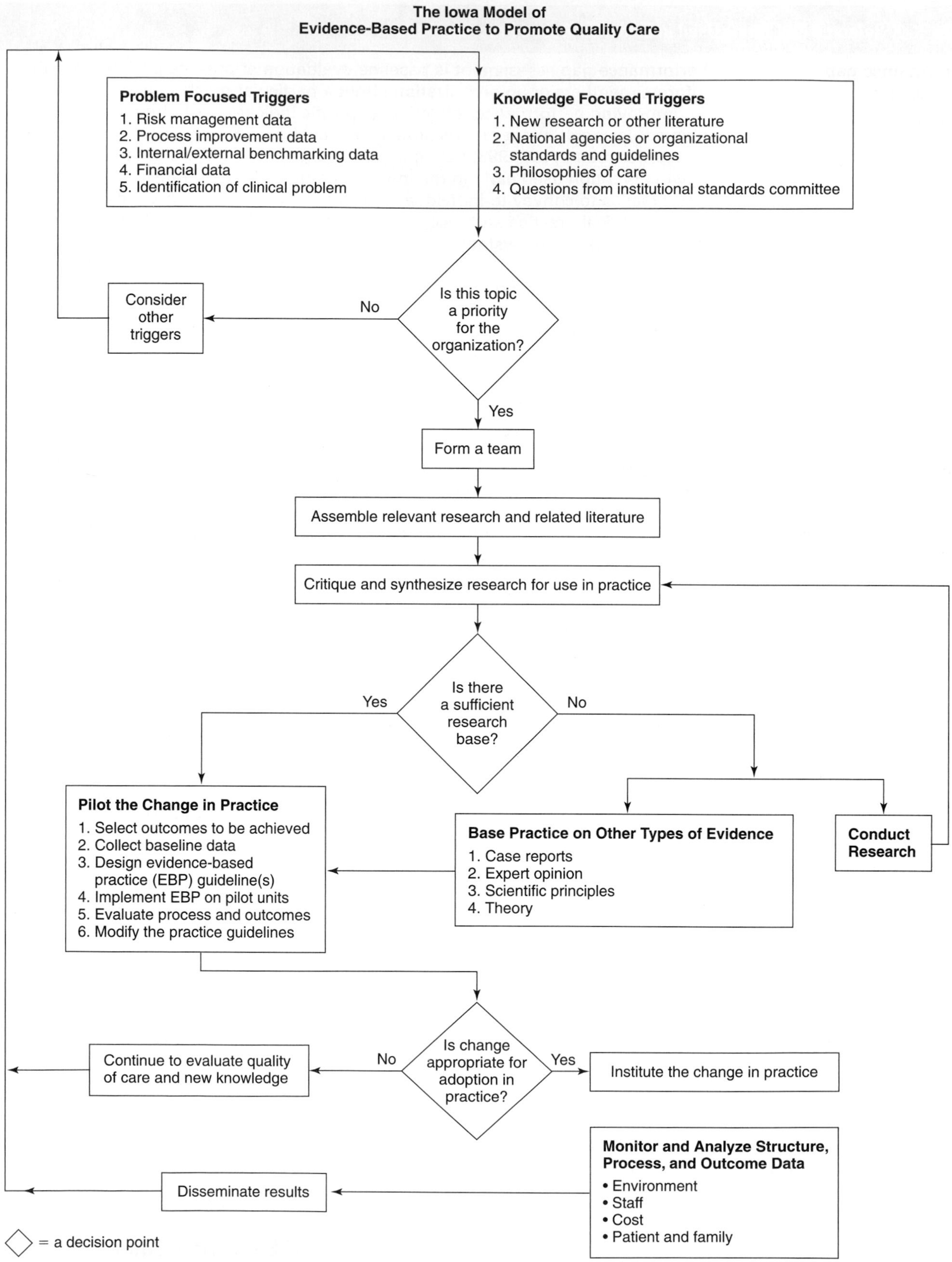

**The Iowa Model of
Evidence-Based Practice to Promote Quality Care**

Problem Focused Triggers

1. Risk management data
2. Process improvement data
3. Internal/external benchmarking data
4. Financial data
5. Identification of clinical problem

Knowledge Focused Triggers

1. New research or other literature
2. National agencies or organizational standards and guidelines
3. Philosophies of care
4. Questions from institutional standards committee

Is this topic a priority for the organization?

No → Consider other triggers

Yes

Form a team

Assemble relevant research and related literature

Critique and synthesize research for use in practice

Is there a sufficient research base?

Yes / No

Pilot the Change in Practice

1. Select outcomes to be achieved
2. Collect baseline data
3. Design evidence-based practice (EBP) guideline(s)
4. Implement EBP on pilot units
5. Evaluate process and outcomes
6. Modify the practice guidelines

Base Practice on Other Types of Evidence

1. Case reports
2. Expert opinion
3. Scientific principles
4. Theory

Conduct Research

Is change appropriate for adoption in practice?

No → Continue to evaluate quality of care and new knowledge

Yes → Institute the change in practice

Monitor and Analyze Structure, Process, and Outcome Data

• Environment
• Staff
• Cost
• Patient and family

Disseminate results

◇ = a decision point

Figure 5-2 The Iowa Model of Evidence-Based Practice to Promote Quality Care. (From Titler, M. G., Kleiber, C., Steelman, V. J., Rakel, B. A., Budreau, G., Buckwalter, K. C., et al. [2001]. The Iowa Model of Evidence-Based Practice to Promote Quality Care. *Critical Care Nursing Clinics of North America, 13*(4), 497-509. For permission to use or reproduce, please contact Dr. Titler.)

& Derksen, 2004; Titler et al., 2001). Since the original publication of this model in 1994 (Titler et al., 1994), the authors have received 165 written requests to use the model for publications, presentations, graduate and undergraduate research courses, and clinical research programs. It has been cited 52 times in journal articles (Web of Science, 2006). This organizational, collaborative model incorporates conduct of research, use of research evidence, and other types of evidence (Titler et al., 2001). Authors of the Iowa Model of Evidence-Based Practice adopted the definition of EBP as the conscientious and judicious use of current best evidence to guide health care decisions (Sackett, Rosenberg, Gray, Haynes, & Richardson, 1996). Levels of evidence range from randomized clinical trials to case reports and expert opinion. Knowledge- and problem-focused "triggers" lead staff members to question current nursing practice and whether patient care can be improved through the use of research findings. If the literature review and the critique of studies result in an insufficient number of scientifically sound studies to use as a base for practice, consideration is given to conducting a study. Nurses in practice collaborate with scientists in nursing and other disciplines to conduct clinical research that addresses practice problems encountered in the care of patients. Findings from such studies are then combined with findings from existing scientific knowledge to develop and implement these practices. If there is insufficient research to guide practice, and conducting a study is not feasible, other types of evidence (e.g., case reports, expert opinion, scientific principles, theory) are used or combined with available research evidence to guide practice. Priority is given to projects in which a high proportion of practice is guided by research evidence. Practice guidelines usually reflect research and nonresearch evidence and therefore are considered EBP guidelines.

Clinical Topics of Evidence-Based Practice for Care of Older Adults

Many clinical topics for care of older adults have an evidence base to guide clinical decision making. These include prevention and treatment of pressure ulcers, fall prevention, prompted voiding for persons with urinary incontinence, management of constipation, exercise promotion, hypertension detection and treatment, and acute pain management (Table 5-1) (Mezey, Fulmer, & Abraham, 2003; Tang & Titler, 2003). Although many of these topics will benefit from further empirical study, the current evidence base should be applied in clinical care. For example, an incontinence management protocol resulted in decreasing pressure ulcer incidence in a long-term care setting (Frantz, Xakellis, Harvey, & Lewis, 2003). The challenge is using this evidence base in day-to-day care delivery.

Steps of Evidence-Based Practice

The Iowa Model of Evidence-Based Practice to Promote Quality Care (Titler et al., 2001) (see Figure 5-2), in conjunction with Rogers' Diffusion of Innovation Model (Rogers, 2003; Titler & Everett, 2001), provides guiding steps in actualizing EBP. A team approach is most helpful in fostering a specific EBP, with one person in the group providing the leadership for the project (Titler, 2002).

The first step in carrying out an EBP project is to select a topic. Ideas for EBP come from several sources categorized as problem- and knowledge-focused triggers. Problem-focused triggers are those identified by staff through quality improvement, risk surveillance, benchmarking data, financial data, or recurrent clinical problems. An example of a problem-focused trigger is increased incidence of acute confusion in hospitalized older adults. Knowledge-focused triggers are ideas generated when staff read research, listen to scientific papers at research conferences, or encounter EBP guidelines published by federal agencies or specialty organizations. Examples initiated from knowledge-focused triggers include pain management, prevention of skin breakdown, and risk factors for urinary incontinence. Sometimes topics arise from a combination of problem- and knowledge-focused triggers, such as managing hydration in long-term care. When selecting a topic, nurses and assistive personnel should consider how the clinical topic fits with the organization, department, and unit priorities in order to garner support from organizational leaders and the necessary resources to successfully complete and sustain the practice improvement. It is critical that the staff members who will implement the potential practice changes are involved in selecting the topic and view it as contributing significantly to the quality of care (Titler, 2005).

Forming a team that is responsible for development, implementation, and evaluation of the EBP is the next step. The team or group may be an existing committee such as the quality improvement committee, the practice council, or the research committee. A task force approach also may be used, in which a group is appointed to address a specific practice issue and uses research findings or other evidence to improve practice. The composition of the team is directed by the topic selected and should include interested stakeholders in the delivery of care. For example, a team working on evidence-based pain management should be interdisciplinary and include pharmacists, nurses, physicians, and psychologists. In contrast, a team working on the EBP of bathing might include a nurse expert in skin care (e.g., gerontological advanced practice nurse), assistive nursing personnel, and staff nurses. In addition to forming a team, key stakeholders who can facilitate the EBP project or put up barriers against successful implementation

Table 5-1 *Evidence-Based Practice Guidelines for Care of Older Adults*

Title	Author/Year	Brief Description
Acute Confusion/Delirium	Rapp, C. G. (1998; revised 2005)	Describes the assessment and management practices for older patients with acute confusion/delirium. This includes screening and ongoing surveillance for acute confusion/delirium based on identified risk factors with a focus on preventing or minimizing acute confusion/delirium.
Acute Pain Management with Quick Reference Guides	Herr, K., Titler, M., Sorofman, B., Ardery, G., Schmitt, M., & Young, D. (2000; reviewed 2003)	Helps providers manage acute pain in older patients. The outcomes of effective management include reduced pain levels, minimization or elimination of complications of pain treatment, and increased patient satisfaction with pain management. It includes guides for baseline pain assessment, patient/family education, acute pain monitoring, and pharmacological and nonpharmacological treatments.
Advance Directives (with Quick Reference Guide and Consumer Insert)	Garand, L. & Weiler, K. (1999; reviewed 2001)	Provides guidance in end-of-life health care decision making through education and discussion about preparation of an advance directive. Assists health care personnel to facilitate informed decision making by patients choosing end-of-life care. Includes "Quick Reference Guide" algorithm chart to help in selecting the appropriate advance directive choices. The set also includes a "Consumer Information Sheet" that contains possible reference material that may be helpful to use in conjunction with the advance directives protocol.
Bathing Persons with Dementia	Hall, G., & Buckwalter, K. C. (1995; revised 2004)	Provides strategies for minimizing fear, agitation, combative behavior, and development of secondary behavioral symptoms during and after personal hygiene. The goal is to reduce the frequency and severity of negative bathing episodes in patients with chronic dementing illness.
Changing the Practice of Physical Restraint Use in Acute Care (formerly Restraints with Quick Reference Guide)	Park, M., Tang, J., & Ledford, L. (1995; revised 1997, 2005)	An interdisciplinary protocol that provides guidelines for the appropriate use of protective devices, chemical restraints, and physical restraints.
Detection of Depression in the Cognitively Intact Older Adult (with Quick Reference Guide and Consumer Insert)	Piven, M. (1998; reviewed 2001)	The purpose of this guideline is to improve detection of depression in medically compromised, cognitively intact older adults. Identification of depression in the older adult is critical in reducing the negative impact of depression on quality of life, health care utilization, adherence with treatment regimens, and functional status.
Elder Abuse Prevention	Daly, J. (2005)	Facilitate health care professionals to assess older persons in domestic and institutional settings who are at risk for elder abuse and recommend interventions to reduce the incidence of mistreatment.
Elderly Suicide: Secondary Prevention	Holkup, P. (2002)	Provides information that will assist the nurse or other health care provider in recognizing at-risk suicidal behavior in older adults and providing appropriate and effective crisis intervention. The goal is to decrease the occurrence of suicide among older individuals who have contact with nurses or other health care providers.
Exercise Promotion: Walking in Elders (with Consumer Insert)	Jitramontree, N. (2001)	Encourages providers in all settings to enhance or maintain exercise behavior of elders. Regular walking and moderate-intensity physical activity improve health, enhance independent living, decrease depression, and increase overall quality of life.

*Available from the Research Translation and Dissemination Core of the Gerontological Nursing Interventions Research Center at the University of Iowa Hospitals and Clinics (www.nursing.uiowa.edu/centers/gnirc/). For permission to use or reproduce, please contact Dr. Titler.

Table 5-1 *Evidence-Based Practice Guidelines for Care of Older Adults—cont'd*

Title	Author/Year	Brief Description
Fall Prevention for Older Adults	Lyons, S. (1995; revised 2004)	Describes strategies for identifying persons at risk for falling and for preventing falls in older adults, while maintaining autonomy and independence. Includes information regarding risk factors, assessment tools, interventions, and outcome evaluations.
Family Bereavement and Support Before and After the Death of a Nursing Home Resident	Davidson, K. (2002)	Provides an intervention guideline designed to assist family members before and after the death of their loved one in nursing home settings. The guideline is intended for front-line staff (registered nurses, care attendants, social workers, chaplains) who care for older adults and provide support to the elders' families in nursing homes.
Family Involvement in Care (FIC)	Kelly, L., Specht, J., & Maas, M. (1999; reviewed 2001)	Focuses on a program to involve family members in the care of their relative with dementia through partnerships with other, both formal and informal, care providers. Successful care partnerships result in the establishment of meaningful and satisfactory caregiving roles regardless of the care setting.
Hydration Management (with Quick Reference Guide and Consumer Insert)	Mentes, J. (1998; revised 2004)	Helps health care providers determine adequate oral fluid intake for elders and provides strategies to maintain hydration and to prevent conditions associated with dehydration, such as acute confusion/delirium.
Identification, Referral, and Support of Elders with Genetic Conditions	Schutte, D. (1999; reviewed 2001)	Describes assessment and management practices related to the genetic aspects of health conditions in elders. This guideline is meant for non–genetic specialist gerontological nurses as the integration of new genetic information into clinical nursing care of the older adult evolves.
Improving Medication Management for Older Adult Clients	Bergman-Evans, B. (2004)	Helps registered nurses, nurse practitioners, and pharmacists to improve medication management practices for older adults. The goals are to reduce inappropriate prescribing, decrease polypharmacy, avoid adverse events, and maintain function.
Individualized Music (with Quick Reference Guide and Consumer Insert)	Gerdner, L. (1996; revised 2001)	Describes strategies for alleviating agitation in chronically confused older persons through use of individualized music. The goal is to reduce and prevent the frequency and severity of agitation episodes by assessing music preferences and playing music for the elder at designated times.
Interpreter Facilitation for Persons with Limited English Proficiency	Enslein, J., Tripp-Reimer, T., Kelley, L. S., Choi, E., & McCarty, L. (2001)	Provides information to assist in the effective use of interpreter services in health care settings. The goals are to increase the use of interpreters, enhance the communication process between clients and providers, and improve the satisfaction of clients and providers with health care encounters.
Management of Constipation with Consumer Insert	Hinrichs, M., & Huseboe, J. (1996; revised 2001)	The purpose of this protocol is to reduce the frequency and severity of constipation among older adults. It is applicable to older adults who are hospitalized, residing in long-term care or skilled care facilities, or living in the community.
Non-Pharmacologic Management of Agitated Behaviors in Persons with Alzheimer Disease and other Chronic Dementing Conditions	McGonigal-Kenney, M. L., & Schutte, D. L. (1995; revised 2004)	Presents intervention activities designed to minimize secondary symptoms in patients with Alzheimer's disease and related disorders (ADRD). The goal is to increase the functional quality of life and reduce incidence of problems related to dementia.

Continued

Table 5-1 *Evidence-Based Practice Guidelines for Care of Older Adults—cont'd*

Title	Author/Year	Brief Description
Nurse Retention	Tang, J. (2002)	Retaining expert nurses has a positive effect on quality patient care. Nurse managers are critical to promoting job satisfaction and diminishing turnover of nurses working in their area. This administrative protocol is a helpful guide for nurse managers who are striving to improve retention of staff in various health care settings.
Oral Hygiene Care for Functionally Dependent and Cognitively Impaired Older Adults	Johnson, V., & Chalmers, J. (2002)	Provides practical information to assist health care providers with the provision and documentation of oral hygiene care for functionally dependent and cognitively impaired older adults to prevent plaque-related oral diseases.
Prevention of Deep Vein Thrombosis	Blondin, M. (1999; reviewed 2001)	Describes a standard method for the assessment of risk for development of deep vein thrombosis in older surgical patients. Suggestions and options regarding modes of prophylaxis are described as applicable in the acute care setting.
Prevention of Pressure Ulcers	Folkedahl, B., Frantz, R., & Goode, C. (1997; revised 2002)	Assists health care providers in determining those patients at risk for development of pressure ulcers, and describes prevention activities that will reduce patients' risk for pressure ulcers.
Progressive Resistance Training	Mobily, K., & Mobily, P. (1998; revised 2004)	Describes a training program to improve and maintain the functional fitness of older adults through progressive resistance training, with the intent of improving their prospects for independent living, reducing fall risk, and enhancing commitment to regular exercise.
Promoting Spirituality in the Older Adult	Gaskamp, C., Sutter, R., & Meraviglia, M. (2004)	Provides guidelines for promoting spirituality for health care providers working with older adults in community and institutional settings, from a holistic perspective. The ultimate goal for promoting spirituality is to support and enhance quality of life.
Prompted Voiding—Urinary Incontinence (with Quick Reference Guide and Consumer Insert)	Lyons, S., & Specht, J. (1999; reviewed 2001)	Provides information for implementing a treatment program of prompted voiding for older persons with urinary incontinence.
Quality Improvement in Nursing Homes	Dyck, M. (2003)	Provides knowledge and evidence-based strategies for quality and performance improvement in nursing homes. Departments can use this administrative guideline as a team to develop, define, implement, and evaluate their own quality improvement program.
Split Thickness Skin Graft Donor Site Care	Abbott, L. (1998; reviewed 2001)	Outlines the care of split-thickness skin graft donor sites. Use of this protocol will aid in the management of donor sites through the use of various dressings to promote healing rate and quality, reduce infection and pain, and decrease associated costs.
Treatment of Pressure Ulcers	Folkedahl, B., Frantz, R., & Goode, C. (1997; revised 2002)	Provides guidelines for the treatment of pressure ulcers among older patients. Assists in the assessment of patients for skin alterations and describes interventions to aid in the healing of ulcers.
Wandering (with Consumer Insert)	Futrell, M., & Melillo, K. (2002)	Assists formal caregivers of older adults with dementia who wander, with a guideline for dealing with problem wandering behavior.
Wheelchair Biking for the Treatment of Depression	Fitzsimmons, S., & Buettner, L. (2003)	Describes a specific recreation therapy program, wheelchair biking, for the treatment of depression in older adults, with and without cognitive impairments. The goal is to reduce depressive mood in older adults and to provide a complementary or alternative treatment to medications.

should be identified. A stakeholder is a key individual or group of individuals who will be directly or indirectly affected by the implementation of the EBP. Some of these stakeholders are likely to be members of the team. Others may not be team members but are key individuals within the organization or unit who can adversely or positively influence adoption of the EBP. An example of a key stakeholder in a long-term care setting is the director of nursing (formal/positional power) or a nursing assistant who is seen as an informal leader by his or her peer group (informal power) (Jones et al., 2004). Questions to consider in identification of key stakeholders include the following:

■ How are decisions made in the practice areas where the EBP will be implemented?
■ What types of system changes will be needed?
■ Who is involved in decision making?
■ Who is likely to lead and champion implementation of the EBP?
■ Who can influence the decision to proceed with implementation of an EBP?
■ What type of cooperation do you need from which stakeholders to be successful?
■ Who is likely to facilitate sustainability of the change in practice?
■ What system changes are necessary to sustain the change in practice?

An important early task for the EBP team is to formulate the evidence-based practice question. This helps set boundaries around the project and assists in retrieval of the evidence. A clearly defined question should specify the types of people/patients (e.g., adults older than 65 years of age with acute pain), interventions or exposures (e.g., pain assessment), outcomes (e.g., less pain intensity; early ambulation), and relevant study designs that are likely to provide reliable data to address the clinical question (e.g., descriptive designs; randomized controlled trials) (Alderson, Green, & Higgins, 2003).

Retrieving the evidence is the next step and should include clinical studies, meta-analyses, integrative literature reviews, and EBP guidelines. As more evidence is available to guide practice, professional organizations and federal agencies are developing and making available EBP guidelines and synthesis reports (Titler, 2005). It is important that these are accessed as part of the literature retrieval process. For example, AHRQ funds 13 Evidence-Based Practice Centers (Box 5-3) that develop evidence reports on selected clinical topics. AHRQ also sponsors a National Guideline Clearinghouse where abstracts of EBP guidelines are set forth on its Web site. Other professional organizations that have EBP guidelines or synthesis reports include the American Pain Society; the Oncology Nursing Society; the American Association of Critical-Care Nurses; the Association for Women's Health, Obstetrics, and Neonatal Nursing; the Gerontological Nursing Interventions Research Center; the American Thoracic Society; the American Geriatric Society (AGS); the Gerontological Society of America; and Sigma Theta Tau International (STTI). Current best evidence from specific studies of clinical problems can be found in an increasing number of electronic databases such as the Cochrane Library, the Centers for Health Evidence, and Best Evidence. Another electronic database, Evidence-Based Medicine Reviews (EBMR) from Ovid Technologies, combines several electronic databases, including the Cochrane Database of Systematic Reviews, Best Evidence, Evidence-Based Mental Health, Evidence-Based Nursing, Cancerlit, Healthstar, AIDSline, Bioethicsline, and MEDLINE, plus links to over 200 full-text journals. EBMR links these databases to one another; if a study on a topic of interest is found on MEDLINE and also has been included in a systematic review in the Cochrane Library, the review can be readily and easily accessed (Sackett et al., 2000). In using these sources, it is important to identify key search terms and to use the expertise of health science

---

BOX 5-3 Agency for Healthcare Research and Quality Evidence-Based Practice Centers

1. Blue Cross and Blue Shield Association, Technology Evaluation Center (TEC), Chicago, Illinois
2. Duke University, Durham, North Carolina
3. ECRI, Plymouth Meeting, Pennsylvania
4. Johns Hopkins University, Baltimore, Maryland
5. McMaster University, Hamilton, Ontario, Canada
6. Oregon Evidence-Based Practice Center, Portland, Oregon
7. RTI International—University of North Carolina at Chapel Hill, Chapel Hill, North Carolina
8. Southern California Evidence-Based Practice Center—RAND, Santa Monica, California
9. Stanford University—University of California, San Francisco, California
10. Tufts University—New England Medical Center, Boston, Massachusetts
11. University of Alberta, Edmonton, Alberta, Canada
12. University of Minnesota, Minneapolis, Minnesota
13. University of Ottawa, Ottawa, Ontario, Canada

Data from www.ahrq.gov/clinic/epc/.

librarians in locating publications relevant to the project. Additional information about locating the evidence is available from other sources (DiCenso, Ciliska, Cullum, & Guyatt, 2004; LoBiondo-Wood & Haber, 2005; Sackett et al., 2000).

Critiquing the evidence is the next step and includes critique of research, synthesis reports, and EBP guidelines. There is no consensus among professional organizations or across health care disciplines regarding the best system to use for denoting the type and quality of evidence, or the grading schemas to denote the strength of the body of evidence (West et al., 2002). In "grading the evidence," two important areas are essential to address: (1) the quality of the individual research; and (2) the strength of the body of evidence (West et al., 2002). Important domains and elements of any system used to rate quality of individual studies are listed in Box 5-4 by type of study. The important domains and elements to include in grading the strength of the evidence are defined in Box 5-5. The AHRQ technology report is necessary reading for those undertaking synthesis of evidence for practice and public policy; the scholars reviewed 121 systems (checklists, scales, guidance documents) as the basis of this report (West et al.,

2002). From this set, 19 systems fully addressed the key domains for assessing study quality and 7 systems fully addressed all 3 domains for grading the strength of the evidence. Resources are available to assist with critique of research and other evidence, including books (Brown, 1999; Craig & Smyth, 2002; DiCenso et al., 2004; LoBiondo-Wood & Haber, 2004; Melnyk & Fineout-Overholt, 2004; Sackett et al., 2000) and the Toolkit for Promoting Evidence-Based Practice (Titler, 2002).

As EBP guidelines proliferate, it becomes increasingly important that nurses critique these guidelines with regard to the methods used for formulating them and consider how they might be used in their practice (Brown, 1999; Cluzeau & Littlejohns, 1999; Cluzeau, Littlejohns, Grimshaw, & Feder, 1997; Liddle, Williamson, & Irwig, 1996). Critical areas that should be assessed when critiquing EBP guidelines include the following: (1) date of publication or release; (2) authors of the guideline; (3) endorsement of the guideline; (4) a clear purpose of what the guideline covers and patient groups for which it was designed; (5) types of evidence (research, nonresearch) used in formulating the guideline; (6) types of research included in formulating the guideline (e.g., "We considered only randomized and

---

BOX 5-4 Important Domains and Elements for Systems to Rate Quality of Individual Articles

SYSTEMATIC REVIEWS	RANDOMIZED CLINICAL TRIALS	OBSERVATIONAL STUDIES	DIAGNOSTIC TEST STUDIES
Study question	Study question	Study question	*Study population*
Search strategy	*Study population*	Study population	*Adequate description of test*
Inclusion and exclusion criteria	*Randomization*	*Comparability of subjects*	*Appropriate reference standard*
Interventions	*Blinding*	*Exposure or intervention*	*Blinded comparison of text and reference*
Outcomes	*Interventions*	Outcome measurement	
Data extraction	*Outcomes*	*Statistical analysis*	*Avoidance of verification bias*
Study quality and validity	*Statistical analysis*	Results	
Data synthesis and analysis	Results	Discussion	
Results	Discussion	*Funding or sponsorship*	
Discussion	*Funding or sponsorship*		
Funding or sponsorship			

From Agency for Healthcare Research and Quality. (2002). *Systems to rate the strength of scientific evidence. Summary.* Evidence Report/Technology Assessment Report no. 47, pub. no. 02-E015. Bethesda, MD: U.S. Department of Health and Human Services, Agency for Healthcare Research and Quality.
NOTE: Key domains are in *italics*.

BOX 5-5 Important Domains and Elements for Systems to Grade the Strength of Evidence

Quality	The aggregate of quality ratings for individual studies, predicated on the extent to which bias was minimized
Quantity	Magnitude of effect, numbers of studies, and sample size or power
Consistency	For any given topic, the extent to which similar findings are reported using similar and different study designs

From Agency for Healthcare Research and Quality. (2002). Systems to rate the strength of scientific evidence. Evidence Report/Technology Assessment no. 47. AHRQ pub. no. 02-E016. Rockville, MD: Agency for Healthcare Research and Quality, U.S. Department of Health and Human Services.

BOX 5-6 Consistency of Evidence from Critiqued Research, Appraisals of Evidence-Based Practice Guidelines, and Critiqued Systematic Reviews

1. Are there replication of studies with consistent results?
2. Are the studies well designed?
3. Are recommendations consistent among systematic reviews, EBP guidelines, and critiqued research?
4. Are there identified risks to the patient by applying EBP recommendations?
5. Are there identified benefits to the patient?
6. Have cost analysis studies been conducted on the recommended action, intervention, or treatment?
7. What are the summary recommendations about assessments, actions, interventions/treatments from the research, systematic reviews, and evidence-based guidelines with an assigned evidence grade?

From Titler, M. G. (2002). *Toolkit for promoting evidence-based practice.* Iowa City: Department of Nursing Services and Patient Care, University of Iowa Hospitals and Clinics. For permission to use or reproduce, please contact Dr. Titler.)

---

other prospective controlled trials in determining efficacy of therapeutic interventions . . ."); (7) a description of the methods used in grading the evidence; (8) search terms and retrieval methods used to acquire research and nonresearch evidence used in the guideline; (9) well-referenced statements regarding practice; (10) comprehensive reference list; (11) review of the guideline by experts; and (12) whether the guideline has been used or tested in practice, and if so, with what types of patients and in what types of settings. Evidence-based guidelines that are formulated using rigorous methods provide a useful starting point for nurses to understand the evidence base of certain practices. However, more research may be available since the publication of the guideline, and refinements may be needed. Although information in well-developed, national, evidence-based guidelines is a helpful reference, it is usually necessary to localize the guideline using institution-specific evidence-based policies, procedures, or standards before application within a specific setting. A useful tool for critiquing guidelines is available from the Appraisal of Guidelines Research and Evaluation (AGREE) collaboration (2001).

The critique process should be a shared responsibility, using the same methodology. It is helpful, however, to have one individual provide leadership for the critique of the evidence and design strategies for completing critiques. A group approach is recommended because it distributes the workload, helps those responsible for implementing the changes to understand the scientific base for the change in practice, arms nurses with citations and research-based sound bites to use in effecting practice changes with peers and other disciplines, and provides novices an environment to learn critique and application of evidence.

The next step is setting forth evidence-based practice recommendations, based on critique and synthesis of the evidence. The type and strength of evidence used to support the practice need to be clearly delineated. Box 5-6 provides questions to assist with this activity. The following are examples of practice recommendation statements:

- Older people who have recurrent falls should be offered long-term exercise and balance training (strength of recommendation = B) (American Geriatrics Society et al., 2001).
- Apply dressings that maintain a moist wound environment. Examples of moist dressings include, but are not limited to, hydrogels, hydrocolloids, saline-moistened gauze, and transparent film dressings. The ulcer bed should be kept continuously moist (evidence grade = B) (Folkedahl, Frantz, & Goode, 2002).

After the evidence is critiqued and EBPs are set forth, the next step is to decide if findings are appropriate for use in practice. Criteria to consider in making these decisions include the following:

- Relevance of evidence for practice
- Consistency in findings across studies or guidelines
- A significant number of studies or EBP guidelines with sample characteristics similar to those for which the findings will be used
- Consistency among evidence from research and other nonresearch evidence
- Feasibility for use in practice
- The risk/benefit ratio (risk of harm; potential benefit for the patient)

Practice changes should be based on knowledge/evidence derived from several sources (e.g., several research studies) that demonstrate consistent findings. Synthesis of study findings and other evidence may result in supporting current practice, making minor practice modifications, undertaking major practice changes, or developing a new area of practice.

The next step is writing an EBP standard (e.g., policy, procedure, guideline) specific to the health care setting, using the grading schema that has been agreed on (Haber et al., 1994). This is necessary so that individuals in the setting know (1) that the practices are based on evidence and (2) the type of evidence (e.g., randomized clinical trial, expert opinion) used in developing the EBP standard. Several different formats can be used to document the evidence base of the standard; use a consistent approach to writing EBP standards and referencing the research and related literature. The format chosen is influenced by what and how the document will be used. Written EBPs should be part of the organizational policy and procedure manual and should include linkages to the references for the parts of the policy and procedure that are based on research and other types of evidence.

Clinicians (e.g., nurses, physicians, pharmacists) who adopt EBPs are influenced by the perceived participation they have had in developing and reviewing the EBP standard (Baker & Feder, 1997; Bauchner & Simpson, 1998; Bero et al., 1998; Shortell et al., 1995; Soumerai et al., 1998; Titler, 2004a). Therefore it is imperative that key stakeholders have an opportunity to review the written EBP standard and provide feedback. Use of focus groups is a useful way to provide discussion about the EBP standard and to identify key areas that may be potentially troublesome during the implementation phase.

When a practice change is warranted, the next steps are to implement the EBP changes in practice. This goes beyond writing a policy or procedure that is evidence based; it requires interaction among direct care providers to champion and foster evidence adoption, leadership support, and system changes. Strategies for implementation are discussed later in this chapter.

Evaluation is a critical component of EBP; it provides information to determine if the EBP should be retained, modified, or eliminated. A desired outcome achieved in a more controlled environment, when a researcher is implementing a study protocol with a homogeneous group of patients (conduct of research), may not result in the same outcome when the practice is implemented in the natural clinical setting, by several caregivers, to a more heterogeneous patient population. Steps of the evaluation process are summarized in Box 5-7.

Evaluation should include both process and outcome measures (Lepper & Titler, 1999; Rosswurm & Larrabee, 1999; Titler, 2005). The process component focuses on use of the EBP by staff in care delivery.

BOX 5-7 Steps of the Evaluation Process

1. Identify process and outcome variables of interest. Example:
   Process variable—Patients older than 65 years of age will have a Braden scale completed on admission.
   Outcome variable—Presence/absence of nosocomial pressure ulcer; if present, determine stage as I, II, III, or IV.
2. Determine methods and frequency of data collection. Example:
   Process variable—Chart audit of all patients older than 65 years of age, 1 day a month.
   Outcome variable—Patient assessment of all patients older than 65 years of age, 1 day a month.
3. Determine number of patient assessments and chart audits for baseline and follow-up.
4. Design data collection forms. Example:
   Chart audit abstraction form (process).
   Outcome variable—Pressure ulcer assessment form.
5. Establish content validity of data collection forms.
6. Educate data collectors.
7. Assess interrater reliability of data collectors.
8. Collect data at specified intervals.
9. Provide "on-site" feedback to staff regarding the progress in achieving the practice change.
10. Provide feedback of analyzed data to staff.
11. Use data to assist staff in modifying or integrating the evidence-based practice change.

Evaluation of the process should also note (1) barriers that staff encounter in carrying out the practice (e.g., lack of information, skills, or necessary equipment), (2) differences in opinions among health care providers, and (3) difficulty in carrying out the steps of the practice as originally designed (e.g., shutting off tube feedings 1 hour before aspirating contents for checking placement of nasointestinal tubes). Process data can be collected from staff or patient self-reports, medical record audits, or observation of clinical practice. Examples of process and outcome questions are shown in Figure 5-3.

Outcome data are an equally important part of evaluation to assess whether the patient, staff, and fiscal outcomes expected are achieved. The outcome variables measured should be those that are projected to change as a result of changing practice (Rosswurm & Larrabee, 1999; Soukup, 2000; Titler, 2005). It is important that baseline data be used for a pretreatment/posttreatment comparison (Cullen, 2005; Titler et al., 2001). Outcome measures should be measured before the change in practice is implemented, after implementation, and

EXAMPLE PROCESS QUESTIONS					
NURSES' SELF RATING	**SD**	**D**	**NA/D**	**A**	**SA**
1. I feel well prepared to use the Braden Scale with older patients.	1	2	3	4	5
2. Malnutrition increases patient risk for pressure ulcer development	1	2	3	4	5

EXAMPLE OUTCOME QUESTION

PATIENT

1. On a scale of 0 (no pain) to 10 (worst possible pain), how much pain have you experienced over the past 24 hours? _____

(pain intensity)

SD, strongly disagree; *D*, disagree; *NA/D*, neither agree nor disagree; *A*, agree; *SA*, strongly agree

Figure 5-3 Examples of evaluation measures. (From Titler, M. [2005]. Developing an evidence-based practice. In G. LoBiondo-Wood & J. Haber [Eds.], *Nursing research* [5th ed.]. St. Louis: Mosby. For permission to use or reproduce, please contact Dr. Titler.)

every 6 to 12 months thereafter. Findings must be provided to clinicians to reinforce the impact of the changes in practice and to ensure that they are incorporated into quality improvement programs. Feedback to staff includes verbal or written appreciation for the work and visual demonstration of progress in implementation and improvement in patient outcomes. The key to effective evaluation is to ensure that the evidence-based change in practice is warranted (e.g., will improve quality of care) and that the intervention does not bring harm to patients (Lepper & Titler, 1999). For example, when instituting a change in practice for assessing return of bowel motility following abdominal surgery in older adults, it was important to inform staff that using other markers for return of bowel motility, rather than bowel sound assessment, did not result in increased paralytic ileus or bowel obstruction (Madsen et al., 2005).

Implementation Strategies. Rogers' seminal work on diffusion of innovations (Rogers, 2003) is extremely useful in selecting strategies for promoting adoption of EBPs. Other investigators describing barriers and facilitators of EBPs have used Rogers' (2003) model (Camiletti & Huffman, 1998; Carroll et al., 1997; Funk, Champagne, Tornquist, & Wiese, 1995; Rutledge et al., 1996; Sackett et al., 2000; Schnelle et al., 1998; Shively et al., 1997; Wells & Baggs, 1994). According to this model, adoption of innovations such as EBPs is influenced by the nature of the innovation (e.g., the type and strength of evidence; the clinical topic) and the manner in which it is communicated (disseminated) to members (nurses) of a social system (organization, nursing profession) (Rogers, 1995; Titler & Everett, 2001). Strategies for promoting adoption of EBPs must address these four areas within a context of participative, planned change (Figure 5-4).

Nature of the Innovation/Evidence-Based Practice. The strength of the evidence alone does not guarantee that the EBP will be adopted (Grimshaw et al., 2004). Implementation processes that encourage practitioner adaptation/reinvention of EBP guidelines for use in practitioners' local agency increase adherence to the guideline (Bero et al., 1998; Berwick, 2003; Titler & Everett, 2001). Studies funded by AHRQ (Farquhar et al., 2002) and others suggest that clinical systems, computerized decision support, and prompts that support practice (e.g., decision-making algorithms, equianalgesic chart) have a positive effect on aligning practices with the evidence base (Cook, Greengold, Ellrodt, & Weingarten, 1997; Hunt, Haynes, Hanna, & Smith, 1998; O'Connor et al., 1996; Oxman, Thomson, Davis, & Haynes, 1995; Titler et al., 2003). To move evidence from the "book to the bedside," information from EBPs must have perceived benefits for patients, nurses, physicians, and administrators; be "reinvented" and integrated into daily patient care processes; impart evidence in a readily available format; and make EBPs observable for practitioners (Berwick, 2003; Rogers, 2003). Those responsible for implementing the EBP standard need to consider use of practice prompts, decision support systems, and quick reference guides as part of the implementation process. An example of a quick reference guide is shown in Figure 5-5.

Methods of Communication. Methods of communicating the EBP to those delivering care affect adoption of the practice (Carroll et al., 1997; Funk, Tornquist, & Champagne, 1995; Rogers, 2003; Wells & Baggs, 1994). Education of staff, use of opinion leaders, change champions, core groups, and consultation by experts in the content area are essential components of the implementation process. Continuing education alone does little to change practice behavior (Thomson

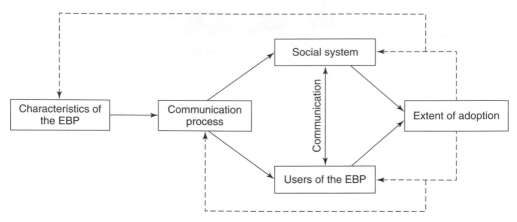

Figure 5-4   Implementation model. (Redrawn from Rogers, E. M. [2003]. *Diffusion of innovations* [5th ed.]. New York: Free Press; and Titler, M. G., & Everett, L. Q. [2001]. Translating research into practice: Considerations for critical care investigators. *Critical Care Nursing Clinics of North America, 13*[4], 587-604. For permission to use or reproduce, please contact Dr. Titler.)

O'Brien et al., 2004a). Interactive and didactic education, used in combination with other practice-reinforcing strategies, has more positive effects than education alone (Bero et al., 1998; Schneider & Eisenberg, 1998; Thomson O'Brien et al., 2004b). It is important that staff know the scientific basis for the changes in practice and the improvements in quality of care anticipated by the change. Disseminating this information to staff needs to be done creatively using various educational strategies. A staff inservice may not be the most effective method and may not reach the majority of the staff. Although it is unrealistic for all staff members to have participated in the critique process or to have read all studies used to develop the EBP, it is important that they know evidence-based myths and realities of the practice. Education of staff members also must include ensuring that they are competent in the skills necessary to carry out the new practice. For example, if a pain assessment tool is being implemented to assess pain in cognitively impaired elders in the long-term care setting, it is essential that caregivers have the knowledge and skill to use the tool in their practice setting.

One method of communicating information to staff is through use of colorful posters that identify myths and realities or describe the essence of the change in practice (Titler et al., 2001). Visibly identifying those who have learned the information and are using the EBP (e.g., buttons, ribbons, pins) stimulates interest in others who may not have internalized the change. As a result, the "new" learner may begin asking questions about the practice and be more open to learning. Other educational strategies such as train-the-trainer programs, computer-assisted instruction, and competency testing are helpful in education of staff (Titler, 2005).

Several studies have demonstrated that opinion leaders are effective in changing behaviors of health care practitioners (Berner et al., 2003; Bero et al., 1998;

Cullen, 2005; Locock, Dopson, Chambers, & Gabbay, 2001; Oxman et al., 1995; Soumerai et al., 1998; Thomson O'Brien et al., 2002), especially in combination with (1) outreach or (2) performance feedback. Opinion leaders are from the local peer group, are viewed as respected sources of influence, are considered by associates as technically competent, and are trusted to judge the fit between the EBP and the local situation (Oxman et al., 1995; Soumerai et al., 1998; Thomson O'Brien et al., 2004b). They use the EBP, influence peers, and alter group norms (Collins, Hawks, & Davis, 2000; Rogers, 2003). The key characteristic of an opinion leader is that he or she is trusted to evaluate new information in the context of group norms. To do this, an opinion leader must be considered by associates as technically competent and a full and dedicated member of the local group (Oxman et al., 1995; Rogers, 2003; Soumerai et al., 1998). Social interactions such as "hallway chats," one-on-one discussions, and addressing questions are important yet often overlooked components of translation (Berwick, 2003; Rogers, 2003). Thus having local opinion leaders (early adopters) discuss the EBPs with members of their peer group is necessary to translate research into practice. If the EBP change that is being implemented is interdisciplinary in nature (e.g., pain management), it is recommended that an opinion leader be selected for each discipline (nursing, medicine, pharmacy).

Change champions are also helpful for implementing EBP changes in practice (Rogers, 2003; Shively et al., 1997; Titler, 2004a; Titler & Mentes, 1999). They are practitioners within the local group setting (e.g., clinical, patient care unit) who are expert clinicians, are passionate about the clinical topic, are committed to improving quality of care, and have a positive working relationship with other health professionals (Harvey et al., 2002; Rogers, 2003; Titler, 1998; Titler & Mentes,

DETECTION OF DEPRESSION IN THE COGNITIVELY INTACT OLDER ADULT

QUICK REFERENCE GUIDE

USE THIS GUIDE TO:
- Assess older adults (age 60 or older) for their risk of depression (see Table 1 for risk factors)
- Detect symptoms of major depression (see Table 2)
- Determine appropriate referral and follow-up for persons identified as being at-risk for depression

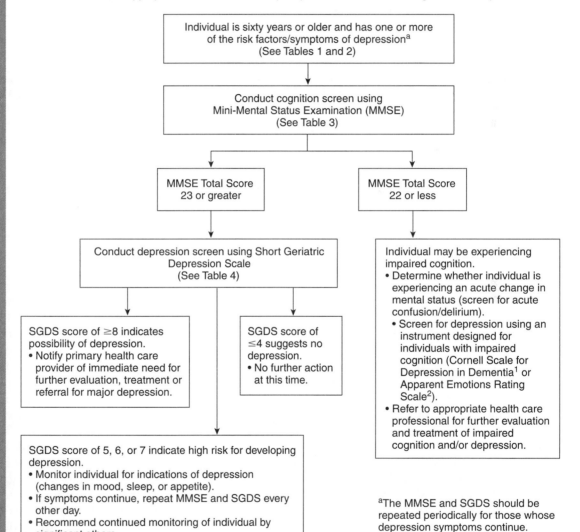

Individual is sixty years or older and has one or more of the risk factors/symptoms of depression[a]
(See Tables 1 and 2)

Conduct cognition screen using Mini-Mental Status Examination (MMSE)
(See Table 3)

MMSE Total Score 23 or greater

MMSE Total Score 22 or less

Conduct depression screen using Short Geriatric Depression Scale
(See Table 4)

SGDS score of ≥8 indicates possibility of depression.
- Notify primary health care provider of immediate need for further evaluation, treatment or referral for major depression.

SGDS score of ≤4 suggests no depression.
- No further action at this time.

Individual may be experiencing impaired cognition.
- Determine whether individual is experiencing an acute change in mental status (screen for acute confusion/delirium).
- Screen for depression using an instrument designed for individuals with impaired cognition (Cornell Scale for Depression in Dementia[1] or Apparent Emotions Rating Scale[2]).
- Refer to appropriate health care professional for further evaluation and treatment of impaired cognition and/or depression.

SGDS score of 5, 6, or 7 indicate high risk for developing depression.
- Monitor individual for indications of depression (changes in mood, sleep, or appetite).
- If symptoms continue, repeat MMSE and SGDS every other day.
- Recommend continued monitoring of individual by significant others.
- Notify primary health care provider of individual's high risk for developing depression.

[a]The MMSE and SGDS should be repeated periodically for those whose depression symptoms continue.

Figure 5-5 Quick reference guide to detection of depression in the cognitively intact older adult. (From Piven, M. [2001]. *Detection of depression in the cognitively intact older adult with QRG and consumer insert.* Iowa City, IA: Research Dissemination Core of the Gerontological Nursing Interventions Research Center, University of Iowa College of Nursing.)

1999). They circulate information, encourage peers to align their practice with the best evidence, arrange demonstrations, and orient staff to the EBP (Shively et al., 1997; Titler, 2004a). The change champion believes in an idea; will not take "no" for an answer; is undaunted by insults and rebuffs; and above all, persists (Greer, 1988). For potential research-based changes in practice to reach direct care, it is imperative that one or two "change champions" be identified for each patient care unit or service where the change is being made (Titler, 2003). Staff nurses or nursing assistants can be some of the best change champions for EBP.

Using a "core group" in conjunction with change champions is also helpful for implementing the practice change (Barnason, Merboth, Pozehl, & Tietjen, 1998; Schmidt, Alpen, & Rakel, 1996; Titler et al., 2001). A core group is a select group of practitioners with the mutual goal of disseminating information regarding a practice change and facilitating the change in practice by other staff in their unit or peer group. Success of the core group approach requires that core group members work well with the change champion and represent various shifts, days of the week, and tenures in the practice setting. Core group members become knowledgeable about the scientific basis for the practice, assist with disseminating the EBP information to other staff, and reinforce the practice change on a daily basis. The change champion educates the core group members and assists them in changing their practices. Each member of the core group, in turn, takes the responsibility for effecting the change in two to three of his or her peers. Core group members provide positive feedback to their assigned staff who are changing their practices and encourage those reluctant to change to try the new practice. Core group members also are able to assist the change champion in identifying the best way to teach staff about the practice change and to proactively solve issues that arise (Schmidt et al., 1996; Titler et al., 2001). Using a core group approach in conjunction with a change champion results in a critical mass of practitioners promoting adoption of the EBP (Rogers, 2003).

Outreach and consultation by an expert promotes positive changes in practice behaviors of nurses and physicians (Hendryx et al., 1998; Thomson O'Brien et al., 2003b). In *outreach* (academic detailing), an expert meets one-on-one with practitioners in their setting to provide information about the EBP and feedback on provider performance (Davis, Thomson, Oxman, & Haynes, 1995; Hendryx et al., 1998; Hulscher et al., 1997; Oxman et al., 1995; Thomson O'Brien et al., 2003a, 2003b). This strategy, alone or in combination with other strategies, results in positive changes in health care practices (Davis et al., 1995; Hendryx et al., 1998; Jiang, Fieselmann, Hendryx, & Bock, 1997;

Pippalla, Riley, & Chinburapa, 1995; Thomson O'Brien et al., 2003a, 2003b; White, 1999). Geriatric nurse practitioners or advanced practice nurses (APNs) with expertise in gerontology can provide one-on-one consultation to staff regarding use of the EBP with specific patients, assist staff in troubleshooting issues in application of the practice, and provide feedback on provider performance regarding use of the EBPs. Studies have demonstrated that use of APNs as facilitators of change promotes adherence to the EBP (Bauchner & Simpson, 1998; Hendryx et al., 1998; Titler, 2003; Watson, 2004).

Users of the Innovation/Evidence-Based Practice. Members of a social system influence how quickly and widely EBPs are adopted (Rogers, 2003). Audit and feedback, performance gap assessment (PGA), and trying the EBP are strategies that have been tested (Berwick & Coltin, 1986; Lomas et al., 1991; Rogers, 2003; Thomson O'Brien et al., 2003a; Titler, 2003, 2004a; Titler et al., 2001). PGA and audit and feedback have consistently shown a positive effect on changing practice behavior of providers (Berwick & Coltin, 1986; Lomas et al., 1991; McCartney, Macdowall, & Thorogood, 1997; Thomson O'Brien et al., 2003a). PGA (baseline practice performance) informs members, at the beginning of change, about a practice performance and opportunities for improvement. Specific practice indicators selected for PGA are related to the practices that are the focus of EBP change, such as every-4-hour pain assessment for acute pain management.

Audit and feedback is ongoing auditing of performance indicators (e.g., every-4-hour pain assessment) throughout the implementation process, and discussing the findings with practitioners during the practice change (Jamtvedt et al., 2004; Titler, 2004a). This strategy helps staff know and see how their efforts to improve care and patient outcomes are progressing throughout the implementation process. Audit and feedback should be done at regular intervals throughout the implementation process (e.g., every 4 to 6 weeks) (Jamtvedt et al., 2004; Thomson O'Brien et al., 2003a). Performance gap assessment and audit and feedback data can be provided in run charts, statistical process control charts, or bar graphs (Carey, 2002).

Characteristics of users such as educational preparation, practice specialty, and views on innovativeness influence adoption of an innovation (Retchin, 1997; Rogers, 2003; Rutledge et al., 1996; Salem-Schatz, Gottlieb, Karp, & Feingold, 1997; Schneider & Eisenberg, 1998; Shively et al., 1997). Users of an innovation usually try it for a period of time before adopting it in their practice (Meyer & Goes, 1988; Rogers, 2003). When "trying an EBP" (piloting the change) is incorporated as part of the implementation process, users have an opportunity to use it for a period of time, provide feedback to those in charge of implementation, and modify the practice if necessary. Piloting the EBP as part of implementation has a positive influence on the extent of adoption of the new practice (Rogers, 2003; Shively et al., 1997; Titler, 2003; Titler et al., 2001).

Social System. The social system (context) has a high degree of influence on adoption of an innovation (Ciliska et al., 1999; Fraser, 2004a, 2004b; Institute of Medicine, 2001; Morin et al., 1999; Rogers, 2003; Thompson, 2001; Vaughn et al., 2002). Leadership support is critical for promoting use of EBPs (Antrobus & Kitson, 1999; Baggs & Mick, 2000; Berwick, 2003; Carr & Schott, 2002; Jadad & Haynes, 1998; Katz, 1999; Morin et al., 1999; Nagy, Lumby, McKinley, & Macfarlane, 2001; Omery & Williams, 1999; Retsas, 2000; Stetler, 2003), and is expressed verbally, as well as by providing necessary resources, materials, and time to fulfill assigned responsibilities (Omery & Williams, 1999; Rutledge & Donaldson, 1995). Additional organizational variables that influence adoption include (1) access to inventors/researchers, (2) authority to change practice, and (3) support from and collaboration with peers, other disciplines, and administrators to align practice with the evidence base (Bach, 1995; Barnason et al., 1998; Crane, 1995; Funk et al., 1995; Funk, Tornquist, & Champagne, 1995; Leatt, Baker, Halverson, & Aird, 1997; Nutley & Davies, 2000; Rodgers, 1994; Shortell et al., 1995; Thomson O'Brien et al., 2002; Titler, 1998; Tranmer et al., 1998; Walshe & Rundall, 2001). As part of the work of implementing the change, it is important that the social system—unit, service line, or clinic—ensure that policies, procedures, standards, clinical pathways, and documentation systems support the use of the EBPs (Rutledge & Donaldson, 1995; Titler, 2004a). Documentation forms or clinical information systems may need revision to support changes in practice; documentation systems that fail to readily support the new practice thwart change. For example, if staff members are expected to reassess and document pain intensity within 30 minutes following administration of an analgesic agent, documentation forms must reflect this practice standard. It is the role of upper- and middle-level leadership to ensure that organizational documents and systems are flexible and supportive of the EBPs.

In summary, making an evidence-based change in practice involves a series of steps and a process that is often nonlinear. Implementing the change will take several weeks to months, depending on the nature of the practice change. It is important that senior leadership and those leading the project are aware of change as a process and continue to encourage and teach peers about the change in practice. The new practice must be continually reinforced and sustained or the practice change will be intermittent and soon fade, allowing more traditional methods of care to return (Titler, 2005).

Sites of Care Delivery. Care of older adults occurs in a variety of settings, such as the home health, ambulatory, hospital, and skilled and long-term care settings. Clearly, organizational context matters when implementing EBPs (Denis et al., 2002; Fleuren, Wiefferink, & Paulussen, 2004). For example, investigators have demonstrated the effectiveness of prompted voiding for urinary incontinence in nursing homes, but sustaining the intervention in day-to-day practice was limited when the responsibility of carrying out the intervention was shifted to nursing home staff (rather than the investigative team) and required staffing levels greater than those in a majority of nursing home settings (Engberg, Kincade, & Thompson, 2004). A number of factors influence the organizational context for EBP.

The mission and vision of the organization lay the foundation for the integration of EBPs. For EBPs to be manifested in everyday work, it is necessary to incorporate specific action statements that promote and foster EBPs into the organization's or department's strategic plan. Such actions might include offering an annual EBP staff nurse internship program; integrating educational content about EBP into orientation of new staff; monitoring and acting on the results of key indicators for selected EBPs (acute pain management, prevention of pressure ulcers, fall prevention); and initiating two to three new EBPs per year that are triggered by operational or quality improvement data. Clarity about the following is also helpful: (1) the definition and meaning of EBP in the organization, (2) the organizational process or model of EBP, and (3) a philosophy of care that embraces clinical inquiry and questioning of the status quo (Titler, 2005).

The chief nurse executive sets the tone for EBP and explicates role expectations of others regarding the knowledge, skills, and behaviors necessary to promote adoption of EBPs. Enactment of EBP includes providing resources for EBP such as easy access to EBP Web sites, retaining personnel with expertise in EBP, supporting programs that develop a critical mass of staff nurses with expertise in EBP (e.g., EBP staff nurse internship program) (Cullen & Titler, 2004), providing access to assistance with analysis of data and transforming data into information, and ensuring staffing ratios that promote use of the EBP. More explicitly, to sustain a vision of providing evidence-based health care, the work and accountability for EBP must be integrated into the governance structure. This includes interdisciplinary collaboration across departments and services, as well as coordination within discipline-specific areas of practice. For example, in nursing, the process and evaluation of evidence-based changes in practice should be coordinated with professional nursing practice, quality improvement, research, policy and procedure, and staff education committees or councils (Titler, 2005).

Both recognition of and reward for EBP behaviors are essential. Such recognition can range from submitting staff projects and names to national and international professional organizations that have recognition programs for excellence in EBP (e.g., STTI), to recognizing specific staff members in their unit at the change of shift for the care they provide based on evidence. Some organizations integrate EBP expectations into the clinical ladder system, and others provide staff release time from direct patient care to do the work of EBP. Recognition by peers, as well as senior administrators, is important (Titler, 2005).

Although these strategies help create an EBP culture, their feasibility in different types of settings is not well understood. Little research to date has been done to expand our understanding of organizational context

(Denis et al., 2002; Fleuren et al., 2004; Foxcroft & Colen, 2004; Greenhalgh et al., 2004). "Context is displayed as an important (and poorly understood) mediator of the diffusion of innovations" (Dopson et al., 2002, p. 43). Research is necessary to understand how to measure and improve organizational capacity and system readiness for innovations such as EBPs (Greenhalgh et al., 2004). This is particularly important in long-term, skilled, and home health care settings (Feldman & McDonald, 2004; Jones et al., 2004; Roe et al., 2004; Watson, 2004).

Role of Nurses in Promoting Evidence-Based Practice

Sample performance criteria for various nursing roles are listed in Box 5-8. Chief nurse executives and their leadership staff set the stage and culture for EBP in their settings. Providing this leadership is a continuous

---

BOX 5-8 Sample EBP Performance Criteria for Nursing Roles

STAFF NURSE (RN)	ADVANCED PRACTICE NURSE (APN)	NURSE MANAGER (NM)	ASSOCIATE DIRECTOR FOR CLINICAL SERVICES	CHIEF NURSE EXECUTIVE
Questions current practices	Serves as coach and mentor in EBP	Creates a microsystem that fosters critical thinking	Hires and retains NMs and APNs with knowledge and skills in EBP	Ensures the governance reflects EBP if initiated in the councils and committees
Participates in implementing changes in practice based on evidence	Facilitates locating evidence	Challenges staff to seek out evidence to resolve clinical issues and improve care	Provides learning environment for EBP	Assign accountability for EBP
Participates as a member of an EBP project team	Synthesizes evidence for practice		Uses evidence in leadership decisions	Ensures explicit articulation of organizational and department commitment to EBP
Reads evidence related to one's practice	Uses evidence to write/modify practice standards	Role models EBP		
Participates in quality improvement initiatives	Role models use of evidence in practice	Uses evidence to guide operations and management decisions	Sets strategic directions for EBP	Modifies mission and vision to include EBP language
	Facilitates system changes to support use of EBPs	Uses performance criteria about EBP in evaluation of staff	Provides resources for EBP	Provides resources to support EBPs by direct care providers
Suggests resolutions for clinical issues based on evidence			Integrates EBP processes into division/service line governance	Articulates value of EBP to CEO and governing board
				Role models EBP in administrative decision making

process that involves the following (Titler, Cullen, & Ardery, 2002):

- Incorporating EBP terminology into the mission, vision, strategic plan, and philosophy of care delivery
- Establishing explicit performance expectations about EBP for staff at all levels of the organization
- Integrating the work of EBP into the governance structure of nursing departments and the health care system
- Recognizing and rewarding EBP behaviors

Performance expectations of nurses in advanced practice roles (e.g., APN, GNP) include leading a team, finding the evidence, and synthesizing the evidence for practice. Advanced practice nurses assist staff members with focusing their clinical question about improving practice, finding and evaluating the research evidence, and maneuvering through governance structures to implement and sustain the changes in practice. Nurses in advanced practice roles are critical to helping staff retrieve and critique the studies and other evidence on the selected topic. Although staff nurses are often willing to participate, nurses in advanced practice roles provide significant leadership in the process by facilitating synthesis of the research and other evidence, critically analyzing what practices should be changed, assisting staff members to communicate these changes to their peers, and role modeling changes in practice (Titler, 2005).

Nurse managers set the tone, value, and work culture for the microsystems they lead. The role of the nurse manager is critical in making EBP changes a reality for staff providing direct care. Performance expectations include creating a culture that fosters interdisciplinary quality improvement based on evidence. Nurse managers must expect that staff members will participate in EBP activities, role model the change in their practice, and provide written and verbal support for the practice change. When selecting a potential topic, it is important that the nurse manager values the idea and supports the potential changes. Nurse managers also foster EBPs in their units by allocation of resources, an important element for staff nurse enactment of EBP. Staff migrate to microsystems that foster professional growth, professional nursing practice, data-based decision making, and innovative practices, all of which are characteristics of cultures that promote adoption of evidence-based nursing practices (Titler, 2005).

Associate directors of nursing who hire, retain, and value, via performance appraisals, nurse managers and APNs skilled in EBP are more likely to observe development of clinical innovations and adoption of EBPs in the multiple units and sites of care delivery for which they are responsible. They must expect that their direct reports will foster EBP in their roles and reward these behaviors through performance appraisals and other forms of recognition (Titler, 2005).

Staff nurses are key to improving care delivery through use of evidence and serve key roles in influencing their peers in implementation of EBP standards. The role of staff nurses in EBP include challenging the status quo of care delivery, asking clinical questions, bringing forward problem- or knowledge-focused triggers that might be addressed through the use of evidence, serving as change champions, and learning the evidence-based knowledge and skills to carry out the EBPs. Additionally, staff nurses should keep abreast of new knowledge generated through research and think critically about application of this evidence in practice (Cullen & Titler, 2004; Titler, 2005).

The role of nursing assistants/assistive personnel is less well developed, and little attention has been given to engagement of nursing assistants in EBP work (Frantz et al., 2003; Jones et al., 2004; Watson, 2004). Role expectations of nursing assistants for EBP are, to date, not available, nor do EBP experts agree on their role. It is imperative, however, that nursing assistants have basic knowledge and skills for carrying out the EBPs and that leadership staff work with them to clarify their role. For example, nursing assistants can do initial screening for pain assessment and work with licensed personnel to develop an effective, evidence-based plan of care.

Educators in clinical practice are important resources for teaching components of the EBP process and for the evidence base of specific clinical topics. In addition, staff educators should think critically about the content they teach in orientation and staff education programs to determine if it is evidence based. They should also be using evidence-based educational strategies.

Educators in academic settings have significant responsibilities: teaching clinical content from an evidence-based perspective, teaching the process of EBP, and providing learning opportunities with an EBP project. This requires that learning objectives for EBP are identified for undergraduate, master's, and doctoral students, and that corresponding learning activities are incorporated throughout the curriculum. For example, a learning objective of knowing where to find the evidence is essential for undergraduate students. A learning experience might include finding and applying the evidence for a clinical patient assignment (e.g., prevention of pressure ulcers) or reading and critiquing a research article or EBP guideline applicable to their clinical assignment.

Resources for Evidence-Based Practice

A number of resources for EBP have been outlined in the preceding discussions. In addition, resources in your local area may include an academic health care setting with individuals knowledgeable about EBP or gerontology (e.g., colleges of nursing, schools of public health); local librarians, who can assist with finding the evidence;

national centers, such as the Gerontological Nursing Interventions Research Center at the University of Iowa; and other written resources, such as *Geriatric Nursing Protocols for Best Practice* (Mezey et al., 2003).

Individuals should also contact nurse researchers conducting research on a specific topic that is the focus of EBP work. Because professional organizations such as AGS and federal agencies such as AHRQ have made commitments to synthesis of evidence on clinical topics, the process is less of a challenge today than 10 years ago. Focus and expertise on implementation strategies specific to types of organizations (e.g., acute care, long-term care) is less well understood, and there is not one "well-worn path" to implementation. However, several excellent written and human resources can assist with this process (Cullen & Titler, 2004; DiCenso et al., 2004; Feldman & McDonald, 2004; Frantz et al., 2003; Melnyk & Fineout-Overholt, 2004; Nursing Knowledge International, 2005; Registered Nurses Association of Ontario, 2004; Titler, 2002).

FUTURE TRENDS IN EVIDENCE-BASED PRACTICE AND TRANSLATION SCIENCE

Education of nurses must include knowledge and skills in the use of research findings and other types of evidence in practice. Nurses are increasingly being held accountable for practices based on scientific evidence. Thus we must communicate and integrate into our profession the expectation that it is the professional responsibility of all nurses to read and use research in their practice and to communicate with nurse scientists the many and varied clinical problems for which we do not yet have a scientific base.

Future trends in EBP include creating organizational practice cultures that support EBP; teaching graduate and undergraduate students the knowledge and skills necessary to practice, based on evidence; redesigning health care work to have evidence readily available for direct care providers; and providing human and monetary resources that support EBP. Given the limited number of resources available, it seems likely that decision makers will need to prioritize which EBP guidelines to implement based on considerations of local burden of disease, availability of effective and efficient health care interventions, and local evidence of suboptimal performance (Grimshaw et al., 2004). As federal agencies such as the Center for Medicare and Medicaid Services (CMS) start expecting and reimbursing for care based on evidence, EBP will no longer be an option but an expectation.

Although there are a myriad of initiatives aimed at increasing use of evidence in practice, there is little systematic evidence of the effectiveness of these initiatives (Greenhalgh et al., 2004; Grimshaw et al., 2004; Nutley et al., 2003). Translation science is the investigation of methods, interventions, and variables that influence adoption of EBPs by individuals and organizations to improve clinical and operational decision making in health care (Kovner, Elton, & Billings, 2000; Titler & Everett, 2001; Walshe & Rundall, 2001). Examples of translation studies include describing facilitators of and barriers to knowledge uptake and use, testing the effect of implementation strategies on promoting and sustaining adoption of EBPs, organizational predictors of adherence to ambulatory care guidelines, attitudes toward EBPs, and defining the structure of the scientific field (Dykes, 2003; Estabrooks, 2004; Feldman & McDonald, 2004; Jones et al., 2004; Kirchhoff, 2004; Pineros, Sales, Yu-Fang, & Sharp, 2004; Titler, 2004a). To advance knowledge regarding the best mechanisms for promoting and sustaining adoption of EBPs in health care, translation science needs more experimental studies that test translating research into practice interventions (Tang & Titler, 2003; Titler, 2004a; Titler & Everett, 2001). Partnership models, which encourage ongoing interaction between researchers and practitioners, may be the way forward to carry out such studies (Nutley et al., 2003). The state of the science and the challenges, issues, methods, and instruments used in translation research are described elsewhere (Dawson, 2004; Donaldson, Rutledge, & Ashley, 2004; Dufault, 2004; Feldman & McDonald, 2004; Fraser, 2004a, 2004b; Kirchhoff, 2004; Pineros et al., 2004; Titler, 2004a, 2004b; Tripp-Reimer & Doebbeling, 2004; U.S. Invitational Conference, 2004; Watson, 2004; Williams, 2004).

For organizations to take advantage of EBP projects from various sites throughout the country, a national center for EBP and translation science is needed. Such a center could facilitate networking among health care professionals working on similar EBP topics and provide helpful educational materials and consultation services for EBP and translation science (Titler, 1997). This center would also provide data regarding the interventions/strategies that have been tested to translate research into practice and provide a "tool kit" of these interventions for use by all types of health care agencies (QUERI, 2004; Registered Nurses Association of Ontario, 2004; Titler, 2002). For example, a tool kit on use of opinion leaders to translate research into practice might include a definition, characteristics, and function of opinion leaders; methods for selecting an opinion leader; types of settings and projects in which opinion leaders have been used effectively; and methods to evaluate the effect of using opinion leaders in promoting adoption of certain EBPs. Last, such a center would also conduct translation research and provide consultation regarding research methods and design specifically for translation science (Titler, 2004a).

SUMMARY

EBPs have the potential to improve care for older adults in all settings by increasing the use of research findings in practice. This chapter provides an overview of the EBP process and the Iowa Model of Evidence-Based Practice to Promote Quality Care (Titler et al., 2001). Steps in the process include selecting a topic, forming a team, retrieving and critiquing the evidence, developing practice recommendations, implementing the EBPs, and evaluating the EBPs and their impact. Rogers' Diffusion of Innovation Model (Rogers, 2003) is used to discuss issues in implementing changes in practice. Gerontological nurses can play many roles in the development and implementation of EBPs and promote a practice environment that supports use of evidence to provide quality care.

REFERENCES

Agency for Healthcare Research and Quality. (2002). *Systems to rate the strength of scientific evidence. Summary.* Evidence Report/Technology Assessment Report no. 47, pub. no. 02-E015. Bethesda, MD: U.S. Department of Health and Human Services, Agency for Healthcare Research and Quality.

Alderson, P., Green, S., & Higgins, J. P. T. (2003). Cochrane reviewers' handbook 4.2.1. Retrieved March 30, 2004, from www.cochrane .org/resources/handbook/handbook.pdf.

American Geriatrics Society, British Geriatrics Society, American Academy of Orthopaedic Surgeons, & Panel on Falls Prevention. (2001). Guideline for the prevention of falls in older persons. *JAGS, 49*(5), 664-672.

Antrobus, S., & Kitson, A. (1999). Nursing leadership: Influencing and shaping health policy and nursing practice. *Journal of Advanced Nursing, 29*(3), 746-753.

Appraisal of Guidelines Research and Evaluation. (2001). Retrieved June 5, 2005, from www.agreecollaboration.org/instrument.

Atkins, D. M., Kamerow, D. M., & Eisenberg, J. M. M. (1998, March-April). Evidence-based medicine at the Agency for Health Care Policy and Research. *ACP Journal Club, 128*, A1214.

Bach, D. M. (Ed.). (1995). *Implementation of the Agency for Health Care Policy and Research postoperative pain management guideline* (vol. 30). Philadelphia: W. B. Saunders.

Baggs, J. G., & Mick, D. J. (2000). Collaboration: A tool addressing ethical issues for elderly patients near the end of life in intensive care units. *Journal of Gerontological Nursing, 26*(9), 41-47.

Baker, R., & Feder, G. (1997). Clinical guidelines: Where next? *International Journal for Quality in Health Care, 9*(6), 399-404.

Barnason, S., Merboth, M., Pozehl, B., & Tietjen, M. J. (1998). Utilizing an outcomes approach to improve pain management by nurses: A pilot study. *Clinical Nurse Specialist, 12*(1), 28-36.

Barnsteiner, J. H., Ford, N., & Howe, C. (1995). Research utilization in a metropolitan children's hospital. *Nursing Clinics of North America, 30*(3), 447-455.

Bauchner, H., & Simpson, L. (1998). Specific issues related to developing, disseminating, and implementing pediatric practice guidelines for physicians, patients, families, and other stakeholders. *Health Services Research, 33*(4), 1161-1177.

Berg, A. O., Atkins, D., & Tierney, W. (1997, April). Clinical practice guidelines in practice and education. *JGIM, 12*(suppl 2), S25-S33.

Berner, E. S., Baker, C. S., Funkhouser, E., Heudebert, G. R., Allison, J. J., Fargason, C. A., et al. (2003). Do local opinion leaders augment hospital quality improvement efforts? A randomized trial to pro-mote adherence to unstable angina guideline. *Medical Care, 41*(3), 420-431.

Bero, L. A., Grilli, R., Grimshaw, J. M., Harvey, E., Oxman, A. D., & Thomson, M. A. (1998). Closing the gap between research and practice: An overview of systematic reviews of interventions to promote the implementation of research findings. *BMJ, 317*, 465-468.

Berwick, D. M. (2003). Disseminating innovations in health care. *JAMA, 289*(15), 1969-1975.

Berwick, D. M., & Coltin, K. L. (1986). Feedback reduces test use in a health maintenance organization. *JAMA, 255*, 1450-1454.

Bostrom, J., & Suter, W. (1993). Research utilization: Make the link to practice. *Journal of Nursing Staff Development, 9*, 28-34.

Bottrell, M., Abraham, I., Fulmer, T., & Mezey, M. (1999). *Geriatric nursing protocols for best practice.* New York: Springer.

Brown, S. J. (1999). *Knowledge for health care practice: A guide to using research evidence.* Philadelphia: W. B. Saunders.

Brown, S. J. (2002). Focus on research methods. Nursing intervention studies: A descriptive analysis of issues important to clinicians. *Research in Nursing and Health, 25*, 317-327.

Burns, R., Pahor, M., & Shorr, R. I. (1997). Evidence-based medicine holds the key to the future for geriatric medicine. *JAGS, 45*(10), 1268-1272.

Camiletti, Y. A., & Huffman, M. C. (1998). Research utilization: Evaluation of initiatives in a public health nursing division. *Canadian Journal of Nursing Administration, 11*(2), 59-77.

Carey, R. A. (2002). *Improving healthcare with control charts: Basic and advanced SPC methods and case studies.* Milwaukee, WI: American Society for Quality.

Carr, C. A., & Schott, A. (2002). Differences in evidence-based care in midwifery practice and education. *Journal of Nursing Scholarship, 34*(2), 153-158.

Carroll, D. L., Greenwood, R., Lynch, K. E., Sullivan, J. K., Ready, C. H., & Fitzmaurice, J. B. (1997). Barriers and facilitators to the utilization of nursing research. *Clinical Nurse Specialist, 11*(5), 207-212.

Ciliska, D., Hayward, S., Dobbins, M., Brunton, G., & Underwood, J. (1999). Transferring public-health nursing research to health-system planning: Assessing the relevance and accessibility of systematic reviews. *Canadian Journal of Nursing Research, 31*(1), 23-36.

Cluzeau, F., Littlejohns, P., Grimshaw, J., & Feder, G. (1997). *Appraisal instrument or clinical guidelines, version 1 user guide.* London: St. George's Hospital Medical School.

Cluzeau, F. A., & Littlejohns, P. (1999). Appraising clinical practice guidelines in England and Wales: The development of a methodologic framework and its application to policy. *Joint Commission Journal on Quality Improvement, 25*(10), 514-521.

Collins, B. A., Hawks, J. W., & Davis, R. L. (2000, July). From theory to practice: Identifying authentic opinion leaders to improve care. *Managed Care*, pp. 56-62.

Cook, D. (1998). Evidence-based critical care medicine: A potential tool for change. *New Horizons, 6*(1), 20-25.

Cook, D. J., Greengold, N. L., Ellrodt, A. G., & Weingarten, S. R. (1997). The relation between systematic reviews and practice guidelines. *Ann Intern Med, 127*(3), 210-216.

Craig, J. V., & Smyth, R. L. (2002). *The evidence-based practice manual for nurses.* London: Churchill Livingstone.

Crane, J. (1995). The future of research utilization. *Nursing Clinics of North America, 30*, 566-579.

Cronenwett, L. R. (1995). Effective methods for disseminating research findings to nurses in practice. *Nursing Clinics of North America, 30*, 429-438.

Cullen, L. (2005). Evidence-based practice: Strategies for nursing leaders. In D. Huber (Ed.), *Leadership and nursing care management* (3rd ed). Philadelphia: Elsevier.

Cullen, L., & Titler, M. G. (2004). Promoting evidence-based practice: An internship for staff nurses. *Worldviews on Evidence-Based Practice, 1*(4), 215-223.

Davis, D. A., Thomson, M. A., Oxman, A. D., & Haynes, R. B. (1995). Changing physician performance: A systematic review of the effect of continuing medical education strategies. *JAMA, 274*(9), 700-705.

Dawson, J. D. (2004). Quantitative analytical methods in translation research. *Worldviews on Evidence-Based Nursing, 1*(S1), S60-S64.

Denis, J.-L., Hebert, Y., Langley, A., Lozeau, D., & Trottier, L.-H. (2002). Explaining diffusion patterns for complex health care innovations. *Health Care Management Review, 27*(3), 60-73.

DiCenso, A., Ciliska, D., Cullum, N., & Guyatt, G. (2004). *Evidence-based nursing: A guide to clinical practice.* St. Louis: Mosby.

Dickersin, K., & Manheimer, E. (1998). The Cochrane Collaboration: Evaluation of health care and services using systematic reviews of the results of randomized controlled trials. *Clinical Obstetrics and Gynecology, 41*(2), 315-331.

Doebbeling, B. N., Vaughn, T. E., Woolson, R. F., Peloso, P. M., Ward, M. M., Letuchy, E., et al. (2002). Benchmarking Veterans Affairs Medical Centers in the delivery of preventive health services: Comparison of methods. *Medical Care, 40*(6), 540-554.

Donaldson, N. E., Rutledge, D. N., & Ashley, J. (2004). Outcomes of adoption: Measuring evidence uptake by individuals and organizations. *Worldviews on Evidence-Based Nursing, 1*(S1), S41-S51.

Dopson, S., FitzGerald, L., Ferlie, E., Gabbay, J., & Locock, L. (2002). No magic targets! Changing clinical practice to become more evidence based. *Health Care Management Review, 27*(3), 35-47.

Dufault, M. A. (2001). A program of research evaluating the effects of collaborative research utilization model. *Online Journal of Knowledge Synthesis for Nursing, 8*(3), 7.

Dufault, M. A. (2004). Testing a collaborative research utilization model to translate best practices in pain management. *Worldviews on Evidence-Based Nursing, 1*(S1), S26-S32.

Dykes, P. C. (2003). Practice guidelines and measurement: State-of-the-science. *Nursing Outlook, 51*, 65-69.

Eliopoulos, C. (1997). *Gerontological nursing.* Philadelphia: Lippincott-Raven.

Engberg, S., Kincade, J., & Thompson, D. (2004). Future directions for incontinence research with frail elders. *Nursing Research, 53*(6S), S22-S29.

Estabrooks, C. A. (1998). Will evidence-based nursing practice make practice perfect? *Canadian Journal of Nursing Research, 30*(1), 15-36.

Estabrooks, C. A. (2004). Thoughts on evidence-based nursing and its science: A Canadian perspective. *Worldviews on Evidence-Based Nursing, 1*(2), 88-91.

Estabrooks, C. A., Winther, C., & Derksen, L. (2004). Mapping the field: A bibliometric analysis of the research utilization literature in nursing. *Nursing Research, 53*(5), 293-303.

Farquhar, C. M., Stryer, D., & Slutsky, J. (2002). Translating research into practice: The future ahead. *International Journal for Quality in Health Care, 14*(3), 233-249.

Feldman, P. H., & McDonald, M. V. (2004). Conducting translation research in the home care setting: Lessons from a just-in-time reminder study. *Worldviews on Evidence-Based Nursing, 1*, 49-59.

Fleuren, M., Wiefferink, K., & Paulussen, T. (2004). Determinants of innovation within health care organizations: Literature review and Delphi study. *International Journal for Quality in Health Care, 16*(2), 107-123.

Folkedahl, B., Frantz, R., & Goode, C. (2002). *Evidence-based protocol: Treatment of pressure ulcers.* Iowa City: Research Dissemination Core, Gerontological Nursing Interventions Research Center, University of Iowa College of Nursing.

Foxcroft, D. R., & Colen, N. (2004). Organisational infrastructures to promote evidence based nursing practice (protocol for a Cochrane Review). *Cochrane Library, 4.*

Frantz, R. A., Xakellis, G. C., Jr., Harvey, P. C., & Lewis, A. R. (2003). Implementing an incontinence management protocol in long-term care: Clinical outcomes and costs. *Journal of Gerontological Nursing, 29*(8), 46-53.

Fraser, I. (2004a). Organizational research with impact: Working backwards. *Worldviews on Evidence-Based Nursing, 1*(S1), S52-S59.

Fraser, I. (2004b). Translation research: Where do we go from here? *Worldviews on Evidence-Based Nursing, 1*(S1), S78-S83.

Funk, S. G., Champagne, M. T., Tornquist, E. M., & Wiese, R. A. (1995). Administrators' views on barriers to research utilization. *Applied Nursing Research, 8*(1), 44-49.

Funk, S. G., Tornquist, E., M., & Champagne, M. T. (1995). Barriers and facilitators of research utilization: An integrative review. *Nursing Clinics of North America, 30*, 395-408.

Geyman, J. P. (1998). Evidence-based medicine in primary care: An overview. *Journal of the American Board of Family Practice, 11*(1), 46-56.

Goode, C. J., & Piedalue, F. (1999). Evidence-based clinical practice. *JONA, 29*(6), 15-21.

Greenhalgh, T., Robert, G., MacFarlane, F., Bate, P., & Kyriakidou, O. (2004). Diffusion of innovations in service organizations: Systematic review and recommendations. *Milbank Quarterly, 82*(4), 581-629.

Greer, A. L. (1988). The state of the art versus the state of the science. *International Journal of Technology Assessment in Health Care, 4*, 5-26.

Grimshaw, J. M., Thomas, R. E., MacLennan, G., Fraser, C., Ramsay, C. R., Vale, L., et al. (2004). Effectiveness and efficiency of guide dissemination and implementation strategies. *Health Technology Assessment, 8*(6), i-xi, 1-72.

Haber, J., Feldman, H. R., Penney, N., Carter, E., Bidwell-Cerone, S., & Hott, J. R. (1994). Shaping nursing practice through research-based protocols. *Journal of the New York State Nurses Association, 25*(3), 4-12.

Harvey, G., Loftus-Hills, A., Rycroft-Malone, J., Titchen, A., Kitson, A., McCormack, B., & Seers, K. (2002). Getting evidence into practice: The role and function of facilitation. *Journal of Advanced Nursing, 37*(6), 577-588.

Health Grades, Inc. (2004). *Health Grades quality study: Patient safety in American Hospitals.* Golden, CO: Health Grades, Inc.

Hendryx, M. S., Fieselmann, J. F., Bock, M. J., Wakefield, D. S., Helms, C. M., & Bentler, S. E. (1998). Outreach education to improve quality of rural ICU care. Results of a randomized trial. *American Journal of Respiratory and Critical Care Medicine, 158*(2), 418-423.

Herr, K., Titler, M. G., Schilling, M. L., Marsh, J. L., Xie, X., Ardery, G., et al. (2004). Evidence-based assessment of acute pain in older adults: Current nursing practices and perceived barriers. *Clinical Journal of Pain, 20*(5), 331-340.

Hodes, R. (2005). Director's message. Retrieved September 24, 2005, from www.nia.nih.gov/aboutnia/strategicplan/directorsmessage.htm.

Hulscher, M. E., van Drenth, B. B., van der Wouden, J. C., Mokkink, H. G., van Weel, C., & Grol, R. P. (1997). Changing preventive practice: A controlled trial on the effects of outreach visits to organise prevention of cardiovascular disease. *Quality in Health Care, 6*(1), 19-24.

Hunt, D. L., Haynes, R. B., Hanna, S. E., & Smith, K. (1998). Effects of computer-based clinical decision support systems on physician performance and patient outcomes: A systematic review. *JAMA, 280*(15), 1339-1346.

Institute of Medicine. (2001). *Crossing the quality chasm: A new health system for the 21st century.* Washington, DC: National Academy Press.

Institute of Medicine. (2003). *Priority areas for national action: Transforming health care quality.* Washington, DC: National Academy Press.

Jadad, A. R., & Haynes, R. B. (1998). The Cochrane collaboration: Advances and challenges in improving evidence-based decision making. *Medical Decision Making, 18*, 2-9.

Jamtvedt, G., Young, J. M., Kristoffersen, D. T., Thomson O'Brien, M. A., & Oxman, A. D. (2004). *Audit and feedback: Effects on professional practice and health care outcomes (Cochrane Review). Cochrane Library, Issue 1.* Chichester, UK: John Wiley & Sons, Ltd.

Jiang, H. J., Fieselmann, J. F., Hendryx, M. S., & Bock, M. J. (1997). Assessing the impact of patient characteristics and process performance on rural intensive care unit hospital mortality rates. *Critical Care Medicine, 25*(5), 773-778.

Joanna Briggs Institute. (2000). Appraising systematic review. *Changing Practice, 1*(1), 1-6. Retrieved September 19, 2005, from www.joannabriggs.edu.au/pubs/cpmenu.php.

Joanna Briggs Institute. (2001). An introduction to systematic reviews. *Changing Practice, 2*(1), 1-6. Retrieved September 19, 2005, from www.joannabriggs.edu.au/pubs/cpmenu.php.

Jones, J. (2000). Performance improvement through clinical research utilization: The linkage model. *Journal of Nursing Care Quality, 15*(1), 49-54.

Jones, K. R., Fink, R., Vojir, C., Pepper, G., Hutt, E., Clark, L., et al. (2004). Translation research in long-term care: Improving pain management in nursing homes. *Worldviews on Evidence-Based Nursing, 1*(S1), S13-S20.

Kamerow, D. B. (1997). Before and after guidelines. *Journal of Family Practice, 44*(4), 344-346.

Katz, D. A. (1999). Barriers between guidelines and improved patient care: An analysis of AHCPR's unstable angina clinical practice guideline. *HSR, 34*(1), 337-389.

Kirchhoff, K. T. (2004). State of the science of translational research: From demonstration projects to intervention testing. *Worldviews on Evidence-Based Nursing, 1*(S1), S6-S12.

Kitson, A., Harvey, G., & McCormack, B. (1998). Enabling the implementation of evidence based practice: A conceptual framework. *Quality in Health Care, 7*(3), 149-158.

Kovner, A. R., Elton, J. J., & Billings, J. (2000). Evidence-based management. *Frontiers of Health Services Management, 16*(4), 3-24.

Lavis, J. N., Robertson, D., Woodside, J. M., McLeod, C. B., Abelson, J., & Knowledge Transfer Study Group. (2003). How can research organizations more effectively transfer research knowledge to decision makers? *Milbank Quarterly, 81*(2), 221-248.

Leatt, P., Baker, G. R., Halverson, P. K., & Aird, C. (1997). Downsizing, reengineering, and restructuring: Long-term implications for health care organizations. *Frontiers of Health Services Management, 13*, 3-37.

Lepper, H. S., & Titler, M. G. (1999). Program evaluation. In M. A. Mateo & K. T. Kirchhoff (Eds.), *Using and conducting nursing research in the clinical setting* (2nd ed.). Philadelphia: W. B. Saunders.

Liddle, J., Williamson, M., & Irwig, L. (1996). *Improving health care and outcomes: Method for evaluating research guideline evidence.* State Health pub. no. (CEB) 96-204. Sydney: NSW Health Department.

LoBiondo-Wood, G., & Haber, J. E. (2005). *Nursing research: Methods and critical appraisal for evidence-based practice* (6th ed.). St. Louis: Mosby.

Locock, L., Dopson, S., Chambers, D., & Gabbay, J. (2001). Understanding the role of opinion leaders in improving clinical effectiveness. *Social Science and Medicine, 53*, 745-757.

Logan, J., Harrison, M. B., Graham, I. D., Dunn, K., & Bissonnette, J. (1999). Evidence-based pressure-ulcer practice: The Ottawa Model of Research Use. *Canadian Journal of Nursing Research, 31*(1), 37-52.

Lomas, J., Enkin, M., Anderson, G. M., Hannah, W. J., Vayda, E., & Singer, J. (1991). Opinion leaders vs. audit and feedback to implement practice guidelines: Delivery after previous cesarean section. *JAMA, 265*, 2202-2207.

Lubarsky, D. A., Glass, P. S. A., Ginsberg, B., Dear, G. L., Dentz, M. E., Gan, T. J., et al. (1997). The successful implementation of pharmaceutical practice guidelines: Analysis of associated outcomes and cost savings. *Anesthesiology, 86*(5), 1145-1160.

Madsen, D., Sebolt, T., Cullen, L., Folkedahl, B., Mueller, T., Richardson, C., & Titler, M. (2005). Listening to bowel sounds: An evidence-based practice project: Nurses find that a traditional practice isn't the best indicator of returning gastrointestinal motility in patients who've undergone abdominal surgery. *American Journal of Nursing, 105*(12), 40-49.

Mateo, M. A., & Kirchhoff, K. T. (1999). *Conducting and using nursing research in the clinical setting* (2nd ed.). Philadelphia: W. B. Saunders.

McCartney, P., Macdowall, W., & Thorogood, M. (1997). Feedback to general practitioners: Increased prescribing of aspirin to patients with ischaemic heart disease. *BMJ, 315*, 35-36.

McCormick, K. A., Cummings, M. A., & Kovner, C. (1997). The role of the Agency for Health Care Policy and Research in improving outcomes of care. *Nursing Clinics of North America, 32*(3), 521-542.

McCurren, C. (1995). Research utilization: Meeting the challenge. *Geriatric Nursing, 16*(5), 132-135.

Melnyk, B. M., & Fineout-Overholt, E. (2004). *Evidence-based practice in nursing and healthcare: A guide to best practice.* Hagerstown, MD: Lippincott Williams & Wilkins.

Meyer, A. D., & Goes, J. B. (1988). Organizational assimilation of innovations: A multilevel contextual analysis. *Academy of Management Journal, 31*, 897-923.

Mezey, M., Fulmer, T., & Abraham, I. (2003). *Geriatric nursing protocols for best practice* (2nd ed.). New York: Springer.

Mion, L. C. (1998). Evidence-based health care practice. *Journal of Gerontological Nursing, 24*(12), 5-6.

Morin, K. H., Bucher, L., Plowfield, L., Hayes, E., Mahoney, P., & Armiger, L. (1999). Using research to establish protocols for practice: A statewide study of acute care agencies. *Clinical Nurse Specialist, 13*(2), 77-84.

Mount Sinai Hospital—University Health Network: Centre for Evidence-Based Medicine. (2001). Retrieved September 24, 2005, from www.library.utoronto.ca/medicine/ebm/glossary/.

Nagy, S., Lumby, J., McKinley, S., & Macfarlane, C. (2001). Nurses' beliefs about the conditions that hinder or support evidence-based nursing. *International Journal of Nursing Practice, 7*(5), 314-321.

Newman, K., Pyne, T., Leigh, S., Rounce, K., & Cowling, A. (2000). Personal and organizational competencies requisite for the adoption and implementation of evidence-based healthcare. *Health Services Management Research, 13*, 97-110.

NHS Research and Development: Centre for Evidence Based Medicine. (2001). Retrieved September 24, 2005, from http://cebm.jr2.ox.ac.uk/docs/glossary.html.

Nursing Knowledge International. (2005). Retrieved January 19, 2005, from www.nursingknowledge.org/Portal/main.aspx.

Nutley, S., Davies, H., & Walter, I. (2003). Evidence based policy and practice: Cross sector lessons from the UK. Keynote paper for the Social Policy Research and Evaluation Conference, Wellington, NZ.

Nutley, S., & Davies, H. T. O. (2000, October-December). Making a reality of evidence-based practice: Some lessons from the diffusion of innovations. *Public Money and Management*, pp. 35-42.

O'Connor, P. J., Solberg, L. I., Christianson, J., Amundson, G., & Mosser, G. (1996). Mechanism of action and impact of a cystitis clinical practice guideline on outcomes and costs of care in an HMO. *Joint Commission Journal on Quality Improvement, 22*, 673-682.

Olade, R. A. (2004). Evidence-based practice and research utilization activities among rural nurses. *Journal of Nursing Scholarship, 36*(3), 220-225.

Omery, A., & Williams, R. P. (1999). An appraisal of research utilization across the United States. *Journal of Nursing Administration, 29*(12), 50-56.

Oxman, A. D., Thomson, M. A., Davis, D. A., & Haynes, R. B. (1995). No magic bullets: A systematic review of 102 trials of interventions to improve professional practice. *Canadian Medical Association Journal, 153*(10), 1423-1431.

Pettengill, M., Gilles, D., & Clar, C. (1994). Factors encouraging and discouraging the use of nursing research. *Image: Journal of Nursing Scholarship, 26*(2), 143-147.

Pineros, S. L., Sales, A. E., Yu-Fang, L., & Sharp, N. D. (2004). Improving care to patients with ischemic heart disease: Experiences in a single network of the Veterans Health Administration. *Worldviews on Evidence-Based Nursing, 1*(S1), S33-S40.

Pippalla, R. S., Riley, D. A., & Chinburapa, V. (1995). Influencing the prescribing behavior of physicians: A metaevaluation. *Journal of Clinical Pharmacy and Therapeutics, 20,* 189-198.

Piven, M. (2001). *Detection of depression in the cognitively intact older adult with QRG and consumer insert.* Iowa City, IA: Research Dissemination Core of the Gerontological Nursing Interventions Research Center, University of Iowa College of Nursing.

QUERI. (2004). Retrieved November 30, 2004, from www.hsrd .research.va.gov/queri/implementation/section_2/default.cfm.

Registered Nurses Association of Ontario. (2004). Implementation of clinical practice guidelines. Retrieved November 30, 2004, from www.rnao.org/bestpractices/completed_guidelines/BPG_Guide_C1 _Toolkit.asp.

Retchin, S. M. (1997). The modification of physician practice patterns. *Clinical Performance and Quality Health Care, 5,* 202-207.

Retsas, A. (2000). Barriers to using research evidence in nursing practice. *Journal of Advanced Nursing, 31*(3), 599-606.

Rochon, P. A., Dikinson, E., & Gordon, M. (1997). The Cochrane Field in health care of older people: Geriatric medicine's role in the collaboration. *JAGS, 45*(2), 241-243.

Rodgers, S. (1994). An exploratory study of research utilization by nurses in general medical and surgical wards. *Journal of Advanced Nursing, 20,* 904-911.

Roe, B., Watson, N. M., Palmer, M. H., Boyington, A. R., O'Dell, K. K., & Wooldridge, L. (2004). Translating research on incontinence into practice. *Nursing Research, 53*(6S), S56-S60.

Rogers, E. M. (1995). *Diffusion of innovations.* New York: Free Press.

Rogers, E. M. (2003). *Diffusion of innovations* (5th ed.). New York: Free Press.

Rosswurm, M. A., & Larrabee, J. H. (1999). A model for change to evidence-based practice. *Image: Journal of Nursing Scholarship, 31*(4), 317-322.

Rutledge, D. N., & Donaldson, N. E. (1995). Building organizational capacity to engage in research utilization. *JONA, 25*(10), 12-16.

Rutledge, D. N., Greene, P., Mooney, K., Nail, L. M., & Ropka, M. (1996). Use of research-based practices by oncology staff nurses. *Oncology Nursing Forum, 23*(8), 1235-1244.

Rycroft-Malone, J., Kitson, A., Harvey, G., McCormack, B., Seers, K., Titchen, A., & Estabrooks, C. A. (2002). Ingredients for change: Revisiting a conceptual framework. *Quality and Safety in Health Care, 11,* 174-180.

Sackett, D., Rosenberg, W., Gray, J., Haynes, R., & Richardson, W. (1996). Evidence based medicine: What it is and what it isn't. *BMJ, 312,* 71-72.

Sackett, D. L., Straus, S. E., Richardson, W. S., Rosenberg, W., & Haynes, R. B. (2000). *Evidence-based medicine: How to practice and teach EBM.* London: Churchill Livingstone.

Salem-Schatz, S. R., Gottlieb, L. K., Karp, M. A., & Feingold, L. (1997). Attitudes about clinical practice guidelines in a mixed model HMO: The influence of physician and organizational characteristics. *HMO Practice, 11*(3), 111-117.

Schmidt, K. L., Alpen, M. A., & Rakel, B. A. (1996). Implementation of the Agency for Health Care Policy and Research pain guidelines. *AACN Clinical Issues, 7*(3), 425-435.

Schneider, E. C., & Eisenberg, J. M. (1998). Strategies and methods for aligning current and best medical practices: The role of information technologies. *Western Journal of Medicine, 168*(5), 311-318.

Schnelle, J. F., Cruise, P. A., Rahman, A., & Ouslander, J. G. (1998). Developing rehabilitative behavioral interventions for long-term care: Technology transfer, acceptance, and maintenance issues. *Journal of the American Geriatrics Society, 46*(6), 771-777.

Schoenbaum, S. C., Sundwall, D. N., Bergman, D., Buckle, J. M., Chernov, A., George, J., et al. (1995). *Using clinical practice guidelines to evaluate quality of care.* Volume 2: *Methods.* Rockville, MD: U.S. Department of Health and Human Services, Public Health Service, Agency for Health Care Policy and Research.

Shively, M., Riegel, B., Waterhouse, D., Burns, D., Templin, K., & Thomason, T. (1997). Testing a community level research utilization intervention. *Applied Nursing Research, 10*(3), 121-127.

Shortell, S. M., O'Brien, J. L., Carman, J. M., Foster, R. W., Hughes, E. F., Boerstler, H., & O' Connor, E. J. (1995). Assessing the impact of continuous quality improvement/total quality management: Concept versus implementation. *Health Services Research, 30,* 377-401.

Soukup, S. M. (2000). The center for advanced nursing practice evidence-based practice model. *Nursing Clinics of North America, 35*(2), 301-309.

Soumerai, S. B., McLaughlin, T. J., Gurwitz, J. H., Guadagnoli, E., Hauptman, P. J., Borbas, C., et al. (1998). Effect of local medical opinion leaders on quality of care for acute myocardial infarction: A randomized controlled trial. *JAMA, 279*(17), 1358-1363.

Stetler, C. B. (2003). Role of the organization in translating research into evidence-based practice. *Outcomes Management, 7*(3), 97-105.

Tang, J. H. C., & Titler, M. G. (2003). Evidence-based practice: Residency program in gerontological nursing. *Journal of Gerontological Nursing, 29*(11), 9-14.

Thompson, C. J. (2001). The meaning of research utilization: A preliminary typology. *Critical Care Nursing Clinics of North America, 13*(4), 475-485.

Thomson O'Brien, M., Freemantle, N., Oxman, A., Wolf, F., Davis, D., & Herrin, J. (2004a). Continuing education meetings and workshops (Systematic Review). Cochrane Effective Practice and Organisation of Care Group. *Cochrane Database of Systematic Reviews,* 4.

Thomson O'Brien, M., Oxman, A., Haynes, R., Davis, D., Freemantle, N., & Harvey, E. (2004b). Local opinion leaders: Effects on professional practice and health care outcomes (Cochrane Review). *Cochrane Library,* 4.

Thomson O'Brien, M. A., Oxman, A. D., Davis, D. A., Haynes, R. B., Freemantle, N., & Harvey, E. L. (2003a). Audit and feedback versus alternative strategies: Effects on professional practice and health care outcomes. *Cochrane Library,* Issue 2. Oxford: Update Software.

Thomson O'Brien, M. A., Oxman, A. D., Davis, D. A., Haynes, R. B., Freemantle, N., & Harvey, E. L. (2003b). Educational outreach visits: Effects on professional practice and health care outcomes. *Cochrane Library,* 2.

Thomson O'Brien, M. A., Oxman, A. D., Haynes, R. B., Davis, D. A., Freemantle, N., & Harvey, E. L. (2002). Local opinion leaders: Effects on professional practice and health care outcomes (Cochrane Review). *Cochrane Library,* 2.

Titler, M. (2003). TRIP intervention saves healthcare dollars and improves quality of care (abstract/poster). Paper presented at Translating Research into Practice: What's Working? What's Missing? What's Next? Sponsored by Agency for Healthcare Research and Quality, Washington, DC, July 22-24, 2003.

Titler, M. G. (1997). Research utilization: Necessity or luxury? In J. C. McCloskey & H. Grace (Eds.), *Current issues in nursing* (5th ed.). St. Louis: Mosby.

Titler, M. G. (1998). Use of research in practice. In G. LoBiondo-Wood & J. Haber (Eds.), *Nursing research* (4th ed.). St. Louis: Mosby.

Titler, M. G. (2002). *Toolkit for promoting evidence-based practice.* Iowa City: Department of Nursing Services and Patient Care, University of Iowa Hospitals and Clinics.

Titler, M. G. (2004a). Methods in translation science. *Worldviews on Evidence-Based Nursing, 1,* 38-48.

Titler, M. G. (2004b). Overview of the U.S. Invitational Conference "Advancing Quality Care through Translation Research." *Worldviews on Evidence-Based Nursing, 1*(S1), S1-S5.

Titler, M. G. (2005). Developing an evidence-based practice. In G. LoBiondo-Wood & J. Haber (Eds.), *Nursing research: Methods and critical appraisal for evidence-based practice* (6th ed.). St. Louis: Mosby.

Titler, M. G., Cullen, L., & Ardery, G. (2002). Evidence-based practice: An administrative perspective. *Reflections of Nursing Leadership, 28*(2), 26-27, 46.

Titler, M. G., & Everett, L. Q. (2001). Translating research into practice: Considerations for critical care investigators. *Critical Care Nursing Clinics of North America, 13*(4), 587-604.

Titler, M. G., Herr, K., Schilling, M. L., Marsh, J. L., Xie, X., Ardery, G., et al. (2003). Acute pain treatment for older adults hospitalized with hip fracture: Current nursing practices and perceived barriers. *Applied Nursing Research, 16*(4), 211-227.

Titler, M. G., Kleiber, C., Steelman, V., Goode, C., Rakel, B., Barry-Walker, J., et al. (1994). Infusing research into practice to promote quality care. *Nursing Research, 43*(5), 307-313.

Titler, M. G., Kleiber, C., Steelman, V. J., Rakel, B. A., Budreau, G., Buckwalter, K. C., et al. (2001). The Iowa Model of Evidence-Based Practice to Promote Quality Care. *Critical Care Nursing Clinics of North America, 13*(4), 497-509.

Titler, M. G., & Mentes, J. C. (1999). Research utilization in gerontological nursing practice. *Journal of Gerontological Nursing, 25*(6), 6-9.

Tranmer, J. E., Coulson, K., Holtom, D., Lively, T., & Maloney, R. (1998). The emergence of a culture that promotes evidence based clinical decision making within an acute care setting. *Canadian Journal of Nursing Administration, 11*(2), 36-58.

Tripp-Reimer, T., & Doebbeling, B. N. (2004). Qualitative perspectives in translational research. *Worldviews on Evidence-Based Nursing, 1*(S1), S65-S72.

U.S. Census Bureau. (2000a). Census 2000 summary file 1, matrices P13 and PCT 12. Retrieved June 23, 2003, from www.census.gov/main/www/cen2000.html.

U.S. Census Bureau. (2000b). Projections of the total resident population by 5-year age groups, and sex with special age categories: Middle series, 2016 to 2020. Retrieved June 23, 2003, from www.census.gov/popest/estimates.php.

U.S. Invitational Conference. (2004). Advancing quality care through translation research. Set of two CD-ROMs. Conference Proceedings.

Vaughn, T. E., McCoy, K. D., Bootsmiller, B. J., Woolson, R. F., Sorofman, B., Tripp-Reimer, T., et al. (2002). Organizational predictors of adherence to ambulatory care screening guidelines. *Medical Care, 40*(12), 1172-1185.

Wagner, E. H., Austin, B. T., Davis, C., Hindmarsh, M., Schaefer, J., & Bonomi, A. (2001). Improving chronic illness care: Translating evidence into action. *Health Affairs (Millwood), 20*, 64-78.

Walshe, K., & Rundall, T. G. (2001). Evidence-based management: From theory to practice in health care. *Milbank Quarterly, 79*(3), 429-457.

Watson, N. M. (2004). Advancing quality of urinary incontinence evaluation and treatment in nursing homes through translation research. *Worldviews on Evidence-Based Nursing, 1*(S2), S21-S25.

Web of Science. (2006). Retrieved January 20, 2006 from www.scientific.thomson.com/products/wos.

Wells, N., & Baggs, J. G. (1994). A survey of practicing nurses' research interests and activities. *Clinical Nurse Specialist, 8*, 145-151.

West, S., King, V., Carey, T. S., Lohr, K. N., McKoy, N., Sutton, S. F., & Lux, L. (2002). Systems to rate the strength of scientific evidence. Evidence Report/Technology Assessment no. 47 (prepared by the Research Triangle Institute—University of North Carolina Evidence-based Practice Center under contract no. 290-97-0011). AHRQ pub. no. 02-E016. Rockville, MD: Agency for Healthcare Research and Quality.

White, C. L. (1999). Changing pain management practice and impacting on patient outcomes. *Clinical Nurse Specialist, 13*(4), 166-172.

Williams, C. A. (2004). Preparing the next generation of scientists in translation research. *Worldviews on Evidence-Based Nursing, 1*(S1), S73-S77.

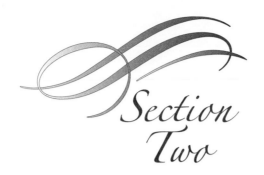

Section Two

Foundations of Gerontological Nursing Practice

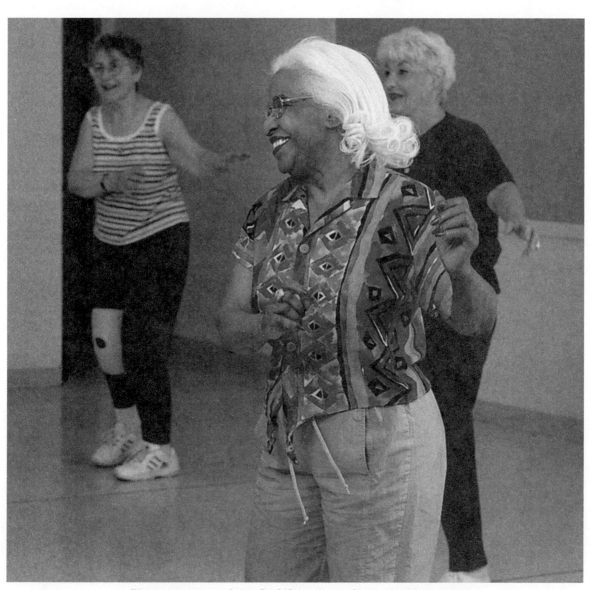

Photo courtesy of the OASIS Institute, St. Louis, Missouri.

Chapter 6

Gerontology: The Study of Aging

Helen W. Lach

Objectives

Define gerontology.
Define aging *and* senescence.
Explore challenges in gerontological research.
List and describe theories of aging.
Identify changes associated with aging at the cellular, tissue, and organ levels.

The purpose of this chapter is to provide background information on gerontology as a foundation for nursing practice. The first part of the chapter examines the field of gerontology and explores challenges in the study of aging. The second half of the chapter presents key elements from the biological sciences, including current theories of aging. Details about the impact of the aging process on each of the body systems are provided in the following chapters in Section 3 of the text, as well as information from the medical, psychological, and social sciences.

Gerontology is the study of the processes of aging and challenges of older people. Although observations about the nature of aging are as old as written history, gerontology is considered a young science. Most research in gerontology has occurred since 1950. Gerontological research is conducted at all levels of living system organization: from the subcellular level through the organ system levels and the human organism level to the social-cultural levels of organization.

Gerontology is an applied science; gerontologists use no unique investigative tools. Biochemists, physiologists, pharmacologists, psychologists, epidemiologists, physicians, sociologists, anthropologists, physicians, nurses, and a host of other professionals are involved in the study of aging. Although nurses often collaborate with scientists in other specialties, nurses are increasingly learning how to use the wide variety of tools available to study aging. Findings from gerontological research enhance understanding of the nature of aging and older adults and help remove stereotypic ideas from clinical practice. Relevant findings from the gerontology literature are summarized throughout this text as they apply to the health care of older people.

Gerontology seeks to understand the processes and effects of normal aging. *Geriatrics*, in contrast, is the study and practice of the medical problems and care of older people with diseases. Geriatric research seeks to understand the causes, consequences, and factors that modify disease expression in the elderly. *Gerontological nursing* as defined in Chapter 1 is the practice and study of adapting and applying generic nursing methods to the older adult patient, using specialized knowledge about aging, including information derived from gerontology and geriatrics.

As nursing research expands and becomes more interdisciplinary, nurses are looking to methods from all fields of gerontology to support their work. Nurse researchers use epidemiological techniques, as well as methods from the clinical and bench sciences. Even genetic research has implications for gerontological nursing. The reflections of a gerontological nurse conducting genetic research related to Alzheimer's disease are explored in Box 6-1. As we expand our scope of research, nurses can ask and answer a broad range of questions to help people.

DEFINITIONS OF OLD AGE

Although there is no commonly accepted definition of aging, definitions of old age and related terms reflect the variety of meanings and connotations of the words *aged, aging, old,* and *elderly* held by lay people. The term *old* can be used to mean "wise," "familiar," or, in a less positive light, "declining in vigor and strength." Scientific definitions offer similar variety in tone. Biological

125

Box 6-1 *Reflections on Genetic Research and Nursing*

The availability of the human genome sequence, information related to the organization and function of the human genome, and increasingly accessible genetic and genomics technologies are valuable new tools for nurse scientists (Jenkins, Grady, & Collins, 2005; Loescher & Merkle, 2005), including nurse researchers in the area of gerontology and geriatrics. Professional nurses provide interventions for the prevention and management of many diseases and associated health problems that are prevalent among elders, including alterations in cognition and concomitant behavioral symptoms, incontinence, alterations in skin integrity, and altered immune response, to name a few. A better understanding of the molecular basis of these problems has the potential to greatly influence the care that we provide (Schutte, 2004).

At one level, an understanding of the role that genes play in the etiology of disease and other health problems provides the foundation for the development of cures, perhaps through genetic or pharmaceutical therapies. On another level, the identification of genetic and environmental factors that predict the onset, progression, or particular clinical features of a disease or other health problem may be helpful in targeting biobehavioral or pharmaceutical interventions to improve outcomes. Will the integration of genetic variables into predictive models increase our ability to provide the best interventions in the most effective manner to our patients? Can we use genetic variables to identify clinical subgroups that may respond better to a particular intervention than other subgroups? Can we use this information to provide improved anticipatory guidance to individuals and their families about the likely progression of a disease or health problem to improve planning and resource utilization?

Until recently, nurse researchers primarily relied on collaborations with basic scientists in other disciplines to provide the molecular genetics data required to answer these questions. Today, nurse researchers are increasingly prepared to independently conduct basic and clinical molecular genetics research to move the scientific foundation of our discipline forward. My own doctoral preparation involved crafting a program of study that included didactic and laboratory training in molecular genetics research in conjunction with training in gerontological nursing. Although collaboration with genetic scientists across disciplines remains essential, this training allows me to maintain an independent molecular genetics laboratory and to independently pursue a program of research that examines the relationship between genetic variants and the cognitive, behavioral, and functional phenotypes of Alzheimer's disease (Schutte, Maas, & Buckwalter, 2003). Increasingly, more formal preparation in genetics is available to nurse scientists through nursing doctoral programs, postdoctoral opportunities, and research institutes. Regardless of the preparatory path chosen, nurse scientists are in powerful positions to harness emerging genetics and genomics information and technologies to answer key questions related to the health of aging populations toward the goal of improved outcomes and quality of life.

Debra L. Schutte

Debra L. Schutte, PhD, RN
Assistant Professor
Adult and Gerontology Area of Study
University of Iowa College of Nursing
Iowa City, Iowa

definitions often emphasize decline in structure or function of cells and organs, but some are more neutral in tone, defining aging as merely the changes that accrue with the passage of time. Because there is diversity in definitions of *old*, clinicians should be alert to the possibility for miscommunication when generalizations are made about "old" people or the "aging process."

In a landmark study, Butler (1975) drew attention to the ambivalent notions of old age held by Americans, which range from the "golden ager" to the "old geezer" or "old biddy" stereotypes. He contended that these conflicting stereotypes combine "wishful thinking and stark terror." The terror is grounded in a natural fear of death and disability; the wishful thinking is based on reluctance to confront the impact of current lifestyle choices on function in later life. Most people do not realize that important factors influencing the quality of life in old age are as numerous as physical health, personality,

earlier life experiences, the environment surrounding late life events, and social support, including finances, housing, health care, social roles, recreation, and spiritual pursuits. Butler proposed a more realistic view of aging as "neither inherently miserable nor inherently sublime—like every stage of life it has problems, joys, fears, and potentials" (p. 2). His insights about stereotypes of aging remain salient over three decades later.

The fact that aging has cultural, social, psychological, and biological meanings makes definitions of descriptive terms difficult to fit all cases. The segment of life referred to as "old age" can span over 40 years; it is therefore misleading to try to characterize people in this age-group as homogeneous. Terms such as *young-old* are used to describe those 55 to 74 years of age and *old-old* to refer to those 75 years of age and older. Caranasos (1993) has proposed a nomenclature using the terms *early old age* to denote those age 65 to 74, *middle old age* for those age 75 to 84, and *late old age* for those over 84.

The term *frail elderly,* once used to refer to those over 75, is now used to mean something quite specific about vulnerability to disease.

Two classic approaches to defining people as old are the chronological approach and the functional approach (Schroots & Birren, 1990). The *chronological method* defines a certain age as old—for example, 65 years—and compares the number of years an individual has lived against this standard. It is the most popular approach because it is economical and objective. Use of chronological age to establish who is elderly may be convenient, but it tells little about function or performance.

The *functional approach* to defining old age evaluates the functional performance of the individual against standard adult performance. This is analogous to the use of developmental screening tests commonly used in children. Those adults who are unable to meet the criteria for performance are considered "old." A commonly used performance standard for adults is employment. Because it is normal for adults to engage in paid employment, retired adults are thus considered "old." In another example, states use functional criteria such as ability to perform certain activities of daily living to determine if Medicaid enrollees are eligible for nursing home placement.

Sometimes the chronological and functional methods are used together. Chronological age criteria are first applied, and then a functional test of age is used. The combined approach is being used increasingly to make decisions about employment of people over 65. It is also used when scarce or expensive resources must be allocated. For example, Medicare uses the concept of "home-bound" status (a judgment of functional ability) to determine which Medicare recipients are eligible for home health benefits. Functional criteria are thus used to subdivide the chronologically defined "elderly" population in order to determine who receives certain costly resources.

For the purposes of this text, the term *older adult* refers to those age 65 years and older, unless otherwise specified. The semantic difficulties in defining older age are important, for they reflect the power of labels in defining social opportunities for old people. Although this may seem only tangentially related to health, most definitions of health are related to ability to carry out social role expectations.

CHALLENGES IN GERONTOLOGICAL RESEARCH

Controversy exists over which changes associated with aging are caused by physiological aging, which are caused by lifestyle factors, and which are caused by disease processes. These difficulties are only exacerbated by the problem of arriving at a generally accepted definition of "aging" and "old." However, research over the past few decades is helping to identify the underlying mechanisms of many aging changes.

Many of the early studies of aging were based on cross-sectional studies of ill and institutionalized old people. Conclusions drawn from these studies tend to portray the elderly and the aging process in a very negative manner. The validity of these conclusions has been questioned for two reasons. First, an institutionalized population is not representative of all older people, and second, results from cross-sectional studies cannot be used to determine whether the differences between young and old are due to aging or to some other factor, such as disease or a cohort effect.

Intelligence is frequently measured by standardized tests. In the past it was concluded on the basis of cross-sectional studies using standardized tests that intelligence declined with age (Stuart-Hamilton, 2003). Critics now question this conclusion. It is difficult to determine if differences between young people and old people in "intelligence" are due to aging or to some other factor, such as differences in educational level, nutritional status during the formative years, or cultural bias within the test itself. Tests may also measure different aspects of intelligence. More recent research has concluded that some kinds of intelligence remain stable or even improve with age (Stuart-Hamilton, 2003).

Studies employing a longitudinal design circumvent the problem of a cohort effect leading to erroneous conclusions. However, such studies are expensive and time-consuming to conduct. Additionally, these studies may be biased by a "survivor effect." The survivor effect refers to the problem that results from not knowing whether the individuals who live to *complete* the longitudinal study represent the "average" individual or an especially advantaged subpopulation. This limits the generalizability of study results. Therefore both longitudinal and cross-sectional studies are useful. It is important to understand the limitations of both research designs, and to be open to revising long-standing opinions or generalizations about the effects of aging, as results from newer studies become available. The challenge for gerontological nurses is to remain abreast of the new information being generated about the aging process and older people.

Several significant programs of study have helped build the base of gerontological research. First are the Duke Longitudinal Studies on Aging (Palmore, 1970) and the Baltimore Longitudinal Study on Aging (Schock, Greulich, Costa, Andres, & Lakatta, 1984). These two sets of studies followed groups of healthy older adults with a goal of differentiating normal aging from disease processes. These studies helped describe the decline in health and functional ability with age, as well as the variability among individuals and among subjects, contributing to development of geriatrics as a specialty (Blazer, 2004).

The National Institute on Aging has also funded a set of Alzheimer's Disease Research Centers across the country over the past two decades to help understand the development of and potential treatment for this growing disease of aging. These research programs have led to current understanding of both genetic and nongenetic factors that increase the risk of developing Alzheimer's disease, as well as increasing knowledge of the mechanisms that lead to changes in the brain (Rodgers, 2003).

Another series of studies sought to understand why some people seem to age well, through the MacArthur Foundation Study of Successful Aging (Rowe & Kahn, 1998). These studies identified the concept of "usual aging" as what we normally think of as aging, usually implying decline and sickness. "Successful aging," on the other hand, was described as having three important characteristics: (1) low risk of disease and disease-related disability, (2) high mental and physical function, and (3) active engagement with life. Rowe and Kahn went on to describe the role of exercise, nutrition, and other lifestyle factors that play important roles in aging well.

Other major nationally funded programs have included the Claude D. Pepper Older Americans Independence Centers. The purpose of these research centers is to increase independence in older Americans. Edward R. Roybal Centers are designed to move promising social and behavioral basic research findings out of the laboratory and into programs, practices, and policies that will improve the lives of older people and the capacity of society to adapt to societal aging. These and many other research programs have increased our understanding of aging.

Thus, although the breadth and scope of research in gerontology is impressive and growing with time, significant gaps still exist in the scientific base for understanding changes with age. The next section explores the current thinking as to the biological processes of aging.

AGING AND THE LIFE SPAN

Life span is defined as the average maximum length of time an organism can be expected to survive or last (Venes, 2001). In human beings, the life span is thought to be about 110 to 115 years, in spite of reports, which have tended to be inaccurate, of groups living well beyond those years. *Life expectancy* is defined as the average observed years of life from birth or any stated age, and depends on both biological and environmental influences (Katic & Kahn, 2005). The present life expectancy at birth in the United States is 74.7 years in men and 79.9 years in women (Administration on Aging, 2004), up about 30 years from 1900 (Figure 6-1).

These increases are primarily due to improvements in sanitation and medical care resulting in reductions in premature death among younger individuals. This elimination of premature death has resulted in the "rectangularization of the survival curve," where fewer people are dying early and more are living into older age and closer to the natural life span (Fries & Crapo, 1981). However, scientists report that "even eliminating all

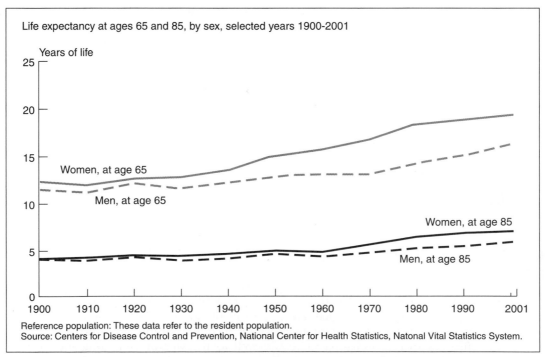

Figure 6-1 Changes in life expectancy in the United States. (Reprinted from Federal Interagency Forum on Aging-Related Statistics. [2004]. *Key indicators of well-being.* Washington, DC: Author.)

aging-related causes of death currently written on the death certificates of the elderly will not increase human life expectancy by more than 15 years" (Olshansky, Hayflick, & Carnes, 2002).

The human life span can be divided into three stages: (1) embryonic development, which occurs from conception to birth; (2) growth and maturity, which occur from birth through adulthood; and (3) senescence, which occurs at the last stages of adulthood through

death. The terms *aging* and *senescence* are frequently used interchangeably, and both are considered fundamental and intrinsic properties of most living organisms. *Aging* can be defined as "the sum of all the changes that normally occur in an organism with the passage of time." Senescence is the progressive deterioration of the body and its processes. The process is common to all members of a given species (i.e., it is universal); the process is progressive over time; and the

---

BOX 6-2 Characteristics of Aging in Mammals

Increased mortality rate with age after maturation	In the early nineteenth century, Gompertz first described the exponential increase in mortality rate with aging due to various causes, a phenomenon that still exists today. In 1995, the death rate from all causes for people in the United States between 25 and 44 years of age was 189.5/100,000 and for those age 65 years and over was 5069.0/100,000, a 25-fold increase. The pattern of age-related survival is similar across species, including invertebrates and singe-cell organisms.
Changes in biochemical composition in tissues with age	There are notable age-related decreases in lean body mass and total bone mass in humans. Although the amount of subcutaneous fat is either unchanged or decreases, total fat remains the same. Consequently the percentage of adipose tissue increases with age. At the cellular level, many markers of aging have been described in various tissues from different organisms. Two of the first to be described were increases in lipofuscin (age pigment) and increased crosslinking in extracellular matrix molecules such as collagen. Additional examples include age-related changes in both the rates of transcription of specific genes and the rate of protein synthesis and numerous age-related alterations in posttranslational protein modifications, such as glycation and oxidation.
Progressive decrease in physiological capacity with age	Many physiological changes have been documented in both cross-sectional and longitudinal studies. Examples include declines in glomerular filtration rate, maximum heart rate, and vital capacity. These decreases occur linearly from about age 30; however, the rate of physiological decline is heterogeneous from organ to organ and individual to individual.
Reduced ability to respond adaptively to environmental stimuli with age	A fundamental feature of senescence is diminished ability to maintain homeostasis. This is manifest not primarily by changes in resting or basal parameters, but in the altered response to an external stimulus such as exercise or fasting. The loss "reserve" can result in blunted maximum responses, as well as delays in reaching peak levels and in returning to basal levels. For example, the induction of hepatic tyrosine aminotransferase activity by fasting is both attenuated and delayed in old rodents.
Increased susceptibility and vulnerability to disease	The incidence and mortality rates for many diseases increase with age and parallel the potential increase in mortality rate with age. For the five leading causes of death for people over 65, the relative increase in death rates compared with the rates for people age 24 to 44 are as follows: heart disease 92-fold, cancer 43-fold, stroke greater than 100-fold, chronic lung disease greater than 100-fold, and pneumonia and influenza 89-fold. The basis for these dramatic rises in mortality rates is incompletely understood, but presumably involves changes in the function of many types of cells, which lead to tissue/organ dysfunction and systemic illness. Interestingly, a retrospective study of centenarians demonstrated that they lived 90%-95% of their lives in very good health and with a high level of functional independence. The centenarians do suffer a 30%-50% annual mortality rate at the end of their lives, but this represents a marked compression of morbidity toward the end of life and is close to the idealized survival curve.

Adapted from Troen, B. R. (2003). The biology of aging. *Mount Sinai Journal of Medicine, 70*(1), 3-23.

process is deleterious, ultimately leading to death. Troen (2003) describes five characteristics of the aging process in mammals (Box 6-2):

- Increased mortality rate with age after maturation
- Changes in biochemical composition in tissues with age
- Progressive decrease in physiological capacity with age
- Reduced ability to respond adaptively to environmental stimuli with age
- Increased susceptibility and vulnerability to disease

In spite of the fact that all humans are aging, aging is a complex and variable phenomenon. Not only do organisms of the same species age at different rates, the rate of aging varies within a single organism of a given species. Reasons for this variability are not fully known, but a variety of theories of aging have been proposed and are discussed in this chapter. Because aging takes place at many levels within the human organism, it is likely that several mechanisms are responsible for aging changes.

Aging is a highly individualized process that affects each person in unique ways. Aging is the result of the interaction among genetic endowment, environmental influences, lifestyles, and the effects of disease processes. Therefore people become increasingly diverse as they age, and it is difficult to predict with certainty a person's health or functional level on the basis of chronological age alone. A biomarker or set of biomarkers for aging or mortality risk would be helpful, but so far has not been identified (Warner, 2004). However, much progress has been made in understanding the various mechanisms involved in aging, advancing the theories of aging that are discussed next.

THEORIES OF AGING
Historical Approaches

The earliest theories of aging were highly speculative and frequently had a philosophical basis. The Greeks were the first people to speculate on the cause of aging. Several hundred years before the birth of Christ, Hippocrates characterized aging as an irreversible and natural event caused by a decrease in body heat. Later, Galen elaborated on this idea by saying that aging was caused primarily by changes in the body's "humors" that produced increased dryness and coldness. He also stated that aging was a lifetime process rather than an event occurring at the end of the life span.

Late in the twelfth century, Maimonides, a Jewish philosopher, postulated that life was predetermined and unalterable but that the life span could be prolonged by taking suitable precautions. Early in the thirteenth century, Roger Bacon, a European, wrote prolifically about the aging process, so much so that he was imprisoned for his philosophical views. He adhered to the Greek model of decreased heat and dryness related to aging, but added that aging was a pathological process that

could be halted by good hygiene. He further postulated that aging was a result of the wear and tear of living; however, the Catholic Church ultimately determined one's life span.

Leonardo da Vinci (1452-1519) was the first person to attempt to identify physiological changes associated with aging by performing autopsies on old men and young children. Later, Santorio theorized that aging was manifested through a hardening of fibers and a progressive consolidation of earthy material within one's body. However, it was not until the eighteenth and nineteenth centuries that scientists began to investigate seriously the physiological and anatomical processes of aging. According to Darwin, aging was due to a decrease in irritability of nervous and muscular tissues resulting in a failure of the body to respond to stimuli. Other theorists claimed that life was a vital force or an intrinsic energy that gradually decreased over time and diminished to the point of death (Wallace, 1977).

After 1900, few scientists and researchers studied aging as a primary interest. In the early 1900s, C. S. Minot studied mortality rates with the use of statistical analysis. The "autointoxication" theory, which stated that age was attributed to particular physiological systems or conditions, and the "wear and tear" theory, which claimed that organisms had fixed amounts of energy available to them, were predominant at that time. Not until recently did science begin to display a renewed interest in researching biological theories of the aging process, which continue to develop along with our understanding of the intrinsic and extrinsic causes of aging changes. The latter half of the twentieth century saw the growth of geriatrics and gerontology both in the United Kingdom and in the United States (Morley, 2004a).

Recent Theories of Aging

Current developments in our understanding of the aging process have grown out of the research done over the past few decades, much supported by the National Institute on Aging (NIA), which was created in 1974 (Manton, 2003). Research on twins who have identical genes suggests that aging is determined by both genetic and environmental factors, with genetics responsible for about 35% of the aging process (NIA, 2002). It is likely that no one theory will completely explain how we age, but the mechanisms currently being explored likely affect aging and health. In addition, there may be some overlap among theories, with the effects of some aging changes resulting in other changes. The following provides an overview of current theories of aging, including the evolutionary, molecular, cellular, and system theories as classified by Weinert and Timiras (2003) (Box 6-3).

Evolutionary Theories. Research has not supported early ideas of the presence of a biological clock

BOX 6-3 Classification and Brief Description of the Main Theories of Aging

Evolutionary

Mutation accumulation	Mutations that affect health at older ages are not selected against
Disposable soma	Somatic cells are maintained only to ensure continued reproductive processes; after reproduction, soma becomes disposable
Antagonistic pleiotropy	Genes beneficial at younger age become deleterious at older ages

Molecular

Gene regulation	Aging is caused by changes in the expression of genes regulating both development and aging
Codon restriction	Fidelity/accuracy of mRNA translation is impaired due to inability to decode codons in mRNA
Error catastrophe	Decline in fidelity of gene expression with aging results in increased fraction of abnormal proteins
Dysdifferentiation	Gradual accumulation of random molecular damage impairs regulation of gene expression

Cellular

Cellular senescence—telomere theory	Phenotypes of aging are caused by an increase in frequency of senescent cells. Senescence may result from telomere loss (replicative senescence) or cell stress (cell senescence)
Free radical	Oxidative metabolism produces highly reactive free radicals that subsequently damage lipids, proteins, and DNA
Protein modification	Protein changes result in advanced glycation end products (AGEs) that crosslink with other molecules, impairing function
Wear and tear	Accumulation of normal injury
Apoptosis	Programmed cell death from genetic events or genome crisis

System

Neuroendocrine	Alterations in neuroendocrine control of homeostasis result in aging-related physiological changes
Immunological	Decline of immune function with aging results in decreased resistance to infectious diseases and increased incidence of autoimmunity
Rate of living	Assumes a fixed rate of metabolic potential for every living organism

Adapted from Weinert, B. T., & Timiras, P. S. (2003). Theories of aging. *Journal of Applied Physiology, 95,* 1706-1716. Used with permission.

that regulates aging (Kirkwood, 2003), but evolution clearly plays a role in determining the life span. The evolutionary or developmental theories explore the human life span as affected by the forces of natural selection. Natural selection encourages reproduction of the species; as a result, genes that encourage healthy life until successful reproduction are selected and the population is increased. This selection in turn affects aging either directly or through mechanisms that are helpful early in life, yet affect the aging process later. The first is

the mutation accumulation theory, which suggests that genes that have negative effects in later life gradually increase in the population, because they are not weeded out by natural selection. Although this theory seems logical, there has been little support for it from research (Weinert & Timiras, 2003).

Two other evolutionary theories are explored. The disposable soma theory proposes that once the organism has reproduced, it is disposable. As a result, humans are not programmed to continue maintenance and repair of the body after reproduction, and become more susceptible to disease with age. The antagonistic pleiotropy theory (*pleiotropy* is defined as having more than one genetic effect) says that genes may be selected because they positively influence early life through reproduction, but just happen to have negative affects on health in later life. Aging may ultimately result from evolutionary neglect rather than an active process that causes aging. There is some research support for these latter two theories, which may help provide a general framework for explaining aging, even though they do not point to the specific mechanisms at work.

Molecular Theories. The molecular theories explore genetic influences on aging. Yeast, nematodes, fruit flies, and mice have genes that scientists have directly related to the life span (Box 6-4). By altering these genes, researchers have been able to extend the life span of the *C. elegans* nematode (NIA, 2002). Fruit flies with a certain mutation of a gene humorously named INDY (I'm Not Dead Yet) live longer than other flies (Rogina, Reenan, Nilsen, & Helfand, 2000). Studies in animals have shown that genes can affect other genes, the stress response, nutritional effects, and metabolic capacity, which in turn affects the aging process. Ongoing research will help determine if these genes found in animal models have the same effects in humans.

The gene regulation theory proposes that genes regulate aging and development through differential actions throughout the life span. Studies of how genes express themselves over time are being done through microarrays, a technology that allows researchers to track the activity of a large number of genes throughout the life span. Studies comparing the expression of genes from young and old cells have shown limited differences, but the impact of these changes is not known and could be significant (NIA, 2002).

Researchers are further making the link between genetics and environmental factors. From pharmacogenetics to the behavioral sciences, research is developing to help explain the complex interactions between genetic disposition and the physical, behavioral, and social environment (Harris, 2005). For example, caloric restriction has been shown to prolong life in a variety of species, perhaps because it changes genetic activity (NIA, 2002).

According to the error catastrophe theory of aging, inappropriate information is intermittently emitted from the cell nucleus causing a buildup of abnormal proteins, which eventually interferes with normal cell functioning. It is thought that this process may occur through changes in the base pairing or coding of deoxyribonucleic acid (DNA) or through increased levels of error in ribonucleic acid (RNA) transcription or protein synthesis. Information may be lost from the DNA as a result of an accumulation of a certain number of somatic mutations, macromolecular damage, or chromosomal abnormalities. In addition, there may be

---

BOX 6-4 Tracking Down a Longevity Gene

Investigators are finding clues to aging and longevity in yeast, one-celled organisms that have some intriguing genetic similarities to human cells. In a laboratory at Louisiana State University Medical Center in New Orleans, Michael Jazwinski, Ph.D., has found genes that seem to promote longevity in these rapidly dividing, easy to study organisms.

Yeast normally have about 21 cell divisions or generations. Jazwinski observed that over the course of that life span, certain genes in the yeast are more active or less active as the cells age; in the language of molecular biology, they are differentially expressed. So far, Jazwinski has found 14 such genes in the yeast.

Selecting one of these genes, Jazwinski tried two different experiments. First, he introduced the gene into yeast cells in a form that allowed him to control its activity. When the gene was activated to a greater degree than normal, or overexpressed, some of the yeast cells went on dividing for 27 or 28 generations; their period of activity was extended by 30 percent. In his second experiment, Jazwinski mutated the gene. When he introduced this non-working version into a group of yeast cells, they had only about 12 divisions.

The two experiments made it clear that the gene, now called LAG-1, influences the number of divisions in yeast or, according to some researchers' way of thinking, its longevity. (LAG-1 is short for longevity assurance gene.) But how it works is still a mystery. One small clue lies in its sequence of DNA bases—its genetic code—which suggests that it produces a protein found in cell membranes. One next step is to study the function of that protein. Similar sequences have been found in human DNA, so a second investigative path is to clone the human gene and study its function. If there turns out to be a human LAG-1 counterpart, new insights into aging may be uncovered.

In another laboratory, Leonard Guarente, Ph.D., of the Massachusetts Institute of Technology found that mutation of a silencing gene—a gene that "turns off" other genes—delayed aging by 30 percent in yeast. This gene is also found in *C. elegans* and other animals; it produces an enzyme that alters the structure of DNA, which, in turn, alters patterns of gene expression.

From National Institute on Aging. (2002). *Under the microscope: A biological quest.* Bethesda, MD: Author.

a decreased ability of the cells to clear abnormal proteins with age (Troen, 2003).

Other molecular theories involve damage to the molecules or genes. These theories include the codon restriction theory, in which messenger RNA (mRNA) translation is impaired; the somatic mutation theory, which is caused by damage to DNA; and the dysdifferentiation theory, which is caused by random molecular damage that impairs gene expression.

Cellular Theories. Cellular theories of aging explore factors that affect cell division and cumulative damage to cells that result in cell senescence. All of the cells can divide initially, but with age, many stop dividing, although they continue to function well. When studied in vitro, researchers have found that cells have a finite number of cell divisions, called the *Hayflick limit* (NIA, 2002). For example, fibroblasts will divide about 50 times in the test tube. After they stop dividing, these senescent cells also change their function, releasing enzymes that could increase risk of cancer in later life. It is unclear if these senescent cells accumulate throughout the body or how they affect aging. The cellular theories explore mechanisms that result in cell damage. When this damage reaches a certain level, *apoptosis,* or cell death, can result. This mechanism can be adaptive, but excessive cell loss may be responsible for diseases related to aging such as Alzheimer's disease (Warner, 2003).

The telomere theory looks at the role of telomeres, which are the ends of chromosomes involved in stabilizing and protecting the chromosome. They do not carry genetic information; however, the ends of the telomeres are not completely reproduced when chromosomes divide. Telomeres become shorter with cell division, and ultimately cells stop dividing or reach cell senescence, which has been related to altered life span in animals (Katic & Kahn, 2005). Some cells use the enzyme telomerase to restore the telomeres so that they continue dividing. Telomeres may also play a role in cancer as they regulate cell replication, and if they act abnormally, they may produce immortal cells that divide endlessly.

According to the protein modification theory, crosslinking occurs; this is a chemical reaction that produces altered proteins called *advanced glycation end products* (AGEs) (Holliday, 2004a). An accumulation of these compounds over a lifetime produces the random, irreparable binding together of essential molecules in the cells. The crosslinked network interferes with normal cell functioning and impedes intracellular transport. It is thought that the irreversible aging of proteins such as collagen is responsible for the ultimate failure of tissues and organs. Collagen is an important connective tissue support for the lungs, heart, muscle, and lining of the vessel walls. Age-related changes in the structure of collagen are partially responsible for arteriosclerosis and the concomitant loss of elasticity in the tissues (Troen, 2003).

The free radical theory has enjoyed a long history of support since it was proposed by Harman (1957). Free radicals are highly reactive cellular components called *reactive oxygen species* (ROS) that cause molecular damage. Generated by mitochondrial respiration, ROS compounds have a large amount of free energy and oxidatively attack adjacent molecules. The O_2 molecule most commonly generates free radicals, and the most vulnerable sites are the mitochondria. Chemical and structural changes are progressive, particularly in the mitochondria, with a potential for a chain reaction in which free radicals generate other free radicals. Free radicals do not contain useful biological information and replace genetic order with randomness; thus faulty molecules and cellular debris accumulate in the nucleus and cytoplasm over the lifetime of a cell. This debris can cause cumulative cell damage and cell senescence. Fortunately, new studies have found that cells are able to use antioxidants from vitamins such as C and E and enzymes they produce such as superoxide dismutase, catalase, and glutathione peroxidase to help prevent damage from free radicals (NIA, 2002).

According to the wear and tear theory, aging is a physiological process determined by the amount of stress and damage to which one has been exposed. The process is similar to the mechanical breakdown that is inevitable with an automobile or piece of machinery. Cells wear out from normal use, ultimately resulting in cell death.

The body has *repair mechanisms* to help repair and maintain itself against the various processes that may cause cellular aging (Holliday, 2004a). However, it is clear that even the repair mechanisms become inefficient over time. This could explain the variability in the expression of aging among individuals. Rates of aging may depend on both the type of damage and the repair processes that fail, resulting in increased vulnerability to pathology and disease (Hayflick, 2004).

System Theories. The system theories explore the impact of the body's regulatory systems on aging, including the neurological-endocrine systems and immune system. These systems help the body respond and adapt to both internal and external stimuli by their impact on other body systems. Declines in the organs and functions of these systems may play a role in aging.

The neuroendocrine theory explores the effect of hormonal and nerve regulatory systems on aging. Signals from these systems control growth and development, as well as reproduction and physiological responses to the environment. Changes over time may affect aging through the hypothalamic-pituitary-adrenal axis, ultimately affecting hormones and growth factors. This axis signals the body to make developmental changes, maintain homeostasis, and respond to stress. The decreased efficiency in responding to stress may increase aging processes. Declines in reproductive hormones are examples of aging changes related to this system, as well as reduced sympathetic responses with age (Weinert & Timiras, 2003).

Using hormonal therapies to prevent or treat aging is not a new approach (Morley, 2004b), but clear benefits of therapy have yet to be definitively proven. In addition to the reproductive hormones, growth hormone, melatonin, and dehydroepiandrosterone (DHEA) levels decline with age, and research using supplementation is ongoing (Box 6-5). Another key hormone is insulin-like growth factor I (IGF-I), which stimulates cell activities that may affect aging through impact on the stress response (Weinert & Timiras, 2003).

The immunity theory proposes that changes in the immune system affect aging. The immune system protects the body by seeking out and destroying foreign agents such as viruses, bacteria, fungi, and possibly

---

BOX 6-5 Hormones and Research on Aging

Produced by glands, organs, and tissues, hormones are the body's chemical messengers, flowing through the bloodstream and searching out cells fitted with special receptors. Each receptor, like a lock, can be opened by the specific hormone that fits it and also, to a lesser extent, by closely related hormones. Here are some of the hormones and growth factors of special interest to gerontologists.

Estrogen
Among its many roles, estrogen slows the bone thinning that accompanies aging and may help prevent frailty and disability. After menopause, fat tissue is the major source of a weaker form of estrogen than that produced by the ovaries. Although women may be helped by estrogen replacement therapy after menopause, some are placed at higher risk of certain diseases if they take it. As research yields more information about this carefully studied hormone, it may help clarify who should take estrogen replacement supplements and who should not.

Growth Hormone
This product of the pituitary gland appears to play a role in body composition and muscle and bone strength. It is released through the action of another trophic factor, growth hormone–releasing hormone, which is produced in the brain. It works, in part, by stimulating the production of insulin-like growth factor, which comes mainly from the liver. All three hormones are being studied for their potential to strengthen muscles and bones and prevent frailty among older people. For now, there is no convincing evidence that growth hormone supplements will improve the health of those who do not suffer a profound deficiency of this hormone.

Melatonin
Contrary to some claims, secretion of this hormone, made by the pineal gland, does not necessarily diminish with age. Instead, a number of factors, including light, can affect production of this hormone, which seems to regulate various seasonal changes in the body. Currently, research indicates that melatonin in low dosages may help some older individuals with their sleep, but a physician should be consulted. Claims that melatonin can slow or reverse aging are far from proven.

Testosterone
Testosterone is produced in the testes and peaks in early adulthood. However, the range of normal testosterone production is vast. So although there are some declines in production with age, most older men stay within normal limits. The NIA is investigating the role of testosterone supplementation in delaying or preventing frailty. Preliminary results have been inconclusive, and it remains unclear if this hormone can sharpen memory or help men maintain stout muscles, sturdy bones, and robust sexual activity. Investigators are also looking at its side effects, which can include an increased risk of cancers, particularly prostate cancer. A small percentage of men with profound deficiencies may be helped by supplementation.

DHEA
Short for dehydroepiandrosterone, DHEA is produced in the adrenal glands. It is a precursor to some other hormones, including testosterone and estrogen. Production peaks in the midtwenties and gradually declines with age. What this drop means or how it affects the aging process, if at all, is unclear. Investigators are working to find more definite answers about DHEA's effects on aging, muscles, and the immune system. DHEA supplements, even when taken briefly, may cause liver damage and have other detrimental effects on the body.

Adapted from National Institute on Aging. (2002). *Under the microscope: A biological quest.* Bethesda, MD: Author.

one's own somatic cells that undergo neoplastic changes. Changes in the immune system with age lead to increased mortality risk, due to increased risk of infection, increased rates of cancer, and an increase in autoimmune disease (Weinert & Timiras, 2003).

Immune responses depend on a number of different cells and tissues and the complex interactions among them. When an antigen, such as a virus or bacteria, enters the body, two types of immunological reactions may occur. First, the antigen may induce the formation of lymphocytes, which stimulate the synthesis and release of antibodies principally involved in the neutralization of bacterial toxins and the destruction of bacteria. Aging individuals have reduced antibody production (Troen, 2003).

Second, the antigen may induce lymphocytes to produce cell-mediated reactions such as delayed hypersensitivity or destruction of foreign tissue grafts and tumors. The primary organs of the immune system (bone marrow and thymus) may be most affected by the aging process. The immune response declines steadily after young adulthood when the thymus begins to decrease both in weight and in its ability to produce T cells (Gravenstein, Fillit, & Erschler, 2003).

According to some scientists, the decrease in immunological function may result in alterations in the body's autoimmune response. With aging, the body becomes less able to recognize or tolerate "self" antigens, so that the immune system produces antibodies that act to destroy body cells. This is evidenced by an increased level of autoantibodies and an increased accumulation of lymphocytes and plasma cells in various tissues of normal, healthy older people, and the increase in autoimmune diseases with age, such as rheumatoid arthritis and multiple sclerosis (Gravenstein, Fillit, & Ershler, 2003). Approaches to preventing the effects of "immune aging" and preventing infection may be to improve nutrition, avoid overuse of medications, decrease stress, and minimize the use of immunizations (Gravenstein, Fillit, & Ershler, 2003).

The body's metabolic rate may have a role in aging as proposed by the rate of living theory, as species that have a shorter life span have faster metabolic rates (Katic & Kahn, 2005). The shorter life span may be related to faster cell respiration, which causes the development of free radicals that may ultimately be responsible for aging.

Antiaging Movement

Interest in preventing aging has led to a burgeoning industry of "antiaging medicine" that proposes a variety of methods to slow down the biological clock. Although many theories exist to explain the mechanisms of aging, "there is no empirical evidence to support the claim that aging in humans can be modified by any means, nor is

there evidence that it is possible to measure biological age, or that anti-aging products extend the duration of life" (Olshansky, Hayflick, & Perls, 2004, p. 513). The false promises of this industry may be damaging and detract from the public's understanding of the real progress in the science of aging, besides preying on the public's fears of growing old. Professionals should take an active role in educating consumers about potentially harmful and fraudulent claims (Mehlman et al., 2004).

AGING AT THE CELLULAR, TISSUE, AND ORGAN LEVELS

Scientists have observed aging changes in the cells, tissues, organs, and organ systems that tend to have an effect on body functioning. Generally there is a slowing down of functioning at all levels, beginning at the cellular level. This section provides a brief overview of aging of the cells and tissues. Organs and organ systems are discussed in detail in later chapters.

Cells

A *cell* is defined as a minute protoplasmic mass that, together with other cells, makes up organized tissue. All living matter is composed of cells, all cells arise from other cells, and all metabolic reactions of a living organism take place within cells. There are many different kinds of cells, more than 100 types in the human body; however, all cells have basically the same structure.

A typical cell is made up of two parts, the nucleus and the cytoplasm. The nucleus controls the chemical reactions and reproduction of the cell and contains chromosomes, which are composed of *deoxyribonucleic acid (DNA)* and protein. The nucleus also contains the *nucleolus*, composed of DNA and protein, which is the principal site of RNA formation. The *nuclear envelope* surrounds the nucleus; it is a porous membrane that separates the nucleus from the cytoplasm.

The cytoplasm contains organelles important to cell functioning, including the *endoplasmic reticulum, ribosomes, mitochondria, microsomes, lysosomes,* and *Golgi bodies.* The cytoplasm is surrounded by the *cell membrane,* separating it from the surrounding fluids. Substances that make up the cell are collectively called *protoplasm,* which is composed mainly of water, electrolytes, proteins, lipids, and carbohydrates.

The Aging Cell. Several age-related changes have been noted in both the nucleus and cytoplasm of aging cells. The nucleus appears to enlarge with aging, although there is no noticeable increase in the amount of DNA. The nucleolus also increases in size and number, and, whereas there is an increase in RNA content, there seems to be a decrease in RNA synthesis and protein metabolism. Chromosomal changes have been observed in the nucleus, with clumping, shrinkage, fragmentation, and shortening of the telomeres. Although cells may cease to replicate, this does not always indicate impending cell death. The nuclear membrane tends to invaginate with aging, and there is an appearance of intranuclear inclusions (Griffiths & Meecham, 1990).

In the cytoplasm there is fragmentation of the Golgi apparatus, and the mitochondria show alterations and increasing damage. Vacuole formation increases with an accumulation of lysosomes. It is thought that lysosomes, which are associated with digestion and the breakdown of cell products, may accumulate owing to alterations in the rates of protein turnover or deficiencies in the protein disposal process. Protoplasmic changes associated with cellular aging include an increase in abnormal protein content, but a decrease in protein synthesis; an increase in cellular lipids; an accumulation of pigments or lipofuscin, especially in the fixed, postmitotic cells of the nervous tissue and muscle; and a depletion of glycogen.

Although the body contains many different cell populations, *all* types of cells show age changes. Not only are cells from older populations larger, but they also tend to decrease in the capacity to divide and reproduce as already described. This decrease in the ability of the cell to proliferate with aging is thought to be a major factor in senescence.

Tissues

Tissues are defined as groups or layers of similarly specialized cells that together perform certain special functions. Various kinds of tissues unite structurally and coordinate activities to form organs, which in turn make up organ systems. There are four basic types of tissues in the body: (1) epithelial tissue, (2) connective tissue, (3) muscle tissue, and (4) nervous tissue. Epithelial tissue forms the covering and lining membranes of the entire body, internal organs, cavities, and passageways. Connective tissue binds together and supports other tissues and includes bone, blood, and lymph tissues. Muscle tissue is divided into two types: striated and smooth. Striated, or voluntary, muscle moves the skeleton, usually at will; smooth, or involuntary, muscle surrounds the walls of the internal organs, such as the heart and stomach. Nerve cells and tissues carry nerve impulses from one part of the body to another. A brief discussion of tissue aging changes follows.

Aging in the Tissues. One of the most noticeable changes in aging tissue is the accumulation of the pigmented material *lipofuscin*, especially in the postmitotic tissue of the muscle and nervous tissues. There is also an accumulation of lipids and fat in the tissues, which tends to increase until middle age, stabilize, and gradually decline in older adults. Many lipids are stored in the endothelial tissues of artery walls, as well as extracellular

tissues between the elastic lamella and collagen fibers. Epithelial tissues decrease in subcutaneous tissue, resulting in wrinkles, and also develop age spots and heal less efficiently with age (Holliday, 2004b).

Connective tissues are widely distributed throughout the body and are diverse in composition. They contain an *extracellular matrix* made up of ground substance and fibrous proteins, such as *collagen* and *elastin*. Age changes in the tissues are best observed in the extracellular matrix, although changes result from alterations in the cells, which synthesize most of the extracellular material.

Collagen is found in all connective tissues and shows changes in structure with aging, perhaps due to crosslinking proteins. Because of the altered structure and degradation of elastin and collagen, the tissues become stiffer, less elastic and pliable, and less efficient in their functioning (Holliday, 2004b).

Muscle mass decreases with age, up to 23% (NIA, 2002). This loss of muscle mass is called *sarcopenia* and contributes to muscle weakness and frailty. Factors that may be involved with sarcopenia include loss of motor neurons, hormone loss with age, nutrition, and declines in physical activity (Borst, 2004). Nervous tissues experience shrinkage of the neurons, and tangles and plaques develop in the nervous tissues, thought to play a role in the development of Alzheimer's disease (Rodgers, 2003). Sensory tissues, in particular those affecting vision and hearing, are also influenced by environmental damage and injury over the lifetime (Mobbs, 2003). All of these tissue changes occur as a result of the molecular and cellular changes, as well as wear and tear.

Aging at the Organ Level

As with cells and tissues, the organs experience a decrease in functional capacity with older age, perhaps because of the cumulative aging changes. Physiological reserves show a linear decline beginning at age 30 years, especially in the cardiac, respiratory, and renal organs, so that maintenance of homeostasis becomes increasingly difficult (Masoro, 2002). Although these changes appear slowly and over a long period of time, moderate or severe stressors can precipitate unexpected problems or failures of bodily functions as a result of compromised reserve capacity and homeostatic mechanisms. Age-related changes at the system and organ level are discussed in greater detail in Section 3.

SUMMARY

Gerontology is the broad interdisciplinary study of aging, providing a strong base for gerontological nursing. Aging and senescence are fundamental and intrinsic properties of most living organisms. Since the beginning of time, humans have attempted to unlock the secrets of aging and prolonging life. Some recent theories of aging are related to biological programming, error in DNA and RNA coding, immune and endocrine responses, free radicals, and stress. Research is continuing to explore and test these theories, and it is likely that a combination of processes ultimately results in aging.

Scientists have observed aging changes in molecules, cells, tissues, organs, and organ systems, all affecting body functioning. Molecules may experience wear and tear or changes resulting from chemical processes in the body. Cells experience damage and change leading to senescence. In the tissues, there is an accumulation of lipofuscin, lipids, and fat. There are also changes in the structure of collagen and a degradation of elastin, so that the tissues become stiffer, less elastic and pliable, and less efficient in their functioning. The organs undergo a decline in functional capacity and ability to maintain homeostasis with aging. Aging occurs slowly and is a complex and dynamic process involving many internal and external influences, including genetics and the physical, psychological, and social environment. Research is ongoing to try to unlock the mysteries that may ultimately lead to healthier, longer lives.

REFERENCES

Administration on Aging. (2004). Life expectancy continues to grow. Retrieved June 10, 2005, from www.aoa.gov/press/did_you_ know/2004/march.asp.

Blazer, D. G. (2004). Longitudinal studies on aging and development of geriatrics in North America. *Journal of Gerontology, 89A*(11), 1155-1156.

Borst, S. E. (2004). Interventions for sarcopenia and muscle weakness in older people. *Age and Ageing, 33,* 548-555.

Butler, R. N. (1975). *Why survive? Growing old in America.* New York: Harper & Row.

Caranasos, G. J. (1993). A more opportune description of the stages of aging. *Journal of the American Geriatrics Society, 41,* 888.

Fries, J. F., & Crapo, L. M. (1981). *Vitality and aging.* San Franciso: W. H. Freeman.

Gravenstein, S., Fillit, H. M., & Erschler, W. B. (2003). Clinical immunology of aging. In R. C. Tallis & H. M. Fillit (Eds.), *Brocklehurst's textbook of geriatric medicine and gerontology* (6th ed.). London: Churchill Livingstone.

Griffiths, T. D., & Meecham, P. J. (1990). Biology of aging. In K. F. Farraro (Ed.), *Gerontology: Perspectives and issues.* New York: Springer.

Harman, D. (1957). Aging: A theory based on free radical and radiation chemistry. *Journal of Gerontology, 2,* 298-300.

Harris, J. R. (2005). Introduction: Research on environmental effects in genetic studies of aging. *Journal of Gerontology, Special Issue, 60B,* 5-6.

Hayflick, L. (2004). The not-so-close relationship between biological aging and age-associated pathologies in humans. *Journal of Gerontology, 59A,* B547-B500.

Holliday, R. (2004a). The multiple and irreversible causes of aging. *Journal of Gerontology, 59A,* B568-572.

Holliday, R. (2004b). The close relationship between biological aging and age-associated pathologies in humans. *Journal of Gerontology, 59A,* B543-546.

Jenkins, J., Grady, P. A., & Collins, F. S. (2005). Nurses and the genomics revolution. *Journal of Nursing Scholarship, 37*(2), 98-101.

Katic, M., & Kahn, C. R. (2005). The role of insulin and IGF-1 signaling in longevity. *Cellular and Molecular Life Sciences, 62,* 320-343.

Kirkwood, T. B. L. (2003). Evolutionary theory and the mechanisms of aging. In *Brocklehurst's textbook of geriatric medicine and gerontology* (6th ed.). London: Churchill Livingstone.

Loescher, L. J., & Merkle, C. J. (2005). The interface of genomic technologies and nursing. *Journal of Nursing Scholarship, 37*(2), 111-119.

Manton, K. G. (2003). The future of old age. In R. C. Tallis & H. M. Fillit (Eds.), *Brocklehurst's textbook of geriatric medicine and gerontology* (6th ed.). London: Churchill Livingstone.

Masoro, E. J. (2002). Physiology of aging. In R. C. Tallis & H. M. Fillit (Eds.), *Brocklehurst's textbook of geriatric medicine and gerontology* (6th ed.). London: Churchill Livingstone.

Mehlman, M. J., Binstock, R. H., Juengst, E. T., Ponsaran, R. S., & Whitehouse, P. J. (2004). Anti-aging medicine: Can consumers be better protected? *Gerontologist, 44*(3), 304-310.

Mobbs, C. V. (2003). Neurobiology of aging. In *Brocklehurst's textbook of geriatric medicine and gerontology* (6th ed.). London: Churchill Livingstone.

Morley, J. E. (2004a). A brief history of geriatrics. *Journal of Gerontology, 59A,* M1132-M1152.

Morley, J. E. (2004b). Is the hormonal fountain of youth drying up? *Journal of Gerontology, 59A,* M458-460.

National Institute on Aging. (2002). *Under the microscope: A biological quest.* Washington, DC: Author.

Olshansky, S. J., Hayflick, L., & Carnes, B. A. (2002). Position statement on human aging. Retrieved June 10, 2005, from www.sciam.com/article.cfm?articleID=0004F171-FE1E-1CDF-B4A8809EC588EEDF.

Olshansky, S. J., Hayflick, L., & Perls, T. T. (2004). Anti-aging medicine: The hype and reality—part 1. *Journal of Gerontology, 59A,* B513-B514.

Palmore, E. (1970). *Normal aging.* Durham, NC: Duke University Press.

Rodgers, A. B. (2003). *Alzheimer's disease: Unraveling the mystery.* Washington, DC: National Institute on Aging.

Rogina, B., Reenan, R. A., Nilsen, S. P., & Helfand, S. L. (2000). Extended lifespan conferred by contransporter gene mutations in Drosphila. *Science, 290,* 2137-2140.

Rowe, H. W., & Kahn, R. L. (1998). *Successful aging.* New York: Pantheon.

Schock, N., Greulich, R., Costa, P., Andres, R., & Lakatta, E. (1984). *Normal human aging: The Baltimore Longitudinal Studies of Aging.* Washington, DC: U.S. Government Printing Office.

Schroots, J. J. F., & Birren, J. E. (1990). Concepts of time and aging in science. In J. E. Birren & K. W. Schaie (Eds.), *Handbook of the psychology of aging* (3rd ed.). San Diego: Academic Press.

Schutte, D. L. (2004). The evolving role of genomics in shaping care for persons with dementia. *Nursing Clinics of North America, 39*(3), 581-592.

Schutte, D. L., Maas, M., & Buckwalter, K. C. (2003). A LRPAP1 intronic insertion/deletion polymorphism and phenotypic variability in Alzheimer disease. *Research and Theory for Nursing Practice: An International Journal, 17*(4), 301-319.

Stuart-Hamilton, I. A. (2003). Normal cognitive aging. In R. C. Tallis & H. M. Fillit (Eds.), *Brocklehurst's textbook of geriatric medicine and gerontology* (6th ed.). London: Churchill Livingstone.

Troen, B. R. (2003). The biology of aging. *Mount Sinai Journal of Medicine, 70*(1), 3-23.

Venes, D. (2001). *Taber's cyclopedic medical dictionary.* Philadelphia: F. A. Davis.

Wallace, D. J. (1977). The biology of aging: An overview. *Journal of the American Geriatrics Society, 25,* 104-111.

Warner, H. R. (2003). Biology of aging. In R. C. Tallis & H. M. Fillit (Eds.), *Brocklehurst's textbook of geriatric medicine and gerontology* (6th ed.). London: Churchill Livingstone.

Warner, H. R. (2004). Current status of efforts to measure and modulate the biological rate of aging. *Journal of Gerontology, 59a*(7), 692-696.

Weinert, B. T., & Timiras, P. S. (2003). Theories of aging. *Journal of Applied Physiology, 95,* 1706-1716.

Pharmacological Considerations

Adrianne Dill Linton

Objectives

Discuss psychosocial factors that affect drug responses in older adults and describe their impact on nursing care.

Describe age-related changes in pharmacokinetics and pharmacodynamics.

Analyze the basis of common adverse drug reactions in older adults, including confusion, falls, incontinence, and immobility.

Describe the components of a drug assessment with an older adult.

Develop a plan of care for safe and effective administration of medications for an older adult.

Drugs are potent therapeutic agents with the potential to cause great harm in older adults, as well as alleviate symptoms and cure disease. Nurses have tremendous opportunities through assessment, monitoring, teaching, and evaluation to intervene so that maximum benefit and minimal harm come to the older adult undergoing drug therapy.

Safe and effective drug therapy for older adults requires an understanding of the psychological and social influences on drug utilization in this population, the effects of aging on pharmacokinetics and pharmacodynamics, and the potential drug-related health problems.

PSYCHOSOCIAL INFLUENCES ON DRUG USAGE AND RESPONSES OF OLDER ADULTS

Individual and system factors are among the psychosocial variables that affect drug usage and responses in older adults.

Personal Values

Value systems influence individual patterns of drug usage. Consider the miracles of pharmacotherapy that today's older adults have witnessed first hand! Medical care has been transformed through the development of drugs such as antibiotics, insulin, antihypertensive agents, and psychotropic medications. Against this background, it is not surprising that many older adults expect to receive "a pill for every ill." Indeed, some people feel slighted if they leave the physician's or advance practice nurse's office *without* a prescription. Unfortunately, health care practitioners sometimes foster this expectation by substituting medications for time in dealing with a person's problems. The practice is common even though it may lead to new or greater problems for the person.

Older adults are more likely to receive a prescription during an outpatient visit to a physician than any other age-group, yet the length of time spent in an office visit with older persons is *less* than that of any other age-group. As a result, less time is spent educating individuals about drugs in a population that uses more drugs and requires more time to learn new information. Nurses may contribute to this problem when they seek sedation for disruptive persons rather than taking the time to determine the underlying cause of the problem.

A different situation that may be encountered is the older adult who declines to use drug therapy when it is indicated and offered. This may occur when the patient tries to be stoic, fears adverse drug effects, or believes that various symptoms are just a part of aging that should be endured.

Health Care System

Many aspects of the health care system reinforce the tendency to use drugs as the first line of therapy for diseases, which can lead to suboptimal utilization of drugs. Drug marketing to professionals and to the public, the emphasis on technological rather than human solutions to the problems associated with chronic disease, as well as ageism, affects drug utilization in older adults.

Drug Marketing. Profit is an important incentive in drug marketing. Regardless of the health care setting, drugs are featured prominently. In clinics, long-term care, and acute care facilities, drug advertising is subtle but ever present. Basic tools such as rulers, tape measures, pens, and note pads are emblazoned with drug names. In the home, television, radio, and print media all contain drug advertisements for various products. Many of the drugs advertised are designed to treat ailments common among older adults, such as constipation, urinary incontinence, pain, and insomnia. Over-the-counter (OTC) laxatives, analgesics, sleep aids, and cold preparations often are taken without the knowledge of the individual's health care provider, and they are not benign agents. Significant problems for older persons may develop as a result of interactions with other drugs and age-related variables that predispose to adverse drug reactions. Marketing strategies of pharmaceutical companies are a controversial topic. In 1998, the industry invested $12.724 million in promotions that included free drug samples to physicians, office promotions, direct-to-consumer (DTC) advertising, hospital promotions, and advertising in medical journals (Ma, Stafford, Cockburn, & Finkelstein, 2003). Annual spending on DTC advertising reached nearly $2.5 billion in 2000 (Rosenthal, Berndt, Donohue, Frank, & Epstein, 2002; Vogel, Ramachandran, & Zachry, 2003).

The multiple names given to the same drug produced by different companies create confusion for consumers. In addition, some drugs are compounds with several ingredients. A classic example of the harm this may cause is the individual who comes to the clinic complaining of "ringing ears." Her drug history reveals that she takes Bufferin, Anacin, B.C. powders, and Pepto-Bismol for indigestion. The individual has unwittingly become the victim of salicylate intoxication, without ever having taken an "aspirin."

For professionals, drug advertising is even more pervasive. Few professional journals could exist without pharmaceutical advertising. Many professional meetings and continuing education offerings are in part (or in whole) underwritten by the pharmaceutical industry. Although no coercion is involved, the degree of oversimplification expressed in some drug advertisements borders on the unethical. For example, one laxative advertisement chides professionals for "complicating a simple problem." The solution suggested is a saline cathartic, which has the potential for inducing fluid and electrolyte imbalance, not to mention laxative dependency, in older adults.

Technological versus Human Responses to Chronic Disease. American society values technological solutions to problems over more mundane remedies that may involve greater expenditures of time. Note the proliferation of weight reduction products and plans to which people willingly subscribe. Prescriptions for lifestyle change, counseling, or exercise regimens are seldom as well received as plans for elaborate diagnostic studies or prescriptions.

Ageism. Ageism on the part of health care providers also may contribute to the overprescription of drugs to the elderly. This concern is not new. In 1980, Besdine noted that older persons "often bear the brunt of reflexive prescribing for uninvestigated symptoms." He noted that the average older American filled 13 prescriptions per year and took three times the number of drugs as the average younger American. More recent studies continue to reflect a high rate of prescribing for older adults.

Economics. Attempts by the insurance industry to manage rising drug costs have led to the increasing use of incentive-based formularies. Under this system, drugs are classified into tiers. Generic drugs typically require the lowest copayments; preferred brand name drugs (as identified by the company) require a higher copayment; and drugs not on the preferred list require the highest copayment (Thomas, 2003). Despite this system, copayments have been rising steadily.

Increasing drug costs may pose a hardship for older adults on limited incomes who sometimes cannot purchase prescribed drugs or may be forced to choose among those they need to be taking. One U.S. study of 387 older adults with limited incomes found 80% to be below the federal poverty level. The average number of medications taken by subjects in this sample was 8.9 (Upchurch, Menon, Levin, Catellier, & Conlisk, 2001).

Impact on Care of Older Adults

In the United States, where only 13% of the population is over age 65 years, older people are reported to consume 30% to 33% of all prescription drugs and to take two to three times as many drugs as younger people (Arslan, Gookce-Kutsal, & Atalay, 2002; Guay, Artz, Hanlon, & Schmader, 2003; Patel, 2003). The Slone survey of prescription and OTC medication use in the ambulatory adult population assessed the number of medications taken in 1 week before a telephone interview. In this sample, older women used the greatest number of medications, with 94% taking 1 or more medications, 57% taking 5 or more, and 12% taking 10 or more. In terms of race/ethnicity for all age-groups, whites and Native Americans had the highest use (84%), and Asians/Pacific Islanders had the lowest use (57%). Data on prescription drug use by older adults revealed that 23% of women had taken five or more prescription drugs in the preceding week whereas 19% of men had taken at least five prescription drugs in the same time frame.

The categories of drugs most commonly prescribed for the elderly are cardiovascular (including diuretics), gastrointestinal, central nervous system, analgesic, and endocrine-metabolic agents, and vitamins (Guay et al., 2003; Kaufman, Kelly, Rosenberg, Anderson, & Mitchell, 2002). In the United States, Centers for Disease Control and Prevention (CDC) data on prescribing patterns for women in ambulatory care settings in 2000 found antidepressants to be the most frequently used drug class. Estrogens and progestins were next, followed by antiarthritics and gastrointestinal drugs. Over the 5-year interval studied, the total number of medications prescribed to women in outpatient settings increased by 13% (Burt & Bernstein, 2003). Slone survey data showed that for women age 65 or older, the most common prescription drugs were conjugated estrogens, levothyroxine, and hydrochlorothiazide; for older men, furosemide was by far the most common (Kaufman et al., 2002). Using the minimum data set, researchers

in Kansas found a pattern of increasing antidepressant use among nursing facility residents from 1994 to 1997 (Rigler et al., 2003) (Box 7-1). The reasons cited by ambulatory adults for taking various medications are summarized in Table 7-1.

The use of OTC medications also is important because of the potential for drug-drug interactions and the lack of public awareness of their potential for harm. Among people age 65 and older, an average of 1.8 OTC drugs are taken daily, with highest rates among whites and women. Analgesics, laxatives, and nutritional supplements were the most commonly used OTCs among community-dwelling older adults in a study by Hanlon, Fillenbaum, Ruby, Gray, and Bohannon (2001). From the Slone survey, it was determined that the OTCs most often used by both older women and men were acetaminophen, aspirin, and ibuprofen (Kaufman et al., 2002). These data are congruent with another study in which 90% of older adults reported taking pain medication (Amoako, Richardson-Campbell, & Kennedy-Malone, 2003) (see Box 7-1).

Use of complementary and alternative therapies has received increasing attention in recent years as the potential for adverse effects and for interactions with conventional drugs has come under study. In the Slone survey, 14% of the sample had taken at least one herbal agent or supplement in the preceding week. Of 10 common products reported, older men were most likely to have used glucosamine and saw palmetto; older women were more likely to have taken *Ginkgo biloba* (Kaufman et al., 2002) (see Box 7-1).

BOX 7-1 Pharmacologic Agents Most Commonly Used by Community-Dwelling Ambulatory Older Adults

Prescription Drugs
Analgesics
Endocrine-metabolic agents
  Estrogens
  Thyroid replacement
Cardiovascular drugs
Diuretics
Central nervous system agents
Gastrointestinal agents

Over-the-Counter Drugs
Analgesics
Laxatives
Nutritional supplements

Vitamins and Minerals
Multivitamin
Vitamin E
Vitamin C
Calcium

Herbal Supplements
Ginkgo biloba extract
Allium sativum
Glucosamine
Chondroitin
Serenca repens

Data from Kaufman, D. W., Kelly, J. P., Rosenberg, L., Anderson, T. E., & Mitchel, A. A. (2002). Recent patterns of medication use in the ambulatory adult population of the United States: The Slone survey. *Journal of the American Medical Association, 287*(3), 337-344.

Table 7-1 *Most Common Reasons Given by Ambulatory Adults for Taking Various Medications*

Medication	Reasons
Prescription/over the counter	Hypertension Headache Heart Allergy Pain
Vitamins/minerals	Good for you Dietary supplement Vitamin/mineral supplement Prevent osteoporosis Physician recommended
Herbal supplements	Good for you Arthritis Memory improvement

Data from Kaufman, D. W., Kelly, J. P., Rosenberg, L., Anderson, T. E., & Mitchel, A. A. (2002). Recent patterns of medication use in the ambulatory adult population of the United States: The Slone survey. *Journal of the American Medical Association, 287*(3), 337-344.

Few studies report the number of medicines used in hospitalized older adults; however, several investigators have reported the average number of medicines used as between four and five per day. More important, as many as 75% of older persons have one or more medicines discontinued and new ones started during a hospital stay. The most common types of drugs given to hospitalized older adults are not well documented; however, some small studies have reported the high use of antimicrobials and laxatives in addition to cardiovascular, gastrointestinal, central nervous system, and analgesic drugs.

In U.S. long-term care facilities, the average number of routine medications per resident is 6 to 7; more than 75% of the residents receive 4 or more medications, and 33% take 7 to 10 medications. Medication patterns of residents of long-term care facilities are similar to those of hospitalized persons, with the most common medications being cardiovascular and central nervous system drugs, laxatives, and analgesics (Guay et al., 2003). In the United Kingdom, Kennerfalk, Ruigomez, Wallander, Wilhelmsen, and Johansson (2002) found the prevalence of polypharmacy (concurrent use of four or more drugs) to be the same in men and women. The most commonly used drugs in the sample of 5000 were cardiovascular, neurological, and gastrointestinal medications.

The widespread use of drugs by older adults, along with their enhanced vulnerability to adverse effects, provides a strong rationale for gerontological nurses to study drug utilization patterns, age-related variables that affect drug effects, and potential adverse effects in older adults. Armed with such knowledge, the gerontological nurse can help optimize drug effects and prevent or promptly recognize adverse drug reactions (Box 7-2).

AGE-RELATED CHANGES IN PHARMACOKINETICS AND PHARMACODYNAMICS

An understanding of pharmacokinetics and pharmacodynamics is necessary to select the most appropriate drug for maximal therapeutic efficacy and minimal risk

---

BOX 7-2 Drugs Commonly Associated with Adverse Drug Reactions in Older Adults

Older psychotropics
Digoxin
Phenytoin
Warfarin
Theophylline
Morphine
Meperidine
Metamizole

---

of adverse effects. This is particularly important when caring for older adults because it often is difficult to determine whether observed changes are due to age alone, to chronic diseases, or to drug actions.

Altered Pharmacokinetics

Pharmacokinetics, defined as the study of drug movement, includes four processes: absorption, distribution, metabolism, and elimination (Lehne, 2004). The following summarizes what is known about how aging affects each of the four major processes. Of course, this summary reflects common changes that occur over many years. The extent to which these changes are present in a particular person is highly individualized; therefore drug responses are highly individualized.

Absorption. A number of age-related changes in the stomach, including increased gastric pH, delayed gastric emptying, and decreased splanchnic blood flow, could potentially affect drug absorption. However, except for drugs such as calcium that require an acid environment for absorption, these changes appear to have little influence on the total amount of drug absorbed. Whereas the percentage of a drug that is absorbed remains stable with aging, the *rate* of absorption is slower (Lehne, 2004).

Distribution. The distribution of medications in the body depends on blood flow, plasma protein binding, and body composition. Age-related changes that can alter drug distribution include a relative decrease in body water and lean body weight, an increase in percent of body fat, and reduced serum albumin.

Drug characteristics also influence drug distribution. For example, water-soluble drugs are more concentrated in body fluids because of reduced total body water, resulting in more intense effects. On the other hand, lipid-soluble drugs are readily stored in body fat, which reduces their concentration in the plasma thereby reducing their physiological effects.

The two major plasma proteins that medications can bind to are albumin and alpha-1-acid glycoprotein. Acidic drugs bind with albumin, and basic drugs bind with alpha-1-acid glycoprotein. Deficiencies in the serum proteins are important because only unbound ("free") drug molecules are available to interact with tissue receptors. If a drug is normally bound highly to a protein, a deficiency of that protein will result in a higher level of free drug. Consequently, the drug will exert a more intense effect.

A slight decrease in serum albumin has been observed in older adults, but it is unclear whether this is a "normal" age-related change or if it is caused by chronic disease, poor nutrition, or some other factor (Sarkozi &

Ramanathan, 2003). An example of a drug that is affected by hypoalbuminemia is phenytoin. With decreased serum albumin, a person's free fraction of phenytoin is increased resulting in an enhanced pharmacological effect. For other acidic drugs such as naproxen, tolbutamide, and warfarin, decreased serum albumin also may lead to increased drug intensity (Guay et al., 2003).

Alpha-1-acid glycoprotein levels remain the same or increase with age. The level is increased in the presence of inflammatory disease, burns, and cancer. An increase in alpha-1-acid glycoprotein may bind a higher proportion of drug molecules, leading to a decreased free fraction of basic medications such as lidocaine, beta blockers, quinidine, and tricyclic antidepressants (Guay et al., 2003).

Changes in serum proteins should be considered when interpreting serum drug levels because generally only total concentrations (i.e., free and bound drug) are reported (Ahronheim, 2000). The extent to which distribution of a drug is affected by altered plasma proteins has a direct impact on drug half-life and the amount of a drug needed as a loading dose.

Metabolism. The liver is the major organ responsible for drug metabolism. Hepatic metabolism can be divided into either phase I or phase II. Phase I comprises preparative reactions that include oxidation and reductive and hydrolytic biotransformations. Cytochrome P450 mono-oxygenase enzymes are the primary mediators of phase I reactions. Phase II comprises conjugative/synthetic reactions, including glucuronidation, sulfation, and acetylation biotransformations. Advancing age does not appear to alter phase II reactions; however, changes in phase I reactions are more detectable. Specifically, there is a decline in drug oxidation attributed to reduced liver volume (Crome, 2003; Guay et al., 2003). In older people, decreased drug metabolism and clearance with associated increased half-life have been reported for medications such as diazepam, piroxicam, theophylline, and quinidine. Age-related decreases in hepatic blood flow also could significantly decrease the metabolism of drugs that undergo extensive first-pass metabolism, such as imipramine, lidocaine, and propranolol.

Despite the decrease in liver size and apparent altered metabolism of some drugs, most sources agree that age *alone* has little effect on drug metabolism (Crome, 2003). A number of confounding factors including race, gender, frailty, smoking, diet, and drug interactions can significantly affect hepatic metabolism (Guay et al., 2003). For example, theophylline metabolism is increased by smoking and phenytoin, whereas theophylline metabolism is decreased by cimetidine (Skidmore-Roth, 2004).

Elimination. Renal excretion is the primary route of elimination for many drugs or their active metabolites. Whether declining renal function is part of normal aging or represents pathology is unclear (Lamb, O'Riordan, & Delaney, 2003). Among the changes that have been attributed to age are reductions in renal mass, size and number of nephrons, renal blood flow, glomerular filtration, and tubular secretion. These changes can significantly impair the excretion of water-soluble drugs.

One problem in determining the impact of normal aging on drug elimination is the difficulty assessing glomerular filtration rate (GFR) in older adults. Serum creatinine alone is not considered an acceptable measure of renal function because it remains in the reference range until significant function has been lost (Lamb et al., 2003). Furthermore, measures of serum creatinine do not accurately reflect renal function in the elderly because muscle mass, the source of creatinine, declines with age (Ahronheim, 2000; Guay et al., 2003). Measures of urinary creatinine often are inaccurate because the process of specimen collection is inconvenient and patients may not follow instructions. As with serum creatinine, urinary creatinine excretion is reduced in older adults because of decreased muscle mass.

A number of equations have been developed to estimate the GFR using serum creatinine while correcting for confounding variables. Though less than perfect, these estimates are appropriate screening tools. One of the most commonly used equations, created by Cockcroft and Gault (1976), is:

$$\text{Creatinine clearance (men)} = \frac{(140 - \text{age})(\text{lean body weight in kg})}{(72)(\text{serum creatinine})}$$

For women, the result is multiplied by 0.85.

A second formula to estimate GFR, and a later abbreviated version, was developed in the Modification of Diet in Renal Disease Study by scientists who believe it is more accurate than the Cockcroft and Gault formula. Its accuracy with older people, however, has not yet been demonstrated (Lamb et al., 2003).

An important finding from the Baltimore Longitudinal Study of Aging was the correlation of declining GFR with hypertension. In the absence of diseases known to impair kidney function (including hypertension), GFR remained stable in one third of older adults over a 24-year period (Lamb et al., 2003).

Cystatin C is a protein that is produced at a constant rate by all nucleated cells and catabolized and excreted in the urine. The measurement of serum cystatin C is reportedly superior to serum creatinine in detecting mild to moderate renal disease. The clinical usefulness of serum cystatin C measurements to assess GFR in older adults is under study (Lamb et al., 2003).

The doses of medications that are excreted primarily by the kidneys generally should be reduced to compensate for decreased clearance. Examples of drugs eliminated by renal excretion are angiotensin-converting enzyme (ACE) inhibitors, acetazolamide, amantadine, aminoglycosides, digoxin, furosemide, metformin, ranitidine, and vancomycin (Guay et al., 2003). An example of a drug that is metabolized by the liver and yield metabolites that must be excreted by the kidneys is morphine sulfate. The elimination process should be considered in dosage regimens for older adults with impaired renal function.

Implications of Altered Pharmacokinetics.

As a generalization, the most significant age-related changes in pharmacokinetics are decreased hepatic metabolism and renal excretion (Guay et al., 2003). The importance of this depends on the pharmacokinetics for specific drugs. Of course, the prescriber must base decisions about drug therapy for individuals on the unique combinations of factors that predict drug responses in that person.

Altered Pharmacodynamics

Drug *pharmacodynamics*, defined broadly, is the effect that medications have on the body. A narrower definition is the pharmacological effect that results from a drug interacting with receptors at the site of action. There is evidence in older adults of enhanced responses, or "sensitivity," to some drugs and diminished responses to other drugs. This may be due to changes in receptor numbers or affinity (Lehne, 2004). It also is possible that some effects are blunted because of age-related impairment in physiological responses or homeostatic mechanisms (Guay et al., 2003).

Older adults have been found to have diminished responses to beta blockers and beta agonists, furosemide, and vaccines. They demonstrate enhanced responses to benzodiazepines, H1 blockers, neuroleptics, opioids, and warfarin. The exaggerated effects of central nervous system depressants may contribute to an increased risk of falls, hip fractures, incontinence, and cognitive impairment in older persons. Knowledge of medications that demonstrate altered pharmacodynamic sensitivity can allow clinicians and persons to use these drugs safely by making the appropriate adjustments in dosage. Many prescribers start with the lowest possible dose and only increase it if the medication is tolerated. The rule of thumb is "start low, go slow."

Interestingly, some drugs simultaneously demonstrate both enhanced and decreased sensitivity. For example, with calcium channel blockers, enhanced sensitivity is evident in greater reduction in blood pressure, and decreased sensitivity is evident in reduced

atrioventricular node blockade. This information leads the clinician to anticipate different side and adverse effects in older persons. There may be a smaller therapeutic window where the drug is effective, yet does not cause untoward effects.

Another example of altered response in older adults is the absence of reflex tachycardia that commonly is seen with vasodilators in younger people. It is possible that this is due to dampened baroreceptor response in the older person.

DRUG-RELATED PROBLEMS

Although drug therapy offers many benefits to older adults, the potential for drug-related problems exists. These problems include adverse drug reactions (ADRs), also referred to as adverse drug events (ADEs), and triggering or exacerbation of common geriatric syndromes such as cognitive impairment, falls, dysmobility, and incontinence. The epidemiology of ADRs follows, along with a discussion of predisposing factors. Not only do ADRs present physical threats, they also significantly add to the cost of health care. For the year 2000, the cost of drug-related problems in the United States was estimated to exceed $177 billion in the ambulatory population and $4 billion in nursing homes (Rodriguez-Monguio, Otero, & Rovira, 2003).

Epidemiology

An *adverse drug reaction* can be defined as "an undesired effect produced by a drug at standard doses, which typically necessitates reducing or stopping the suspected agent and may require treatment for the noxious effect produced" (Diasio, 2000). Most ADRs in older adults are dose related (Lehne, 2004).

ADRs can be classified as either predictable or unpredictable. Predictable reactions represent exaggerated pharmacological effects and are dose dependent. Unpredictable reactions cannot be anticipated based on the known pharmacological effects and include toxic, idiosyncratic, and immunological reactions (Diasio, 2000).

Estimates of the incidence of ADRs hover around 20% for outpatients and from 2% to 7% for inpatients (Diasio, 2000). The incidence of ADRs in older adults is seven times that of young adults. An estimated 16% of hospital admissions of older adults are related to ADRs (Lehne, 2004). A review of emergency medical admissions for falls, hypotension, heart failure, and delirium found that 30.4% may have been related to ADRs (Chan, Nicklason, & Vial, 2001). Drugs most often implicated are anticoagulants, antiarrhythmics, anticonvulsants, digoxin, lithium carbonate, oral hypoglycemics, theophylline, long-acting benzodiazepines, and phenothiazine derivatives (Diasio, 2000; Patel, 2003). A review of ADEs published from 1977 to 1997 revealed that the drug classes most often associated with life-threatening events for all ages were antimicrobials and central nervous system drugs (Marcellino & Kelly, 2001). From the same database, Kelly (2001) determined that drug-induced permanent disabilities were most often associated with antimicrobials, vaccines, central nervous system drugs, and antineoplastics. The types of resultant disabilities in this review included hearing loss, tardive dyskinesia, brain damage, blindness, and quadriplegia.

Few investigations of ADRs in older adults in outpatient settings have been reported. A study of all Medicare enrollees ($n = 30,397$) cared for in a multispecialty group practice over a 1-year period confirmed that ADEs were common in older adults seen in ambulatory settings. Adverse drug events occurred at a rate of 50.1 per 1000 person-years. Thirty-eight percent of the ADEs were serious, life-threatening, or fatal. The rate of ADEs deemed preventable was 13.8 per 1000 person-years. Examination of the preventable occurrences revealed that most were related to prescribing or monitoring. Drug categories most often associated with ADEs in this sample were cardiovascular drugs, diuretics, nonopioid analgesics, hypoglycemics, and anticoagulants. The most common types of ADEs considered preventable were classified as electrolyte/renal, gastrointestinal, hemorrhagic, metabolic/endocrine, and neuropsychiatric (Gurwitz et al., 2003). A sample assessed by Forster, Murff, Peterson, Gandhi, and Bates (2003) comprised 400 persons discharged home after hospitalization. In telephone interviews conducted 3 weeks after discharge, 12.8% of the participants reported ADEs. In another survey with 661 respondents, 25% of ambulatory care patients reported adverse drug events most often involving selective serotonin reuptake inhibitors (SSRIs), beta blockers, ACE inhibitors, and nonsteroidal antiinflammatory drugs (NSAIDs) (Gandhi et al., 2003).

An evaluation of 15,000 ADRs among hospitalized persons in the western United States discovered the rate of preventable ADRs to be higher among older adults (0.63) than among younger people (0.17) (Thomas & Brennan, 2000). Though not confined to older adults, the results of a study of ADRs in a surgical intensive care unit in Spain emphasizes one aspect of the cost of ADRs. In a sample of 401 people, 9.2% experienced an ADR. The resultant extended length of stay was estimated at 2.3 days (Vargas et al., 2003). In the United Kingdom, the National Service Framework for Older People reports that 5% to 17% of hospital admissions are necessitated by ADRs and that 6% to 17% of older persons experience ADRs when hospitalized (Bretherton, Day, & Lewis, 2003).

In a review of drug use by 1354 nursing home residents in Norway, 2445 potential medication problems were identified. Psychoactive drugs accounted for 38% of the potential problems, most of which were classified

as risk of ADRs, inappropriate drug choice, or probable undertreatment (Ruths, Straand, & Nygaard, 2003).

Collectively, the studies document that ADRs are a common phenomenon in older people regardless of the setting of care. Table 7-2 presents the most common drugs found to cause ADRs in older people. These drugs also are among the most commonly prescribed for them. Unfortunately, older adults have more medical conditions, many of which are best treated pharmacologically.

Risk Factors

A number of factors may predispose older adults to ADRs: the presence of multiple diseases, inappropriate drug use, and polypharmacy. Polypharmacy is the concurrent use of multiple medications, sometimes defined as four or five or more, by a single person. An alternative definition of polypharmacy is "the administration of more medications than are clinically indicated" (Hanlon, Lindblad, Maher, & Schmader, 2003, p. 1290). Recognition of polypharmacy as a risk factor for ADRs is important because multiple medication use is potentially modifiable, unlike some other risk factors.

The extent to which age and gender are independently associated with ADRs is controversial. Early studies demonstrated that older adults, especially women, were at greater risk for ADRs. However, more recent studies that control for other known risk factors, such as number of medications, comorbidity, and disease severity, have not supported the relationship of ADRs to age and gender. Other factors that are suspected of being associated with ADRs include previous history of an ADR, inappropriate prescribing, drug interactions, and

Table 7-2 *Common Adverse Drug Reactions in Older Adults*

Affected System	Adverse Reactions
Gastrointestinal	Diarrhea Constipation Dry mouth
Circulatory	Dizziness Cardiac dysrhythmias Orthostatic hypotension
Central nervous system	Sleep disturbances Neuropsychiatric symptoms
Fluids and electrolytes	Leg edema
Metabolic	Hypoglycemia
Hematological	Bleeding, bruising Hemorrhage

medication dispensing and administration errors. The three latter subjects deserve further discussion.

Inappropriate Prescribing. An inappropriate prescription is one that does not agree with accepted medical standards (Hanlon et al., 2003). Prescribing errors involve incorrect drug selection, dose, dosage form, quantity, route, concentration, rate of administration, and instructions for use (American Hospital Formulary Service, 1994).

The preceding discussion cites numerous specific drugs or drug classes that commonly contribute to adverse effects in older adults. The list is so long that the clinician may wonder what drugs older adults *can* take safely. A useful resource for prescribers is the Beers criteria. The Beers criteria classifies potentially inappropriate drug use in older adults as follows:

- Medications that generally should be avoided in ambulatory older adults
- Doses, frequencies of administration, or therapy duration of drugs that generally should not be exceeded for older adults
- Medications that should be avoided in older adults with specific common conditions

The criteria are to be used as guidelines to alert prescribers to potential problems, and are not applicable in all cases. The Beers and other criteria often are used in epidemiological studies, in drug utilization review systems, by health care providers, and in educational offerings (Beers, 1997). The criteria were updated in 2003. Table 7-3 lists drugs that are potentially inappropriate for older adults independent of diagnoses. Table 7-4 lists potentially inappropriate medications for older adults with specific diagnoses or conditions.

A comprehensive review of the literature on inappropriate prescribing for the older adult yielded disturbing results. The prevalence of older adults using at least one inappropriate drug was 21.3% in the community and 40% in nursing home residents. In most cases, the most significant predictors of inappropriate prescribing were polypharmacy, poor health status, and female gender (Liu & Christensen, 2002). The most frequently prescribed inappropriate drugs were propoxyphene, amitriptyline, long-acting benzodiazepines, and dipyridamole. Among the causes cited for inappropriate prescribing were provider knowledge deficit, multiple prescribers and pharmacies serving the same people, ageism, cost issues, patient demands, and restrictive formularies (Liu & Christensen, 2002; Mort & Aparasu, 2002). Analysis of the National Ambulatory Medical Care Survey for 1997 determined that during 191 million visits to physicians' offices, approximately 10% of older adults received at least one inappropriate prescription. The data also revealed that four or more prescriptions were issued per visit for 17.7% of female patients and 16.4% of male patients (Huang et al., 2002).

A study of medications prescribed to over 2000 older adults in residential care/assisted living settings revealed that inappropriate prescribing was associated with polypharmacy (the majority of the participants were taking five or more medications), smaller facilities, moderate licensed practical nurse turnover, low monthly fees, absence of dementia, and absence of weekly physician visits (Sloane, Zimmerman, Brown, Ives, & Walsh, 2002).

Analysis of medication records for older adults admitted to nursing homes in Canada over a 2-year period revealed an inappropriate prescribing rate of 25.4% on admission. After admission, the rate fell to 20.8%. Drugs involved were long-acting benzodiazepines and strongly anticholinergic antidepressants (Dhalla et al., 2002).

Among hospitalized adults, 14% reportedly received at least one potentially inappropriate medication; most commonly ticlopidine, digoxin, or amytriptyline. The greatest risk factor was the number of drugs taken (Onder et al., 2003).

Computerized drug alert systems are in place to reduce medication errors; however, a study by Weingart and colleagues (2003) found that few physicians in primary care changed their prescription in response to a drug allergy or interaction alert. The researchers noted that the low occurrence of ADRs incurred despite the override may indicate that the alert threshold was set too low. The magnitude of the risk of ADRs or negative consequences of inappropriate prescribing is unclear. In this study, inappropriate prescriptions were defined as those that could result in drug interactions, contraindicated drugs, and unnecessary drugs.

Drug Interactions. A *drug interaction* can be defined as the effect that the administration of one medication has on another drug. Drug interactions also can be considered in a broader sense as involving medications that can affect and be affected by patients' diseases, nutrition, and biochemical status. Mechanisms by which one drug might affect the actions or effects of another drug include inhibition of absorption, hepatic enzyme induction or inhibition, inhibition of excretion, displacement from plasma protein binding sites, and altered pharmacodynamics at the tissue level (Bressler & Bahl, 2003).

Polypharmacy places the patient at risk for drug-drug interactions, with the likelihood of interactive effects increasing with each additional medication (Patel, 2003). One factor that contributes to polypharmacy and drug interactions is the tendency of prescribers to treat side effects of one drug by prescribing another drug instead of finding an alternative to the first drug (Patel, 2003). Some examples of drug-drug interactions are enhancement of anticoagulants by aspirin and

Table 7-3 *2002 Criteria for Potentially Inappropriate Medication Use in Older Adults: Independent of Diagnoses or Conditions*

Applicable Medications*	Summary of Prescribing Concern	Severity Rating (High or Low)
Propoxyphene (Darvon) and combination products (Darvon with ASA, Darvon-N, Darvocet-N)	Offers few analgesic advantages over acetaminophen, yet it has the side effects of other narcotic drugs.	Low
Indomethacin (Indocin, Indocin SR)	Of all available nonsteroidal, antiinflammatory drugs, indomethacin produces the most central nervous system side effects.	High
Pentazocine (Talwin)	Narcotic analgesic that causes more central nervous system adverse effects, including confusion and hallucinations, more commonly than other narcotic drugs. Additionally, it is a mixed agonist and antagonist.	High
Trimethobenzamide (Tigan)	One of the least effective antiemetic drugs, yet it can cause extrapyramidal side effects.	High
Muscle relaxants and antispasmodics: methocarbamol (Robaxin), carisoprodol (Soma), chlorzoxazone (Paraflex), metaxalone (Skelaxin), cyclobenzaprine (Flexeril), and oxybutynin (Ditropan); do not consider the extended-release Ditropan XL	Most muscle relaxants and antispasmodic drugs are poorly tolerated by older adults because they cause anticholinergic adverse effects, sedation, and weakness. Additionally, their effectiveness at doses tolerated by older adults is questionable.	High
Flurazepam (Dalmane)	This hypnotic has an extremely long half-life in older adults (often days), producing prolonged sedation and increasing the incidence of falls and fractures. Medium- or short-acting benzodiazepines are preferable.	High
Amitriptyline (Elavil), chlordiazepoxide-amitriptyline (Limbitrol), and perphenazine-amitriptyline (Triavil)	Because of its strong anticholinergic and sedating properties, amitriptyline is rarely the antidepressant of choice for older adults.	High
Doxepin (Sinequan)	Because of its strong anticholinergic and sedating properties, doxepin is rarely the antidepressant of choice for older adults.	High
Meprobamate (Miltown, Equanil)	Highly addictive and sedating anxiolytic to be avoided in older patients. Those using meprobamate for prolonged periods may become addicted and may need to be withdrawn slowly.	High

Modified from Beers M. H. (1997). Explicit criteria for determining potentially inappropriate medication use by the elderly, *Archives of Internal Medicine, 157,* 1531-1536; and Fick, D. M., Cooper, J. W., Wade, W. E., Waller, J. L., Maclean, R., & Beers, M. H. (2003). Updating the Beers criteria for potentially inappropriate medication use in older adults, *Archives of Internal Medicine, 163,* 2719-2720.
Most package circulars produced by drug manufacturers do not include language identical to the statements presented herein. Although adverse effects that these drugs can produce are generally listed in the package circulars, these as well as warnings and contraindications must be approved by regulatory agencies and in general are not based on consensus or surveys.
*Dose limits are total daily dose.

Table 7-3 *2002 Criteria for Potentially Inappropriate Medication Use in Older Adults: Independent of Diagnoses or Conditions—cont'd*

Applicable Medications*	Summary of Prescribing Concern	Severity Rating (High or Low)
Doses of short-acting benzodiazepines: doses > lorazepam (Ativan), 3 mg; oxazepam (Serax), 60 mg; alprazolam (Xanax), 2 mg; temazepam (Restoril), 15 mg; and triazolam (Halcion), 0.25 mg	Because of increased sensitivity to benzodiazepines in older adults, smaller doses may be effective as well as safer. Total daily doses should rarely exceed the suggested maximums.	High
Long-acting benzodiazepines: chlordiazepoxide (Librium), chlordiazepoxide-amitriptyline (Limbitrol), clidinium-chlordiazepoxide (Librax), diazepam (Valium), quazepam (Doral), halazepam (Paxipam), and chloazepate (Tranxene)	These drugs have a long half-life in older adults (often several days), producing prolonged sedation and increasing the risk of falls and fractures. Short- and intermediate-acting benzodiazepines are preferred if a benzodiazepine is required.	High
Disopyramide (Norpace, Norpace CR)	Of all antiarrhythmic drugs, this is the most potent negative inotrope and therefore may induce heart failure in older adults. It is also strongly anticholinergic. Other antiarrhythmic drugs should be used.	High
Digoxin (Lanoxin) (should not exceed 0.125 mg daily except when treating atrial arrhythmias)	Decreased renal clearance may lead to increased risk of toxic effects.	Low
Short-acting Dipyridamole (Persantine); do not consider long-acting Dipyridamole (which has better properties than the short-acting in older adults) except for patients with artificial heart valves	This may cause orthostatic hypotension in older adults.	Low
Methyldopa (Aldomet) and methyldopa/hydrochlorothiazide (Aldoril)	May cause bradycardia and exacerbate depression in older adults.	High
Reserpine at doses >0.25 mg	May induce depression, impotence, sedation, and orthostatic hypotension.	Low
Chlorpropamide (Diabinese)	Has a prolonged half-life in older adults and can cause prolonged hypoglycemia. Additionally, it is the only oral hypoglycemic agent that causes SIADH.	High
Gastrointestinal antispasmodic drugs: dicyclomine (Bentyl); hyoscyamine (Levsin, Levsinex), propantheline (Pro-Banthine), belladonna alkaloids (Donnatal and others), and clidinium-chlordiazepoxide (Librax)	Gastrointestinal antispasmodic drugs are highly anticholinergic and have uncertain effectiveness. These drugs should be avoided in older adults, especially for long-term use.	High
Anticholinergics and antihistamines: chlorpheniramine (Chlor-Trimeton), diphenhydramine (Benadryl), hydroxyzine (Vistaril, Atarax), cyproheptadine (Periactin), promethazine (Phenergan), tripelennamine, and dexchlorpheniramine (Polaramine)	All nonprescription and many prescription antihistamines have potent anticholinergic properties. Many cough and cold preparations are available without antihistamines, and these are safer substitutes in older adults.	High

SIADH, Syndrome of inappropriate antidiuretic hormone.

Continued

Table 7-3 *2002 Criteria for Potentially Inappropriate Medication Use in Older Adults: Independent of Diagnoses or Conditions—cont'd*

Applicable Medications*	Summary of Prescribing Concern	Severity Rating (High or Low)
Diphenhydramine (Benadryl)	May cause confusion and sedation. Should not be used as a hypnotic. When used to treat or prevent allergic reactions, it should be used in the smallest possible dose.	High
Ergot mesyloids (Hydergine) and cyclospasmol	Have not been shown to be effective in the doses studied.	Low
Iron supplements >325 mg	Iron supplements rarely need to be given in doses exceeding 325 mg of ferrous sulfate daily. When doses are higher, total absorption is not substantially increased, but constipation is more likely to occur.	Low
All barbiturates (except phenobarbital), except when used to control seizures	Cause more side effects than most other sedative or hypnotic drugs in older adults and are highly addictive.	High
Meperidine (Demerol)	Not an effective oral analgesic in the doses commonly used. It may cause confusion and has many disadvantages to other narcotic drugs.	High
Ticlopidine (Ticlid)	Has been shown to be no better than aspirin in preventing clotting and may be considerably more toxic. Safer, more effective alternatives exist.	High
Ketorolac (Toradol)	Immediate and long-term use should be avoided in older adults because a significant number have asymptomatic GI pathological conditions.	High
Amphetamines and anorexic agents	These drugs have the potential for causing dependence, hypertension, angina, and myocardial infarction.	High
Long term use of full dosage, longer half-life, non-COX-selective NSAIDs: naproxen (Naprosyn, Avaprox, Aleve), oxaprozin (Daypro), and piroxicam (Feldene)	Have the potential to produce GI bleeding, renal failure, high blood pressure, and heart failure.	High
Daily fluoxetine (Prozac)	Long half-life of drug and risk of producing excessive CNS stimulation, sleep disturbances, and increasing agitation. Safer alternatives exist.	High
Long-term use of stimulant laxatives: cascara sagrada, bisacodyl (Dulcolax), and Neoloid, except in the presence of opiate analgesic use.	May exacerbate bowel dysfunction.	High
Amiodarone (Cordarone)	Associated with QT interval problems and risk of provoking torsades de pointes, and has a lack of efficacy in older adults.	High

CNS, Central nervous system; *COX*, cyclooxygenase; *GI*, gastrointestinal; *NSAIDs*, nonsteroidal antiinflammatory drugs.

Table 7-3 *2002 Criteria for Potentially Inappropriate Medication Use in Older Adults: Independent of Diagnoses or Conditions—cont'd*

Applicable Medications*	Summary of Prescribing Concern	Severity Rating (High or Low)
Orphenadrine (Norflex)	Causes more sedation and anticholinergic adverse effects than safer alternatives.	High
Guanethidine (Ismelin)	May cause orthostatic hypotension.	High
Guanadrel (Hylorel)	May cause orthostatic hypotension. Safer alternatives exist.	High
Cyclandelate (Cyclospasmol)	Lack of efficacy.	Low
Isoxsurpine (Vasodilan)	Lack of efficacy.	Low
Nitrofurantoin (Macrodantin)	Potential for renal impairment. Safer alternatives exist.	High
Doxazosin (Cardura)	Potential for dry mouth, hypotension, and urinary problems.	Low
Methyltestosterone (Android, Virilon, Testrad)	Potential for prostatic hypertrophy and cardiac problems.	High
Thioridazine (Mellaril)	Greater potential for CNS and extrapyramidal adverse effects.	High
Mesoridazine (Serentil)	CNS and extrapyramidal adverse effects.	High
Short-acting nifedipine (Procardia, Adalat)	Potential for hypotension and constipation.	High
Clonidine (Catapres)	Potential for orthostatic hypotension and CNS adverse effects.	Low
Mineral oil	Potential for aspiration and adverse effects. Safer alternatives are available.	High
Cimetidine (Tagamet)	CNS adverse effects, including confusion.	Low
Ethacrynic acid (Edecrin)	Potential for hypertension and fluid imbalances. Safer alternatives exist.	Low
Dessicated thyroid	Concerns about cardiac effects. Safer alternatives exist.	High
Amphetamines (excluding methylphenidate hydrochloride and anorexics)	CNS stimulant adverse effects.	High
Estrogens only (oral)	Evidence of carcinogenic (breast and endometrial cancer) potential of these agents and lack of cardioprotective effect in older women.	Low

CNS, Central nervous system.

Table 7-4 2002 Criteria for Potentially Inappropriate Medication Use in Older Adults: Considering Diagnoses or Conditions

Disease or Condition	Drug	Concern	Severity Rating (High or Low)
Heart failure	Disopyramide (Norpace), and drugs with high sodium content (sodium and sodium salts [alginate bicarbonate, biphosphate, citrate, phosphate, salicylate, and sulfate])	Negative inotropic effect; potential to promote fluid retention and exacerbation of heart failure	High
Hypertension	Phenylpropanolamine hydrochloride (removed from the market in 2001) and pseudoephedrine, diet pills, and amphetamines	May produce elevation of blood pressure secondary to sympathomimetic activity	High
Gastric or duodenal ulcers	NSAIDs and aspirin (>325 mg) (coxibs excluded)	May exacerbate existing ulcers or produce new or additional ulcers	High
Seizures or epilepsy	Clozapine (Clorazil), chlorpromazine (Thorazine), thioridazine (Mellaril), and thiothixene (Navane)	May lower seizure thresholds	High
Blood clotting disorders or receiving anticoagulant therapy	Aspirin, NSAIDs, dipyridamole (Persantin), ticlopidine (Ticlid), and clopidogrel (Plavix)	May prolong clotting time and elevate INR values or inhibit platelet aggregation, resulting in an increased potential for bleeding	High
Bladder outflow obstruction	Anticholinergics and antihistamines, gastrointestinal antispasmodics, muscle relaxants, oxybutynin (Ditropan), flavoxate (Urispas), anticholinergics, antidepressants, decongestants, and tolterodine (Detrol)	May decrease urinary flow, leading to urinary retention	High
Stress incontinence	α-blockers (Doxazosin, Prazosin, and Terazosin), anticholinergics, tricyclic antidepressants (imipramine hydrochloride, doxepin hydrochloride, and amitriptyline hydrochloride), and long-acting benzodiazepines	May produce polyuria and worsening of incontinence	High
Arrhythmias	Tricyclic antidepressants (imipramine hydrochloride, doxepin hydrochloride, and amitriptyline hydrochloride)	Concern due to proarrhythmic effects and ability to produce QT interval changes	High
Insomnia	Decongestants, theophylline (Theodur), methylphenidate (Ritalin), MAOIs, and amphetamines	Concern due to CNS stimulant effects	High

Reproduced with permission from Fick, D. M., Cooper, J. W., Wade, W. E., Waller, J. L., Maclean, R., & Beers, M. H. (2003). Updating the Beers criteria for potentially inappropriate medication use in older adults. *Archives of Internal Medicine, 163,* 2721.
CNS, Central nervous system; *INR,* international normalized ratio; *MAOIs,* monoamine oxidase inhibitors; *NSAIDs,* nonsteroidal antiinflammatory drugs.

increased risk of digitalis toxicity with potassium-wasting diuretics.

Although potential drug interactions may be common, research has yet to document clinically significant adverse outcomes in most cases (Hanlon et al., 2003).

That is not to say that health care professionals should not be vigilant about this issue, as older people are more vulnerable to serious consequences if a clinically significant interaction does occur. To reduce the risk of drug interactions, the prescriber needs to take a thorough

Table 7-4 *2002 Criteria for Potentially Inappropriate Medication Use in Older Adults: Considering Diagnoses or Conditions—cont'd*

Disease or Condition	Drug	Concern	Severity Rating (High or Low)
Parkinson disease	Metoclopramide (Reglan), conventional antipsychotics, and tacrine (Cognex)	Concern due to their antidopaminergic/cholinergic effects	High
Cognitive impairment	Barbiturates, anticholinergics, antispasmodics, and muscle relaxants. CNS stimulants: dextroAmphetamine (Adderall), methylphenidate (Desoxyn), and pemolin	Concern due to CNS-altering effects	High
Depression	Long-term benzodiazepine use. Sympatholytic agents: methyldopa (Aldomet), reserpine, and guanethidine (Ismelin)	May produce or exacerbate depression	High
Anorexia and malnutrition	CNS stimulants: DextroAmphetamine (Adderall), methylphenidate (Ritalin), methamphetamine (Desoxyn), pemolin, and fluoxetine (Prozac)	Concern due to their appetite-suppressing effects	High
Syncope and falls	Short- to intermediate-acting benzodiazepine and tricyclic antidepressants (imipramine hydrochloride, doxepin hydrochloride, and amitriptyline hydrochloride)	May produce ataxia, impaired psychomotor function, syncope, and additional falls	High
SIADH/hyponatremia	SSRIs (fluoxetine [Prozac], citalopram [Celexa], fluvoxamine [Luvox], paroxetine [Paxil], and sertraline [Zoloft])	May exacerbate or cause SIADH	Low
Seizure disorder	Bupropion (Wellbutrin)	May lower seizure threshold	High
Obesity	Olanzapine (Zyprexa)	May stimulate appetite and increase weight gain	Low
COPD	Long-acting benzodiazepines (chlordiazepoxide [Librium], chlordiazepoxide-amitriptyline [Limbitrol], clidinium-chlordiazepoxide [Librax], diazepam [Valium], quazepam [Doral], halazepam [Paxipam], and chlorazepate [Tranxene]) and β-blockers (propanolol)	Adverse CNS effects; may induce respiratory depression; may exacerbate or cause respiratory depression	High
Chronic constipation	Calcium channel blockers, anticholinergics, and tricyclic antidepressants (imipramine hydrochloride, doxepin hydrochloride, and amitriptyline hydrochloride)	May exacerbate constipation	Low

COPD, Chronic obstructive pulmonary disease; *SIADH,* syndrome of inappropriate antidiuretic hormone secretion; *SSRIs,* selective serotonin reuptake inhibitors.

medication history, including prescription drugs, OTC drugs, vitamins and minerals, and herbal supplements (Patel, 2003).

Medication Errors. Medication errors can be defined as drug misadventures that involve the prescribing, dispensing, or administration of medications. The 1999 report issued by the Institute of Medicine (IOM) focused attention on medication errors by estimating that 98,000 deaths each year resulted from medical errors. Seven thousand of these deaths were attributed to medication errors. This startling announcement has been the impetus for many additional studies designed at identifying both the source of the problem and solutions. The figures are reinforced by Phillips and Bredder (2002), who reported 9856 deaths from acknowledged prescription errors in 1998. One reason for the variance in statistics is the variety of data collection procedures. Flynn, Barker, Pepper, Bates, and Mikeal (2002) examined methods of data collection and concluded that direct observation was more efficient and accurate than chart review or incident reports in detecting medication errors.

Although this problem has been most extensively examined for persons in institutional settings, it is pertinent to older adults in all settings of care. The possibility of medication errors should be considered when evaluating the effects of drug regimens in older people. Bond, Raehl, and Franke's (2002) review of data from 1081 hospitals determined that 5.22% of the patients admitted were recipients of medication errors. A British study of intravenous (IV) drug errors discovered that at least one error occurred in 49% of IV drug doses—mostly involving bolus administration or preparing drugs that required multiple steps. Fortunately, only 1% of those was potentially serious (Taxis & Barber, 2003). In a U.S. study, 19% of medication doses in hospitals and nursing homes were in error: wrong time, omission, wrong dose, or unauthorized drug. About 7% of those were considered potentially harmful (Barker, Flynn, Pepper, Bates, & Mikeal, 2002).

Case reports of life-threatening ADEs published in *Clin-Alert* from 1977 to 1997 attributed 4% of the events to medication errors (Marcellino & Kelly, 2001). From the same database, medication errors were blamed in 55% of drug-induced permanent disabilities (Kelly, 2001).

Nursing errors have been categorized as follows: lack of attentiveness, lack of agency/fiduciary concern, inappropriate judgment, lack of intervention on the patient's behalf, medication errors, lack of prevention, missed or mistaken prescriber orders, and documentation errors (Benner et al., 2002). McGillis Hall, Doran, and Pink (2004) examined nurse staffing and demonstrated that the rate of medication errors was inversely related to the proportion of professional nursing staff on a unit.

U.K. researchers interviewed physicians whom pharmacists identified as having made a potentially serious prescribing error. The physicians' errors included slips in attention, workload, whether they were prescribing for their own patients, team communication, mental and physical well-being, and lack of knowledge (Dean, Schachter, Vincent, & Barber, 2002).

Interventions that have been recommended to decrease medication errors include improved written and oral communication, better patient education, computerized integrated medication delivery with adequate training of professionals, computerized medical orders, and replacement of abbreviations and outdated terminology with plain English (Benjamin, 2003); pharmacist participation in patient rounds (LaPointe & Jollis, 2003); and better training in use of IV therapy equipment (Amoore & Adamson, 2003). One randomized controlled study showed that the error rate was not reduced by having dedicated medication nurses (Greengold et al., 2003).

Nonadherence. Adverse drug reactions may occur as a result of nonadherence. Failure to adhere to prescribed regimens, intentionally or unintentionally, is thought to be common among older persons. However, there is no consistent evidence from the literature that age per se increases the risk of medication nonadherence. Nonadherence tends to be associated with underuse rather than overuse of medicines. In fact, overuse of drugs seems to be less common in elderly than in younger people. A systematic review of studies of adherence to therapy among psychotic patients revealed a nonadherence rate of 25.78%. Notably, nonadherence was associated with younger age (Nose, Barbui, & Tansella, 2003). Similarly, a systematic review of drug therapy in people with schizophrenia found a mean nonadherence rate of 42%; however, age was not a consistent predictor in this review (Lacro, Dunn, Dolder, Leckband, & Jeste, 2002).

Choo and colleagues (2001) compared self-report and electronic monitoring in persons on single-drug antihypertensive therapy. Electronic monitoring revealed a mean nonadherence rate of 42%, compared with a self-report rate of 21%. People who overreported their adherence were more likely to be taking more than one daily dose, perceived a lower health risk from nonadherence, and had lower annual income. Another study assessed adherence to newly prescribed antihypertensive drugs over an 18-month period. By the end of the study period, 43.3% of those studied had stopped taking the drug either because of side effects or cost (Gregoire et al., 2002).

Among adults with disabilities, Kennedy and Erb (2002) reported that many are nonadherent because of drug costs, despite resultant health problems. Data from the Survey of Asset and Health Dynamics among the Oldest Old revealed that skipping doses or omitting drugs because of costs was reported by 8% of those with no prescription coverage, 3% of those with partial coverage, and 2% of those with full coverage (Steinman, Sands, & Covinsky, 2001). An interesting study that assessed reading difficulties among older adults found no correlation between nonadherence and difficulty reading and understanding prescription labels (Moisan, Gaudet, Gregoire, & Bouchard, 2002). Among rural older adults, those most likely to mismanage prescription medications were African American, younger, in poorer mental health, and having trouble paying for their medications (Mitchell, Mathews, Hunt, Cobb, & Watson, 2001).

Research results on polypharmacy and adherence have yielded contradictory results. A study that relied on patient self-report concluded that the total number of drugs prescribed did not correlate with medication adherence rates. Those on multiple drugs who were less adherent generally were nonadherent with a single drug. Reasons cited for nonadherence with specific drugs included unreported side effects and lack of confidence in benefits of the drug (Grant, Devita, Singer, & Meigs, 2003). Similarly, a Portuguese study of polypharmacy in older hypertensive adults reported a nonadherence rate of only 14% despite relatively high costs (Fonseca & Clara, 2000). In contrast, Barat, Andreasen, and Damsgaard's (2001) study of community-dwelling older adults found nonadherence to be associated with the use of three or more drugs, number of doses per day, multiple physician prescribers, and probable dementia.

In some cases, underuse of drugs may prevent adverse reactions. Problems may occur, however, if the patient is hospitalized and administered the drug dose that the physician believed was being taken at home. For example, a person who has been nonadherent with antihypertensive medicines at home may become hypotensive and sustain a fall-related injury if dosage is increased or additional antihypertensive drugs are given during hospitalization.

The concept of nonadherence has limited usefulness unless it is considered as a symptom of an underlying problem to be discovered and addressed rather than as a label to apply to a person. The failure of the term to give meaningful guidance to care is highlighted by use of the term *intelligent nonadherence*, which distinguishes failure to adhere to medication regimens that have clear objective benefits from nonadherence with regimens that serve little apparent purpose or that are actually harmful.

Although the range of ADRs is enormous, it is particularly important to recognize that certain common geriatric syndromes may be triggered or exacerbated by ADRs. These syndromes include cognitive impairment, falls, dysmobility, and incontinence, discussed next. Box 7-3 describes the challenges of managing medications in the nursing home setting by geriatric nurse practitioners.

Drug-Related Pathology

Delirium. Disturbed thought processes are a common adverse effect of medication use in older adults. Unfortunately, changes in mentation often go undiagnosed because of the erroneous belief that mental impairment is normal in older persons. Symptom reporting by older people themselves and their families is affected by this belief, and many health care professionals fail to consider drugs as the source of cognitive impairment.

Risk factors for delirium include both baseline vulnerability and precipitating factors. Baseline characteristics that affect risk for delirium and precipitating events have been summarized by Pompei (2003). Baseline characteristics include cognitive impairment, illness severity or burden of comorbidity, infection, renal abnormalities, metabolic derangement, social stress, advanced age, vision impairment, depression, and alcoholism. Factors found to precipitate delirium during hospitalization are the addition of more than three new medications, use of a bladder catheter, physical restraints, malnutrition, and iatrogenic events. Drug intoxication sometimes presents as delirium. The *Diagnostic and Statistical Manual of Mental Disorders* (American Psychiatric Association, 1994) classifies disturbances in consciousness and changes in cognition that are associated with medication side effects, as well as substance intoxication or withdrawal, as substance-induced delirium.

The drugs most commonly associated with altered mental function are tricyclic antidepressants, benzodiazepines, lithium, anticholinergics, digitalis, analgesics, histamine-2 antagonists, NSAIDs, and steroids (Pompei, 2003). A more complete list is found in Table 7-5.

Although many persons cannot function without some of these drugs, thoughtful drug choice and dosage in light of the age-related changes in pharmacokinetics and pharmacodynamics can alleviate drug-induced mental alterations in many cases. The high incidence of mental confusion associated with ADRs points to the need for baseline mental status testing in older persons before new regimens are instituted. Failure to do so results in an inadequate database with which to evaluate possible drug side effects. Many simple, valid screening tests are available (see Chapter 3 for further details). Careful choice of drugs, especially in people who are vulnerable to delirium, may make the difference between an effective therapy and one that creates new problems or exacerbates the problem for which it was initially prescribed.

Sometimes hypnotic medications are prescribed for depressed persons who have sleep difficulties. If the person subsequently is placed on an antidepressant, the hypnotic may no longer be required, because many antidepressants have sedative effects. Failure to discontinue the hypnotic before beginning the antidepressant may result in depressed mental function. Tapering and discontinuation of the hypnotic when the antidepressant is started should prevent the unwanted side effect. In any case, hypnotics should be prescribed only for short periods of time.

When mental alterations caused by drug side effects are suspected, nurses should report the domains of impaired function to the prescriber. Data related to nature of the symptom, duration of symptom relative to starting the new medication, severity of the symptom,

Box 7-3 *Reflections on Managing Medications*

Nurses and advanced practice nurses often assist with monitoring or managing complicated medication regimens for older adults. Because older patients have multiple health conditions, undergo multiple treatments, and have various levels of frailty, managing their medications is particularly challenging. My clinical practice is in a long-term care setting. The complexities of the patients and the setting create some interesting challenges. Careful attention to medication management is crucial to the older adults' health and well-being. I will use the example of warfarin management in the long-term care setting to illustrate the many factors at play in good medication management and demonstrate some of the common pitfalls.

Warfarin is a medication commonly used in the long-term care setting to prevent strokes in patients with atrial fibrillation and for treatment of pulmonary embolus and deep vein thrombosis, as well as other conditions. Warfarin is a protein-bound drug that is dependent on the patient's nutritional status, diet, and other medications. Drug-drug interactions and food-drug interactions are common. In addition, warfarin has a narrow therapeutic window, so it is easy for a patient to have subtherapeutic levels or toxic levels after any change in condition or treatments for other medical problems.

Patients on warfarin require frequent monitoring of their blood levels. In healthy older adults in the community, blood levels are often checked monthly. However, most nursing home and subacute residents need to have their prothrombin and international normalized ratio (INR) levels checked and dosages adjusted weekly or biweekly. This requires teamwork, with good communication on the part of the physician or advanced practice nurse and the nursing staff.

The patient and family are important partners in medication management, and decision to take medications should be discussed with them. For example, patients and families should be made aware of the risks and benefits of taking warfarin, as well as precautions that will be taken to maintain safety. These discussions and decisions should be documented in the patient's medical record. Patients or families may decide they do not want to take the risk of a particular medication and ask to explore alternative therapies. More and more patients and family members are becoming active partners in the decisions regarding their health.

Communication among staff members is another crucial step to managing medications. Simple techniques to facilitate this include documenting on the allergy section of the chart and kardex that the patient is taking warfarin. Staff are then reminded and can readily notify the physicians, advanced practice nurses, and others that the patient takes warfarin. This notification is important in order to prevent drug-drug interactions and to facilitate

closer monitoring of the prothrombin time (PT)/INR when antibiotics or other interfering medications are ordered.

For example, a patient develops a urinary tract infection with positive sensitivities to trimethaprim sulfa, so the nursing staff notifies the health professional on call. The health professional on call asks about allergies but doesn't necessarily ask if the patient is on warfarin. Trimetheprim sulfa is ordered, and a week later the patient has bruising (and, luckily, no worse effects). The PT/INR is markedly elevated. If the staff had been triggered by a system in the chart and reminded the health professional on call that the patient was on warfarin, a level might have been checked sooner and the dose adjusted before any serious side effects occurred. Ideally the same person prescribes all the medications for a patient and monitors and adjusts drug dosages, but this is not always feasible in a group practice.

Staff must also be diligent in monitoring the patient for signs and symptoms of medication side effects or toxic levels. For example, warfarin can result in bruising, hematuria, or gastrointestinal bleeding. In addition, some drugs like warfarin require safety precautions and careful attention if the patient has a fall or an accident in which he or she hits their head. Excessive bruising at the site of a contusion or a subdural hematoma should be monitored for up to a week after a fall or injury. Effects of drug-drug interactions and drug-food interactions should also be monitored. Staff often overlook alcohol intake as a reason for poorly controlled PT/NR levels. This can even be a problem for long-term care residents, who may go out on pass to visit friends or relatives and have a drink. Many things can influence the patient's response to warfarin. Successful management of warfarin can be difficult particularly with long-term care elders, but it can be accomplished well if everyone knows what to do and plays their part.

Tips for managing medications well are to start low and go slow with new medications, watch closely for changes after any medication adjustments, and always be suspect of potential side effects or toxic reactions. Stay up to date on all new medications and new evidence for the use of old ones. Be aware of clinical tools to help you, such as practice guidelines that outline care for patients on different medications. For example, the American Geriatrics Society (AGS) has a Clinical Practice Guideline for Oral Anticoagulation for Older Adults (AGS, 2002). These tips and tools can help you become skilled at managing monitoring patient's medications.

Pamela Z. Cacchione
Pamela Z. Cacchione, PhD, RN, GNP, BC
Associate Professor
Saint Louis University School of Nursing
St. Louis, Missouri

Table 7-5 *Common Medications Associated with Altered Mental Staus in Older Adults*

Type of Disorder	Medication Class	Common Examples
Cardiovascular	Antidysrhythmics	Procainamide, propranolol, quinidine, lidocaine
	Antihypertensives	Clonidine, methyldopa, reserpine
	Cardiac glycosides	Digitalis
Gastrointestinal	Antidiarrheals	Atropine, belladonna, homatropine, hyoscyamine
	Antinauseants	Phenothiazines
	Antispasmodics	Phenothiazines, scopolamine
	Antiulcer agents	Propantheline, cimetidine, ranitidine, metoclopromide
Musculoskeletal	Antiinflammatory agents	Corticosteroids, indomethacin, phenylbutazone, salicylates
	Muscle relaxants	Carisoprodol, diazepam
Neurological-psychiatric	Anticonvulsants	Barbiturates, phenytoin
	Antiparkinson agents	Amantadine, benzotropine, bromocriptine, levodopa, trihexyphenidyl, selegiline
	Hypnotics and sedatives	Barbiturates, bromides, chloral hydrate, glutethimide, hydroxyzine
	Psychotropics	Benzodiazepines, lithium salts, neuroleptics, antidepressants
Respiratory/allergic	Antihistamines	Brompheniramine, chlorpheniramine, cyproheptadine, diphenhydramine
	Bronchodilators	Theophylline
Miscellaneous	Analgesics	Opioids
	Antidiabetic agents	Insulin, oral hypoglycemics
	Antineoplastic agents	Methotrexate, mitomycin, procarbazine
	Antiinfectives	Acyclovir, amphotericin B, co-trimoxazole, isoniazid, ketoconazole, rifampin

and aggravating factors are most important. Have information regarding suitable alternative treatments in hand before discussing the case with the prescriber to make the consultation process more efficient. Examples of alternatives include (1) use of different drugs with lower potential for adverse side effects, (2) dosage reductions to produce the same therapeutic effect but with fewer adverse side effects, and (3) use of nonpharmacological interventions, such as environmental modification or relaxation techniques.

Falls. Falls are an important source of both morbidity and death among older adults. Smith (2003) analyzed 169 most often prescribed medications for reported side effects including, or potentially contributing to, falls in older adults. For 9.5% of the drugs reviewed, traumatic injuries and falls were documented. In addition, 92.9% of the drugs had adverse effects on the nervous, circulatory, or muscular system that could contribute to falls.

Psychotropic drugs, including both tricyclic and SSRI antidepressants, antipsychotics, and both long- and short-acting benzodiazepines, are related to falls in older adults. Other drugs that have been implicated, but for which less conclusive evidence exists, are class 1a

antiarrhythmics, digoxin, diuretics, opioid analgesics, and anticonvulsants (Kallin, Jensen, Olsson, Nyberg, & Gustafson, 2004; Neutel, Perry, & Maxwell, 2002).

A rehabilitation center in the United Kingdom implemented a pharmaceutical intervention program aimed at assessing effects of the intervention on the number of patient falls. In a sample of 200 subjects randomly selected from the study population, the number of falls had decreased by 47% after 1 year. Drug classes that were used less often after the intervention included cardiovascular drugs, analgesics, psychoactive drugs, and sedatives and hypnotics (Haumschild, Karfonta, Haumschild, & Phillips, 2003). A study of falls in healthy older persons identified a number of correlates, including medication use. Benzodiazepines specifically were implicated for women (de Rekeneire et al., 2003). Box 7-4 summarizes drugs commonly associated with syncope, falls, and hip fractures.

A number of etiological mechanisms have been postulated to explain the relationship between drug use and falls. They include impaired postural control, impaired balance and reaction time, hypotension, diminished perceptual ability, impaired judgment, and memory impairment.

Drugs that interfere with postural control by acting on the autonomic nervous system include beta blockers,

---

BOX 7-4 Drugs Associated with Syncope, Falls, and Hip Fractures

Anticonvulsants
Antilipemics
Antihypertensives
Analgesics
Antidiabetic agents
Hormone replacement agents
Antidepressants (SSRIs and tricyclics)
Sedatives and hypnotics: benzodiazepines
Psychotropics: neuroleptics (especially during initial therapy)

---

antidepressants, and antipsychotics. Postural hypotension may occur with antihypertensives, nitrates, tricyclic antidepressants, and antipsychotics. Hypoglycemics can cause acute hypoglycemia with weakness, confusion, and impaired consciousness. Volume depletion caused by diuretics may also interfere with postural control.

Dizziness and syncope are important causes of falls in the elderly. Dizziness was identified as an adverse effect of all but 8 of 157 drugs included in the review of most frequently prescribed medications by Smith (2003). Syncope can be associated with arrhythmias and with hypotension caused by vasodilators, antihypertensives, antidepressants, neuroleptics, diuretics, and dopaminergics. Ototoxic drugs such as diuretics, salicylates, and some antibiotics may produce disturbances in balance. Digitalis, quinidine, and tricyclic antidepressants can cause arrhythmias, with a resulting decrease in cardiac output and cerebral perfusion. The phenothiazines and diltiazem may cause drug-induced parkinsonism, with impaired motor function and muscle rigidity.

Diminished mental acuity may result in diminished perception of obstacles to ambulation. Impaired judgment may cause older people to overestimate their abilities, resulting in falls when the environment is too challenging for their capabilities. Sedative medications may reduce the older person's ability to remember to use assistive devices, resulting in diminished competence and falls. Any drug that produces sedation may cause excessive drowsiness and contribute to falls.

With the addition of a new medication to the older adult's therapeutic regimen, the risk for falls must be reassessed. If the risk is considered to be substantial, the need for the new drug should be closely evaluated. If the drug is essential, appropriate measures should be taken to reduce the possibility of injury. The patient should be instructed in measures that may reduce the likelihood of falls, including instructions regarding gradual postural changes. For more detail on prevention of fall-related injury, see Chapter 11.

Urinary Incontinence and Retention. Incontinence related to drug therapy can be due to either therapeutic action such as smooth muscle relaxation or to adverse effects such as sedation, confusion, and motor impairment. Numerous drug classes have been implicated in causing or contributing to urinary retention. The list includes diuretics, sedatives, alpha-receptor antagonists, anticholinergics, opioids, calcium channel blockers, antipsychotics, tricyclic and SSRI antidepressants, antiparkinsonian drugs, vincristine, anesthetics, and ACE inhibitors (Hsu et al., 2000; Malone-Lee, 2003; Ouslander, 2000; Schultz, 2002).

Some studies have focused on specific drugs or subclasses. In a large Italian study of people in home care, 21% of subjects age 60 to 74 and 38% of those age 75 or older reported urinary incontinence. The incidence was determined to be greater in those taking oxidative benzodiazepines than in those taking nonoxidative benzodiazepines (Landi et al., 2002). Hsu and colleagues (2000) have published several studies that explored the mechanisms by which clozapine contributes to urinary incontinence. Newman (2003) points out that drugs that can induce cough, such as ACE inhibitors and alpha blockers, can aggravate stress incontinence. A study of SSRIs revealed that 15 of 1000 persons develop urinary incontinence, with the greatest risk in older adults and users of sertraline (Movig, Leufkens, Belitser, Lenderink, & Egberts, 2002). Finkelstein (2002) examined gender differences and found that psychoactive drugs were associated more often with incontinence in women, and antidepressants were associated more often with incontinence in men. Antipsychotics and alpha antagonists aggravate sphincter weakness with stress incontinence; anticholinergics, anesthetics, and analgesics can cause urinary retention that is due to failure of bladder contraction (Drake, Nixon, & Crew, 1998). Some drugs do not directly affect the bladder, but may indirectly contribute to incontinence because they cause sedation or confusion (Newman & Giovannini, 2002).

Drugs that diminish mental acuity may interfere with the perception of the need to void or defecate and may prevent an appropriate response. Impairment in sensation, alertness, judgment, memory, or problem solving as a result of a drug side effect may precipitate incontinence. Drugs that may contribute to decreased mental acuity include long-acting benzodiazepines, sedative-hypnotics, alcohol, and others listed in the previous section of this chapter.

Mobility is a critical factor in maintaining continence. Older persons are predisposed to mobility problems because of age-related chronic illness such as arthritis, stroke, Parkinson's disease, and dementing disorders. With decreased mobility, the time needed to respond to the urge to urinate or defecate is increased. An important mechanism for drug-induced incontinence is that the

Table 7-6 *Medications Implicated in Altering Urinary Continence in Older Adults*

Class of Medication	Site of Action	Mechanism	Potential Consequences
Adrenergic agents			
■ Alpha-agonists	Prostatic urethra	Increase urethral closing pressure	Urinary retention
■ Alpha-antagonists	Urethra in women	Decrease urethral closing pressure	Stress leakage
Anticholinergic agents	Detrusor	Decrease bladder contractility; some also lead to confusion, rigidity, immobility	Urinary retention, overflow incontinence
■ Neuroleptics			
■ Tricyclic antidepressants			
■ Antiparkinsonians			
■ Antispasmodics			
■ Antiarrhythmics			
■ Opiates			
Calcium channel blockers	Detrusor	Decrease bladder contraction	Urinary retention
Diuretics	Renal	Increase bladder volume	Urgency, incontinence
Sedative/hypnotics	CNS		
■ Benzodiazepines		Delirium, sedation, immobility	Urgency, incontinence
■ Alcohol		Delirium, sedation, diuresis	Frequency, urgency, incontinence

From Brandeis, G. H., & Resnick, N. M. (1998). Urinary incontinence. In E. H. Duthie & P. R. Katz (Eds.), *Practice of geriatrics* (3rd ed.). Philadelphia: W. B. Saunders, p. 191.
CNS, Central nervous system.

speed required to respond to the urge to urinate or defecate exceeds the individual's capacity to respond because of a drug effect.

Drugs that increase the frequency of excretion or the amount of excrement may precipitate incontinence in elderly people who are unable to reach the toilet quickly enough. Such drugs may include diuretics, Kayexalate (potassium binding/exchange resin), laxatives, and antibiotics that cause diarrhea. Also, antipsychotic and antiparkinsonian drugs can indirectly affect continence by causing sedation, rigidity, and immobility (Table 7-6).

NURSING PROCESS AND PHARMACOLOGICAL INTERVENTIONS

Nurses often are responsible for administering medications and always are responsible for assessing individual responses to drugs. Safe and effective drug therapy requires knowledge of drug actions, effects, and the conditions that influence the outcomes of therapy. The nurse applies this knowledge when administering drugs and when teaching individuals and family members who are responsible for drug administration.

Assessment

Assessment of drug therapy for the older adult should include (1) the drug name and class, dose, schedule, and purpose of each medication taken; (2) the individual's

ability to take drugs independently; (3) the potential for drug interactions and adverse drug reactions; and (4) a baseline from which to evaluate effectiveness of the therapeutic regimen.

Drug Inventory. The drug inventory should include prescription medications, OTC drugs, social drugs (alcohol, caffeine, tobacco, "street drugs"), herbal remedies, and dietary supplements. An incomplete drug assessment may result in inaccurate diagnosis of patient problems. For example, laxatives may have dangerous side effects, such as fluid and electrolyte disturbances, cathartic colon, and fat-soluble vitamin deficiency. Therefore it is important to consider the use or misuse of laxatives by the older adult who has diarrhea, constipation, dehydration, electrolyte imbalance, or vitamin deficiency. Social drugs should be documented because they may inhibit or potentiate the effects of pharmacological agents, and often are overlooked because of aging biases.

Patient Perception of Purpose of Drug Therapy. Determining the older adult's perception of the purpose of the medication is a key aspect of the drug assessment because the older adult may use medications for purposes other than those for which they are intended. Misconceptions about the purpose of a drug may lead to tragic results. Consider the following case. An elderly woman was found to be taking a phenothiazine to relieve "heartburn." She had borrowed the medicine from a friend and then talked her physician into prescribing this for her. It is unlikely that the drug relieved her heartburn, yet she was exposed to the potentially irreversible adverse effects of extrapyramidal reactions and tardive dyskinesia. When the drug actions and the potential for adverse effects of the drug were explained to her, the patient willingly gave up the medicine.

Ability to Administer Medications Safely.
Not all persons are able to take their own drugs correctly. Factors affecting self-medication include vision, reading ability, memory, reasoning ability, judgment, motivation, and fine motor coordination. When patients take multiple medications on multiple schedules, ask what approaches they use to help them take the medications accurately. Have them demonstrate key steps of medication taking, including reading labels, opening medication containers, and measuring dosage.

Baseline Measures.
The medication assessment should include baseline measures of functions that may be affected by medications. Standard ongoing assessments should evaluate both therapeutic and adverse drug effects. For example, it is standard practice to assess the apical heart rate before each dose of digitalis to monitor the drug effects. However, a history of nausea or a mental status assessment is seldom elicited before the person starts to take digitalis preparations. These evaluations are important because nausea and mental status impairment are two signs of digitalis toxicity often seen in older adults. If the individual has chronic problems with nausea, digitalis toxicity may be incorrectly inferred. If the person's mental status is not evaluated before the initiation of the drug, impairment may be overlooked or incorrectly attributed to digitalis toxicity.

Problems encountered by those taking drugs with anticholinergic properties also highlight the need for accurate baseline assessment. Once again, mental status assessment is important because anticholinergics may precipitate delirium. Elimination problems also are especially important because constipation and urinary retention caused by prostate enlargement are aggravated by anticholinergics. These medications also may induce or enhance Parkinson's symptoms such as gait disturbance.

Planning

The key aspects of planning pharmacological interventions in older adults are (1) supervision of drug regimens, (2) reducing the risk of ADRs, (3) early identification of ADRs, (4) formulating new nursing diagnoses related to ADRs, and (5) monitoring the day-to-day responses to the medication regimen. If the person cannot manage independently, a designated person should manage medication administration and patient monitoring.

When drug therapy in older adults is complicated by psychosocial factors such as cognitive impairment, affective disorders, multiple prescribers, multiple daily dosage regimens, and poverty, the care plan requires further individualization.

Supervision of Drug Regimen.
Every drug regimen requires ongoing supervision. In most cases, older adults themselves are capable of carrying out this function independently. Effective management of one's drug regimen requires (1) ability to procure the drugs, (2) ability to comprehend instructions about dosage and schedule, (3) ability to select the proper drugs and dosages from a stock supply, (4) ability to follow a schedule, and (5) ability to recognize adverse or toxic effects and take appropriate action.

For individuals who lack any of these abilities, some level of assistance is vital to ensure that the regimen is followed as prescribed. All of these abilities require intact memory and judgment. For the older adult who has some cognitive impairment, the use of a drug calendar or other memory aids such as pill boxes may suffice. The number of drugs and the complexity of the medication schedule should be considered. Fewer drugs and fewer scheduled dosage times simplify the process and increase the chance of correct implementation (e.g., changing to medications with once-per-day preparations). For those with more severe impairments, support personnel may be necessary, such as family or paid helpers. The caregiver's availability should be considered in the selection of dosage schedules.

Risk Reduction and Early Identification of Adverse Drug Reactions.
Some ADRs are predictable on the basis of known drug actions; however, others are less readily explained. Knowledge of common ADRs and interactions allows nurses to educate patients and to detect many unwanted drug effects early. Periodic, systematic assessments are essential to detect untoward drug effects.

New Nursing Diagnoses.
Many nursing diagnoses are related to the effects of pharmacotherapy. Table 7-7 summarizes common nursing diagnoses with pharmacological etiologies and suggestions for treatment. The list is not intended to be exhaustive, but to serve as a quick summary of the more common drug-related problems. In-depth material about these diagnoses and their treatments is contained in appropriate chapters throughout this book. Because older adults often are excluded from drug studies, some adverse effects become apparent in this segment of the population only after the drugs reach the market. Therefore the gerontological nurse must be alert for both known and previously unrecognized ADRs in older adults.

Table 7-7 *Common Nursing Diagnoses Associated with Pharmacotherapy in Older Adults*

Category	Common Etiologies	Possible Interventions
Disturbed body image	Weight gain secondary to antidepressant use	Assess motivation to modify diet. Teach methods of weight reduction. Be alert for noncompliance; instruct about the dangers of sudden withdrawal of antidepressants.
Risk for deficient fluid volume	Iatrogenic effect of diuretic therapy. Diarrhea or vomiting secondary to drug side effect	Monitor hydration status, including intake and output. Hold diuretic if dehydrated and consult with prescriber. Obtain order for antiemetic or antidiarrheal if drug will only be taken for short term; if long-term drug therapy is indicated, consider changing to another drug.
Disturbed thought processes	Anticholinergic delirium secondary to polypharmacy with anticholinergic agents. Sedative effects of medication. Depression secondary to drug effect (e.g., adrenergic drugs such as reserpine and methyldopa)	Consider reduced dosage. Consider alternative drug. Instruct caregivers regarding limitations and assistance needed to prevent injury. Monitor emotional status.
Constipation	Anticholinergic effects of medications. Mobility-reducing effects of medications. Dehydration secondary to overly aggressive diuresis	Consider alternative medication or reduced dosage; consider use of laxatives. Institute exercise regimen to enhance mobility, especially around trunk and abdominal muscles. Increase fluid intake unless contraindicated because of cardiac or renal problems.
Diarrhea	Reduced gastrointestinal flora secondary to broad-spectrum antibiotic use. Cholinergic stimulation secondary to medication side effect	Try replacing flora through dietary means such as yogurt or buttermilk or pharmacy-supplied agents such as Lactinex granules. If medication needed on ongoing basis, consider use of bulk formers while restricting fluid intake to provide bulkier stool. Use antidiarrheal medications if drug is to be used for the short term to prevent excessive fluid loss and promote comfort.
Impaired physical mobility	Extrapyramidal side effects of neuroleptic drugs. Sedative effects of drugs or adverse effects on balance	Consider reduced dosage. Consider alternative drug. Instruct caregivers regarding limitations and assistance needed to prevent injury.
Functional urinary incontinence	Decreased time to respond secondary to diuretic use. Sedative effects of medications. Pharmacological effects on micturition	Evaluate need for diuretic therapy. Schedule diuretics in morning. Is patient now motivated to try sodium restriction to eliminate need for diuretic and hence incontinence? Evaluate need for medications. Is therapeutic benefit worth induction of incontinence? Consider alternative medications that may be less sedating. Institute toilet scheduling. Consider alternative medication. Institute toilet scheduling.

Continued

Table 7-7 *Common Nursing Diagnoses Associated with Pharmacotherapy in Older Adults—cont'd*

Category	Common Etiologies	Possible Interventions
Urinary retention	Secondary to anticholinergic effects of medication	Consider alternative medication. Consider altered dose. If on other anticholinergics, could some of those be discontinued or changed to medication with fewer anticholinergic side effects?
Risk for injury	Orthostatic hypotension	If possible, give medication at bedtime, because peak effect will be felt shortly after dosage. Teach patient to get up slowly (especially from reclining position), to use assistive devices, such as furniture or walker, and to re-equilibrate before moving. Consider another drug with less propensity to cause orthostatic hypotension.
	Dizziness	Consider reducing dosage to see if therapeutic effect can be obtained without dizziness. Consider different drug. Instruct family or paid caregivers of temporary hazard due to drug therapy and instruct them on ways to provide assistance with ambulation and transfer appropriate to the patient's functional capacity.
	Visual disturbances	Consider reducing dose to see if therapeutic effect can be obtained without side effect. Consider different drug. Instruct family or paid caregivers of temporary hazard due to drug therapy and instruct them on ways to assist with ambulation and transfer appropriate to the patient's functional capacity.
	Impaired judgment	Consider reduced dosage. Consider alternative drug. Instruct caregivers regarding limitations and assistance needed to prevent injury.
	Disturbance in balance or postural control	Consider reduced dosage. Consider alternative drug. Instruct caregivers regarding limitations and assistance needed to prevent injury.
	Sedation	Consider reduced dosage. Consider alternative drug. Instruct caregivers regarding limitations and assistance needed to prevent injury.
Noncompliance	Too many medications	Review medications for possibility of discontinuing some (e.g., dietary potassium supplements, tranquilizers, antihypertensives).
	Noxious side effects	Consider alternative agent within the same class of drug or a different type of drug to accomplish the desired effect (e.g., antihypertensives, antidepressants, NSAIDs). Consider nonpharmacological interventions (e.g., relaxation exercises, psychotherapy, massage).
	Complex or frequent dosing regimen	For drugs with long half-lives (e.g., many psychotropic medications, Dilantin), consider fewer doses per day. Can drug dosage be reduced to maintenance schedule, allowing for less frequent dosing?

Table 7-7 *Common Nursing Diagnoses Associated with Pharmacotherapy in Older Adults—cont'd*

Category	Common Etiologies	Possible Interventions
Noncompliance— cont'd	Complex or frequent dosing regimen	Consider changing to similar drug that allows for less frequent dosage. Use drug calendar or prepoured medications to simplify task of preparing medications.
	Insufficient funds	Consider less expensive drugs that accomplish same therapeutic objective. Consider nonpharmacological interventions. If therapy is short term, consider drug samples.
	Insufficient understanding of medications	Explain time is needed to see full therapeutic effect. Explain purpose, time it will require to take effect, importance of dosage schedule, and common side effects. Consider linking patient with another individual with similar problems but with successful drug therapy.
Imbalanced nutrition: less than body requirements	Anorexia secondary to gastrointestinal side effects of drug	Consider administering medications with meals to decrease gastric irritation, unless contraindicated because of drug-food interaction Evaluate for possibility of toxic drug reaction (e.g., digitalis). Monitor severity of nutritional alteration by assessing weight changes, actual food intake, and frequency and amount of vomiting and diarrhea. Consider alternative medication. If medication is short term, teach patient/family about temporary nature of symptoms. If patient has borderline adequate nutritional status, consider supplementation between meals.
	Hypoglycemia or hyperglycemia	Monitor serum blood glucose levels on periodic basis and increase frequency of monitoring during initiation and with dose increases.
Impaired oral mucous membranes	Side effects of anticholinergic medications	Consider reduction in dosage or change in medication. Use oral lubricant. Teach regarding use of sugarless candy to relieve symptoms of dry mouth.
	Dehydration	Evaluate continued need for diuretic if taking one. Monitor hydration status. Encourage fluid intake unless contraindicated by cardiac or renal status. Pay scrupulous attention to mouth care in dependent patients until dehydration is resolved.
Sensory/perceptual alterations: visual, auditory, sensory	Neurotoxic side effects of drugs	Teach about risk of side effect and encourage patient to notify when changes occur. Monitor for changes in sensory perception. If symptoms develop, consider using different drug. Teach patient compensatory responses to alteration (e.g., peripheral neuropathy, to examine feet daily for ulceration).

Financial Issues. Economic factors influence drug taking in the older adult, because many live on fixed incomes and take increasingly higher numbers of drugs with advancing age. Most people economize on medications before more basic necessities, such as food or shelter. The prescriber should consider costs and patient resources when selecting specific drugs. Several sources are available that provide average wholesale prices (AWPs) of drugs, which helps in making comparisons. The AWP is the price a pharmacy can expect to pay a wholesaler for the drug. It is not possible to predict an individual prescription price from this figure; however, the AWP is useful when contrasting the relative cost of various therapeutic agents within the same class. Similar information is available in sources such as *Medical Letter* and *Facts and Comparisons.* Thus consideration of the price of a medication and its impact on the older person's budget should be routine practice. In one survey of 109 physicians, 78% indicated that they were unaware of drug cost, and only 22% asked patients about their out-of-pocket drug costs when prescribing (Korn, Reichert, Simon, & Halm, 2003).

Several general strategies for containing the costs of drug therapy are worthy of consideration. First, encourage patients to request the use of generic brand drugs when there is no evidence that a particular brand of drug affects bioavailability. Second, for patients who are on stable doses of medicines for chronic illnesses, encourage the prescriber to order larger quantities for each refill, such as a 90-day supply instead of a 1-month supply. This saves the patient the cost of the filling fee for 2 months. Third, avoid the use of newer agents, unless the therapeutic advantages are clear. Fourth, encourage the patient to request a review of medicines with his or her prescriber every 6 months, so that obsolete prescriptions can be discontinued. Finally, encourage patients to review their drug regimens with a clinical pharmacist if one is not already a regular member of the team. The pharmacist may be able to suggest methods of simplifying the drug regimen or be able to propose less costly alternatives.

The Medicare Modernization Act of 2003 (MMA) provides new prescription drug benefits with extra assistance for people with low incomes. Medicare participants who wish to do so can choose a prescription drug plan from an approved list that requires a monthly fee predicted to be around $32 . After the enrollee has paid a $250 deductible, Medicare will pay 75 percent of costs up to $2250. Thereafter the enrollee will pay 100% until out-of-pocket expenses reach $3600. After the $3600 level is reached, Medicare will pay about 95% of costs. Both brand name and generic drugs are covered. The MMA includes a plan to offer additional assistance to individuals whose income falls below $14,355 (single) and 19,245 (married) (Centers for Medicare and Medicaid Services [CMS], 2006).

Using mail order pharmacies as the primary approach to cost containment may yield considerable savings. However, this practice has some drawbacks. In the high-volume business of mail order pharmacies, the patient loses access to a personal relationship with a clinical pharmacist who can provide medication counseling on such important matters as the rationale for the drug, administration directions, potential interactions (especially if multiple pharmacies are used), and common side effects. Moreover, when using a mail order pharmacy, reordering of medicines must be planned carefully and adjustments in dosage or short-term medication use may not be accommodated easily.

Multiple Prescribers. Many older people must contend with multiple prescribers because they have multiple chronic diseases treated by multiple specialists. Undiagnosed and preventable drug interactions are one risk of having multiple prescribers. Nurses in ambulatory care and home health settings especially should be alert to the possibility of multiple prescribers and be prepared to intervene when possible adverse drug interactions are identified. When obtaining a drug inventory from an older person, ask about the various health care providers seen regularly who may prescribe drugs, including dentists and podiatrists. Counsel the older person to maintain a medication list to share with all care providers at each visit.

Outcomes of Drug Therapy

Outcomes vary with the nursing diagnosis, but might include the following: Adherence Behavior, Motivation, Symptom Control, Treatment Behavior: Illness or Injury, Knowledge: Treatment Regimen, Self-Care: Non-parenteral Medication, and Self-Care: Parenteral Medication.

Intervention

Nursing interventions related to drug therapy using the Nursing Intervention Classification System (NIC) are addressed in Medication Management (NIC 2380) and Medication Administration (NIC 2300), with interventions for specific routes being further detailed under NIC 2301, 2302, 2303, 2304, 2307, 2308, 2310, 2311, 2312, 2313, 2314, 2315, 2316, 2317, 2318, 2319, and 2320. Interventions generally fall into the following areas: (1) the procedure for administration by each route; (2) monitoring responses to therapy, including identifying ADRs and titrating dosage; (3) patient teaching about medications; (4) documentation; and (5) collaboration with prescribers regarding alternative forms of treatment. For the advanced practice nurse, Medication Prescribing (NIC 2390) is applicable.

Medication Administration. Nurses are experts in medication administration techniques. They can teach patients and families about ways to promote comfort and drug effectiveness, as well as prevent or ameliorate side effects. Maximizing the effectiveness of drug therapy requires knowledge of drug pharmacokinetics and pharmacodynamics, as well as understanding of the nonpharmacological factors that potentiate or inhibit drug effects. For example, knowing that absorption of tetracycline is diminished by calcium leads the nurse to administer this drug with water rather than milk. Likewise, knowing that ethanol potentiates the sedative effects of benzodiazepines and antihistamines, the nurse cautions patients to abstain from alcohol while using these drugs. Lower dosages of central nervous system depressants may be recommended or avoided altogether for individuals who habitually drink alcohol. Administering regular doses of analgesics and antianxiety agents rather than waiting until the patient experiences symptoms also may decrease dosage requirements.

Physiological disturbances in some older adults complicate drug therapy. In addition to the pharmacokinetic changes described earlier, many older adults have dysphagia, tremor, constipation, decreased muscle mass, and ineffective tissue perfusion. Nurses should be alert for these problems and knowledgeable about their impact and successful remedies. For example, difficulty in swallowing pills may be the result of decreased esophageal motility, poor positioning, anxiety, or a combination of these. Use of liquid medications rather than pills may alleviate swallowing problems. However, if positioning is incorrect, both pills and liquids will present problems. Hyperextension of the neck puts the individual at risk for aspiration and makes swallowing of any substance difficult. Demented individuals with swallowing difficulty may not tell a caregiver about their problem but may spit out the pill instead.

When a patient has difficulty swallowing or has a feeding tube, the nurse must make a decision about whether or not it is acceptable to crush a tablet or open a capsule and dissolve its contents. Although charts listing medicines that should not be crushed or opened are available, it is possible to make this decision by considering several characteristics of the tablet or capsule. Tablets or capsules often are prepared with special coatings to delay the release of the medication in the gut. This generally is done either to promote absorption, as in the case of omeprazole; to protect the gastric lining from irritation, as in the case of bisacodyl tablets or enteric-coated aspirin; or to prolong the release of the active medication to allow less frequent dosing intervals, as in the case of sustained-release theophylline. Many classes of drugs have at least one medication available as a liquid. Lists of medicines that should not be crushed and alternative preparations are available in professional literature, as well as from pharmacy organ-

izations and pharmaceutical manufacturers. When in doubt, consult a pharmacist.

Monitoring Responses to Therapy. As noted earlier, nurses often are the main caregivers responsible for noting patient responses to drug therapy. As such, it is imperative that they be knowledgeable about drug actions, therapeutic goals, and common ADRs. Nurses also must draw on their knowledge of patient behaviors, pathophysiology, and other factors affecting the symptom under treatment to titrate medication dosages for maximum effectiveness with minimum adverse effects.

Patient Education. Because physiological changes often are subtle in older persons, it is particularly important that someone who has frequent contact with the individual understands drug effects and toxicity. Furthermore, some practicing physicians, pharmacists, and nurses are not knowledgeable about the increased risk for ADRs in older adults. Nurses, therefore, should focus particular attention on teaching older adults and their caregivers about drugs and be prepared to educate other health professionals about the special considerations for older adults who are on drug therapy.

Documentation. Documentation of drug therapy not only provides a legal record of medications administered, but also assessments performed before and during drug therapy, patient teaching, and how adverse events were reported and managed.

Collaboration with Prescribers on Alternative Forms of Therapy. Nurses often are in a position to educate older adults about the use of alternative and complementary therapies for chronic diseases or symptom relief. Deep breathing and relaxation techniques and massage are examples of nonpharmacological interventions that may be used to enhance the relief provided by sedatives or analgesics. These complementary therapies may also reduce the doses required for symptom relief. Techniques that promote relaxation also may diminish the discomfort associated with invasive routes of administration such as injections, venipuncture, and rectal administration.

Many chronic diseases can be managed with a multifaceted approach that includes dietary management, psychosocial care, and activity modifications in addition to pharmacotherapy. For example, constipation sometimes can be managed by modifying diet, fluid intake, and activity level rather than medications. Another clinical problem of older people that often benefits from nonpharmacological interventions is chronic pain. However, unless a clinician advocates their use, pharmacotherapy often is the only treatment offered. The establishment of a division in the National Institutes of Health to study complementary and alternative medicine will result in increasing evidence on which to base recommendations about such interventions. Nurses need to become better educated on alternatives to pharmacotherapy, and share their knowledge with other care providers. When patients choose alternative therapies, the nurse should assess patients' responses, including both positive and negative outcomes. At times, the nurse may need to seek modifications in drug therapy because of the alternative therapies used.

Evaluation

Drug therapy requires ongoing evaluation of the impact of the drug regimen on the health status and self-care abilities of patients. Although the prescribing physician or advanced practice nurse ultimately is responsibility for evaluating the efficacy of medications, other nurses function collaboratively with prescribers to evaluate patients' responses and manage side effects. In many settings, nurses are responsible for titrating dosage within preestablished parameters according to patient

---

BOX 7-5 Medication Appropriateness Index*

To assess the appropriateness of the drug, please answer the following questions and circle the applicable score:

	1	2	3	9
1. Is there an indication for the drug? Comments:	Indicated		Not Indicted	DK†
2. Is the medication effective for the condition? Comments:	Effective		Ineffective	DK
3. Is the dosage correct? Comments:	Correct		Incorrect	DK
4. Are the directions correct? Comments:	Correct		Incorrect	DK
5. Are the directions practical? Comments:	Practical		Impractical	DK
6. Are there clinically significant drug-drug interactions? Comments:	Insignificant		Significant	DK
7. Are there clinically significant drug-disease/condition interactions? Comments:	Insignificant		Significant	DK
8. Is there unnecessary duplication with other drug(s)? Comments:	Necessary		Unnecessary	DK
9. Is the duration of therapy acceptable? Comments:	Acceptable		Unacceptable	DK
10. Is this drug the least expensive alternative compared with others of equal utility? Comments:	Least expensive		Most expensive	DK

From Schmader, K. E., Hanlon, J. T., Weinberger, M., Lordsman, P. B., Samsa, G. P., Lewis, I., et al. (1994). Appropriateness of medication prescribing in ambulatory elderly patients. *Journal of the American Geriatrics Society, 42*, 1241-1247.
*Complete instructions for use are available upon written request from Joseph T. Hanlon, MS PharmD, Duke University Center for the Study of Aging and Human Development, Box 3003, Duke University Medical Center, Durham, NC 27710.
†Don't know.

response. The overlapping roles among health care professionals necessitate clear communication.

Many models of evaluation of drug therapy are available. A sample appears in Box 7-5. It can be followed before initiating drug therapy or whenever a patient's drug regimen is reviewed. Pagliaro and Pagliaro (1983, p. 269) offer a helpful algorithm for evaluating drug

therapy (Figure 7-1). Both models should be viewed as part of an ongoing process of assessment, planning, and intervention, as well as evaluation.

Timing of the evaluation depends on the nature of the patient's problems and therapy. Some conditions require daily or more frequent monitoring (e.g., unstable diabetes, newly initiated anticoagulant therapy,

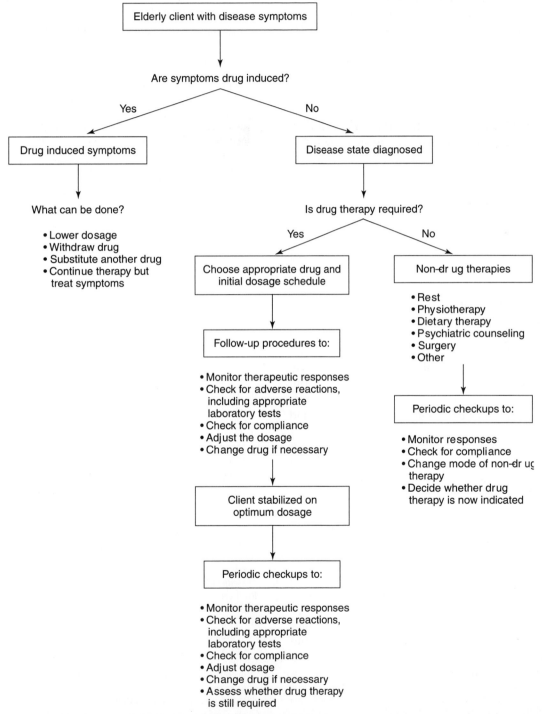

Figure 7-1 A process for ongoing drug evaluation in the elderly. (From Pagliaro, L. A., & Pagliaro, A. M. [1983]. *Pharmacologic aspects of aging.* St. Louis: Mosby, p. 269.)

acute pain, or titration of psychotropic medications for an acute behavioral disturbance). Less frequent monitoring is required for more stable conditions and those treated with drugs that have less serious adverse effects or adverse effects that are seen only with long-term therapy.

An aspect of drug evaluation that often is overlooked is assessment of whether the drug is still necessary. When the patient is functioning at baseline and not complaining about drug therapy, the tendency is to follow the old adage, "If it ain't broke, don't fix it!" However, because older persons experience more ADRs, especially with multiple drugs, opportunities to stop medications should not be overlooked. In the past the use of "drug holidays" (a day during which most or all of a person's drugs are withheld) was advocated. However, current knowledge suggests that drug holidays are not helpful and may be harmful. A more reasonable approach is regular review of medications, and a supervised withdrawal of certain medications, particularly if the indication for the medication is not clear or if the side effects are no longer tolerated.

Most medications can be discontinued abruptly without adverse complications. However, certain medications are associated with withdrawal syndromes, or exacerbation of underlying disease. Safe withdrawal of a drug requires understanding of the risks of withdrawal syndromes. A withdrawal syndrome is a clinically significant set of symptoms that occurs when a drug is discontinued. The syndrome may reflect exacerbation of conditions or symptoms that had been under control. For example, abrupt withdrawal of an antihypertensive may precipitate possibly severe rebound hypertension. Withdrawal from corticosteroids can result in weakness and nausea unrelated to the condition for which it had been prescribed.

Medications commonly used by older adults that have been associated with withdrawal syndromes or exacerbations include alpha-antagonist antihypertensives, antianginals, anticonvulsants, antiparkinsonians, antipsychotics, muscle relaxants, benzodiazepines, beta-adrenergic blockers, corticosteroids, opioids, sedative-hypnotics, and tricyclic antidepressants.

Case reports of withdrawal reactions are common, but few studies have addressed the phenomenon of withdrawal syndromes in a systematic manner. Slow, systematic withdrawal from a medication is thought to decrease or eliminate the risk of adverse effects. The lack of specific guidelines on withdrawal of most drugs requires the practitioner to devise a withdrawal schedule based on the pharmacokinetics of the drug.

SUMMARY

Although only advanced practice nurses prescribe drug therapy, all nurses have important responsibilities in monitoring and sometimes titrating or modifying drug regimens in older adults. Given the high rate of ADRs in older persons and the serious implications of these reactions, this is a responsibility that nurses must take very seriously. Armed with an understanding of the interrelationships between physical and psychosocial aging, pharmacokinetics, and pharmacodynamics, the nurse can play a major role in drug therapy with maximum benefit and minimum adverse effects.

REFERENCES

Ahronheim, J. C. (2000). Special problems of the geriatric patient. In L. Goldman & J. C. Bennett (Eds.), *Cecil textbook of medicine* (21st ed.). Philadelphia: W. B. Saunders.

American Geriatrics Society (AGS). (2002). Anticoagulation for older adults. Retrieved January 13, 2006, from www.americangeriatrics. org/education/cp_index.shtml.

American Hospital Formulary Service. (1994). *Drug information.* Bethesda, MD: American Society of Hospital Pharmacists.

American Psychiatric Association. (1994). *Diagnostic and statistical manual of mental disorders, 4th edition (DSM- IV).* Washington, DC American Psychiatric Association.

Amoako, E. P., Richardson-Campbell, L., & Kennedy-Malone, L. (2003). Self-medication with over-the-counter drugs among elderly adults. *Journal of Gerontological Nursing, 29*(8), 10-15.

Amoore, J., & Adamson, L. (2003). Infusion devices: Characteristics, limitations and risk management. *Nursing Standard, 17*(28), 45-52.

Arslan, S., Gookce-Kutsal, Y., & Atalay, A. (2002). Drug use in older people. *Journal of the American Geriatrics Society, 50*(6), 1163-1164.

Barat, I., Andreasen, F., & Damsgaard, E. M. (2001). Drug therapy in the elderly: What doctors believe and patients actually do. *British Journal of Clinical Pharmacology, 51*(6), 615-622.

Barker, K. N., Flynn, E. A., Pepper, G. A., Bates, D. W., & Mikeal, R. L. (2002). Medication errors observed in 36 health care facilities. *Archives of Internal Medicine, 162*(16), 1897-1903.

Beers, M. H. (1997). Explicit criteria for determining potentially inappropriate medication use by the elderly: An update. *Archives of Internal Medicine, 157*(14), 1531-1536.

Benjamin, D. M. (2003). Reducing medication errors and increasing patient safety: Case studies in clinical pharmacology. *Journal of Clinical Pharmacology, 43*(7), 768-783.

Benner, P., Sheets, V., Uris, P., Malloch, K., Schwed, K., & Jamison, D. (2002). Individual, practice, and system causes of errors in nursing: A taxonomy. *Journal of Nursing Administration, 32*(10), 509-523.

Besdine. R. (1980). Geriatric medicine: An overview. In C. Eisdorfer (Ed.), *Annual review of geriatrics and gerontology* (volume 1). New York: Springer.

Bond, C. A., Raehl, C. L., & Franke, T. (2002). Clinical pharmacy services, hospital pharmacy staffing, and medication errors in United States hospitals. *Pharmacotherapy, 22*(2), 134-147.

Bressler, R., & Bahl, J. J. (2003). Principles of drug therapy for the elderly patient (symposium on geriatrics). *The Mayo Foundation for Medical Education and Research, 78*(12), 1564-1577.

Bretherton, A., Day, L., & Lewis, G. (2003). Polypharmacy and older people. *Nursing Times, 99*(17), 54-55

Burt, C. W., & Bernstein, A. F. (2003). Observations from the CDC: Trends in use of medications associated with women's ambulatory care visits. *Journal of Women's Health, 12*(3), 213-217.

Centers for Medicare and Medicaid Services (CMS). (2006). Medicare prescription drug coverage. Retrieved January 25, 2006, from *www.cms.gov.*

Chan, M., Nicklason, F., & Vial, J. H. (2001). Adverse drug events as a cause of hospital admission in the elderly. *Internal Medicine Journal, 31*(4), 199-205.

Choo, P. W., Rand, C. S., Inui, T. S., Lee, M. L., Canning, C., & Platt, R. (2001). A cohort study of possible risk factors for over-reporting of antihypertensive adherence. *BMC Cardiovascular Disorders, 1*(1), 6.

Cockcroft, D. W., & Gault, M. H. (1976). Prediction of creatinine clearance from serum creatinine. *Nephron, 16,* 31.

Crome, P. (2003). What's different about older people? *Toxicology, 192*(1), 49-54.

Dean, B., Schachter, M., Vincent, C., & Barber, N. (2002). Causes of prescribing errors in hospital inpatients: A prospective study. *Lancet, 359*(9315), 1373-1378.

de Rekeneire, N., Visser, M., Peila, R., Nevitt, M. C., Cauley, J. A., Tylavsky, F. A., Sinomsick, E. M., & Harris, T. B. (2003). Is a fall just a fall: Correlates of falling in healthy older persons. The Health, Aging, and Body Composition Study. *Journal of the American Geriatrics Society, 51*(6), 841-846.

Dhalla, I. A., Anderson, G. M., Mandani, M. M., Bronskill, S. E., Sykora, K., & Rochon, P. A. (2002). Inappropriate prescribing before and after nursing home admission. *Journal of the American Geriatrics Society, 50*(6), 995-1000.

Diasio, R. B. (2000). Principles of drug therapy. In L. Goldman & J. C. Bennett (Eds.), *Cecil textbook of medicine* (21st ed.). Philadelphia: W. B. Saunders.

Drake, M. J., Nixon, P. M., & Crew, J. P. (1998). Drug induced bladder and urinary disorders: Incidence, prevention, and management. *Drug Safety, 19*(1), 45-55.

Fick, D. M., Cooper, J.W., Wade, W. E., Waller, J. L., Maclean, J. R., & Beers, M. H. (2003). Updating the Beers criteria for potentially inappropriate medication in older adults: Results of a U.S. consensus panel of experts. *Archives of Internal Medicine, 163*(22), 2716-2724.

Finkelstein, M. M. (2002). Medical conditions, medications, and urinary incontinence: Analysis of a population based survey. *Canadian Family Physician, 48,* 96-101.

Flynn, E. A., Barker, K. N., Pepper, G. A., Bates, D. W., & Mikeal, R. L. (2002). Comparison of methods for detecting medication errors in 36 hospitals and skilled nursing facilities. *American Journal of Health-System Pharmacy, 59*(5), 436-446.

Fonseca, T., & Clara, J. G. (2000). Polypharmacy and non-compliance in the hypertensive elderly patient [abstract]. *Revista Portuguesa de Cardiologia, 19*(9), 855-872. Retrieved March 20, 2004, from OVID.

Forster, A. J., Murff, H. J., Peterson, J. F., Gandhi, T. K., & Bates, D. W. (2003).The incidence and severity of adverse events affecting patients after discharge from the hospital. *Annals of Internal Medicine, 138*(3), 1-16.

Ghandi, T. K., Weingart, S. N., Borus, J., Seger, A. C., Peterson, J., Burdick, E., et al. (2003). Advrse drug events in ambulatory care. *New England Journal of Medicine, 348*(16), 1556-1564.

Grant, R. W., Devita, N. G., Singer, D.E., & Meigs, J. B. (2003). Polypharmacy and medication adherence in patients with type 2 diabetes. *Diabetes Care, 26*(5), 1408-1412.

Greengold, N. L., Shane, R., Schneider, P., Flynn, E., Elashoff, J., Hoying, C. L., et al. (2003). The impact of dedicated medication nurses on the medication administration error rate: A randomized controlled trial. *Archives of Internal Medicine, 163*(19), 2359-2367.

Gregoire, J. P., Moisan, J., Guibert, R., Ciampi, A., Milot, A., Gaudet, M., & Cote, I. (2002). Determinants of discontinuation of new courses of antihypertensive medications. *Journal of Clinical Epidemiology, 55*(7), 728-735.

Guay, D. R. P., Artz, M. B., Hanlon, J. T., & Schmader, K. (2003). The pharmacology of aging. In R. C. Tallis & H. M. Fillit (Eds.), *Brocklehurst's textbook of geriatric medicine and gerontology* (6th ed.). London: Churchill-Livingstone.

Gurwitz, J. H., Field, T. S., Harrold, L. R., Rothschild, J., Debellis, K., Seger, A. C., Cadoret, C., Fish, L. S., Garber, L., Kelleher, M., & Bates, D. W. (2003). Incidence and preventability of adverse drug events among older persons in the ambulatory setting. *Journal of the American Medical Association, 289*(9), 1107-1116.

Hanlon, J. T., Fillenbaum, G. G., Ruby, C. M., Gray, S., & Bohannon, A. (2001). Epidemiology of over-the-counter drug use in community dwelling elderly: United States perspective. *Drugs and Aging, 18*(2), 123-131.

Hanlon, J. T., Lindblad, C., Maher, R. L., & Schmader, K. (2003). Geriatric pharmacotherapy. In R. C. Tallis & H. M. Fillit (Eds.), *Brocklehurst's textbook of geriatric medicine and gerontology* (6th ed.). London: Churchill-Livingstone.

Haumschild, M. J., Karfonta, T. L., Haumschild, M. S., & Phillips, S. E. (2003). Multidisciplinary medication review in nursing home residents: What are the most significant drug-related problems? *Quality and Safety in Health Care, 12*(3), 176-180.

Hsu, J. W., Wang, Y. C., Lin, C. C., Bai, Y. M., Chen, J. Y., Chiu, H. J., et al. (2000). No evidence for association of alpha 1a adrenoreceptor gene polymorphism and clozapine-induced urinary incontinence. *Neuropyschobiology, 42*(2), 62-65.

Huang, B., Bachmann, K. A., He, X., Chen, R., McAllister, J. S., & Wang, T. (2002). Inappropriate prescription for the aging population of the United States: An analysis of the National Ambulatory Medical Care Survey, 1997. *Pharmacoepidemiology and Drug Safety, 11*(2), 127-134.

Institue of Medicine (IOM). (1999). To err is human: Builing a safer health care system. Retrieved January 13, 2006, from www.iom.edu/?id=5575&redirect=0.

Kallin, K., Jensen, J., Olsson, L. L., Nyberg, L., & Gustafson, Y. (2004). Why the elderly fall in residential care facilities, and suggested remedies. *Journal of Family Practice, 53*(1), 41-52.

Kaufman, D. W., Kelly, J., Rosenberg, L., Anderson, T. E., & Mitchell, A. A. (2002). Recent patterns of medication use in the ambulatory adult population of the United States: The Slone survey. *Journal of the American Medical Association, 287*(3), 337-344. Retrieved March 16, 2004, from OVID.

Kelly, W. N. (2001). Potential risks and prevention, part 2: Drug-induced permanent disabilities. *American Journal of Health-System Pharmacy, 58*(14), 1325-1329.

Kennedy, J., & Erb, C. (2002). Prescription noncompliance due to cost among adults with disabilities in the United States. *American Journal of Public Health, 92*(7), 1120-1124.

Kennerfalk, A., Ruigomez, A., Wallander, M., Wilhelmsen, J., & Johansson., S. (2002). Geriatric drug therapy and healthcare utilization in the United Kingdom. *Annals of Pharmacotherapeutics, 36*(5), 797-803.

Korn, L. M., Reichert, S., Simon, T., & Halm, E. A. (2003). Improving physicians' knowledge of the costs of common medications and willingness to consider costs when prescribing. *Journal of General Internal Medicine, 18*(1), 31-37.

Lacro, J. P., Dunn, L. B., Dolder, C. R., Leckband, S. G., & Jeste, D. V. (2002). Prevalence of and risk factors for medication nonadherence in patients with schizophrenia: A comprehensive review of recent literature. *Journal of Clinical Psychiatry, 63*(10), 892-909.

Lamb, E. J., O'Riordan, S. E., & Delaney, M. P. (2003). Kidney function in older people: Pathology, assessment and management. *Clinica Chimica Acta, 334*(1-2), 25-40.

Landi, F., Cesari, M., Russo, A., Onder, G., Bernabei, R., & Silvernet-HC Study Group. (2002). Benzodiazepines and the risk of urinary incontinence in frail older persons living in the community. *Clinical Pharmacology and Therapeutics, 72*(6), 729-734.

LaPointe, N. M., & Jollis, J. G. (2003). Medication errors in hospitalized cardiovascular patients. *Archives of Internal Medicine, 163*(12), 1461-1466.

Lehne, R. A. (2004). *Pharmacology for nursing care* (5th ed.). Philadelphia: W. B. Saunders.

Liu, G. G., & Christensen, D. B. (2002). The continuing challenge of inappropriate prescribing in the elderly: An update of the evidence. *Journal of the American Pharmaceutical Association, 42*(6), 847-857.

Ma, J., Stafford, R. S., Cockburn, I. M., & Finkelstein, S. N. (2003). A statistical analysis of the magnitude and composition of drug promotion in the United States in 1998. *Clinical Therapeutics, 25*(5), 1503-1517.

Malone-Lee, J. (2003). Urinary incontinence. In R. C. Tallis & H. M. Fillit (Eds.), *Brocklehurst's textbook of geriatric medicine and gerontology* (6th ed.). London: Churchill-Livingstone.

Marcellino, K., & Kelly, W. N. (2001). Potential risks and prevention, part 3: Drug-induced threats to life. *American Journal of Health-System Pharmacy, 58*(15), 1399-1405.

McGillis Hall, L., Doran, D., & Pink, G. H. (2004). Nurse staffing models, nursing hours, and patient safety outcomes. *Journal of Nursing Administration, 34*(1), 41-45.

Mitchell, J., Mathews, H. F., Hunt, L. M., Cobb, K. H., & Watson, R. W. (2001). Mismanaging prescription medications among rural elders: The effects of socioeconomic status, health status, and medication profile indicators. *Gerontologist, 41*(3), 348-356.

Moisan, J., Gaudet, M., Gregoire, J. P., & Bouchard, R. (2002). Non-compliance with drug treatment and reading difficulties with regard to prescription labeling among seniors. *Gerontology, 48*(1), 44-51.

Mort, J. R., & Aparasu, R. R. (2002). Prescribing of psychotropics in the elderly: Why is it so often inappropriate? *CNS Drugs, 16*(2), 99-109.

Movig, K. L., Leufkens, H. G., Belitser, S. V., Lenderink, A. W., & Egberts, A. C. (2002). Selective serotonin reuptake inhibitor-induced urinary incontinence. *Pharmacoepidemiology and Drug Safety, 11*(4), 271-279.

Neutel, C. I., Perry, S., & Maxwell, C. (2002). Medication use and risk of falls. *Pharmacoepidemiology and Drug Safety, 11*(2), 97-104.

Newman, D. K. (2003). Stress urinary incontinence in women. *American Journal of Nursing, 103*(8), 46-56.

Newman, D. K., & Giovannini, D. (2002). The overactive bladder: A nursing perspective. *American Journal of Nursing, 102*(6), 36-46.

Nose, M., Barbui, C., & Tansella, M. (2003). How often do patients with psychosis fail to adhere to treatment programmes? A systematic review. *Psychological Medicine, 33*(7), 1149-1160.

Onder, G., Landi, F., Cesari, M., Gabmassi, G., Carbonin, P., & Bernabei, R. (2003). Inappropiate medication use among hospitalized older adults in Italy: Results from the Italian Group of Pharmacoepidemiology in the Elderly. *European Journal of Clinical Pharmacology, 59*(2), 157-162.

Ouslander, J. (2000). Urinary incontinence. In L. Goldman & J. C. Bennett (Eds.), *Cecil textbook of medicine* (21st ed.). Philadelphia: W. B. Saunders.

Pagliaro, L. A., & Pagliaro, A. M. (1983). *Pharmacologic aspects of aging*. St. Louis: Mosby.

Patel, R. B. (2003). Polypharmacy and the elderly. *Journal of Infusion Nursing, 26*(3), 166-169. Retrieved March 16, 2004, from OVID.

Phillips, D. P., & Bredder, C. C. (2002). Morbidity and mortality from medical errors: An increasingly serious public health problem. *Annual Review of Public Health, 23*, 135-150.

Pompei, P. (2003). Delirium. In R. C. Tallis & H. M. Fillit (Eds.), *Brocklehurst's textbook of geriatric medicine and gerontology* (6th ed.). London: Churchill-Livingstone.

Rigler, S. K., Perera, S., Redford, L., Studenski, S., Brown, E. F., Wallace, D., & Webb, M. (2003). Urban-rural patterns of increasing antidepressant use among nursing facility residents. *Journal of the American Medical Directors Association, 4*(2), 67-73.

Rodriguez-Monguio, R., Otero, M. J., & Rovira. J. R. (2003). Assessing the economic impact of adverse drug effects. *Pharmacoeconomics, 21*(9), 623-650.

Rosenthal, M. B., Berndt, E. R., Donohue, J. M., Frank, R. G., & Epstein, A. M. (2002). Promotion of prescription drugs to consumers. *New England Journal of Medicine, 346*(7), 498-505.

Ruths, S., Straand, J., & Nygaard, H. A. (2003). Multidisciplinary medication review in nursing home residents: What are the most significant drug-related problems? The Bergen District Nursing Home (BEDNURS) Study. *Quality & Safety in Health Care, 12*(3), 176-180.

Sarkozi, L., & Ramanathan, L. (2003). Biochemical tests. In R. C. Tallis & H. M. Fillit (Eds.), *Brocklehurst's textbook of geriatric medicine and gerontology* (6th ed.). London: Churchill-Livingstone.

Schultz, J. M. (2002). Urinary incontinence. *Nursing 2002, 32*(11), 53-55.

Skidmore-Roth, L. (2004). *Mosby's nursing drug reference*. St. Louis: Mosby.

Sloane, P. D., Zimmerman, S., Brown, L. C., Ives, T. J., & Walsh, J. F. (2002). Inappropriate medication prescribing in residential care/assisted living facilities. *Journal of the American Geriatrics Society, 50*(6), 1001-1011.

Smith, R. G. (2003). Fall-contributing adverse effects of the most frequently prescribed drugs. *Journal of the American Podiatric Medical Association, 93*(1), 42-50.

Steinman, M. A., Sands, L. P., & Covinsky, K. E. (2001). Self-restriction of medications due to cost in seniors without prescription coverage. *Journal of General Internal Medicine, 16*(12), 864-866.

Taxis, K., & Barber, N. (2003). Ethnographic study of incidence and severity of intravenous drug errors. *BMJ, 326*(7391), 684.

Thomas, C. P. (2003). Incentive-based formularies. *New England Journal of Medicine, 349*(23), 2186-2188.

Thomas, E. J., & Brennan, T. A. (2000). Incidence and types of preventable adverse events in elderly patients: Population based review of medical records. *BMJ, 320*, 741-744.

Upchurch, G. A., Menon, M. P., Levin, K. S., Catellier, D. J., & Conlisk, E. A. (2001). Prescription assistance for older adults with limited incomes: Client and program characteristics. *Journal of Pharmacy Technology, 17*(1), 6-12.

Vargas, E., Terleira, A., Hernando, F., Perez, E., Cordon, C., Moreno, A., & Portoles, A. (2003). Effect of adverse drug reactions on length of stay in surgical intensive care units. *Critical Care Medicine, 31*(3), 694-698.

Vogel, R. J., Ramachandran, S., & Zachry, W. M. (2003). A 3-stage model for assessing the probable economic effects of direct-to-customer advertising of pharmaceuticals. *Clinical Therapeutics, 25*(1), 309-329.

Weingart, S. N., Toth, M., Sands, D. Z., Aronson, M. D., Davis, R. B., & Phillips, R. S. (2003). Physicians' decision to override computerized drug alerts in primary care. *Archives of Internal Medicine, 163*(21), 2625-2631.

Chapter 8

Nutritional Considerations

Anna J. Biggs

Objectives

Identify physiological and psychosocial factors affecting the nutritional status of older adults.

Discuss the impact of selected health problems on nutritional status.

Describe techniques for assessment of nutritional problems.

Examine common nutritional disorders and management techniques.

OVERVIEW OF NUTRITION

Along with air and water intake, food intake is fundamental to health promotion and maintenance as people age. Good nutritional status throughout life helps prevent the development and progression of diseases and disabilities in later life, as well as promoting successful medical treatment outcomes, thereby significantly contributing to the quality of life. Goals and objectives in *Healthy People 2010* link nutritional status with health status for all U.S. citizens, including older adults (Office of Disease Prevention and Health Promotion, 2004).

At the same time, making eating an enjoyable and pleasant experience also contributes to quality of life, so a balanced approach to managing nutrition in the older adult is important. Nurses are often in the position to assess nutritional problems and initiate interventions. Box 8-1 describes the important role nurses can play in nutritional support through the eyes of one gerontological nurse.

Factors affecting nutritional status are multidimensional and interrelated at any age. For older adults, age-related changes in body composition and function, lifestyle, medication use, and the prevalence of chronic disease challenge maintenance of good nutrition. Lifetime eating habits and heredity, as well as psychosocial factors such as income, social interactions, and access to transportation, can all affect an older adult's

nutritional status. Measures to promote good nutrition must specifically address the needs and problems of older adults in order to be effective.

This chapter provides an overview of general nutritional needs of older adults and dietary guidelines for healthful eating; physiological changes with aging; and psychosocial, mobility, and safety issues. Relevant nursing measures for managing problems of eating and undernutrition and overnutrition are discussed.

GENERAL ISSUES IN NUTRITION
Recommendations for Healthful Eating

Generally the "young-old" are those in their sixties, those in their seventies are considered old (or "middle-old"), and those over 80 are the "old-old." Although these distinctions are made in chronological age, fewer distinctions are made with regard to nutritional needs of those who are aging robustly, those who have chronic illnesses or are "less robust," and those who are very frail, for whom few dietary recommendations are available (Sherer, 2000). Younger, healthy older adults should probably follow the usual adult guidelines (with some differences that are noted later in this chapter), whereas the frail older individual with chronic disease may be at risk for nutritional deficiencies and special monitoring or interventions may be needed.

The U.S. Department of Agriculture (USDA) recommendations for the types and servings of foods for a healthy diet are laid out in the Food Guide Pyramid. The Food Guide Pyramid is now provided in a form individualized by age and activity level (USDA, 2005a). The 2005 Dietary Guidelines (USDA, 2005b) described the ABCs of nutrition:

- Aim for fitness
- Build a healthy body
- Choose sensibly

Box 8-1 *Reflections on the Role of Nurses in Nutritional Support*

The selection, preparation, and sharing of food arguably plays an important role in all our lives. The sight and smell of certain foods connects us to our past with memories of meals shared, special treats, and life's milestones. Over food we have all laughed and cried, talked out issues, listened to troubles and joys, and passed some time in the simple pleasure of eating together. Food is not just about keeping the body alive but about sustaining the whole person.

One of my favorite tasks as a young trainee nurse was to "do the lunches." This involved serving each patient's food from a large mobile hot box in the kitchen and delivering all the trays. I paused one day to sit with an older man who, despite his failing abilities, knew what smelt and tasted good and thus was worth eating. He was a strong critic of hospital food, refused many offerings, and often regaled me with tales of his mother's cakes and desserts. He had two sterling pieces of advice: "If it doesn't smell good and look good don't eat it!" and "Never eat alone."

Later in my career, in psychiatric practice, we routinely ate lunch with patients. This was the time when we talked and said some of the most important things to each other. The meal itself was not the focus of the event, but rather the exchanges that took part over the sharing of food and conversation. The normalizing effect of such a meal in the midst of the vulnerability and chaos of mental illness was tangible and potent. I will always remember one man emerging from the hell of a first schizophrenic breakdown telling me, "When you sat and ate with me I felt normal for a while."

Now, in gerontology, as care settings have changed, we have been challenged to provide nutritious meals in more stimulating and attractive dining settings for residents living in long-term care. We have come far in understanding dentition and the mechanics of eating. We understand much about weight loss, frailty and vulnerability, nutritional status, and healing. Yet as caregivers we still struggle daily with the notion of "independence" in eating and what it means to truly help another person to eat well with dignity and pleasure. Caregivers are so pressed for time, and there are often not enough caregivers to supervise the mealtime for many residents.

What I see repeatedly is physically and cognitively impaired residents who are left with food access but without feeding help. The containers are opened, the food cut or pureed, the utensils set out—but the resident does not get the level of help needed to enjoy the mealtime event. I have watched residents struggle to lift a spoon to the mouth, drag a cup closer, suck on a straw that will never deliver, slump exhausted in the chair waiting for help to arrive as the food congeals. In our urge to avoid learned helplessness and excess disability, the bar we set for giving help may be too high. Excellent feeding assessment skills are required to learn what a resident is actually able to do, and consistently will do, alone and what is needed from caregivers to systematically support sound nutrition. Once we get the assessment right we can begin to provide the interactive mealtime environment in which eating becomes a social event associated with pleasure.

I was in a special care dementia unit recently. A resident came up to me and said, "Smell that bread . . . it's going to be so good." There was no bread baking nearby and no smell of crusty loaves fresh from the oven. But we had a great conversation about his family bakery over a cup of coffee on the porch. When you work with older adults, conjure up your own memories of food and smells and eating pleasure and bring them to the caregiving table with you.

Elizabeth R. A. Beattie

Elizabeth R.A. Beattie, PhD, RN, FGSA
Assistant Research Scientist
University of Michigan
School of Nursing
Ann Arbor, Michigan

Nine major messages for healthy eating are conveyed by the 2005 Report of the Dietary Guidelines Advisory Committee and are applicable to all older adults:
- Consume a variety of foods within and among the basic food groups while staying within energy needs.
- Control caloric intake to manage body weight.
- Be physically active every day.
- Increase daily intake of fruits and vegetables, whole grains, and nonfat or low-fat milk and milk products.
- Choose fats wisely to decrease the amount of trans fats.
- Choose carbohydrates wisely—more whole grains and complex carbohydrates.
- Choose and prepare foods with little salt.
- If you drink alcoholic beverages, do so in moderation.
- Keep food safe to eat.

Tufts University (Amersbach, 1999) proposed a modified pyramid for older adults (with several modifications to address the special needs of this population) that has gained wide acceptance (Figure 8-1). First is the addition of water or other liquids as the base of the pyramid. Water is an essential component of body tissues and the metabolic and excretory processes necessary to sustain life. The reminder to maintain fluid intake is important for older adults without fluid intake restrictions, who often have an age-related decreased sense of thirst. Dehydration is a common problem in frail older adults, and is discussed in more detail later in the chapter.

A second recommendation suggests that older adults tend to be less active than younger people, and therefore

T U F T S

Food Guide Pyramid for Older Adults

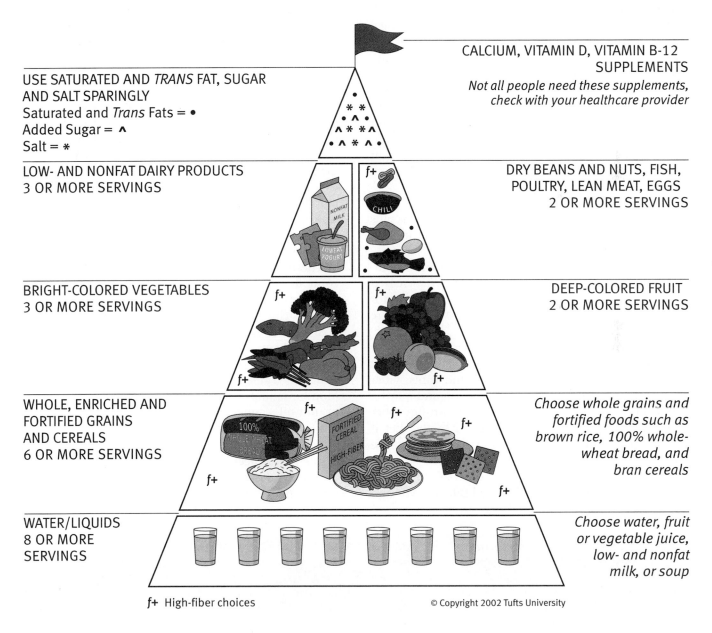

CALCIUM, VITAMIN D, VITAMIN B-12
SUPPLEMENTS
*Not all people need these supplements,
check with your healthcare provider*

USE SATURATED AND *TRANS* FAT, SUGAR
AND SALT SPARINGLY
Saturated and *Trans* Fats = •
Added Sugar = ∧
Salt = *

LOW- AND NONFAT DAIRY PRODUCTS
3 OR MORE SERVINGS

DRY BEANS AND NUTS, FISH,
POULTRY, LEAN MEAT, EGGS
2 OR MORE SERVINGS

BRIGHT-COLORED VEGETABLES
3 OR MORE SERVINGS

DEEP-COLORED FRUIT
2 OR MORE SERVINGS

WHOLE, ENRICHED AND
FORTIFIED GRAINS
AND CEREALS
6 OR MORE SERVINGS

*Choose whole grains and
fortified foods such as
brown rice, 100% whole-
wheat bread, and
bran cereals*

WATER/LIQUIDS
8 OR MORE
SERVINGS

*Choose water, fruit
or vegetable juice,
low- and nonfat
milk, or soup*

f+ High-fiber choices   © Copyright 2002 Tufts University

For additional copies, visit us on the web at http://nutrition.tufts.edu.

Figure 8-1 Food Guide Pyramid for Older Adults. (Copyright 2002 by Tufts University.)

need fewer calories. In addition, metabolic rate decreases with age. Older adults usually require between 1600 and 2200 calories per day, with men at the higher end of this range, but this should be individualized based on size and activity level. Obesity is a major problem in the United States, and obesity is expected to increase in the older population over the next decade (Arterburn, Crane, & Sullivan, 2004). This is significant because of the potential impact of obesity on chronic health conditions and quality of life. As a result, it is important to get the most nutrients per serving of food in later life to avoid excessive weight gain.

Weight loss may be an important goal for younger seniors who are overweight and those who are very obese, but Wilson and Morley (2003) would add a cautionary note for the frail elderly, who may be at risk for undernutrition. It may be healthier to maintain a little extra weight in the older years because of the negative health consequences (morbidity and mortality risk) for older adults who may lose weight during an acute illness. Studies suggest that being somewhat overweight becomes less of a risk factor for death in later life (Heiat, Voaccarino, & Krumholz, 2001).

A standard method of calculating energy requirements is to multiply 13.5 times weight in kilograms plus 487 for men over age 60, and 10.5 times weight in kilograms plus 596 for women over age 60 (Reuben et al., 2005). However, patients who are stressed from acute illness or who have healing wounds may have increased caloric requirements. Add 25% in basic requirements for mild physiological stress, and up to 100% for severe stress.

Another recommendation for older adults is to increase the amount of fiber consumed by eating more whole grains and cereals, vegetables, and fruits. Fiber can help prevent problems of constipation and may be beneficial in maintaining a healthy lipid profile. Fiber supplements or additives can be added to the diet if needed, but require additional fluid intake to be safe and effective.

The final recommendation is for older adults to supplement their food intake with added calcium, vitamin D, folate, and vitamin B_{12}, which are discussed later. These general guidelines provide the basis for more in-depth discussion of the older adult's need for macronutrients and micronutrients.

Macronutrients

The macronutrients are carbohydrates, proteins, and fats. The recommended intake of these nutrients remains the same as individuals age, with considerations given to activity or health conditions. Older adults need approximately 130 grams (520 kilocalories) of carbohydrate for each kilogram of body weight. Other guidelines recommend that about 45% to 65% of the diet should come from carbohydrates (USDA, 2005b). Foods that are higher in fiber are better sources of carbohydrates, and foods with added sugars are less desirable.

Intake of protein should be about 0.8 grams of protein for each kilogram of body weight (or about 56 grams of protein per day for men and about 46 grams for women). This would account for 20% to 30% of the diet, making 0.8 grams per kilogram slightly low at 12% to 13%. Given normal renal function, additional protein in the 20% to 30% range is reasonable to maintain lean muscle mass and avoid dietary-related sarcopenia and protein-energy malnutrition. The typical American diet usually includes plenty of protein.

The remaining calories, about 25% to 30%, would come from fat (USDA, 2005b). At 9 calories per gram, this would account for about 60 to 70 grams of fat per day (Mitchell, 2003; Williams & Schlenker, 2003). The goal is to avoid trans fats and have most fat intake come from polyunsaturated and monounsaturated fats in nonanimal products. Cholesterol intake should be maintained at less than 300 mg per day (USDA, 2005b). Monounsaturated fats (olive oil, peanut butter and peanut oil, canola oil, and avocados, along with other nut meats and nut oil) are a good choice.

Eating some saturated fats or animal fats (butter, whole milk, cheese, and beef tallow) provides cholesterol needed for the body to make hormones (testosterone, progesterone, estrogen, etc.) and for cell wall

Table 8-1 *Dietary Reference Intakes* for Vitamins: Middle and Older Adults*

Gender/Age Range	Vitamin A (mcg/day)	Vitamin C (mg/day)	Vitamin D (mcg/day)	Vitamin E (mg/day)	Vitamin K (mcg/day)	Vitamin B$_1$ (Thiamin) (mg/day)	Vitamin B$_2$ (Riboflavin) (mg/day)
Male/51-70	900	90	10	15	120	1.2	1.3
Male/>70	900	90	15	15	120	1.2	1.3
Female/51-70	700	75	10	15	90	1.1	1.1
Female/>70	700	75	15	15	90	1.1	1.1

From National Academy of Sciences. (2004). Dietary Reference Intakes (DRIs): Recommended intakes for individual, vitamins. Retrieved July 10, 2005, from *www.iom.edu/Object.File/Master/21/372/0.pdf.*
*Dietary Reference Intakes are Recommended Daily Allowances or Adequate Intakes.

synthesis and maintenance. Moderation and balance in the diet, including adequacy of fiber intake, will help maintain a serum cholesterol level around 200 mg/dl as recommended for adults over age 65 to 70 years in the absence of diagnosed hyperlipidemia and heart disease (Sardesai, 2003). Overuse of polyunsaturated fats may not be healthy, so the use of monounsaturated fats is preferred.

Diets low in carbohydrates and high in protein and fat are recommended for health and weight loss by Atkins (1998), as well as a variety of authors describing spin-off diets that build on this principle. These low-carbohydrate diets have been shown to help with weight loss, and there is some indication of decreased cardio-vascular risk factors (Acheson, 2004; Foster et al., 2003). However, researchers agree that long-term studies are needed to evaluate the safety and impact of low-carbohydrate and high-protein diets over time, and the USDA guidelines are still considered the gold standard for nutritional health. Overall, older adults need to maintain balance in their consumption of proteins, fats, carbohydrates, and fiber for both nutritional health and overall health, while attending to recommended alterations required because of health conditions.

Micronutrients

Vitamins and minerals are the micronutrients from the foods we eat, and in the past, guidelines for all adults have been the same. In the late 1990s the Dietary Reference Intakes (DRIs) were developed; the DRIs provide four reference values for the various nutrients: the Recommended Dietary Allowance (RDA), the Estimated Average Requirement (EAR), the Tolerable Upper Intake Level (UL), and Adequate Intake (AI) (USDA, 2005b). The RDA for each specific nutrient is the goal toward which individuals should strive in their daily food intake. The UL is provided to advise individuals who take multiple food supplements, so that they can avoid overdoses of specific nutrients. The DRIs for vitamins (Table 8-1) and minerals (Table 8-2) now make some distinctions for gender and age ranges (51 to 70 and

over 70 years of age). Additional information is available from the National Academy of Sciences and in clinical nutrition texts.

Of particular note is the recommendation for increased intake of vitamin D and riboflavin for older men and women in comparison with younger adults. Older adults may have less exposure to sunshine with age, which can reduce the body's production of vitamin D, as well as cause changes in absorption. Riboflavin supports metabolic processes that were formerly thought to have declined. Suboptimal intakes of other vitamins and minerals have also been reported, including vitamin B_{12}, folate, selenium, and zinc (deJong et al., 2001; deJong et al., 2003). Future research may result in new recommendations for other micronutrients for older adults.

Vitamin and mineral supplementation recommendations vary among health care providers. Nurses working with older adults and their families can suggest a multiple-vitamin supplement that contains the additional B vitamins, vitamin D, and folate that even a balanced diet may fall short on. Vitamins and minerals designed for those over age 50 (e.g., the "silver" vitamins) contain recommended allowances without adding iron (Fleming et al., 2002). Although it is often suggested that individuals will get all the nutrients they need from eating a balanced diet, the fact is that many older adults do not eat a healthful diet all the time; therefore taking a general multiple vitamin is probably a good idea.

Calcium supplementation above and beyond a multiple vitamin is also recommended. Older adults should have an intake of 1500 mg of calcium per day, which can be hard to achieve with a regular diet, especially for those who do not consume a variety of milk products. Calcium from calcium-rich mineral water (and by extraction, calcium-enriched fruit juices) is an acceptable way to increase calcium intake (Bohmer, Muller, & Resch, 2000). Some studies suggest that supplements with calcium citrate have better bioavailability than calcium carbonate (Kenny et al., 2004), but other studies have shown no difference (Heaney et al., 2001; Heller, Poindexter, & Adams-Huet, 2002). A study in Korea

Vitamin B_3 (Niacin) (mg/day)	Vitamin B_6 (Pyridoxine) (mg/day)	Folate (mcg/day)	Vitamin B_{12} (Cobalamin) (mcg/day)	Pantohenic Acid (mg/day)	Biotin (mcg/day)	Choline (mg/day)
16	1.7	400	2.4	5	30	550
16	1.7	400	2.4	5	30	550
14	1.5	400	2.4	5	30	425
14	1.5	400	2.4	5	30	425

Table 8-2 *Dietary Reference Intakes* for Minerals: Middle and Older Adults*

Gender/Age Range	Calcium (mg/day)	Chromium (mcg/day)	Copper (mcg/day)	Fluoride (mg/day)	Iodine (mcg/day)	Iron (mg/day)	Magnesium (mg/day)
Male/51-70	1200	30	900	3	150	8	420
Male/>70	1200	30	900	3	150	8	420
Female/51-70	1200	20	900	3	150	8	320
Female/>70	1200	20	900	3	150	8	320

From National Academy of Sciences. (2004). Dietary Reference Intakes (DRIs): Recommended intakes for individual, elements. Retrieved July 10, 2005, from *www.iom.edu/Object.File/Master/21/372/0.pdf*.
*Dietary Reference Intakes are Recommended Daily Allowances or Adequate Intakes.
†Upper limits.

(Kim, Kim, & Song, 2003) validated the higher lead levels in calcium supplements made of bone meal about which U.S. studies have also raised concern (Ross, Szabo, & Tebbett, 2000; Roberts, 2000) and that were confirmed by an Australian study (Gulson et al., 2001).

The National Osteoporosis Foundation (1999) states that the best calcium supplement is the one that meets the individual's needs based on tolerance, convenience, cost, and availability. The National Osteoporosis Foundation further suggests avoiding calcium supplements from unrefined oyster shells, bone meal, or dolomite if they do not carry the symbol of the *United States Pharmacopeia* (USP), a nonprofit certifying agency, for purity and safety. A simple test to see if a brand of calcium tablets will be easily absorbed is to put one in a glass of warm water for 30 minutes: if it does not dissolve in that amount of time, it probably would not dissolve in the stomach. Chewable and liquid calcium supplements dissolve well and are absorbed well because they are broken down before entering the stomach.

Nurses working with older adults should also be aware of additional studies regarding calcium supplementation. For example, dose timing (morning, evening, or smaller doses throughout the day) is less important than it had been thought to be (Karkkainen, Lamberg-Allardt, Ahonen, & Valimaki, 2001). In addition, postmenopausal women may need vitamin C in addition to calcium, even if they take estrogen supplements to prevent bone loss and hip and vertebral fractures (Morton, Barrett-Connor, & Schneider, 2001). Women should take calcium supplementation while attempting to lose weight to protect their bones (Jensen, Kollerup, Quaade, & Sorensen, 2001). Calcium and vitamin D supplementation may also protect against colon cancer (Holt et al., 2001), and supplemental calcium may reduce the incidence of calcium oxalate renal calculi (Williams et al., 2001).

Older adults and families may also ask nurses for advice on other minerals such as sodium, potassium, and magnesium as they relate to food intake. Nurses can evaluate available laboratory data for sodium, potassium, and magnesium in particular, along with

prescribed and over-the-counter medications and vital signs, particularly blood pressure. The USDA (2005b) recommends less than 2300 mg of sodium per day (1 teaspoon of table salt). Moderation in the consumption of sodium and with consideration to climate/weather and activity levels of older adults is probably the "best" advice. Omitting the use of salt, both while cooking and at the table, helps avoid excess sodium intake without sacrificing taste.

A diet high in fruits and vegetables should provide an adequate intake of potassium for older adults who are not on potassium-depleting diuretics, for whom potassium supplementation may be required. Good sources of potassium are orange juice, bananas, greens, beets, tomatoes, and soybeans. Nurses working with older adults may be among the first to recognize possible nutritional insufficiencies or deficiencies because of their holistic approach and their focus on health promotion and protection. For suspected vitamin or mineral deficiencies, further blood tests, comprehensive nutritional assessments, or referrals to dietitians may be required.

Nutrition Education

Nurses can provide guidance to older adults, their families, and caregivers by maintaining and updating their knowledge of current trends and research on nutrition for older adults and in the dietary management of chronic health conditions, such as cardiovascular disease and diabetes. Techniques for health promotion and education are described in Chapter 27. In addition, fad diets and nutritional supplements can be a problem.

Nutritional information in the lay media may be misleading. It seems that every month there is a new diet craze that promises to help people lose weight or stay young. In addition, nutritional and herbal supplements of all kinds are constantly marketed to older adults. Educate older adults to use supplements cautiously and let their health care providers know what they are taking. Later chapters include information about complementary therapies, including nutritional

Manganese (mg/day)	Molybendum (mcg/day)	Phosphorus (mg/day)	Selenium (mcg/day)	Zinc (mg/day)	Boron (mg/day)	Nickel (mg/day)	Vanadium (mg/day)
2.3	45	700	55	11	20[†]	1[†]	1.8[†]
2.3	45	700	55	11	20[†]	1[†]	1.8[†]
1.8	45	700	55	8	20[†]	1[†]	1.8[†]
1.8	45	700	55	8	20[†]	1[†]	1.8[†]

supplements when there is evidence supporting their use. If nutritional supplements are not harmful or overly expensive, their use is a personal choice by individuals. Nurses can help educate older adults by maintaining an awareness of both the lay literature on nutrition and research concerning nutrition, foods, medications, herbal supplements, or other nutritional supplements.

PHYSIOLOGICAL FACTORS IN NUTRITION
Aging Changes

Aging changes and other physiological factors may affect the nutritional status of older adults negatively. These include changes in the gastrointestinal system, senses, metabolism, health conditions, medications, and other factors, which are described in detail in later chapters and briefly discussed here.

Loss of teeth and changes in the jaw and gums are common, and having fewer than 20 natural teeth, or being edentulous even with removable dentures, places older adults at nutritional risk (Bailey et al., 2004; Walls et al., 2000). Food choices may be altered to avoid chewing (such as avoiding tougher or drier meats, fresh vegetables, and fresh fruits), putting the older adult at risk for undernutrition. Measures to ensure continued food and fiber intake with missing teeth include serving shredded vegetables and fruits, such as radishes, turnips, carrots, apples, fresh pears, or soft fruits such as cantaloupe and watermelon. Shredded or food-processed meats with vegetable juices, gravy, or canned cream soups to moisten the meat can help maintain protein intake along with cottage cheese or other soft cheeses, or tofu.

In addition to changes in dentition with aging, good oral hygiene is important for taste and enjoyment of food. This is often overlooked, particularly in the institutional setting. Dry mouth, or *xerostomia*, is not a normal change with aging, but may be related to medications or other conditions, and can affect nutrition. Nurses working with older adults in all settings can assess oral health, make referrals for needed dental or oral care,

and teach and provide good oral hygiene to help maintain nutritional status.

Other changes occur in the gastrointestinal system. The prevalence of gastric atrophy and atrophic gastritis increases with age, so that secretion of intrinsic factor, hydrochloric acid, and pepsin is impaired, but usually does not affect vitamin B_{12} absorption (Morley, Glick, & Rubenstein, 1995). Delayed gastric emptying is not a normal change with aging (Tougas et al., 2000), but some may report feeling "full" before meals and may be candidates for a trial of metoclopramide. A low-fat diet may also increase gastric emptying time (Tougas et al., 2000). Peristalsis is decreased with age, but constipation usually results from other problems such as poor nutrition, immobility, or medications.

Basal metabolism (basal metabolic rate [BMR]) is controlled by thyroid hormones necessary to the activation of the sodium pump and protein balance (turnover and synthesis). Triiodothyronine (T3) stimulates release of insulin and growth hormone and is required for healthy function of the sympathetic nervous system. There is a gradual decline in the BMR with advancing age, which may be related to the loss of muscle mass as one ages, and in turn, BMR helps maintain muscle tone in old age. Thus maintaining muscle strength through physical activity and exercise and maintaining optimal nutrition, along with maintaining or supplementing thyroid function if needed, go hand in hand in caring for aging individuals to maintain their metabolic rate (Russell, 2002).

A progressive decline in sensory acuity occurs with aging. Taste and smell perceptions can affect both appetite and food intake and therefore nutritional status in the elderly (Nordin, Razani, Markison, & Murphy, 2003). Comparisons between young and older adults suggest that the sense of smell declines more than the sense of taste. About one fourth of older adults have alterations in the sense of smell, rising to about half those over age 80 (Murphy et al., 2002). Alterations in taste of food from diminished sense of smell or taste can diminish the enjoyment or pleasure of eating and lead to decreased food intake.

To maximize taste, food seasonings can help compensate for this loss of smell and taste. These seasonings should have strong odors and flavors such as garlic, lemon, basil, and oregano, rather than those containing salt or monosodium glutamate. Smelling food cooking also can help stimulate an older adult's appetite.

Appetite seems to decrease somewhat, particularly in the frail elderly. It was once thought that the decline of the opioid feeding system and increased satiety action of cholecystokinin might account for anorexia and hypophagia in advanced age (Chapman, MacIntosh, Morley, & Horowitz, 2002). More recent evidence suggests that there is a decrease in basal hunger and that changes observed in cholecystokinin are less likely to be responsible for diminished appetite or "anorexia of aging" (Sturm et al., 2003).

Chronic Diseases

Chronic diseases are more prevalent with age, including diabetes, arthritis, heart disease, pulmonary disease, kidney and liver disease, and others. Nutritional problems can result from changes in function, energy level, mood, or direct impact on intake or absorption. In addition, many conditions require drug therapy, which may affect nutrition. General factors related to chronic disease and nutrition are discussed here, as well as a few specific conditions that commonly affect nutrition in older people.

Dietary restrictions can decrease interest in food and in turn lead to nutritional problems. In most circumstances, therapeutic diets should be liberalized for older adults who have chronic diseases that are treated with diet modification (Chernoff, 2003). Restrictive diets frequently are not palatable and differ markedly from long-standing eating habits. The dependent older adult who finds eating less enjoyable because of dietary restrictions will likely consume less food. An adequate intake of essential nutrients is necessary to maintain maximal functional ability and to prevent complications that occur with immobility. Nurses can work with older adults to approach dietary changes with moderation, explore changes in diet gradually, and seek options that are healthy while keeping eating an enjoyable experience.

Pharmacotherapy. Older adults are more likely to take medications, which can play a role in poor nutrition causing anorexia, especially digoxin, selective serotonin reuptake inhibitor antidepressants, pain medications, and cancer drugs (Johnson, 2002). Medications such as antimicrobials, antidepressants, antiepileptics, antiinflammatories, and chemotherapeutic agents can affect taste sensation (Schiffman et al., 2000a; Schiffman et al., 2000b), making foods taste bitter, metallic, or sour.

Drugs can affect nutritional status by altering food intake or absorption, metabolism, and excretion of nutri-

ents (Table 8-3). Factors that increase the risk of adverse drug-nutrient interactions include the following:

- Inadequate or marginal nutrient intake
- Increased nutritional needs caused by catabolic illness
- Impaired ability to absorb, metabolize, or excrete drugs and nutrients
- Long-term drug therapy
- Multiple-drug use

Drug-nutrient interactions can also alter drug efficacy. For example, grapefruit or grapefruit juice may interact with certain antihypertensive and cardiovascular medications. Vitamin supplements can affect anticonvulsants, anticoagulants, and corticosteroids.

Cancer. Unintentional weight loss is often the first sign of an occult malignancy. Individuals undergoing treatment for cancer are therefore likely to have marginal or depleted nutritional reserves. Cancer treatments such as chemotherapy and radiation therapy are frequently associated with anorexia and weight loss, and the pathophysiology of weight loss in cancer is not well understood (Crown et al., 2002). People undergoing cancer therapies may complain of nausea, changes in taste and smell, and feelings of fullness early in a meal. Foods not tolerated are often reported as tasting sour, bitter, salty, or spoiled. Treatment-induced stomatitis also increases the risk of inadequate intake, as well as xerostomia (Amosson et al., 2003).

A systematic regimen of oral hygiene has been shown to reduce the incidence and severity of stomatitis associated with chemotherapy and radiation therapy. A rinse of $1/4$ teaspoon of salt and $1/4$ teaspoon of baking soda is one option. Other measures to provide nutritional support are often necessary, ranging from creative menu planning to nutritional supplementation. Nurses can provide nutritional counseling or refer patients as needed, which has been shown to be effective (Ravasco, Monteiro-Grillo, & Camilo, 2003).

Dementia. Dementia can affect nutritional intake in many ways across the course of the disease. Even early in the disease, the loss of judgement and functional capacity can cause difficulty in obtaining, preparing, and eating healthy foods. The impact can include overeating of sweets resulting in weight gain, or not eating enough food resulting in weight loss. For the older adult with dementia who lives at home or in assisted living, supervision and assistance with meals as previously described and monitoring of eating and weight are indicated.

As the disease progresses, other factors come into play, including anorexia, decreased attention span, and wandering (Amella, 2002; Beattie & Algase, 2002). Later, difficulty recognizing food, agitation, apraxia, fatigue,

Table 8-3 *Influence of Some Drugs on Nutritional Status*

Drug	Effect on Nutritional Status
ANTACIDS	
Magnesium hydroxide and aluminum hydroxide	Decreased absorption of folacin, B_{12}, calcium, phosphate, and iron Orange juice may increase absorption of aluminum
ANTI-ALZHEIMER'S AGENTS	
Donepezil	Anorexia, nausea, vomiting, diarrhea, and weight loss
Rivastigmine	Anorexia, nausea, vomiting, diarrhea or constipation, abdominal pain, dysphagia, flatulence, eructation, and weight loss
Galantamine	Anorexia, nausea, vomiting, diarrhea, weight loss, infrequent hyperglycemia, and increased alkaline phosphatase
Mementine	Nausea, vomiting, and constipation
ANTIARRYHTHMIC AGENTS	
Digoxin	Anorexia, marked nausea with high doses, electrolyte changes, diarrhea, and abdominal pain, (these effects must be considered as signs of possible toxicity); need added vitamin D intake, avoid large intake of oatmeal or other high fiber cereals (which interfere with drug absorption).
Qunidine	Anorexia, nausea, vomiting, diarrhea, and abdominal cramps/pain
ANTIBIOTICS	
Gentamicin	Decreased appetite and increased urinary excretion of potassium and magnesium
Tetracycline	Decreased absorption of calcium with long-term therapy; avoid milk/milk products
Neomycin	Decreased absorption of folacin, B_{12}, fat-soluble vitamins, calcium, iron, sodium, potassium and lactose
ANTICOAGULANTS	
Coumadin/warfarin	Nausea, vomiting, diarrhea, abdominal cramps/pain, and vitamin K depletion (bleeding, including gastrointestinal); high vitamin A, and E and herbal supplements intake may increase the anticoagulant effect; large amounts of dark green leafy vegetables can decrease the effect of anticoagulants
ANTICONVULSANTS	Decreased absorption of calcium (folate in phenytoin)
ANTIDEPRESSANTS	
Tricyclics	Increased appetite; avoid high vitamin C intake (which reduces drug absorption)
MAOI's	Constipation, gastrointestinal upset/distress, appetite changes, weight changes, dry mouth, and possibly B_6 deficiency; certain foods must be avoided (foods high in tyramine, caffeine, alcohol, and chocolate)
Selective Serotonin Reuptake Inhibitors	Gastrointestinal distress and increase or decrease in appetite
Lithium	Anorexia, nausea, vomiting, and diarrhea (signs of toxicity); bloated feeling, dry mouth, thirst, metallic taste, weight changes, altered glucose tolerance test, and hypercalcemia
ANTIHYPERTENSIVES	
Hydralazine	Increased excretion of B_6; anorexia, nausea, vomiting, diarrhea, rarely constipation, gastrointestinal distress, weight changes, dry mouth, and thirst
Methyldopa	Decreased absorption of B_{12}
Nitroprusside	Decreased absorption of B_{12}
ANTIINFLAMMATORIES	
Colchicine	Decreased absorption of folacin, B_{12}, carotene, calcium, sodium, potassium, lactose, and fat
Sulfasalazine	Decreased absorption of folacin, and iron
Aspirin/indomethicin	Increased urinary excretion of ascorbic acid; iron deficiency due to gastrointestintal blood loss
Penicillamine	Anorexia due to impaired taste acuity secondary to chelation of zinc, copper, and inhibited B_6 metabolism
Other NSAIDs	Stomach ulcers, gastrointestinal bleeding; and iron deficiency anemia or anemia of chronic illness; avoid high fat intake, associated with kidney damage

Continued

Table 8-3 *Influence of Some Drugs on Nutritional Status—cont'd*

Drug	Effect on Nutritional Status
ANTILIPIDEMICS	
Cholestyramine	Decreased absorption of folacin, B_{12}, fat-soluble vitamins, calcium, iron, and fat; anorexia and weight changes
Atorvastatin	May interact with grapefruit or grapefruit juice; upset stomach and flatulence
ANTI-PARKINSONIANS	
Levodopa	Nausea, vomiting, diarrhea or constipation, and epigastric pain/distress
ANTITUBERCULARS	
Isoniazid	Decreased absorption of B_6
Para-aminosalicylic acid	Decreased absorptioin of folacin, B_{12}, and fat
Cycloserine	B_6 antagonist
BETA-ADRENERGIC BLOCKING AGENTS	Nausea, vomiting, diarrhea, stomach discomfort, constipation, dry mouth, and impaired glycogenolysis; should be taken consistently with food to achieve optimum bioavailability
BRONCHODILATORS	
Theophylline	High protein/low carbohydrate (related to Krebs' cycle); may increase the clearance of the drug, requiring dosage adjustment; avoid high caffeine or other CNS stimulant foods/drugs; respiratory distress may make eating difficult; avoid grilled meats which may decrease the effectiveness of theophylline
CALCIUM-CHANNEL BLOCKERS	Increased appetite; may interact with grapefruit or grapefruit juice
CORTICOSTEROIDS	
Prednisone	Increased urinary excretion of ascorbic acid; decreased absorption of calcium with long-term therapy
DIURETICS	
Thiazides	Increased urinary excretion of sodium, potassium, magnesium, zinc, and water; anorexia, vomiting, diarrhea, gastrointestinal upset/pain, gastrointestinal irritation/ulcers, constipation (loss of water from bowel/stools harden), dry mouth, and thirst
Furosemide	Increased urinary excretion of potassium, magnesium, and calcium; anorexia, diarrhea, dehydration, and dry mouth
Ethacrynic acid	Increased urinary excretion of potassium, magnesium, and zinc
Spironolactone	Hyperkalemia, abdominal cramps, nausea, vomiting, diarrhea, and dry mouth
H_2 RECEPTOR ANTAGONISTS	
Cimetidine	Decreased absorption of B_{12} from decreased gastric acid and intrinsic factor, calcium, iron, and diarrhea
LAXATIVES	
Phenolphthalein	Decreased absorption of vitamin D, calcium, potassium, and fat
Bisacodyl	Decreased absorption of vitamin D, calcium, potassium, and fat; hyperperistalsis; avoid milk/milk products
Senna	Decreased absorption of vitamin D, calcium, potassium, and fat; hyperperistalsis
Mineral oil	Decreased absorption of fat-soluble vitamins, and flatulence
Bulk-forming (psyllium)	Reduced appetite, feeling of fullness, decreased food intake, flatulence, and possible hypokalemia with prolonged use
Potassium supplement (slow release)	Decreased absorption of folate and B_{12}
THYROID PREPARATIONS	Avoid iodine-rich foods, which lower effectiveness of thyroid medications

Table 8-3 *Influence of Some Drugs on Nutritional Status—cont'd*

Drug	Effect on Nutritional Status
TRANQUILIZERS	
Benzodiazepines	Increased appetite
Phenothiazines	Increased appetite
Haloperidol	Anorexia, nausea, vomiting, dyspepsia, constipation or diarrhea, and increased salivation
Risperidone	Nausea, vomiting, dry mouth, dyspepsia, constipation, abdominal pain, and toothache

From Kee, J., & Hayes, E. (2003). *Pharmacology: A nursing process approach.* Philadelphia: W. B. Saunders; and Smith, C. H. (1999). Drug-food/drug-drug interactions. In J. E. Morley, Z. Glick, and L. Z. Rubenstein (Eds.), *Geriatric nutrition: A comprehensive review.* New York: Raven.

extreme slowness, inability to feed self, and swallowing problems may result. Assessment of nutrition and interventions may be needed to support healthy eating. At the stage when institutionalization is common, it is critical for the nurse to take a leadership role in maintaining nutrition because as many as 50% of nursing home residents with dementia are malnourished (Bronner, 2003). An interdisciplinary approach to assessing, planning, and intervening may be needed to maintain food intake.

Many techniques assist with self-feeding in people with dementia and skillful feeding when individuals can no longer feed themselves. Verbal and nonverbal prompting, physical guidance, modified utensils, and small frequent meals with few choices are helpful. In addition, a nondistracting and pleasant eating environment that is well lit is important. Creativity in meal planning and food provision might include finger foods for those who are distracted or wandering, or providing a larger meal at midday when cognitive abilities tend to peak. Adequate feeding time is particularly important.

Controversy remains about the use of artificial hydration and feeding, with enteral tubes, during late-stage dementia (Manthorpe & Watson, 2003). Nurses can help older adults in early stages make decisions regarding advance directives and can assist family caregivers and caregivers in long-term care in maintaining careful hand-feeding even into final stages. Although tube-feeding may "cost less" in nursing homes than hand-feeding, because of nursing assistant time involved (Mitchell, Buchanan, Littlehale, & Hamel, 2003), tube-feeding does not prevent weight loss or the development of pressure ulcers, and may be more uncomfortable for the older adult (Ina, 2002). Tube-feeding may also be a predictor of death (Alvarez-Fernandez, Garcia-Ordonez, Martinez-Manzanares, & Gomez-Huelgas, 2005). There is little evidence that feeding tubes are beneficial in this population, and their use may result in restraints, cellulites, or decreased social opportunities at meals (Breier-Mackie, 2005). Giving small amounts of food, ice chips, sips of water, or other liquids and using mouth swabs and mouth and lip lubricants were found to be effective and likely sufficient to prevent and alleviate hunger and thirst in the last stages of dementia (Ina, 2002). See also the sections on dysphagia or impaired swallowing and on enteral feedings later in this chapter.

Diabetes. Diabetes affects 15% of older adults (Administration on Aging [AOA], 2004) and presents special challenges, including higher rates of hospitalizations and complications such as renal, visual, and cardiovascular problems (Damush et al., 2004). Older adults most often have type 2 diabetes, and the nutritional recommendations for diabetes management must be tailored to the older adult's age and health status (Huang, Gorawara-Bhat, & Chin, 2004). For the younger and healthier patient, tight glucose control may have long-term benefits in preventing complications. However, for the frail older adult this may have greater risks and effects on quality of life.

Although a "no concentrated sweets" diet has been widely used in the past, particularly in long-term care settings, it is no longer recommended by the American Dietetic Association or the American Diabetes Association (Baron, 2003). There is little evidence that sucrose- or sugar-containing foods are any more likely to raise blood sugar than starches or complex carbohydrates. The restriction does, however, affect food choices and enjoyment. Both organizations now recommend a "regular" diet for frail or older adults in long-term care.

Pulmonary Disease. Pulmonary diseases, such as chronic obstructive pulmonary disease, are not easily treated with dietary prescriptions to increase caloric intake (Thomas, 2002). Reducing carbohydrates and increasing proteins and fat may have some effect on reducing the amount of carbon dioxide produced in the Krebs cycle, and increasing the amount of vitamin A may aid in cell maintenance and regeneration (Bronner, 2003). Providing a diet that is easily masticated and digested may help an older adult who has dyspnea and fatigue that interfere with eating and who therefore eats less.

PSYCHOSOCIAL AND FUNCTIONAL FACTORS IN NUTRITION

A number of nonphysiological factors affect nutritional intake in the older adult. Many activities are involved in maintaining nutrition: planning meals, shopping for food, meal preparation, actually eating the food, and cleaning up and storing food and leftovers. Older adults who have difficulty in any of these areas may be at risk nutritionally. Nursing assessment, plans, and interventions can address these activities with older adults and their informal caregivers.

Planning Meals

Planning for meals includes planning menus based on nutritional needs, likes and dislikes, and any dietary prescriptions. Habit, cultural influences, and functional abilities often influence the kinds of foods older adults consider. Women who have been planning menus for their families all their lives may find it a challenge to plan menus for only one or two, or may find that it no longer interests them after many years of meeting family needs. Older adult men may have limited experience in meal planning and preparation. Safe food handling and storage is also part of the planning: will the food be used by any expiration dates or before spoilage? In general, a 3- to 5-day supply of food is recommended, with weather and other considerations influencing the amount and kind of food kept on hand.

Availability of storage (refrigerator, freezer, or pantry) also influences the kind and quantity of food that can be kept, as well as remembering or listing food available so duplication is limited. Planning meals also requires giving thought to time and energy available for meal preparation. Nutritional adequacy and appropriateness of prepared foods may need to be addressed with older adults.

Shopping

After planning for meals and preparing a shopping list, getting to the grocery store may be an area of concern for older adults. Can the individual drive safely to do the shopping? If public transportation is required, is it available, safe, and affordable? Is transportation available from friends, from family, as part of a congregate living facility, or through community services?

Once at the store, the next step is to purchase healthy foods. Reduced visual acuity makes reading fine print on food labels difficult, and older adults may need information on making sense of label information so that they can make good food choices. Cost can pose a challenge for low-income older adults who have difficulty affording healthy foods, especially with the high cost of medications or utility bills. Instead some choose foods that are high calorie, cheap, and easy to fix and eat. This can result in a higher-calorie diet and weight gain, despite the presence of actual malnourishment (Guthrie & Lin, 2002; Klesges et al., 2001). Older adults may need education on the many low-cost, healthy choices that are available from the wide range of foods that are easy to cook and eat, including frozen meals.

Once the shopping is done, the older adult needs to be able to carry the shopping bags and put away the food in a timely manner. Those who have access to phone or online shopping and delivery and can afford any additional charges for the delivery service may find that this approach saves them time and energy. However, this method may also diminish the social interaction of "going shopping."

Meal Preparation

Functional problems, low vision, impaired hearing, and problems with mobility can all contribute to issues regarding safety in meal preparation by older adults. Fire and burn prevention is one of the major concerns. Independently living older adults may need evaluation of their safety in the kitchen:

- Kitchen fire extinguisher and household smoke detector available and in working order
- Usual attire worn in the kitchen (no nylon nightgowns or bathrobes, no loose-fitting clothing while cooking); not reaching over or above cooking surface while cooking
- Flammable materials kept away from cooking areas and appliances: paper of any kind (paper towels, newspapers, paper bags), pizza boxes or other prepackaged food containers, pot holders, cloth towels, or clothing
- Oil spills or grease buildup cleaned; covering burning oil or grease with a larger lid or pan rather than using water or flour to put out the fire
- Storing frequently used foods/items away from the stove so not reaching over the stove for anything while cooking
- Keeping pot handles turned inward so not accidentally bumped or tipped when cooking
- Checking for frayed cords and keeping cords on the countertop; repairing or replacing frayed or broken cords or appliances
- Never leaving cooking unattended; if must leave, turn heat/burner off and take an item (pot holder or spoon) along as a reminder that something is cooking
- Shielding self from steam when uncovering food or pouring hot liquids, including when using the microwave
- Knife safety: clean, sharp, handles/grips for safe holding (adaptive equipment or enlarged rubber handles); use fork, tongs, or other food holder rather than other hand when cutting foods

- Spills on floors cleaned; drawers, cupboard, oven, and dishwasher doors closed to prevent falls; safe, sturdy stepladder available for reaching items from shelves if absolutely necessary
- Care in transporting hot liquids from tea or coffee pot, stove, or microwave

If an older adult cannot see adequately, food preparation may also become difficult and even hazardous. Low-vision food preparation equipment may be needed, such as talking food scales or timers or page-size magnifiers; many of these items are available at low-vision centers or through the Internet.

Eating

Psychosocial factors have a strong influence on how well older adults actually eat. Older adults living alone may be deprived of stimulating interaction with others and thus lack incentive to cook and eat meals (Choi & Smith, 2004; Hendy, Nelson, & Greco, 1998). This is of particular concern with rural elderly. Lack of interest in eating and anorexia, common symptoms of depression, can result in limited food intake. Hearing loss interferes with participation in conversation, possibly creating embarrassment or frustration, resulting in social isolation and increased risk of inadequate dietary intake. Opportunities for social interaction and a lifestyle of varied social and physical activities have a positive impact on morale, life satisfaction, and food intake (Huffman, 2002).

Cleanup

Independent community-dwelling older adults also need to be able to clean up after meal preparation and consumption. Water safety (water heater temperature) needs to be balanced with sanitation of food preparation equipment and surfaces, dishes and utensils, tables, and floors. Convenience items (e.g., cleaning wipes) and antibacterial dish detergents can help with maintaining a sanitary food environment. Dishwashers may not be available in the homes of all older adults and even if available may not be used if perceived as more difficult than hand washing dishes and utensils. Disposable dishware might be an option, though perhaps more costly than regular dishes and detergents. Cost, time, energy, and ease of use are all considerations in this aspect of maintaining food intake.

Options for Assistance

For older adults who are not able to plan, prepare, and clean up after meals, home-delivered meals are often available. Low-cost meals may be available at senior centers and nutrition sites sponsored by the Area Agencies on Aging, as well as other institutions (local schools and restaurants). For some older adults, meal preparation may be provided by moving to senior apartments or assisted living facilities. In addition, other formal or informal caregivers might be needed to help provide nutritional assistance. Family, friends, neighbors, and church groups can provide support by doing the shopping, meal preparation, and cleanup. Some family members provide home-prepared frozen meals. Other older adults or their families may hire companion personal care assistants who will do shopping and meal preparation. Family caregivers of frail elderly need continued nursing support and guidance for nutritional care to prevent weight loss and nutritional deficiencies (Biggs & Freed, 2000).

Nutritional Assessment

Nutritional assessment is the evaluation of dietary and other nutrient-related indicators to determine the need for interventions. A complete nutritional assessment includes a nutritional history, anthropometric measurements, physical examination, and laboratory analysis. General components of nutrition screening include general assessment questions, physical examination, and laboratory assessment, which are described in Chapter 2. These help identify those with nutritional problems or at risk for developing problems. The following discusses some additional methods for more detailed nutritional assessment and norms for the older adult.

Nutritional History

Actual food intake is an essential component of a nutritional history. Methods for obtaining dietary intake include 24-hour recall, food frequency questionnaires, food records, and observation of food intake. The 24-hour recall method requires remembering food consumption from the previous day, whereas a food frequency questionnaire requires remembering the number of times per day, week, or month that particular foods are eaten. The 24-hour recall and food frequency methods are sometimes used together to gather more complete information about intake. The food record or diary involves recording all food eaten for at least 3 days, to include 2 weekdays and 1 weekend day if different, which is then calculated to provide an average daily intake. Methods of food recall, food frequency questionnaires, and food records/diaries are sometimes criticized for their reliability (Kaczkowski, Jones, Feng, & Bayley, 2000). However, they are still used in research with elderly, who tend to underreport actual food intake (Westerterp & Goris, 2002). Because research finds an acceptable level of use of self-reported food recall and recording among the elderly, these methods are also useful in a food intake history for nurses working with older adults.

The method of observation of food intake is time-consuming and most easily used in an institutional setting. It involves unobtrusive observation and recording of actual intake and enables identification of factors affecting intake, such as mealtime milieu and inappropriate feeding or assistive techniques used by caregivers, or other problems of feeding, such as difficulty swallowing or pocketing. Dietary intake is evaluated by food group or nutrient composition (RDAs) for macronutrients, micronutrients, and calories consumed. Computer software programs are available to enable rapid calculation of nutrients. Observation can be an important tool when accurate nutrition information is needed, However, intake may be overreported by staff, particularly in the nursing home setting (Simmons & Reuben, 2000), so the nurse may want to double-check meal trays when evaluating a patient's intake.

A nutritional history should also include the following information:

- Adequacy of income to purchase food
- Educational level
- Religious and cultural dietary practices
- Food shopping accessibility
- Adequacy of food preparation facilities
- Physical mobility and activity level
- Functional ability
- Food allergies and intolerances, likes and dislikes
- Intentional or unintentional recent weight changes
- Problems with chewing and swallowing
- Gastrointestinal problems such as anorexia, heartburn, indigestion, nausea, vomiting, bloating, flatulence, diarrhea, and constipation
- Medical and psychiatric conditions
- Over-the-counter and prescription medication use

Nutrition Screening Tools

Three measures are commonly used to evaluate nutritional disorders and are discussed here. First is Determine Your Nutritional Health (Figure 8-2) (Gallagher-Allred, 1993), which is a general screening instrument for community-dwelling older adults and can be completed by the older adult. The checklist includes 10 risk factors for nutritional problems and provides a score of nutritional risk. Information about each of the items is provided with the tool, so that it can be used for nutrition education for older adults.

A helpful clinical tool that can be used to support a focused clinical assessment of nutritional problems is the Mini Nutritional Assessment (MNA) (Figure 8-3) (Guigoz, Vellas, & Garry, 1996). The tool includes assessment of function, food intake, and a number of other factors, and it has been validated in many studies.

Another nutrition questionnaire useful for assessing food and water intake of dependent or frail older adults is shown in Box 8-2 (Biggs & Freed, 2000). A review of these items may help caregivers identify nutritional problems and plan interventions. Other tools are available and should be matched to the setting and purpose of nutritional screening.

Anthropometric Measurement

Anthropometric measurement includes height, weight, skinfold thickness, and circumferences. These measurements provide estimates of body fat and muscle mass for determining nutritional status when compared with available standards. The usefulness of these values depends on accurate measurement technique. The *Anthropometric Standardization Reference Manual* (Lohman, Martorell, & Roche, 1988) provides detailed descriptions of standard techniques. Other sources of information concerning accurately taking these measurements based on this classic source can be found in current clinical nutrition texts (Mitchell, 2003; Williams & Schlenker, 2003).

Height and Weight. If possible, height should be measured with the person standing erect against a wall without shoes. Because arm span approximates height at maturity and changes little with aging, it has been used as an alternative method to estimate true height (Mitchell, 2003; Williams & Schlenker, 2003). Measurement is taken from fingertip to fingertip with the measuring tape passing over the clavicles. Although some sources do not recommend arm span for the nonambulatory person because it is difficult to obtain reliable measurements, others find arm span to be accurate even in immobile older persons. If there is limited mobility of one arm, doubling the distance from fingertip to midline of the supraclavicular notch is an alternative. Comparing arm span with measured height also gives an approximation of height loss, an indication of osteoporosis.

Knee height is another measure used to estimate true height for the nonambulatory adult, or when standing erect is not possible. Knee height in the adult does not change with age and is believed to be more highly correlated with stature than total arm length or other length measurements (Mitchell, 2003; Williams & Schlenker, 2003). Knee height (KH) is measured from the floor to the tip of the tibia with both the knee and ankle at 90-degree angles, and estimation of height is made using the formula for deriving height equivalents (Williams & Schlenker, 2003):

$$\text{Height (women) cm} = [(1.833 \times KH) - (0.24 \times age)] + 84.88$$

$$\text{Height (men) cm} = [(2.02 \times KH) - (0.04 \times age)] + 64.19$$

Weight should be tested in light clothing without shoes. A bed or chair scale should be used for persons who are nonambulatory or unable to safely stand unsupported and without their shoes. Weight, along

The Warning Signs of poor nutritional health are often overlooked. Use this checklist to find out if you or someone you know is at nutritional risk.

Read the statements below. Circle the number in the yes column for those that apply to you or someone you know. For each yes answer, score the number in the box. Total your nutritional score.

DETERMINE YOUR NUTRITIONAL HEALTH

	YES
I have an illness or condition that made me change the kind and/or amount of food I eat.	2
I eat fewer than 2 meals per day.	3
I eat few fruits or vegetables, or milk products.	2
I have 3 or more drinks of beer, liquor or wine almost every day.	2
I have tooth or mouth problems that make it hard for me to eat.	2
I don't always have enough money to buy the food I need.	4
I eat alone most of the time.	1
I take 3 or more different prescribed or over-the-counter drugs a day.	1
Without wanting to, I have lost or gained 10 pounds in the last 6 months.	2
I am not always physically able to shop, cook and/or feed myself.	2
	TOTAL

Total Your Nutritional Score. If it's —

0-2 **Good!** Recheck your nutritional score in 6 months.

3-5 **You are at moderate nutritional risk.** See what can be done to improve your eating habits and lifestyle. Your office on aging, senior nutrition program, senior citizens center or health department can help. Recheck your nutritional score in 3 months.

6 or more **You are at high nutritional risk.** Bring this checklist the next time you see your doctor, dietitian or other qualified health or social service professional. Talk with them about any problems you may have. Ask for help to improve your nutritional health.

Implementing Nutrition Screening and Intervention Strategies

These materials developed and distributed by the Nutrition Screening Initiative, a project of:

AMERICAN ACADEMY OF FAMILY PHYSICIANS

THE AMERICAN DIETETIC ASSOCIATION

NATIONAL COUNCIL ON THE AGING, INC.

Remember that warning signs suggest risk, but do not represent diagnosis of any condition. Turn the page to learn more about the Warning Signs of poor nutritional health.

The Nutrition Checklist is based on the Warning Signs described below.
Use the word DETERMINE to remind you of the Warning Signs.

DISEASE
Any disease, illness or chronic condition which causes you to change the way you eat, or makes it hard for you to eat, puts your nutritional health at risk. Four out of five adults have chronic diseases that are affected by diet. Confusion or memory loss that keeps getting worse is estimated to affect one out of five or more of older adults. This can make it hard to remember what, when or if you've eaten. Feeling sad or depressed, which happens to about one in eight older adults, can cause big changes in appetite, digestion, energy level, weight and well-being.

EATING POORLY
Eating too little and eating too much both lead to poor health. Eating the same foods day after day or not eating fruit, vegetables, and milk products daily will also cause poor nutritional health. One in five adults skip meals daily. Only 13% of adults eat the minimum amount of fruit and vegetables needed. One in four older adults drink too much alcohol. Many health problems become worse if you drink more than one or two alcoholic beverages per day.

TOOTH LOSS/MOUTH PAIN
A healthy mouth, teeth and gums are needed to eat. Missing, loose or rotten teeth or dentures which don't fit well or cause mouth sores make it hard to eat.

ECONOMIC HARDSHIP
As many as 40% of older Americans have incomes of less than $6,000 per year. Having less—or choosing to spend less—than $25-30 per week for food makes it very hard to get the foods you need to stay healthy.

REDUCED SOCIAL CONTACT
One-third of all older people live alone. Being with people daily has a positive effect on morale, well-being and eating.

MULTIPLE MEDICINES
Many older Americans must take medicines for health problems. Almost half of older Americans take multiple medicines daily. Growing old may change the way we respond to drugs. The more medicines you take, the greater the chance for side effects such as increased or decreased appetite, change in taste, constipation, weakness, drowsiness, diarrhea, nausea, and others. Vitamins or minerals when taken in large doses act like drugs and can cause harm. Alert your doctor to everything you take.

INVOLUNTARY WEIGHT LOSS/GAIN
Losing or gaining a lot of weight when you are not trying to do so is an important warning sign that must not be ignored. Being overweight or underweight also increases you chance of poor health.

NEEDS ASSISTANCE IN SELF CARE
Although most older people are able to eat, one of every five have trouble walking, shopping, buying and cooking food, especially as they get older.

ELDER YEARS ABOVE AGE 80
Most older people lead full and productive lives. But as age increases, risk of frailty and health problems increase. Checking your nutritional health regularly makes good sense.

The Nutrition Screening Initiative, 1010 Wisconsin Avenue, NW, Suite 800, Washington, DC 20007
The Nutrition Screening Initiative is funded in part by a grant from Ross Laboratories, a division of Abbott Laboratories

The Nutrition Screening Initiative

Figure 8-2 Nutrition checklist. (From Gallagher-Allred, C. R. [1993]. Implementing nutrition screening and intervention strategies. Washington, DC: Nutrition Screening Initiative. Used with permission of Ross Products Division, Abbott Laboratories, Columbus, Ohio 43125. Copyright 1995.)

NESTLÉ NUTRITION SERVICES

Nestlé

Mini Nutritional Assessment
MNA®

Last name:	First name:	Sex:	Date:
Age:	Weight, kg:	Height, cm:	I.D. Number:

Complete the screen by filling in the boxes with the appropriate numbers.
Add the numbers for the screen. If score is 11 or less, continue with the assessment to gain a Malnutrition Indicator Score.

Screening

A   Has food intake declined over the past 3 months
    due to loss of appetite, digestive problems,
    chewing or swallowing difficulties?
    0 = severe loss of appetite
    1 = moderate loss of appetite
    2 = no loss of appetite   ☐

B   Weight loss during last months
    0 = weight loss greater than 3 kg (6.6 lbs)
    1 = does not know
    2 = weight loss between 1 and 3 kg (2.2 and 6.6 lbs)
    3 = no weight loss   ☐

C   Mobility
    0 = bed or chair bound
    1 = able to get out of bed/chair but does not go out
    2 = goes out   ☐

D   Has suffered psychological stress or acute
    disease in the past 3 months
    0 = yes   2 = no   ☐

E   Neuropsychological problems
    0 = severe dementia or depression
    1 = mild dementia
    2 = no psychological problems   ☐

F   Body Mass Index (BMI) (weight in kg) / (height in m)²
    0 = BMI less than 19
    1 = BMI 19 to less than 21
    2 = BMI 21 to less than 23
    3 = BMI 23 or greater   ☐

Screening score (subtotal max. 14 points)   ☐ ☐

12 points or greater   Normal – not at risk –
                         no need to complete assessment

11 points or below   Possible malnutrition – continue assessment

Assessment

G   Lives independently (not in a nursing home or hospital)
    0 = no   1 = yes   ☐

H   Takes more than 3 prescription drugs per day
    0 = yes   1 = no   ☐

I   Pressure sores or skin ulcers
    0 = yes   1 = no   ☐

J   How many full meals does the patient eat daily?
    0 = 1 meal
    1 = 2 meals
    2 = 3 meals   ☐

K   Selected consumption markers for protein intake
    • At least one serving of dairy products
      (milk, cheese, yogurt) per day?   yes ☐   no ☐
    • Two or more servings of legumes
      or eggs per week?   yes ☐   no ☐
    • Meat, fish or poultry every day   yes ☐   no ☐
    0.0 = if 0 or 1 yes
    0.5 = if 2 yes
    1.0 = if 3 yes   ☐ ☐

L   Consumes two or more servings
    of fruits or vegetables per day?
    0 = no   1 = yes   ☐

M   How much fluid (water, juice, coffee, tea, milk...)
    is consumed per day?
    0.0 = less than 3 cups
    0.5 = 3 to 5 cups
    1.0 = more than 5 cups   ☐ ☐

N   Mode of feeding
    0 = unable to eat without assistance
    1 = self-fed with some difficulty
    2 = self-fed without any problem   ☐

O   Self view of nutritional status
    0 = view self as being malnourished
    1 = is uncertain of nutritional state
    2 = views self as having no nutritional problem   ☐

P   In comparison with other people of the same age,
    how do they consider their health status?
    0.0 = not as good
    0.5 = does not know
    1.0 = as good
    2.0 = better   ☐.☐

Q   Mid-arm circumference (MAC) in cm
    0.0 = MAC less than 21
    0.5 = MAC 21 to 22
    1.0 = MAC 22 or greater   ☐.☐

R   Calf circumference (CC) in cm
    0 = CC less than 31   1 = CC 31 or greater   ☐

Assessment (max. 16 points)   ☐ ☐.☐

Screening score   ☐ ☐

Total Assessment (max. 30 points)   ☐ ☐.☐

Malnutrition Indicator Score

17 to 23.5 points   at risk of malnutrition   ☐

Less than 17 points   malnourished   ☐

Ref.:   Guigoz Y, Vellas B and Garry PJ. 1994. Mini Nutritional Assessment: A practical assessment tool for
        grading the nutritional state of elderly patients. *Facts and Research in Gerontology.* Supplement
        #2:15-59.
        Rubenstein LZ, Harker J, Guigoz Y and Vellas B. Comprehensive Geriatric Assessment (CGA) and
        the MNA: An Overview of CGA, Nutritional Assessment, and Development of a Shortened Version
        of the MNA. In: "Mini Nutritional Assessment (MNA): Research and Practice in the Elderly". Vellas
        B, Garry PJ and Guigoz Y , editors. Nestlé Nutrition Workshop Series. Clinical & Performance Pro-
        gramme, vol. 1. Karger, Bâle, in press.

08.98 USA

Figure 8-3   Mini Nutritional Assessment. (Copyright by Nestle USA, Inc. Used with permission.)

BOX 8-2 Biggs' Elderly Self-Care Assessment Tool (BESCAT) of Water and Food Intake

Review the following information with caregiver or family member for community-dwelling, dependent elderly.

Water Intake
Does the older adult you are caring for:
1. Drink 4 to 8 glasses (cups) of water, juice, milk, tea, coffee, or other beverages, or eat soups, gelatin, ice cream, or pudding, each day?
2. Have a mouth and tongue that is moist in appearance?
3. Get and drink fluids when thirsty?
4. Drink water or other fluids when they are offered?
5. Accept and drink extra fluids on hot days?

Food Intake
Does the older adult you are caring for:
1. Have a weight change of more than 2 or 3 pounds in the past month?
2. Assist with planning meals based on nutritional needs and likes/dislikes?
3. Help with meal preparation, including table setting?
4. Eat without spilling or making a mess, or in an amount that is accepted by other members of the household?
5. Eat foods from each of the following food groups every 24 hours?
   a. Proteins: meat, eggs, fish, poultry, peanut butter or other nuts, dried beans or peas (when mixed with other foods for a complete protein)
   b. Milk/dairy: milk, cheese, yogurt, ice cream
   c. Grains/cereals: bread, rolls, donuts, cookies, cereals, popcorn, potatoes, pasta (whole grains with higher fiber for all cereals and grains; other highly processed and potentially high trans fat cereals, grains, breads in moderation)
   d. Fruits: fresh, canned, or frozen/thawed, or juices
   e. Vegetables: fresh, canned, or frozen/cooked or juices
   f. Fats: moderation in saturated (animal fats) and polyunsaturated fats and oils (soybean, safflower, corn or sesame); more emphasis on monounsaturated fats (olive oil, canola oil, nuts and nut oils, avocados) and limited trans fats (partially hydrogenated oils/fats found in processed foods and baked goods)
6. Follow a special diet to limit fats, salt, or calories if told to do so by the physician?
7. Get enough calcium each day, in milk, cheese, yogurt, ice cream, broccoli, or green beans, or take a daily calcium supplement?
8. Take a vitamin/mineral supplement?
9. Enjoy eating?
10. Say that foods taste bad or different?
11. Have dentures or a removable partial bridge? Is so, do they fit comfortably? Do they help with chewing food?

Review problem areas and develop a nutritional plan to address them.

From Biggs, A., & Freed, P. E. (2000). Nutrition and older adults: What do family caregivers know and do? *Journal of Gerontological Nursing, 26*(8), 6-14.

---

with height, is used to calculate body mass index (BMI) or Quetelet index (weight in kilograms divided by the square of height in meters) (Williams & Schlenker, 2003). Nurses should keep in mind that it is better for older people to carry some extra weight (and therefore a higher BMI) into old age than to be underweight. The desirable BMI for adults over 65 may be 24 to 29 (Chernoff, 2003) rather than the usual 18.5 to 25 (see the BMI chart, Chapter 2), and the risks associated with BMI of 25 to 29 for older adults are minimal (Arterburn, Crane, & Sullivan, 2004).

Skinfold Thickness and Circumference Measures. Triceps and subscapular skinfold thicknesses provide measures of subcutaneous fat on the arm and trunk that significantly correlate with total body fat,

indicating energy or caloric reserves. These reserves are important into older age as protection from chronic health conditions when appetite and eating may be problematic. Subscapular skinfold thickness is measured 1 cm below the inferior angle of the scapula. Triceps skinfold (TSF) thickness is measured with calipers at midpoint between the olecranon and acromion processes on the posterior aspect of the arm (Mitchell, 2003; Sardesai, 2003). Percentile norms for TSF thickness are presented in Table 8-4.

Circumference measures are another method of monitoring nutritional health in older adults (Mitchell, 2003; Sardesai, 2003; Williams & Schlenker, 2003). Calf circumference measurement is recommended to monitor muscle loss from reduced physical activity. Measurement is done at the largest circumference of the calf

Table 8-4 Norms for Upper Arm Anthropometric Measurements: Ages 60 to 89

Site/Percentile	Men	Women
MID UPPER ARM CIRCUMFERENCE (CM)		
10th	26.6	25.1
50th	30.4	29.7
95th	36.3	38.1
MID UPPER ARM MUSCLE CIRCUMFERENCE (CM)		
10th	18.1	17.7
50th	23.4	21.9
95th	29.7	28.3
MID UPPER ARM MUSCLE AREA		
10th	26.2	25.0
50th	43.6	38.0
95th	70.4	63.8
TRICEPS SKINFOLD (MM)		
10th	7.6	14.4
50th	20.4	24.0
95th	45.8	43.6

Modified from Falciglia, G., O'Connor, J. O., & Gadling, E. (1988). Upper arm anthropometric norms in elderly white subjects. *Journal of the American Dietetic Association, 88*(5), 569-574.

with an inelastic tape measure. Midarm circumference is measured halfway between the olecranon and acromion processes using an insertion tape. Midarm circumference and TSF thickness are used to calculate midarm muscle circumference (MAMC [cm] = arm circumference [cm] − [π × triceps skinfold thickness in mm]). Midarm muscle area (MAMA = $MAMC^2/4$). Both MAMC and MAMA are estimates of the amount of body muscle, an indication of muscle protein reserve. Waist circumference is considered important as a risk factor for cardiovascular disease, but most individuals who are at risk can be identified using BMI (Kiernan & Winkleby, 2000).

NUTRITIONAL DISORDERS

Four nutritional disorders common in older adults are addressed in this chapter: dehydration, impaired swallowing, obesity, and malnutrition. Other relevant problems are discussed in later chapters.

Dehydration

Definition and Scope. Dehydration, or fluid volume deficit, is a frequent problem in older age because of aging changes, functional problems, and decreased thirst sensation. Dehydration results in unnecessary hospitalizations and resulting health care costs, particularly in community-dwelling older adults (Steen, 2004;

Xiao, Barber, & Campbell, 2004). In addition, dehydration increases the risk for acute confusion/delirium, which can further impair water intake and mobility, increasing the risk of pressure sores (Stotts & Hopf, 2003) and pneumonia (van der Steen et al., 2002).

Etiology. Although required water intake does not change with age, total body water decreases significantly with age because of reduced lean body mass and increased body fat. The older adult needs 30 ml of water per kilogram of body weight, or six to eight glasses of water daily, enough to produce about 1.5 liters of urine (Mitchell, 2003; Posthauer, 2005). The following formula is a method for estimating fluid needs (Chidester & Spangler, 1997):

$$(Body\ weight\ [kg] - 20) \times 15 + 1500\ ml$$

Risks for dehydration include impaired cognition, swallowing difficulties, poor oral intake, receiving enteral feedings, diarrhea, undiagnosed diabetes mellitus, use of diuretics, and abuse of laxatives (Stotts & Hopf, 2003). Older adults in the community and those in nursing homes are also at risk for dehydration from inappropriately limiting fluid intake to control urinary incontinence. Diminished thirst drive is a normal alteration in aging (Morley et al., 1995), as well as a decreased ability to concentrate urine.

Most older adults, both community-dwelling adults and (especially) those residing in nursing homes, do not get enough water, with many in long-term care getting less than 1000 ml per day in total fluids and water (Kayser-Jones et al., 1999). Most fluid consumed in a nursing home is from fluids on trays or in foods, and not enough is from plain water, contributing to dehydration and health problems, including dehydration-associated confusion and hyperosmolarity (Chernoff, 2003). The high prevalence of functional problems limits older adults from accessing adequate water themselves, and the issue is rarely recognized or managed.

Management of Dehydration. Assessment of hydration status includes the basics of monitoring for adequacy of fluid/water intake and balance of output, along with color and concentration of urine and consistency of stools (diarrhea or constipation with dry, hard stools). Daily weight is a relatively sensitive way to monitor for fluid retention in congestive heart failure, and trends, such as weight loss of 3% in 1 month's time, may indicate both malnutrition and dehydration, as the two often go hand in hand (Zembrzuski, 2003). Bioelectrical impedance (Culp et al., 2004) is a more expensive but effective means of monitoring intracellular water, extracellular water, and total body water. Monitoring of serum osmolality, sodium, and blood urea nitrogen can be helpful (Posthauer, 2005).

Zembrzuski's (2003) hydration assessment checklist can also be used as a guide for addressing symptoms of dehydration; associated factors; vulnerability; dietary prescriptions/restrictions; medications with risk for dehydration; nothing-by-mouth status for laboratory, radiological, or surgical procedures (including dental or eye surgeries); and trends in biochemical laboratory results. Assessment also requires monitoring adequacy and commitment of nursing home staff to provide this fundamental care (Kayser-Jones et al., 1999; Rantz & Zwygart-Stauffacher, 2004).

Maintenance of hydration and prevention of dehydration for community-dwelling older adults includes teaching and guiding older adults to maintain adequate water intake. Suggestions include having a favorite water glass and knowing and planning how many glasses of water need to be consumed each day along with other usual beverages or fluid-containing foods. Another method is to fill a liter bottle with water each day, keep it in the refrigerator, and drink all of its contents each day. Older adults can also be encouraged to carry water bottles with them when walking or working outdoors to maintain a sufficient intake of water. Flavoring water with lemon or lime or crystal flavorings, or purchasing flavored waters, is an option for those who do not like to drink "plain water." In addition to water, liquids can include fruit or vegetable juices, milk, ice cream, and soup with care counted toward the daily servings of liquids. This can be an important clarification, because drinking eight glasses of water each day can be difficult.

Maintaining water intake and preventing dehydration among older adults in long-term care facilities is on ongoing challenge throughout the world (Porock et al., 2005). Nursing interventions include providing prompts and reminders along with preferred beverages (Simmons, Alessi, & Schnelle, 2001). Nursing assistants in nursing homes must be taught the importance of assisting immobile and cognitively impaired older adults to safely drink water, and must be given positive reinforcement from professional nurses for their important work in this regard, including litigation risk reduction (Iyer, 2004). In a study by Robinson and Rosher (2002), a hydration program that included regular passing of a variety of fluids to residents improved hydration status, as well as constipation and falls. For nursing home residents who become dehydrated (or are in danger of becoming dehydrated with an cute illness), Walsh (2005) describes an "old" but effective treatment of hypodermoclysis, or the provision of fluid into the tissues rather than intravenously. Nurses play a key role in preventing and managing dehydration.

Dysphagia/Impaired Swallowing

Definition and Scope. Dysphagia refers to difficulty in swallowing and affects a significant number of older adults (Schindler & Kelly, 2002). Persons with swallowing problems are at risk for nutritional deficiency because of their inability to ingest sufficient amounts of essential nutrients. Dysphagia can also lead to aspiration and pneumonia, even when symptoms have not been apparent. As many as 40% to 50% of older adults in nursing homes may have dysphagia (Chen, Schilling, & Lyder, 2001).

Etiology. Dysphagia may be divided into two types: oropharyngeal or transfer dysphagia and esophageal dysphagia (Schindler & Kelly, 2002). Oropharyngeal dysphagia is trouble initiating a swallow or difficulty with voluntary transfer of food or fluid from the mouth into the esophagus (deglutition). Concurrent xerostomia, fatigue or activity intolerance, and decreased chewing ability further complicate this problem. Other symptoms associated with transfer dysphagia are nasal regurgitation, coughing during swallowing, and dysarthria caused by weakness of palatal muscles. Drooling, spitting, or retaining food in the mouth may be symptoms as well. Stroke and Parkinson's disease are common causes of oropharyngeal dysphagia, although other neuromuscular disorders, mechanical conditions, and cognitive dysfunction can contribute. Although many stroke patients recover, a small number develop dysphagia some time after the acute event, so swallowing should be monitored for some time (Schindler & Kelly, 2002). Diagnostic tests for oropharyngeal dysphagia include radiological swallowing examinations, including video fluoroscopic swallow studies with varying consistencies of barium from thin to thick or barium-coated cookie chew and swallow.

Difficulty with food or fluid transport down the esophagus after swallowing is termed *esophageal dysphagia*. A characteristic of esophageal dysphagia is a sensation of food stopping or sticking after it has been swallowed. Esophageal strictures, esophagitis, and esophageal muscle spasms with motility disturbances are common causes that must be evaluated. Medications that can damage the esophagus especially in the presence of reflux disease should be evaluated. Other causes of esophageal dysphasia include sphincter disorders, diseases affecting the esophagus, or mechanical problems such as a tumor. Diagnostic examinations include radiological swallowing examinations and esophagoscopy to determine a diagnosis.

Management of Dysphagia. The goals of dysphagia management are to treat any underlying conditions; enhance swallowing ability to meet fluid, calorie, and other essential nutrient needs; and prevent aspiration. Achievement of these goals requires a collaborative effort by the nursing staff, physician, speech therapist, and dietitian. Modifying food and liquid consistency and amount may be an important approach. The ability of the patient to swallow different consistencies of food and liquids may be identified through swallowing studies and evaluation by a speech therapist.

Identifying and providing food preferences is important in maintaining enjoyment of food.

Preventing aspiration is an important goal in the care of patients with dysphagia, but there is some research regarding prevention of pneumonia, even in those who may aspirate on their own saliva. Providing frequent oral care may help decrease the risk of pneumonia in older adults in the institutional setting, even those who receive tube-feedings (Marik & Kaplan, 2003). The use of tube-feedings has not been shown to decrease the risk of pneumonia.

Family caregivers of community-dwelling older adults and nurse aides or restorative aides who may be assigned to feed older adults in nursing homes need to be taught methods of hand-feeding to prevent aspiration. A number of techniques helpful for safe feeding are noted in Box 8-3. It is possible to hand-feed even severely cognitively impaired older adults with dysphagia. Caregivers or family members can be taught feeding strategies for even the most frail, dependent, and demented older adults. Careful feeding by a caring caregiver provides the comfort of feeding, in addition to the nutrients and fluids that are required (Ina, 2002). Combined with discussions concerning advance directives, these measures can prevent inappropriate feeding tube placement in late stages of dementia.

BOX 8-3 Feeding Techniques for Older Adults with Dysphagia

The following steps can help promote safe feeding and optimal nutrition for all older adults, including those with dysphagia:

- Provide mouth care before the meal to remove any dried secretions or debris and freshen the mouth before eating.
- Position the older adult sitting up. If the older adult must remain in bed, the person needs to be correctly positioned in the bed and the head of the bed elevated to 90 degrees (Metheny, 2004), which may require the foot to be slightly elevated to keep the person from sliding down.
- Flex the head slightly (for "chin tuck" swallowing) with a small pillow or folded towel to help open the oropharynx for swallowing (Shanahan et al., 1993).
- Offer small bites sized to the ability of the person to chew and swallow; avoid forcing food into the mouth. Place food in the mouth on the side unaffected by a stroke or other muscular weakness. Meat that is "chopped" in a food processor or moistened with vegetable juice, creamed soup, or gravy will provide enough texture to allow for easier mastication and may be easier to feel and manage in the older adult's mouth than pureed meat. Food-processed meat mixed with mashed potatoes and gravy is also easier for some older adults with dysphagia to manage.
- Most adults take 15 to 20 minutes to eat a meal (Stanner, 2003), so avoid rushing. A pace that is too rapid may lead to choking or refusing to eat.
- Use thickened liquids (nectar, honey, or pudding consistency) as prescribed or needed following swallow studies (Castellanos, Butler, Gluch, & Burke, 2004). Milk is considered to be "nectar" consistency and may not need additional thickening; milk can promote viscosity of sputum in some individuals, so end the meal with a more astringent beverage (citrus juice, lemonade) or water.
- Address food preferences and use condiments as appropriate and desired. Combining all the food on a plate may not be palatable and is inappropriate.
- Alternate solid foods with liquid foods.
- Caregivers should feed only a few older adults at a time (upper limit is probably three older adults being fed by one person at a time).
- Keep distractions to a minimum. Encourage even dependent elderly to participate in feeding, such as holding toast, helping to hold an adaptive spoon or "spork," and using handled cups with lips for controlled fluid flow.
- Try to be social during meals, but avoid asking questions during chewing/swallowing. The older adult may choke and aspirate while attempting to be sociable and answer.
- Pay attention to the person rather than other staff, television, and so on, and watch for swallowing difficulties or changes (Kayser-Jones & Pengilly, 1999).
- Mouth inspection should be done at the end of each meal for older adults who pocket food or are unable to determine when food is left in their mouth. Provide oral hygiene to remove any pocketed food and to ensure there is no food left in the mouth to be aspirated later; this will also help remove milk residue that might contribute to sputum production.
- Allow a rest period before lunch and dinner, making sure the older adult is rested, awake, and alert, and also free from the effects of sedatives, hypnotics, or sedating analgesics.
- Staff training and supervision of feeding should be an ongoing process.

Obesity

Definition and Scope. Obesity refers to excess body fat and is generally defined as a BMI above 30 or as a weight of 20% or more than ideal or desirable (Sardesai, 2003). The nursing diagnosis is *altered nutrition: more than body requirements.* Although weight for height is the most frequently used criterion to define obesity in elderly people, skinfold thickness and abdominal/gluteal ratio provides additional information for defining degree of obesity. The prevalence of obesity among people over 60 in 2000 was 32.0%, and this is expected to increase at least 5% by 2010 (Arterburn et al., 2004). This increase is alarming because obesity (not just overweight, considered BMI of 25 to 29) is associated with a number of physical problems for older adults. These can include mobility and functional problems, hypertension, diabetic management, and cardiovascular disease. Obesity is also a risk factor for poor quality of life and health care use. Unexpectedly, 10% to 15% of people entering nursing homes are obese (Johnson, 2002).

Etiology. Obesity results when caloric intake is greater than energy expenditure. Factors contributing to obesity in older people include inactivity, reduced metabolic rate, lifelong patterns, limited social contacts, psychological issues, poor dentition, reduced mobility, and appetite-stimulating medications. Other causes, such as endocrine or hypothalamic disorders, rarely account for obesity in the older adult (Mitchell, 2003; Williams & Schlenker, 2003). Recent surveys show that Americans are more likely to be overweight than underweight at retirement age and obesity to be more prevalent among persons of lower socioeconomic status (Sardesai, 2003). Most often, the individual has carried excess weight into older age.

Management of Obesity. Weight reduction is achieved by reducing calorie intake and increasing energy expenditure through exercise and behavior modification. To be sustained, changes must be integrated into the older adult's lifestyle. The plan for weight reduction in older adults must be undertaken very carefully because dieting can be dangerous. Older adults who are more than 130% of ideal body weight are the most appropriate patients for weight reduction (Morley et al., 1995). Older adults who are over 110% of ideal body weight may also be encouraged to lose weight if they have coexisting diabetes or are experiencing other problems with function or health related to weight.

Weight loss counseling should help the older adult establish appropriate personal weight goals and identify the support needed to achieve those goals. Many find support groups and planned programs very helpful. Evaluation of weight loss should not occur too frequently, because day-to-day fluctuations in weight may be discouraging. An evaluation form completed by the older adult provides a concrete record of goal achievement. Dieting and weight loss should be monitored closely by health professionals in older adults to ensure that calories are not reduced to excess (below 1000 kcal per day).

A balanced, reduced-calorie diet designed to promote weight loss of no more than 2 pounds per week is recommended for the seriously overweight or obese older adult. The goal is weight reduction while conserving lean body mass. A cut in calorie intake of 500 to 1000 calories per day will promote a safe weight loss of 1 to 2 pounds per week. The recommended balance of foods discussed earlier in the chapter continues to be helpful for meal planning. A diet consisting of the lowest number of servings from the Food Guide Pyramid and emphasizing low-fat foods will provide 1600 calories a day. Increasing fiber and water intake also benefits older adults attempting to lose weight.

Combined with diet, moderate exercise is important to conserve lean body mass. Exercise also improves muscle tone, cardiovascular condition, and body image. Encourage older adults to work toward 30 minutes of moderate exercise most days of the week to maximize weight loss. This should be adjusted depending on the individual's fitness level. Using weights for resistance will help maintain lean muscle mass and improve metabolism. More details on exercise and behavior change are discussed in Chapter 27.

Malnutrition

Definition and Scope. Malnutrition is a serious and common concern and threatens the health of older adults. It is associated with increased morbidity and mortality rates, development of pressure sores and poor wound healing in general, impaired immunity and increased risk for infection, longer hospital stays, and higher health care costs (Sardesai, 2003). Several terms are used for the problem, including the nursing diagnosis of *nutrition: less than body requirements, undernutrition, protein-calorie malnutrition,* and *failure to thrive.* Inadequate intake of protein and calories to meet metabolic requirements results in a progressive loss of lean body mass and body fat. A definition of malnutrition in the older adult is provided by Chen, Schilling, and Lyder (2001, p. 138):

Faulty or inadequate nutritional status; undernourishment characterized by insufficient dietary intake, poor appetite, muscle wasting and weight loss. In the elderly, malnutrition is an ominous sign. Without intervention it presents as a downward trajectory leading to poor health and decreased quality of life. Malnutrition in the elderly is a multidimensional concept encompassing physical and psychosocial elements. It is precipitated by loss, dependency, loneliness and chronic illness.

Major indicators of protein-calorie undernutrition (PCU) include the following (Beck, Ovesen, & Schroll, 2001; Collins, 2004; Sardesai, 2003):

- Unintended loss of 5% or more of body weight in 1 month (10% in 6 months) or body weight less than 90% of reference standard; or BMI below 20
- Loss of appetite or refusal of food and fluids; chewing or swallowing difficulties; difficulty self-feeding
- Serum albumin less than 3.5 g/dl or prealbumin less than 18 mg/L; transferrin 2 g/L; total lymphocyte count less than 1800 n/mm; serum cholesterol less than 160 mg/dl; low or decreased hemoglobin
- Nonhealing wounds; pressure ulcers

The exact prevalence of PCU among older adults is not known. Population surveys have indicated that 15% of older adults experience PCU, whereas the incidence of PCU has been reported to range from 25% to 65% in acute care settings and 40% to 85% in long-term care facilities (Chen et al., 2001; Crogar & Pasvogel, 2003). Regardless of where it is found, undernutrition is an ominous sign in older adults, and it warrants immediate evaluation and intervention. Older adults in long-term care are at higher risk of protein-calorie (or protein-energy) malnutrition related to their problems with chewing, dry mouth, and difficulty swallowing (Nordenram, Ljunggren, & Cederholm, 2001).

Etiology. Usually more than one factor contributes to PCU in older adults. Age-related physical changes may alter food intake and the ability to utilize and metabolize essential nutrients. Social factors such as poverty, isolation, and lack of knowledge about nutritional requirements and appropriate food selection contribute to inadequate intake. Acute and chronic diseases may cause anorexia, increase energy utilization, cause nitrogen loss, alter vitamin and mineral metabolism, or alter the ability to self-feed. Medical treatments such as surgery and chemotherapy may alter intake while simultaneously increasing metabolic demands. Drug-nutrient interactions and anorexia associated with medications may also contribute to undernutrition. Anticipatory guidance and early intervention to reduce risk can prevent many causes of PCU.

Management of Malnutrition. Adequate assessment of the older adult is necessary to identify risk and causative factors, as well as the degree of PCU. Screening and assessment have been discussed earlier in the chapter. Intervention for undernutrition must address specific contributory and causative factors. Nutritional support will vary depending on the older adult's medical condition and degree of PCU. Interventions include improving access to appropriate foods, use of nutritional supplements, and addressing any contributing causes such as medications or health problems. Promoting self-feeding is often the best way to maintain adequate food intake. When oral intake is insufficient despite conservative measures and supplementation, enteral and parenteral nutrition may be considered as alternative means for feeding.

CONGREGATE NUTRITION PROGRAMS AND HOME-DELIVERED MEALS. Two resources in the community that address the problem of access to food are congregate nutrition programs and home-delivered meals. Most congregate nutrition programs have been developed for socially isolated, urban or rural, older adults whose nutritional problems are related more to access (financial and transportation) and social stimulation than to mechanical eating difficulties. Many are funded through the Older Americans Act (AOA, 2005). Nutrition education has been successfully included in many congregate meal sites (Ellis, Johnson, Fischer, & Hargrove, 2005; Rosenbloom, Kicklighter, Patacca, & Deshpande, 2004).

For older adults lacking the ability to go to nutrition sites, many communities also have home-delivered meal programs for homebound older adults. They usually deliver one hot meal per day, which provides one third of the daily nutrient requirements for older adults (Balsam, Sullivan, Millen, & Rogers, 2000; Krondl, Lau, Coleman, & Stocker, 2003; Sharkey et al., 2002). Weekends, holidays, and inclement weather can interfere with home meal delivery, putting the older adult at risk, because many programs are staffed with volunteers. Researchers have shown that adding a breakfast portion to home-delivered meals improves the nutritional status of homebound older adults (Gollub & Weddle, 2004). Others have suggested increasing the amount of protein in the home-delivered meals (Dasgupta, Sharkey, & Wu, 2005). There is concern about the future of nutrition programs with the increasing older population, many of whom will need nutritional support services (Balsam et al., 2000).

Some older adults have the option of moving to supportive apartments or assisted living situations that have congregate meal plans included as part of the rent or for an additional fee. Facilities may provide one to three meals and serve restaurant-style meals with choices for entrees (Weatherspoon, Worthen, & Handu, 2004). However, these facilities may be costly and unavailable to lower-income older adults.

NUTRITIONAL SUPPLEMENTATION. High-calorie/high-protein supplementation can be an effective means of increasing calories and protein for community-dwelling older adults (Payette, Boutier, Coulombe, & Gray-Donald, 2002; Wouters-Wesseling et al., 2003). Many specialty products are available as nutritional supplements (e.g., prepared beverages, food bars, and puddings). Other products to increase protein and calories that may cost less than the specialty products are instant powdered preparations that can be added to milk or adding powdered milk or protein powders (whey and soy are commonly available) to cooked cereals, puddings, liquids, semiliquids, or soft foods (soups or mashed potatoes). The unflavored protein powders do not alter the taste of foods and make only minor texture changes to most foods; flavored powders can be added to many foods. Another effective means to increase calories is to add healthful oils (monounsaturated oils, such as olive oil, peanut butter and peanut oil, canola oil, and nut oils, or flax oil) to food. Liberal use of cream, butter, whole milk, and other dairy products (e.g., ice cream, whole milk cottage cheese) is also good, because many malnourished older adults also have low serum cholesterol.

Prescribed supplements are also effective in acute care and long-term care of older adults, using either the specialty products available over the counter, or higher-calorie/higher-protein (therefore smaller quantity to be ingested) liquid supplements (Bender et al., 2000; Potter, Roberts, McColl, & Reilly, 2001). Improved Mini Nutritional Assessment scores and increased weight followed the improved dietary intake with the oral supplementation (Lauque et al., 2000). Increasing nurses' and nursing assistants' knowledge of nutrition, along with instructions and support for maintaining nutritional status and feeding older adults, is imperative for preventing and reversing malnutrition in vulnerable older adults (Crogan, Shultz, & Massey, 2001).

PROMOTING SELF-FEEDING. The nursing diagnosis of *feeding self-care deficit* applies to the inability to feed oneself when food is available and can be coupled with the Nursing Intervention Classification (NIC) of Self-Care Assistance: Feeding (McCloskey & Bulechek, 1996). In rehabilitation settings, where PCU may affect 49% to 67% of older adults (Strakowski, Strakowski, & Mitchell, 2002), special attention should be placed on promoting independence in self-feeding. Adaptive equipment may be helpful, along with restorative aides and nursing aides who are trained in patiently promoting self-feeding. The institutional long-term care environment may contribute to reduced self-feeding behavior (Morley, Thomas, & Kamel, 2004), including the lack of nutrition knowledge among nurses in long-term care (Crogan, Shultz, Adams, & Massey, 2001). Therefore measures to enhance the self-feeding capacities of nursing home residents are advocated, recognizing that this is a time-consuming and labor-intensive task (Thomas, Kamel, & Morley, 2004). These measures include the following:

- Attention to making the social environment of a meal more homelike through the use of small groups, removal of trays, and use of tablecloths and centerpieces and appropriate/adequate lighting, noise control, and family-style food service

- Individualized adaptive equipment to promote self-feeding, such as plate guards, built-up utensil handles, universal cuffs, and proper setup of plates
- Staff training to emphasize techniques that promote self-feeding, such as proper positioning, the use of finger food, enhancing social exchange during the meal, and avoiding feeding the older adult unless absolutely necessary to ensure adequate nutritional intake
- When assistance with feeding is needed, use (by specially trained aides or volunteers) of techniques discussed earlier for dysphagia

The older adult is more likely to have a positive attitude toward food and mealtime when self-feeding is fostered, thereby reducing the risk of inadequate intake and nutritional deficiency. Family caregivers and staff in long-term care facilities should also maintain a positive attitude and continue to encourage participation in self-feeding, periodically retrying attempts to allow and encourage the dependent older adult to hold foods, utensils, and cups. These principles of maintaining or restoring self-feeding ability apply to homebound older adults as well. Home health agencies provide assistance by teaching caregivers how to compensate for disabilities and create an environment conducive to eating.

For older adults who lack the capacity to feed themselves, it is important to make feeding as risk free and pleasant as possible. Relinquishing the self-care task of eating may have devastating psychological consequences. Failure to pay meticulous attention to position, pace of feeding, food preferences, and nonverbal communication during feeding is likely to result in the person's refusal to eat or increase the risk of aspiration and undernutrition (Shimizu, Otsuka, Kanai, & Oki, 2004; Swann, 2005;). Safe feeding techniques are described in Box 8-3. In addition, mealtime provides an opportunity to engage the older adult socially and to send messages that strengthen self-esteem. A depersonalized or threatening feeding environment discourages optimal food intake and minimizes self-worth (Westergren et al., 2001).

ENTERAL NUTRITION. Enteral nutritional therapy is an option when the older adult is unable to meet nutritional needs orally but has normal gastrointestinal function. Enteral feeding may be used to supplement oral intake or to provide total nutrient requirements. Families and other caregivers may seek enteral feedings for older adults who are near the end of life and need guidance and support from advanced practice nurses when making decisions (Eggenberger & Nelms, 2004). Ethical and end-of-life issues, including advance directives, need to be considered in planning for placing an enteral feeding tube, along with purported effectiveness.

The most common sites for enteral feeding are stomach and jejunum. Placement of a feeding tube will depend on the older adult's medical condition and the length of time that enteral therapy will be used. Naso-gastric and other transnasal tubes are used only for short-term therapy. Feeding tubes placed in the stomach or jejunum either surgically or by percutaneous endoscopy are preferred for permanent or long-term enteral feeding. A jejunostomy tube is indicated for the older adult who has a diminished or absent gag reflex to reduce the risk of aspiration. Care should be taken to prevent contamination of tube-feedings (Padula, Kenny, Planchon, & Lamoureux, 2004). In addition, careful testing/verification of placement or location of feeding tubes is important (Metheny & Meert, 2004; Metheny & Titler, 2001).

A number of commercially prepared formulas are available. Selection depends on the patient's nutrient and fluid needs, ability to digest and absorb nutrients, other health conditions (such as diabetes or renal disease), and the type of feeding tube used. Standard formulas are available in isotonic and hypertonic forms. Nurses are encouraged to seek current nutrient information on prescribed products from the manufacturer. In addition, nurses should determine the caloric and fluid needs of patients to verify that adequate nutrition and water are being provided by tube-feedings.

Tube-feedings can be delivered by continuous drip, intermittent infusion, and bolus administration. The method of delivery depends on the location of the feeding tube, type of formula used, and tolerance for the feeding. Bolus administration is used only with naso-gastric and gastrostomy tube-feeding. Formula is given by gravity with a large barrel syringe over 15 to 30 minutes, four to six times a day. Bolus feeding is not well tolerated by some older adults. Intermittent feeding by slow gravity drip or infusion pump over 30 to 60 minutes helps alleviate some of the problems of intolerance encountered with bolus administration. The preferred method is continuous drip over 16 to 24 hours using an infusion pump to maintain consistent flow rate, thus minimizing feeding intolerance. Feedings delivered to the small intestine, duodenum, and jejunum require use of an infusion pump to prevent dumping syndrome.

Isotonic formulas are started at full strength at a rate of 25 to 50 ml per hour, increased by 25 ml per hour over 12 to 24 hours as tolerated until the desired rate to meet nutrient needs is achieved. Hypertonic formulas should be diluted to isotonic strength when initiated. The concentration is increased every 8 to 12 hours as tolerated to full strength; the rate is then increased 25 ml per hour every 8 to 12 hours until the desired rate to meet nutrient needs is achieved. The rate and concentration should never be advanced at the same time (Williams & Schlenker, 2003).

Complications of enteral therapy may be mechanical, gastrointestinal, or metabolic. These complications and related management measures are presented in Table 8-5.

TOTAL PARENTERAL NUTRITION. Total parenteral nutrition (TPN) is indicated when oral intake or enteral feeding is inadequate to meet metabolic needs for more than 3 to 5 days and is most often used in the acute care setting. Other indications for TPN include conditions in which bowel rest is desirable or the gastrointestinal tract is nonfunctioning. The solutions are administered through a central line inserted into the superior vena cava via the subclavian or internal jugular vein, where a high rate of blood flow enables rapid dilution to avoid irritation of venous endothelium.

TPN solutions are prepared under aseptic conditions and individualized based on nutrient needs and laboratory tests. Nutrients provided include dextrose, amino acids, electrolytes, vitamins, minerals, and fat emulsions. Solutions are delivered at a continuous rate via an infusion pump to prevent metabolic complications. TPN infusion rates are gradually advanced to the desired caloric intake, allowing body adaptation, and gradually decreased before discontinuing therapy to avoid rebound hypoglycemia. Frequent monitoring of catheter patency and gastrointestinal and metabolic status is required with TPN (Williams & Schlenker, 2003).

Mechanical, metabolic, and sepsis complications can occur with TPN. These complications are mostly avoidable with proper care and well-defined protocols. Patients should be carefully monitored for signs of infection. In addition, monitoring of blood glucose and electrolytes should be ongoing.

Home enteral nutrition and TPN are now common modes of therapy for persons who do not need to be hospitalized but can benefit from continued nutritional support, such as older adults during chemotherapy or following head and neck or gastrointestinal surgeries, or recovering from acute pancreatitis. With adequate instruction and supportive follow-up, an older adult or caregiver can successfully manage enteral nutrition or TPN at home.

SUMMARY

Nurses have many opportunities to promote nutritional health in older adults. The growing body of knowledge about the impact of nutritional alterations in later life, along with improved and sophisticated methods of assessment and treatment, has expanded nutritional therapy into an interdisciplinary endeavor. To serve older adults best, nurses in all care settings should routinely conduct nutritional assessments and intervene when possible to promote optimal nutritional status.

Table 8-5 *Complications of Enteral Tube-Feeding*

Complication	Management
MECHANICAL Nasoparyngeal irritation	▪ Use the smallest pliable tube possible ▪ Provide nose and mouth care ▪ Monitor for nasopharyngeal bleeding and infection
TUBE OBSTRUCTION	▪ Flush tube with 30 to 60 ml warm water after each feeding, every 4 hours with continous feedings, and before and after medication administration ▪ Use liquid medications when possible; crush tablets and dissolve in 10 to 15 ml water before administration; do not mix medications with formula ▪ Use infusion pump for high-viscosity formula; switch formula ▪ Use pancreatic enzymes to break up an obstruction
ASPIRATION	▪ Keep head of bed elevated 30-45 degrees ▪ Check tube placement before feeding ▪ Use small-bore pliable feeding tubes to minimize gastropharyngeal relaxation ▪ Assess regularly for distention, residual volume of greater than 500 ml, bowel sounds
TUBE MIGRATION	▪ Stabilize the tube position appropriately ▪ Mark tube at insertion site; check marking before feeding ▪ Check abdominal tube insertion site for drainage ▪ Notify physician of signs of tube migration
INFECTION	▪ Clean abdominal tube insertion sites daily ▪ Stabilize the tube appropriately ▪ Monitor for local signs of skin infection
GASTROINTESTINAL Dry mouth	▪ Provide regular mouth care
DISTENTION/BLOATING	▪ Measure abdominal girth; assess regularly for distention, residual volume of greater than 500 ml, bowel sounds ▪ Keep tube clamped between intermittent feedings, remove air from delivery system before connection
NAUSEA, VOMITING	▪ Assess bowel sounds, check for distention and rigidity; measure abdominal girth ▪ Stop feeding and notify primary care provider ▪ Check residual
DIARRHEA (5 STOOLS/24 HOURS)	▪ Give formula at room temperature ▪ Prevent contamination of formula: wash hands, wear gloves, and use aseptic technique with formula preparation ▪ Hang formula no longer than recommended by manufacturer; change tubing every 24 hours ▪ Use a lactose-free formula or switch to a different formula ▪ Check placement of gastric tube for migration to small intestine ▪ Assess medications ▪ Obtain diagnostic studies, stool culture for *Clostridium difficile*
CONSTIPATION	▪ Use fiber-enriched formula ▪ Add free water if intake is not adequate ▪ Encourage ambulation and activity ▪ Monitor intake and output
METABOLIC Hyperglycemia	▪ Monitor for signs of hyperglycemia and infection ▪ Check blood glucose level and administer insulin as prescribed

Continued

Table 8-5 *Complications of Enteral Tube-Feeding—cont'd*	
Complication	**Management**
METABOLIC—*cont'd*	
Hyperglycemia—*cont'd*	■ Use infusion pump to ensure consistent flow rate ■ Reduce flow rate; change to lower calorie content
HYPOGLYCEMIA	■ Monitor for signs of hypoglycemia ■ Check glucose levels, notify physician
HYPERNATREMIA/DEHYDRATION	■ Monitor for signs of hypernatremia and dehydration ■ Monitor serum sodium, blood urea nitrogen, hematocrit, urine output ■ Assess medications ■ Increase fluid intake ■ Use lower-protein formula
HYPONATREMIA/OVERHYDRATION	■ Monitor for signs of hyponatremia and fluid overload ■ Monitor intake and output ■ Assess medications ■ Decrease free water to minimum of 30 to 50 ml ■ Change to more nutrient-dense formula

Sources: Chernoff, R. (2003). *Geriatric nutrition: The health professionals handbook*. Boston: Jones & Bartlett; Williams, S. R., & Schlenker, E. D. (2003). *Essentials of nutrition and diet therapy*. St. Louis: Mosby; Keithley, J. K., & Sanson, B. (2004). Enteral nutrition: An update on practice recommendations. *Medsurg Nursing, 13*(2), 131-134; Padula, C. A., Kenny, A., Planchon, C., & Lamoreux, C. (2004). Enteral feedings: What the evidence says. Avoid contamination of feedings and its sequelae with this research-based protocol. *American Journal of Nursing, 104*(7), 62-69; and Sanko, J. S. (2004). Aspiration assessment and prevention in critically ill enterally fed patients: Evidence-based recommendations for practice. *Gastroenterology Nursing, 27*(6), 279-285.

REFERENCES

Acheson, K. F. (2004). Carbohydrate and weight control: Where do we stand? *Current Opinion in Clinical Nutrition and Metabolic Care, 7*(4), 485-492.

Administration on Aging. (2004). A profile of older Americans: 2004. Retrieved July 10, 2005, from www.aoa.gov/prof/Statistics/profile/2004/profiles2004.asp.

Administration on Aging. (2005). Older Americans Act. Retrieved July 10, 2005, from www.aoa.gov/about/legbudg/oaa/legbudg_oaa.asp.

Alvarez-Fernandez, B., Garcia-Ordonez, M. A., Martinez-Manzanares, C., & Gomez-Huelgas, R. (2005). Survival of a cohort of elderly patients with advanced dementia: Nasogastric tube feeding as a risk factor for mortality. *International Journal of Geriatric Psychiatry, 20*(4), 363-370.

Amella, E. J. (2002). Resistance at mealtimes for persons with dementia. *Journal of Nutrition, Health and Aging, 6*(2), 117-122.

Amersbach, G. (1999). More water, more fiber, fewer calories: Reinventing the food pyramid for older adults. *Tufts Nutrition Magazine*. Retrieved July 10, 2005, from www.nutrition.tufts.edu/magazine/1999fall/pyramid.html.

Amosson, C., Teh, B., Van, T., Uy, N., Huang, E., Mai, W. Y., et al. (2003). Dosimetric predictors of xerostomia for head-and-neck cancer patients treated with the SMART (Simultaneous Modulated Accelerated Radiation Therapy) boost technique. *International Journal of Radiation Oncology, Biology, Physics, 56*, 1.

Arterburn, D. E., Crane, P. K., & Sullivan, S. D. (2004). The coming epidemic of obesity in elderly Americans. *Journal of the American Geriatrics Society, 52*, 1907-1912.

Atkins, R. C. (1998). *Dr. Atkins' new diet revolution*. New York: Avon Books.

Bailey, R. L., Ledikwe, J. H., Smiciklas-Wright, H., Mitchell, D. C., & Jensen, G. L. (2004). Persistent oral health problems associated with comorbidity and impaired diet quality in older adults. *Journal of the American Dietetic Association, 104*(8), 1273-1276.

Balsam, A. L., Sullivan, A. F., Millen, B. E., & Rogers, B. L. (2000). Service innovations in the elderly nutrition program: Two decades of accomplishments. *Journal of Nutrition for the Elderly, 19*(4), 41-48.

Baron, M. (2003). Is the NCS diet obsolete? *Health Care Food and Nutrition Focus, 20*(8), 1, 3-8.

Beattie, E. R., & Algase, D. L. (2002). Improving table-sitting behavior of wanderers via theoretic substruction: Designing an intervention. *Journal of Gerontological Nursing, 10*(6), 6-11.

Beck, A. M., Ovesen, L., & Schroll, M. (2001). Validation of the Resident Assessment Instrument triggers in the detection of undernutrition. *Age and Ageing, 30*, 161-165.

Bender, S., Pusateri, M., Cook, A., Ferguson, M., & Hall, J. C. (2000). Malnutrition: For prosthetic therapy. *Journal of Public Health Dentistry, 60*(4), 308-312.

Biggs, A., & Freed, P. E. (2000). Nutrition and older adults: What do family caregivers know and do? *Journal of Gerontological Nursing, 26*(8), 6-14.

Bohmer, H., Muller, H., & Resch, K. L. (2000). Calcium supplementation with calcium-rich mineral waters: A systematic review and meta-analysis of its bioavailability. *Osteoporosis International, 11*(11), 938-943.

Breier-Mackie, S. (2005). PEGs and ethics revisited: A timely reflection in the wake of the Terri Schiavo case. *Gastroenterology Nursing, 28*(4), 292-297.

Bronner, F. (2003). *Nutritional aspects and clinical management of chronic disorders and diseases*. Boca Raton, FL: CRC Press.

Castellanos, V. H., Butler, E., Gluch, L., & Burke, B. (2004). Use of thickened liquids in skilled nursing facilities. *Journal of the American Dietetic Association, 104*(8), 1222-1226.

Chapman, I., MacIntosh, C., Morley, J. E., & Horowitz, M. (2002). The anorexia of ageing. *Biogerontology, 3,* 67-71.

Chen, C. C., Schilling, L. S., & Lyder, C. H. (2001). A concept analysis of malnutrition in the elderly. *Journal of Advanced Nursing, 36*(1), 131-142.

Chernoff, R. (2003). *Geriatric nutrition: The health professionals handbook.* Boston: Jones & Bartlett.

Chidester, J. C., & Spangler, A. A. (1997). Fluid intake in the institutionalized elderly. *Journal of the American Dietetic Association, 97,* 23-28.

Choi, N., & Smith, J. (2004). Reaching out to racial/ethnic minority older persons for elderly nutrition programs. *Journal of Nutrition for the Elderly, 24*(1), 89-104.

Collins, N. (2004). Nutrition and wound healing: Strategies to improve patient outcomes. *Wounds, 16*(9, suppl), 12s-18s.

Crogan, N., Shultz, J. A., Adams, C. E., & Massey, L. K. (2001). Barriers to nutrition care for nursing home residents. *Journal of Gerontological Nursing, 27*(12), 25-31.

Crogan, N. L., Shultz, J. A., & Massey, L. K. (2001). Nutrition knowledge of nurses in long-term care facilities. *Journal of Continuing Education in Nursing, 32*(4), 171-176.

Crogar, N. L., & Pasvogel, A. (2003). The influence of protein-calorie malnutrition on quality of life in nursing homes. *Journals of Gerontology Series A: Biological Sciences and Medical Sciences, 58*(2), 159-164.

Crown, A. L., Cottle, K., Lightman, S. L., Falk, S., Mohamed-Ali, V., Armstrong, L., et al. (2002). What is the role of insulin-like growth factor system in pathophysiology of cancer cachexia and how is it regulated? *Clinical Endocrinology, 56*(6), 723-733.

Culp, K. R., Wakefield, B., Dyck, M. J., Cacchione, P. Z., DeCrane, S., & Decker, S. (2004). Bioelectrical impedence analysis and other hydration parameters as risk factors for delirium in rural nursing home residents. *Journals of Gerontology Series A: Biological and Medical Sciences, 59*(8), 813-817.

Damush, T. M., Smith, D. M., Perkins, A. J., Dexter, P. R., & Smith, F. (2004). Risk factors for nonelective hospitalization in frail and older adults, inner city outpatients. *Gerontologist, 44*(1), 68-75.

Dasgupta, M., Sharkey, J. R., & Wu, G. (2005). Inadequate intakes of indispensable amino acids among homebound older adults. *Journal of Nutrition for the Elderly, 24*(3), 85-99.

deJong, N., Gibson, R., Thomson, C. D., Ferguson, E. L., McKenzie, J. E., Gree, T. J., et al. (2001). Selenium and zinc status are suboptimal in a sample of older New Zealand women in a community-based study. *Journal of Nutrition, 131*(10), 2677-2684.

deJong, N., Green, T. J., Skeaff, C. M., Gibson, R., McKenzie, J. E., Ferguson, E. L., et al. (2003). Vitamin B-12 and folate status of older New Zealand women. *Asia Pacific Journal of Clinical Nutrition, 12*(1), 85-91.

Eggenberger, S. K., & Nelms, T. P. (2004). Artificial hydration and nutrition in advanced Alzheimer's disease: Facilitating family decision-making. *Journal of Clinical Nursing, 13*(6), 661-667.

Ellis, E., Johnson, M. A., Fischer, J. G., & Hargrove, J. L. (2005). Nutrition and health education intervention for whole grain foods in the Georgia older Americans nutrition programs. *Journal of Nutrition for the Elderly, 24*(3), 67-83.

Falciglia, G., O'Connor, J. O., & Gadling, E. (1988). Upper arm anthropometric norms in elderly white subjects. *Journal of the American Dietetic Association, 88*(5), 569-574.

Fleming, D. J., Tucker, K. L., Jacques, P. F., Dallal, G. E., Wilson, P. W. F., & Wood, R. J. (2002). Dietary factors associated with the risk of high iron stores in the elderly Framingham Heart Study cohort. *American Journal of Clinical Nutrition, 76*(6), 1375-1384.

Foster, G. D., Wyatt, H. R., Hill, J. O., Mcguuckin, B. G., Brill, C., Mohammed, B. S., et al. (2003). A randomized trial of a low-carbohydrate diet for obesity. *New England Journal of Medicine, 348*(21), 2082-2090.

Gallagher-Allred, C. R. (1993). *Implementing nutrition screening and intervention strategies.* Washington, DC: Nutrition Screening Intiative.

Gollub, E. A., & Weddle, D. O. (2004). Improvements in nutritional intake and quality of life among frail homebound older adults receiving home-delivered breakfast and lunch. *Journal of the American Dietetic Association, 104*(8), 1227-1235.

Guigoz, Y., Vellas, B., Garry, P. J. (1996). Assessing the nutritional status of the elderly: The Mini Nutritional Assessment as part of the geriatric assessment evaluation. *Nutritional Review, 54,* S59-S60.

Gulson, B. L., Mizen, K. J., Palmer, J. M., Korsch, M. J., & Taylor, A. J. (2001). Contribution of lead from calcium supplements to blood lead. *Environmental Health Perspectives, 109*(3), 283-288.

Guthrie, J. F., & Lin, B. H. (2002). Overview of the diets of lower- and higher-income elderly and their food assistance options. *Journal of Nutrition Education and Behavior, 34*(suppl 1), S31-41.

Heaney, R. P., Dowell, S., Bierman, J., Hale, C. A., & Bendich, A. (2001). Absorbability and cost effectiveness in calcium supplementation. *Journal of the American College of Nutrition, 20*(3), 239-246.

Heiat, A., Voaccarino, V., & Krumholz, H. M. (2001). An evidence-based assessment of the federal guidelines for obesity as they apply to elderly persons. *Archives of Internal Medicine, 161*(9), 1194-1203.

Heller, H. J., Poindexter, J. R., & Adams-Huet, B. (2002). Effect of estrogen treatment and vitamin D status on differing bioavailabilities of calcium carbonate and calcium citrate. *Journal of Clinical Pharmacology, 42*(11), 1251-1256.

Hendy, H., Nelson, G., & Greco, M. (1998). Social cognitive predictors of nutritional risk in rural elderly adults. *International Journal of Aging and Human Development, 47*(4), 299-327.

Holt, P., Wolper, C., Moss, S. F., Yang, K., & Lipkin, M. (2001). Comparison of calcium supplementation of low-fat dairy foods on epithelial proliferation and differentiation. *Nutrition and Cancer, 41,* 150-155.

Huang, E. S., Gorawara-Bhat, R., & Chin, M. H. (2004). Practical challenges of individualizing diabetes care in older patients. *Diabetes Educator, 30*(4), 558-570.

Huffman, G. B. (2002). Evaluating and treating unintentional weight loss in the elderly. *American Family Physician, 65*(4), 551-553.

Ina, L. (2002). Feeding tubes in patients with severe dementia. *American Family Physician, 65*(8), 1605-1609.

Iyer, P. (2004). Liability in the care of the elderly. *JOGNN, 33*(1), 124-131.

Jensen, L. B., Kollerup, G., Quaade, F., & Sorenson, O. H. (2001). Bone mineral changes in obese women during a moderate weight loss with and without calcium supplementation. *Journal of Bone and Mineral Research, 16*(1), 141-147.

Johnson, L. E. (2002). Nutrition. In R. J. Ham, P. D. Sloane, & G. A. Warshaw (Eds.), *Primary care geriatrics: A case-based approach* (4th ed.). St. Louis: Mosby.

Kaczkowski, C. H., Jones, P. J., Feng, J., & Bayley, H. S. (2000). Four-day multimedia diet records underestimate energy needs in middle-aged and elderly women as determined by doubly-labeled water. *Journal of Nutrition, 130*(4), 802-805.

Karkkainen, M. U., Lamberg-Allardt, C. J., Ahonen, S., & Valimaki, M. (2001). Does it make a difference how and when you take your calcium? *American Journal of Clinical Nutrition, 74*(3), 335-342.

Kayser-Jones, J., & Pengilly, K. (1999). Dysphagia among nursing home residents. *Geriatric Nursing, 20*(2), 77-82.

Kayser-Jones, J., Schell, E. S., Porter, C., Barbaccia, J. C., & Shaw, H. (1999). Factors contributing to dehydration in nursing homes: Inadequate staffing and lack of professional supervision. *Journal of the American Geriatrics Society, 47*(10), 1187-1194.

Kee, J., & Hayes, E. (2003). *Pharmacology: A nursing process approach.* Philadelphia: W. B. Saunders.

Keithley, J. K., & Sanson, B. (2004). Enteral nutrition: An update on practice recommendations. *Medsurg Nursing, 13*(2), 131-134.

Kenny, A., Prestwood, K., Biskup, B., Robbins, B., Zayas, E., Kleppinger, A., et al. (2004). Comparison of the effects of calcium loading with calcium citrate or calcium carbonate on bone turnover in post-menopausal women. *Osteoporosis International, 15*(4), 290-294.

Kiernan, M., & Winkleby, M. A. (2000). Identifying patients for weight-loss treatment: An empirical evaluation of the NHLBI obesity education initiative expert panel treatment recommendations. *Archives of Internal Medicine, 160*(14), 2169-2176.

Kim, M., Kim, C., & Song, I. (2003). Analysis of lead in 55 brands of dietary calcium supplements by graphite furnace atomic absorption spectrometry after microwave digestion. *Food Additives and Contaminants, 20*(2), 149-153.

Klesges, L. M., Pahor, M., Shorr, R. I., Wan, J. Y., Williamson, J. D., & Guralnick, J. M. (2001). Financial difficulty in acquiring food among elderly disabled women: Results from the women's health and aging study. *American Journal of Public Health, 91*(1), 68-75.

Krondl, M., Lau, D., Coleman, P., & Stocker, G. (2003). Tailoring of nutritional support for older adults in the community. *Journal of Nutrition for the Elderly, 23*(2), 17-32.

Lauque, S., Arnaud-Battandier, F., Mansourian, R., Guigoz, Y., Paintin, M., Nourhashemi, F., et al. (2000). Protein-energy oral supplementation in malnourished nursing-home residents: A controlled trial. *Age and Ageing, 29*(1), 51-56.

Lohman, J., Martorell, R., & Roche, A. F. (1988). *Anthropometric standardization reference manual.* Champaign, IL: Human Kinetics.

Manthorpe, J., & Watson, R. (2003). Poorly served? Eating and dementia. *Journal of Advanced Nursing, 41*(2), 162-169.

Marik, J. P. E., & Kaplan, D. (2003). Aspiration pneumonia and dysphagia in the elderly. *Chest, 124*(1), 328-336.

McCloskey, J. C., & Bulechek, G. M. (1996). *Nursing intervention classification (NIC): Iowa intervention project* (2nd ed.). St. Louis: Mosby.

Metheny, N. A. (2004, Fall). Preventing aspiration in older adults with dysphagia. *Best Practices in Nursing Care to Older Adults.* The Hartford Institute for Geriatric Nursing. Retrieved September, 19, 2005, from *www.hartfordign.org/publications/trythis/issue_20.pdf.*

Metheny, N. A., & Meert, K. L. (2004). Monitoring feeding tube placement. *Nutrition in Clinical Practice, 19*(5), 487-495, 542.

Metheny, N. A., & Titler, M. G. (2001). Assessing placement of feeding tubes. *American Journal of Nursing, 101*(5), 36-45.

Mitchell, M. (2003). *Nutrition across the lifespan.* Philadelphia: W. B. Saunders.

Mitchell, S., Buchanan, J. L., Littlehale, S., & Hamel, M. B. (2003). Tube-feeding versus hand-feeding nursing home residents with advanced dementia: A cost comparison. *Journal of American Medical Directors Association, 4*(1), 27-33.

Morley, J., Glick, Z., & Rubenstein, L. (1995). *Geriatric nutrition: A comprehensive review.* New York: Raven Press.

Morley, J. E., Thomas, D. R., & Kamel, H. (2004). Nutritional deficiencies in long-term care. *Supplement to Annals of Long-Term Care, 6*(5), 183-191.

Morton, D. J., Barrett-Connor, E. L., & Schneider, D. L. (2001). Vitamin C supplement use and bone mineral density in postmenopausal women. *Journal of Bone and Mineral Research, 16*(1), 135-140.

Murphy, C., Schubert, C. R., Cruickshanks, K., Klein, B. E., Klein, R., & Nondahl, D. (2002). Prevalence of olfactory impairment in older adults. *JAMA, 288*(18), 2307-2312.

National Academy of Sciences. (2004a). Dietary Reference Intakes (DRIs): Recommended intakes for individual, vitamins. Retrieved July 10, 2005, from www.iom.edu/Object.File/Master/21/372/0.pdf.

National Academy of Sciences. (2004b). Dietary Reference Intakes (DRIs): Recommended intakes for individual, elements. Retrieved July 10, 2005, from www.iom.edu/Object.File/Master/21/372/0.pdf.

National Osteoporosis Foundation. (1999). Calcium supplements. Retrieved July 10, 2005, from www.nof.org/prevention/calcium_supplements.htm.

Nordenram, G., Ljunggren, G., & Cederholm, T. (2001). Nutritional status and chewing capacity in nursing home residents. *Aging: Clinical and Experimental Research, 13*(5), 370-377.

Nordin, S., Razani, L. J., Markison, S., & Murphy, C. (2003). Age-associated increases in intensity discrimination for taste. *Experimental Aging Research, 29*(3), 371-381.

Office of Disease Prevention and Health Promotion. (2004). *Healthy people 2010.* Retrieved July 10, 2005, from www.healthypeople.gov/About/.

Padula, C. A., Kenny, A., Planchon, C., & Lamoreux, C. (2004). Enteral feedings: What the evidence says. Avoid contamination of feedings and its sequelae with this research-based protocol. *American Journal of Nursing, 104*(7), 62-69.

Payette, H., Boutier, V., Coulombe, C., & Gray-Donald, K. (2002). Benefits of nutritional supplementation in free-living, frail, under-nourished elderly people: A prospective randomized community trial. *Journal of the American Dietetic Association, 102*(8), 1088-1095.

Porock, D., Oliver, D. P., Zweig, S., Rantz, M., Mehr, D., Madsen, B., et al. (2005). Predicting death in the nursing home: Development and validation of the 6-month Minimum Data Set mortality risk index. *Journals of Gerontology Series A: Biological Sciences and Medical Sciences, 60*(4), 491-498.

Posthauer, M. E. (2005). Hydration: An essential element. *Advances in Skin and Wound Care, 18*(1), 32-33.

Potter, J. M., Roberts, M. A., McColl, J. H., & Reilly, J. J. (2001). Protein energy supplements in unwell elderly patients—a randomized controlled trial. *Journal of Parenteral and Enteral Nutrition, 25*(6), 323-329.

Rantz, M. J., & Zwygart-Stauffacher, M. (2004). Back to the fundamentals of care: A roadmap to improve nursing home care quality. *Journal of Nursing Care Quality, 19*(2), 92-94.

Ravasco, P., Monteiro-Grillo, I., & Camilo, M. E. (2003). Does nutrition influence quality of life in cancer patients undergoing radiotherapy? *Radiotherapy and Oncology, 67*(2), 213-220.

Reuben, D. B., Herr, K., Pacala, J. T., Pollock, B. G., Potter, J. F., & Semla, T. P. (2005). *Geriatrics at your fingertips.* New York: American Geriatrics Society.

Roberts, H. J. (2000). Lead in calcium supplements. *JAMA, 284*(24), 3126.

Robinson, S. B., & Rosher, R. B. (2002). Can a beverage cart help improve hydration? *Geriatric Nursing, 23*(4), 208-211.

Rosenbloom, C. A., Kicklighter, J. R., Patacca, D., & Deshpande, K. (2004). Nutrition education in six congregate meal sites improves participants' nutrition knowledge. *Journal of Nutrition for the Elderly, 23*(3), 73-83.

Ross, E. A., Szabo, N. J., & Tebbett, I. R. (2000). Lead content of calcium supplements. *Journal of the American Medical Association, 284*(11), 1425-1429.

Russell, R. M. (2002). The aging process as a modifier of metabolism. *American Journal of Clinical Nutrition, 72*(suppl), 529S-532S.

Sanko, J. S. (2004). Aspiration assessment and prevention in critically ill enterally fed patients: Evidence-based recommendations for practice. *Gastroenterology Nursing, 27*(6), 279-285.

Sardesai, V. M. (2003). *Introduction to clinical nutrition.* New York: Marcel Dekker.

Schiffman, S., Zervakis, J., Westall, H., Graham, B., Metz, A., Bennett, J. L., et al. (2000a). Effect of antimicrobials and anti-inflammatory medications on the sense of taste. *Physiology and Behavior, 69*(4-5), 413-424.

Schiffman, S. S., Zervakis, J., Suggs, M. S., Budd, K. C., & Iuga, L. (2000b). Effect of tricyclic antidepressants on taste response in humans and gerbils. *Pharmacology, Biochemistry and Behavior, 65*(4), 599-609.

Schindler, J. S., & Kelly, J. H. (2002). Swallowing disorders in the elderly. *Laryngoscope, 112,* 589-602.

Shanahan, T. K., Logemann, J. A., Rademaker, A. W., Pauloski, B. R., & Kahrlas, P. J. (1993). Chin-down posture effect on aspiration in dysphasic patients. *Archives of Physical Medicine and Rehabilitation, 74*(7), 736-739.

Sharkey, J. R., Branch, L. G., Zohoori, N., Guiliani, C., Busby-Whitehead, J., & Haines, P.S. (2002). Inadequate nutrient intakes among homebound elderly and their correlation with individual characteristics and health-related factors. *American Journal of Clinical Nutrition, 76*(6), 1435-1445.

Sherer, R. A. (2000). Focusing on the nutritional needs of older Americans. *Geriatric Times, 1*(2), 1-5.

Shimizu, M. E., Otsuka, A., Kanai, S., & Oki, S. (2004). The therapeutic effects of independent eating for severely physically disabled. *Journal of Physical Therapy Science, 16*(2), 73-79.

Simmons, S. F., Alessi, C., & Schnelle, J. F. (2001). An intervention to increase fluid intake in nursing home residents: Prompting and preference compliance. *Journal of the American Geriatrics Society, 49*(7), 926-933.

Simmons, S. F., & Reuben, D. (2000). Nutritional intake monitoring for nursing home residents: A comparison of staff documentation, direct observation, and photography methods. *Journal of the American Geriatrics Society, 48*, 209-213.

Smith, C. H. (1999). Drug-food/drug-drug interactions. In J. E. Morley, Z. Glick, and L. Z. Rubenstein (Eds.), *Geriatric nutrition: A comprehensive review.* New York: Raven.

Stanner, S. (2003). Preparing food and assisting clients at mealtimes. *Nursing and Residential Care, 5*(2), 56-62.

Steen, B. (2004). Maximizing outcome of dementia care: The role of nutrition. *Archives of Gerontology and Geriatrics, Suppl 9*, 413-417.

Stotts, N. A., & Hopf, H. W. (2003). The link between tissue oxygenation and hydration in nursing home residents with pressure ulcers: Preliminary data. *Journal of Wound, Ostomy and Continence Nursing, 30*(4), 184-190.

Strakowski, M. M., Strakowski, J. A., & Mitchell, M. C. (2002). Malnutrition in rehabilitation. *American Journal of Physical Medicine and Rehabilitation, 81*(1), 77-78.

Sturm, K., MacIntosh, C., Parker, B., Wishart, J., Horowitz, M., & Chapman, I. (2003). Appetite, food intake, and plasma concentrations of cholecystokinin, ghrelin, and other gastrointestinal hormones in undernourished older women and well-nourished younger and older women. *Journal of Clinical Endocrinology and Metabolism, 88*(8), 3747-3755.

Swann, J. (2005). Food for thought: Providing solutions to feeding problems. *Nursing and Residential Care, 7*(3), 118-121.

Thomas, D. R. (2002). Dietary prescription for chronic obstructive pulmonary disease. *Clinics in Geriatric Medicine, 18*(4), 835-839.

Thomas, D. R., Kamel, H. K., & Morley, J. E. (2004). Management of protein energy malnutrition and dehydration. *Supplement to Annals of Long-Term Care, 6*(8), 250-258.

Tougas, G., Eaker, E., Abell, T., Abrahamsson, H., Boivin, M., Chen, J., et al. (2000). Assessment of gastric emptying using a low fat mean: Establishment of international control values. *American Journal of Gastroenterology, 95*(6), 1456-1462.

U.S. Department of Agriculture. (2005a). My pyramid. Retrieved July 10, 2005, from www.mypyramid.gov.

U.S. Department of Agriculture. (2005b). *Dietary guidelines for Americans.* Retrieved July 10, 2005, from www.health.gov/dietaryguidelines/.

van der Steen, J. T., Ooms, M. E., Mehr, D. R., van der Wal, G., & Ribbe, M. W. (2002). Severe dementia and adverse outcomes of nursing home-acquired pneumonia: Evidence for mediation by functional and pathophysiological decline. *Journal of American Geriatrics Society, 50*(3), 439-448.

Walls, A. W., Steele, J. G., Sheiham, A., Marcenes, W., & Moynihan, P. J. (2000). Oral health and nutrition in older people. *Journal of Public Health Dentistry, 60*(4), 304-307.

Walsh, G. (2005). Hypodermoclysis: An alternative method for rehydration in long-term care. *Journal of Infusion Nursing, 28*(2), 123-129.

Weatherspoon, L. J., Worthen, H., & Handu, D. (2004). Nutrition risk and associated factors in congregate meal participants in northern Florida: Role of Elder Care Services. *Journal of Nutrition for the Elderly, 24*(2), 37-54.

Westergren, A., Karlsson, S., Andersson, P., Ohlsson, O., & Hallberg, I. (2001). Eating difficulties, need for assisted eating, nutritional status and pressure ulcers in patients admitted for stroke rehabilitation. *Journal of Clinical Nursing, 10*(2), 257-269.

Westerterp, K. R., & Goris, A. H. C. (2002). Validity of the assessment of dietary intake: Problem of misreporting. *Current Opinion in Clinical Nutrition and Metabolic Care, 5*(5), 489-493.

Williams, C. P., Child, D. F., Hudson, P. R., Davies, M. G., John, R., Anandaram, P. S., et al. (2001). Why oral calcium supplements may reduce renal stone disease: Report of a clinical pilot study. *Journal of Clinical Pathology, 54*(1), 54-62.

Williams, S. R., & Schlenker, E. D. (2003). *Essentials of nutrition and diet therapy.* St. Louis: Mosby.

Wilson, M. M., & Morley, J. E. (2003). Invited review: Aging and energy balance. *Journal of Applied Physiology, 95*(4), 1728-1736.

Wouters-Wesseling, W., Van Hooijdonk, C., Wagenaar, L., Bindels, J., de Groot, L., & Van Staveren, W. (2003). The effect of liquid nutrition supplement on body composition and physical functioning in elderly people. *Clinical Nutrition, 22*(4), 371-377.

Xiao, H., Barber, J., & Campbell, E. S. (2004). Economic burden of dehydration among hospitalized elderly patients. *American Journal of Health-System Pharmacy, 61*(23), 2534-2540.

Zembrzuski, C. D. (2003). Try this: Nutrition and hydration. *Best Practice in Nursing Care to Older Adults, Hartford Institute for Geriatric Nursing, 15*(5), 475-476.

Chapter 9

Ethical Considerations

Kathleen T. Lucke

Objectives

Define and describe professional ethics and ethical
dilemmas related to nursing care of older adults.

Employ ethical models and principles as frameworks for
ethical decision making in gerontological nursing.

Use specific processes and techniques to promote ethical
decision making in the care of older patients.

Relate community and societal ethical problems, such as
rationing of services, euthanasia, and rights of
institutionalized patients, to standards of nursing care of
the older adults.

Analyze individual and family ethical dilemmas and
formulate appropriate nursing care measures.

THE NURSE'S RESPONSIBILITY FOR ETHICAL ACTION

Nursing is the protection, promotion, and optimization of
health and abilities, prevention of illness and injury, alleviation of suffering through the diagnosis and treatment of
human response, and advocacy in the care of individuals, families, communities, and populations. (American Nurses
Association [ANA], 2003)

Nursing is fundamentally a moral endeavor. Our social
contract requires that each person be treated with dignity
and that nurses work to improve the health of people.
This moral imperative becomes increasingly challenging as the problems facing society and health care
become ever more complex: aging of the population,
burgeoning chronic illness, increased technology,
declining resources, widening economic and health disparities, and globalization of health. It is essential that
advanced practice nurses possess the requisite ethical
knowledge and skills to be leaders in shaping health
policy to address these issues in the local, national, and
international arenas.

The collision of three factors in particular creates
unique ethical challenges for gerontological nurses

today. An aging population, coupled with our rapidly
expanding biological and technological knowledge and
widening gulf of access to and resources for health care
among segments of society, poses quandaries never
before experienced in society. It is now possible to identify and replace defective body parts with hardware or
cells that can extend life. At the same time, it is also possible to prematurely end life. Nurses must ensure that
patients, families, communities, and policymakers have
the necessary knowledge to make informed decisions.
Nurses must also be committed to partnering with marginalized groups to empower them to have their voices
heard at all levels of society to shape a more responsive
health care system.

Ethics Defined

Ethics is the reflective, deliberative process of examining
our values and beliefs and choosing a course of action
that upholds those values. The study of ethics provides
the philosophical underpinnings and language to systematically analyze issues faced by nurses today. An
increasingly diverse society, interdisciplinary health care
decision making, and burgeoning legislation with growing complexity require nurses to skillfully participate in
dialogue with patients, families, colleagues, communities, and legislators about the multitude of issues facing
health care today. To participate in the discourse, nurses
need to have a deep appreciation and discernment of
their own values and beliefs, the theories and concepts
used, relevant cultural nuances, and the values and
motivation of the other parties involved.

Racial and ethnic diversity continues to increase at a
rapid pace in the United States. Nurses must recognize the
implications of this growing cultural diversity. Cultural
knowledge, sensitivity, competence, and proficiency are
prerequisites for the nurse to provide respect and dignity
to patients and families. This poses special challenges
for gerontological nurses because many elderly family
members from other cultures continue to hold their values and beliefs dear. The nurse must recognize that the

values of the dominant culture may not be congruent with those of other cultures. For example, individual self-determination regarding health care decision making, a standard to which we aspire, may not be compatible across cultural boundaries. In many cultures, decision making involves the entire family, which includes extended family members. Careful reflection can elucidate the basis of one's own moral values and beliefs and provide a foundation for openness to other perspectives and serve to initiate meaningful dialogue. This iterative process of critical reflection and thoughtful dialogue engenders nursing practice that communicates authentic respect for the dignity of those we encounter from multiple diverse backgrounds.

Decision making in the current health care environment is no longer singular. In many cases, a team of health care professionals contributes to the care of patients. Improved health outcomes result from interdisciplinary collaboration. However, each team member brings his or her own professional values and codes of ethics, as well as his or her own personal moral beliefs, to the encounter. As patient advocates, nurses serve in central roles coordinating care and fostering collaboration among team members to achieve the desired outcomes. This often requires thoughtful deliberation and skillful communication with the patient, family, and team members. Personal awareness, professional integrity, and sensitivity to the values of others will contribute to successful navigation of these often ethically troubling issues.

Today legislation is placing constraints on health care environments and consumers at an ever-increasing rate. Often legislation is crafted with special interests in mind, with little time for input or awareness on the part of consumers or health care professionals. Many times laws impose further hardships on already marginalized or vulnerable populations seeking health care. In addition, health care professionals are often left with the challenge of attempting to provide care with fewer resources and less time. Gerontological nurses must remain informed and recognize that legal and ethical practice may not always be congruent. Many times the law guides ethical practice; sometimes ethical dilemmas serve as the impetus for new legislation, because ethical standards and codes often exceed the law. Nurses must always strive to provide a professional level of care that is consistent with personal and professional ethical and practice standards while challenging the system to meet the moral ideal of being responsive to the health care needs of all people.

Nursing Ethics

Nursing ethics is systematic analysis of ethical issues emanating from nursing practice, education, and research. Situated within the larger context of the discipline of bioethics, nursing ethics encompasses the values, standards, and ideals of the profession. Nursing ethics is the core of professional integrity in the practice of nursing.

The evolution of nursing ethics is stimulated by forces in the health care environment, maturity of a distinct nursing philosophy, and emerging significance of relational and narrative ethics within the discipline of bioethics. The discipline of nursing ethics is the study of (1) the foundational values of nursing, (2) their philosophical underpinnings, (3) ethical theories, (4) moral principles, (5) common ethical problems, and (6) analytical frameworks for resolution of ethical quandaries in nursing. Each is discussed in this chapter.

Foundational Values. Historically, foundational values of nursing ethics include holistic care, virtue, respect for the dignity of persons, caring relationships, a commitment to the most vulnerable populations, and an obligation to improve the health of people. Beginning in 1859, Nightingale (1859, 1992) described nursing as encompassing the whole person, well or ill, including the environment in which the person is situated. Inherent in the holistic conception of nursing is moral practice that embodies the art and science of nursing. Each nurse acts as a moral agent when applying aesthetic, empirical, personal, and ethical knowledge (Carper, 1978), as well as political knowledge, to meet the unique needs of patients, families, or communities (Heath, 1998; White, 1995).

The character of the nurse holds the highest importance in nursing ethics. Nightingale alluded to the moral nature of the profession of nursing by noting that it should be considered a "calling" (Gadow, 1999; Jameton, 1984; Rodney et al., 2002). According to Henderson (1982, p. 30), "Ethics involves clarifying one's own idea: Who I ought to be, as a nurse: What is my commitment to my patient? The fundamental issue of who the nurse is precedes the issue of what the nurse does." The quality of the character of the moral agent, in part, determines the quality of the decisions made. As moral agents, nurses are required to possess the highest ethical standards and ideals to make the best possible decisions.

Watson (1985) characterizes the moral ideal of nursing practice as caring. The ideal nurse-patient interaction is embedded in a caring relationship (Erlen, 2002; Lucke, 1999). Attention to the contextual elements and individual nuances discerned through connectedness with others distinguishes caring from more traditional objective, distanced professional relationships. Moral discernment with accompanying responsibility and responsiveness can liberate nurses from the constraints of impersonal detachment. Nursing practice that is committed to the caring ideal results in patient outcomes more congruent with the patient's values because of the insights gained from a deep understanding of the patient's needs and goals.

Because nursing arose from a strong commitment to the needs of the most vulnerable populations, this obligation remains central to the profession. Nursing is steadfast in its dedication to improve the health of people through advocacy, empowerment, and political activism (Drevdahl, Kneipp, Canales, & Dorcy, 2001; White, 1995). Partnerships formed with patients, families, and communities help ensure that nurses impart the necessary knowledge and skills to members of the community to act on their own behalf to attain their desired outcomes. Ethical care often involves rule bending by nurses to provide care in a health care system that is frequently unresponsive and inflexible concerning the needs of those with the greatest health disparities (Lucke, 1999).

Respect for the inherent dignity of each person is the fundamental guiding principle of nursing ethics (ANA, 2001). Valuing the uniqueness and intrinsic worth of each human being is the fundamental belief and expectation in nursing. Two assumptions flow from the value of respect for persons in nursing: human beings are self-determining and humans are relational beings.

Philosophical Underpinnings.
The philosophical basis of nursing is now explored. Respect for persons is an underlying principle in nursing ethics; this principle forms the basis of the ANA Code of Ethics (2001) and is based on three philosophical perspectives. First is the notion put forward by Kant (Volbrecht, 2002) that persons must be treated as valuable in themselves. A unique feature of being human is the ability to reason, that is, rational will, self-determination, or the ability to freely choose a path in life. The capacity for determining the course of one's life must be allowed to flourish in each person. A second philosophical perspective is that of liberty. Each person is free to choose an individual course of action, without interference from others, except when those actions interfere with another's liberty or freedom. Respect for the uniqueness of persons is grounded in a third philosophical view, that of equality or justice. This perspective requires that no distinction in treatment between persons exist, except when based on *morally* relevant grounds.

Existentialist philosophy forms the basis for the belief that humans exist in relationship with others. In this conception of being human, the discovery of meaning occurs in the context of an open, engaged dialogue between persons. Our basic humanity involves uncovering meaning in our experiences with others (Gadow, 1999). These philosophical perspectives, which form the foundation of the deep respect for people held by nurses, necessitate that all people participate in decision making, to the extent possible, in a way that supports their values, beliefs, needs, and expectations (Cameron, 2003).

Authentic caring, the moral imperative of nursing, embraces nursing practice that fosters self-determined choices, enhances desired quality of life, and advocates for those who do not have a voice or are disenfranchised.

Gerontological nurses should be knowledgeable of different ethical theories that can be used to assist with ethical reasoning. Nurses also need to recognize that values of the patient, family, and members of the health care team may differ, which contributes to complexity of ethical decision making. Familiarity with the ethical literature is essential to remain current in the ethical deliberation involved in today's complex health care decisions.

Traditional Ethical Theories.
Ethics as a discipline dates back to the time of Hippocrates (Volbrecht, 2002). Bioethics, however, has a fairly recent history in the United States. The discipline of ethics is historically rooted in philosophy and theology. As Western thought developed, there was interest in discerning right thought and conduct to guide society and individuals. Four major theories have been developed to guide the process of decision making about what is right or best: duty-based ethics, or deontology; goal-based ethics, or utilitarianism; virtue ethics; and social justice. More recent is the development of relational or care ethics (Table 9-1).

DUTY-BASED ETHICAL THEORY. Duty-based, or deontological, ethical theory was largely shaped by the work of the eighteenth-century philosopher, Immanuel Kant (Erlen, 2002). There are two major tenets of Kant's theory. The first of Kant's tenets is based on his belief that human beings have free will that is grounded in reason. Because people have rational powers they have a moral obligation, or duty, to perform the right action. Accepted moral rules form the basis for right actions, which are freely chosen and justified, based on our obligations to mankind. Further, these moral rules are generalizable across situations; that is, the same rule applies to situations that have similar circumstances (Botes, 2000).

A second major tenet of Kant's theory is that every person should be treated as an end and never as a means only (Erlen, 2002). This means that, whenever possible, we should avoid treating another solely as a means to our ends. To the extent possible, people should exercise choice and maintain control over their lives. In research where study participants are in fact a means to an end (that is, a means to gain knowledge to improve the care or outcomes for future patients), they should always be treated with respect and dignity, harm should be minimized, and they should participate only on a voluntary basis.

Several duties must be upheld by nurses in the care of the elderly: autonomy, beneficence, nonmaleficence,

Table 9-1 *Ethical Theories and Moral Principles*

Theory/Principle	Description
THEORIES	
Duty-based ethics (deontology)	Human beings have a duty to do the moral or right thing for others
Goal-based ethics (utilitarian)	Focuses on the outcome of providing the greatest good for the greatest number of people
Virtue ethics	Moral character of the individual determines the right course
Social justice	Moral imperative is to act for equal distribution of benefits and burdens among others
Relational or care ethics	Actions are based on a caring relationship and anticipated to meet the individual goals and needs of others
PRINCIPLES	
Right to quality health care	Adequate access to quality health care for all
Respect for the individual person	Respect for others as individuals
Autonomy or self-determination	Individuals have the right to make decisions about their own care
Confidentiality	Respect for privacy of personal information
Beneficence	Doing the best thing to maximize benefits and minimize harm
Distributive justice	Equal treatment and allocation of resources

justice, confidentiality, privacy, fidelity, and veracity. In addition, nurses have duties to the profession, to their colleagues, and to society. At any one time it may be difficult to balance multiple competing duties.

In its application to the care of the elderly, a duty-based approach to ethics requires that each person be treated with respect and dignity by fully participating in decision making regarding his or her care, based on the individual's values, beliefs, goals, expectations, and desires. When the capacity for full participation in decision making is limited, family members, the health care team, or other surrogate decision makers must try to respect the intentions of the elderly person to the extent possible or to the extent they are known. A right or wrong action is judged by the duties upheld in the provision of care and the degree to which these are consistent with similar situations in the past or future.

There are three major criticisms of the duty-based approach to ethical decision making. First, there may be multiple competing duties that simultaneously apply in a situation. Second, how these duties are prioritized may differ between individual practitioners. And third, generalizing to other situations often leads to the contextual nuances of particular circumstances being ignored.

GOAL-BASED ETHICAL THEORY. In contrast to the duty-based approach to ethical problems, a goal-based or utilitarian approach to ethical decision making focuses on the outcome or consequences of an action. Based primarily on the work of Jeremy Bentham and John Stuart Mill (Erlen, 2002), this ethical theory relies on the single ethical principle of utility. This guide to action demands that the right outcome is one that results in the greatest good for the greatest number. In other words, the right course of action is one that creates the best overall outcomes.

Applied to a practice situation, a goal-based ethical theory would support a plan of care that maximizes benefit and minimizes harm in the care of the elderly. A utilitarian or goal-based approach to ethical decision making could also support decisions that result in the best outcomes for all involved, such as the elderly person and his or her family caregiver. Although the code of ethics indicates that the primary responsibility of the nurse is to the patient, this often includes the patient's family members, who may provide care or pay for the care of their elderly family member.

Several criticisms of the goal-based approach to ethical decision making are presented. Because our society values individual self-determination, consequentialist ethical reasoning is criticized for placing the needs of the individual secondary to those of a group. Another criticism is that it is often difficult for those involved to determine a single goal or to agree on one goal. Additionally, we may not be able to accurately predict outcomes, thereby making the selection of a goal difficult or the desired outcome potentially not achievable.

VIRTUE ETHICS. Since the time of Aristotle, moral virtues have been esteemed. Virtue ethics addresses the character of the nurse or health care provider. Until the 1960s the ANA Code of Ethics largely addressed the moral character of the nurse and was based primarily on virtue ethics. In this conception of ethics, the motivation to pursue the right action comes from within the nurse, based on the nurse's moral character. Today, a virtuous nurse is expected to be compassionate, trustworthy, conscientious, and courageous, as well as possess integrity and discernment (Beauchamp & Childress, 2001).

One of the major criticisms of virtue ethics is that what is valued in the moral character of the nurse varies with time and culture. For example, in the early part of the twentieth century, when the role of women in society was viewed as subservient, virtues reflective of the passive or "handmaiden" role were valued. Another criticism is that an ethical theory that addresses the moral character of the individuals in the profession does not necessarily serve as a guide to ethical decision making. Last, strictly adhering to moral virtues without using judgment can lead to wrong actions or outcomes despite laudable motivations.

SOCIAL JUSTICE. A theory of social justice was developed in the twentieth century by John Rawls. Social justice refers to the equal distribution of the benefits and burdens of society. That is, members of society should share in both the benefits and burdens such as education and health care (Drevdahl et al., 2001). However, tremendous health disparities exist today for segments of society. Nurses have a moral imperative to improve the health of all people; this requires that efforts be undertaken to address the inequities that exist in health care and access to health care.

With the aging of society and diminishing financial resources, social justice seems like an elusive ideal. Older adults in particular are vulnerable to inequities in health care because of fixed incomes and mobility problems, which may limit accessibility. Nurses must work to eliminate health disparities for this age group and others in order to improve health outcomes and enhance quality of life.

RELATIONAL OR CARE ETHICS. An ethic of care developed from the work of Gilligan (1993), Noddings (2003), and other feminist ethicists. Because caring is a value in nursing, nursing philosophers and ethicists were also major contributors to the development of an ethic of care, or *relational ethics* (Benner, 1994; Gadow, 1999). Although not as well developed as other ethical theories, care ethic is evolving as a contrast to the objective, distanced, principled approach. Relationships and context are central to an ethic of care. As with other ethical theories, respect for persons is foundational. Responsiveness to the other and mutual responsibility are the hallmarks of care ethics. Within the nurse-patient relationship, the nurse is responsive and attentive to the needs and goals of the patient; each has a responsibility in the relationship to work toward the patient's desired goals. From this connected relationship, reciprocity occurs for both the nurse and patient; that is, both derive benefit from the relationship.

Several major criticisms of care ethics are found. First, deep, committed relationships with patients may result in the nurse becoming self-sacrificing. Second, if the nurse is not truly open to listening to the patient's goals and expectations, the nurse's actions or plan could become paternalistic. Finally, the feasibility of an ethic of care in an era of a nursing shortage, diminishing resources, and an aging population is challenging.

Moral Principles Applicable to Care of Older Adults.
Some moral principles that undergird standards of care for older people include the following:

(1) the right to quality health care, (2) respect for the personhood of the aged, (3) the principle of autonomy or self-determination, (4) confidentiality, (5) the principle of beneficence, and (6) the principle of distributive justice (see Table 9-1). Application of each principle to care of the elderly is discussed next.

THE RIGHT TO QUALITY HEALTH CARE. A major challenge facing not only older adults in the United States is whether there is a general right to health care. Two major routes to health care services are based on the ability to pay or services for which one qualifies, which include Medicare, Medicaid, and military or veterans' benefits. Debate continues in the United States about what constitutes a minimal level of health care, as well as what if any component of health care is a right, and what is a privilege. According to Callahan (2002, p. 885),

> the drive for new knowledge and the technological application...become(s) the source of ever worsening cost pressures and eventually pose a threat to the equitable distribution of health care. This argument...could turn out to be a source of serious problems...to those who think all of life must be downhill if not constantly getting better.

The right to quality health care for older adults means that they have adequate access to quality care. Practically speaking, this means that older citizens have a right to the same high standards of health care as those in any other age-group. For example, older individuals have a right to complete evaluation of a problem, information on treatment options, and participation in the decision making about the best course of treatment. If a terminally ill patient develops a new problem, the health care team, including the patient, may elect not to assess the problem using invasive techniques. However, the decision to elect a less aggressive course of assessment and treatment should not be based on age alone, or mean that quality of care should be compromised.

The prevailing standard of health care for older people in the United States is based on an inadequate understanding of the aging process and their care needs. Current inadequacies of the U.S. health care system for the aged are well known. Problems regarding high-quality health care pervade acute, long-term, and community care, although the nature of the problem in each setting is somewhat different. In acute care, the primary problems are expense, lack of expert care, the difficulties of obtaining individualized care despite great expense, and the difficulty of retaining personal autonomy in the hospital (Callahan, 2002). Abuses, as well as the poor standard of care, in nursing homes have been well documented for many years. The problems of care at home include inadequate intensity of rehabilitative services, inadequate reimbursement of in-home services, waiting list, and unreliability of services.

Older adults are particularly vulnerable to overtreatment and undertreatment. The large multicenter SUPPORT study (Study to Understand Prognoses and Preferences for Outcomes and Risks of Treatment) (SUPPORT Principal Investigators, 1995) demonstrated that even with advance directives, many older people admitted to hospitals in their final days received treatment they did not desire or request, yet suffered unrelieved pain in their last days. In addition, older adults are less likely to receive ventilator support, surgery, or dialysis than younger patients (Hamel et al., 1999).

Technology's subtle influence on shaping our values has yet to be recognized. Callahan (2003) contends that the use of technology has become confused with the sanctity of life. That is, some believe that if we do not use all the technology available to us to extend life, we have failed to respect the sanctity of life. Because evidence-based medicine is population based rather than individual oriented, health care providers are still required to make judgments on how to treat each individual patient. Wisdom in these decisions requires the practitioner to incorporate the patient's values into the decision of whether or not to incorporate technology in a particular situation.

From the other perspective, advance directives not to undertake advanced life support should not be interpreted by clinicians to mean that all curative therapies should be abandoned. Such a stance oversimplifies the issues at stake. Mezey and colleagues (2002) discuss a range of technology available in health care for the aged and suggest that high-quality care can often be provided with low-technology services. The issue of rationing certain technologies using chronological age as the criterion is extremely controversial, partly because of the serious limitations of using chronological age as a predictor of functional status or quality of life. Because age alone is a poor predictor of health status, older people should receive individualized care in consideration of their unique life situations as suggested by the ANA Code of Ethics for Nurses (2001).

RESPECT FOR THE INDIVIDUAL PERSON. Older adults deserve respect for their personhood. Inherently they are worthy and valuable, especially in ways that make them unique individuals. They are not merely a means to some other end (Volbrecht, 2002). Kant (1964, p. 96) explicates this fundamental principle in ethics as follows: "So act that you treat humanity in your own person and in the person of everyone else...as an end and never merely as a means."

Although it has been argued that an older person is "an irrepeatable amalgam of experience and hope, a center of freedom and love" (Jonsen, 1976, p. 98), older people are often treated stereotypically and thus are depersonalized. One example of depersonalization and ageism is in the derogatory generalizations made about older adults. Proclamations that all older people are set in their ways and not open to change indicate disrespect for older adults as persons.

In contrast, respect for older persons involves appreciation of the special characteristics and needs that are more common in this population. For example, as a group, older people have less income and increasing health care needs. A respectful response to this dilemma would be for society to provide an adequate safety net for the most vulnerable. Respect for personhood in the aged means treating them with quality health care that is specifically designed to meet their particular needs. It means respecting older adults as decision makers who deserve to be informed and allowed to make decisions about their living and dying, including participation or nonparticipation in research and teaching efforts.

May (1982) contends that the aged should not be excluded from expectations of their own moral responsibility. He provides a novel description of virtues called for by advanced age, including courage, humility, patience, simplicity, benignity, and hilarity. Although not all would agree with these virtues, the point that respect for the individual includes consideration of the older person's moral responsibilities to others is valid and sometimes overlooked.

AUTONOMY OR SELF-DETERMINATION. The principle of autonomy or self-determination is critical in caring for older people. Respecting the principle of autonomy means that older patients will be respected as decision makers about their own care. All competent older persons have a perspective on their own best interests, shaped by their values and beliefs developed over a lifetime, that defines each individual as a unique person. Based on this unique set of values and beliefs, individuals assess alternatives, arrive at preferences, and try to implement those preferences, either individually or with the assistance of others.

In health care situations, frail older persons have varying abilities to exercise autonomy, and therefore clinicians have specific responsibilities to an older patient in order to respect autonomy. These include (1) recognizing and acknowledging the validity of the values and beliefs of the older person, especially when the clinician differs with those values and beliefs; (2) assisting the older person to identify relevant values and beliefs; (3) assisting the older person to express a value-based preference; and (4) refraining from interfering with the implementation of that preference by the older person, or assisting with its implementation as necessary, given the limitations on the older person's ability (Mezey et al., 2002). Although autonomy is a complex, multidimensional concept that has eluded simple definitions, an underlying theme among all definitions is the presumption that individuals are the best judges of what is in their interest (Callahan, 2003).

Ironically, it is in the care of people with questionable capacity to make decisions that autonomy becomes such a predominant issue. Gadow (1996) suggests that if a patient is not self-determining, the principle of autonomy requires action that will most likely facilitate or restore autonomy or that has "the least possibility of permanently precluding it." For those patients who wish to waive their autonomy in deference to their care provider's advice, it must be clear that this decision was consciously and freely made. When there is a possible clash between what the health care professionals feel is most beneficial and what the patient wants, the principle of autonomy dictates that the patient's wishes should supersede the care provider's recommendation.

Legally, all adults are presumed to be competent to make their own decisions unless a court of law has been convinced that an individual is unable to make rational decisions or to care for self or property adequately, usually as the result of mental illness, developmental disabilities, or cognitive impairment. However, health care professionals cannot consider a consent or refusal of treatment valid if they have reason to believe that the individual is incapable of making a rational decision.

Ethicists and clinicians recognize that individuals may have varying capacity to make different types of decisions. For example, although a person in the early stages of a dementing illness may not be able to handle all business affairs, he or she may be fully capable of voicing values and opinions about treatment decisions and preferences about daily routines and activities. The principle of autonomy requires that an older patient be allowed, and in fact encouraged, to function at the highest level of decision making possible. Often, if a person is given the pertinent information at a time when thinking ability is clearest and patiently allowed the time necessary to process the information and make a decision, he or she can express helpful advice to caregivers regarding a treatment plan. Drane (1985) described a "sliding scale" model of competency, in which the standards for determining competence are based on the type of decision required regarding health care. The greater the potential for harm from the decision, the more rigorous the standard for competency.

CONFIDENTIALITY. Respect for persons also requires respecting the individual's confidentiality, and older adults should be given the same consideration as any other age-group. Adult children often put pressure on health care professionals to tell them their parent's diagnosis and prognosis and options for treatment before sharing the information with the older patient. The temptation is for the clinicians and adult children to make decisions, supposedly in the best interest of the patient, instead of respecting the patient's autonomous decision-making ability. An autonomous person must be able to control his or her personal information.

Clinicians must ensure patient confidentiality. There may also be instances when a clinician may be obligated to override the duty to maintain confidentiality, for instance when an older person may be at risk of harming himself or herself (or others), or when decision-making capacity is impaired.

BENEFICENCE. The principle of beneficence, or "doing good," means that the highest good will be done for older people in a particular situation. Obviously, use of this principle must involve providing an interpretation of what is "good." According to Keenan (2004), in medicine, the criteria for defining benefit relate to the alleviation of suffering and the preservation of life. Although these are generally accepted benefits of care, they are still subject to interpretation and weighing of benefits to define the highest value. The best thing to do in the case of a terminally ill patient who wants to die may be to alleviate suffering by withholding antibiotic therapy rather than prolonging life. Some ethicists claim that this action would violate the principle of doing no harm (nonmaleficence), whereas others would contend that inappropriately aggressive treatment of this person in this situation would be harmful. Deciding with the patient or family (or both) what is most beneficial given the particular circumstances and then facilitating that action is an example of "doing good" in the care of the aged.

The establishment of programs to enable older persons to stay as healthy and independent as possible could be regarded as beneficent. Beneficence relies on the sensitivity of the provider to detect and interpret the needs of a patient and then to respond in a caring and helpful way. Beneficence also requires looking at the long-term benefits or harms of treatment. In certain situations, immediate beneficial results are realized for the patient and family when lives are saved. However, the disability that sometimes ensues may not be judged beneficial by the individual. It can be argued that society has an obligation to provide long-term quality of life for those who "benefit" from aggressive treatment in acute situations. Ethical decisions thus have long-term implications, however difficult it may be to predict certain outcomes.

DISTRIBUTIVE JUSTICE. Distributive justice deals with problems of allocation and equitable distribution of scarce resources. Although there are several bases for claims in distributive justice, the two that apply most aptly to older adults are contribution and need. Jonsen, Seigler, and Winslade (2002, p. 102) interpret Hobhouse's rule for distribution as follows: "Distributive justice is the equal satisfaction of equal need, subject to the adequate maintenance of useful functions."

Callahan (2002) warns that methods of distributing medical resources, such as measuring the worth of an individual in terms of present earning capability or absence of disability, have a built-in bias against older persons. Many people think of older adults as unproductive parasites that drain societal resources. They forget that older people have been contributing to our society all their lives in various ways, including working in paying jobs and birthing and raising children who are now productive. The nature of their contribution may be different now from when they were younger, but they continue to contribute their knowledge, wisdom, and experiences to others as grandparents, volunteers, consultants, and church members. They are therefore due their share of societal goods and services. Some societies expect productivity according to one's abilities, and then share goods and services according to the needs of the people. In such a system, older adults are due whatever they need to maintain their health and autonomy. Given that health care resources are finite, how will priorities be determined? Jonsen, Siegler, and Winslade (1998, p. 102) contend that:

If, in fact, it could be shown that the provision of health services to the elderly becomes so costly, in money and energy, that the health of those by whose taxable productivity the health system exists is compromised, it would not be unjust to reduce care for the elderly until equity is restored. But...only if this is the case would such a policy be just.

"Lifeboat ethics," or making decisions based on who will be sacrificed for the greater good, should be a last resort, used only after all other measures to meet existing needs have been exhausted. It is possible that if all decisions to use (or not use) costly, high-technology measures were judiciously made, sufficient funds would be added to the health care resource pool to pay for some chronic disease needs that are currently neglected. The implication of distributive justice is that all health care needs of older individuals would receive attention, not just those acute needs that are amenable at certain times to inpatient medical manipulation. Distributive justice would not allow curtailment of services using chronological age alone as a criterion.

In this age of anticipated rationing because of high costs and the necessity for cost containment, Callahan (2002) suggests that "essential" care be defined for all citizens to set minimum standards of care. This would entail identifying specific interventions; patient indications; estimation and evaluation of benefits, harms, and costs; and a comparison with alternative treatments. Using outcome criteria to justify costly interventions will become increasingly commonplace in all age-groups. It may become evident through proper research into effectiveness of interventions that some high-technology procedures and treatments in the acute care setting are less beneficial than some less costly outpatient rehabilitative and maintenance interventions that would apply to many of the chronically ill at home. A related basic

ethical question is whether a society is obligated to provide the appropriate long-term maintenance therapies to patients whose lives have been prolonged through aggressive interventions in the hospital.

Common Ethical Dilemmas in Gerontological Nursing. As society ages, health care of older people presents the nurse as ethicist particularly challenging problems. Ethical dilemmas in the care of older people can be identified on many levels, including societal, family, and individual (e.g., ability to participate or refuse to participate as a research subject). Nurses and their patients feel the effects of unresolved ethical dilemmas in their practice almost daily. The result of many poorly resolved dilemmas is frustration about the quality of care given and the quality of life left to the older person. Explicit consideration of the issues underlying moral dilemmas in health care helps the gerontological nurse achieve greater understanding of the forces that shape the practice world and may also provide direction for a new, more satisfying, course of action.

DECISIONAL CAPACITY. Decisional capacity comprises four elements: comprehension of the information presented or available, understanding the options and their possible consequences, deliberating among the choices consistent with one's life values and beliefs, and communicating a choice (Mezey et al., 2002). Decision-making capacity can vary from time to time. Additionally, decisional capacity in the various aspects of one's life is not an all-or-none phenomenon. That is, a person may have the capacity to make decisions regarding some aspects of his or her life, but not others.

Determining decision-making capacity may be difficult. The primary component of decisional capacity is the ability to understand the consequences of a decision. Some validated standardized measures are now being used to assess decisional capacity (Marson, Ingram, Cody, & Harrell, 1995). Determining the capacity for decision making must be established before obtaining informed consent for treatment.

When older individuals are unable to make decisions for themselves, surrogate decision makers, usually family members, can respect the patient's wishes by making decisions in accordance with the patient's general values and past choices. This practice is based on the principle of "substituted judgment," which means trying to decide as the patient would decide if he or she were capable. "Best interest" is another principle of decision making that directs the surrogate to decide what seems optimal for the patient's good, when specific wishes may be unknown, and perhaps includes factors such as the relief of suffering, the quality of life presently and in the future, and the return of function (Flaherty, Fulmer, & Mezey, 2003).

END-OF-LIFE ISSUES. Issues surrounding end-of-life care in older patients are becoming increasingly complex. Technology advances and genetic enhancements will make the extension of life possible, but a focus on treatment that fosters the older person's goals and freely determined choices, as well as enhances quality of life, is essential. We will consider some common ethical issues in end-of-life care, including withholding or withdrawing treatment, assisted suicide, and euthanasia.

Withholding or Withdrawing Treatment. Since the landmark Quinlan case in 1976, withdrawing life-sustaining treatment has been legally acceptable provided there is clear and convincing evidence of the patient's wishes to avoid prolonging the dying process. Since the sixteenth century, forgoing and discontinuing life-prolonging treatment has been morally acceptable based primarily on religious grounds. A competent patient's right to choose or refuse treatment is the current standard of care. Recent developments, however, may make following the patient's wishes difficult.

In Florida, the governor requested the legislature to pass a law to have a feeding tube reinserted in a woman who was in a persistent vegetative state for 13 years, after the courts finally granted her husband's request to have the feeding tube removed, reflecting the patient's wishes. Recently, the Pope issued an address in which he characterized the use of feeding tubes as part of "normal care" and declared the removal of feeding tubes as "euthanasia by omission." These troubling actions deviate from long-standing opinions held by the courts and Roman Catholic bioethical positions. Traditionally, a decision to forgo or withdraw treatment that may prolong the dying process was made by weighing the benefits against the harms to the patient, family, and community (Shannon & Walter, 2004). Artificial means were not considered part of medical intervention when a patient was terminally or irreversibly ill. Rather, the goal of care became the relief of pain and suffering and the provision of comfort.

Assisted Suicide. The role of health care professionals in assisting a person to take his or her own life is increasingly controversial. Currently, Oregon is the only state in which physician-assisted suicide is legal. The major debate over assisted suicide is whether individuals have the right to choose when and how they die, and whether health care professionals should play a role in individuals' choice to end their life prematurely. Participation in assisted suicide is viewed as contrary to the first precept of the Hippocratic oath: "First, do no harm." Many people consider assisted suicide because of fear of inadequate pain relief and unbearable suffering at the end of their lives. The ANA has a position statement recommending that nurses not participate in assisted suicide (ANA, 1994). Both the nursing and medical organizations have major educational and practice initiatives to improve end-of-life care. Discussion of

end-of-life values, goals, and preferences needs to include older people, their families, and their health care providers while they possess decisional capacity.

Euthanasia. Euthanasia, an action taken to terminate someone's life, is currently considered legally and ethically unacceptable in the United States. What makes this issue controversial is the desire for a comfortable death and evidence that patients' wishes are often not followed at the end of life. Two major objections to euthanasia prevail. The first equates the termination of another's life with homicide; it is considered immoral and illegal. Second is the fear that we may begin down the slippery slope of deciding for others when their life is no longer of value. Older adults, people with significant disabilities, and those with impaired cognitive functioning could be primary targets.

RATIONING OF SERVICES. Health care costs consume an increasing proportion of the gross domestic product. As the population ages, costs for older people consume a disproportionate amount of health care spending. Increasing pressure is being placed on clinicians to reduce health care spending. Evidence suggests that health disparities exist because of socioeconomic inequities, differential access to health care, and a different level of care offered to members of vulnerable populations. Older people are often not offered the standard level of care because of an inherent bias that they have lived their lives and resources could be better used in a younger population.

Evidence suggests that there are steadily increasing numbers of older people who are uninsured or underinsured and lack access to health care (Schmidt, 2000). Additionally, the number of emergency department visits for serious medical problems in the elderly is on the rise (Rosenblatt et al., 2000). This is exacerbated by the fact that in many communities or regions, the number of generalists and specialists accepting Medicare patients is declining. Fee-for-service and capitated payment structures offer disincentives to provide services not covered and to undertreat medical problems. Clinicians have an ethical obligation to provide care that is consistent with the acceptable standard (Flaherty et al., 2003).

RIGHTS OF INSTITUTIONALIZED PATIENTS. Older people in long-term care facilities create unique ethical challenges for their care providers. They experience diminished choice, control, dignity, and privacy in an institutionalized setting. Particular attention must be paid to factors that will decrease the vulnerability of those who are institutionalized. Special ethical problems arise in the following situations: a setting where decisions are often made by someone else; well-meaning staff may restrict self-determination; and multiple levels of regulations and laws often challenge privacy, confidentiality, and autonomy.

Inherent in satisfactory nursing home life is resolution of the "dialectic between autonomy and security needs," a dialectic that requires continual renegotiation for satisfactory function (Mezey et al., 2002). Recognition of this difficult reality has spawned a thought-provoking study of "everyday ethics" in nursing homes that raises the startling prospect that for some individuals, the "morality of the mundane" may be a determining factor in quality of life (Kane & Caplan, 1990). Realizing the importance of the potential for violations of autonomy in everyday living in institutions is a particularly important function for nurses, because they are frequently in a position to enforce decisions about everyday routines. They often decide whether or not an individual's choice, even one that may be contrary to conventional wisdom or one that may disrupt ward routine, should be upheld.

Today, because of recent changes in reimbursement, the number of older adults who are in long-term care (LTC) facilities for short-term rehabilitation and care is growing. This growing trend presents a challenge to our traditional approach to two issues in particular: cardiopulmonary resuscitation and the use of enteral feeding tubes.

Successful outcomes for cardiopulmonary resuscitation (CPR) in LTC patients occur in few cases (Applebaum, King, & Finucare, 1990). Traditionally, nursing home residents were not considered candidates for CPR; consequently, CPR was usually not initiated. With the increase in healthy older adults living in LTC facilities or there for rehabilitation, this approach may need to be reconsidered. With the advent of the Patient Self-Determination Act, inquiries about advance directives are made of every patient entering an institution receiving federal funds. This should stimulate discussions about the desire for resuscitation efforts if an untoward event occurs. Sensitivity and skill are required on the part of the clinician to handle these discussions well. Most people do not have an accurate understanding of what is involved in CPR (Mueller, Hook, & Fleming, 2004). The effectiveness of CPR outside an acute care setting is not encouraging. Careful and thoughtful discussion of this issue includes a description of what happens during CPR, the risk and benefits, and the expected outcomes, to facilitate informed decision making. These discussions should take place within the context of the patient's overall life goals, values, expectations, and preferences.

Another issue that requires careful and thoughtful deliberation is the use of enteral feeding tubes. Regulatory agencies have encouraged the use of enteral feeding tubes in LTC facilities to prevent nutritional deficits in the elderly, who may not take in adequate nutrition by mouth (Flaherty et al., 2003). Recent research indicates that the utility of this approach may be questionable, especially in people with advanced dementia. Nutrition therapy is used for three goals of treatment: "increased survival, prevention of aspiration and pressure sores, and increased comfort and amelioration of symptoms associated with malnutrition and dehydration" (Ersek, 2003). These goals have not been supported by research findings. Survival is increased in some populations, but it is not associated with improved functional outcomes or enhanced quality of life.

Prevention of pressure sores by improving nutritional status is not accomplished with enteral feedings. And finally, palliative care and hospice research findings do not support the goal that tube feedings relieve symptoms of hunger and dehydration. In fact, hunger is not experienced by terminally ill patients, and enteral feedings actually contribute to complications when used for rehydration. Comfort measures traditionally used by nurses to treat thirst and dry mouth include frequent oral care, ice chips, sips of fluids, and artificial saliva (Ersek, 2003).

Research findings contradict the regulatory basis for using enteral feeding tubes in LTC. The use of enteral feeding tubes increases complications and morbidity in the majority of LTC patients. Gerontological, hospice, and palliative care nurses are actively seeking legislative change to policies that encourage the appropriate use of feeding tubes in patients. It is ethically problematic to be required to participate in care that is potentially harmful to the majority of older patients (Shannon & Walter, 2004).

COGNITIVE IMPAIRMENT. Particular ethical problems arise when an older person is cognitively impaired. Assessing decisional capacity, advance directives, and guardianship are discussed in other sections of this chapter. The focus here is on three issues: truth-telling, protection from harm, and the definition of personhood. Implications for truth-telling occur at two distinct time periods for persons with cognitive impairment (CI): at the time of diagnosis and, with more advanced CI, when the person may become agitated and aggressive. Disclosing a diagnosis of dementia requires skill and sensitivity. Persons with dementia have a right to know their diagnosis and help in understanding what is happening to them, so future planning and necessary legal and family preparations can be addressed. Throughout the course of the disease, it is imperative that the person with CI be informed of his or her treatment options and participate in decision making to the extent possible; later in the course of the disease, it may simply be having the opportunity to voice preferences. The overarching goal is to preserve the dignity and autonomy of the older person for as long as possible.

As CI progresses, persons with dementia may not be aware that certain behaviors may be potentially harmful, both to themselves and to others (Flaherty et al., 2003). For example, people with CI may not recognize when their driving ability is impaired or when their behavior is inappropriate or unsafe. At other times, the care of the person with CI may be emotionally and physically beyond what the family caregiver may be capable of providing. In this case, families may need help at home, they may need respite care, or the point may arise when placement is necessary for the health of the family member. Health care providers must recognize when these situations are evolving and be supportive of the patient and family if measures must be taken to protect the patient, family, or others, as in the case of driving.

The essence of who a person is changes with the progression of dementia. Although careful and thoughtful planning of care occurred at the time of diagnosis, based on goals, values, beliefs, and preferences of the person with CI, the person who made these plans changes considerably over time as the dementia progresses. Family members and health care providers may experience conflict when faced with what is in the best interest of the person with CI. The demands of the situation and the safety of the patient and family may conflict with the vision the person with CI had of themselves before the progression of the symptoms. Weighing benefits (safety) and potential harms (injury) to the patient and others requires careful consideration when caring for persons with dementia (Mueller et al., 2004).

RESEARCH IN OLDER ADULTS. Special emphasis must be placed on the ethical problems in conducting research with vulnerable populations such as older adults. There is a tension between the need to include older people in appropriate research and the possibility of coercion. Likewise, the ability to understand the research, the possible consequences, and the alternatives must be weighed in light of the person's capacity to provide informed consent. Research designed to provide benefit to the older population and improve their health status and quality of life must be well designed and of importance to them.

Certain aspects of research warrant scrutiny in relation to older adults (American Geriatrics Society, 2001). Whenever possible, respecting the wishes and intentions of the person before the loss of decisional capacity should occur. Even those who cannot be considered competent to provide legal consent can be asked to provide assent at the time of testing or participation in a research procedure. Only research that offers minimal risk or direct benefit should be offered to persons with CI. Surrogates can withdraw consent or refuse participation if there is a determination that the research is not what the person intended. And last, only in rare situations would the refusal of an incapacitated person to participate in research be overridden.

Research involving institutionalized older people warrants special precautions. Because they are easily accessible for the researcher, close monitoring of research for the protection of human subjects is indicated. Also, being in a constrained environment may create an atmosphere of subtle coercion for those who are institutionalized. They may feel pressure to "go along," fearing loss of privileges or services if they do not conform. Research in institutions should have some relationship to their condition or circumstances, rather than for the convenience of the researcher. Long-term care facilities have an obligation to review and oversee research to ensure that there is some benefit, or at least minimal risk, and that research subjects are protected (Boult et al., 2003). In addition, information given should facilitate informed consent or an indication of preference for participation, and the privacy of study participants and confidentiality of information should be protected.

Specific Techniques to Promote Ethical Decision Making. Because the care of older adults presents many unique issues, special attention is paid to techniques that can facilitate communication and ethical decision making. The uses and limitations of several techniques are analyzed next.

VALUES HISTORY. Doukas and McCullough (1991) developed the Values History form so that individuals could record a summary of their ideas and wishes for care. Individuals identify their values and beliefs and then determine preferences about whether they would want various health care procedures. Ideally, the Values History is obtained when the individual is fully competent, but some cultural groups may not understand the need for discussing end-of-life decisions well in advance of their occurrence (Sotnik & Jezewski, 2005). If completed, the Values History can preserve patient autonomy and respect for personhood if later faced with dilemmas involving impaired competence (Doukas & McCullough, 2000). A sophisticated history would allow the patient to rank values between length of life and quality of life. An example of items might be, "(1) I want to maintain my capacity to think clearly; (2) I want to avoid unnecessary pain and suffering; (3) I want to be treated in accord with my religious beliefs and traditions." The information is then used in determining advance directives.

If a patient is not able to give a Values History, the next best option is to construct one with the help of family members or significant others. The contention is made that a Values History can inform the practitioner and families' decisions about aggressiveness of care when the older individual is no longer able to reason.

There are two major limitations to the use of these histories. First, most clinicians are not trained in eliciting information about patients' values. Second, the patient is not questioned about values and preferences until there is some crisis, when it may be too late for patients to express themselves and significant others may not be sure about the specifics of the patient's values.

PATIENT SELF-DETERMINATION LEGISLATION. With the advancement of technology that enables prolongation of life, the increased interest in autonomy and self-determination by consumers, and the increased consciousness of the high cost of technological aggressiveness at the end of life, special attention is now being paid to end-of-life decisions. Specifically, there is increased interest in having older adults prepare advance directives declaring what kind of care they want at the end of life. Advance directives often are used to limit the amount of aggressive treatment in terminal illness, although they can serve the broader purpose of clearly indicating care wishes, to remove the burden of decision making from a family member.

A long history of case law, beginning with the initial Karen Ann Quinlan ruling in 1976, established that a competent person could determine the extent of medical treatment should he or she become incapacitated. A second legal point from the Quinlan case clearly established who the surrogate decision maker would be when a person becomes incapacitated. These rulings have been reinforced over the past three decades through other situations, namely Cruzan, Wanglie, and most recently the tragic Schiavo case (Volbrecht, 2002). A few states, however, have adopted a strict approach to advance directives, requiring "clear and convincing evidence" of a person's intent. This is interpreted to mean a written, legal document (Lo & Steinbrook, 2004).

Another landmark event in this area of end-of-life decisions, growing out of the Cruzan case, was the passage of the Patient Self-Determination Act (Cate & Gill, 1991) by the federal government in 1990, which became effective in December 1991. The Patient Self-Determination Act was passed as part of the Omnibus Budget Reconciliation Act of 1990. According to one of the architects of the legislation,

It is the purpose of this act to ensure that a patient's right to self-determination in health care decisions be communicated and protected...The traditional right to accept or reject medical or surgical treatment should be available to an adult while competent, so that in the event that such adult becomes unconscious or otherwise incompetent to make decisions, such adult would more easily continue to control decisions affecting their [*sic*] health care. (Cate & Gill, 1991, p. 7)

The Patient Self-Determination Act requires that any health care institution accepting Medicare or Medicaid monies must inform all patients of their right to make decisions about their care, including the right to accept or reject medical or surgical treatment. Patients must be given written information about their right to have advance directives according to state law, which can vary in requirements. Institutions must have written policies about patients' rights and document on their charts whether or not they have executed an advance directive.

ADVANCE DIRECTIVES. Advance directives allow individuals to designate their wishes in writing so that they are available in case they become unable to express themselves or develop diminished decision-making capacity. Advance directives are an extension of a fully autonomous person, recognized by all 50 states. There are two forms of advance directives: the living will and the durable power of attorney for health care. Often, people who have an advance directive do not discuss their wishes with their primary care provider or with family members. In addition, advance directives are frequently not found when they are needed (Mueller et al., 2004). To fully execute advance directives, they must be discussed and given to health providers and family members, and kept easily accessible.

How to increase the frequency of patients executing advance directives has been investigated. For about a decade only approximately 15% of people had an advance directive, but more recent evidence indicates that the prevalence of a written advance directive is currently near 25% (Lo & Steinbrook, 2004). A number of different approaches have been developed to help elderly persons and their family members understand the concept and to consider carefully the issues involved in making advance directives. These include creating possible end-of-life scenarios, counseling models, and written materials. Educational materials are widely available through organizations such as the American Association of Retired Persons (2005), health care organizations, legal agencies, and bioethics centers, which often are located in universities.

Despite the increased attention to the need for more formalized approaches to decision making about aggressiveness of care for seriously ill patients, initiating, documenting, and implementing a coordinated team effort in this area can be challenging. The first step is to give the patient and family the information and opportunity to discuss advance directives in the context of an individual's particular situation. Experts point out the paramount role of the patient in decision making when aggressive treatment is considered to be death prolonging and there is a medical indication to diminish aggressiveness (Callahan, 2002; Keenan, 2004).

Cultural differences may influence not only the specific decision made but also a patient's or family's willingness to formalize these arrangements (Stone, 2005).

Health care providers need to provide information and care that is culturally competent to ensure sensitivity to patient and family wishes and be aware of the differences in cultural influences on decisions.

It is difficult to get patient and family preferences discussed and documented, but also there is often disagreement among staff members as to the best decision for patients. Some nursing staff members may disagree with the physician (Lo & Steinbrook, 2004), and house officers may disagree with the attending physicians. Team consensus about ethical decisions can be facilitated if differing value systems of providers are recognized, disagreements are openly aired, there is an increase in formal ethics teaching, ethics consultants are used to help resolve differences, and a plan is formulated and reevaluated periodically (Keenan, 2004).

Once decisions are made, they must be communicated. For example, the information that a patient has do-not-resuscitate orders in effect must be available to all caregivers at all times. Innovative ways of identifying patients who do not wish to be resuscitated have been reported, such as family conferences (McDonagh et al., 2004).

Living Wills. The living will is the oldest and most common form of advance directive. A living will generally stipulates what the individual would want in the event of a terminal illness, and generally identifies when the person does not desire any life-prolonging treatment. In most states, this document does not have to be written by a lawyer, but must have two disinterested witnesses, that is, people who will not benefit from the patient's estate and who do not work for the institution providing care. It must also be notarized. Patients can be as general or specific as they choose, and they can address specific measures such as surgery, antibiotics, feeding tubes, CPR, respirators, cancer treatments, and so on. The living will may also stipulate that decisions could depend on the circumstances at the time, such as the individual's chances for full recovery (Missouri Bar, 2005).

Durable Power of Attorney for Health Care Decisions. The durable power of attorney is another type of advance directive that allows individuals to appoint a legal surrogate for health care decisions. The surrogate serves as a spokesperson for the individual in case he or she becomes incapable of making the necessary choices about treatment. The surrogate should know the person well, having paid particular attention to understanding the person's values, philosophy, and preferences regarding end-of-life treatment decisions, and have a copy of the person's living will.

Many nursing home residents who are offered the opportunity to appoint a durable power of attorney elect to execute this document; most choose a close relative, such as a spouse or a son or daughter (Hayley, Cassel, Snyder, & Rudberg, 1996). A majority of residents never

discuss their wishes for future medical care with anyone, fearing they will upset their family members by engaging in these discussions (Mueller et al., 2004). Interest in life-sustaining treatment declines significantly when cognitive function is perceived as declining in the future and as the treatment becomes permanent instead of temporary.

ETHICS COMMITTEES. Interdisciplinary ethics committees are now mandated by the Joint Commission on Accreditation of Healthcare Organizations (JCAHO) (2003) in health care organizations. A number of factors have led to their need in health care, including (1) the growing sophistication of medical technology, (2) an increasing recognition that there is usually a range of acceptable options in patient care rather than just one best way, (3) a desire to be protected from litigation in controversial situations, (4) a growing awareness that factors other than medical criteria influence clinical decisions, (5) an increasing need for arbitration between patient desires and health care institutions, (6) an increasing likelihood that certain technologies or services will be rationed, (7) a need for religious groups to have a forum for discussing the conflicts between religious beliefs and health care practices, and (8) a need for a forum where the conflicting values of various parties with a stake in the outcome of clinical decisions can be aired. The most common reasons for ethics committee consultations include end-of-life decisions, issues of patient autonomy, and conflict (DuVal et al., 2001). Box 9-1 provides the reflections of a nurse serving on a hospital ethics committee.

The functions of ethics committees are generally education, policy development, and consultation or case review. Newly formed ethics committees often spend the first several months of their meetings educating their members regarding their purpose, ethical theories and principles, and process, and deciding on how they would like to function. They then broaden their educational efforts to include workshops for staff and conducting ethics conferences. Interdisciplinary ethics committees that view themselves as successful are long-standing, are large, and have experienced members (Guo & Schick, 2003). That is, diverse, ongoing, experienced membership is beneficial for an effective clinical ethics committee. It is also essential that some members have geriatric-specific knowledge about patient care and outcomes. In the past few years, institutions have been requesting ethics committees to become involved in organizational ethics, a role for which most clinicians feel unprepared.

Policy development is an important function of ethics committees because it fills a void between the macro-level of policy dictated by the government and other third-party payers and the microlevel of individual

Box 9-1 *Reflections on Ethics and Nursing*

Ethics and nursing are intrinsically interwoven. Nurses touch lives in so many ways and at so many poignant junctures for patients and families. The opportunity to practice "with compassion and respect for the inherent dignity, worth and uniqueness of every individual..." (ANA, 2001, p. 3) is particularly significant when caring for the elderly and their families. This is a nonnegotiable standard for all nurses, regardless of personal values and beliefs. It is our common thread.

Nationally, the general public relies heavily on nurses adhering to high ethical standards. Nurses have topped the list of the Gallup Organization's annual survey on the honesty and ethical standards of various professions for many years (Moore, 2004). It becomes all nurses' collective responsibility to maintain this proud ethical heritage that has been handed down to them for generations.

It is quite common for nurses to face challenging ethical issues when caring for the elderly in the hospital. Common ethic issues that are encountered with the elderly population are often those related to end-of-life care, and include decision-making capacity, advance directives, and surrogate decision making. Nurses are often dealing with patient and families at their most vulnerable times.

Nurses need not face ethical dilemmas alone. Health care organizations have interdisciplinary ethics committees to provide consultation on challenging ethical cases. Ethics consultation committees typically support patients, families, and the health care team in addressing ethical issues related to patient care.

In my experiences on a hospital ethics committee, ethical dilemmas often arise for family members making decisions for elderly patients. Surrogates often lose focus on their task of providing substitute judgment for the person and instead make decisions that they themselves are comfortable with. This is understandable in that the emotional stress of a loved one's illness makes it very difficult to make decisions. Sadness, denial, and feelings of guilt further complicate the ability to make decisions on behalf of someone else. It is often very difficult for the surrogate to "let go" of a loved one in spite of the belief that every person has the right to die peacefully and with dignity. One of the most valuable things that an ethics consultation committee can do is help clarify the goals of an older adult's treatment for the family members. Asking goal-related questions can achieve this. For example, family members may be asked, "What would your loved one want? What would he consider a good quality of life?" These questions are typically easy for families to answer. The tougher follow-up question is, "If they wouldn't want this quality of life, then are you ready to let go?"

Nurses will continue to uphold high ethical standards and support patients and families respectfully and faithfully throughout time. This is something we can always count on.

Catherine C. Powers
Catherine C. Powers, MSN, APRN, BC
Clinical Nurse Specialist
Heart Services
Ethics Committee Member
Barnes-Jewish Hospital
St. Louis, Missouri

decisions. Singer, Pellegrino, and Siegler (1990) call this the *mesolevel*, where policies help define the moral mission of the institution, promote fair treatment by explicating criteria that pertain to similar clinical situations, and foster institutional discussions when management is unclear. Policies regarding CPR, palliative care, end-of-life care, and withdrawing and withholding treatment are essential to eliminating ethically and legally marginal practices, enhancing the quality of patient care, and reducing legal liability.

Consultation is usually the last and most difficult function that ethics committees provide. There are several models for consultation on individual cases, where providers usually seek advice: (1) full committee review of a case; (2) a consultant or team reviewing the case and presenting it to the committee for input; (3) a consultant or team reviewing and advising on the case, and then bringing it back to the committee for post hoc discussion; and (4) a team from the ethics committee advising on the case alone. There is no consensus as to which is the most effective method for case consultation. An evaluation of ethics committee case consultations, however, revealed that earlier consultations regarding end-of-life care result in improved patient outcomes and cost savings by focusing on the patient's quality of life (Daly, 2000).

Membership of institutional ethics committees varies from one institution to another and often is dictated by the express purposes of the committee. The JCAHO requires a variety of disciplines. Often attorneys and community representatives are part of an ethics committee. If lawyers for the organization are included, conflict of interest may arise between the attorney's role as representative of the organization versus counsel to the committee. Using an attorney from outside the institution is beneficial for the plethora of legal questions arising. Some voice concern that including members of the community on the committee will increase the risk of breaches in confidentiality of patient information, although one could argue that the benefits of diversifying the committee with public representation far outweigh the risks.

Anyone involved in the care of a patient should be able to initiate an ethics committee consultation, including family members. The committee's responsibility for balancing conflicts and seeking the best decision is helpful in considering whether to include the patient/family as part of the committee meeting. Patient and family input is essential to any case discussion, but this might most easily and comfortably be obtained in a one-to-one discussion with a consultant or committee member and shared with the committee later.

Ethics committees are not as common in nursing homes; one small study reported that 29% of homes had a committee, although many were interested (Hogstel, Curry, Walker, & Burns, 2004). Size and religious affiliation may be factors (Lo & Steinbrook, 2004). The most frequent cases reviewed by long-term care committees included treatment decisions, capacity for decision making, and formulating a professional code of ethics. Facilities without ethics committees often used institutional policies or legal advice to help in ethical dilemmas. Nine percent sought the advice of a philosopher or an ethics expert.

The increase in technology and the complexity of care in nursing homes, as well as the lack of guidelines regarding appropriateness of certain treatments such as resuscitation and tube feedings, make ethical decision making increasingly difficult. Ethics committees or policies regarding treatment are needed. Ethical issues in the care of patients with dementia in nursing homes fall into four major areas: learning the limits of interventions, tempering the culture of surveillance and restraint, preserving the integrity of the individual, and defining community norms and values (Powers, 2000).

Nurses must be involved in such ethical decisions for nursing home patients because they know these patients and their families well. More widespread establishment of ethics committees in nursing homes would help ensure that an ethical reasoning approach is applied to these difficult decisions.

A final consideration in the development of an institutional ethics committee is the degree to which the institution expects its providers to consult with and abide by the decisions of the committee. In most organizations, the role of the interdisciplinary ethics committee is advisory to clinicians and administration. A second model involves mandatory review of certain decisions, for example, review of do-not-resuscitate orders in incompetent patients or surrogate decision makers (DeRenzo & Olick, 2000), but the professionals retain the authority for the final decision. A third model calls for mandatory review and compliance with the committee's recommendations. The third model is not recommended, because of the dilution of responsibility for decisions and the potential negative legal ramifications of using the ethics committee as a decision-making body.

Although not all health care institutions have formalized ethics committees, the plethora of ethical dilemmas in the care of the aged make them a worthwhile consideration for any institution or agency caring for large numbers of older people.

LEGAL ISSUES. Decision-making capacity is a critical issue in the care of older adults. People who are confused, have dementia, or are mentally impaired are often encountered in the health care setting. Persons who are mentally incompetent are not capable of giving informed consent. Several options are available for people who lack decision-making capacity.

Guardianship. Legal guardianship is a mechanism that allows a surrogate to exercise individual rights for an older person who is no longer mentally competent (Mezey et al., 2002). When incompetence is established through court proceedings, a guardian is appointed by the court to be responsible for the care of the incompetent person and his or her estate. Other terms used for guardian include *conservator, committee,* and *curator.* A conservator is appointed to manage the individual's property and finances, and the guardian is usually also appointed conservator. The guardian may be an individual or a corporation.

Limited or full guardianship may be granted. In *limited guardianship* or conservatorship, the court specifies the particular types of decisions the individual is incapable of making, and the guardian is empowered to act as surrogate only in financial matters. Guardian of person involves decisions pertaining to consent for treatment or refusal of health care. Plenary guardians are empowered to make all types of decisions about the incompetent person, including financial assets, where and with whom the incompetent person will live, and consent or refusal of medical treatment. The durable power of attorney already discussed comes into play only after someone becomes incapable of making decisions.

Payee Status. The Social Security Administration recognizes a *"payee" status* for relatives of elderly individuals who are unable to manage their financial affairs because of physical or mental infirmity. This procedure does not require court proceedings and has no impact on the rights of the individual to make decisions in other domains. It merely allows another individual to cash the older person's social security check and, by implication, manage a major source of income (Gallo, Fulmer, Paveza, & Reichel, 2000). Some elderly people establish joint ownership of checking accounts or assets to allow a friend or family member to assist in financial management or set up legal trusts. These are options for assisting older people in financial management when their abilities are limited without going through court proceedings, or for transferring assets after death.

Elder Abuse. All states have mandatory reporting laws for suspected abuse of older persons in domestic and institutional settings. In 1 year, a study reported nearly 1 million cases of elder abuse; this is thought to reflect about one quarter of the number of actual cases

(Jogerst et al., 2003). Abuse of the elderly is associated with increased morbidity and mortality rates and decreased quality of life and functional status.

Increased reporting of elder abuse is associated with public education programs required by states, mandatory reporting laws, penalties for failing to report abuse, and professional awareness of state statutes. Greater incidence of elder abuse was thought to be related to greater population density and increased poverty levels, but this was not substantiated by the research. In fact, in areas where there are greater numbers of elderly people, the confirmed cases of abuse were lower. This could also be explained, however, by work overload by the caseworkers and their inability to follow up on reported cases.

Restraint Use. The work of nurses brought to light the ethical problems with the use of physical and chemical restraints (Strumpf & Evans, 1991) resulting in legislation dramatically reducing their use (Flaherty et al., 2003). Research demonstrated the limited value of restraints and the increased risk of injury associated with their use, particularly from falls. Instead the emphasis is placed on maintaining function and promoting rehabilitative aspects of care using the least restrictive environment. Strategies for environmental modification and supervision reduce the need for the use of restraints.

When considering the use of restraints, several factors need to be weighed. Autonomy and nonmaleficence are the major ethical considerations. An assessment includes the resident's capabilities; weighing the risks versus the benefits of restraint use; evaluation of less restrictive alternatives; the potential for harm to other residents; thoughtful consideration and discussion of the options with the caretakers, family, and friends; and obtaining informed consent (Hayley et al., 1996). Occasionally the use of restraints is the least harmful option. If the patient's surrogate does not agree, the surrogate may be able to help provide continued observation to keep the patient safe, or to pay for assistance.

ETHICAL DECISION-MAKING FRAMEWORKS FOR GERONTOLOGICAL NURSES

A formalized (systematic) framework for ethical decision making is extremely useful in guiding the consideration of the various ethical problems encountered by older people and their caregivers. Although the process for ethical decision making is systematic, it is not necessarily linear. The analytical approach used in nursing embraces an engaged dialogue that seeks to elucidate the values, beliefs, and goals of all involved. Because dialogue and discussion are paramount for good ethical analysis and decision making, the process is often iterative. It is also important that nurses analyze ethical issues from a perspective that reflects the values, assumptions, and beliefs of the profession.

Two frameworks for ethical reasoning in clinical decision making are presented here. Each outlines a systematic process to ensure complete and relevant information required for analysis of the situation. In addition, through the process of dialogue and information gathering, the pertinent issues can be distilled to elucidate the salient ethical concerns.

First, the nurse must determine whether the issue at hand is truly an ethical dilemma (Cassells et al., 2003). Many times communication difficulties or differences of professional opinion in areas where practice guidelines are unclear may initially seem like an ethical challenge. Sometimes it may require extended discussion with members of the health care team, family members, and the patient to determine if the situation at hand is an ethical problem.

Ethical challenges arise when there is not a clear course of action, usually in a complex clinical situation. There may be two equally desirable or undesirable choices and the decision is not clear to those involved. When these ethical dilemmas occur, a guide to ethical reasoning can assist by adding clarity to the goals or issues involved.

The first framework for ethical analysis is presented in Box 9-2. This approach may be helpful to the gerontological nurse who is part of an interdisciplinary team working with elderly persons and their families. It must be recognized that ethical decision making is often an iterative process in which additional information gained helps to further inform the ethical reasoning process (Cassells & Gaul, 1998). The questions outlined in the framework allow the nurse or health care team to work through all the relevant information and issues to help inform a decision.

A second model also may be helpful to guide ethical decision making for the gerontological nurse in clinical practice. Originally proposed for medical residents, this model was developed by Jonsen and colleagues (2002). This framework for ethical analysis involves thinking through a series of questions in four areas: medical indications, patient preferences, quality of life, and contextual features (Box 9-3).

The discussions that follow provide examples of specific ethical problems that nurses may encounter. Each problem is considered within one of the ethical decision-making frameworks presented. The cases highlight the use of philosophical and ethical principles in evaluating a problem and making a decision.

EXAMPLES OF ETHICAL DILEMMAS

Ethical quandaries arise on a daily basis in gerontological nursing practice. The confluence of societal and economic pressures can affect individual and family choices, as well as their values and those of their caregivers. Three case studies are presented for consideration and analysis using the decision-making frameworks

BOX 9-2 A Decision-Making Approach to Ethical Problems Arising in Clinical Practice

1. Determine the problem.
   a. What is the health problem?
   b. What are the ethical issues arising from the health situation?
   c. What is known about the health issue?
   d. What available scientific evidence is there that can help inform this situation?
2. Identify the appropriate decision maker(s).
   a. Who is involved in the decision making?
   b. Who should be involved in assisting with this decision?
   c. What is the role of each person involved?
   d. What are the values of those involved in the situation?
3. Determine the context (what is known).
   a. What is known about the current situation?
   b. What do we need to know?
   c. What are the relevant contextual factors in the case?
   d. How do we obtain any additional information needed to inform the ethical quandary?
4. Frame the issue.
   a. What ethical perspective will help inform decision making based on the patient's values and goals?
   b. Is this problem primarily a question of benefit versus burden, quality of life, relief of pain and suffering, the value of life, or maintaining dignity and independence for as long as possible?
   c. What is clinically and ethically relevant information within this ethical frame?
5. Determine the possible options and implications.
   a. What are all the possible choices for a course of action within the relevant ethical frame?
   b. What are the implications of each option?
   c. Which are morally acceptable and congruent with the values of the patient, family, team members, and organization?
6. Select a course of action.
   a. What is the best or right decision in this patient situation?
   b. What is the ethical justification for this choice?
   c. What is the desired outcome?
   d. How, when, and by whom will the decision and outcomes be reevaluated?
7. Evaluate the decision and the outcomes.
   a. Were the desired outcomes achieved? If so, why? If not, why not?
   b. Knowing what is known now, would the choice have been different? What would change?
   c. If similar circumstances were to arise again, would the decision be the same or different?

Adapted from Cassells, J. M., & Gaul, A. L. (1998). An ethical assessment framework for nursing practice. *Maryland Nurse*, *17*(1), 9-12.

BOX 9-3 A Case Analysis Approach to Ethical Decision Making in Clinical Practice

Medical Indications
1. What is the patient's medical problem? History? Diagnosis? Prognosis?
2. Is the problem acute? Chronic? Critical? Emergent? Reversible?
3. What are the goals of treatment?
4. What are the possibilities of success?
5. What are plans in case of therapeutic failure?
6. In sum, how can this patient be benefited by medical and nursing care, and how can harm be avoided?

Patient Preferences
1. What has the patient expressed about preferences for treatment?
2. Has the patient been informed of benefits and risks, understood, and given consent?
3. Is the patient mentally capable and legally competent? What is the evidence of incapacity?
4. Has the patient expressed prior preferences (e.g., advance directive)?
5. If incapacitated, who is an appropriate surrogate? Is the surrogate using appropriate standards?
6. Is the patient unwilling or unable to cooperate with medical treatment? If so, why?
7. In sum, is the patient's right to choose being respected to the extent possible in ethics and law?

Quality of Life
1. What are the prospects, with or without treatment, for a return to the patient's normal life?
2. Are there biases that might prejudice a provider's evaluation of the patient's quality of life?
3. What physical, mental, and social deficits is the patient likely to experience if treatment succeeds?
4. Is the patient's present or future condition such that continued life might be judged undesirable by him or her?
5. Is there any plan and rationale to forgo treatment? What plans are there for comfort and palliative care?

Contextual Features
1. Are there family issues that might influence treatment decisions?
2. Are there provider issues that might influence treatment decisions?
3. Are there financial and economic factors?
4. Are there religious or cultural factors?
5. Is there any justification to breach confidentiality?
6. Are there problems of allocation of resources?
7. What are the legal implications of treatment decisions?
8. Is clinical research or teaching involved?
9. Is there any provider or institutional conflict of interest?

From Jonsen, A. R., Siegler, M., & Winslade, W. J. (2002). *Clinical ethics* (5th ed.). New York: McGraw-Hill. Reprinted with permission from McGraw-Hill.

presented in Boxes 9-1 and 9-2. Difficult ethical problems facing older adults, their families, and health care professionals are illustrated in these case examples.

Conflict with a Do-Not-Resuscitate Order

Mr. B., an 82-year-old man, is seen in the emergency department (ED) for chest pain, possibly related to a myocardial infarction (MI). The ED physician inquires whether Mr. B. desires CPR if he should experience a cardiopulmonary arrest. Mr. B. tells the physician that he "wants everything done." Following admission for an extensive MI, Mr. B. develops several complications that extend his hospitalization and require admission to the intensive care unit (ICU). Following a "code" in the next room, Mr. B. asks the nurse what happened. When the nurse explains that the patient in the next room coded, Mr. B. becomes concerned and asks what is done to a person during a code. After the nurse describes what typically happens during a code, Mr. B. states that he does not want to go through that. He states that he has lived a good life, he is tired, and he would not want to end up in a nursing home or be a burden for his family. Following discussion with his physician, a do-not-resuscitate (DNR) order is written for Mr. B. At the next family visit, Mr. B. explains to his wife and daughter that he requested a DNR order. The family becomes upset and asks the nurse what is going on. They explain to the nurse that their father would want everything possible done.

Several factors are of concern in this case study. Did Mr. B. make an informed choice when he initially expressed his desire to have everything done? Were there ongoing discussions with Mr. B. and his family members to ascertain their comprehension of the situation and the facts? What are their values, beliefs, goals, expectations, and preferences regarding the current circumstances and possible future events? Are Mr. B. and his family informed of the treatment options and their possible outcomes based on his circumstances and the available scientific information?

Using the framework presented in Box 9-1, an analysis of this case follows:

1. Determine the problem.
   a. What is the health problem? Mr. B., who is 82 years old, suffered a severe MI and is now experiencing several complications, such as congestive heart failure and borderline renal failure, which are minimally responsive to medical intervention.
   b. What are the ethical issues? It is questionable whether Mr. B. made a truly informed choice in the ED when he determined that he wanted everything done. Now, after receiving more complete information, Mr. B. obtained a DNR order from his physician. However, his family does not believe this is in his best interest because they were not included as part of the discussions. Does Mr. B.

have the capacity to provide informed consent given his medical condition? Did he give informed consent when he requested the DNR order?
   c. What is known about the health issue? There is little likelihood that Mr. B. will return to his pre-MI state of health and independence. Whether he will be able to return home to the care of his wife and family is unknown at this time.
   d. What is the available scientific evidence? In men, mean age of 81, the 1-year survival rate for congestive heart failure associated with MI was 80% in a prospective study (Aronow, Ann, & Kronzon, 2000). A meta-analysis of outcomes following CPR in hospitalized patients revealed the survival rate to be 13% at discharge (Ebell, Becker, Barry, & Hagen, 1998).
2. Identify the decision makers.
   a. Who is involved? Mr. B. made the decision to obtain a DNR order after discussions with the nurse and his physician.
   b. Who should be involved? His wife and family (to the extent that he desires their involvement) should also be included in the discussions about his condition, complications, prognosis, and likely outcomes given various scenarios.
   c. What are their roles? Mr. B. and his family have been very involved in his hospitalization. They visit at least daily and interact mostly with the nurses because the physicians usually make rounds at hours when families are not there. Mrs. B. will likely be the primary family caregiver if Mr. B. returns home after hospitalization.
   d. What are their values and beliefs? These are unknown because discussions have not occurred with the family members present. Interactions at the bedside have primarily focused on the events of the day and any changes in orders.
3. Determine the context.
   a. What is known about the situation? Currently Mr. B. receives health care coverage from Medicare. He and his wife live on his retirement and social security income, which provides a comfortable living.
   b. What do we need to know? Since Mr. B. has been relatively healthy until now, what is not known is the extent of medical care and support that will be needed at discharge and whether his current health care coverage will be adequate for those needs.
   c. What are the relevant contextual factors (cultural, spiritual, social, economic, etc.)? Currently, little is known about Mr. B.'s lifestyle, cultural, and spiritual preferences except that he was relatively healthy and independent until this hospitalization.
   d. How do we obtain additional information? The social worker and case manager will need to

become involved in Mr. B.'s case, and discussions with the health care team will need to include Mrs. B.

4. Frame the issue.
   a. What ethical perspective will best inform this situation? Mr. B. indicated that he did not want to go to a nursing home or be a burden to his family following his hospitalization.
   b. Is this problem primarily a question of benefit versus burden? Mr. B.'s stated wish not to be a burden to his family places the situation in a benefit versus burden frame. What is the benefit versus the burden of the various options? We do not know Mrs. B.'s or the rest of the family's feelings on these issues.
   c. What is the clinically and ethically relevant information within this frame? The chances of survival for Mr. B., based on the best available evidence, should he experience a cardiopulmonary arrest are less than 20% of leaving the hospital alive. If he survives, his quality of life will be unknown.
5. Identify options and implications.
   a. What are all the possible options? At this point, aggressive medical and nursing interventions are being implemented. Should Mr. B. suffer an arrest, the options are to institute CPR or not to institute CPR.
   b. What are the implications of each option? If Mr. B. were to experience an arrest, his chances of survival without CPR are nonexistent. If CPR were initiated, there is about a 13% chance that he may survive to be discharged from the hospital, but the quality of his life is unknown.
   c. Which are morally congruent with the values of the decision makers? After receiving more information, the decision for a DNR order seems congruent with Mr. B.'s values and preferences at this time. Based on the available scientific information, this decision is supported by the staff involved. It is not known whether his family supports this choice.
6. Select a course of action.
   a. What is the best decision? At this point, Mr. B.'s decision regarding DNR status seems to be based on informed consent and congruent with his values and preferences. However, family members were not included in the decision-making process. Mr. B. needs to be encouraged to discuss this with his family. If Mr. B. desires, the physician and nurse can also discuss these issues with his family.
   b. What is the ethical reasoning? Based on self-determination and informed consent, Mr. B. requested a DNR order after obtaining more information. Based on an ethic of care, Mr. B.'s family members, who are close and attentive, should also be included in these discussions for everyone to

be informed about the values and preferences expressed by Mr. B. through this decision.
   c. What is the desired outcome? Mr. B. wants to live and to have a good quality of life.
   d. How, when, and by whom will the decision and outcomes be evaluated? After discussing these issues with the family and encouraging Mr. B. to talk with his family thoroughly about his decision, this issue should be revisited periodically as his medical condition changes and before any major procedures.
7. Evaluate the decision.
   a. Were the desired outcomes achieved? If so, why? If not, why not? After thoroughly discussing the extent of Mr. B.'s medical condition, prognosis, and treatment preferences with his family, a determination can be made whether the decision for a DNR is consistent with Mr. B.'s values, beliefs, expectations, and preferences. After discussing whether this decision is consistent with Mr. B.'s life plan, the health care team and family can determine whether this decision was truly informed.
   b. Knowing what is known now, would the choice have been different? Probably not if Mr. B. gave an informed choice. What would change? A more thorough discussion of the issues in the initial conversation or soon after admission, including the family, would have avoided the confusion and anguish in this case.
   c. Would the decision be the same in the future? More in-depth conversations about what is actually involved in a "code," including other options, outcomes, and experiences, should occur with elderly patients to ensure a truly informed choice.

Conflict of Questioning a Patient's Competence

Ms. T. is referred to a community-based long-term care program by her neighbor to obtain in-home services. Ms. T. has early dementia and has received meals on wheels and extensive support from her neighbor. She has no children, and her nearest relative, an elderly sister, lives 150 miles away. To receive needed in-home services, Ms. T. must keep careful financial records to qualify for Medicaid. Until now, the neighbor has handled Ms. T.'s finances for her and provided numerous other services, such as visiting, phoning, daily checking, and assistance with meal preparation. Now that the financial record keeping is becoming more complex, the neighbor is reluctant to remain involved.

Ms. T. has repeatedly stated that she wants to stay at home. However, safety is a major concern because she often leaves the stove on unattended. Her neighbor feels that a rest home would be the best place for Ms. T. The local adult protective services unit has a history of routinely institutionalizing incompetent elderly patients with cognitive and functional impairments.

The nurse case manager sees two options available: (1) to suggest that the neighbor obtain power of attorney so that she has legal authority to act for Ms. T., or (2) to pursue an incompetence proceeding, which involves petitioning the court and removing all rights of self-determination from Ms. T. The dilemma is which course of action to pursue, because Ms. T.'s cognitive capabilities may be such that she cannot be found incompetent, yet she has difficulty understanding complex matters (such as power of attorney).

Using the framework presented in Box 9-2, an analysis of this case follows.

Medical Indications

1. What is the patient's medical problem? History? Diagnosis? Prognosis? Ms. T. has early dementia and has been living independently with extensive support from her neighbor. With time, a continued decline in Ms. T.'s mental and physical functioning is expected.
2. Is the problem acute? Chronic? Critical? Emergent? Reversible? This is a chronic, irreversible problem that will progress with time.
3. What are the goals of treatment? The goal has been for Ms. T. to maintain her independence for as long a safely possible.
4. What are the possibilities of success? Unless the neighbor is willing to obtain power of attorney, it seems unlikely that Ms. T. will be able to remain safely in her home.
5. What are plans in case of failure? Ms. T. is unable to live independently unassisted. A determination must be made whether Ms. T. could live with her elderly sister, or her sister could live with Ms. T. If either of these is not possible a referral will need to be made to adult protective services.
6. In sum, how can this patient be benefited by medical and nursing care, and how can harm be avoided? An assessment can be made by the nurse about the possibility of Ms. T.'s sister, a friend, or her neighbor coming to live with her or the possibility of Ms. T. relocating to live with one of them. A referral to a social worker can be made to assist with these evaluations. If none of these is an option, adult protective services will need to be notified to make arrangements for Ms. T. to be moved to an assisted living facility.

Patient Preferences

1. What has the patient expressed about preferences for treatment? Ms. T. has no desire to be institutionalized. Her expressed desire is to remain in her own home.
2. Has the patient been informed of benefits and risks, understood, and given consent? At the time these discussions took place, Ms. T. was capable of expressing her choice. In the present, Ms. T. is no longer able to understand the potential harm to herself or make an informed choice because of her diminished decisional capacity.
3. Is the patient mentally capable and legally competent? What is the evidence of incapacity? Ms. T. does not have the mental capacity, nor is she legally competent, to make decisions. She is unable to weigh the risks of a situation or understand the consequences of her actions. She does not have insight into the potential harm of living alone.
4. Has the patient expressed prior preferences (e.g., advance directive)? Ms. T. does not have an advance directive but has stated her preference in the past to live independently for as long as possible.
5. If incapacitated, who is an appropriate surrogate? Is the surrogate using appropriate standards? Ms. T. does not have a legal surrogate. If Ms. T.'s neighbor could obtain assistance with managing the financial aspects of her affairs, perhaps Ms. T. could remain independent a while longer with in-home supportive services.
6. Is the patient unwilling or unable to cooperate with medical treatment? If so, why? Ms. T. is unwilling to consider living anywhere other than her home.
7. In sum, is the patient's right to choose being respected to the extent possible in ethics and law? To this point, yes, but without increasing assistance in her home and with her financial affairs, and continued support from her neighbor, Ms. T. will need a referral to adult protective services.

Quality of Life

1. What are the prospects, with or without treatment, for a return to the patient's normal life? There are none; her disease is progressive and irreversible.
2. Are there biases that might prejudice a provider's evaluation of the patient's quality of life? No; the nurse has tried to maintain Ms. T.'s independence for as long as possible.
3. What physical, mental, and social deficits is the patient likely to experience if treatment succeeds? If Ms. T. is admitted to a nursing home, she will lose her independence and some autonomy that she currently has.
4. Is the patient's present or future condition such that continued life might be judged undesirable by her? Based on Ms. T.'s past expressed desires, moving from her home would be unacceptable to her.
5. Is there any plan and rationale to forgo treatment? What plans are there for comfort and palliative care? Care would be provided for her in an assisted living facility.

Contextual Features

1. Are there family issues that might influence treatment decisions? Whether or not Mrs. T.'s sister would be able to assist with living arrangements could influence a decision for a referral to adult protective services.

2. Are there provider issues that might influence treatment decisions? No.

3. Are there financial and economic factors? Ms. T. needs someone to manage her financial affairs to receive increased in-home supportive services.

4. Are there religious or cultural factors? None known.

5. Is there any justification to breach confidentiality? Seeking further assistance for Ms. T. may require sharing information about her medical condition.

6. Are there problems of allocation of resources? Ms. T. has adequate financial resources for her care.

7. What are the legal implications of treatment decisions? Guardianship for Ms. T. would need to be obtained.

8. Is clinical research or teaching involved? No.

9. Is there any provider or institutional conflict of interest? Unknown.

The nurse case manager sees three options: (1) attempt to have Ms. T.'s sister or a friend move in with her; (2) encourage the neighbor to obtain power of attorney to manage Ms. T.'s financial affairs, thus maintaining her independence for a while longer, and her sister to obtain durable power of attorney to manage medical decisions; or (3) obtain a competency hearing for Ms. T., which would result in her losing her right of self-determination. Preventing harm to Ms. T. is the nurse's primary objective, and secondarily, preserving her independence for as long as possible.

Conflict over Aggressiveness of Care for a Depressed Elderly Woman

Ms. W. is an 83-year-old woman living in an intermediate care facility with chronic pain secondary to nonunion of a clavicular fracture, heart block, depression, and mild dementia. She has lost 17 pounds in the past month. A hospital admission to insert a feeding tube or to address her nutritional status is being considered. During two previous hospitalizations, her family has elected not to have a pacemaker put in to treat her heart block. It is not clear whether the patient has been consulted about the pacemaker. The patient, when approached by anyone, keeps repeating, "Just leave me alone!"

She is currently being treated with antidepressants prescribed by the consulting geropsychiatrist and has shown some small increase in interaction with others, but she continues to lose weight. The nurse caring for Ms. W. is aware of the following limitations of the care environment: volunteer services at the facility are limited and psychotherapy is not an option because of reimbursement and transportation issues.

Using the framework presented in Box 9-2, an analysis of this case follows.

Medical Indications

1. What is the patient's medical problem? History? Diagnosis? Prognosis? Ms. W. suffers from chronic pain, depression, and mild dementia. As a result, she has had a 10% weight loss in the past month. If this continues it will become life threatening.

2. Is the problem acute? Chronic? Critical? Emergent? Reversible? The depression may be reversible, but the dementia is irreversible. Without further treatment of the depression or socialization and assistance with eating, the weight loss will continue.

3. What are the goals of treatment? Ms. W. is requesting to be left alone; however, the health care team wants to treat the depression with a subsequent return of appetite. The family refused to consent for a pacemaker for her heart block, so it is unclear whether they would consent to aggressive treatment for her depression.

4. What are the possibilities of success? The depression may be treatable; a referral or involuntary commitment would be required.

5. What are plans in case of therapeutic failure? If the depression is not abated and nutrition restored, consideration of placement of a feeding tube would be an option. If the family and patient are not in agreement, the patient will die.

6. In sum, how can this patient be benefited by medical and nursing care, and how can harm be avoided? This situation would need to be discussed in depth with the family. A determination would then need to be made whether to pursue more aggressive treatment for the depression or to obtain an involuntary commitment. A decision about the placement of a feeding tube to maintain nutrition would also need to be made to avoid continued weight loss.

Patient Preferences

1. What has the patient expressed about preferences for treatment? The patient continually states that she wants to be left alone. It is unclear whether this is due to the depression or the dementia.

2. Has the patient been informed of benefits and risks, understood, and given consent? Ms. W. is unable to give informed consent because of her severe depression and early dementia.

3. Is the patient mentally capable and legally competent? What is the evidence of incapacity? Ms. W. is not legally competent at this time because of her early dementia and severe depression. It is unclear whether she is mentally capable of indicating her treatment preferences, because she says only that she

wants to be left alone. However, legal proceedings have not been initiated.

4. Has the patient expressed prior preferences (e.g., advance directive)? Ms. W. does not have an advance directive. The family indicated in the past that they would not agree to aggressive treatment because of her dementia.

5. If incapacitated, who is an appropriate surrogate? Is the surrogate using appropriate standards? The family is the appropriate surrogate unless there is some indication of secondary gain by not treating her medical problems.

6. Is the patient unwilling or unable to cooperate with medical treatment? If so, why? The patient is unwilling and unable to cooperate because of her severe depression and dementia. This is evidenced by her weight loss over the past month.

7. In sum, is the patient's right to choose being respected to the extent possible in ethics and law? The potential for further harm is great because of continued weight loss resulting from severe depression.

Quality of Life

1. What are the prospects, with or without treatment, for a return to the patient's normal life? Without treatment and a spontaneous return of appetite and relief of her depression, Ms. W. will die.

2. Are there biases that might prejudice a provider's evaluation of the patient's quality of life? No, the health care providers are very concerned about Ms. W.'s health state. Because of her limited financial coverage, however, more aggressive psychotherapy may not be available.

3. What physical, mental, and social deficits is the patient likely to experience if treatment succeeds? There is the potential for greater benefit than harm if psychotherapy services are obtained.

4. Is the patient's present or future condition such that continued life might be judged undesirable by her? Due to severe depression, Ms. W. is not eating and states that she wishes to be left alone. It is unclear whether the consequences of these actions are evident to Ms. W.

5. Is there any plan and rationale to forgo treatment? If psychiatric services are not available because of limited financial resources, and someone is not able to provide social interaction and assistance with eating on a regular basis, there are no other options other than to insert a feeding tube or do nothing. What plans are there for comfort and palliative care? Discussions with the family are indicated.

Contextual Features

1. Are there family issues that might influence treatment decisions? It is not known if there are additional family resources for psychotherapy if Ms. W.'s plan does not cover those services. It is also not known what the reasons are for not pursuing aggressive treatment, considering that her dementia is in the early stages.

2. Are there provider issues that might influence treatment decisions? Reimbursement for further psychiatric services may not be available.

3. Are there financial and economic factors? Family resources other than Ms. W.'s are unknown.

4. Are there religious or cultural factors? Unknown.

5. Is there any justification to breach confidentiality? Discussion of Ms. W.'s health status with her family would require disclosure of her health information.

6. Are there problems of allocation of resources? The limits of Ms. W.'s Medicare.

7. What are the legal implications of treatment decisions? Obtaining a surrogate decision maker for health care decisions is an option.

8. Is clinical research or teaching involved? No.

9. Is there any provider or institutional conflict of interest? The only potential conflict of interest may be if there is secondary gain for the institution from either continuing to have Ms. W. as a patient or a benefit from her demise.

Because the reason for Ms. W.'s refusal to eat is unclear in this case, a referral to psychiatry for treatment of her depression should be considered, which may benefit her. The nurse can also discuss the option of having a family member or friend visit at meal times for socialization and assistance with meals. If nothing is done and Ms. W. continues to experience weight loss, additional harm will come to her and she will eventually die. More aggressive treatment, such as the insertion of a feeding tube, would require the consent of Ms. W. or her family and probably require the use of restraints, which would further compromise Ms. W.'s autonomy. If Ms. W. or her family refuses further treatment, involuntary commitment can be sought to treat her depression, and ideally her desire to eat will return.

SUMMARY

Ethical issues involving the care of older adults continue to grow more complex. With the aging of our society, the growing diversity of our population, increasing technological advances, and declining resources, the recognition of ethical concerns is essential. The gerontological nurse requires a background in ethics and a working knowledge of the analysis of ethical problems. As a member of an interdisciplinary team, an awareness of the values and beliefs that underpin the nurse's decision making, as well as understanding of and sensitivity to the personal and professional values of other team members, is necessary.

As nurses, our moral imperative is to treat each individual with dignity and to respect the value and worth of each person. Preserving the autonomy and self-determination of the elderly for as long as possible, while sometimes implementing measures to protect them from harm, presents interesting challenges. Our code of ethics also demands that we work to improve the health of all people. Working collaboratively and collectively are skills that nurses traditionally have in the workplace that must be transferred to the community arena to bring about change in the laws and policies that affect older people. Political activism is a skill that gerontological nurses must acquire to share their knowledge and expertise with legislators and administrators to bring about change that will improve the conditions and health of the elderly and promote ethical care.

REFERENCES

American Association of Retired Persons. (2005). Resources on end of life, living wills, dying and death. Retrieved July 10, 2005, from www.aarp.org/families/end_life/recent_resources_on_end_of_life_living_wills_dying.html.

American Geriatrics Society. (2001). AGS position statement: The responsible conduct of research. Retrieved July 10, 2005, from www.americangeriatrics.org/products/positionpapers/respcondresearch.shtml.

American Nurses Association. (1994). Ethics and human rights position statements: Assisted suicide. Silver Springs, MD: Author.

American Nurses Association. (2001). *Code of ethics for nurses with interpretive statements.* Washington, DC: Author.

American Nurses Association. (2003). *Nursing's social policy statement* (2nd ed.). Washington, DC: Author.

Applebaum, G. E., King, J. E., & Finucare, T. E. (1990). The outcome of CPR initiated in nursing homes. *Journal of the American Geriatrics Society, 38*(3), 197-200.

Aronow, W. S., Ann, C., & Kronzon, I. (2000). Prognosis of congestive heart failure after prior myocardial infarction in older men and women with abnormal versus normal left ventricular ejection fraction. *American Journal of Cardiology, 85*(11), 1382-1384.

Beauchamp, T. L., & Childress, J. F. (2001). *Principles of biomedical ethics* (5th ed.). Oxford: Oxford University Press.

Benner, P. (1994). *Interpretive phenomenology: Embodiment, caring, and ethics in health and illness.* Thousand Oaks, CA: Sage.

Botes, A. (2000). An integrated approach to ethical decision-making in the health team. *Journal of Advanced Nursing, 32*(5), 1076-1082.

Boult, L., Dentler, B., Volicer, L., Mead, S., & Evans, J. (2003). Ethics and research in long-term care: A position statement from the American Medical Directors Association. *Journal of the American Medical Directors Association, 4*(3), 171-174.

Callahan, D. (2002). How much medical progress can we afford? Equity and the cost of health care. *Journal of Molecular Biology, 319,* 885-890.

Callahan, D. (2003). Living and dying with medical technology. *Critical Care Medicine, 31*(5), s344-s346.

Cameron, M. E. (2003). Legal and ethical issues: Our best ethical and spiritual values. *Journal of Professional Nursing, 19*(3), 117-118.

Carper, B. A. (1978). Fundamental patterns of knowing in nursing. *Advances in Nursing Science, 1,* 13-23.

Cassells, J. M., & Gaul, A. L. (1998). An ethical assessment framework for nursing practice. *Maryland Nurse, 17*(1), 9-12.

Cassells, J. M., Jenkins, J., Lea, D. H., Calzone, K., & Johnson, E. (2003). An ethical assessment framework for addressing global genetic issues in clinical practice. *Oncology Nursing Forum, 30*(3), 383-390.

Cate, F. H., & Gill, B. A. (1991). *The Patient Self-Determination Act: Implementation issues and opportunities: A white paper of the Annenberg Washington Program.* Evanston, IL: Northwestern University Press.

Daly, G. (2000). Ethics and economics. *Nursing Economics, 18*(4), 194-201.

DeRenzo, E. G., & Olick, R. S. (2000). Should it be mandated that an HEC review a physician's decision not to honor a patient's or surrogate's refusal of treatment? *HEC Forum, 12*(2),161-165.

Doukas, D. J., & McCullough, L. B. (1991). The Values History: The evaluation of the patient's values and advance directives. *Journal of Family Practice, 31*(1), 145-153.

Doukas, D. J., & McCullough, L. B. (2000). Using the Values History to enhance advance directive communication. In J. J. Gallo, T. Fulmer, G. J. Paveza, & W. Reichel (Eds.), *Handbook of geriatric assessment.* Gaithersburg, MD: Aspen.

Drane, J. F. (1985). The many faces of competency. *Hastings Center Report, 14,* 17-21.

Drevdahl, D., Kneipp, S. M., Canales, M. K., & Dorcy, K. S. (2001). Reinvesting in social justice: A capital idea for public health nursing? *Advances in Nursing Science, 24*(2), 19-31.

DuVal, G., Sartorius, L., Clarridge, B., Gensler, G., & Danis, M. (2001). What triggers requests for ethics consultations? *Journal of Medical Ethics, 27*(suppl, 1), 24-29.

Ebell, M. H., Becker, L. A., Barry, H. C., & Hagen, M. (1998). Survival after inhospital cardiopulmonary resuscitation: A meta-analysis. *Journal of General Internal Medicine, 13,* 805-816.

Erlen, J. A. (2002) Ethics in chronic illness. In I. M. Lubkin & P. D. Larsen (Eds.), *Chronic illness: Impact and interventions* (5th ed.). Sudbury, MA: Jones & Bartlett.

Ersek, M. (2003). Artificial nutrition and hydration: Clinical issues. *Journal of Hospice and Palliative Nursing, 5*(4), 221-230.

Flaherty, E., Fulmer, T., & Mezey, M. (2003). *Geriatric nursing review syllabus: A core curriculum in advanced practice geriatric nursing.* New York: American Geriatrics Society.

Gadow, S. (1996). Aging as death rehearsal: The oppressiveness of reason. *Journal of Clinical Ethics, 7*(1), 35-40.

Gadow, S. (1999). Relational narrative: The postmodern turn in nursing ethics. *Scholarly Inquiry for Nursing Practice, 13*(1), 57-70.

Gallo, J. J., Fulmer, T., Paveza, G. J., & Reichel, W. (2000). *Handbook of geriatric assessment* (3rd ed.). Gaithersburg, MD: Aspen.

Gilligan, C. (1993). *In a different voice: Psychological theory and women's development.* Cambridge, MA: Harvard University Press.

Guo, L., & Schick, I. C. (2003). The impact of committee characteristics on the success of healthcare ethics committees. *HEC Forum, 15*(3):287-299.

Hamel, M. B., Teno, J. M., Goldman, L., Davis, L. J., Galanos, A. N., Desbienss, N., et al. (1999). Patient age and decisions to withhold life-sustaining treatments from seriously ill, hospitalized adults. *Annals of Internal Medicine, 130*(2), 116-125.

Hayley, D. C., Cassel, C. K., Snyder, L., & Rudberg, M. (1996). Ethical and legal issues in nursing home care. *Archives of Internal Medicine, 156*(3), 249-256.

Heath, H. (1998). Reflections and patterns of knowing in nursing. *Journal of Advanced Nursing, 27*(5), 1054-1059.

Henderson, M. (1982). Ethical considerations for the nurse as primary provider. In M. L. Lynch (Ed.), *On your own: Professional growth through independent nursing practice.* Monterey, CA: Wadsworth Health Sciences.

Hogstel, M. O., Curry, L. C., Walker, C. A., & Burns, P. G. (2004). Ethics committees in long-term care facilities. *Geriatric Nursing, 25*(6), 364-369.

Jameton, A. (1984). *Nursing practice: The ethical issues.* Englewood Cliffs, NJ: Prentice-Hall.

Jogerst, G. J., Daly, J. M., Brinig, M. F., Dawson, J. D, Schmuch, G. A., & Ingram, J. G. (2003). Domestic elder abuse and the law. *American Journal of Public Health, 93*(12), 2131-2136.

Joint Commission on Accreditation of Healthcare Organizations. (2003). *Joint Commission: 2003 hospital accreditation standards.* Oakbrook Terrace, IL: Author.

Jonsen, A. R. (1976). Principles for an ethics of health services. In B. Neugarten (Ed.), *Social ethics and the aging society.* Chicago: Committee on Human Development, University of Chicago.

Jonsen, A. R., Siegler, M., & Winslade, W. J. (1998). *Clinical ethics* (4th ed.). New York: McGraw-Hill.

Jonsen, A. R., Seigler, M., & Winslade, W. J. (2002). *Clinical ethics* (5th ed.). New York: McGraw-Hill.

Kane, R. A., & Caplan, A. L. (1990). *Everyday ethics: Resolving delimmas in nursing home life.* New York: Springer.

Kant, I. (1964). In H. J. Paton (Ed.), *Groundwork of the metaphysics of morals.* New York: Harper & Row, p. 96.

Keenan, S. P. (2004). Improving end-of-life care: Targeting what we can. *Critical Care Medicine, 32*(5), 1230-1231.

Lo, B., & Steinbrook, R. (2004). Resuscitating advance directives. *Archives of Internal Medicine, 164,* 1501-1506.

Lucke, K. T. (1999). Outcomes of caring as perceived by spinal cord injured individuals during rehabilitation. *Rehabilitation Nursing, 24*(6), 247-253.

Marson, D. C., Ingram, K. K., Cody, H. A., & Harrell, L. E. (1995). Assessing the competency of patients with Alzheimer's disease under different legal standards: A prototype instrument. *Archives of Neurology, 52,* 949-954.

May, W. F. (1982). Who cares for the elderly? *Hastings Center Report, 12*(6), 31-37.

McDonagh, J. R., Elliot, T. B., Engleberg, R. A., Treece, P. D., Shannon, S. E., Rubenfeld, G. D., et al. (2004). Family satisfaction with family conferences about end-of-life care in the intensive care unit: Increased proportion of family speech is associated with increased satisfaction. *Critical Care Medicine, 32*(7), 1609-1611.

Mezey, M. D., Cassel, C. K., Bottrell, M. M., Hyer, K., & Howe, J. L. (2002). *Ethical patient care: A casebook for geriatric health care teams.* Baltimore: Johns Hopkins University Press.

Missouri Bar. (2005). Durable power of attorney and health care directive: Questions and answers, instructions and sample forms. Retrieved June 5, 2005, from www.mobar.org/pamphlet/livewill.htm.

Moore, D. W. (2004). Nurses top list in honesty and ethics poll. The Gallup Organization. Retrieved September 24, 2005, from www.gallup.com/poll/content/login.aspx?ci=14236.

Mueller, P. S., Hook, C., & Fleming, K. C. (2004). Ethical issues in geriatrics: A guide for clinicians. *Mayo Clinic Proceedings, 79*(4), 554-562.

Nightingale, F. (1859). *Notes on nursing: What it is and what it is not.* Philadelphia: J. B. Lippincott.

Nightingale, F. (1992). *Notes on nursing* (commemorative ed.). Philadelphia: J. B. Lippincott.

Noddings, N. (2003). *Caring: A feminine approach to ethics and moral education* (2nd ed.). Berkeley: University of California Press.

Powers, B. A. (2000). Everyday ethics of dementia care in nursing homes: A definition and taxonomy. *American Journal of Alzheimer's Disease, 15*(3), 143-151.

Rodney, P., Varcoe, C., Storch, J. L., McPherson, G., Mahoney, K., Brown, H., et al. (2002). Navigating towards a moral horizon: A multisite qualitative study of ethical practice in nursing. *Canadian Journal of Nursing Research, 35*(3), 75-102.

Rosenblatt, R. A., Wright, G. E., Baldwin, L., Chan, L., Clitherow, P., Chen, F. M., & Hart, L. G. (2000). The effect of the doctor-patient relationship on emergency department use among the elderly. *American Journal of Public Health, 90*(1), 97-102.

Schmidt, W. C. (2000). Health care financing and delivery for the elderly: A planned regulated system in counterpoint to a competitive marketplace approach. *Ethics, Law, and Aging Review, 6,* 53-65.

Shannon, T. A., & Walter, J. J. (2004). Implications of the papal allocution on feeding tubes. *Hastings Center Report, 34*(4), 18-20.

Singer, P. A., Pellegrino, E. D., & Siegler, M. (1990). Ethics committees and consultants. *Journal of Clinical Ethics, 1*(4), 263-267.

Sotnik, P., & Jezewski, M. A. (2005). Culture and the disability services. In J. H. Stone (Ed.), *Culture and disability.* Thousand Oaks, CA: Sage.

Stone, J. H. (Ed.). (2005). *Culture and disability: Providing culturally competent services.* Thousand Oaks, CA: Sage.

Strumpf, N. E., & Evans, L. K. (1991). The ethical problems of prolonged physical restraint. *Journal of Gerontological Nursing, 27*(3), 27-30.

SUPPORT Principal Investigators. (1995). A controlled trial to improve care for seriously ill hospitalized patients. The Study to Understand Prognoses and Preferences for Outcomes and Risks of Treatments (SUPPORT). *JAMA, 274,* 1591-1598.

Volbrecht, R. M. (2002). *Nursing ethics: Communities in dialogue.* Upper Saddle River, NJ: Prentice Hall.

Watson, J. (1985). *Nursing: Human science and human care.* Norwalk, CT: Appleton-Century-Crofts.

White, J. (1995). Patterns of knowing: Review, critique and update. *Advances in Nursing Science, 17*(4), 73-86.

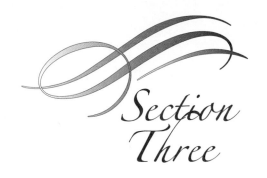

Section Three

Aging Changes and Health Deviations

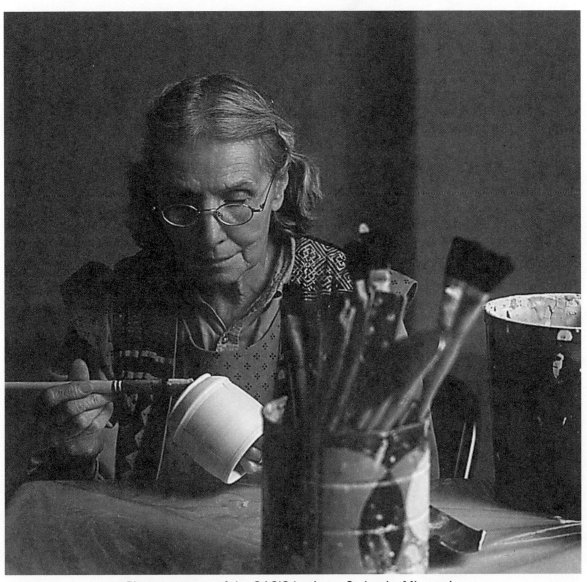

Photo courtesy of the OASIS Institute, St. Louis, Missouri.

Chapter 10

Integument System

Adrianne Dill Linton

Objectives

Describe normal skin, hair, and nail changes associated with aging.

Discuss causes of normal skin changes in older persons.

Describe measures to maintain healthy, intact skin in the older adult.

Identify the causes and treatment of skin disorders that are common in older persons.

Describe the components of skin assessment in the older adult.

Formulate nursing diagnoses for older adults with skin disorders.

Develop management plans for older adults with skin problems (actual or potential).

The primary functions of the skin are protection from environmental stresses, regulation of temperature, maintenance of fluid and electrolyte balance, excretion of metabolic wastes, and sensory reception (touch, pain, pressure). The skin is composed of three layers: the epidermis, or outer layer; the dermis, or middle layer; and subcutaneous tissue that lies beneath the dermis. The epidermis receives its nourishment from the underlying dermis and is divided into four strata (in order from the outer to the inner layer): (1) keratin layer or stratum corneum; (2) granular layer; (3) spinous layer or prickle layer; and (4) basal layer. The outer horny layer contains dead keratinized cells; the inner cellular layers produce melanin (pigment) and keratin (protein). Essentially, the epidermis grows from the basal layer, structures itself in the spinous or prickle layer, establishes the permeability barrier in the granular layer, and sheds itself in the outer cornified layer. The dermis contains blood vessels, nerves, hair follicles, and sebaceous glands. The subcutaneous tissue contains eccrine or sweat glands, some hair follicles, blood vessels, and fat (Figure 10-1). The three layers are supported by an underlying network of collagen fibers and associated elastin fibers. The collagen fibers attach the skin to the underlying tissues, and the elastin fibers give the skin flexibility, elasticity, and strength. Hair, nails, and sweat glands are considered to be dermal appendages, or accessory structures of the skin (Farmer & Hood, 1990).

NORMAL CHANGES WITH AGING

The changes in the appearance and function of the skin, perhaps more than any other organ system, reflect the continuous aging process. One needs only to look at a person to determine an approximate age. Observations considered to be evidence of advancing age include wrinkles, sagging skin, gray hair, and baldness. Aging changes can be categorized as either intrinsic or extrinsic (Table 10-1). Intrinsic factors are related to a decrease in proliferative capacity that leads to cellular senescence resulting in altered biosynthetic activity of skin-derived cells (Jenkins, 2002). Genetics plays a role in intrinsic aging, although it is difficult to determine how much variation is explained by genetics. Extrinsic factors are environmental, with sunlight being the primary culprit.

Cumulative changes related to environmental factors are referred to as *photoaging*, which is dependent on the degree of exposure and skin pigment (Fisher et al., 2002). The effects of ultraviolet light on the skin, which have been studied extensively, include long-term growth arrest in dermal fibroblasts and alterations in enzymes in the stratum corneum that make it vulnerable to oxidative damage (Batisse, Bazin, Baldeweck, Querleux, & Leveque, 2002; Hellmans, Corstjens, Neven, Declercq, & Maes, 2003; Ma, Wlaschek, Hommel, Schneider, & Scharffetter-Kochanek, 2002). Ultraviolet light affects the dermal connective tissue that maintains tensile strength, resilience, and stability of the skin. This explains the effects of prolonged exposure which include wrinkling, laxity, fragility, a leathery appearance, and impaired healing (Ma, et al., 2001). Photoaging is most apparent in people who reside in sunny climates and

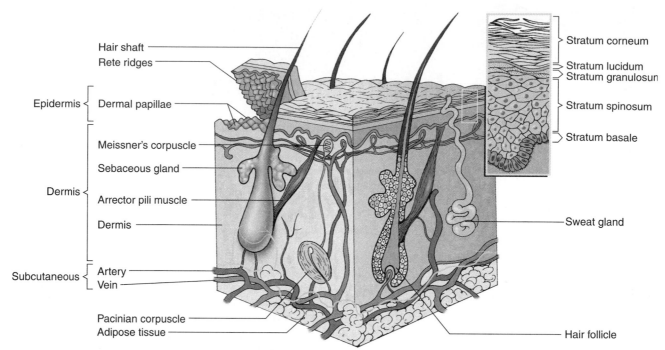

Figure 10-1 Anatomy of the skin. (From Monahan, F. D., Sands, J. K., Neighbors, M., Marek, J. F., & Green C. J. [2007]. *Phipps' medical surgical nursing* [8th ed.]. St. Louis: Mosby, p. 1860.)

have light skin pigmentation. The effect of sunlight on skin aging is obvious when the skin in exposed areas is compared with nonexposed skin. Skin that usually is covered shows far less change with age (Figure 10-2). Giacomoni and Rein (2001) report that the mechanisms by which intrinsic and extrinsic factors trigger aging changes in the skin are essentially the same. Both induce a step of the microinflammatory cycle that causes breakdown of the extracellular matrix. The effect is random damage to cells, which leads to the secretion of prostaglandins and leukotrienes.

Table 10-1 *Clinical Features of Intrinsic and Extrinsic Aging*

Change with Time	Intrinsic or Chronological Aging	Extrinsic or Photoaging
Fine wrinkles	Yes	Yes
Skin laxity	Yes	Yes
Skin thinning	Yes	No
Xerosis (dryness)	Yes	Minimal
Coarse wrinkles	Minimal	Yes
Solar lentigines (age or liver spots)	No	Yes
Mottled dyspigmentation	No	Yes
Actinic keratoses	No	Yes

From Brooke, R. C. C., & Griffiths, C. E. M. (2003). Aging of the skin. In *Brocklehurst's textbook of geriatric medicine and gerontology* (6th ed.). London: Churchill Livingstone, p. 1269.

In addition to ultraviolet light, smoking has been implicated in accelerated skin aging, although not all researchers have reached the same conclusions. Aizen and Gilhar (2001) reported more prominent facial wrinkling among smokers than among nonsmokers. Based on visual assessment of subjects' skin with a 10-point rating scale, Leung and Harvey (2002) concluded that smoking 20 cigarettes a day was equivalent to nearly 10 years of chronological aging. In contrast, Knuutinen, Kallioinen, Vahakangas, and Oikarinen (2002) studied the physical qualities and histology of skin in male smokers and nonsmokers and found no significant differences between the groups in dermal elastic fibers or skin elasticity.

Epidermis (Stratum Corneum, Keratinocytes, Melanocytes, Langerhans Cells)

With advancing age the *epidermis* generally thins in protected areas and thickens in sun-exposed areas. Despite variations in epidermal thickness, the average number of cell layers remains unchanged. The prickle cells of the inner layer of the epidermis show greater variation in nuclear and cytoplasmic size and a less orderly arrangement of cells than in younger people. Cells reproduce more slowly and are larger and more irregular; however, exposed epidermal cells may divide more frequently than unexposed cells. The main skin cell type involved in photoaging may be keratinocytes (Bosset, et al., 2003).

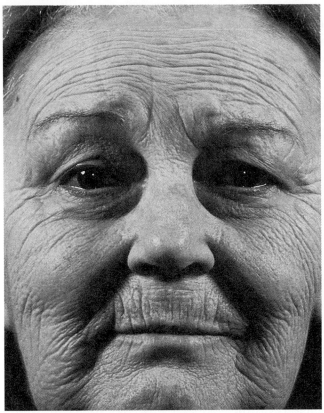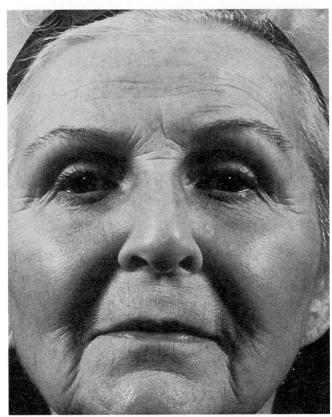

Figure 10-2 Faces of two 71-year-old women. The woman on the right has avoided sun exposure over most of her life and the changes are mostly intrinsic. In contrast, the woman on the left had a great deal of sun exposure and shows evidence of wrinkling and skin thickening associated with photoaging. (From Brooke, R. C. C., & Griffiths, C. E. M. [2003]. Aging of the skin. In *Brocklehurst's textbook of geriatric medicine and gerontology* [6th ed.]. London: Churchill Livingstone.)

Melanocytes, the cells in the basal layer of the epidermis responsible for the production of melanin, decrease in number and function as an effect of intrinsic aging. Intrinsically aged skin is less likely to tan when exposed to ultraviolet light. In contrast, photoaged skin has an increased number of melanocytes (Brooke & Griffiths, 2003).

The turnover rate of epidermal cells declines 30% to 50% by the eighth decade, and the replacement rate of stratum corneum cells may be prolonged as much as 100%. Repair of injured skin takes longer in older persons. Hypersensitivity reactions are delayed and less dramatic because of decreases in circulating thymus-derived lymphocytes, cytokines, and epidermal Langerhans cells (cells responsible for skin immunosurveillance) (Berger & Gilchrest, 1998). The decrease in epidermal immune surveillance may explain the decreased incidence of allergic contact dermatitis in older adults (Brooke & Griffiths, 2003).

Decreased vitamin D precursor in the epidermis may reduce vitamin D production, which may be a factor in the development of osteomalacia (Brooke & Griffiths, 2003).

Dermis (Fibroblasts, Endothelium, Mast Cells) and Subcutaneous Tissue

The *dermis* contains blood vessels, nerves, hair follicles, and sebaceous glands, but the major portion (79%) is made up of collagen. This layer of the skin thins by as much as 20% with aging and may explain the transparent quality of aged skin (Berger & Gilchrest, 1998). The strength and elasticity of the skin are largely due to dermal collagen, and decreased skin strength and elasticity with aging are attributed to collagen changes. Collagen and elastic fibers are affected by both intrinsic and extrinsic factors. By the fourth decade, the architecture of collagen fibers becomes disorganized (El-Domyati, et al., 2002). In facial skin areas where collagen is lost, elastin accumulates. The number of fibroblasts, which are the cells underlying the dermis that are responsible for the synthesis of protein and collagen, tends to decrease (Kulozik & Krieg, 1989; Lapiere, 1990). These changes, along with exposure to sunlight, cause *elastosis*, which is characterized by a weather-beaten or tanned appearance.

With aging the vascularity of the dermal skin decreases, as evidenced by fewer epithelial cells and blood vessels. There is greater vascular fragility, leading to the frequent appearance of hemorrhages (senile purpura), cherry angiomas, venous stasis, and venous lakes on the ears, face, lips, and neck. The thinning cells and vessels have a slower rate of repair with aging, resulting in a higher and more severe incidence of decubitus ulcers and slower healing of damaged skin (Fenske & Lober, 1990; Jones & Millman, 1990; Lober & Fenske, 1990). Delayed healing also may be due to other factors, such as circulatory changes, poor nutritional state, sun-induced damage, and lowered resistance to infection (Lober & Fenske, 1991).

Decreased vascular responsiveness compromises thermal regulation (Brooke & Griffiths, 2003). Decreased vascularity and decreased circulation in the dermis and the underlying *subcutaneous tissue* also affect drug absorption. Drugs administered subcutaneously are absorbed more slowly, thus prolonging the half-life of the drug. The amount of subcutaneous fat tissue also decreases, especially in the extremities, so that arms and legs appear to be thinner.

Another important change that makes older skin vulnerable to injury is flattening of the dermoepidermal junction. In younger people, the interface between the two layers is strengthened by an interlaced structure. With age the adjacent layers flatten so that the epidermis is more easily damaged by shearing force (Berger & Gilchrest, 1998; Brooke & Griffiths, 2003).

Skin Glands

The two major types of skin glands are *sebaceous glands* and *sweat glands*. Sebaceous glands originate in the dermis and secrete *sebum*, an oily, colorless, odorless fluid, through hair follicles. Sebaceous glands show increased size with age; however, their function tends to diminish, as seen by a decrease in sebum secretion. In men, the decrease is minimal and does not begin until after age 70 years, but in women, there is a gradual diminution in sebum secretion after menopause, and no significant changes occur after the seventh decade. Research has not demonstrated a direct relationship between decreased sebum and xerosis or seborrheic dermatitis (Berger & Gilchrest, 1998).

Sweat glands originate in the subcutaneous tissue and are of two major types: *eccrine* and *apocrine*. Eccrine sweat glands are unbranched, coiled, tubular glands that are widely distributed and open directly onto the skin surface. They promote body cooling by allowing the sweat secretions to evaporate from the skin surface. The apocrine sweat glands are large, branched, specialized glands located chiefly in the axillary and genital regions that empty into hair follicles. They are responsible for body odor through bacterial decomposition of the sweat secretions.

Sweat glands generally decrease in size, number, and function with age. In the eccrine glands, the secretory epithelial cells become uneven in size, ranging from normal to small, and there is a progressive accumulation of lipofuscin in the cytoplasm. In the very old, the secretory coils of many eccrine glands are replaced by fibrous tissue, which drastically diminishes their capacity to produce sweat. However, recent studies have found that there is little decrease in sweat production in persons younger than 70 years. Apocrine glands do not decrease in number or size, but they do decrease in function. An accumulation of lipofuscin has also been noted in apocrine glands. The diminished functioning of sweat glands in the elderly impairs the ability to maintain body temperature homeostasis (Berger & Gilchrest, 1998; Brooke & Griffiths, 2003).

Box 10-1 summarizes the morphological features of aging human skin, and Figure 10-3 illustrates the histological changes associated with aging in normal human skin (Gilchrest, 1986).

Hair

Changes in hair color, growth, and distribution are associated with aging. The most obvious change in aging hair is the gradual loss of color to gray or white. Half of the population older than 50 years has at least 50% gray body hair, regardless of sex or hair color. Graying usually begins at the temples of the head and extends to the vertex of the scalp. It may not occur in the axilla, presternum, or pubis, especially in women. Gray

---

BOX 10-1 Morphological Features of Aging Human Skin

Epidermis	Dermis	Appendages
Flat dermoepidermal junction	Atrophy	Graying of hair
Variable thickness	Fewer fibroblasts	Loss of hair
Variable cell size and shape	Fewer blood vessels	Conversion of terminal to vellus hair
Occasional nuclear atypia	Shortened capillary loops	Abnormal nail plates
Loss of melanocytes	Abnormal nerve endings	Fewer glands

From Gilchrest, B. A. (1982). Skin. In J. W. Rowe & R. W. Besdine (Eds.), *Health and disease in old age.* Boston: Little, Brown, p. 383.

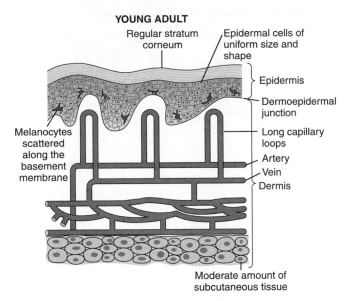

YOUNG ADULT

Regular stratum corneum

Epidermal cells of uniform size and shape

Epidermis

Dermoepidermal junction

Long capillary loops

Artery

Vein

Dermis

Melanocytes scattered along the basement membrane

Moderate amount of subcutaneous tissue

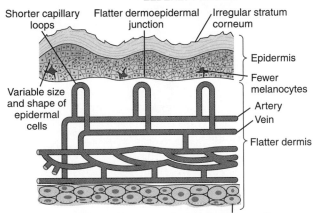

ELDERLY PERSON

Shorter capillary loops

Flatter dermoepidermal junction

Irregular stratum corneum

Epidermis

Fewer melanocytes

Artery

Vein

Flatter dermis

Variable size and shape of epidermal cells

Less subcutaneous tissue

Figure 10-3 Histological changes associated with aging in normal human skin. (From Copstead-Kirkhorn, L., & Banasik, J. [2005]. *Pathophysiology* [3rd ed.]. St. Louis: Elsevier.)

hair is determined by an autosomal dominant gene and results from a decreased rate of melanin production by the hair follicle. Pure white hair is seen in people who lack alpha-melanocyte–stimulating hormone binding sites (Brooke & Griffiths, 2003).

The amount and distribution of hair are determined by racial, genetic, and sex-linked factors; however, almost all older people have a diminution of body hair except on the face. Adults develop a full terminal hair pattern by age 40, and this is followed by a progressive loss of hair in reverse order of development. Postmenopausal white women lose trunk hair first, then pubic and axillary hair. Unopposed adrenal androgens produce coarse facial hair in 50% of white women older than 60 years of age, especially on the chin and around the lips (Coni, Davison, & Webster, 1980). Women also tend to have some thinning of scalp hair and frontal recession of the hairline.

Although men experience general thinning of their hair, the hairs of the eyebrows, ears, and nose become longer and coarser. Frontal recession of the hairline occurs in 100% of older men. Scalp hair loss commonly is more dramatic among men than women. Baldness in men is inherited through the mother and occurs only in the presence of testosterone. The onset of baldness most often is characterized by an M-shaped pattern of hair loss on either side of the midline or by a thinning patch over the vertex (Dalziel & Bickers, 1992; Kligman & Balin, 1989).

Nails

With aging, nails become dull, brittle, hard, and thick. Factors thought to contribute to nail changes are diminished blood supply to the nailbed and changes in the lipid composition of the nail plate (Brooke & Griffiths, 2003). Thickening of the nail also results from nutritional disturbances, repeated trauma, inflammation, and local infection. There is approximately a 30% to 50% decrease in the growth rate of nails, from 0.83 mm per week in 30-year-olds to 0.52 mm per week in 90-year-olds. Aging nails show an increase in longitudinal striations, which can cause splitting of the nail surface and lead to infection.

Toenails are particularly prone to thickening, perhaps as a result of constant trauma and pressure from shoe coverings. Along with thickening, the toenails may become discolored and grooved, and debris may accumulate under the nail. This condition may be exacerbated as the distal portion of the nail works free from the underlying nailbed, accumulating more debris; fungal infections may also follow. Treatment usually consists of periodic debridement of the nail plate; however, return to normal nail structure rarely occurs after thickening (Helfand, 1983).

Tumors involving the nails include both benign and malignant cancers. Malignant melanoma is the most serious of these. It most commonly appears as a pigmented area at the base of the nail or as a longitudinal streak in the nail. Although similar pigmentation can be related to trauma, nevi, and some medications, the possibility of melanoma warrants a matrix biopsy (Parker, 2000).

Psychological Effects

The cosmetic effects of aging changes in the skin and hair are troublesome for many older persons. Because it is highly valued in society, appearance is closely related to self-esteem and to the way others respond to an individual (Brooke & Griffiths, 2003). Many older adults seek treatment to help them look younger. Box 10-2 describes skin changes and cosmetic treatments currently in use.

Box 10-2 *Age-Related Changes and Selected Treatment Options: Integument*

COSMETIC SKIN CHANGE	TREATMENT
Wrinkles	Photoprotection Tretinoin (Retin-A) Soft tissue augmentation (Zyderm, Artefill) Chemical peel Dermabrasion Blepharoplasty Face-lift Fat transplant (lipoaugmentation) Botulinum toxin (Botox) Laser resurfacing/photorejuvenation Intense pulsed light
Hair loss	Minoxidil (Rogaine) Antiandrogens Hair transplantation
Gray hair	Hair coloring
Unwanted facial hair	Facial bleaches Tweezing Depilatories Shaving Waxing Electrolysis Intense pulsed light
Skin tags	Scissor excision Electrodesiccation and curettage
Cherry angiomas	Electrodesiccation and curettage Cryosurgery Shave excision
Seborrheic keratoses	Cryosurgery Electrodesiccation and curettage Alpha-hydroxy acids Glycolic acid
Sebaceous hyperplasia	Photoprotection Electrodesiccation and curettage Cryosurgery
Solar lentigines	Photoprotection 3% hydroquinone (Melanex) Cryosurgery
Telangiectasia	Photoprotection Electrodesiccation Intense pulsed light

Modified from Fenske, N. A., & Albers, S. E. (1990). Cosmetic modalities for aging skin: What to tell patients. Geriatrics, 45(9), 59-60.

COMMON DISORDERS

Skin disorders are extremely common among the elderly. Estimates of the prevalence of dermatological disorders (excluding "normal" aging) among older adults range from 40% to 67% (Berger & Gilchrest, 1998; Brooke & Griffiths, 2003). Possible consequences of untreated skin problems include discomfort, disfigurement, systemic infection, functional impairments, and even loss of limbs. Extensive disruption of skin integrity can affect temperature regulation, vitamin D production, and fluid and electrolyte balance.

Dermatological disorders may be hereditary or related to other internal or external factors. Among the internal disorders that may have skin manifestations are diabetes, gout, malignancies, liver disease, and some neurological, vascular, and metabolic disorders. Adverse skin effects, including allergic reactions, are common with both drugs and cosmetics. Other external factors that are related to skin disorders include sunlight, climate, industrial contaminants, indoor heating systems, clothing, and plants. Psychological factors such as stress have been implicated in some disorders as causative or aggravating factors.

The major cause of pathological skin changes is sunlight. In addition to the photoaging described earlier, other effects of sunlight on the skin include elastotic syndromes, keratoacanthomas, premalignant diseases, basal cell epitheliomas, squamous cell epitheliomas, and cutaneous malignant melanomas (Veierod et al., 2003).

Common skin disorders in the elderly that are addressed here include pruritus, neoplasms, infections, inflammatory conditions, and psoriasis. Older adults with severe mobility impairments also are at increased risk for pressure ulcers. Other common findings that usually are of limited clinical significance are comedones (blackheads), asteatosis (scaling), cherry angiomas (small, red, benign tumors), nevi (moles), skin tags (pedunculated fleshy growths), and lentigos ("liver spots").

Pruritus

Pruritus, or generalized itching, is an extremely common geriatric disorder. It may occur with or without a rash and may be caused by internal, external, or psychological factors. Because of the diminished immune response of aged skin, skin rashes may be very subtle. Therefore the nurse should examine the affected area closely for evidence of primary skin disorders such as eczema or scabies. When there is no rash, the possibility of internal causes should be investigated. Possible internal causes of pruritus are renal, hematopoietic, and endocrine disorders; hepatic disorders with cholestasis; malignancies such as Hodgkin's disease and multiple myeloma; drug effects, especially with opiates; psychosis; and acquired immunodeficiency syndrome (AIDS). With hepatic disease, itching may precede jaundice (Berger & Gilchrest, 1998; Gilchrest, 1982) (Box 10-3).

Some clinicians use the term *senile pruritus* when no causative factor can be found. Proposed explanations for senile pruritus include age-related alterations in the barrier functions of the skin, sensory nerve endings, and the physiology of dermal neuropeptides (Stitt & Gilchrest, 2003).

Dryness and itching often are relieved by restricting the amount of bathing and soap use and by applying topical emollients. Oily emollients and those containing alpha-hydroxy acids relieve symptoms by improving the barrier function of the skin. Topical lotions that contain menthol and camphor help relieve itching. Even without xerosis, emollients usually are recommended

---

BOX 10-3 Clinical Associations with Pruritus

Skin Diseases
Dermatitis, including contact dermatitis
Bullous disorders, especially dermatitis herpetiforms and bullous pemphigoid
Drug effects (opiates, aspirin, quinidine)
Urticaria and angioedema
Lichen planus
Sunburn
Seborrheic dermatitis
Infestations (e.g., scabies, pediculosis)
Xerosis (dry skin)
Irritant particles (e.g., fiberglass, "itching powder")

Systemic Diseases
Uremia
Obstructive biliary disease (primary biliary cirrhosis, cholestatic hepatitis, cholestasis of pregnancy, extrahepatic biliary obstruction)
Hematological and myeloproliferative disorders (lymphoma, polycythemia vera, iron-deficiency anemia)
Endocrine disorders (thyrotoxicosis, hypothyroidism, diabetes, carcinoid)
Carcinomas (breast, stomach, or lung)
Psychiatric disorders (e.g., delusional states, stress, psychosis)
Neurological disorders (e.g., multiple sclerosis, notalgia paresthetica, neuropathy)
Mastocytosis (urticaria pigmentosum, telangiectasia macularis eruptive perstans)

From Norris, D. A. (2004). Structure and function of the skin. In L. Goldman & D. Ausiello (Eds.), *Cecil textbook of medicine* (22nd ed.). Philadelphia: Saunders, p. 2449.

---

to avoid episodes of dry skin that exacerbate pruritus. The effectiveness of emollients and ointments lies in their ability to coat the skin surface, thereby reducing evaporation and building up the underlying moisture content (Banov, Epstein, & Grayson, 1992; Duncan & Fenske, 1990). Topical corticosteroids are useful in treating inflammation and itching. They can have a drying or emollient effect depending on the preparation (vehicle) used (Lehne, 2001).

Traditional systemic antihistamines may provide some relief from itching, but their use is controversial in older adults because of the adverse effects that include urinary retention, impaired psychomotor function, and drowsiness. If used, the nonsedating antihistamines such as loratidine (Claritin) are preferred (Abrams, 2004; Lilley, Aucker, & Albanese, 2001; Stitt & Gilchrest, 2003). Nilsson, Psouni, and Schouenborg (2003) demonstrated that transcutaneous electrical stimulation could inhibit itching. However, only one other study on this therapy for pruritus in the older population was found (Monk, 1993).

Xerosis is the term used to describe dry, rough skin. It is the most common cause of itching in older persons and is almost universal in persons older than 70 years. The skin may be mildly inflamed, with fine scaling, dryness, and flakiness, and slight fissuring. Contrary to common belief, xerosis does not reflect overall skin dehydration. Only the superficial stratum corneum has reduced water content. Xerosis more likely is due to minor abnormalities in epidermal maturation that cause the surface of the stratum corneum to be uneven and change the makeup of the stratum corneum (Stitt & Gilchrest, 2003). Xerosis is exacerbated by dry heat during cold weather and excessive washing with soaps and detergents. Pruritus associated with xerosis most often occurs on the lower legs, hands, and forearms, but also may occur in skinfolds and in the genital and anal regions. In addition to xerosis, conditions associated with pruritus are eczema, allergic reactions, and stasis dermatitis with leg ulcers. When patients have xerosis, the following actions are recommended:

- Avoid using rough-textured bed linens.
- Encourage or assist patient to wear loose-fitting clothing.
- Apply lubricant to moisten lips and oral mucosa as needed.
- Loosely apply incontinent garments (if used).
- Refrain from using alkaline soap on the skin.
- Keep bed linens clean, dry, and free of wrinkles.

Rashes

Rashes are a common manifestation of many skin conditions, including infections, allergic reactions, chemical irritations, psychological stressors, and poor hygiene. Rashes associated with poor hygiene commonly are seen in older adults who are not independent in bathing. Underlying factors that predispose to fungal infection include immunosuppressant drug use, diabetes mellitus, and antibiotic therapy. The most common sites for these rashes are underneath the breasts in women and in the groin for both men and women.

Assessment of Rashes. Assessment of rashes includes inspection of the entire body for distribution and careful description. The color, configuration, and symptoms associated with the rash should be described. Drug reactions are commonly distributed over the trunk and face, whereas cellulitis is generally confined to the locale of prior ulceration, although erysipelas may involve an entire extremity and not have continuous distribution. Other important parts of the assessment include historical information, such as the following:

- Recent changes in drug regimen
- Recent skin trauma or ulceration
- History of chronic skin problems, such as eczema or seborrheic dermatitis

- Associated symptoms, such as itching, pain
- Ability to perform skin hygiene routines independently
- Patient's perception of the problem and its impact

It is important to distinguish potentially life-threatening rashes, such as those from drug reactions and cellulitis, from those with more benign courses, because physicians often rely on nursing judgment regarding the urgency of treating a rash.

Planning and Intervention. Treatment of the various rashes experienced by older people depends on the causative agent. Therapy is directed toward eliminating the cause and alleviating associated problems such as itching and infection. Proper hygiene of rashes includes gentle cleansing to remove exudate and gentle drying to prevent further skin trauma. Tender skin can be dried either by patting gently with a towel or using a hair dryer on cool or warm setting after washing and rinsing. When the rash is related to dry skin, moisturizing agents should be applied to the skin immediately after a bath, while the skin is still damp, to seal water within the hydrated epidermis (Stitt & Gilchrest, 2003). Efforts to ensure adequate systemic hydration should also be made.

Itching is sometimes a major source of discomfort with a rash. Local counterirritation, such as massage, or the use of cool compresses is sometimes effective. If the discomfort is severe, short-term use of antihistaminic drugs or topical corticosteroids is warranted, but attention should be paid to other drugs the patient is taking—both to establish the correct dosage and to prevent adverse drug interactions.

Senile Purpura

The incidence of senile purpura significantly increases with age, especially in the very old. Senile purpura, which occurs mainly on the hands and extensor surfaces of the forearms, is related to the loss of subcutaneous fat and connective tissue that supports the skin capillaries. Shearing forces, even when minor, can cause rupture of small blood vessels. Extravasated blood tracks into surrounding tissues where it may remain for several weeks because of the older person's poor phagocytic response (Nierodzik, Sutin, & Freedman, 2003). Figures 10-4 to 10-6 illustrate several of the common skin lesions associated with aging. The color plates in this chapter illustrate additional skin changes and disorders.

Inflammatory Conditions

Eczema/Dermatitis. Excessive scratching associated with pruritus can lead to acute or chronic *dermatitis* (skin inflammation). In *acute dermatitis*, all four signs of acute inflammation are present: erythema (redness),

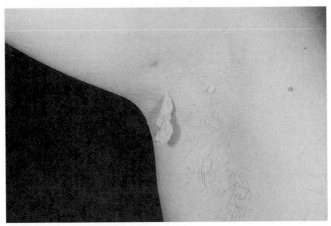

Figure 10-4 Acrochordon (skin tag). (From Callen, J. P., Greer, K. E., Paller, A., & Swinyer, L. [2000]. *Color atlas of dermatology* [2nd ed.]. Philadelphia: Saunders, p. 107).

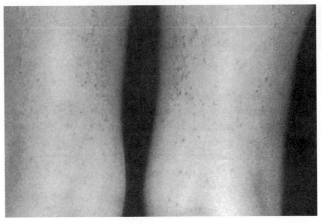

Figure 10-6 Papular eczema. (From Callen, J. P., Greer, K. E., Hood, A. F., et al. [1993]. *Color atlas of dermatology*. Philadelphia: Saunders, p. 192).

edema, heat, and pain (which may result from the itching and scratching). *Chronic dermatitis* is less obviously inflammatory, and the skin is scalier, darker, thickened, and leathery, with exaggerated normal skin markings.

Eczema is a term often used interchangeably with the term *dermatitis*. Eczema is characterized by round

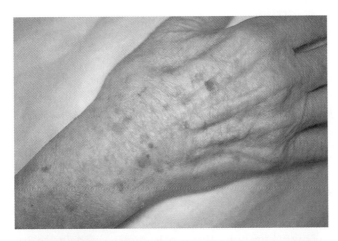

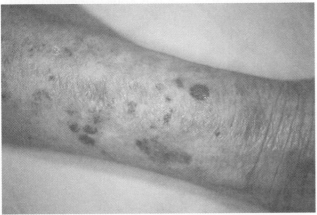

Figure 10-5 Purpura. (From Copstead-Kirkhorn, L., & Banasik, J. [2005]. *Pathophysiology* [3rd ed.]. St. Louis: Saunders.)

patches of inflammation that are reddened, scaly, and extremely itchy. The patches usually are located on the fingers, the dorsa of the hands, the forearms, and the anterior tibial area (see Figure 10-6). Drying agents, such as soap and water, are the main causes of eczema, so treatment consists of avoidance of the drying agent and application of moisturizers and topical immunosuppressants. Topical corticosteroids decrease inflammation but can cause skin atrophy, hypopigmentation, and teleangiectasis. Alternatives to corticosteroids are tacrolimus (Prograf) ointment and pimecrolimus (Elidel) cream. These alternatives usually are well tolerated, but both increase sensitivity to ultraviolet light. Therefore patients should avoid exposure to sunlight, sun lamps, and tanning beds (Lehne, 2004). Box 10-4 lists measures for treatment and prevention of dry skin.

Seborrheic Dermatitis. This eczematous condition often is bothersome to older people, not only because it causes itching and discomfort but also because of the appearance of erythema and greasy-appearing scales affecting the scalp, eyebrows, sides of the nose, hairline, sternum, and axilla (Figure 10-7). Seborrheic dermatitis is believed to be an inflammatory response to *Malassezia* yeasts (Gupta, Bluhm, Cooper, Summerbell, & Batra, 2003). *Pitysporum ovale* is present in a greater number in people with seborrheic dermatitis, but its role is controversial (Berger & Gilchrest, 1998). Among those at increased risk for seborrheic dermatitis are people with Parkinson's disease, spinal cord injury, and human immunodeficiency virus (HIV) infection, and people taking drugs with Parkinson's-like side effects (Stitt & Gilchrest, 2003).

Depending on the body areas affected, cream or shampoo containing ketoconazole is recommended for initial treatment. Topical glucocorticoids can be used concurrently. Among the topical preparations that have

1. Artificial humidification can be done with a home humidifier.
2. The patient may bathe less frequently, using warm rather than hot water.
3. The use of a mild superfatted soap or cleansing cream is helpful, especially in older adults.
4. The patient should wear protective clothing in cold weather.
5. Moisturizers can be used for restoration of the epidermal water barrier. Occlusive moisturizers coat the surface of the skin, reducing the evaporative loss of moisture from the surface. Vaseline is an excellent moisturizer. A petrolatum-glycerin combination is especially effective in the treatment of dry skin.
6. The use of bath oils for bathing can be extremely hazardous for the elderly because of the increased possibility of slipping in the tub. Creams and moisturizers should be applied after getting out of the bathtub or shower. At that time, the body should be patted dry with a towel and the moisturizing preparation applied. Under these conditions, the skin is fully hydrated, and the moisturizing preparation is more effective in preventing epidermal water loss.

From Callen, J. P., Greer, K. E., Hood, A. F., et al. (1993). *Color atlas of dermatology.* Philadelphia: Saunders, pp. 100-101.

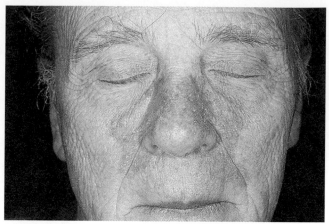

Figure 10-7 Severe seborrheic dermatitis. (From Callen, J. P., Greer, K. E., Paller, A., & Swinyer, L. [2000]. *Color atlas of dermatology* [2nd ed.]. Philadelphia: Saunders, p. 98.)

demonstrated effectiveness in the treatment of this condition in clinical trials are ciclopirox olamine cream (Tarmed) (Unholzer et al., 2002) and ketoconozole with desonide gel (Pierard-Franchimont & Pierard, 2002). A comparative study of ciclopirox olamine alone and in combination with coal tar, coal tar alone, and ketoconazole with 274 subjects achieved similar results for all except the coal tar alone, which was less effective (Davies, Boorman, & Shuttleworth, 1999). For seborrheic dermatitis of the scalp, commonly called dandruff, effects usually can be maintained with a shampoo that contains a yeast suppressant such as ketoconazole, pyrithione zinc, selenium sulfide, salicylic acid, or tar. A steroid solution can be applied to the scalp if it does not respond to other treatments (Stitt & Gilchrest, 2003; Lehne, 2001). One study in the United Kingdom reported rapid and highly significant improvement in AIDS-associated facial seborrheic dermatitis with the use of lithium succinate (Efalith) ointment (Langtry et al., 1997).

Positive results have been reported in single studies with several alternative therapies. Among the therapies that have been studied are an oral homeopathic medication consisting of potassium bromide, sodium bromide, nickel sulfate, and sodium chloride (Smith, Baker, &

Williams, 2002), aloe vera crude extract emulsion (Vardy, Cohen, Tchetov, Medvedovsky, & Biton, 1999), and 90% honey diluted in warm water (Al-Waili, 2001).

Intertrigo. Intertrigo is an erythematous skin eruption with inflammation in the skinfolds under the breasts, the groin, the transverse abdominal folds, and the axilla. The main symptom is intense pruritus. Intertrigo is more common in obese elderly persons who do not maintain an appropriate level of cleanliness. Risk factors for intertrigo include the following:

1. Adductor spasticity of the lower extremities, making perineal hygiene difficult to achieve, leaving a chronically moist environment ideal for the growth of fungal organisms
2. Incontinence, providing both a chemical irritant to the skin and a chronically moist environment that supports the growth of fungi
3. Low energy or motivation, leading to inadequate drying under breasts or in the perineal area during baths
4. Staff or family members with inadequate training or motivation to adequately dry patients under breasts or in the perineum

Inflammation is due to a combination of friction and moisture. Bacterial or candidal infection of the compromised tissue is common. The importance of differential diagnosis has been emphasized by Wolf, Orion, and Matz (2003), who described 11 cases of intertrigonous eruptions that eventually were attributed to adverse drug effects.

Research on cutaneous fungal infections has focused primarily on the feet in adults and the diaper area in infants. Although many principles of treatment of intertrigo may be the same as for other cutaneous fungal infections, research is needed to determine the most appropriate care. Generally accepted recommendations emphasize the importance of keeping affected areas clean and dry and separating adjacent tissues (Evans & Gray, 2003). Folds should be washed with tepid water and dried thoroughly. Soft gauze may be used to separate adjacent surfaces. Undergarments and positioning have a role in treatment and prevention of fungal infections. For breast candidiasis, a well-fitting cotton brassiere will help absorb moisture and reduce chafing. In perineal candidiasis, an adductor block pillow may improve air circulation to the affected area, reducing moisture accumulation. Appropriate treatment of the rash with antifungal agents and good hygiene often reduce the discomfort and anxiety associated with rashes. However, itching sometimes persists as a major source of discomfort.

Superficial fungal infections usually are treated first with topical antifungals. Topical antifungal agents include polyene antibiotics (nystatin), azoles (ketoconazole, clotrimazole, ciclopirox olamine, and others), and allylamines (terbinafine, butenafine). Over-the-counter agents such as clotrimazole are generally considered first-line drugs, whereas prescription drugs are used if initial therapy is unsuccessful (Evans & Gray, 2003). Nystatin cream or powder is effective against *Candida* in immunocompetent patients, but it has not been shown to be effective against dermatophytes or bacteria. Combination antifungal-corticosteroid preparations are available; however, the risk of complications increases with long-term use. The antiinflammtory actions of the imidazoles, allylamines, and butenafine may preclude the need for steroids (Aly, Forney, & Bayles, 2001).

Oral therapy usually is reserved for chronic or extensive skin involvement and for patients who do not respond to topical therapy (Aly, Forney, & Bayles, 2001). Ketoconazole and the newer antifungals (itraconazole, fluconazole, terbinafine) all are effective against *Candida*, dermatophytes, and *Malassezia furfur*. All are generally safe, but the newer drugs are thought to be somewhat more effective. Hepatic function should be monitored in patients who take antifungal drugs on a long-term basis.

Lichen Simplex Chronicus.

Lichen simplex chronicus (neurodermatitis) is characterized by erythematous papules that coalesce to form plaques (Bielan, 2002). The thickened patches of skin vary in size and appear scaly, leathery, and darker than normal (Figure 10-8). The lesions cause intense itching. The condition may be localized, especially on the dorsal forearms, lateral tibial areas, and posterior neck, or it may be generalized over the entire body. When the condition is localized, the constant scratching and rubbing of a particular area produces *lichenification*—a thickening of the skin. This leads to chronic inflammation and itching, which in turn produce further scratching and rubbing—a

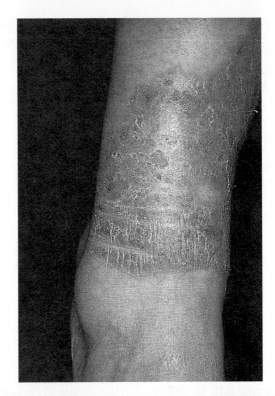

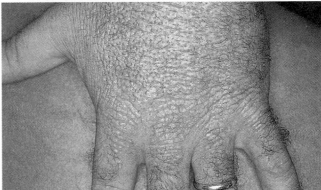

Figure 10-8 Lichen simplex chronicus. (From Callen, J. P., Greer, K. E., Paller, A., & Swinyer, L. [2000]. *Color atlas of dermatology* [2nd ed.]. Philadelphia: Saunders, p. 14.)

self-perpetuating cycle. When assessing vulvar lichen simplex chronicus, Vigili, Bacilieri, and Corazza (2003) recommend patch tests to assess sensitization that may contribute to the symptoms.

The condition is treated with steroid creams and antihistamines for the itch. Even if the condition improves, it will recur unless scratching is controlled. Bedtime oral antihistamines are prescribed to prevent nighttime scratching. The dosage should be titrated, starting with a low dose, until satisfactory results are achieved. The patient is encouraged to keep the fingernails very short. The application of a dressing such as DuoDERM may protect the plaque from scratching. Mittens may be needed for confused older adults. For localized lesions, a tape that is impregnated with a topical steroid

(Cordran) can be applied for a maximum of 24 hours. Caution patients not to apply occlusive dressings over corticosteroids because they greatly increase the absorption of the medication. Some patients find that a cold pack is helpful (Bielan, 2002). Other treatments that often are employed include oatmeal baths, moisturizers, menthol, and ultraviolet B light. Excoriated areas may require topical antiseptics (Rogers, 2003).

An open pilot study in Germany evaluated the intralesional injection of botulinum toxin type A to control itching. In a sample of three subjects, itching subsided within 1 week and all treated lesions cleared completely within 4 weeks (Heckmann, Heyer, Brunner, & Plewig, 2002). In a double-blind crossover placebo study, researchers in Singapore determined that a topical aspirin/dichloromethane solution was superior to placebo in reducing the intensity of itching of localized circumscribed lesions (Yosipovitch et al., 2001).

Lichen Sclerosis. Lichen sclerosis is characterized by white plaques of keratin around the vulva with purple areas where keratin is reduced. Tissues fuse so that introital stenosis sometimes occurs. Chronic scratching causes the skin to thicken (lichenification). A topical antiinflammatory steroid such as betamethasone valerate 0.1% is the usual treatment. Topical estrogen is not beneficial. Because there is a 5% to 10% risk of the lesions undergoing change to squamous cell carcinoma, patients should be examined at least twice each year (Brown & Cooper, 2003).

Pruritus Ani. This dermatitis, which affects the perianal area, is caused by irritation from heat, swelling, hemorrhoids, or fissures. Rubbing and scratching leads to thickening of the perianal skin. Itching frequently occurs at night, causing the appearance of scratch marks in the morning. The condition is complicated by urinary or fecal incontinence and is especially troublesome for chronically ill or confused older persons. Measures employed to treat pruritus ani include avoidance of irritating medications and the use of warm compresses or baths, application of mild steroid creams, and administration of oral antipruritic medications (Bornstein, Pascal, & Abramovici, 1993; Ensebio, Graham, & Moody, 1990; Origoni, Garcia, & Sideri, 1990; Silverman et al., 1989). In a double-blind, placebo-controlled crossover study comparing topical capsaicin with a placebo (topical menthol 1%) in the treatment of pruritus ani, 70% of the subjects experienced relief of discomfort with capsaicin but not with menthol (Lysy et al., 2003).

Drug Eruptions

Any drug can cause an adverse cutaneous reaction, called a *drug eruption*. Drugs are the most common cause of allergic reactions in older persons, and the most frequent drug side effects are skin eruptions

(Hari et al., 2001). Not only are older adults at greater risk for skin reactions to drugs, they also are at greater risk for major morbidity and for mortality than younger persons (Sullivan & Shear, 2002). The morbilliform or exanthematous (maculopapular) eruption is the most common form of drug eruption. This eruption typically consists of discrete and coalescing erythematous macules and papules that are distributed symmetrically on the trunk and extremities. Most drug eruptions appear within a week of exposure; however, delayed reactions can occur weeks to months later. Other types of drug eruption include photosensitivity, a lichenoid or lichen planus-like eruption, urticaria, fixed drug eruption, vasculitis, and serum sickness reaction (Table 10-2). Uncommon but serious skin reactions are hypersensitivity, anaphylaxis/angioedema, exfoliative erythroderma, erythema multiforme major (Stevens-Johnson syndrome), and toxic epidermal necrolysis (Stitt & Gilchrest, 2003).

Withdrawal of the drug is the primary treatment. Patients who are taking multiple medications should have all nonessential drugs withdrawn or replaced until the culprit is identified. Topical corticosteroids, antipruritic lotions, and antihistamines commonly are used to relieve symptoms until eruptions resolve (Stitt & Gilchrest, 2003).

This section has addressed cutaneous adverse effects that are caused by drugs. However, the practitioner should be aware that drugs also can worsen primary skin diseases. Examples include a psoriasis exacerbation triggered by a beta blocker and pemphigus associated with captopril (Stitt & Gilchrest, 2003).

NEOPLASTIC DISORDERS
Keratoses

Seborrheic Keratoses. Seborrheic keratoses are pigmented, hyperkeratotic papules that look as if they could be scraped off easily (Lebwohl, 2004). They are extremely common among older adults. The lesions originate from the horny layer of the epidermis. They commonly are seen on the trunk, but may affect sun-exposed skin as well (Jarvis, 2000; Parker, 2000). Seborrheic keratoses typically have comedo-like openings and milia-like cysts. Other common characteristics are fissures that create a "brainlike" appearance, hairpin blood vessels, "moth-eaten" borders, a pigment pattern that resembles a fingerprint, sharply demarcated borders, and a specific wobble pattern elicited during dermoscopic examination. A wobble pattern is discerned by touching a device to a lesion and moving it horizontally. A seborrheic keratosis moves with the instrument while surrounding skin remains in place. The appearance of the lesion is unchanged during this assessment because of the rigidity of the lesion (Braun, Rabinovitz, Oliviero, Kopf, & Saurat, 2002). Based on the detection of human papillomavirus (HPV) DNA in some nongenital

Table 10-2 *Drug Eruptions*

Type of Eruption	Manifestations	Drugs/Classes Implicated
Morbilliform	Discrete and coalescing erythematous macules and papules. Distributed symmetrically on trunk and extremities.	Penicillins, trimethoprim-sulfamethoxazole, cephalosporin, gentamycin sulfate, acetylcysteine, allopurinol, quinidine, dipyrone
Photosensitivity	Redness and swelling of sun-exposed skin, burning sensation. Skin darkens and peels after several days.	Doxycycline, thiazides, amiodarone
Lichenoid or lichen planus-like eruption	Wide, flat, purplish, shiny papules in circumscribed patches	Gold, phenothiazines
Urticaria	Elevated patches that may appear red or paler than surrounding skin. Pruritus common.	Penicillin, contrast media containing iodine
Fixed drug eruption	Small number of round red to purplish plaques. Reappear in same location with second exposure to causative agent.	Tetracyclines, nonsteroidal antiinflammatory agents
Cutaneous vasculitis	Palpable purpura in lower extremities. Clustered lesions of hemorrhagic bullae.	Phenothiazines, barbiturates, sulfonamides
Serum sickness reaction	Urticaria, fever, arthritis, nephritis, neurological symptoms (sometimes)	Penicillins, sulfonamides, streptomycin

Data from Stitt, W. Z. D., & Gilchrest, B. A. (2003). Skin diseases and old age. In R. C. Tallis & H. M. Fillit (Eds.), *Brocklehurst's textbook of geriatric medicine and gerontology* (6th ed., 1277-1289). London: Churchill Livingstone; O'Toole, M. T., (2003). *Miller-Keane encyclopedia and dictionary of medicine, nursing, and allied health* (7th ed.). Philadelphia: Saunders; and Huether, S. E. (2000). Structure, function, and disorders of the integument. In S. E. Huether & K. L. McCance (Eds.), *Understanding pathophysiology* (2nd ed.). St. Louis: Mosby.

seborrheic keratoses, it is postulated that HPV may play a role in the pathogenesis of these lesions (Gushi, Kanekura, Kanzaki, & Eizuru, 2003). Although seborrheic keratoses are benign, noninvasive lesions some have been associated with skin malignancies. A retrospective analysis of the results of 23,000 histological examinations of clinically apparent seborrheic keratoses revealed that 11.9% were in fact basal cell carcinomas, 3.4% were squamous cell carcinomas, and 1.01% were malignant melanomas. An analysis of 9204 lesions submitted for study found 61 cases of melanoma that resembled serborrheic keratoses (Izikson, Sober, Mihm, & Zembowicz, 2002). This underscores the importance of differential diagnoses when assessing lesions that resemble keratoses.

Seborrheic keratoses can be removed for microscopic study or for cosmetic reasons. Biopsy, shave, or excision procedures may be used to remove complete lesions or specimens for examination (Duque et al., 2003). Mehrabi and Brodell (2002) described the use of the alexandrine laser to treat patients with multiple lesions, and they reported that excellent cosmetic results were achieved and that the procedure was well tolerated.

Actinic Keratoses. These lesions also are known as *senile* or *solar keratoses*. Because actinic keratoses are associated with excessive exposure to sun, they usually appear on the forehead, cheeks, and dorsal hands and forearms, and on the ears and balding scalp of older men. The keratotic patches begin as small, reddened areas of light-damaged skin (Figure 10-9). They become well demarcated, gradually losing normal skin surface markings. They appear yellow to brown in color with a rough surface; the patches are often most easily identified by touch.

A small percent of actinic keratoses develop into squamous cell carcinomas; however, very few metastasize (Stitt & Gilchrest, 2003). Decreased exposure to sunlight may cause the lesions to regress, but because they are potentially malignant, treatment usually is recommended. Topical agents used to treat actinic keratoses include fluorouracil, diclofenac sodium, and aminolevulinic acid with blue light photoactivation after 14 to 18 hours. All topical treatments tend to cause local skin irritation and photosensitivity. During treatment, patients should avoid direct sun exposure. Sunscreens are not adequate to prevent adverse effects (Lehne, 2004).

Nonmelanoma Skin Cancer

The prevalence of skin cancer is increasing, with more than 1 million cases of skin cancer diagnosed in the United States every year. Although skin cancers are

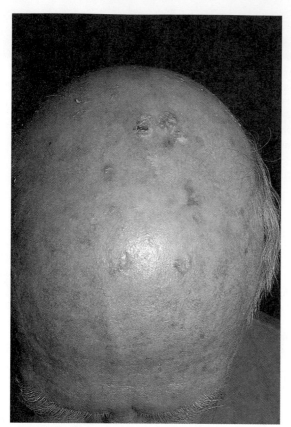 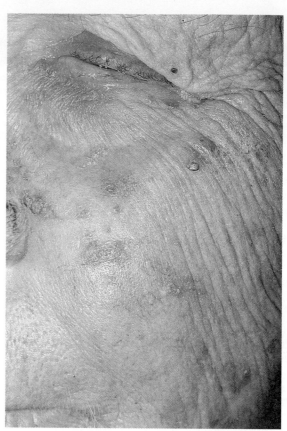

Figure 10-9 Actinic keratoses. (From Callen, J. P., Greer, K. E., Paller, A., & Swinyer, L. [2000]. *Color atlas of dermatology* [2nd ed.]. Philadelphia: Saunders, pp. 88, 294.)

associated with lower morbidity and mortality rates than other malignancies, these lesions are among the five most costly cancers to Medicare (Housman et al., 2003). Skin cancers are classified as nonmelanoma skin cancer (NMSC) and malignant melanoma (MM). NMSC includes basal cell carcinoma (BCC), which is the most common type, and squamous cell carcinoma (SCC).

Risk factors for skin cancer include sun exposure, male gender, cigarette smoking, fair skin with freckling, light-colored eyes, red or blond hair, and a tendency to sunburn easily (Stitt & Gilchrest, 2003). It is estimated that 90% of all skin cancers result from long-term ultraviolet light exposure (Schober-Flores, 2001). Solid organ transplant recipients who are receiving immunosuppressant therapy also are at increased risk for cancers, with skin cancer being the most common (Berg & Otley, 2002; Clayton & Stasko, 2003). Cumulative exposure to sunlight is related to NMSC, whereas sunburn severity is better correlated with MM (Stitt & Gilchrest, 2003). Whereas fair-skinned people are at increased risk for all types of skin cancer, African Americans are more likely to have SCC than BCC.

The role of tanning beds is a topic of debate because few epidemiological data exist. Interviews of people with NMSC led to the conclusion that tanning lamp

exposure may contribute to the development of NMSC (Karagas et al., 2002). As a result, the U.S. Preventive Services Task Force recommends avoidance of sun lamps and tanning beds as one strategy to prevent skin cancer (U.S. Preventive Services Task Force, 2003). In a survey of 50 tanning facilities, Hornung, Magee, Lee, Hansen, and Hsieh (2003) found that 95% of their patrons exceeded the exposure limits for tanning beds recommended by the Food and Drug Administration. Another study found that half of sunbathing beachgoers used tanning beds as well as natural sunlight, therefore exposing themselves to two forms of ultraviolet light (Ramirez, Warthan, Uchida, & Wagner, 2003).

Most NMSCs are highly treatable. However, once regional metastasis has occurred, the prognosis for NMSC is poor even with aggressive treatment (Chu & Osguthorpe, 2003). Regardless of the initial treatment outcome, patients with a history of skin cancer must be monitored long-term. When a person has had an NMSC, the risk of a second skin cancer of the same type within 5 years may be as high as 50% (Stitt & Gilchrest, 2003). Likewise, individuals who have had one MM are at risk for a second MM (Goggins & Tsao, 2003).

Current NMSC treatment options include surgical excision, electrodissection and curettage, and Moh's micrographic surgery. The efficacy of imiquimod, a topical immune response modifier, is under study (Gaspari & Sauder, 2003; Urosevic & Dummer, 2002). The best way to prevent skin cancer is to protect oneself from prolonged or intense exposure to sunlight.

Basal Cell Carcinoma

BCC is the most common form of skin cancer in whites. The lesion arises from the cells of the epidermis or hair follicles and most often occurs on the face or neck. The classic early lesion starts as a small, smooth, hemispherical, translucent papule covered by thinned epidermis, through which dilated blood vessels and occasional specks of brown or black pigment can be seen. The papule gradually enlarges into a mass of pearly nodules or a papular plaque that may be darkly pigmented, resembling a malignant melanoma. It also can become an ulcerated lesion surrounded by a nodular rim ("rodent ulcer"), resembling a keratoacanthoma or squamous cell carcinoma. Variations in lesion appearance exist among the subtypes, which include nodular, superficial, morpheiform, and pigmented BCCs.

Although metastasis is rare, BCCs can be locally invasive and can cause mutilation or death if untreated. Treatment options include removal of the lesion by electrodessication and curettage, cryosurgery, excision, micrographic surgery, radiotherapy, and topical treatment with 5-fluorouracil and intralesional/perilesional cytokines. Newer therapies that are being studied are photodynamic therapy and imiquimod, an immune response modifier (Stitt & Gilchrest, 2003; Stockfleth & Sterry, 2002). A systematic review of interventions for cutaneous BCC concluded that surgery and radiotherapy were more effective than cryotherapy. Preliminary studies suggest that imiquimod 5% cream may be highly successful in treating superficial BCCs (Bath, Bong, Perkins, & Williams, 2003). Depending on the size, location, and type of lesion, skin grafting may be required after excision. The treatment success rate is extremely high. However, long-term follow-up is essential because of the possibility of recurrence, the development of new lesions, or both (Stitt & Gilchrest, 2003).

Squamous Cell Carcinoma

Cutaneous SCC occurs most often in middle-aged and older persons, and twice as often in men as in women. It arises from the epidermis and mucosa of sun-exposed, damaged skin, especially from areas such as actinic keratoses, scars, and sites exposed to oils and tars. Its exact appearance depends on the preceding lesion, but the tumor usually begins as a small, hard, red nodule that may appear wartlike. The lesion may also appear ulcerated with a raised, rolled, gray-yellow edge.

This form of cancer is locally invasive and has a higher incidence of metastasis than BCC. Estimates of rates of metastasis range from 2% to 10% (Stitt & Gilchrest, 2003). The risk of metastasis is greatest with lesions on the lip or in scarred or irradiated areas, with lesions larger than 1 cm in diameter and more than 4 mm in thickness, and in immunosuppressed people (Stitt & Gilchrest, 2003). A deep incisional biopsy is necessary for diagnosis, and treatment consists of removal by cautery, curettage, deep cryotherapy, excision, or radiotherapy. Regional metastases are treated with surgery and adjuvant radiotherapy. The high risk of regional recurrence after regional metastasis justifies long-term follow-up (Jol et al., 2003).

Malignant Melanoma

Malignant melanoma is the most common cause of death from skin cancer (Geller & Annas, 2003). The incidence increased at a rate of 6% per year from 1973 to 1995 (Stat bite, 2003). In 1992, there were approximately 32,000 new cases and 6700 deaths from melanoma (Drake, Ceilley, & Cornelison, 1993; National Institutes of Health Consensus Development Panel on Early Melanoma, 1992). In 2003, 54,200 new cases of melanoma and 7600 deaths related to melanoma were predicted (Stat bite, 2003).

The melanoma lesions are pigmented macules, papules, nodules, patches, or tumors with any of the ABCD warning signs:
1. Asymmetry
2. Border irregularity
3. Color variegation
4. Diameter greater than 6 mm

In some cases, malignant melanomas may be mistaken for rapidly enlarging, deeply pigmented warts, so that biopsy is often necessary for a definitive diagnosis.

The interaction of genetic and environmental factors (particularly solar ultraviolet radiation) that transforms melanoctyes into malignant melanomas is not yet understood (Jhappan, Noonan, & Merlino, 2003). Because lesions appear on both exposed and unexposed skin, it has been proposed that there may actually be two different pathways leading to cutaneous melanomas, one associated with sunlight and the other with melanocyte proliferation (Whiteman et al., 2003).

Major subtypes of melanoma are
1. *Lentigo maligna melanoma*, found on exposed skin of fair-complexioned elderly whites
2. *Superficial spreading melanoma*, found on all body surfaces
3. *Nodular melanoma*, found on all body surfaces
4. *Acral lentiginous melanoma*, found on palms, soles, and under the tongue

The disease is highly malignant, producing rapid metastasis through the lymphatic system. Early detection improves prognosis; therefore older persons should be particularly sensitive to changes in the shape, size, or texture of nevi. Diagnosis is through biopsy, and treatment is through surgical excision. Immunotherapy has become an increasingly popular treatment for high-risk patients with diffuse nodules, particularly the combination of bacillus Calmette-Guérin with chemotherapy. Trials continue in order to demonstrate effectiveness of this therapy (Brozena, Waterman, & Fenske, 1990; Drake et al., 1993; National Institutes of Health Consensus Development Panel on Early Melanoma, 1992; Physicians and Scientists, University College London Medical School, 1992).

Older men are at increased risk for melanoma, as are white persons of European descent who are fair complexioned, are redheaded, and sunburn easily or have a history of severe sunburn. Additionally, people with a family or personal history of skin cancer and those with many nevi or clinically atypical nevi are at risk. Some epidemiologists have suggested that topical sunscreens are associated with increased risk of melanoma. These conclusions have been controversial (Bastuji-Garin & Diepgen, 2002; Huncharek & Kupelnick, 2002).

The keys to reducing mortality rates from melanoma are believed to be modified ultraviolet exposure and early detection and treatment (Brenner & Tamir, 2002; Desmond & Soong, 2003; Freedman et al., 2003). In addition to avoiding sun exposure, sunscreens with a sun protection factor (SPF) of 15 or higher are still recommended (Bastuji-Garin & Diepgen, 2002).

INFECTIOUS DISORDERS
Herpes Zoster

Herpes zoster (HZ), also known as *shingles,* is an acute infection caused by varicella-zoster virus (VZV), the virus that causes chickenpox. The incidence of HZ in individuals age 80 and older is 10 times that in adolescents and young adults (Stitt & Gilchrest, 2003).

HZ is thought to arise from a reactivation of the VZV that has lain dormant in the sensory root ganglia for many years after a primary varicella infection. Age-related decreased immunity may permit reactivation of the virus. Pathological immunosuppression, whether associated with disease or with therapies, and trauma also are recognized as contributing factors (Stitt & Gilchrest, 2003).

Herpes zoster most commonly is located in the thoracic area in a unilateral dermatomal or linear distribution, or in the trigeminal, cervical, lumbar, or lumbosacral areas (Schmader, 1990). The classic symptoms begin with burning pain, followed after several days by the eruption of a papular rash distributed along a single dermatome. The rash becomes edematous, then becomes vesicular and pustular or hemorrhagic, and finally exhibits erosions and crusting. The lesions typically are unilateral. The term *disseminated zoster* is used when 20 or more lesions appear outside the primary and adjacent dermatomes. Temporary voiding dysfunction has been reported among some patients who have HZ involving the lumbosacral dermatomes (Chen, Hsueh, & Hong, 2002). After the eruption fades, the skin may be permanently scarred or discolored. Particularly among older adults, chronic pain at the site may persist for many years, a phenomenon termed *postherpetic neuralgia.*

The most effective treatment of acute herpes zoster is antiviral therapy. Available agents include acyclovir (Zovirax), famciclovir, and valacyclovir (Valtrex). An alternative to acyclovir is foscarnet. Valcyclovir is approved only for immunocompetent patients because it can cause a potentially fatal syndrome in immunocompromised patients. Drug therapy should be initiated within 72 hours after the onset of the rash to be effective for relief of pain and to promote healing. Although controversial, opioid analgesics may be justified for severe pain (Raja et al., 2003). For antiviral therapy, the oral route is effective unless the patient is immunocompromised, in which case intravenous therapy is indicated (Lehne, 2004). Options for topical treatments during the acute phase include compresses of hypertonic solutions such as Burow's and gentle washing with antibacterial soaps. After lesions have crusted, a topical antibiotic such as mupirocin ointment can be applied two to three times daily (Stitt & Gilchrest, 2003). Systemic corticosteroids have been used alone and with antiviral agents with varying results. Based on a review of the literature, Santee (2002) concluded that oral corticosteroids were helpful in treating acute pain, but no more effective than placebo in preventing postherpetic neuralgia.

Some studies have found antivirals to be helpful in reducing the incidence or duration of postherpetic neuralgia. When postherpetic neuralgia occurs, systemic management employs analgesics, anticonvulsants (carbamazepine, gabapentin), and antidepressants (amitriptyline). Topical treatments include capsaicin cream, antiinflammatory agents, and topical anesthetics (Curran & Wagstaff, 2003; Nickkels & Pierard, 2002; Reisner, 2003; Singh & Kennedy, 2003; Stitt & Gilchrest, 2003). Acupuncture, nerve blocks, transcutaneous electrical nerve stimulation, and deep brain stimulation also have been used for pain relief.

Psoriasis

Psoriasis (including psoriatic arthritis) significantly affects some 1.4 million people in the United States and imposes a cost estimated at $649.6 million each year (Javitz, Ward, Farber, Nail, & Vallow, 2002). The incidence of psoriasis peaks around age 30, but it can appear at any age, even over 100 years. There is a second peak in the sixth decade. In an interesting parallel with diabetes mellitus, early onset appears to be more strongly associated with a positive family history.

The disorder is now understood to be an inflammatory disease—one that is immune mediated with skin-directed T cells playing a key role (Cameron, Kirby, Fei, & Griffiths, 2002; Mehrabi, DiCarlo, Soon, & McCall, 2002; Prinz, 2003). Activation of T lymphocytes with a subsequent release of cytokines leads to proliferation of keratinocytes (Lebwohl, 2003). The keratinocytes reproduce more rapidly than normal, both in the lesions and in normal-appearing skin. Both the dermis and the epidermis thicken and plaques of loosely cohesive keratin create a silvery appearance. Erythema results from capillary dilation and increased vascularity in response to increased cellular metabolism (Huether, 2000).

Exactly what triggers the disease process is the topic of much study; however, there is considerable evidence of a genetic influence (Bowcock & Barker, 2003). There may have been a previous history of dandruff or scaling around the ears. The incidence is increased in people with Crohn's disease (Najarian & Gottlieb, 2003; Rahman et al., 2003). Psoriasis may exacerbate after emotional stress, drug ingestion (such as lithium, antimalarials, and some beta blockers), or sun exposure; however, some people note improvement during the summer months. In some cases, the patches develop after trauma.

Psoriatic plaques vary in size and shape and appear as red, elevated areas of skin covered by a fine scale. Many people complain of mild to moderate itching. They may affect any part of the body, including the scalp, ears, face, trunk, external genitalia, perineal area, limbs, hands and feet, and nails. The appearance of the lesions may vary according to their location. Psoriasis may have a profound effect on the quality of life (Weiss, Bergstrom, Weiss, & Kimball, 2003). Specific psychosocial effects of the disease were incorporated into an assessment tool developed by McKenna and colleagues (2003). They included fear of negative reactions from others; self-consciousness; poor self-confidence; problems with socialization, physical contact, and intimacy; limitations on personal freedom; and impaired relaxation, sleep, and emotional stability.

Diagnosis of the disease is accomplished through history, observation, and skin biopsy. Because psoriasis is a chronic, lifelong disease, treatment must involve the patient's support and cooperation. Patients should be taught that the condition is not contagious and that a healthy lifestyle (good diet, exercise, and avoidance of smoking and heavy alcohol intake) is important. Stress management also is helpful. Topical medications that decrease local inflammation or slow keratinocyte proliferation are recommended for initial treatment of mild to moderate psoriasis. These agents include corticosteroids, tazarotene, anthralin, tars, dithranol, and vitamin D derivatives (calcipotriene). Keratolytic agents such as salicylic acid may be used in combination with topical steroids. Side effects of topical agents usually are local and not severe (Bruner, Feldman, Ventrapragada, & Fleischer, 2003). Ultraviolet B (UVB) light exposure can be used to enhance topical therapy with tar and anthralin (Lehne, 2004). Dawe and colleagues (2003) report that the narrow-band UVB is replacing UVA and that it is more efficacious.

Moderate to severe psoriasis may require photochemotherapy with UVA (PUVA) and systemic agents. PUVA employs UVA in combination with oral methoxsalen. Systemic drugs include oral retinoids (acitretin), biological agents (alefacept), and cytotoxic drugs (methotrexate). PUVA has been found to increase the risk of SCC, a risk that may be reduced with oral retinoids (McClure, Valentine, & Gordon, 2002; Nijsten & Stern, 2003). Systemic corticosteroids usually are reserved for short-term use in severe psoriasis (Lehne, 2004; McClure, Valentine, & Gordon, 2002). Other systemic therapies carry various risks. For example, methotrexate can cause liver fibrosis and cirrhosis, and both oral retinoids and methotrexate are teratogenic (McClure, Valentine, & Gordon, 2002).

The future of psoriasis treatment is predicted by many to lie in monoclonal antibodies, recombinant cytokines, fusion proteins (alefacept), and tumor necrosis factor inhibitors (infliximab, etanercept) (Andreakos, Taylor, & Feldmann, 2002; Leone, Rolston, & Spaulding, 2003; Villadsen, Skov, & Baadsgaard, 2003; Vizcarra, 2003). Proponents anticipate that the biological agents will be more effective and have fewer side effects. Immunosuppressants such as tacrolimus and cyclosporine have been reported to be safe and effective in small studies (Freeman et al., 2002; Geilen & Orfanos, 2002). Freeman and colleagues (2002) specifically tested the use of tacrolimus ointment on the face and intertriginous areas. However, Zackheim (2002) cautions that prolonged therapy with cyclosporine A can cause renal toxicity and malignancy.

A study that investigated the use of commercial bed tanning (UVB) with acitretin concluded that the treatments were effective and convenient, but that variability in the light and quality of tanning salon equipment merits caution (Carlin, Callis, & Krueger, 2003).

Dermal Ulcers

Dermal ulcers include pressure ulcers, ulcers that are due to venous stasis or arterial insufficiency, and ulcers from trauma. The three major contributors to dermal ulcers are arterial insufficiency, venous insufficiency, and chronic unrelieved pressure. In all three categories, ischemia produces cellular necrosis and ulceration. Patients with arterial insufficiency have ischemia because of inadequate arterial circulation to the affected body part—usually a distal part of a lower extremity. Venous insufficiency interferes with blood flow to the extremities by producing chronic peripheral edema, which interferes with exchange of nutrients at the cellular level. Chronic pressure impedes blood flow to and from affected tissues.

Ulcers associated with vascular insufficiency and chronic pressure are discussed here. Arterial insufficiency is covered in Chapter 13.

Leg Ulcers and Stasis Dermatitis. Stasis dermatitis is the result of venous stasis and edema. Varicosities, phlebitis, and trauma lead to erythema and pruritus followed by scaling, petechiae, and hyperpigmentation (Figure 10-10). Ulcers may develop, most commonly on the ankles and tibia (Huether & McCance, 2000; Ward, Kosinski, & Markinson, 2003).

Leg ulcers are the most common chronic wound in the United States, and the incidence increases with age. The prevalence rises from 1% in people age 70 years to 5% in those age 90 years, with women outnumbering men 2.8:1. Chronic leg ulcers not only impose a significant financial burden (estimated at $3 billion per year in the United States); they also reduce patient quality of life (Franks, McCullagh, & Moffatt, 2003; McGuckin et al., 2002). The ulcers are caused by venous insufficiency, arterial insufficiency, neuropathic diabetes, or a combination of these factors. Venous insufficiency is by far the most common cause, representing approximately 70% of all cases (Nelson & Bradley, 2003).

In venous insufficiency, chronic venous distention and loss of valve competence allow blood to pool, causing edema in the lower extremities. Sluggish circulation interferes with the distribution of oxygen and nutrients and the removal of wastes in the skin and supporting tissues (Huether & McCance, 2000). An eczematous reaction occurs that may be aggravated by scratching or by topical ointments used to alleviate the discomfort. Skin breakdown, in the form of a venous leg ulcer, may occur spontaneously or may be precipitated by even minor trauma. Delayed healing invites chronic infection and cellulitis. The recurrence rate for healed ulcers has been reported as high as 59% (Huether & McCance, 2000). Older adults with venous reflux in combination with local or systemic disease have a greater risk of recurrence (Fassiadis, Kapetanakis, & Law, 2002). The relationship of psychosocial factors to the healing of chronic wounds has received little attention. However, Cole-King and Harding (2001) found a statistically significant relationship between anxiety and depression and wound healing in 53 subjects with chronic wounds.

The first step in the management of a leg ulcer is to determine the cause of the ulcer because the treatment varies with the cause. Peripheral pulses and sensation should be assessed to rule out arterial disease and neuropathy, respectively. The application of compression to a limb with arterial insufficiency could lead to gangrene. On the other hand, failure to apply compression with venous insufficiency could lead to extension and failure of the ulcer to heal (Hofman, 2000). Adam, Naik, Hartshorne, Bello, and London (2003) recommend a full clinical assessment, ankle/brachial pressure index, and lower limb venous duplex scan to guide the selection of treatment options.

Treatment of leg ulcers has become increasingly successful when a multidisciplinary, holistic approach has been used. Bed rest is no longer necessary, and many outpatient clinics (including some that are run by nurses) are devoted exclusively to leg ulcer care. The goals of treatment are to alleviate swelling, eliminate infection, and promote healing. When venous disease is confirmed, the mainstay of conservative management is compression bandages or hosiery (Moore, 2002; Roberts, Hammad, Collins, Shearman, & Mani, 2002). Debate exists over which level of pressure is most appropriate (Moore, 2002). Treatment of ulcers requires class 2 compression stockings. Class 1 stockings and TED compression hosiery do not exert adequate compression. For patients who cannot manage stockings, a four-layer compression dressing is recommended. A compression pump is another option, but it must be used for 6 hours a day, which makes it impractical for many people (McMullin, 2001).

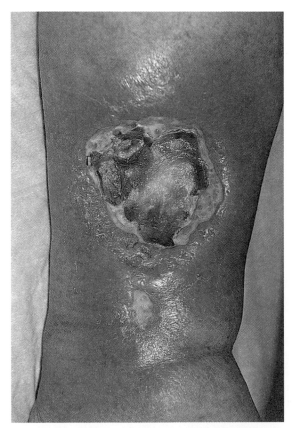

Figure 10-10 Stasis dermatitis. (From Callen, J. P., Greer, K. E., Paller, A., & Swinyer, L. [2000]. *Color atlas of dermatology* [2nd ed.]. Philadelphia: Saunders, p. 209.)

Other treatment options include superficial venous surgery, occlusive dressings, topical ointments, corticosteroid therapy, and antibiotics if infection is present. Topical negative pressure is a relatively new therapy that appears to hold promise for chronic wound healing. One study used the vacuum-assisted closure (VAC) system with 17 patients who had nonhealing diabetic and dysvascular lower extremity wounds; 14 of the 17 wounds healed successfully in an average treatment period of 8.2 weeks (Clare et al., 2002).

The prevalence of this problem justifies considerable research aimed at identifying effective treatment measures. The Cochrane Database of Systematic Reviews has published summaries of studies that address an array of treatments for chronic leg ulcers. Among the approaches that were supported by the literature are compression (Cullum, Nelson, Fletcher, & Sheldon, 2003) and pentoxyfylline as an adjunct to compression bandaging (Jull, Waters, & Arroll, 2003). In relation to compression, the systematic review concluded that multilayered systems are more effective than single-layered systems and that high compression is superior to low compression (Cullum, Nelson, Fletcher, & Sheldon, 2003). Therapies lacking adequate research evidence of effectiveness include ultrasound therapy (Flemming & Cullum, 2003a), oral zinc sulfate (Wilkinson & Hawke, 2003), low-level laser therapy (Flemming & Cullum, 2003a), and electromagnetic therapy (Flemming & Cullum, 2003a). Therapies that may be effective but require further research include topical negative pressure (Evans & Land, 2003), skin grafts (Jones & Nelson, 2003), intermittent pneumatic compression (Mani, Vowden, & Nelson, 2003), and horse chestnut seed extract (Pittler & Ernst, 2003). Novel treatments that have received limited attention include the application of honey-medicated dressings (Ahmed, Hoekstra, Hage, & Karim, 2003), a flexible transparent chamber applied over the ulcer to maintain moisture (Vranckz et al., 2002), maggot therapy (Wollina, Liebold, Schmidt, Hartmann, & Fassler, 2002), and bioengineered skin (Badiavas, Paquette, Carson, & Falanga, 2002). The impact of individualized nutrition plans on healing of chronic wounds has not been clearly demonstrated. However, it is recommended that malnourishment be addressed in patients with nonhealing wounds (Wissing, Ek, Wengstron, Skold, & Unosson, 2002).

Pressure Ulcers (Decubitus Ulcers)

DESCRIPTION. Pressure ulcers, or decubitus ulcers, are localized areas of cellular necrosis resulting from prolonged pressure between any bony prominence and an external object, such as a bed, chair, or cast. Pressure occludes capillaries and produces local edema and hemorrhage that disrupts nutrient exchange and removal of toxic metabolites. Areas frequently affected in older persons include the heels, greater trochanter, sacrum, dorsal spine (especially in thin, kyphotic persons), scapular spines, and elbows. Long-term pressure increases vulnerability to decubitus ulcer development, as evidenced by the fact that high pressure maintained for a short time is less dangerous than low pressure continued for a long time. Predisposing factors include poor nutrition, aging, immobility, altered level of consciousness, superficial sensory loss, and disturbed autonomic function (loss of bowel and bladder control). Older adults are particularly prone to development of pressure ulcers because of arteriosclerotic changes in the vessels, loss of subcutaneous tissue, and loss of tissue elasticity.

The National Pressure Ulcer Long-Term Care Study (NPULS) analyzed data on 2420 adults who were considered to be at risk for developing pressure ulcers (defined as a Braden Scale score of 17 or less). About 22% had a pressure ulcer at the beginning of data collection (group 3). Over a 12-week period, 19% of those with no ulcer at baseline (group 2) developed an ulcer, and 6% of those who had ulcers at baseline (group 4) developed new ones. Residents in group 2 were more likely to be female, older, cognitively impaired, and immobile. Group 4 had the greatest number of pressure ulcers per resident and had the highest percentage of males. In order of frequency of occurrence, the ulcers occurred on the heel, buttocks, coccyx, sacrum, ankle, foot, toe, trochanter, and ischial tuberosities (Horn et al., 2002).

The two types of pressure ulcers are superficial (benign) and deep (malignant). Superficial ulcers are reddened areas involving only the outer skin layers and are less dangerous than deep ulcers. They are caused by friction, shearing stresses, trauma, infection, and saturation with urine or other moisturizing agents. The lesions are frequently painful.

Deep ulcers develop quickly as a result of thrombosis of the vessels in deep tissue overlying the bony prominences. The muscle and fat layers are more vulnerable than the dermis, causing deep, large ulcers. The ulcer begins as a reddening of the skin with unobservable necrosis in the deep underlying tissues. In 1 to 2 days, the lesion bursts through the skin like an abscess, revealing a deep cavity full of black or infected slough, which may go through to the bone. There is a large area of skin loss, resulting in extensive scarring. The development of deep pressure ulcers during an illness can delay recovery and may even be fatal.

RISK ASSESSMENT. Among the factors that affect tissue tolerance for pressure are age, vascular competency, glycemic control in diabetes mellitus, and body weight/malnutrition. Assessment of the older adult with a high potential for dermal ulcers should include ability to perceive pressure, continence, activity level, ability to reposition, and nutritional status. Individuals with any abnormalities, such as absent dorsalis pedis pulses; reduced sensitivity to light touch, pressure, pain, and temperature; greater than 2+ edema in feet; cyanosis, erythema, or pallor; and bony deformities, are at high risk for impaired skin integrity related to vascular insufficiency. Functional and environmental factors such as poorly fitting shoes, hazardous foot care practices, and inability to cut own toenails may interact with vascular and sensory factors to further increase risk.

Instruments used to assess severity of pressure ulcer risk are the Braden Scale (Bergstrom & Braden, 1988), the Norton Scale (Norton, McLaren, & Exton-Smith, 1962), and the Waterlow Scale (Waterlow, 1985). Dependent older adults should be assessed with one of the risk assessment tools on a regular basis (Figures 10-11 and 10-12). Patients with Braden scores less than 16 or Norton scores less than 15 should have plans for pressure ulcer prevention in place. Vap and Dunaye (2000) collected data from 555 resident charts in eight long-term care facilities and compared the predictive abilities of the Braden Scale and the Minimum Data Set (MDS). In this sample, the Braden Scale rated 172 residents at risk and correctly predicted 46 of 66 pressure ulcers. In contrast, the MDS identified 311 at-risk residents and correctly predicted 62 of 66 ulcers. The authors concluded that concurrent use of both tools was unnecessary. Further, an evidenced-based review of the risk assessment scales determined that most risk indicators used in the Braden Scale and the Waterlow Scale (Figure 10-13) were poorly suited for assessing wheelchair users (Anthony, Barnes, & Unsworth, 1998).

PREVENTION. Good nursing care is the key to preventing pressure ulcers. Pressure ulcer prevention protocols include activities that maintain and improve tissue tolerance of pressure and those that protect against the adverse effects of the external mechanical forces of pressure, friction, and shear (Agency for Health Care Policy and Research Panel for the Prediction and Prevention of Pressure Ulcers in Adults, 1992). An algorithm for pressure ulcer prediction, as well as specific intervention strategies, appears in Figure 10-14 (Inman, Sibbald, Rutledge, & Clark, 1993).

Prevention of pressure ulcers is more difficult in the elderly. The risk of developing deep pressure ulcers is greatest during the 10 days after the onset of illness or admission to the hospital, whichever coincides with the period of greatest immobility. Of special concern is the hospice patient in whom measures to prevent or treat pressure ulcers cause discomfort (Eisenberger & Zeleznik, 2003). A deep ulcer that develops early and penetrates deeply is most dangerous to the older person.

Norton Scale

A Physical condition	B Mental state	C Activity	D Mobility	E Incontinence	Total Score
4 Good	4 Alert	4 Ambulant	4 Full	4 Not	_____
3 Fair	3 Apathetic	3 Walks with help	3 Slightly limited	3 Occasional	
2 Poor	2 Confused	2 Chairbound	2 Very limited	2 Usually urine	
1 Bad	1 Stupor	1 Bedrest	1 Immobile	1 Double incontinence	

Norton Plus Scale
(For determining high risk for pressure sores)

Check ONLY if YES	**YES**
Diagnosis of diabetes	
Diagnosis of hypertension	_____
Hematocrit (M) <41%	_____
(F) <36%	_____
Hemoglobin (M) <14 g/dl	_____
(F) <12 g/dl	_____
Albumin level <3.3 g/dl	_____
Febrile >99.6F	_____
5 or more medications	_____
Changes in mental status to confused, lethargic within 24 hours	_____

TOTAL Number of Checkmarks
Norton Scale Score	
Minus total from above	_____
Norton Plus Score	_____

Figure 10-11 The Norton Scale and Norton Plus Scale for measuring the risk of pressure sore formation. Patients scoring 15 to 20 have little risk of pressure sore development, whereas patients with scores between 12 and 15 have a moderately high risk of developing a pressure sore, and patients scoring below 12 are at high risk. Pressure sore prevention methods should be instituted for those with scores less than 15. (From Norton, D., McLaren, R. S., & Exton-Smith, A. N. [1962]. Pressure sores. In *Investigation of geriatric nursing problems in hospitals.* London: National Corporation for the Care of Old People.)

Client's Name _____

Evaluator's Name _____

Date of Assessment

	1	2	3	4
Sensory perception Ability to respond meaningfully to pressure-related discomfort	**1. Completely limited** Unresponsive (does not moan, flinch, or grasp) to painful stimuli because of diminished level of consciousness or sedation OR limited ability to feel pain over most of body surface	**2. Very limited** Responds only to painful stimuli; cannot communicate discomfort except by moaning or restlessness OR has a sensory impairment that limits the ability to feel pain or discomfort over 1/2 of the body	**3. Slightly limited** Responds to verbal commands but cannot always communicate discomfort or need to be turned OR has some sensory impairment that limits ability to feel pain or discomfort in 1 or 2 extremities	**4. No impairment** Responds to verbal commands; has no sensory deficit that would limit ability to feel or voice pain or discomfort
Moisture Degree to which skin is exposed to moisture	**1. Completely moist** Skin is kept moist almost constantly by perspiration, urine; dampness is detected every time the client is moved or turned	**2. Moist** Skin is often but not always moist; linen must be changed at least once a shift	**3. Occasionally moist** Skin is occasionally moist, requiring an extra linen change approximately once a day	**4. Rarely moist** Skin is usually dry; linen requires changing only at routine intervals
Activity Degree of physical activity	**1. Bedfast** Confined to bed	**2. Chairfast** Ability to walk severely limited or nonexistent; cannot bear own weight and must be assisted into chair or wheelchair	**3. Walks occasionally** Walks occasionally during the day but for very short distances, with or without assistance; spends the majority of each shift in bed or chair	**4. Walks frequently** Walks outside the room at least twice a day and inside the room at least once every 2 hours during walking hours
Mobility Ability to change or control body position	**1. Completely immobile** Does not make even slight changes in body or extremity position without assistance	**2. Very limited** Makes occasional slight changes in body or extremity position but unable to make frequent or significant changes independently	**3. Slighted limited** Makes frequent though slight changes in body or extremity position independently	**4. No limitations** Makes major and frequent changes in position without assistance
Nutrition Usual food intake pattern	**1. Very poor** Never eats a complete meal; rarely eats more than 1/3 of any food offered; eats 2 servings or less of protein (meat or dairy products) per day; takes fluids poorly; does not take a liquid dietary supplement OR is NPO or maintained on clear liquids or IV for more than 5 days	**2. Probably inadequate** Rarely eats a complete meal and generally eats only about 1/2 of any food offered; protein intake includes only 3 servings of meat or dairy products per day; occasionally will take a dietary supplement OR receives less than optimal amount of liquid diet or tube feeding	**3. Adequate** Eats over half of most meals; eats a total of 4 servings of protein (meat, dairy products) each day; occasionally will refuse a meal, but will usually take a supplement if offered OR is receiving tube feeding or total parenteral nutrition, which probably meets most nutritional needs	**4. Excellent** Eats most of every meal; never refuses a meal; usually eats a total of 4 or more servings of meat and dairy products; occasionally eats between meals; does not require supplementation
Friction and shear	**1. Problem** Requires moderate to maximum assistance in moving; complete lifting without sliding against sheets is impossible; frequently slides down in bed or chair, requiring frequent repositioning with maximum assistance; spasticity, contractures, or agitation leads to almost constant friction	**2. Potential problem** Moves feebly or requires minimum assistance; during a move, skin probably slides to some extent against sheets, chair, restraints, or other devices; maintains relatively good position in chair or bed most of the time but occasionally slides down	**3. No apparent problem** Moves in bed and in chair independently and has sufficient muscle strength to lift up completely during move; maintains good position in bed or chair at all times	

Total score _____

Figure 10-12 The Braden Scale. (Source: Barbara Braden and Nancy Bergstrom. Copyright 1988. Reprinted with permission.)

WATERLOW PRESSURE ULCER PREVENTION/TREATMENT POLICY
RING SCORES IN TABLE, ADD TOTAL. MORE THAN 1 SCORE/CATEGORY CAN BE USED

BUILD/WEIGHT FOR HEIGHT	◆	SKIN TYPE VISUAL RISK AREAS	◆	SEX AGE	◆	MALNUTRITION SCREENING TOOL (MST) (Nutrition Vol.15, No.6 1999 - Australia

BUILD/WEIGHT FOR HEIGHT		SKIN TYPE		SEX/AGE		MST
AVERAGE BMI = 20-24.9	0	HEALTHY	0	MALE	1	A - HAS PATIENT LOST WEIGHT RECENTLY B - WEIGHT LOSS SCORE
ABOVE AVERAGE BMI = 25-29.9 OBESE BMI > 30	1 / 2	TISSUE PAPER DRY OEDEMATOUS CLAMMY, PYREXIA	1 / 1 / 1 / 1	FEMALE 14 - 49 50 - 64	2 / 1 / 2	YES - GO TO B 0.5 - 5kg = 1
BELOW AVERAGE BMI < 20 BMI=Wt(Kg)/Ht (m)^2	3	DISCOLOURED GRADE 1 BROKEN/SPOTS GRADE 2-4	2 / 3	65 - 74 75 - 80 81 +	3 / 4 / 5	NO - GO TO C 5 - 10kg = 2 / UNSURE - GO TO C AND SCORE 2 10 - 15kg = 3 / > 15kg = 4 / unsure = 2

A - HAS PATIENT LOST WEIGHT RECENTLY
- YES - GO TO B
- NO - GO TO C
- UNSURE - GO TO C AND SCORE 2

B - WEIGHT LOSS SCORE
- 0.5 - 5kg = 1
- 5 - 10kg = 2
- 10 - 15kg = 3
- > 15kg = 4
- unsure = 2

C - PATIENT EATING POORLY OR LACK OF APPETITE
'NO' = 0; 'YES' SCORE = 1

NUTRITION SCORE
If > 2 refer for nutrition assessment / intervention

CONTINENCE	◆	MOBILITY	◆	SPECIAL RISKS
COMPLETE/ CATHETERISED	0	FULLY	0	
URINE INCONT.	1	RESTLESS/FIDGETY	1	
FAECAL INCONT.	2	APATHETIC	2	
URINARY + FAECAL INCONTINENCE	3	RESTRICTED	3	
		BEDBOUND e.g. TRACTION	4	
		CHAIRBOUND e.g. WHEELCHAIR	5	

SPECIAL RISKS

TISSUE MALNUTRITION	◆	NEUROLOGICAL DEFICIT	◆
TERMINAL CACHEXIA	8	DIABETES, MS, CVA	4-6
MULTIPLE ORGAN FAILURE	8	MOTOR/SENSORY	4-6
SINGLE ORGAN FAILURE (RESP, RENAL, CARDIAC,)	5	PARAPLEGIA (MAX OF 6)	4-6
PERIPHERAL VASCULAR DISEASE	5	**MAJOR SURGERY or TRAUMA**	
ANAEMIA (Hb < 8)	2	ORTHOPAEDIC/SPINAL	5
SMOKING	1	ON TABLE > 2 HR#	5
		ON TABLE > 6 HR#	8

MEDICATION - CYTOTOXICS, LONG TERM/HIGH DOSE STEROIDS, ANTI-INFLAMMATORY   MAX OF 4

SCORE
10+ AT RISK
15+ HIGH RISK
20+ VERY HIGH RISK

© J Waterlow 1985 Revised 2005*
Obtainable from the Nook, Stoke Road, Henlade TAUNTON TA3 5LX
* The 2005 revision incorporates the research undertaken by Queensland Health.
www.judy-waterlow.co.uk

Scores can be discounted after 48 hours provided patient is recovering normally

---

REMEMBER TISSUE DAMAGE MAY START PRIOR TO ADMISSION, IN CASUALTY. A SEATED PATIENT IS AT RISK
ASSESSMENT (See Over) IF THE PATIENT FALLS INTO ANY OF THE RISK CATEGORIES, THEN PREVENTATIVE NURSING IS REQUIRED A COMBINATION OF GOOD NURSING TECHNIQUES AND PREVENTATIVE AIDS WILL BE NECESSARY
ALL ACTIONS MUST BE DOCUMENTED

PREVENTION
PRESSURE REDUCING AIDS
Special Mattress/beds:
10+ Overlays or specialist foam mattresses.
15+ Alternating pressure overlays, mattresses and bed systems
20+ Bed systems: Fluidised bead, low air loss and alternating pressure mattresses
Note: Preventative aids cover a wide spectrum of specialist features. Efficacy should be judged, if possible, on the basis of independent evidence.

Cushions: No person should sit in a wheelchair without some form of cushioning. If nothing else is available - use the person's own pillow. (Consider infection risk)
10+ 100mm foam cushion
15+ Specialist Gell and/or foam cushion
20+ Specialised cushion, adjustable to individual person.

Bed clothing: Avoid plastic draw sheets, inco pads and tightly tucked in sheet/sheet covers, especially when using specialist bed and mattress overlay systems
Use duvet - plus vapour permeable membrane.

NURSING CARE
General HAND WASHING, frequent changes of position, lying, sitting. Use of pillows
Pain Appropriate pain control
Nutrition High protein, vitamins and minerals
Patient Handling Correct lifting technique - hoists - monkey poles Transfer devices
Patient Comfort Aids Real Sheepskin - bed cradle
Operating Table
Theatre/A&E Trolley 100mm(4ins) cover plus adequate protection

Skin Care General hygene, NO rubbing, cover with an appropriate dressing

WOUND GUIDELINES
Assessment odour, exudate, measure/photograph position

WOUND CLASSIFICATION - EPUAP
GRADE 1 Discolouration of intact skin not affected by light finger pressure (non-blanching erythema)
This may be difficult to identify in darkly pigmented skin
GRADE 2 Partial thickness skin loss or damage involving epidermis and/or dermis
The pressure ulcer is superficial and presents clinically as an abrasion, blister or shallow crater
GRADE 3 Full thickness skin loss involving damage of subcutaneous tissue but not extending to the underlying fascia
The pressure ulcer presents clinically as a deep crater with or without undermining of adjacent tissue
GRADE 4 Full thickness skin loss with extensive destruction and necrosis extending to underlying tissue.

Dressing Guide Use Local dressings formulary and/or www.worldwidewounds

IF TREATMENT IS REQUIRED, FIRST REMOVE PRESSURE

Figure 10-13 The Waterlow Card. (Courtesy of Judy Waterlow, SRN, RCNT, Henlade, Taunton. Copyright 2005. www.judy-waterlow.co.uk.)

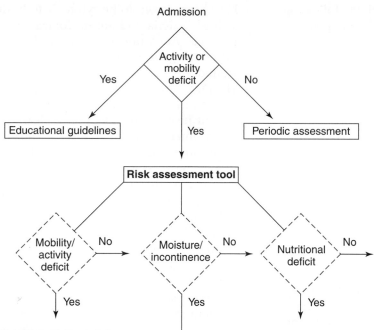

Admission

Activity or mobility deficit

Yes → Educational guidelines

No → Periodic assessment

Yes → **Risk assessment tool**

Mobility/activity deficit — No →

Moisture/incontinence — No →

Nutritional deficit — No →

Yes ↓ (Mobility/activity deficit)

Yes ↓ (Moisture/incontinence)

Yes ↓ (Nutritional deficit)

Mobility/activity deficit:

Mechanical loading and support surface guideline

For bed-bound individuals:
- Reposition at least every 2 hours.
- Use pillows or foam wedges to keep bony prominences from direct contact.
- Use devices that totally relieve pressure on the heels.
- Avoid positioning directly on the trochanter.
- Elevate the head of the bed as little and for as short a time as possible.
- Use lifting devices to move rather than drag individuals during transfers and position changes.
- Place at-risk individuals on a pressure reducing mattress. **Do not use donut-type devices.**

For chair-bound individuals:
- Reposition at least every hour.
- Have patient shift weight every 15 minutes if able.
- Use pressure-reducing devices for seating for seating surfaces. **Do not use donut-type devices.**

Skin care and early treatment guideline

- Inspect skin at least once a day.
- Individualize bathing schedule. Avoid hot water. Use mild cleansing agent.
- Minimize environmental factors such as low humidity and cold air. Use moisturizers for dry skin.
- Avoid massage over bony prominences.
- Use proper positioning, transferring, and turning techniques.
- Use lubricants to reduce friction injuries.
- Institute a rehabilitation program.
- Monitor and document interventions and outcomes.
- Consider postural alignment, distribution of weight, balance and stability, and pressure relief when positioning individuals in chairs or wheelchairs.
- Use a written plan.

Nutritional deficit:

Skin care and early treatment guideline

- Investigate factors that compromise an apparently well-nourished individual's dietary intake (especially protein or calories) and offer him or her support with eating.
- Plan and implement a nutritional support and/or supplementation program for nutritionally compromised individuals.

Moisture/incontinence:

Skin care and early treatment guideline

- Cleanse skin at time of soiling.
- Minimize skin exposure to moisture. Assess and treat urinary incontinence. When moisture cannot be controlled, use underpads or briefs that are absorbent and present a quick-drying surface to the skin.

Figure 10-14 Pressure ulcer prediction and prevention algorithm. (Adapted from Agency for Health Care Policy and Research [AHCPR] Panel for the Prediction and Prevention of Pressure Ulcers in Adults. [1992]. *Pressure ulcers in adults: Prediction and prevention.* Clinical practice guideline no. 3. Rockville, MD: AHCPR, Public Health Services, pp. 16-17.)

Although high-quality research is limited, the following measures are generally believed to help prevent pressure ulcers:

1. Change position at least every 2 hours.
2. Protect feet from pressure from bedcovers.
3. Keep vulnerable areas clean and dry.
4. Avoid oversedation and undersedation.
5. Promote good nutrition.
6. Promote good hydration.
7. Use an alternating-pressure airbed or waterbed.
8. Use high-specification foam mattresses rather than standard hospital mattresses.
9. Use pressure-relieving mattresses in the surgical suite.

ASSESSMENT OF EXISTING ULCERS. Appropriate treatment of pressure ulcers requires an accurate description of the lesions. The description should include location, size, depth, presence of granulation or necrotic tissue, characteristics of drainage, odor, presence of inflammation, extent of undermining, and aggravating factors.

Pressure ulcers should be classified using the staging system described in Figure 10-15. If necrotic tissue or eschar is extensive, the ulcer cannot be staged because the depth of the lesion cannot be determined until the eschar is removed. After the initial assessment, documentation of changes in the ulcer should be made at least every 3 days.

TREATMENT. Pressure ulcer treatment consists of the following components:

■ *Assessment*, including that described previously, plus wound culture if the patient shows signs of infection such as fever, increased white blood count, inflammation or edema around the ulcer, or purulent drainage. The procedure for obtaining a wound culture varies according to the amount of exudate and the type of wound.
■ *Debridement* to remove necrotic tissue, such as slough and eschar. When the ulcer bed is pink with granulation tissue, debridement should be discontinued.
   ■ *Sharp debridement.* The most rapid and effective technique is sharp debridement, using scalpel and scissors.
   ■ *Enzymatic debridement.* A German study comparing wound debridement with collagenase and with fibrinolysin/deoxyribonuclease found no difference between the two (Pullen, Popp, Volkers, & Fusgen, 2002).
   ■ Whirlpool and wet-to-dry dressings.
   ■ Biotherapy using maggots is an ancient treatment that has been subjected to modern study and found to be effective (Sherman, 2002).
■ Gentle *cleansing* with tepid normal saline. Antiseptic solutions such as povidone-iodine and hypochlorite

have been shown to be cytotoxic to healthy tissue as well as bacteria and are no longer routinely recommended. Antiseptic solutions followed by normal saline irrigation may be indicated for infected wounds.

■ The *dressing* chosen for the ulcer should provide an environment that supports healing. Research on wound healing suggests that a clean, moist wound environment is more conducive to healing than a dry environment, because epithelial cells proliferate and migrate more readily.
   ■ Occlusive dressings that produce a moist healing environment include occlusive dressings such as DuoDERM. Occlusive dressings should not be used if wound infection is present, because vapor-impermeable dressings may promote growth of anaerobic organisms. Kohr (2001) recommends moist wound healing instead of wet-to-dry dressings.
   ■ Semipermeable transparent films such as Opsite.
   ■ Absorptive gels such as karaya powder, Debrisan, and Bard absorptive dressings are useful with deep wounds that have a large amount of exudate because they absorb the excess drainage and necrotic tissue without overly drying the wound.
   ■ Belmin, Meaume, Rabus, and Bohbot (2002) found more rapid healing with calcium alginate dressings applied for 4 weeks, followed by hydrocolloid dressings for 4 weeks, than the use of hydrocolloid dressing for the entire treatment period.
   ■ A study comparing topical phenytoin, DuoDERM, and triple antibiotic ointment revealed healing progress with all three, but the most rapid healing with phenytoin (Rhodes, Heyneman, Culbertson, Wilson, & Phatak, 2001).
   ■ Noncontact normothermic wound therapy (NNWT) that involved warming the dressing to 38° C for 1 hour three times a day was determined to significantly increase healing rate when compared with moisture-retentive dressings (Whitney, Salvadelena, Higa, & Mich, 2001). When used with pressure-reducing surfaces and repositioning, NNWT was found to decrease the surface areas of stages 3 and 4 pressure ulcers by 2.5 times, with a savings of nearly $7000 over a 40-month time frame (Macario & Dexter, 2002).
■ Intensified *pressure relief* efforts for stage 3 and stage 4 pressure ulcers. A systematic review of studies of pressure-relieving devices concluded that air-fluidized and low-air-loss devices were effective in treating pressure ulcers. The relative value of alternating and constant low pressure could not be determined. Insufficient data were available on the benefits of seat cushions (Cullum, Deeks, Sheldon, Song, & Fletcher, 2003).

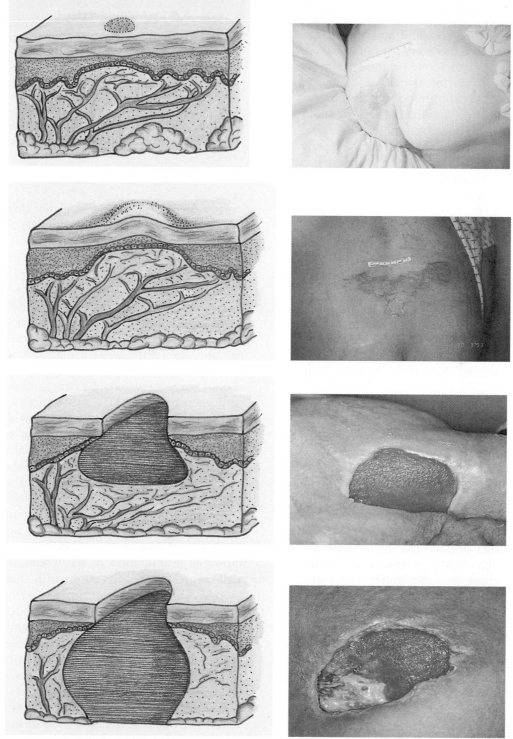

Figure 10-15   Staging of pressure ulcers. (From Lewis, S. M., & Ayello, E. A. [2004]. Inflammation, infection, and healing. In S. M. Lewis, M. M. Heitkemper, & S. R. Dirksen (Eds.), *Medical-surgical nursing: Assessment and management of clinical problems* [6th ed.]. St. Louis: Mosby, p. 226.)

- New treatments:
    - Growth factors used to stimulate angiogenesis, epithelial cell migration, and fibroblast activity are available in selected centers with physician supervision. Growth factors hold promise for improving the treatment of chronic dermal ulcers.
    - VAC devices apply continuous negative pressure to the wound bed. A limited number of studies of devices on VAC effectiveness were found. One study that compared the VAC and Healthpoint (HP) systems concluded that the VAC was more effective in increasing the rate of wound healing (Ford et al., 2002).
    - Hyperbaric oxygen has been shown to facilitate healing and full closure in patients with diabetes mellitus. A study conducted in the United Kingdom found no added benefit to using electrical stimulation in conjunction with the hyperbaric oxygen (Edsberg, Brogan, Jaynes, & Fries, 2002).
- Therapies that have been tested on a limited scale and not yet shown to be beneficial include ultrasound (Flemming & Cullum, 2003b, 2003c).

The outcomes of nursing care with pressure ulcers include tissue integrity, skin; and wound healing: secondary intention.

FOOT PROBLEMS

Skin problems affecting the feet are numerous in older persons and therefore deserve special mention. The range of problems includes dry skin, onychogryphosis, diminished sensation, deformities of feet and nails, inadequate hygiene from reduced ability to reach or see feet, and improperly fitting footwear. Foot ulcers and infections are particularly devastating, because if vascular supply is compromised, wound healing and prevention of infection become much more difficult. Nonhealing ulcers of the foot are a significant source of dysfunction in the elderly, for they may later necessitate amputation because of osteomyelitis or gangrene. The older person then experiences pain and disability associated with the loss of a lower extremity. Nurses, therefore, should pay particular attention to the integrity of skin on the feet of older people.

NURSING CARE FOR SKIN CONDITIONS

Impairments in skin integrity have many manifestations. Adverse consequences from untreated skin problems in the aged include discomfort, disfigurement, systemic infection, and loss of limbs and subsequent functional impairment. Older adults are at increased risk for impaired skin integrity and the associated adverse effects for a variety of reasons. Therefore the

---

BOX 10-5 *TOWARD BETTER INTEGUMENT HEALTH*

- Avoid friction, irritation, and mechanical injury.
- Limit baths to 2 to 3 per week.
- Avoid soap, rubbing alcohol, and very hot water.
- Apply lubricants directly to the skin rather than putting them in the bathwater.
- Adequate intake of vitamins A and C and protein is needed for healthy skin and connective tissue.
- Limit exposure to sun, wind, and cold.

---

nurse plays a critical role in promoting and restoring health integument. Box 10-5 summarizes measures to promote healthy skin.

Nursing Assessment

History. The nursing history can help clarify whether a skin condition is normal or pathological. It also can indicate whether or not an older person is at risk for developing a particular condition and what measures are necessary for prevention. The history should cover all aspects of living and functioning that could affect the skin. The nurse should investigate the onset, development, and pattern of all skin conditions, accompanying symptoms, recent skin trauma, past or present systemic diseases, and medications taken. Finally, the general state of health, nutritional status, allergies, functional status, and physical and social environments should be determined, as well as the patient's perception of the problem and its impact.

Physical Assessment. Perform a systematic and thorough examination of the integument in a warm, well-lighted room (preferably with indirect daylight). Examine the entire skin surface, skinfolds, mucous membranes, hair, and nails. Progress from head to toe, comparing the left and right sides of the body for symmetry. Inspect the extremities for edema, erythema, cyanosis, pallor, hair loss, dry skin, nail abnormalities, presence of bony deformities, and evidence of poorly fitting footwear. Palpate the extremities for edema, peripheral pulses, and temperature, and test sensation. If a rash is present, describe the distribution, color, configuration, and associated symptoms such as itching or pain. Box 10-6 outlines the components of the integument history and physical assessment. Box 10-7 defines terms used to describe skin lesions.

It is important to distinguish potentially life-threatening rashes, such as those from drug reactions and cellulitis, from those with more benign courses, because physicians often rely on nursing judgment regarding the urgency of treating a rash. Distribution provides diag-

Box 10-6 Skin Assessment

Health History
- Past and present skin conditions: onset, development, pattern, duration, symptoms
- Past and present systemic diseases: history and treatment
- Drug history: topical, systemic, prescription, nonprescription, allergies
- Nutrition: malnourished, obese, diet and eating habits
- Functional status: mobility, mental status, activities of daily living capacity
- Environment:
  - Physical (temperature, climate, use of soaps or other drying agents)
  - Social (support system, work, family interactions)

Physical Examination
- Color: red, jaundiced, brown, gray, cyanotic, pale, blotchy
- Temperature: hot, warm, cool
- Moisture: dry, oily, or combination of both; moist, clammy
- Texture: rough, smooth, scaly, flaky
- Edema: location, extent
- Thickness: differences among various parts of the body, relationship to itching or redness
- Mobility and turgor: supple, pliable, flexible, creases and folds
- Lesions: color, size, texture, identifying characteristics, distribution
- Hair: amount, distribution, texture, color, dandruff or scaling, odor
- Nails: color, length, thickness, splitting, swelling, accumulations

BOX 10-7 Dermatological Terms

Macule	Flat, nonpalpable lesion differing in color from the surrounding skin
Papule	Small, raised, solid, superficial lesion, usually less than 0.5 cm in diameter
Plaque	Raised, solid, plateau-like lesion, usually more than 0.5 cm in diameter, greater in its diameter than in its depth
Nodule	Raised, solid lesion greater than 0.5 cm in both width and depth
Vesicle	Small (less than 0.5 cm), fluid-filled lesion
Bulla	Large (greater than 0.5 cm), fluid-filled lesion
Pustule	Fluid-filled sack containing cloudy or purulent material
Erosion	Loss of superficial surface epidermis often occurring after the natural breakage of a vesicle, bulla, or papule
Ulcer	Loss of epidermis extending into the dermis or subcutaneous tissue, usually as broad as it is deep
Fissure	Crack in the skin that is usually narrow but deep
Crust	Dried serum or purulent material overlying an erosion or ulcer
Wheal (hive)	Papule or plaque caused by dermal edema
Neoplasm (tumor)	New growth
Excoriation	Scratch marks indicating pruritis
Scale	Thickened stratum corneum
Lichenification	Thickening of the epidermis

nostic clues. For example, drug reactions are commonly distributed over the trunk and face, whereas cellulitis is generally confined to the locale of prior ulceration, although erysipelas may involve an entire extremity and not have continuous distribution. Other important parts of the assessment include historical information (see Box 10-6).

NURSING DIAGNOSES: AGE-RELATED CHANGES AND COMMON DISORDERS OF THE INTEGUMENT

1. Impaired skin integrity, related to itching, related to physical immobilization, related to alterations in turgor
2. Risk for impaired skin integrity related to physical immobilization, related to pressure, related to skeletal prominence, related to alterations in skin turgor

3. Impaired tissue integrity related to impaired physical mobility, related to pressure, related to altered circulation
4. Disturbed sleep pattern related to pain or itching
5. Risk for infection related to impaired tissue integrity

Nursing Management

The goals of nursing care related to the older adult's integument include preservation or restoration of skin integrity without complications, relief of discomfort, and implementation of measures to reduce the risk of ulcers.

Nursing interventions related to skin care for the older adult are aimed at preserving skin integrity and preventing disease and injury. Stress good personal grooming and cleanliness, not only to promote healthy skin but also for well-being and comfort. Because the skin of older persons is dry and fragile, handle it gently. Avoid friction, irritation, or mechanical injury when bathing, dressing, moving, or turning an older patient. Baths are not necessary every day for older people, and complete baths two or three times a week supplemented by partial baths are sufficient. The bath water temperature should not exceed 105° F. Avoid soap and rubbing alcohol because they tend to dry the skin. Do not put oily lubricants in the bathtub, because they could make the tub surface slippery. Instead, apply lubricants directly to the skin. Include hair and nail care in personal hygiene. Soak the feet to loosen debris under the nails and make the nails easier to cut.

Encourage a diet high in vitamins and nutrients to help maintain healthy skin in the older adult. Vitamins A and C and protein are necessary for healthy skin cells and supportive tissues. Teach the patient about foods high in these nutrients and help ensure that they are included in the diet.

Environmental modifications also can be made to promote healthy skin. To preserve moist and younger looking skin, advise the older adult to stay out of the sun, keep the air moist with a humidifier, and avoid exposure to wind and cold. Soft, unwrinkled clothing next to the skin minimizes skin irritation and pruritus. Encourage ambulatory patients to wear supportive shoes that protect the feet from trauma.

Evaluation

Timing of the evaluation in skin conditions deserves special note. The evaluation of responses to therapy for acute skin conditions that produce discomfort or threaten life is done much more frequently than evaluation of chronic, basically clean skin ulcers. Frequent evaluation of treatment regimens for chronic ulcers may cause the patient to become frustrated and inappropriately change treatments before an adequate trial.

Although observation for a sudden increase in the amount of wound drainage or a sudden change in appearance should be done daily, evaluation of treatment regimens should be less frequent—for example, weekly.

Criteria for evaluation of patients with impaired skin integrity include the following:
1. The patient's wound heals or rash resolves.
2. The patient remains free of signs and symptoms of preventable consequences such as infection.
3. The patient reports that discomfort accompanying the skin problem is relieved.
4. The patient adopts appropriate measures to prevent skin problems or complications.
5. Caregivers implement measures to prevent skin breakdown in at-risk individuals.

COLLABORATIVE PRACTICE ISSUES

Nurses have long had a prominent role in the treatment of skin problems in patients. However, some ambiguity regarding the responsibilities of nurses and physicians in treating some skin conditions exists, particularly in the case of pressure ulcers and foot problems.

Nursing care plays a critical role in prevention of pressure ulcers, yet in some institutions nurses may not independently order pressure-relieving devices, such as foam mattresses. In contrast, in practice settings where older people predominate, physicians often consider the patient's skin to be the nurse's domain of practice, unless a specific pathological lesion is present other than pressure or irritation from urine. Nurses should clarify their responsibilities regarding prevention and treatment of skin disorders where they work.

SUMMARY

Normal skin changes, almost more than any other body system, reflect the aging process. Changes generally seen in the skin in older people include thinning of the skin layers, decreased strength and elasticity, decreased vascularity, and delayed healing. The secretions of both the sebaceous and the sweat glands tend to diminish. Hair becomes thinner and grayer, and nails become thicker, more brittle, and hard, with diminished growth rates.

Common skin disorders associated with older age include pruritus, neoplastic disorders, herpes zoster, psoriasis, and pressure ulcers. Skin tags, cherry angiomas, nevi, venous lakes, and lentigos also are common; these cause little discomfort, but the appearance of mottled and spotty skin that they produce may be troublesome to the elderly. Dryness is perhaps the most significant skin problem with aging. It may cause itchiness and scaling and may even lead to other lesions. Treatment with moisturizers and emollients is useful for lubrication.

History and assessment of the skin should focus on past conditions and systemic diseases; drug use; nutrition; the environment; observation of the color, temperature, texture, and thickness of the skin; and any lesions or abnormalities. Nursing care should include the proper use of equipment, encouragement of proper nutrition, avoidance of injury, good hair and nail care, and instruction in self-care and preventive techniques. Prevention is the key to good skin care for older adults.

Nursing Care Plan: The Older Adult with a Pressure Ulcer

Data

87-year-old woman with history of stroke 1 month ago. Admitted to nursing facility from acute care hospital.

Assessment

Responds to touch and voice by opening eyes; no verbal response. Right hemiplegia. Incontinent. PEG tube in place. Height estimated at 5 ft 3 in. Weight before stroke was 123 lb. Current weight is 107 lb. Score on Braden Scale of 13. In bed most of the day. Transferred to chair for 2 hours three times daily.

Skin is dry and thin. Purpura on forearms, skin tear on left wrist with edges approximated with Steri-Strips. Stage 2 pressure ulcer on coccyx, 4 cm in diameter, 1 cm deep, base dark pink. No tunneling. Serosanguineous drainage, no odor. Stage 1 pressure ulcer on left scapula.

Nursing Diagnoses

Impaired skin integrity related to immobility

Goals/Outcomes

Patient's skin integrity is restored as evidenced by healed ulcers on coccyx and scapula.

NOC Suggested Outcomes

Wound Healing by Secondary Intention (1103)
Tissue Integrity, Skin and Mucous Membranes (1101)

NIC Suggested Interventions

Major interventions: Pressure Ulcer Care (3520), Pressure Ulcer Prevention (3540), Wound Care (3660)

- Document skin status on admission and daily.
- Use an established risk assessment tool to monitor individual's risk factors.
- Monitor for sources of pressure and friction.
- Inspect skin over bony prominences and other pressure points when repositioning at least daily.
- Monitor any reddened areas closely.
- Use methods of measuring skin temperature to determine pressure ulcer risk, per agency protocol.
- Document weight and shifts in weight.
- Turn every 1 to 2 hours.
- Post turning schedule at bedside.
- Turn with care (avoid shearing) to prevent injury to fragile skin.
- Position with pillows to elevate pressure points off the bed.
- Avoid hot water and use mild soap when bathing.
- Remove excessive moisture on the skin resulting from perspiration and fecal or urinary incontinence.
- Apply protective barriers, such as creams or moisture-absorbing pads, to remove excess moisture as appropriate.
- Moisturize dry, unbroken skin.
- Apply elbow and heel protectors as appropriate.
- Avoid massaging over bony prominences.
- Use specialty bed and mattress as appropriate.
- Keep bed linens clear, dry, and wrinkle free.
- Make bed with toe pleats.
- Use sheepskin on bed.
- Avoid use of "donut"-type devices in sacral area.
- Describe characteristics of ulcer at regular intervals, including size (length by width by depth), stage (1 through 4), location, exudates, granulation of necrotic tissue, and epithelialization.
- Monitor color, temperature, edema, moisture, and appearance of surrounding skin.
- Cleanse the ulcer with the appropriate nontoxic solution, working in a circular motion from the center.
- Monitor for signs and symptoms of infection in the wound.
- Apply dressing as prescribed by physician or enterostomal therapy nurse.
- Keep the ulcer moist to aid in healing.
- Cleanse the skin around the ulcer with mild soap and water.
- Monitor nutritional status in collaboration with dietitian.
- Institute consultation services of the enterostomal therapy nurse.

Other relevant interventions: Bed rest care, circulatory precautions, infection protection, nutrition management, positioning, urinary incontinence care, and positioning in chair.

Evaluation Parameters

Absence of purulent drainage from ulcer, decreased size of pressure ulcer, and absence of redness over left scapula and other bony prominences.

REFERENCES

Abrams, A. C. (2004). *Clinical drug therapy* (7th ed.). Philadelphia: Lippincott.

Adam, D. J., Naik, J., Hartshorne, T., Bello, M., & London, N. J. (2003). The diagnosis and management of 689 chronic leg ulcers in a single-visit assessment clinic. *European Journal of Vascular and Endovascular Surgery, 25*(5), 462-468.

Agency for Health Care Policy and Research Panel for the Prediction and Prevention of Pressure Ulcers in Adults. (1992). *Pressure ulcers in adults: Prediction and prevention.* Clinical practice guideline no. 3. AHCPR publication No. 92-0047. Rockville MD: RHCPR, Public Health Services, US Department of Health and Human Services.

Ahmed, A. K., Hoekstra, M. J., Hage, J. J., & Karim, R. B. (2003). Honey-medicated dressing: Transformation of an ancient remedy into modern therapy. *Annals of Plastic Surgery, 50*(2), 143-147.

Aizen, E., & Gilhar, A. (2001). Smoking effect on skin wrinkling in the aged population. *Isr Medical Association Journal, 3*(10), 734-738.

Al-Waili, N. S. (2001). Therapeutic and prophylactic effects of crude honey on chronic seborrheic dermatitis and dandruff. *European Journal of Medical Research, 6*(7), 306-308.

Aly, R., Forney, R., & Bayles, C. (2001). Treatments for common superficial fungal infections. *Dermatology Nursing, 13*(2), 91-94, 98-101.

Andreakos, E., Taylor, P. C., & Feldmann, M. (2002). Monoclonal antibodies in immune and inflammatory diseases. *Current Opinion in Biotechnology, 13*(6), 615-620.

Anthony, D., Barnes, J., & Unsworth, J. (1998). An evaluation of current risk assessment scales for decubitus ulcers in general inpatients and wheelchair users. *Clinical Rehabilitation, 12*(2), 136-142.

Badiavas, E. V., Paquette, D., Carson, P., & Falanga, V. (2002). Human chronic wounds treated with bioengineered skin: Histologic evidence of host-graft interactions. *Journal of the American Academy of Dermatology, 46*(4), 524-530.

Banov, C. H., Epstein, J. H., & Grayson, L. D. (1992). When an itch persists. *Patient Care, 26*, 75-81, 84-88.

Bastuji-Garin, S., & Diepgen, T. L. (2002). Cutaneous malignant melanoma, sun exposure, and sunscreen use: Epidemiological evidence. *British Journal of Dermatology, 146*(suppl 61), 24-30.

Bath, F. J., Bong, J., Perkins, W., & Williams, H. C. (2003). Interventions for basal cell carcinoma of the skin. *Cochrane Database of Systematic Reviews, 2*, CD003412.

Batisse, D. Bazin, R., Baldeweck, T., Querleux, B., & Leveque, J. L. (2002). Influence of age on the wrinkling capacities of skin. *Skin Research and Technology, 3*(8), 148-154.

Belmin, J., Meaume, S., Rabus, M., & Bohbot, S. (2002). Sequential treatment with calcium alginate dressings and hydrocolloid dressings accelerates pressure ulcer healing in older subjects: A multicenter randomized trial of sequential versus nonsequential treatment with hydrocolloid dressings alone. *Journal of the American Geriatrics Society, 50*(2), 269-274.

Berg, D., & Otley, C. C. (2002). Skin cancer in organ transplant recipients: Epidemiology, pathogenesis, and management. *Journal of the American Academy of Dermatology, 47*(1), 1-17.

Berger, R., & Gilchrest, B. A. (1998). Skin disorders. In E. H. Duthie & P. R. Katz (Eds.), *Practice of geriatrics* (3rd ed.). Philadelphia: W. B. Saunders.

Bergstrom, N., & Braden, B. (1988). A prospective study of pressure sore risk among institutionalized elderly. *Journal of the American Geriatrics Society, 40*, 747-758.

Bielan, B. (2002). What's your assessment? *Dermatology Nursing, 14*(4), 247, 256.

Bornstein, J., Pascal, B., & Abramovici, H. (1993). The common problem of vulvar pruritus. *Obstetrics and Gynecology Survey, 48*, 111-118.

Bosset, S., Bonnet-Duquennoy, M., Barre, P., Chalon, A., Kurfurst, R., Bonte, F., Schnebert., S., LeVarlet, B., & Nicolas, J. F. (2003). Photoageing shows histological features of chronic skin inflamma-tion without clinical and molecular abnormalities. *British Journal of Dermatology, 149*(4), 826-835.

Bowcock, A. M., & Barker, J. N. (2003). Genetics of psoriasis: The potential impact on new therapies. *Journal of the American Academy of Dermatology, 49*(2 suppl), S51-56.

Braun, R. P., Rabinovitz, H., Oliviero, M., Kopf, A. W., & Saurat, J. H. (2002). Dermoscopic diagnosis of seborrheic keratosis. *Clinics in Dermatology, 20*(2), 270-272.

Brenner, S., & Tamir, E. (2002). Early detection of melanoma: The best strategy for a favorable prognosis. *Clinics in Dermatology, 20*(3), 203-211.

Brooke, R. C. C., & Griffiths, C. E. M. (2003). Aging of the skin. In R. C. Tallis & H. M. Fillit (Eds.), *Brocklehurst's textbook of geriatric medicine and gerontology* (6th ed.). London: Churchill Livingstone.

Brown, A. D. G., & Cooper, T. K. (2003). Gynecological disorders. In R. C. Tallis & H. M. Fillit (Eds.), *Brocklehurst's textbook of geriatric medicine and gerontology* (6th ed.). London: Churchill Livingstone.

Brozena, S. J., Waterman, D. O., & Fenske, N. A. (1990). Malignant melanoma: Management guidelines. *Geriatrics, 45*, 55-62.

Bruner, C. R., Feldman, S. R., Ventrapragada, M., & Fleischer, A. B., Jr. (2003, February). A systematic review of adverse effects associated with topical treatments for psoriasis. *Dermatology Online Journal, 9*(1), 2.

Cameron, A. L., Kirby, B., Fei, W., & Griffiths, C. E. (2002). Natural killer and natural killer-T cells in psoriasis. *Archives of Dermatological Research, 294*(8), 363-369.

Carlin, C. S., Callis, K. P., & Krueger, G. G. (2003). Efficacy of acitretin and commercial tanning bed therapy for psoriasis. *Archives in Dermatology, 139*(4), 436-442.

Chen, P. H., Hsueh, H. F., & Hong, C. Z. (2002). Herpes zoster-associated voiding dysfunction: A retrospective study and literature review. *Archives of Physical Medicine and Rehabilitation, 83*(11), 1624-1628.

Chu, A., & Osguthorpe, J. D. (2003). Nonmelanoma cutaneous malignancy with regional metastasis. *Otolaryngology—Head and Neck Surgery, 128*(5), 663-673.

Clare, M., Fitzgibbons, T. C., McMullen, S. T., Stice, R. C., Hayes, D. F., & Henckel, L. (2002). Experience with the vacuum assisted closure negative pressure technique in the treatment of non-healing diabetic and dysvascular wounds. *Foot and Ankle International, 23*(10), 896-901.

Clayton, A. S., & Stasko, T. (2003). Treatment of nonmelanona skin cancer in organ transplant recipients: Review of responses to a survey. *Journal of American Academic Dermatology, 49*(3), 413-416.

Cole-King, A., & Harding, K. G. (2001). Psychological factors and delayed healing in chronic wounds. *Psychosomatic Medicine, 63*(2), 216-220.

Coni, N., Davison, W., & Webster, S. (1980). *Lecture notes on geriatrics.* Boston: Blackwell Scientific Publications.

Cullum, N., Deeks, J., Sheldon, T. A., Song, F., & Fletcher, A. W. (2003). Beds, mattresses, and cushions for pressure ulcer prevention and treatment. *Cochrane Database of Systematic Reviews, 3*.

Cullum, N., Nelson, E. A., Fletcher, A. W., & Sheldon, T. A. (2003). Compression for leg ulcers. *Cochrane Database of Systematic Reviews, 3*.

Curran, M. P., & Wagstaff, A. J. (2003). Gabapentin: In postherpetic neuralgia. *CNS Drugs, 17*(13), 975-982.

Dalziel, K. L., & Bickers, D. R. (1992). Skin aging. In J.C. Brocklehurst, R. C. Tallis, & H. M. Fillit (Eds.), *Textbook of geriatric medicine and gerontology* (4th ed.). Edinburgh: Churchill Livingstone.

Davies, D. B., Boorman, G. C., & Shuttleworth, D. (1999). Comparative efficacy of shampoos containing coal tar (4.0% w/w; Tarmed™), coal tar (4.0% w/w) plus ciclopirox olamine (1.0% w/w; Tarmed™ AF) and ketoconazole (2.0% w/w; Nizoral™) for the treatment of dandruff/seborrheic dermatitis. *Journal of Dermatological Treatment, 10*(3), 177-183.

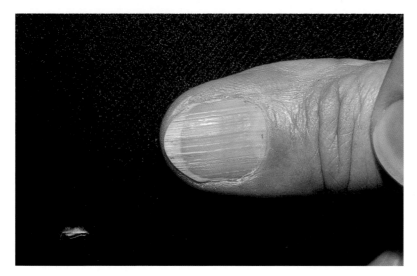

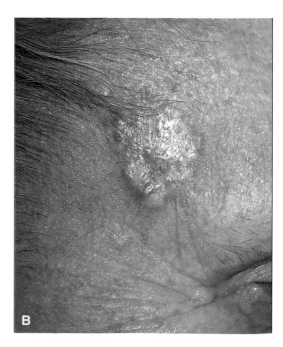

Plate 1 Ridges of the nails are common in older patients. The ridges may have a longitudinal beaded appearance, resembling a row of sausages. (From White, G. M., & Cox, N. H. [2006]. *Diseases of the skin: A color atlas and text* [2nd ed.]. St. Louis: Elsevier.)

Plate 2 Multiple skin tags of the axilla. Patients often want these tags removed as they are irritating. (From White, G. M., & Cox, N. H. [2006]. *Diseases of the skin: A color atlas and text* [2nd ed.]. St. Louis: Elsevier.)

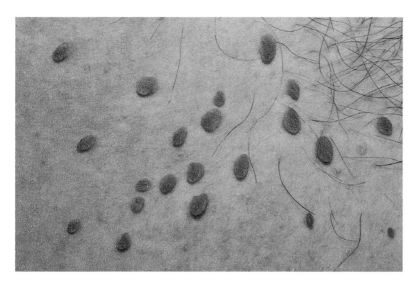

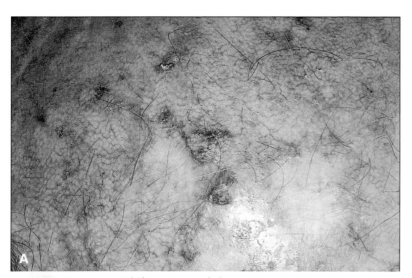

Plate 3 Close-up of **(A)** scalp and **(B)** temple actinic keratosis, showing the typical hard scale and stuck-on appearance. (From White, G. M., & Cox, N. H. [2006]. *Diseases of the skin: A color atlas and text* [2nd ed.]. St. Louis: Elsevier.)

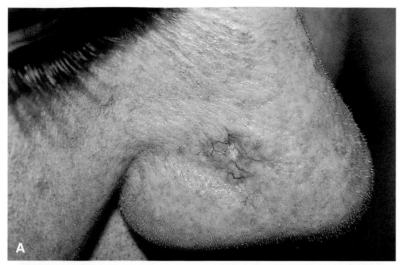

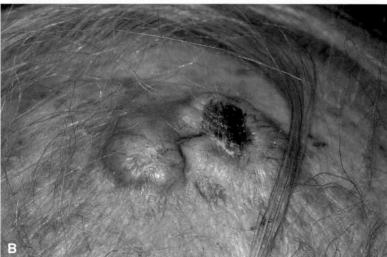

Plate 4 Nodular basal cell carcinomas **(A)** on the sidewall of the nose and **(B)** on the forehead. Both have typical morphology and telangiectasia. (From White, G. M., & Cox, N. H. [2006]. *Diseases of the skin: A color atlas and text* [2nd ed.]. St. Louis: Elsevier.)

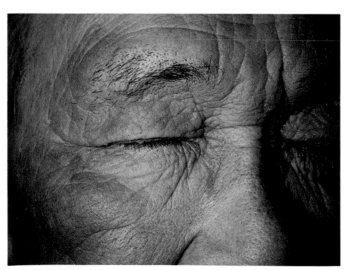

Plate 5 Chronic actinic dermatitis. (From James, W. D., Berger, T. G., & Elston, D. M. [2006]. *Andrews' diseases of the skin: Clinical dermatology* [10th ed.]. St. Louis: Elsevier.)

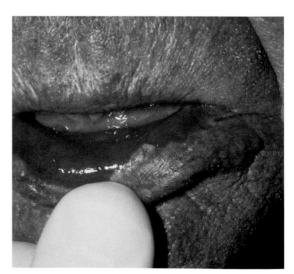

Plate 6 Actinic cheilitis. (From James, W. D., Berger, T. G., & Elston, D. M. [2006]. *Andrews' diseases of the skin: Clinical dermatology* [10th ed.]. St. Louis: Elsevier.)

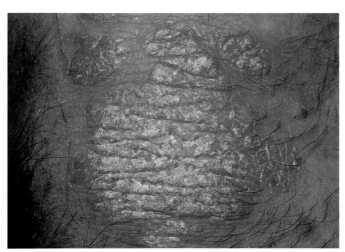

Plate 7 Psoriasis plaque: red plaque with silver scale on the knee. (From James, W. D., Berger, T. G., & Elston, D. M. [2006]. *Andrews' diseases of the skin: Clinical dermatology* [10th ed.]. St. Louis: Elsevier.)

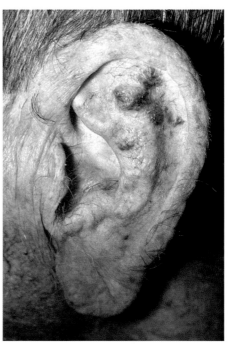

Plate 9 Venous lake. (From James, W. D., Berger, T. G., & Elston, D. M. [2006]. *Andrews' diseases of the skin: Clinical dermatology* [10th ed.]. St. Louis: Elsevier.)

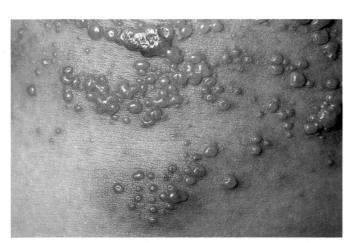

Plate 8 Herpes zoster. (From James, W. D., Berger, T. G., & Elston, D. M. [2006]. *Andrews' diseases of the skin: Clinical dermatology* [10th ed.]. St. Louis: Elsevier.)

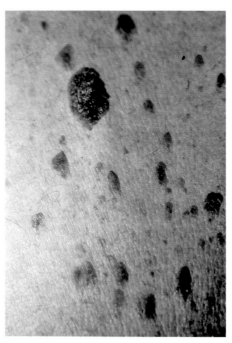

Plate 10 Seborrheic keratosis. (From James, W. D., Berger, T. G., & Elston, D. M. [2006]. *Andrews' diseases of the skin: Clinical dermatology* [10th ed.]. St. Louis: Elsevier.)

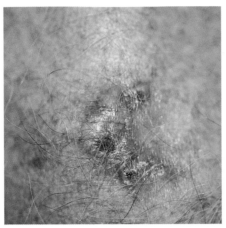

Plate 11 Basal cell carcinoma. (From James, W. D., Berger, T. G., & Elston, D. M. [2006]. *Andrews' diseases of the skin: Clinical dermatology* [10th ed.]. St. Louis: Elsevier.)

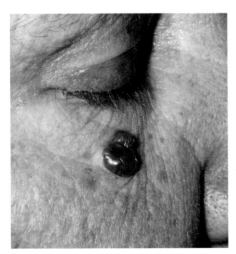

Plate 12 Basal cell carcinoma: cystic. (From James, W. D., Berger, T. G., & Elston, D. M. [2006]. *Andrews' diseases of the skin: Clinical dermatology* [10th ed.]. St. Louis: Elsevier.)

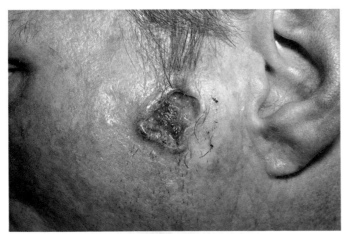

Plate 13 Squamous cell carcinoma: preauricular ulceration in a patient with AIDS. (From James, W. D., Berger, T. G., & Elston, D. M. [2006]. *Andrews' diseases of the skin: Clinical dermatology* [10th ed.]. St. Louis: Elsevier.)

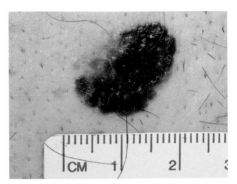

Plate 14 Superficial spreading malignant melanoma. (From James, W. D., Berger, T. G., & Elston, D. M. [2006]. *Andrews' diseases of the skin: Clinical dermatology* [10th ed.]. St. Louis: Elsevier.)

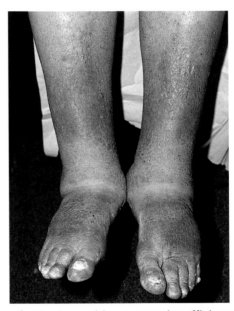

Plate 15 Statis dermatitis, venous insufficiency. (From James, W. D., Berger, T. G., & Elston, D. M. [2006]. *Andrews' diseases of the skin: Clinical dermatology* [10th ed.]. St. Louis: Elsevier.)

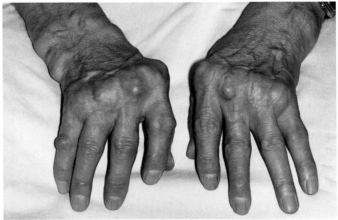

Plate 16 Rheumatoid nodules. (From James, W. D., Berger, T. G., & Elston, D. M. [2006]. *Andrews' diseases of the skin: Clinical dermatology* [10th ed.]. St. Louis: Elsevier.)

Dawe, R. S., Cameron, H., Yule, S., Man, I., Wainwright, N. J., Ibbotson, S. H., & Ferguson, J. (2003). A randomized controlled trial of narrowband ultraviolet B vs bath-psoralen plus ultraviolet A photochemotherapy for psoriasis. *British Journal of Dermatology, 148*(6), 1194-1204.

Desmond, R. A., & Soong, S. J. (2003). Epidemiology of malignant melanoma. *Surgical Clinics of North America, 83*(1), 1-29.

Drake, L. A., Ceilley, R. I., & Cornelison, R. L. (1993). Guidelines for malignant melanoma. *Journal of American Academy of Dermatology, 28*, 638-641.

Duncan, W. C., & Fenske, N. A. (1990). Cutaneous signs of internal disease in the elderly. *Geriatrics, 45*, 24-30.

Duque, M. I., Jordan, J. R., Fleischer, A. B., Jr., Williford, P. M., Teuschler, H., & Chen, G. J. (2003). Frequency of seborrheic keratosis biopsies in the United States: A benchmark of skin lesion care quality and cost effectiveness. *Dermatologic Surgery, 29*(8), 796-801.

Edsberg, L. E., Brogan, M. S., Jaynes, C. D., & Fries, K. (2002). Topical hyperbaric oxygen and electrical stimulation: Exploring potential synergy. *Ostomy Wound Management, 48*(11), 42-44.

Eisenberger, A., & Zeleznik, J. (2003). Pressure ulcer prevention and treatment in hospices: A qualitative analysis. *Journal of Palliative Care, 19*(1), 9-14.

El-Domyati, M. Attia, S., Salen, F., Brown, D., Birk, D. E., Gasparro, F., Ahmad, H., & Uittio, J. (2002). Intrinsic aging vs. photoaging: A comparative histopathological, immunohistochemical, and ultrastructural study of skin. *Experimental Dermatology, 11*(5), 398-405.

Ensebio, E. B., Graham, J., & Moody, N. (1990). Treatment of intractable pruritus ani. *Diseases of the Colon and Rectum, 33*, 770-772.

Evans, E. C., & Gray, M. (2003). What interventions are effective for the prevention and treatment of cutaneous candidiasis? *JWOCN, 30*, 11-16.

Evans, E. C., & Land, L. (2003). Topical negative pressure for treating chronic wounds. *Cochrane Database of Systematic Reviews, 3*.

Farmer, E.R., & Hood, A.F. (1990). . *Pathology of the skin*. East Norwalk, CT: Appleton & Lange.

Fassiadis, N., Kapetanakis, E., & Law, N. (2002). Etiology of leg ulcers, healing and recurrence rates in octo- and nonagenarians. *International Angiology, 21*(2), 193-195.

Fenske, N.A., & Lober, C.S. (1990). Skin changes of aging: Pathological implications. *Geriatrics, 45*, 27-35.

Fisher, G. J., Kang, S., Varani, J., Bata-Csorgo, Z., Wan, Y., Datta, S., & Vorhees, J. J. (2002). Mechanisms of photoaging and chronological skin aging. *Archives of Dermatology, 138*(11), 1462-1470.

Flemming, K., & Cullum, N. (2003a). Laser therapy for venous leg ulcers. *Cochrane Database of Systematic Reviews, 3*.

Flemming, K., & Cullum, N. (2003b). Therapeutic ultrasound for venous leg ulcers. *Cochrane Database of Systematic Reviews, 3*.

Flemming, K., & Cullum, N. (2003c). Electromagnetic theapy for treating venous leg ulcers. *Cochrane Database of Systematic Reviews, 3*.

Ford, C. N., Reinhard, E. R., Yeh, D., Syrek, D., DeLas Morenas, A., Bergman, S. B., et al. (2002). Interim analysis of a prospective, randomized trial of vacuum-assisted closure versus the healthpoint system in the management of pressure ulcers. *Annals of Plastic Surgery, 49*(1), 55-61.

Franks, P. J., McCullagh, L., & Moffatt, C. J. (2003). Assessing quality of life in patients with chronic leg ulceration using the Medical Outcomes Short Form-36 Questionnaire. *Ostomy Wound Management, 49*(2), 26-37.

Freedman, D. M., Sigurdson, A., Rao, R. S., Hauptmann, M., Alexander, B., Mohan, A., Doody, M. M., & Lundt, M. S. (2003). Risk of melanoma among radiologic technologists in the United States. *International Journal of Cancer, 103*(4), 556-562.

Freeman, A. K., Linowski, G. J., Brady, C., Lind, L., Vanveldhuisen, P., Singer, G., & Lebwohl, M. (2003). Tacrolimus ointment for the treatment of psoriasis on the face and intertriginous areas. *Journal of the American Academy of Dermatology, 48*(4), 564-568.

Gaspari, A. A., & Sauder, D. N. (2003). Immunotherapy of basal cell carcinoma: Evolving approaches. *Dermatologic Surgery, 29*(10), 1027-1034.

Geilen, C. C., & Orfanos, C. E. (2002). Standard and innovative therapy of psoriasis. *Clinical and Experimental Rheumatology, 20*(6 suppl 28), S81-S87.

Geller, A. C., & Annas, G. D. (2003). Epidemiology of melanoma and nonmelanoma skin cancer. *Seminars in Oncology Nursing, 19*(1), 2-11.

Giacomoni, P. U., & Rein, G. (2001). Factors of skin ageing share common mechanisms. *Biogerontology, 2*(4), 219-229.

Gilchrest, B. A. (1982). Pruritus: Pathogenesis, therapy and significance in systemic disease states. *Archives in Internal Medicine, 142*, 101.

Gilchrest, B.A. (1986). The aging skin. *Dermatology Clinics, 4*, 345-531.

Goggins, W. B., & Tsao, H. (2003). A population-based analysis of risk factors for a second primary cutaneous melanoma among melanoma survivors. *Cancer, 97*(3), 639-643.

Gupta, A. K., Bluhm, R., Cooper, E. A., Summerbell, R. C., & Batra, R. (2003). Seborrheic dermatitis. *Dermatologic Clinics, 21*(3), 401-412.

Gushi, A., Kanekura, T., Kanzaki, T., & Eizuru, Y. (2003). Detection and sequences of human papillomavirus DNA in nongenital seborrheic keratosis of immunopotent individuals. *Journal of Dermatological Science, 31*(2), 143-149.

Hari, Y., Frutig-Schnyder, K., Hurni, M., Yawalkar, N., Zanni, M. P., Schnyder, B., et al. (2001). T cell involvement in cutaneous drug eruptions. *Clinical and Experimental Allergy, 31*(9), 1398-1408.

Heckmann, M., Heyer, G., Brunner, B., & Plewig, G. (2002). Botulinum toxin type A injection in the treatment of lichen simplex: An open pilot study. *Journal of the American Academy of Dermatology, 46*(4), 617-619.

Helfand, A. (1983). Foot health for the elderly patient. In W. Reichel (Ed.), *Clinical aspects of aging* (2nd ed.). Baltimore: Williams & Wilkins.

Hellmans, L., Corstjens, H., Neven, A., Declercq, L., & Maes, D. (2003). Antioxidant enzyme activity in human stratum corneum shows seasonal variation with an age-dependent recovery. *Journal of Investigational Dermatology, 120*(3), 434-439.

Hofman, D. (2000, April 5-11). Quick reference guide 15: Management of leg ulcers. *Nursing Standard, 14*(29), insert 2p.

Horn, S. D., Bender, S. A., Bergstrom, N., Cook, A. S., Ferguson, M. L., Rimmasch, H. L., et al. (2002). Description of the National Pressure Ulcer Long-term Care Study. *Journal of the American Geriatrics Society, 50*(11), 1816-1825.

Hornung, R. L., Magee, K. H., Lee, W. J., Hansen, L. A., & Hsieh, Y. C. (2003). Tanning facility use: Are we exceeding Food and Drug Administration limits? *Journal of the American Academy of Dermatology, 49*(4), 655-661.

Housman, T. S., Feldman, S. R., Williford, P. M., Fleischer, A. B. Jr., Goldman, N. D., Acostamadiedo, J. M., & Chen, G. J. (2003). Skin cancer is among the most costly of all cancers to treat for the Medicare population. *Journal of the American Academy of Dermatology, 48*(3), 425-429.

Huether, S. E. (2000). Structure, function, and disorders of the integument. In S. E. Huether & K. L. McCance (Eds.), *Understanding pathophysiology* (2nd ed.). St. Louis: Mosby.

Huether, S. E., & McCance, K. L. (2000). *Understanding pathophysiology* (2nd ed.). St. Louis: Mosby.

Huncharek, M., & Kupelnick, B. (2002). Use of topical sunscreens and the risk of malignant melanoma: A meta-analysis of 9067 patients from 11 case-control studies. *American Journal of Public Health, 93*(1), 1173-1177.

Inman, K. J., Sibbald, W. J., Rutledge, F. S., & Clark, B. J. (1993). Clinical utility and cost-effectiveness of an air suspension bed in the prevention of pressure ulcers. *Journal of the American Medical Association, 269*, 1139-1143.

Izikson, L., Sober, A. J., Mihm, M. C., Jr., & Zembowicz, A. (2002). Prevalence of melanoma clinically resembling seborrheic keratosis: Analysis of 9204 cases. *Archives of Dermatology, 138*(12), 1562-1566.

Jarvis, C. (2000). Physical examination and health assessment (4th ed.). Philadelphia: Saunders.

Javitz, H. S., Ward, M. M., Farber, E., Nail, L., & Vallow, S. G. (2002). The direct cost of care for psoriasis and psoriatic arthritis in the United States. *Journal of the American Academy of Dermatology, 46*(6), 850-860.

Jenkins, G. (2002). Molecular mechanisms of skin ageing. *Mechanisms of Ageing and Development, 123*(7), 801-810.

Jhappan, C., Noonan, F. P., & Merlino, G. (2003). Ultraviolet radiation and cutaneous malignant melanoma. *Oncogene, 22*(20), 3099-3112.

Jol, J. A., van Velthuysen, M. L., Hilgers, F. J., Keus, R. B., Neering, H., & Balm, A. J. (2003). Treatment results of regional metastasis from cutaneous head and neck squamous cell carcinoma. *European Journal of Surgical Oncology, 29*(1), 81-86.

Jones, J. E., & Nelson, E. A. (2003). Skin grafting for venous leg ulcers. *Cochrane Database of Systematic Reviews, 3.*

Jones, P.L., & Millman, A. (1990). Wound healing and the aged patient. Nursing Clinics of North America, 25, 263-277.

Jull, A. B., Waters, J., & Arroll, B. (2003). Pentoxyfylline for treating venous leg ulcers. *Cochrane Database of Systematic Reviews, 3.*

Karagas, M. R., Stannard, V. A., Mott, L. A., Slattery, M. J., Spencer, S. K., & Weinstock, M. A. (2002). Use of tanning devices and risk of basal cell carcinoma and squamous cell skin cancers. Journal of the National Cancer Institute, 94(3), 224-226.

Kligman, A.M., & Balin, A.K. (1989). Aging of human skin. In A. K. Balin, and A. M. Kligman (Eds.), *Aging and the skin.* New York: Raven Press.

Knuutinen, A., Kallioinen, M., Vahakangas, K., & Oikarinen, A. (2002). Smoking and skin: a study of the physical qualities and histology of skin in smokers and non-smokers. *Acta Dermato Venereologica, 82*(1), 36-40.

Kohr, R. (2001). Moist healing versus wet-to-dry. *Canadian Nurse, 97*(1), 17-19.

Kulozik, M., & Krieg, T. (1989). Changes in collagen connective tissue and fibroblasts in aging. *Zeitschrift Hautkrankheiten, 64*(11), 1003-1004, 1007-1009.

Langtry, J. A., Payne, C. M. R., Staughton, R. C., Stewart, J. C., & Horrobin, D. F. (1997). Topical lithium succinate ointment (Efalith) in the treatment of AIDS-related seborrheic dermatitis. *Clinical and Experimental Dermatology, 22*(5), 216-219.

Lapiere, C.M. (1990). The ageing dermis: The main cause for the appearance of "old" skin. *British Journal of Dermatology, 122*(35, suppl), 5-11.

Lebwohl, M. G. (2003). Psoriasis. Lancet, 361(9364), 1197-1204.

Lebwohl, M. G. (2004). *The skin and systemic disease* (2nd ed.). London: Churchill Livingstone.

Lehne, R. A. (2001). *Pharmacology for nursing care* (4th ed.). St. Louis: Mosby.

Lehne, R. A. (2004). *Pharmacology for nursing care* (5th ed.). St. Louis: Mosby

Leone, G., Rolston, K., & Spaulding, G. (2003). Alefacept for chronic plaque psoriasis: A selective therapy with long-lasting disease remissions and an encouraging safety profile. *Dermatology Nursing, 15*(3), 216-220.

Leung, W. C., & Harvey, I. (2002). Is skin ageing in the elderly caused by sun exposure or smoking? *British Journal of Dermatology, 147*(6), 1187-1191.

Lilley, L. L., Aucker, R. S., & Albanese, J. A. (2001). *Pharmacology and the nursing process* (3rd ed.). St. Louis: Mosby.

Lober, C.W., & Fenske, N.A. (1990). Photoaging and the skin: Its clinical differentiation and meaning. *Geriatrics, 45,* 36-42.

Lober, C.W., & Fenske, N.A. (1991). Cutaneous aging: Effect of intrinsic changes on surgical considerations. *Southern Medical Journal, 84*(12), 1444-1446.

Lysy, J., Sistiery-Ittah, M., Israelit, Y., Shmueli, A., Strauss-Liviatan, N., Mindrul, V., et al. (2003). Topical capsaicin—a novel and effective treatment for idiopathic intractable pruritus ani: A randomized, placebo controlled, crossover study. *Gut, 52*(9), 1233-1256.

Ma, W., Wlaschek, M., Hommel, C., Schneider, L. A., & Scharffetter-Kochanek, K. (2002). Psoralen plus UVA (PUVA) induced premature senescence as a model for stress-induced premature senescence. *Experimental Gerontology, 37*(10-11), 1197-1201.

Ma, W., Wlaschek, M., Tantcheva-Poor, I., Schneider, L. A., Naderi, L., Razi-Wolf, Z., Schuller, J., & Scharffetter-Kochanek, K. (2001). Chronological ageing and photoageing of the fibroblasts and the dermal connective tissue. *Clinical and Experimental Dermatology, 26*(7), 592-599.

Macario, A., & Dexter, F. (2002). Is noncontact normothermic wound therapy cost effective for the treatment of stages 3 and 4 pressure ulcers? *Wounds, 14*(3), 93-106.

Mani, R., Vowden, K., & Nelson, E. A. (2003). Intermittent pneumatic compression for treating venous leg ulcers. *Cochrane Database of Systematic Reviews, 3.*

McClure, S. L., Valentine, J., & Gordon, K. B. (2002). Comparative tolerability of systemic treatments for plaque-type psoriasis. *Drug Safety, 25*(13), 913-927.

McGuckin, M., Waterman, R., Brooks, J., Cherry, G., Porten, L., Hurley, S., & Kerstein, M. D. (2002). Validation of venous leg ulcer guidelines in the United States and United Kingdom. *American Journal of Surgery, 183*(2), 132-137.

McKenna, S. P., Cook, S. A., Whalley, D., Doward, L. C., Richards, H. L., Griffiths, C. E., Van Assche, D. (2003). Development of the PSORIQol, a psoriasis-specific measure of quality of life designed for use in clinical practice and trials. *British Journal of Dermatology, 149*(2), 323-331.

McMullin, G. M. (2001). Improving the treatment of leg ulcers. *Medical Journal of Australia, 175*(7), 375-378.

Mehrabi, D., & Brodell, R. T. (2002). Use of the alexandrite laser for treatment of seborrheic dermatitis. *Dermatologic Surgery, 28*(5), 437-439.

Mehrabi, D., DiCarlo, J. B., Soon, S. L., & McCall, C. O. (2002). Advances in the management of psoriasis: Monoclonal antibody therapies. *International Journal of Dermatology, 41*(12), 827-835.

Moore, Z. (2002). Compression bandaging: Are practitioners achieving the ideal sub-bandage pressures? *Journal of Wound Care, 11*(7), 265-268.

Monk, B. E. (2003). Transcutaneous electronic nerve stimulation in the treatment of generalized pruritus. *Clinical and Experimental Dermatology, 18*(1), 67-68.

Najarian, D. J., & Gottlieb, A. B. (2003). Connections between psoriasis and Crohn's disease. *Journal of the American Academy of Dermatology, 48*(6), 805-821.

National Institutes of Health Consensus Development Panel on Early Melanoma. (1992). Diagnosis and treatment of early melanoma. *Journal of the American Medical Association, 268,* 1314-1319.

Nelson, E. A., & Bradley, M. D. (2003). Dressings and topical agents for arterial leg ulcers. *Cochrane Database of Systematic Reviews, 1,* CD001836.

Nickkels, A. F., & Pierard, G. E. (2002). Oral antivirals revisited in the treatment of herpes zoster: What do they accomplish? *American Journal of Clinical Dermatology, 3*(9), 591-598.

Nierodzik, M. L. R., Sutin, D., & Freedman, M. L. (2003). Blood disorders and their management in old age. In R. C. Tallis & H. M. Fillit (Eds.), *Brocklehurst's textbook of geriatric medicine and gerontology* (6th ed.). London: Churchill Livingstone.

Nijsten, T. E., & Stern, R. S. (2003). Oral retinoid use reduces cutaneous squamous cell carcinoma risk in patient with psoriasis treated with psoralen-UVA: A nest cohort study. *Journal of the American Academy of Dermatology, 49*(4), 644-650.

Nilsson, H. J., Psouni, E., & Schouenborg, J. (2003). Long term depression of human nociceptive skin senses induced by thin fibre stimulation. *European Journal of Pain, 7*(3), 225-233.

Norton, D., McLaren, R. S., & Exton-Smith, A. N. [1962]. Pressure sores. In *Investigation of geriatric nursing problems in hospitals.* London: National Corporation for the Care of Old People.

Origoni, M., Garsia, S., & Sideri, M. (1990). Efficacy of topical oxatomide in women with pruritus vulvae. *Drugs Experimental and Clinical Research, 16,* 591-596.

Parker, F. (2000). Skin diseases of general importance. In L. Goldman & J. C. Bennett (Eds.), *Cecil textbook of medicine* (21st ed.). Philadelphia: W. B. Saunders.

Physicians and Scientists, University College London Medical School. (1992). Malignant melanoma. *Lancet, 340,* 948-951.

Pierard-Franchimont, C., & Pierard, G. E. (2002). A double-blind placebo-controlled study of ketoconazole + desonide gel combination in the treatment of facial seborrheic dermatitis. *Dermatology, 204*(4), 344-347.

Pittler, M. H., & Ernst, E. (2003). Horse chestnut seed extract for chronic venous insufficiency. *Cochrane Database of Systematic Reviews, 3.*

Prinz, J. C. (2003). The role of T cells in psoriasis. *Journal of the European Academy of Dermatology and Venereology, 17*(3), 257-270.

Pullen, R., Popp, R., Volkers, P., & Fusgen, I. (2002). Prospective randomized double-blind study of the wound debriding effects of collagenase and fibrinolysin/deoxyribonuclease in pressure ulcers. *Age and Aging, 31*(2), 126-130.

Rahman, P., Bartlett, S., Siannis, F., Pellett, F. J., Peddle, L., Schentag, C. T., et al. (2003). CARD15: A pleiotropic autoimmune gene that confers susceptibility to psoriatic arthritis. *American Journal of Human Genetics, 73*(3), 677-681.

Raja, S. N., Haythornthwaite, J. A., Pappagallo, M., Clark, M. R., Travison, T. G., Sabeen, S., et al. (2003). Opioids versus antidepressants in postherpetic neuralgia: A randomized, placebo-controlled trial. *Neurology, 59*(7), 1015-1021.

Ramirez, M. A., Warthan, M. M., Uchida, T., & Wagner, R. F., Jr. (2003). Double exposure: Natural and artificial ultraviolet radiation exposure in beachgoers. *Southern Medical Journal, 96*(7), 652-655.

Reisner, L. (2003). Antidepressants for chronic neuropathic pain. *Current Pain and Headache Reports, 7*(1), 24-33.

Rhodes, R. S., Heyneman, C. A., Culbertson, V. L., Wilson, S. E., & Phatak, H. M. (2001). Topical phenytoin treatment of stage II decubitus ulcers in the elderly. *Annals of Pharmacotherapy, 35*(6), 675-681.

Roberts, G., Hammad, L., Collins, C., Shearman, C., & Mani, R. (2002). Some effects of sustained compression on ulcerated tissues. *Angiology, 53*(4), 451-456.

Rogers, C. (2003). Lichen simplex chronicus. *Dermatology Nursing, 15*(3), 271.

Santee, J. A. (2002). Corticosteroids for herpes zoster: What do they accomplish? *American Journal of Clinical Dermatology, 3*(8), 517-524.

Schmader, K.E. (1990). New weapons against herpes zoster. *Geriatrics, 45,* 21-23.

Schober-Flores, C. (2001). The sun's damaging effects. *Dermatology Nursing, 13*(4), 279-286.

Sherman, R. A. (2002). Maggot versus conservative debridement therapy for the treatment of pressure ulcers. *Wound Repair and Regeneration, 10*(4), 208-214.

Silverman, S.H., Young, D.J., Allan, A., Ambrose, N. S., & Keighley, M. R. (1989). The fecal microflora in pruritus ani. *Diseases of the Colon and Rectum, 32,* 466-468.

Singh, D., & Kennedy, D. H. (2003). The use of gabapentin for the treatment of postherpetic neuralgia. *Clinical Therapeutics, 25*(3), 852-889.

Smith, S. A., Baker, A. E., & Williams, J. H. (2002). Effective treatment of seborrheic dermatitis using a low dose oral homeopathic medication consisting of potassium bromide, sodium bromide, nickel sulfate, and sodium chloride in a double-blind, placebo-controlled study. *Alternative Medicine Review, 7*(1), 59-67.

Stat bite. (2003). Incidence and mortality from melanoma of the skin, 1975-2000. *Journal of the National Cancer Institute, 95*(13), 933.

Stitt, W. Z. D., & Gilchrest, B. A. (2003). Skin diseases and old age. In R. C. Tallis & H. M. Fillit (Eds.), *Brocklehurst's textbook of geriatric medicine and gerontology* (6th ed.). London: Churchill Livingstone.

Stockfleth, E., & Sterry, W. (2002). New treatment modalities for basal cell carcinoma. *Recent Results in Cancer Research, 160,* 259-268.

Sullivan, J. R., & Shear, N. H. (2002). Drug eruptions and other adverse effects in aged skin. *Clinics in Geriatric Medicine, 18*(1), 21-42.

Unholzer, A., Varigos, G., Nicholls, D., Schinzel, S., Nietsch, K. H., Ulbricht, H., & Korting, H. C. (2002). Ciclopirox olamine cream for treating seborrheic dermatitis: A double blind parallel group comparison. *Infection, 30*(6), 373-376.

Urosevic, M., & Dummer, R. (2002). Immunotherapy for nonmelanoma skin cancer: Does it have a future? *Cancer, 94*(2), 477-485.

U.S. Preventive Services Task Force. (2003). Counseling to prevent skin cancer: Recommendations and rationale of the U.S. Preventive Services Task Force. *Morbidity and Mortality Weekly Report. Recommendations and Reports, 52*(RR-15), 13-17.

Vap, P. W., & Dunaye, T. (2000). Pressure ulcer risk assessment in long-term care nursing. *Journal of Gerontological Nursing, 26*(6), 37-45.

Vardy, D. A., Cohen, A. D., Tchetov, T., Medvedovsky, E., & Biton, A. (1999). A double-blind, placebo-controlled trial of an aloe vera (A. Barbadensis) emulsion in the treatment of seborrheic dermatitis. *Journal of Dermatological Treatment, 10*(1), 7-11.

Veierod, M. B., Weiderpass, E., Thorn, M., Hansson, J., Lund, E., Armstrong, B., & Adami, H. O. (2003). A prospective study of pigmentation, sun exposure, and risk of cutaneous malignant melanoma in women. *Journal of the National Cancer Institute, 95*(20), 1530-1538.

Vigili, A., Bacilieri, S., & Corazza, M. (2003). Evaluation of contact sensitization in vulvar lichen simplex chronicus. A proposal for a battery of selected allergens. *Journal of Reproductive Medicine, 48*(1), 33-36.

Villadsen, L. S., Skov, L., & Baadsgaard, O. (2003). Biological response modifiers and their potential use in the treatment of inflammatory skin diseases. *Experimental Dermatology, 12*(1), 1-10.

Vizcarra, C. (2003). New perspectives and emerging therapies for immune-mediated inflammatory disorders. *Journal of Infusion Nursing, 26*(5), 319-325.

Vranckz, J. J., Slama, J., Preuss, S., Perez, N., Svensjo, T., Visovatti, S., et al. (2002). Wet wound healing. *Plastic and Reconstructive Surgery, 110*(7), 1680-1687.

Ward, K., Kosinski, M. A., & Markinson, B. (2003). In R. C. Tallis & H. M. Fillit (Eds.), *Brocklehurst's textbook of geriatric medicine and gerontology* (6th ed.). London: Churchill Livingstone.

Waterlow, J. (1985). Risk assessment card. *Nursing Times, 81,* 49-55.

Weiss, S. C., Bergstrom, K. G., Weiss, S. A., & Kimball, A. B. (2003). Quality of life considerations in psoriasis treatment. *Dermatology Nursing, 15*(2), 120, 123-127.

Whiteman, D. C., Watt, P., Purdie, D. M., Hughes, M. C., Hayward, N. K., & Green, A. C. (2003). Melanocytic nevi, solar keratoses, and divergent pathways to cutaneous melanoma. *Journal of the National Cancer Institute, 95*(11), 806-812.

Whitney, J. D., Salvadalena, G., Higa, L., & Mich, M. (2001). Treatment of pressure ulcers with noncontact normothermic wound therapy healing and warming effects. *Journal of WOCN, 28*(5), 244-252.

Wilkinson, E. A. J., & Hawke, C. (2003). Oral zinc for arterial and venous leg ulcers. *Cochrane Database of Systematic Reviews, 3.*

Wissing, U. E., Ek, A. C., Wengstrom, Y., Skold, G., & Unosson, M. (2002). Can individualized nutritional support improve healing in therapy-resistant leg ulcers? *Journal of Wound Care, 11*(1), 15-20.

Wolf, R., Orion, E., & Matz, H. (2003, August). The baboon syndrome or intertriginous drug eruption: A report of eleven cases and a second look at its pathomechanism. *Dermatology Online Journal, 9*(3), 2.

Wollina, U., Liebold, K., Schmidt, W. D., Hartmann, M., & Fassler, D. (2002). Biosurgery supports granulation and debridement in chronic wounds—clinical data and remittance spectroscopy measurement. *International Journal of Dermatology, 41*(10), 635-639.

Yosipovitch, G., Sugeng, M. W., Chan, Y. H., Goon, A., Ngim, S., & Goh, C. L.. (2001). The effect of topically applied aspirin on localized circumscribed neurodermatitis. *Journal of the American Academy of Dermatology, 45*(6), 910-913.

Zackheim, H. S. (2002). The FDA guidelines for the treatment of psoriasis using cyclosporine A: Are they adequate? *Cutis, 70*(5), 288-290.

Chapter 11
Musculoskeletal System

Adrianne Dill Linton

Objectives

Describe normal changes in the structure and function of bones, joints, and muscles associated with aging.

Describe measures to maintain musculoskeletal health in the older adult.

Explain the cause and treatment of musculoskeletal disorders that are common in older persons.

Describe the components of the musculoskeletal assessment in the older adult.

Formulate nursing diagnoses for older adults with musculoskeletal disorders.

Develop management plans for older adults with actual or potential musculoskeletal problems.

The musculoskeletal system functions to support and protect internal organs, provide for voluntary movement, and serve as a mineral reservoir. Age-related changes in this system can have a profound effect on the older adult's function and general well-being. Changes in the bones and muscles contribute to the characteristic age-related changes in stature and posture. Musculoskeletal aches and pains are the most common complaints of older adults and require considerable attention from primary health care providers (Calkins & Vladutiu, 1998).

ALTERATIONS IN STRUCTURE AND FUNCTION
Skeleton

Stature and Posture. With advancing years, stature progressively decreases, especially among older women (Figure 11-1). This decrease mainly is attributed to compression of the spinal column, the result of progressive narrowing of the intervertebral discs and loss of height of individual vertebrae. Disc changes begin during midlife, whereas vertebral changes tend to occur in later life. Height diminishes by approximately 1.2 cm

per 20 years, and this tendency toward a smaller stature appears to be universal among all races and sexes. Although aging changes cause shortening of the trunk, the long bones of the extremities remain the same length throughout adult life. Thus the arms and legs may appear longer in relation to the shortened torso.

Other changes that affect the general appearance are a lengthening and broadening of the nose and ears, probably as a result of the continued growth of cartilage into older age. The shoulders become narrower, and the pelvis becomes wider, producing a "pear-shaped" appearance that is enhanced by an increase in the anteroposterior diameter of the chest.

Changes in the distribution of fat and lean body mass with advancing age alter body contours, appearance, and function. Lean body mass decreases primarily because of *sarcopenia* (decreased skeletal muscle mass). Diminished muscle mass is significant in that it is responsible for decreased muscle strength, basal metabolic rate, and activity levels in older adults (Evans, 2003). Body fat mass increases and gradually is redistributed with a loss in the face and extremities and a gain in the abdomen and hips. With the loss of subcutaneous fat, bony landmarks such as the tips of the vertebrae, iliac crests, ribs, scapulae, and bones of the extremities become more prominent. Even in athletes, some loss of lean mass and increase in fat mass occurs. However, physical exercise can reduce the extent of lost muscle mass and improve functional capacity in older adults (Masoro, 2003).

Bone Mass and Metabolism. Skeletal bone provides support, protection, calcium storage, and blood cell production for the body. As with muscle tissue, metabolic processes slow down, and changes in structure occur in bone tissue with older age.

Skeletal bone is made up of three major components: *organic matrix, minerals,* and *cells.* The organic matrix is composed predominantly of collagen fibers that provide the bone's great tensile strength. Deposits

259

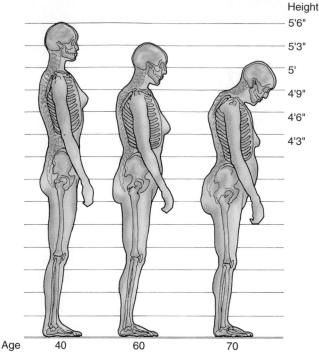

Figure 11-1 Normal spine at age 40 years and osteoporotic changes at ages 60 and 70. These changes can cause a loss of as much as 6 to 9 inches in height. Note the exaggerated thoracic and lumbar curves at age 70 years. (From Ignatavicius, D. D., Workman, M. I., & Michler, M. A. [2006]. *Medical-surgical nursing: A nursing process approach* [5th ed.]. Philadelphia: Saunders.)

of the minerals calcium and phosphate further strengthen the organic matrix. Calcium, phosphorus, alkaline phosphatase, and the proper pH are essential for bone mineralization. The cellular component of bone tissue is made up of *osteoblasts, osteocytes,* and *osteoclasts.* Osteoblasts synthesize bone collagen, which makes up the organic matrix, forming new bone tissue. As the osteoblasts synthesize new bone tissue, they become imbedded in the organic matrix and are then known as osteocytes. Osteoclasts promote bone tissue resorption or destruction. All bones have a compact outer shell called the *cortex.* The cortex surrounds the spongy bone-containing sheets of tissue termed *trabeculae.* Cortical bone is chiefly responsible for providing support, whereas the function of trabecular bone is to provide sites for bone formation and hemopoiesis.

Bone tissue continuously undergoes change, called *remodeling,* even into older age. Various mechanical and hormonal mechanisms, such as physical stress, serum levels of vitamin D, parathyroid hormone, estrogens, androgens, and calcium, stimulate bone formation and resorption. Bone formation and resorption are dynamic processes that occur simultaneously; however, the rate of activity in each process changes with age. From birth to adolescence, bone formation exceeds bone absorption and then equalizes into the mid- to late twenties.

Beginning around age 30, bone absorption begins to exceed bone formation, particularly in trabecular bone. Genetic factors probably govern the onset of bone loss. Other related factors are low body weight, smoking, excess alcohol consumption, and hormonal influences (Francis, 2003).

Although bone loss begins about the same time in both sexes, women experience accelerated loss during the decade after the menopause. The amount of trabecular bone shows a linear decrease beginning in the early thirties and continuing into older age (Figure 11-2). With advancing age, men lose 15% to 45% of trabecular bone whereas women lose 35% to 50%. Because loss of trabecular bone begins earlier than cortical bone loss, the ratio of cortical bone to trabecular bone increases with age. At age 15, the average cortical-trabecular bone ratio is 55 to 45; by age 85, it is 70 to 30.

The areas of the skeleton containing the largest amount of trabecular bone are the vertebral bodies and the ends of long bones, including the wrist and the hip. Because these areas have the highest rate of bone loss with aging, older persons are at risk for sustaining vertebral body compression fractures, Colles' fractures, and femoral neck fractures (Tobias & Sharif, 2003) (Figure 11-3). Cortical bone loss, though less profound, also occurs as a result of an expanded intermedullary cavity and increased haversian canal number and size (Tobias & Sharif, 2003). Cortical loss begins around age 45 in women and age 50 in men, and progresses more rapidly in women. Women lose 25% to 30% of cortical bone mass compared with 5% to 15% in men (Francis, 2003).

Among the factors that may elevate osteoclast activity in older adults are decreased vitamin D intake and reduced exposure to sunlight, which can produce a mild state of hyperparathyroidism. Insufficient intake of

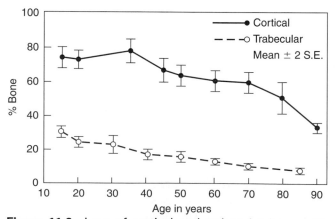

Figure 11-2 Loss of cortical and trabecular bone with age. The relative decrease in cortical and trabecular bone with age in apparently normal persons. Note the relatively rapid loss early in life in trabecular bone and comparatively little loss at this age in cortical bone. The situation is reversed after age 35. (From Jowsey, J. [1977]. *Metabolic diseases of the bone.* Philadelphia: Saunders.)

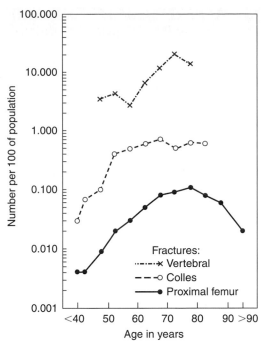

Figure 11-3 Fracture rate in females in relation to age. Vertebral fractures appear early and are more frequent than either Colles' or femoral fractures. (From Jowsey, J. [1977]. *Metabolic diseases of the bone.* Philadelphia: Saunders.)

dietary calcium combined with decreased absorption of calcium in the intestines may further impede bone formation (Tobias & Sharif, 2003). However, a clear correlation between calcium intake and bone mass in postmenopausal women has not been demonstrated (Francis, 2003). Reduced physical activity may contribute to bone loss by removing the mechanical stimulus for osteoblast activity (Tobias & Sharif, 2003).

Because a primary metabolic function of bone tissue is to maintain calcium homeostasis, the roles of parathyroid hormone and calcitonin should be mentioned. Bone tissue provides a storage depot for calcium. When serum calcium falls below normal, parathyroid hormone, which stimulates release of calcium from bone tissue into the blood, is released. When serum calcium is above normal, calcitonin is released from the thyroid to negate the effect of parathyroid hormone and to promote calcium storage in the bone. Parathyroid hormone, along with vitamin D metabolites, also promotes absorption of dietary calcium through the intestinal tract and the reabsorption of calcium in the kidneys.

Musculature

Muscle Mass and Structure of Muscle Fibers. A decrease in lean body mass is related to changes in muscle composition and function. Muscle wasting occurs as a result of a decrease in the number of

muscle fibers. The loss is greatest for type II fibers, which are fast twitch and have a high glycolytic capacity, compared with type I (slow-twitch, fatigue-resistant) fibers, which have greater oxidative capacity. The increased proportion of type I fibers occurs with aging regardless of activity level (Greenlund & Nair, 2003). There may be variation in the extent of fiber loss in specific muscles. For example, Klein, Marsh, Petrella, and Rice (2003), using magnetic resonance imaging (MRI) and muscle biopsy, determined that age was not a factor in the number of muscle fibers in the biceps brachii of young and old men. Box 11-1 lists factors thought to be related to sarcopenia. In addition, significant amounts of lipofuscin (age-related waste material) and fat are deposited within the muscle tissue. The density of capillaries per motor unit diminishes; however, oxygen utilization per unit of muscle tissue remains constant.

Like bone, healthy muscle tissue constantly undergoes remodeling as muscle proteins are synthesized and broken down. Regeneration of muscle tissue slows with age, and atrophied tissue is replaced with fibrous tissue. This change is most noticeable in the muscles of the hands, which become thin and bony, with deep interosseous spaces. The arm and leg muscles also become thin and flabby.

Muscle Function. The age-related changes in muscle affect voluntary and involuntary movement, strength and endurance, and reflexes.

VOLUNTARY MOVEMENT. Movement slows with older age as a result of changes in both the musculoskeletal and the nervous systems. Slower movement is attributed to a decrease in the number of motor nerve units and to prolongation of the contraction time, latency period, and relaxation period of the remaining motor units in the muscle tissue. Impairment of the extrapyramidal nervous system also can cause slow movements and a decrease in spontaneous and associated movements. The ability to stabilize the body with postural changes also may be less efficient.

Joints such as the hips, knees, elbows, wrists, neck, and vertebrae become mildly flexed with older age. The increased flexion is caused by changes in the vertebral column, ankylosis (stiffening) of the ligaments and joints, shrinkage and sclerosis of the tendons and muscles, and degenerative changes in the extrapyramidal system. Limited movement results from increased muscle rigidity, especially in the neck, shoulders, hips, and knees.

INVOLUNTARY MOVEMENT. Examples of involuntary movements associated with aging are *resting tremors* and *muscular fasciculations.* Resting tremors are manifestations of an impaired extrapyramidal system. Involuntary movements may appear in the extremities or head and neck when an older person is sitting quietly. There may be no obvious cause for these tremors, or

---

BOX 11-1 Factors Related to Sarcopenia in the Aging Process

FACTOR	MECHANISM
Reduced protein synthesis	Amount of messenger ribonucleic acid (mRNA) for translation of myosin heavy chain (MHC) is reduced so that mixed muscle protein synthesis declines. Slowed MHC synthesis rate is associated with decreased muscle strength.
Mitochondrial dysfunction	Reduction in the number or activity of mitochondria affects muscle fatigability, endurance capacity, and possibly muscle strength. Because mitochondria generate adenosine triphosphate (ATP), they are vital to the generation of contractile force.
Nutrition	Without adequate intake of protein and calories, negative nitrogen balance occurs with resulting muscle breakdown.
Testosterone	Decline in free testosterone in aging men correlates with decreased lean muscle mass and loss of strength.
Growth hormone (GH) and immunoglobulin F-1 (IGF-1) (GH peripheral mediator)	Circulating level of growth hormone decreases with age; deficiency is known to cause decreased muscle mass and increased adipose mass.
Dehydroepiandrosterone (DHEA)	May affect IGF-1 bioavailability and mass of selected muscles.
Perfusion	Adequate blood flow and oxygenation are essential for muscle endurance, and may be related to muscle protein synthesis and mitochondrial function.
Age-associated neuromuscular changes	Loss of motor neurons, innervation, and muscle stimulation contribute to age-related muscle dysfunction and atrophy.

Data from Greenlund, L. J. S., & Nair, K. S. (2002). Sarcopenia—Consequences, mechanisms, and potential therapies. *Mechanisms of Aging and Development, 124,* 287-299.

---

they may be associated with drug side effects (especially from psychotropic medications) or neurological disorders. Muscular fasciculations are characterized as flickering movements of muscles in the calves, eyelids, hands, and feet. Fatigue and excessive loss of sodium chloride may exacerbate this phenomenon, but loss of muscle strength and function is the primary cause.

Older persons who are inactive or relatively immobile may experience weakness or paresthesia in the legs as a result of decreased movement. In "restless legs," irresistible leg movements occur when trying to get to sleep. Restless leg syndrome has been associated with various neurological disorders, anemia, renal failure, and some drugs (lithium, tricyclic antidepressants). Drugs that sometimes are effective in relieving this condition are levodopa, dopamine agonists, clonazepam, and codeine (Meara, 2003).

STRENGTH AND ENDURANCE. The age-related decrease in muscle strength is directly related to the decrease in muscle mass. This is significant because reduced strength is a major cause of disability in older adults. The decrease in the size or number of muscle fibers, particularly type II muscle fibers, results in a reduction in isometric strength, especially in the proximal lower extremities. A study of arm strength in older women showed that age-related loss of strength contributed to wrist injuries because the elbows buckled when the women tried to brace themselves in a forward fall (De Goede & Ashton-Miller, 2003).

The extent to which the decline in muscle mass affects endurance is a source of disagreement among experts, possibly because of differences in experimental approaches. Some assert that decreased endurance is a normal age-related change. Certainly, decreased muscle mass requires that the older person use a greater percentage of the remaining muscle mass and a higher percentage of the maximal capacity to perform a task of a given intensity than a younger person. Factors that may decrease endurance, in addition to reduced muscle mass, are reduced blood flow, impaired glucose transport, lower mitochondrial density, decreased oxidative enzyme activity, and decreased phosphocreatine repletion rate (Frontera & Larsson, 1999).

REFLEXES. Diminished reflexes usually result from the shrinkage and sclerosis of muscles and tendons rather than from changes in the spinal reflex arc. The extent to which reflexes change with normal aging is difficult to determine because many studies have not excluded conditions such as diabetes and alcoholism. Diminution or absence of tendon jerks, especially in the ankles, has been reported in healthy older adults. In addition, arm, abdominal, and plantar reflex responses tend to decrease. A positive Babinski response has been considered abnormal. However, it has been reported by Assal and Cummings (2002) in 5% to 11.8% of normal older subjects. Much attention has been given to the emergence of primitive reflexes in some older adults. It is important to note that any one of these reflexes, taken in isolation, is neither characteristic nor predictive of dementia. However, the concurrent presence of the snout, suck, and grasp reflexes is more common in dementia and correlates with the severity of cognitive impairment (Assal & Cummings, 2002).

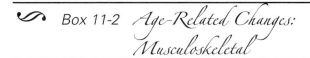

Box 11-2 *Age-Related Changes: Musculoskeletal*

- Skeleton
  - Compression of spinal column
  - Narrower shoulders
  - Wider pelvis

- Body mass
  - Diminished muscle mass
  - Increased body fat mass
  - Body fat redistribution
  - Increased prominence of bony landmarks

- Bone mass and metabolism
  - Bone absorption exceeds bone formation
  - Increased ratio of cortical bone to trabecular bone

- Musculature
  - Muscle wasting
  - Slowed regeneration
  - Atrophic tissue replaced with fibrous tissue
  - Slowed voluntary movement
  - Involuntary movements more common
  - Decreased muscle mass and strength
  - Possible decreased endurance

- Reflexes: diminished

- Joints
  - Mild flexion
  - Deterioration of joint capsule

Joints

Joints, the sites in the body where two or more bones meet, provide motion and flexibility for the human frame. Freely movable joints are made up of bones, synovial membrane, cartilage, synovial cavity, tendons, and ligaments. Examples of freely movable joints are elbows, knees, and wrists. The bones are not in direct contact with each other but are protected by articular cartilage, which forms a cushion between the bony surfaces. The synovial membrane, attached at the margins of the articular cartilage, is pouched or folded to allow for joint movement. The membrane surrounds the synovial cavity and secretes synovial fluid (viscous lubricating fluid) into it. The synovial membrane is surrounded by a fibrous joint capsule, which is strengthened by ligaments extending from bone to bone. Bursae are disc-shaped, fluid-filled synovial sacs that develop at points of friction around the joints. Their purpose is to decrease friction and to promote ease of motion. Slightly movable joints are found between the vertebral bodies. They are separated by fibrocartilaginous discs that contain the nucleus pulposa, a fibrogelatinous material that cushions the movements between the vertebrae.

All of these articulating joint surfaces are subject to changes in structure and function with aging. Breakdown of components of the joint capsule results in inflammation, pain, stiffness, and deformity (Box 11-2).

COMMON DISORDERS OF THE AGING MUSCULOSKELETAL SYSTEM
Metabolic Bone Disease

Osteoporosis. Osteoporosis is so ubiquitous in older age that it generally is considered a normal, age-related phenomenon rather than a disease. It is characterized by a decrease in bone mass per unit volume, producing a porous-looking skeletal frame that fractures easily when stressed.

Senile osteoporosis results from an imbalance in the activity of osteoblasts and osteoclasts. Because more bone is resorbed than is formed, there is a net loss of bone (Mankin & Mankin, 2003; Seeman, 2003) (Figure 11-4).

Bone mass peaks around age 30, is stable for a period, and then begins to decline. Based on the rate, two types of bone loss are recognized. When the activity of both osteoclasts and osteoblasts increases, but bone resorption exceeds bone formation, the individual is said to have *high-turnover osteoporosis* (or *rapid bone loss*). *Low-turnover osteoporosis*, which is more common in older persons, occurs when osteoclast activity is normal but osteoblasts fail to fill the cavities completely (Navas & Lyles, 1998). Low-turnover bone loss affects men and women equally and involves both trabecular and cortical bone. In contrast, rapid bone loss is not

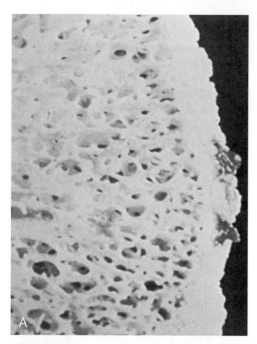

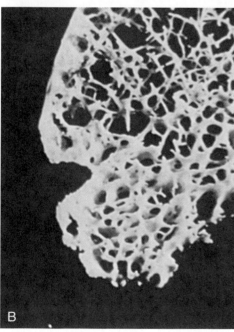

Figure 11-4 Microscopic view of normal and osteoporotic bone. **A,** Normal bone. **B,** Osteoporotic bone. (From Maher, A. B., Salmond, S. W., & Pellino, T. A. [1998]. *Orthopedic nursing* [2nd ed.]. Philadelphia: Saunders.)

universal, occurring in about one third of women and in some men with hypogonadism. Postmenopausal rapid bone loss usually stabilizes after 5 to 8 years (Navas & Lyles, 1998).

ETIOLOGY. The cause of osteoporosis is unknown, but numerous variables have been indicated. The relationship to estrogen deficiency is well documented. (Other contributing factors include genetics,

developmental factors, lifestyle, dietary patterns, low body weight, other pathological states, and drug therapy.

Genetics is believed to account for 60% to 80% of the variance in peak bone mass (Francis, 2003; Navas & Lyles, 1998). Osteoporosis occurs four times more frequently in women than in men, and most often in whites and Northern Europeans. Women also suffer bone loss at a faster rate than men. The difference in incidence among sexes and races is thought to be due to the varying amounts of skeletal bone mass at maturity; men tend to have a denser bone mass than women, and blacks tend to have a denser bone mass than nonblacks. Female whites, Asians, and Eskimos are at greater risk for osteoporosis than African American and Hispanic women (Navas & Lyles, 1998).

Despite the higher incidence of osteoporosis in women, 30% of hip fractures occur in men, and the mortality rate 1 year after injury is nearly twice that of women. Osteoporotic fractures of the hip, vertebral body, and distal wrist generally occur a decade later in men than in women. Risk factors for men, in addition to advancing age, include glucocorticoid use exceeding 6 months, evidence of osteopenia on plain radiographs, history of a nontraumatic fracture, and hypogonadism (Campion & Maricic, 2003).

Developmental factors that appear to play a role in determining the risk of osteoporosis in later years are peak bone mass (Cameron & Demerath, 2002) and birth weight (Antoniades, MacGregor, Andrew, & Spector, 2003). Nutritional factors that affect bone mass are calcium, protein, and vitamin D. Lactose intolerance would seem to a predictor of bone loss associated with decreased calcium intake. However, an Austrian study of bone loss and vertebral fractures in lactose-intolerant individuals did not confirm a relationship between lactose intolerance and accelerated bone loss, although a disproportional number of vertebral fractures occurred in a few individuals with severe lactose intolerance (Kudlacek, Freudenthaler, Weissboeck, Schneider, & Willvonseder, 2002). Several studies have found low-protein diets to be associated with low bone density, possibly because low protein intake induces secondary hyperparathyroidism (Kerstetter, O'Brien, & Insogna, 2003). Protein has both positive and negative effects on calcium balance. Dietary protein provides a substrate for bone matrix and promotes bone formation; however, it also increases the loss of calcium in the urine (Dawson-Hughes, 2003). Changes in bone density are dependent on the net effects of gain and loss. Dawson-Hughes (2003) proposes that bone mass can be increased with protein supplements if supplemental calcium and vitamin D are taken also. One study established a link between vitamin B_{12} deficiency and osteoporosis in frail elderly women, suggesting that this vitamin also may be essential to bone health (Dhonukshe-Rutten et al., 2003). Low body weight also is a risk factor for osteoporosis and for fractures (Cifuentes et al., 2003). Lifestyle contributors include smoking and inadequate physical activity (Geller & Derman, 2001).

Medical conditions that commonly are associated with osteoporosis are Cushing's syndrome, androgen deficiency, Crohn's disease, and rheumatoid arthritis (Von Tirpitz et al., 2003). Adult growth hormone deficiency (Ahmad et al., 2003) and occlusive arterial disease also have been examined in relation to osteoporosis (Laroche et al., 2003). Interestingly, in a Canadian study of over 5000 individuals age 50 and older, no relationship was found between low bone density and vertebral fracture and 12 common medical conditions, including diabetes mellitus, hypertension, rheumatoid arthritis, and inflammatory bowel disease. In this sample, bone mineral density actually was increased in individuals with type 2 diabetes and with hypertension (Hanley et al., 2003). Medical treatments that may contribute to bone mass loss are hemodialysis and drug therapy with corticosteroids. Other drugs under study for possible adverse effects on bone mass are loop diuretics and long-term antipsychotic therapy (Naidoo, Goff, & Klibanski, 2003; Rejnmark et al., 2003).

Riggs and colleagues (1982) identified two syndromes: type I or *postmenopausal* osteoporosis and type II or *senile* osteoporosis. Postmenopausal osteoporosis affects mainly the trabeculae of the vertebral column in a certain group of women during the early postmenopausal period. This condition seems to be associated with compression-type vertebral fractures, distal radial fractures, and, less often, hip fractures. Senile osteoporosis affects both trabecular and cortical bone of the vertebrae and articulating bones of the hip in all aging persons. Bone resorption takes place primarily in the trabeculae rather than in the cortex because remodeling occurs at a higher rate in trabecular bone than in cortical bone. Senile osteoporosis seems to be associated with fractures of the hip, proximal humerus, and tibia, and wedge fractures of the vertebrae (Marek, 2003).

MANIFESTATIONS. Osteoporosis typically is asymptomatic until a fracture occurs. It should always be suspected in an older adult who experiences a low-impact fracture (Simonelli, Chen, Morancey, Lewis, & Abbott, 2003). Major signs and symptoms of osteoporosis due to vertebral fractures are skeletal deformities, pain, and loss of height. Fractures occur when the vertebral bodies become stressed during flexion of the spine and break easily as a result of the loss of the supporting trabecular matrix. Vertebral fractures associated with low bone density typically are wedged anteriorly, compared with posterior involvement, which is more characteristic of malignancy (Sculco, 1998). They usually are associated with sudden movement, lifting,

bending, or falls, and produce acute episodes of sharp pain. The most common sites are the thoracic and upper lumbar regions, which produce radiating pain around the flank and the abdomen. Collapse of the vertebral bodies may also be gradual, accompanied by aching spinal pain or tenderness on percussion and palpation (Navas & Lyles, 1998).

Spinal osteoporosis produces changes in height and posture with advancing years (Figure 11-5). Collapse fractures occurring in the upper thoracic vertebrae may be asymptomatic, but height may diminish by 1 to 1.5 inches. Painful collapse of the vertebrae of the lower spine can reduce height by 2 to 2.5 inches per episode. *Kyphosis* in the upper dorsal spine produces a "hunchback" or "dowager's hump" and, together with downward angulation of the ribs, produces horizontal folds of skin over the chest and abdomen (Navas & Lyles, 1998). Whereas some fractures are asymptomatic or symptoms decrease over time, many result in chronic pain, functional decline, physiological disorders, psychosocial dysfunction, and early death (Truumees, 2003).

Conservative treatment options for vertebral fractures include hormone replacement therapy, calcitonin, bisphosphonates, and activity limitation that may include bracing and bed rest (Kim, Silber, & Albert, 2003). A Korean study reported effective pain relief using nerve-root injections of lidocaine, bupivacaine, and Depo-Medrol (Kim, Yun, & Wang, 2003).

Relatively new surgical options include two minimally invasive procedures: vertebroplasty and kyphoplasty. Vertebroplasty is the percutaneous injection of bone cement into the fractured vertebral body. Kyphoplasty corrects spinal deformity by using an inflatable balloon to expand the fractured vertebral body, removing the balloon, and filling the cavity with cement. Rates of pain relief have been reported at 70% to 92% with vertebroplasty and 90% with kyphoplasty. Most

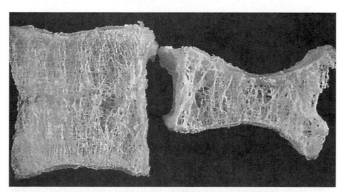

Figure 11-5 Normal versus osteoporotic vertebral body. The vertebra on the left is normal. The one on the right has been shortened by compression fractures. (From Cotran, R. S., Kumar, V., & Collins, T. [1999]. *Robbins pathologic basis of disease* [6th ed.]. Philadelphia: Saunders.)

patients who benefit report immediate relief whereas others report improvement within the first 4 weeks (Tanner, 2003). Less than 10% of patients have short-term complications with vertebroplasty. They include pain and nerve damage caused by epidural cement leakage, transient foreign body reaction (to the cement), rib fractures, and venous thrombosis. A 4-year follow-up after vertebroplasty found an 18% rate of fractures in vertebrae adjacent to treated vertebrae. This may be the result of increased stress transferred to untreated vertebrae by the ones made stiffer by treatment. Although kyphoplasty is newer and therefore the subject of fewer studies, the complication rate has been reported to be between 0.4% and 1.2% (Tanner, 2003).

The extremities also are increasingly susceptible to fracture, especially the hip and the wrist. Overall, for women the lifetime risk of fractures is three times greater than for men (Tobias & Sharif, 2003). About 1 million hip fractures occur each year among women older than 45 years of age. Like vertebral fractures, hip fractures occur as a result of decreased resistance to stress and loss of bone mass. Older women tend to fall more frequently as a result of decreased muscle strength, poor coordination, syncopal episodes, and cardiovascular disease. In addition, reduced bone turnover and poor repair of microfractures contribute to the high incidence of fractures.

Aging increases the mortality risk associated with hip fracture, and the incidence doubles every 5 years after age 50. The excess mortality rate over a 5-year period after hip fracture is 17%; most related deaths occur in the first 6 months after the fracture (Francis, 2003). In some cases, the possibility of femoral neck fracture is overlooked in older persons who have sustained falls because they are sometimes able to walk after the fracture has occurred. The pain associated with the fracture also may go unnoticed if other injuries are associated with the trauma. Increased pain or general decline after the injury may indicate an undiagnosed fractured hip.

DIAGNOSIS. The history and the presence of secondary causes should lead the practitioner to suspect osteoporosis in the older adult. Secondary causes include hyperparathyroidism, hyperthyroidism, acromegaly, Cushing's disease, diminished physical activity, paralysis, alcoholism, nutritional deficiencies (calcium, vitamin D, phosphate), neoplastic disorders, and renal tubular acidosis. Results of blood tests, including calcium, phosphorus, and alkaline phosphatase levels, commonly are normal. Radiographic studies may reveal vertebral compression fractures and a decrease in bone density; however, there must be a 30% to 50% loss of bone mass before bone loss shows up on the radiograph. When a significant loss of bone mass is apparent on the radiograph, the condition is known as osteopenia.

Dual-energy X-ray absorptiometry (DEXA) is the most accurate means of assessing bone mineral density (BMD) of the femur and lumbar spine (Francis, 2003). Newman, Ayoub, Starkey, Diehl, and Wood (2003) in a 5-year study demonstrated the value of routine assessment of BMD and preventive pharmacological treatment of individuals with low bone density. Treatment resulted in a significant decrease in hip fractures. Because the value of BMD studies is to guide treatment decisions, it generally is considered unnecessary in frail older adults with fractures because the results are unlikely to alter management. Similarly, individuals on long-term oral corticosteroid therapy are likely to be treated for osteoporosis regardless of BMD results (Francis, 2003).

MANAGEMENT. Goals for the prevention and treatment of osteoporosis or osteopenia are to inhibit bone resorption and to stimulate bone formation. The National Osteoporosis Foundation has issued practice guidelines with specific recommendations for postmenopausal osteoporosis risk assessment and management (Wei, Jackson, & O'Malley, 2003). Data from the Women's Health Initiative have demonstrated a modest benefit in preserving bone mass (1% in hip bone density) and preventing hip fractures in certain groups. Only the group of women over age 60 and those who took the full daily dose of 1000 mg of calcium carbonate and 400 IU of vitamin D_3 had a statistically significant decrease in hip fractures. The number of fracture in other bones remained the same. Whereas calcium and vitamin D supplements offer modest bone improvement, they provide no benefits for colorectal cancer, (National Institutes of Health [NIH], 2006).

Exercise. Patients are encouraged to exercise by either walking or swimming to slow bone loss. Exercise can reduce fracture risk not only by preventing bone loss but also by decreasing the risk of falling and the force of impact by improving strength, flexibility, balance, and reaction time. The benefits of vigorous exercise on strength, endurance, and bone density in early postmenopausal women with low bone density have been demonstrated (Kemmler, Engelke, Weineck, Hensen, & Kalender, 2003). They also are encouraged to avoid strain on the spine, such as occurs with lifting or bending, to prevent compression fractures of the vertebrae. Smoking is discouraged, as is excessive alcohol intake.

Drug Therapy. Types of drugs that are employed for both the *prevention and treatment* of osteoporosis include calcium salts, vitamin D, estrogen, bisphosphonates, and selective estrogen receptor modulators (SERMs) such as raloxifene (Lehne, 2004). Agents that are used only for *treatment* of established postmenopausal osteoporosis are calcitonin-salmon and teriparatide (human recombinant parathyroid hormone) (Lehne, 2004). Table 11-1 summarizes these agents, their actions, adverse effects, and special considerations.

Estrogen replacement can prevent the loss of bone mass after menopause; however, some women fail to respond to hormone replacement therapy (HRT) at all, and others respond to HRT for a limited period of time after which no benefit is obtained. Morishige and colleagues (2003) reported an increase in bone density after adding alendronate to HRT in a sample of HRT "nonresponders." In another study of over 500 postmenopausal women, Greenspan, Resnick, and Parker (2003) found alendronate superior to HRT in increasing bone mass, and found that alendronate-HRT combination therapy was superior to either agent alone. A decision to use HRT must consider the 2002 findings that it offers fewer benefits and poses greater risks than once thought (Lehne, 2004).

Plant-based phytoestrogens are being studied as possible alternatives to conjugated estrogens in postmenopausal women. However, at this time well-controlled studies on the benefits and risks of alternatives such as black cohosh are limited (Fetrow & Avila, 2001).

Bisphosphonates are antiresorptive agents that inhibit the function of osteoclasts (Rogers et al., 2000). Dosing options include daily and weekly preparations. In a study of 324 women, 86% preferred weekly dosing and believed it would be more compatible with long-term compliance (Simon et al., 2002). A comparison of daily and weekly dosing of alendronate over a 2-year period found equivalent therapeutic effects. However, it is not known if the effects would be equivalent over a longer period of time (Hernandez, Beaupre, Marcus, & Carter, 2002). The most serious adverse effect of the

Table 11-1 *Drug Therapy for the Prevention and Treatment of Postmenopausal Osteoporosis*

Classification	Specific Agents	Action on Bone	Adverse Effects	Considerations
Calcium	Oral calcium salts: acetate, carbonate, citrate, glubionate, gluconate, lactate, and tricalcium phosphate	Essential component of bone structure	Hypercalcemia: nausea, vomiting, constipation, renal dysfunction, lethargy, depression, cardiac dysrhythmias	Recommened daily intake for persons over age 50: 1200 mg/day. Thiazide diuretics increase risk of hypercalcemia. Oxalic and phytic acids in foods such as spinach and whole-grain cereals impair calcium absorption. Calcium citrate is best absorbed, and calcium carbonate has the highest percentage of calcium.
Vitamin D		Increases intestinal absorption of calcium and phosphorus; mobilizes calcium and phosphorus from bone.	Toxicity: nausea, headache, hypercalcemia, hyperphosphatemia, calcification of soft tissues	Recommended daily intake is 400 IU for persons ages 51 to 70 and 600 IU for persons over 70.
Estrogen	Conjugated estrogens Conjugated synthetic A estrogens	Suppresses bone resorption; reduces risk of fractures	Breast tenderness, vaginal bleeding, headache, nausea Increased risk of endometrial and breast cancer, cholecystitis, myocardial infarction, and stroke	Prolonged replacement therapy no longer advised. Most effective if initiated immediately after menopause. Progestin needed with intact uterus. Forms: oral, parenteral, intravaginal, transdermal.

Continued

Table 11-1 _Drug Therapy for the Prevention and Treatment of Postmenopausal Osteoporosis—cont'd_

Classification	Specific Agents	Action on Bone	Adverse Effects	Considerations
Calcitonin-salmon	Calcimar, Miacalcin, Osteocalcin, Salmonine	Decreases bone resorption	Flushing of face and hands Nasal spray: dryness and irritation Parenteral form: nausea	Therapeutic effect requires supplemental calcium and adequate vitamin D. For nasal spray, use alternate nostrils daily. Resistance may develop after a year or more.
Human recombinant parathyroid hormone	teriparatide	Increases bone mineral density; decreases risk of vertebral and nonvertebral fractures	Nausea, headache, back pain, leg cramps, orthostatic hypotension Rare bone cancer in rats	Very expensive (>$7000/year) daily subcutaneous injections. Serum calcium, phosphorus, and uric acid rise initially, then return to normal.
Selective estrogen receptor modulators	raloxifene	Preserve and increase bone density; decrease risk of spinal fractures Reduce LDL cholesterol	Increased risk of venous thrombosis, abortion, fetal harm, hot flushes	Discontinue at least 72 hours before prolonged immobilization
Bisphosphonates	alendronate risedronate	Inhibits bone resorption	Esophagitis Esophageal and gastric ulceration	Compliance may be better with weekly preparations. Instruct patient to take before breakfast, on empty stomach, with full glass of water, and to remain upright afterwards for at least 30 minutes.

_IU,_ International units; _LDL,_ low-density lipoprotein.

bisphosphonates is esophagitis that rarely leads to ulceration. In a study comparing the gastrointestinal effects of risedronate and alendronate after 14 days of therapy, 6% of subjects on risedronate and 12.1% of subjects on alendronate had gastric ulcers confirmed by endoscopy (Thomson et al., 2002). Esophageal inflammation and ulceration result from prolonged exposure of esophageal tissues to the drug. Therefore the patient is instructed to take the bisphosphonate before breakfast on an empty stomach with a full glass of water and to remain in an upright position for at least 30 minutes after taking the drug (Lehne, 2004). The bisphosphonates are contraindicated in patients with esophageal disorders that extend the contact of the drug with the esophagus.

SERMs such as raloxifene exert estrogenic effects on some tissues and antiestrogenic effects on others. Like estrogen, SERMs can preserve or increase bone mineral density, decrease the risk of spinal fractures, reduce serum low-density lipoprotein cholesterol, and increase the risk of venous thrombosis. Unlike estrogens, they do not increase the risk of breast and endometrial cancer. Adverse effects include venous thromboembolism, abortion and fetal harm, and hot flushes. Because of the risk of deep vein thrombosis, raloxifene should be discontinued at least 72 hours before prolonged immobilization (surgery, bed rest, travel) (Lehne, 2004).

Calcitonin-salmon, which reduces bone resorption and inhibits tubular reabsorption of calcium, is indicated for treatment of established osteoporosis. For postmenopausal osteoporosis, either a nasal spray or a parenteral preparation may be used. Calcitonin-salmon usually is safe and well tolerated. In some individuals, antibodies form, rendering the drug ineffective after a year or more of use (Lehne, 2004).

Teriparatide (human recombinant parathyroid hormone) increases bone mineral density and decreases the risk of vertebral and nonvertebral fractures (Marcus, Wang, Satterwhite, & Mitlak, 2003). It currently is the only drug that actually increases bone formation (Lehne, 2004). Adverse effects include nausea, headache, back pain, leg cramps, and orthostatic hypotension. In laboratory studies, a rare form of bone cancer has occurred in rats given teriparatide. Therefore the drug is contraindicated with current or past skeletal cancer and in patients who are at increased risk for bone cancer (Lehne, 2004).

Research continues to develop additional pharmacological agents for the prevention and treatment of postmenopausal osteoporosis. One substance under study is strontium ranelate, which has been shown to decrease bone resorption and promote bone formation (Marie, 2003). Phase 2 dose-ranging studies have confirmed its effectiveness in preventing bone loss in early postmenopausal nonosteoporotic women and postmenopausal osteoporotic women. Phase 3 studies now are underway (Meunier & Reginster, 2003).

CORTICOSTEROID-INDUCED OSTEOPOROSIS.
A special situation is the risk of osteoporosis in individuals taking high-dose corticosteroids. Recommended agents to prevent corticosteroid-induced osteoporosis (CIO) include calcium and vitamin D supplements, postmenopausal hormone replacement, and bisphosphonates (Lafage-Proust, Boudignon, & Thomas, 2003). A study that compared various pharmacological options concluded that alendronate was superior to both vitamin D and calcitriol in reducing bone loss in CIO (Sambrook et al., 2003).

Osteomalacia. Osteomalacia is a softening of the bones with an excessive accumulation of bone matrix (osteoid) resulting from impaired mineralization with calcium and phosphorus (Francis, 2003). Abnormalities that can cause osteomalacia include vitamin D deficiency (most commonly), renal failure, and hypophosphatemia. Causes of vitamin D deficiency in older adults include reduced sunlight exposure, inadequate nutritional intake, poor absorption, and impaired hepatic metabolism.

Vitamin D promotes calcium absorption through the small bowel. Exactly how it enhances the mineralization of bone is unknown (Guyton & Hall, 2000). Vitamin D deficiency delays mineralization, leading to an increase in the amount of osteoid (bone matrix). This phenomenon occurs because mineralization proceeds more slowly than osteoid formation. The result in osteomalacia is an increased amount of *unmineralized matrix.* Figure 11-6 shows the proportions of unmineralized

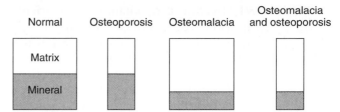

Figure 11-6 Proportions of unmineralized matrix and mineralized bone in the normal bone and bones affected by osteomalacia and osteoporosis. (From Rosse, C., & Clawson, D. [1970]. *Introduction to the musculoskeletal system.* New York: Harper & Row, p. 118.)

matrix and mineralized bone in osteoporosis, osteomalacia, and the two conditions together. Note that the level of mineralized bone in osteoporosis is normal, but it is lower in the other two conditions.

The decreased absorption of ingested calcium that occurs with vitamin D deficiency causes a decrease in serum calcium levels. Lowered serum calcium levels trigger release of parathyroid hormone, which not only causes release of calcium from bone tissue but also promotes reabsorption from the renal tubules. Thus there is a decrease in urinary calcium excretion and an increase in serum calcium. In addition, parathyroid hormone promotes excretion of phosphorus from the kidneys, resulting in a decreased level of phosphorus in the bloodstream. Eventually, parathyroid hormone is unable to keep up with the fall in serum calcium, so calcium levels also drop.

MANIFESTATIONS. Persons with osteomalacia usually experience vague symptoms of pain, tenderness, and weakness. Pain and tenderness occur in skeletal areas, especially the shoulder bones, thorax, hips, thighs, forearms, and feet. Symptoms are aggravated by exercise and active movement. Hip pain may result in an ataxic, waddling gait. Muscle weakness usually occurs proximally and may be mistaken for muscle disorders.

DIAGNOSIS. A diagnosis of osteomalacia is based on histological, serum, and radiographic findings, as well as the health history and physical examination. Histologically, bone tissues show excessive amounts of osteoid and increased bone resorption. Blood studies may reveal hypocalcemia, hypophosphatemia, and increased serum alkaline phosphatase associated with increased bone remodeling (Francis, 2003). Classical radiographic findings (large areas of osteoid) often are absent, especially in the early stage of osteomalacia. Radiographs also may show decreased bone density as a result of osteoporosis, which frequently accompanies osteomalacia. Deformities of the rib cage, pelvis, and long bones caused by softening of bones may be apparent (Francis, 2003).

TREATMENT. Treatment of vitamin D deficiency osteomalacia generally consists of calcium and vitamin D supplements. Foods high in vitamin D such as oily fish and margarine are encouraged. The daily intake of calcium should be increased by 1000 mg. During treatment, patients still are at increased risk for fractures and should take safety precautions. Bone pain gradually diminishes and biochemical and radiological signs eventually return to normal. Alkaline phosphatase typically rises during treatment and may remain elevated for many months. Treatment will not correct existing skeletal deformities (Francis, 2003).

Paget's Disease

Paget's disease, described by Sir James Paget in 1877, is a condition associated with older age in which there is excessive resorption and deposition of bone. The disease is characterized by periods of increased bone resorption, which result in replacement of original bone with fibrous material, alternating with periods of increased bone formation, which result in the appearance of "sclerotic" or osteoblastic lesions. Typically, only a few bones are affected in an individual, most commonly the pelvis, spine, femur, tibia, or skull. The effects usually are not symmetrical. Over time the affected bones become weak, more vascular, and prone to fractures (Francis, 2003). Skeletal deformities may occur. Joints adjacent to affected bones are prone to secondary degenerative arthritis. A complication is osteosarcoma arising in affected bones (Cheng, Wright, Walstad, & Finn, 2002). When the skull is affected, compression of the auditory nerve can lead to deafness. Complications specifically related to spinal involvement include spinal stenosis, compression fractures, and sarcomatous degeneration (Saifuddin & Hassan, 2003).

Approximately 4% of individuals over age 55 are affected with Paget's disease, which most often is diagnosed in the sixth decade of life (Francis, 2003). The cause of the disease is unknown, but there appears to be a genetic influence perhaps triggered by some environmental factor or a slow virus, possibly the measles virus (Bender, 2003; Francis, 2003; Keen, 2003). A Paget's disease registry in New England reported a familial history of Paget's disease in 20% of those enrolled. The registry data have yet to elucidate the role of environmental factors; however, those with a family history of Paget's disease tended to have grandparents born abroad (Seton, Choi, Hansen, Sebaldt, & Cooper, 2003).

MANIFESTATIONS. Although Paget's disease usually is asymptomatic, the most common symptom is bone pain. The pain frequently occurs at rest, under pressure, and during the night, and is relieved by movement. This is unlike arthritis pain, which may occur with movement during the day and is relieved by rest. Disease involving the weight-bearing bones produces the most severe symptoms (Figure 11-7).

DIAGNOSIS. The diagnosis often is an incidental finding on radiological or imaging studies. Radiological findings include enlargement of affected bones,

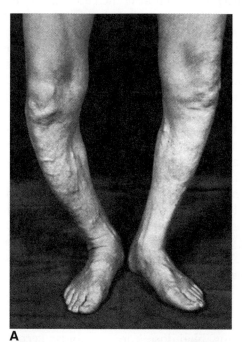

A

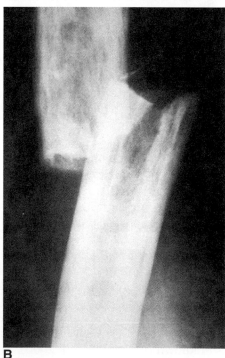

B

Figure 11-7 Manifestations of Paget's disease in the lower extremities. **A,** Severe bowing of the right tibia. **B,** Chalkstick fracture characteristic of Paget's disease. The fracture is transverse with little comminution, similar to a broken piece of chalk. (Courtesy of The Paget Foundation, New York, New York.)

characteristic changes in texture, skeletal deformities, and degeneration of adjacent joints. MRI is useful in assessing complications of Paget's disease, especially sarcomatous degeneration (Whitten & Saifuddin, 2003). Isotope bone scanning is diagnostic and permits determination of the extent of disease (Hain & Fogelman, 2002). Serum calcium and phosphorus levels typically are normal. Increased osteoblast activity is reflected in increased serum phosphatase, and increased osteoclast activity is evidenced by elevated urine deoxypyridinoline/creatinine (Francis, 2003). Serum osteoprotegerin has been found to rise with Paget's disease and to fall in response to tiludronate treatment (Alvarez et al., 2003).

MANAGEMENT. Bisphosphonates have replaced calcitonin as the treatment of choice for Paget's disease (Cremers et al., 2003; Francis, 2003; Keen, 2003). The most effective agents are oral risedronate, intravenous pamidronate, and tiludronate. Clodronate, the only bisphosphonate available in both oral and parenteral preparations, also has demonstrated effectiveness in treating Paget's disease (Ghinoi & Brandi, 2002). Patients who fail to respond to one bisphosphonate may respond to another (Joshua, Epstein, & Major, 2003). Etidronate has been found to cause impaired mineralization when used for more than 6 months. Further, the effectiveness of etidronate decreases over time (Francis, 2003). Bisphosphonate therapy may not reverse hearing impairment incurred with Paget's disease of the skull (Donath, Krasznai, Fornet, Gergely, & Poor, 2004). When selecting a bisphosphonate, the ulcerogenic potential must be considered. Risedronate is believed to be safer than etidronate in this characteristic (Graham, 2002). One advantage of calcitonin over bisphosphonates is that calcitonin has some direct analgesic effect on bone pain (Mehta, Malootian, & Gilligan, 2003).

Muscular Disorders

Polymyalgia Rheumatica and Giant Cell Arteritis. Polymyalgia rheumatica (PMR) and giant cell arteritis (GCA) are two closely related inflammatory disorders that frequently are seen together, usually in people over 50 years of age. PMR is a rheumatic disease characterized by muscular pain and stiffness that lasts a month or more and affects the shoulders, neck, hips, and pelvic girdle (Kennedy-Malone & Enevold, 2001).

GCA is an immune-mediated condition that involves large and medium-sized arteries, especially the extracranial branches of the carotid arteries (Calvo-Romero, 2003; Weyand & Goronzy, 2003). Inflammation causes hyperplasia of the intima leading to occlusion of vessel lumina and tissue ischemia (Weyand & Goronzy, 2003). With GCA, inflammation of the temporal artery results in a unilateral headache, local tenderness, and diminution of the temporal artery pulse. Visual disturbances

and even permanent blindness can result from occlusion of the ophthalmic artery (Scott, 2003). The cause of PMR is unknown; however, genetic and environmental factors are being explored. A suspected relationship with parvovirus B19 has not been supported by immunoglobulin M (IgM) serologies or deoxyribonucleic acid (DNA) studies of biopsied tissue (Helweg-Larsen, Tarp, Obel, & Baslund, 2002; Peris, 2003).

MANIFESTATIONS. The onset of PMR may be abrupt or insidious. Muscle pain (myalgia) begins in the posterior neck muscles and spreads to the muscles of the shoulders and pelvic girdle. Pain may interfere with sleep and is aggravated by exercise. Morning stiffness may last for at least an hour, and resulting weakness can make getting out of bed or a chair difficult (Box 11-3). Synovitis of the knees, wrists, and hands may occur. Tenderness may be reported on palpation of the posterior neck, shoulder, and pelvic musculature, and over the flexor surfaces of the elbows, wrists, and knees. Muscle atrophy and joint deformities are not characteristic, though people with PMR may also have deforming joint disorders concurrently. Accompanying symptoms are low-grade fever, anorexia, weight loss, depression, malaise, and apathy (Scott, 2003).

A throbbing temporal headache is characteristic of GCA, although initial symptoms frequently are the same as those of PMR. The headache usually is unilateral and is accompanied by fever and visual disturbances. When an individual has symptoms of PMR and symptoms of headache, fever, and visual disturbances, suspect GCA. No specific diagnostic test for PMR or GCA exists; however, erythrocyte sedimentation rate (ESR) and C-reactive protein (CRP) usually are elevated in both diseases. The value of assessing cytokines as more specific

---

BOX 11-3 Criteria for Diagnosis of Polymyalgia Rheumatica

- Age greater than 50 years
- Shoulder girdle or pelvic girdle symptoms of pain or stiffness
- Morning stiffness of longer than 1 hour's duration
- Duration of symptoms of at least 4 weeks if untreated
- No actual muscle weakness found on objective examination
- No evidence of intrinsic muscle disease, infection, or other collagen-vascular disease
- Elevated erythrocyte sedimentation rate
- Relief of symptoms within several days of initiating low-dose corticosteroid therapy

Adapted from Goodwin, J. S. (1992). Progress in gerontology: Polymyalgia rheumatica and temporal arteritis. *Journal of the American Geriatrics Society, 40,* 516.

markers is under study (Weyand & Goronzy, 2003). A biopsy of the temporal arteries is advised when clinical symptoms of GCA are present (Scott, 2003; Weyand & Goronzy, 2003). The presence of a dark halo on ultrasonography has been used as a diagnostic indicator; however, its value is debated (Salvarani et al, 2002; Schmidt & Gromnica-Ihle, 2002).

MANAGEMENT. Both PMR and GCA are treated with oral corticosteroids; GCA requires a higher daily dose than PMR (Hunder, 2000; Scott, 2003). Dosage increases may be required to bring about relief of symptoms. Corticosteroids produce such a dramatic clinical improvement that this is thought to be diagnostic of the disease. If a good clinical response is obtained, the drug dosage eventually is tapered off. In one study of persons with both PMR and GCA, 95% required corticosteroid therapy for longer than 2 years (Myklebust & Gran, 2001). In addition to corticosteroids, some patients require nonsteroidal antiinflammatory drugs (NSAIDs) or disease-modifying drugs (Scott, 2003). Leeb and colleagues (2003) propose the following response criteria for treatment of PMR: ESR or CRP, pain, physician's global assessment, morning stiffness, and elevation of upper limbs. Frearson, Cassidy, and Newton (2003) caution that guidelines for management of PMR and GCA have been developed from studies that excluded older people. Studies are lacking to guide the management of these conditions in older adults. Pharmacological doses of corticosteroids can have serious adverse effects on anyone, but older adults may be especially vulnerable because of altered pharmacokinetics, comorbidity, and polypharmacy. Management of common conditions such as diabetes, hypertension, and gastroesophageal reflux disease may be complicated by corticosteroid side effects (e.g., hyperglycemia, fluid retention, and decreased gastric mucus).

Muscle Cramps. Older adults frequently experience muscle cramps after unusual exercise. The cramps occur at night after a day's activity and are characterized by sustained, involuntary, and painful contractions of muscle groups of the calf, foot, thigh, hand, or hip. They result primarily from peripheral vascular insufficiency but may also be related to sodium deprivation or loss, low serum calcium, toxins, hypoglycemia, or peripheral nerve disease. The pain may be relieved by passive stretch and often can be prevented by soaking in a hot bath at bedtime (Grob, 1989).

Joint Diseases

Osteoarthritis. Osteoarthritis, also known as degenerative joint disease (DJD), is a noninflammatory disorder of movable joints. It clearly is associated with age as the prevalence is less than 1% before age 30,

about 30% by age 64, and about 68% in those over age 65 (Schnitzer, 2000; Scott, 2003). Factors that contribute to the development of osteoarthritis include the effects on the joint of mechanical stress, trauma, and infectious, inflammatory, endocrine, or metabolic disease (Scott, 2003). Cartilage deterioration that occurs with aging generally is a result of accumulated trauma. Major areas affected are the weight-bearing joints (knees, hips, lumbar spine), the cervical spine, and the terminal interphalangeal joints of the hands. Among individuals age 70 and older who were enrolled in the Framingham study, 13% of men and 26% of women reported symptoms of hand osteoarthritis (Arthritis Foundation, 2003b). Osteoarthritis rarely is found in the wrists, elbows, ankles, or feet except after trauma. Joint involvement is unilateral in more than half of all cases. The typical course of the disease is slow and progressive, without exacerbations or remissions. An exception is rapidly progressing osteoarthritis, a subgroup that can progress to complete joint destruction in only 1 to 2 years (Scott, 2003).

Osteoarthritis affects all joint structures, not cartilage alone (Brandt, 2004; Felson, 2004). It is characterized by fibrillation and loss of articular cartilage, bone exposure, and a clinical syndrome of pain and disability (Scott, 2003). Most sources agree that the disease process begins when cartilage loses its elasticity and then becomes soft and frayed. Loss of water from the cartilage may cause narrowing of the joint spaces. Continuous abrasion results in a progressive loss of cartilaginous surface, leaving the underlying (subchondral) bone exposed. Ulceration of the cartilage and exposure of subchondral bone promote new bone formation and thickening of the cortical bone. *Osteophytes*, or bony spurs, form at the joint margins, and *subchondral cysts* frequently develop. Small pieces of cartilage may break off, resulting in loose bodies in the joint. The synovial membrane may become fibrous, hypertrophic, or inflamed as a result of changes in the cartilage, bony spurs, or loose bodies. Figure 11-8 shows pathological changes in osteoarthritis.

An alternative explanation of the pathophysiology of osteoarthritis is that the triggering event is abnormal bone cell metabolism that causes enhanced bone remodeling. According to this hypothesis, cartilage damage follows the bone changes. Attempts by the body to repair the cartilage produce additional biochemical changes that subsequently cause further sclerosis and damage (Lajeunesse, 2004).

MANIFESTATIONS. Classic manifestations of osteoarthritis include pain, stiffness, and joint hypertrophy. Pain usually is aggravated by joint motion or weight bearing. Transient episodes of stiffness, especially after periods of inactivity, are common. Palpation may reveal tenderness and swelling around affected joints.

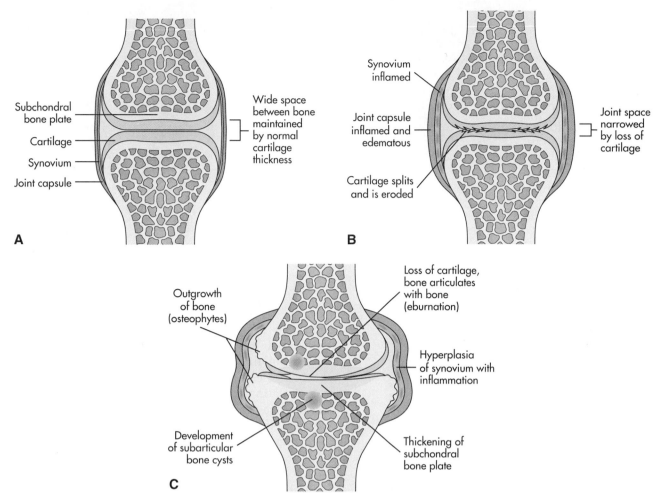

Figure 11-8 Pathological changes in osteoarthritis. **A,** Normal synovial joint. **B,** Early osteoarthritis with destruction of articular cartilage and narrowing of joint space. The joint capsule and synovium are inflamed and thickened. **C,** Advanced osteoarthritis with thickened subarticular bones caused by friction of bone surfaces and osteophytes around the periphery. (Modified from Lewis, S. M., Heitkemper, M. M., & Dirksen, S. R. [2004]. *Medical-surgical nursing: Assessment and management of clinical problems* [6th ed.]. St. Louis: Mosby.)

Crepitation, a dry, crackling, grating sound or sensation, is a characteristic associated with movement of an affected joint. There may be some limitation of movement as a result of pain, muscle spasm, muscle contracture, malalignment of joints, or osteophyte formation. Abnormal posture and gait can produce muscle pain and soreness.

Other characteristic signs of osteoarthritis, especially in older women, are *Heberden's nodes*, which are bony protuberances located at the distal interphalangeal joints. Early nodes are soft and cystlike, developing into bony enlargements with angular deformities in which the joints become flexed or displaced laterally (Figure 11-9). Generally, the nodes are painless, but they may produce local aching, redness, tenderness, clumsiness, and a tight feeling over the area. An inherited trait found chiefly in women, Heberden's nodes sometimes are associated with trauma.

The knee is one of the joints most frequently affected by osteoarthritis, particularly in women. Because it makes ambulation painful, it is a major cause of disability. Another potentially disabling site for DJD is the hip joint. Compared with other sites, risk factors for osteoarthritis of the hip are more likely to include congenital and developmental abnormalities. Degenerative hip disease produces pain on motion or weight bearing that radiates to the groin and anterior thigh or knee. It sometimes is difficult to determine whether hip pain is caused by osteoarthritis of the hip or the lumbar spine (Schnitzer, 2000). Hip range of motion, especially internal rotation, is limited with osteoarthritis. Progressively declining range of motion with subsequent functional decline often necessitates surgery.

Degenerative disease of the spine, known as *spondylosis*, often is observed on radiographic studies of middle-aged and older persons (Figure 11-10). The cervical and

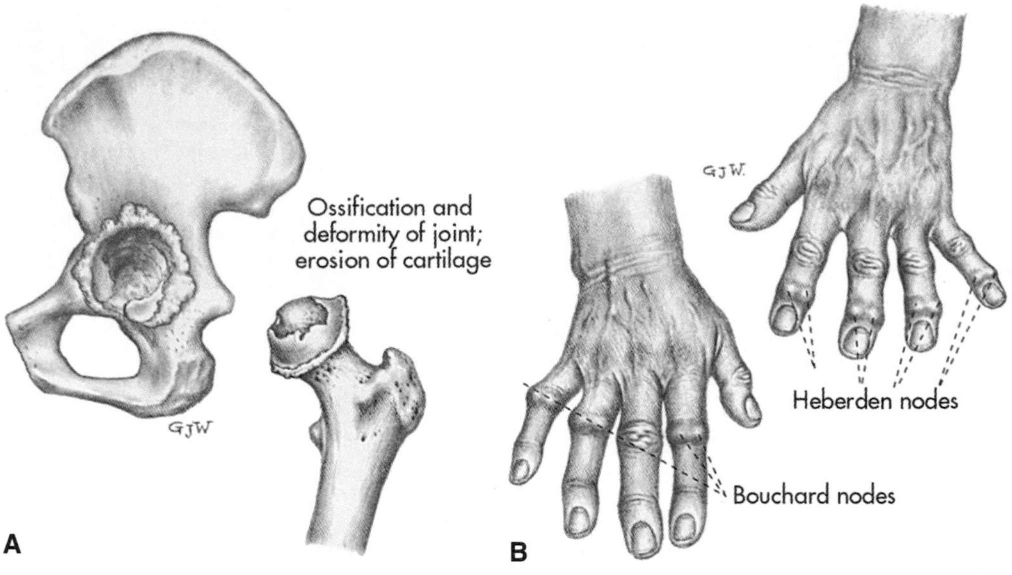

Figure 11-9 Osteoarthritis. **A,** Cartilage and bone changes in the hip. **B,** Heberden's nodes and Bouchard's nodes. (From Huether, S., & McCance, K. (2004). Understanding pathophysiology [3rd ed.]. St. Louis: Mosby.)

Ossification and deformity of joint; erosion of cartilage

Heberden nodes

Bouchard nodes

A

B

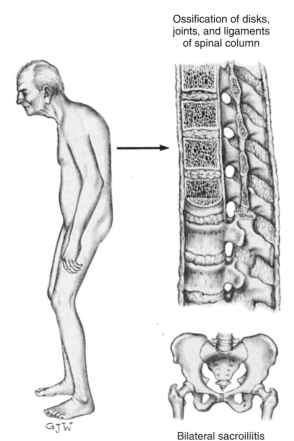

Ossification of disks, joints, and ligaments of spinal column

Bilateral sacroiliitis

Figure 11-10 Ankylosing spondylosis. Characteristic posture. Affected verbebrae are square, and the spine has lost the normal thoracic and lumbar curvatures. (From J. M. Thompson, G. K. McFarland, J. E. Hirsch, & S. M. Tucker [Eds.] [2002]. *Mosby's clinical nursing* [5th ed.]. St. Louis: Mosby.)

lumbar regions of the spine are most frequently involved, producing symptoms such as backache, stiffness, and limitation of motion. Degeneration of the vertebrae affects primarily the intervertebral discs and the articulating edges of adjacent vertebral bodies. Degeneration of the discs increases the stress on the vertebral bodies, producing osteophyte formation and narrowing of the intervertebral foramina. Osteophyte formation and protrusion of the discs cause compression of the nerve roots or spinal cord in the cervical or lumbar spines in severe cases (Schnitzer, 2000).

In the cervical spine, the greatest stress is placed on C4 to C6 vertebrae. Because the nerve roots are close to the articulating joints, they are vulnerable to irritation or compression. Persons may experience pain in the shoulders, arms, hands, head, neck, and chest, which is aggravated by active or passive spinal movement, especially rotation and lateral bending. The pain often is accompanied by muscle spasm. Burning sensations or numbness may occur, accompanied by muscle wasting and weakness, decreased tendon reflexes, and occasional fasciculations.

Cervical spondylosis can produce signs of cerebral ischemia, particularly on extension, rotation, or flexion of the neck. This movement causes blockage of the vertebral arteries, which enter at C6 and pass upward through the canal in the transverse processes. The person may exhibit transient episodes of giddiness, syncope, or drop attacks, which are characterized by sudden falling without loss of consciousness. Older persons with this problem should be encouraged to avoid sudden movement of the head and neck to prevent cerebral ischemic events.

Vertebral degeneration of the lumbar spine occurs at L5 to S1 in 90% of cases. Prolapse or protrusion of the lumbar intervertebral discs accounts for most low back pain in older persons. The pain is preceded by either an injury from lifting or bending or chronic, intermittent low back pain. Other signs and symptoms include pain in the legs and feet, decreased sensation in the legs and feet, decreased or absent patellar reflex, and weak knee and toe extension. Back pain may respond to a properly fitted brace used in conjunction with muscle strengthening exercises (Schnitzer, 2000).

DIAGNOSIS. Diagnostic tests generally are not definitive in diagnosing osteoarthritis. Results of laboratory studies usually are normal. Plain radiographs may demonstrate narrowing of the joint space and the presence of osteophytes at the joint margins. However, the degree of degenerative disease seen on radiography is a poor indicator of the degree of symptoms manifested in older persons (Scott, 2003). Some older persons with radiographic evidence of degeneration experience mild symptoms or none at all. A limitation of radiography is the inability to assess cartilage damage. MRI has greater potential sensitivity to detect changes in cartilage (Schnitzer, 2000).

MANAGEMENT. Treatment of osteoarthritis varies according to the joints affected, severity of symptoms, and degree of joint deformity. Currently, treatment is aimed toward symptomatic relief of pain and prevention of further damage. Therapeutic measures include physical therapy, exercise programs, rest, reduced joint load, diet therapy, drug therapy, and surgery.

Physical Therapy and Exercise Programs. Although rest is useful for the relief of stress on affected joints, a mild exercise program, particularly isometric exercise or walking, helps to maintain muscle strength and joint motion and to prevent muscle atrophy. With mild osteoarthritis, exercise to strengthen muscle groups around affected joints is advised. Older adults with moderate osteoarthritis may be reluctant to participate in exercise programs, but they should be encouraged to do so. Some may find aquatic exercise more comfortable. With advanced disease, weight-bearing exercises are not recommended (Loeser, 2003). Other physical measures that may relieve symptoms are heat and cold applications and transcutaneous nerve stimulation. Recent systematic reviews concluded that ice massage improved range of motion, function, and knee strength, and that cold packs reduced swelling. Additional well-designed studies are needed to determine the value of heat therapy and ultrasound (Brosseau et al., 2003; Welch et al., 2004).

Rest and Reduced Joint Load. The use of rest as a therapeutic measure for osteoarthritis is chiefly associated with relief of stress on the affected joints. Work forces and weight bearing should be minimized, and normal joint alignment and motion should be maintained. When there is hip or knee involvement, a sensible modification of strenuous activities is appropriate. The use of a cane or crutch can reduce the force of weight bearing by as much as 50%. Although periods of rest are recommended, too much rest can lead to stiffness and muscle atrophy. Poor body mechanics associated with faulty work habits can be corrected with proper teaching. Supportive, cushioned shoes help with balance and absorb shock on hard surfaces. Persons with vertebral involvement should avoid hyperflexion and hyperextension.

Diet Therapy. Obesity is an identified risk factor for osteoarthritis of the knee, and there is evidence that weight loss in obese persons can greatly decrease the risk of developing symptomatic osteoarthritis. Further, weight loss of as little as 10 lb can reduce painful symptoms of knee osteoarthritis in obese older adults (Henderson, 2004). Therefore it is appropriate to advise obese older adults that weight reduction can reduce both risk and symptoms of osteoarthritis of the knees. Based on a review of the evidence, Henderson (2004) concluded that glucosamine may be beneficial with osteoarthritis whereas support is lacking for boswellia serrata, ginger, s-adenosylmethionine (SAM-e), and unsaponifiable part of avocado and soybean (ASU). McAlindon's (2001) meta-analysis further supports the use of glucosamine and chondroitin for modest efficacy. McAlindon notes the possibility that these products may have disease-modifying effects in osteoarthritis. Some recent studies have shown glucosamine with chondroitin to be more effective for severe pain than for mild pain.

Drug Therapy. A combination of nonpharmacological and pharmacological measures is recommended for management of osteoarthritis. The goal of drug therapy is pain relief because only symptomatic treatments are available. The most commonly used drugs are over-the-counter analgesics such as NSAIDs and acetaminophen. Many patients experience similar degrees of pain relief with NSAIDs or acetaminophen.

NONSTEROIDAL ANTIINFLAMMATORY DRUGS. NSAIDs are classified as salicylates (aspirin), propionic acid derivatives (ibuprofen, naproxen), and the cyclooxygenase-2 (COX-2) inhibitors. All NSAIDs reduce pain and suppress inflammation by inhibiting cyclooxygenase, the enzyme that is responsible for the synthesis of chemical mediators of inflammation, including prostaglandins (Lehne, 2004). COX-1 is the form of the enzyme that is widely distributed in body tissues. Among the functions of COX-1 are the synthesis of prostaglandins that protect the gastric mucosa and the synthesis of thromboxane (TXA), which stimulates platelet aggregation. COX-2 is produced mainly at the site of tissue injury where it mediates inflammation and enhances pain sensitivity. Nonselective COX inhibitors suppress pain and inflammation, but also inhibit protective gastric mechanisms and interfere with blood coagulation.

It is especially important to observe older patients for toxic effects of these drugs, which include nausea and vomiting, epigastric distress, upper gastrointestinal bleeding, rash, edema, anemia, leukopenia, nephrotoxicity, hypertension, and thrombocytopenia. Because of high-frequency hearing impairment, older adults may be unaware of tinnitus associated with salicylate toxicity; therefore you should monitor for other signs or symptoms that indicate toxicity, including dizziness, hearing loss without tinnitus, drowsiness or feelings of excitement, and hyperpnea. In fewer than 1% of subjects in controlled trials, ibuprofen produced mental confusion, depression, or insomnia (Mosby, 2004). The nurse must be aware of these drug side effects when an acute confusional state or depression occurs in an older person with osteoarthritis.

The COX-2 inhibitors spare COX-1 so they relieve pain and inflammation with less effect on the gastric mucosa and on platelet activity (Lehne, 2004). Although many people tolerate NSAIDs well, the possibility of gastrointestinal, cardiovascular, hepatic, and renal adverse effects must be considered with older adults. The newer COX-2 inhibitors, especially rofecoxib, have been well received because they have fewer gastrointestinal adverse effects but, like other NSAIDs, cause retention of sodium and water. This is a concern for patients with hypertension, heart failure, and edema. There is no evidence that selective COX inhibitors are more effective than their nonselective counterparts (Brandt, 2004). Although COX-2 inhibitors have been widely used, they are being reevaluated because of evidence that linked rofecoxib with an increased risk of myocardial infarction. When NSAIDs fail to relieve symptoms, the occasional addition of acetaminophen may be helpful (Loeser, 2003).

ACETAMINOPHEN. Acetaminophen is the most frequently ingested drug in the United States. Its analgesic and antipyretic properties are similar to aspirin, but it lacks antiinflammatory activity, possibly because it inhibits prostaglandins only in the central nervous system. Therefore it does not pose a threat to the gastric mucosa or to platelet function. The most serious adverse effect of acetaminophen is liver toxicity. Recent studies have found that bleeding may occur in patients who take warfarin and four or more acetaminophen tablets daily. It is conjectured that acetaminophen inhibits the metabolism of warfarin, causing the blood level to rise beyond the therapeutic level (Lehne, 2004).

TRAMADOL HYDROCHLORIDE. Moderate to moderately severe pain associated with osteoarthritis that is not managed well with NSAIDs or acetaminophen may respond to tramadol, a centrally acting mu-opioid agonist that prevents the uptake of neurotransmitters. Adverse effects of tramadol include sedation, headache, and constipation. This drug is not classified as a controlled substance because the risk of abuse is very low

(Lehne, 2004; Mosby, 2004). A randomized, placebo-controlled trial demonstrated that osteoarthritis pain could be safely and more effectively treated with tramadol/acetaminophen (Ultracet) along with COX-2 inhibitors than with either drug alone (Emkey, Rosenthal, Wu, Jordan, & Kamin, 2004).

CORTICOSTEROIDS. Systemic corticosteroid therapy is not recommended for osteoarthritis. Some short-term benefit (1 to 6 weeks) can be achieved with intraarticular injections. Best results have been reported with less severe radiographic findings, the presence of effusion, and the successful aspiration of fluid at the time of injection. (Wise, 2003-2004). A single joint should not be injected more than three to four times in a year because the drug may potentiate cartilage deterioration (Schnitzer, 2000).

INTRAARTICULAR HYALURONAN. When injected into the knee, hyaluronan temporarily increases the viscosity of the synovial fluid, and may produce improvement over several months (Schnitzer, 2000). The injections are expensive and have been described as "only moderately beneficial" (Brandt, 2004, p. 118).

Joint Lavage. Tidal irrigation of the knee and arthroscopic debridement and lavage have been used commonly over the past decade, and anecdotally are reported to bring pain relief for some patients. However, the work of Moseley and colleagues (2002) has cast doubt on the value of such procedures. In a widely publicized randomized controlled study, the researchers treated 180 patients with either irrigation/lavage or a sham procedure. The results showed that debridement was no more effective than placebo in relieving symptoms or producing measurable functional outcomes.

Surgery. When pain is persistent and disabling despite physical and pharmacological interventions, and severe structural damage is evident radiographically, surgery is probably the best option (Loeser, 2003). Severe restriction of joint movement or severe pain in the hip and knees can be relieved by total joint replacement (arthroplasty), often called the "happy operation" because of its high success rate in the relief of pain and immobility. This type of surgery has typically been reserved for adults older than 60 years because they are less likely to wear out or damage implants. Total joint replacement surgery has more than a 95% success rate in older adults. Although revision may be possible, the outcomes often are less satisfactory. Improved prostheses have made older age less important because there now is an 80% chance that a prosthesis will last at least 20 years (Branson & Goldstein, 2003). Some evidence exists that delaying surgery until the older adult has serious functional disability results in poorer outcomes (Arthritis Foundation, 2003a).

Under ideal circumstances, surgery is planned so that the patient can be prepared mentally and physically. Specific preoperative and postoperative exercises may be taught, although effects of various perioperative exercise programs have had conflicting results (Crowe & Henderson, 2003; Jesudason & Stiller, 2002; Wang, Gilbey, & Ackland, 2002). Medication and nutritional supplements that affect blood coagulation usually are discontinued at least 14 days before surgery. The patient may be instructed to scrub the operative site with chlorhexidine daily for the week preceding surgery. Decisions must be made about blood replacement in the event it is necessary. Oral iron supplements or epoetin may be ordered preoperatively to boost hemoglobin. Intravenous antibiotics usually are administered within an hour of the beginning of the surgical procedure.

Priorities during the immediate postoperative period include pain control, hydration, prevention of infection, and maintenance of proper joint alignment. For example, with a hip replacement, the hip must be maintained in a position of abduction to prevent dislocation. With procedures on the hips and knees, deep vein thrombosis (DVT) is the most common serious complication (Hanna, 2002). Strategies to reduce the risk of DVT include antiembolism stockings, pneumatic compression devices, and warfarin therapy adjusted to maintain an international normalized ratio (INR) of 1.8 to 2.5. The risk of DVT after hip replacement is greatest between the seventh and fourteenth postoperative days (Branson & Goldstein, 2003). Because older persons have a tendency to develop postoperative urinary tract infections, use of urethral catheters should be minimized or avoided if possible. Sterile technique should be used when changing wound dressings. Prevention of infection is critical because it almost always requires removal of the prosthesis (Hanna, 2002). Loosening of the prosthesis is another complication that varies with the type of prosthesis and the method of securing it into the bone.

The progression of activity varies with the specific procedure. To illustrate, after hip replacement, the patient is advanced from sitting in a chair to ambulating with a walker with weight bearing as specified by the surgeon. Patients may be discharged as early as the third postoperative day. Depending on the patient's condition and the amount of assistance available, the older adult may go home or to an extended care or rehabilitation facility. Physical and occupational therapy help the patient regain function and avoid complications after joint replacement (Branson & Goldstein, 2003). A recent development in hip and knee replacement is the use of a much smaller incision—a procedure referred to as "minimally invasive." Some facilities perform this procedure on an outpatient basis. Evaluation of these new approaches is pending. Alternatives to total knee replacement for some patients are unicompartmental knee arthroplasty, in which either the medial or the lateral compartment is replaced, and implantation of the unispacer knee, which allows for smooth articulation of the femur and the tibia (Hanna, 2002). Total joint replacements for the treatment of arthritis in the shoulders, hands, ankles, and feet are used less frequently. Preoperative and postoperative measures and considerations are similar to those associated with total knee and hip replacements.

Individuals who are not candidates for arthroplasty or those who reject that option may benefit from water exercise and strengthening activities with minimal joint impact (Loeser, 2003).

Education of the Older Adult with Osteoarthritis. The value of education in the management of symptoms of osteoarthritis cannot be underestimated. Ultimately, it is the older adult who must carry out measures to protect and strengthen joints, to reduce discomfort, and to make adaptations in daily living. Good patient education is a combination of providing knowledge, developing skills, and motivating the individual (Brandt, 2004). Group osteoarthritis management programs have been especially helpful in enabling patients to gain confidence in their ability to live fully with this condition.

Future Directions in Osteoarthritis Management. Products that are being studied for potential benefits in osteoarthritis include glucosamine and chondroitin, and topical capsaicin. Licofelone, which is currently being tested in Europe, inhibits COX-1, COX-2, and LOX (5-lipoxygenase), and is anticipated to be as effective as celecoxib without causing fluid retention (Alvaro-Gracia, 2004). Other drug development is focusing on disease-modifying antirheumatic drugs (DMARDs) that will prevent or arrest joint damage, or restore damaged cartilage (Brandt, 2004; Schnitzer, 2000). Gene therapy offers several treatment approaches. For example, local gene transfer to synovium and cartilage may provide a way to enhance synthesis of cartilage or inhibit its breakdown (Evans, 2004; Evans, Gouze, Gouze, Robbins, & Ghivizzani, 2004). Another approach being explored is the transplantation of cultured chondrocytes (Morehead & Sack, 2003).

Table 11-2 lists the points in differential diagnosis of rheumatoid arthritis and osteoarthritis.

Rheumatoid Arthritis. Rheumatoid arthritis (RA) is a chronic, systemic, progressive disease of unknown origin. The onset of the disease can occur at any age, but it usually begins after age 35 in women and after age 45 in men (Scott, 2003). Women are affected two to three times more frequently than men.

Although the cause is unknown, the factors under study are host genetic factors, immunoregulatory abnormalities and autoimmunity, and microbial infection (Arnett, 2000). The pathogenesis of RA begins when lymphocytes stimulate the release of cytokines that cause chronic inflammation of the synovium

Table 11-2 *Points in Differential Diagnosis of Rheumatoid Arthritis and Osteoarthritis*

	Rheumatoid Arthritis	Osteoarthritis
Joints most commonly involved	Proximal interphalangeal Metacarpophalangeal Metatarsophalangeal Knees, hips, wrists, etc. Spine may be involved.	Distal interphalangeal Carpometacarpal of thumb Knee, hip Cervical and lumbar spine
Duration of morning stiffness	1 hr to all day	10-30 minutes
Time when pain is most severe	Morning	Evening
Constitutional symptoms	Present	Absent
Tenderness and thickening of synovium	Characteristically present May be severe	May be present May be severe in localized areas (point tenderness)
Synovial fluid	Increased cells Decreased viscosity	Few cells Viscosity normal
X-ray (early changes)	Synovium thickened Erosions at joint margin Subchondral osteoporosis	Cartilage loss Subchondral condensation Osteophytes Cysts

Adapted from Calkins, E., Ford, A. B., & Katz, J. R. (1992). Practice of geriatrics (2nd ed.). Philadelphia: Saunders, p. 383.

(Anderson, 2004). The synovium thickens and adheres to the adjacent margins of the articular cartilage. The thickened synovium, called *pannus,* is composed of fibrous tissue containing chronic inflammatory cells. The pannus penetrates the underlying cartilage and underlying bone, forming scar tissue that immobilizes the joint (Figure 11-11).

MANIFESTATIONS. The onset of RA usually is insidious, although some people have a dramatic sudden occurrence of symptoms. In either case, the manifestations of synovitis are joint swelling, tenderness, and stiffness. Notably, morning stiffness can persist for more than an hour after awakening. Over time, the articular cartilage, fibrous joint capsule, and surrounding ligaments and tendons become inflamed, eventually causing joint deformity and loss of function (Huether & McCance, 2000). Small peripheral joints usually are affected symmetrically. The hands typically are affected first, followed by the feet. Other joints that may be affected are the wrists, knees, ankles, elbows, neck, and shoulders. Unlike osteoarthritis, RA usually affects proximal (metacarpophalangeal) rather than distal (distal interphalangeal) joints in the hands and feet (Scott, 2003).

Extraarticular (systemic) involvement in RA is related to the formation of rheumatoid nodules that can invade the skin, the heart valves and pericardium, the pleura and lung parenchyma, and the spleen. Nodules are cores of fibrinoid and cellular debris surrounded by clumps of inflammatory cells that most often occur over extensor surfaces of the hands and wrists (Huether & McCance, 2000). Involvement of small and medium-sized blood vessels is termed *rheumatoid vasculitis.* Resulting thrombosis can cause myocardial infarction, cerebrovascular occlusion, mesenteric infarction, kidney damage, and vascular insufficiency of the hands and fingers known as Raynaud's phenomenon. Because vasculitis is most common in people taking steroids, it is possible that these drugs play some contributing role (Huether & McCance, 2000). Among the manifestations of systemic involvement are peripheral neuropathy, leg ulcers, anemia, enlarged spleen, leukopenia, xerostomia, pleuritis, and pericarditis. Though not common, complications can include right-sided heart failure, cardiac conduction abnormalities, valvular stenosis or incompetence, respiratory insufficiency, and necrotizing bronchiolitis. Dryness of the eyes can lead to scleral inflammation and corneal damage. Pleural involvement usually is asymptomatic (Arnett, 2000). Nonspecific manifestations include malaise, weight loss, and intermittent fever (Scott, 2003).

Pain on movement may be relieved by rest early in the disease, but later pain may occur spontaneously,

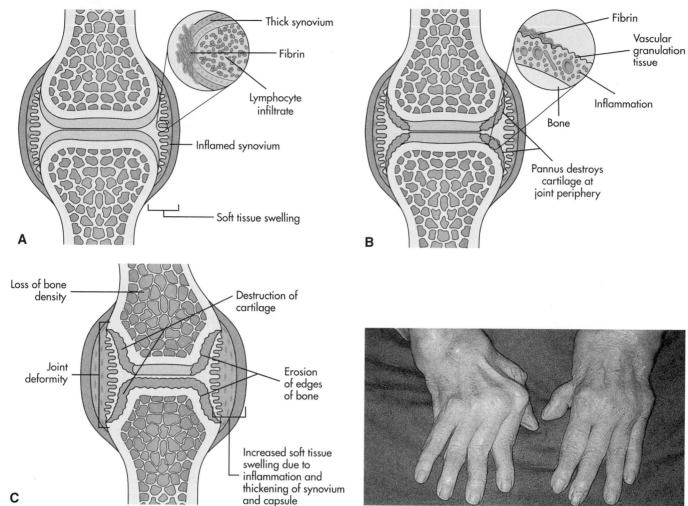

A

Thick synovium

Fibrin

Lymphocyte infiltrate

Inflamed synovium

Soft tissue swelling

B

Fibrin

Vascular granulation tissue

Inflammation

Bone

Pannus destroys cartilage at joint periphery

C

Loss of bone density

Destruction of cartilage

Joint deformity

Erosion of edges of bone

Increased soft tissue swelling due to inflammation and thickening of synovium and capsule

Figure 11-11 Stages in progression of rheumatoid arthritis. **A,** Early pathological change: inflamed synovium, increased lymphocytes. **B,** Progressive changes: articular cartilage destruction, vascular granulation tissue (pannus) grows across the cartilage surface. **C,** Bone destruction and joint deformity. **D,** Characteristic deformity and soft tissue swelling associated with longstanding rheumatoid disease of the hands. (Modified from Lewis, S. M., Heitkemper, M. M., & Dirksen, S. R. [2004]. *Medical-surgical nursing: Assessment and management of clinical problems* [6th ed.]. St. Louis: Mosby.)

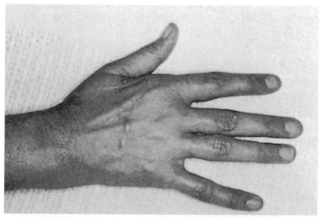

Figure 11-12 Early rheumatoid arthritis spindling of the fingers. (From Kelley, W. N., Harris, E. D., Ruddy, S., & Sledge, C. B. [1985]. *Textbook of rheumatology* [2nd ed.]. Philadelphia: Saunders, p. 934.)

even at rest. Synovitis and synovial effusion produce swelling, warmth, tenderness, edema, and a "boggy" feeling around the joints. A phenomenon called "spindle fingers" results from swelling of the interphalangeal joints (Figure 11-12). Limited motion is due to synovial effusions, muscle spasms, and contractures. Dominance of flexor muscles causes flexion contractures, and fibrosis of the joint capsule, ligaments, and tendons produces joint deformities of the knees, hips, elbows, and toes. Ulnar deviation of the metacarpophalangeal joints, swan neck deformity, boutonnière (buttonhole) deformity, and flexion deformities of the knee are most common. In older persons, pain or limitation of movement in the shoulders is more common than in younger people (Figure 11-13).

The course of the disease usually is marked by remissions and exacerbations in a downhill, stepwise progression.

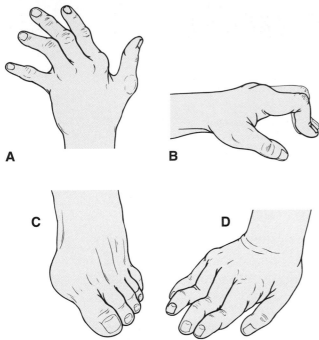

Figure 11-13 Typical deformities of rheumatoid arthritis. **A,** Ulnar drift. **B,** Boutonnière deformity. **C,** Hallus valgus. **D,** Swan neck deformity. (From Lewis, S. M., Heitkemper, M. M., & Dirksen, S. R. [2004]. *Medical-surgical nursing: Assessment and management of clinical problems* [6th ed.]. St. Louis: Mosby.)

DIAGNOSIS. In addition to the standard history and physical examination, assessment data are obtained from the functional examination, laboratory studies, and imaging procedures. Laboratory tests of significance measure rheumatoid factor, ESR, and CRP. Findings associated with a poor prognosis are increased rheumatoid factor in early RA and high ESR or CRP levels. Plain radiographic studies are sufficient for diagnostic purposes, but MRI, bone scans with isotopes, and DEXA scans provide more detailed information that may be useful in monitoring disease progression and response to therapy. Aspirated synovial fluid is inflamed with a poor mucin clot test and an increased white blood cell count with 50% to 70% polymorphonuclear leukocytes (Arnett, 2000; Scott, 2003). The importance of an early, accurate diagnosis is supported by evidence that irreversible damage occurs in the first 1 to 2 years. More aggressive early treatment, especially with disease-modifying agents, is believed to improve outcomes (Arnett, 2000; El-Miedany, 2002; Palferman, 2003; Williams & Fye, 2003). Points in differentiating rheumatic and osteoarthritis are listed in Table 11-2.

MANAGEMENT. Any treatment plan of the person with rheumatoid arthritis should include patient and family education and psychological support. The goals of therapy for RA are maintenance or restoration of joint function, management of pain, reduction of inflammation, and management of generalized symptoms

such as fatigue. For most patients, these goals can be achieved initially with rest, antiinflammatory therapy, and measures to maintain joint function (Arnett, 2000). Interventions include rest, physical therapy, drug therapy, occupational therapy, and surgery.

Rest. The term *rest* commonly appears in care plans for people with RA, but exactly what that implies is not defined. Arnett (2000) suggests that an afternoon rest period helps reduce midafternoon fatigue. Although it is important to avoid immobilization in the elderly, rest is imperative during flare-ups to enhance the action of antiinflammatory medications and to prevent further damage to the joint. Bed rest decreases systemic inflammation and may be necessary during acute episodes. With bed rest, range-of-motion exercises are needed to maintain function.

Splinting is used to rest specific joints. A review of research on the use of splints and orthotic devices with RA concluded the following: (1) there is insufficient evidence that wrist splints decrease pain or increase function, (2) resting hand and wrist splints did not seem to affect pain or range of motion, (3) patients preferred wearing a resting hand or wrist splint to not wearing one, and (4) extra-depth shoes with molded insoles decreased pain during weight-bearing activities (Egan et al., 2003). Li-Tsang, Hung, and Mak (2002) compared the effect of dynamic and static splints used to correct flexion contractures in rheumatoid fingers. Both devices produced significant improvements in finger contractures, grip strength, and hand function. Overall results were similar; however, patients with dynamic splints had better flexion. Another small study compared static, hinged, and spiral wrist splints with no splint. The results showed decreased grip strength with hinged splints and improved pinch and dexterity with the spiral splint (Burtner et al., 2003).

Physical Therapy/Exercise. It once was thought that exercise was harmful to arthritic joints. Indeed, overexertion increases inflammation in joints affected by RA (Arnett, 2000). However, various forms of exercise are now known to be safe and beneficial (Stenstrom & Minor, 2003). Community-based occupational therapy education and functional training programs for older adults have been shown to improve occupational performance and quality of life in people with RA (Wilkins, Jung, Wishart, Edwards, & Norton, 2003). A randomized controlled multicenter trial compared the effectiveness and safety of a 2-year intensive exercise program for persons with RA with usual physical therapy. Subjects in the intensive program showed greater improvement in functional ability. Neither group had significant increases in radiographic damage to the large joints. However, individuals who had more serious joint damage at baseline showed slightly more progression in damage (de Jong et al., 2003). In another study the long-term benefits of exercise were assessed. RA patients who participated in a 2-year home-based strength training

Table 11-3 *Drugs Used To Treat Rheumatoid Arthritis*

Classification	Action	Specific Agents	Major Adverse Effects
NONSTEROIDAL ANTIINFLAMMATORY DRUGS (NSAIDs)			
First generation (nonselective)	Inhibit synthesis of prostaglandins	Salicylates (aspirin) Ibuprofen (Motrin) Naproxen (Naprosyn)	All nonselective NSAIDs can cause gastric irritation and renal damage and impair coagulation
Second generation (COX-2 inhibitors)	Inhibit synthesis of prostaglandins	Celecoxib (Celebrex) Rofecoxib (Vioxx) Valdecoxib (Bextra)	Fatigue, anxiety, depression, tachycardia, GI disturbances, dry mouth, GI bleeding (less than first generation), blood dyscrasias, nephrotoxicity
Corticosteroids	Suppress migration of polymorpho-nuclear leukocytes and fibroblasts; stabilize lyosomes	Prednisone Prednisolone	Systemic therapy: osteoporosis, hyperglycemia, poor resistance to infection, metabolic disturbances Intraarticular injection: may damage cartilage if used more than 2 to 4 times/year
DISEASE-MODIFYING ANTIRHEUMATIC DRUGS (DMARDs)			
Antimalarials	Action in relation to RA is unknown	Hydroxychloroquine (Plaquenil)	Retinal lesions, blood dyscrasias, GI disturbances
Antineoplastic-antimetabolite	Most rapid-acting DMARD	Methotrexate	Liver toxicity, oral and gastrointestinal ulcers, bone marrow suppression, pneumonitis
Pyrimidine antagonist	Inhibits activated T-lymphocytes	Leflunomide (Arava)	GI disturbances, headache, elevated liver function tests (LFTs)
Antibiotics		Sulfasalazine	Headache, GI disturbance, skin rash, pruritus
Immunosup-pressants	Inhibit purine synthesis in cells	Azathroprine (Imuran)	Pancreatitis, hepatotoxicity, blood dyscrasias, decreased resistance to infection.
	Inhibit synthesis of amino acids in protein	Cyclophosphamide (Cytoxin)	Blood dyscrasias, GI disturbances, hepatotoxicity, genitourinary (GU) disorders, pulmonary fibrosis, syndrome of inappropriate antidiuretic hormone (SIADH), alopecia, hemorrhagic cystitis, decreased risk for infection
	Inhibit T-lymphocytes	Cyclosporine	GI disturbances, oral candida, renal and liver toxicity, infection
Gold salts	Action in relation to RA unknown; may suppress lysozymes	Auranofin	Pruritic skin rash, oral ulcers, bone marrow suppression, renal damage
Chelator	Inhibits biosynthesis of DNA, RNA, and protein	Penicillamine (Cuprimine)	Bone marrow suppression, renal damage, other autoimmune disease
Biologic response modifiers (BRMs) (TNF inhibitors)	Inhibit tumor necrosis factor (TNF)	Etanercept (Enbrel) Infliximab (Remicade) Adalimumab (Humira)	All BRMs: serious infections, injection site reactions, malignancies (particularly lymphoma) Rare: seizures and demyelinating disease, blood dyscrasias, autoimmunity
Interleukin-1 receptor antagonist	Blocks the proinflam-matory cytokine involved in synovial inflammation and joint destruction	Anakinra (Kineret)	Injection site reactions, increased risk of serious infections, neutropenia

Data from Anderson, D. L. (2004). TNF inhibitors: A new age in rheumatoid arthritis treatment. *American Journal of Nursing, 104*(2), 60-68; Arnett, F. C. (2000). Rheumatoid arthritis. In L. Goldman & J. C. Bennett (Eds.), *Cecil textbook of medicine* (21st ed.). Philadelphia: Saunders, pp. 1492-1499; Lehne, R. A. (2004). *Pharmacology for nursing care* (5th ed.). Philadelphia: Saunders; and Skidmore-Roth, L. (2004). *Mosby's nursing drug reference*. St. Louis: Mosby.

program significantly improved the strength of assessed muscle groups and maintained the improvement over a 3-year follow-up period (Hakkinen, Sokka, & Hannonen, 2004).

An evidence-based review by Stenstrom and Minor (2003) concluded that the goal for intensity level of exercise in RA should be moderate to hard (60% to 85% of maximum heart rate) in three sessions of 30 to 60 minutes weekly with the intensity progressively adjusted. Recommended activities were walking, cycling, aerobic class, and aquatics. The same review concluded that the goal for the load level of strengthening exercises in RA should be moderate to hard (50% to 80% of maximum voluntary contraction) performed two to three times per week, static or dynamic, and either against body weight or equipment. Again, progressive load adjustment was recommended. Arnett (2000) points out that appropriate exercise can be facilitated by preceding the activity with heat treatments.

Drug Therapy. Drug treatment for rheumatoid arthritis is aimed toward suppression of inflammation and relief of pain. Because older adults metabolize drugs differently and because they typically have chronic health problems, they are at greater risk for drug side effects, interactions, and toxicities. The drugs most frequently used to treat RA include first- and second-generation NSAIDs, corticosteroids, and DMARDs (Table 11-3). First-generation NSAIDs (aspirin, ibuprofen, etc.) are inexpensive and tolerated well by most people, although they can cause gastric and duodenal ulcers and bleeding. A review of studies conducted to assess the effectiveness of interventions to prevent NSAID-induced upper gastrointestinal toxicity concluded that misoprostol, proton pump inhibitors, and double-dose H-2 receptor blockers effectively prevented ulcers with NSAID therapy (Rostom et al., 2004). Second-generation NSAIDs are less likely to cause serious bleeding, but are more expensive. Systemic corticosteroids are not recommended for long-term use because of the many serious adverse effects. However, intraarticular injections may be done two to four times a year for symptomatic relief. The earliest DMARDs such as gold salts, penicillamine, and azathioprine were first used only after NSAIDs failed. A major problem with these drugs is that they are slow acting. Methotrexate was the first DMARD with relatively rapid onset of action. Despite this advantage, it often has to be discontinued because of its toxic adverse effects (Anderson, 2004). Drug manufacturers continue to work on developing DMARDs in the hope that a drug will be found that will stop or reverse the deterioration of joints in RA. The newest DMARDs are tumor necrosis factor (TNF) inhibitors and interleukin-1 receptor antagonists. The TNF inhibitors can cost thousands of dollars per year, and as of 2003, infliximab was the only TNF covered by Medicare (Anderson, 2004). It must be emphasized that TNF inhibitors can have serious adverse effects, especially infections (Anderson, 2004). Combination therapy is common, especially with newer DMARDs and methotrexate. Table 11-3 summarizes drugs used to treat rheumatoid arthritis.

The variety of drugs available poses a dilemma for the practitioner. Because of the importance of early treatment of RA, a referral to a rheumatologist is recommended. Many clinicians are using a "step-down" approach beginning with aggressive combination DMARD therapy once a diagnosis is made. The number of drugs or drug dosage is reduced when there is radiographic evidence that joint damage is no longer progressing. The most toxic drugs usually are tapered off first (Anderson, 2004). A review of 25 randomized controlled trials from 1966 to 2000 identified nine drugs that were superior to placebo in increasing radiographic scores of joint bone erosion: cyclosporine, infliximab, sulfasalazine, leflunomide, methotrexate, parenteral gold, corticosteroids, auranofin, and an interleukin-1 receptor antagonist (Anonymous, 2003). Another review (Anonymous, 2002) looked at the outcomes when a DMARD was added to methotrexate for RA patients who had an incomplete response to methotrexate alone. The conclusion was that the addition of a DMARD, compared to addition of placebo, produced an improvement of 20% or more in swollen and tender joint counts in two to three times as many patients.

Occupational Therapy. The occupational therapist (OT) teaches people with RA how to perform more easily everyday activities that have become more challenging because of pain or mobility limitations. A major focus for the rheumatology OT is joint protection (Hammond, Jeffreson, Jones, Gallagher, & Jones, 2002). The OT is an excellent resource for assistive devices.

Surgery. Among the surgical options for RA are synovectomy, tenosynovectomy, tendon transfer or repair, and removal of bony spurs. Synovectomy may be recommended if synovitis does not respond to medical treatment in 6 months. Although it is controversial, synovectomy does bring about pain relief in the absence of serious cartilage and bone destruction. The patient with significant tissue destruction is a candidate for arthrodesis (fusion) or arthroplasty (joint replacement). With the wrist, fusion relieves pain but can interfere with activities of daily living (ADLs) if bilateral (Eisler et al., 2003). Hip and knee arthroplasty provide excellent results, and elbow and shoulder replacements are improving (Arnett, 2000). Ankle arthroplasty has improved greatly and now has "excellent results in experienced hands" (Eisler et al., 2003, p. 922). For hand deformities, a combination of fusion, silicone arthroplasty, and rebalancing of tendons and ligaments can be done (Eisler et al., 2003).

Complementary and Alternative Therapies. Balneotherapy (spa therapy) is commonly believed to be helpful; however, scientific evidence of benefit is contradictory at this time. Usichenko, Ivashkivsky, and Gizhko (2003) reported improvement in pain intensity, joint stiffness, and laboratory parameters with electromagnetic millimeter waves applied to acupuncture points. However, a review of studies on acupuncture and electroacupuncture did not find well-designed studies with adequate samples on which to base a recommendation for these therapies. Likewise, the use of transcutaneous electrical nerve stimulation (TENS) has demonstrated conflicting results (Brosseau et al, 2003). For most complementary and alternative therapies, well-designed studies with adequate samples are needed to determine their value (Verhagen et al., 2003). The use of chondroitin is discussed under osteoarthritis.

Treatment Advances. Research is exploring many avenues to improve treatment options for RA (Arthritis Foundation, n.d.). Among the current biological approaches under study are the following:

- Inhibition of cytokines, specifically TNF and interleukin-1 (IL-1), IL-6, and IL-8 with biological response modifiers
- Blocking of blood vessel growth with antiangiogenics
- Inhibition of destructive enzymes in the joints
- Prevention of bone erosion
- Manipulation of the very early stages of the immune process
- Explanation of genetic and environmental triggers
- Management of pain and depression to improve quality of life
- Transfer of local genes to synovium; now in phase I studies (Evans, 2004)

Other studies are focusing on psychosocial factors such as reducing psychological stress, reducing work disability, and promoting physical activity.

Gouty Arthritis. Gout is a syndrome or collection of metabolic disorders in which uric acid crystallizes in body fluids and is deposited in tissues. Increased serum uric acid results from either increased formation or decreased excretion of uric acid. When the concentration of uric acid exceeds a threshold, crystals form that are deposited in connective tissue. The effects of these crystals in the synovium, subcutaneous tissue, and the kidneys account for the clinical manifestations of gout. Uric acid precipitates in synovial fluid producing acutely painful joint inflammation referred to as gouty arthritis. Repeated acute episodes result in damage to joints and other structures. When crystals are deposited in subcutaneous tissue, small white nodules called tophi are visible through the skin. In the kidneys, crystals can form calculi that obstruct tubules and lead to kidney damage (Huether & McCance, 2000).

The chief risk factor for gout is hyperuricemia (elevated serum urate level), which most often results from a hereditary defect in purine metabolism. Other risk factors that have been associated with gout include male gender, obesity, and alcohol consumption. Also, hyperuricemia has been linked with cardiovascular disease, hyperlipidemia, and glucose intolerance (Wortmann, 2002). When hyperuricemia is due principally to an inherited metabolic abnormality, the condition is called *primary gout.* When it is secondary to acquired conditions such as polycythemia vera, leukemia, multiple myeloma, chronic renal insufficiency, or lead poisoning, or to treatment with diuretics or salicylates, it is known as *secondary gout* (Kamienski, 2003). Whereas the onset of gout in men usually is between ages 40 and 50, the onset in women usually is later. Between ages 60 and 80, men and women are equally affected, but after age 80, most newly diagnosed cases of gout are in women (Arnett, 2003; Kim, Schumacher, Hunsche, Wertheimer, & Kong, 2003; Rott & Agudelo, 2003).

MANIFESTATIONS. An acute attack of gouty arthritis most often affects the great toe. The initial attack almost always is confined to a single joint. Acute gout also may appear in other joints such as the feet and ankles, knees, wrists, and hands. The affected joint becomes reddened, tender, swollen, and hot. Individuals may have a sensation of discomfort that develops into excruciating pain over a period of hours. Larger joints, such as the knee, may have accumulations of inflammatory effusion. Acute symptoms may resolve in a day or two, or may persist for more than a week. Each acute episode is followed by an interval during which there is freedom from symptoms. Some people have only one or two attacks during their lifetime, whereas others have repeated occurrences of increasing duration, severity, and frequency, with multiple joints becoming involved. The presentation in older adults is not always typical. Compared with younger people, multiple joints more often are affected, acute attacks are less frequent, and the incidence of tophi is increased (Kim et al., 2003).

Precipitating factors for acute attacks, though not always present, include stress, trauma, alcohol consumption, infection, surgery, and the ingestion of certain drugs (e.g., thiazide and loop diuretics, low-dose salicylates, cyclosporine, niacin, ethambutol, pyrazinamide, and didanosine) (Rott & Agudelo, 2003).

DIAGNOSIS. Gout is suspected on the basis of the history and physical examination. The serum uric acid level will be elevated; however, hyperuricemia can be present for reasons other than gout. Therefore the identification of uric acid crystals in aspirated synovial fluid is a more accurate diagnostic measure (Kamienski, 2003).

MANAGEMENT. Treatment options for an acute attack include NSAIDs, colchicine, corticosteroids, and corticotropin (adrenocorticotropic hormone [ACTH]). In the United States, NSAIDs have replaced colchicine as the initial drug of choice (Kim et al., 2003). For persons who cannot tolerate nonselective NSAIDs, the newer selective COX-2 inhibitors are an option (Rubin et al., 2004; van Doornum & Ryan, 2000). Colchicine, though effective, has a narrow margin of safety and potentially fatal adverse effects. The Food and Drug Administration Office of Drug Safety reported 20 deaths associated with toxicity when colchicine was administered intravenously. Causes of death were blood dyscrasias, acute renal failure, and disseminated intravascular coagulation (Bonnel, Villalba, Karwoski, & Beitz, 2002). Oral prednisone generally is reserved for persons who cannot tolerate NSAIDs or colchicine or who have multiple joint involvement. The intraarticular route may be effective when only a few joints are affected. ACTH has been used for decades to treat acute gout, but it is generally used only when first-line drugs are contraindicated or have failed (Kim et al., 2003). Nonpharmacological measures during the acute phase include rest with no weight bearing on affected joints, increased fluid intake, and abstinence from alcohol (Kamienski, 2003).

Allopurinol is the treatment of choice to prevent further episodes of acute gout; however, it should not be started during an acute flare-up, because it could make the episode worse (Arnett, 2003). Tapering the NSAID or colchicine as the allopurinol is increased reduces the risk of triggering an acute attack (Lehne, 2004). When prescribing for older adults, it is especially important to start at the low end of the dosage range and carefully titrate the dose. An Australian audit of allopurinol prescriptions for people over age 65 found that 47% were receiving more than the recommended dose and 40% were receiving less (Smith, Karlson, & Nair, 2000). An alternative to allopurinol is a uricosuric (probenecid, sulfinpyrazone). Whereas allopurinol is effective in persons who overproduce or underexcrete urate, uricosurics are effective only for underexcretors with good renal function (Kim et al., 2003). Tophi sometimes become infected or ulcerated, requiring surgical treatment. A study of 45 patients in New Zealand who had surgery for tophaceous gout revealed a complication rate of 53%, most commonly delayed wound healing. The authors attributed the high incidence of complications to poor gout control and comorbidities (Kumar & Gow, 2002).

In addition to drug therapy, the patient should be encouraged to lose weight if obese and to maintain a high fluid intake. General dietary guidelines advise avoidance of foods high in purines (liver, kidney, sweetbreads). Based on Cochrane reviews, Schlesinger and Schumacher (2001) recommend a diet low in carbohydrates and high in protein and unsaturated fats. Drug therapy is not recommended for asymptomatic hyperuricemia (Dincer, Dincer, & Levinson, 2002).

MOBILITY AND MOBILITY DISABILITY IN OLDER ADULTS

Musculoskeletal function and mobility are inextricably woven together, and the older adult's mobility status has a profound effect on many aspects of life, including ADLs, interpersonal relationships, occupation, leisure activities, and self-esteem. Physiological subsystems that affect mobility have been identified as the central nervous system, perceptual system, peripheral nervous system, musculoskeletal system, and energy production/delivery (Ferrucci et al., 2000).

Factors That Affect Mobility

Treatment of mobility impairment depends on accurate diagnosis and treatment of the underlying physical, psychological, iatrogenic, or environmental problem.

Musculoskeletal Conditions. Musculoskeletal conditions that can affect mobility can be classified as degenerative conditions, acute inflammatory processes, autoimmune disorders, fractures, or chronic musculoskeletal disorders. Patients with these disorders may be immobilized by pain, joint destruction, muscle weakness, or contractures, or they may be immobilized for therapeutic reasons.

Interventions for the older adult are based on individual characteristics and the specific reason for immobilization. Acute inflammation may be treated with rest, heat or cold, and antiinflammatory drugs. Pain always should be treated because it may cause patients to withdraw and become less active. Fractures require immobilization of the affected bone, but the rest of the patient is immobilized as little as possible. Individuals who must wear casts or who remain in traction for any period of time should be taught isometric exercises to maintain muscle tone and strength in the immobilized body part.

Chronic musculoskeletal impairments include degenerative joint disease (DJD) and contractures. A regular program of exercise and analgesic therapy helps maintain mobility with DJD. Contractures are a consequence of immobility, but they also cause further impairment in mobility. When the contracture involves ligament and tendon shortening, surgical correction is the only available "cure." Flexion contractures of the hips and knees commonly are seen in patients who spend much of their time in a wheelchair. However, hip contractures also occur in patients confined to bed, unless the patient spends part of the time in the supine position. Contractures increase the amount of energy required to maintain an upright position or to walk. They also render the individual much less stable and therefore prone to falls. Range of motion to all joints with three repetitions, two times each day, is recommended to prevent contractures in most patients. Lying in the prone position promotes hip, knee, and back extension for those who are at risk for hip and knee flexion contractures.

Depression and Anxiety. Recognition and treatment of psychoemotional disorders that contribute to impaired mobility is essential. Both drugs and psychotherapy are useful. The decision to use antidepressant or antianxiety drugs requires careful consideration. Both are potent drug classes that must be used cautiously in older adults. Referrals to appropriate therapists may be in order. Along with psychotherapy or pharmacological intervention, physical rehabilitation strategies should continue to prevent new problems and to help the individual compensate for mobility impairments.

Medically Prescribed Treatments. Bed rest, traction, and casts are the three most common prescriptions that result in impaired physical mobility. Question orders for prolonged bed rest and initiate exercise regimens for older adults who must be immobilized. Individuals on bed rest should perform isometric and isotonic exercises that have been shown to maintain muscle strength. Individuals who are in casts should be taught isometric exercises to prevent loss of muscle mass, tone, and strength.

Environmental Factors

PHYSICAL ENVIRONMENT. Hospitalized older adults may be fearful of moving because of numerous tubes, monitor wires, machines, and alarms. To avoid unnecessary restriction of movement, explain the purpose of the tubes and demonstrate what movements are permitted and how to protect the tubes when moving. Encourage discontinuing tubes and appliances that limit mobility as soon as possible. Acute care facilities often are poorly prepared for handling patients who are cognitively impaired or become confused. Sometimes this results in the use of pharmacological or physical restraints. Although this may be justified in limited situations, the routine use of physical restraint to treat behavioral disturbance can no longer be considered an acceptable intervention in care of frail older adults. In the event restraint is used, implement plans for adequate exercise and mobilization.

POLICIES. Some institutions still prescribe restraints for patients who cannot walk unassisted. This practice has not been shown to reduce falls. Moreover, restraints produce considerable mobility impairment and predispose the older person to further impairment. Institutional policies also may enhance mobility. Consider the difference between facility A, in which all patients, including those who require two-person assistance, walk to every meal each day, and facility B, in which patients are always wheeled to the dining room or fed

in their rooms. Which patients do you think have the greatest impairments in mobility?

Caregiver Characteristics. Caregiver attitudes are critical in promoting mobility and in treating mobility disorders. Sometimes it is easier to do something for disabled older adults instead of letting them do it for themselves, but this can lead to excess disability. Patience, willingness to persevere and support patients through their pain and boredom, and a belief that promoting mobility is important in the aged are essential characteristics of the caregiver. It may be difficult to sustain enthusiasm for exercise regimens, because the rewards are in what you do *not* see (the absence of further impairment) rather than in what you do see. However, neglecting the regimen results in functional decline over time.

Effects of Immobility

When mobility is impaired, the well-known consequences may include activity intolerance, self-care deficits, incontinence, pressure ulcers, social isolation, psychological disturbances, contractures, loss of muscle mass and strength, bone demineralization, and increased risk for thromboembolism and respiratory infections. Not only does musculoskeletal function affect mobility, but poor balance and muscle strength have been shown to be long-term predictors of morbidity and death (Rantanen, Guralnik, et al., 2001; Rantanen, Harris, et al., 2000; Rantanen, Volpato, et al., 2003).

Taxonomy of Disability

Leveille, Fried, McMullen, and Guralnik (2004) developed a taxonomy of disability based on five contributing factors: pain, balance, weakness, endurance, and other symptoms. Among older disabled women in the Women's Health and Aging Study (WHAS), disability was classified and individuals grouped according to the specific category. As a result, it became evident which older adults were at greatest risk for disability related to each factor. For example, women with pain-related disability tended to be younger and more often were obese. Balance-related disability was more common among women age 85 or older, Caucasian, and those who performed poorly on tests of standing balance and gait. Women with weakness-related disability more often were sedentary, were African American, had a diagnosis of stroke and diabetes, and performed poorly on the chair-stands and tests of knee strength. Variables associated with endurance-related disability were depressive symptoms, smoking history, and lung and cardiovascular diagnoses. In other analyses of the AHAS data, musculoskeletal pain was found to predict increased risk of falling and disability (Leveille, Bean, et al., 2002; Leveille,

Ling, et al., 2001). Other variables that have been found to be related to disability and declining physical performance are benzodiazepines (Gray et al., 2003), chronic depression (Penninx, Deeg, van Eijk, Beekman, & Guralnik, 2000), lower socioeconomic status (Melzer, Izmirlian, Leveille, & Guralnik, 2001), comorbidity (Rozzini et al., 2002), and anemia (Penninx et al., 2003).

Mobility Status of Older Adults

Difficulty quantifying the extent of mobility problems among older adults exists for several reasons. Data often are reported in terms of diagnoses rather than function, self-report surveys lack validation, an array of assessment instruments are used, and the prevalence of various problems varies with the setting. Longitudinal studies have documented the trend toward declining physical ability as people age. Important to note is that factors associated with continued ability included never having cardiovascular disease, never having arthritic complaints, being younger, not being obese, and having a higher educational level.

Data from a population-based study of 10,263 older adults in three U.S. communities were used to describe the prevalence of mobility disability specifically. In this sample, mobility disability was reported in 22% of women at age 70 and 81% of women at age 90. For men, mobility disability was present in 15% at age 70 and 57% at age 90 (Leveille, Penninx, Melzer, Izmirlian, & Guralnik, 2000).

Falls

Falls are a dreaded occurrence for older adults. Not only can they result in loss of function and confidence, but they are the leading cause of death-related injury among older adults. Studies of the incidence of falls show that 25% to 50% of community-dwelling older persons fall at least once each year, and about half of those who fall do so multiple times. The rates for long-term care residents are reported as falls per bed and range from 0.2 to 3.6 per year. In hospitals, the fall rate has been reported as 0.6 to 3.6 per 1000 patient bed days (Fink, Wyman, & Hanlon, 2003).

Community-dwelling older adults are most likely to fall in the home or outdoors. Activities that displace the base of support are most often at fault. Falls among long-term care residents occur most during ambulation, but also occur with sitting and transferring. Patients in acute care facilities are most likely to fall in the course of using a wheelchair. In all settings, most falls happen during the daytime (Fink, Wyman, & Hanlon, 2003).

Among persons over age 65, 2 out of 1000 falls result in death. Soft tissue injuries are common, with as many as 10% requiring medical attention for lacerations and dislocations. From 2% to 6% of falls in community dwellers result in fractures, one half of which are hip fractures. The risk of fracture is greatest with a straight down or side fall, from standing height or greater, and onto a hard surface. Fallers are not only at risk for physical injury, but they may limit their physical activity and grow progressively weaker because of fear of falling (Fink, Wyman, & Hanlon, 2003).

Evidence-based risk factors for falls include age (greater than 80 years); medical conditions; gait, balance, and functional difficulties; and medication use. Medical conditions that have been implicated are arthritis, dizziness, stroke history, and cognitive impairment. Predictors associated with mobility and function are impaired ability to perform ADLs, lower extremity disability, gait or balance problems, and a history of a previous fall. In addition to polypharmacy, specific drug classes associated with falling are antidepressants, antipsychotics, and benzodiazepines (Fink, Wyman, & Hanlon, 2003; Kallin, Jensen, Olsson, Nyberg, & Gustafson, 2004).

ACTIVITIES OF DAILY LIVING: SELF-CARE DEFICITS IN OLDER ADULTS
Definition and Scope of Problem

Activities of daily living are basic self-care tasks engaged in by adults to maintain health and social acceptability. The North American Nursing Diagnosis Association recognizes the following categories of self-care deficits: feeding, dressing/grooming, bathing/hygiene, and toileting.

Dependence in basic activities of daily living is widespread among older adults. U.S. Census 2000 data estimate that 9.5% of those over age 65 years who live in the community have limitations in self-care (U.S. Census Bureau, 2003). Those over age 85 years have a higher prevalence. Most older adults have at least one chronic condition, with hypertension being the most common. Approximately one third have arthritic symptoms and one third have heart disease, both conditions that may affect self-care abilities. Thirty-one percent of older Americans live alone, including half of women over age 75 (Administration on Aging, 2003). Over half of individuals age 80 and older have one or more severe disabilities; 35% require help as a result of their disabilities. Among noninstitutionalized Medicare recipients in 1999, 27.3% had difficulty performing one or more ADLs; 13% had difficulty with instrumental activities of daily living (IADLs). Among institutionalized Medicare beneficiaries, 76.3% had difficulty with three or more ADLs (Administration on Aging, 2003). Those most likely to have difficulty with two or more ADLs were individuals who were age 85 or older, black (non-Hispanic), female, below the poverty level, and living in the southern United States (Administration on Aging, 2003).

Self-care deficits are important to gerontological nurses because people with functional impairments require considerable nursing assistance to compensate for the lost function, to prevent associated problems, and, when possible, to regain the lost abilities. In addition, without appropriate support/assistance, the older adult is at risk for loss of self-esteem, alterations in skin integrity, inadequate nutrition, constipation, incontinence, and even institutionalization. Fortunately, many self-care deficits in older adults are reversible. Helping older people retain as much independence in self-care as possible should be a high priority.

Theoretical Issues

Meaning of Independence. The ability to perform one's basic personal care tasks is achieved at an early stage in development. Relinquishing control over activities of daily living, therefore, can be devastating to the older person's self-concept. Inability to perform basic self-care tasks means that the individual must rely on others or risk developing the problems associated with self-neglect.

Dependency Conflicts. Assisting another with self-care tasks generally involves intimate body contact. Both the patient and the caregiver must resolve feelings of shame, guilt, and anxiety that may be aroused by such intimate contact. Health care professionals are assisted with the identification and resolution of these feelings during their educational preparation. Paraprofessional and lay caregivers have no formal means of working through feelings aroused by provision of intimate care. Unresolved negative feelings about providing personal care assistance may adversely affect the care rendered.

Complexity of Self-Care Tasks. Most adults perform self-care tasks automatically. The activities of daily living are habitual and routine and require minimal effort. However, analysis of ADLs reveals that the tasks are actually quite complex, requiring intact, integrated function of multiple body systems. The systems most involved include the central and peripheral nervous systems, the special senses, the musculoskeletal system, the cardiorespiratory system, and the psyche. Impairments in any of these systems make performance of basic activities of daily living considerably more complex. Severe impairments in any of the systems may make independent self-care impossible.

Influence of Environment on Self-Care Task Performance. Human factors research, which is based in an engineering perspective, provides an interesting way of looking at human performance in the context of environmental systems (Miller, 2003). In high-risk fields, particularly aviation, the rigorous study of factors that affect job performance has led to redesign of tasks or systems with resulting improved outcomes and reduced errors (Weinger & Slagle, 2002). This approach has great potential for generating interventions for those with self-care deficits. One major tenet of this framework is the notion that functional independence of older adults can be improved by changing the designed physical environment to be more congruent with the capabilities of older adults. A second major principle is the belief that activities such as ADLs can be analyzed systematically for their task demands in a given environment, and the environment modified to lessen task demand. For example, the average hand grip strength of an older adult has been estimated to be 15 pounds. Although the force required to operate sink controls is less than this average (approximately 8 pounds), human factors research has demonstrated that if the controls are at an awkward height, or if the individual has difficulty grasping owing to joint deformity, the required amount of force may not be delivered.

Other examples of human/environmental interactions that may affect functional performance include the amount of reach to clothing in closets and the amount of bending to get into or out of a bathtub or shower. Human factors research delineates many of the anthropometric and biomechanical demands of tasks. Future studies are likely to be helpful in describing the sensory and cognitive demands of everyday tasks.

Contributing Factors

Factors that may also create or exacerbate a self-care deficit include physiological and psychological impairments and environmental barriers.

Intolerance to Activity. Activity intolerance leads to a self-care deficit, because the individual lacks the stamina to perform the necessary tasks. Many older adults have reduced stamina and postural instability. Those who perform activities of daily living independently despite severe activity intolerance are often left with a socially impoverished existence, because they lack the time or resources to engage in other activities, work, or leisure.

Pain. Pain caused by coronary artery disease, arthritis, fracture, or other pathological conditions may so overwhelm the patient that self-care becomes difficult, if not impossible. Pain also may restrict mobility, so that performance is impaired. For example, a patient might have a painful left arm from severe lymphedema. Although technically she is able to dress herself independently (that is, she has the motor skill), she is totally dependent in dressing because the pain in her arm when performing the task unassisted is so great.

Perceptual Impairment. Activities of daily living are considered routine or automatic behaviors, but perceptual impairments may prevent normal performance. Typically, the more complex tasks, such as toileting, grooming, and dressing, are first affected, followed by bathing and feeding. According to the U.S. Census Bureau (2003), 14.2% of noninstitutionalized people age 65 and older reported some type of sensory disability in 2000; 3.6% reported having physical, mental, and sensory disabilities.

Sensory-perceptual impairments affect self-care ability in several ways. First, they interfere with the individual's ability to receive signals that prompt the individual to perform a self-care task. For example, people with visual impairment lack visual cues to tell them if their hair needs combing or they have put their clothes on properly, thus potentially developing self-care deficits in grooming and dressing. Sensory impairments also affect the ability to execute selected tasks. For example, people with severe visual impairment have difficulty locating toilets in strange surroundings, interfering with their toilet independence. They also have difficulty finding the food on a plate, relying on the sense of touch and smell unless guided by another. Visual impairment may result in disturbances in balance and increase the risk of falls during some self-care activities.

Cognitive Impairment. Cognitive impairments affect self-care abilities in many ways. Indeed, one study found cognitive impairment to be the greatest predictor of self-care deficits in the nursing home setting (Schultz, Ellingrod, Turvey, Moser, & Arndt, 2003). People with cognitive disorders may lose the social awareness that it is important to perform activities of daily living and omit these tasks unless prompted to perform. An example is the lack of attention to grooming often noticed in the early stage of dementia. Cognitive impairments also interfere with the reasoning ability needed to perform self-care tasks in new environments. Thus a demented person may be independent in self-care tasks in the home environment, but become unable to perform the tasks when relocated. Those with severe cognitive impairment often become apraxic, unable to perform the steps or properly use devices involved in self-care.

Neuromuscular Impairment. Impaired physical mobility because of neuromuscular impairment is likely to affect self-care abilities. Hemiplegia is a classic example of a neuromuscular disorder common among the elderly that dramatically affects self-care ability. With the use of only one half of the body, all aspects of self-care become extraordinarily complex. Hemiplegia is often associated with other disorders that affect self-care abilities, such as unilateral neglect (a condition in which the individual is unaware of or does not attend to one side of the body), chronic pain syndromes, and

sensory impairments. Other neuromuscular dysfunctions associated with self-care deficits include Parkinson's disease and the demyelinating disorders, such as amyotrophic lateral sclerosis, multiple sclerosis, and degenerative cerebellar disorders.

Musculoskeletal Impairment. Arthritis, contractures, scoliosis, kyphosis, and decreased muscle mass and strength all contribute to self-care deficits in the aged. These disorders contribute primarily by inducing impaired mobility, endurance, strength, or coordination. In one study, lower extremity muscle force and lower extremity range of motion explained 77% of the variance in functional limitations in older adults in independent and dependent living situations. When the two groups were examined separately, a higher percentage of the variance was explained by musculoskeletal measures in the dependent group (Beissner, Collins, & Holmes, 2000).

Depression. Performance of self-care activities requires that individuals value themselves sufficiently to invest the time and energy in performing ADLs. People who are depressed may lose interest in self-care and thus become dependent on others or suffer the effects of neglect. In grooming and hygiene, the effects are not life threatening but certainly reinforce a cycle of negative self-worth. The individual feels too poorly to bathe or dress properly and, in turn, begins to feel worse and lose social contacts because of a socially unacceptable appearance. Going without food is a more life-threatening lapse that calls for prompt intervention to resolve the depression and restore nutritional health.

A large longitudinal study of older adults found that cognitive impairment and depressive symptoms are risk factors for functional decline among individuals who were independent in ADLs at baseline (Mehta, Yaffe, & Covinsky, 2002). A second study of community-dwelling older persons showed that depressive symptoms were associated with episodes of disabling musculoskeletal pain (Reid, Williams, & Gill, 2003).

NURSING CARE OF PATIENTS WITH MUSCULOSKELETAL ALTERATIONS
Health Assessment

Assessment of the musculoskeletal system focuses not only on muscles, bones, and joints, but also on function, including gait, balance, mobility, fall risks, activities of daily living, and self-care. Because of the integrated relationship between the neurological and musculoskeletal systems, there necessarily is some overlap. For details about specific assessment techniques, see an assessment resource. This section takes a holistic approach and discusses modifications and relevant issues when the patient is an older adult. In addition, pathophysiology underlying some findings is discussed.

Health History. Because musculoskeletal problems common in older adults often are associated with pain, this is an important component of the system assessment. Pain assessment in older adults may be complicated for several reasons. First, because many older adults believe pain is "normal" with aging, they may not report it unless specifically asked. Second, cultural differences influence the patient's beliefs about pain and how it should be expressed and managed (or endured). Third, individuals with cognitive or speech disorders may have difficulty expressing or describing pain. Fourth, some older adults deny pain or refuse analgesics because they are excessively concerned about adverse effects, especially addiction and respiratory depression (Welsh, Fallon, & Keeley, 2003). Last, the subjective data may be altered if the patient has taken analgesics before the assessment. Therefore always inquire if and when the patient last took pain medication.

JOINTS. For older adults, the "chief complaint" often is related to the joints—either pain, stiffness, swelling, or limitations of movement. Such complaints often are associated with arthritis. If pain is reported, assess the location, quality, severity, and factors that aggravate and relieve it. Location is especially useful because it can help to differentiate types of joint problems. For example, rheumatoid arthritis typically affects symmetrical joints whereas osteoarthritis more commonly affects isolated joints. Ask if pain is accompanied by the classic signs of inflammation: swelling, warmth, and redness. When joint stiffness is a problem, ask when it occurs and how long it lasts. Again, types of arthritis differ in that rheumatoid arthritis often persists for more than an hour after arising and osteoarthritis usually resolves much more quickly. Record drug therapy and alternative therapies used to manage joint disorders. The social history, including the individual's occupation and hobbies, and current living arrangement often is relevant to joint problems because repetitive stress is one cause of joint injury.

MUSCLES. The most important muscular symptoms are pain, cramping, and weakness. Once again, elicit a detailed description of the pain. Determine what activities, if any, were associated with the onset of pain. If the pain is the result of arterial insufficiency, it typically ceases when activity stops. Back pain and paresthesia of the lower extremties may be symptoms of vertebral or intervertebral lumbar disk degeneration. Muscle cramps can occur during activity or rest and can be caused by overuse, circulatory impairment, or electrolyte imbalances (hypocalcemia, hypokalemia, hyponatremia). A decline in muscle strength compared with a younger person is common, although there is debate over whether this is a normal change or a consequence of disease or inactivity. Nevertheless, when weakness is sudden, marked, unilateral, or affects only one group of muscles, further investigation is indicated. The medication history may reveal drugs that can affect muscle such as antiadrenergics, corticosteroids, diuretics, statins, and muscle relaxants. Drugs that can cause electrolyte imbalances also can affect function.

BONES. To assess skeletal symptoms, inquire about pain, previous and recent injuries, deformity, and related symptoms. When bone pain is present, inquire about any recent injury that could have caused a fracture. Fractures are not always complete or displaced and only can be ruled out radiographically. Back pain specifically should be assessed because the changes in the vertebrae and the intervertebral disks can lead to fractures and nerve compression. Data about the intake of protein, dairy products, calcium supplements, and vitamin D are relevant to bone disorders. Box 11-4 presents a simple screening tool that can be used to assess risk for osteoporosis.

ACTIVITIES OF DAILY LIVING. Any disorder or injury that affects the musculoskeletal system can affect the older adult's ability to perform activities of daily living. Therefore the assessment should seek to identify whether musculoskeletal symptoms interfere with mobility, ADLs, and IADLs. Note the use of assistive devices and other resources. In addition to the physical impact of musculoskeletal disorders, explore the emotional and social impact. Chapter 2 provides a comprehensive discussion of functional assessment, including appropriate tools to use with the older adult.

PHYSICAL ACTIVITY/EXERCISE. Document the usual activity level, and describe any activities that might affect the musculoskeletal system. For example, imagine the possible effects of the following: welding, caring for a toddler grandchild, running marathons, sitting at a computer 8 hours a day, playing tennis twice a week, and gardening. Inquire about an exercise program, listing the type, frequency, and length of each session. Also, ask how well the activity is tolerated and describe any problems reported such as pain, exhaustion, angina, intermittent claudication, or dyspnea.

FALLS. If the individual has a history of falling, use the mnemonic SPLATT to assess aspects of the fall experience (Fink, Wyman, & Hanlon, 2003). "S" stands for symptoms such as dizziness that occurred in relation to the fall. "P" refers to previous falls. "L" is for location— where the fall occurred. "A" is for the activity at the time of the fall. "T" is for timing. Under what circumstances

---

BOX 11-4 Risk Factors for Osteoporosis: Can It Happen To You?

RISK FACTORS YOU CANNOT CHANGE	RISK FACTORS YOU CAN CHANGE
■ Gender: Your chances of developing osteoporosis are greater if you are a women. Women have less bone tissue and lose bone more rapidly than men because of the changes involved in menopause. ■ Age: The older you are, the greater your risk of osteoporosis. Your bones become less dense and weaker as you age. ■ Body size: Small, thin-boned women are at greater risk. ■ Ethnicity: Caucasian and Asian women are at highest risk. African-American and Latino women have a lower, but still significant, risk. ■ Family history: Susceptibility to fracture may be, in part, hereditary. People whose parents have a history of fractures also seem to have reduced bone mass and may be at risk for fractures.	■ Sex hormones: Abnormal absence of menstrual periods (amenorrhea), low estrogen level (menopause), and low testosterone level in men. ■ Anorexia. ■ Lifetime diet low in calcium and vitamin D. ■ Use of certain medications, such as glucocorticoids or some anticonvulsants. ■ An inactive lifestyle or extended bed rest. ■ Cigarette smoking. ■ Excessive use of alcohol.

From Osteoporosis. (2004). Courtesy of the National Center for Health Promotion and Disease Prevention, Durham, NC. Retrieved July 10, 2006, from www.nchpdp.med.va.gov/MonthlyPreventionTopics/2004_10_BJDW/Osteoporosis.doc.

---

did the fall occur? The final "T" is for trauma resulting from the fall. Also, note medication and alcohol use and chronic conditions that might contribute to falling. More specialized evaluation by a physical therapist or an occupational therapist is indicated if significant mobility and strength impairments are present (Fink, Wyman, & Hanlon, 2003).

Physical Examination. The physical examination actually begins when the patient is first seen. Observe the general appearance, stature, posture, ease of movement, symmetry of movements, and gait. Current height and weight compared with those measurements at maturity provide data to help determine shortening of the vertebral column, obesity, edema, and severe muscle wasting. Observation of the patient's movements gives clues to flexibility, agility, and control. Note any involuntary movements such as tremors. Common changes in the posture of the older adult include slight hip and knee flexion, kyphosis, and a backward head tilt. Loss of subcutaneous fat may cause the cheeks to appear more hollow and bony prominences to be more prominent (Jarvis, 2004).

The importance of observing an older person walking cannot be overemphasized. Note the width of the base of support, whether steps are smooth and even, how well balanced the person is, and whether the arms swing symmetrically. Older adults often assume a wider stance, use the arms more for balance, and take shorter, uneven steps. Gait abnormalities may represent musculoskeletal or neurological disorders. Guidelines for the assessment of gait and balance in the older adult are outlined in Tables 3-1 and 3-2 in Chapter 3. Once again,

direct observation by the examiner is preferred so that the patient's true abilities are determined. Otherwise, less sophisticated care providers may provide inappropriate care based on inaccurate assumptions.

The steps of the standard musculoskeletal examination proceed from head to toe and from inspection, to palpation, to range of motion and muscle testing. Tendon reflexes, which are discussed with the neurological system, may actually be performed with the musculoskeletal assessment.

INSPECTION. Inspect each joint for size, contour, color, swelling, masses, and deformity. Swelling and redness signify inflammation. Joint enlargement and nodules can appear with all types of arthritis. Joint deformity is more common with rheumatoid arthritis. Also, the specific pattern of joints affected is characteristic of the types of arthritis. Osteoarthritis usually is unilateral and affects the distal joints of the hands, whereas rheumatoid arthritis is more often symmetrical and affects the proximal joints of the hands.

Look for deformities characteristic of common disease processes. Chronic rheumatoid arthritis (RA) may produce swan neck and boutonnière deformities of the hands and ulnar deviation. Subcutaneous nodules may be visible with RA. Nodules of the distal interphalangeal joints called Heberden's nodes are characteristic of osteoarthritis. When the nodules are located on the proximal interphalangeal joints, they are called Bouchard's nodes. White nodules that are visible under the skin are tophi, which are created by sodium urate crystals deposited under the skin in chronic gout. Inflammation of the first metatarsophalangeal joint is characteristic of gout. Other foot deformities are common in older adults and can have significant impact on mobility. Inspect the feet for bunions, hammer toe, and hallus valgus (lateral deviation of the great toe).

If the patient is able to stand alone, stand behind and inspect the alignment of the spine. The spine should appear straight and the shoulders, scapulae, iliac crests, and gluteal folds should be symmetrical. The spaces between the arms and the thorax on each side should be approximately the same. Move to the patient's side and examine the spinal curvature. Many older adults have an exaggerated convex thoracic curve (kyphosis). Obese patients may have an exaggerated lumbar curve (Jarvis, 2004).

PALPATION. As each joint is inspected, palpate for warmth, tenderness, and masses. Palpation should not elicit pain or tenderness. A thickened synovial membrane feels boggy; however, the membrane normally is not palpable. When nodules are palpable, assess whether they are firm, soft, movable, or tender. The location of subcutaneous nodules provides a clue to specific types of arthritis. With an acute attack of gout, the affected joint is extremely tender to the touch.

RANGE OF MOTION. Have the patient perform active range of motion of each joint to assess for limitations, pain, and crepitation. Limitations may result from joint deformities or muscle weakness; ease of movement is affected by pain in the muscles or joints. When active motion is limited, support the joint and gently attempt to move the joint through passive motion. A goniometer can be used to measure degrees of joint movement precisely. The experienced examiner can recognize deviations from normal ranges.

MUSCLE STRENGTH. To evaluate muscle strength, have the patient perform range of motion again, but now apply opposing force to the motion. The specific joint ranges of motion and techniques for evaluation are detailed in textbooks on health assessment (Welsh, Fallon, & Keeley, 2003).

Mobility. The musculoskeletal assessment would be incomplete without establishing the patient's mobility status. These data enable the practitioner to determine patient and caregiver perceptions of mobility status, the impact of impaired mobility on the individual, the etiology of mobility impairments, and coping or adaptive strategies employed. The individual's perception of mobility problems is important, but the most useful data come from direct observation of performance. Various assessment tools and techniques are available for quantifying each aspect of the assessment. For example, the nursing home Minimum Data Set (MDS) requires only screening level information about mobility and the need for assistive devices. When more precise measures of an individual's physical mobility are needed, more sophisticated tools such as those employed by physical therapists and occupational therapists are needed.

During the mobility assessment, have the patient perform a standardized series of maneuvers, such as those outlined in Tables 3-1 and 3-2 in Chapter 3. Quantify the amount of assistance required, if any, and note any symptoms accompanying those maneuvers such as pain, stiffness, or awkwardness. If impairments are noted, identify the conditions under which they occur and the conditions under which they improve. The term *mobility disability* is defined as "difficulty walking medium distances, typically a quarter or half mile" (Fried & Guralnik, 1997, cited in Melzer, Lan, & Guralnik, 2003, p. 619). For example, people with Parkinson's disease often have several types of mobility impairments, including bradykinesia, cogwheeling rigidity, and decreased joint range of motion. Frequently, after receiving assistance with an activity such as ambulation, the amount of bradykinesia and rigidity is temporarily lessened. Medications also may lessen the symptoms of impaired mobility. Therefore document whether the assessment was conducted before or after exercising and medications currently taken.

When a patient is bedridden, assess bed mobility tasks. Unless medically contraindicated (as with unstable or suspected fracture, unstable vital signs, increased intracranial pressure), instruct the patient to attempt each of the following movements: (1) turn from side to side in bed; (2) flex the knees bilaterally and raise the hips (bridging); (3) move from a supine to a sitting position, with legs dangling over the side of the bed; and (4) assume the prone position in bed.

Observing the performance of each of these tasks can yield considerable information about the patient's muscle strength, joint range of motion, and ability to follow motor commands. This information also provides a basis for interventions aimed at maintaining or improving mobility. For example, patients who can turn from side to side in bed should be encouraged to participate in that task to the maximum extent possible, because this will help maintain trunk flexibility and strength and possibly upper extremity function. In addition, it allows the individual to maintain control of repositioning schedules. Individuals who cannot perform this task are unlikely to be able to accomplish a supine-to-sit transfer unassisted. Raising the hips 2 to 3 inches into the air requires considerable hip extensor muscle strength. Ability to perform this task suggests sufficient leg strength to stand, although the individual may still need support for balance or assistance with other steps in the sit-to-stand transfer. Inability to raise the hips in bed may represent motor planning problems rather than an absence of strength, so manual muscle testing is still indicated in patients who cannot complete the bridging task. Moving from a supine to a sitting position is a key movement required for transferring from bed to chair or from bed to a prewalking position. Retained ability to perform this task is a good sign, because it involves the coordinated movement of many body segments.

Assessing an individual's ability to assume the prone-lying position often is overlooked, yet it is an important maneuver for individuals who spend long periods of time in a bed or chair. Hip and knee flexion contractures, which are common in institutionalized older persons, affect the ability to walk and to transfer. The prone position is the only bed position that eliminates hip flexion. If the patient is able to lie comfortably in this position, it is another turning position for prevention of skin breakdown.

Remember, failure to perform a task may be due to a musculoskeletal problem, but it also may result from other problems such as fear, cognitive impairment, sedation, or aphasia. Each of these potential contributors must be assessed individually.

Risk for Falls. A simple screening test for fall risk is the "get up and go" test. Start with the individual seated in an armless chair and instruct him or her to rise without using the arms, walk a short distance, turn, return to the chair, and sit without using the arms. For those persons who have difficulty with this task, a more complete assessment of fall risk is indicated.

Activities of Daily Living. The musculoskeletal changes that occur with aging are of less concern than the extent to which they interfere with ADLs. Therefore all older adults should be assessed for the ability to perform ADLs. Options for assessing function of ADLs include direct observation, patient report, and proxy report (usually a family member or paid caregiver). Although direct observation provides the most objective and richest data, reported function more commonly is used because it takes less time and is more practical. Evidence exists that patient self-report is more consistent with observed performance than either the family or physician estimates of patient abilities. On some measures of function, such as the Barthel Index of ADLs, self-report ratings and those based on direct observation are highly correlated. Nevertheless, when patients report self-care deficits, direct observation is indicated if feasible. Using both performance-based measures of function and reported function may provide complementary data.

Data obtained by direct observation may support or refute information provided by a caregiver, and this has important implications. If the older adult is observed to perform at a higher level than is reported by a caregiver,

the person may suffer from excess disability and could benefit from intervention. If the older adult functions at a level lower than the caregiver reports, the reason for the discrepancy deserves further evaluation.

A number of instruments are available to assess independence in ADLs. See Chapter 2 for a discussion of functional assessment tools.

To assess mobility, the following activities described by Jarvis (2004) should be done:

- Have the patient walk with shoes on. The older person may have a shuffling gait, sway, hold the arms out for balance, keep the feet wider apart, and watch his or her feet.
- If safe, ask the patient to walk up stairs. The older person may use the handrail to pull up to the next step; may use the stronger leg first to step up to the next step.
- If safe, ask the patient to walk down stairs. Older adults tend to use the handrail. Those who are weak may place both hands on the rail and descend one step at a time with the weaker leg going forward first.
- Ask the patient to pick up an object from the floor. The older person may bend from the waist rather than the knees and hold onto furniture for support.
- Have the patient rise from a sitting to a standing position. Older adults commonly place the feet apart, lean forward, and then push up using the chair arms.
- If appropriate, ask the patient to rise from a reclining to a sitting position. An older person may roll to one side, use the arms to push the torso up, and hold onto a siderail or furniture for leverage.

Assessment of a person's performance of ADLs can be evaluated using this scale:

0 = Completely independent

1 = Requires use of equipment or device

2 = Requires help from another person for assistance, supervision, or teaching

3 = Requires help from another person and equipment or device

4 = Dependent; does not participate in activity

Environment. The environment significantly affects the older adult's mobility and performance of ADLs. Determine the individual's living arrangements and identify barriers and adaptations that interfere with or facilitate function. An on-site assessment of the environment, if possible, is preferred.

Related Data. Other general topics that are relevant to the musculoskeletal system are the medication history and nutritional status. Be sure to inquire about over-the-counter products, as well as prescription drugs. Avoid judgmental statements about nonallopathic products that the older adult reports. Critical remarks may cause the patient to not disclose some information.

The nursing assessment related to changes and common disorders of the musculoskeletal system are summarized in Box 11-5.

Nursing Diagnoses

The following are examples of nursing diagnoses that commonly apply to the older adult who has musculoskeletal disorders. Some possible etiologies are suggested.

1. Activity intolerance: related to weakness, stiffness, and pain secondary to habitual inactivity, fatigue
2. Pain, chronic: related to musculoskeletal disease, injury
3. Diversional activity, deficient: related to loss of ability to perform usual or favorite activities secondary to immobility, pain, and weakness
4. Home maintenance management, impaired: related to inability to perform household tasks secondary to the effects of musculoskeletal limitations
5. Injury, risk for: related to sensory or motor deficits
6. Mobility, impaired physical: related to poor balance, weakness, pain, cognitive impairment, musculoskeletal deformity
7. Knowledge, deficient: of nutritional requirements for musculoskeletal health, disease process, drug therapy
8. Self-care deficit: feeding, bathing/hygiene, dressing/grooming, feeding, toileting: related to weakness, confusion, apraxia, poor coordination, balance or coordination disturbance, motor impairments
9. Self-esteem, chronic low: related to loss of body function
10. Skin integrity, risk for impaired: related to immobility

Box 11-5 Musculoskeletal Assessment

Health History
- Joints
  - Symptoms: pain, stiffness, swelling, limited movement
  - Past injuries
  - Therapy for joint symptoms: drugs, complementary and alternative
  - Social history: occupation, hobbies
- Muscles
  - Symptoms: pain, cramps, weakness
  - Past injuries
  - Therapy for muscle symptoms
- Bones
  - Symptoms: pain, deformity
  - Past injuries
- Activities of daily living
  - Perceived mobility
  - Perceived ability to perform activities of daily living
  - Perceived ability to perform instrumental activities of daily living
  - Assistive devices used
  - Impact of mobility impairments
- Physical activity/exercise
  - Usual activity level
  - Exercise program; type, frequency, length of sessions
  - Activity tolerance
- Falls
  - Related symptoms (e.g., dizziness)
  - Previous falls
  - Location
  - Circumstances
  - Resulting trauma

Physical Examination
- Measurements: height and weight
- General observations:
  - Stature, posture, body alignment
  - Voluntary and involuntary movements
  - Walking
  - Gait
  - Balance
- Inspection
  - Joints: swelling, redness, deformity
  - Muscles: atrophy
  - Extremities: symmetry, deformity
  - Spine: alignment, curvatures
  - Range of motion
    - Active/passive
    - Degree of movement
    - Crepitation
- Palpation
  - Joints
    - Warmth, bogginess
    - Synovial membrane
    - Nodules
    - Crepitation
  - Muscle tone and strength

Mobility Status
- Performance
- Related medical diagnoses, drugs
- Bed mobility tasks
- Ability to lie prone
- Risk for falls screening
- Activities of daily living
- Environment

Overlaps exist among the diagnostic categories of impaired physical mobility, activity intolerance, self-care deficit, and sometimes chronic pain. Do not become overly concerned with finding the single right diagnosis for each patient. Multiple diagnoses often will apply to the older adult, and it is wise to consider the differences in intervention strategies suggested by each of the diagnostic categories.

Nursing Goals

The goals of nursing care related to the older adult's musculoskeletal status include (1) preservation, restoration, or improvement of joint mobility, muscle strength, and skeletal health; (2) maintenance, restoration, or improvement in mobility and self-care; (3) relief of discomfort related to musculoskeletal disorders or injuries; (4) prevention of complications associated with immobility or musculoskeletal disorders; and (5) adaptation to the effects of musculoskeletal disorders.

The care setting is a major factor in the achievement of these goals. In many long-term care settings, it is difficult for patients to regain or compensate for lost function, because the level of staffing does not allow the time for restorative approaches to care. Initially it takes more time to encourage and supervise someone to perform a task than to do the task for the person. In addition, nursing home staff may not have adequate training in restorative care techniques. In contrast, rehabilitation center staff are highly motivated and well trained to assist patients in regaining lost function or in compensating for impairments.

Nursing Interventions

Regardless of the extent of the impairment, the opportunity to prevent further impairment almost always exists. The primary interventions to maintain or preserve musculoskeletal function in the older adult are exercise, nutrition, and patient education. Both pharmacological and nonpharmacological therapy may be needed for relief of discomfort, treatment of depression, or management of symptoms of conditions that affect mobility, such as Parkinson's disease. Numerous other therapeutic options are available, such as massage, application of heat and cold, electrical stimulation, and use of orthothic and prosthetic devices. An interdisciplinary team can provide a variety of services to maximize mobility and self-care and to decrease the risk of injuries to older adults. Although there is some overlap, for purposes of this discussion, interventions are classified as those used to promote mobility, those used to promote self-care, and those used to prevent falls (Box 11-6).

Interventions to Promote Mobility. Exercise is the cornerstone of maintaining mobility. However,

---

BOX 11-6 *TOWARD BETTER MUSCULOSKELETAL HEALTH*

- Individualized activity considering patient abilities and limitations
- Ideally, 20 to 30 minutes of moderate-intensity exercise on most days of the week
- Passive exercise to maintain joint mobility for patients who cannot move unassisted
- Resistive exercise to improve muscle mass, strength, and endurance
- Isometric exercise limited to 10 seconds
- Balance training such as Tai Chi
- Aerobic exercise to reduce risks of type 2 diabetes mellitus, hypertension, cardiac disease, and osteoporosis

---

older adults may interpret the word *exercise* to mean only calisthenics when in fact exercise can include active and passive range of motion, flexion and stretching movements, walking, swimming, jogging, aerobics, and resistance training, depending on the individual's level of fitness and functional abilities. Every older person can benefit from some sort of exercise; however, the program must be tailored to the individual's needs. Benefits extend beyond physical gains to have a positive impact on the older adult's quality of life (Dias, Dias, & Ramos, 2003; Papaioannou et al., 2003). People who are physically active throughout the day may think their activity meets their exercise needs, but research has shown that they do not derive the same benefits in physical function as those who engage in 20 to 30 minutes of moderate-intensity exercise on most days of the week (Brach, Simonsick, Kritchevsky, Yaffe, & Newman, 2004).

Passive exercise, which is needed when the patient is unable to move unassisted, does not result in muscle contraction. It helps maintain joint mobility and, following joint surgery, helps prevent adhesions and stimulates healing. Active exercise, whether independent or assisted, uses active muscle contraction, which strengthens muscles in addition to maintaining joint mobility. Active resistive exercise uses muscle contraction against some type of resistance (weights, equipment, weight bearing). Resistive exercise, also called strength training exercise, includes isometric, isotonic, and isokinetic exercises (Addamo & Clough, 1998).

RANGE-OF-MOTION EXERCISE. General strengthening and conditioning exercises are useful for all patients, but individuals with mobility impairments require specific exercise regimens to prevent contractures and preserve function. Range-of-motion exercises prevent loss of joint motion and help some individuals regain lost motion. When possible, older people should be taught how to perform their own range of motion.

Experience shows that many individuals who require it are unable to do this for a variety of reasons, including cognitive impairment, lack of motivation, and impaired mobility. These patients require someone else to construct an exercise program and assist in conducting it. Family members or friends can be taught range-of-motion exercises. Their successful performance by severely impaired patients requires considerable sophistication. The only way to develop this expertise is to practice the exercises. Emphasize the following points:

1. Move in a gentle, circular motion, not in a jerky, rapid motion.
2. Circular motion is more effective in reducing spasticity than direct opposition.
3. When performing range of motion on upper extremities, mobilize the scapulae first to facilitate relaxation in the remainder of the extremity.
4. When working on the lower extremities, mobilize the hips first, to facilitate relaxation in other lower extremity joints.
5. When working on the back, begin with flexibility of the head and neck.

RESISTIVE EXERCISE. Resistive exercise (resistance/strength training) increasingly is recognized as an important component of both musculoskeletal and cardiovascular fitness. It is credited with improving muscle mass, strength, and endurance. Along with aerobic exercise, it also helps maintain the basal metabolic rate for weight control. Through mechanisms different from aerobic exercise, resistance training has a positive effect on bone density, glucose tolerance, and insulin sensitivity (Pollock et al., 2000). Increased strength can have a significant impact on the ability of the older adult to perform activities of daily living and to remain mobile. Only strength conditioning can increase muscle mass by increasing protein synthesis. One study examined the effects of high-intensity resistance training of knee extensors and flexors in men age 60 to 72 years. The average increase in flexor strength was 227%, and extensor strength average gain was 107%. Computed tomography and muscle biopsies showed an 11% increase in total muscle area with a 33.5% increase in type 1 fibers and a 27.5% increase in type 2 fiber area. The increase in muscle mass equated with an increase in maximal aerobic power. Similar interventions in frail nursing home residents produced similar benefits and also resulted in increased spontaneous physical activity. Frail older women taking hormone replacement therapy who engaged in progressive resistance and endurance exercises over a 9-month period significantly increased lumbar spine BMD (Villareal et al., 2003). Resistance training does not seem to be especially helpful in treating obesity in older people, but it does help preserve muscle mass during weight loss.

Various organizations have offered standards, guidelines, and position statements regarding strength training for older adults and individuals with cardiac disease. For older adults, the recommendation is for one set of 8 to 10 exercises with 10 to 15 repetitions to be done a minimum of 2 days each week; for cardiac patients the recommendation includes one set of 8 to 10 exercises with 10 to 15 repetitions done 2 to 3 days each week (Pollock et al., 2000). Individual response always must be carefully monitored and adjustments made as indicated.

ISOMETRIC EXERCISE. In an isometric exercise, the muscle is contracted without moving the joint. An example of an isometric exercise is quadriceps setting. Contrary to common opinion, isometric exercises generally are safe if the hold time is limited to 10 seconds and the Valsalva maneuver is avoided. Isometric contraction longer than 30 seconds has been shown to affect blood pressure (Kauffman, 1999). An advisory statement issued by the Committee on Exercise, Rehabilitation, and Prevention, Council on Clinical Cardiology, American Heart Association states that cardiac patients who have good aerobic fitness and normal or near-normal left ventricular systolic function can safely perform weight lifting at 8 to 12 repetitions per set (Pollock et al., 2000).

ISOTONIC EXERCISE. An isotonic exercise contracts the muscle against resistance, such as when the elbow is flexed and extended while holding a weight. Isotonic exercise can benefit the older adult because many aspects of ADLs require this type of contraction. The outcomes of isotonic exercise are influenced by the frequency of exercise sessions, the number of repetitions, and the amount of resistance applied (Addamo & Clough, 1998).

ISOKINETIC EXERCISE. Isokinetic exercise uses a device that has a preset dynamic speed that accommodates resistance to muscle tension developed at each point of the range of motion. The machine maintains a constant speed but varies resistance in proportion to the force applied to a lever. An advantage for older adults is that the resistance stops when the patient stops contracting because of weakness or pain. This way, the patient can continue exercising as prescribed without pain or trauma (Addamo & Clough, 1998).

BALANCE EXERCISES. Balance training can be a component of strength training, and may reduce the risk of falls. Tai Chi is a form of exercise that has been demonstrated to reduce falls in older adults (Evans, 2003). A Japanese study compared the benefits of balance and gait exercises for frail older adults. Those who engaged in balance exercises showed gains in static balance function, whereas those who did gait exercises improved more in dynamic balance and gait function (Hiroyuki, Uchiyama, & Kakurai, 2003).

AEROBIC EXERCISE. Aerobic exercise has multiple benefits, including reduced risks of type 2 diabetes mellitus, hypertension, cardiac disease, and osteoporosis (Evans, 2003; Pollock et al., 2000). Endurance exercise alone has not been shown to maintain muscle strength in older athletes (runners and swimmers). The maximal aerobic capacity reportedly declines 1% for each year between ages 20 and 70 regardless of the level of physical activity. Initially, sedentary older adults who perform aerobic exercise regularly show gains in aerobic capacity, increased insulin action, increased glucose tolerance, and increased skeletal muscle glycogen stores. A longitudinal study of individuals with knee osteoarthritis showed that factors which protected against a poor functional outcome included strength and aerobic exercise (Sharma et al., 2003). Ourania, Yvoni, Christos, and Ionannis (2003) demonstrated that the amount of improvement in dynamic balance, muscular endurance and coordination, and sit-and-reach flexibility was proportional to the frequency of training activities. Studies of the effects of endurance training on cardiac output in older individuals have yielded contradictory results. Aerobic exercise commonly is prescribed along with reduced calorie intake for weight reduction.

The Karvonen method for calculating target heart rate range is commonly used for older adults. This formula, which uses the resting heart rate and prescribed range of exercise intensity, is illustrated in Box 11-7. Although target heart rate guidelines are often used to keep intensity of exercise within safe limits, older adults may have difficulty learning to monitor their pulse during exercise. Also, the pulse counted after exercise stops may be different than the pulse during activity. Use of heart rate monitors where available is one option; another is Borg's Revised Perceived Exertion Scale (Borg, 1982, cited in Reynolds, 1999) (Figure 11-14). Monitoring the heart rate is of limited value in older adults who are taking antiadrenergic drugs because these drugs suppress the sympathetic response. Therefore the person's heart rate may not increase in proportion to the amount of exertion, and other data may be more useful.

Other symptoms that may occur during exercise include hypoglycemic episodes in people with diabetes, respiratory decompensation in individuals with chronic lung disease, and cardiac symptoms, such as angina and syncope. A well-understood standard operating procedure for management of these predictable symptoms and potential emergencies is essential for a smoothly run program. In medical settings, an emergency cart containing basic life-support equipment and readily available medications for symptom control will permit

BOX 11-7 Calculating Target Heart Rate Range Using the Karvonen Method	
Maximal heart rate	220
Subtract age	−70
	———
	150
Subtract resting heart rate	−60
	———
Equals heart-rate reserve	90
Multiply by % intensity	×0.40
	———
	36.0
Add resting heart rate	+60
	———
Target heart-rate range for 40% to 60%	96 beats/min

From Reynolds, P. (1999). Exercise considerations for cardiopulmonary disease. In T. L. Kauffman (Ed.), *Geriatric rehabilitation manual.* New York: Churchill Livingstone, p. 201.

prompt treatment of exercise-induced chronic disease symptoms.

INDIVIDUALIZED EXERCISE PLANS. Each person should have an individualized exercise prescription that contains at a minimum (1) the goal of the exercise(s), (2) the type of movement to be performed in each exercise, (3) the intensity of each exercise (often expressed as the number of repetitions of each movement or the amount of resistance to be used on an ergometer), (4) the frequency with which the exercise should be performed, (5) the duration of the exercise, and (6) any precautions the person should observe. Even in group exercise programs, each individual should have a prescription, even if the prescriptions are quite similar among the members of the group. Individual constraints on certain movements or activities should be respected.

Although group exercise activities are efficient, some people prefer solitary exercise. Respect the preference and do not try to force participation in a group. However, the peer support and social interaction available in

6 No exertion at all	14
7 Extremely light	15 Hard (heavy)
8	16
9 Very light	17 Very hard
10	18
11 Light	19 Extremely hard
12	20 Maximal exertion
13 Somewhat hard	

Instructions to the Borg-RPE-Scale®

During the work we want you to rate your perception of exertion, ie. how heavy and strenuous the exercise feels to you and how tired you are. The perception of exertion is mainly felt as strain and fatigue in your muscles and as breathlessness or aches in the chest.

Use this scale from 6 to 20, where **6** means "No exertion at all" and **20** means "Maximal exertion."

   9   Very light. As for a healthy person taking a short walk at his or her own pace.

  13   Somewhat hard. It still feels OK to continue.

  15   It is hard and tiring, but continuing is not terribly difficult.

  17   Very hard. It is very strenuous. You can still go on, but you really have to push yourself and you are very tired.

  19   An extremely strenuous level. For most people this is the most strenuous exercise they have ever experienced.

Try to appraise your feeling of exertion and fatigue as spontaneously and as honestly as possible, without thinking about what the actual physical load is. Try not to underestimate, nor to overestimate. It is your own feeling of effort and exertion that is important, not how it compares to other people's. Look at the scale and the expressions and then give a number. You can equally well use even as odd numbers.

Any questions?

Figure 11-14   Borg-RPE-Scale®. (Copyright Gunnar Borg, 1970, 1985, 1998.)

group settings can be powerful motivators and rein-forcers of regular exercise.

MOTIVATION AND COMPLIANCE. Compliance with physical exercise programs may be problematic for older adults. Failure to adhere to exercise programs may be a problem of motivation, and the traditional structure of supervised exercise programs may not address the highly individualized needs of older adults. Tailoring exercise regimens to meet the goals of the individual can foster motivation and commitment. Data from a study of the benefits of Tai Chi show that older adults were motivated to continue the exercise because it improved their general mental and physical well-being (Evans, 2003). It may be difficult to engage the older adult who has never been physically active.

Some strategies that have been useful in getting older adults to initiate and continue exercise regimens are the use of peer exercise partners and telephone follow-up on absentees. Frail individuals may feel safer if "beginner" classes are held in a medical setting. Once they become more confident, they may be comfortable in a community-based setting (Kinnie, Dinan, & Young, 2003). Kinnie, Dinan, and Young (2003) offer guidelines for structuring physical exercise programs successfully (Box 11-8).

Stimulate the participants' intellectual and physical capabilities through creative approaches to exercise by using music or dance. Verbal cues may enhance the older person's awareness of bodily feelings affected by exercise. For example, "I notice you're breathing more slowly now after walking than when we first started.

From Tallis, R. C., & Fillit, H. M. (2003). *Brocklehurst's textbook of geriatric medicine and gerontology* (ed 6). London: Churchill Livingstone, p. 209.

BOX 11-8 Recommendations for Safe, Successful Exercise Sessions for Elderly People

FOR TEACHERS

- Emphasize posture and technique
- Give more coaching points and repeat more often
- Give earlier warning of directional and step changes
- Break moves and instructions down into step-by-step stages
- Allow longer times for transitions
- Improve own demonstration and communication skills
- Improve own observation, analytical, and correction skills
- Improve own monitoring skills and self-monitoring skills of participants
- Have adaptations/alternatives for all exercises to cater for all functional levels
- Ensure variety
- Integrate information to educate and motivate
- Be polished, patient, punctual, and persistent

FOR PROGRAMMING

- Include older people in planning, staffing, evaluation, and promotional material
- Ensure effective preexercise assessment before participation
- Aim to include an individual functional assessment
- Offer progressive, multilevel, multiactivity programs
- Ensure that facilities meet health and safety and comfort requirements
- Keep registers, follow up absence, and offer telephone support
- Schedule socialization and individual feedback
- Provide and monitor a home exercise program
- Encourage an education program

Can you feel the difference?" Comment on the way improvements are moving the individual toward achievement of personal goals.

Structured exercise programs are not the only way to promote mobility. Encourage each individual to perform as many activities of daily living as is practical. People who can use the toilet should be given the opportunity to do so rather than using a bedpan. Simply moving from a sitting to a standing position, if done using the lower extremities without extensive assistance from the upper extremities or another person, strengthens lower extremity muscles. Standing and bearing weight retard resorption in long bones, prevent contractures, and promote blood return from the extremities. Combing one's own hair enhances shoulder flexibility and range of motion. Dressing uses fine motor coordination and helps preserve joint mobility. Walking is an excellent general conditioning exercise and should be encouraged within the limits of the individual's cardiorespiratory capacity. Encourage any individual who can walk to do so at least three times daily.

EXERCISE PROTOCOLS. Exercise programs may include isometric, isotonic, and isokinetic activities, and may use continuous/sustained or intermittent protocols. A continuous protocol uses large muscle groups for a prolonged period, resulting in a cardiovascular training response. With older adults who have low functional capacities or conditions that limit performance, such as cardiac or pulmonary disease, an intermittent protocol is more appropriate. For example, a continuous protocol might begin with 17 minutes of walking daily either in single or divided sessions. As the time is increased by 2 to 3 minutes each week, the frequency is reduced until the individual is walking 45 to 50 minutes three times a week. In contrast, an intermittent program might begin with 2 minutes of exercise followed by 1 minute of rest with the cycle being repeated three times. The exercise time is increased by 1 minute at a time based on exercise tolerance parameters until the person can exercise for 7 minutes between rest periods (Reynolds, 1999). Readiness to progress to the next level is based on the absence of signs of overexertion, return to within 5 beats per minute of resting heart rate within 5 minutes, and return to preexercise breathing rate and comfort level within 10 minutes (Reynolds, 1999).

General guidelines for exercise programs for older adults are presented in Box 11-9.

RISK FOR EXERCISE-RELATED INJURY. The potential for injury exists in all forms of exercise, and the individual's risk for sustaining various types of injury should be evaluated. The major types of injury associated with exercise include (1) cardiac events, such as myocardial ischemia, dysrhythmias, blood pressure changes, and sudden death; (2) soft tissue injury, either from muscle strain or tendon damage; (3) joint dislocation from improper handling of body parts; (4) fracture, either from stress to brittle bones or trauma from a fall; and (5) exacerbation of symptoms of preexisting chronic diseases, such as degenerative joint disease and chronic pulmonary disease.

Always evaluate when an individual should not engage in a self-care activity because the energy expenditure is too great or because the activity may actually cause harm. For example, patients in the acute phase of heart failure require assistance with activities of daily living to reduce the workload on the myocardium.

PREVENTION OF INJURY. Prevention of injury begins with preexercise evaluation for conditions that contraindicate exercise. Explain to older adults the proper use of exercise to promote joint flexibility, muscle strength, and cardiopulmonary endurance.

Individuals with unstable medical illness, electrolyte imbalances, anemia, or a recent fracture or soft tissue injury should not participate in vigorous exercise programs until cleared by the primary provider. Individuals with poorly compensated chronic disease should begin exercise in a supervised environment, in which their response to exercise can be monitored and treatment implemented promptly if needed. Some conditions require modification of an exercise program so as not to exacerbate a preexisting problem. The American Academy of Sports Medicine recommends medical clearance before increasing activity for individuals who have one or more major symptoms of cardiovascular disease or two or more risk factors for cardiovascular disease (Reynolds, 1999). In addition to vital signs and electrocardiograph monitoring, the physical therapist uses a variety of evaluation tools to establish baseline functional capacity. Preliminary exercise electrocardiograms are recommended by many to rule out silent ischemia in individuals without known cardiac disease.

To minimize the risk for injury, the best-prepared professionals should prescribe and monitor exercise. Team members who consult or directly participate in exercise program planning and implementation include exercise physiologists, occupational and physical therapists, nurses, physicians, and psychologists. Team membership and exercise programs are individualized for the unique needs and capabilities of patients. Exercise group leaders must understand basic exercise physiology and the biomechanics of exercise and must have the ability to recognize and respond promptly to signs or symptoms of complications.

Another strategy for reducing injury risk and maximizing benefit during exercise is careful monitoring of participants' performance to ensure that exercises are done correctly. Participants may require physical cues, as well as verbal instructions, particularly in the early phases of the program. Be certain that patients use proper body mechanics and body alignment. Indications of exercise intolerance are listed in Box 11-9.

BASELINE MEASUREMENTS AND GOALS. Before an exercise regimen is instituted, obtain resting pulse and respiratory rates, orthostatic blood pressures, and estimates of muscle mass and strength. These measures serve as a baseline for establishing goals for the exercise regimen and for recognizing exercise intolerance. An increasing respiratory rate may indicate either anxiety or an ineffective breathing pattern for the new exercise program. The patient may require a slower pace or instruction in deep breathing, because maintaining adequate tissue oxygenation is essential for an effective exercise program.

BOX 11-9 Guidelines for Termination of an Exercise Session

These signs and symptoms are general indicators of exercise intolerance:

- Severe breathlessness: able to speak only in two- or three-word sentences
- Drop in heart rate with an increase in or continuous steady workload greater than 10 beats per minute
- Drop in systolic blood pressure (SBP) while exercising: greater than 20 mm Hg
- Light-headedness, dizziness, pallor, cyanosis, confusion, ataxia
- Loss of muscle control or fatigue
- Onset of angina; tightness or severe pain in chest, arms, or legs
- Nausea or vomiting
- Excessive rise in blood pressure: SBP equal to or greater than 220 mm Hg or diastolic blood pressure (DBP) equal to or greater than 110 mm Hg
- Excessively large rise in heart rate: greater than 50 beats per minute increase with low-level activity
- Severe leg claudication: 8/10 on a 10/10 pain scale
- Electrocardiograph abnormalities: ST-segment changes and multifocal PVCs greater than 30% of complexes
- Failure of any monitoring equipment

From Reynolds, P. (1999). Exercise considerations for cardiopulmonary disease. In T. L. Kauffman (Ed.), *Geriatric rehabilitation manual.* New York: Churchill Livingstone, p. 201. *PVC,* Premature ventricular contraction.

Muscle mass and strength are useful guides to the strenuousness of the activity that can be tolerated. The goals and schedules for therapy must be adjusted in light of the patient's baseline performance.

PAIN AND EXERCISE. Effective management of chronic muscle and joint pain is essential for mobility and well-being. Pain relief measures must be individualized, so various interventions or combinations may be tried and evaluated to attain the best results. Pain often serves as a warning signal of tissue damage. Therefore, before beginning an exercise regimen for individuals who have mobility impairments secondary to pain, determine the location, nature, severity, and etiology of the pain, along with aggravating and alleviating factors. Interventions for individuals with angina and those with osteoarthritis would be different. Patients with coronary artery disease may be prescribed antianginal drugs. Those with pain from degenerative joint disease, disc disease, contractures, and chronic immobility may benefit from analgesics such as NSAIDs or acetaminophen taken before exercise. As the individual's mobility improves, pain is likely to diminish, resulting in further gains in mobility.

Siebens (1992) recommends the following approach to assessment and treatment of pain associated with exercise. First, acute pain syndromes can be treated with rest, but if the pain is more chronic, therapeutic exercises as prescribed by a therapist should be performed. Second, temporary soreness lasting only several hours should be treated by lowering the intensity of the exercise during the next session. If soreness persists or increases despite reduced intensity, seek medical evaluation. Residual soreness, which appears later, may last up to 3 to 4 days. Management of this type of pain is dictated by its location. Pain that is localized to a muscle will probably resolve spontaneously, and continued exercise is not contraindicated, within the patient's tolerance for discomfort. Pain localized to a joint or to the back may represent injury and should receive medical evaluation. If an individual has pain with a specific exercise, it may be a sign of overuse. The exercise should be stopped, and alternative exercises, such as isometric strengthening exercises, substituted to promote strength while the overuse syndrome is treated with rest and medication.

Siebens (1992) notes that chronic pain associated with arthritis or chronic back pain should not be a contraindication to exercise. In these disorders, movement necessary to maintain function often induces pain, but the pain is tolerable and ends when the exercise session is concluded. In these conditions, it is important to maintain muscle strength around the affected joint to prevent joint deformity.

PERCEPTUAL IMPAIRMENT AND EXERCISE.
Teaching an exercise regimen to the older adult who has perceptual impairment may be difficult. Interventions must be highly individualized, capitalizing on the older adult's remaining capabilities and support network. For example, a person with severe visual impairment may have difficulty following an exercise regimen because of difficulty remembering instructions, or fear of injury. In this situation, a tape-recorded set of instructions may help. Fears of injury related to visual impairment during an exercise program might be alleviated by a "buddy system," in which an individual with sensory impairment is consistently paired with someone who is not impaired. Another strategy to promote confidence in people with sensory impairment is to set up a group exercise session for the visually impaired that is sufficiently supervised to prevent injury.

People with hearing deficits also require modified exercise programs. Written instructions and diagrams are more appropriate, with the therapist using touch to guide the person in learning the regimen. Again, supportive family and friends are invaluable in reinforcing exercise programs. Videotaped exercises may be effective because the patient can exercise by following the tape. Group exercise may be less effective for those with hearing impairments because of the difficulty of communicating in a large and diverse group (see Box 11-6).

COGNITIVE IMPAIRMENT AND EXERCISE.
Maintaining musculoskeletal health in individuals with cognitive impairment presents a special challenge to nurses. Some people with dementing illnesses withdraw from activity, which can be the beginning of a cycle of progressive loss of musculoskeletal function. Therefore efforts to maintain physical activity should be a part of the care plan from the earliest stages of dementia. As cognitive skills diminish, exercise must be adapted to the individual's abilities. A person with mild dementia may continue to enjoy activities such as walking, golf, and swimming. Persons with moderate to severe dementia often respond to music and tend to imitate the actions of others. Therefore group exercise sessions may be effective unless an individual is disruptive. Cognitively impaired individuals should not be mixed with unimpaired persons, because they will have difficulty attending and following complex instructions. A special group for older adults with cognitive impairments may be effective, but such a group will require a much smaller leader-to-participant ratio, and the leader must be skilled in effective communication with the cognitively impaired. For the person with severe dementia who no longer participates in active exercise, the caregiver will need to perform range-of-motion exercises.

LONG-TERM IMMOBILIZATION AND EXERCISE.
Orthostatic hypotension is common after long periods of immobilization. The dizziness and instability associated with this syndrome may cause the older person to resist activity. People who have a greater than 20 mm Hg drop in diastolic blood pressure or those who experience severe dizziness with position changes should perform "stir-up" movements before attempting more strenuous exercise. A tilt table may be used or the patient may be assisted to sit at the bedside several times per day until a vertical position can be tolerated. Until baroreceptor function is reestablished, isometric and isotonic in-bed exercises may be done to increase muscle strength and joint flexibility.

Examples of exercises that may be suitable for a bed-bound older adult include the following:
- Deep breathing (slow inhalation and full exhalation)
- Neck rolls (flex neck forward, lateral flex, and rotate)
- Knee to chest (in either supine or side-lying position, bring one knee to chest, wrap arms around, hold and breathe, straighten leg slowly)
- Pelvic tilts (on back, knees bent, feet flat, tuck in abdomen, relax)
- Bridging (on back, feet flat on bed, raise hips, lower slowly)
- Head raising in prone and supine positions
- Unilateral leg lifts

- Ankle circling (or have patient "write" different numbers or letters in the air)
- Rolling from side to side
- Lying prone
- Arms straight over head of bed while lying supine
- Arms out to sides, palms up in supine position
- Hands behind head with elbows bent
- Hands at lower back

The number of repetitions and the pace of an exercise program depend on the individual's endurance and other health problems. However, the exercises just described are not strenuous and will help promote circulation and prevent contractures.

Specific recommendations for physical activity/exercise with osteoarthritis and rheumatoid arthritis are summarized in Table 11-4.

NEUROMUSCULAR IMPAIRMENT AND EXERCISE. The specific nature of the neuromuscular impairment influences the exercise regimen prescribed to prevent further loss of mobility and compensate for dysfunction. For example, individuals with hemiplegia and those with Parkinson's disease require different exercises and adaptive equipment.

ADAPTATIONS FOR IMPAIRMENTS. Adaptive equipment for patients with impaired physical mobility of musculoskeletal or neuromuscular origin must be individualized to the patient and the disorder. Splints preserve joint motion and prevent contractures. Slings hold joints in alignment, redistribute weight, and prevent dependent edema formation. Braces stabilize unsteady joints—for example, when muscles are flaccid. Walking aids—canes, walkers, and crutches—assist in maintaining balance and stability. A wide range of appliances are available. Encourage the older adult to see professionals qualified to prescribe and fit walking aids rather than choosing from their local medical equipment company, so that the most appropriate appliance is selected. Improperly fitted or used adaptive equipment may produce new problems for the older person. A study of frail older adults who had assistive devices determined that the most common reason for not using a device was a perceived lack of need (Mann, Goodall, Justiss, & Tomita, 2002). This study emphasizes the need to include patient perception in the assessment of need for such devices. Consider how often an unused walker or cane is seen collecting dust when the patient no longer needs it or simply resists

Table 11-4 *Work Group Recommendations for Exercise and Physical Activity in Adults with Arthritis*

Type of Arthritis	Type of Exercise/Program	Recommendations
Hip/knee osteoarthritis	Aerobic	30 minutes of moderate intensity physical activity or exercise (50% to 70% maximal heart rate) at least 3 days per week Aerobic activity and venue tailored to individual needs Diet modification combined with activity/exercise if overweight Education for self-management
Knee osteoarthritis	Neuromuscular rehabilitation	Lower extremity exercise program with strengthening, endurance, coordination/balance, and functional exercise Progressive program in duration, intensity, and complexity according to individual needs and preferences Movement from clinical supervision to self-directed community setting Periodic review, revision, and reinforcement

Rheumatoid arthritis	Cardiovascular and neuromuscular conditioning	Safety and dose determination on basis of initial fitness assessment
		Supervised or self-directed setting
		Periodic review, revision, reinforcement
		Cardiovascular:
		  Intensity: 60% to 85% maximal heart rate, progressively adjusted
		  Frequency: 2 to 3 times per week
		  Duration: 30 to 60 minutes
		  Mode: walk, dance, water, stationary cycle
		Neuromuscular:
		  Intensity: 50% to 80% maximal load, progressively adjusted
		  Frequency: 2 to 3 times per week
		  Volume: 8 to 10 exercises, 8 to 12 repetitions, 1 to 2 sets
		  Mode: dynamic (static)

Data from Minor, M., Stenstrom, C. H., Klepper, S. E., Hurley, M., & Ettinger, W. H. (2003). Work group recommendations: 2002 exercise and physical activity conference, St. Louis, Missouri. *Arthritis and Rheumatism, 49*(3), 453-454.

using it. The literature comparing various types of adaptive equipment to improve mobility is likely to continue to increase, and nurses should remain up to date on developments in adaptive equipment to promote mobility. A systematic review is in progress to assess whether walking aids are beneficial after stroke, and if they are, the ideal time to introduce them, which type of aid is best, and which patients benefit most from their use (Dixon & Wellwood, 2003).

Wheelchairs can be tremendous mobility enhancers, but they must be used correctly. Improper propulsion technique has been shown to cause shoulder injuries, particularly among women (Boninger et al., 2003). Some older adults lose their remaining ability to ambulate after receiving a wheelchair, and become its "prisoner." Another consequence of wheelchair use is constant upward tilting of the head, resulting in neck discomfort (Kirby, Fahie, Smith, Chester, & Macleod, 2004).

Wheelchairs must be fitted to the individual; Figure 11-15 shows the effects of poor seating. As with walking aids, wheelchairs come in many different types, and the older person deserves a professional evaluation for the wheelchair. For example, wheelchairs with elevating leg rests and proper back and seat support are essential for people who are inactive and spend many hours each day in the wheelchair. Yet elevating leg rests are not "standard" equipment on wheelchairs, and standard seats and backs are of a sling-type fabric that makes proper posture nearly impossible to maintain. Removable arm and foot rests greatly facilitate transfers and access to tabletops for patients with hemiplegia and leg amputations. These features are not standard either. Wheelchairs with one-sided drive mechanisms are available so that people with hemiplegia can propel them with relative ease. Wheelchair components that can be customized include seat height, angle, and depth; and arm rests, foot rests, and drive (one arm, two arm, motorized). Wheelchair design can be altered to promote safety using anti-tipping devices for those whose transfer techniques cause them to push back in the chair and risk tipping it backward.

Motorized wheelchairs are more available than in the past, although care must be taken to prescribe the appropriate type to maximize mobility. Scooters, power chairs, and transporters offer additional options. Some of these, such as the iBOT system, are able to climb curbs and allow the user to move about at an elevated height—a tremendous advantage in terms of interpersonal contacts, as well as IADLs. Occupational and physical therapists are valuable consultants in identifying appropriate equipment, obtaining proper fit, and instructing in proper use.

Measures to Prevent Falls. Prevention of falls requires a multifaceted approach that begins with assessment of the individual and the environment. If

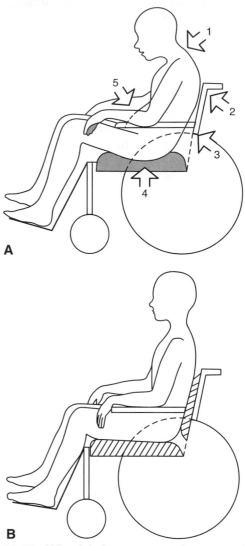

Figure 11-15 Wheelchair support and posture. **A,** Poor support creates strain of upper back and neck, pressure on scapula and sacrum, overstretching of lumbar extensors, and poor lung expansion. **B,** Proper seat and posture improve both function and appearance. (From Kottke, F. J., & Lehman, J. F. [1990]. *Krusen's handbook of physical medicine and rehabilitation* [4th ed.]. Philadelphia: Saunders, p. 554.)

the patient has a history of falls, document the circumstances and location of previous falls. Observe the patient in the home setting if possible to identify behaviors and factors that might lead to falls. Assess gait, balance, and level of fatigue with ambulation. Examine the patient's shoes and advise sturdy, supportive shoes that fit well. If the patient takes drugs that can cause orthostatic hypotension, explain the importance of changing positions slowly. If a drug is very sedating, consult with the prescriber about other options.

Consider a physical therapy evaluation to design an exercise program to improve strength, gait, and balance if appropriate. Exercises that have been shown to reduce fall risk are muscle strengthening and balance training, as well as Tai Chi (Gillespie et al., 2003; Steadman, Donaldson, & Kalra, 2003; Wu, Zhao, Zhou, & Wei, 2002). Generally, a minimum of two to three exercise sessions per week is needed to produce measureable improvement (Carter et al, 2002). Patients who have any type of mobility disability should be evaluated by an expert for use of adaptive devices. If the patient has an assistive device, observe him or her using it to be sure it is used correctly.

In any setting, especially the community, environmental obstacles can pose a threat. Since most falls occur at home, that is the place to start in creating a safer environment. Inside the home, assess lighting, furniture placement, clutter, and potentially dangerous surfaces. Specifically, look for a nightlight along the path from the bed to the bathroom. Also, check for nonslip mats and rugs in the bathroom and ease of accessibility to the tub/shower. If the patient ventures outside, examine walkways, steps, and features of the terrain that could pose a threat. For patients who are confused, safety factors are especially important because the individual lacks judgment about safety. Be sure that access to dangerous areas is controlled and that there is a safe designated area for walking. Enlist the help of relatives, friends, or community service organizations to make needed changes, including the addition of ramps and rails as needed. Rather than restricting the patient's activity, the environment should be altered to enhance it.

Because the angle of a fall affects the likelihood of a fracture, teach the patient to attempt to rotate forward or backward rather than sideways when falling (Rabinovitch, Inkster, Maurer, & Warnick, 2003). Discuss the use of hip protectors by high-risk individuals. Their effectiveness in reducing fall-related fractures is debated, but continuing improvements may support their use. Unfortunately, they often are rejected by patients who consider them uncomfortable, unattractive, and unnecessary (Patel, Ogunremi, & Chinappen, 2003).

Interventions to Promote Activities of Daily Living. Individuals with self-care deficits require assistance with ADLs. Depending on the nature of the deficit, interventions might include teaching, providing adaptive equipment, modifying the environment, supervising or assisting, positioning, or doing for the patient. Each of these approaches is discussed in the context of specific self-care deficits related to musculoskeletal disorders.

SELF-CARE DEFICIT: FEEDING. Self-feeding deficits generally fall into three categories: (1) an inability to ingest sufficient food, (2) an inability to ingest food in a socially acceptable manner, and (3) an inability to ingest food safely. The etiologies of self-feeding deficits include upper extremity sensorimotor impairments, visual impairments, apraxia, and oral-motor dysfunctions.

Teaching. Feeding problems caused by visual impairment may be partly resolved by teaching. The individual is taught to approach the meal place setting as though it were the face of a clock. The meal server can then assist the patient to locate food through a verbal description. Individuals with impaired sensation in the mouth can be taught to sweep the affected side of their mouth with their tongue to dislodge any pocketed food particles, thus reducing the danger of aspiration.

Adaptive Equipment. Patients with upper extremity impairments that interfere with self-feeding often benefit from adaptive equipment. The variety of tools available ranges from simple, easily obtained equipment, such as a drinking straw, to complex apparatus, including motor-driven orthoses. A midrange of equipment in common use includes specialized handles on cutlery for individuals with grasp problems and plate guards for people with poor coordination. Most adaptive equipment requires individualization and instruction, which are best done by an occupational therapist. It is most important that caregivers be instructed in the proper use of adaptive equipment, because misuse of the equipment can impede rather than help a person with self-feeding. For example, a plate guard, if improperly placed on the plate, obscures the patient's view of the plate, making eye-hand-mouth coordination more difficult.

Dietary Modification. Modification of the diet consistency is a common intervention for those who have oral-motor dysfunction. A softer diet is often easier to handle, because the need for extensive manipulation of the food during chewing is eliminated. In extreme cases a puréed or liquid diet may be indicated, although these should be avoided unless absolutely necessary. Food in puréed or liquid form lacks varied texture, an important ingredient in the enjoyment of food.

A useful diet modification for people with upper extremity impairments is a "finger food" menu. Individuals with coordination problems find utensils difficult to control and often messy to use.

Supervision and Assistance. When the patient has upper extremity impairments, supervision of eating is indicated. Supervision of a meal may require varying degrees of assistance—from opening containers and cutting meat to actually placing food in the patient's mouth. Even though it may take longer, it is better for patients to feed themselves if at all possible. Consult with the person who prepares the patient's meals to obtain food that the patient can manage most easily.

Some institutional facilities manage the labor intensiveness of supervision during meals by placing those who require supervision in one dining area and assigning one staff member to provide assistance as needed during the meal. This type of group arrangement can also be used to assess patients with new onset of dysphagia or self-care deficit in eating. Staff members assigned to supervise this area should be knowledgeable about positioning techniques, correct use of adaptive equipment, and use of physical and verbal cues to enhance independence. In addition, staff members should be skilled in providing first aid for choking and aspiration.

Positioning. Proper positioning is essential for safe and comfortable eating. Individuals who have difficulty positioning themselves or maintaining postural control are at risk for aspiration of food during a meal. Some patients require repositioning more than once during a meal. The person with dysphagia should be evaluated by a speech pathologist who will recommend specific positions.

Feeding the Patient. When a patient's motor impairment prevents adequate self-feeding, the caregiver takes over this function. Feeding another person is an intervention that requires great sensitivity on the part of the caregiver. When people are fed, they have no control over the pace of feeding, the type of food ingested, or the order of solid and liquid foods. Few if any people enjoy being fed. Therefore try to make the meal as normal and unhurried as possible. Do not mix dissimilar foods such as oatmeal and scrambled eggs. Using a syringe to instill food or fluid into a person's mouth is dangerous because it may cause aspiration. Engage the patient in pleasant mealtime conversation. The older adult should be assisted with oral hygiene following the meal, to promote comfort and to ensure that no food is pocketed in the mouth, where it might later be aspirated into the respiratory tract. See Chapter 8 for a more detailed discussion of feeding techniques.

SELF-CARE DEFICIT: BATHING/GROOMING.
Mobility impairments—specifically, lack of flexibility, coordination, endurance, or strength—can interfere with self-bathing. Other reasons that patients may neglect bathing and hygiene are environmental barriers, lack of awareness of poor hygiene, and poor self-esteem.

Teaching. Physical and occupational therapists can design interventions to enable the individual to bathe as independently as possible. Both the patient and caregiver require instruction in safe and thorough hygiene practices. Emphasize the importance of good hygiene to maintain skin integrity, reduce the risk of infections, and maintain self-esteem. Encourage energy-saving approaches. For example, if a tub bath is too difficult, a shower or bedside bath may be less tiring.

Adaptive Equipment. Long-handled bath sponges help those with reduced flexibility reach distal parts of the lower extremities and the back without assistance from another person. Special shower chairs and bathtub benches facilitate independent transfer to the shower or

tub. The chairs also reduce energy expenditure and risk of falling for those with limited activity tolerance. Suitably placed grab rails in the bathroom greatly enhance independence and safety of transfers. A handheld shower attachment that can also be fixed to the wall increases the number of bathing options. All equipment should have nonskid grips or bases to prevent unexpected slippage in the wet bathroom environment. Many long-term care facilities have bathing systems that consist of a whirlpool-type bathtub with a hydraulically lifted chair that puts the patient into and out of the tub.

Environmental Modification. To promote independence in bathing for the mobility-impaired person, the accessibility and safety of bathing facilities must be evaluated. If the individual uses a wheelchair or a walker, can it be maneuvered in the bathroom? Can the person reach and manipulate faucet handles and drain plugs? Is there a temperature control on the hot water heater to prevent accidental burns? Can the individual step high enough to get into a standard tub or shower? If the answer to any of these questions is no, modifications are indicated.

Supervision and Assistance. Persons with impaired balance or musculoskeletal problems may be able to bathe independently with minimal supervision or assistance. Some patients can manage washing once in the tub or shower. Others can handle some aspects of the bath, but not all. Encourage patients to do as much as possible for themselves, even if only washing their face. Offer to wash areas the patient cannot reach, such as the feet and back.

Apraxic individuals find bathing a formidable task. The complexity of such activities as undressing, running wash water, getting into the shower or tub, washing, and drying may be completely overwhelming. Caregivers can assist greatly by breaking down the massive, complex task into smaller, easier-to-manage tasks, rather than taking over and bathing the patient. Some patients require extensive verbal and physical prompting to bathe but are then able to perform the task.

Positioning. Environmental resources control the position used for bathing. Some people do not have running water in the home or accessible bathtubs. A sponge bath is the only alternative. People with activity intolerance should be "set up" for their bath, so that the bath is taken in an energy-conserving position—seated, with feet well supported. All necessary toilet items should be within easy reach.

Bathing the Patient. Bathing another person requires great sensitivity. Naked people feel extremely vulnerable. To minimize patient distress, limit exposure as much as possible, use a gentle touch, and engage the patient in conversation or talk soothingly if the patient is unable to communicate.

SELF-CARE DEFICIT: DRESSING/GROOMING.
Dressing and grooming are complex acts that require physical and cognitive skills. This section focuses on the older adult who has difficulty with dressing and grooming because of physical problems.

Teaching. Demonstrate simple methods of dressing to the patient. For example, individuals with hemiplegia will find that it is easier to dress if they begin with their affected side. Larger sizes of clothing also will simplify the task. If adapted clothing or new equipment is introduced, the older person and caregivers will probably require some instruction in its proper use.

Adaptive Equipment. A wealth of adaptive equipment and adapted clothing is available for people who have difficulty dressing themselves. An occupational therapist is an especially good resource for evaluating individual needs and teaching adaptive strategies. Examples of clothing adaptations that make dressing easier are Velcro closures instead of zippers, buttons, and shoelaces; elastic waist pants; dresses that open down the back for wheelchair-bound women; and oversized buttons. Other adaptive equipment includes long-handled shoehorns and combs, zipper pulls, and button hooks. Unfortunately, the cost of most of this equipment is not reimbursed by third-party payers. However, patients and families can be counseled to use birthdays and other celebrations for the giving of needed adapted clothing, and volunteers may be able to adapt already-purchased clothing.

Environmental Modifications. Manipulating the environment can make a significant difference in dressing behavior. If the patient is unsteady, position him or her near a grab rail or other secure device to facilitate standing, and place clothing within easy reach. Clothing stored in drawers and closets must be accessible if the patient is to select and obtain clothing. Everyday clothing should be placed in drawers that the patient can reach. A lower rod in the closet may enable the person who uses a wheelchair to reach hanging garments.

Supervision and Assistance. The verbal and physical prompting described in bathing and feeding deficits apply to supervision of dressing as well. Particularly in institutions, caregivers tend to dress residents rather than providing the time and assistance needed for self-dressing. It is better for the patient to complete this task with as little help as possible, and there is no sound rationale for rushing patients to dress. Getting dressed moves joints, uses muscles, and maintains a sense of independence. Caregivers can supervise dressing while performing other tasks such as making the bed, tidying the room, or assisting the patient's roommate.

Dressing the Patient. When a patient's efforts at dressing and grooming are too time consuming, energy consuming, or discouraging for the patient, dressing the patient is the sensible alternative. Even so, try to find ways in which the patient can participate in the task, such as choosing clothing for the day or helping with a small part, such as fastening buttons.

SELF-CARE DEFICIT: TOILETING. Impaired mobility presents a tremendous barrier to self-toileting. Patients with self-toileting deficits are at risk for skin breakdown and social stigma. For the individual patient, determine exactly what problem exists. It could be difficulty managing clothing before or after toileting, difficulty with self-cleaning, or difficulty getting to the toilet. Like other self-care deficits, toileting problems may be best managed by a team approach. Physical and occupational therapists are especially skilled at designing and teaching strategies to enable maximum possible independence in toileting. The chief interventions include toileting schedules and adaptive equipment.

Teaching. In addition to the patient, family and professional caregivers need to understand the adaptive strategies so they can assist or support the patient appropriately. Otherwise, a continent patient may be left with less desirable alternatives such as incontinence briefs.

Adaptive Equipment. Raised toilet seats and properly placed grab rails in the toilet stall are essential items for most patients with mobility problems, including those with arthritis, hemiplegia, and neurological impairments. Long-handled toilet paper holders can be obtained for those who have flexibility problems that impair the ability to perform perineal hygiene after toileting. If available, a bidet also can be used for effective perineal cleansing. If the patient is wheelchair bound, removable leg rests on the wheelchair often make transfers easier. Bedside commodes are indicated when the toilet cannot be suitably modified or the patient cannot access it. Bedside commodes, like any other piece of adaptive equipment, should be tailored to the individual's situation. Bedside commodes come in adjustable heights, and some are available with arm rests that drop down easily to facilitate transfers.

Supervision and Assistance. Toileting schedules are useful for people who are unable to get to the toilet quickly enough. More independent patients may need only a watch or clock and a written schedule; others require verbal prompting. Even with a schedule, some patients with impaired mobility will require physical assistance in toileting. Toileting schedules send a message that continence is valued and remind staff that the patient is capable of using the toilet. Unfortunately, many long-term care facilities and hospitals do not incorporate toileting into their routines. The routinization of toileting in child day care centers, where there is tremendous emphasis on toileting, could profitably be applied to institutional settings of care. In many child day care centers, before each major activity change (that

Nursing Care Plan: The Older Adult at Risk for Falls

Data

78-year-old woman seen for routine orthopedic follow-up. Only other chronic condition is hypothyroidism. Medications: levothyroxine, raloxifene.

Assessment

Height: 5 ft, 6 in. Weight: 115 lb. Lives at home with spouse of 60 years. Mother of five adult children, four of whom live within 200 miles. Patient reports good general health. Only recent hospitalization was for left total hip replacement following fracture after fall in yard 1 year ago. Before that, had fallen twice at home —once while using a chair to retrieve something from the top of a cabinet, and once when stepping over an obstacle in her home. Has smoked two packs of cigarettes daily for 50 years. Rarely drinks alcohol. Socially active. Skin is dry and thin with purpura on forearms. Range of motion is normal. Muscle strength is weak, especially in upper extremities. Some difficulty rising from chair without using arms.

Nursing Diagnoses

Risk for injury related to falls.

Goals/Outcomes

The patient will remain free of injury related to falls.

NOC Suggested Outcomes

Safety Status: Falls Occurrence
Safety Status: Physical Injury

NIC Suggested Interventions

Major interventions: Fall Prevention (6490), Surveillance: Safety (6654)
Environmental Management: Safety
Risk Identification
Optional interventions: Teaching prescribed activity/exercise
- Identify physical safety hazards in the environment.
- Remove safety hazards from the environment if possible.

- Modify the environment to minimize hazards and risk.
- Provide adaptive devices.
- Identify behaviors and factors that affect risk for falls.
- Review history of falls with patient and family.
- Monitor gait, balance, and level of fatigue with ambulation.
- Ask patient for perception of balance.
- Share with patient observations about gait and balance.
- Suggest changes in gait to patient.
- Provide assistive devices, and encourage patient to use them.
- Instruct patient in use of assistive devices.
- Teach patient how to fall to minimize injury.
- Avoid clutter on floor surface.
- Remove low-lying furniture that presents tripping hazard.
- Provide adequate lighting for increased visibility.
- Provide nightlight at bedside.
- Provide nonslip, nontrip floor surfaces.
- Provide a nonslip surface in bathtub and shower.
- Provide sturdy, nonslip step stools to facilitate easy reaches.
- Suggest safe footwear.
- Institute a physical exercise program that includes walking.
- Determine past and current level of functioning.
- Plan for risk reduction activities, in collaboration with individual.
- Use mutual goal-setting as appropriate.

Evaluation Parameters

NOC outcomes: Ambulation, balance, coordinated movement, endurance, knowledge: fall prevention, mobility, nutritional status, physical injury severity, risk control, risk detection, transfer performance.
Evidence: Evidence of accomplishment of goals might include the following: no falls, environmental hazards removed, patient uses adaptive devices as indicated, patient wears supportive nonslip shoes, patient initiates exercise program.

is, approximately every 2 hours), time is blocked in for toileting. Unfortunately, in many long-term care facilities, the emphasis is on "changing" rounds, rather than on "toileting" rounds. A change in this emphasis would do a great deal to reduce incontinence in institutions.

Interventions to Promote Nutrition. Dietary assessment, modification, and teaching may be needed to help older persons lose weight and maintain good

nutrition for musculoskeletal health. Stress the importance of calcium and other vitamins and minerals to promote strong bones. In one study of older adults with a mean age of 76.3 years, aerobic exercise and vitamin E supplementation reduced oxidative stress, reduced blood pressure and weight, and improved aerobic fitness (Jessup, Horne, Yarandi, & Quindry, 2003). When a patient does not respond to strength training exercises, inadequate caloric and protein intake may be at fault. (Kauffman, 1999). Fluid and electrolyte imbalances, especially fluid volume deficit, hypokalemia, hypophosphatemia, and hyponatremia, may be manifested as weakness.

Evaluation

Ongoing evaluation assesses the achievement of outcomes for the older adult. The outcomes of nursing management include activity tolerance, comfort level, leisure participation, IADLs, risk control, safety behavior, safety status, joint movement (active), muscle function, knowledge (diet, illness care, medication), self-care (ADLs), quality of life, self-esteem, and tissue integrity (skin and mucous membranes).

Examples of indicators of goal achievement for patients with musculoskeletal disorders include the following:

- The patient's vital signs and skin color remain within expected parameters during daily activity.
- The patient reports that discomfort related to musculoskeletal problems is relieved.
- The patient resumes previously enjoyed or new diversional activities.
- The patient accomplishes IADLs as independently as possible.
- The patient takes measures to reduce the risk of injury.
- The patient's range of motion and muscle strength are maintained or improved.
- The patient correctly describes nutritional needs, explains disease process, and describes drug therapy.
- The patient maintains ADLs with adaptations for musculoskeletal disorders.
- The patient's mobility status is maintained or improved.
- The patient verbalizes self-acceptance and acceptance of limitations.
- The patient's skin remains intact.

SUMMARY

Changes and disorders of the musculoskeletal system are associated with altered stature and posture, decreased mobility, self-care deficits, injuries, and pain in older age. Normal age-related changes include decreased height, redistribution of lean body mass and subcutaneous fat, increased porosity of bones, muscle atrophy, slowed movement, diminished strength, and stiffening of joints. Common disorders include metabolic diseases, such as osteoporosis, osteomalacia, Paget's disease, and gouty arthritis; degenerative joint diseases, such as osteoarthritis; autoimmune disorders, such as rheumatoid arthritis; and muscle disorders, such as polymyalgia rheumatica.

Nursing care takes a holistic approach to promoting mobility, comfort, and safety. Patients should be taught to increase their movement and strength through appropriate exercise, relief of pain, and use of necessary aids and adaptive devices. The physical and social environment can be modified to promote safety, mobility, and independence. Evaluation criteria include freedom from injury and improvement or maintenance of function.

REFERENCES

Addamo, S. M., & Clough, J. A. A. (1998). Modalities for mobilization. In A. B. Maher, S. W. Salmond, & T. A. Pellino (Eds.), *Orthopaedic nursing* (2nd ed.). Philadelphia: W. B. Saunders.

Administration on Aging. (2003). A statistical profile of older Americans aged 65+. Retrieved June 22, 2004, from www.aoa.gov.

Ahmad, A. M., Hopkins, M. T., Fraser, W. D., Ooi, C. G., Durham, B. H., & Vora, J. P. (2003). Parathyroid hormone secretory pattern, circulating activity, and effect on bone turnover in adult and growth hormone deficiency. *Bone, 32*(2), 170-179.

Alvarez, L., Peris, P., Guanabens, N., Vidal, S., Ros, I., Pons, F., et al. (2003). Serum osteoprotegerin and its ligand in Paget's disease of bone: Relationship to disease activity and effect of treatment with bisphosphonates. *Arthritis and Rheumatism, 48*(3), 824-828.

Alvaro-Gracia, J. M. (2004). Licofelone-clinical update on a novel LOX/COX inhibitor for the treatment of osteoarthritis. *Rheumatology, 43*(suppl 1), 121-125.

Anderson, D. L. (2004). TNF inhibitors: A new age for rheumatoid arthritis treatment. *American Journal of Nursing, 104*(2), 60-69.

Anonymous. (2002, May-June). Review: Adding newer disease-modifying drugs or biological agents to methotrexate improved rheumatoid arthritis symptoms. *ACP Journal Club, 136*(3), 97. Retrieved May 27, 2004, from http://80-gateway2.ovid.com.

Anonymous. (2003, September-October). Review: 9 drugs prevent an increase in radiographic scores of bone erosion in joints in adult rheumatoid arthritis. *ACP Journal Club, 139*(2), 46. Retrieved May 27, 2004, from http://80-gateway2.ovid.com.

Antoniades, L., MacGregor, A. J., Andrew, T., & Spector, T. D. (2003). Association of birth weight with osteoporosis and osteoarthritis in adult twins. *Rheumatology, 42*(6), 791-796.

Arnett, F. C. (2000). Rheumatoid arthritis. In L. Goldman & J. C. Bennett (Eds.), *Cecil textbook of medicine* (21st ed.). Philadelphia: Saunders.

Arthritis Foundation. (2003a, March-April). Early joint replacement may be better for hip and knee osteoarthritis. *Research Update.* Retrieved May 22, 2004, from www.arthritis.org/research/Research Update/03Mar_Apr.

Arthritis Foundation. (2003b, March-April). Prevalence and impact of hand osteoarthritis among the elderly. *Research Update.* Retrieved May 22, 2004, from www.arthritis.org/research/ResearchUpdate/03Mar_Apr.

Arthritis Foundation. (2003c, July-August). Biotechnology advances provide hope in osteoarthritis. *Research Update.* Retrieved May 22, 2004, from www.arthritis.org/research/ResearchUpdate/03July_Aug.

Arthritis Foundation. (n.d.). Arthritis Foundation research: Delivering on the promise in rheumatoid arthritis. Retrieved May 29, 2004, from www.arthritis.org/Research_Program/RA.

Assal, F., & Cummings, J. L. (2002). Neuropsychiatric symptoms in the dementias. *Current Opinion in Neurology, 15,* 445-450.

Beissner, K. L., Collins, J.E., & Holmes, H. (2000). Muscle force and range of motion as predictors of function in older adults. *Physical Therapy, 80*(6), 556-563.

Bender, I. B. (2003). Paget's disease. *Journal of Endodontics, 29*(11), 720-723.

Boninger, M. L., Dicianno, B. E., Cooper, R. A., Towers, J. D., Koontz, A. M., & Souza, A. L. (2003). Shoulder magnetic resonance imaging abnormalities, wheelchair propulsion, and gender. *Archives of Physical Medicine and Rehabilitation, 84*(11), 1615-1620.

Bonnel, R. A., Villalba, M. L., Karwoski, C. B., & Beitz, J. (2002). Deaths associated with inappropriate intravenous colchicine administration. *Journal of Emergency Medicine, 22*(4), 385-387.

Borg, G. A. (1982). Psychophysical bases of perceived exertion. *Medicine and Science in Sports and Exercise, 14*(5), 377-381.

Brach, J. S., Simonsick, E. M., Kritchevsky, S., Yaffe, K., & Newman, A. B. (2004). The association between physical function and life-style activity and exercise in the health, aging, and body composition study. *Journal of the American Geriatrics Society, 52*(4), 502-509.

Brandt, K. D. (2004). Nonsurgical treatment of osteoarthritis: A half century of "advances." *Annals of Rheumatic Disease, 63*, 117-122.

Branson, J. J., & Goldstein, W. M. (2003). Primary total hip arthroplasty. *AORN Journal, 78*(6), 946-953, 956-959, 961-969, 971-974.

Brosseau, L., Yonge, K. A., Robinson, V., Marchand, S., Judd, M., Wells, G., et al. (2003). Transcutaneous electrical nerve stimulation (TENS) for the treatment of rheumatoid arthritis in the hand. *Cochrane Database of Systematic Reviews, 3*, CD004287.

Burtner, P. A., Anderson, J. B., Marcum, M. L., Poole, J. L., Qualls, C., & Picchiarini, M. S. (2003). A comparison of static and dynamic wrist splints using electromyography in individuals with rheumatoid arthritis. *Journal of Hand Therapy, 16*(4), 320-325.

Calkins, E., & Vladutiu, A. O. (1998). Musculoskeletal disorders. In E. H. Duthie & P. R. Katz (Eds.), *Practice of geriatrics* (3rd ed.). Philadelphia: Saunders.

Calvo-Romero, J. M. (2003). Giant cell arteritis. *Postgraduate Medical Journal, 79*(935), 511-515.

Cameron, N., & Demerath, E. W. (2002). Critical periods in human growth and their relationships to diseases of aging. *American Journal of Physical Anthropology, Supplement, 35*, 159-184.

Campion, J. M., Maricic, M. J. (2003). Osteoporosis in men. *American Family Physician, 67*(7), 1521-1526.

Carter, N. D., Khan, K. M., McKay, H. A., Petit, M. A., Waterman, C., Heinonen, A., et al. (2002). Community based exercise program reduces risk factors for falls in 65 to 75 year old women with osteoporosis: Randomized controlled trial. *Canadian Medical Association Journal, 167*(9), 997-1004.

Cheng, Y. S., Wright, J. M., Walstad, W. R., & Finn, M. D. (2002). Osteosarcoma arising in Paget's disease of the mandible. *Oral Oncology, 38*(8), 785-792.

Cifuentes, M., Johnson, J. A., Lewis, R. D., Heymsfield, S. B., Chowdury, H. A., Modlesky, C. M., & Shapses, S. A. (2003). Bone turnover and body weight relationships differ in normal-weight compared with heavier postmenopausal women. *Osteoporosis International, 14*(2), 116-122.

Cremers, S. C., Eekhoff, M. E., Den Hartigh, J., Hamdy, N. A., Vermeij, P., & Papapoulos, S. E. (2003). Relationships between pharmacokinetics and rate of bone turnover after intravenous bisphosphonate (olpadronate) in patients with Paget's disease of bone. *Journal of Bone and Mineral Research, 18*(5), 868-875.

Crowe, J., & Henderson, J. (2003). Pre-arthroplasty rehabilitation is effective in reducing hospital stay. *Canadian Journal of Occupational Therapy, 70*(2), 88-96.

Dawson-Hughes, B. (2003). Interaction of dietary calcium and protein in bone health in humans. *Journal of Nutrition, 133*(3), 852S-854S.

De Goede, K. M., & Ashton-Miller, J. A. (2003). Biomechanical simulations of forward fall arrests: Effects of upper extremity arrest strategy, gender, and aging-related declines in muscle strength. *Journal of Biomechanics, 36*(3), 413-420.

de Jong, Z., Munneke, M., Zwinderman, A. H., Kroon, H. M., Jansen, A., Ronday, K. H., et al. (2003). Is a long-term high-intensity exercise program effective and safe in patients with rheumatoid arthritis? Results of a randomized controlled trial. *Arthritis and Rheumatism, 48*(9), 2415-2424.

Dhonukshe-Rutten, R. A., Lips, M., deJong, N., Chin, A., Paw, M. J., Hiddink, G. J., et al. (2003). Vitamin B_{12} status is associated with bone mineral content and bone mineral density in frail elderly women but not in men. *Journal of Nutrition, 133*(3), 801-807.

Dias, R. C., Dias, J. M., & Ramos, L. R. (2003). Impact on an exercise and walking protocol on quality of life for elderly people with OA of the knee. *Physiotherapy Research International, 8*(3), 121-130.

Dincer, H. E., Dincer, A. P., & Levinson, D. J. (2002). Asymptomatic hyperuricemia: To treat or not to treat. *Cleveland Clinic Journal of Medicine, 69*(8), 594, 597, 600-602.

Dixon, S. M., & Wellwood, I. (2003). Walking aids for reducing walking impairment and disability after stroke [protocol]. *Cochrane Database of Systematic Reviews, 2*. Retrieved June 16, 2004, from http://gateway.ut.ovid.com.libproxy.uthscsa.edu/ovidweb.cgi.

Donath, J., Krasznai, M., Fornet, B., Gergely, P., Jr., & Poor, G. (2004). Effect of bisphosphonate treatment in patients with Paget's disease of the skull. *Rheumatology, 43*(1), 89-94.

Egan, M., Brosseau, L., Farmer, M., Ouimet, M. A., Rees, S., Wells, G., et al. (2003). Splints/orthoses in the treatment of rheumatoid arthritis. *Cochrane Database of Systematic Reviews, 1*, CD004018.

Eisler, J., Gallina, J., Johnson, E., Shah, A., Wu, K., & Strauss, E. (2003). Orthopedic geriatrics. In R. C. Tallis & H. M. Fillit (Eds.), *Brocklehurst's textbook of geriatric medicine and gerontology* (6th ed.). London: Churchill Livingstone.

El-Miedany, Y. (2002). The evolving therapy of rheumatic diseases, the future is now. *Current Drug Targets—Immune, Endocrine, and Metabolic Disorders, 2*(1), 1-11.

Emkey, R., Rosenthal, N., Wu, S. C., Jordan, D., & Kamin, M. (2004). Efficacy and safety of tramadol/acetaminophen tablets (Ultracet) as add-on therapy for osteoarthritis pain in subjects receiving a COX-2 nonsteroidal anti-inflammatory drug: A multicenter, randomized, double-blind, placebo-controlled trial. *Journal of Rheumatology, 31*(1), 150-156.

Evans, C. H. (2004). Gene therapies for osteoarthritis. *Current Rheumatology Reports, 6*(1), 31-40.

Evans, C. H., Gouze, J. N., Gouze, E., Robbins, P. D., & Ghivizzani, S. C. (2004). Osteoarthritis gene therapy. *Gene Therapy, 11*(4), 379-389.

Evans, W. (2003). Exercise for successful aging. In R. C. Tallis & H. M. Fillit (Eds.), *Brocklehurst's textbook of geriatric medicine and gerontology* (6th ed.). London: Churchill Livingstone.

Felson, D. T. (2004). An update on the pathogenesis and epidemiology of osteoarthritis. *Radiologic Clinics of North America, 42*(1), 1-9.

Ferrucci, L., Bandinelli, S., Benvenuti, E., Di Iorio, A., Macchi, C., Harris, T. B., & Guralnik, J. M. (2000). Subsystems contributing to the decline in ability to walk: Bridging the gap between epidemiology and geriatric practice in the InCHIANTI study. *Journal of the American Geriatrics Society, 48*(12), 1618-1625.

Fetrow, C. W., & Avila, J. R. (2001). *Complementary and alternative medicines* (2nd ed.). Springhouse, PA: Springhouse.

Fink, H. A., Wyman, J. F., & Hanlon, J. T. (2003). Falls. In R. C. Tallis & H. M. Fillit (Eds.), *Brocklehurst's textbook of geriatric medicine and gerontology* (6th ed.). London: Churchill Livingstone.

Francis, R. (2003). Metabolic bone disease. In R. C. Tallis & H. M. Fillit (Eds.), *Brocklehurst's textbook of geriatric medicine and gerontology* (6th ed.). London: Churchill Livingstone.

Frearson, R., Cassidy, T., & Newton, J. (2003). Polymyalgia rheumatica and temporal arteritis: Evidence and guidelines for diagnosis and management in older people. *Age and Aging, 32*(4), 370-374.

Fried L, P., & Guralnik, J. M. (1997). Disability in older adults: Evidence regarding significance, etiology, and risk. *Journal of the American Geriatrics Society. 45*(1), 92-100.

Frontera, W. R., & Larsson, L. (1999). Skeletal muscle function in older people. In T. L. Kauffman (Ed.), *Geriatric rehabilitation manual*. New York: Churchill Livingstone.

Geller, S. E., & Derman, R. (2001). Knowledge, beliefs, and risk factors for osteoporosis among African-American and Hispanic women. *Journal of the National Medical Association, 93*(1), 13-21.

Ghinoi, V., & Brandi, M. L. (2002). Clodronate: Mechanisms of action on bone remodeling and clinical use in osteometabolic disorders. *Expert Opinion in Pharmacotherapy, 3*(11), 1643-1656.

Gillespie, L. D., Gillespie, W. J., Robertson, M. C., Lamb, S. E., Cumming, R. G., & Rowe, B. H. (2003). Interventions for preventing falls in elderly people. *Cochrane Database of Systematic Reviews, 1.*

Graham, D. Y. (2002). What the gastroenterologist should know about gastrointestinal safety profiles of bisphosphonates. *Digestive Diseases and Sciences, 47*(8), 1665-1678.

Gray, S. L., Penninx, B. W., Blough, D. K., Artz, M. B., Guralnik, J. M., Wallace, R. B., et al. (2003). Benzodiazepine use and physical performance in community-dwelling older women. *Journal of the American Geriatrics Society, 51*(11), 1563-1570.

Greenlund, L. J., & Nair, K. S. (2003). Sarcopenia—consequences, mechanisms, and potential therapies. *Mechanisms of Aging and Development, 124*(3), 287-299.

Greenspan, S. L., Resnick, N. M., & Parker, R. A. (2003). Combination therapy with hormone replacement and alendronate for prevention of bone loss in elderly women: A randomized controlled trial. *Journal of the American Medical Association, 289*(19), 2525-2533.

Grob, D. (1989). Common disorders of muscles in the aged. In W. Reichel (Ed.), *Clinical aspects of aging* (3rd ed.). Baltimore: Williams & Wilkins.

Guyton, A. C., & Hall, J. E. (2000). *Textbook of medical physiology* (10th ed.). Philadelphia: W. B. Saunders.

Hain, S. F., & Fogelman, I. (2002). Nuclear medicine studies in metabolic bone disease. *Seminars in Musculoskeletal Radiology, 6*(4), 323-329.

Hakkinen, A., Sokka, T., & Hannonen, P. (2004). A home-based two-year strength training period in early rheumatoid arthritis led to good long term compliance: A five year followup. *Arthritis and Rheumatism, 51*(1), 56-62.

Hammond, A., Jeffreson, P., Jones, N., Gallagher, J., & Jones, T. (2002). Clinical applicability of an educational-behavioural joint protection program for people with rheumatoid arthritis. *British Journal of Occupational Therapy, 65*(9), 405-412.

Hanley, D. A., Brown, J. P., Tenenhouse, A., Olszynski, W. P., Ioannidis, G., Gerger, C., et al. (2003). Associations among disease conditions, bone mineral density, and prevalent vertebral deformities in men and women 50 years of age and older: Cross-sectional results from the Canadian Multicentre Osteoporosis Study. *Journal of Bone and Mineral Research, 18*(4), 784-790.

Hanna, M. W. (2002). Update on hip and knee arthroplasty. *Bulletin on the Rheumatic Diseases, 51*(11). Retrieved May 22, 2004, from www.arthritis.org/research/Bulletin/vol51no11.

Helweg-Larsen, J., Tarp, B., Obel, N., & Baslund, B. (2002). No evidence of parvovirus B19, *Chlamydia pneumoniae,* or human herpes virus infection in temporal artery biopsies in patients with giant cell arteritis. *Rheumatology, 41*(4), 445-449.

Henderson, C. J. (2004). Dietary outcomes in osteoarthritis disease management. *Bulletin on the Rheumatic Diseases, 52*(12). Retrieved May 22, 2004, from www.arthritis.org/research/Bulletin/vol 52no12.

Hernandez, C. J., Beaupre, G. S., Marcus, R., & Carter, D. R. (2002). Long term predictions of the therapeutic equivalence of daily and less than daily alendronate dosing. *Journal of Bone and Mineral Research, 17*(9), 1662-1666.

Hiroyuki, S., Uchiyama, Y., & Kakurai, S. (2003). Specific effects of balance and gait exercises on physical function among the frail elderly. *Clinical Rehabilitation, 17*(5), 472-479.

Huether, S. E., & McCance, K. L. (2000). *Understanding pathophysiology* (2nd ed.). St. Louis: Mosby.

Hunder, G. G. (2000). Polymyalgia rheumatica and giant cell arteritis. In L. Goldman & J. C. Bennett (Eds.), *Cecil textbook of medicine* (21st ed.). Philadelphia: Saunders.

Jarvis, C. (2004). *Physical examination and health assessment* (4th ed.). Philadelphia: Saunders.

Jessup, J. V., Horne, C., Yarandi, H., & Quindry, J. (2003). The effects of endurance exercise and vitamin E on oxidative stress in the elderly. *Biological Research in Nursing, 5*(1), 47-55.

Jesudason, C., & Stiller, K. (2002). Are bed exercises necessary following hip arthroplasty? *Australian Journal of Physiotherapy, 48*(2), 73-81.

Joshua, F., Epstein, M., & Major, G. (2003). Bisphosphonate resistance in Paget's disease of bone. *Arthritis and Rheumatism, 48*(8), 2321-2323.

Kallin, K., Jensen, J., Olsson, L. L., Nyberg, L., & Gustafson, Y. (2004). Why the elderly fall in residential care facilities, and suggested remedies. *Journal of Family Practice, 53*(1), 41-52.

Kamienski, M. (2003). Gout: Not just for the rich and famous: Everyman's disease. *Orthopaedic Nursing, 22*(1), 16-20.

Kauffman, T. L. (1999). Muscle weakness and therapeutic exercise. In T. L. Kauffman (Ed.), *Geriatric rehabilitation manual.* New York: Churchill Livingstone.

Keen, R. W. (2003). The current status of Paget's disease of the bone. *Hospital Medicine, 64*(4), 230-232.

Kemmler, W., Engelke, K., Weineck, J., Hensen, J., & Kalender, W. A. (2003). The Erlangen fitness osteoporosis prevention study: A controlled exercise trial in early postmenopausal women with low bone density—first year results. *Archives of Physical Medicine and Rehabilitation, 84*(5), 673-682.

Kennedy-Malone, L. M., & Enevold, G. L. (2001). Assessment and management of polymyalgia rheumatica in older adults. *Geriatric Nursing, 22*(3), 152-155.

Kerstetter, J. E., O'Brien, K. O., & Insogna, K. L. (2003). Low protein intake: The impact of calcium and bone homeostasis in humans. *Journal of Nutrition, 133*(3), 855S-861S.

Kim, D. H., Silber, J. S., & Albert, T. J. (2003). Osteoporotic vertebral compression fractures. *Instructional Course Lectures, 52,* 541-550.

Kim, D. J., Yun, Y. H., & Wang, J. M. (2003). Nerve-root injections for the relief of pain in patients with osteoporotic vertebral fractures. *Journal of Bone and Joint Surgery—British Volume, 85*(2), 250-253.

Kim, K. Y., Schumacher, H. R., Hunsche, E., Wertheimer, A I., & Kong, S. X. (2003). A literature review of the epidemiology and treatment of acute gout. *Clinical Therapeutics, 25*(6), 1593-1617.

Kinnie, D. C., Dinan, S., & Young, A. (2003). Health promotion and physical activity. In R. C. Tallis & H. M. Fillit (Eds.), *Brocklehurst's textbook of geriatric medicine and gerontology* (6th ed.). London: Churchill Livingstone.

Kirby, R. L., Fahie, C. L., Smith, C., Chester, E. L., & Macleod, D. A. (2004). Neck discomfort of wheelchair users: Effect of neck position. *Disability and Rehabilitation, 26*(1), 9-15.

Klein, C. S., Marsh, G. D., Petrella, R. J., & Rice, C. L. (2003). Muscle fiber number in the biceps brachii muscle of young and old men. *Muscle and Nerve, 28*(1), 62-68.

Kudlacek, S., Freudenthaler, O., Weissboeck, H., Schneider, B., & Willvonseder, R. (2002). Lactose intolerance: A risk factor for reduced bone mineral density and vertebral fractures? *Journal of Gastroenterology, 37*(12), 1014-1019.

Kumar, S., & Gow, P. (2002). A survey of indications, results and complications of surgery for tophaceous gout. *New Zealand Medical Journal, 115*(1158), U109.

Lafage-Proust, M. H., Boudignon, B., & Thomas, T. (2003). Glucocorticoid-induced osteoporosis: Pathophysiological data and recent treatments. *Joint, Bone, Spine: Revue du Rhumatisme, 70*(2), 109-118.

Lajeunesse, D. (2004). The role of bone in the treatment of osteoarthritis. *Osteoarthritis Cartilage, 12*(suppl A), 534-538.

Laroche, M., Moulinier, L., Leger, P., Lefebvre, D., Mazi, A. B., & Boccalon, H. (2003). Bone mineral decrease in the leg with unilateral chronic occlusive arterial disease. *Clinical and Experimental Rheumatology, 21*(1), 103-106.

Leeb, B. F., Bird, H. A., Nesher, G., Andel, I., Hueber, W., Logar, D., et al. (2003). EULAR response criteria for polymyalgia rheumatica: Results of an initiative of the European Collaborating Polymyalgia

Rheumatica Group. *Annals of the Rheumatic Diseases, 62*(12), 1189-1194.

Lehne, R. A. (2004). *Pharmacology for nursing care* (5th ed.). Philadelphia: W. B. Saunders.

Leveille, S. G., Bean, J., Bandeen-Roche, K., Jones, R., Hochberg, M., & Guralnik, J. M. (2002). Musculoskeletal pain and risk for falls in older disabled women living in the community. *Journal of the American Geriatrics Society, 50*(4), 671-678.

Leveille, S. G., Fried, L. P., McMullen, W., & Guralnik, J. M. (2004). Advancing the taxonomy of disability in older adults. *Journal of Gerontology Series A—Biological Sciences and Medical Sciences, 59*(1), 86-93.

Leveille, S. G., Ling, S., Hochberg, M. C., Resnick, H. E., Bandeen-Roche, K. J., Won, A., & Guralnik, J. M. (2001). Widespread musculoskeletal pain and progression of disability in older disabled women. *Annals of Internal Medicine, 135*(12), 1038-1046.

Leveille, S. G., Penninx, B. W., Melzer, D., Izmirlian, G., & Guralnik, J. M. (2000). Sex differences in the prevalence of mobility disability in old age: The dynamics of incidence, recovery, and mortality. *Journals of Gerontology Series B—Psychological Sciences and Social Sciences, 55*(1), S41-S50.

Li-Tsang, C. W., Hung, L. K., & Mak, A. F. (2002). The effect of corrective splinting on flexion contracture of rheumatoid fingers. *Journal of Hand Therapy, 15*(2), 185-191.

Loeser, R. F. (2003). A stepwise approach to the management of osteoporosis. *Bulletin on the Rheumatic Diseases, 52*(5). Retrieved May 22, 2004, from www.arthritis.org/research/bulletin/Vol52No5.

Maher, A. B., Salmond, S. W., & Pellino, T. A. (1998). *Orthopedic nursing* (2nd ed.). Philadelphia: W.B. Saunders.

Mankin, H. J., & Mankin, C. J. (2003). Metabolic bone disease: An update. *Instructional Course Lectures, Harvard Medical School, 52,* 769-784.

Mann, W. C., Goodall, S., Justiss, M. D., & Tomita, M. (2002). Dissatisfaction and nonuse of assistive devices among frail elders. *Assistive technology, 14*(2), 130-139.

Marcus, R., Wang, O., Satterwhite, J., & Mitlak, B. (2003). The skeletal response to teriparatide is largely independent of age, initial bone mineral density, and prevalent vertebral fractures in postmenopausal women with osteoporosis. *Journal of Bone and Mineral Research, 18*(1), 18-23.

Marek, J. F. (2003). Degenerative disorders. In W. J. Phipps, F. D. Monahan, J. K. Sands, J. F. Marek, & M. Neighbors, *Medical-surgical nursing: Health and illness perspectives* (7th ed.). St. Louis: Mosby.

Marie, P. J. (2003). Optimizing bone metabolism in osteoporosis: Insight into the pharmacologic profile of strontium ranelate. *Osteoporosis International, 14*(suppl 3), 9-12.

Masoro, E. J. (2003). Physiology of aging. In R. C. Tallis & H. M. Fillit (Eds.), *Brocklehurst's textbook of geriatric medicine and gerontology* (6th ed.). London: Churchill Livingstone.

McAlindon, T. (2001). Glucosamine and chondroitin for osteoarthritis? *Bulletin on the Rheumatic Diseases, 50*(7). Retrieved May 22, 2004, from www.arthritis.org.

Meara, J. (2003). Parkinsonism and other movement disorders. In R. C. Tallis & H. M. Fillit (Eds.), *Brocklehurst's textbook of geriatric medicine and gerontology* (6th ed.). London: Churchill Livingstone.

Mehta, K. M., Yaffe, K., & Covinsky, K. E. (2002). Cognitive impairment, depressive symptoms, and functional decline in older people. *Journal of the American Geriatrics Society, 50*(6), 1045-1050.

Mehta, N. M., Malootian, A., & Gilligan, J. P. (2003). Calcitonin for osteoporosis and bone pain. *Current Pharmaceutical Design, 9*(32), 2659-2676.

Melzer, D., Izmirlian, G., Leveille, S. G., & Guralnik, J. M. (2001). Educational differences in the prevalence of mobility disability in old age: The dynamics of incidence, mortality, and recovery. *Journals of Gerontology Series B—Psychological Sciences and Social Sciences, 56*(5), S294-S301.

Melzer, D., Lan, T. Y., & Guralnik, J. M. (2003). The predictive validity for mortality of the index of mobility-related limitaion: Results from the EPESE study. *Age and Aging, 32*(6), 619-625.

Meunier, P. J., & Reginster, J. Y. (2003). Design and methodology of the phase 3 trials for the clinical development of strontium ranelate in the treatment of women with postmenopausal osteoporosis. *Osteoporosis International, 14*(3, suppl), 66-76.

Miller, L. A. (2003). Safety promotion and error reduction in perinatal care: Lessons from industry. *Journal of Perinatal and Neonatal Nursing, 17*(2), 128-138.

Minor, M., Stenstrom, C. H., Klepper, S. E., Hurley, M., & Ettinger, W. H. (2003). Work group recommendations: 2002 exercise and physical activity conference, St. Louis, Missouri. *Arthritis and Rheumatism, 49*(3), 453-454.

Morehead, K., & Sack, K. E. (2003). Osteoarthritis: What therapies for the disease of many causes? *Postgraduate Medicine, 114*(5), 11-17.

Morishige, K., Yamamoto, T., Sawada, K., Ohmichi, M., Tasaka, K., & Murata, Y. (2003). Etidronate and hormone replacement therapy (HRT) for postmenopausal women with osteoporosis despite HRT. *Archives of Gynecology and Obstetrics, 268*(2), 105-106.

Mosby. (2004). *Mosby's drug consult.* St. Louis: Mosby.

Moseley, J. B., O'Malley, K., Petersen, N. J., Menke, T. J., Brody, B. A., Kuykendall, D. H., Hollingsworth, J. C., Ashton, C. M., & Wray, N. P. (2002). A controlled trial of arthroscopic surgery for osteoarthritis of the knee. *New England Journal of Medicine. 347*(2), 81-88.

Myklebust, G., & Gran, J. T. (2001). Prednisolone maintenance dose in relation to starting dose in the treatment of polymyalgia rheumatica and temporal arteritis: A prospective two-year study in 273 patients. *Scandinavian Journal of Rheumatology, 30*(5), 260-267.

Naidoo, U., Goff, D. C., & Klibanski, A. (2003). Hyperprolactinemia and bone mineral density: The potential impact of antipsychotic agents. *Psychoneuroendocrinology, 28*(suppl 2), 97-108.

National Institutes of Health (NIH). (2006). Scientists and study participants gather at conference on scientific contributions of the Women's Health Inititative—The largest study of older women's health. Retrieved May 26, 2006 from www.nih.gov/news/pr/feb2006/nhlbi22.htm.

Navas, L. R., & Lyles, K. W. (1998). Osteoporosis. In E. H. Duthie & P. R. Katz (Eds.), *Practice of geriatrics* (3rd ed.). Philadelphia: W. B. Saunders.

Newman, E. D., Ayoub, W. T., Starkey, R. H., Diehl, J. M., & Wood, G. C. (2003). Osteoporosis disease management in a rural health care population: Hip fracture reduction and reduced costs in postmenopausal women after 5 years. *Osteoporosis International, 14*(2), 146-151.

Ourania, M., Yvoni, H., Christos, K., & Ionannis, T. (2003). Effects of a physical activity program: The study of selected physical abilities among elderly women. *Journal of Gerontological Nursing, 29*(7), 50-55.

Palferman, T. G. (2003, August). Principles of rheumatoid arthritis control. *Journal of Rheumatology, Supplement 67,* 10-13.

Papaioannou, A., Adachi, J. D., Winegard, K., Ferko, N., Parkinson, W., Cook, R. J., et al. (2003). Efficacy of home-based exercise for improving quality of life among elderly women with symptomatic osteoporosis-related vertebral fractures. *Osteoporosis International, 14*(8), 677-682.

Patel, S., Ogunremi, L., & Chinappen, U. (2003). Acceptability and compliance with hip protectors in community-dwelling women at high risk of hip fracture. *Rheumatology, 42*(6), 769-772.

Penninx, B. W., Deeg, D. J., van Eijk, J. T., Beekman, A. T., & Guralnik, J. M. (2000). Changes in depression and physical decline in older adults: A longitudinal perspective. *Journal of Affective Disorders, 61*(1-2), 1-12.

Penninx, B. W., Guralnik, J. M., Onder, G., Ferrucci, L, Wallace, R. B., & Pahor, M. (2003). Anemia and decline in physical performance among older persons. *American Journal of Medicine, 115*(2), 104-110.

Peris, P. (2003). Polymyalgia rheumatica is not seasonal in pattern and is unrelated to parvovirus b19 infection. *Journal of Rheumatology, 30*(12), 2624-2626.

Pollock, M. L., Franklin, B. A., Balady, G. J., Bernard, L., Fleg, J. L., Fletcher, B., et al. (2000). Resistance exercise in individuals with and without cardiovascular disease: An advisory from the Committee on Exercise, Rehabilitation, and Prevention, Council on Clinical Cardiology, American Heart Association. *Circulation, 101*(7). Retrieved June 15, 2004, from http://gateway.ut.ovid.com.libproxy.uthscsa.edu/ovidweb.cgi.

Rabinovitch, S. N., Inkster, L., Maurer, J., & Warnick, B. (2003). Strategies for avoiding hip impact during sideways falls. *Journal of Bone and Mineral Research, 18*(7), 1267-1273.

Rantanen, T., Guralnik, J. M., Ferrucci, L., Penninx, B. W., Leveille, S., Sipila, S., & Fried, L. P. (2001). Coimpairments as predictors of severe walking disability in older women. *Journal of the American Geriatrics Society, 49*(1), 21-27.

Rantanen, T., Harris, T., Leveille, S. G., Visser, M., Foley, D., Masaki, K., & Guralnik, J. M. (2000). Muscle strength and body mass index as long-term predictors of mortality in initially healthy men. *Journals of Gerontology Series A—Biological Sciences and Medical Sciences, 55*(3), M168-M173.

Rantanen, T., Volpato, S., Ferrucci, L., Heikkinen, E., Fried, L. P., & Guralnik, J. M. (2003). Handgrip strength and cause-specific and total mortality in older disabled women: Exploring the mechanism. *Journal of the American Geriatrics Society, 51*(5), 636-641.

Reid, M. C., Williams, C. S., & Gill, T. M. (2003). The relationship between psychological factors and disabling musculoskeletal pain in community-dwelling older persons. *Journal of the American Geriatrics Society, 51*(8), 1092-1098.

Rejnmark, L., Vestergaard, P., Pedersen, A. R., Heickendorff, L., Andreasen, F., & Mosekilde, L. (2003). Dose-effect relations of loop and thiazide diuretics on calcium homeostasis: A randomized, double-blinded Latin-square multiple cross-over study in postmenopausal osteopenic women. *European Journal of Clinical Investivation, 33*(1), 41-50.

Reynolds, P. (1999). Exercise considerations for cardiopulmonary disease. In T. L. Kauffman (Ed.), *Geriatric rehabilitation manual.* New York: Churchill Livingstone.

Riggs, B. L., Wahner, H. W., Seeman, E., Offord, K. P., Dunn, W. L., Mazess, R. B., Johnson, K. A., & Melton, L. J. III. (1982). Changes in bone mineral density of the proximal femur and spine with aging: Differences between the postmenopausal and senile osteoporosis syndromes. *Journal of Clinical Investigation, 70,* 716-723.

Rogers, M. J., Gordon, S., Benford, H. L., Coxon, F. P., Luckman, S. P., Monkkonen, J., & Frith, J. C. (2000). Cellular and molecular mechanisms of action of bisphosphonates. *Cancer, 88*(S12), 2961-2978.

Rostom, A., Dube, C., Wells, G., Tugwell, P., Welch, V., Jolicoeur, E., & McGowan, J. (2004). Prevention of NSAID-induced gastroduodenal ulcers. *Cochrane Database of Systematic Reviews, 2.* Retrieved May 27, 2004, from http://80-gateway2.ovid.com.

Rott, K. T., & Agudelo, C. A. (2003). Gout. *Journal of the American Medical Association, 289*(21), 2857-2860.

Rozzini, R., Frisoni, G. B., Ferrucci, L., Barbisoni, P., Sabatini, T., Ranieri, P., et al. (2002). Geriatric index of comorbidity: Validation and comparison with other measures of comorbidity. *Age and Ageing, 31*(4), 277-285.

Rubin, B. R., Burton, R., Navarra, S., Antigua, J., Londono, J., Pryhuber, K. G., et al. (2004). Efficacy and safety profile of treatment with etoricoxib 120 mg once daily compared with indomethacin 50 mg three times daily in acute gout: A randomized controlled trial. *Arthritis and Rheumatism, 50*(2), 598-606.

Saifuddin, A., & Hassan, A. (2003). Paget's disease of the spine: Unusual features and complications. *Clinical Radiology, 58*(2), 102-111.

Salvarani, C., Silingardi, M., Chirarduzzi, A., LoScocco, G., Macchioni, P., Bajocchi, G., et al. (2002). Is duplex ultrasonography useful for the diagnosis of giant-cell arteritis? *Annals of Internal Medicine, 137*(4), 232-238.

Sambrook, P. N., Kotowicz, M., Nash, P., Styles, C. B., Naganathan, V., Henderson-Briffa, K. N., et al. (2003). Prevention and treatment of glucocorticoid-induced osteoporosis: A comparison of calcitriol, vitamin D plus calcium, and alendronate plus calcium. *Journal of Bone and Mineral Research, 18*(5), 919-924.

Schlesinger, N., & Schumacher, H. R., Jr. (2001). Gout: Can management be improved? *Current Opinion in Rheumatology, 13*(3), 240-244.

Schmidt, W. A., & Gromnica-Ihle, E. (2002). Incidence of temporal arteritis in patients with polymyalgia rheumatica: A prospective study using colour Doppler ultrasonography of the temporal arteries. *Rheumatology, 41*(1), 46-52.

Schnitzer, T. J. (2000). Osteoarthritis (degenerative joint disease). In L. Goldman & J. C. Bennett (Eds.), *Cecil textbook of medicine* (21st ed.). Philadelphia: Saunders.

Schultz, S. K., Ellingrod, V. L., Turvey, C., Moser, D. J., & Arndt, S. (2003). The influence on cognitive impairment and behavioral dysregulation on daily functioning in the nursing home setting. *American Journal of Psychiatry, 160,* 582-584.

Scott, D. L. (2003). Arthritis in the elderly. In R. C. Tallis & H. M. Fillit (Eds.), *Brocklehurst's textbook of geriatric medicine and gerontology* (6th ed.). London: Churchill Livingstone.

Sculco, T. P. (1998). Orthopedic disorders. In E. H. Duthie & P. R. Katz (Eds.), *Practice of geriatrics* (3rd ed.). Philadelphia: Saunders.

Seeman, E. (2003). Reduced bone formation and increased bone resorption: Rational targets for the treatment of osteoporosis. *Osteoporosis International, 14*(suppl 3), 2-8.

Seton, M., Choi, H. K., Hansen, M. F., Sebaldt, R. J., & Cooper, C. (2003). Analysis of environmental factors in familial versus sporadic Paget's disease of bone—the New England registry for Paget's disease of bone. *Journal of Bone and Mineral Research, 18*(8), 1519-1524.

Sharma, L., Cahue, S., Song, J., Hayes, K., Pai, Y. C., & Dunlop, D. (2003). Physical functioning over three years in knee osteoarthritis: Role of psychosocial, local mechanical, and neuromuscular factors. *Arthritis and Rheumatism, 48*(12), 3359-3370.

Siebens, H. (1992). Practical issues in physical medicine, rehabilitation, and pain management. In E. Calkins, A. B. Ford, & P. Katz (Eds.), *Practice of geriatrics* (2nd ed.). Philadelphia: W. B. Saunders.

Simon, J. A., Lewiecki, E. M., Smith, M. E., Petruschke, R. A., Wand, L., & Palmisano, J.J. (2002). Patient preference for once-weekly alendronate 70 mg versus once daily alendronate 10 mg: A multicenter, randomized, open-label, crossover study. *Clinical Therapeutics, 24*(11), 1871-1886.

Simonelli, C., Chen, Y. T., Morancey, J., Lewis, A. F., & Abbott, T. A. (2003). Evaluation and management of osteoporosis following hospitalization for low-impact fracture. *Journal of General Internal Medicine, 18*(1), 17-22.

Skidmore-Roth, L. (2004). *Mosby's nursing drug reference.* St. Louis: Mosby.

Smith, P., Karlson, N., & Nair, B. R. (2000). Quality use of allopurinol in the elderly. *Journal of Quality in Clinical Practice, 20*(1), 42-43.

Steadman, J., Donaldson, N., & Kalra, L. (2003). A randomized controlled trial of an enhanced balance training program to improve mobility and reduce falls in elderly patients. *Journal of the American Geriatrics Society, 51*(6), 847-852.

Stenstrom, C. H., & Minor, M. A. (2003). Evidence for the benefit of aerobic and strengthening exercise in rheumatoid arthritis. *Arthritis and Rheumatism, 49*(3), 428-434.

Tanner, S. B. (2003). Back pain, vertebroplasty, and kyphoplasty: Treatment of osteoporotic vertebral compression fractures. *Bulletin on the Rheumatic Diseases, 52*(2). Retrieved May 22, 2004, from www.arthritis.org/research/Bulletin/Vol52No2.

Thomson, A. B., Marshall, J. K., Hunt, R. H., Provenza, J. M., Lanza, F. L., Royer, M. G., et al. (2002). Fourteen day endoscopy study comparing risedronate and alendronate in postmenopausal women stratified by *Helicobacter pylori*. *Journal of Rheumatology, 29*(9), 1965-1974.

Tobias, J. H., & Sharif, M. (2003). In R. C. Tallis & H. M. Fillit (Eds.), *Brocklehurst's textbook of geriatric medicine and gerontology* (6th ed.). London: Churchill Livingstone.

Truumees, E. (2003). Medical consequences of osteoporotic vertebral compression fractures. *Instructional Course Lectures, 52,* 551-558.

U.S. Census Bureau, Census 2000. (2003). Disability status: 2000— Census 2000 brief. Retrieved June 22, 2004, from www.census .gov/hhes.

Usichenko, T. L., Ivashkivsky, O. I., & Gizhko, V. V. (2003). Treatment of rheumatoid arthritis with electromagnetic millimeter waves applied to acupuncture points—a randomized double blind clinical study. *Acupuncture and Electro-Therapeutics Research, 28*(1/2), 11-18.

van Doornum, S., & Ryan, P. F. (2000). Clinical manifestations of gout and their management. *Medical Journal of Australia, 172*(10), 493-497.

Verhagen, A. P., Bierma-Zeinstra, S. M., Cardoso, J. R., de Bie, R. A., Boers, M., & de Vet, H. C. (2003). Balenotherapy for rheumatoid arthritis. *Cochrane Database of Systematic Reviews, 4,* CD000518.

Villareal, D. T., Binder, E. F., Yarasheski, K. E., Williams, D. B., Brown, M., Sinacore, D. R., et al. (2003). Effects of exercise training added to ongoing hormone replacement therapy on bone mineral density in frail elderly women. *Journal of the American Geriatrics Society, 51*(7), 985-990.

Von Tirpitz, C., Klaus, J., Steinkamp, M., Hofbauer, L. C., Kratzer, W., Mason, R., et al. (2003). Therapy of osteoporosis in patients with Crohn's disease: A randomized study comparing sodium fluoride and ibandronate. *Alimentary Pharmacology and Therapeutics, 17*(6), 807-816.

Wang, A. W., Gilbey, H. J., & Ackland, T. R. (2002). Perioperative exercise programs improve early return of ambulatory function after total hip arthroplasty: A randomized, controlled trial. *American Journal of Physical Medicine and Rehabilitation, 81*(11), 801-806.

Wei, G. S., Jackson, J. L., & O'Malley, P. G. (2003). Postmenopausal osteoporosis risk management in primary care: How well does it adhere to national practice guidelines? *Journal of the American Medical Women's Association, 58*(2), 99-104.

Weinger, M. B., & Slagle, J. (2002). Human factors research in anesthesia patient safety: Techniques to elucidate factors affecting clinical task performance and decision making. *Journal of the American Medical Informatics Association, 9*(6, suppl), S58-S63.

Welch, V., Brosseau, L., Peterson, J., Shea, B., Tugwell, P., & Wells, G. (2004). Therapeutic ultrasound for osteoarthritis of the knee. *Cochrane Database of Systematic Reviews, 2.*

Welsh, J., Fallon, M., & Keeley, P. W. (2003). Palliative care. In R. C. Tallis & H. M. Fillit (Eds.), *Brocklehurst's textbook of geriatric medicine and gerontology* (6th ed.). London: Churchill Livingstone.

Weyand, C. M., & Goronzy, J. J. (2003). Giant cell arteritis and polymyalgia rheumatica. *Annals of Internal Medicine, 139*(6), 505-515.

Whitten, C. R., & Saifuddin, A. (2003). MRI of Paget's disease of bone. *Clinical Radiology, 58*(10), 763-769.

Wilkins , S., Jung, B., Wishart, L., Edwards, M., & Norton, S. G. (2003). The effectiveness of community-based occupational therapy education and functional training programs for older adults: A critical literature review. *Canadian Journal of Occupational Therapy, 70*(4), 214-225.

Williams, E. A., & Fye, K. H. (2003). Rheumatoid arthritis. Targeted interventions can minimize joint destruction. *Postgraduate Medicine, 114*(5), 19-28.

Wise, C. (2003-2004). The rational use of steroid injections in arthritis and nonarticular musculoskeletal pain syndromes. *Bulletin on the Rheumatic Diseases, 52*(1). Retrieved May 22, 2004, from www .arthritis.org/research/Bulletin/vol52no1.

Wortmann, R. L. (2002). Gout and hyperuricemia. *Current Opinion in Rheumatology, 14*(3), 281-286.

Wu, G., Zhao, F., Zhou, X., & Wei, L. (2002). Improvement of isokinetic knee extensor strength and reduction of postural sway in the elderly from long-term Tai Chi exercise. *Archives of Physical Medicine and Rehabilitation, 83*(10), 1364-1369.

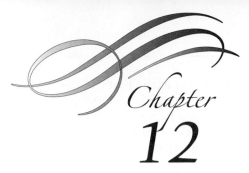

Chapter 12

Cardiovascular System

Mary Ann House-Fancher § Ronald J. Lynch

Objectives

Describe normal changes in the structure and function of the heart and blood vessels associated with aging.

Describe measures to maintain cardiovascular health in the older adult.

Explain the cause and treatment of cardiovascular disorders that are common in older persons.

Describe the components of the cardiovascular assessment in the older adult.

Formulate nursing diagnoses for older adults with cardiovascular disorders.

Develop management plans for older adults with actual or potential cardiovascular problems.

In the United States, cardiovascular disease, such as atherosclerosis and hypertension that lead to heart failure and stroke, is the leading cause of death in those age 65 years or older. Over 80% of all cardiovascular deaths occur in this age-group (American Heart Association [AHA], 2004). Thus age, per se, is the major risk factor for cardiovascular disease.

The clinical manifestations and prognosis of these cardiovascular diseases likely become altered in older persons with advanced age because interactions occur between age-associated cardiovascular changes in health and specific pathophysiological mechanisms that underlie a disease. Many studies over the last two decades have focused on cardiovascular structure and function as characterizing the multiple effects of aging on health.

AGING

The process of aging is a continuum progressing throughout a person's life. It is a process that is genetically programmed but modified by environmental influences, so the actual process of aging can vary widely among individuals. Physiological aging is characterized

by gradual loss of function in many organ systems. With aging there is also an increased incidence of coronary artery disease (CAD), peripheral vascular disease (PVD), and cerebrovascular, renal, and pulmonary diseases that accelerate the loss of function. The effects of physical conditioning can radically affect the measurements of cardiovascular function in all age-groups. Changes in physical activity, which commonly are decreased in the older adult, can profoundly change cardiovascular function. A major problem in measuring the effect of aging on cardiovascular processes is that of eliminating the effects of latent disease. This is illustrated by the prevalence of CAD in autopsy studies, in which over 60% of the patients dying at age 60 or older had at least one coronary artery that had a 70% or greater occlusion. Studies also have demonstrated that 20% of people over age 80 have asymptomatic obstructive CAD. Therefore when evaluating the findings of many studies reportedly in "healthy" older adult populations, the possibility of latent CAD must be considered (Cheitlin, 2003). The high incidence of cardiovascular diseases in the United States makes it difficult to determine normal age-related changes.

Cardiovascular changes associated with aging may result in alterations in cardiovascular physiology. The changes with age occur in everyone but not necessarily at the same rate, therefore accounting for the difference seen in some people between chronological age and physiological age. Age-related cardiovascular changes include decreased elasticity and increased stiffness of the arterial wall. This causes increased afterload of the left ventricle and increased systolic blood pressure, which results in left ventricular hypertrophy and other changes in the left ventricular wall that prolong relaxation of the left ventricle in diastole (diastolic dysfunction). There is a dramatic loss of atrial pacemaker cells, resulting in a decrease in intrinsic heart rate. Fibrosis of the cardiac skeleton may result in calcification at the base of the aortic valve and cause electrical damage to the His bundle. Finally, there is a decrease in responsiveness to beta-adrenergic receptor stimulation, a

313

decreased reactivity of baroreceptors and chemoreceptors, and an increase in circulating catecholamines. These changes set the stage for isolated systolic hypertension (ISH), diastolic dysfunction, heart failure, atrioventricular conduction defects, and aortic valve calcification (Cheitlin, 2003).

NORMAL CHANGES WITH AGING
Heart

Normal anatomical changes in the heart include an increase in a yellow-brown pigment, lipofuscin, in the myocardial fibers, producing a "brown heart." The physiological effects of this pigment have not been clearly described. Although the overall size of the heart does not increase with age, the thickness of the left ventricular free wall and ventricular septum increases, as does the overall weight. Within the myocardium, there are increases in fat, collagen, elastin, and lipofuscin, and a progressive loss of myocytes (Cheitlin, 2003). All of these factors contribute to increased stiffness and decreased myocardial contractility in the older adult's heart. The stiffness reduces diastolic compliance, thereby limiting the amount of blood that can fill the ventricles, and the reduced contractility further limits the amount of blood ejected with each heartbeat. Thus the physiological effect of these normal age-related changes is a reduction of stroke volume in the older adult.

Left ventricular hypertrophy and increased diastolic pressure, which changes coronary artery perfusion pressures responsible for subendocardial perfusion, create the potential for subendocardial ischemia and interstitial fibrosis (ventricular remodeling) (Cheitlin, 2003). Because increased left ventricular pressure also increases left atrial pressures and results in atrial dilation, the enlarged left atrium has a high risk of atrial dysrhythmias. Secondary to delayed left ventricular relaxation and the stiffer left ventricle, the importance of left atrial contraction (atrial kick) increases and the contribution of the atrial contraction to left ventricular end-diastolic volume increases (Cheitlin, 2003; Fioranelli et al., 2001). Therefore the maintenance of normal sinus rhythm in these individuals with ventricular hypertrophy (decreased diastolic function) becomes increasingly important for subendocardial perfusion.

In old age, the coronary arteries become tortuous and dilated and have areas of focal calcification. Coronary collateral vessels may also increase in number, but it is not known if this increase is related to aging alone or is a result of atherosclerosis with resultant chronic ischemia.

The cardiac valves thicken and stiffen, especially the mitral and aortic valves, which are subject to higher pressures and flows. There is some accumulation of lipids, degeneration of collagen, and calcification of the valve fibrosa at the sites of maximum movement of the valve

cusps. The increased stiffness at the bases of the aortic valve cusps might be the cause of the common ejection systolic murmur that is often heard in older persons.

With normal aging, the conduction system shows marked changes in the sinoatrial (SA) node, located in the right atrium near the vena cava. Pacemaker cells make up about 50% of the mass of the SA node in younger persons but constitute only about 10% of the mass of the SA node in the older adult. There is apoptosis of atrial pacemaker cells, with a loss of 50% to 75% of these cells by age 50 (Cheitlin, 2003). Thus the number of pacemaker cells is decreased, but the amount of fibrous tissue and fat is increased. There are only minor changes in the atrioventricular (AV) node and the right bundle branch of the conduction system with age. However, the left bundle branch passes through connective tissue that is attached to the mitral and aortic valves; the collagen there increases in density and becomes calcified, which contributes to a leftward shift of the electrical axis of the electrocardiogram (ECG) with increased age (Davies, 1992).

Electrocardiographic changes also can be demonstrated with aging. Some of these changes, such as the loss of the normal sinus rhythm and the decline in the inherent rhythmicity of the SA node, may be explained by the anatomical differences noted earlier. Other changes may be attributed to the increase in size of the left ventricle. These changes include a leftward shift in the frontal plane axis, longer PR and QT intervals, and changes in R- and S-wave amplitude (Seals, Monahan, Bell, Tanaka, & Jones., 2001). The QRS complex of adults is wider than that of children (Schwartz, 1999), but it may become somewhat narrower in the older adult. The Cardiovascular Heart Study (Furberg et al. 1992) examined ECGs of 5150 adults older than 65 years for evidence of major ECG abnormalities, which they defined as ventricular conduction defects, isolated major ST-T–wave abnormalities, left ventricular hypertrophy, atrial fibrillation, and first-degree AV block. The prevalence of any major ECG abnormality was 29% overall. However, major ECG abnormalities were found in 37% of those with a history of CAD or hypertension, compared with only 19% of those with no such history.

Atrial premature contractions increase with age and are frequent in up to 95% of older healthy volunteers at rest and during exercise in the absence of detectable cardiac disease. Atrial fibrillation is usually associated with coronary, hypertensive, valvular, or sinus node disease, or thyrotoxicosis, but may occur in older persons with no other detectable diseases (one fifth of older men and one twentieth of older women have atrial fibrillation). Isolated and even multiform ventricular ectopy has been reported in up to 80% of older men and women without detectable cardiac disease (Schwartz, 1999).

The activity of the sympathetic nervous system seems to increase with age, as suggested by higher blood levels of norepinephrine and epinephrine in older than in younger persons during any effort. Because levels of norepinephrine and epinephrine are higher, more beta-adrenergic receptors on cardiac and vascular cell surfaces are occupied. The result is a desensitization of beta-adrenergic receptors, thereby causing a down-regulation of associated intracellular signaling pathways. Such desensitization may account for all or a substantial portion of the age-associated postsynaptic reduction in responsiveness to beta-adrenergic stimulation (Seals et al., 2001). This decreased responsiveness to beta-adrenergic stimulation may cause the decreased heart rate seen during exercise, decreased responsiveness to stimulate the contractile response of the left ventricle, and changes seen in baroreceptors and aortic relaxation. This delay in arterial relaxation in response to exercise increases vascular impedance (Cheitlin, 2003). However, vasoconstriction in response to alpha-adrenergic stimulation remains intact in older persons (Aronow, 2003).

Blood Vessels

With advanced age, the aorta thickens and becomes stiffer and less distensible. The stiffness results from the following degenerative changes: (1) the aortic media thickens, as some elastic tissue is replaced with collagen; (2) calcification occurs; and (3) cholesterol is taken up into the aortic media and the other large arteries (Assey, 1993). The reduced distensibility is partly compensated for by an increase in the size of the aorta. A further compensatory mechanism is the increase in systolic blood pressure (BP), which sends blood into the larger and stiffer aorta with greater force in the older adult than in young people who have more flexible arteries. The loss of elasticity of the aorta and large arteries causes impedance to flow and an increased systemic vascular resistance, so the left ventricle pumps against a greater resistance, contributing to the hypertrophy of the left atria and ventricle (Cheitlin, 2003; Kallaras et al., 2001). This increase in left ventricular afterload causes an increased workload for the left ventricle and therefore over time increases the process of hypertrophy and diastolic dysfunction.

Other arteries also thicken and become less distensible with age. In the very young, leg arteries have been shown to be much more compliant than the aorta. By the sixth decade, the compliance of the iliac, femoral, and other peripheral arteries is the same as that of the aorta. With advancing age, the smooth muscle of the walls of the arteries becomes less responsive to beta-adrenergic stimulation and to other vasoactive hormones. This may explain the blunted cardiovascular heart rate response to the stress of exercise.

The baroreceptors, which regulate BP in various positions, are less sensitive in the older adult. A study was designed to test cardiovascular variability between cardiac output and mean arterial pressure and between mean arterial pressure and heart rate. Subjects over 70 years of age were compared with subjects in their early twenties. It was concluded that cardiac output-mean arterial pressure oscillations were not significantly synchronized or not related in a simply linear fashion. Aging not only diminished mean arterial pressure-heart rate changes with exercise, but also demonstrated that with any volume depletion there was more significant orthostatic intolerance (Guo & Schaller, 2004). This probably explains the fairly common finding of orthostatic hypotension in the older adult, as well as individual responses to vasodilator therapy (Cheitlin, 2003).

Capillary walls also show age-related changes. Capillary endothelial cells lie on a layer of collagen-like material, the basement membrane, which separates these cells from tissue cells. With age, the basement membrane thickens, which may slow the exchange of nutrients and waste products between the blood and tissues (Schwartz, 1999).

Blood

The components of the blood also change slightly with age. Blood volume is reduced owing to the drop in plasma volume. There is a 50% reduction in hemopoietic activity in persons over age 60, probably because the volume of the bone marrow is less, and some of the hemopoietic tissue is replaced by fat and connective tissue. A slight decrease in hemoglobin is present in men and women after age 60. The decline is steeper for black men, and the hemoglobin level is lower in black women of all ages. The red cell mass (mean corpuscular volume [MCV]) is slightly lower in older persons and correlates with a decrease in lean body mass; however, the survival of red blood cells remains the same. Nevertheless, red cell counts, hemoglobin, and hematocrits are within normal ranges for most older adults (Nierodzik, Sutin, & Freedman, 2003). Erythropoiesis is affected more than leukopoiesis, so there is a slight drop in the number of red blood cells and in hemoglobin and hematocrit values. In addition, the red cells have less flexibility and decreased resistance to osmotic changes. Blood coagulability is increased with age, probably because of increased platelet aggregation and decreased fibrinolytic activity. Box 12-1 indicates the changes in blood components (DeNicola & Casale, 1983).

Pumping Ability of the Heart

Both the isometric contraction phase and the relaxation time of the left ventricle are prolonged with age. The heart spends more time in the contraction phase, which provides a slightly longer systole, to more effectively squeeze out the blood from the stiffer left ventricle. Because the aged left ventricle, which is less distensible,

§ Box 12-1 *Age-Related Changes in Blood Components*

COMPONENT	CHANGE	IMPLICATIONS OF CHANGE
Erythrocytes	Reduced	Increased fatigue
Hemoglobin	Reduced	Increased fatigue
Hematocrit	Reduced	
Leukocytes	Same	
Neutrophils	Same	
Eosinophils	Same	
Basophils	Same	
Monocytes	Same	
Lymphocytes	Reduced	Decreased resistance to infection

requires a more active filling, the "atrial kick," which is the result of the contraction of the left atrium late in diastole, takes on a special importance. This may also explain another normal finding with age, a delay in early diastolic filling. The delay in normal filling time may be due to a slowing down of ventricular relaxation or to the increased stiffness of the left ventricle. The delay allows the heart more time to fill, which gives full opportunity for the active filling caused by the atrial kick and provides an adequate stroke volume in spite of the stiffness of the heart.

Formerly, many authors maintained that the left ventricular function of the normal older heart was impaired, leading to age-related reductions in cardiac output. It is now recognized that those studies were performed on older persons without proper screening for the presence of CAD. At present, cardiac physiologists believe that the systolic function of the older heart is not impaired (Cheitlin, 2003). Cardiac output at rest and with exercise is maintained by compensating for a slower heart rate with increasing left ventricular end-diastolic volume. Left ventricular wall stress remains normal in spite of the increased left ventricular diameter and increased systolic pressure because of the already present left ventricular hypertrophy (Cheitlin, 2003).

The Baltimore Longitudinal Study on Aging, which studied 61 volunteers ages 26 to 79 years who were physically active and free of cardiovascular disease, produced data that also provide evidence of normal cardiac output in the older adult. This older but classic study found that with exercise, the heart rate of older persons did not increase as much as that of young subjects, but the stroke volume did increase. As a result, the cardiac output of the older adult subjects was not significantly different from that of the young subjects (Rodeheffer & Gerstenblith, 1985). All subjects with cardiovascular disease were excluded through the use of stress ECGs and stress thallium scintigraphy.

In summary, the normal cardiovascular changes with aging include a moderate increase in blood pressure, especially systolic blood pressure; prolonged contraction time; a slow ventricular filling rate; and increased overall stiffness. There is no evidence for a specific cardiomyopathy of aging. The response of the cardiovascular system to stress, although somewhat blunted in the aged, is still more than adequate in the absence of cardiac pathology (Cheitlin, 2003).

There is a large body of evidence that biological aging is related to a series of long-term catabolic processes resulting in decreased function and structural integrity of several physiological systems, including the cardiovascular system. These changes in the aging phenotype are correlated with a decline in the amplitude of pulsatile growth hormone secretion and the resulting decrease in plasma levels of its anabolic mediator, insulin-like growth factor 1 (IGF-1). The relationship between growth hormone and biological aging is supported by studies demonstrating that growth hormone administration to old animals and humans raises plasma IGF-1 and results in increases in skeletal muscle and lean body mass, a decrease in adiposity, increased immune function, improvements in learning and memory, and increases in cardiovascular function. Since growth hormone and IGF-1 exert potent effects on the heart and vasculature (Khan, Sane, Wannenburg, & Sonntag, 2002), the relationship between age-related changes in cardiovascular function and the decline in growth hormone levels with age has become of interest and is currently under investigation.

Among the age-related changes in the cardiovascular system are decreases in myocyte number, accumulation of fibrosis and collagen, decreases in stress-induced cardiac function through deterioration of the myocardial conduction system and beta-adrenergic receptor function, decreases in exercise capacity, vessel rarefaction, decreased arterial compliance, and endothelial dysfunction leading to alterations in blood flow. Growth hormone has been found to exert potent effects on cardiovascular function in young animals and reverses many of the deficits in cardiovascular function in aged animals and humans (Khan et al., 2002).

CARDIOVASCULAR CHANGES: CAUSED BY AGE OR DISUSE?

Several studies indicate that loss of cardiovascular function may be more related to the lack of conditioning than to the effects of age. A Japanese study that controlled for the effects of aging, training, and myocardial ischemia found that all athletes, regardless of age, had the same response as young subjects. This response was a slight early rise in left ventricular end-diastolic volume and a gradual increase in myocardial contractility and heart rate. Healthy older nonathletes had a similar early response but maintained increased cardiac output only by an increased heart rate. Subjects with heart disease had different patterns of response (Mizutani, Nakano, Ote, Iwase, & Fujinami, 1984).

Aging is associated with reduced maximal aerobic capacity, cardiovascular performance during exercise, and muscle strength, which are signs of reduced physical fitness. Peak exercise capacity and peak oxygen consumption decrease with age, but individual variation is substantial (Beers & Berkow, 2000). The reductions occur at a rate of 3% to 8% per decade after the second decade of life. These reductions are due to the decreases in cardiac output, decreases in oxygen utilization, and associated deductions in muscle mass and strength. Other possible mechanisms include inefficient redistribution of blood flow to working muscles and reduced oxygen extraction and utilization per unit of muscle (Beers & Berkow, 2000).

In another study comparing younger and older males, with upright exercise there was a slower rise in heart rate in the older adult than in the younger subject. Stroke volume was maintained in the older person by an increase in end-diastolic volume through the Frank-Starling mechanism at every exercise (Cheitlin, 2003). With age, heart rate during exhaustive exercise decreases, but heart volume at end-diastole and throughout the cardiac cycle (including end-systole) is larger during exercise in older than in younger persons. Thus, in older persons, the early diastolic left ventricular filling volume increases during exercise. As a result, the end-diastolic volume, even at peak exercise, is not compromised because of a "stiff heart," and stroke volume during exercise is maintained in older persons. The 25% reduction in maximum cardiac index that occurs between ages 25 and 85 is completely due to the age-associated reduction in maximum heart rate (Beers & Berkow, 2000).

Researchers have demonstrated that factors other than age may account for the decline in aerobic power seen in older persons. These additional factors may be concurrent disease or merely physical inactivity. Steinhaus and colleagues (1988) studied 30 healthy young men (ages 20 to 31 years) and 30 healthy older men (ages 50 to 62 years). Half of the men in each group reported sedentary lifestyles in the previous 5 years, and half said they often participated in strenuous physical exercise. The researchers found that the active older men had significantly lower resting heart rates, lower resting systolic and diastolic BPs, higher maximal aerobic power, lower maximal exercise diastolic BP, and lower resting heart rates than the inactive young men. Thus the physiological profiles of the older active men were closer to those of active men who were 30 years younger than to those of older sedentary men. These findings suggest that some of the changes commonly attributed to aging are actually caused by disuse. If this is true, increasing physical exercise could ward off some of the effects of aging.

General and Cardiovascular Benefits of Increased Exercise

The Surgeon General has reported that regular participation in moderate physical activity is an essential component of a healthy lifestyle (Centers for Disease Control and Prevention [CDC], 2004). Despite evidence of the benefits (both physiological and psychological) of physical activity, few Americans engage in regular exercise. It is essential that all health care providers routinely assess and counsel patients about the frequency, duration, type, and intensity of their physical activity. All health care providers can take an active role in meeting the nation's goals of *Healthy People 2010* to improve health, fitness, and quality of life through daily activity (U.S. Department of Health and Human Services, 2002).

Participation in regular activity declines with age, with women experiencing a greater decline in older age-groups than men (Sherwood & Jeffery, 2000). Despite well-documented evidence of the benefits of physical activity, only 30% of individuals over age 65 years exercise routinely. Such inactivity leads to muscle atrophy, decreased blood volume, decreased immunity, and decreased physical fitness. Maintaining muscle mass and bone density and increasing muscle strength and flexibility reduces the risk of falls and fractures and prevents musculoskeletal disabilities. Functional ability can be increased and chronic problems can be prevented by regular physical activity among older adults.

Physical training in the elderly can produce profound improvements in the functions necessary for physical fitness (Wenger, Scheidt, & Weber, 2001). A large body of research supports the beneficial effects of exercise on strength and aerobic power in older adults. However, there may be additional, less obvious, benefits of an active lifestyle. Although further research is needed, intervention studies have shown that exercise may improve gait, balance, and physical function in the older adult. A training program can normalize glucose intolerance in older people and enhance the muscle's sensitivity to insulin. The more physically active a person is, the higher energy intake can be without risking obesity. Because the older adult is at risk for inadequate nutrition, the ability to eat more with less risk of obesity may ensure an adequate intake of essential nutrients. In addition, exercise may promote bone mineral density and thus decrease the risk of fractures in the older adult. It is also possible that regular physical activity can lessen the rate of functional decline in the older adult and possibly improve neurological functioning (Li et al., 2001; Li, Harmer, Fisher, & McAuley, 2002; Vincent et al., 2002).

How do older regular exercisers differ from their sedentary counterparts? Elward, Larson, and Wagner (1992) studied 561 randomly selected people ages 65 years and older who lived in the community. Compared with the nonexercisers, the exercisers had higher perceptions of current health and a more positive outlook regarding their health; they also had higher incomes and higher educational levels. Further, the exercisers were less likely to report having hypertension, arthritis, or two or more of the following medical conditions: heart disease, hypertension, arthritis, and emphysema. A large study of Dutch men showed that physical activity decreased with age but that total weekly physical activity and specific activators, such as gardening and walking, had favorable associations with cholesterol and systolic BP. Data from the Established Populations for Epidemiologic Studies of the Elderly (EPESE) showed that after 3 years of study, the mortality rate of those who were moderately or highly active was one half to two thirds the mortality rate of those who were inactive. The Longitudinal Study of Aging produced similar results: less activity or exercise was associated with a higher risk of mortality (Rakowski & Mor, 1992). The association between walking and reduced mortality rate was particularly strong in women.

In a review of literature including all studies pertaining to exercise and the older adult, Heath and Stuart (2002) concluded that exercise continues to be an underused therapeutic intervention for frail elders as a result of barriers created by patients themselves, their caregivers, and their health care providers. They recommended that family physicians and health care providers prescribe appropriate exercises for all patients. An exercise prescription for frail elders is based on a pragmatic strategy that makes therapeutic exercise both sustainable and safe.

The authors strongly recommended that the clinician elicit information on the patient's regular physical activity, and they provided four simple questions to use to assess activity:

1. Compared to other persons your age, would you say you are physically more active, less active, or about the same? (Follow up to determine the degree of more or less activity.)
2. Do you feel that you get as much exercise as you need, or less than you need?
3. Do you follow a regular routine of physical exercise?
4. How often do you walk a mile or more at a time, without resting? (Probe to determine the number of days per week.)

In 1992, the AHA recognized physical inactivity as a risk factor for coronary artery disease and summarized the benefits of exercise (Fletcher et al., 1992). The AHA also continues to support these benefits and continues to espouse the need for prescriptions for physical activity at all ages (AHA, 2002a). Exercise training results in decreased myocardial oxygen demand for the same level of external work; it favorably alters lipid and carbohydrate metabolism, especially if it is accompanied by weight loss; and it enhances the beneficial effects of a low–saturated fat and low-cholesterol diet. "Persons of all ages should include physical activity in a comprehensive program of health promotion and disease prevention, and should increase their habitual physical activity to a level appropriate to their capacities, needs and interest" (Fletcher et al., 1992, p. 341). The physiological advantages produced by exercise are summarized in Box 12-2.

Astrand (1992) recommended the following prescription for exercise: at least 60 minutes of physical activity daily, not necessarily vigorous, and not necessarily continuous. This regimen can be incorporated into the daily routine of such activities as moving and walking, whether for 1 minute 60 times a day, 12 minutes 5 times a day, or any combination that totals 60 minutes. Three times a week, more strenuous exercises should be performed for 30 to 45 minutes. Examples of these activities are brisk walking, jogging, cycling, swimming, and aerobic dancing. One of the best exercises for ambulatory older persons is walking.

New recommendations for physical activity have caused a shift from an exercise-fitness paradigm to a physical activity–health paradigm. Previously, it was thought that in order to achieve benefit, one had to exercise strenuously and sustain a target heart rate for at least 20 minutes, 3 times a week. Later these guidelines were changed to include 60 minutes per day, 7 days a week (as previously described). Current recommendations are to increase physical activity to a total of 30 minutes or more every day. The CDC (2004) and the American College of Sports Medicine (ACSM) now recommend 30 to 60 minutes of moderate activity (heart rate 65% of maximum, age determined) each day of the week for adults of all ages (Roitman, 2001).

Before beginning an activity program, the patient should be carefully evaluated, with emphasis on a

BOX 12-2 Effects of Habitual Physical Exercise

Increase in maximal oxygen uptake and cardiac output

Reduced heart rate at given oxygen uptake

Reduced blood pressure

Reduced heart rate $\times$ blood pressure product

Improved efficiency of heart muscle

Improved myocardial vascularization (possibly)

Favorable trend in incidences of cardiac morbidity and mortality

Increased capillary density in skeletal muscle

Increased mitochondrial density in skeletal muscle

Reduced lactate production at given percentage of maximal oxygen uptake

Reduced perceived exertion at given oxygen uptake

Enhanced ability to utilize free fatty acids as substrate during exercise, which saves glycogen

Improved endurance during exercise

Increases metabolism, which is advantageous from a nutritional viewpoint

Counteracts obesity

Increases high-density lipoprotein concentrations in blood

Improved structure and function of ligaments, tendons, and joints

Increased muscular strength

Increased production of endorphins

Enhances nerve fiber sprouting to reinnervate muscle fibers

Enhances tolerance to hot environment, resulting in increased sweat production

Reduced platelet aggregation (possibly)

Counteracts osteoporosis

Can normalize glucose tolerance

Adapted from Astrand, P. O. (1992). Why exercise? *Medicine and Science in Sports and Exercise* 24(2), 153-162.

cardiovascular, musculoskeletal, or neurological condition that would preclude exercise or require treatment before the program is begun. Box 12-3 lists guidelines for safe exercise for older adults.

Nurses should be aware that hospitalized older patients also need physical activity. A study of 500 older patients in five hospitals showed that no activity order was in effect for 13% of the 3500 patient days reviewed, and when activity was ordered, the patient activity was different from that permitted by the doctor on 41% of the days. Patients who remained in bed or a chair rarely received physical therapy, never had physician orders for exercises, and never performed exercises with the nurses (Lazarus, Murphy, Coletta, McQuade, & Culpepper, 1991). These results demonstrate the need for health care staff to consult with nurse practitioners/physician assistants and doctors to recommend and initiate activity orders.

Risk Factor Modification in the Older Adult

The leading cause of mortality and morbidity in the older adult is CAD. CAD risk factor modification has been a major focus for the primary health care provider. Hypertension, dyslipidemia, obesity, diabetes, and smoking are major risk factors in this paradigm of care and require intervention.

Hypertension

There was once a widely prevalent notion that hypertension in older adults was a "normal and natural" response to aging, and that treating it likely would lead to harm. One of the reasons for widespread acceptance of the time-honored term *essential hypertension* was the mistaken notion that vital organs (heart, brain, and kidney) require a higher pressure to function efficiently in older, hypertensive individuals. During the last 30 years, there has been an impressive body of work, from both epidemiological studies and clinical trials, showing that lowering BP in older adults is one of the most beneficial and cost-effective strategies for preventing costly cardiovascular events (strokes, myocardial infarction, heart failure, and renal failure). Although hypertension becomes more prevalent with increasing age in most developed nations, perhaps as a consequence of the reduced arterial compliance that accompanies aging, reducing elevated BP in older individuals has now become a universal recommendation in all national and international guidelines (Chobanian et al., 2003; Hiwada et al., 1999; Ramsay et al., 1999). Further, Asmar (2003) stresses that no evidence exists of an age threshold beyond which treatment is not considered beneficial. This view was supported by the findings of the Prospective Study Collaboration (PSC), which showed

BOX 12-3 Guidelines for Safe Exercise

- Pre-exercise screening should be done for any individual with a significant health problem and for people with unstable or recent cardiovascular disease.

- Absolute contraindications to physical training include recent electrocardiograph changes or myocardial infarction, unstable angina, acute congestive heart failure, third-degree heart block, and uncontrolled dysrhythmias.

- Relative contraindications are hypertension, cardiomyopathy, valvular heart disease, complex ventricular ectopy, and uncontrolled metabolic disease.

- Men over age 40 and women over age 50 should be screened before commencing vigorous activities such as jogging, tennis, or cycling.

- Preconditioning exercises may be prescribed before beginning a program of active exercise.

- The duration and intensity of exercise should be gradually increased under proper supervision.

- Because medications that affect a person's coordination, blood pressure, heart rate, or alertness may alter the response to exercise, people taking medications should ask their care provider about necessary modifications in exercises.

- A care provider should be consulted if a person experiences dizziness, light-headedness, or pain during physical activity.

- Assistive devices can improve safety and reduce energy costs during exercise for frail and very old individuals.

- Exercise may be temporarily contraindicated during treatment for hernia, cataract, retinal bleeding, and joint injury.

- To reduce the risk of injury, inactive older people should avoid:
  - Activities that unnecessarily strain the shoulders
  - Jogging on hard surfaces
  - High-impact sports
  - Sports that require sudden jerky movements (e.g., tennis)

Data from *Healthy ageing and physical activity*. (1999, January). NSW Health. State health pub. no. (HP) 980195.

that the absolute benefit of medical treatment was greater among older persons (Adab, Cheng, Jiang, Zhang, & Lam, 2003). Nevertheless, many older adults with hypertension are not being treated. One study of hypertensive non-Hispanic whites, blacks, and Hispanics ($n = 281$) revealed respective pharmacological treatment rates of 62.9%, 60.2%, and 45.2%. Even after controlling for numerous sociodemographic and health variables, the difference between Hispanics and others remained significant. Notably, lack of Medicaid insurance was characteristic of more Hispanics than the other ethnic groups (Raji, Kuo, Salazar, Satish, &, Goodwin, 2003).

Older persons with hypertension are unique because they have (1) a higher absolute risk of cardiovascular events, compared to younger individuals with the same risk factor profile, (2) higher systolic BP and a greater prevalence of isolated systolic hypertension, and (3) concomitant medical conditions that directly affect the choice of antihypertensive drug therapy (Elliott & Black, 2002).

Sufficient data have now been collected that implicate hypertension as one of the primary risk factors for cardiovascular disease. The results of many randomized clinical trials have proven the benefits of lowering BP in older hypertensive individuals. In 1994, two meta-analyses of nine treatment trials in 15,559 older hypertensives showed, compared with placebo, clear and significant reductions in stroke (35%), stroke deaths (34%), CAD events (15%), CAD deaths (25%), all cardiovascular events (29%), cardiovascular deaths (25%), and even all-cause mortality rate (12%) (Mulrow, Lau, Cornell, & Brand, 2000b). These meta-analyses drew attention to the fact that treating hypertension in older adults was much more cost-effective than treating the same level of BP in younger people (Elliot & Black, 2002).

A review of 15 studies with a total of 21,908 older adults clearly demonstrated reduced cardiovascular and overall mortality rates among individuals with either diastolic or systolic antihypertensive drug therapy. Most of these studies employed diuretics or beta blockers and were conducted in industrialized Western countries (Mulrow, Lau, Cornell, & Brand, 2000b).

Attention has shifted to treating isolated systolic hypertension (ISH), which is related to increased stiffness of large arteries and is more prevalent among older persons (Asmar, 2003). Eight treatment trials have addressed this condition, comparing active treatment with placebo; these trials included 15,693 subjects with an average initial BP of 174/83 mm Hg. Although the average BP lowering with active treatment in these studies was only 10.4/4.1 mm Hg, across all trials, drug treatment was associated with highly significant benefits. Stroke was reduced by 30%, CAD events by 23%, all cardiovascular events by 26%, and cardiovascular deaths by 13% (Staessen et al., 2000). Likewise, Waeber's (2003) review of trials in ISH concluded that lowering systolic blood pressure is associated with a decrease in cardio-vascular events, especially stroke. Patients with diabetes were found to have the greatest benefit. Adequate control of hypertension often required combination therapy.

Most authorities now recommend that before the decision to begin antihypertensive drug therapy is made, an estimate of the absolute risk of cardiovascular events be performed, based on the presence of various cardiovascular risk factors, evidence of target organ damage, or the presence of concomitant cardiovascular disease (Elliot & Black, 2002). Table 12-1 is a modification (pertaining only to older adults) of the recommendations in the Seventh Report of the Joint National Committee on Prevention, Detection, Evaluation, and Treatment (JNC7) (Chobanian et al., 2003). People with diabetes and individuals with either target organ damage or previously diagnosed cardiovascular disease should be started on drug therapy (along with lifestyle modifications) when hypertension is confirmed.

Lifestyle modification and nonpharmacological treatment should be stressed; however, there are no data showing that these changes reduce event rates or change mortality or morbidity rates (Elliot & Black, 2002). Several randomized studies have demonstrated the benefits of reducing salt intake, adopting a regular exercise habit, and keeping body weight under control (maintaining ideal body weight) (Appel et al., 1997; Kokkinos et al., 1995; Whelton et al., 1998) for people with hypertension. However, these methods alone do not reduce cardiovascular events or reach the target goal of antihypertensive therapy (Elliot & Black, 2002).

The PREMIER Study that is now in progress may shed some light on the impact of a comprehensive behavioral lifestyle intervention on BP in individuals with above optimal BP through stage 1 hypertension prevention. This study, which is supported by the National Heart, Lung and Blood Institute, is examining behavior as it relates to control of hypertension. Subjects in the multicenter randomized trial have been assigned to one of three groups: (1) advice only standard of care group, (2) standard clinical practice guidelines that include reduced sodium, increased physical activity, limited alcohol intake, and weight loss if overweight, and (3) Dietary Approaches to Stop Hypertension (DASH) diet in addition to interventions for group 2 (Svetkey et al., 2003).

Sodium restriction has long been recommended as a measure to lower BP. Several systematic reviews of research on this topic are available. A review of studies of varying durations that compared low and high sodium intake concluded that the effect of reduced sodium intake was useful in hypertensive Caucasians, but not in those with normal BP. Although too few studies of blacks and Asians were found on which to base conclusions, both of these ethnic groups appeared to respond better to reduced sodium intake. To address the question about sustained benefits of sodium reduction, He and MacGregor (2004) reviewed studies with modest salt reduction that extended over 4 weeks or more. Based on a meta-analysis, it was concluded that this strategy had a significant effect on BP in both hypertensive and normotensive individuals. This is often referred to as "salt-sensitive" hypertension.

A third review of interventions ranging from 6 months to 7 years concluded that intensive interventions provided only minimal long-term reductions in blood pressure. An important finding was that reduced sodium intake helped maintain lower BP in individuals who stopped taking antihypertensive drugs (Hooper, Bartlett, Davey Smith, & Ebrahim, 2004).

A major difference between older and younger hypertensive individuals is the greater likelihood of the presence of other concomitant medical problems. Compared to younger persons with hypertension, older individuals are more likely to have arthritis, heart failure, renal dysfunction, diabetes, dyslipidemia, osteoporosis, benign prostatic hypertrophy, and many other conditions. These

Table 12-1 *Recommended Initial Treatment and Risk Stratification in Older Individuals with Hypertension*

Diabetes, Evidence of TOD, or Previously Diagnosed CVD	Absent	Present
"High-normal" blood pressure (130-139/85-89 mm Hg)	Lifestyle modifications alone	Lifestyle modifications and antihypertensive drug therapy
Stage 1 hypertension (140-159/90-99 mm Hg)	Lifestyle modifications alone 6 months before starting antihypertensive drug therapy	Lifestyle modifications and antihypertensive drug therapy
Stage 2 or 3 hypertension (≥160/100 mm Hg)	Lifestyle modifications and antihypertensive drug therapy	Lifestyle modifications and antihypertensive drug therapy

Adapted from Chobanian, A., Bakris, G., Black, H., Cushman, W. C., Green, L. A., Izzo, J. L., et al. (2003). The seventh report of the Joint National Committee on Prevention, Detection, Evaluation and Treatment of High Blood Pressure: THE JNC report. *Journal of the American Medical Association, 289*(19), 2560-2572.
CVD, Cardiovascular disease; TOD, target organ damage.

medical problems often directly influence the choice of initial antihypertensive therapy, because it often is possible to treat both the hypertension and the other condition with a single medication (Chobanian et al., 2003). Similarly, there are some conditions for which specific antihypertensive therapy might worsen the concomitant condition. This would change the choice of the initial agent for a person affected. Some of the contraindications for specific classes of antihypertensive agents when treating older individuals are shown in Table 12-2 (Elliot & Black, 2002).

Many restrictive managed care organizations in the United States have allowed a broadening of choice of antihypertensive agents by adopting "prescribing by indication." This process requires the health care provider to note on each prescription the medical condition for which the drug is indicated. By doing so, a patient with heart failure and hypertension can be initially prescribed an angiotensin-converting enzyme (ACE) inhibitor, because it is indicated for the former condition.

First-line antihypertensive drug therapy in the elderly is usually diuretics; beta blockers are also used. Thiazide diuretics have been found to be just as efficacious for initial treatment of hypertension than other more costly medications. Both of these types of drugs have been shown in controlled trials to reduce cardiovascular morbidity and mortality rates. Alternative drugs are calcium antagonists, ACE inhibitors, alpha$_1$-receptor blockers, and alpha-beta blockers. Drug therapy should be carried out more cautiously in older patients because they may be more sensitive to volume depletion and sympathetic inhibition than are younger patients (Elliot & Black, 2002). Profound or sudden diuresis may lead to urinary retention or incontinence. Long-acting diuretics may cause excessive nocturia and insomnia. Diuretic therapy may result in hypokalemia, increased blood glucose level, and hyperuricemia, which may exacerbate concomitant problems.

Adverse reactions to antihypertensive drugs are more common in older adults. Nurses must be aware of the

Table 12-2 *Initial Drug Therapy for Hypertension in Older Individuals, According to Concomitant Medical Conditions*

Condition	Diuretic	Beta Blocker	Calcium Antagonist	ACE Inhibitor	ARB
COPD/asthma	−	− − − −	±	± or − (?)	±
Heart failure (systolic type)	+++	− − or +	+ or -	+++	++
Heart failure (diastolic type)	++	++	+ or ++	±	±
Diabetes mellitus	−	− −	+	++	+
■ Prone to hypoglycemia	±	− − −	±	++	+
■ With renal impairment	++	±	±	+++	++
■ With proteinuria	±	±	±	+++	++
Dysrhythmias	− (?)	+++	+++ or ±	+	±
Angina pectoris	+	+++	+++	+	±
Post–myocardial infarction	+(?)	+++	+ or − (?)	+ or +++	±
"Silent ischemia"	+ or − (?)	++	++	+	±
Degenerative joint disease (likely NSAID use)	− −	− −	±	− − −	− − −
Renal impairment	++	+	+	++	+
Renovascular hypertension	±	±	+	− − − −	− − − −
Benign prostatic hypertrophy	− −	−	±	±	±

+, Positive effect; −, negative effect; ?, questionable or no available data.
ACE, Angiotensin-converting enzyme; *ARB,* angiotensin receptor blocker; *COPD,* chronic obstructive pulmonary disease; *NSAID,* nonsteroidal antiinflammatory drug.

potential problems related to these drugs, such as electrolyte disturbances, glucose intolerance, depression, orthostatic hypotension, and sexual dysfunction. In addition, BP in the older adult often falls after meals. Therefore, to prevent postural hypotension, older patients should not take antihypertensives with meals. The typical strategies for treating the older adult should include starting with lower doses and titrating slowly. The end point should be treating to the goal BP. A summary of the key points about caring for hypertensive older patients is given in Box 12-4.

Because of the many potential side and adverse effects of antihypertensive drugs, numerous studies have examined quality of life among individuals who are taking these drugs on a long-term basis. The most common effects found to have an impact on quality of life were male sexual dysfunction with some diuretics; depression, memory impairment, and erectile dysfunction with nonselective beta blockers; and adverse cognitive effects with first-generation calcium channel blockers. A review by Fogari and Zoppi (2004) concluded that antihypertensive drugs in general had no negative impact on quality of life and, in some instances, even resulted in improvement. It appears that ACE inhibitors and angiotensin II receptor antagonists may have advantages in relation to cognitive function and sexual activity.

A study of the effectiveness of the ACE inhibitor perindropril in older adults who had been nonresponsive to other antihypertensive drugs demonstrated improvements in BP. Response was rated satisfactory in 73.8% of the participants; 40% of the subjects achieved pressures below 140/90 mm Hg. The effects were significant not just among older subjects, but also among blacks and individuals with ISH, concomitant cardiovascular disease, and a history of nonresponse to other ACE inhibitors (Guo et al., 2004).

Another trial assessed the efficacy of perindropril in whites and African Americans. Significant reductions were reported in both ethnic groups, with whites having a greater response. Nevertheless, 32.1% of older African Americans reached the target BP of less than 140/90 mm Hg (Cohn et al., 2004).

Calcium channel blockers effectively reduce blood pressure in older persons, and have been shown to reduce cardiovascular and cerebrovascular morbidity and mortality rates. The dihydropyridines (e.g., felodipine, nifedipine), a subcategory of calcium channel blockers, are available to accommodate patient comorbidities, though they are not recommended as first-line drugs in hypertensive individuals with heart failure. These drugs generally are well tolerated although adverse effects include edema, flushing, and headache (Israili, 2003).

According to McInnes (2003), an important advantage of angiotensin receptor blockers is that they are better tolerated than many other drugs and can be used

BOX 12-4 Key Points about Hypertension

1. Elderly hypertensive patients benefit from antihypertensive drug therapy.
2. Systolic hypertension is especially prevalent and dangerous in the elderly and should be treated even when diastolic blood pressure is below 90 mm Hg.
3. There is no absolute upper age limit for treatment of hypertension in otherwise relatively healthy elderly persons.
4. Multiple blood pressure determinations are necessary before confirming a diagnosis of hypertension in the elderly, whose blood pressure is often labile.
5. Nonpharmacologic interventions should be instituted in all hypertensive patients and should be the mainstay of therapy in those with borderline and mild hypertension.
6. Drug therapy should be initiated at lower doses and increased in smaller increments and at longer intervals in older compared with younger patients to avoid abrupt and marked falls in blood pressure.
7. Blood pressure should be monitored in the standing as well as seated or supine position in elderly patients, especially when initiating or changing drug therapy, to avoid postural hypotension. Drugs that frequently cause postural hypotension should be avoided.
8. The benefits of antihypertensive therapy have been proven only in relatively healthy, carefully selected elderly patients, and the study results may not be applicable to the frail elderly with multiple medical problems.
9. The principal therapeutic goal in the elderly is maintaining quality of life rather than extending its duration. Therefore, therapy may not be justified if troublesome side effects cannot be avoided.
10. Low doses of diuretics are almost equal in effectiveness to high doses, produce fewer symptomatic and metabolic side effects, and may be associated with improved outcomes.
11. Diuretics and β-blockers are the principal drugs used in studies of hypertension in the elderly to date. It is not known whether newer drugs such as α-blockers, calcium channel blockers, and angiotensin-converting enzyme inhibitors will produce outcomes that are better, worse, or equal to those achieved so far.
12. Step-down therapy (reduction of the number and dosage of medications) should be attempted after 6 to 12 months of successful treatment. However, complete withdrawal of treatment is rarely possible.

From Burris, J. F. (1994). Hypertension management in the elderly. *Heart Disease and Stroke 3*, 77-83. Reproduced with permission. Copyright 1994, American Heart Association.

despite comorbidities. Describing women as a neglected risk group for cardiovascular disease, Erhardt (2003) advises that some types of antihypertensive drugs, specifically angiotension receptor blockers, may be more appropriate and beneficial for women than some other types of antihypertensive agents.

For older adults with resistant ISH, Stokes (2004) recommends the use of a combination of isosorbide mononitrate with an ACE inhibitor or an angiotensin II receptor blocker. The author theorizes that the combinations address both nitric oxide deficiency and endothelial dysfunction, thereby inducing vasodilation; however, no randomized trials were detailed.

Despite an increasing number of classes of antihypertensive drugs, beta blockers and diuretics continue to play an important role in treating older persons. Moser and Setaro (2004) note that few studies have directly compared these drugs with other agents. An advantage of diuretics and beta blockers is that they are less expensive than many other antihypertensives.

Cleophas and van Marum (2003) contend that long-term beta blocker treatment may actually prevent orthostatic impairment by opposing alpha-adrenergic–mediated vasoconstriction associated with sympathetic dysfunction in older persons. Messerli and Grossman (2004) note that most studies of beta blockers have used beta$_1$-selective blockers. They contend that newer vasodilating beta blockers such as carvedilol have both alpha$_1$ and beta$_1$ effects that may increase their appropriateness in older persons.

An Italian study compared losartan and atenolol in subjects age 75 to 89 years with mild to moderate hypertension. Although the drugs were equally effective in lowering BP, only losartan was associated with significant increases in two out of three tests of memory (Fogari et al., 2003). A second study that compared valsartan with amlodipine in the treatment of ISH among older adults concluded that valsartan, used alone or with hydrochlorothiazide (HCTZ), was similar to amlodipine in efficacy, but was better tolerated (Malacco et al., 2003).When the effectiveness of valsartan and enalapril were compared in hypertensive older adults, valsartan proved to be superior in reducing BP and also was associated with improved episodic memory (Fogari et al., 2003).

Nurses must also be aware of the potential problems of older hypertensive patients. These patients are at high risk for target organ damage to the kidneys, brain, and eyes. This means that they have the potential for complications of hypertension, especially renal failure, transient ischemic attacks (TIAs), cerebrovascular accidents, cerebral hemorrhage, and retinal hemorrhage. Additional nursing diagnoses include the following: noncompliance related to negative side effects of prescribed therapy versus the belief that no treatment is needed in the absence of symptoms; ineffective individual management of therapeutic regimen related to lack of knowledge of condition, diet restrictions, medications, risk factors, and follow-up care; and risk for fluid volume deficit related to diuretic therapy (Johnson, Bulechek, Dochterman, Maas, & Moorhead, 2001).

Dyslipidemia

Should the older patient be treated as aggressively as the younger patient for dyslipidemia? In reference to primary prevention, the majority of first-time coronary events and deaths related to CAD occur in the older adult. According to the third report of the National Cholesterol Education Program (NCP ATP III) guidelines, "for primary prevention, therapeutic lifestyle changes are first line therapy for older persons. However, LDL lowering drugs can also be considered when older persons are at higher risk" (Executive Summary of the Third Report of the National Cholesterol Education Program, 2001). Studies such as the Heart Protection Study, 2002 (HPS), and the Prospective Study of Pravastatin in the Elderly at Risk (PROSPER) (Shepherd et al., 2002) included patients who were at risk but who had not suffered cardiac events. The decreased risk of future events in the older adult was similar to that observed in the younger primary prevention population studies. However, the number of events avoided is actually higher in the older adult because more events occur in this age-group. Data pertaining to primary prevention in the older adult with low high-density lipoprotein (HDL) syndrome is scarce. HDL levels of more than 60 are considered protective and reduce risk of cardiovascular events.

Secondary prevention in the older patient is much more straightforward. A multitude of studies, including HPS, 2002; the Scandinavian Simvastatin Survival Study (Miettinen et al., 1997); and the Long-Term Intervention with Pravastatin in Ischemic Disease Study (LIPID) (1998), all demonstrated significant benefit in treating low-density lipoprotein (LDL) cholesterol for secondary prevention. The overwhelming benefit of treatment in the older adult was similar to the younger cohort. The Veterans Affairs High-Density Lipoprotein Cholesterol Intervention Trial (Rubins et al., 1999) included older patients with CAD and low HDL cholesterol. The treated group had a significant reduction in events. The Third National Health and Nutrition Examination Survey (Burt et al., 1995) indicated significantly inadequate treatment of the older adult with respect to primary or secondary prevention. The survey found that patients were not being treated to goal according to the NCEP ATP III guidelines. Therapeutic lifestyle changes should be stressed in the older adult. When lipid-lowering therapy is indicated in the older adult, consider the principles outlined previously. Start with low doses and titrate slowly over time. Unless problems arise, medications should be titrated until NCEP ATP III goals are met. Assess lipid and liver profiles as recommended in the package insert. The older patient is often troubled by arthritic-type pain complaints. It is often difficult to discern arthritic complaints from myalgias potentially secondary to lipid-lowering therapy. A creatine phosphokinase (CPK) level can be checked, and if elevated, the etiology of this needs to be investigated. Often the patient will complain of myalgias and the CPK level will be within normal limits. In this situation, the lipid-lowering drug can be held for 2 to 4 weeks to assess whether the medication is responsible for the symptoms.

It is important to impress on the patient the significance of the medication in preventing future cardiovascular events. Consider resuming the medication if symptoms persist. If the medication is possibly associated with the symptoms, consider a trial of another medication in the same class. A lower dose of the medication (with a lower incidence of side effects) can be used and still attain the treatment goal.

Obesity

Obesity and sedentary lifestyle are considered significant risk factors for cardiovascular disease. Few data are available specifically addressing obesity in the older adult. However, obesity is often closely tied to dyslipidemia, hypertension, diabetes, and metabolic syndrome. This is especially true of abdominal obesity. One large study of women age 60 to 85 years confirmed that peripheral fat mass negatively correlated with atherogenic metabolic risk factors. In contrast, women with a high percentage of central fat and low percentage of peripheral fat were found to have the most severe insulin resistance—dyslipidemic syndrome and aortic calcification (Tanko, Bagger, Alexandersen, Larsen, & Christiansen, 2003).

There are no data to suggest significant variation from the rest of the population in relation to success with diet and exercise programs. A systematic review of studies that employed dieting for weight loss as a means of reducing hypertension concluded that weight reduction in overweight hypertensive individuals produced weight loss in the range of 3% to 9%. The concomitant reduction in both systolic and diastolic BP was about 3 mm Hg. Studies that compared dieting versus pharmacological therapy generally demonstrated greater increases with a stepped care approach to drug therapy than to diet (Mulrow et al., 2000a).

There is no body of evidence to support the current fad of low-carbohydrate diets in the older adult or in the general population. The Mediterranean-style diets have been studied in the secondary prevention population (de Lorgeril et al., 1999). These studies include the Lyon Diet Heart Study, the Diet and Re-infarction Trial, and the GISSI-Prevention Trial (Burr et al., 1989; Gruppo Italiano per lo Studio della Sopravvivenza nell-Infarto Miocardio, 1999). A reduction in cardiovascular events or death was noted in the treatment groups.

Diabetes Mellitus

Diabetes is the leading risk factor in the development of cardiovascular disease in the United States today. The development of this systemic disease can cause changes in lipids and potentiate the further progress of CAD, renal disease, and blindness. The management of diabetes, more than any other cardiac risk factor, requires significant collaboration with the patient and family for success. The incidence of diabetes, metabolic syndrome, and insulin resistance increases with age. Eighteen percent of the American population over 60 years of age has diabetes. From 15% to 20% of the Veterans Administration (VA) population has diabetes (CDC, 2003). Studies that address the older diabetic patient are limited. Conventional goals of treatment are the same for the older adult as the general population. The United Kingdom Prospective Diabetes Study Group, in a study reviewing types of blood sugar control, included patients only up to 65 years of age (United Kingdom Prospective Diabetes Study Group, 1995). A strategy of tighter blood sugar control was superior to conventional therapy in prevention of diabetic complications. The goal is to achieve a hemoglobin A_{1c} level of 7% or less. Lifestyle changes, including weight loss and exercise, can be of great benefit in reducing insulin sensitivity, treating metabolic syndrome, and treating diabetes. Patients should be strongly encouraged to exercise to whatever degree they are physically able. Many of the new serum glucose monitors on the market are simple to use and have large, easy-to-read numbers.

Pharmacological therapy for treatment of diabetes continues to evolve. A variety of medication strategies are available and need to be individualized to each patient. Starting with low-dose regimens with gradual titration is prudent in the older population. Hypoglycemia is especially troubling in the older adult. Differentiating symptoms of hypoglycemia from dementia is often difficult. Older patients may have erratic eating patterns, may inadvertently be noncompliant, and may be isolated from others. Thiazolidinediones may be an attractive option because of the decreased likelihood of hypoglycemia. Renal or liver impairment limits the use of metformin. Fluid retention associated with thiazolidinediones can limit their use in patients with left ventricular dysfunction. With slow titration of doses, gradual addition of medications as needed, and close monitoring; success in the management of diabetes is possible. Diabetes is discussed in detail in Chapter 17.

Orthostatic Hypotension

Although orthostatic hypotension is not strictly a disease, this symptom, which is characterized by dizziness and light-headedness on rising from a supine or seated position, is a major cause of morbidity in the older adult. It can cause confusion, falls, and a tendency to avoid activity as a result of insecurity and fear of falling. The baroreceptor reflex is intact in the older adult, but it often is blunted. Even a modest cardiovascular abnormality may produce orthostatic hypotension in a person confined to bed with a subacute or chronic illness.

Many conditions can produce this problem. Disorders of the central or peripheral nervous system, cardiovascular problems, and many medications can cause postural hypotension. Box 12-5 lists some conditions that should alert the nurse to the fact that the person may be at risk for injury related to postural hypotension.

Orthostatic hypotension is a drop in systolic BP, when moving to a standing position, of 20 to 30 mm Hg that is sustained for at least 1 to 2 minutes. Assuming an upright posture produces a pooling of blood in the lower body, which, if unopposed by autonomic responses, results in hypotension. The older adult is particularly prone to postural hypotension because of the age-related loss of elasticity of the carotid sinuses,

which combines with hypertension to reduce the sensitivity of the baroreceptors. In addition, there is a reduction in the responsiveness of the sympathetic autonomic system (as previously described). A third factor that may cause orthostatic hypotension is reduced intravascular volume. As a result of impaired sympathetic activation, the secretion of renin, vasopressin, and aldosterone declines so that more water and sodium are excreted by the kidneys (Kaufmann & Biaggioni, 2003). It is possible that individuals with orthostatic hypotension may have become volume depleted and may not be getting enough sodium in their diet. In persons older than 75 years, the prevalence of orthostatic hypotension is 30% to 45%. Cardiovascular drugs that can cause orthostatic hypotension are alpha and beta blockers, diuretics, vasodilators, and calcium channel blockers.

Treatment of the person with this problem should begin with a review of all medications being taken and must include a careful measure of BP in various positions. Ideally, the BP should be taken after the person has been lying flat for 1 hour and then after he or she has been standing for 1 or 2 minutes. Isometric exercises and elastic stockings, put on before the person gets out of bed, may help prevent orthostatic hypotension. These patients must be cautioned to get up slowly and to sit on the edge of the bed for a few minutes before standing.

BOX 12-5 Causes of Orthostatic Hypotension

Primary Autonomic Failure Syndromes
Pure autonomic failure

Multiple system atrophy (Shy Drager syndrome)

Autonomic failure associated with idiopathic Parkinson's disease, possibly aggravated by: antiparkinsonian drugs, autonomic neuropathy complicating coexisting diabetes mellitus, and drug therapy for comorbidity (e.g. vasodilators, alpha adrenergic antagonists)

Secondary Autonomic Dysfunction
Multiple sclerosis

Brainstem lesions

Compressive and noncompressive spinal cord lesions

Demyelinating polyneuropathies

Diabetic polyneuropathy

Chronic renal failure

Chronic liver disease

Connective tissue disorders

Data from Kenny, R. A., & Dey, A. B. (2003). Syncope. In R. C. Tallis and H. M. Fillit (Eds.). *Brocklehurst's textbook of geriatric medicine and gerontology* (6th ed.). London: Churchill Livingstone, pp. 441-461.

Anemia

Anemia is fairly common in the older adult, but it is not due to aging per se. Rather, it is probably due to the increase in underlying conditions, such as apathy, neglect, and dementia, which can lead to malnutrition and development of chronic infections that predispose to anemia. Although anemia may be suspected by a clinical finding of pale conjunctiva, it is easily verified by measuring the hemoglobin and hematocrit. Normal values are shown in Table 12-3. A word of caution is in order in relation to diagnosing anemia on the basis of hemoglobin and hematocrit alone. Correct interpretation assumes constant plasma volume. In fact, plasma volume is affected by many factors, including activity level, altitude, time of day, water and salt intake, plasma proteins, and diuretic and antihypertensive drugs. Inactivity initially is associated with decreased antidiuretic hormone and subsequent decrease in plasma volume; with prolonged bed rest, oxygen demand falls and erythropoiesis decreases. Suspected anemia should be further investigated with a peripheral blood smear, complete blood count, and reticulocyte count. This battery of studies usually is sufficient to determine the type of anemia. In most cases, bone marrow studies are unnecessary (Nierodzik, Sutin, & Freedman, 2003).

Even mild anemia may be a clue to an underlying disorder. Diseases that produce anemia include gastrointestinal disturbances (caused by malabsorption of

Table 12-3 *Anemia in the Elderly*

	Normal Hemoglobin	Anemic Hemoglobin	Hematocrit
Women aged 62-80	13.5 g/100	Less than 12 g/100	41%
Men aged 62-80	14.8 g/100	Less than 13 g/100	44.8%

From Adler, S. S. (1980). Anemia in the aged: Causes and considerations. *Geriatrics 35*, 49-59.

nutrients or chronic blood loss through the gastrointestinal tract), chronic inflammatory disorders, autoimmune diseases, cardiac valvular diseases or valve replacement, and drug treatment for chronic diseases. Other possible causes that should be evaluated are hemolysis, malignancy, infection, and renal disease (Nierodzik et al., 2003).

Management of anemia in the older adult depends on the underlying cause. One specific hematinic such as iron, vitamin B_{12}, folic acid, or sometimes ascorbic acid or pyridoxine is recommended instead of multiple agents. This simplifies treatment and helps confirm that the correct diagnosis has been made. If a blood transfusion is indicated (hematocrit less than 25% or hemoglobin less than 8 g/dL), precautions must be taken to prevent circulatory overload. The volume should be small (0.5 L) and delivered slowly (6 to 8 hours) (Nierodzik et al., 2003).

Atherosclerosis

Atherosclerosis, the principal cause of death in Western civilization, is a progressive systemic disease that generally begins in childhood but may not have clinical manifestations until middle to late adulthood. Our knowledge of the pathogenesis of atherosclerosis has changed greatly in the past 10 years. It is now believed that the development of advanced lesions, that is, atheromatous plaques, is a many-faceted process that requires extensive proliferation of vascular smooth muscle cells within the intima of the artery and inflammation that leads to clinical disease. Although the initial response-to-injury theory did not even hint at inflammation in the original hypothesis, it had become clear during the late 1980s and early 1990s that inflammation was as important as smooth muscle proliferation. Three fundamental biological processes are involved:

1. Proliferation of the smooth muscle cells of the intimal lining of the artery, plus accumulation of macrophages and T lymphocytes (inflammatory process)
2. Formation (by the smooth muscle cells) of large amounts of connective tissue matrix, which includes collagen, elastic fibers, and proteoglycans
3. Accumulation of lipids within the cells and the surrounding connective tissue (the lipids mainly being in the form of cholesterol esters and free cholesterol)

All of this is occurring within the intimal layer of the arterial wall (Libby, 2002a). The structure of a normal artery is shown in Figure 12-1.

The new view of atherosclerosis is that the formation of early atherosclerotic lesions involves the recruitment of monocytes and T lymphocytes. In the intima, the monocytes mature into active macrophages and trigger the production of multipotent proinflammatory cytokines, such as interleukin-1, tumor necrosis factor alpha, and CD40 ligand. The macrophages, altered to the presence of LDL cholesterol within the artery wall, turn into foam cells as they become filled with cholesterol ester. These foam cells and T lymphocytes constitute the fatty streak, the earliest form of the atherosclerotic plaque (Libby, 2002a).

The earliest signs of changes in the lumen of arteries are fatty streaks, which have been shown to be present by age 10 years. Autopsy studies of children who died of other causes have shown that these fatty streaks are located at places in the aorta and the coronary and other arteries where atheromatous plaques develop in adults, that is, at branching areas. Over many years, some of these fatty streaks may progress to foam cells filled with lipid droplets, and then to an atheromatous plaque. An advanced plaque typically contains large amounts of intimal smooth muscle cells, surrounded by collagen and elastic fibers; many, but not all, plaques

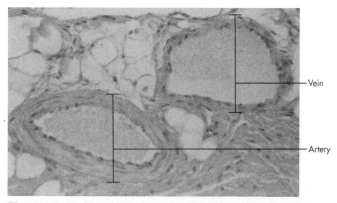

Figure 12-1 Photomicrograph showing a normal artery seen in cross-section. (From Thibodeau, G. A., & Patton, K. T. [2003]. *Anatomy & physiology* (5th ed.). St. Louis: Mosby.

also contain lipids. These lesions do not cause symptoms or clinical events until the lesion has grown to partially or totally occlude the lumen of the artery or until cracks or fissures develop in the lesions (Libby, 2002b).

The risk factors for the atherosclerotic diseases have been well established. For adults, the major risk factors are glucose intolerance, hypertension, smoking, low serum levels of HDL, high serum levels of LDL, a family history of cardiovascular disease, physical inactivity, and high fibrinogen (Kannel, 2002). Hypertension, dyslipidemia, impaired glucose tolerance, and obesity remain the major modifiable risk factors for most of the coronary disease afflicting the older adult (Kannel, 2002). The relative risk associated with these established risk factors diminishes with advancing age, but this is offset by a greater absolute and attributable risk. Diabetes is increasing alarmingly in prevalence and operates more powerfully in women, eliminating their coronary disease resistance. Interest in this entity now focuses on the insulin resistance syndrome promoted by abdominal obesity that has become so common in the older adult. The isolated systolic hypertension and large pulse pressure that predominate in the elderly are now recognized as coronary disease hazards (Kannel, 2002).

The three major categories of atherosclerotic disease are coronary, cerebral, and peripheral artery disease. All of the major risk factors are important in the development of coronary heart disease; however, for stroke, hypertension is particularly important, whereas lipids play a small role. For peripheral arterial disease, cigarette smoking and glucose intolerance are the most important risk factors. In the older adult, some risk factors are not as important as others. For instance, the impact of blood lipid levels and fibrinogen are less in the older adult. However, because the older adult has an increased overall risk of cardiovascular disease, these factors still should be considered.

Coronary Artery Disease

In developed countries, cardiovascular disease is the most common cause of death and hospitalization in the older adult, and coronary atherosclerosis is the most common underlying pathology. Autopsy data have shown that 65% to 75% of men age 50 to 80 years and 60% to 65% of women age 70 to 80 years have significant coronary stenoses (greater than 75% occlusion) (Rodeheffer & Gerstenblith, 1985), yet less than half this number have clinical evidence of coronary disease. The prevalence and severity of coronary atherosclerosis increase so dramatically with age that more than half of all deaths in people age 65 years or older are due to coronary disease and about three fourths of all deaths from ischemic heart disease occur in the older adult.

Treatment of CAD in the United States has come under the direct guidance of the AHA and the American College of Cardiology (ACC). The guidelines set forth by the AHA and the ACC for the treatment of CAD include the following: modification of risk factors (modification of these risk factors is effective in reducing the risk of atherosclerosis in older patients); use of aspirin; use of beta blockers; use of ACE inhibitors; use of lipid-lowering agents (statins); and smoking cessation.

The approach to diagnosis in the older adult is similar to that in the younger patient. The history may be somewhat more difficult to interpret because exercise may be limited by other factors, and chest discomfort may be atypical because of the prevalence of diabetes (10% of the elderly) and greater preponderance of women in the older populations. ECG criteria for the diagnosis of CAD are also not as reliable in women of any age as in men. Nuclear imaging (usually thallium) with or without pharmacological stress is often used to overcome the limits of ECG interpretation, but again is not as good in women as men (estimated 20% false positives) (Schwartz, 1999). Because the prevalence of CAD is high in older adults, the goal of diagnostic testing may be to quantify the amount of ischemia rather than to diagnosis its presence. Perfusion imaging thus allows for localization, quantification, and differentiation between infarcted and ischemic myocardium. Pharmacological stress testing combined with echocardiography may also have some advantages in the older patient because it can provide assessment of valvular function, left ventricular function, and the presence and extent of wall motion abnormalities indicative of ischemia or infarction. Other noninvasive diagnostic tests for CAD include ultrafast computed tomography, which relies on calcium scoring to determine extent of atherosclerosis, and cardiovascular magnetic resonance imaging with or without contrast, which provides distinct images of valvular structures and myocardial scarring. Angiography is of value both for assessment and as a prelude to interventions. Slightly greater complications are seen in older patients than in younger patients (local bleeding, stroke) but remain low. This should be recognized but should not preclude procedures. The risk of a procedure should be weighted against the risk of death from angina, acute coronary syndrome, and acute myocardial infarction in this older population (Schwartz, 1999). A disadvantage of coronary angiogram is that it does not reveal atheromatous plaques within vessel walls unless they impinge on the lumen. Therefore intravascular ultrasound (IVUS) sometimes is recommended to provide a more complete assessment of the state of the coronary vessels (Kendall & Nuttall, 2003).

Treatment considerations for CAD in the older patient do not differ from those in the younger patient with CAD with the exception of the elderly diabetic patient (in the elderly diabetic with multivessel disease, surgical intervention has a more favorable outcome than angioplasty) (Schwartz, 1999). The therapeutic choices include medications (nitrates, beta blockers, ACE inhibitors, and calcium channel blockers), lipid-lowering regimens (effective in both older and younger patients), antiplatelet therapy (aspirin and clopidogrel), and revascularization procedures. Note that resting heart rates should not be used as either an indication or a contraindication of beta blockade. Revascularization procedures (angioplasty, stent, or surgery) may be of greater benefit than pharmacological therapy in patients with multivessel disease and decreased left ventricular function.

Angina. Angina is chest pain caused by a temporarily insufficient supply of blood to the heart muscle. It commonly occurs with exertion, but a variant of angina occurs at rest. The incidence of angina drops after age 80, possibly because of the reduction of physical activity in the very old. The major symptoms may be similar to those seen in the young. There may be mild, pressure-like discomfort, with a suffocating, strangling, crushing, or heavy sensation located under the sternum. This sensation often radiates down the inside of the left arm, and it may or may not radiate to the right arm, neck, jaw, or throat. Because of the increased tolerance to pain, the older patient may not experience chest pain at all but may have what has been called "anginal equivalents": breathlessness, faintness, or extreme fatigue. Dyspnea is a common anginal equivalent in the older adult.

Angina may be either stable or unstable. Stable angina usually indicates a pattern of symptoms that recur in a regular fashion, rather predictably. Stable angina may occur for many years, and patients usually have medications or interventions prescribed that are effective. ECG findings of stable angina include ST segment depression in the leads associated with ischemia.

Unstable angina, or angina that is characterized by a change in frequency, type, or severity of symptoms, usually requires immediate medical attention. Pain may now occur at rest, or there may be a change in the predictability of the pain or pain relief. ECG findings also include ST segment depression in the leads consistent with ischemia. Unstable angina, or acute coronary syndrome (ACS), carries a greater risk of mortality and morbidity. ACS presents a major challenge to clinicians because of the frequency and high risk of early recurrent cardiovascular events (Braunwald, 2001). After presentation with non-ST segment elevation ACS, a patient's 6-month risk of death or recurrent nonfatal acute myocardial infarction (AMI) is approximately 10%, and the risk of death, AMI, or recurrent unstable ischemia is approximately 20% (Schwartz, 2004). At present, patients with ACS are admitted to the emergency department, triaged, diagnosed, and sent to the heart catheterization laboratory for further diagnostics and treatment, such as direct angioplasty or stent placement.

The treatment for angina pectoris in the older patient is similar to that given to younger patients. It is designed to improve the myocardial oxygen supply-demand ratio. To reduce myocardial oxygen consumption and increase coronary blood flow, sublingual, nasal, or epidermal nitroglycerin is given for attacks, and long-acting nitrates are often given to prevent or reduce the frequency of angina. Because of loss of vasomotor and baroreceptor reactivity, the older patient is more likely to have orthostatic hypotension, so a lower dose of nitrates may be indicated. Nitroglycerin should be taken in the sitting position to reduce the chance of postural hypotension. If it is taken when supine, there is an increase in venous side effects and a decrease in the desired cardiac benefits.

Long-acting nitroglycerin is frequently prescribed as a topical ointment or in the form of transdermal paste patches that are applied topically. Nurses must teach patients to remove previous patches when the next one is applied to avoid an accidental overdose. In addition, patients should be instructed to place the patch in an area that will allow for maximum absorption. Some patients put the patch on their feet, under their stockings. Although this may be convenient, it could impede absorption in patients who have peripheral vascular disease, which is associated with reduced circulation to the extremities. A better location would be the chest or the inner aspect of the upper arm. Nitroglycerin also has the property of tachyphylaxis, or dose dependency. Nitroglycerin patches are removed at night and replaced in the early morning to reduce drug tolerance.

Beta blockers, such as lopressor, metoprolol, or carvedilol, are used to decrease myocardial oxygen consumption by reducing the heart rate, BP, and myocardial contractility. Beta blockers have been shown to decrease the incidence of reinfarction and reduce postinfarction angina. Patients must be carefully monitored because resting heart rate is often lower, and the incidence of sinus and AV node dysfunction is greater in the older adult. There is a greater risk of provoking symptomatic bradyarrhythmias, including heart block, with beta blockade. The side effects, such as central nervous system depression, excessive fatigue, and hypoglycemia, may be more common in older than in younger patients.

The calcium antagonists act as direct coronary vasodilators. Verapamil (Calan, Isoptin) and diltiazem (Cardizem) are examples of calcium antagonists that have been used successfully in older patients for hypertension, as well as for myocardial ischemia. However, when the older person also has reduced left ventricular function, the use of calcium channel blockers may be restricted. These calcium antagonists increase serum digitalis levels, often requiring digitalis dosage reductions when used concurrently. Whereas verapamil and diltiazem block calcium channels in the heart, nifedipine (Procardia) does not. Therefore it has no effect on cardiac rhythm and will not exacerbate heart failure or AV block. Nifedipine is more likely than verapamil or diltiazem to cause reflex tachycardia (Lehne, 2004).

ACE inhibitors have been shown to decrease ventricular remodeling during and after myocardial ischemia. It is now recommended for any person with angina, ACS, or AMI to begin a low-dose ACE inhibitor. This class of drugs also decreases BP, vascular smooth muscle contraction, and inflammation of the endothelial layer.

Some lifestyle changes are also recommended for patients with angina. Smoking may exacerbate angina because cigarettes contain nicotine, which stimulates catecholamine release. This phenomenon increases cardiac work and myocardial irritability and causes coronary vasoconstriction and platelet aggregation. Smokers also may have high levels of carbon monoxide in their blood, which reduces the ability of the blood to deliver oxygen to the myocardium.

Patients with angina should also avoid heavy meals, cold weather, and caffeine. They should avoid emotional and physical strain. If sexual activity brings on anginal symptoms, prophylactic nitroglycerin may be used just before maximal exertion to prevent the pain. The use of Viagra has been contraindicated for patients who also require nitroglycerin for myocardial ischemia. Patients who also have chronic lung disease should be told that drugs such as sympathomimetics given for an asthma attack may aggravate angina. These agents include some over-the-counter preparations that contain beta-adrenergic drugs. Excessive thyroid replacement also may aggravate angina.

Acute Myocardial Infarction. People over 70 years of age account for one third to one half of the patients admitted with AMI. Furthermore, 80% of myocardial infarction deaths occur in those over age 65. Sixty percent of total deaths occur in those over age 75. Despite these impressive statistics, the majority of clinical trials have excluded patients who are 75 years or older (Barron, 2003), which makes clinical management and care according to evidence-based practice difficult in this age-group.

Physical examination and history taking do not differ depending on the age of the person being treated for chest pain. The same differential information is required for correct diagnosis: history, physical examination, 12-lead ECG, cardiac enzymes, chest x-ray, and complete laboratory information. The symptoms must be carefully documented and continually assessed. Patients must be placed on cardiac monitoring with rhythm analysis, as well as vital signs, including oxygenation saturations.

The clinical presentation of an AMI in the older adult may be quite different from that in the young. As in the young, some older patients may have the typical picture of acute, crushing, substernal chest pain that is not relieved by nitroglycerin and rest and may be accompanied by hypotension and diaphoresis. However, often the clinical features of AMI in the older adult are quite subtle. Rather than pain, dyspnea and symptoms related to decreased cardiac output, including confusion and mental status changes, may be prominent. Not only is the clinical presentation different, but the clinical course can be much more complicated, and the mortality rate from AMI is higher in older adults, as is the risk of heart failure, pulmonary edema, dysrhythmias, and ventricular rupture.

The older patient with myocardial infarction also benefits from the same therapies as the younger patient, and age greater than 75 years alone should not be a contraindication to treatment. The goals of AMI treatment are to reperfuse the myocardium and preserve ventricular function. Pharmacological therapy, thrombolytic therapy, percutaneous coronary intervention (PCI) therapy, and coronary artery bypass graft (CABG) are reperfusion strategies. Aspirin and beta blockers should be administered early in the diagnosis stage and in the postinfarction period. Even though aspirin has been shown to decrease short-term mortality rates by 20% to 25% (Barron, 2003), the Cooperative Cardiovascular Project database showed that only 66% of those persons 65 to 74 years of age and only 54% of those over 84 years of age received aspirin early in the infarction period. Beta blockers have a class I indication in the ACC/AHA guidelines (AHA, 2005) for AMI management, and only 27% to 40% of those patients who would be candidates for therapy received it (Barron, 2003). Ironically, those who could benefit the most from beta blockers, that is, those with transient heart failure and low ejection fraction, are even less likely to receive them. ACE inhibitors, in conjunction with beta blockers, are also of benefit if given in lower doses.

Medical management of AMI has changed greatly in the past 10 years, but includes pharmacological therapy, thrombolytic therapy, PCI, and CABG. Thrombolytic therapy is recommended as soon as possible after infarction, when cardiac catheterization and PCI are not available. Unfortunately, studies indicate that many physicians may not consider relatively aggressive treatment for patients older than 70 years (Barron, 2003). The main cause of death and complications with thrombolytic therapy is hemorrhage, intracerebral hemorrhage being a devastating complication. Increased age alone should not be a major consideration in the choice of therapy. House (1992) provided guidelines to assess the potential risks related to thrombolytic therapy (Box 12-6). Meta-analyses indicate a reduced benefit of thrombolytic therapy in persons older than 74 years of age, and thrombolytic therapy has been given a class IIA indication for those 75 years of age or older in the

BOX 12-6	Risk Assessment: Measuring Potential Risks for Thrombolytic Therapy
POTENTIAL	**RISK FACTORS**
Potential for increased mortality	History of angina pectoris, history of previous myocardial infarction, hypertension, congestive heart failure, diabetes mellitus, heart block, bundle branch block
Potential for bleeding complications	Female, low body weight, hypertension, older than 75 years
Potential for heparin complications	Altered bleeding times
Potential for compromise of patient's coagulation system	Altered fibrinogen levels, increased fibrin-degradation products
Potential for allergic reaction	Exposure to streptococci bacteria, exposure to streptokinase
Potential for drug-related hemodynamic compromise	Hypotension, risk of hypotension
Potential for reinfarction	High-grade stenotic lesion, three-vessel disease

From House, M. A. (1992). Thrombolytic therapy for acute myocardial infarction: The elderly population. *AACN Clinical Issues* 3(2), 106-113.

ACC/AHA guidelines for AMI management (AHA, 2006). The National Registry of Myocardial Infarction (NRMI) database indicates that age is the third most important predictor of failure to receive any reperfusion (lytic or angioplasty) therapy, following only lack of chest pain and the presence of left bundle branch block (Barron, 2003).

The most common treatment plan if the patient is admitted to a hospital that has an interventional cardiac catheterization laboratory is PCI, including angioplasty, directional atherectomy, and stent placement. This invasive procedure is particularly useful for those who are at increased risk for a poor outcome from revascularization surgery. Numerous studies in recent years have shown a similar outcome for PCI compared with CABG as a reperfusion strategy. Percutaneous transluminal coronary angioplasty (PTCA), or stent placement, does not require surgery or the prolonged convalescence associated with surgery. Early clinical trials showed that the elderly had more complications and a higher mortality rate from PTCA than did younger patients, but more recent data indicate that increased age itself is not a contraindication or a predictor of complications. The older adult has similar long-term benefits from the procedure as younger patients (Barron, 2003). Recent data also support the benefit of immediate revascularization with PCI if accomplished with a "door to needle" time of less than 90 minutes.

A substantial number of older patients who have AMI do not receive lifesaving therapies, the use of aspirin, beta blockers, and ACE inhibitors. This problem is most marked in the sickest individuals, who would be expected to benefit most. One of the most important challenges, therefore, is to translate the findings of clinical trials to the large population of patients with AMI. Evidence-based practice for older adults is one of the most important challenges of our times.

Another strategy for patients who sustain a large AMI with reduced ventricular function, ejection fraction less than 40%, is the placement of an implantable cardiac defibrillator (ICD). The newest guidelines from the ACC and AHA (AHA, 2002b) state that the use of an ICD may decrease mortality and morbidity rates in those patients with decreased heart function.

The management of older AMI patients in the coronary care or progressive care unit may be difficult. Management may be complicated by changes in BP and perfusion pressures of the brain, lungs, and kidneys that affect mentation and behavior. In addition, confusion may be made worse in the elderly by displacement to an unfamiliar environment, disorientation, and the typical presence of disease in other major organ systems. Nursing interventions are similar to those used in younger patients. However, some measures to prevent disorientation are needed, such as more frequent visits by relatives, providing glasses and hearing aids, and keeping a few personal items in the room, even in special care units.

Cardiac Rehabilitation for the Older Adult.
Rehabilitation is very important to the older cardiac patient. Rehabilitation goals include the preservation

and maintenance of physical functional capacity, strength, and coordination, which provide for mobility and self-sufficiency. Mental functional integrity must also be maintained so that the older cardiac patient can remain alert and maintain self-respect and self-confidence. A well-planned cardiac rehabilitation program promotes both physical and mental functional capacity and limits or prevents anxiety and depression. It also encourages readjustment to family, community, and society (Padden, 2002).

Teaching about cardiac disease, recommendations of lifestyle modifications, diet, signs and symptoms of possible complications, and the expected actions and possible side effects of drugs should be part of a rehabilitation program. Education regarding community resources for individuals and families is also an integral part of rehabilitation. In addition, such a program should include emotional support of the patient and family, as well as information about when to call the health care professional and the importance of continuing physical activity. Group classes are particularly helpful with older patients because they provide an opportunity to share experiences and make suggestions.

Physical training begins in the hospital with early ambulation. Nursing research has shown that it requires more energy to use a bedpan than to get on a commode. Patients are usually allowed out of bed soon after an uncomplicated AMI and may walk in the halls within a few hours of treatment, depending on the type of reperfusion therapy. This early ambulation reduces some of the complications of immobility and prevents deconditioning. It also provides the nurse with an opportunity to teach the patient how to monitor the heart rate and to use that information for self-monitoring.

A cardiac rehabilitation program can safely improve cardiac functional capacity, reduce ischemic episodes during ordinary activities, improve psychological outlook, modify cardiovascular risk factors, improve health habits, and decrease morbidity and mortality risk. A study of the effects of exercise on left ventricular function in 79 patients with coronary artery disease showed that age did not influence left ventricular function at rest or in response to exercise. Heart function was related to the extent of the disease, not to the age of the subjects (Kallaras et al., 2001). Unfortunately, not all patients who have had an AMI participate in cardiac rehabilitation. Studies have shown that older women are less likely to be referred for cardiac rehabilitation, although they can have improvements in functional capacity similar to those seen in men (Padden, 2002).

Carroll and Pollock (1992) divided the exercise portion of cardiac rehabilitation into three phases. Phase I, the inpatient program, begins as soon as the patient is stable after the event. Many older patients with an uncomplicated AMI are admitted, are taken to the cardiac catheterization laboratory, receive reperfusion therapy,

and are discharged home within 24 to 48 hours. Activities during this short hospital time include progression from self-care activities and range-of-motion exercises to low-level ambulation and stair climbing by the time the patient is discharged from the hospital. An important part of this phase of rehabilitation is education about myocardial ischemia and medications.

Phase II of rehabilitation begins at discharge and lasts for 8 to 12 weeks. This is a transitional time in which the patient progresses from a restricted, low-level program to a less restricted, moderate-level training program. The intensity of the training gradually increases so that by the third or fourth week after AMI or cardiac surgery, the patient's heart rate during exercise is 20 beats above that during standing rest. (Remember that patients may be on beta blockers and heart rate may not be elevated with exercise.) After an exercise stress test is performed, the intensity of activity is based on reaching 60% to 70% of the predicted maximal heart rate reserve. Exercises include walking, biking, arm ergometry, mild calisthenics, and, in the later stages of phase II, swimming and jogging.

Phase III, the long-term program, is often performed in a community-based program. The exercises are more varied, and intensity can increase somewhat, up to 80% to 85% of maximal heart rate. Table 12-4 gives sample target heart rates based on the age and the conditioning of the patient.

Although the components of the exercise prescription are the same for the older adult as for the healthy younger adult, there is a difference in the application of the principles of exercise prescription. Older adults need a longer warm-up period because they take longer to reach steady-state levels of heart rate and blood pressure than do younger subjects. They also need a more prolonged cool-down period because of potential problems with orthostatic hypotension and heat dissipation. Low-level aerobic activities and stretching should be included in the cool-down period.

Surgery for Coronary Artery Disease. Older patients with CAD that cannot be treated with angioplasty or stent placement, or those patients who have failed percutaneous reperfusion and continue to have ischemia, may be candidates for a coronary artery bypass graft (CABG). In this operation, a blood vessel from another part of the body—the saphenous vein, the internal mammary artery, or radial artery—is removed and used as a homograft to carry blood directly from the aorta to the coronary artery distal to the atheromatous plaque that is obstructing the flow of blood, as shown in Figure 12-2.

Improvements in the preoperative, intraoperative, and postoperative periods have decreased mortality and morbidity rates across the populations of people requiring surgery. The most devastating complication

Table 12-4 *Maximum Heart Rate*

Maximum Heart Rate, %	Age (Years)														
	20	25	30	35	40	45	50	55	60	65	70	75	80	85	90
UNCONDITIONED															
100%	197	195	193	191	189	187	184	182	180	178	176	174	172	170	168
90%	177	175	173	172	170	168	166	164	162	160	158	157	155	153	152
75%	148	146	144	143	142	140	138	137	135	134	132	131	129	128	127
60%	118	117	115	114	113	112	110	109	108	107	106	104	103	102	101
CONDITIONED															
100%	190	188	186	184	182	180	177	175	173	171	169	167	165	163	161
90%	171	169	167	166	164	162	159	158	156	154	152	150	149	147	145
75%	143	141	140	138	137	135	133	131	130	128	127	125	124	122	121
60%	114	113	112	110	109	108	106	105	104	103	101	100	99	98	97

From Anderson, J. M. (1991). Rehabilitating elderly cardiac patients. *Western Journal of Medicine, 54*(5), 573-578.

postoperatively, excluding death, is intracerebral hemorrhage or infarction. The incidence of this complication is related to the cardiopulmonary bypass (CBP) circulation and the presence of preexisting carotid disease in the patient. Careful preoperative assessments, often including carotid ultrasound, pulmonary function testing, complete laboratory testing—including chemistries, complete blood count and coagulation parameters—are often helpful in determining mortality and morbidity risks.

Off-pump CABG (CABG performed on a beating heart without the use of CBP), minimally invasive

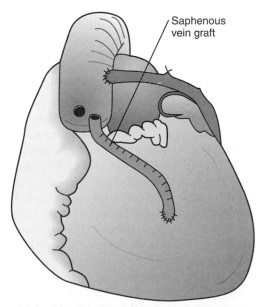

Figure 12-2 Nearly completed aortocoronary saphenous vein bypass of the circumflex and anterior descending branches of the left coronary artery.

Saphenous vein graft

CABG, shorter CBP times, improved cardiac preservation during surgery, improved anesthesia, and the use of pharmacology based on hemodynamic monitoring, as well as the patient's renal and pulmonary function, have in general been very helpful in reducing complications in the older population. Techniques of surgical procedures, as well as preoperative interventions, have opened the opportunity of surgery to previously denied older patients.

Hospital mortality rates in older patients who undergo CABG have declined significantly in recent years. Typically, mortality rates are greater in patients older than 75 years, particularly in-hospital mortality rates. Women in this age-group are at even higher risk of hospital death than men. Variables that predict perioperative mortality rates are the same as in younger patients: angina at rest, presence of 70% or more severe stenosis of the left main coronary artery, severe left ventricular dysfunction, renal insufficiency or failure, the presence of diabetes, and the presence of one or more associated medical disorders. Compared with younger patients, older adults spend more time in the hospital and are more prone to complications, which include stroke, atrial fibrillation, sternal wound dehiscence, and respiratory failure. However, angina is relieved or diminished in about 80% to 90% of patients older than 65. Thus advanced age by itself is not a contraindication to surgery (Hirose et al., 2000; Porter, 2003).

Researchers at Glasgow Royal Infirmary University analyzed approximately 25,000 CABG operations performed in Scottish hospitals between 1981 and 1996. Over the course of the study, the number of operations per year increased more than sevenfold, from 68 to 490 per 1 million population. The investigators found that the percentage of operations conducted in patients older than age 65 increased from 2% to 30% among men over the study period, and from 16% to 45% among women. It was found that the patients' risk of death decreased over the 15-year period. There was a 37% reduction in the age-adjusted risk of death among men. The risk reduction was not as significant in women (Pell et al., 2002).

Another study that supports the notion that heart surgery is getting less risky for older patients was conducted by Rosengart and colleagues (2002). They reviewed the outcomes of 100 patients age 85 to 94 years who had undergone elective open-heart surgery such as CABG or valve replacement at New York Presbyterian Hospital—Weill Medical College of Cornell University between 1994 and 1997. Significant improvements in postoperative death rates were seen compared with outcomes reported 10 years ago for the patients in the same age-group. After an average follow-up period of 2 years, the researchers found that all 100 patients in their study survived their operations, and about 50% lived at least another 40 months. Among the 45 patients available for follow-up interviews, 71% reported major improvements in function, such as reductions in shortness of breath. In addition, the researchers found that the risk of major complications dropped from 24% to 14% over the study period.

Research has shown that nursing care can significantly improve recovery from cardiac surgery. In a study of 156 patients at two hospitals, patients and spouses assigned to an experimental group received two interventions: (1) supplemental in-hospital education on emotional reactions to surgery and methods of conflict resolution and (2) weekly telephone coaching after discharge to provide support and information. As compared with the control subjects, patients in the experimental group reported significantly greater self-efficacy expectations for walking, and more were walking, lifting, climbing stairs, and returning to work (Gilliss et al., 1993).

Patients who are older may require more complicated surgical procedures and have more medical problems as they are admitted for CABG surgery. With "fast track" protocols for earlier extubation, earlier ambulation, and earlier discharge from the hospital, nursing care and interventions with social workers and case managers are increasingly important to the continued improved outcomes of this patient population.

Dysrhythmias

Cardiac dysrhythmias are more common in the older adult, are more often accompanied by cardiac decompensation, and may be harder to treat than in younger patients. Dysrhythmias are more serious in the older adult because they compromise the blood supply of organs that may already be seriously impaired by aging

and disease and may cause further deterioration of heart function, as well as heart failure. Generally, electrophysiology of dysrhythmias and the principles of diagnosis and management are the same in the aged as in others.

For any dysrhythmia in an older patient, the first action is to evaluate the immediate electrical and hemodynamic effects of the dysrhythmia on the individual. A rapid identification of the dysrhythmia should be made to determine if it is life threatening. If it is identified as ventricular tachycardia, ventricular fibrillation, asystole, complete heart block, or a precursor of these, immediate action is required to terminate the arrhythmia. The next step is to determine how well the patient is tolerating the rhythm. A very rapid heart rate, even if it is sinus tachycardia, may be poorly tolerated in the older adult because the rapid rate reduces the amount of time for cardiac filling, causing a drop in cardiac output. If the person has CAD or cerebrovascular disease, this drop in output could trigger chest pain, dyspnea, syncope, or change in level of consciousness. Because the person may become hypotensive, the BP should be monitored at intervals during the dysrhythmia. An extremely low heart rate could also produce a significant drop in cardiac output, with similar results.

Possible causes of dysrhythmias in the older adult are enlargement of the heart chambers and other anatomical changes associated with chronic ischemic heart disease, hypertensive heart disease, cardiomyopathy, or valvular disease. In addition, drug toxicity, heart failure, infection, endocrine dysfunction (thyroid dysfunction), and electrolyte imbalance, especially low serum potassium level, can all induce dysrhythmias.

Older adults have normal sinus rhythm (Schwartz, 1999). The incidence of ectopic activity of the heart increases with age, but dysrhythmias and very frequent ectopic beats in the older adult indicate underlying cardiac disease, not normal changes with aging. The most common dysrhythmias are premature atrial beats, premature ventricular beats, and atrial fibrillation. Precipitating factors for premature ventricular complexes are heavy intake of caffeine, smoking, excessive ingestion of alcohol, and ingestion of heavily spiced foods.

Atrial fibrillation (AF) is the most common sustained dysrhythmia affecting older people. It can have particularly severe consequences in the older adult because of the loss of the active contraction of the atrium, the "atrial kick" producing a decrease in subendocardial perfusion. In the older adult, chronic atrial fibrillation is associated with a significant risk of systemic emboli, notably stroke. This complication is reduced by long-term anticoagulation with warfarin (Coumadin). Furthermore, AF may complicate other conditions, such as hypertension and heart failure. AF is associated with an increased risk of death (Berry & Rae, 2003).

The management of AF can be a difficult problem, particularly in symptomatic, older patients. Results from recent large, multicenter clinical trials in sustained AF have demonstrated that a rate control strategy with conventional drugs is at least as effective as, and possibly superior to, rhythm control by chemical or electrical cardioversion over a 3-year period. Whether these results can be extrapolated to longer time periods than the trials' durations is not known (Fuster et al., 2001).

The management strategies for AF include either to attempt to control the ventricular rate, or to restore and maintain sinus rhythm. Rate-limiting drug therapies, such as beta blockers, digoxin, or verapamil, can be used to achieve a normal heart rate during rest and daily activities. In some symptomatic patients, the ventricular rate may still not be well controlled; in this case, an invasive strategy, involving implantation of a permanent pacemaker and AV nodal ablation, or pulmonary artery ablation (the MAZE procedure, so named because the surgical concept is based on a puzzle) may be needed. Figure 12-3 shows management strategies for AF.

Older patients are less likely to tolerate antidysrhythmic drugs, such as amiodarone and sotalol. These drugs should be used with caution, and in conjunction with a cardiologist. Flecainide carries a risk of provoking ventricular dysrhythmias and sudden death in patients with CAD. It should not be used in patients with coronary disease. CAD is common in older patients and is often subclinical. If other drugs have failed and flecainide is being considered, a stress test should be performed to exclude inducible myocardial ischemia, together with an echocardiogram to establish normal left ventricular function (Berry & Rae, 2003).

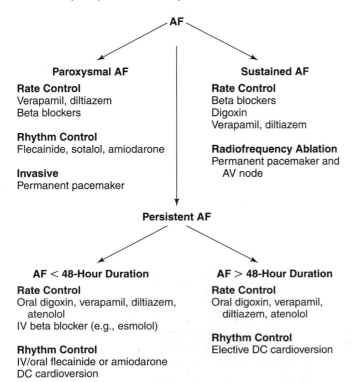

Figure 12-3 Management strategies for atrial fibrillation.

Treatment of cardiac dysrhythmias is the same in the older adult as in other patients. However, the effect of aging and the presence of concurrent disease may affect the action of antidysrhythmic drugs, as well as the choice of antidysrhythmic drug.

Bradyarrhythmias and conduction disturbances are common in the older adult as well. The incidence of bundle branch block increases with age. Right bundle branch block, which occurs in about 3.5% of the elderly, is almost twice as common as left bundle branch block. Uncomplicated right bundle branch block is not associated with increased prevalence of heart disease, but left bundle branch block is nearly always associated with preexisting organic heart disease. Complete, or third-degree, heart block occurs in about 1% of older adults and is an indication for insertion of a permanent cardiac pacemaker (Bexton, 1992).

Sick sinus syndrome is a dysrhythmia that is more common in the older adult, usually occurring in those in their sixties and seventies. It is characterized either by instances of a very slow heart rate or by the sudden occurrence of a very rapid heart rate alternating with a slow rate. About 60% of older adults with sick sinus syndrome experience a form of tachycardia, which is often accompanied by dizziness or syncope. It may be caused by many drugs, such as digoxin, propranolol, lithium, and most sympathetic agents. Sick sinus syndrome is treated by insertion of a permanent pacemaker that provides atrial demand pacing (Rials, Marinchak, & Kowey, 1992).

Heart Failure

Heart failure (HF) in the older adult is recognized as a national public health priority; however, clinical diagnosis can be problematic in older persons, many of whom have a history of heart failure in the presence of normal or only minimally decreased ejection fraction (Mathew, Gottdiener, Kitzman, & Aurigemma, 2004). The outcome for HF in older adults is poor both for systolic and diastolic heart failure. Because most clinical trials have studied younger patients with predominantly systolic heart failure, the appropriate therapy for HF in elderly persons remains to be determined.

HF is a clinical syndrome that is defined as an inadequate contraction of the heart muscle, which results in insufficient cardiac output to meet body needs and in circulatory congestion. HF should be viewed as a neurohormonal model in which heart failure progresses as a result of the overexpression of biologically active molecules that are capable of exerting effects on the heart and circulation.

HF may be due to systolic or diastolic ventricular dysfunction. The long-term prognosis of HF depends on the underlying conditions; however, mortality rate is approximately 50% for 5-year survival. In the older adult, the most common cause of heart failure is coronary heart disease; other causes are hypertension, valvular heart disease, cardiomyopathy, and ventricular aneurysm. The prevalence of HF has increased greatly since 1980, and it is now common in the very old.

Almost 80% of the nearly 5 million people in the United States with HF are 65 years of age or older. Aging of the population, enhanced susceptibility of older hypertensives to HF, and improved survival after AMI in middle age have increased the number of older adults at risk for HF (Rich, 1997).

There are several possible explanations for this marked increase in HF as people age. First, the normal changes of the heart with aging, which slow ventricular filling, may compromise diastolic function and become especially significant during tachycardia, ischemia, or volume stress. Thus the left atrial pressure could be increased, and this increased pressure could be transmitted to the pulmonary vessels, producing pulmonary hypertension, with symptoms of shortness of breath and pulmonary edema. Second, there is an increased incidence of diseases in the older adult that predispose them to cardiac failure. Coronary artery disease is the main cause of HF, but mitral stenosis and insufficiency, calcific aortic stenosis, pulmonary embolism, chronic fibrotic and hemorrhagic pericarditis, subacute bacterial endocarditis, congenital heart disease, thyrotoxicosis, myxedema, bronchitis, and pneumonia can all produce HF.

The symptoms of HF in the older adult include wheezing, cough, dyspnea, orthopnea, and paroxysmal nocturnal dyspnea, often leading to insomnia and nocturnal wandering. In some patients, the predominating symptoms may be anorexia, early satiety, and nausea. In others, weakness, made worse by chronic malnutrition, may be the major complaint. Weight gain may also be noted as fluid accumulates in the lungs in left-sided heart failure and in the extremities in right-sided heart failure. Auscultation might reveal moist crackles, or rales, heard best at the end of inspiration. A third heart sound may be heard, caused by the dilation and noncompliance of the ventricle during rapid filling. Tachycardia is almost invariably present.

The diagnosis and etiology of HF may be difficult in the older adult because some of the symptoms, such as dyspnea and ankle edema, may be due to other diseases. Abnormalities of the thoracic cage displace the cardiac apex and complicate palpation. A fourth heart sound is often heard normally in the elderly, and crackles or rales are often heard with chronic lung disease. In addition, there may be no apparent clinical cause for the heart failure. Unfortunately, HF often has atypical signs and symptoms. Nonspecific signs, such as somnolence, confusion, disorientation, weakness, and fatigue, may be the initial signs, without dyspnea. In some patients, worsening of preexisting dementia is an important sign of HF. Peripheral edema is not a reliable sign of HF in the elderly, because dependent edema is often seen with immobility (Mathew et al., 2004).

In patients with HF caused by systolic dysfunction, treatment consists of rest, minimizing sodium and fluid intake, and reduction of afterload and preload. Because prolonged bed rest is dangerous, chair rest with legs elevated is preferred because it enhances diuresis and oxygenation. Preload is reduced with diuretics. If renal function is normal, the use of nesiritide (Natrecor) (brain natriuretic peptide [BNP]) in the decompensated HF patient is now widely accepted for diuresis, as well as afterload reduction. Afterload may be reduced with vasodilators, particularly nitrates and ACE inhibitors. ACE inhibitors, such as captopril and enalapril, have now been shown to be effective in treating HF; they reduce mortality rate and may have beneficial synergistic effects with other drugs. Digitalis is useful in chronic HF and may minimize symptoms but has no impact on mortality rate. Digoxin has been shown to reduce the number of HF hospitalizations.

In patients with HF caused solely by diastolic dysfunction, the goal is to enhance ventricular filling. For these patients, beta-adrenergic antagonists and ACE inhibitors may be beneficial (Mathew et al., 2004). Fluid status and renal function become extremely important considerations in this patient population. Decreased filling pressures may further reduce cardiac output. Lusitropic drugs, those that have a relaxation effect on ventricular muscle, may improve function. Lusitropic drugs include beta blockers, ACE inhibitors, and nesiritide (Natrecor).

The patient should restrict salt intake to 2 g per day or less and eat foods and fruits high in potassium to prevent hypokalemia secondary to the large doses of diuretics that may be required. The older person receiving diuretic therapy is also susceptible to calcium and magnesium depletion. Serum levels of potassium, calcium, and magnesium should be monitored regularly. The impact of HF on the older adult is severe because it is associated with functional disability resulting from activity intolerance, long-term drug therapy, and frequent hospitalizations.

Nursing interventions to improve activity tolerance are particularly important because of the diminished cardiac reserve of many older adults, especially those who have led inactive lives. Because prolonged bed rest and inactivity can further reduce that reserve, it is important to encourage some activities but to space them well. During and after activity, the nurse should evaluate the patient's heart rate and watch for shortness of breath, fatigue, or other symptoms.

The concept of a team approach for the care of the patient with HF is rapidly gaining favor. The team compositions vary but usually consist of physicians and nurses, dietitians, social workers, physical therapists, or exercise trainers who all focus not only on medication prescribing but also on patient and family education. Close follow-up of weight and symptoms of patients in the home focuses on the goals of slowing progression of the disease, improving symptoms and quality of life, and preventing hospitalizations.

Valvular Disease

Aortic stenosis is by far the most common and most important valvular lesion in the older adult. Progressive degenerative calcification is now the most common cause, as opposed to rheumatic disease. The calcification occurs along the margins of the valve leaflet and thus does not affect valve opening or closing during the early stages but will produce a murmur. Progression to critical aortic stenosis is often gradual and unpredictable. Therefore diagnostic testing is essential for the diagnosis or evaluation of a symptomatic older patient with an aortic systolic murmur. About 20% of older patients with aortic disease have a rheumatic etiology; these patients usually have associated mitral valve disease and should receive antibiotic prophylaxis before all invasive procedures, including dental procedures. The only effective treatment for critical aortic stenosis is surgical. Aortic valve replacement, even in older patients, improves survival and quality of life. Experience with aortic balloon valvuloplasty has shown that restenosis occurs frequently within months, and it has thus been largely abandoned (Schwartz, 1999).

Calcific aortic stenosis is caused by degenerative changes in the aortic cusps, sometimes with fusion of the cusps. In patients in whom the degenerative changes are severe, the clinical presentation is one of palpitations, fatigue, exertional syncope or near-syncope, and angina that may be clinically identical to the angina of CAD. On auscultation, there is a systolic ejection murmur, which is loudest at the right upper sternal border and is conducted to the neck vessels and above the clavicles. The intensity of the murmur is *not* related to the severity of the disease, because this murmur may be heard in the absence of clinically significant disease. A fourth heart sound is common, whereas the S_2 is soft or absent. Peripheral signs are often misleading in the older adult.

The most common cause of aortic regurgitation in the older adult is aortic root dilation secondary to the age-related rise in BP and increased peripheral resistance. With the advent of widespread echocardiography, mild degrees of aortic regurgitation are diagnosed frequently and are usually not of clinical significance. Aortic regurgitation caused by rheumatic valvular disease or associated with disease of a bicuspid valve is more likely to progress to clinically significant disease. When significant aortic regurgitation is present, therapy is aimed at afterload reduction and clinical symptom relief. Definitive surgical intervention before left ventricular failure is preferred (Schwartz, 1999).

Mitral regurgitation accounts for two thirds of mitral valve disease in the older adult. The etiologies include rheumatic disease, papillary muscle dysfunction caused by ischemia or infarction, calcification of the mitral annulus, and myxomatous degeneration causing mitral valve prolapse. Medical management centers on maintenance of sinus rhythm or control of AF, afterload reduction, and prevention of infection by use of prophylactic antibiotic regimens before all invasive procedures (including dental). The subset of patients with significant mitral regurgitation and mitral valve prolapse may have an increased risk for stroke and should be considered for anticoagulation therapy. Acute symptoms may also benefit from preload reduction.

As the disease progresses, the ventricle dilates and pulmonary hypertension develops, making medical treatment ineffective. Surgical interventions have the best results before the development of ventricular dysfunction or marked dilation. Operative results to date show return toward normal pressures and ventricular size, but improvement is not as marked as that seen after aortic valve replacement. Therefore optimal surgical timing has not been identified, but morbidity and mortality rates are high once left ventricular failure occurs. Surgical repair as opposed to replacement is currently being used and evaluated for patients with regurgitation and noncalcified, nonstenotic valves (Schwartz, 1999).

The management of the less common mitral stenosis in the older adult also targets control of heart rate and symptoms, anticoagulation to prevent emboli, and antibiotic prophylaxis to prevent infections (endocarditis). Surgical therapy is the only definitive therapy. Valvuloplasty is seldom of long-term benefit for this older population (Schwartz, 1999). Sutaria, Elder, and Shaw (2000) completed a study that demonstrated the safety and benefit of mitral balloon valvotomy (MBV) in patients greater than 80 years of age. This was a retrospective study of 20 octogenarians in whom MBV was performed as a definitive or palliative treatment for severe mitral stenosis. Dilation of the mitral valve was achieved in all patients without major complications. One month after MBV, all patients were alive, and 16 of the 20 patients were improved by at least one New York Heart Association (NYHA) class. This improvement was sustained in 7 of the 20 patients followed for 1 year. More severe mitral valve degenerative change, determined by echocardiography, was associated with poorer results. Conclusions of this study again suggest that surgical intervention remains the most effective treatment with the best overall outcomes. However, in those older adults with multiple medical problems and high-risk assessment for anesthesia, MBV offers short-term palliation.

Remember that many people have both stenosis and regurgitation of the affected valve and have symptoms of HF, AF, and decreased exercise tolerance.

Cerebrovascular Disease

One of the most important health care problems in the United States today is stroke. Stroke is the third leading cause of death in the United States. The mortality rate associated with the approximately 750,000 strokes per year is 40% to 50%. Magnetic resonance imaging studies have suggested that as many as 22 million "silent strokes" may occur each year. Of those who survive, 40% require skilled nursing services at discharge and 10% are transferred to inpatient rehabilitation facilities. Stroke is also the most common cause of mental disability and nursing home admissions, and two thirds of stroke patients are left with persistent physical deficits. It is estimated that strokes account for $46 billion in direct and indirect costs to society (Leary & Saver, 2001).

In the past, stroke has been regarded as an inevitable result of aging and little attention was paid to reduction of risk factors. Strokes occur at all ages, but even when they afflict the older adult, the risk factors began much earlier in life, and preventive measures cannot begin too early. Surveys of the public have shown very little awareness of either stroke risk factors or warning signs (Kirshner, 2003).

Transient Ischemic Attack. A transient ischemic attack (TIA), called a "ministroke" by some, is characterized by transient focal neurological signs and symptoms that occur suddenly and last a short time, usually less than an hour, and never longer than 24 hours. In about 90% of the aged who have this syndrome, it is caused by a microembolism to the brain from atherosclerotic plaques in the aortocranial arteries. In the remainder, it is caused by mural thrombi; valvular diseases of the heart, especially mitral valve prolapse; vegetations on the heart valves; polycythemia; or some other blood clotting disorder. The presence of a TIA is indicative of an impending stroke in about 25% to 35% of those with this syndrome, but at present, there is no way to clearly identify those who go on to develop a stroke.

The specific signs and symptoms of a TIA vary depending on which vessel is involved, the degree of obstruction of the vessel, and the collateral blood supply. If the anterior (carotid) system is involved, the person may experience ipsilateral blindness, monocular blurring, gradual obscuration of vision, flashes of light, and headaches that may simulate a migraine. If the posterior (vertebrobasilar) system is involved, symptoms may include tinnitus and vertigo, simultaneous bilateral sensory and motor symptoms, and signs of brainstem pathology, including diplopia, facial weakness, ataxia, and "drop attacks" (falling without losing consciousness).

Older persons who have a TIA may ignore the episode because the symptoms completely resolve.

However, they should be seen by a physician so that a major disabling stroke may be prevented. Patients who have a TIA need a complete medical evaluation to determine its cause and to rule out intracranial tumors. One of the most important diagnostic tests for detection of carotid artery stenosis is the carotid ultrasound duplex scan.

Studies have shown that carotid endarterectomy is more beneficial than aspirin in patients with TIAs (Perler, 2003). In a completed clinical trial of 659 patients with TIAs and incomplete strokes, those randomly assigned to medical treatment (aspirin and anticoagulants) had a 26% occurrence of stroke over 2 years, whereas those who received carotid endarterectomy had only a 9% occurrence of stroke (North American Symptomatic Carotid Endarterectomy Trial [NASCET] Collaborators, 1991). In the search for safe and effective treatments for carotid disease, several large trials in North America and Europe have defined carotid endarterectomy (CEA) as the standard treatment for symptomatic and asymptomatic carotid artery disease (European Carotid Surgery Trialists' Collaborative Group, 1998).

Patients most likely to benefit from CEA are those with a greater than 80% diameter reduction at the carotid bifurcation. In the Asymptomatic Carotid Atherosclerosis Study, the procedure was beneficial in asymptomatic patients with at least a 60% internal carotid artery stenosis (Perler, 2003). At Johns Hopkins University Medical Center, for example, 63 procedures were performed over a 12-month period in patients age 75 to 92. There were no perioperative deaths and three perioperative strokes, one of which was secondary to a postoperative intracerebral hemorrhage and one of which was secondary to a cardiogenic embolus. There were two myocardial infarctions, and one patient developed unstable angina. At the 5-year follow-up examination, the rate of survival and of freedom from stroke was 80% (Perler, 2003).

Perler (2003) concluded in a discussion of the management of carotid and peripheral vascular disease in the older adult that CEA is a safe and effective stroke-prevention intervention in the older population and that advanced age is a marker for those who would most benefit from the procedure. CEA also carries a significant risk of postoperative complications in certain subsets of patients that were excluded in all of the aforementioned trials (patients with prior neck radiation, prior CEA, or age greater than 80 years). Recently, catheter-based percutaneous transluminal angioplasty (PTA) and stenting techniques have become well-accepted alternatives for treating arterial stenosis throughout the circulation (Paniagua et al., 2001). Older adults who would not meet the criteria for surgery may be candidates for carotid artery angioplasty and stenting (CAS).

Paniagua and colleagues (2001) demonstrated that CAS is a safe and feasible alternative to CEA in patients unable to undergo surgery. The study was completed in 62 patients age 32 to 89, with a mean age of 67 ± 9 years. All 69 CAS procedures were technically successful, and long-term follow-up revealed restenosis in only four patients.

The major role of the nurse in caring for older persons with this syndrome is the early identification and referral of people who have these transient symptoms. The nurse may be the first person to whom such vague symptoms are reported. Including auscultation for carotid bruits in the routine assessment of the aged would also lead to early identification of potential problems. The older patient also needs support and teaching through the diagnostic process, treatment, and possible surgery.

Stroke

Stroke is a syndrome characterized by a sudden or gradual onset of neurological deficits caused by a compromise of the blood supply to a part of the brain. It is the third leading killer in the United States, after heart disease and cancer.

The incidence of stroke increases exponentially with age after 55 years of age. In addition to advanced age, the most important risk factor for stroke is hypertension. Other risk factors are a history of TIAs or previous stroke; atherosclerosis, especially in the heart, neck, and legs; and atrial fibrillation. Lifestyle risk factors for stroke are smoking and a high alcohol intake (Kirshner, 2003).

Strokes can be classified as thrombotic, embolic, or hemorrhagic. The most common type of stroke in the older adult is the thrombotic stroke, which is associated with atherosclerosis. The most common sites of cerebrovascular atherosclerotic deposits are the bifurcation of the common carotid artery, the origin of the vertebral arteries, and the middle cerebral artery.

A survey of stroke patients of all ages found that almost one in three was dead at 3 weeks after the event, with mortality rate being highest in patients with intracerebral hemorrhage (66%) and subarachnoid hemorrhage (52%) and lower in those with ischemic stroke (15% to 20%). Clinical signs and symptoms on admission that are associated with a poor prognosis are coma, papillary disturbances, Cheyne-Stokes respirations, dysphagia, and urinary incontinence.

In a major stroke, the symptoms are severe and do not disappear. The maximal neurological deficits are present at the onset of the stroke. The specific symptoms depend on the location and amount of the brain involved. Symptoms include motor deficits (hemiplegia, dysarthria, dysphagia), sensory deficits (perceptual deficits), language deficits (aphasia), visual deficits

(defects in the visual fields, diplopia, decreased acuity), decreased level of consciousness, intellectual or emotional deficits, and bowel and bladder dysfunction. Other specific symptoms depend on the site of occlusion and which side of the body is involved. Box 12-7 illustrates the symptoms that may vary with left-sided and right-sided brain damage.

During the initial history and physical examination, a determination of the type of stroke must be made in order to direct the most effective therapy. A computed tomography scan of the head with contrast dye is necessary to determine if the stroke is hemorrhagic or embolic in nature. If the stroke is embolic, the possibility of whether this patient is a candidate for thrombolytic therapy is considered. If there are no contraindications, tissue plasminogen activator (tp-a) is administered intravenously for reperfusion of the cerebral artery. This therapy may cause complete remission of all stroke symptoms with great improvement in patient outcomes. However, if the stroke is hemorrhagic in nature, there is no interventional therapy noted to help with reperfusion. The interventions used in caring for the neurologically injured patient, such as body alignment, BP control, oxygenation, reduction of arterial CO_2 to low-normal levels, and fluid management, are all continued.

Recovery may take days or months, depending on the amount of brain damage and cerebral edema that has occurred. Eventually, a plateau is reached, usually in 3 to 6 months after the event. The focus of nursing care in the first days after the episode includes a complete

---

BOX 12-7 Possible Consequences of Left- and Right-Brain Injury

Damage to the Left Side of the Brain
Right-side paralysis

Speech and language deficits

Slow, cautious behavior

Memory problems related to language

Right-side neglect (less common than left-side neglect; see below)

Damage to the Right Side of the Brain
Left-side paralysis

Spatial-perceptual problems

Left-side neglect

Quick, impulsive behavior

Memory problems related to performance

From Brass, L. M. (1992). Stroke. In B. Zaret, M. Moser, & L. Cohen (Eds.), Yale University School of Medicine Heart Book. New Haven, CT: Yale University School of Medicine.

physical and neurological status examination to provide a baseline measurement and maintenance of life support functions by preventing aspiration and reducing intracranial pressure. Immediate action should be taken to prevent future complications of immobility, deep vein thrombosis, and pneumonia. Later, after the initial "shock" of the stroke is receding, brain edema begins to resolve, and blood flow to the ischemic area begins to improve through collateral circulation. The patient is more attentive to people and the environment and may begin to participate in self-care activities and to learn the extent of his or her deficits. Emotional support for the patient and family is especially crucial at this time.

By 2 to 4 weeks after the stroke, cerebral edema should be completely resolved and collateral circulation should be improving. The neurological deficits gradually improve, leaving those that are permanent.

The nursing needs of a stroke patient are complex and varied. Nursing care can be made more precise by recognition of the differences in behavioral responses of patients with left-sided and right-sided brain damage. If the left side of the brain is damaged, right hemiplegia results. Right hemiplegics often have problems with speech and language because the speech center is in the left side of the brain in most people. These patients also tend to be somewhat cautious, anxious, and disorganized when attempting a new task. The AHA (Fowler & Fordyce, 1974) makes these suggestions about caring for a right hemiplegic:

1. Do not underestimate the patient's ability to learn and communicate even if he or she cannot use speech.
2. If he or she cannot use speech, try other forms of communication. Pantomime and demonstration are often useful.
3. Do not overestimate the patient's understanding of speech and overload the patient with "static."
4. Do not shout. Keep messages simple and brief.
5. Do not use special voices.
6. Divide tasks into simple steps.
7. Give much feedback and many indications of progress.

If the right side of the brain is damaged, the left side of the body will be paralyzed. Left hemiplegics often have spatial-perception deficits, which can impair their ability to judge distance, size, position, rate of movement, form, and the relation of parts to wholes. These deficits are subtler than loss of the ability to speak and are often overlooked. In fact, the left hemiplegic can often talk better than he or she can perform. These spatial-perception deficits may have profound effects on the self-care ability of the elderly stroke patient and the family. Patients may not recognize potentially dangerous situations and may overestimate their capacities. They may also have visual field abnormalities and do not "see" things on the affected (left) side of the body.

AHA suggestions for working with left hemiplegic patients with significant spatial-perceptual deficits include the following:

1. Do not overestimate their abilities. Spatial-perceptual deficits are easy to miss.
2. Use verbal cues if the patients have difficulty with demonstration.
3. Break tasks into small steps and give much feedback.
4. Watch to see what they can do safely rather than taking their word for it.
5. Minimize clutter around them.
6. Avoid rapid movement around them.
7. Highlight visual reference points.

The older stroke patient is subject to many complications. Nursing care should focus on prevention of these complications. Table 12-5 provides a list of potential problems, factors that might aggravate the problems, and measures to prevent and treat these complications.

The major rehabilitation goals for older stroke victims are to prevent complications from inactivity and to prevent additional strokes and other vascular events. Thus it is vital to have ways to safely increase activity in these patients. A nursing study of 33 older stroke patients during ambulation validated that they are at risk for activity intolerance but also showed that subjective symptoms, such as dyspnea and weakness, were good predictors of activity intolerance. Other predictors were changes in heart rate and rhythm and in respiratory rate and pattern. The authors concluded that older stroke patients can be taught to recognize signs of activity intolerance so they can begin low-risk rehabilitation exercise programs (Mol & Baker, 1991).

Peripheral Vascular Disease: Claudication

Peripheral arterial disease (PAD) is a common manifestation of systemic atherosclerosis. The most frequent symptom is intermittent claudication, which results from poor oxygenation of the muscles of the lower extremities and is experienced typically as an aching pain, cramping, or numbness in the calf, buttock, hip, thigh, or arch of the foot. Symptoms are induced by walking or exercise and are relieved by rest.

A German study of over 6000 individuals age 65 and older in primary care settings found prevalence rates of 19.8 (males) and 16.8 (females) based on an ankle-brachial index less than 90. Comorbidities that were higher in the groups with PAD included diabetes, hypertension, lipid disorders, cerebrovascular events, and cardiovascular events (Diehm et al., 2004).

Patients can be stratified into groups according to symptom severity. One half of all PAD patients older than 55 years are asymptomatic (Weitz, Byrne, & Clagett, 1996). Of the symptomatic patients, approximately 40% experience intermittent claudication, and 10% have critical limb ischemia. Intermittent claudication is

Table 12-5 *Possible Complications of Stroke*

	Inciting Factor(s)	Aggravating Factor(s)	Prevention	Therapy
Pressure sores	Prolonged pressure over bony prominences	Poor bed positioning Incontinence	Identify high-risk patient Prescribe regular turning and repositioning	Prescribe intensive nursing care
Peripheral nerve palsy	Traction or pressure injury of peripheral nerve or nerve plexus	Bed and wheelchair positioning Hemiparesis and hemisensory loss	Position properly	Initiate intensive rehabilitation program
Urinary incontinence	Neurogenic bladder	Environmental access Coexisting gynecological or urological disease Medication toxicity	Provide easy access to toilet or commode	Institute bladder schedule Provide incontinence aids Treat coexisting disease
Fecal incontinence	Fecal stasis	Neurogenic bowel Immobility Low fiber diet Dehydration	Encourage early mobilization Increase dietary fiber and fluid intake	Institute bowel program
Adjustment to disability	Brain injury Depression	Inadequate information about deficits and abilities	Ensure early communication regarding prognosis	Provide patient and family education Institute active rehabilitation program
Withdrawal of family support	Stress secondary to impact of illness	Poor premorbid family relationships Inadequate education and involvement of family in therapeutic process	Promote active communication with family Provide programs to involve family in care	Initiate family conferences or family therapy
Depression	Multiple losses Brain injury	Premorbid personality Unrealistic expectations about recovery	Provide early information regarding deficits and prognosis	Set up rehabilitation program to assure sense of progress
Sensory deprivation	Environmental isolation	Dysphasia Hemianopsia Preexisting cognitive and sensory deficits	Provide stimulating environment	Augment sensory input
Medication toxicity	Altered pharmacokinetics and pharmacodynamics	Multiple medications	Review medications Use lowest dosage	Discontinue offending medications
Spasticity	Brain injury	Pain Contractures Anxiety	Position properly	Initiate definitive measures to treat spasticity
Contractures	Immobility	Spasticity Pain	Position properly Prescribe range-of-motion exercises	Institute physical therapy program

Continued

Table 12-5 *Possible Complications of Stroke—cont'd*

	Inciting Factor(s)	Aggravating Factor(s)	Prevention	Therapy
Shoulder problems	Hemiparesis	Improper lifting and positioning of flaccid shoulder	Lift and position shoulder properly	Treat specific conditions
Falls	Hemiparesis	Orthostatic hypotension Coexisting musculoskeletal, neurological, or cardiovascular disease Medication toxicity	Institute environmental safety program	Increase environmental safety measures Eliminate possible offending medications
Physical deconditioning	Hemiparesis Immobility	Coexisting chronic diseases	Encourage early rehabilitation	Institute a graded exercise program

From Kelly, J., & Winograd, C. H. (1985). A functional approach to stroke management in elderly patients. *Journal of the American Geriatrics Society 33*, 48-60.

usually accurately diagnosed based on the vascular history and physical examination, which should include palpation of the abdomen and peripheral pulses. Because palpation of the peripheral pulses alone is too insensitive a measure of PAD and many older adults with PAD are symptomatic, noninvasive vascular tests, such as determining the ankle-brachial index, should be performed to quantify the degree of limb ischemia. The ankle-brachial index, which is the ratio of the ankle systolic pressure to the brachial artery systolic pressure, is useful in assessing disease severity. An ankle-brachial index of 0.90 or greater is considered normal; 0.70 to 0.89 is considered mild disease, 0.5 to 0.69 is considered moderate disease, and less than 0.5 is considered severe disease (Cimminiello, 2002; Tabet & Berg, 1996).

Risk factors for the development of PAD include smoking, hypertension, diabetes, lipid abnormalities, elevated serum homocysteine levels, age, increased fibrinogen and blood viscosity, male gender, and elevated triglycerides. Many older adults also have these risk factors. PAD is not a disease of older adults; however, as seen in the preceding discussions, many older adults have these recurrent risk factors.

The main cause of claudication in the older adult is atherosclerosis. Because this is a systemic problem, the person with claudication is likely to have other related problems, such as angina, a history of ACS, or cerebrovascular disease. The location of the atherosclerotic obstruction determines the location of pain. An obstruction in the femoral artery usually causes calf pain; pain in the gluteal region and thigh or even in the back could be caused by an obstruction higher in the arterial system, perhaps at the bifurcation of the aorta.

Some other, less common, causes of ischemia of the legs are diabetes; venous stasis with ulceration; arterial embolization; trauma, especially a fractured femur; and polyarteritis.

Symptoms that may make a nurse suspect that an older patient has peripheral vascular disease include complaints of cold feet on warm days, a burning pain in the feet when they are warmed, and intermittent claudication. This latter symptom is highly characteristic. The person has leg pain and cramps when walking that are completely relieved with rest. Typically, walking a specific distance, such as two blocks, induces the pain. This distance is fairly consistent for an individual. If leg pain is present at rest, there is probably advanced obstructive disease complicated by poor collateral flow.

On physical examination, there are diminished or absent peripheral pulses. In addition, a bruit may be heard over the obstructed artery. The affected leg may have a red or violaceous skin color with mottling. It may show pallor when elevated and redness when dependent and may feel cool to the touch. There is an increased venous filling time. Color is slow to return to the leg after pressure is applied. In addition, trophic changes may be seen in the leg. These include thinning of the skin, loss of hair, thick nails, and decreased muscle mass.

In managing PAD, it is critically important to deal with the high risk of developing severe and often fatal cardiovascular complications. The first priority is to aggressively modify risk factors that enhance the progression of atherosclerosis and atherosclerotic complications. It is also important, however, to relieve the symptoms of intermittent claudication. Unlike risk reduction, symptomatic improvement is apparent to the patient, often within a matter of weeks or a few months, and can enhance a patient's quality of life considerably (Schainfeld, 2001).

Most patients with chronic arterial occlusive disease and intermittent claudication are treated conservatively and do not require surgery. In these patients, it is vital to control risk factors, especially cigarette smoking. Patients should be told that if they continue to smoke, their arterial disease will progress, and they may lose a limb. Patients who stop smoking, lose weight (if overweight), and start a regular exercise program can see significant improvement in their symptoms. Diabetes, if present, should be rigidly controlled, because peripheral vascular disease is more common and progresses much faster in those with diabetes.

Antiplatelet and lipid-lowering therapies are effective in decreasing the risk of cardiovascular morbidity and improving long-term survival. Some agents can also improve symptoms of claudication. Emerging therapies, such as carnitine and propionyl-L-carnitine, prostaglandins, angiogenic growth factors, and L-arginine, are under investigation. Antiplatelet drugs are commonly used in the treatment of PAD primarily to decrease the occurrence of clot formation, but have not been shown to improve intermittent claudication, as measured by pain-free walking distance or maximum walking distance. Cilostazol is of proven benefit and pentoxifylline of questionable benefit in the treatment of intermittent claudication. In fact, only these drugs are approved by the Food and Drug Administration for treatment of this condition.

If the older patient is severely disabled and cannot carry out daily activities because of leg pain, surgical correction may be considered. Surgery can take the form of vascular reconstruction by percutaneous transluminal angioplasty (PTA). Surgical reconstruction with aortobifemoral grafts or femoral-femoral grafts is also an option. The 5-year patency of aortobifemoral grafts is more than 90%, and the surgical mortality rate is about 1% to 2%. PTA is most effective in cases in which surgery cannot be justified either because of the location of the lesion or because the patient is a poor surgical risk.

Some local treatments are important to preserve tissue. The feet must be kept clean and protected from trauma because healing would be severely compromised in the absence of adequate arterial flow. Thickened nails or skin calluses should be treated by a podiatrist because of the danger of ulceration. Infections should be promptly treated with an appropriate antibiotic. If ulcers develop as a complication of peripheral vascular disease, skillful nursing care is required, involving regular, gentle cleansing of the ulcer. The ulcer can be firmly bandaged, allowing the blood supply to improve with walking.

Venous Disease

Varicose veins, the simplest of venous disorders, may develop in the older adult as the veins lose their elasticity and the muscles supporting them weaken. The treatment consists simply of consistent use of elastic stockings to counteract stasis and swelling. Vein ligation and stripping may not be necessary if support hose are worn. Other conservative measures are periodic leg elevation, weight loss if needed, and avoidance of prolonged standing and constrictive clothing. Exercise such as walking, cycling, and swimming is recommended.

Thrombophlebitis is the inflammation of superficial or deep veins, the incidence of which increases with advanced age. The symptoms of superficial thrombophlebitis are red, warm, painful, or tender areas under the skin along the course of a vein. Thrombophlebitis can occur in varicose as well as in normal veins. There is no edema and no danger of emboli, so no anticoagulant therapy is needed. Treatment consists of the application of moist heat, rest, elevation of the extremity, and possibly antibiotics.

Deep vein thrombosis (DVT) is more difficult to diagnose. There may be minimal physical findings, or edema may be present with distended superficial veins, a reddish cyanotic color of the leg, pain, and tenderness. Unfortunately, about half of the patients with clinical signs of DVT have normal veins, whereas others with the problem may have no clinical signs.

The danger of DVT is the association with emboli and the possibility of a fatal pulmonary embolus. DVT and pulmonary emboli are the leading causes of morbidity and death in hospitalized patients, especially older adults.

There are three primary predisposing factors to DVT: venous stasis, hypercoagulability, and injury to the endothelial structure. Effects of these factors are increased by advanced age, surgery, prolonged bed rest, prolonged crossing or strapping of the legs, obesity, and a previous history of DVT. Box 12-8 lists some factors in the older adult that may predispose to DVT.

Some of these factors, such as dehydration and immobility, can be diagnosed and treated by nurses. Other factors cannot be treated directly, but their presence can increase the nurse's awareness of the potential problem of DVT and pulmonary emboli and the need to continue nursing interventions to prevent DVT occurrence.

Prevention of DVT begins with treatment of the underlying disorder, prescribing sequential hose therapies for the patient on bed rest for any duration, and anticoagulation therapy with heparin or low-molecular-weight heparin.

Diagnosis of DVT can be difficult. The most sensitive test is contrast phlebography, in which the venous system is visualized by the injection of contrast material, or dye, into the superficial veins of the foot or ankle. Other, less invasive, methods are available. These include Doppler ultrasound studies, plethysmography, and fibrinogen scanning.

Treatment of DVT consists of aggressive anticoagulation, pain control, and bed rest. Heparin is the initial anticoagulant used, followed by an oral anticoagulant

---

BOX 12-8 Factors That Predispose to Deep Vein Thrombosis

Hypercoagulability
Postoperative state

Fever

Abrupt discontinuation of anticoagulants

Some malignancies, such as cancer of the pancreas

Dehydration

Acute or chronic inflammation (e.g., urinary tract infections, cellulitis, bronchopneumonia)

Changes in the Vessel Wall
Trauma, especially hip fractures

Peripheral vascular disease

Degenerative disease

Pooling

Varicose veins

Venous Stasis
Obesity

Congestive heart failure

Arrhythmias, especially atrial fibrillation

Long-term immobility

---

for 3 to 6 months. Because aging increases sensitivity to oral anticoagulants, lower doses of warfarin may be given to the older adult. In addition to managing symptoms of DVT, nursing care must include careful observation for any signs of bleeding in the older adult, who often is taking multiple other drugs that can either antagonize or potentiate the oral anticoagulant.

SPECIAL ISSUES: CARDIOVASCULAR DISEASE IN WOMEN

Recently, health professionals have become more aware of the importance of cardiovascular disease in women, especially older women. Cardiovascular diseases, especially CAD and stroke, are the leading causes of death in women in the United States and cause more deaths than cancer, accidents, and diabetes combined. The age-adjusted death rates from heart diseases in women are four times higher in white women and six times higher in black women than the death rates from breast cancer. By 75 to 84 years of age, the death rate from coronary heart disease (CHD) in women is approximately 500,000 per year (AHA, 2004).

Although the risk factors for cardiovascular disease are the same in women as in men, those risk factors may affect women differently. For example, there is some evidence that diabetes, hypertriglyceridemia, low levels of HDL cholesterol, obesity, and sedentary lifestyle seem to be stronger risk factors for women than for men. However, more research is needed. Unfortunately, the prevalence of smoking in women has increased, so more older women are now likely to be smokers, thus further increasing their risk for cardiovascular disease.

Diagnosis and treatment of cardiovascular disease is more complicated in older women than in older men. Shortness of breath and fatigue are the predominant initial symptoms of CAD in women, but an exercise-based diagnostic test may not be conclusive. Many women, even young women, are unable to exercise to sufficient intensity for a conclusive result, and many older women have concomitant diseases that make such a test impossible. The onset of CAD is about 7 to 10 years later in women than in men. Although the clinical presentation of AMI is similar for men and women, more women have shortness of breath and fatigue. Treatment tends to be more conservative in women. Mortality rates from AMI are higher in women than in men; mortality rate is highest in black women. Women have greater operative and postoperative mortality rates from CABG surgery, and they have lower graft patency.

Based on epidemiological studies demonstrating mainly positive biological effects of estrogen on cardiovascular risk factors and outcomes, earlier recommendations suggested that most if not all women should be treated with long-term postmenopausal hormone replacement (Wilson, 1966; Wilson & Wilson, 1963). A review of recent controlled clinical trials demonstrates that previously held clinical evidence might not be accurate (Manson & Martin, 2001; Mosca et al., 2001; Rossouw, 2001; Simon et al., 2001). For older women, the decision to begin hormone replacement therapy should not be based on an assumption of protection from cardiovascular diseases. A careful assessment of the risks and benefits, as well as acknowledgement of the outcomes for which hormone replacement therapy has unknown impact, is needed for any decision to begin, continue, or stop hormone replacement therapy.

For all of these reasons, prevention of cardiovascular disease is extremely important in women. Prevention should include avoidance of obesity through an active lifestyle, healthful eating (low-fat foods, with plenty of fruits, vegetables, and complex carbohydrates), and no smoking.

CARDIOVASCULAR NURSING ASSESSMENT OF THE OLDER ADULT
History

Obtaining a detailed history from an older patient may be difficult. The older patient may have a poor memory and may have had so many health problems that a history could be very long and complicated. Often, older individuals have diminished pain perception or have learned to ignore or live with symptoms for so long that they may no longer recognize them as important. They may have altered their normal lifestyle to avoid important cardiovascular symptoms, such as dyspnea on exertion, pain, and fatigue.

Because of this, it is often helpful to get a picture of the typical daily activities, such as how often the person leaves the house to shop, how often he or she takes walks and how far, and what type of work the individual does around the house. It is important to ask if the person's usual activity level has changed in the previous 5 to 10 years to determine whether alterations in exercise tolerance may be the result of cardiovascular problems. Ask if the patient needs to take breaks during activities of daily living and if he or she can climb a flight of stairs without stopping.

A nutritional history is also important. Obtain a description of all the food eaten in a day (24-hour dietary recall), including condiments, such as bouillon cubes, garlic salt, and other sources of sodium. A smoking history is very important for the older adult. The pack-year smoking history can be determined by multiplying the number of packs of cigarettes smoked daily by the total number of years the person has been smoking.

A family history, including brothers, sisters, and children, as well as parents, may give some clues to potential cardiovascular problems. It also gives the older patient a chance to reminisce and helps establish the rapport that is necessary to help the person relax and promote a climate of trust. Determine whether there is a family history of coronary or cerebrovascular disease, renal vascular hypertension, varicose veins, peripheral vascular disease, or pulmonary emboli.

Ask specific questions to determine the presence or absence of cardiovascular problems. Does the person have a history of high BP? If so, for how long, and what treatment was prescribed (and was the prescription followed? If not, why not?). If the patient is hypertensive, has he or she experienced any headaches or epistaxis?

Dyspnea is a common symptom of cardiac disease in the older adult, so a detailed description of typical episodes of shortness of breath is warranted. Dyspnea may be an important pain-equivalent symptom of a myocardial infarction in the older adult, especially with women. Does labored breathing occur with exertion or at rest? Does it occur suddenly? Is nocturnal dyspnea or orthopnea present? How many pillows does the person need at night, and has this number changed recently? If orthopnea is present, has it worsened recently? Is there a history of heart failure? Because the presence of right-sided heart failure or venous insufficiency may produce edema, ask if the patient's shoes, rings, or clothes seem tight at the end of the day. If so, how much swelling is present, where is it, and does it disappear with rest? Also ask if edema is present on awakening.

Have there been any episodes of chest pain or tightness in the chest? Did the pain radiate to the arms, the shoulders, or the jaw? This type of pain, or pain in the throat and epigastrium, may be due to cardiac ischemia and may be confused with arthritis, hiatal hernia, peptic ulcer, or other common problems of the older adult. Is there any pain in the legs with walking? The location, intensity, duration, and onset of pain should be described, along with any aggravating factors or associated sensory or motor disturbances.

Have there been any dizzy spells, light-headedness, or vertigo? Do these occur when the patient is standing up, and is any medication being taken for them? Have there been any transient changes in vision or other signs of cerebral insufficiency? Does the person cough or wheeze? If so, when? If a cough is present, what are the amount, color, and consistency of the sputum?

Has the person had any episodes of thumping or racing heart or markedly irregular heartbeats? When do these occur, what seems to bring them on, and how long do the episodes last? Most important, are there any associated symptoms, such as weakness, dyspnea, and faintness?

Finally, it is important to find out all the medications the person is currently taking for any reason, both prescribed and over-the-counter drugs. Try to find out which of the drugs the person is actually taking, and how often. Many older adults take drugs only when they feel sick and try to "do without" as long as possible. Many try to "stretch" medications because of financial constraints.

Physical Examination

Inspection and palpation of the neck is particularly important in the older adult. A prominent arterial pulsation above the right clavicle, caused by kinking of the right common carotid artery, is often found. If the neck veins are distended when they are inspected with the patient sitting at a 45-degree angle, heart disease and congestive heart failure may be present. Auscultate the carotid arteries for bruits, which may indicate arterial stenosis and increased risk of stroke. As in all patients, it is important to palpate only one carotid artery at a time and gently, to avoid stimulating the vagal receptors in the neck or dislodging any atherosclerotic plaques that may be present.

Assessment of the heart and chest of older patients is more difficult because of the greater incidence of pulmonary emphysema, kyphoscoliosis, and other rib cage deformities. The precordial pulsations should be examined, but these are often difficult to see or palpate. In addition, the heart borders are harder to palpate or percuss, and the heart sounds may be distant or diminished. Because of the difficulty in localizing heart murmurs in the elderly, it is essential to palpate the chest for a thrill, the palpable component of a murmur.

On auscultation, extra sounds may be heard in the normal older person. Alterations in the heart sounds have the same significance in the older adult as in younger patients. An easily heard S_4 gallop, especially when it is accompanied by a palpable presystolic lift, is an abnormal finding in an older patient. It suggests that the left ventricle is noncompliant, and it may be caused by hypertension, aortic stenosis, cardiomyopathy, or left ventricular ischemia. An S_3 gallop is always abnormal. It can occur with volume overload of the left ventricle and thus is a sign of heart failure.

When a murmur is heard, it is important to carefully describe the location where it was heard; whether the sound radiated; and the timing (in systole or diastole), pitch, duration, character, and intensity. The intensity of a murmur is indicated by grade, measured on a scale of I to VI. Grade I/VI is the softest audible sound, V/VI is the loudest heard with a stethoscope on the chest, and VI/VI is so loud it is heard with the stethoscope off the chest. The character of the murmur is described as harsh, blowing, rumbling, crescendo, or decrescendo.

A soft systolic ejection murmur, occurring late in systole and heard best at the base of the heart, is often found. As many as 60% to 80% of very old patients may have systolic murmurs. These murmurs generally originate from the aortic area and may be due to the dilation of the aortic annulus and ascending aorta or to the thickening or calcification of the aortic cusps. This type of murmur is short in duration, peaks early in systole, and is soft, usually grade I to grade II/VI. If such a murmur is heard, it is important to ask about associated symptoms. Other, more serious, causes of systolic murmurs are aortic stenosis, mitral regurgitation, and idiopathic hypertrophic subaortic stenosis (Fields, 1991).

A diastolic murmur is always abnormal in the older adult. A diastolic decrescendo blowing murmur heard best along the left sternal border almost always indicates aortic regurgitation, which may not be clinically significant. A diastolic rumble, heard best at the apex of the heart, indicates mitral stenosis, a condition that may be first diagnosed when the patient is elderly. This rumble may be accompanied by atrial fibrillation.

Peripheral pulses, including brachial, radial, femoral, popliteal, posterior tibial, and dorsalis pedis, should be carefully examined. The arteries may be quite firm as a result of atherosclerotic changes in the vessel walls, or peripheral pulses may be very faint, or even absent. Pulses are commonly graded as follows: 0 = absent, 1+ = greatly diminished, 2+ = slightly diminished, 3+ = normal, and 4+ = bounding. Note the skin temperature and any atrophic changes, such as thin, shiny, taut skin; decreased hair distribution; and nail changes. If these are found, elevate the affected leg for about a minute, then lower it to the floor. If the foot turns pale or gray when elevated, and dark red, dusky, and mottled

when dependent, the person may have significant peripheral vascular disease.

Carefully inspect the legs for stasis dermatitis, varicosities, and leg ulcers. To detect dependent "pitting" edema, apply pressure *over a bone* in the foot or lower leg.

Finally, take a BP measurement in both arms while the patient is lying, sitting, and standing. The normal range is 100/60 to 140/90 mm Hg, with less than 10 mm Hg difference between arms and less than 20 mm Hg difference between standing and sitting. Because of the common presence of peripheral vascular abnormalities, the BP is often different in the arms. Note this difference, and document which arm has the highest pressure so that it can be consistently used for routine BP checks. Box 12-9 outlines the nursing assessment of the cardiovascular system.

Box 12-9 Cardiovascular Assessment

Health History
History of cardiovascular problems (e.g., hypertension, heart attacks, congestive heart failure)
Family history of cardiovascular problems
Typical daily activities and changes in exercise tolerance
Symptoms: dyspnea, edema, chest pain, tightness in chest, pain in legs with walking, dizziness, lightheadedness, transient changes in vision, thumping or racing heart, irregular heart rate or palpitations, confusion, blackouts, syncope, fatigue, shortness of breath, dyspnea, and orthopnea
Medications
Diet
Life stressors

Physical Assessment
Inspection and palpation
   Neck vein distention
   Carotid artery bruits
   Trophic changes in legs
Palpation of arterial pulses
   Radial, brachial, femoral, popliteal, dorsalis pedis, and posterior tibialis
Auscultation of blood pressure
   Both arms
   Lying, sitting, and standing
Auscultation of the heart
   Systole and diastole (extra sounds and murmurs)
   Rhythm
   Extra sounds and murmurs
Percussion
   Heart size

NURSING DIAGNOSES

1. Acute pain related to cardiac ischemia, impaired circulation in the extremities, and cardiac surgery
2. Activity intolerance related to decreased cardiac output, fear of recurrent angina, impaired ability of peripheral vessels to supply tissue with oxygen, arterial spasms, pain, hemiplegia, physical deconditioning, and fatigue
3. Anticipatory grieving or Ineffective denial, related to actual or perceived losses secondary to cardiac condition
4. Sexual dysfunction related to decreased libido or erectile dysfunction secondary to medication side effects
5. Deficient knowledge about disease, prognosis, course, treatment, risk factors (obesity, smoking, alcohol), postoperative and follow-up care, and cognitive deficits
6. Ineffective tissue perfusion related to thrombus, compromised circulation, and venous congestion
7. Ineffective tissue perfusion related to interruption of cerebral blood flow, fall in blood pressure, orthostatic hypotension, and cerebral edema
8. Decreased cardiac output related to increased preload or impaired myocardial contractility, or excessively increased afterload
9. Impaired gas exchange related to immobility, ventilation/perfusion imbalance, or fluid in alveoli
10. Risk for impaired skin integrity related to compromised peripheral circulation
11. Potential for injury related to decreased sensation in superficial tissues
12. Imbalanced nutrition: less than body requirements related to nausea and anorexia secondary to venous congestion of gastrointestinal tract and fatigue
13. Impaired home maintenance management related to inability to perform activities of daily living secondary to breathlessness and fatigue
14. Fluid volume excess related to compensatory kidney mechanisms and excessive sodium intake in diet
15. Risk for deficient fluid volume related to excessive diuresis
16. Disturbed thought processes related to impaired cerebral circulation and damage to brain structures
17. Self-care deficits related to neuromuscular impairment, indifference, decreased attention span, and fatigue
18. Risk for constipation related to immobility and interruption of normal lifestyle and schedule, drug therapy
19. Impaired physical mobility related to neuromuscular impairment, activity intolerance, and fatigue
20. Impaired verbal communication related to damage to left hemisphere brain structures and impairment of left hemisphere cerebral circulation
21. Ineffective therapeutic regimen management related to insufficient knowledge of low-salt diet, drug therapy, activity program, and signs and symptoms of complications
22. Powerlessness related to progressive nature of condition

NURSING INTERVENTIONS AND EVALUATION

Nursing interventions should begin with strategies to prevent the development of cardiovascular disease and to promote a healthy lifestyle. Exercise, especially walking, is beneficial to people of all ages and can be tailored to the abilities of each older individual. Improvements in diet, such as minimizing saturated fats and salt intake, can also help fight cardiovascular disease. Older people should be encouraged to stop smoking, if possible, and to drink alcohol in moderation. The adage that "you can't teach an old dog new tricks" is not always true for older people, and many are able to change habits if they believe it is to their benefit (Box 12-10). Strategies to encourage smoking cessation are discussed in Chapter 13.

For older patients with cardiovascular disease, the goal is to maximize functional abilities, thereby increasing mobility and independence in carrying out activities of daily living. Older patients and their families should be taught strategies for management of medication, management of diet and stress, and maintenance of a proper balance of rest and activity. Concerns, both spoken and unspoken, about the effects of the illness on sexuality should be explored. Health professionals cannot assume that because people are older they do not have an active sex life. Informal and formal support systems in many cases make the difference between living relatively independently in the community and living relatively dependently in a nursing home. Referrals to social service agencies can facilitate the process of obtaining formal supports, such as meals-on-wheels,

---

BOX 12-10 *TOWARD BETTER CARDIOVASCULAR HEALTH*

- Engage in physical activity for a minimum of 60 minutes (total) every day or as recommended by your primary health care provider.
- Have a physical examination before beginning a new program of exercise.
- Consume a low-saturated fat, low-cholesterol diet.
- Avoid smoking.
- Attain and maintain an appropriate weight.
- Monitor your blood pressure.
- Follow prescribed therapy for hypertension, elevated serum lipids, and diabetes.

Nursing Care Plan: The Older Adult With Chronic Heart Failure

Data

78-year-old retired nurse with history of long-standing hypertension and heart failure over past 5 years. Lives at home with husband who is a retired teacher. They enjoy church activities and traveling. Medications: beta blocker, ACE inhibitor, diuretic.

Assessment

When seen in nurse practitioner's office, is alert and pleasant. States she is doing "pretty well," but tires more quickly since last visit 3 months ago. When visiting daughter in another city, needed to rest after several hours. Concerned that she was irritable and not able to enjoy activities planned during the visit. Has noticed more ankle edema and reports gaining 5 lb in past 2 weeks.

Height: 5 ft 4 in; weight: 165 lb; BP: 124/66 mm Hg; heartbeat: 66 beats per minute, regular; respiratory rate: 24 breaths per minute; temperature: 37° C

Head, eyes, ears, nose, and throat: pupils equal, round, react to light, accommodate (PERRLA); extraocular movements full; teeth in good repair

Neck: full range of motion, supple, trachea midline, jugular vein normal at 90 degrees, no bruit

Chest: decreased breath sounds bilaterally with rales in both bases, regular rate and rhythm, II/VI systolic murmur over apex

Abdomen: round, soft, nontender, no organomegaly noted, positive bowel sounds

Neurological: cranial nerves II through XII grossly intact, no neurological deficits

Extremities: no cyanosis, clubbing has 2+ pitting edema both legs; feet cool with poor venous return, multiple varicosities both legs, 1+ dorsalis pedis, posterior tibial pulses

Nursing Diagnoses

Decreased cardiac output related to altered contractility

Activity intolerance related to imbalance between oxygen supply and demand and decreased cardiac output

Goals/Outcomes

Patient's cardiac output will improve as evidenced by increased activity tolerance, maintenance of euvolumic weight, and less ankle edema.

Patient's activity tolerance will be improved as evidenced by daily journal of activity.

NOC Suggested Outcomes

Cardiac pump effectiveness (0400)
Tissue perfusion: peripheral (0407)
Vital signs (0802)

NIC Suggested Interventions

Major interventions: Hemodynamic Regulation (4150), Vital Signs Monitoring (6680), Energy Management (0180)

- Auscultate lung sounds for crackles or other adventitious sounds.
- Recognize presence of blood pressure alterations.
- Auscultate heart sounds.
- Monitor and document heart rate, rhythm, and pulses.
- Monitor electrolyte levels.
- Administer neurohormonal medications: beta blockers, ACE inhibitor, and diuretics.
- Monitor peripheral pulses, capillary refill, and temperature and color of extremities.
- Monitor for peripheral edema, jugular vein distention, and S_3 and S_4 heart sounds.
- Monitor effects of medications.
- Determine patient's physical limitations.
- Determine patient's/significant other's perception of causes of fatigue.
- Encourage verbalization of feelings about limitations.
- Determine causes of fatigue.
- Determine what and how much activity is required to build endurance.
- Monitor cardiorespiratory response to activity.
- Encourage alternating rest and activity periods.
- Arrange physical activities to reduce competition for oxygen supply to vital body functions.
- Encourage an afternoon nap if appropriate.
- Assist patient to schedule rest periods.
- Plan activities for periods when patient has the most energy.
- Encourage physical activity.
- Monitor patient's oxygen response.
- Teach patient and significant others techniques of self-care that will minimize oxygen consumption.
- Instruct patient/significant other to recognize signs and symptoms of fatigue that require reduction of activity.
- Instruct patient/significant other to notify health care provider if signs and symptoms of fatigue persist.
- Assist the patient to identify tasks that family and friends can perform in the home to prevent/relieve fatigue.
- Teach activity organization and time management techniques to prevent fatigue.
- Assist the patient in assigning priority to activities to accommodate energy levels.

Nursing Care Plan—cont'd

- Assist the patient/significant other to establish realistic activity goals.
- Assist patient to identify preferences for activity.
- Monitor blood pressure, pulse, and respirations before, during, and after activity, as appropriate.
- Monitor for a widening of pulse pressure.
- Monitor cardiac rate and rhythm.

- Monitor heart tones.
- Monitor lung sounds.

Evaluation Parameters

Patient report of improved exercise tolerance and reduced fatigue, vital signs within normal ranges, peripheral pulses present, skin color normal.

---

homemaker services, home health services, and telephone services. The AHA provides information and support for older patients with cardiovascular diseases and their families.

Evaluation of nursing care is based on whether the goals of functional independence, or at least prevention of deterioration, are met. The nurse should determine whether medications are managed correctly, the diet is appropriate, and a proper balance of exercise and rest is achieved. Stress and anxiety should be minimized, and adequate support systems should be maintained for older patients.

SUMMARY

Normal age-related changes occur in the heart, the blood vessels, the blood, and in the pumping ability of the heart. Generally, there is a stiffening and decreased elasticity of the tissues and a decrease in cardiac output and blood volume. Several studies have shown that regular physical exercise can retard the changes in the cardiovascular system that occur with age.

Commonly occurring cardiovascular diseases in older age include hypertension, anemia, atherosclerosis, ACS, cardiac arrhythmias, heart failure, valvular disease, cerebrovascular disease, and peripheral vascular disease. In some cases, the classic symptoms of the diseases are altered or absent in the older adult, so that accurate assessment and diagnosis are imperative. Older people should not be ruled out of active rehabilitation programs solely because of age, because they often respond well to treatment. Nursing interventions should focus on prevention of further disease by helping older people to minimize risk factors by stopping smoking, eating a balanced diet low in salt and cholesterol, maintaining an active lifestyle, exercising regularly, and managing stress.

REFERENCES

Adab, P., Cheng, K. K., Jiang, D. Q., Zhang, W. S., & Lam, T. H. (2003). Age-specific relevance of usual blood pressure to vascular mortality. *Lancet, 361*(9366), 1391.

American Heart Association. (2006). ACC/AHA 2005 guideline update for percutaneous intervention. ACC/AHA Task Force on Practice Guidelines. Retrieved February 25, 2006, from www.americanheart.org/downloadable/heart/11317477032425summary.pdf.

American Heart Association. (2005). Fact sheet: Beta-blockers for acute myocardial infarction. Retrieved February 24, 2006, from www.americanheart.org.

American Heart Association. (2004). *2004 heart and stroke statistical update.* Retrieved January 5, 2004, from www.americanheart.org.

American Heart Association. (2002a). AHA scientific position: Exercise. Retrieved January 22, 2002, from www.americanheart.org/presenter.jhtml?identifier=4563.

American Heart Association. (2002b). *2002 heart and stroke statistical update.* Retrieved January 22, 2002, from www.americanheart.org.

Appel, L. J., Moore, T. J., Oberzanek, E., Vollmer, W. M., Svetkey, L. P., Sachs, F. M., et al. for the DASH Collaborative Research Group. (1997). A clinical trial of the effects of dietary patterns on blood pressure. *New England Journal of Medicine, 336,* 1117-1124.

Aronow, W. S. (2003). Effects of aging on the heart. In R. C. Tallis & H. M. Fillit (Eds.), *Brocklehurst's textbook of geriatric medicine and gerontology* (6th ed.). London: Churchill Livingstone.

Asmar, R. (2003). Benefits of blood pressure reduction in elderly patients. *Journal of Hypertension, 21*(suppl), S25-S30.

Assey, M. E. (1993). Heart disease in the elderly. *Heart Disease and Stroke, 2,* 330-334.

Astrand, P. O. (1992). Physical activity and fitness. *American Journal of Clinical Nutrition, 55,* 1231S-1236S.

Barron, H. V. (2003, November 10). Management of patients over age 75 with cardiovascular disease. 72nd Scientific Sessions of the American Heart Association. Retrieved from www.medscape.com/viewarticle/426383?src=search.

Beers, M. H., & Berkow, R. (Eds.). (2000). *The Merck manual of geriatrics* (3rd ed.). Philadelphia: John Wiley & Sons.

Berry, C., & Rae, A. (2003). Atrial fibrillation in the elderly. *British Journal of Cardiology, 10*(5), 373-378.

Bexton, R. S. (1992). Cardiac arrhythmias. In J. C. Brocklehurst, R. C. Tallis, & H. M. Fillet (Eds.), *Textbook of geriatric medicine and gerontology* (4th ed.). Edinburgh: Churchill Livingstone.

Braunwald, E. (2001). *A textbook of cardiovascular medicine.* Philadelphia: Saunders.

Burr, M. L., Fehily, A. M., Gilbert, J. F., Rogers, S., Holliday, R. M., Sweetnam, P. M., et al. (1989). Effect of changes in fat, fish, and fibre intakes on death and myocardial reinfarction: Diet and reinfarction (DART). *Lancet, 2*(8666), 757-761.

Burt, V. L., Whelton, P., Roccella, E. J., Brown, C., Cutler, J. A., Higgins, M., et al. (1995). Prevalence of hypertension in the U.S. adult population: Results from the Third National Health and Nutrition Examination Survey, 1988-1991. *Hypertension, 25,* 305-313.

Carroll, J. F., & Pollock, M. L. (1992). Rehabilitation and lifestyle modification in the elderly. *Cardiovascular Clinics, 22,* 209-227.

Centers for Disease Control and Prevention. (2003). *Diabetes fact sheet.* Atlanta: CDC.

Centers for Disease Control and Prevention. (2004). Physiologic responses and long-term adaptations to exercise. Retrieved September 2004 from www.cdc.gov/nccdphp/sgr/chap3.htm.

Cheitlin, M. D. (2003). Cardiovascular physiology—Changes with aging. *American Journal of Geriatric Cardiology, 12*(1), 9-13.

Chobanian, A., Bakris, G., Black, H., Cushman, W. C., Green, L. A., Izzo, J. L., et al. (2003). The seventh report of the Joint National Committee on Prevention, Detection, Evaluation, and Treatment of High Blood Pressure: The JNC 7 report. *JAMA, 289*(19), 2560-2572.

Cimminiello, C. (2002). PAD: Epidemiology and pathophysiology. *Thrombosis Research, 106*(6), V295-301.

Cleophas, T. J., & van Marum, R. (2003). Age-related decline in autonomic control of blood pressure: Implications for the pharmacological management of hypertension in the elderly. *Drugs and Aging, 20*(5), 313-319.

Cohn, J. N., Julius, S., Neutel, J., Weber, M., Turlapaty, P., Shen, Y., et al. (2004). Clinical experience with perindropril in African American hypertensive patients: A large U.S. community trial. *American Journal of Hypertension, 17*(2), 134-138.

Davies, M. J. (1992). Pathology of the aging heart. In J. C. Brocklehurst, R. C. Tallis, & H. M. Fillet (Eds.), *Textbook of geriatric medicine and gerontology* (4th ed.). Edinburgh: Churchill Livingstone.

de Lorgeril, M., Salen, P., Martin, J. L., Monjaud, I., Delaye, J., Mamelle, N., et al. (1999). Mediterranean diet, traditional risk factors, and the rate of cardiovascular complications after myocardial infarction. Final report of the Lyon Diet Heart Study. *Circulation, 99,* 779-785.

DeNicola, P., & Casale, G. (1983). Blood in the aged. In Platt, D. (Ed.), *Geriatrics.* New York: Springer-Verlag.

Diehm, C., Schuster, A., Allenberg, J. R., Darius, H., Haberl, R., Lange, S., et al. (2004). High prevalence of peripheral arterial disease and co-morbidity in 6880 primary care patients: Cross sectional study. *Atherosclerosis, 172*(1), 95-105.

Elliott, W. J., & Black, H. R. (2002). Treatment of hypertension in the elderly. *American Journal of Geriatric Cardiology, 11*(1), 11-21.

Elward, K., Larson, E., & Wagner, E. (1992). Factors associated with regular aerobic exercise in an elderly population. *Journal of the American Board of Family Practice, 5,* 467-474.

Erhardt, L. R. (2003). Women—a neglected risk group for atherosclerosis and vascular disease. *Scandinavian Cardiovascular Journal, 37*(1), 3-12.

European Carotid Surgery Trialists' Collaborative Group. (1998). Randomized trial of endarterectomy for recently symptomatic carotid stenosis: Final results of the MRC European Carotid Surgery Trial (ECST). *Lancet, 351,* 1379-1387.

Executive Summary of the Third Report of the National Cholesterol Education Program. (2001). Expert Panel on Detection, Evaluation, and Treatment of High Blood Cholesterol in Adults (Adult Treatment Panel III). *JAMA, 285,* 2486-2497.

Fields, S. D. (1991). Special considerations in the physical exam of older patients. *Geriatrics, 46*(8), 39-44.

Fioranelli, M., Piccoli, M., Mileto, G. M., Risa, M. P., Sgreccia, F., Azzolini, A. P., et al. (2001). Modifications in cardiovascular functional parameters with aging. *Minerva Cardioangiologica (Torino), 49*(3), 169-178.

Fletcher, G. F., Blair, S. N., Blumenthal, J., Caspersen, C., Chaitman, B., Epstein, S., et al. (1992). Statement on exercise: Benefits and recommendations for physical activity programs for all Americans. *Circulation, 86*(1), 340-344.

Fogari, R., Mugellini, A., Zoppi, A., Derosa, G., Pasotti, C., Fogari, E., et al. (2003). Influence of losartan and atenolol on memory function in very elderly hypertensive patients. *Journal of Human Hypertension, 17*(11), 781-785.

Fogari, R., Mugellini, A., Zoppi, A., Marasi, G., Pasotti, C., Poletti, L., et al. (2004). Effects of valsartan compared with enalapril on blood pressure and cognitive function in elderly patients with essential hypertension. *Journal of Clinical Pharmacology, 59*(12), 863-868.

Fogari, R., & Zoppi, A. (2004). Effect of antihypertensive agents on quality of life in the elderly. *Drugs and Aging, 21*(6), 377-393.

Fowler, R. S., & Fordyce, W. E. (1974). *Stroke: Why do they behave that way?* Dallas: American Heart Association.

Furberg, C. D. , Coletta, E. M., Manolio, T. A., Psaty, B. M., Bild, D. E., Borhani, N. D., Newman, A., et al. (1992). Major electrocardiographic abnormalities in persons aged 65 and older (the Cardiovascular Health Study). *American Journal of Cardiology, 69,* 1329-1335.

Fuster, V., Ryden, L. E., Asinger, R. W., Cannom, D. S., Crijns, M., J., Fryer, L., et al. (2001). ACC/AHA/ESC guidelines for the management of patients with atrial fibrillation. *European Heart Journal, 22,* 1852-1923.

Gilliss, C. L., Gortner, S. R., Hauck, W. W., Shinn, J. A., Sparacino, P. A., Tompkins, C., et al. (1993). A randomized clinical trial of nursing care for recovery from cardiac surgery. *Heart and Lung, 22,* 125-133.

Gruppo Italiano per lo Studio della Sopravvivenza nell-Infarto Miocardio. (1999). Dietary supplementation with n-3 polyunsaturated fatty acids and vitamin E after myocardial infarction: Results of the GISSI-Prevenzione trial. *Lancet, 354,* 447-455.

Guo, H., & Schaller, F. (2004). Cardiovascular function with aging— transfer function analysis. Updated March 15, 2004. Retrieved September 18, 2004, from www.hsc.unt.edu/RAD/abstracts/viewabstract.cfm?ID=102.

Guo, W., Turlapaty, P., Shen, Y., Dong, V., Batchelor, A., Barlow, D., & Lagast, H. (2004). Clinical experience with perindropril in patients nonresponsive to previous antihypertensive therapy: A large U.S. trial. *American Journal of Therapeutics, 11*(3), 199-205.

He, F. J., & MacGregor, G. A. (2004). Effect of longer-term modest salt reduction on blood pressure. *Cochrane Database of Systematic Reviews, 3.*

Heath, J. M., & Stuart, M. R. (2002). Prescribing exercise for frail elders. *Journal of the American Board of Family Practice, 15*(3), 218-228.

Hirose, H., Amano, A., Yoshida, S., Takahashi, A., Nagano, N., & Kohmoto, T., (2000). Coronary artery bypass grafting in the elderly. *Chest, 117*(5), 1336-1344.

Hiwada, K., Ogihara, T., Matsumoto, M., Matsuoko, H., Takishita, S., Shimamoto, K., et al. (1999). Guidelines for hypertension in the elderly—1999 revised version. Ministry of Health and Welfare of Japan. *Hypertension Research, 22,* 231-259.

Hooper, L., Bartlett, C., Davey Smith, G., & Ebrahim, S. (2004). Advice to reduce dietary salt for prevention of cardiovascular disease. *Cochrane Database of Systematic Reviews, 3.*

House, M. A. (1992). Thrombolytic therapy for acute myocardial infarction: The elderly population. *AACN Clinical Issues, 3*(2), 106-113.

Israili, Z. H. (2003). The use of calcium antagonists in the therapy of hypertension in the elderly. *American Journal of Therapeutics, 10*(6), 383-395.

Johnson, M., Bulechek, G., Dochterman, J. M., Maas, M., & Moorhead, S. (2001). *Nursing diagnoses, outcomes, and interventions: NANDA, NOC, and NIC linkages.* St. Louis: Mosby.

Kallaras, K., Sparks, E. A., Schuster, D. P., Osei, K., Whooley, C. F., & Boudoulas, H. (2001). Cardiovascular effects of aging: Interrelationships of aortic, left ventricular, and left atrial function. *Herz, 26*(2), 129-139.

Kannel, W. B. (2002). Coronary heart disease risk factors in the elderly. *American Journal of Geriatric Cardiology, 11*(2), 101-107.

Kaufmann, H., & Biaggioni, I. (2003). Disorders of the autonomic nervous system. In R. C. Tallis & H. M. Fillit (Eds.), *Brocklehurst's textbook of geriatric medicine and gerontology* (6th ed.). London: Churchill Livingstone.

Kendall, M. J., & Nuttall, S. L. (2003). Coronary artery disease—more disease, more patients, better treatment. *Journal of Clinical Pharmacy and Therapeutics, 28,* 1-4.

Khan, A. S., Sane, D. C., Wannenburg, T., & Sonntag, W. E. (2002). Growth hormone, insulin-like growth factor-1 and the aging cardiovascular system. *Cardiovascular Research, 54*(1), 25-35.

Kirshner, H. S. (2003). Medical prevention of stroke, 2003. *Southern Medical Journal, 96*(4), 354-358.

Kokkinos, P.F., Narayan, P., Colleran, J. A., Pittaras, A., Notargiacomo, A., Reda, D., et al. (1995). Effects of regular exercise on blood pressure and left ventricular hypertrophy in African-American men with severe hypertension. *New England Journal of Medicine, 333,* 1462-1467.

Lazarus, B. A., Murphy, J. B., Coletta, E. M., McQuade, W. H., & Culpepper, L. (1991). The provision of physical activity to hospitalized elderly patients. *Archives of Internal Medicine, 151,* 2452-2456.

Leary, M. C., & Saver, J. L. (2001). Incidence of silent stroke in the United States. Poster presented at the 26th American Heart Association Stroke Meeting, February 2001, Fort Lauderdale, Florida.

Lehne, R. A. (2004). *Pharmacology for nursing care* (5th ed.). Philadelphia: W. B. Saunders.

Li, F., Harmer, P., Fisher, K. J., Harmer, P., McAuley, E., Duncan, T. E., & Duncan, S. C., et al. (2001). An evaluation of the effects of Tai Chi exercise on physical function among older persons: A randomized controlled trial. *Annals of Behavioral Medicine, 23,* 139-146.

Li, F., Harmer, P., Fisher, K. J., & McAuley, E. (2002). Delineating the impact of Tai Chi training on physical function among elderly. *American Journal of Preventive Medicine, 23*(2S), 92-97.

Libby, P. (2002a). Inflammation in atherosclerosis. *Nature, 286*(6917), 868-874.

Libby, P. (2002b). Atherosclerosis: The new view. *Scientific American, 286*(5), 46-55.

Malacco, E., Vari, N., Capuano, V., Spagnuolo, V., Borgnino, C., Palatini, P., et al. (2003). A randomized, double-blind, active-controlled, parallel group comparison of valsartan and amlodipine in the treatment of isolated systolic hypertension in elderly patients: The Val-Syst study. *Clinical Therapeutics, 25*(11), 2765-2780.

Manson, J. E., & Martin, K. A. (2001). Postmenopausal hormone-replacement therapy. *New England Journal of Medicine, 346,* 34-40.

Mathew, S. T., Gottdiener, J. S., Kitzman, D., & Aurigemma, G. (2004). Congestive heart failure in the elderly: The cardiovascular health study. *American Journal of Geriatric Cardiology, 13*(2), 61-68.

McInnes, G. T. (2003). The expanding role of angiotensin receptor blockers in the management of the elderly hypertensive. *Current Medical Research and Opinion, 19*(5), 452-455.

Messerli, F. H., & Grossman, E. (2004). Beta-blockers in hypertension: Is carvedilol different? *American Journal of Cardiology, 93*(9A), 7B-12B.

Miettinen, T., Pyorala, K., Olsson, A. G., Musliner, T. A., Cook, T. J., Faergeman, O., et al. (1997). Cholesterol lowering therapy in women and elderly patients with myocardial infarction or angina pectoris: Findings from the Scandinavian Simvastatin Survival Study (4S). *Circulation, 96*(12), 4211-4218.

Mizutani, Y., Nakano, S., Ote, N., Iwase, T., & Fujinami, T. (1984). Evaluation of effects of aging, training and myocardial ischemia on cardiac reserve by exercise echocardiography. *Japanese Circulation Journal, 48*(9), 969-979.

Mol, V. J., & Baker, C. A. (1991). Activity intolerance in the geriatric stroke patient. *Rehabilitation Nursing, 16*(6), 337-343.

Mosca, L., Collins, P., Herrington, D. M., Mendelsohn, M. E., Pasternak, R. C., Robertson, R. M., et al. (2001). Hormone replacement therapy and cardiovascular disease: A statement for health care professionals from the American Heart Association. *Circulation, 104,* 499-503.

Moser, M., & Setaro, J. (2004). Continued importance of diuretics and beta-adrenergic blockers in the management of hypertension. *Medical Clinics of North America, 88*(1), 167-187.

Mulrow, C. D., Chiquette, E., Angel, L., Cornell, J., Summerbell, C., Anagnostelis, B., et al. (2000a). Dieting to reduce body weight for controlling hypertension in adults. *Cochrane Database of Systematic Reviews, 2,* CD000484.

Mulrow, C., Lau, J., Cornell, J., & Brand, M. (2000b). Pharmacotherapy for hypertension in the elderly. *Cochrane Database of Systematic Reviews, 2,* CD000028.

Nierodzik, M. L. R., Sutin, D., & Freedman, M. L. (2003). Blood disorders and their management in old age. In R. C. Tallis & H. M. Fillit (Eds.), *Brocklehurst's textbook of geriatric medicine and gerontology* (6th ed.). London: Churchill Livingstone.

North American Symptomatic Carotid Endarterectomy Trial (NASCET) Collaborators. (1991). Beneficial effect of carotid endarterectomy in symptomatic patients with high-grade carotid stenosis. *New England Journal of Medicine, 325,* 445-453.

Padden, D. L. (2002). The role of the advanced practice nurse in the promotion of exercise and physical activity. *Topics in Advanced Practice Nursing eJournal, 2*(1). Retrieved May 5, 2005, from www.medscape.com/viewarticle/421475.

Paniagua, D., Howell, M., Strickman, N., Velasco, J., Dougherty, K., Skolkin, M., et al. (2001). Outcomes following extracranial carotid artery stenting in high-risk patients. *Journal of Invasive Cardiology, 13*(5), 375-381.

Pell, J. P., MacIntyre, K., Walsh, D., Capewell, S., McMurray, J. J., Chalmars, J. W., et al. (2002). Time trends in survival and readmission following coronary artery bypass grafting in Scotland, 1981-1996: Retrospective observational study. *BMJ, 324,* 201-202.

Perler, B. A. (2003, November 10). Management of patients over age 75 with cardiovascular disease. 72nd Scientific Sessions of the American Heart Association. Retrieved May 5, 2005, from www.medscape.com/viewarticle/426383?src=search.

Porter, V. (2003). Cardiac surgery. Part I: Improved surgical techniques expand patient population to include elderly. *Medscape Cardiology, 7*(1), 29-35.

Raji, M. A., Kuo, Y. F., Salazar, J. A, Satish, S., & Goodwin , J. S. (2003). Ethnic differences in antihypertensive medication use in the elderly. *Annals of Pharmacotherapy, 38*(2), 209-214.

Rakowski, W., & Mor, V. (1992). The association of physical activity with mortality among older adults in the longitudinal study of aging (1984-1988). *Journal of Gerontology: Medical Sciences, 47*(4), M122-M129.

Ramsay, L. E., Williams, B., Johnston, G. D., MacGregor, C. A., Poston, L, Potter, J. F., et al. (1999). British Hypertension Society guidelines for hypertension management. Summary. *BMJ, 319,* 630-635.

Rials, S. J., Marinchak, R. A., & Kowey, P. R. (1992). Arrhythmias in the elderly. *Cardiovascular Clinics, 22,* 139-157.

Rich, M. W. (1997). Epidemiology, pathophysiology, and etiology of congestive heart failure in older adults. *Journal of the American Geriatrics Society, 45*(8), 968-974.

Rodeheffer, R. J., & Gerstenblith, G. (1985). Effect of age on cardiovascular function. In H. A. Johnson (Ed.), *Relations between normal aging and disease.* New York: Raven Press.

Roitman, J. L. (Ed.). (2001). *ACSM's resource manual of guidelines for exercise testing and prescription* (4th ed.). Philadelphia: W. B. Saunders.

Rosengart, T. K., Finnin, E. B., Kim, D. Y., Samy, S. A., Tanhehco, Y., Ko, W., et al. (2002). Open heart surgery in the elderly: Results from a consecutive series of 100 patients aged 85 years or older. *American Journal of Medicine, 112,* 143-147.

Rossouw, J. E. (2001). Early risk of cardiovascular events after commencing hormone replacement therapy. *Current Opinion in Lipidology, 12,* 371-375.

Rubins, H. B., Robins, S. J., Collins, D., Fye, C. L., Anderson, J. W., Elam, M. B., et al. (1999). Gemfibrozil for the secondary prevention of coronary artery disease in men with low levels of high-density lipoprotein cholesterol. Veterans Affairs High-Density Lipoprotein

Cholesterol Intervention Trial Study Group. *New England Journal of Medicine, 341*(6), 410-425.

Schainfeld, R. M. (2001). Management of peripheral arterial disease and intermittent claudication. *Journal of the American Board of Family Practice, 14*(6), 443-445.

Schwartz, G. G. (2004). Lipid management after acute coronary syndromes and percutaneous coronary interventions. *Baylor College of Medicine Reports on Dyslipidemias, 3*(2), 1-8.

Schwartz, J. B. (1999, June 9). Cardiovascular function and disease in the elderly. Retrieved from www.galter.northwester.edu/geriatrics/chapters/cardiovascuar_function_disease.cfm.

Seals, D. R., Monahan, K. D., Bell, C., Tanaka, H., & Jones, P. P. (2001). The aging cardiovascular system: Changes in autonomic function at rest and in response to exercise. *International Journal of Sport Nutrition, Exercise and Metabolism, 11*(suppl), S189-S195.

Shepherd, J., Blauw, G., Murphy, M. B., Bollen, E. L., Buckley, B. M., Cobbe, S. M., et al. (2002). Pravastatin in elderly individuals at risk of vascular disease (PROSPER): A randomized controlled trial. *Lancet, 360*(9346), 1623-1630.

Sherwood, N. E., & Jeffery, R. W. (2000). The behavioral determinants of exercise: Implications for physical activity interventions. *Annual Review of Nutrition, 20*, 21-44.

Simon, J. A., Hsia, J., Cauley, J. A., Richards, C., Harris, F., Fong, J., et al. (2001). Postmenopausal hormone therapy and risk of stroke: The Heart and Estrogen-Progestin Replacement Study (HERS). *Circulation, 103*, 638-642.

Staessen, J. A., Gasowski, J., Wang, J. G., Thijs, L., Dentlond, E., Boissel, J. P., et al. (2000). Risks of untreated and treated isolated systolic hypertension in the elderly: Meta-analysis of outcome trials. *Lancet, 355*, 865-872.

Steinhaus, L. A., Dustman, R. E., Ruhlings, R. O., Emmerson, R. Y., Johnson, S. C., Shearer, D. E., et al. (1988). Cardio-respiratory fitness of young and older active and sedentary men. *British Journal of Sports Medicine, 22*(4), 163-166.

Stokes, G. S. (2004). Systolic hypertension in the elderly: Pushing the frontiers of therapy—a suggested new approach. *Journal of Clinical Hypertension, 6*(4), 192-197.

Sutaria, N., Elder, A. T., & Shaw, T. R. (2000). Mitral balloon valvotomy for the treatment of mitral stenosis in octogenarians. *Journal of the American Geriatrics Society, 48*(8), 971-974.

Svetkey, L. P., Harsha, D. W., Vollmer, W. M., Stevens, V. J., Obarzanek, E., Elmer, P. J., et al. (2003). Premier: A clinical trial of comprehensive lifestyle modification for blood pressure control: Rationale, design, and baseline characteristics. *Annals of Epidemiology, 13*, 462-471.

Tabet, S., & Berg, A. O., for the U.S. Preventive Services Task Force. (1996). Screening for peripheral arterial disease. In *Guide to clinical preventive services: Report of the U.S. Preventive Services Task Force.* Baltimore: Williams & Wilkins.

Tanko, L. B., Bagger, Y. Z., Alexandersen, P., Larsen, P. J., & Christiansen, C. (2003). Peripheral adiposity exhibits an independent dominant antiatherogenic effect in elderly women. *Circulation, 107*(12), 1626-1631.

United Kingdom Prospective Diabetes Study Group. (1995). United Kingdom Prospective Study. *Diabetes, 44*, 1249-1258.

U.S. Department of Health and Human Services. (2002). Healthy people 2010: Physical activity and fitness. Retrieved April 5, 2006, from www.health.gov/healthypeople/document/html/volume2/22physi cal.htm.

Vincent, K. R., Braith, R. W., Feldman, R. A., Magyari, P. M., Cutler, R. B., Persin, S. A., et al. (2002). Resistance exercise and physical performance in adults aged 60 to 83. *Journal of the American Geriatrics Society, 50*, 1100-1107.

Waeber, B. (2003). Trials in isolated systolic hypertension: An update. *Current Cardiology Reports, 5*(6), 427-434.

Weitz, J. L., Byrne, J., & Clagett, G. P. (1996). Diagnosis and treatment of chronic arterial insufficiency of the lower extremities: A critical review. *Circulation, 94*, 3026-3049.

Wenger, N. K., Scheidt, S., & Weber, M. A. (2001). Exercise and elderly persons. *American Journal of Geriatric Cardiology, 10*(5), 241-242.

Whelton, P. K., Appel, L. J., Espeland, M. A., Applegate, W. B., Ettinger, W. H. Jr., Kostis, J. B., et al. (1998). Sodium reduction and weight loss in the treatment of hypertension in older persons: A randomized controlled trial of nonpharmacologic interventions in the elderly (TONE). TONE Collaborative Research Group. *Journal of the American Medical Association, 179*, 878-879.

Wilson, R. A. (1966). *Feminine forever.* New York: M. Evans.

Wilson, R. A., & Wilson, T. A. (1963). The fate of the nontreated postmenopausal woman: A plea for the maintenance of adequate estrogen from puberty to grave. *Journal of the American Geriatrics Society, 11*, 347-362.

Chapter 13

Respiratory System

Adrianne Dill Linton

Objectives

Describe normal changes in the structure and function of the respiratory system associated with aging.

Describe measures to maintain respiratory health in the older adult.

Explain the cause and treatment of respiratory disorders that are common in older persons.

Describe the components of the respiratory assessment in the older adult.

Formulate nursing diagnoses for older adults with respiratory disorders.

Develop plans to manage older adults with actual or potential respiratory problems.

The respiratory system, like the skin, is exposed continually to the environment. Smoke, bacteria, and multiple irritants are inhaled daily. Therefore it sometimes is difficult, if not impossible, to differentiate the effects of environmental exposures and disease from the effects of age. Many of the studies of the effects of aging have been cross-sectional rather than longitudinal, and many early studies included smokers, so some of the effects attributed to "normal aging" of the respiratory system may in fact have resulted from smoke-related pathology. Also, many older adults have neuromuscular and cardiovascular conditions that affect respiratory function. So, having acknowledged the uncertainty about normal versus disease-induced changes, this section addresses changes that commonly are found in the respiratory system of older adults.

CHANGES WITH AGING
Anatomical Changes

Aging produces changes in the respiratory system itself and in related systems that collectively result in a moderate decline in pulmonary function.

Extrapulmonary Changes. Changes in the thorax that affect respiratory status include ossification of costal cartilage, loss of vertebral disk space, and increased anteroposterior diameter. The reduction of type IIA fibers in the muscles of respiration (diaphragm, intercostals, anterior abdominal muscles, and accessory muscles) diminishes muscle strength and endurance. The extent to which the loss of strength is related to atrophy associated with a sedentary lifestyle is a topic of debate. All of these common changes might have no functional impact under stable conditions, but with deconditioning, certain medications, or acute infection, the older adult's lack of reserve becomes apparent (Connolly, 2003).

Intrapulmonary Changes. With aging, opposite processes are occurring in the lung parenchyma and the conducting airways. The elastic recoil that normally opposes the elastic forces in the chest wall declines with age. Because both of these forces are reduced in the aged, the effects balance each other. The lungs become more compliant because of the loss of elastic forces, which partially compensates for the decreased chest wall compliance, making it somewhat easier for the weakened respiratory muscles to move the stiffer chest wall.

Bronchial structure generally is unchanged. The number of glandular epithelial cells in the large airways declines, resulting in a decrease in the mucus that normally protects the lungs against infection. Changes in elastin and collagen reduce the support in the small airways so they collapse more readily during expiration. The number of alveoli remains constant in the healthy aging person, but alveolar changes occur. Whereas the alveoli and alveolar ducts enlarge, the alveolar surface for gas exchange is reduced by the breakdown of intraalveolar septa. This change in alveolar structure gives aged lungs some of the microscopic characteristics of emphysematous lungs and sometimes is called "senile lung." A person can lose up to 20% of the alveolar surface area without compromising function. In healthy older adults, blood flow toward the apices of the lungs increases, partially because of an increase in pulmonary artery pressure (Connolly, 2003).

Functional Changes

As a result of the changes described, the mechanics of breathing are modified with age. As the chest wall becomes less mobile, chest wall compliance is reduced, and the older adult is less able to provide adequate force to *move air rapidly*. The maximal force available for both inspiration and expiration decreases. Because the work of breathing is increased, the older person tends to make greater use of all respiratory muscles, especially the diaphragm. This increased reliance on the diaphragm makes the older person more sensitive to changes in intraabdominal pressure, such as those caused by a large meal or body position.

An increase in blood flow to the apices of the lungs while ventilation remains greater in the bases creates a tendency toward ventilation-perfusion mismatch. Although the cough reflex appears to remain intact, older adults do have reduced mucociliary clearance. Possibly because of altered chemoreceptor sensitivity, the ability to perceive acute bronchoconstriction declines. Respiratory and cardiovascular changes result in a decline in maximal oxygen uptake—a change that can be attenuated by regular aerobic exercise.

Measures of Pulmonary Function.
Lung volumes are measured with pulmonary function tests (PFTs). The commonly measured volumes are defined in Table 13-1. Normal adult values and comparable values for older adults are shown. Although total lung volume remains fairly constant, age influences the subdivisions of this volume. Residual volume (RV), which is the volume of air remaining in the lung after a maximal expiration, increases with age, probably because of the diminished elastic forces in the lung. This increased RV encroaches on and reduces the vital capacity (VC). Tidal volume (VT), which is simply the amount of air moved with a normal breath, should be relatively unchanged with age.

Not only do lung volumes change with age, but the rate at which air is moved also is reduced. Airflow is dependent on airway size and resistance, muscle strength, and elastic recoil. Indices of airflow that decrease with age are forced vital capacity (FVC), forced expiratory volume in 1 second (FEV_1), forced expiratory flow (FEF), forced expiratory volume (FEV), and maximal voluntary ventilation (MVV). Some FEV_1 change appears to be inevitable with age as demonstrated by a decline of 8.5% over 10 years in young adults who had never smoked and did not have asthma (Apostol et al., 2002).

The FEV_1/FVC ratio, which normally is 70% in individuals age 40 to 45 years, falls by approximately 0.2% each year. This ratio declines more rapidly in women, whereas maximal expiratory flow and maximum voluntary ventilation decline more rapidly in men.

The lung volume when the airways collapse is termed *closing volume*. Closing volume increases with early collapse of airways related to degeneration of airway support structures. Impaired ventilation can cause a ventilation-perfusion mismatch, which, along with small airway closure and structural alveolar changes, results in reduced resting arterial oxygen tension (Connolly, 2003).

Changes in pulmonary function measurements are summarized in Table 13-1.

Control of Ventilation.
Cumulative age-related changes appear to decrease the efficiency of mechanisms that monitor and control ventilation (Connolly, 2003). Various studies have reported impaired ventilatory responses to hypoxia and hypercapnia at rest, whereas others have found normal responses to eucapnic hypoxia but an impaired response to hypoxia during sustained hypercapnia. Most current studies support the finding of a decreased homeostatic response to lowered oxygen content and increased carbon dioxide (Lucy, Kowalchuk, Hughson, Paterson, & Cunningham, 2003). The response to exercise-induced carbon dioxide production has been shown to increase (Connolly, 2003). In one study of healthy older people (59 to 72 years), the heart rate response to hypoxemic stress was 25% that of younger persons (22 to 29 years) (Lucy et al., 2003). Another interesting study compared the hypoxic ventilatory response (HVR) of young and old climbers to high-altitude hypoxia. Serum levels of dopamine (DA) and dihydroxyphenylalanine (DOPA, a dopamine precursor) were measured at sea level, after passive transport to 2200 meters, and after climbs to 4200 and 5642 meters. The changes in HVR, DA, and DOPA indicated decreased DA receptor sensitivity and enhanced DA reuptake in older adults during altitude adjustment (Serebrovskaya et al., 2000). A small study assessed the ventilatory response and venous lactate levels of older and younger men during incremental exercise on a bicycle ergometer. The investigators concluded that the ventilatory response of older subjects was greater than that of younger subjects and that the increase was influenced by increased serum lactate (Prioux, Ramonatxo, Hayot, Mucci, & Prefaut, 2000).

Diminished response to hypoxia and hypercarbia has great clinical significance for nurses. The usual clinical signs of increased need for oxygen include increases in respiratory rate and volume and increased heart rate and blood pressure. These responses all are blunted to varying degrees in older adults. Therefore additional cues to impaired gas exchange, such as changes in mentation and affect, must be used. An older patient who normally has a low arterial oxygen level could have clinically

Table 13-1 *Air Flow Rates, Lung Volumes, and Capacities: Changes in Older Adults*

Parameter	Definition	Normal Change with Age
VOLUMES		
Tidal volume (VT)	Volume of air inhaled with each breath	Unchanged
Expiratory reserve volume (ERV)	Additional air that can forcefully exhaled after completion of a normal exhalation	Decreased
Residual volume (RV)	Amount of air remaining in the lungs after forced expiration	Increased
Inspiratory reserve volume (IRV)	Maximum volume of air that can be inhaled forcefully after a normal inhalation	Decreased
CAPACITIES		
Total lung capacity (TLC)	Maximum volume of air the lungs can contain	Unchanged
Functional residual capacity (FRC)	Volume of air remaining in the lungs at the end of normal exhalation	Increased
Vital capacity (VC)	Maximum volume of air that can be exhaled after maximum inspiration	Decreased
Inspiratory capacity (IC)	Maximum volume of air that can be inhaled after normal expiration	Decreased
Forced vital capacity (FVC)	Amount of air that can be quickly and forcefully exhaled after maximum inspiration	Decreased
Forced expiratory volume in first second of expiration (FEV_1)	Amount of air exhaled in first second of FVC	Decreased
FEV_1/FVC	Proportion of FVC exhaled in first second	Decreased
Forced midexpiratory flow rate ($FEF_{25\%-75\%}$)	Airflow rate in middle half of forced expiration	Decreased
Maximal voluntary ventilation (MVV)	Rapid deep breathing for specified period of time	Decreased
Peak expiratory flow rate (PEFR)	Maximum airflow rate during forced expiration	Decreased

Data from Hagler, D. A. (2004). Nursing assessment: Respiratory system. In S. M. Lewis, M. M. Heitkemper, & S. R. Dirksen (Eds.). *Medical surgical nursing* (6th ed.). St. Louis: Mosby, p. 558.

significant arterial hypoxemia (PO_2 less than 60 mm Hg) with a relatively minor pulmonary insult. In addition, these patients may respond more slowly to treatment.

Lung Host Defense. Serious respiratory infections are more common in older adults probably because of changes in defense mechanisms along with various pathological changes. Especially among institutionalized persons, the pharynx often becomes colonized by pathogenic organisms that reach the lungs through microaspiration. Also, bacteria can be transported toward the pharynx by reflux of gastric contents,

and aspirated into the lungs. Normally, hydrochloric acid in the stomach helps eliminate ingested bacteria. However, older persons often have less gastric acid, so this protective mechanism is impaired. Tracheal intubation and nasogastric tubes also appear to provide avenues for organisms to access the pharynx. Patients with dysphagia are at increased risk for aspiration, which is a risk factor for pulmonary infection. Some drugs have been implicated in the increased incidence of respiratory infections among older persons. Gastric acid neutralizers and inhibitors raise the pH of the stomach, which may provide a more hospitable environment for pathogens. Widespread use of antibiotics such as amoxicillin may contribute to growth of gram-negative organisms that subsequently cause infection.

Other changes in the pulmonary defenses that increase the risk of infection are reduced mucociliary clearance, alterations in the mucous layer caused by smoking or chronic lung disease, and age-related changes in immune function. Changes have been identified in both cell-mediated and humoral immunity. The number of active peripheral T cells declines while there is an increase in the proportion of circulating immature T cells. The T-cell response to interleukins and to mitogens is reduced along with a reduction in thymic mass and reduced generation of cytotoxic T cells (Connolly, 2003).

In summary, multiple changes in the older adult as a result of normal aging or the effects of environment and disease affect pulmonary function (Box 13-1). For the healthy older person, these changes seem to have no impact on daily functional status, but they can be important when physiological demands exceed capacity (Zeleznik, 2003).

Exercise Effects

The capacity to exercise is determined by many factors in addition to pulmonary function. A decrease in cardiac output and muscle mass, the presence of joint and circulatory and respiratory system diseases, and an overall decrease in physical activity all contribute to the decrease in exercise tolerance that is commonly seen in the elderly. Declining muscle power and muscle coordination increases the energy expenditure for a given load. Various exercises require a certain percentage of a person's maximum aerobic power, which declines with age, even among elite veteran endurance athletes (Kennie, Dinan, & Young, 2003). The body of evidence is growing that older adults can benefit significantly from both strength and endurance training, thereby mitigating to some extent the changes in the respiratory system. See Chapter 12 for a more detailed discussion of other benefits of exercise.

Factors That May Further Decrease Lung Function

Smoking, obesity, and immobility are common problems that can further decrease lung function in older adults. In addition, the older person undergoing surgery is at increased risk of pulmonary complications.

Smoking. The 2002 National Health Interview Survey data indicated that approximately 9.3% of adults age 65 and older were smokers. The overall prevalence rate for adult smokers in the United States was 22.5%, a significant decline since 1998, when the rate was

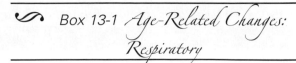

Box 13-1 *Age-Related Changes: Respiratory*

- Thorax
  - Ossification of costal cartilage
  - Loss of vertebral disk space
  - Increased anteroposterior diameter
  - Decreased chest wall compliance

- Muscles of respiration
  - Fewer type IIA fibers
  - Decreased strength

- Lung tissue
  - Decreased elasticity
  - Increased compliance

- Large airways
  - Decreased glandular epithelial cells
  - Decreased mucus production

- Small airways
  - Altered elastin and collagen
  - Earlier collapse during expiration
  - Increased closing volume

- Alveoli and alveolar ducts
  - Enlargement
  - Breakdown of intraalveolar septa
  - Decreased surface for gas exchange
  - Reduced resting arterial oxygen tension

- Pulmonary blood flow
  - Increased flow to apices of lungs
  - Tendency toward ventilation-perfusion mismatch

- Lung host defenses
  - Decreased mucociliary clearance
  - Reduced immune response

- Control mechanisms
  - Blunted response to hypoxemia
  - Increased ventilatory response to increased serum lactate

24.1%. However, public health officials are concerned that the target of 12% by 2010 is unlikely to be met at this rate (Centers for Disease Control and Prevention [CDC], 2004b).

The adverse effects of smoking tobacco are well known. Worldwide, it is responsible for 5 million deaths each year. In the United States, smokers have a reduced life expectancy with a loss of 13.2 years for men and 14.5 years for women (CDC, 2004a). It has long been recognized as a risk factor for pulmonary, cardiovascular, and cerebrovascular disease. The most recent Surgeon General's report on smoking and health (CDC, 2004b) added the following to the list of disease caused by smoking: abdominal aortic aneurysm, acute myeloid leukemia, cataract, cervical cancer, kidney cancer, pancreatic

CHAPTER 13 § Respiratory System **357**

cancer, pneumonia, periodontitis, and stomach cancer. Even nonsmokers may be significantly harmed by long exposure to cigarette smoke. "Secondhand" smoke has been linked with sudden infant death syndrome and with new cases of asthma, and with bronchitis among children (CDC, 2004b).

Smoking greatly increases the age-related decline in FEV_1, inhibits mucociliary clearance, and increases airway resistance and closing volume. A study of the effects of cigarette smoking in older adults with asthma demonstrated an increased immunoglobulin E (IgE) antibody production, enhanced bronchial hyperresponsiveness, and the generation of leukotriene by leukocytes (Mitsunobu et al., 2004). A 10-year longitudinal study that included FEV_1 measurements showed that individuals who had never smoked and did not have asthma had a decline of 8.5% in FEV_1, compared with 10.1% in nonsmoking individuals who had asthma. Individuals who smoked 15 or more cigarettes a day had an 11.1% decline, and heavier smokers with asthma had a 17.8% decline in FEV_1 (Apostol et al., 2002).

Smoking also has been linked to a decreased health-related quality of life (Bass, Wilson, & Griffith, 2004). A study of quality of life in smokers and former smokers (over 20 years without smoking) used the St. George's Respiratory Questionnaire (SGRQ), pulmonary function tests, and a 6-minute walk distance. Cough and phlegm were two variables related to decreased quality of life among smokers who did not have chronic obstructive pulmonary disease (Heijdra, Pinto-Plata, Kenney, Rassulo, & Celli, 2002).

Fortunately, it has been shown that smoking cessation can mitigate many of these harmful effects. Even long-time smokers may show a significant improvement in lung function after they stop. Research on smoking cessation, mostly done with younger people, has shown motivation to be the most important predictor of success (Connolly, 2000). Unfortunately, older smokers tend to dismiss evidence that smoking is harmful so that other motivators need to be sought. Evidence exists that smoking cessation does not reverse changes in lung function, but slows the rate of change to that occurring in nonsmoking older adults. Smoking cessation has been shown to reduce the risk of myocardial infarction in women, and may reduce the risk of ischemic, but not embolic, stroke. The rate of bone loss does not appear to be affected by smoking cessation (British Thoracic Society, 1997, cited in Connolly, 2000).

The ideal situation would be to discourage individuals from starting to smoke at any age. The influence of smokers in a family cannot be denied, as the likelihood of an individual smoking has been shown to increase significantly as the number of smokers in that person's family increased (Apostol et al., 2002). Community education should attempt to impress on adults the influence of their smoking behavior on their children.

Obesity. Lung and chest wall compliance and some lung volumes (functional residual capacity [FRC], expiratory reserve volume [ERV], and vital capacity [VC]) are markedly reduced by obesity, further increasing the work of breathing, which is already compromised by age. Amara, Koval, Paterson, and Cunningham (2001) studied factors related to the decline in FEV_1 in independently living adults ages 55 to 86 years. Both age and fat free mass were identified as important influences. Individuals with lung function values above average were those with more fat free mass and a higher level of physical activity. Another study that evaluated the relationship between body composition and lung function in Italian men ages 67 to 78 years demonstrated negative correlations between adiposity and FVC and FEV_1. Fat free mass and FVC were correlated positively (Santana et al., 2001).

In a study of obese hospitalized adults, 31% of those with severe obesity (defined as a body mass index of $35 kg/m^2$ or greater) had hypoventilation. This group had higher rates of intensive care, long-term care after discharge, and mechanical ventilation. They also were found to have decreased objective attention/concentration and increased subjective sleepiness. Over a period of 18 months, the mortality rate for those with obesity-related hypoventilation was 23% compared with 9% for those classified as having simple obesity (Nowbar et al., 2004).

Immobility. The inactivity that accompanies certain diseases, such as stroke and arthritis, can further jeopardize lung function in the aged. Bed rest is particularly harmful because the supine position increases the closing volume in adults and predisposes to early airway closure and atelectasis in the dependent parts of the lung.

Surgery. Surgery in older adults has become increasingly common. Whereas some procedures are lifesaving, many others such as cataract extraction and total joint replacement may be done to improve the quality of life. Technological advances such as minimally invasive surgery that have had a major impact in urology, gynecology, and general surgery explain some of the increase in surgical procedures on older persons (Seymour, 2003). A major challenge is to change the perception that all older adults are equally poor surgical risks. Factors that are associated with increased risk in older patients are emergency surgical procedures and coexisting major medical problems such as cardiac or pulmonary disease. It is true that older persons have diminished reserve to respond to extreme stress situations, but the adaptability is extremely variable among individuals. Seymour (2003) summarizes the issues of surgery and older adults by saying, "it appears to be age-associated illness rather than the aging process itself that is the main reason for the increase in morbidity and mortality following surgery and anesthesia in old age" (p. 321). Age usually does not independently predict postoperative outcome. What must be assessed in each case is whether the potential benefits of a surgical procedure outweigh the potential risks for the individual.

The two predominant concerns in the surgical experience are the response to anesthesia and the incidence of postoperative complications. Seymour (2003) stresses that postoperative deaths caused solely by anesthesia are very rare, regardless of age. Dodds (cited in Seymour, 2003) outlined the following considerations related to anesthesia and older patients:

- Polypharmacy presents a multitude of potentially adverse drug interactions.
- Increased shunting in the lungs and decreased cardiac output affect the uptake of volatile gases; effects are reduced with less soluble gases.
- Ischemic heart disease increases vulnerability to cardiac depressants.
- Decreased hepatic metabolism and renal clearance increase the risk of drug toxicity; insoluble agents that are not metabolized by the liver are safer.
- Reduced neuronal density, slowed metabolic rate, and delayed circulation time increase risk of overdosage; small doses and slower infusion or small boluses reduce risk.
- The nondepolarizing neuromuscular blocking agent atracurium is preferred for older adults because it is not dependent on renal and hepatic function.
- Increased sensitivity to opioids can contribute to late postoperative hypoxemia.
- Nonsteroidal antiinflammatory drugs can cause nephrotoxicity, fluid retention, and gastric irritation, which are more troubling adverse effects in older persons.

Respiratory complications are the most common postoperative problem in older patients. The prevalence rises with the number of preoperative medical problems. Various studies of respiratory complications have identified variables that increased the risk in older adults. They include age 60 and over, preexisting lung disease, smoking in previous 8 weeks, volume depletion, upper abdominal incisions, emergency procedures, prolonged anesthesia, greater body mass index, and pancreatitis (Seymour, 2003).

Contrary to popular belief, postoperative atelectasis commonly is initiated not by retained secretions but by the collapse of basal airways. This is related partly to the increased closing volume common in older adults, but is enhanced by surgical incisions near the diaphragm, supine posture, and postoperative sedation. Activity that encourages deep inhalation such as incentive spirometry, intermittent positive pressure breathing, and deep breathing exercises may be helpful in reducing atelectasis caused by airway collapse. Methods that emphasize expiratory maneuvers such as coughing and

---

BOX 13-2 A Pragmatic Approach to Perioperative Pulmonary Management

- Several weeks before surgery:
  - Try to get the patient to stop smoking (but 8 weeks of abstinence is probably required).
  - Consider 2 weeks of nutritional support in very malnourished patients (nutritional depletion may decrease respiratory muscle function).
  - In the very obese, weight reduction can improve arterial oxygen levels.

- 48 to 96 hours before elective surgery:
  - In patients with known lung disease, consider drug therapy with bronchodilators, antibiotics if sputum is infected, and possibly corticosteroids.
  - Emphasize preoperative and postoperative "inspiratory" physiotherapy techniques unless there is significant sputum.

- During anesthesia:
  - The use of warm humidified gases is logical, as is the avoidance of very high concentrations.
  - The introduction of periodic full lung expansions should reduce atelectasis.

- In the postoperative period:
  - In high-risk cases continue "inspiratory" physiotherapy into the postoperative period (but note that the most severe cases may require therapy every 1 to 2 hours while awake for 3 to 5 days).
  - Continuous positive airway pressure administered by mask may have a role.
  - Adequate analgesia, early removal of nasogastric tubes, and early mobilization should be beneficial.
  - Be vigilant for signs of atelectasis or pneumonia. Pulse oximeters can be used to monitor for oxygen desaturations, but blood gases are required to monitor carbon dioxide levels and absolute arterial oxygen levels.
  - To reduce the risk of postoperative hypoxemia on the second to fourth postoperative night, consider giving prophylactic oxygen via nasal cannula for 3 days and 5 nights postoperatively.

From Seymour, D. G. (2003). Surgery and anesthesia in old age. In R. C. Tallis & H. M. Fillit (Eds.), *Brocklehurst's textbook of geriatric medicine and gerontology* (6th ed.). London: Churchill Livingstone, p. 324.

---

percussion probably are less helpful. Unless patients are producing at least 30 mL of sputum, some experts say that coughing and percussion may do more harm than good in older persons (Seymour, 2003).

The risk of hypoxemia in the early postoperative period is commonly known; however, there also is a risk of *late postoperative hypoxemia* that occurs 2, 3, 4, or even more days after surgery. This phenomenon was recognized when the use of pulse oximetry became commonplace. The mechanism behind this phenomenon is thought to be related to rapid eye movement (REM) sleep suppression in the first few postoperative days caused by surgical stress and opioids. When REM sleep reappears, there is a disturbance in the respiratory mechanism and episodes of desaturation occur (Seymour, 2003). The administration of continuous oxygen by nasal cannula for several days after surgery almost always prevents late hypoxemic episodes.

Possibly related is a study by Wong, Tsui, Yung, Chan, and Cheng (2004) that employed continuous pulse oximeter monitoring and daily intermittent arterial blood gases (ABGs) in patients hospitalized with long bone fractures. The measurements were taken over a 72-hour period after the fracture, or after surgical intervention if done. All but 1 of 20 patients with fractures had recurrent desaturations below 90% SaO_2. ABG analyses did not detect the phenomena, which in most cases were asymptomatic. The investigators concluded that patients with long bone fractures should have routine continuous pulse oximetry to detect inapparent hypoxia.

A treatment algorithm for perioperative pulmonary management is presented in Box 13-2. Box 13-3 outlines risk reduction measures for respiratory disorders.

RESPIRATORY DISEASES COMMON TO THE AGED

Respiratory disorders are among the most common reasons that older adults seek medical care. It now is recognized that many older adults have atypical and nonspecific manifestations of respiratory problems. These differences make it especially important for the practitioner to do a thorough assessment of the respiratory status of older patients. Common conditions that are addressed in this section are obstructive pulmonary disease, including asthma, chronic bronchitis, and emphysema; pneumonia; tuberculosis; lung cancer; and sleep apnea.

Obstructive Pulmonary Disease

Obstructive pulmonary diseases include asthma, emphysema, chronic bronchitis, bronchiectasis, and cystic fibrosis. The prevalence of the first three merits coverage here. Although life expectancy with cystic fibrosis has greatly improved, these patients are not yet represented in the older adult population.

Asthma. Asthma is a clinical syndrome characterized by three phenomena: recurrent episodes of airway obstruction that resolve spontaneously or in response to treatment, airway hyperresponsiveness (hyperreactivity), and airway inflammation. *Airway hyperresponsiveness* is defined as exaggerated bronchoconstriction in response to stimuli that elicit no or minimal response in nonasthmatics (Drazen, 2000).

EPIDEMIOLOGY AND STATISTICS. Asthma has been considered a disease of the young, and chronic obstructive pulmonary disease (COPD) a disease of the elderly. However, asthma now is recognized as relatively common in older adults with prevalence rates estimated between 6.5% and 17% (Connolly, 2003). Although childhood asthma is a risk factor for asthma in adulthood, most older asthmatics develop the condition as adults. Other risk factors for asthma in U.S. adults as determined by the 2000 Behavioral Risk Factor Surveillance System include female gender, age 18 to 34, lower socioeconomic status, overweight/obesity, and current or former smoker (Gwynn, 2004).

PATHOLOGY AND PATHOGENESIS. Mild asthma is characterized by mucosal edema and hyperemia. Lymphocytes, mast cells, and eosinophils infiltrate the mucosa, produce interleukins, and promote the synthesis of immunoglobulin E (IgE). Epithelial and inflammatory cells produce chemokines that amplify and perpetuate the inflammatory process. Inflammation causes collagen to be deposited below the basement membrane, resulting in thickening of the airway wall. In chronic, severe asthma, the airway walls are further thickened by hypertrophy and hyperplasia of airway glands and secretory cells, and by hyperplasia of airway smooth muscle. Patchy areas of the airway epithelium shed, leaving denuded surfaces. Thickening of the airway walls causes increased airflow resistance and airway responsiveness. Also, in severe asthma, hyperviscous mucus and shed epithelial cells contribute to airway obstruction.

An acute exacerbation of asthma is characterized by bronchoconstriction, tracheobronchial mucosal edema, and increased secretion of thick, tenacious mucus. The physiological effects of these events include increased resistance to airflow and decreased flow rates. During an acute attack, severe airway narrowing can decrease elastic recoil, which depresses expiratory flow rates even more. Tachypnea is common during an acute attack. The combination of increased respiratory rate and airway narrowing increases the work of breathing and can lead to fatigue of the muscles of ventilation. Airway narrowing is not evenly distributed so that a maldistribution of ventilation to perfusion exists, and there may even be complete obstruction of airways by large mucous plugs. The result is hypoxemia and, as a result of hyperventilation, a low P_{CO_2} (Drazen, 2000).

Asthma in older adults is generally thought to be "intrinsic," meaning it does not have allergic or environmental triggers; as opposed to "extrinsic" asthma, which is more common in children. This distinction is difficult to confirm because IgE level, which rises with atopic asthma, generally is lower to begin with in older people. The relationship between IgE and bronchial responsiveness has not been as clearly defined among older subjects as it has among younger individuals with asthma. A possible imbalance between beta-adrenergic, cholinergic, and alpha-adrenergic receptor pathways may be a factor in the development of asthma in older adults. Possibly, beta-adrenergic receptor activity is exaggerated in older persons with late-onset asthma, resulting in disturbed autonomic regulation of airway smooth muscle and increased leukocyte activation—a factor in airway inflammation. Genetic studies are pursuing the possibility that late-onset asthma may represent the delayed expression of the same phenotype that is found in younger people with asthma (Connolly, 2003).

Regardless of the pathogenesis, both intrinsic and extrinsic asthma are characterized by airway inflammation. Several explanations for the inflammation have been proposed. The role of environmental pollutants is variously described as causative or as a factor that exacerbates a condition that already is present (Connolly, 2003). Respiratory infections are common precipitating factors of acute episodes, but exposure to dust, cigarette smoke, polluted air, or even a change in temperature can precipitate an attack. Workplace air pollution, especially damp and moldy conditions, also is associated with an increased risk of adult-onset asthma (Flodin & Jonsson, 2004). Numerous patient variables have been studied to elucidate additional causes or contributing factors. Based on self-report data, the prevalence of asthma was found to increase among women as body mass index (BMI) increased. For men, the prevalence increased with both the lowest and the highest BMI (Luder, Ehrlich, Lou, Melnik, & Kattan, 2004).

The role of emotional status in acute asthmatic episodes is less well understood. A small study classified asthmatic subjects as suggestible and suggestion resistant and administered sham bronchoconstrictors.

Subjects identified as suggestible were more likely to respond to the "drug" with dyspnea and reduced FEV_1 than those who were suggestion resistant (Leigh, MacQueen, Tougas, Hargreave, & Bienenstock, 2003). Not only can emotional factors affect asthma, but asthma can also affect the mental-emotional state and quality of life of older adults. Among the problems identified in people with asthma are depression and anxiety (Krommydas et al., 2004).

CLINICAL MANIFESTATIONS. Like younger persons, the older adult with asthma may experience breathlessness, wheezing, intermittent cough, and tightness in the chest, often in response to viral infection, inhaled irritants, exercise, or emotions. Paroxysms of dyspnea may occur, especially at night. Other clinical manifestations are the use of accessory muscles of respiration, intercostal retractions, chest hyperinflation, and prolonged expiratory phase of respirations. Percussion elicits hyperresonance, and auscultation detects wheezing that typically is loudest on expiration, and possibly rales and rhonchi. The absence of breath sounds indicates severe obstruction to airflow (Drazen, 2000).

The problem with recognizing the symptoms of asthma in the older person is that similar symptoms occur with COPD, heart failure, angina, and even myasthenia gravis and gastroesophageal reflux disease. Further, asthma symptoms in older adults tend to be worse during winter, the opposite of young people. A misdiagnosis of COPD often is based on findings of right-sided heart failure and continued bronchoconstriction even with maximal asthma treatment. Clinicians should remember that both asthma and COPD may be present. Failure to recognize and treat asthma can have fatal consequences (Connolly, 2003).

DIAGNOSIS. Asthma is believed to be both underdiagnosed and undertreated in older persons for several reasons. The incidence of symptoms may be reduced because older adults tend to be less active. Also, the lack of typical symptoms may mislead the practitioner (Connolly, 2003).

The primary diagnostic tests for asthma are PFTs and, except for mild attacks, ABG measurement (preferably on room air). The cardinal pulmonary function changes during an asthma attack are decreased peak expiratory flow rate (PEFR), FEV_1, and FEF_{25-75}. If abnormalities are noted in the standard PFTs, a methacholine challenge test may be done to detect hyperactive airway disease and to assess reversibility in response to inhaled or nebulized bronchodilators. The methacholine challenge test uses increasing doses of methacholine, a bronchoconstrictor, to detect airway hyperreactivity. Because severe bronchospasm can occur, an inhalant bronchodilator must be available (Pagana & Pagana, 2003). A person with asthma typically reacts to the bronchoconstrictor at a lower dose than a person who does not have asthma. Although airway hyperresponsiveness is characteristic of asthma, it is not always demonstrated in this test (Drazen, 2000). Reversibility in the older person with asthma commonly is less than in younger persons, but usually it exceeds 20%. If immediate reversibility is not significant, a course of corticosteroids (6 weeks per inhaler or 2 weeks orally) may be ordered followed by reassessment of reversibility. Challenge testing is *not* done if the patient already has been diagnosed with asthma.

Blood gas values depend on the duration and severity of the episode. Initially, respiratory alkalemia is common with a PaO_2 of 55 to 70 mm Hg and a $PaCO_2$ of 25 to 35 mm Hg. With a prolonged attack, the pH normalizes as compensatory mechanisms respond. A normal or rising $PaCO_2$ in an individual with moderate to severe airflow obstruction is cause for alarm as the patient may be approaching respiratory failure (Drazen, 2000). The severity of an asthma attack is judged by the pulmonary function changes and symptoms (Table 13-2).

Other diagnostic tools that may assist in the differential diagnosis are chest radiographs, serum eosinophil and IgE levels, electrocardiogram, and sputum studies. Because chest radiographs usually are normal in people with asthma, they are most useful in ruling out other conditions such as pneumothorax, pulmonary edema, and infection. Findings that are consistent with asthma are elevated serum eosinophil and IgE levels, radiographic evidence of chest hyperinflation and a depressed diaphragm, and eosinophils in the sputum (Drazen, 2000). Sputum color is not informative; therefore studies for pathogens are advised if infection is suspected.

One reason that most asthma deaths occur in older people is that they often do not recognize or seek prompt treatment for acute exacerbations. When seen by a health care provider, the older adult's impaired cardiac response to acute bronchoconstriction may cause the provider to underestimate the severity of the condition. An accurate assessment of the severity of the attack requires measurement of peak expiratory flow and comparison with the patient's predicted or previous known best level. Patients being treated in the emergency department should have ABG measurements done, preferably on room air, and chest radiographs should be taken (Connolly, 2003).

Table 13-2 *Classification of Asthma Severity Based on Clinical Features before Treatment**

Severity	Symptoms†	Nighttime Symptoms	Lung Function
Mild intermittent	Between exacerbations, asymptomatic with normal PEFR Exacerbations Frequency: 2 or less times per week Duration: several hours to a few days Intensity: varies	No more than twice a month	FEV_1 or PEFR = or >80% predicted PEFR variability <20%
Mild persistent	Exacerbations Frequency: >2 times a week, <1 time per day May affect activity	More than twice a month	FEV_1 or PEFR = or >80% predicted PEFR variability 20% to 30%
Moderate persistent	Daily symptoms requiring use of inhaled short-acting $beta_2$ agonists Exacerbations Frequency: 2 or more times per week Duration: may last for days Affect activity	More than once a week	FEV_1 or PEFR >60% but <80% predicted PEFR variability >30%
Severe persistent	Continual symptoms Limited physical activity Frequent exacerbations	Frequent	FEV_1 or PEFR = or <60% predicted PEFR variability >30%

Modified from National Institutes of Health, National Heart, Lung, and Blood Institute. (1997, July). Stepwise approach for managing asthma in adults and children older than 5 years of age. *Guidelines for the diagnosis and management of asthma* (NIH pub. no. 97-4051.). Bethesda, MD: National Institutes of Health, National Heart, Lung, and Blood Institute. Modified from Figure 3-4a.

*The presence of one of the features of severity is sufficient to place a patient in that category. An individual should be assigned to the most severe grade in which any feature occurs. The characteristics noted in this table are general and may overlap because asthma is highly variable. Furthermore, an individual's classification may change over time.

†Patients at any level of severity can have mild, moderate, or severe exacerbations. Some patients with intermittent asthma experience severe and life-threatening exacerbations separated by long periods of normal lung function and no symptoms.

FEV₁, Forced expiratory volume in 1 second; *PEFR*, peak expiratory flow rate.

The National Heart, Lung, and Blood Institute (NIHLB) guidelines recommend a short course of oral corticosteroids as a means of assessing reversibility, which helps rule out obstructive lung disease other than asthma.

LONG-TERM MANAGEMENT. The goals of asthma therapy are to prevent chronic and troublesome symptoms, maintain nearly normal pulmonary function, maintain normal activity levels, prevent recurrent exacerbations, provide optimal pharmacotherapy with minimal adverse effects, and meet expectations of patients and families in relation to asthma care (National Institutes of Health [NIH], 1997).

Drug Therapy. Pharmacological therapy employs various agents classified as relievers and controllers. Relievers ("rescue" drugs) are used to reverse acute airway obstruction and include beta agonists and anticholinergics. Controllers are inhaled corticosteroids, leukotriene modifiers, long-acting beta-adrenergic agonists, methylxanthines, mast cell stabilizers, and systemic corticosteroids. They are used on a regular basis to prevent inflammation and bronchoconstriction.

Selection of specific drugs can be based on a stepwise approach such as the one presented in the *Guidelines for the Diagnosis and Management of Asthma* (NIH, 1997), and summarized in Table 13-3. Note that the guidelines were updated in 2002, but the information in Table 13-3 did not change. The first step in using this approach is to classify the severity of the patient's symptoms. The guidelines advise initiation of therapy at a higher step of drug therapy with cautious step-down therapy to identify the minimum drug needed to maintain control. However, some practitioners may choose to begin treatment at the step deemed appropriate to the patient's symptoms, and then gradually move up until control is achieved.

The British Thoracic Society (BTS) also recommends a stepped care approach to treatment that includes the following: step 1, on-demand bronchodilators; step 2, regular inhaled corticosteroids; step 3, increased dosage of inhaled corticosteroids; step 4, additional regular beta agonists; and step 5, oral corticosteroids. Connolly (2003) recommends the following alterations in the BTS guidelines for older adults:

- Initial treatment should employ the prophylactic use of inhaled corticosteroids on a regular basis instead of as-needed ("reliever") bronchodilators because of the older adult's impaired perception of bronchoconstriction.
- Instead of increasing the corticosteroid dose as in the BTS step 3, the low-dose inhaled steroid should be continued with the addition of a long-acting beta-agonist bronchodilator. Regular beta agonists can be added, as can ipratropium or oxitropium—both inhaled muscarinic antagonists.

BETA-ADRENERGIC AGONISTS. Beta-adrenergic agonist bronchodilators are widely used in the management of asthma. Inhaled short-acting forms are used as relievers. They include albuterol, bitolterol, levalbuterol, and pirbuterol. Inhaled long-acting beta-adrenergic agonists, including salmeterol and formoterol, are used as controllers because the duration of action is much longer (Lehne, 2004). The safety of beta agonists in asthma management has been the focus of many studies as reviewed by Abramson, Walters, and Walters (2003). Among the important findings in their review were the following:

1. Salbutamol (albuterol) has not been associated with increased asthma mortality risk and has been shown to have a positive antiinflammatory effect.
2. Nebulized and oral beta agonists have been associated with cardiovascular complications.
3. In general, regular use of long-acting beta agonists has been shown to have significant advantages over regular use of short-acting beta agonists.

In the older adult, regular use of controllers is advised because of the decreased perception of bronchoconstriction. The older patient on reliever therapy only may fail to recognize the need for the medication, which could lead to worsening of bronchospasm and increases the mortality risk.

A comparative study of the safety and effectiveness of salbutamol and formoterol in over 18,000 children and adults demonstrated that the safety profiles of both drugs were similar and that formoterol as a reliever was associated with fewer symptoms and exacerbations (Pauwels et al., 2003).Older adults reportedly respond poorly to salbutamol.

The issue of adjustable maintenance dosing versus fixed-dose therapy has been the topic of several studies. One large study reported more effective asthma control with adjustable dosing with budesonide/formoterol when compared with fixed-dose salmeterol/fluticasone (Aalbers et al., 2004).

ANTICHOLINERGICS. Inhaled anticholinergic agents such as ipratropium bromide effectively relieve bronchospasm by antagonizing acetylcholine in the airway smooth muscle. Systemic effects are minimal when taken by oral inhalation. For patients who use both ipratropium and albuterol, combination agents are available as Combivent for metered-dose inhalers and DuoNeb for nebulizers.

CORTICOSTEROIDS. Inhaled corticosteroids suppress the inflammatory response in the airways, which reduces hyperreactivity, decreases mucus production, and increases the number and responsiveness of beta-2 receptors (Lehne, 2004). A study using computed tomography demonstrated that a 12-week course of inhaled corticosteroids decreased the thickness of airway walls, decreased the serum eosinophil cationic protein, and increased FEV_1 (Niimi et al., 2004). A 5-year study of

Table 13-3 *Stepwise Approach for Managing Asthma in Adults and Children Older than 5 Years of Age: Treatment*

	Classify Severity: Clinical Features Before Treatment or Adequate Control		Medications Required to Maintain Long Term Control
	Symptoms/Day — Symptoms/Night	PEF or FEV, PEF Variablity	Daily Medications
Step 4: Severe persistent	Continual — Frequent	≤60% — >30%	Preferred treatment: ■ High-dose inhaled corticosteroids AND ■ Long-acting inhaled beta$_2$-agonists AND, if needed ■ Corticosteroid tablets or syrup long term (2 mg/kg/day, generally do not exceed 60 mg per day). (Make repeat attempts to reduce systemic corticosteroids and maintain control with high-dose inhaled corticosteroids.)
Step 3: Moderate persistent	Daily — >1 night/week	>60% to <80% — >30%	Preferred treatment: ■ Low-to-medium dose inhaled corticosteroids and long acting inhaled beta$_2$-agonists Alternative treatment (listed alphabetically): ■ Increase inhaled corticosteroids within medium-dose range OR ■ Low-to-medium dose inhaled corticosteroids and either leukotriene modifier or theophylline. If needed (particularly in patients with recurring severe exacerbations): ■ Preferred treatment: Increase inhaled corticosteroids within medium-dose range and add long-acting inhaled beta$_2$-agonists. ■ Alternative treament (listed alphabetically): Increase inhaled corticosteroids within medium-dose range and add either leukotriene modifier or theophylline.
Step 2: Mild persistent	>2/week but <1 ×/day — >2 nights/month	≥80% — 20%-30%	Preferred treatment: ■ Low-dose inhaled corticosteroids. Alternative treatment (listed alphabetically): cromolyn, leukotriene modifier, nedocromil, OR sustained-release theophylline to serum concentration of 5 to 15 mcg/mL.
Step 1: Mild intermittent	≤2 days/week — ≤2 nights/month	≥80% — <20%	No daily medication needed. Severe exacerbations may occur, separated by long periods of normal lung function and no symptoms. A course of systemic corticosteroids is recommended.
Quick Relief: All patients	■ Short-acting bronchodilator: 2 to 4 puffs short-acting inhaled beta$_2$-agonists as needed for symptoms. ■ Intensity of treatment will depend on severity of exacerbation: up to 3 treaments at 20-minute intervals of a single nebulizer treatment as needed. Course of systemic corticosteroids may be needed. ■ Use of short-acting beta$_2$-agonists >2 times a week in intermittent asthma (daily, or increasing use in persistent asthma) may indicate the need to initiate (increase) long-term-control therapy.		

Continued

Table 13-3 *Stepwise Approach for Managing Asthma in Adults and Children Older than 5 Years of Age: Treatment—cont'd*

⇓ Step down
Review treatment every 1 to 6 months; a gradual stepwise reduction in treatment may be possible.

⇑ Step up
If control is not maintained, consider step up. First, review patients medication technique, adherence, and environmental control.

Goals of Therapy: Asthma Control
- Minimal or no chronic symptoms day or night
- Minimal or no exacerbations
- No limitations on activities; no school/work missed
- Maintain (near) normal pulmonary function
- Minimal use of short-acting inhaled beta₂-agonist
- Minimal or no adverse effects from medications

Note
- The stepwise approach is meant to assist, not replace, the clinical decision making required to meet individual patient needs.
- Classify severity: assign patient to most severe step in which any feature occurs (PEF is % of personal best; FEV_1 is % predicted).
- Gain control as quickly as possible (consider a short course of systemic corticosteroids); then step down to the least medication necessary to maintain control.
- Minimize use of short-acting inhaled beta₂-agonists. Overreliance on short-acting inhaled beta₂-agonists (e.g., use of approximately one canister a month even if not using it every day) indicates inadequate control of asthma and the need to initiate or intensify long-term control therapy.
- Provide education on self-management and controlling environmental factors that make asthma worse (e.g., allergens, irritants).
- Refer to an asthma specialist if there are difficulties controlling asthma or if step 4 care is required. Referral may be considered if step 3 care is required.

From National Heart, Lung, and Blood Institute. (2002). *NAEPP expert panel report: Guidelines for the diagnosis and management of asthma—update on selected topics 2002 (EPR—update 2002)* (NIH pub. no. 02-5075.). Bethesda MD: NHLBI Health Information Network.

more than 400 subjects showed that those who began treatment with inhaled corticosteroids within 2 years of the onset of symptoms had significantly better airway function and asthma control at lower maintenance doses than individuals who began the therapy later. This finding makes a case for prompt intervention rather than waiting until symptoms worsen. Despite widely accepted treatment guidelines, an analysis of outpatient medication reports revealed that an inhaled corticosteroid was prescribed for only 49% of individuals diagnosed with asthma, and inhaled beta agonists were prescribed for only 67.1% (Gilberg, Laouri, Wade, & Isonaka, 2003). Cho and Lee (2003) reported that some older patients with severe bronchial asthma respond poorly to corticosteroid therapy, possibly because of decreased binding affinity of the drug with receptors in these individuals.

Various inhaled corticosteroid preparations are available in a variety of dispensers. Hoarseness and oropharyngeal candidiasis are the most common adverse effects of inhaled corticosteroids. These local effects are preventable by gargling after each dose and using a spacer to reduce the amount of drug deposited in the oropharynx (Lehne, 2004). A large study of adults with persistent asthma compared the effectiveness of budesonide inhalation powder via dry-powder inhaler and triamcinolone acetonide via pressurized metered-dose inhaler. The budesonide dry-powder inhaler proved to be significantly more effective as measured by multiple variables, including change in the number of symptom-free days, FEV_1, FVC, and breakthrough bronchodilator use (Weiss, Liljas, Schoenwetter, Schatz, & Luce, 2004).

One concern when treating older adults with corticosteroids is the possibility of significant bone demineralization. The harmful effect of systemic corticosteroids on bone mass density is well known; however, the potential adverse effects of inhaled forms of these drugs are less clear. A review of the data on clinical efficacy and tolerability of budesonide with mild to moderate persistent asthma concluded that the doses required to treat these patients did not pose a risk in terms of hypothalamic-pituitary-adrenal axis function, bone mineral density, cataract formation, or (in children) final adult height (Banov, 2004). On the other hand, a Finnish study that measured serum DHEA-S, the most abundant precursor to adrenal androgen and estrogen, in asthmatic subjects using the inhaled corticosteroid budesonide found evidence of adrenocortical suppression. The investigators concluded that reduced estrogen and androgen precursors could increase the risk of osteoporosis, especially in postmenopausal women (Kannisto et al., 2004). Also, an 8-year study of long-term inhaled and nasal corticosteroid use showed the rate of hip and upper extremity fractures to be elevated only among individuals who took daily doses in excess of 2000 mcg (Suissa, Baltzan, Kremer, & Ernst, 2004). After reviewing evidence regarding potential complications of inhaled corticosteroid use in asthma, an expert panel concluded that the benefits of this therapy outweigh the proven risks (Leone, Fish, Szefler, & West, 2003).

LEUKOTRIENE MODIFIERS. Leukotriene modifiers suppress chemical mediators that cause bronchoconstriction, eosinophil infiltration, mucus production, and airway edema. The three leukotriene modifiers are zileuton, zafirlukast, and montelukast. They represent the newest category of antiasthma drugs, and have been tested primarily in younger people, so their usefulness for older adults has not yet been confirmed. One study compared the relative efficacy of a leukotriene modifier (zafirlukast) and an inhaled corticosteroid (flutacasone) in patients of various ages. Subjects treated with flutacasone showed significant improvement. The older adults treated with zafirlukast showed small improvements in symptoms and lung function, but they had more exacerbations (Creticos, Knobil, Edwards, Rickard, & Dorinsky, 2002). A small study that compared the effects on airway blood flow of montelukast and fluticasone (a corticosteroid) concluded that the two were equally beneficial, and no additional benefit was gained from combining them (Mendes, Campos, Hurtado, & Wanner, 2004).

Elevated liver enzymes and hepatitis have been reported in some patients who were taking zileuton or zafirlukast. Advantages of montelukast over other leukotriene modifiers are that it does not appear to be harmful to the liver and it does not interact with warfarin or theophylline (Lehne, 2004). Although leukotriene modifiers seem to be well tolerated, several cases of Churg-Strauss syndrome have been attributed to montelukast in asthma patients after corticosteroids had been withdrawn. Churg-Strauss syndrome is a disseminated small vessel vasculitis with late-onset asthma, upper airway disease, eosinophilia, and peripheral neuropathy (Boccagni et al., 2004; Michael & Murphy, 2003).

MAST CELL STABILIZERS. Mast cell stabilizers including cromolyn sodium and nedocromil sodium have been shown most effective in managing mild to moderate persistent asthma in children or other individuals in whom a specific known stimulus induces symptoms (Drazen, 2000).

METHYLXANTHINES. Methylxanthines, including theophylline and aminophylline, are moderately potent bronchodilators whose usefulness is limited by the risk for toxicity. Theophylline formulations are available for once- or twice-daily dosing. Its use generally is limited to patients whose asthma is inadequately controlled despite controller drugs. Monitoring of serum theophylline levels is vital because its metabolism is highly variable and toxic levels (above 20 mcg/mL) can cause seizures and potentially fatal cardiac arrhythmias. Severe toxicity may occur without warning; therefore serum levels should be assessed after any dosage adjustments

and every 6 to 12 months in clinically stable patients. However, more frequent monitoring is warranted in the older adult because reduced theophylline clearance has been demonstrated in persons over age 55, especially men and those with chronic lung disease. A common target for therapeutic blood levels is 10 to 14 mcg/mL (Mosby, 2004). Hospitalized patients receiving intravenous aminophylline require especially close monitoring.

Table 13-4 summarizes drugs used in the treatment of asthma and COPD.

Peak Flow Monitoring. Connolly (2003) acknowledges the value of diurnal peak flow monitoring and assessment of reversibility, but notes that some older adults have difficulty reading the meters and graphing the results. Therefore he recommends that older persons be taught to use peak flow meters with a range of 50 to 350 L/min and to simply record the results on a table. Variability in readings normally is greatest between the early morning and late afternoon; however, such variability may not be seen in the older person with asthma.

Management of Acute Exacerbations. Treatment of an acute exacerbation is initiated with high-flow oxygen, nebulized beta agonists, and ipratroprium. If the patient has glaucoma, the ipratropium should be omitted. High-dose intravenous corticosteroids are given initially, followed by daily oral doses. The patient's response is monitored by peak flow rates and repeated blood gas measurements. Individuals who do not respond to these drugs may be treated with intravenous salbutamol or aminophylline (or both). Endotracheal intubation and intermittent positive pressure ventilation may be indicated. Antibiotic therapy is appropriate in the presence of infection (Connolly, 2003).

Complementary and Alternative Asthma Therapies. Older adults may use complementary and alternative therapies to treat asthma symptoms. Investigators in one study queried hospitalized asthma patients in a Mexico-U.S. border city regarding their use of herbal products. Forty-two percent reported treating asthma with herbs, including oregano, chamomile, garlic, eucalyptus, and lime. It is especially noteworthy that no documentation of herbal usage was found on review of those patients' charts (Rivera, Hughes, & Stuart, 2004). Scientific review of traditional remedies is increasing, and probably will identify therapeutic benefits of some herbal products, as well as other complementary and alternative therapies. However, some studies are sure to discover serious adverse effects and interactions that should discourage the use of those therapies. A systematic review of complementary and alternative therapies for asthma failed to find support for homeopathy, air ionizers, manual therapy, or acupuncture (Gyorik & Brutsche , 2004). A second review published in *Swiss Medical Weekly* also concluded that evidence of the

Table 13-4 *Drugs Used to Treat Asthma and COPD*

Classification	Specific Drugs	Therapeutic Effect	Considerations

Corticosteroids	Inhaled:
	   Budesonide (Pulmicort)
	   Flunisolide (Aerobid)
	   Fluticasone (Flovent)
	   Triamcinolone (Azmacort)
	   Advair Diskus is a combination of fluticasone and salmeterol
		Antiinflammatory, increases number and responsiveness of $beta_2$ receptors	May have long-term benefits when started before symptoms become severe. However, some older patients reportedly respond poorly. Spacer and gargling after each dose reduce oral-pharyngeal irritation and candidiasis.
			Benefits judged to outweigh risks.
			With COPD, should be continued only with evidence of clinical improvement.

	Systemic:
	   Prednisone
	   Prednisolone
		Antiinflammatory	Severe adverse effects with systemic therapy over 10 days.

Beta-adrenergic agonists	Inhaled, short-acting:
	   Albuterol (Proventil, Ventolin)
	   Bitolterol (Tornalate)
	   Levalbuterol (Xopenex)
	   Pirbuterol (Maxair)
		Relief of acute bronchoconstriction	Early symptoms may not be recognized by older person.
			Nonselective beta agonists may increase mortality risk caused by acute asthma attacks.

	Inhaled, long-acting:
	   Salmeterol (Serevent)
	   Formoterol (Foradil Aerolizer)
		Prevention of acute bronchoconstriction	Preferred over short-acting forms for older adults because of their decreased perception of bronchoconstriction.
			Older adults may respond better to formoterol than to salbutamol.
			Compliance may be better with long-acting drugs.

Anticholinergics	Inhaled:
	   Ipratropium (Atrovent)
	   Tiotropium (Spirava)
		Spiriva is a maintenance bronchodilator for COPD	Older adults may respond to anticholinergics better than to beta agonists.
			Ipratropium: rapid onset of action. Approved only for COPD though is being used for asthma. Minimal systemic effects. Dispensed in MDI.
			Tiotropium: serious allergic reactions and paradoxical bronchospasm can occur. Dispensed as capsules for use with HandiHaler.

Leukotriene modifiers	Zileuton (Zyflo) Zafirlukast (Accolate) Montelukast (Singulair)	Antiinflammatory	Limited data on efficacy in older adult. Montelukast appears to have less risk of liver damage and fewer drug-drug interactions than others in this class.
Mast cell stabilizers	Cromolyn sodium (Intal) Nedocromil sodium (Tilade)	Antiinflammatory	Both taken by inhalation. Most effective in management of mild-moderate asthma in which specific triggers are known. Not effective for acute bronchospasm.
Methylxanthines	Theophylline	Oral route usual for maintenance	Usefulness limited by risk for toxicity. Serum level should be monitored; clearance is reduced in older persons.
	Aminophylline	Oral, IV, rectal routes	Must be given slowly IV.

COPD, Chronic obstructive pulmonary disease; *IV,* intravenous; *MDI,* metered-dose inhaler.

effectiveness of alternative treatments is lacking. These reviewers reminded readers that lack of evidence does not mean a treatment is ineffective, but that its effectiveness has not been confirmed through high-quality research (Steurer-Stey, Russi, & Steurer, 2002). However, a Chinese study compared the effects on quality of life when people with asthma received standard treatment alone, and with acupuncture or acupressure. In this study, both complementary treatments resulted in significant improvements in quality of life among patients with clinically stable, chronic obstructive asthma (Maa et al., 2003).

Nonpharmacological Management. In addition to drug therapy, treatment of asthma in the older adult includes cessation of smoking, removal of animals if the person is allergic to them, and good bronchial hygiene to improve airway clearance because many patients with advanced disease may have problems mobilizing airway secretions. Hygiene measures include adequate oral hydration and humidification of inspired air. Education for self-management is a critical factor. Individuals who have completed asthma education classes have demonstrated increased asthma knowledge in addition to an improved quality of life (Yang, Chiang, Yao, & Wang, 2003). When nurse asthma specialists conducted an asthma clinic and collaborated with primary health care providers to provide education and support and to promote use of guidelines for asthma management, the frequency of unscheduled care decreased for white patients, but not patients of other ethnic groups in the study (Griffiths et al., 2004).

ASTHMA AND COMORBIDITY. A problem for many older adults with asthma is comorbidity. Cardiovascular disease, COPD, and myasthenia gravis, for example, all complicate the diagnosis and management of asthma and vice versa. The hypoxemia characteristic of moderate to severe asthma may exacerbate cardiac ischemia. Also, beta-adrenergic antagonists such as propranolol (Inderal) that commonly are used for cardiac conditions should be avoided if possible because they can cause bronchial constriction. Some individuals have an allergic response to aspirin that could be a problem because aspirin commonly is used for arthritis. Finally, the older adult's mental status may be adversely affected, especially if the asthma is poorly controlled. The cognitively impaired older adult with asthma is at special risk for inadequate asthma management. Confused patients may be unable to communicate symptoms, to perform self-assessments, or to take appropriate self-care action. Special care is needed to foster compliance and efficacy. Because less frequent dosing simplifies self-care and improves adherence, a long-acting beta agonist can be taken twice daily and inhaled corticosteroids in a single daily dose.

Chronic Obstructive Pulmonary Disease. The term *chronic obstructive pulmonary disease* (COPD) commonly is used when a person has both emphysema and chronic bronchitis (Heuther & McCance, 2000). COPD is common in older adults, typically becoming apparent between ages 50 and 60 after a period of asymptomatic decline in respiratory function.

EPIDEMIOLOGY AND STATISTICS. The U.S. prevalence rate of COPD in men has remained fairly stable, but it has increased among women (Connolly, 2003). In fact, in 2000 the number of women dying from COPD in the United States exceeded the number of men for the first time. Data from the National Health Interview Survey indicate that 10 million Americans reported having COPD that was diagnosed by a physician. However, the National Health and Nutrition Examination Surveys reported that approximately 24 million Americans have evidence of impaired lung function. The conclusion based on the difference in these numbers is that COPD, like asthma, often goes undiagnosed (Mannino, Homa, Akinbami, Ford, & Redd, 2002). In 2000, COPD necessitated 8 million office and outpatient visits, 1.5 million visits to the emergency department, and 726,000 hospitalizations, and was the cause of 119,000 deaths (Mannino et al., 2002). The direct and indirect costs of COPD in the United States in 2002 totaled $32.1 billion (Pauwels et al., 2003).

Other costs that are more difficult to quantify are the decline in quality of life and the increase in depression. Studies of general health status in older adults show that COPD is associated with more severe impairment as measured by the Barthel Index, the 6-minute walking test, and the Mini-Mental State Examination (Antonelli-Incalzi et al., 2004). Another study of older adults with COPD found that health status declined dramatically when the FEV_1 fell below 50% of predicted. This measurement correlates with the GOLD stage IIb, which is discussed later (Antonelli-Incalzi et al., 2003).

PATHOPHYSIOLOGY: EMPHYSEMA. *Emphysema* is defined as abnormal and permanent dilation of the terminal air spaces of the lungs, combined with destruction of the alveolar wall. Air trapping occurs as a result of decreased elastic recoil in the alveoli and narrowing of the bronchiole. The alveoli become hyperinflated and produce air spaces called *bullae* and *blebs* in which gas exchange is not effective. A ventilation-perfusion mismatch and hypoxemia occur. The muscles of respiration are taxed by the hyperexpansion of the chest, which increases the work of breathing, resulting in hypoventilation and hypercapnia. Depending on the extent to which the acini are involved, emphysema is classified as centriacinar or panacinar. The *acinus* (plural: *acini*) refers to the gas-exchange unit: respiratory bronchiole, alveolar duct, and alveoli. In centriacinar emphysema, which is typical among smokers and persons with chronic bronchitis, destruction occurs in the septa of respiratory bronchioles and alveolar ducts. Bronchioles are inflamed, but alveoli are intact. Panacinar emphysema, which is more common in older adults and people with alpha-1 antitrypsin deficiency, is characterized by more randomly distributed damage involving primarily the lower lobes of the lungs (Heuther & McCance, 2000; Rodarte, 2000).

When alveoli are lost in emphysema, so are the capillaries that served them. Therefore the distribution of ventilation and perfusion is relatively well maintained. The patient with pure emphysema is not cyanotic and does not have hypoxemia (PO_2 below 60 mm Hg) or carbon dioxide retention until the disease is terminal. In spite of this, the dyspnea experienced is profound.

Cigarette smoking is the primary risk factor for emphysema; however, other inhaled pollutants and frequent childhood respiratory infections have been implicated as well. An analysis of the respiratory health, general health status, and occupational history of over 2000 individuals in the United States led investigators to conclude that one in five cases of COPD may be attributable to occupational exposures (Trupin et al., 2003). An inherited deficiency of enzyme alpha-1 antitrypsin often is the culprit in individuals who develop emphysema despite never having smoked and those who develop it during younger or middle adult years (Heuther & McCance, 2000).

PATHOPHYSIOLOGY: CHRONIC BRONCHITIS. Chronic bronchitis is diagnosed when an individual has a chronic productive cough on most days for at least 3 consecutive months in a year for 2 successive years (Connolly, 2003). The pathological process is triggered by inspired irritants in the form of smoke or other pollutants that stimulate mucus production and damage cilia. The mucous glands and goblet cells in the airway epithelium increase in number and size and produce thick mucus that is not easily cleared. Chronic bronchospasm leads to hypertrophy of bronchial smooth muscle, which combines with inflammation to cause thickening of the bronchial walls and narrowing of the inner diameter of the airways. Large airways are affected first, then the smaller airways. Airway closure occurs early in expiration so that gas is trapped. Over time there is a ventilation-perfusion mismatch with hypoventilation and hypoxemia (Heuther & McCance, 2000).

COPD COMPLICATIONS. Acute exacerbations of COPD may be triggered by infection, pulmonary or peripheral edema, or pulmonary embolism. Hospitalization is indicated in the presence of severe breathlessness, poor or deteriorating general condition, cyanosis, increasing peripheral edema, confusion or impaired consciousness, and inability to manage at home, as well as in individuals already receiving long-term oxygen therapy (Connolly, 2003). Hypoxia is the usual cause of death in acute exacerbations.

With severe COPD, arterial hypoxia and destruction of the pulmonary capillary bed produce pulmonary hypertension leading to right ventricular failure. Heart failure under these circumstances is called *cor pulmonale*. Individuals who predominantly have bronchitis tend to have more ventilation-perfusion abnormalities and worse hypoxia and tend to develop cor pulmonale earlier than individuals with pure emphysema. In addition, patients with COPD are at increased risk for pneumonia, which carries a higher than usual mortality risk for these patients (Rodarte, 2000).

CLINICAL MANIFESTATIONS. Chronic bronchitis and emphysema can exist independently, but more often occur together. Therefore this section addresses findings associated with both. In the earliest phases, clinical signs and symptoms of COPD are minimal. A chronic productive cough, commonly reported as a "smoker's cough," is the classic sign of chronic bronchitis. Patients also may report frequent "chest colds" that resolve slowly. There are no characteristic physical findings of emphysema early in the disease. As COPD progresses, however, complaints include general fatigue and increasing breathlessness and wheezing on exertion (Connolly, 2003). PFTs show large lung volumes because of overdistention. Residual volume is increased because of trapping of air on expiration due to the loss of elastic recoil in the large, floppy alveoli. Obstruction is evidenced by reduced FEV_1 and FEV_1/FVC ratio. Generally, breathing symptoms are not noticed until the FEV_1 falls below 60% of predicted, though older adults may tolerate even lower levels before becoming symptomatic. Late in the course of emphysema, when FEV_1 falls below 40% of predicted, symptoms worsen and classic signs appear: chest hyperinflation, cyanosis, and right-sided heart failure. Pursed-lip breathing may be used in an unconscious effort to get rid of the excess trapped air. The patient has a prolonged expiratory phase of breathing, often with wheezes. Polycythemia, nocturnal hyperventilation, hypoxia, and sleep disturbances are common. The increased work of breathing and breathlessness that interferes with eating cause gradual weight loss (Connolly, 2003; Heuther & McCance, 2000; Rodarte, 2000). When the FEV_1 falls to less than one third of predicted, patients typically are completely incapacitated (Rodarte, 2000).

DIAGNOSIS. A history of exposure to risk factors and airflow limitation that is not fully reversible provide the basis for a presumptive diagnosis of COPD, regardless of the presence or absence of symptoms. Exposure risk factors include tobacco smoke, occupational dust and chemicals, and smoke from home cooking and heating fuels. Any patient with a history of exposure to risk factors who has a chronic cough with sputum production should be evaluated for airflow limitation. In addition to chronic cough and sputum production, dyspnea that is progressive, persistent, or worse during exercise or with respiratory infections should prompt the practitioner to consider COPD. The recommended means of assessing for airflow limitations is spirometry. A diagnosis of airflow limitation that is not fully reversible is justified when FEV_1/FVC is less than 70% and a post-bronchodilator FEV_1 is less than 80% of predicted (Pauwels, Buist, Calverley, Jenkins, & Hurd, 2001).

Several severity scales exist. The GOLD classification scale was developed by the NHLBI/World Health Organization (WHO) Global Initiative for Chronic Obstructive Lung Disease and endorsed by the American Thoracic Society. It provides guidelines for classifying the severity of COPD as *at risk*, *mild*, *moderate*, or *severe* based on symptoms, FEV_1, and FEV_1/FVC (Table 13-5). It also recommends additional diagnostic procedures depending on the degree of severity. The validity of the GOLD scale was supported by a study that compared various scales and the frequency of hospitalization for COPD exacerbations. Of the four scales compared, the highest correlation was achieved with the GOLD scale (Tsoumakidou et al., 2004).

MANAGEMENT OF COPD. The goals of COPD management as defined in the GOLD workshop report are to
- Prevent disease progression
- Relieve symptoms
- Improve exercise tolerance
- Improve health status
- Prevent and treat complications
- Prevent and treat exacerbations
- Reduce mortality risk

Interventions for COPD are designed to reduce risk factors, manage stable COPD, and manage exacerbations.

Reduce Risk Factors. The patient must be encouraged to avoid continued exposure to known risk factors. The single most important measure is smoking cessation, which may be achieved through education, counseling, social support, and pharmacotherapy. Antonelli-Incalzi and colleagues (2004) note that smoking cessation is the only strategy, in addition to continuous oxygen therapy for respiratory insufficiency, that can delay the progression of COPD and prolong life expectancy. By positively affecting inflammatory and remodeling processes, smoking cessation interrupts the accelerated decline in FEV_1 (Willemse, Postma, Timens, & ten Hacken, 2004). Strategies recommended by the Public Health Service to help the person who is willing to quit smoking are outlined in Box 13-4. Pharmacological options include nicotine replacement (gum, inhaler, nasal spray, transdermal patch, sublingual tablet, lozenge) and antidepressants (bupropion, nortriptyline, clonidine) (Pauwels et al., 2001).

Manage Stable COPD. Because COPD is not curable, patient education is essential to help the patient take steps to improve function and delay progression of the disease. Key factors in managing stable COPD are exercise and drug therapy. The GOLD report (Pauwels et al., 2001) recommends a stepwise approach to the management of COPD based on severity as follows:
- At-risk individuals:
  - Avoid risk factors
  - Regular influenza vaccinations
- Mild COPD: bronchodilators as needed
- Moderate COPD:
  - Regular bronchodilator(s)
  - Inhaled corticosteroids for significant symptoms that respond to steroids
  - Rehabilitation
- Severe COPD:
  - Regular bronchodilator(s)
  - Inhaled corticosteroids
  - Rehabilitation
  - Treatment of complications
  - Long-term oxygen therapy for respiratory failure

Table 13-5 *Classification of COPD by Severity*

Stage	Characteristics
0. At Risk	Normal spirometry Chronic symptoms (cough, sputum production)
I. Mild COPD	FEV_1/FVC <70% 30% <FEV_1 <80% predicted With or without chronic symptoms (cough, sputum production)
II. Moderate COPD	FEV_1/FVC <70% FEV_1 <80% predicted IIA: 50% <FEV_1 <80% predicted IIB: 30% <FEV_1 <50% predicted With or without chronic symptoms (cough, sputum production)
III. Severe COPD	FEV_1/FVC <70% FEV_1 <30% predicted, or the presence of respiratory failure,* or clinical signs of right-sided heart failure

From Pauwels, R. A., Buist, S., Calverley, P. M. A., Jenkins, C. R., & Hurd, S. S. (2001). Global strategy for the diagnosis, management, and prevention of chronic obstructive pulmonary disease. *American Journal of Respiratory and Critical Care Medicine, 163*, 1256-1276. Official journal of the Thoracic Society. Copyright American Thoracic Society.
*Respiratory failure: Pao_2 <8.0 kPa (60 mm Hg) with or without $Paco_2$ >6.7 kPa (50 mm Hg) while breathing air at sea level.

BOX 13-4 Strategies to Help the Patient Willing to Quit Smoking

Ask

Systematically identify all tobacco users at every visit. Implement an office-wide system that ensures that, for every patient at every clinic visit, tobacco use status is queried and documented.

Advise

Strongly urge all tobacco users to quit. In a clear, strong, and personalized manner, urge every tobacco user to quit.

Assess

Determine willingness to make a quit attempt. Ask every tobacco user if he or she is willing to make a quit attempt at this time (e.g., within the next 30 days).

Assist

Aid the patient in quitting. Help the patient with a quit plan; provide practical counseling; provide intratreatment social support; help the patient obtain extratreatment social support; recommend use of approved pharmacotherapy except in special circumstances; provide supplementary materials.

Arrange

Schedule follow-up contact. Schedule follow-up contact, either in person or via telephone.

From Pauwels, R. A., Buist, S., Calverley, P. M. A., Jenkins, C. R., & Hurd, S. S. (2002). Global strategy for the diagnosis, management, and prevention of chronic obstructive pulmonary disease. *American Journal of Respiratory and Critical Care Medicine, 163,* 1256-1276. Official journal of the Thoracic Society. Copyright American Thoracic Society.

In addition to drug therapy, exercise training programs are advised to improve exercise tolerance and symptoms of dyspnea and fatigue.

DRUG THERAPY. The same classes of drugs used to treat asthma are used for COPD, although the specifics are different. An inhaled anticholinergic such as ipratropium or tiotropium commonly is used in older COPD patients. There is some evidence that older adults respond to anticholinergics better than to beta-adrenergic agonists (Rodarte, 2000). Tiotropium is a long-acting drug that has been shown to be superior to the shorter acting ipratropium (Tashkin & Cooper, 2004). However, some studies have shown that the maximal bronchodilating effect of anticholinergics is achieved only with doses that are much higher than the current standard dose (Connolly, 2003). If anticholinergics are prescribed, the inhalation route is recommended because systemic doses can cause urinary retention, constipation, tachycardia, and increased intraocular pressure with glaucoma—all common in older adults.

The benefits of beta-adrenergic agonists in older adults with COPD must be weighed against some risks. Some evidence exists that relatively nonselective beta agonists are associated with increased mortality rates because of acute asthma attacks. It appears that the more selective drugs such as albuterol pose less threat (Connolly, 2003). Many COPD management guidelines were developed before long-acting adrenergic bronchodilators such as formoterol and salmeterol were available. Although some guidelines do not yet reflect their use, research supports the benefits of these agents in effectively improving lung function, compliance, and exercise endurance, and in reducing exacerbation rates (Lipson, 2004; Man et al., 2004; Yohannes & Hardy, 2003). Additional study is needed to assess the advantages and disadvantages of the long-acting drugs in older persons.

Inhaled corticosteroids are appropriate only for individuals who demonstrate objective improvement in lung function. For those who show no objective benefit, the drug (inhaled as well as oral) should be gradually withdrawn to prevent exacerbation of symptoms. High-dose, long-term, inhaled corticosteroids have been shown to reduce the rate of functional lung decline with severe COPD (Connolly, 2003). Claims that inhaled corticosteroids reduce mortality rates in COPD are refuted by Suissa (2004), who contends that those conclusions resulted from a bias in the cohort design and analysis. Two new drugs that are under investigation for the treatment of airway inflammation are the soft steroid loteprednol etabonate (now an ophthalmic preparation), and a pro-drug soft steroid, ciclesonide. Researchers hope to market ciclesonide in an inhaler formulation that would be used only once daily and have a low profile of side effects (Belvisi & Hele, 2003).

As noted with asthma, methylxanthines are beneficial as bronchodilators but pose a special risk of toxicity to the older person. For that reason, they are not often used on a routine basis except in patients with cognitive impairment who cannot use inhalation drugs successfully (Connolly, 2003).

The use of mucolytics is controversial. Some sources, including the GOLD report, indicate that the benefits are very small with the exception of a few patients with viscous sputum. Others indicate that they help reduce exacerbations and improve symptoms, especially with chronic bronchitis but to some extent with COPD as well (Halpin, 2004).

Inhaled medications are widely used for obstructive pulmonary disease, but they must be used, and used properly, to benefit the patient. Older adults are thought to be less compliant with inhaled medications than with those taken by other routes. Use of a long-acting beta$_2$ agonist such as salmeterol or formoterol may promote better compliance (Connolly, 2003).

Yohannes and Hardy (2003) point out that most treatments are unlikely to improve pulmonary function in most patients with severe COPD. Therefore treatment outcomes are better evaluated by tests of dynamic exercise such as the 6-minute walk and assessment of quality of life than by pulmonary function testing.

IMMUNIZATIONS. Older people, especially those with chronic pulmonary disease, are at increased risk for respiratory infections. Therefore both influenza and pneumococcal vaccinations generally are recommended for COPD patients. Many older adults decline influenza immunizations because of erroneous beliefs about side effects. Although healthy older persons usually achieve acceptable antibody titers after vaccination, the chronically ill person may not respond as well. Some experts recommend supplemental doses of pneumococcal and influenza vaccines (Gravenstein, Fillit, & Ershler, 2003).

PULMONARY REHABILITATION. Pulmonary rehabilitation aims to reduce symptoms of COPD, improve quality of life, and increase participation in daily activities. It has been shown to improve exercise tolerance and reduce symptoms of dyspnea and fatigue regardless of the stage of COPD severity. Some of the problems encountered in initiating rehabilitation programs are physical deconditioning, social isolation, depression, muscle wasting, and weight loss. A multidisciplinary approach is needed to address these problems in a coordinated manner. Goals must be individualized and records maintained to document responses. Data to be tracked include spirometry before and after a bronchodilator, exercise capacity, health status and impact of breathlessness, inspiratory and expiratory muscle strength, and lower limb strength in patients with muscle wasting (Pauwels et al., 2001). The benefits of pulmonary rehabilitation have been demonstrated in various settings, including patients' homes; home settings may be the most appropriate for some older persons (Connolly, 2003; Ferrari et al., 2004). However, Connolly (2003) cites a lack of data on the impact of pulmonary rehabilitation on quality of life in older persons.

OXYGEN THERAPY. *Long-term oxygen therapy* (LTOT) is defined as the delivery of oxygen for at least 15 hours per day. This therapy has been shown to prolong survival in people with COPD. By relieving chronic hypoxia, it prevents pulmonary hypertension and subsequent right ventricular failure. Criteria for selection for LTOT developed by the British Thoracic Society are listed in Box 13-5 (Connolly, 2003, p. 501). The GOLD report recommends that LTOT be started at severity stage 3 or when there is evidence of heart failure, pulmonary hypertension, or polycythemia (Pauwels et al., 2001). LTOT for patients who meet standard criteria has been associated with significant improvements in health-related quality of life that were sustained or improved further over a study period of 6 months (Eaton et al., 2004).

SURGICAL TREATMENTS. Procedures that have been used to treat COPD include bullectomy, lung volume reduction surgery (LVRS), and lung transplantation. Bullectomy reduces dyspnea and improves lung function in selected patients. The effectiveness and comparative cost

---

BOX 13-5 British Thoracic Society Criteria for Selection for Long-Term Oxygen Therapy (LTOT)

- Persistent irreversible airflow obstruction (FEV_1 less than 1.5 L)
- Nonsmoker
- With or without hypercapnia
- Po_2 less than 55 mm Hg on two sequential estimations at least 1 month apart, and not during an acute exacerbation
- LTOT leads to increased Po_2 without a dangerous fall in pH or rise in Pco_2

From Connolly, M. J. (2003). Asthma and chronic obstructive pulmonary disease. In R. C. Tallis & H. M. Fillit (Eds.), *Brocklehurst's textbook of geriatric medicine and gerontology* (6th ed.). London: Churchill Livingstone.

---

of LVRS versus conventional therapy is under study and remains controversial at this time. Some patients with very advanced COPD are candidates for lung transplantation, which has been shown to improve functional capacity and quality of life. To be considered for transplantation, a patient should meet the following criteria: FEV_1 less than 35% of predicted, Pao_2 of 55 to 60 mm Hg, $Paco_2$ less than 50 mm Hg, and secondary pulmonary hypertension (Pauwels et al., 2001).

Management of Exacerbations. Acute exacerbations, which are common in COPD patients, most often are triggered by airway infection or air pollution. Differential diagnosis is important because an acute exacerbation may mimic pneumonia, heart failure, pneumothorax, pleural effusion, pulmonary embolism, and cardiac arrhythmias.

Pharmacological therapy employs inhaled short-acting bronchodilators, or intravenous theophylline, and systemic corticosteroids. Aminophylline has traditionally been used, but its limited benefits must be weighed in light of a tendency to worsen gas exchange and hypoxemia. Antibiotics are appropriate with clinical signs of airway infection.

Noninvasive positive pressure ventilation (NIPPV) may improve blood gases and pH, reduce in-hospital mortality rates, and decrease the need for intubation and mechanical ventilation. A Cochrane Review cited sufficient good-quality randomized studies to support the use of this therapy as an adjunct to usual medical care, and recommended that it be initiated early in the course of respiratory failure and before severe acidosis develops (Ram, Picot, Lightowler, & Wedzicha, 2004). Unfortunately, this therapy is not suitable for all patients. Exclusion criteria include respiratory arrest, cardiovascular instability, somnolence, impaired mental state, uncooperative behavior, high risk for aspiration, viscous or copious secretions, recent facial or gastroesophageal surgery, craniofacial trauma, nasopharyngeal abnormalities, and extreme obesity.

The major indications for invasive mechanical venti-lation are severe dyspnea with use of accessory muscles and paradoxical abdominal motion, respiratory rate greater than 35 breaths per minute, life-threatening hypoxemia, and severe acidosis. Decisions to initiate invasive mechanical ventilation can be difficult and are best made with patient input when possible. COPD patients can be especially difficult to wean from mechanical ventilation. Sometimes NIPPV is used to facilitate weaning, and it has been reported to decrease the incidence of nosocomial infection and to improve survival rates (Ferrer et al., 2003; Girou, Brun-Buisson, Taille, Lemaire, & Brochard, 2003; Pauwels et al., 2001). Conflicting results were obtained in a randomized trial comparing NIPPV with standard medical support after discontinuation of mechanical therapy. The trial was stopped early when it was found that NIPPV did not prevent the need for reintubation or reduce mortality rate after extubation. In this study, the mortality rate was higher for the NIPPV group than for those receiving standard treatment (25% versus 14%) (Esteban et al., 2004). Therefore continued study is indicated to deter-mine if and when NIPPV should be used to facilitate weaning.

An acute exacerbation requires not only management of oxygenation, but also maintenance of fluid balance and nutritional intake. Low-molecular-weight heparin may be used to reduce the risk of embolism created by immobilization, polycythemia, and dehydration. If spu-tum clearance is a problem, stimulated coughing, low-volume forced expirations, and chest percussion and postural drainage may be employed (Pauwels et al., 2001).

Pneumonia

Epidemiology and Statistics. Pneumonia is a global health problem, particularly among older per-sons. Along with influenza, it is the fifth leading cause of death in people older than 65 in the United States. A review of all Medicare recipients who were hospitalized with community-acquired pneumonia (CAP) in a single year revealed an incidence rate of 18.3 per 1000; 10.6% of those admitted died. Both the incidence and the mor-tality rates rose dramatically between individuals age 65 to 69 and those over age 90. In 1997, hospitalization for pneumonia cost $4.4 billion, which was 6.3% of the total expenditure for hospital care of older adults in the United States. Nearly half of the cost was incurred by cases managed in intensive care units (Kaplan et al., 2003). A study of adults in Canada who were hospital-ized with CAP reported 8500 cases per year with an overall mortality rate of 12%. Although the length of hospitalization increased with age, total costs for those age 85 and older were similar to the costs of patients age

65 to 74, presumably because of limitations in care provided for the oldest patients (Carriere, Jin, Marrie, Predy, & Johnson, 2004). The Polish city of Lodz has the oldest population among large cities in that country. A review of persons admitted to the hospital internal medicine department there showed that over half were age 65 or older. Approximately 20% of these admis-sions were for respiratory diseases; 11.5% with pneu-monia (Kardas & Ratajczyk-Pakalska, 2003). Expressing concern about the increasing incidence of severe CAP in the rising older population, Kaplan and Angus (2003) called for preventive efforts and standardization of cri-teria for hospital admission and management decisions.

Pathogenesis. Pneumonia can be classified as community-acquired pneumonia (CAP) or nosocomial pneumonia (NP). Nosocomial infections sometimes are further classified as hospital acquired, ventilator associated, or nursing-home acquired. The microorgan-isms that cause CAP and NP tend to differ in identity, virulence, and mortality rate. The organism most often responsible for CAP in older adults is *Streptococcus pneu-moniae. Mycoplasma pneumoniae* is common in the gen-eral population, but not among older people (Connolly & Gosney, 2003). Both have relatively low mortality rates. Among individuals with other health problems, such as COPD and viral infections, infecting organisms may include *Staphylococcus aureus, Haemophilus influen-zae,* and *Klebsiella pneumoniae. Legionella* is less common among older adults and tends to be associated with spo-radic outbreaks of pneumonia (Connolly & Gosney, 2003). Influenza viruses are the usual cause of viral pneumonia (Heuther & McCance, 2000). Generally, Asian countries report having the same causative organ-isms for CAP as found in Western countries, but report a higher frequency of macrolide-resistant *Streptococcus pneumoniae* (Matsushima, Miyashita, & File, 2002).

Nosocomial infections have much higher mortality and complication rates and are more often caused by gram-negative organisms, including *Escherichia coli, Klebsiella pneumoniae,* and *Pseudomonas aeruginosa. Staph-ylococcus aureus* has been identified as the second most common cause of nosocomial infection (after gram-negative enterobacteria) in Britain (Connolly & Gosney, 2003).

According to Dent (2004), early-onset ventilator-associated pneumonia (VAP) occurs within 5 days of initiation of mechanical ventilation and usually is caused by *Streptococcus pneumoniae, Haemophilus influen-zae,* or *Moraxella catarrhalis.* Late-onset VAP more likely is caused by *Pseudomonas aeruginosa, Acinetobacter, Enterobacter,* or methicillin-resistant *Staphylococcus aureus* (MRSA). In a study of VAP in India, *Pseudomonas aeruginosa* and *Escherichia coli* were the most common causes (Pawar et al., 2003).

Organisms implicated in nursing-home-acquired pneumonia are *Streptococcus pneumoniae, Haemophilus influenzae, Staphylococcus aureus* (including MRSA), *Escherichia coli, Klebsiella pneumoniae, Pseudomonas aeruginosa,* and *Moraxella catarrhalis* (Coleman, 2004; Marrie, 2002; Mylotte, 2002). Fungal pneumonia, though not common, is being seen with increasing frequency among immunocompromised individuals and is most often caused by *Aspergillus,* dimorphic fungi, and *Cryptococcus neoformans* (Pound, Drew, & Perfect, 2002). Table 13-6 lists organisms that have been associated with nosocomial pneumonia.

Differences have been found in epidemiological studies of older adults hospitalized with pneumonia. As expected, hospitalization rates for pneumonia rose with age, especially for men. Among males, black males had more aspiration, unspecified, *Klebsiella,* other gram-negative, and staphylococcal pneumonias, whereas white males had more *Haemophilus* and pneumococcal pneumonias. Among females, black females had more aspiration and *Klebsiella* pneumonias and white females had higher rates of *Haemophilus* and bronchopneumonia (Baine, Yu, & Summe, 2001).

Pathophysiology. When pathogens successfully invade the lungs despite protective mechanisms, they release toxins that trigger local inflammatory and immune responses. Bronchial mucous membranes and alveolocapillary membranes are damaged, and terminal bronchioles fill with debris and exudates. Red hepatization occurs, followed by leukocyte infiltration, and then gray hepatization. Red hepatization is consolidation of lung tissue in which pulmonary exudates are blood stained. The term *gray hepatization* is used once the red blood cells have disintegrated, but a fibrinosuppurative exudate remains. Fibrin is deposited on pleural surfaces, and phagocytosis takes place in the alveoli. As the process resolves, debris in the alveoli are ingested by macrophages and lung function improves (Heuther & McCance, 2000).

MODE OF TRANSMISSION. Bacterial pulmonary infections can result when bacteria are introduced into the lung by way of microaspiration of oropharyngeal secretions (most bacterial pneumonias), inhalation of airborne organisms (tuberculosis), the bloodstream (staphylococcal endocarditis), and direct extension (amebic liver abscess). Aspiration of contaminated oropharyngeal secretions occurs routinely in healthy people but in small quantities that are handled by defensive mechanisms. However, acute infection is more likely if the host defenses are impaired by ineffective mucociliary clearance, inadequate neutrophils or antibodies, and an ineffective reticuloendothelial system (Johanson, 2000). Following hospitalization, oropharyngeal colonization with gram-negative organisms is common (Connolly & Gosney, 2003).

Sources of VAP include pooled secretions above an inflated endotracheal tube cuff, contaminated bedside resuscitative bag-valve equipment, contaminated tubing and condensate, improperly cleaned and stored small-volume medication nebulizers, unnecessary suctioning, saline instilled in the airway, contaminated in-line suction catheters, and neglected oral hygiene (Dent, 2004).

RISK FACTORS. The risk factors for pneumonia are age related, pathological, and environmental. Common age-related changes that increase the risk of pneumonia in older adults are decreased cough reflex and reduced lung elasticity and respiratory muscle strength (Coleman, 2004). Chronic and disabling conditions that are more common with age also increase risk. These include neurological conditions (especially those that affect swallowing and mobility), alcoholism, malnutrition, and cardiovascular or respiratory disease (Connolly & Gosney, 2003). Social and environmental variables that

Table 13-6 *Organisms Associated with Nosocomial Pneumonias*

	Hospital Acquired	Ventilator Associated	Nursing-Home Acquired
Enterobacter	X	X	
Escherichia coli	X	X	X
Proteus	X		
Klebsiella	X		X
Serratia marcescens	X		
Haemophilus influenzae	X	X	X
Methicillin-sensitive *Staphylococcus aureus*	X		
Streptococcus pneumoniae	X	X	X
Anaerobes	X		
Staphylococcus aureus	X		X
Acinetobacter species	X	X	
Legionella	X		
Pseudomonas aeruginosa	X	X	X
Methicillin-resistant *Staphylococcus aureus*	X	X	X
Moraxella catarrhalis		X	X

increase the risk of CAP are low socioeconomic status and exposure to tobacco smoke or air pollution. Older adults who do not receive influenza or pneumococcus vaccinations also are at increased risk for pneumonia (Loeb, 2003).

Risk factors identified in a French geriatric hospital included a history of NP in the past 6 months, oxygen therapy, severe malnutrition, heart failure, antibiotics in the preceding month, eating dependency, and nasogastric tube feedings (Rothan-Tondeur et al., 2003). Additional risk factors for nursing-home-acquired pneumonia are the presence of a tracheostomy and multiple medication use, especially sedative-hypnotics, immunosuppressants, and gastric acid inhibitors (Coleman, 2004).

Studies of various specific patient populations have demonstrated the increased risk for complications, including pneumonia, in older persons. Among patients recovering from intact abdominal aortic aneurysm, increasing age was associated with the increased incidence of pulmonary insufficiency and pneumonia. Patients 51 to 60 years old had an overall complication rate of 18.8% compared with a rate of 34.3% in patients over age 80 (Vemuri et al., 2004). Based on the assumption that gastric acids control pathogens in the stomach, it is theorized that gastric acid suppressive therapy would be associated with an increased risk for respiratory infections. A survey of community-dwelling older adults confirmed that individuals taking gastric acid suppressants reported having more respiratory infections than those not taking the drugs (Laheij, Van Ijzendoorn, Janssen, & Jansen, 2003).

Clinical Manifestations.

Initial symptoms in the elderly may differ from those in younger patients. High-spiking fevers, productive cough, and an elevated white blood cell count may not be present. Instead, the initial cues may be confusion, tachypnea (greater than 24 breaths per minute), and evidence of dehydration. Signs of heart failure may be present, but pleuritic chest pain is uncommon. Core temperature is almost always elevated even when oral and axillary temperatures are normal. With pneumonia, localizing crackles often are heard on chest auscultation, whereas isolated basal crackles are less specific (Connolly & Gosney, 2003). Assessment of dehydration in the older adult is more difficult than in younger patients. However, Connolly's work showed that the presence of axillary sweating indicates the older person is not dehydrated (Connolly & Gosney, 2003). Leukocytosis is not always present in older adults with pneumonia. The absence of typical symptoms in an older person with pneumonia has been associated with a higher mortality rate because of the delay in seeking care and initiating treatment.

Diagnosis.

When confusion is the only symptom present, the practitioner must begin with a general assessment because many causes are possible. When pneumonia is suspected, the diagnostic process for older adults is the same as for younger persons. Useful data include serum urea nitrogen and electrolytes, complete blood count, chest radiograph, blood culture, blood gas estimation, and estimation of peak flow rate. The specimen for blood culture should be collected before the initiation of antibiotic therapy, but antibiotics should not be delayed pending sputum results. Although sputum analysis may be useful, patients often are unable to produce a specimen in the initial stages of pneumonia. A Gram stain will provide some information about the dominant pathogen. Interestingly, in controlled clinical trials with older persons, a pathogenic organism could not be identified in 30% to 60% of all cases (Connolly & Gosney, 2003). Some experts have questioned the value of routine microbiological diagnostics, citing lack of evidence that it improves outcomes (Lidman, Burman, Lagergren, & Ortqvist, 2002).

The clinical presentations of bacteremic and nonbacteremic CAP are not sufficiently different for diagnosis. Some manifestations are different, but there is much overlap in the presentations of the two (Marrie, Low, & De Carolis, 2003).

Prognosis.

Pneumonia mortality rates in older adults have been reported between 15% and 35%. Patients who survive may require lengthy hospitalization. Radiologic abnormalities resolve slowly, and recovery may take several months (Connolly & Gosney, 2003). Factors associated with pneumonia mortality rates in inpatients and outpatients include hypothermia, altered mental status, elevated serum urea nitrogen, chronic liver disease, leukopenia, and hypoxemia. Respiratory failure has been identified as the most common immediate cause of death; underlying causes include neurological conditions, malignancy, and cardiac conditions (Mortensen et al., 2002).

Management.

An important decision in managing the older person with CAP is whether to treat at home or to admit to the hospital. Patient categories developed by the American Thoracic Society can be used to guide this decision. Category 1 includes outpatients with no history of cardiopulmonary disease and no modifying factors (age greater than 65, alcoholism, multiple medical comorbidities, immunosuppression). Outpatients with a history of cardiopulmonary disease or modifying factors make up category 2. Individuals in category 1 or 2 with mild to moderate CAP usually are treated as outpatients. Category 3 patients have moderately severe pneumonia; hospitalization is recommended, but intensive care unit (ICU) care is not required. Patients with severe infections are considered category 4 and require ICU care (Crimlisk, 2004).

DRUG THERAPY. Decisions about antimicrobial therapy ideally are based on laboratory results of culture and sensitivity. However, it is not always easy to isolate the causative organism(s) and it is risky to delay initiating therapy in these patients. Prompt recognition and treatment of pneumonia with appropriate empiric drugs yields better outcomes in older adults (Mehta & Niederman, 2003; Mehta & Niederman, 2002; Reichmuth & Meyer, 2003). Furthermore, when initial treatment includes coverage for atypical pathogens, the length of stay has been shown to decrease (Trowbridge et al., 2002). Therefore the practitioner makes choices based on knowledge of the most likely pathogens in a given setting, the drugs most likely to be effective, and local resistance patterns. Other factors that influence the choice are patient allergies, cost, potential interactions with other drugs, and the patient's general status (especially renal and hepatic function). Dosages of some drugs must be reduced in older persons with renal or hepatic impairment to prevent toxicity. The primary types of drugs used to treat CAP are aminopenicillins, macrolides, fluoroquinolones, cephalosporins, oxazolidinones, and carbapenems. Guidelines for treatment of CAP are outlined in Table 13-7. Among the many drugs employed to treat nosocomial pneumonia are the fluoroquinolones, aminoglycosides, cephalosporins, carbapenems, oxazolidinones, aztreonam, and vancomycin. Some additional drugs are used in specific circumstances.

It is important to recognize that antimicrobial resistance can vary from one locale to another. For example, a study of the prevalence of local antimicrobial resistance in France demonstrated that amoxicillin/erythromycin was effective in 67.8% of patients with pneumonia and erythromycin/levofloxacin was effective in 48.6%. In the United Kingdom, the effectiveness for the same drug combinations were 71.7% and 65.3%, respectively (Singer, Harding, Jacobs, & Jaffe, 2003). The use of granulocyte colony-stimulating factor (G-CSF) as an adjunct to antibiotic therapy was the subject of a recent systematic review that concluded that there was no current evidence to support routine use of G-CSF in treatment of pneumonia (Cheng, Stephens, & Currie, 2004). Macrolides are widely used for CAP; however, macrolide-resistant *Streptococcus pneumoniae* emerged in the past decade, reminding us that the battle against microorganisms is a continuous one (File & Tan, 2003). Fortunately, in 2000 the rate of clinical macrolide resistance was still low (McCarty, 2000). Also, some macrolides have many drug-drug interactions, a factor to consider with the older person, who may take multiple medications. Generally, clarithromycin has fewer interactions than

erythromycin (Zhanel et al., 2001). On the horizon is telithromycin, the first of a new class of antimicrobials called ketolides, which is showing effectiveness against resistant respiratory pathogens (Clark & Langston, 2003).

OXYGEN THERAPY. Oxygen therapy may be ordered for hospitalized patients. The patient's response can be monitored by continuous oxygen saturation measurements and periodic arterial blood gas analyses. The goal is to maintain SpO_2 of 94% or greater (Ayers & Lappin, 2004). A flow rate of 2 L/min may be adequate. Support the patient who has a productive cough to try to clear the airway. Regardless of the setting, instruct patients to use disposable tissues and discard them properly to avoid exposing others. Suctioning may be necessary if the patient has secretions but cannot clear them from the airway.

The usefulness of mucolytics and expectorants is a topic of debate. Mucolytics react directly with mucus to make it more watery, which should help make it easier to expectorate. Available mucolytics are given only by inhalation and can trigger bronchospasm (Lehne, 2004). An expectorant is a drug that stimulates mucus production. The value of most, except guaifenesin, is doubtful (Lehne, 2004).

ENERGY CONSERVATION. During acute illness, the older adult may have very low activity tolerance. Organize care to reduce energy demands. Remember that the older adult does not need a complete bath every day. Inform patients that recovery can take several months, so activities will need to be resumed gradually.

HYDRATION AND NUTRITION. In general, a patient with pneumonia should take in at least 3 L of fluid each day to maintain normal hydration. Depending on the setting of care and the patient's condition, fluids may be given intravenously, orally, or both. "Forcing fluids" can be dangerous in the older adult whose cardiovascular and renal systems respond more slowly to changes in fluid volume. A frail older person or one with heart failure or renal insufficiency can quickly develop fluid volume excess. Therefore it is especially important to monitor intake and output and vital signs, and to assess for pulmonary and peripheral edema. One other consideration is that the older person may need to void more often during rehydration. A bedside commode may save energy and avoid incontinent episodes. Monitor the patient's nutritional intake as well. A frail older person who was marginally nourished before this illness may benefit from high-calorie, high-protein supplements in addition to small, frequent meals. Provide as much assistance as needed to facilitate adequate intake.

Table 13-7 *Patient Categories and Treatment for Community-Acquired Pneumonia*

	Severity of Illness			
	Category 1 **Mild to Moderate**	**Category 2** **Mild to Moderate**	**Category 3** **Moderately Severe**	**Category 4** **Severe**
Hospitalization	No	No	Yes, not ICU	ICU
Cardiopulmonary disease	No	Yes	Yes or no	
Modifying factors	No	Yes	Yes or no	
Risk for *Pseudomonas*				Yes and no
Antibiotic therapy	Advanced-generation macrolide (azithromycin [Zithromax], clarithromycin [Biaxin]) *or* doxycycline	Beta-lactam* *plus* Macrolide or doxycycline *or* Antipseudomonal fluoroquinolone[†] (used alone)	*If cardiopulmonary disease and with or without modifying factors:* IV beta lactam[‡] *plus* IV or oral macrolide or doxycycline *or* IV antipseudomonal fluoroquinolone alone *If no cardiopulmonary disease, no modifying factors:* IV azithromycin alone *or* Monotherapy with antipseudomonal fluoroquinolone	*No risk for P. aeruginosa:* IV beta-lactam (cefotaxime, caftriaxone) *plus either* IV macrolide (azithromycin) *or* IV fluoroquinolone *Risk for P. aeruginosa:* IV antipseudomonal beta-lactam[§] *plus* Antipseudomonal fluoroquinolone (ciprofloxacin) *or* Selected IV antipseudomonal beta-lactam *plus* IV aminoglycoside *plus either* IV macrolide (azithromycin) *or* IV nonpseudomonal fluoroquinolone

From American Thoracic Society. (1995, November). Hospital-acquired pneumonia in adults: Diagnosis, assessment of severity, initital antimicrobial therapy, and preventative strategies. A consensus statement. *American Journal of Respiratory and Critical Care Medicine, 153,* 1711-1725. Official journal of the Thoracic Society. Copyright American Thoracic Society.

*Oral cefpodoxime (Vantin), cefuroxime (Ceftin), high-dose amoxicillin, amoxicillin /clavulanate (Augmentin); or parenteral ceftriaxone (Rocephin) followed by oral cefpodoxime.

[†]Antipseudomonal fluoroquinolones include ciprofloxacin (Cipro), levofloxacin (Levaquin), sparfloxacin (Zagam), gatifloxacin (Tequin), moxifloxacin (Avelox).

[‡]Cefotaxime (Claforan), ceftriaxone, amoxicillin/sulbactam, high-dose ampicillin.

[§]Cefepime (Maxipime), imipenem (Primaxin), meropenem (Merrem), piperacillin/tazobactam (Zosyn).

ICU, Intensive care unit; *IV,* intravenous.

COMFORT. Comfort is an important consideration with pneumonia, which may be manifested by fever, persistent cough, and chest pain. The patient who is critically or terminally ill may suffer from severe dyspnea, which may be relieved by morphine.

Prevention. Because pneumonia in older adults is so prevalent and exacts such a heavy toll, prevention should be a priority in all settings from the home to the hospital to long-term care. Many age-related changes cannot be modified, but measures still can be taken to

reduce the risk of complications. For example, defenses in the respiratory tract and the immune system diminish with aging, but vaccinations can reduce the risk of influenza and pneumococcal pneumonia.

INFLUENZA IMMUNIZATION. Because influenza can lead to pneumonia, especially in older persons, influenza vaccinations are highly recommended for this population. Research support for this strategy is building. Vaccinations have been found to reduce the risk of hospitalization for pneumonia and death from all causes during influenza seasons (Nichol et al., 2003). Strongly negative correlations have been found between vaccination coverage rates and pneumonia rates requiring hospitalization (Jin, Carriere, Predy, Johnson, & Marrie, 2003). In the Netherlands, vaccination significantly reduced morbidity and mortality rates in older adults during an influenza epidemic (Voordouw et al., 2003). It should be noted that the peak antibody response to immunization is lower in older people and the duration of antibody response is shorter (Connolly, 2003). Nevertheless, the benefits generally are believed to be sufficient to justify immunizing older persons.

Reports of influenza vaccination rates among older adults in the United States show that many vulnerable people remain unprotected. For example, one study found a 60% vaccination rate among older blacks and 79% among older whites (Zimmerman, Mieczkowski, & Wilson, 2002). Various explanations have been proposed for the reluctance of many people to be immunized. One problem is the common belief that the vaccine actually makes people sick and that it is not effective in preventing influenza. Interestingly, it has been demonstrated that vaccination of staff may have a greater impact on reducing mortality rates in long-term care facilities than vaccinating the residents (Carman et al., cited in Kennie, Dinan, & Young, 2003).

PNEUMOCOCCAL IMMUNIZATION. The pneumococcal vaccination is another potential lifesaver, although benefits for frail older adults have not been clearly demonstrated. In the United States, pneumococcal vaccination rates are 59% for older blacks and 70% for older whites (Zimmerman, Mieczkowski, & Wilson, 2002). With so many organisms responsible for pneumonia, 100% prevention is not possible. However, a study of patients hospitalized with pneumonia found that 66% had not been vaccinated for pneumococcus, and the risk of death from pneumonia was lower among those who had been vaccinated (Wagner, Popp, Posch, Vlasich, & Rosenberger-Spitzy, 2003). Whereas influenza vaccination must be repeated annually, the pneumococcal vaccination usually is given only once. Repeat vaccination within a 3-year period has resulted in severe allergic reactions in some people. Therefore revaccination is recommended only for individuals at highest risk for fatal pneumococcus who were first vaccinated at least 4 years previously with no serious or severe adverse effects (Mosby, 2004).

The incidence of upper respiratory infections such as the common cold, pharyngitis, and acute laryngitis is less in older than in younger persons. Nevertheless, these conditions should be treated early because they predispose the individual to pneumonia. Influenza may be a serious threat to life in the elderly, primarily because of the complications of bronchitis and pneumonia. The symptoms of uncomplicated flu are the same in the

elderly as in the young: sudden onset, chills, fever, headache, cough, sore throat, myalgia, and malaise.

At this time, there is no "cure" for influenza or the common cold. However, several pharmacological options exist that have been shown to decrease the severity and duration in older adults. The first generation of these drugs, which includes amantadine (Symmetrel) and rimantadine (Flumadine), is effective only against influenza type A. Resistance to these drugs develops rapidly. The second-generation drugs used to treat influenza are the neuraminidase inhibitors, which include oseltamivir (Tamiflu) and zanamivir (Relenza). They are effective against both influenza A and B, and pose a lower risk of resistance. Prompt treatment after the onset of symptoms (within 2 days) is critical for maximum benefit with these drugs. When started within 12 hours, the duration of influenza can be reduced by more than 3 days. Some studies are in progress to assess whether these drugs are effective prophylactically in a long-term care setting (Lehne, 2004).

A Japanese study confirmed the investigators' observations that Asian patients taking angiotensin-converting enzyme (ACE) inhibitors seemed to have a significantly reduced risk of pneumonia. The effect was not true for non-Asians (Ohkubo et al., 2004). This interesting finding could have considerable value in selected populations.

PREVENTION OF NOSOCOMIAL PNEUMONIA. The first step in decreasing nososcomial pneumonia is to follow procedures known to reduce patient risk. The *Guidelines for Prevention of Nosocomial Pneumonia and Prevention of Health Care Associated Pneumonia* issued by the CDC is a detailed document that can be accessed at www.cdc.gov.

Most of the deaths from hospital-acquired pneumonia occur in individuals who have been on ventilators. Based on survey data, Sole and colleagues (2003) concluded that the implementation of research-based policies and procedures for suctioning and airway management might reduce ventilator-associated pneumonia.

Basic nursing courses emphasize the need to mobilize patients to prevent the hazards of immobility. Keep the older adult up and as active as appropriate for the individual. For the nonambulatory person, turning, coughing, and deep breathing reduce pooling of secretions. Keep in mind that sedated patients are unable to cooperate with these activities, and use sedatives sparingly.

People who are in bed most of the time and those fed by hand or by feeding tube are at increased risk for aspiration pneumonia and must be carefully and frequently observed for early changes in pulmonary function, such as cough, and especially for an increase in respiratory rate and changes in respiratory pattern. Patients with dysphagia should be evaluated by a speech therapist to see if swallowing can be improved. General measures to decrease the risk of aspiration are as follows:

- For meals, seat the patient upright with the chin tilted slightly downward.
- When feeding, offer small bites and allow sufficient time for chewing and swallowing.
- Keep recently extubated patients on nothing-by-mouth status until cough, gag, and swallowing reflexes return (Coleman, 2004).
- After meals, including tube feedings, elevate the head of the bed 30 to 45 degrees (Coleman, 2004).
- Maintain good oral hygiene to reduce microaspiration of pathogens (Mehta & Niederman, 2002; Mylotte, 2002).
- Avoid unnecessary or excessive use of hypnotics and sedatives.

Prophylactic antibiotic therapy for adults in ICUs has been proposed. A systematic review showed significant reduction in respiratory infection and mortality rates when a combination of topical and systemic prophylactic antibiotics was used (Liberati et al., 2004). Antibiotic rotation policies also have been proposed as a strategy to reduce the development of resistant strains (Mehta & Niederman, 2002).

The effectiveness of oral antiseptics, along with basic oral hygiene, in reducing respiratory infections has been explored. A study that demonstrated that the use of chlorhexidine spray or swabs decreased growth of oral pathogens in ventilator patients suggested that it could mitigate or delay VAP (Grap, Munro, Elswick, Sessler, & Ward, 2004). In another study of post-cardiac surgery patients, the overall rate of nosocomial pneumonia was reduced by 52% when chlorhexidine rinse was used for oral care. However, the difference between the chlorhexidine group and a control group that used Listerine was significant only in patients who were intubated more than 24 hours and who had the highest degree of bacterial colonization (Houston et al., 2002).

Noninvasive ventilation (NIV) is believed to pose less risk of pneumonia. It was identified as an independent factor linked with a decreased rate of ICU-acquired pneumonia from 20% to 8% in patients ventilated for acute COPD exacerbation or cardiogenic pulmonary edema (Girou et al., 2003). Also, NIV has been shown to reduce the incidence of nosocomial pneumonia when used in patients with persistent weaning failure (Ferrer et al., 2003).

Clearly, measures to decrease exposure to pathogens and to boost patients' defenses are critical to reducing all nosocomial infections, including pneumonia. However, it is important to consider other factors that may affect infection rates. For example, it has been shown that there is a correlation between pain intensity and postoperative pulmonary complications after abdominal surgery. The implication is that good pain management could reduce the risk of pulmonary complications

(Shea, Brooks, Dayhoff, & Keck, 2002). Another consideration is the availability of adequate staff to provide both preventive and supportive care. Adequate nurse staffing is associated with lower risks of adverse events, including pneumonia, in hospitalized patients (Nurse staffing, 2004; Unruh, 2003).

Tuberculosis

Tuberculosis (TB) is an infection caused by the *Mycobacterium tuberculosis* bacillus. It is classified as pulmonary (the most common site) or extrapulmonary. Extrapulmonary TB can affect many structures, including the kidneys, bones and joints, lymph nodes, meninges, and colon (Connolly & Gosney, 2003). Because pulmonary TB is by far the most common, it is the focus of this section.

Epidemiology and Statistics. TB is a global problem. A review of professional literature reflects efforts to control this communicable disease in every region of the world. In the United States, TB is not the major health hazard that it was in the first half of the twentieth century; however, it still occurs, and 21% of cases occur in patients age 65 and older. Even more significant is the fact that the prevalence rate (8.8 per 100,000) in this age-group is higher than any other age-group. The prevalence rate by race/ethnicity is highest in Asians/Pacific Islanders, followed by blacks, Hispanics, American Indians/Alaskan Natives, and whites (CDC, 2003). In Quebec, Canada, TB rates were 10 to 20 times higher in the Arctic Inuit communities than the national average (Nguyen et al., 2003).

Tuberculosis in older adults often represents reactivation of an earlier infection that may or may not have been diagnosed and treated (Connolly & Gosney, 2003). Factors that may precipitate reactivation are malnutrition, diabetes mellitus, corticosteroid therapy, gastrectomy, alcoholism, cigarette smoking, and even an age-related decline in immunity. An additional risk factor is living in close quarters such as nursing homes with other susceptible individuals (CDC, 2003; Connolly & Gosney, 2003; Gajalakshmi, Peto, Kanaka, & Jha, 2003).

One population at increased risk for TB comprises the many health care workers who come in contact with known and undiagnosed TB patients. Therefore education of personnel is as important as public education. In a study of tuberculin skin test positivity and conversions among health care workers in New York City, 36.2% were positive at baseline. The conversion rate after 6 years was 1.3 per 100 person-years. It was higher among those who worked in high-risk occupational settings (the Office of the Chief Medical Examiner), were of Asian ethnicity, and were older (Cook, Maw, Munsiff, Fujiwara, & Frieden, 2003).

Clinical Manifestations. The classic clinical picture of TB is familiar: fever, night sweats, weight loss, anorexia, and hemoptysis. However, this typical picture may not be seen in the older adult. Some older persons have only fever of unknown origin or other vague symptoms. The older person with TB is less likely to have hemoptysis, but more likely to have lymphopenia, hypoalbuminemia, abnormal liver function tests, hypokalemia, and hyponatremia. An analysis of causes of hemoptysis discovered that the source was more likely to be bronchiogenic carcinoma in older persons and more likely to be TB in younger persons (Wong, Lim, & Liam, 2003). Dyspnea and night sweats are not commonly associated with TB in the elderly. In the absence of classic manifestations, TB may be overlooked. When an older patient complains of cough, fever, and general fatigue, the practitioner may focus on other chronic diseases with similar manifestations.

Diagnosis. Diagnosis is based on chest x-rays or on demonstration of acid-fast bacilli in the sputum. X-rays show shadows in the upper lobes, as in younger patients, but older individuals also are likely to have involvement of the middle and lower lobes (Connolly & Gosney, 2003; Rivzi, Shah, Inayat, & Hussain, 2003). Peripheral calcified primary complexes, calcified hilar nodes, upper zone patchy calcification, and sometimes pleural thickening are common findings associated with old healed disease (Connolly & Gosney, 2003). Cavitation is present in less than one third of older TB patients, and pleural effusion is even less common.

When the diagnosis is uncertain, a computed tomography (CT) scan may be helpful. Among the features evident on CT with pulmonary TB are multifocal airspace consolidation in multiple lobes, cavitary pulmonary nodular shadows, pleural effusion, TB empyema, and lymphadenopathy (Wei et al., 2004). However, atypical patterns have been reported in older adults (van Dyck, Vanhoenacker, Van den Brande, & De Schepper, 2003). High-resolution CT has demonstrated high sensitivity and specificity in predicting the activity of pulmonary TB (Wang et al., 2003). Japanese researchers are exploring the utility of positron emission tomography (PET) scanning in differentiating lung cancer, pulmonary TB, and atypical mycobacterial infection (Hara, Kosaka, Suzuki, Kudo, & Niino, 2003).

A positive Mantoux test is consistent with either present or past TB; however, recent conversion from negative to positive suggests active disease. Even so, the "booster effect" phenomenon can account for a negative response even with a TB history followed by a positive response that is stimulated by the repeated skin testing itself. False-negative results can be associated with several factors, including corticosteroid use and massive TB infection (Connolly & Gosney, 2003).

The only way to obtain a definitive diagnosis of active disease is to isolate *Mycobacterium tuberculosis*. For best results, a sputum culture is recommended. The best process to isolate the organism and identify sensitivity is to obtain at least three good sputum specimens for microscopy and culture before initiating antitubercular drug therapy. For patients who have difficulty providing a sputum specimen, ultrasonic nebulized saline with physiotherapy, bronchoscopy and washings, or aspiration of pleural fluid with pleural biopsy may be employed. A study in the United Kingdom compared the utility of gastric washing and bronchoscopy in the diagnosis of smear-negative pulmonary TB. Bronchoscopy proved to be the superior of the two methods, but a combination of the two proved to be optimal (Dickson, Brent, Davidson, & Wall, 2003). In contrast, New Zealand investigators found that culture-positive specimens were obtained in 52% of subjects by bronchoscopy and 96% of the same subjects in three induced sputum tests. The cost of obtaining induced sputum specimens also was considerably less than bronchoscopy (McWilliams et al., 2002).

Management. The goals of TB treatment, according to the CDC (2003), are to cure the individual patient and to minimize transmission to other persons. Critical components of the treatment plan are drug therapy, infection control measures, and patient education. The drug protocols presented here were developed for use in the United States. Other guidelines such as those developed by WHO and International Union Against Tuberculosis and Lung Disease (IUATLD) differ in certain aspects because of differences in the populations and health care systems throughout the world.

Drug Therapy. Because of the adaptability of the *Mycobacterium tuberculosis* bacillus, resistance develops rapidly when a single drug is used. Therefore active TB is treated with various combinations of drugs depending on the organism sensitivity and patient variables such as comorbidity and other drug therapy.

The document "Treatment of Tuberculosis" issued by the American Thoracic Society, the CDC, and the Infectious Diseases Society of America (Treatment of tuberculosis, 2003) is available on the CDC Web site and provides detailed information for selection of specific drug regimens in various situations.

The first-line drugs for TB in the United States are isoniazid (INH), rifampin, rifapentine, rifabutin, pyrazinamide, and ethambutol. Fixed combinations of INH and rifampin (Rifamate) and INH, rifampin, and pyrazinamide (Rifater) are available, and may improve patient acceptability and adherence and prevent accidental monotherapy. Second-line drugs approved by the Food and Drug Administration for TB treatment are cycloserine, ethionamide, para-aminosalicylic acid, streptomycin, and capreomycin. Additional second-line drugs that had not been approved for TB treatment when the guidelines were published are levofloxacin, moxifloxacin, gatifloxacin, and amikacin/kanamycin.

"Treatment of Tuberculosis" describes four different regimens that are recommended for patients who have drug-susceptible organisms. The practitioner uses the guidelines to select the regimen that is most appropriate for an individual patient. Each regimen begins with a 2-month course of therapy (phase I) followed by one of several combinations for an additional 4 to 7 months (phase II).

Phase I therapy for adults with previously untreated TB employs INH, rifampin, pyrazinamide, and ethambutol. Ethambutol can be omitted if the susceptibility test results are available and show the pathogens to be fully susceptible. Dosing patterns in the initial phase may require daily, twice-weekly, or three-times-weekly therapy. Comorbidities, allergies, and drugs for other conditions may require alterations in the usual regimens. For example, patients with severe liver disease or gout should not take pyrazinamide.

An example of a phase II regimen is INH and rifampin daily for 18 weeks or 5 days a week for 18 weeks. Another regimen prescribes twice-weekly dosing for 18 weeks, and a third example prescribes daily or 5 times per week dosing for 31 weeks. If the patient's organisms are not susceptible to INH or rifampin (alone or in combination), different first-line or second-line drugs are selected.

Treatment of Latent Tuberculosis. Individuals with latent TB are at risk for reactivation of the disease. Among individuals with an induration of 10 mm or more on a tuberculin skin test and either human immunodeficiency virus (HIV) infection or evidence of old, healed TB, the lifetime risk of reactivaton is 20%. Among recent converters, the lifetime risk is 10% to 20%. Intensive efforts should be made to ensure full treatment of these individuals to prevent reactivation (Horsburgh, 2004). The American Thoracic Society recommends a 9-month course of INH therapy for individuals who have latent TB and are at high risk for reactivation. An alternative treatment is a 2-month course of pyrazinamide and rifampin. A comparison of the two regimens in a community setting found that the risk for hepatitis was three times greater with the pyrazinamide/rifampin combination than with INH (McNeill, Allen, Estrada, & Cook, 2003). Another review of records of 148 patients treated with pyrazinamide and rifampin revealed that 9.4% had serious hepatotoxicity and less than 60% completed the course of therapy (Lee, Mennone, Jones, & Paul, 2002).

Drug Resistance. A huge ongoing challenge in the global management of TB has been the emergence of multidrug-resistant strains of *M. tuberculosis* (MDR-TB). Individuals with MDR-TB require extended treatment with expensive and toxic regimens and have higher treatment failure and mortality rates (Chan et al., 2004;

Quy et al., 2003). One region in South Africa reported that at least 55% of previously treated and 19% of new cases were resistant to one or more of the drugs tested (Lin, Sattar, & Puckree, 2004). The resistance rate was much lower in Poland, but doubled between 1997 and 2000 (Augustynowicz-Kopec, Zwolska, Jaworski, Kostrzewa, & Klatt, 2003). The prevalence of MDR-TB is disproportionately high in persons who are HIV positive (Campos et al., 2003).

Accurate susceptibility tests, multidrug therapy in the correct dosage for the correct duration, and a high level of patient adherence are factors that contribute to effective treatment and discourage development of resistant strains. Because patient adherence with long-term therapy is problematic, a strategy that is recommended is directly observed therapy (DOT). DOT may employ a health care provider, family member, lay caregiver, or "buddy," depending on the patient's living arrangements, to observe each dose being taken. This process is simplified by combination drugs and less frequent dosing. Protocols for dealing with MDR-TB are complex and beyond the scope of this text.

Ongoing assessment of response during TB treatment includes monthly sputum examinations and culture until two consecutive negative cultures are obtained. To assess the early response to treatment, more frequent acid fast bacillus (AFB) smears may be useful. Routine assessments of hepatic and renal function and platelet count are advised only if baseline abnormalities were present or the patient has increased risk factors. Patients who are taking ethambutol should have monthly testing of visual acuity and color discrimination because of the risk of optic neuritis (Treatment of tuberculosis, 2003).

Adverse Effects. Antitubercular drugs have significant adverse effects, with hepatitis being the most serious effect common to many of them. Drug-induced hepatitis is defined as "a serum AST [aspartate aminotransferase] level more than three times the upper limit of normal in the presence of symptoms, or more than five times the upper limit of normal in the absence of symptoms" (Treatment of tuberculosis, 2003, p. 7). INH, rifampin, and pyrazinamide all are hepatotoxic, and must be stopped if hepatitis occurs. Nonhepatotoxic drugs must be substituted until the AST level falls to twice the upper limit of normal and symptoms improve, at which time the original drugs can be restarted. Symptoms of hepatitis that may occur early are anorexia, nausea, vomiting, fatigue, malaise, and weakness. Oral therapy is appropriate and effective for most patients; however, parenteral forms of most antitubercular drugs are available for severely ill patients who cannot take oral drugs.

Gastrointestinal adverse effects, which are common, include nausea, vomiting, anorexia, and abdominal pain. If measurement of the AST level rules out hepatitis, the problem may be managed by changing the time of administration (closer to meals or at bedtime) or having the patient take the drug with food.

All antitubercular drugs can cause a rash with a wide range of severity. A minor rash with itching can be treated with antihistamines. Other rashes require more thorough investigation. For example, a petechial rash may be related to thrombocytopenia caused by rifampin and requires discontinuation of that drug. If a generalized erythematous rash with fever or mucous membrane involvement occurs, all drugs must be stopped immediately. Detailed steps to resume treatment are outlined in the "Treatment of Tuberculosis" (2003) guidelines and include temporary use of alternative drugs and the systematic reintroduction of the suspect drugs.

Drug fever is manifested by a high fever in a patient who looks and feels well. It most often occurs after several weeks of therapy to which the patient seems to be responding positively. With TB treatment, superinfection or worsening TB infection should be ruled out before stopping drug therapy. Like management of rash, a protocol details steps to resume treatment with drug fever.

Each drug has additional specific adverse effects that must be monitored. For example, INH can cause peripheral neuropathy, especially in malnourished, bedridden older individuals and in those predisposed to neuritis by diabetes or alcoholism. Daily pyridoxine can prevent neuropathy. Ethambutol can cause optic neuritis, which is manifested by blurred vision, constriction of the visual field, and disturbed color discrimination. Patients should be evaluated by an ophthalmologist before and after being prescribed this drug. Because vision disturbances can be permanent, visual symptoms require discontinuation of ethambutol. When the patient is an older adult, it is significant that this drug also can cause confusion and elevated serum uric acid levels (Lehne, 2004).

A 9-year study assessed the occurrence of major adverse effects in 430 persons who were being treated for active TB with first-line drugs. In this sample, pyrazinamide had the highest incidence of major adverse effects, followed by INH, rifampin, and ethambutol. Risk factors for any major adverse effects were female gender, age over 60 years, and birthplace in Asia (Yee et al., 2003).

Drug Interactions. The fact that antitubercular drugs have many interactions with other drugs has important implications for the older adult who commonly takes drugs for other reasons. In the case of first-line antitubercular drugs, taking them together as a single dose produces higher blood levels. Patients who experience epigastric distress or nausea can take the drugs with meals because food does not adversely affect serum concentrations. Also, antacids do not significantly interfere with absorption of first-line drugs. First-line drugs increase theophylline clearance significantly, which could result in bronchospasm in patients with asthma or COPD (Ahn & Lee, 2003). However, the potential for interactions between most second-line drugs and antacid or food is uncertain. It is possible that antacids and food interfere with absorption of these drugs, so it is best to take them on an empty stomach. It is known that the absorption of fluoroquinolones is markedly decreased by antacids and other drugs that contain divalent cations (didanosine, sucralfate, iron, magnesium, calcium, zinc, and some vitamin and dietary supplements).

SURGICAL INTERVENTION. Spanish researchers analyzed the indications for surgery in individuals with pulmonary TB over an 8-year period. Indications in their sample included pulmonary aspergilloma, pneumothorax, pulmonary nodes and masses without histological diagnosis, bronchiectasis, massive hemoptysis, and pleural empyema. Procedures performed for these conditions were lobectomy, pneumonectomy, pleuropulmonary decorticaton, mediastinoscopy, and thoracoscopy. The most frequent surgical complication was persistent air leakage after pulmonary resection (Freixinet et al., 2002).

INFECTION CONTROL. Formerly, all patients with TB were hospitalized for long periods. This is no longer necessary unless it is likely that the patient will not take the prescribed drugs or there are complications. Patients may be in the hospital for 1 to 2 weeks while therapy is instituted. The patient usually is placed in isolation for the first 2 weeks of therapy. In addition, when an active case of TB is detected, household and other close contacts must be tested for infection. For nursing home residents, this often means that other residents and most of the staff should be tested.

EDUCATION. Most older adults being treated for TB reside in the community and manage their own drug therapy or are assisted by a family member, caregiver, or friend. Nursing care includes teaching the patient and family about the disease and drugs and providing psychological support. One important aspect of the nursing care of the older person with TB is assessment of adherence with the drug regimen. Nurses often are in a position to find out whether the patient is actually taking all the drugs prescribed and in the way they were recommended. Close adherence to the drug regimen for a long time is difficult but essential if the disease is to be cured.

Health beliefs affect a person's willingness to seek treatment and to follow through with the long treatment process. A study of acculturation and health beliefs in Mexican Americans found that more traditional Mexican Americans perceived higher susceptibility to TB than those who were highly integrated. Further, higher perceived susceptibility was associated with greater intent to engage in TB health behaviors (Rodriguez-Reimann, Nicassio, Reimann, Gallegos, & Olmedo, 2004). The patient may view this diagnosis as a stigma and feel like an outcast, because TB patients formerly were placed in sanatoriums, far removed from family and friends.

Because TB is a communicable disease, contacts of individuals diagnosed with active disease need to be notified and assessed. In the United States, contacts are managed through public health agencies. Patients need to understand the importance of identification and follow-up of at-risk contacts. Information gleaned from focus groups has shown that participants are willing to report contacts but did not always understand what constituted a "contact," and they also want the opportunity to personally inform the contacts before the health department contacts them (Shrestha-Kuwahara, Wilce, DeLuca, & Taylor, 2003).

Nutrition. Weight loss and anorexia are common with active TB, yet good nutrition is essential to recovery. A study of the body composition changes during recovery showed that patients gained 10% in body weight during 6 months of therapy. The change was mostly due to increased fat mass; protein mass, total body water, and bone mass did not change significantly (Schwenk et al., 2004). Patients often need nutritional support and may require consultation from a dietitian and a social worker.

Pulmonary Rehabilitation. A study in which post-TB patients, many of whom were postthoracotomy, and COPD patients matched for age and FEV_1 participated in a 9-week pulmonary rehabilitation program demonstrated that both groups benefited equally in terms of dyspnea, activity scores, and 6-minute walking distance (Ando et al., 2003).

Research Directions. Researchers are seeking other markers that could be used to diagnose and treat TB and to assess the response to treatment. For example, vascular endothelial growth factor reflecting intense angiogenesis is increased with active pulmonary TB (Alatas et al., 2004). U.S. researchers are attempting to devise immunoassays for TB based on antibodies that might be present in the serum or urine (Singh et al., 2003). Another procedure under study for the rapid diagnosis of TB is the use of the AMPLICOR assay, a direct amplification test (Lim, Zhu, Gough, Lee, & Kumarasinghe, 2002).

In relation to treatment, many avenues are being explored. Published studies of the fluoroquinolones for TB treatment look promising (Gosling et al., 2003; Valerio et al., 2003). The use of aerosolized interferon-gamma to boost the local immune response is under study. Early, small experiments resulted in conversion of sputum smears in five patients with MDR-TB (Condos, Hull, Schluger, Rom, & Smaldone, 2004).

Cancer of the Lung

Epidemiology and Statistics. Lung cancer, a major disease of the elderly, was predicted to be responsible for more than 160,000 deaths in the United States in 2004. Since 1991, lung cancer death rates in males have continued to decline significantly whereas they have increased in females (American Cancer Society, 2004). A similar pattern is seen in many European countries as well (Janssen-Heijnen & Coebergh, 2003; Tyczynski et al., 2004). Some experts contend that women do not appear to be more susceptible to lung cancer than men given equal smoking exposure (Bain et al., 2004).

The probability of developing lung cancer increases dramatically with age. Up to age 39, the probability for males is 1 in 3439 and for females is 1 in 3046. Between ages 60 and 79, the probability for males is 1 in 17 and for females is 1 in 25. The cohort of women born from 1931 to 1940, in which the prevalence of smoking peaked at about 44%, is likely to have the highest prevalence of lung cancer. Thus the death rate from lung cancer in elderly women will no doubt continue to rise. The increasing incidence of cancer in older age is attributed to three factors: the considerable length of time for carcinogenesis to occur, age-related changes that mimic carcinogenesis, and physical changes that favor cancer progression (Repetto & Balducci, 2002).

In contrast to statistics in Western countries, the incidence and mortality rates for lung cancer among Japanese men is lower despite a high prevalence of cigarette smoking. This phenomenon, called "the Japanese paradox," has been attributed to congenital resistance and to low carcinogenic ingredients in Japanese cigarettes (Nakaji et al., 2003). Likewise, in the United Kingdom smoking patterns appear to be similar to those in the United States, but the lung cancer rates in men declined during a period when U.S. rates more than doubled. The rates among U.S. women increased sevenfold, compared to threefold in the United Kingdom. This study suggests that lung cancer may be associated with multiple smoking and environmental variables that were not assessed (Lee & Forey, 2003).

Types of Bronchogenic Carcinoma. The major histologic types of bronchogenic carcinoma are squamous cell, large cell, and adenocarcinoma, which collectively are referred to as non–small cell lung cancer (NSCLC) and small cell lung cancer (SCLC) (Heuther & McCance, 2000). Non–small cell cancer accounts for 80% of all cases, and SCLC accounts for the remaining 20% (Connolly & Gosney, 2003). Forty percent of patients in the United States diagnosed with NSCLC are

70 years of age or older (Lilenbaum, 2003). Some changes have been noted in the proportions of the various types of lung cancer over recent decades. The proportion of adenocarcinoma to other types of lung cancer has been increasing in both men and women in the United States and the Netherlands. One proposed explanation is the increased use of low-tar filter cigarettes (Janssen-Heijnen & Coebergh, 2003). Also, between 1979 and 1998, squamous cell carcinoma and SCLC increased in women, but decreased in men (Hatcher & Dover, 2003). A review of Australian data for about the same time frame revealed increased proportions of adenocarcinomas and large cell lesions (Nguyen, Luke, & Roder, 2003).

Prognosis. Among men and women over age 75, lung cancer causes the greatest number of cancer deaths. The 3-year survival rate is 6.3%, and the median duration of survival is 7 months (Cataldo, 2003).

Clinical Manifestations. Common signs and symptoms of lung cancer are shown in Box 13-6. These may be related to the primary lung tumor or to the spread of the tumor. Initial symptoms often include cough, dyspnea, and blood-tinged sputum. Pain is uncommon in the early stage unless there is pressure on a nerve or bone involvement (Kreamer, 2003). In addition, paraneoplastic syndromes such as hypercalcemia or inappropriate antidiuretic hormone secretion may be present (Kreamer, 2003). With the exception of hemoptysis, these symptoms often are ignored by the elderly. More severe dyspnea, weight loss, fatigue, pain, and obstructive pneumonia usually are seen later in the disease when the possibility of cure has diminished.

Diagnosis. The first requirement for diagnosing lung cancer is recognizing the possibility of this diagnosis. Classic symptoms such as cough and breathlessness can easily be confused with other conditions. When lung cancer is suspected, a comprehensive geriatric assessment will provide a basis for the treatment plan. Components of the assessment should include function, comorbidity, cognition, depression, social support, nutrition, and polypharmacy (Repetto & Balducci, 2002). Even if no intervention is anticipated, a thorough evaluation may provide direction for palliative and support therapies (Connolly & Gosney, 2003).

Primary diagnostic tests and procedures include radiography, CT or magnetic resonance imaging (MRI) (or both), PET, bronchoscopy, and histological sputum studies. Additional studies that may be done include mediastinoscopy, video-assisted thoracoscopy, pulmonary angiography, lung scans, thoracentesis, and fine-needle aspiration (Crimlisk, 2004). Some practitioners have reservations about the safety and efficacy of bronchoscopy for the older adult. However, Connolly and

---

BOX 13-6 Common Signs and Symptoms of Lung Cancer

Symptoms Due to Central or Endobrachial Growth of the Primary Tumor
Cough
Hemophysis
Wheeze and stridor
Dyspnea from obstruction
Pneumonitis from obstruction (fever, productive cough)

Symptoms Due to Peripheral Growth of the Primary Tumor
Pain from pleural or chest wall involvement
Cough
Dyspnea on a restrictive basis
Lung abscess syndrome from tumor cavitation

Symptoms Related to Regional Spread of the Tumor in the Thorax by Contiguity or by Metastasis to Regional Lymph Nodes
Tracheal obstruction
Esophageal compression with dysphagia
Recurrent laryngeal nerve paralysis with hoarseness
Phrenic nerve paralysis with hemidiaphragm elevation and dyspnea
Sympathetic nerve paralysis with Horner's syndrome
Eighth cervical and first thoracic nerves with ulnar pain and Panacoast's syndrome
Superior vena cava syndrome from vascular obstruction
Pericardial and cardiac extension with resultant tamponade, arrhythmia, or cardiac failure
Lymphatic obstruction with pleural effusion
Lymphangitic spread through lungs with hypoxemia and dyspnea

From Cohen, M. H. (1977). Signs and symptoms of bronchogenic carcinoma. In M. J. Straus (Ed.), *Lung cancer: Clinical diagnosis and treatment.* New York: Grune & Stratton, pp. 85-94.

Gosney (2003) contend that there is a dearth of research to confirm or allay these fears.

Screening. The idea of screening high-risk individuals is appealing because the odds of survival may be improved by early detection. Japanese investigators examined the results of low-dose CT screening for the detection of lung cancer in smokers and nonsmokers. Cancers detected in nonsmokers were more often slow-growing adenocarcinomas that had a faint ground-glass appearance on CT. Smokers were more likely to have rapidly growing cancers that appeared on CT as solid nodules (Li, Sone, Abe, MacMahon, & Doi, 2003). Italian investigators used low-dose spiral CT to detect early lung cancer in high-risk individuals (1035 individuals age 50 and older with a 20 or more pack-year smoking history). PET scans were selectively used for further evaluation. Twenty-two cases of lung cancer were diagnosed, 21 were completely resected, and 17 were at stage 1. Over the subsequent 2.5-year follow-up, no interval lung cancers were found. The investigators concluded that screening with low-dose CT and selective use of PET scans effectively detected early lung cancer (Pastorino et al., 2003). Another screening study, this one conducted at the Mayo Clinic, also concluded that CT can detect early-stage lung cancers (Swensen et al., 2003).

Pathogenesis. Factors implicated in the pathogenesis of lung cancer include smoking, exposure to other carcinogenic agents, and genetic factors. Smoking is by far the most significant risk factor for lung cancer (American Cancer Society, 2004; Kreamer, 2003). Lung cancer also is associated with long-term exposure to a number of other carcinogenic pollutants such as asbestos, arsenic, radon, uranium, nickel, chlormethyl ether, and chromium. Asbestos and uranium exposure apparently act synergistically with cigarette smoke. High-risk occupations increase the risk of lung cancer by 2% for every 10 years in the profession. Combined with smoking, the risk over 20 years might be tripled (Ruano-Ravina, Figueiras, Barreiro-Carracedo, & Barros-Dios, 2003). In a Turkish study, occupations associated with increased risk of lung cancer included textile workers, firefighters, drivers, water treatment plant workers, and highway construction workers (Elci, Akpinar-Elci, Alavanja, & Dosemeci, 2004). Brooks, Palmer, Strom, and Rosenberg (2003) determined that menthol versus nonmenthol cigarettes did not affect the risk of lung cancer.

Environmental, medical, or occupational exposure to radiation also is considered a risk factor for lung cancer (American Cancer Society, 2004). An MD Anderson study showed that smoking was an independent risk factor for lung cancer in women who had had breast cancer. In this sample, radiotherapy alone (for breast cancer) did not present the same risk as smoking. However, radiotherapy combined with smoking posed a risk greater than that from either alone (Ford et al., 2003). Another study found that the increased risk of lung cancer in women who had had breast cancer was related to the volume of lung tissue exposed to radiation and the dose administered (Deutsch et al., 2003).

The etiology of lung cancer in nonsmokers is unknown, although exposure to secondhand smoke is believed to be one factor (Kreamer, 2003). Some other possible contributing factors are mutation of tumor suppression genes caused by exposure to indoor cooking oil fumes and heavy outdoor air pollution. Researchers in Taiwan report a relationship between human papillomavirus and lung cancer in females (Chiou et al., 2003; Wen Cheng & Lee, 2003). The role of genetics in conveying susceptibility or resistance to lung cancer is a topic of current research.

Management. Selecting the best treatment can be difficult because of the common practice of excluding older adults from clinical trials of cancer therapy. This limits knowledge of the best curative and palliative treatment options for the older person. Treatment options include surgery, radiotherapy, and chemotherapy. Surgery is the treatment of choice for NSCLC, but many lung tumors are not resectable when detected and some others prove to be nonresectable in surgery. Unfortunately, many older patients delay seeking diagnosis or are not referred for surgery when their tumors still are operable (Connolly & Gosney, 2003). In one study of 27 patients age 70 and older who had pneumonectomy, the operative mortality rate was 22%, and the 5-year survival rate was 11.5%. Statistics for younger patients with pneumonectomy were 3.2% and 30.5%, respectively. In a review of 1830 patient records, patients over age 70 had a postoperative mortality rate of 17.8% with the main predictors of mortality being age, extent of surgery, and side affected. The mortality rate was higher for right pneumonectomy (van Meerbeeck, Damhuis, & Vos de Wael, 2002). A study in the Netherlands followed 126 patients older than 70 years of age who had resection for NSCLC. The hospital mortality rate was 3.2%, and only 13% had major complications. The survival rate at 5 years was 37% and at 10 years was 15%. The best predictor of complications in this study was comorbidity (Birim et al., 2003). Van Meerbeeck, Damhuis, and Vos de Wael (2002) concluded that the risks of surgery were acceptable and that older persons should not be denied this option. According to Balducci (2004), decisions about options must be based on appropriate patient assessment and selection. Clinical research needs to help us determine which older persons are most likely to benefit from surgical intervention.

Radiotherapy may be used with surgery and is also an important alternative for those who are unable or unwilling to have surgery. For NSCLC, it may be used preoperatively to shrink the tumor and postoperatively for tumors that have extended beyond the resected margins (Kreamer, 2003). With both SCLC and NSCLC, radiotherapy may provide some relief of pain, cough, and dyspnea and reduce neurological symptoms caused by brain metastases (Kreamer, 2003). Radiotherapy is particularly helpful in those with squamous cell cancer and is tolerated by older persons, as well as by younger patients.

Chemotherapy alone or with radiation is the treatment of choice for SCLC (American Cancer Society, 2004; Kreamer, 2003). In addition to traditional antineoplastics, various other drugs are being studied for treatment of lung cancer. Gefitinib (Iressa), which blocks activity of growth factor receptors, has been approved for treatment of NSCLC (American Cancer Society, 2004). The National Comprehensive Cancer Network (NCCN) issued evidence-based guidelines for the treatment of cancer in older persons (Repetto et al., 2003). Key points include the following:

- Safe and effective treatment depends on proper patient selection based on a comprehensive geriatric assessment.
- Drugs that are excreted by the kidneys should be given in reduced dosages.
- Hematopoietic growth factors should be given beginning with the first chemotherapy cycle to maintain hemoglobin levels at or above 12 g/L.

Sometimes older adults are deprived of optimal treatment because of a stereotype that they are too frail to have chemotherapy. Lilenbaum (2003) refutes this generalization and recommends that patients be evaluated on the basis of performance status and comorbidities, not on age alone. Combination carboplatin-based regimens are recommended for fit older persons, and single-agent therapy is recommended for those with less than optimum performance or significant comorbidities (Lilenbaum, 2003). Older adults are more susceptible to chemotherapy complications, including bone marrow toxicity, mucositis, cardiotoxicity, and neurotoxicity. Neutropenia is a common adverse effect of chemotherapy that is even more common among older adults. A study of fatigue in older adults receiving chemotherapy for various types of cancer showed that it was a common symptom, especially among women. A positive correlation existed between fatigue and depression whereas there was a negative correlation between fatigue and hemoglobin (Respini, Jacobsen, Thors, Tralongo, & Balducci, 2003). Balducci and Carreca (2003) recommend the following to reduce the risk of chemotherapy complications in older adults:

- Neutropenic fever: filgrastim and pegfilgrastim have been shown to reduce the risk of neutropenic fever by 50% to 75% in older patients treated with CHOP (cyclophosphamide, doxorubicin, prednisone, and vincristine) or CHOP-like regimens.
- Mucositis: risk can be reduced by using oral capecitabine when feasible instead of intravenous fluorinated pyrimidines.
- Cardiotoxicity: dexrazoxane or liposomal compounds should be used rather than anthracyclines.

Citing neutropenia as the primary dose-limiting toxicity of cancer therapy in older patients, a systematic review of the use of colony-stimulating factors (CSFs) concluded that primary prophylaxis with CSFs should be considered for older persons receiving moderately intensive chemotherapy with responsive malignancies (Lyman, Kuderer, Agboola, & Balducci, 2003). A retrospective study of Canadian patients with limited-stage SCLC showed that older persons had poorer treatment responses and survival rates, which might be explained by poorer baseline performance status and suboptimal treatment. In this sample, older persons were less likely to be treated with combined-modality chemotherapy, intensive chemotherapy, or prophylactic cranial irradiation (Ludbrook et al., 2003).

Nursing Care. Nursing care of the older adult with lung cancer must pay special attention to the increased risk factors imposed by age. Increased risks of adverse effects of therapy require special care to prevent infection, oral lesions, and skin breakdown and to manage fatigue.

The high mortality rate among older patients with lung cancer means that most of these individuals eventually will be faced with recognition that they will not recover. The idea of dying of lung cancer may be particularly frightening because of the fear of pain or severe dyspnea and the possibility that there may be no family and few friends to provide support. The patient needs to be reassured that excessive pain is not common in most cancers, and that the pain that is present can be controlled without significantly changing the ability to function and think. Hospice care is particularly helpful for the elderly patient with lung cancer. End-of-life care is discussed in Chapter 22.

Risk Reduction. The extent to which smoking cessation reduces the risk of lung cancer in older persons has been debated. A Mayo Clinic study used data on over 37,000 women ages 55 to 69 years to address this issue. Not surprisingly, the risk of lung cancer was higher in current and former smokers than in women who had never smoked. For former smokers, the risk declined with the duration of abstinence (Ebbert et al., 2003). Evidence exists that motivated older persons can quit smoking, and, with nicotine replacement therapy, the success rate has been reported around 20% (Connolly, 2000). Unfortunately, few intervention studies target older adults. After smoking cessation, the rate of decline in lung function reverts to the normal, more gradual change. Admittedly, the benefits of cessation decline with age, but they are believed to continue up to age 80, particularly in women (Connolly, 2000). In relation to lung cancer, for every year of smoking, an individual's risk rises by an amount that is equal to the decline in risk after smoking cessation. The work of Ruano-Ravina and colleagues (2003) suggests that there is a saturation effect for lifetime tobacco consumption of around 25,000 to 30,000 packs.

Other variables that have been the focus of research include nutrition and physical activity. A European study of nutrition and cancer analyzed data from 478,021 individuals to assess the relation between intake of fruits and vegetables and incidence of lung cancer. Lung cancer risk and fruit consumption had a significant inverse relationship, whereas there was no association with vegetable consumption. The investigators recommended enhanced fruit consumption, but acknowledge that the effect would be small compared to possible benefits of smoking cessation (Miller et al., 2004). Italian researchers assessed the relationship between the consumption of food items in a typical Mediterranean diet and lung cancer. Two items that were judged to have a protective effect against lung cancer were exclusive olive oil use and sage (Fortes et al., 2003). The Missouri Women's Health Study report concluded that total vegetable intake was predictive of lower cancer risk, in models adjusted for total carotenoids (Wright, Mayne, Swanson, Sinha, & Alavanja, 2003).

A study by the Canadian Centre for Chronic Disease Prevention and Control showed that recreational physical activity reduced lung cancer risk in men and women, with the most profound effect among smokers and people with low and medium body mass indexes (Mao, Pan, Wen, & Johnson, 2003).

Obstructive Sleep Apnea

Pathophysiology. By definition, an apneic episode is the cessation of airflow for longer than 10 seconds. Sleep apnea is a serious condition characterized by repeated upper airway collapse and cessation of breathing during sleep. The most common type is *obstructive sleep apnea* (OSA), in which the airway closes, thereby inhibiting airflow in spite of persistent ventilatory effort. The apneic episode is associated with hypoventilation (hypopnea) and results in decreased oxygen saturation. The brain responds by stimulating arousal so the patient awakens and resumes breathing. In some people, these episodes occur hundreds of time each night.

Clinical Manifestations. The effect of OSA is poor sleep quality leading to complaints such as fatigue, sleepiness, irritability, and problems with memory and judgment that may pose problems in occupational and social settings. It also has been documented as a factor in motor vehicle accidents and has been associated with diminished quality of life (Young, Peppard, & Gottlieb, 2002). Cardiovascular effects may include hypertension, arrhythmias (usually bradycardia), and myocardial ischemia (National Institutes of Health, 1995). The relationship with hypertension is not fully understood, but it has been shown that treatment of OSA lowers blood pressure. Some hypothesized mechanisms are sympathetic activation, hyperleptinemia, insulin resistance, elevated angiotensin I and II and aldosterone, oxidative and inflammatory stress, endothelial dysfunction, impaired baroreflex function, and effects on renal function (Wolk, Shamsuzzaman, & Somers, 2003). Of particular concern with older adults is that OSA has been associated with cognitive dysfunction in inductive and deductive thinking and constructive ability (Antonelli-Incalzi, Marra et al., 2004).

The severity of OSA is rated on a sleep apnea–hypopnea index (AHI) based on the average number of apnea-hypopnea events per hour of sleep. An AHI score of 5 or more per hour accompanied by patient reports of excessive sleepiness is consistent with a diagnosis of OSA. Some clinicians use the term *respiratory disturbance index* (RDI) instead (Tate & Tasota, 2002).

Epidemiology. OSA is estimated to affect 15 million Americans. As many as one half of older Americans are believed to suffer from some type of sleep disorder, most commonly sleep apnea or restless legs syndrome (Barthlen, 2002). The increasing prevalence has been attributed to increasing obesity. Based on reports of snoring and witnessed periods of apnea, the peak prevalence among men is between ages 55 and 59 years; for women the peak is between ages 60 and 64 years (Larsson, Lindberg, Franklin, & Lundback, 2003). The prevalence of OSA usually is greater among men, but the gender difference disappears around age 55, suggesting a role for menopause in OSA among women (Resta et al., 2003).

Diagnosis. Gerontological nurses often are in an ideal position to assess sleep patterns and abnormalities in older persons. Snoring and periods of apnea should be documented and follow-up encouraged. Patients who complain of excessive daytime sleepiness can be screened with a tool such as the Epworth Sleepiness Scale. A score greater than 10 warrants additional investigation. An overnight polysomnogram in a sleep laboratory is the most definitive diagnostic tool (Tate & Tasato, 2002). Polysomnographic measures and subjective measures of OSA do not necessarily correlate; therefore both should be considered in the assessment (Weaver, Kapur, & Yueh, 2004). Cardiac monitoring and continuous pulse oximetry also can provide evidence of changes characteristic of OSA. Cranial radiographs are not diagnostic for OSA, but may reveal abnormalities commonly found with OSA. Volumetric MRI allows measurements of tissue volume of the tongue and pharynx (Schwab et al., 2003).

Risk Factors. Among the established risk factors for OSA are overweight and obesity, central body fat distribution, large neck girth, and craniofacial and upper airway abnormalities. Other suspected factors are genetics, smoking, menopause, alcohol use before sleep, and nighttime nasal congestion. Common comorbid conditions are diabetes, hypertension, coronary artery disease, myocardial infarction, congestive heart failure, and stroke (Young, Skatrud, & Peppard, 2004). Knowledge of risk factors and comorbidities should prompt the practitioner to investigate the possibility of OSA.

Volumetric MRI has confirmed the relationship between OSA and increased volume of the tongue, lateral pharyngeal walls, and total soft tissue (Schwab et al., 2003).

The role of leptin in OSA has been investigated. In one study of 86 patients, leptin levels declined in patients who were effectively treated for OSA, but increased in patients who were not treated effectively (Sanner, Kollhosser, Buechner, Zidek, & Tepel, 2004). In contrast, another study concluded that leptin concentration was not related to the degree of OSA after controlling for body fat (Schafer et al., 2002). The significance of these findings remains to be seen.

In a sample of community-dwelling older adults with symptoms of nocturia and sleep-disordered breathing, investigators found that nighttime urine production was increased in subjects with an AHI greater than 15 (Umlauf et al., 2004).

Management. Sometimes fairly basic interventions are effective. These include avoidance of alcohol and other drugs that relax the pharyngeal muscles, smoking cessation, allergy medications, and weight loss. Patients with mild OSA related to a supine sleep position can sew a small, harmless object into the back of the nightclothes to prevent lying in the supine position (Tate & Tasota, 2002). When measures such as these are not achieved, or are not effective, options include continuous positive airway pressure, oral appliances, surgical intervention, radiofrequency ablation of excess or enlarged tissue, and drug therapy to treat daytime drowsiness.

CONTINUOUS POSITIVE AIRWAY PRESSURE. Continuous positive airway pressure (CPAP) involves the delivery of air under positive pressure that keeps the airway open. To be effective, a mask properly fitted to cover the nose and mouth must be worn during sleep. Despite significant improvement in symptoms when used properly, compliance rates are not good. Some people find the mask to be uncomfortable and restrictive; others report nasal irritation and chest or back discomfort. People with congestive heart failure (CHF) often do not tolerate CPAP well. Alternatives to the standard CPAP are machines that have adjustable inspiratory and expiratory pressures and machines that titrate pressures based on airflow and snoring (Tate & Tasota, 2002).

ORAL APPLIANCES. Various appliances are available that improve airflow during sleep by moving the tongue or mandible forward. Periodic adjustments of the appliance are necessary. Complaints associated with these appliances are excessive salivation and temporomandibular joint discomfort (Tate & Tasota, 2002).

SURGICAL INTERVENTION. Tracheotomy, once the only surgical option, is now reserved for selected patients for whom other treatments are not an option. More common procedures are laser-assisted uvulopalatopharyngoplasty (UPP), radiofrequency ablation, and maxillary and mandibular osteotomies and advancement (Tate & Tasota, 2002). The patient with mild OSA and snoring whose obstruction is confined to the oropharynx may respond well to UPP. However, a good outcome may require a series of surgeries. UPP is done under general anesthesia and is associated with considerable postoperative pain. Radiofrequency ablation reduces excess pharyngeal tissue by coagulating tissue in the upper airway. Like UPP, repeated treatments are required, but recovery is faster and less painful. Mandibular advancement, which inhibits pharyngeal airway obstruction, may be more appropriate than CPAP with CHF (Eskafi, Cline, Petersson, Israelsson, & Nilner, 2004).

DRUG THERAPY. Modafinil, a cerebral stimulant, may be prescribed as an adjunct to nasal CPAP to treat daytime sleepiness in individuals with OSA. It is reported to be effective and well tolerated, with the most common adverse effects being headache, anxiety, and nervousness (Dinges & Weaver, 2003; Schwartz, Hirshkowitz, Erman, & Schmidt-Nowara, 2003). However, it may be inappropriate for some older adults because cautious use is advised with hypertension, glaucoma, severe arteriosclerosis, and cardiovascular disease. Also, reduced renal or hepatic function warrants decreased dosage (Mosby, 2004).

Patients with OSA who are having surgery for other reasons may be at increased risk for postextubation airway obstruction, negative pressure pulmonary edema, and opioid-induced airway obstruction (Harrison, Childs, & Carson, 2003).

EDUCATION. Sleep disorders frequently are accompanied by insomnia; as a result, the older person may use hypnotics or alcohol to help induce sleep. Inform patients that alcohol has been found to increase the occurrence, duration, and severity of sleep apnea events and therefore should be avoided. Sedative and hypnotic drugs also have been implicated in these disorders. Benzodiazepines have less of an impact on respiration than barbiturates or other hypnotics, but they can cause or worsen sleep apnea.

NURSING CARE

Nursing Assessment

Health History. The health history for the respiratory system assesses symptoms of dysfunction or disease, and the impact of the symptoms on function. Because some of these symptoms can be related to more than one system, a complete health history is needed for a meaningful assessment. However, for simplicity of presentation, this section focuses only on the respiratory considerations.

The patient's general well-being is closely linked to respiratory status. Be particularly alert to complaints of severe fatigue with a recent onset because this often signals acute infection. Explore the reason for seeking care, which often is one or more of the following: dyspnea, cough, chest pain, sputum production, or hemoptysis. In addition to describing symptoms in detail, determine the presence of environmental factors that interfere with respiratory function, especially smoking. Also, assess the extent to which the person's usual lifestyle and activities of daily living are affected.

DYSPNEA. Dyspnea, or breathlessness, is one of the most frequent respiratory complaints in older patients. If the patient reports dyspnea, determine precipitating, aggravating, and relieving factors. The distance the person can walk on a flat surface, at a reasonable pace without stopping, is a good measure of breathlessness. Caird and Judge (1979) suggest a simple grading system, shown in Box 13-7. Nocturnal dyspnea and orthopnea usually, but not always, have a cardiac basis.

COUGH. When the patient complains of cough, clarify whether the cough occurs daily or is intermittent and whether it has lasted for months or years. How long do the periods of coughing last? When do they occur? What brings them on? Are they debilitating? Most important, do they produce sputum? The patient should also be asked whether phlegm is brought up from the chest, because many patients who deny cough will admit to producing phlegm, and it has the same clinical significance. The amount, color, and consistency of the sputum should be documented. Although it has long been thought that infection could be determined by color, this is no longer believed to be true. Remember that the diagnosis of chronic bronchitis is made primarily on the basis of the history of cough and sputum.

BOX 13-7 Grades of Dyspnea

- Shortness of breath hurrying on level or walking up hills or stairs
- Shortness of breath walking on level with people of same age
- Shortness of breath walking on level at own pace
- Shortness of breath on washing and dressing
- Shortness of breath while sitting quietly

From Caird, F. I., & Judge, T. G. (1979). *Assessment of the elderly patient.* Philadelphia: Lippincott, p. 34.

CHEST PAIN. Chest pain associated with the respiratory system in the older person may be pleuritic and may be seen in pneumonia, pulmonary embolism, rib fractures, costochondritis, and pulmonary hypertension, or it may be simply muscle pain after severe coughing. Complaints of pleuritic pain are not common in the elderly, even with severe pneumonia. The reason for this blunted pain sensation in the elderly is not clear. The pain of rib fractures, however, can be intense. Ask specific questions if there is a complaint of pain. What brings it on? What relieves it? Is it dull, sharp, stabbing, constant, or intermittent? Is it related to breathing cycles? How long has it been a problem?

WHEEZING. Another symptom that requires attention is wheezing. Many people with chronic bronchitis complain of wheezing, which may vary from week to week with infectious processes but does not vary much from day to day or hour to hour. It often is worse in winter. The wheezing of asthma, however, is more episodic, tends to vary from day to day; and frequently disturbs sleep.

REVIEW OF SYSTEMS. Inquire whether the patient has ever been diagnosed with a lung disease, including asthma, emphysema, chronic bronchitis, pneumonia, TB, lung cancer, or other less common conditions. It also is important to know if the older adult has any other chronic conditions because cardiovascular, endocrine, immune, renal, and hepatic disorders can affect pulmonary function and symptoms, as well as responses to treatment. The review of symptoms should include questions about recent or chronic oral problems, including infections and dental problems, because the oropharynx can be a reservoir for pathogens.

MEDICATION HISTORY. Document all drugs being taken regularly or as needed, including prescription and over-the-counter agents. This information may be relevant to the respiratory condition. For example, beta-adrenergic antagonists can trigger bronchoconstriction in individuals with a hyperreactive airway. Corticosteroids may be given to reduce airway inflammation, but they also reduce resistance to infection. Antidysrhythmics and other drugs that depress the myocardium can lead to heart failure and pulmonary edema. ACE inhibitors, commonly used as antihypertensive agents, can induce a chronic cough.

SELF-CARE BEHAVIORS. Inquire whether the patient has been given influenza and pneumococcal immunizations. Also, document the date of the last chest radiograph and tuberculin skin test.

RISK FACTORS. Inhaled pollutants, including tobacco smoke, are the most significant risk factors for respiratory disease. For smokers, quantify the smoking history in pack-years, a figure that is based on the number of years smoked and the average number of cigarette packs smoked each day. If the person has been smoking for 50 years and has averaged 1.5 packs a day, the person has a 75 pack-year history of smoking. Such a long history is not uncommon in older adults. If they do not smoke, ask if they live with someone who does.

Environmental conditions that could have an impact on respiratory function are living in a highly industrial area with air pollution, a history of working with asbestos in any form, and working as a miner. Note any previous occupation that involved prolonged exposure to dust, smoke, or fumes. Even farming is associated with the development of a variety of respiratory diseases. Ask whether the patient has any pets because they can exacerbate some respiratory diseases.

ACTIVITIES OF DAILY LIVING. Activity and respiratory status are closely intertwined. The person who is inactive is at risk for pulmonary complications, and activity can be affected profoundly by pulmonary disease. A description of a "usual day" provides clues as to risk factors, as well as the impact of pulmonary symptoms. Numerous tools are used to assess activity tolerance, a simple one being to measure how far the patient can walk in 6 minutes. The functional assessment, discussed in Chapter 2, is especially pertinent to the respiratory assessment.

Physical Examination. The pulmonary examination typically is presented in four phases: inspection, palpation, percussion, and auscultation.

INSPECTION (OBSERVATION). Although the oral examination is done with the head and neck assessment, it is relevant to the respiratory assessment because the oropharynx is known to be a reservoir for pathogens that may be aspirated into the lungs. If the patient wears dentures, they should be removed for examination of the oral tissues.

Skin color should be normal, but the thorax of the older person typically reveals some changes. Inspect the curvatures of the spine and the anterior-posterior diameter. Kyphosis is common, especially in women. This accentuation of the thoracic curve, caused by osteoporotic collapse of the spinal vertebrae, makes the person appear to be leaning forward. There also may be a widening of the anterior-posterior distance of the chest, giving a barrel-chest appearance. In the absence of other abnormal pulmonary findings, these may be considered normal findings with age. Patients with COPD may have hypertrophied neck muscles, and may be observed to sit in a "tripod" position: leaning forward with arms braced on knees, chair, or bed (Jarvis, 2004).

Observe the quality, rate, and rhythm of the respirations with the patient at rest. Opinions vary as to whether respiratory rate remains the same or tends to increase with age. Many factors probably account for individual differences. With inpatients and long-term care residents, respirations should be evaluated during sleep for abnormal patterns. Obstructed breathing is seen in patients with COPD and is characterized by a slow rate and increased volume, perhaps with wheezing also present. Gasping respiration consists of irregular, quick inspirations associated with an extension of the neck, followed by a long expiratory pause. This is characteristic of severe cerebral hypoxia and is common in patients with severe cardiac failure. Cheyne-Stokes respiration is a cyclic pattern of alternating apnea and hyperpnea. Though it sometimes is seen in healthy older persons, it is more common during sleep in patients with COPD, cardiac failure, or cerebrovascular insufficiency. Sleep apnea, which was described earlier, is fairly common in older adults and may cause oxygen desaturation, as well as sleep disturbance.

If the patient coughs during the examination, assess the strength of the cough reflex. A weak cough may signal a greater potential for serious trouble from a respiratory infection. If sputum is produced, note the amount, color, and consistency.

PALPATION. The trachea often is deviated in the older adult, but this may be due to scoliosis and so does not have the same significance as when it is found in a younger person. Also, because chest expansion is limited in the older person by calcification of costal cartilage, using a tape measure to try to determine it is ineffective. Rib fractures are common; therefore it is important to palpate for areas of point tenderness. A relatively minor blow can fracture a rib in the person with severe osteoporosis. In the patient with atelectasis or pneumonia, chest expansion may be unequal (Jarvis, 2004). Tactile fremitus is decreased with emphysema and may be increased with lobar pneumonia.

PERCUSSION. Percussion is similar in the young and the old, except that the lungs of the older patient may sound more resonant. Impairment of percussion—that is, dull or flat sounds—indicates consolidation or effusion. Hyperresonance is common in the patient with emphysema, although it may be muted if the patient is obese.

AUSCULTATION. The sounds heard over the normal lung are no different in younger and older adults. However, auscultation may be difficult because the patient may not be able to take deep and frequent breaths. If structural deformities such as kyphosis or barrel chest are present, the breath sounds may be distant in those areas. Crackles, also called rales and rhonchi, and wheezes are heard only if disease is present.

Assessment of the respiratory system is summarized in Box 13-8.

Nursing Diagnoses

Many North American Nursing Diagnosis Association (NANDA) nursing diagnoses apply to the older adult who has or is at risk for respiratory disorders. Examples include the following:

1. Activity intolerance related to compromised respiratory function, dyspnea, and fatigue

2. Airway clearance, ineffective, related to pain, tenacious tracheobronchial secretions, weak cough, bronchospasm, and increased pulmonary secretions

3. Breathing pattern, ineffective, related to increased pulmonary secretions, stiff chest wall, reduced physiological responses to decreased Po_2 and increased Pco_2, and shortness of breath with exercise (and obesity, if present)

4. Gas exchange, impaired, related to carbon dioxide retention, airway obstruction, and excess mucus production

5. Risk for respiratory infection related to decreased cough mechanism, impaired mucociliary escalator,

---

Box 13-8 **Respiratory Assessment**

Health History
- Past history of respiratory disease
  - Infection: frequency, severity
  - Chronic bronchitis, emphysema, COPD, asthma, pneumonia, other
  - Tuberculosis: known exposure, last skin test, results, treatment if any
- Allergies
- Habits
  - Use of tobacco: current or formerly
  - Cigarette pack-years (number of packs per day × number of years smoked)
  - Cessation attempts, strategies
  - Interest in smoking cessation
  - Use of alcohol
- Environment
  - Live in household with smoker
  - Occupational exposure to respiratory irritants
- Symptoms
  - Nasal discharge, frequent colds, epistaxis, change in sense of smell
  - Sinus pain, postnasal drip
  - Throat soreness, hoarseness, dysphagia
  - Cough
    - Duration, frequency
    - Precipitating events and alleviating measures
    - Phlegm, sputum, hemoptysis
    - Associated symptoms
  - Shortness of breath
    - Precipitating events and alleviating measures
    - Relationship to position or time of day/night
    - Severity, impact on daily life
  - Chest pain with breathing: location, characteristics
- Change in sense of taste
- Habits: tobacco, alcohol
- Self-care
  - Exercise: type, frequency, duration, tolerance
  - Nutrition: change in appetite, weight gain or loss

- Health screenings
- Immunizations: influenza, pneumococcal, tetanus
- Medical therapy
  - Drugs
  - Oxygen

Physical Examination
- Measurements
  - Peak expiratory flow rate if indicated
  - 6-minute walk distance
- General observations
  - Facial expression
  - Posture
  - Skin color
  - Respiratory distress
- Inspection
  - Nose
    - External nose: symmetry, lesions
    - Nares: inspect mucosa, septum, turbinates; test patency
  - Chest
    - Shape and symmetry of thorax; anteroposterior diameter
    - Spinal deformity: kyphosis, scoliosis
    - Respiratory effort
    - Use of accessory muscles
- Palpation
  - Nares: patency
  - Sinuses: pain
  - Chest
    - Lumps, tenderness
    - Fremitus
    - Symmetry of expansion
- Percussion over lung fields
  - Resonance
  - Diaphragmatic excursion
- Auscultation of breath sounds

diminished immune response, and less efficient alveolar macrophages

6. Sleep pattern, disturbed, related to sleep apnea, cough, orthopnea
7. Deficient knowledge related to lack of understanding about disease, prognosis, course, treatment, risk factors (smoking, environmental hazards), and complications
8. Anxiety related to breathlessness, fear of suffocation, and fear of recurrence
9. Communication, impaired verbal, related to dyspnea
10. Pain, acute or chronic, related to cough and pulmonary disease
11. Nutrition, imbalanced: less than body requirements, related to anorexia and dyspnea
12. Oral mucous membrane, impaired, related to mouth breathing and frequent expectoration
13. Powerlessness related to loss of control and the restrictions that the condition may place on lifestyle
14. Fluid volume, risk for deficient, related to increased insensible fluid loss secondary to fever and hyperventilation, inadequate oral intake

Nursing Goals

The goals of nursing care for the older adult with respiratory disorders might include (1) maintenance of a patent airway, (2) improved gas exchange, (3) effective breathing pattern, (4) improved activity tolerance, (5) reduced risk for infection, and (6) patient knowledge of self-care and health promotion. Additional goals must be formulated for individual patients with other related diagnoses such as pain or imbalanced nutrition.

Nursing Interventions

An array of nursing interventions to maintain or improve respiratory function in the older adult are available. The selection of specific interventions will depend on the individual's general health status, available resources, medical conditions, and prescribed therapies. This section addresses specific interventions for each of the goals stated previously.

Interventions to Maintain a Patent Airway.
Ineffective airway clearance is the "inability to clear secretions or obstructions from the respiratory tract to maintain a clear airway" (Johnson, Bulechek, Dochterman, Maas, & Moorhead, 2001, p. 48). Standard nursing measures include turning, coughing, and deep breathing to mobilize secretions for expectoration. Good hydration is believed to reduce viscosity of secretions so they can be more easily cleared. Remember that the older person adapts to changes in fluid volume more slowly, so increased fluid intake must be accompanied by monitoring for signs of fluid volume excess. The diminished effectiveness of the cough reflex in

some older adults poses a special challenge. Interestingly, a recent systematic review concluded that there was inadequate evidence to support or refute the use of chest physiotherapy (with chest percussion and postural drainage) in COPD and bronchiectasis (Jones & Rowe, 2004). Nevertheless, chest physiotherapy commonly is employed to enhance removal of secretions. Especially when the level of consciousness is decreased, suctioning may be necessary to clear the airway. The prevention of aspiration is relevant here, and includes proper feeding techniques and positioning after meals or tube feedings.

Positive expiratory pressure (PEP) therapy uses a device that requires the patient to exhale against a fixed-orifice resistor, thereby generating pressure during expiration. The patient is encouraged to perform 3 sets of 10 expirations. Several types of devices are available that assist in clearing mucus. One type of PEP system not only creates positive expiratory pressure, but also controls expiration so that it creates vibration to the airways (Schultz, 2001). Consult with the respiratory therapist about these options.

Interventions to Improve Gas Exchange.
Impaired gas exchange is "excess or deficit in oxygenation and/or carbon dioxide elimination at the alveolar capillary membrane" (Johnson et al., 2001, p. 139). The first requirement for improving gas exchange is to ensure a patent airway by measures discussed previously.

OXYGEN THERAPY. Oxygen therapy is indicated for many respiratory conditions and is available through various delivery systems that can be used in just about any setting. Compact portable devices have done much to improve the quality of life for persons who require continuous oxygen therapy. Some, but not all, COPD patients have "hypoxic drive," meaning low oxygen levels rather than elevated carbon dioxide is the stimulus for respirations. Raising the blood oxygen level too much in these patients can result in significant slowing of respirations. Therefore liter flow commonly is restricted to 2 L/min for COPD patients.

BREATHING EXERCISES. Breathing exercises are intended to increase the depth and strength of respirations. Incentive spirometry encourages full lung expansion and can be done by alert, oriented older persons. For surgical patients, having a baseline preoperative level helps provide a reasonable postoperative goal for the patient to achieve with spirometry. The target volume for incentive spirometry can initially be set at about a quarter to a third of the preoperative VC and gradually raised.

To study the effects of deep breathing on atelectasis and oxygenation after cardiac surgery, investigators compared the results of taking 30 deep breaths without a mechanical device, with a blow bottle device, and with an inspiratory resistance-positive expiratory pressure mask. All decreased atelectasis, increased the lung area aerated, and increased Pao_2 as measured by pre–spiral CT and post–spiral CT and arterial blood gas analyses. There were no differences among the three techniques (Westerdahl, Lindmark, Eriksson, Hedenstierna, & Tenling, 2003).

Breathing training techniques with feedback are intended to help patients learn to control their pattern of breathing during activities that can improve gas exchange and decrease dyspnea. It has been noted that techniques practiced in a resting state do not automatically transfer to an active state (Collins, Langbein, Fehr, & Maloney, 2001).

DRUG THERAPY. Patients with asthma or COPD may be receiving oral, parenteral, or inhaled drugs to prevent or treat acute episodes of bronchoconstriction. Because these drugs are prescribed for long-term use, patient education is critical to ensure proper use. The use of systemic corticosteroids usually is restricted to short-term courses of therapy, although some patients require longer treatments. Remind nursing staff and patients that these patients are at increased risk for infection. Patient teaching related to drug therapy is addressed later in this section.

AVOIDANCE OF IRRITANTS. Older patients who are motivated to stop smoking should be helped in their attempts to do so, either by behavior modification methods or smoking cessation programs. Nicotine replacement therapy should be offered because it has been shown to increase the likelihood of success. The older adult should not be eliminated from these programs simply because of age. Many people have quit after decades of smoking. When the patient is a nonsmoker who lives with a smoker, the smoker should be encouraged to stop smoking or at least to reduce the exposure of the patient to the smoke.

The environment should be modified, if necessary, to prevent exacerbations of existing lung diseases. Examples are the use of air conditioners and filters to remove pollutants, humidifiers or dehumidifiers (whichever is appropriate), and temperature control. Advise patients whose job or hobby brings them in contact with noxious substances to use appropriate protective measures such as respirators that filter inspired air.

POSTOPERATIVE CARE. Good nursing care is vital to prevent postoperative pulmonary complications in the elderly. A stir-up regimen that includes frequent turning, coughing, deep breathing, and incentive spirometry commonly is recommended. Pulse oximetry detects early or late hypoxemia so that treatment can be instituted. Because gas exchange is improved in the seated position, the patient should be up and ambulating as

soon as possible. Surprisingly, when breathing exercises were removed from the usual postoperative physiotherapy program, one study found that patient outcomes were no different between those who did breathing exercises and those who did not (Brasher, McClelland, Denehy, & Story, 2003).

Interventions for Ineffective Breathing Pattern. Ineffective breathing pattern is "inspiration and expiration that does not provide adequate ventilation" (Johnson et al., 2001, p. 65).

BREATHING EXERCISES. Over the years, various types of breathing exercises have been promoted as a means of improving breathing patterns or gas exchange. Basic deep breathing exercises continue to show up on care plans, blow bottles have been abandoned, and incentive spirometry is a mainstay of postoperative care. Numerous other strategies are available that commonly are thought to have pulmonary benefits. However, like many entrenched practices in nursing and medical care, research evidence of their effectiveness often is lacking.

Inspiratory muscle training (IMT) is intended to correct the muscle weakness associated with chest hyperinflation in COPD patients (Larson, Covey, & Corbridge, 2002). Muscle weakness is thought to be a central component of dyspnea in COPD (McConnell & Romer, 2004). A meta-analysis concluded that IMT significantly increases inspiratory muscle strength and endurance and decreases dyspnea at rest and during exercise for COPD patients. The benefits were greatest for individuals with inspiratory muscle weakness at baseline (Lotters, van Tol, Kwakkel, & Gosselink, 2002). In a double-blind study, Spanish investigators implemented a 6-month IMT program with COPD patients. Compared with a control group at the end of the study period, patients in the training group demonstrated increased walking capacity and improved health-related quality of life (Sanchez Riera et al., 2001). To determine the long-term benefits of IMT, 38 COPD patients completed a 12-week IMT program after which half received maintenance training for the next year while the other half had only low-intensity training. The initial training resulted in improved performance, exercise capacity, and sensation of dyspnea. However, at the end of the year, it was clear that benefits of IMT were retained over a 1-year period only when maintenance training was continued (Weiner, Magadle, Beckerman, Weiner, & Berar-Yanay, 2004). No additional benefit was found when expiratory muscle training was added to an IMT program (Weiner, Magadle, Beckerman, Weiner, & Berar-Yanay, 2003).

Diaphragmatic breathing (DB) has been reported to have both beneficial and detrimental effects in people with COPD. Cahalin, Braga, Matsuo, and Hernandez (2002) advise that the most appropriate patient for DB has an elevated respiratory rate, a low tidal volume that increases with DB, and abnormal arterial blood gases with adequate diaphragmatic movement. It should be terminated if a patient develops any abdominal paradoxical breathing pattern with worsening dyspnea and fatigue.

Pursed-lip breathing has been taught for years as a way to relieve dyspnea in COPD. Proposed explanations for its benefits are that it slows the respiratory rate and establishes a more controlled pattern, inhibits dynamic expiratory airway collapse, or shifts the inspiratory work of breathing from the diaphragm to the intercostal muscles. It is assumed to decrease hyperinflation with physical activity, but this effect has not been proven (Collins et al., 2001).

It has been suggested that patients with severe asthma, especially those who have been on corticosteroids, might have a similar weakness of inspiratory muscles that would benefit from IMT. However, a systematic review of the literature concluded that there is insufficient evidence of clinical benefit of IMT in asthma patients (Ram, Wellington, & Barnes, 2003). Likewise, Ritz and Roth (2003) cite lack of clinical evidence that abdominal breathing or pursed-lip breathing and nasal breathing have significant benefits. Another systematic review concluded that breathing retraining in asthma may be helpful, but that current research does not permit any firm conclusions to that effect (Ram, Holloway, & Jones, 2003).

COMPLEMENTARY AND ALTERNATIVE THERAPIES. Various complementary and alternative therapies are touted to improve breathing patterns or reduce symptoms of respiratory disorders. Among the practices that focus on breathing techniques are yoga, Qigong, and the Buteyko method. The Buteyko method claims to correct "overbreathing" by using breath control, breathing exercises, and education (Harris, n.d.). Qigong (pronounced *chee gung*) strives to improve health through regulation of body and mind (Lee et al., 2003). It integrates physical postures, breathing techniques, and focused intentions to reduce stress, build stamina, increase vitality, and enhance the immune system (National Qigong Association, USA, 2004).

A search reveals some research on the effects of these practices, but they have not yet established a body of evidence to support their usefulness in the treatment of asthma (al-Delaimy, Hay, Gain, Jones, & Crane, 2001; Cooper et al., 2003; Steurer-Stey, Russi, & Steurer, 2002). We must remember that management of chronic disorders should take a holistic approach. It may be that these practices do not alter the pathophysiological processes, but they may enhance coping, reduce stress, and improve general well-being. All of these are worthy outcomes. However, we need to caution patients against relying solely on unproven practices for symptom management.

A Chinese study compared the cardiorespiratory responses to exercise among older Tai Chi Chuan practitioners, Qigong participants, and normal sedentary controls. The investigators concluded that both Tai Chi and Qigong improved aerobic capacity, with Tai Chi having the greatest training effect (Lan, Chou, Chen, Lai, & Wong, 2004).

POSITIONING. Various strategies of positioning traditionally are recommended to increase ventilation and to normalize ventilation/perfusion matching. Positioning also can be helpful in promoting airway clearance, as in the use of postural drainage. Leaning forward in a sitting position commonly is used by patients with dyspnea and is thought to improve ventilation by permitting the abdominal organs to drop away from the diaphragm, resulting in better excursion and decreased accessory muscle use. Position change has been shown in laboratory studies to affect pulmonary perfusion. Clinical studies on postoperative patients show beneficial effects of position change, but specific clinical guidelines for older adults are not found.

A recent search of the literature yielded a number of studies related to positioning after cardiac surgery and in patients with adult respiratory distress syndrome (ARDS). However, little new work was found to confirm or refute our long-held beliefs about the benefits of turning and positioning in other situations. Nursing resources typically continue to recommend "turn, cough, and deep breathe at least every 2 hours." Periodic prone positioning of patients with ARDS has been the topic of many recent studies, but has not achieved full acceptance. There is general agreement that this position improves oxygenation and promotes drainage of secretions, but it is not clear whether it improves outcomes. Among the potential complications of prone positioning are facial edema, accidental extubation, increased intracranial pressure, and hemodynamic instability (Davies, 2002; Piedalue & Albert, 2003; Rowe, 2004). An Italian study placed 225 patients with acute lung injury or ARDS in the prone position for 6 hours daily over a 10-day period. Patients who responded to the prone position with decreased $PaCO_2$ showed an increased survival rate over those whose $PaCO_2$ did not improve (Gattinoni et al., 2003). Similar benefits were reported in a study of patients with witnessed pulmonary aspiration (Easby, Abraham, Bonner, & Graham, 2003). Another study determined that prone positioning and positive end-expiratory pressure had additive benefits on oxygenation (Gainnier et al., 2003). Even among acutely ill patients on mechanical ventilation, position changes have been shown to improve arterial oxygen pressure (Kim, Hwang, & Song, 2002).

The effects of body positioning on inspiratory and expiratory muscle strength have been demonstrated in studies that showed that the maximal negative inspiratory pressure and maximal positive expiratory pressure were highest in more erect positions than in recumbent positions (Badr, Elkins, & Ellis, 2002; Ogiwara & Miyachi, 2002). This has relevance for older adults whose baseline respiratory muscle strength commonly is diminished. Kinetic therapy uses a special bed to maintain continuous side-to-side turning as a measure to prevent atelectasis. One study used kinetic therapy with mechanical percussion in adult patients with respiratory failure and some degree of atelectasis. Compared with a control group that received manual positioning and manual percussion, the experimental group had significantly greater partial or complete resolution of atelectasis. Oxygenation improved also, but did not achieve significance (Raoof et al., 1999).

A review of clinical data related to the prevention of hospital-acquired and ventilator-associated pneumonia determined that semierect positioning (45 degrees) reduced the risk of aspiration of gastric contents, thereby reducing the risk of pneumonia (Kollef, 2004).

Interventions to Improve Activity Tolerance.

Activity intolerance is "a state in which an individual has insufficient physiological or psychological energy to endure or complete required or desired daily activities" (Johnson et al., 2001, p. 41). Nursing focuses on helping the patient who has chronic respiratory disease to develop a lifestyle that minimizes energy expenditure while allowing as much activity as possible. Teach the patient to be aware of breathing and not to hold the breath at intervals when shaving or putting on makeup, as most people do. Patients with COPD may be embarrassed by their obvious dyspnea and may avoid going out in public. Advise them to plan ahead when going out because rushing only increases dyspnea. Offer information about discussion groups of people with the same problem. Participation in these groups can help patients feel less alone and give them an opportunity to share coping strategies.

General physical conditioning exercises that improve muscle tone may be necessary because the patient may suffer from extreme breathlessness and disability. It is important to maintain activity at the highest possible level for the patient's psychological and physical benefit. Pulmonary rehabilitation is discussed in the section on COPD.

Interventions to Reduce the Risk for Infection.

Risk for infection is "a state in which an individual is at increased risk for being invaded by pathogenic organisms" (Johnson et al., 2001, p. 406). Older people who are at risk, particularly those with chronic respiratory disease, should be urged to have flu and pneumonia vaccinations. Colds and upper respiratory infections should be evaluated promptly so that treatment can be initiated. Early and aggressive treatment of respiratory infections is especially important for people with COPD. Remind the at-risk older adult to avoid crowds and people with infections, and to practice good hygiene. Advise patients to report fever, unusual fatigue, or an increase in the amount of sputum, which may indicate an infection. It is not unusual for an older adult to have only a slight temperature elevation with infection, so do not rule out infection on the basis of the temperature alone.

Interventions to Improve Patient Knowledge Base for Self-Care and Health Promotion.

Nursing interventions for pulmonary problems are focused on teaching and counseling related to risk factors, medication management, and keeping the airway as clear as possible. Nursing care includes finding ways to help patients adapt to this chronic illness and live their lives as fully as possible in spite of the disability. Helping patients and families find ways to lessen symptoms and cope with the disease can have a major impact on their lives. Some coping techniques that have been suggested for COPD patients are relaxation techniques, activity modification and energy conservation, social support, and contracting for goals.

Another major focus for nursing care is prevention of the exacerbation of symptoms. Adequate hydration is important for those with chronic bronchitis because mucus tends to be thick and difficult to expectorate. If modified postural drainage is required, a family member may be taught to help the patient with simple exercises over pillows in bed. When patients with chronic bronchitis require oxygen at home, instruct the patient and family in the safe use of oxygen. Be certain that they understand the correct liter flow and the potential suppression of breathing with higher flow rates. Abdominal breathing and pursed-lip breathing commonly are recommended with COPD, and many patients use these maneuvers automatically. As noted previously, the effects of these activities need more study. See Box 13-3 for additional interventions.

METERED-DOSE INHALERS. The ability to deliver medicines via inhalation rather than orally has been a tremendous advance, because it reduces the likelihood of systemic side effects from medicines designed to improve pulmonary function. However, correct use of metered-dose inhalers (MDIs) requires not only cognitive function, but also hand-eye coordination, use of the wrist and fingers, and the ability to control the breathing pattern. The major problem with the use of MDIs is improper inhalation technique. Patients must be taught carefully and reinforced at frequent intervals.

Table 13-8 *Interventions Commonly Used to Prevent and Treat Altered Respiratory Function*

Interventions	Intended Effect on Respiratory Function	Indicated for Treatment or Prevention of these Nursing Diagnoses
Deep breathing	Promotes alveolar expansion Enhances O_2-CO_2 exchange Assists in developing effective cough	Ineffective breathing patterns Impaired gas exchange Risk for infection Activity intolerance Acute pain
Encourage effective coughing	Clears respiratory passages of secretions Enhances O_2-CO_2 exchange Prevents bacterial proliferation	Ineffective airway clearance Activity intolerance Risk for infection
Adequate hydration 2000 ml/day unless on fluid restriction: evaluate for signs of fluid overload Frequent offering of fluids or room humidification may be necessary	Reduces viscosity of secretions Reduces energy expenditure required to clear secretions	Ineffective airway clearance Risk for infection Risk for inbalanced fluid volume Activity intolerance
Encourage and increase activity May have to begin with encouraging bed-to-chair rather than bedrest Systematically and regularly increase activity Consider formal exercise program as adjunct to ADLs	Improves respiratory rate and depth Improves tissue perfusion by increasing cardiac output Promotes alveolar expansion by increasing depth of respiration Promotes better positioning for coughing	Impaired physical mobility Activity intolerance Ineffective tissue perfusion Decreased cardiac output
Positioning Discover most comfortable positions for patient Develop routine for changing resting positions: sitting, side-lying, prone, supine, semi-Fowler's, etc. and teach rationale to patient and family	Frequent repositioning prevents pooling of secretions and thus enhances gas exchange and airway clearance, prevents infection Maintaining proper body alignment reduces the effort of breathing by not interfering with musculature involved in lung expansion Necessary for adequate lung perfusion	Impaired physical mobility Acute pain Impaired gas exchange Ineffective airway clearance
Adequate nutrition Consider small, frequent feedings so as to not compromise ventilatory effort and thus conserve energy Look for specific correctable nutritional deficiencies, e.g., iron, protein, vitamins, trace elements, calories	Needed for activity tolerance Malnutrition increases fatigue Severe anemia may precipitate CHF, which contributes to impaired gas exchange	Ineffective tissue perfusion Activity intolerance Imbalanced nutrition: less than body requirements Ineffective breathing patterns Impaired gas exchange
Prevent and identify pulmonary infections Control environmental toxins, e.g., cigarette smoke, paint fumes Monitor sputum production in those at high risk for infection for changes in color, consistency, amount, odor	Reduces environmental irritants Early identification simplifies treatment	Risk for infection
Suctioning	Stimulates cough Removes some secretions	Ineffective airway clearance
Monitoring of ABGs and vital signs	Assessment data about respiratory patterns, effectiveness of treatment	Impaired gas exchange Ineffective airway clearance
Percussion	Helps loosen secretions	Ineffective airway clearance

Continued

Table 13-8 *Interventions Commonly Used to Prevent and Treat Altered Respiratory Function—cont'd*

Interventions	Intended Effect on Respiratory Function	Indicated for Treatment or Prevention of these Nursing Diagnoses
Postural drainage	Helps drain secretions	Risk for infection
Pain medication	In postsurgical patients or those with pleurisy, enables coughing and deep breathing without severe pain	Ineffective airway clearance Impaired gas exchange related to atelectasis Ineffective breathing pattern Ineffective airway clearance Impaired gas exchange related to CHF
Oxygen	Increases oxygen supply to respiratory system	Impaired gas exchange
Intake and output	Helps monitor adequacy of hydration or overhydration	
Ambulation	Helps mobilize secretions Encourages increased rate and depth of respirations	Ineffective airway clearance Impaired gas exchange
Encouraging self-care	Increases mobility	Ineffective breathing pattern Ineffective airway clearance
Comfort measures	Reduces anxiety, which promotes more effective breathing patterns	Ineffective breathing pattern
Patient/family teaching	Re: work simplification and energy conservation reduce fatigue Re: positioning to facilitate air exchange reduces anxiety	Impaired gas exchange related to CHF Ineffective breathing pattern

According to Lilley and Aucker (2001), the proper technique is as follows:

1. Shake the MDI. Attach spacer if used.
2. Tilt head slightly back.
3. Breathe out slowly, but not forcibly.
4. Position the inhaler with the technique that is recommended.
   a. Hold the mouthpiece in the mouth.
   b. Hold the mouthpiece 1 to 2 inches from the mouth.
   c. If a spacer is used, hold the mouthpiece on the spacer in the mouth.
5. Begin to inhale slowly through the mouth and *then* activate the inhaler.
6. Breathe in slowly for 2 to 3 seconds.
7. Hold breath for at least 10 seconds.
8. If two puffs are ordered, wait at least 1 minute between puffs.

A large-volume spacer device is preferred by older patients and is easier to handle than the standard MDI. Some confused persons may be able to use breath-actuated devices more easily. When possible, the same type of device should be used for all inhaled medications.

Allen, Jain, Ragab, and Malik (2003) have studied the ability of dementia patients to use various types of inhalers. They found that frail older adults with abnormal Mini-Mental State Examination or EXIT25 test scores were unlikely to be able to use properly a metered-dose inhaler or Turbohaler. Of the two tests, the EXIT25, which assesses executive function, was the superior predictor. Thus it is important to teach the proper use of the equipment and have the patient regularly demonstrate the use of all prescribed inhalers. For patients who are unable to use inhalers, a nebulizer is an option.

Table 13-8 contains a list of nursing interventions that can be used with various nursing diagnoses.

Evaluation

Ongoing evaluation assesses the achievement of outcomes for the older adult. The outcomes of nursing management include a patent airway, gas blood measurements within desired parameters, effective breathing pattern, less dyspnea, increased activity tolerance,

Nursing Care Plan: The Older Adult with Pneumonia

Data

An 82-year-old man is accompanied to the emergency department by his son. The son reports that his father has had a cold for several days. This morning he did not want to get out of bed and drank only half a cup of coffee for breakfast. He told his son to call the office to report that he was sick, even though he has been retired for 6 years. The son observed that he had a noisy cough and seemed to be breathing faster than usual.

Assessment

A brief health history reveals declining health with medical diagnoses of congestive heart failure, hypertension, and arthritis in his knees. He reports having taken the "flu shot" this year, but does not know if he has been immunized for pneumonia. The physical examination findings include the following: use of accessory muscles of respiration, bronchial breath sounds and crackles on auscultation, increased fremitus, and dullness to percussion. His cough is weak and ineffective. The patient's skin and mucous membranes are dry. A voided urine specimen is dark amber. Vital signs are as follows: temperature, 100.8° F; pulse, 94 beats per minute, regular; respiratory rate, 26 breaths per minute, using accessory muscles of respiration; blood pressure, 116/66 mm Hg.

A chest radiograph confirms pneumonia. An infusion of intravenous fluid is started and empiric antibiotic therapy is ordered. Oxygen therapy is initiated. Because of his declining health and the fact that he is alone during the day, he is admitted to the hospital.

Nursing Diagnoses (Johnson, Bulechek, Dochterman, Maas, & Moorhead, 2001)

Airway clearance, ineffective, related to tenacious tracheobronchial secretions, weak cough, and increased pulmonary secretions

Breathing pattern, ineffective, related to increased pulmonary secretions, stiff chest wall, and reduced physiological responses to hypoxemia

Gas exchange, impaired, related to retained tenacious secretions and fluid in lungs

Goals/Outcomes

The patient's airway will be patent as evidenced by clear breath sounds.

The patient's breathing pattern will be effective as evidenced by normal breath sounds throughout lung fields, respiratory rate less than 20 breaths per minute, and measures of oxygenation within normal limits.

The patient will maintain adequate gas exchange as evidenced by measures of oxygenation within normal limits, resolution of confusion.

NOC Suggested Outcomes (Moorhead, Johnson, & Maas, 2004)

Respiratory Status: Airway Patency
Respiratory Status: Gas Exchange
Respiratory Status: Ventilation
Vital Signs Status

NIC Suggested Interventions (Dochterman & Bulechek, 2004)

Major interventions: Airway Management (3140), Respiratory Monitoring (3350), Vital Signs Monitoring (6680), Positioning (0840), Oxygen Therapy (3320), Cough Enhancement (3250), Acid-Base Management (1913), Electrolyte Management (2000), Laboratory Data Interpretation (7690)

- Monitor rate, rhythm, depth, and effort of respirations.
- Note chest movement, watching for symmetry, use of accessory muscles, and supraclavicular and intercostal muscle retractions.
- Monitor breathing patterns.
- Auscultate breath sounds, noting areas of decreased/absent ventilation and presence of adventitious sounds.
- Monitor for increased restlessness, anxiety, and air hunger.
- Monitor patient's ability to cough effectively.
- Monitor patient's respiratory secretions.
- Monitor chest x-ray reports.
- Monitor blood pressure, pulse, temperature, and respiratory status as appropriate.
- Monitor pulse oximetry.
- Position patient to maximize ventilation potential.
- Encourage slow, deep breathing; encourage coughing.
- Remove secretions by encouraging coughing or by suctioning.
- Instruct how to cough effectively (see NIC 3250 for details).
- Assist with incentive spirometer as appropriate.
- Administer humidified oxygen as appropriate.
- Institute respiratory therapy treatments as appropriate.
- Regulate fluid balance to optimize fluid balance.
- Position to alleviate dyspnea.
- Monitor respiratory and oxygenation status as appropriate.
- Obtain ordered specimen for laboratory analysis of acid-base balance as appropriate.

Nursing Care Plan: The Older Adult with Pneumonia—cont'd

- Monitor ABG levels for decreasing pH level as appropriate.
- Monitor determinants of tissue oxygen delivery (SaO_2) if available.
- Monitor for symptoms of respiratory failure.
- Monitor neurological status.
- Give fluids as appropriate.
- Maintain intravenous solution containing electrolytes as appropriate.
- Maintain accurate intake-and-output record.
- Promote orientation.
- Monitor for manifestations of electrolyte imbalance.
- Recognize physiological factors that can affect laboratory values, including gender, age, and diet.
- Monitor sequential test results for trends or gross changes.
- Report sudden changes in laboratory values to physician immediately.

- Administer supplemental oxygen as ordered.
- Monitor the oxygen flow rate.
- Monitor the effectiveness of oxygen therapy.
- Instruct patient about the importance of leaving the oxygen delivery device on.
- Change oxygen delivery device from mask to nasal prongs during meals as tolerated.
- Position to alleviate dyspnea as appropriate.
- Monitor oxygenation status before and after position change.
- Encourage the patient to get involved in positioning changes as appropriate.

Evaluation Parameters

Vital signs, measures of oxygenation, cognitive status, chest x-ray findings, ease of breathing, respiratory rate and rhythm, moves sputum out of airway, symmetrical chest expansion, depth of inspiration, and auscultated breath sounds (Moorhead, Johnson, & Maas, 2004).

measures taken to reduce the risk for infection, and patient demonstration of self-care and health promotion behaviors. Indicators of goal achievement for patients with musculoskeletal disorders include the following:

- The patient reports being (more) comfortable.
- The patient has no signs of hypoxia, such as alterations in thought process, tachypnea, tachycardia, or cyanosis.
- The patient's vital signs are within his or her usual parameters.
- The patient's arterial blood gas levels are within normal limits.
- No respiratory irritants are present in the patient's immediate environment.
- The patient follows a recommended pulmonary toilet regimen.
- The patient uses MDIs properly.
- The patient's breath sounds are clear on auscultation; no wheezing is heard.
- The patient maintains or improves the level of physical functioning.
- The patient is independent in activities of daily living.
- The patient engages in meaningful social activities.
- The patient's goals are met.

SUMMARY

Because the lungs are constantly exposed to the environment and lung diseases are common in older age, it is difficult to distinguish the effects of the environment and disease from normal aging changes. Changes that

occur with normal aging include reduction of alveolar surface area, loss of elastic recoil, decrease in vital capacity and oxygen saturation, decline in lung host defense, and reduction in exercise tolerance. Risk factors that further decrease lung function are smoking, obesity, immobility, and surgery. Respiratory conditions common in older adults are COPD, asthma, pneumonia, tuberculosis, cancer of the lung, and sleep apnea. Nursing interventions should focus on minimizing risk factors, managing medications, and keeping the airway as clear as possible.

REFERENCES

Aalbers, R., Backer, V., Kava, T. T., Omenaas, E. R., Sandstrom, T., Jorup, C., & Welte, T. (2004). Adjustable maintenance dosing with budesonide/formoterol compared with fixed-dose salmaterol/fluticasone in moderate to severe asthma. *Current Medical Research and Opinion, 20*(2), 225-240.

Abramson, M. J., Walters, J., & Walters, E. H. (2003). Adverse effects of beta-agonists: Are they clinically relevant? *American Journal of Respiratory Medicine, 2*(4), 287-297.

Ahn, H. C., & Lee, Y. C. (2003). The clearance of theophylline is increased during the initial period of tuberculosis treatment. *International Journal of Tuberculosis and Lung Disease, 7*(6), 587-591.

Alatas, F., Alatas, O., Metintas, M., Ozarslan, A., Ergnel, S., & Yildirim, H. (2004). Vascular endothelial growth factor levels in active pulmonary tuberculosis. *Chest, 125*(6), 2156-2159.

Al-Delaimy, W. K., Hay, S. M., Gain, K. R., Jones, D. T., & Crane, J. (2001). The effects of carbon dioxide on exercise-induced asthma: An unlikely explanation for the effects of Buteyko breathing training. *Medical Journal of Australia, 174*(2), 72-74.

Allen, S. C., Jain, M., Ragab, S., & Malik, N. (2003). Acquisition and short-term retention of inhaler techniques require intact executive function in elderly subjects. *Age and Ageing, 32*(3), 299-302.

Amara, C. E., Koval, J. J., Paterson, D. H., & Cunningham, D. A. (2001). Lung function in older humans: The contribution of body composition, physical activity, and smoking. *Annals of Human Biology, 28*(5), 522-536.

American Cancer Society. (2004). Cancer facts and figures. Retrieved July 15, 2004, from www.acs.org.

Ando, M., Mori, A., Esaki, H., Shiraki, T., Uemura, H., Okazawa, M., & Sakakibara, H. (2003). The effect of pulmonary rehabilitation in patients with post-tuberculosis lung disorder. *Chest, 123*(6), 1988-1995.

Antonelli-Incalzi, R., Imperiale, C., Bellia, V., Catalano, F., Scichilone, N., Pistelli, R., et al. (2003). Do GOLD stages of COPD severity really correspond to differences in health status? *European Respiratory Journal, 22*(3), 444-449.

Antonelli-Incalzi R., Marra, C., Salvigni, B. L., Petrone, A., Gemma, A., Selvaggio, D., & Mormile, F. (2004). Does cognitive dysfunction conform to a distinctive pattern in obstructive sleep apnea? *Journal of Sleep Research, 13*(1), 79-86.

Antonelli-Incalzi, R., Pistelli, R., Imperiale, C., Catalano, F., Scichilone, N., Bellia, V., & Sa, R. A. (2004). Effects of chronic airway disease on health status of geriatric patients. *Aging—Clinical and Experimental Research, 16*(1), 26-33.

Apostol, G. G., Jacobs, D. R., Jr., Tsai, A. W., Crow, R. S., Williams, O. D., Townsend, M. C., & Beckett, W. S. (2002). Early life factors contribute to the decrease in lung function between ages 18 and 40: The Coronary Artery Risk Development in Young Adults study. *American Journal of Respiratory and Critical Care Medicine, 166*(2), 166-172.

Augustynowicz-Kopec, E., Zwolska, Z., Jaworski, A., Kostrzewa, E., & Klatt, M. (2003). Drug resistant tuberculosis in Poland in 2000: Second national survey and comparison with the 1997 survey. *International Journal of Tuberculosis and Lung Disease, 7*(7), 645-651.

Ayers, D. M., & Lappin, J. S. (2004). Act fast when your patient has dyspnea. *Nursing2004, 34*(7), 36-42.

Badr, C., Elkins, M. R., & Ellis, E. R. (2002). The effect of body position on maximal expiratory pressure and flow. *Australian Journal of Physiotherapy, 48*(2), 95-102.

Bain, C., Feskanich, D., Speizer, F. E., Thun, M., Hertzmark, E., Rosner, B. A., & Colditz, G. A. (2004). Lung cancer rates in men and women with comparable histories of smoking. *Journal of the National Cancer Institute, 96*(11), 826-834.

Baine, W. B., Yu, W., & Summe, J. P. (2001). Epidemiologic trends in the hospitalization of elderly Medicare patients for pneumonia, 1991-1998. *American Journal of Public Health, 91*(7), 1121-1123.

Balducci, L. (2004). Believing is seeing. *Cancer, 100*(5), 881-882.

Balducci, L., & Carreca, I. (2003). Supportive care of the older cancer patient. *Critical Reviews in OncologyHematology, 48*(suppl), S65-S70.

Banov, C. H. (2004). The role of budesonide in adults and children with mild to moderate persistent asthma. *Journal of Asthma, 41*(1), 5-17.

Barthlen, G. M. (2002). Sleep disorders. *Geriatrics, 57*(11), 34-39.

Bass, P. R., 3rd, Wilson, J. F., & Griffith, C. H. (2004). The association of health-related quality of life and age of initiation of smoking. *Journal of the Kentucky Medical Association, 102*(3), 96-101.

Belvisi, M. G., & Hele, D. J. (2003). Soft steroids: A new approach to the treatment of inflammatory airways diseases. *Pulmonary Pharmacology and Therapeutics, 16*(6), 321-325.

Birim, O., Zuydendorp, H. M., Maat, A. P., Kappetein, A. P., Eijkemans, M. J., & Bogers, A. J. (2003). Lung resection for non–small cell lung cancer in patients older than 70: Mortality, morbidity, and late survival compared with the general population. *Annals of Thoracic Surgery, 76*(6), 1796-1801.

Boccagni, C., Tesser, F., Mittino, D., Terazzi, E., Naldi, P., Colombi, S., et al. (2004). Churg-Strauss syndrome associated with the leukotriene antagonist montelukast. *Neurological Sciences, 25*(1), 21-22.

Brasher, P. A., McClelland, K. H., Denehy, L., & Story, L. (2003). Does removal of deep breathing exercises from a physiotherapy program including preoperative education and early mobilization after cardiac surgery alter patient outcomes? *Australian Journal of Physiotherapy, 49*(3), 165-171.

British Thoracic Society. (1997). BTS guidelines for the management of chronic obstructive pulmonary disease. *Thorax, 52*(suppl 5), S1-S28. Cited in Connolly, M. J. (2000). Smoking cessation in old age: Closing the stable door? *Age and Ageing, 29*, 193-195.

Brooks, D. R., Palmer, J. R., Strom, B. L., & Rosenberg, L. (2003). Menthol cigarettes and risk of lung cancer. *American Journal of Epidemiology, 158*(7), 609-616.

Cahalin, L. P., Braga, M., Matsuo, Y., & Hernandez, E. D. (2002). Efficacy of diaphragmatic breathing in persons with chronic obstructive pulmonary disease: A review of the literature. *Journal of Cardiopulmonary Rehabilitation, 22*(1), 7-21.

Caird, F. I., & Judge, T. G. (1979). *Assessment of the elderly patient.* Philadelphia: Lippincott.

Campos, P. E., Suarez, P. G., Sanchez, J., Zavala, D., Arevalo, J., Ticona, E., et al. (2003). Multidrug resistant *Mycobacterium tuberculosis* in HIV-infected persons, Peru. *Emerging Infectious Diseases, 9*(12), 1571-1578.

Carman, W. F., Elder, A. G., Wallace, L. A., McAuley, K., Walker, A., Murray, G. D., et al. (2000). Effects of influenza vaccination of health-care workers on mortality of elderly people in long-term care: A randomized controlled trial. *Lancet 2000, 355*, 93-97. Cited in Kennie, D. C., Dinan, S., & Young, A. (2003). Health promotion and physical activity. In R. C. Tallis & H. M. Fillit (Eds.), *Brocklehurst's textbook of geriatric medicine and gerontology* (6th ed.). London: Churchill Livingstone.

Carriere, K. C., Jin, Y., Marrie, T. J., Predy, G., & Johnson, D. H. (2004). Outcomes and costs among seniors requiring hospitalization for community-acquired pneumonia in Alberta. *Journal of the American Geriatrics Society, 52*(1), 31-38.

Cataldo, J. K. (2003). Smoking and aging: Clinical implications part 1: Health consequence. *Journal of Gerontological Nursing, 29*(9), 15-20.

Centers for Disease Control and Prevention. (2003). New draft guideline for prevention of healthcare-associated pneumonia, 2003, issued 9/3/02. *Legal Eagle Eye Newsletter for the Nursing Profession, 10*(10), 6.

Centers for Disease Control and Prevention. (2004a). Cigarette smoking among adults—U.S., 2002. *MMWR, 53*, 427-431.

Centers for Disease Control and Prevention. (2004b). Publication of Surgeon General's report on smoking and health. *MMWR, 53*, 435-436.

Chan, E. D., Laurel, V., Strand, M. J., Chan, J. F., Huynh, M. L., Goble, M., & Iseman, M. D. (2004). Treatment and outcome analysis of 205 patients with multidrug-resistant tuberculosis. *American Journal of Respiratory and Critical Care Medicine, 169*(10), 1103-1109.

Cheng, A.C., Stephens, D. P., & Currie, B. J. (2004). Granulocyte colony stimulating factor as an adjunct to antibiotics in the treatment of pneumonia in adults. *Cochrane Database of Systematic Reviews (3)*, CD004400.

Chiou, H. L., Wu, M. F., Liaw, Y. C., Cheng, Y. W., Wong, R. H., Chen, C. Y. et al. (2003). The presence of human papillomavirus type 16/18 DNA in blood circulation may act as a risk marker for lung cancer in Taiwan. *Cancer, 97*(6), 1558-1563.

Cho, Y. J., & Lee, K. E. (2003). Decreased glucocorticoid binding affinity to glucocorticoid receptor is important in the poor response to steroid therapy of older-aged patients with severe bronchial asthma. *Allergy and Asthma Proceedings, 24*(5), 353-358.

Clark, J. P., & Langston, E. (2003). Ketolides: A new class of antibacterial agents for treatment of community acquired respiratory tract infections in a primary care setting. *Mayo Clinic Proceedings, 78*(9), 1113-1124.

Coleman, P. R. (2004). Pneumonia in the long term care setting: Etiology, management, and prevention. *Journal of Gerontological Nursing, 30*(4), 15-23.

Collins, E. G., Langbein, W. E., Fehr, L., & Maloney, C. (2001). Breathing pattern retraining and exercise in persons with chronic obstructive pulmonary disease. *AACN Clinical Issues, 12*(2), 202-209.

Condos, R., Hull, F. P., Schluger, N. W., Rom, W. N., & Smaldone, G. C. (2004). Regional deposition of aerosolized interferon-gamma in pulmonary tuberculosis. *Chest, 125*(6), 2146-2155.

Connolly, M. J. (2000). Smoking cessation in old age: Closing the stable door? *Age and Ageing, 29,* 193-195.

Connolly, M. J. (2003). Asthma and chronic obstructive pulmonary disease. In R. C. Tallis & H. M. Fillit (Eds.), *Brocklehurst's textbook of geriatric medicine and gerontology* (6th ed.). London: Churchill Livingstone.

Connolly, M. J., & Gosney, M. (2003). Nonobstructive lung disease and thoracic tumors. In R. C. Tallis & H. M. Fillit (Eds.), *Brocklehurst's textbook of geriatric medicine and gerontology* (6th ed.). London: Churchill Livingstone.

Cook, S., Maw, K. L., Munsiff, S. S., Fujiwara, P. I., & Frieden, T. R. (2003). Prevalence of tuberculin skin test positivity and conversion among healthcare workers in New York City, New York. *Infection Control and Hospital Epidemiology, 24*(11), 807-813.

Cooper, S., Oborne, J., Newton, S., Harrison, V., Thompson Coon, J., Lewis, S., & Tattersfield, A. (2003). Effect of two breathing exercises (Buteyko and pranayama) in asthma: A randomized controlled trial. *Thorax, 58*(8), 674-679.

Creticos, P., Knobil, K., Edwards, L. D., Rickard, K. A., & Dorinsky, P. (2002). Loss of response to treatment with leukotriene receptor antagonists but not inhaled corticosteroids in patients over 50 years of age. *Annals of Allergy, Asthma, and Immunology, 88*(4), 401-409.

Crimlisk, J. T. (2004). Lower respiratory problems. In S. M. Lewis, M. M. Heitkemper, & S. R. Ruff (Eds.), *Medical-surgical nursing: Assessment and management of clinical problems* (6th ed.). St. Louis: Mosby.

Davies, P. (2002). Guarding your patient against ARDS. *Nursing2002, 32*(3), 36-42.

Dent, M. (2004). Hospital-acquired pneumonia. *Nursing2004, 34*(2), 48-51.

Deutsch, M., Land, S. R., Begovic, M., Wieand, H. S., Wolmark, N., & Fisher, B. (2003). The incidence of lung carcinoma after surgery for breast carcinoma with and without postoperative radiotherapy. *Cancer, 98*(7), 1362-1368.

Dickson, S. J., Brent, A., Davidson, R. N., & Wall, R. (2003). Comparison of bronchoscopy and gastric washings in the investigation of smear-negative pulmonary tuberculosis. *Clinical Infectious Diseases, 37*(12), 1649-1653.

Dinges, D. F., & Weaver, T. E. (2003). Effects of modafinil on sustained attention performance and quality of life in OSA patients with residual sleepiness while being treated with nCPAP. *Sleep Medicine, 4*(5), 393-402.

Dochterman, J. M., & Bulechek, G. M. (Eds.). (2004). *Nursing interventions classification (NIC)* (4th ed.). St. Louis: Mosby.

Drazen, J. M. (2000). Asthma. In L. Goldman & J. C. Bennet (Eds.), *Cecil textbook of medicine* (21st ed.). Philadelphia: W. B. Saunders.

Easby, J., Abraham, B. K., Bonner, S. M., & Graham, S. (2003). Prone ventilation following witnessed pulmonary aspiration: The effect on oxygenation. *Intensive Care Medicine, 29*(12), 2303-2306.

Eaton, T., Lewis, C., Young, P., Kennedy, Y., Garrett, J. E., & Kolbe, J. (2004). Long-term oxygen therapy improves health-related quality of life. *Respiratory Medicine, 98*(4), 285-293.

Ebbert, J. O., Yang, P., Vachon, C. M., Vierkant, R. A., Cerhan, J. R., Folsom, A. R., et al. (2003). Lung cancer risk reduction after smoking cessation: Observations from a prospective cohort of women. *Journal of Clinical Oncology, 21*(5), 921-926.

Elci, O. C., Akpinar-Elci, M., Alavanja, M., & Dosemeci, M. (2004). Occupation and the risk of lung cancer by histological types and morphologic distribution: A case control study in Turkey. *Monaldi Archives for Chest Disease, 59*(3), 183-188.

Eskafi, M., Cline, C., Petersson, A., Israelsson, B., & Nilner, M. (2004). The effect of mandibular advancement device on pharyngeal airway dimension in patients with congestive heart failure treated for sleep apnea. *Swedish Dental Journal, 28*(1), 1-9.

Esteban, A., Frutos-Vivar, F., Ferguson, N. D., Arabi, Y., Apezteguia, C., Gonzalez, M., et al. (2004). Noninvasive positive-pressure ventilation for respiratory failure after extubation. *New England Journal of Medicine, 350*(24), 2452-2460.

Ferrari, M., Vangelista, A., Vedova, E., Falso, M., Segattini, C., Brotto, E., et al. (2004). Minimally supervised home rehabilitation improves exercise capacity and health status in patients with COPD. *American Journal of Physical Medicine and Rehabilitation, 83*(5), 337-343.

Ferrer, M., Esquinas, A., Arancibia, F., Bauer, T. T., Gonzalez, G., Carrillo, A., et al. (2003). Noninvasive ventilation during persistent weaning failure: A randomized controlled trial. *American Journal of Respiratory and Critical Care Medicine, 168*(1), 70-76.

File, T. M., Jr., & Tan, J. S. (2003). International guidelines for the treatment of community acquired pneumonia in adults: The role of macrolides. *Drugs, 63*(2), 181-205.

Flodin, U., & Jonsson, P. (2004). Non-sensitising air pollution at workplaces and adult onset asthma. *International Archives of Occupational and Environmental Health, 77*(1), 17-22.

Ford, M. B., Sigurdson, A. J., Petrulis, E. S., Ng, C. S., Kemp, B., Cooksey, C., et al. (2003). Effects of smoking and radiotherapy on lung carcinoma in breast carcinoma survivors. *Cancer, 98*(7), 1457-1464.

Fortes, C., Forastiere, F., Farchi, S., Mallone, S., Trequattrinni, T., Anatra, F., et al. (2003). The protective effect of the Mediterranean diet on lung cancer. *Nutrition and Cancer, 46*(1), 30-37.

Freixinet, J. G., Rivas, J. J., Rodriguez DeCastro, F., Caminero, J. A., Rodriguez, R., Serra, M., et al. (2002). Role of surgery in pulmonary tuberculosis. *Medical Science Monitor, 8*(12), CR782-CR786.

Gainnier, M., Michelet, P., Thirion, X., Arnal, J. M., Sainty, J. M., & Papazian, L. (2003). Prone position and positive end-expiratory pressure in acute respiratory distress syndrome. *Critical Care Medicine, 31*(12), 2719-2726.

Gajalakshmi, V., Peto, R., Kanaka, T. S., & Jha, P. (2003). Smoking and mortality from tuberculosis and other diseases in India: Retrospective study of 43,000 adult male deaths and 35,000 controls. *Lancet, 362*(9383), 507-515.

Gattinoni, L., Vagginelli, F., Carlesso, E., Taccone, P., Conte, V., Chiumello, D., et al. (2003). Decrease in $PaCO_2$ with prone position is predictive of improved outcome in acute respiratory distress syndrome. *Critical Care Medicine, 31*(12), 2727-2733.

Gilberg, K., Laouri, M., Wade, S., & Isonaka, S. (2003). Analysis of medication use patterns: Apparent overuse of antibiotics and underuse of prescription drugs for asthma, depression, and CHF. *Journal of Managed Care Pharmacy, 9*(3), 232-237.

Girou, E., Brun-Buisson, C., Taille, D., Lemaire, F., & Brochard, L. (2003). Secular trends in nosocomial infections and mortality associated with noninvasive ventilation in patients with exacerbations of COPD and pulmonary edema. *JAMA, 290*(22), 2985-2991.

Gosling, R. D., Uiso, L. O., Sam, N. E., Bongard, E., Kanduma, E. G., Nyindo, M., et al. (2003). The bactericidal activity of moxifloxacin in patients with pulmonary tuberculosis. *American Journal of Respiratory and Critical Care Medicne, 168*(11), 1342-1345.

Grap, M. J., Munro, C. L., Elswick, R. K., Jr., Sessler, C. N., & Ward, K. R. (2004). Duration of action of a single, early oral application of chlorhexidine on oral microbial flora in mechanically ventilated patients: A pilot study. *Heart and Lung, 33*(2), 83-91.

Gravenstein, S., Fillit, H. M., & Ershler, W. B. (2003). Clinical immunology in aging. In R. C. Tallis & H. M. Fillit (Eds.), *Brocklehurst's textbook of geriatric medicine and gerontology* (6th ed.). London: Churchill Livingstone.

Griffiths, C., Foster, G., Barnes, N., Eldridge, S., Tate, H., Begum, S., et al. (2004). Specialist nurse intervention to reduce unscheduled asthma care in a deprived multiethnic area: The east London randomized controlled trial for high risk asthma. *BMJ, 328*(7432), 144.

Gwynn, R. C. (2004). Risk factors for asthma in U.S. adults: Results from the 2000 Behavioral Risk Factor Surveillance System. *Journal of Asthma, 41*(1), 91-98.

Gyorik, S. A., & Brutsche, M. H. (2004). Complementary and alternative medicine for bronchial asthma: Is there new evidence? *Current Opinion in Pulmonary Medicine, 10*(1), 37-43.

Halpin, D. (2004). NICE guidelines for COPD [editorial]. *Thorax, 59*(3), 181-182.

Hara, T., Kosaka, N., Suzuki, T., Kudo, K., & Niino, H. (2003). Uptake rates of 18F-fluorodeoxyglucose and 11C-choline in lung cancer and pulmonary tuberculosis: A positron emission tomography study. *Chest, 124*(3), 893-901.

Harris, J. (n.d.). What is the Buteyko method? Retrieved August 14, 2004, from www.pnc.com.au/~breatheasy/butmeth.htm.

Harrison, M. M., Childs, A., & Carson, P. E. (2003). Incidence of undiagnosed sleep apnea in patients scheduled for elective total joint arthroplasty. *Journal of Arthroplasty, 18*(8), 1044-1047.

Hatcher, J., & Dover, D. C. (2003). Trends in histopathology of lung cancer in Alberta. *Canadian Journal of Public Health, 94*(4), 292-296.

Heijdra, Y. F., Pinto-Plata, V. M., Kenney, L. A., Rassulo, J., & Celli, B. R. (2002). Cough and phlegm are important predictors of health status in smokers without COPD. *Chest, 121*(5), 1427-1433.

Heuther, S. E., & McCance, K. L. (2000). *Understanding pathophysiology* (2nd ed.). St. Louis: Mosby.

Horsburgh, C. R., Jr. (2004). Priorities for the treatment of latent tuberculosis infection in the United States. *New England Journal of Medicine, 350*(20), 2060-2067.

Houston, S., Hougland, P., Anderson, J. J., LaRocco, M., Kennedy, V., & Gentry, L. O. (2002). Effectiveness of 0.12% chlorhexidine gluconate oral rinse in reducing prevalence of nosocomial pneumonia in patients undergoing heart surgery. *American Journal of Critical Care, 11*(6), 567-570.

Janssen-Heijnen, M. L., & Coebergh, J. W. (2003). The changing epidemiology of lung cancer in Europe. *Lung Cancer, 41*(3), 245-258.

Jarvis, C. (2004). *Physical examination and health assessment* (4th ed.). Philadelphia: W. B. Saunders.

Jin, Y., Carriere, K. C., Predy, G., Johnson, D. H., & Marrie, T. J. (2003). The association between influenza immunization coverage rates and hospitalization for community-acquired pneumonia in Alberta. *Canadian Journal of Public Health, 94*(5), 341-345.

Johanson, W. G., Jr. (2000). Overview of pneumonia. In L. Goldman & J. C. Bennet (Eds.), *Cecil textbook of medicine* (21st ed.). Philadelphia: W. B. Saunders.

Johnson, M., Bulechek, G., Dochterman, J. M., Maas, M., & Moorhead, S. (2001). *Nursing diagnoses, outcomes, and interventions.* St. Louis: Mosby.

Jones, A. P., & Rowe, B. H. (2004). Bronchopulmonary hygiene physical therapy for chronic obstructive pulmonary disease and bronchiectasis. *Cochrane Database of Systematic Reviews, 2,* CD000045.

Kannisto, S., Laatikainen, A., Taivainen, A., Savolainen, K., Tukainen, A., & Voutilainen, R. (2004). Serum dehydroepiandrosterone sulfate concentration as an indicator of adrenocortical suppression during inhaled steroid therapy in adult asthmatic patients. *European Journal of Endocrinology, 150*(5), 687-690.

Kaplan, V., & Angus, D. C. (2003). Community acquired pneumonia in the elderly. *Critical Care Clinics, 19*(4), 729-748.

Kaplan, V., Angus, D. C., Griffin, M. F., Clermont, G., Scott-Watson, R., & Linde-Zwirble, W. T. (2003). Hospitalized community acquired pneumonia in the elderly: Age and sex-related patterns of care and outcome in the United States. *American Journal of Respiratory and Critical Care Medicine, 165*(6), 766-772.

Kardas, P., & Ratajczyk-Pakalska, E. (2003). Reasons for elderly patient hospitalization in departments of internal medicine in Lodz. *Aging—Clinical and Experimental Research, 15*(1), 25-31.

Kennie, D. C., Dinan, S., & Young, A. (2003). Health promotion and physical activity. In R. C. Tallis & H. M. Fillit (Eds.), *Brocklehurst's textbook of geriatric medicine and gerontology* (6th ed.). London: Churchill Livingstone.

Kim, M. J., Hwang, H. J., & Song, H. H. (2002). A randomized trial on the effects of body positions on lung function with acute respiratory

failure patients. *International Journal of Nursing Studies, 39*(5), 549-555.

Kollef, M. H. (2004). Prevention of hospital-associated pneumonia and ventilator-associated pneumonia. *Critical Care Medicine, 32*(6), 1396-1405.

Kreamer, J. M. (2003). Getting the lowdown on lung cancer. *Nursing 2003, 33*(11), 36-43.

Krommydas, G. C., Gourgoulianis, K. I., Angelopoulos, N. V., Kotrotsiou, E., Raftopoulos, V., & Molyvday, P. A. (2004). Depression and pulmonary function in outpatients with asthma. *Respiratory Medicine, 98*(3), 220-224.

Laheij, R. J., Van Ijzendoorn, M. C., Janssen, M. J., & Jansen, J. B. (2003). Gastric acid suppression therapy and community acquired respiratory infections. *Alimentary Pharmacology and Therapeutics, 18*(8), 847-851.

Lan, C., Chou, S. W., Chen, S. Y., Lai, J. S., & Wong, M. K. (2004). The aerobic capacity and ventilatory efficiency during exercise of Qigong and Tai Chi Chuan practitioners. *American Journal of Chinese Medicine, 32*(1), 141-150.

Larson, J. L., Covey, M. K., & Corbridge, S. (2002). Inspiratory muscle strength in chronic obstructive pulmonary disease. *AACN Clinical Issues, 13*(2), 320-332.

Larsson, L. G., Lindberg, A., Franklin, K. A., & Lundback, B. (2003). Gender differences in symptoms related to sleep apnea in a general population and in relation to referral to sleep clinic. *Chest, 124*(1), 204-211.

Lee, A. M., Mennone, J. Z., Jones, R. C., & Paul, W. S. (2002). Risk factors of hepatotoxicity associated with rifampin and pyrazinamide for the treatment of latent tuberculosis infections: Experience from three public health tuberculosis clinics. *International Journal of Tuberculosis and Lung Disease, 6*(11), 995-1000.

Lee, M. S., Hong, S. S., Lim, H. J., Kim, H. J., Woo, W. H., & Moon, S. R. (2003). Retrospective survey on therapeutic efficacy of Qigong in Korea. *American Journal of Chinese Medicine, 31*(5), 809-815.

Lee, P. N., & Forey, B. A. (2003). Why are lung cancer rate trends so different in the United States and United Kingdom? *Inhalation Toxicology, 15*(9), 909-949.

Lehne, R. A. (2004). *Pharmacology for nursing care* (5th ed.). Philadelphia: W. B. Saunders.

Leigh, R., MacQueen, G., Tougas, G., Hargreave, F. E., & Bienenstock, J. (2003). Change in forced expiratory volume in one second after sham bronchoconstrictor in suggestible but not suggestion-resistant asthmatic subjects: A pilot study. *Psychosomatic Medicine, 65*(5), 791-795.

Leone, F. T., Fish, J. E., Szefler, S. J., & West, S. L. (2003). Systematic review of the evidence regarding potential complications of inhaled corticosteroid use in asthma: Collaboration of American College of Chest Physicians, American Academy of Allergy, Asthma, and Immunology, and American College of Allergy, Asthma, and Immunology. *Chest, 124*(6), 2329-2340.

Li, F., Sone, S., Abe, H., MacMahon, H., & Doi, K. (2003). Low-dose computer tomography screening for lung cancer in a general population: Characteristics of cancer in non-smokers versus smokers. *Academic Radiology, 10*(9), 1013-1020.

Liberati, A., D'Amico, R., Pifferi Torri, V., Brazzi, L., & Tinazzi, A. (2004). Antibiotic prophylaxis to reduce respiratory tract infections and mortality in adults receiving intensive care. *Cochrane Database of Systematic Reviews, 1,* CD000022.

Lidman, C., Burman, L. G., Lagergren, A., & Ortqvist, A. (2002). Limited value of routine microbiological diagnostics in patients hospitalized for community acquired pneumonia. *Scandinavian Journal of Infectious Diseases, 34*(12), 873-879.

Lilenbaum, R. (2003). Management of advanced non–small-cell cancer in elderly populations. *Clinical Lung Cancer, 5*(3), 169-173.

Lilley, L. L., & Aucker, R. S. (2001). *Pharmacology and the nursing process* (3rd ed.). St. Louis: Mosby.

Lim, T. K., Zhu, D., Gough, A., Lee, K. H., & Kumarasinghe, G. (2002). What is the optimal approach for using a direct amplification test in the routine diagnosis of pulmonary tuberculosis? A preliminary assessment. *Respirology, 7*(4), 351-357.

Lin, J., Sattar, A. N., & Puckree, T. (2004). An alarming rate of drug-resistant tuberculosis at Ngwelezane Hospital in northern KwaZulu Natal, South Africa. *International Journal of Tuberculosis and Lung Disease, 8*(5), 568-573.

Lipson, D. A. (2004). Redefining treatment in COPD: New directions in bronchodilator therapy. *Treatments in Respiratory Medicine, 3*(2), 89-95.

Loeb, M. B. (2003). Community-acquired pneumonia in older people: The need for a broader perspective. *Journal of the American Geriatrics Society, 51*(4), 539-543.

Lotters, F., van Tol, B., Kwakkel, G., & Gosselink, R. (2002). Effects of controlled inspiratory muscle training in patients with COPD: A meta-analysis. *European Respiratory Journal, 20*(3), 570-576.

Lucy, S. D., Kowalchuk, J. M., Hughson, R. L., Paterson, D. H., & Cunningham, D. A. (2003). Blunted cardiac autonomic responsiveness to hypoxemic stress in healthy older adults. *Canadian Journal of Applied Physiology, 28*(4), 518-535.

Ludbrook, J. J., Truong, P. T., MacNeil, M. V., Lesperance, M., Webber, A., Joe, H., et al. (2003). Do age and comorbidity impact treatment allocation and outcomes in limited stage small-cell lung cancer? A community-based population analysis. *International Journal of Radiation Oncology, Biology, Physics, 55*(5), 1321-1330.

Luder, E., Ehrlich, R. I., Lou, W. Y., Melnik, T. A., & Kattan, M. (2004). Body mass index and the risk of asthma in adults. *Respiratory Medicine, 98*(1), 29-37.

Lyman, G. H., Kuderer, N., Agboola, O., & Balducci, L. (2003). Evidence-based use of colony stimulating factors in elderly cancer patients. *Cancer Control, 10*(6), 487-499.

Maa, S. H., Sun, M. F., Hsu, K. H., Hung, T. J., Chen, H. C., Yu, C. T., et al. (2003). Effect of acupuncture or acupressure on quality of life of patients with chronic obstructive asthma: A pilot study. *Journal of Alternative and Complementary Medicine, 9*(5), 659-670.

Man, W. D., Mustfa, N., Nikoletou, D., Kaul, S., Hart, N., Rafferty, G. F., et al. (2004). Effect of salmeterol on respiratory muscle activity during exercise in poorly reversible COPD. *Thorax, 59*(6), 455-457.

Mannino, D. M., Homa, D. M., Akinbami, L. J., Ford, E. S., & Redd, S. C. (2002). Chronic obstructive pulmonary disease surveillance—United States, 1971-2000. *Respiratory Care, 47*(10), 1148-1149.

Mao, Y., Pan, S., Wen, S. W., & Johnson, K. C. (2003). Physical activity and risk of lung cancer in Canada. *American Journal of Epidemiology, 158*(6), 564-575.

Marrie, T. J. (2002). Topics in long term care. *Infection Control and Hospital Epidemiology, 23*(3), 159-164.

Marrie, T. J., Low, D. E., & De Carolis, E. (2003). A comparison of bacteremic pneumococcal pneumonia with nonbacteremic community-acquired pneumonia of any etiology—results from a Canadian multicentre study. *Canadian Respiratory Journal, 10*(7), 368-374.

Matsushima, T., Miyashita, N., & File, T. M., Jr. (2002). Etiology and management of community acquired pneumonia in Asia. *Current Opinion in Infectious Diseases, 15*(2), 157-162.

McCarty, J. M. (2000). Clarithromycin in the management of community acquired pneumonia. *Clinical Therapeutics, 22*(3), 281-294.

McConnell, A. K., & Romer, L. M. (2004). Dyspnoea in health and obstructive pulmonary disease: The role of respiratory muscle function and training. *Sports Medicine, 34*(2), 117-132.

McNeill, L., Allen, M., Estrada, C., & Cook, P. (2003). Pyrazinamide and rifampin vs isoniazid for the treatment of latent tuberculosis: Improved completion rates but more hepatotoxicity. *Chest, 123*(1), 102-106.

McWilliams, T., Wells, A. U., Harrison, A. C., Lindstrom, S., Cameron, R. J., & Foskin, E. (2002). Induced sputum and bronchoscopy in the diagnosis of pulmonary tuberculosis. *Thorax, 57*(12), 1010-1014.

Mehta, R. M., & Neiderman, M. S. (2002). Nosocomial pneumonia. *Current Opinion in Infectious Diseases, 15*(4), 387-394.

Mehta, R. M., & Neiderman, M. S. (2003). Nosocomial pneumonia in the intensive care unit: Controversies and dilemmas. *Journal of Intensive Care Medicine, 18*(4), 175-188.

Mendes, E. S., Campos, M. A., Hurtado, A., & Wanner, A. (2004). Effect of montelukast and fluticasone propionate on airway mucosal blood flow in asthma. *American Journal of Respiratory and Critical Care Medicine, 169*(10), 1131-1134.

Michael, A. B., & Murphy, D. (2003). Montelukast-associated Churg-Strauss syndrome. *Age and Ageing, 32*(5), 551-552.

Miller, A. B., Altenburg, H. P., Bueno-de-Mesquita, B., Boshuizen, H. C., Agudo, A., Berrino, F., et al. (2004). Fruits and vegetables and lung cancer: Findings from the European Prospective Investigation into Cancer and Nutrition. *International Journal of Cancer, 108*(2), 269-276.

Mitsunobu, F., Ashida, K., Hosaki, Y., Tsugeno, H., Okamoto, M., Nishida, N., et al. (2004). Influence of long-term cigarette smoking on immunoglobulin E–mediated allergy, pulmonary function, and high-resolution computed tomography lung densitometry in elderly patients with asthma. *Clinical and Experimental Allergy, 34*(1), 59-64.

Moorhead, S., Johnson, M., & Maas, M. (Eds.). (2004). *Nursing outcomes classification (NOC)* (3rd ed.). St. Louis: Mosby.

Mortensen, E. M., Coley, C. M., Singer, D. E., Marrie, T. J., Obrosky, D. S., Kapoor, W. N., & Fine, M. J. (2002). Causes of death for patients with community acquired pneumonia: Results from the Pneumonia Patient Outcomes Research Team cohort study. *Archives of Internal Medicine, 162*(9), 1059-1064.

Mosby. (2004). *Mosby's drug consult.* St. Louis: Mosby.

Mylotte, J. M. (2002). Nursing home acquired pneumonia. *Clinical Infectious Diseases, 35*(10), 1205-1211.

Nakaji, S., Yoshioka, Y., Mashiko, T., Yamamoto, Y., Kojima, A., Baxter, G. D., et al. (2003). Explanation for the smoking paradox in Japan. *European Journal of Epidemiology, 18*(5), 381-383.

National Institutes of Health. (1995). *Sleep apnea: Is your patient at risk?* NIH Pub. No. 95-3803. Bethesda, MD: National Heart, Lung and Blood Institute.

National Institutes of Health. (1997). Expert panel report 2: Guidelines for the diagnosis and management of asthma. NIH Pub. No. 97-4051. Bethesda, MD: National Heart, Lung and Blood Institute.

National Institutes of Health. (2002). NAEPP expert panel report: Guidelines for the diagnosis and management of asthma—update on selected topics 2002. NIH Pub. No. 02-5075. Bethesda, MD: National Heart, Lung and Blood Institute.

National Qigong Association, USA. (2004). What is quigong? Retrieved August 14, 2004, from www.nqa.org/qigong.html.

Nguyen, A. M., Luke, C. G., & Roder, D. (2003). Time trends in lung cancer incidence by histology in south Australia: likely causes and public health implications. *Australian and New Zealand Journal of Public Health, 27*(6), 596-601.

Nguyen, D., Prouix, J. F., Westley, J., Thibert, L., Dery, S., & Behr, M. A. (2003). Tuberculosis in the Inuit community of Quebec, Canada. *American Journal of Respiratory and Critical Care Medicine, 168*(11), 1353-1357.

Nichol, K. L., Nordin, J., Mullooly, J., Lask, R., Fillbrandt, K., & Iwane, M. (2003). Influenza vaccination and reduction in hospitalizations for cardiac disease and stroke among the elderly. *New England Journal of Medicine, 348*(14), 1322-1332.

Niimi, A., , H., Amitani, R., Nakano, Y., Sakai, H., Takemura, M., et al. (2004). Effect of short-term treatment with inhaled corticosteroid on airway wall thickening in asthma. *American Journal of Medicine, 116*(11), 775-777.

Niimi, A., Matsumoto, H., Takemura, M., Ueda, T., Chin, K., & Mishima, M. (2003). Relationship of airway wall thickness to airway sensitivity and airway reactivity in asthma. *American Journal of Respiratory and Critical Care Medicine, 168*(8), 983-988.

Nowbar, S., Burkart, K. M., Gonzales, R., Fedorowicz, A., Gozansky, W. S., Gaudio, J. C., et al. (2004). Obesity-associated hypoventilation in hospitalized patients: Prevalence, effects, and outcome. *American Journal of Medicine, 116*(1), 1-7.

Nurse staffing: Fewer nurses = poor outcomes. *Nursing2004, 34*(7), 33-34.

Ogiwara, S., & Miyachi, T. (2002). Effect of posture on ventilatory muscle strength. *Journal of Physical Therapy Science, 14*(1), 1-5.

Ohkubo, T., Chapman, N., Neal, B., Woodward, M., Omae, T., & Chalmers, J. (2004). Effects of an angiotensin-converting enzyme inhibitor–based regimen on pneumonia risk. *American Journal of Respiratory and Critical Care Medicine, 169*(9), 1041-1045.

Pagana, K. D., & Pagana, T. J. (2003). *Mosby's diagnostic and laboratory test reference* (6th ed.). St. Louis: Mosby.

Pastorino,U., Bellomi, M., Landoni, C., De Fiori, E., Amaldi, P., Picchio, M., et al. (2003). Early lung cancer detection with spiral CT and positive emission tomography in heavy smokers: Two year study results. *Lancet, 362*(9384), 588-589.

Pauwels, R. A., Buist, S., Calverley , P. M. A., Jenkins, C. R., & Hurd, S. S. (2001). Global strategy for the diagnosis, management, and prevention of chronic obstructive pulmonary disease. *American Journal of Respiratory and Critical Care Medicine, 163*, 1256-1276.

Pauwels, R. A., Sears, M. R., Campbell, M., Villasante, C., Huang, S., Lindh, A., et al. (2003). Formoterol as relief medication in asthma: A worldwide safety and effectiveness trial. *European Respiratory Journal, 22*(5), 787-794.

Pawar, M., Mehta, Y., Khurana, P., Chaudhary, A., Kulkarni, V., & Trehan, N. (2003). Ventilator-assisted pneumonia: Incidence, risk factors, outcome, and microbiology. *Journal of Cardiovascular and Vascular Anesthesia, 17*(1), 22-28.

Piedalue, F., & Albert, R. K. (2003). Prone positioning in acute respiratory distress syndrome. *Respiratory Care Clinics of North America, 9*(4), 495-509.

Pound, M. W., Drew, R. H., & Perfect, J. R. (2002). Recent advances in the epidemiology, prevention, diagnosis, and treatment of fungal pneumonia. *Current Opinion in Infectious Diseases, 15*(2), 183-194.

Prioux, J., Ramonatxo, M., Hayot, M., Mucci, P., & Prefaut, C. (2000). Effect of ageing on the ventilatory response and lactate kinetics during incremental exercise in man. *European Journal of Applied Physiology, 81*(1-2), 100-107.

Quy, H. T., Lan, N. T., Borgdorff, M. W., Grosset, J., Linh, P. D., Tung, L. B., et al. (2003). Drug resistance among failure and relapse cases of tuberculosis: Is the standard re-treatment regiment adequate? *International Journal of Tuberculosis and Lung Disease, 7*(7), 631-636.

Ram, F. S., Holloway, E. A., & Jones, P. W. (2003). Breathing retraining for asthma. *Respiratory Medicine, 97*(5), 501-507.

Ram, F. S., Picot, J., Lightowler, J., & Wedzicha, J. A. (2004). Non-invasive positive pressure ventilation for treatment of respiratory failure due to exacerbations of chronic obstructive pulmonary disease. *Cochrane Database of Systematic Reviews, 1.*

Ram, F. S., Wellington, S. R., & Barnes, N. C. (2003). Inspiratory muscle training for asthma. *Cochrane Database of Systematic Reviews, 4*, CD003792.

Raoof, S., Chowdhrey, N., Raoof, S., Feuerman, M., King, A., Sriraman, R., & Khan, F. A. (1999). Effect of combined kinetic therapy and percussion theapy of the resolution of atelectasis in critically ill patients. *Chest, 115*(6), 1658-1666.

Reichmuth, K. J., & Meyer, K. C. (2003). Management of community-acquired pneumonia in the elderly, part 2. *Annals of Long Term Care, 11*(10), 19-22.

Repetto, L., & Balducci, L. (2002). A case for geriatric oncology. *Lancet Oncology, 3*(5), 289-297.

Repetto, L., Carreca, I., Maraninchi, D., Aapro, M., Calabresi, P., & Balducci, L. (2003). Use of growth factors in the elderly patient with cancer: A report from the Second International Society for Geriatric Oncology (SIOG) 2001 meeting. *Critical Reviews in Oncology Hematology, 45*(2), 123-128.

Respini, D., Jacobsen, P. B., Thors, C., Tralongo, P., & Balducci, L. (2003). The prevalence and correlated of fatigue in older cancer patients. *Critical Reviews in OncologyHematology, 47*(3), 273-279.

Resta, O., Caratozzolo, G., Pannucciulli, N., Stefano, A., Giliberti, T., Carpagnano, G. E., & De Pergola, G. (2003). Gender, age, and menopause effects on the prevalence and the characteristics of obstructive sleep apnea in obesity. *European Journal of Clinical Investigation, 33*(12), 1084-1089.

Ritz, T., & Roth, W. T. (2003). Behavioral interventions in asthma. Breathing training. *Behavior Modification, 27*(5), 710-730.

Rivera, J. O., Hughes, H. W., & Stuart, A. G. (2004). Herbals and asthma: Usage patterns among a border population. *Annals of Pharmacotherapy, 38*(2), 220-225.

Rizvi, N., Shah, R. H., Inayat, N., & Hussain, N. (2003). Differences in clinical presentation of pulmonary tuberculosis in association with age. *Journal of the Pakistan Medical Association, 53*(8), 321-324.

Rodarte, J. R. (2000). Chronic bronchitis and emphysema. In L. Goldman & J. C. Bennet (Eds.), *Cecil textbook of medicine* (21st ed.). Philadelphia: W. B. Saunders.

Rodriguez-Reimann, D. I., Nicassio, P., Reimann, J. O., Gallegos, P. I., & Olmedo, E. L. (2004). Acculturation and health beliefs of Mexican Americans regarding tuberculosis prevention. *Journal of Immigrant Health, 6*(2), 51-62.

Rothan-Tondeur, M., Meaume, S., Girard, L., Weill-Engerer, S., Lancien, E., Abdelmalak, S., et al. (2003). Risk factors for nosocomial pneumonia in a geriatric hospital: A control-case one-center study. *Journal of the American Geriatrics Society, 51*(7), 997-1001.

Rowe, C. (2004). Development of clinical guidelines for prone positioning in critically ill adults. *Nursing in Critical Care, 9*(2), 50-57.

Ruano-Ravina, A., Figueiras, A., Barreiro-Carracedo, M. A., & Barros-Dios, J. (2003). Occupation and smoking as risk factors for lung cancer: A population-based case-control study. *American Journal of Industrial Medicine, 43*(2), 149-155.

Sanchez Riera, H., Montemayor Rubio, T., Ortega Ruiz, F., Cejudo Ramos, P., Del Castillo Otero, D., Elias Hernandez, T., et al. (2001). Inspiratory muscle training in patients with COPD: Effect on dyspnea, exercise performance, and quality of life. *Chest, 120*(3), 748-756.

Sanner, B. M., Kollhosser, P., Buechner, N., Zidek, W., & Tepel, M. (2004). Influence of treatment on leptin levels in patients with obstructive sleep apnea. *European Respiratory Journal, 23*(4), 601-604.

Santana, H., Zoico, E., Turcato, P., Bissoli, L., Olivieri, M., Bosello, O., & Zamboni, M. (2001). Relation between body composition, fat distribution, and lung function in elderly men. *American Journal of Clinical Nutrition, 73*(4), 827-831.

Schafer, H., Pauleit, D., Sudhop, T., Gouni-Berthold, I., Ewig, S., & Berthold, H. K. (2002). Body fat distribution, serum leptin, and cardiovascular risk factors in men with obstructive sleep apnea. *Chest, 122*(3), 829-839.

Schultz, T. R. (2001). Breathing easy. *Nursing Management, 32*(12), 73-76.

Schwab, R. J., Pasirstein, M., Pierson, R., Mackley, A., Hachadoorian, R., Arens, R., et al. (2003). Identification of upper airway anatomic risk factors for obstructive sleep apnea with volumetric magnetic resonance imaging. *American Journal of Respiratory and Critical Care Medicine, 168*(5), 522-530.

Schwartz, J. R., Hirshkowitz, M., Erman, M. K., & Schmidt-Nowara, W. (2003). Modafinil as adjunct therapy for daytime sleepiness in obstructive sleep apnea: A 12 week, open-label study. *Chest, 124*(6), 2192-2199.

Schwenk, A., Hodgson, L., Wright, A., Ward, L. C., Rayner, C. F., Grubnic, S., et al. (2004). Nutrient partitioning during treatment of tuberculosis: Gain in body fat mass but not in protein mass. *American Journal of Clinical Nutrition, 79*(6), 1006-1012.

Serebrovskaya, T. V., Karaban, I. N., Kolesnikova, E. E., Mishunina, T. M., Swanson, R. J., Beloshitsky, P. V., et al. (2000). Geriatric men at altitude: Hypoxic ventilatory sensitivity and blood dopamine changes. *Respiration, 67*(3), 253-260.

Seymour, D. G. (2003). Surgery and anesthesia in old age. In R. C. Tallis & H. M. Fillit (Eds.), *Brocklehurst's textbook of geriatric medicine and gerontology* (6th ed.). London: Churchill Livingstone.

Shea, R. A., Brooks, J. A., Dayhoff, N. E., & Keck, J. (2002). Pain intensity and postoperative pulmonary complications among the elderly after abdominal surgery. *Heart and Lung: Journal of Acute and Critical Care, 31*(6), 440-449.

Shrestha-Kuwahara, R., Wilce, M., DeLuca, N., & Taylor, Z. (2003). Factors associated with identifying tuberculosis contacts. *International Journal of Tuberculosis and Lung Disease, 7*(12 suppl 3), S510-S516.

Singer, M. E., Harding, I., Jacobs, M. R., & Jaffe, D. H. (2003). Impact of antimicrobial resistance on health outcomes in the outpatient treatment of adult community-acquired pneumonia: A probability model. *Journal of Antimicrobial Chemotherapy, 51*(5), 1269-1282.

Singh, K. K., Dong, Y., Hinds, L., Keen, M. A., Belisle, J. T., Zolla-Pazner, S., et al. (2003). Combined use of serum and urinary antibodies for diagnosis of tuberculosis. *Journal of Infectious Diseases, 188*(3), 371-377.

Sole, M. L., Byers, J. F., Ludy, J. E., Zhang, Y., Banta, C. M., & Brummel, K. (2003). A multisite survey of suctioning techniques and airway management practices. *American Journal of Critical Care, 12*(3), 220-230.

Steurer-Stey, C., Russi, E. W., & Steurer, J. (2002). Complementary and alternative medicine in asthma: Do they work? *Swiss Medical Weekly, 132*(25-26), 338-344.

Suissa, S. (2004). Inhaled steroids and mortality in COPD: Bias from unaccounted immortal time. *European Respiratory Journal, 23*(3), 391-395.

Suissa, S., Baltzan, M., Kremer, R., & Ernst, P. (2004). Inhaled and nasal corticosteroid use and the risk of fracture. *American Journal of Respiratory and Critical Care Medicine, 169*(1), 83-88.

Swensen, S. J., Jett, J. R., Hartman, T. E., Midthun, D. E., Sloan, J. A., Sykes, A. M., et al. (2003). Lung cancer screening with CT: Mayo Clinic experience. *Radiology, 226*(3), 756-761.

Tashkin, D. P., & Cooper, C. B. (2004). The role of long-acting bronchodilators in the management of stable COPD. *Chest, 125*(1), 9-11.

Tate, J., & Tasota, F. J. (2002). More than a snore: Recognizing the danger of sleep apnea. *Nursing2002, 32*(8), 46-49.

Treatment of tuberculosis. (2003). Retrieved July 23, 2004, from www.cdc.gov/mmwr/preview/mmwrhtml/rr5211al.htm.

Trowbridge, J. F., Artymowicz, R. J., Lee, C. E., Brown, P. D., Farber, M. S., Kernan, W., et al. (2002). Antimicrobial selection and length of hospital stay in patients with community acquired pneumonia. *Journal of Clinical Outcomes Management, 9*(11), 613-619.

Trupin, L., Earnest, G., San Pedro, M., Balmes, J. R., Eisner, M. D., Yelin, E., et al. (2003). The occupational burden of chronic obstructive pulmonary disease. *European Respiratory Journal, 22*(3), 462-469.

Tsoumakidou, M., Tzanakis, N., Voulgaraki, O., Mitrouska, I., Chrysofakis, G., Samiou, M., & Siafakas, N. M. (2004). Is there any correlation between the ATS, BTS, ERS and GOLD COPD's severity scales and the frequency of hospital admissions? *Respiratory Medicine, 98*(2), 178-183.

Tyczynski, J. E., Bray, F., Aareleid, T., Dalmas, M., Kurtinaitis, J., Plesko, I., et al. (2004). Lung cancer mortality patterns in selected central, eastern, and southern European countries. *International Journal of Cancer, 109*(4), 598-610.

Umlauf, M. G., Chasens, E. R., Greevy, R. A., Arnold, J., Burgio, K. L., & Pillion, D. J. (2004). Obstructive sleep apnea, nocturia and polyuria in older adults. *Sleep, 27*(1), 139-144.

Unruh, L. (2003). Licensed nurse staffing and adverse events in hospitals. *Medical Care, 41*(1), 142-152.

Valerio, G., Bracciale, P., Manisco, V., Quitadamo, M., Legari, G., & Bellanova, S. (2003). Long-term tolerance and effectiveness of

moxifloxacin therapy for tuberculosis: Preliminary results. *Journal of Chemotherapy, 15*(1), 66-70.

van Dyck, P., Vanhoenacker, F. M., Van den Brande, P., & De Schepper, A. M. (2003). Imaging of pulmonary tuberculosis. *European Radiology, 13*(8), 1771-1778.

van Meerbeeck, J. P., Damhuis, R. A., & Vos de Wael, M. L. (2002). High postoperative risk after pneumonectomy in elderly patients with right-sided lung cancer. *European Respiratory Journal, 19*(1), 141-145.

Vemuri, C., Wainess, R. M., Dimick, J. B., Cowan, J. A., Jr., Henke, P. K., Stanley, J. C., & Upchurch, G. R., Jr. (2004). Effect of increasing patient age on complication rates following intact abdominal aortic aneurysm repair in the United States. *Journal of Surgical Research, 118*(1), 26-31.

Voordouw, B. C., van der Linden, P. D., Simonian, S., van der Lei, J., Sturkenboom, M. C., & Stricker, B. H. (2003). Influenza vaccination in community-dwelling elderly: Impact on mortality and influenza-associated mortality. *Archives of Internal Medicine, 163*(9), 1089-1094.

Wagner, C., Popp, W., Posch, M., Vlasich, C., & Rosenberger-Spitzy, A. (2003). Impact of pneumococcal vaccination on morbidity and mortality of geriatric patients: A case controlled study. *Gerontology, 49*(4), 246-250.

Wang, Y. H., Lin, A. S., Lai, Y. F., Chao, T. Y., Liu, J. W., & Ko, S. F. (2003). The high value of high-resolution computed tomography in predicting the activity of pulmonary tuberculosis. *International Journal of Tuberculosis and Lung Disease, 7*(6), 563-568.

Weaver, E. M., Kapur, V., & Yueh, B. (2004). Polysomnography vs self reported measures in patients with sleep apnea. *Archives of Otolaryngology—Head and Neck Surgery, 130*(4), 453-458.

Wei, C. J., Tiu, C. M., Chen, J. D., Chou, Y. H., Chang, C. Y., & Yu, C. (2004). Computed tomography features of acute pulmonary tuberculosis. *American Journal of Emergency Medicine, 22*(3), 171-174.

Weiner, P., Magadle, R., Beckerman, M., Weiner, M., & Berar-Yanay, N. (2003). Comparison of specific expiratory, inspiratory, and combined muscle training programs in COPD. *Chest, 124*(4), 1357-1364.

Weiner, P., Magadle, R., Beckerman, M., Weiner, M., & Berar-Yanay, N. (2004). Maintenance of inspiratory muscle training in COPD patients: One year follow-up. *European Respiratory Journal, 23*(1), 61-65.

Weiss, K. B., Liljas, B., Schoenwetter, W., Schatz, M., & Luce, B. R. (2004). Effectiveness of budesonide administered via dry-powder inhaler versus triamcinolone acetonide administered via pressurized metered-dose inhaler for adults with persistent asthma in managed care settings. *Clinical Therapeutics, 26*(1), 102-114.

Wen Cheng, Y., & Lee, H. (2003). Environmental exposure and lung cancer among nonsmokers: An example of Taiwanese female lung cancer. *Journal of Environmental Science and Health, 21*(1), 1-28.

Westerdahl, E., Lindmark, B., Eriksson, T., Hedenstierna, G., & Tenling, A. (2003). The immediate effects of deep breathing exercises on atelectasis and oxygenation after cardiac surgery. *Scandinavian Cardiovascular Journal, 37*(6), 363-367.

Willemse, B. W., Postma, D. S., Timens, W., & ten Hacken, N. H. (2004). The impact of smoking cessation on respiratory symptoms, lung function, airway hyperresponsiveness and inflammation. *European Respiratory Journal, 23*(2), 464-476.

Wolk, R., Shamsuzzaman, A. S., & Somers, V. K. (2003). Obesity, sleep apnea, and hypertension. *Hypertension, 42*(6), 1067-1074.

Wong, C. M., Lim, K. H., & Liam, C. K. (2003). The causes of haemoptysis in Malaysian patients aged over 60 and the diagnostic yield of different investigations. *Respirology, 8*(1), 65-68.

Wong, M. W., Tsui, H. F., Yung, S. H., Chan, K. M., & Cheng, J. C. (2004). Continuous pulse oximeter monitoring for inapparent hypoxemia after long bone fractures. *Journal of Trauma—Injury Infection and Critical Care, 56*(2), 356-362.

Wright, M. E., Mayne, S. T., Swanson, C. A., Sinha, R., & Alavanja, M. C. (2003). Dietary carotenoids, vegetables, and lung cancer risk in women: The Missouri Women's Health Study. *Cancer Causes and Control, 14*(1), 85-96.

Yang, M. L., Chiang, C. H., Yao, G., & Wang, K. Y. (2003). Effect of medical education on quality of life in adult asthma patients. *Journal of the Formosan Medical Association, 102*(11), 768-774.

Yee, D., Valiquette, C., Pelletier, M., Parisien, I., Rocher, I., & Menzies, D. (2003). Incidence of serious side effects from the first-line anti-tuberculosis drugs among patients treated for active tuberculosis. *American Journal of Respiratory and Critical Care Medicine, 167*(11), 1472-1477.

Yohannes, A. M., & Hardy, C. C. (2003). Treatment of chronic obstructive pulmonary disease in older patients: A practical guide. *Drugs and Aging, 20*(3), 209-228.

Young, T., Peppard, P. E., & Gottlieb, D. J. (2002). Epidemiology of obstructive sleep apnea: A population health perspective. *American Journal of Respiratory and Critical Care Medicine, 165*(9), 1217-1239.

Young, T., Skatrud, J., & Peppard, P. E. (2004). Risk factors for obstructive sleep apnea in adults. *JAMA, 291*(29), 2013-2016.

Zeleznik, J. (2003). Normative aging of the respiratory system. *Clinics in Geriatric Medicine, 19*(1), 1-18.

Zhanel, G. G., Dueck, M., Hoban, D. J., Vercaigne, L. M., Embil, J. M., Gin, A. S., & Karlowsky, J. A. (2001). Review of macrolides and ketolides: Focus on respiratory tract infections. *Drugs, 61*(4), 443-498.

Zimmerman, R. K., Mieczkowski, T. A., & Wilson, S. A. (2002). Immunization rates and beliefs among elderly patients of inner city neighborhood health centers. *Health Promotion Practice, 3*(2), 197-206.

Chapter 14

Neurological System

Pamela Millsap

Objectives

Describe the normal age-related changes in the structure of the neurological system.

Discuss the normal age-related changes in the functional abilities of the neurological system, including cognition, reaction time, proprioception, thermoregulation, and sleep patterns.

Describe measures to maintain neurological health in the older adult.

Explain the cause and treatment of neurological disorders that are common in older persons.

Describe the components of the neurological assessment in the older adult.

Formulate nursing diagnoses for older adults with neurological disorders.

Develop management plans for older adults with actual or potential neurological problems.

The aging neurological system is a complex puzzle that challenges even the most experienced nurse. Many factors account for this complexity, including the vague and atypical presentation of disease in older adults, the interdependence on other body systems, the complications of preexisting comorbidities, and the effects of medications. The nurse who is grounded with a sound knowledge of the neurological system, normal aging changes, and disease processes common in the older adult will be ready to meet this challenge. A systematic and comprehensive assessment will enable the nurse and older adult to plan interventions that can have a dramatic impact on quality of life. "Successful aging," as defined by the individual, is an important goal.

ORGANIZATION OF THE NEUROLOGICAL SYSTEM

Only a brief review of the physiology of the nervous system is provided in this chapter; textbooks on the anatomy and physiology of the nervous system should be consulted for a comprehensive study of the organization of the nervous system. The major function of the nervous system is integrative, seamlessly selecting incoming sensory information and channeling it to cause appropriate motor responses. On the basis of anatomical features the nervous system is divided into two parts: the central nervous system (CNS), consisting of the brain and the spinal cord, and the peripheral nervous system (PNS), consisting of the cranial, spinal, and peripheral nerves. Although it is helpful to divide the nervous system by structure, functionally the anatomical circuits do not pay attention to the boundaries of the CNS and PNS. For example, motor neurons of the spinal nerves are considered to be part of the PNS, but their sensory neurons are within the CNS. The CNS and the PNS have both somatic (innervate and control movements and sensory organs) and autonomic (innervation of internal organs) functions. Communicating networks within the nervous system process incoming sensory information in order to direct appropriate conscious and unconscious responses.

Peripheral efferent nerve fibers distributed to smooth muscle, cardiac muscle, and glands are known as the autonomic nervous system (ANS). The ANS consists of the sympathetic and parasympathetic systems and is involved in regulation of behavioral and neuroendocrinological mechanisms of the body with responsibilities for maintaining a constant internal environment (temperature, fluid balance, and ionic composition of the blood). The parasympathetic system is concerned with body functions such as digestion, excretion, and intermediary metabolism. The sympathetic system is involved in the regulation of stress reactions.

The functional units of the nervous system, the neurons, receive, conduct, and transmit information via nerve impulses throughout the body. The glial cells provide a supportive structure for neurons and serve metabolic and phagocytic roles. Nerves vary greatly in size and shape specific to their function, but each has a cell body, an axon, dendrites, and synapses. The dendrites are the receiving processes of the neuron, and usually there are many. The axon conducts information away from the cell body. Usually a neuron has only one axon and it ends in small branches called axon terminals. These axon terminals make contact with other nerves or organs at the synapse, where the information is transmitted. Some axons are insulated with a lipoprotein sheath called the myelin sheath. Transmission of impulses at the synapse requires the intervention of chemical mediators, or neurotransmitters, and other cell-mediated signals. Examples of neurotransmitters include acetylcholine, dopamine, serotonin, and norepinephrine.

NORMAL CHANGES IN STRUCTURE AND FUNCTION
Structure

There is rapid change in the growing body of knowledge regarding the nervous system of older adults. Box 14-1 summarizes the commonly accepted changes in the structure of the nervous system of the older adult. Important factors to put in perspective when considering structural changes in the nervous system are the complex cellular and molecular changes occurring throughout all body systems and the interrelationships between the nervous system and changes caused by disease states (Duckett, 2002).

These structural changes in the nervous system result in the decreased ability to react quickly to stimuli, diminished nerve conduction velocity, and prolonged muscle action potentials. There is decreased efficiency of the automatic functions of the CNS. Body homeostasis becomes more difficult so that recovery from stress is prolonged and incomplete. Stressors such as heat, cold, and extreme exercise can be particularly harmful, even life-threatening.

Neuronal losses do not necessarily affect brain function, but they may have an influence on brain weight. Current studies do not support the notion of extensive generalized brain atrophy in normal aging. Recent studies of comparisons of brain weight and atrophy at postmortems found little difference between healthy older adults and their younger counterparts. Longitudinal studies of computed tomography (CT) and magnetic resonance imaging (MRI) brain scans have revealed atrophy primarily in only selected areas that begins in the fifth and sixth decades of life and progresses very slowly (Duckett, 2002).

Changes in Functional Abilities of the Neurological System

Cognition. It must be noted that changes in the brain composition, cells, and synapses associated with aging do not necessarily have an effect on thinking and cognition. Little correlation has been noted between cerebral atrophy and cognitive loss. Healthy older

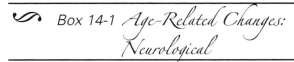

Box 14-1 *Age-Related Changes: Neurological*

- Mild, gradual decline in number of neurons and glial cells
- Structural changes of neurons and glial cells
- Decrease in overall number of synapses (may be compensated by increased synaptic size)
- Changes in the vessels that supply the nervous system caused by age-related atherosclerosis and arteriosclerosis
- Decreased lipids
- Increased accumulation of lipofuscin granules in nerve cells
- Reduced ability to cope with oxidative and metabolic stress
- Alterations of the cellular signaling pathways
- Increased production and accumulation of oxyradicals in all body systems
- Protein aggregation/accumulation (plaques) that are diffuse, nonfibrillar beta-amyloid not associated with neuronal degeneration
- Decreased muscle strength (decreased muscle mass)
- Decreased speed of muscle movement
- Decreased muscle endurance
- Changes in the muscular vasculature caused by age-related vessel changes

Data from Mattson, M. P. (2002). Molecular biology of the aging nervous system. In S. Duckett & J. C. da la Torre (Eds.), Pathology of the aging human nervous system (2nd ed.). New York: Oxford University Press; and Hawkins, C., & Shannon, P. (2002). Pathology of the skeletal muscle in aging. In S. Duckett & J. C. da la Torre (Eds.), Pathology of the aging human nervous system (2nd ed.). New York: Oxford University Press.

adults maintain their cognitive ability despite the physiological changes. Longitudinal studies of cognition in older adults reveal some decline in the ability to concentrate on more than one task at a time, decreased reaction time in processing information, and increased time needed to learn and process new information (Craft, Cholerton, & Reger, 2003; Insel & Badger, 2002). The information is still there, but the speed of retrieval has diminished. A frequent complaint of older adults is the struggle with *word-finding,* or the "tip of the tongue" phenomenon. This phenomenon is not associated with storing information but rather in accessing information and is improved with prompting, unlike the word-finding changes noted in dementia (Craft et al., 2003).

Lifestyle factors, physical activity, and intellectually stimulating activities, as well as diet, are currently under investigation for possible beneficial impact on the cognitive ability of older adults (National Institutes of Health [NIH], 2004). A prospective study of leisure activities among community-dwelling older adults found that reading, playing board games, playing musical instruments, and dancing were associated with reduced risk of dementia (Verghese et al., 2003). Another prospective study of community-dwelling older adults compared no exercise to physical activity and reported that physical exercise was associated with lower risk of cognitive impairment or dementia of any type (Laurin, Verreault, Lindsay, MacPherson, & Rockwood, 2001). Controlling cardiovascular risk factors for heart disease and stroke, reducing stress, and preventing social isolation are other factors being investigated for potential benefit in reducing risk of cognitive decline. See Chapter 20 for additional discussion of cognition, memory, and learning.

Reaction Time. Physically and cognitively, the reaction time of older adults is slower than that of their younger counterparts. Speed of brain processing as measured on psychomotor performance tests is slower, yet just as accurate, in older adults than in younger adults. If there is no time limit to a task, older adults perform as well as younger adults. Accuracy of performance is not altered in normal aging. Reaction times are slower as the complexity or number of tasks increases. These changes in reaction times do not interfere with the function of the normal healthy older adult, although they may be very frustrating. Older adults with sensory impairments or underlying illness, particularly dementia or depression, will experience functional losses related to slower reaction times. Vision changes accompanied by normal slowed reaction times will interfere with driving, for example. Disease, such as dementia, further delays reaction times, impairing functional ability. Medication also plays a potentially important role in reaction times because side effects may further delay reaction times and affect the functional ability of the older adult.

Proprioception. Proprioception is the awareness of body position and limb movement. Integration of sensory input by the cerebral cortex and cerebellum maintains balance and equilibrium by directing the motor responses of the musculoskeletal system. This sensory input is received from the proprioceptive and vestibular systems, as well as the visual and auditory systems. Receptors in the joints, peripheral nerves, muscles, and tendons provide sensory impulses to the cerebral cortex and cerebellum. Although there are age-related changes in these sensory systems, they alone are not sufficient to cause disequilibrium but may predispose the older adult to postural instability and falls in the

presence of disease or other impairments (Nanda & Tinetti, 2003). Masdeu and Rodriguez-Oroz (2003) state that postural instability in older adults is seldom due to one etiology but rather is a result of multiple system impairments. Hill and Schwarz (2004) suggest that medications play an important role in postural stability in the older adult. Psychoactive drugs (antipsychotics, antidepressants, and sedatives), digoxin, diuretics, and antiarrythmics are examples of medications that affect the sensory and neuromuscular systems related to proprioception (Hill & Schwarz, 2004). Although there are well-documented age-related changes in the vestibular, auditory, and visual systems, there are conflicting reports regarding age-related changes in the proprioceptive system. There is reported change in joint-position sense in the normal older adult in active movement, but no change at rest.

BALANCE. The three mechanisms of the nervous system responsible for balance are sensory function, motor function, and the central coordination of sensory and motor function. Postural control decreases in aging are due in part to loss of sensory cues. Decreased vibratory sense in the feet is an example of altered sensory function, as is decreased vision. Postural control is also altered by decreased righting reflex ability (motor responses to maintain supine posture or recover balance). Additionally, changes in gait, decreased stride, and less height in foot lift are motor function changes that negatively affect posture in the older adult. These sensory and motor mechanisms are further affected by chronic diseases such as dementia, stroke, Parkinson's disease, arthritis, cardiac arrhythmias, peripheral neuropathies, and orthostatic hypotension. Medications can also play a role in postural control and balance (Baum, Capezuti, & Driscoll, 2002). Examples of such medications that are commonly used by older adults include psychotropic drugs, insulin and oral hypoglycemics, antidepressants, antihypertensives, and anticholinergics (Baum et al., 2002). These age-related changes, as well as the contributions of other physical conditions, contribute to the risk for falls in older adults.

DIZZINESS. The central nervous system is constantly integrating sensory input in order to provide information required for maintaining balance and movement to allow the individual to interface with the environment. Sensory messages are received through vision, vestibular sensation, joint position sense, touch-pressure (cutaneous) sensation, and hearing. When this sensory input is not integrated correctly or insufficient information is provided, dizziness may occur. Nanda and Besdine (2003, p. 1543) define *dizziness* as "an abnormal sensation of unsteadiness or motion in space." It may result from visual, proprioceptive, vestibular, or CNS disorders. Older adults who are prone to decreased sensory input are especially likely to develop dizziness. Dizziness prevalence ranges from 4% to 30% in adults over age 65 and is the most frequent complaint to physicians by adults over age 75 (Hill-O'Neill & Shaughnessy, 2002; Nanda & Besdine, 2003). Dizziness is associated with negative effects on quality of life, social interactions, and overall mood. Dizziness also plays a role in fear of falling. Dizziness can be categorized into four types: (1) vertigo, (2) pre-syncope, (3) disequilibrium (imbalance), and (4) nonspecific dizziness (Nanda & Besdine, 2003).

Vertigo. *Vertigo* produces a rotational sensation in which persons feel that either they or the environment is spinning. Vertigo is related to disorders of the vestibular system. Vestibular diseases are reported to represent up to 70% of dizziness in older adults (Nanda & Besdine, 2003). Common forms of vertigo include benign positional vertigo, vertebrobasilar insufficiency, and Ménière's disease. The onset of vertigo is often instantaneous, and it may be accompanied by nausea, vomiting, staggering gait, tinnitus, hearing loss, or visual changes, depending on vestibular system impairment.

Pre-Syncope. *Pre-syncope* (light-headedness) produces a sensation of impending faint or loss of consciousness. Pre-syncope is frequently caused by orthostatic hypotension, but hypoglycemia, arrhythmias, and oxygen deprivation are also causes. Occasionally, light-headedness is accompanied by pallor, roaring in the ears, and diaphoresis (Hill-O'Neill & Shaughnessy, 2002).

Disequilibrium. *Disequilibrium* is the persistent sense of unsteadiness that is prominent when standing or walking. This dizziness is a mechanism of impaired sensory signals (relay or reception) resulting in inability to maintain proper motor responses. The causes are vestibular impairment, sensory loss, and motor or cerebellar lesions.

Nonspecific Dizziness. *Nonspecific dizziness* is described as vague descriptions of dizziness. Panic, anxiety, and depression are frequent causes of this type of dizziness.

SYNCOPE. Syncope is a transient loss of consciousness and postural tone with spontaneous and complete recovery. Onset is rapid, with occasional warning symptoms of light-headedness, nausea, sweating, or generalized weakness. Syncopal episodes result from a sudden loss of blood flow to the brainstem's reticular activating system, which is responsible for consciousness (Kapoor, 2003; Kenny, 2003).

Multiple chronic illnesses, medications, and age-related changes predispose the older adult to syncopal episodes. Many syncopal episodes are not due to one single cause but rather have a multifactorial etiology. The causes of syncopal episodes are frequently classified as neurally mediated syndromes, orthostatic causes, cardiac arrhythmias, and mechanisms that cause decreased cardiac output. Neurally mediated syndromes refer to those etiologies that cause bradycardia and inappropriate

vasodilation. Examples are a vasovagal episode, situational factors (large-volume micturition, cough, swallow, or defecation), anxiety disorders, and high altitude. Medications that contribute to syncopal episodes include diuretics, alcohol, psychoactive drugs, antihypertensives, vasodilators, and digoxin (Kapoor, 2003; Kenny, 2003).

Orthostatic Hypotension. *Orthostatic hypotension* is defined as a 20 mm Hg drop in systolic blood pressure or a 10 mm Hg drop in diastolic blood pressure after changing from a supine position to a standing position. Orthostatic hypotension represents the cause of 14% of syncopal episodes in older adults, and Kane, Ouslander, and Abrass (2004) report that up to 20% of community-dwelling older adults have orthostatic hypotension. Syncopal episodes caused by orthostatic hypotension are the result of pooling of blood in lower extremities and splanchnic circulation with resultant decreased venous return to the heart, causing a decrease in cardiac output. Decreased cardiac output stimulates the aortic, carotid, and cardiopulmonary baroreceptors, which are often blunted as a result of age-related changes (Kapoor, 2003; Kenny, 2003) such that blood pressure homeostasis is altered; this can result in decreased cerebral blood flow and syncope.

Many medications play a significant role in orthostatic hypotension. As well as considering a single medication as the cause, the synergistic effects of different medications must also be considered as a cause of hypotension. Systolic hypertension and volume depletion are other significant causes of orthostatic hypotension, as well as diseases that affect the autonomic nervous system (Kapoor, 2003).

Older adults are often hospitalized following an initial syncopal event to evaluate potential causes. Understanding the cause or possible causes is an important first step in planning interventions to prevent further syncopal episodes. Education would include understanding the precipitating factors and behavioral changes to prevent syncope. Simple examples of these interventions would include the following: arising slowly from bed or chair, dorsiflexing the ankles several times before standing, and maintaining fluid intake sufficient for adequate hydration. Careful medication review followed by cautious addition of new medications, with frequent assessment of orthostatic blood pressure measurements to monitor medication effect on blood pressure homeostasis, is another important intervention to prevent further syncopal episodes. See Chapter 11 for additional discussion of falls.

MOTOR ACTIVITY. As discussed in Chapter 11, motor activity tends to change with aging, especially posture, movement, and reflexes. Reflexes are less brisk, primarily in proximal areas of the lower extremities, where ankle jerks may be completely absent. Motor activity slows, and there may be some difficulty with fine motor movement. Joints become more rigid in a flexed position, and muscle strength declines. The gait is often characterized by a shortened stride and mild symmetrical decreased arm swing. Also, older adults often do not pick their feet up as high. Older men have a wide-based, short-stepped gait. Older women may develop a "waddling," narrow-based gait (Kane et al., 2004; Seidel, Ball, Dains, & Benedict; 1999).

Benign essential tremor affecting the upper extremities, head, and voice occurs with increasing age and is common among older adults. These action tremors occur with sustained arm extension and with voluntary movements such as writing or drinking. These tremors usually remain mild with no interference of function. Infrequently they can progress to a point of causing social embarrassment or disability. These age-related tremors are intermittent, are exaggerated by movement, and rarely appear at rest. Nervousness, anxiety, and embarrassment can exacerbate the tremor. When there is a strong family history of essential tremor, these tremors are called *familial tremors*. Older adults should be reassured that this tremor does not represent Parkinson's disease.

Thermoregulation. Because of decreased homeostatic regulation in advancing age, older adults are much more susceptible to hypothermia and hyperthermia during temperature extremes. Additionally, older adults who are alone, have dementia, or have chronic illness are particularly at risk for temperature dysregulation states.

HYPOTHERMIA. *General hypothermia* is defined as a core temperature of 35° C (95° F) or below. It is so prevalent among older adults that it is one of the most important causes of death in Great Britain in the winter. Older adults who live in mild climates, however, are also susceptible to hypothermia during the cooler months, and hypothermia is a common occurrence in homes not heated above 21° C (70° F) (Abrass, 2003; Kane et al., 2004). The etiology of hypothermia is multifactorial. Social factors that may play an important role in cold exposure include inadequate income, social isolation, inadequate housing, and inability to maintain heating appliances. Disorders that may decrease heat production in the older adult include hypothyroidism, hypoglycemia, malnutrition, and conditions that decrease mobility such as stroke or arthritis. Impaired thermoregulation factors that predispose older adults to hypothermia include loss of fat and subcutaneous tissue, decreased shivering and vasoconstriction, trauma, hypoxia, cerebrovascular disease, and medications. Other factors that predispose the older adult to hypothermia include infection, alcoholism, and cardiovascular diseases (Kane et al., 2004). The drugs most commonly thought to predispose the older adult to

hypothermia are alcohol, barbiturates, phenothiazines, benzodiazepines, anesthetics, opioids, salicylates, and acetaminophen (Abrass, 2003).

Early clinical signs of hypothermia include fatigue, apathy, slurred speech, confusion, possible shivering, and cool skin. When body temperature falls below 30° C (86° F), the clinical presentation is cold skin; bradycardia with atrial and ventricular arrhythmias; a slow, shallow respiratory pattern with cyanosis; hypotension; semicoma to coma; generalized edema; and slowed reflexes. As the core temperature continues to fall, the presentation is that of rigidity, apnea, pulselessness, and unresponsiveness (Abrass, 2003).

Mild-to-moderate hypothermia (body temperature of 32° to 35° C) is treated with passive rewarming of the body with a warm environment and wrapping the person in blankets. Active external rewarming (electric blankets or submersion in a warm bath) can be dangerous, because cold blood is shunted to the core, possibly triggering cardiac dysrhythmias and precipitation of hypovolemic shock as peripheral vasodilation decreases the circulatory blood volume. Severe hypothermia (body temperature lower than 32° C) is treated more vigorously as a medical emergency, and core warming is necessary. The patient should be handled gently and central lines should be avoided because of myocardial irritability. Practical methods of core rewarming include peritoneal dialysis and inhalation rewarming (Abrass, 2003; Kane et al., 2004). The emergency priority in treating severe hypothermia is to rewarm and then treat the other serious complications of hypothermia (arrhythmias, acidosis, and fluid and electrolyte abnormalities), because these respond to treatment only after rewarming as a result of delayed metabolism. The underlying medical condition causing hypothermia must also be treated (Kane et al., 2004). The prognosis depends more on the severity of the underlying clinical condition than on temperature at the time of diagnosis or the rate of rewarming. The mortality rate of severe hypothermia is reported to be 50% (Kane et al., 2004).

HYPERTHERMIA. In the United States, 5000 people die from heatstroke each year—two thirds of them over age 60 years. Deaths are greatest during prolonged heat waves (Abrass, 2003). Heatstroke is due to an impairment of the thermoregulatory function and physiological change and is defined as a core temperature greater than 40.6° C (105° F). Transfer of body heat from the core to the periphery decreases owing to an inability to make circulatory adjustments. It has long been thought that older people sweat less than younger people. Recent studies suggest that less sweating is not a consequence of normal aging but is due to deconditioning that leads to decreased response to thermal and neurochemical stimulations in older adults compared with their younger counterparts (Abrass, 2003). Medications that place older adults at increased risk for hyperthermia include phenothiazines, anticholinergics, antidepressants, diuretics, and beta blockers (Abrass, 2003).

Heat exhaustion, which generally precedes heatstroke, is manifested by dizziness, weakness, nausea and vomiting, diarrhea, feelings of warmth, headache, and dyspnea. As the temperature rises above 40.6° C, the classic signs and symptoms of heatstroke appear: psychosis, delirium, loss of consciousness, and hot, dry skin (Abrass, 2003). There is a widening pulse pressure, decreased cardiac output, and low peripheral resistance, progressing to circulatory failure and eventual death. The complications of heatstroke in older adults are seizures and focal neurological deficits caused by cerebral edema, liver failure, hypokalemia, respiratory alkalosis, metabolic acidosis, and shock (Abrass, 2003; Kane et al., 2004).

Heat exhaustion is treated by moving the person to a cooler environment, removing excess clothing, and using fans. The priority in treating severe hyperthermia is immediate rapid cooling using ice packs or ice-water baths. Estimates of mortality rates range from 17% to 80%, depending on the duration and severity of the hyperthermia. The risk for death from heatstroke is greatest for those who are in shock or coma or who have underlying congestive heart failure, diabetes mellitus, obstructive lung disease, obesity, and previous central nervous system lesion.

Sleep Changes. Sleep disturbance is a common occurrence in older adults, with a reported incidence of greater than 50% in adults 65 and older. Lack of restful nights can result in daytime sleepiness, impairments in attention and decision making, memory problems, falls, and depression. Poor sleep can be a contributing factor in the development of cardiovascular disease; it is associated with higher mortality rates and may also contribute to disorders of the immune system (Kryger, Monjan, Bliwise, & Ancoli-Israel, 2004).

Many complex mechanisms regulate sleep. The circadian drive is a primary mechanism for sleep. The suprachiasmatic nucleus within the hypothalamus regulates this complex drive for sleep and wakefulness, synchronizing with the light-dark environmental cycle. Melatonin, produced by the pineal gland during dark hours, is another factor in the sleep cycle. Melatonin is important to sleep induction because it is released in response to light changes and inhibits neurotransmitters involved in arousal. Body temperature fluctuations, release of cortisol, and release of growth hormone are other biological factors that regulate sleep patterns (Hoffman, 2003).

The normal sleep cycle is outlined in Box 14-2. The usual sleep cycle consists of non–rapid-eye-movement (NREM) sleep stage 1 followed by NREM stages 2, 3, and 4 with possible drifting through NREM stage 2 and

---

BOX 14-2 Normal Sleep Cycle

Non–Rapid-Eye-Movement (NREM) Sleep

Stage 1
Transitional period of drifting off to sleep

Lightest sleep stage with easy arousal

Lasts only a few minutes, about 5% of sleep time in adults

Stage 2
Period of greater relaxation

Light sleep, not easily aroused

Accounts for about 50% to 55% of sleep time in adults

Stage 3
Deeper sleep, difficult to arouse

Vital signs, body temperature, and metabolism gradually decline

Constitutes about 10% to 15% of sleep time in adults

Stage 4
Deepest sleep with very difficult arousal

Vital signs and body temperature at lowest point

Represents about 5% to 10% of normal sleep time in adults

Rapid-Eye-Movement (REM) Sleep
Follows stage 4 NREM sleep and occurs about 90 minutes after falling asleep

Deepest level of relaxation

Vital signs (respiratory rate, heart rate, blood pressure) are variable, irregular, and frequently elevated

Rapid eye movements are visible

Characterized by vivid dream activity

Constitutes 20% to 25% of sleep time in adults

Adapted from Hoffman, S. (2003). Sleep in the older adult: Implications for nurses. *Geriatric Nursing, 24*(4), 210-216; and Burke, M. M., & Laramie, J. A. (2004). *Primary care of the older adult* (2nd ed.). St. Louis: Mosby, p. 566.

---

stage 3 before initiation of rapid-eye-movement (REM) sleep. REM sleep is followed by NREM stage 2 and then repeating of the cycle through the night. The sleep cycle typically lasts 90 minutes, and a person would experience three to five sleep cycles during a normal night's sleep (Burke & Laramie, 2004; Hoffman, 2003).

Changes in the sleep cycle that occur with aging include the following: lighter, more easily interrupted sleep; increased time spent in stage 1 of NREM sleep, that transition period between sleep and wakefulness; and decreased time spent in stages 3 and 4 of NREM sleep, the deepest and most restorative sleep. REM sleep remains the same but occurs earlier in the sleep cycle of older adults. These changes alone usually do not interfere with the quality of sleep, but in the presence of other comorbidities older adults are predisposed to insomnia. Illnesses such as stroke, diabetes, chronic pain, heart and respiratory disease, Parkinson's disease, Alzheimer's disease, and depression have a profound influence on the sleep cycle of older adults. It is not only the illness that affects the sleep cycle but also the medications used to treat the condition (Hoffman, 2003). Classes of drugs that are stimulating include alcohol (may be sedating initially but later cause wakefulness and poor sleep), nicotine, CNS stimulants, thyroid supplements, corticosteroids, calcium channel blockers, beta blockers, and some bronchodilators. Some drugs taken during the day cause daytime drowsiness and napping, which contributes to nighttime insomnia. These include antihypertensives, antihistamines, antidepressants, and tranquilizers (Cohen-Zion & Ancoli-Israel, 2003; Kryger et al., 2004).

Insomnia is the most frequent sleep problem cited by older adults. Older adults typically experience either difficulty falling asleep, trouble staying asleep, or early morning awakening (Hoffman, 2003). Older adults also experience disrupted sleep due to obstructive sleep apnea, discussed in Chapter 13. Assessment of sleep disturbances should center on inquiry of regular sleep habits; quality of sleep; use of alcohol, caffeine, and medications; review of medical history; and exercise habits. A sleep diary is a good tool to use to gather sleep information and is a valuable tool in facilitating behavior change for the older adult (Cohen-Zion & Ancoli-Israel, 2003; Hoffman, 2003).

Interventions that promote sleep and preserve the circadian rhythm include encouraging a consistent bedtime routine, being exposed to bright light later in the day by getting out in the late afternoon/early evening before sunset, and regular exercise. Progressive relaxation techniques and using guided imagery or relaxing music are also methods that may promote sleep in older adults. Other interventions that assist the sleeping environment include only going to bed when fatigued, getting out of bed after 15 to 20 minutes if unable to fall asleep to complete a quiet activity and returning to bed when sleepy, and arising each day at the same time. Efforts should be made to retain usual sleep patterns or rituals in hospital and nursing home settings. Sleep patterns are often disrupted in these settings. Nurses can play an important role in ensuring an environment that is conducive to sleep in these settings, understanding that noise is a major hindrance to sleep (Cohen-Zion & Ancoli-Israel, 2003; Hoffman, 2003). Medication intervention typically used would include antidepressants or short-acting hypnotics, used intermittently and for a limited time. Medications should be gradually reduced to decrease the risk of rebound insomnia (Cohen-Zion & Ancoli-Israel, 2003).

Music and exercise are examples of nonpharmacological interventions for sleep that have been investigated. Lai and Good (2005) recently reported that the use of soothing music played for 45 minutes at bedtime significantly improved sleep quality in community-dwelling older adults with sleeping difficulty. In this study, sleep improved weekly over the 3-week intervention, demonstrating a cumulative effect of music on perceived sleep quality (Lai & Good, 2005). Fuzhong and colleagues (2004) demonstrated that a 6-month low- to moderate-intensity Tai Chi program was effective in improving sleep quality in community-dwelling older adults.

COMMON NEUROLOGICAL DISORDERS IN THE OLDER ADULT
Delirium

Delirium is a frequently occurring geriatric syndrome that often goes undetected by health care professionals, even by nurses who are at the patient-side 24 hours a day (Inouye, Foreman, Mion, Katz, & Cooney, 2001; Roche, 2003). It is associated with many adverse outcomes: increased mortality rate, poor physical function and cognitive status, transfer to nursing home, increased severity of comorbid illness, and increased hospital stay. Delirium has been identified as an important measure of quality of care because of the potential impact on the health outcomes of older adults.

Delirium is defined as an abrupt change in attention and cognition. The essential features of delirium, as defined in the *Diagnostic and Statistical Manual of Mental Disorders* (fourth edition, text revision) (DSM-IV-TR) (American Psychiatric Association, 2000), are disturbances in consciousness and cognition that are not explained by a known or evolving dementia. These disturbances manifest over a short period of time, hours to days, and fluctuate over the course of 24 hours. Delirium is differentiated based on etiology: medical condition, substance-induced etiology, or multiple etiologies (American Psychiatric Association, 2000). Delirium is seen in all health care areas but is most prevalent in emergency departments and hospitals. During hospitalization for general medical conditions, approximately 14% to 24% of people over age 65 years have delirium on admission, and another 6% to 56% develop delirium during hospitalization (Agostini & Inouye, 2003; Inouye, 2003). Up to 50% of older adults develop delirium following a surgical procedure, and in recent research 70% of older adults who spent any time in the intensive care unit had delirium during that hospital stay (McNicoll et al., 2003). The American Psychiatric Association (2000) estimates that 60% of adults over 75 years in the nursing home setting have delirium at any given time.

Delirium manifests as the inability to focus, sustain, or shift attention in a normal manner. The individual is easily distracted and difficult to engage in meaningful activity. The level of consciousness may fluctuate from drowsiness to stupor or coma, or the individual may be restless or hyperactive. Perceptual disturbances may precipitate misinterpretation of environmental cues, causing illusions or hallucinations (usually visual). Cognitive changes may also appear as memory impairment, disorientation, or language disturbance. Wandering attention is closely linked with an inability to maintain goal-directed thinking and behavior, leading to disorganized thinking, incoherent speech, and perseveration of speech and behavior. Features also associated with delirium include disturbed sleep-wake cycle and disturbed psychomotor behaviors. Clinical delirium is described as hyperactive, hypoactive, or mixed psychomotor behaviors. Individuals with hyperactive delirium are restless, irritable, and physically agitated. This often interferes with healthcare interventions. Individuals with hypoactive delirium are lethargic and apathetic, and are often not identified as having delirium or are misdiagnosed as having depression. A mixed presentation fluctuates between hyperactive and hypoactive delirium (Inouye, 2003; Kurlowicz, 2002). Other symptoms associated with delirium include anxiety, depression, irritability, anger, apathy, euphoria, sudden mood changes, and fear.

Although in some cases a single cause of delirium may be identified, most often delirium is due to many interrelated factors. Inouye (2003) discusses delirium in the context of the interrelationship between the vulnerabilities or predisposing factors of the individual and precipitating factors. Each individual has a threshold for development of delirium. Key predisposing factors of delirium are listed in Box 14-3. Precipitating factors of delirium are identified in Box 14-4. Effects of medications are reported to be the most common precipitating factor of delirium in older adults (Inouye, 2003; Kane et al., 2004; Kurlowicz, 2002). The most common medications that precipitate delirium in older adults are outlined in Box 14-5. It is important to note that many medical conditions can cause delirium in older adults. Acute myocardial infarction, congestive heart failure, infection, and metabolic disorders (including thyroid disorders, hypoglycemia and hyperglycemia, hyponatremia and hypernatremia, and acid-base disorders) can cause delirium without the usual attendant symptoms of disease in older adults (Inouye, 2003). Delirium can also be a symptom of fecal impaction or urinary retention in older adults.

Differential diagnosis is important so that proper treatment can be initiated. Cognitive assessment is the first step in the differential diagnosis. Knowledge of the individual's baseline cognitive status is an important aspect of the assessment. This is particularly important if

---

BOX 14-3 Key Predisposing Factors of Delirium in Older Adults

- Age (particularly over 80)
- Dementia or underlying cognitive impairment
- Multiple medical comorbid diseases
- Functional impairments
- Vision or hearing impairment
- Chronic renal insufficiency
- Depression

Adapted from Inouye, S. K. (2003). Delirium. In C. K. Cassel (Ed.), *Geriatric medicine: An evidence-based approach.* New York: Springer-Verlag; Roche, V. (2003). Etiology and management of delirium. *American Journal of Medical Science, 325*(1), 20-30; and American Psychiatric Association (APA). (2000). *Diagnostic and statistical manual of mental disorders* (4th ed., text revision). Washington, DC: American Psychiatric Association.

BOX 14-4 Precipitating Factors of Delirium in Older Adults

Medications

Infection

Immobilization (think also of interventions that immobilize, e.g., bed rest, Foley catheters, physical restraints, surgical procedures)

Dehydration

Malnutrition

Electrolyte disorders

Metabolic disorders

Iatrogenic events

General anesthesia

Change in health status—medical conditions (not inclusive):
- CNS disorders: head trauma, seizures, stroke, infection
- Metabolic disorders: renal/hepatic disease, fluid/electrolyte imbalance—dehydration
- Cardiovascular disorders: myocardial infarction, congestive heart failure
- Systemic changes: infection, trauma

Adapted from Tullmann, D. F., & Dracup, K. (2000). Creating a healing environment for elders. *AACN Clinical Issues, 11*(1), 34-50; Inouye, S. K. (2003). Delirium. In C. K. Cassel (Ed.), *Geriatric medicine: An evidence-based approach.* New York: Springer-Verlag; Roche, V. (2003). Etiology and management of delirium. *American Journal of Medical Science, 325*(1), 20-30; and American Psychiatric Association (APA). (2000). *Diagnostic and statistical manual of mental disorders* (4th ed., text revision). Washington, DC: American Psychiatric Association.

BOX 14-5 **Common Medications that Precipitate Delirium in Older Adults**

Anticholinergic medications—furosemide, digoxin, nifedipine, theophylline, oxybutynin, Parkinson's disease medications, and over-the-counter medications (nonsteroidal antiinflammatory drugs, nasal sprays, and cold/flu remedies)

Benzodiazepines/hypnotics

Sedatives—zolpidem, buspirone

Narcotic analgesics

H_2-blocking agent

Any three medications added in 24 hours

Adapted from Kurlowicz, L. H. (2002). Delirium and depression. In V. T. Cotter & N. E. Stumpf (Eds.), *Advanced practice nursing with older adults: Clinical guidelines.* New York: McGraw-Hill; Inouye, S. K. (2003). Delirium. In C. K. Cassel (Ed.), *Geriatric medicine: An evidence-based approach.* New York: Springer-Verlag; and American Psychiatric Association (APA). (2000). *Diagnostic and statistical manual of mental disorders* (4th ed., text revision). Washington, DC: American Psychiatric Association.

---

there is underlying dementia. The individual's family or someone who knows the individual well will be very helpful in assessing baseline function. The Mini-Mental State Examination (MMSE) and the short Blessed test (SBT) are two helpful screening tests to assess cognition (Folstein, Folstein & McHugh, 1975; Katzman et al., 1983). The MMSE is the most universally used screening tool and assesses memory, orientation, concentration, language, and praxis. The SBT is a quick assessment, administered in about 5 minutes, and is a test of memory and concentration. Comprehensive medical history should be focused on change from baseline function, course of mental status changes, recent medical changes/illnesses, and prescription and over-the-counter medication review. The physical examination should be comprehensive and focus on any focal neurological signs, evidence of falls, trauma, infection, or other system abnormalities. Laboratory studies are tailored to the clinical evidence and setting; targeted baseline laboratory tests include complete blood count, chemistries, glucose, renal and liver function tests, urinalysis, and oxygen saturation. Other laboratory work might include vitamin B_{12}, thyroid function studies, and a toxicology screen. Clinical evidence for cardiac changes would warrant electrocardiogram, chest films, and arterial blood gases. Clinical evidence of neurological changes might lead to further investigation with neuroimaging or cerebrospinal fluid collection for assessment of infection.

Two assessment tools developed for quick patient-side assessments that are specific and sensitive to delirium detection are the Confusion Assessment Method (CAM) and the NEECHAM Confusion Scale. The NEECHAM is a structured assessment done as part of routine nursing care that can be repeated at frequent intervals and detects either hypoactive or hyperactive forms of delirium in the early stages (Neelon, Champagne, Carlson, & Funk, 1996). The CAM is a standardized screening diagnostic algorithm based on the cardinal features of delirium (Inouye et al., 1990). A CAM for the intensive care unit (ICU) setting has also been developed and validated, the CAM-ICU, for cases in which the individual is critically ill and often unable to verbally communicate (McNicoll et al., 2003). Use of these tools will aid the gerontological nurse in early detection and treatment of the causes of delirium.

Treatment of underlying conditions may reverse the confusional state, but it may be several weeks to months before normal mental and physical functioning is restored. Early identification and treatment of delirium and prevention are the cornerstones of intervention in delirium. If there are behavioral symptoms of severe agitation in the patient with delirium, the use of neuroleptics is warranted while the cause of delirium is being corrected. Currently the safety and effectiveness of the newer neuroleptic agents, risperidone, olanzapine, and quetiapine, is being investigated for the treatment of the agitation symptoms of delirium (Hwang, Yang, Lee, & Tsai, 2003; Kurlowicz, 2002). These newer atypical antipsychotics have fewer extrapyramidal side effects and may be better tolerated by older adults than the older antipsychotics such as haloperidol. Haloperidol, which has a long history of safe use in a diverse group of patients with severe illness and has various routes of administration, is still used to treat severe agitation in delirium. Careful assessment for extrapyramidal side effects is important when using haloperidol. The goal of treatment is an awake, manageable patient who poses no threat of harm to self or staff (Inouye, 2003).

Nonpharmacological interventions suggested by research focus on identifying modifiable precipitating factors in older adults at risk for developing delirium and modifying the environment to prevent or minimize the effects of delirium. The 1999 Delirium Prevention Trial targeted six precipitating factors that are modifiable: cognitive impairment, sleep deprivation, immobility, vision impairment, hearing impairment, and dehydration (Inouye, Bogardus, Williams, Leo-Summers, & Agostini, 2003). Older adults at high risk for delirium received interventions by protocols (primarily nursing care) or usual care on separate hospital units. Although the rates of delirium were lower in the intervention group, there were no differences in the severity of delirium when it occurred in either group. In this study the lowest rates of delirium occurred in the group in which adherence to the intervention was highest. This study identified no single intervention that was statistically significant in preventing delirium; rather, adherence, as implemented by nursing staff, to all interventions was statistically significant (Inouye et al., 2003). Another research group is exploring the use of a dedicated "delirium room" (DR) in the hospital as a model of care for the management of older adults with delirium (Flaherty et al., 2003). In this model, the multidisciplinary staff received in-service education in providing nonpharmacological interventions to prevent and reduce the complications of delirium. The DR was able to provide 24-hour observation in a setting as free of physical and chemical restraints as possible. This descriptive study did not present any evidence-based conclusions but does demonstrate that an innovative and flexible healthcare system is necessary to provide care for delirious individuals (Flaherty et al., 2003).

A summary of nonpharmacological interventions is outlined in Box 14-6. Nurses in every setting are in a position to identify delirium early and implement interventions to reduce the complications of delirium.

Dementia

Dementia is a syndrome of progressive global cognitive decline that results in functional impairment. Memory impairment, accompanied by one or more deficits in other cognitive domains (e.g., organization, judgment, and language) that significantly interfere with usual work or social activities, is the basis of the diagnosis of dementia. Specific criteria for a diagnosis of dementia as defined by the DSM-IV are in Box 14-7.

BOX 14-6 Summary of Nonpharmacological Interventions for Delirium	
GOAL	**INTERVENTIONS**
Communication to provide orientation and cognitive stimulation	Use clocks and calendars
	Provide frequent reminders of time, location, health care provider names, and daily schedule
	Based on individual preferences, engage in activities: discuss current events, structured reminiscence, word games
	Involve family/friends in care to orient and provide support
Facilitate sleep	Provide adequate sleep/rest times
	Maintain normal night/day patterns—open blinds during the day, turn off lights at night
	Schedule procedures/medications to allow uninterrupted sleep at night
	Provide a nightlight in the bathroom
	Reduce noise levels at night
Facilitate mobility	Encourage or facilitate ambulation to normal routine as much as possible
	Provide active range-of-motion exercises
	Limit use of devices that immobilize: catheters, restraints
Prevent sensory misperceptions	Daily reinforcement of use of glasses, hearing aids (magnifying glass, amplification devices as needed)
	Individualized use of special communication techniques for vision or hearing impaired
	Validate communication
Prevent dehydration	Monitor fluid status
	Encourage oral intake

Adapted from Tullmann, D. F., & Dracup, K. (2000). Creating a healing environment for elders. *AACN Clinical Issues, 11*(1), 34-50; and Inouye, D. K., Bogardus, S. T., Williams, C. S., Leo-Summers, L., & Agostini, J. V. (2003). The role of adherence on the effectiveness of nonpharmacologic interventions. *Archives of Internal Medicine, 163*(4), 958-964.

BOX 14-7 DSM-IV Diagnostic Criteria for Dementia

A. The development of multiple cognitive deficits manifested by both
   (1) Memory impairment (impaired ability to learn new information or to recall previously learned information)
   (2) One (or more) of the following cognitive disturbances:
      (a) Aphasia (language disturbance)
      (b) Apraxia (impaired ability to carry out motor activities despite intact motor function)
      (c) Agnosia (failure to recognize or identify objects despite intact sensory function)
      (d) Disturbance in executive functioning (i.e., planning, organizing, sequencing, abstracting)
B. The cognitive deficits in criteria A(1) and A(2) each cause significant impairment in social or occupational functioning and represent a significant decline from previous level of functioning.
C. The deficits do not occur exclusively during the course of a delirium episode.

Reprinted with permission from *Diagnostic and statistical manual of mental disorders*. (2000). (4th ed.). Text revision. Washington, DC: American Psychiatric Association.

Dementia is a common problem in older adults, and prevalence increases with age. The prevalence of dementia is estimated as 10% of adults over 65 years of age and 30% of those over 85 years of age (Kennedy, 2003; Knopman, Boeve, & Petersen, 2003). For individuals over 85 years of age with a first-degree relative with dementia, prevalence approaches 50% (Kennedy, 2003).

Dementia is not an inevitable consequence of aging. Although there are age-related changes of memory function (delay in memory retrieval), given time the ability to recall newly learned information is no different for older and younger adults. The change in cognitive ability in dementia is due to disease, not age.

Mild cognitive impairment (MCI) is a term that has recently been used to describe cognitive impairment that is greater than expected for normal age-related change but does not meet criteria for dementia. A 2001 practice parameter for the Academy of Neurology described the criteria for MCI as objective informant–corroborated memory impairment with otherwise normal cognitive ability that does not interfere with activities of daily living (Petersen et al., 2001). Although there are many potential causes of MCI, some researchers believe that many cases of MCI represent a transition phase between normal aging and very mild Alzheimer's disease (Petersen et al., 1999). Other researchers who follow volunteers with informant-based interviews longitudinally have reliably been able to diagnosis very

early Alzheimer's disease in individuals who meet MCI criteria (Morris et al., 2001). Morris and colleagues (2001) reported a series of autopsy-confirmed Alzheimer's disease in 84% of individuals who met criteria for MCI. Because of the frequency with which this group of individuals progresses to dementia (10% to 15%, compared with 1% to 2% for cognitively intact older adults under 80), clinical monitoring for early recognition and possible treatment to delay the onset of dementia has been recommended. Delay of the onset of dementia could mean significant healthcare cost savings annually. The Alzheimer's Disease Cooperative Study (ADCS) recently reported the results of a multicenter, placebo-controlled study to test the effectiveness of vitamin E or donepezil, current treatment recommendations for Alzheimer's disease, in delaying the diagnosis of Alzheimer's disease in patients with MCI. Petersen and colleagues (2005) reported no significant difference in the probability of progression to Alzheimer's disease in the groups treated with vitamin E, donepezil, or placebo. The group treated with donepezil, as compared with the placebo group, did not have the same rate of decline on cognitive measures during the first 12 months of the 36-month study, but did decline at about the same rate as the placebo group thereafter. These results could not support the recommendation of treating individuals with MCI with standard Alzheimer's disease treatments.

Dementia is a general term that describes a syndrome with a common symptom presentation but not the same etiology (American Psychiatric Association, 2000). Dementias are classified by the DSM-IV-TR by diagnostic features as dementia of the Alzheimer's type, vascular dementia, dementia due to human immunodeficiency virus (HIV) disease, dementia due to head trauma, dementia due to Parkinson's disease, dementia due to Huntington's disease, dementia due to Pick's disease, dementia due to Creutzfeldt-Jakob disease, dementia due to other general medical conditions, substance-induced persisting dementia, dementia due to multiple etiologies, and dementia not otherwise specified. An American Academy of Neurology work group has further defined the diagnostic features of dementia due to frontotemporal lobe pathology (McKhann et al., 2001).

The most common causes of dementia are Alzheimer's disease, vascular dementia, frontotemporal dementia, and dementia with Lewy bodies. Reversible causes of dementia, such as vitamin B_{12} deficiency, hypothyroidism, infection, tumor, subdural hematoma, medication toxicity, and depression, represent less than 10% of dementia cases. Depression is a common comorbidity in dementia, particularly in those who have Alzheimer's disease, and can worsen dementia severity. Screening and treatment of depression is important in the assessment and management of dementia. Individuals with dementia are at high risk for developing

BOX 14-8 Key Features of Delirium and Dementia	
DELIRIUM	**DEMENTIA**
Acute onset, hours to days	Slow, insidious onset
Acute illness, variable duration	Chronic, progressive illness
Usually reversible	Rarely reversible
Acute fluctuations	Gradual decline of abilities
Wandering attention with disorganized thinking prominent feature	Memory impairment that interferes with function prominent feature
Disturbed sleep-wake cycle and psychomotor behaviors	Behavioral changes later in the course

delirium. Whereas dementia and delirium can coexist, dementia cannot be diagnosed when cognitive changes occur only in the presence of delirium. Key features differentiating delirium and dementia are presented in Box 14-8.

Dementia Assessment. An informant-based history of cognitive and functional ability, baseline ability, and any decline is key to the dementia assessment. Often the individual with dementia does not have insight of the cognitive or functional changes and so cannot give an accurate history of change. Changes in memory and one or more of the following cognitive domains are the prominent features of dementia: language, orientation (time and geographical), executive function (organizing and carrying out complex tasks), judgment and problem solving, and praxis (the ability to carry out motor tasks). Changes in ability to handle finances, drive, function in the community (shop, work, or volunteer), prepare meals, and maintain usual hobbies and housekeeping are important functional abilities to assess. History of personality or behavior change is also important in the assessment of dementia. Careful attention to these changes will differentiate the dementia's etiology. Other areas of assessment include review of past medical history, medications (prescription and over-the-counter drugs), family history, physical examination, laboratory evaluation, and neuroimaging.

Standardized assessment tools are helpful in identifying dementia, objectively assessing progression of dementia, and measuring response of dementia symptoms

to treatment (Cotter, 2002; Morris, 2005). There are many standardized tools to assess cognitive function. The MMSE (Folstein et al., 1975), discussed earlier, is the most widely used brief screening test. The MMSE can be used in any setting; can be administered in about 10 minutes; and assesses memory, orientation, concentration, language, and praxis. Two widely used standardized instruments to measure global dementia severity are the Clinical Dementia Rating (CDR) and the Global Deterioration Scale (GDS). The CDR (Hughes, Berg, Danziger, Coben, & Martin, 1982; Morris, 1993) assesses cognitive and functional ability in a structured informant interview and patient testing in six domains (memory, orientation, judgment and problem solving, community affairs, home and hobbies, and personal care) with descriptors for each level of dementia severity. Global CDR scores increase with disease severity: CDR 0 is normal, CDR 0.5 is very mild dementia, CDR 1 is mild dementia, CDR 2 is moderate dementia, and CDR 3 is severe dementia. The GDS (Reisberg, Ferris, & deLeon, 1982) is a seven-point scale with global clinical descriptors for dementia severity. The GDS was expanded to the Functional Assessment Staging (FAST) (Reisberg, Ferris, deLeon, & Crook, 1988) to assess the functional changes of dementia through very severe and end-stage levels of dementia. FAST is the assessment tool currently used to determine Medicare eligibility for hospice with a diagnosis of dementia (Cotter, 2002). FAST stage 7, which encompasses the range of functional abilities of intelligible speech limited to a few words, nonambulatory, unable to sit independently, unable to smile, and unable to hold head up, is the stage that would meet Medicare eligibility for hospice services. A standardized tool that is widely used to assess behavioral changes of dementia is the Neuropsychiatric Inventory (NPI). The NPI is an informant-based interview to assess for 12 behavioral disturbances, noting the frequency, severity, and caregiver distress associated each identified behavior (Cummings, 1997). The 12 behaviors assessed are delusions, hallucinations, agitation, dysphoria, anxiety, apathy, irritability, euphoria, disinhibition, aberrant motor behavior, nighttime behavior disturbances, and appetite/eating changes (Cummings, 1997). Depression assessment tools would also be helpful; further discussion of depression is found in Chapter 20.

Dementia Management. The primary symptom domains of dementia that require management include cognition, activities of daily living, and inappropriate behavior. Dementia care is provided in many settings and by many types of caregivers. An overall goal of nursing care is to promote a meaningful life for individuals with dementia and their caregivers. Interventions to achieve this goal include activities that maximize the cognitive abilities of the individual and provision of an enriched, stimulating environment that is free from emotional and physical harm. Support of the appropriate completion of activities of daily living (ADLs) and instrumental activities of daily living (IADLs) and provision of education, support, and resources for the individual and caregiver are key to this goal.

An important general principle for dementia care is the concept of personhood. In providing dementia care it is important to protect the individual's sense of identity. Care is provided for the person, not the disease. Individualized interventions for dementia management are based on the biography of the individual (employment, volunteerism, hobbies, and family), personality traits, habits, current sensory and cognitive abilities, and physical capabilities. Caregivers must be flexible in adjusting intervention strategies to the individual and making accommodations to meet the needs of the individual while preventing harm to self and others.

Cognitive loss does not mean the individual does not have feelings or emotional responses. Everyone, regardless of illness, needs to be engaged in meaningful activity and to have the assurance that comfort will be provided when necessary. Examples of caregiver behaviors that are detractors to sense of personhood include the following: labeling (thinking of someone by his or her behavior, diet, or treatment as the basis for interacting with the person); ignoring (talking to others while providing care as if the person is not there); disruption (interrupting an activity without explanation); and accusation (blaming the individual for actions that are due to lack of ability) (Moore, 2003).

The specific medical management of dementia is discussed further in this chapter by dementia etiology. General principles of nonpharmacological interventions for dementia are presented here.

COGNITION. To maximize cognitive ability in dementia, there must be careful management of physical health. Poorly controlled chronic illness will worsen dementia symptoms, as will uncompensated sensory impairments. New onset of acute physical illness may cause altered cognitive ability in the individual with dementia. Minimizing medications that affect cognition is another important intervention. Medications outlined in Box 14-5, mentioned earlier, are those that will have a negative effect on cognition and so should be eliminated or minimized. Use of memory aids (written lists, calendars, daily information/activity boards) may support cognitive functions. Orientation techniques such as clocks, calendars, newspapers, labels, visual cues, and organization of belongings are other interventions that may maximize cognitive ability. However, frequently correcting the person with dementia and reciting the day, date, time, and place may cause agitation. Whereas the individual with dementia is unable to learn new material, interventions that make use of preserved implicit memory (activities/tasks carried out without conscious recognition of learning the task) can be used until the severe stages of dementia. For example, a stop sign may reduce exit attempts because the individual recognizes the familiar symbol. Communication techniques, including one on one, active listening, repeated simple commands, gestures, and nonverbal communication, can help maximize cognitive performance. Choices and decision making should be limited based on level of impairment and should lend a sense of mastery and control for the individual. Providing a structured environment and routine is another intervention to help support cognitive function in dementia.

Current research studies of nonpharmacological interventions have demonstrated the ability to improve or delay decline of cognition. These studies of nonpharmacological interventions have demonstrated effect sizes equal to the cholinesterase inhibitors currently used to manage cognitive symptoms of dementia (Beck, 2004). One such study compared 30 minutes of music therapy twice a week to 30 minutes of conversation for 2 weeks in a small sample of nursing home residents. The intervention of music therapy demonstrated a statistically significant improvement of speech content and fluency in demented individuals (Brotons & Koger, 2000). Cognitive stimulation therapy, provided 45 minutes twice a week for 7 weeks, is another intervention that demonstrated improved MMSE scores and quality of life compared with controls (Spector et al., 2003). There was no follow-up evaluation of the interventions in either of these studies, which illustrates a problem in seeking research-based interventions. Many single studies have been reported but not corroborated. Also, the range of abilities of persons with dementia is extremely variable so that an intervention may be effective at one stage, but not another.

ACTIVITIES OF DAILY LIVING. Assessment of need and providing information about resources for meals, transportation, home maintenance (home repairs and cleaning), management of finances, and medication supervision are interventions in the mild stages of dementia. Assessment and assistance for completion of ADLs is more necessary in the later stages of the dementing illness. There are various levels of assistance strategies for completion of ADLs, from providing the stimulus—cueing, laying out clothes, changes in the environment that cue the individual to bathe, dress, or use the toilet—to verbally prompting to complete task, using physical gestures or modeling the desired activity, physically guiding to complete assistance. Providing the individual with the information in a way that is understood to allow the person to complete the task as independently as possible is the goal. Modifications to the environment may be necessary, for example, controlling temperature, light, noise, and activity levels. Adaptive equipment might be used to accommodate individual needs. Strategies that are organized and consistently used are important, as is being alert to the cues the individual is giving about his or her response to the assistance. Simple one-step commands with limited choices and frequent praise are other strategies to employ to assist in completion of ADLs. An occupational therapy evaluation of the home environment may provide recommendations for adaptations to the physical and social environment to enhance the individual's ability to complete IADLs and ADLs safely and as independently as possible.

BEHAVIOR. Inappropriate behaviors commonly occur in dementia and are a great emotional burden to the individual with dementia and his or her caregivers. Inappropriate behaviors can lead to harm of self or others and inhibit meaningful interactions. For the purposes of description and intervention, inappropriate behavior is divided into subtypes: physically aggressive (striking out at self or others); physically nonaggressive (repetitive motor behaviors such as pacing, handling objects); verbally nonaggressive (repetitive words, phrases); and verbal aggression (screaming, hostile or accusatory language) (Cohen-Mansfield, 2001). Nursing literature often describes inappropriate verbal behaviors as problematic vocal behavior (Beck & Vogelpohl, 1999). Employing nonpharmacological interventions

to manage these behaviors is important because they address the reason for the behavior and increase overall quality of life for the individual. Medication management may reduce the behavior, but the effectiveness is limited and presents the risk of side effects (Cohen-Mansfield, 2001). Beck (2004) reports that nonpharmacological interventions have effects equal to those of medication management, typically the use of atypical antipsychotics.

Several theoretical models provide the foundation for the application of nonpharmacological interventions for inappropriate behavior. Three relevant nursing models, the Need-driven Dementia-compromised Behavior (NDB) model, the Progressively Lowered Stress Threshold (PLST) model, and the Cognitive Developmental Approach, are discussed here.

The NDB model conceptualizes disruptive inappropriate dementia behaviors as unmet needs. If these unmet needs are identified and understood, individualized intervention will manage the behavior (Kolanowski, 1999). The inappropriate behavior is meaningful and directs the intervention, improving the quality of life. The NDB model is depicted in Figure 14-1 and describes the interaction between background and proximal factors that result in inappropriate behaviors. Background factors, such as dementia-compromised functions, health status, demographic variables, and psychosocial variables, place the individual at risk for

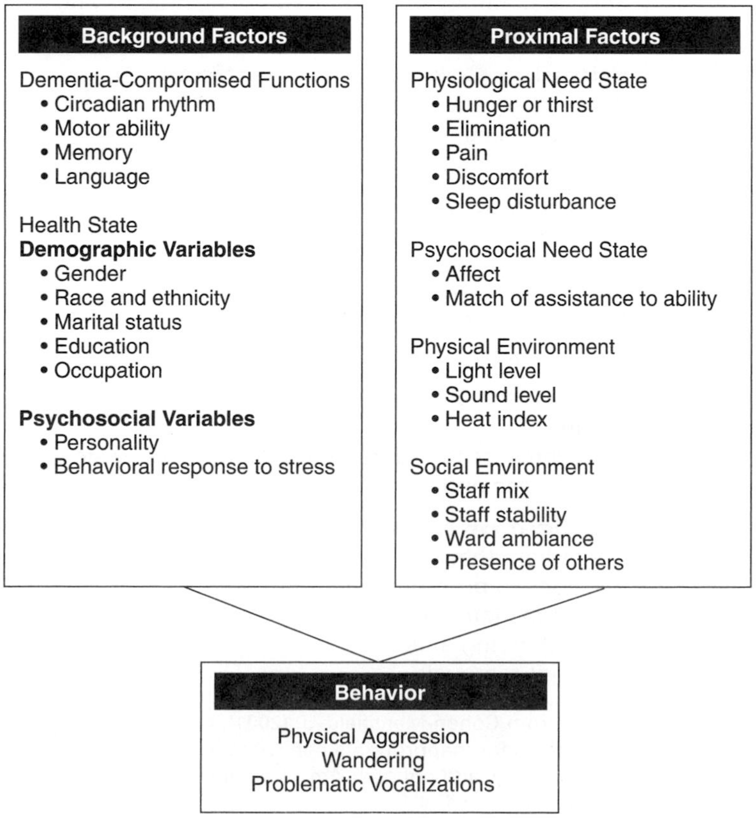

Figure 14-1 Need-driven dementia-compromised behavior model. (From Kolanowski, A. M. [1999]. An overview of the need-driven dementia-compromised behavior model. *Journal of Gerontological Nursing, 25*[9], 7-9.)

inappropriate behaviors (Kolanowski, 1999). Proximal factors, such as physiological needs, psychosocial needs, the physical environmental, and the social environment, precipitate inappropriate behaviors (Kolanowski, 1999). Nursing interventions for managing inappropriate behaviors are developed by identifying the proximal factors associated with the behavior and altering them in an individualized, meaningful way to meet the need (Kolanowski, 1999). Cohen-Mansfield (2001) advocates interventions that would prevent the behavior by preventing the individual from reaching the point of unmet need and assisting the individual in meeting his or her own needs. An example of these interventions would be to ensure use of hearing aids to prevent sensory deprivation, providing an environment with activity and sensory stimulation that meets individual needs.

The PLST model is based on the concept that inappropriate behavior is the response to overwhelming stress (Hall & Buckwalter, 1987). As a result of declining cognitive function, the individual with dementia is progressively less able to perceive and interact with the environment, leading to unsuccessful person-environment interactions and inappropriate behavior. As the dementia progresses, the individual is progressively less able to manage stress, and less exposure to the trigger stimulus produces stress (Smith, Gerdner, Hall, & Buckwalter, 2004). Examples of stressors for the individual with dementia include fatigue; physical illness; pain; change in environment, caregiver, or routine; multiple and competing stimuli in the environment; and demands that exceed the individual's ability to function (Smith et al., 2004). Assessment and interventions that modify the environment and stress triggers may decrease or prevent inappropriate behaviors (Cohen-Mansfield, 2001; Smith et al., 2004).

The Cognitive Developmental Approach (Matteson, Linton, & Barnes, 1996) is a theoretical model based on Piaget's cognitive developmental stages classification system. This approach is based on the belief that the cognitive abilities of the individual with dementia are lost in a predictable sequence that is the opposite of the order in which they were acquired. Therefore approaches to ADLs and behavioral symptoms need to be adapted to the individual's cognitive level of function. This brings expectations and communication in line with the patient's abilities, which reduces frustration and uncooperative behavior. A 3-year study of the Cognitive Developmental Approach demonstrated that behavioral and environmental interventions were effective in reducing behavioral symptoms of dementia even while psychotropic drug therapy was being reduced (Matteson, Linton, Cleary, Barnes, & Lichtenstein, 1997).

Research reviews by Cohen-Mansfield (2001) and Beck (2004) demonstrate that nonpharmacological interventions are effective in managing inappropriate behaviors. Examples of interventions employed in research

studies to manage inappropriate behavior are shown in Box 14-9. Cohen-Mansfield's (2001) review purports that future intervention studies should focus on health care that addresses functional limitations, pain, sleep problems, and limitations of autonomy. Future interventions should be tailored to the individual and provide meaningful stimulation and social contact. Interventions that increase relaxation or decrease stress during care activities would also be important.

Inappropriate behavior management is challenging for the individual with dementia and the caregiver. The same intervention will not work for everyone, and the intervention that works one day may not be the intervention that works the next. Careful investigation to discover the reason for or meaning of the behavior,

---

BOX 14-9 Examples of Interventions Employed in Research Studies to Manage Inappropriate Behavior

Sensory Enhancement
Massage
Therapeutic touch
Music
White noise
Aromatherapy

Social Contact Interventions
Pet therapy
One-on-one interaction
Simulated family interactions with videotapes and audio recordings

Stimulus Control Interventions
Cues to prevent exiting a door
Cues for toileting
Cues to reinforce desirable behaviors

Structured Activity Interventions
Recreational activity
Music or reading
One-to-one supervision in an outdoor garden
Strength and flexibility programs
Exercise programs

Enhanced Environments
Nature
Environments to reduce stimulation (no television; quiet voices and reduced fast movement)

Medical or Nursing Care Interventions
Bright-light therapy
Activities to promote nighttime sleep
Pain management
Use of hearing aids
Restraint removal

Adapted from Cohen-Mansfield, J. (2001). Nonpharmacologic interventions for inappropriate behaviors in dementia; a review, summary, and critique. *American Journal of Geriatric Psychiatry, 9*(4), 361-381.

tailoring meaningful strategies based on the individual's functional and cognitive abilities, and learning by trial and error are tools that will help. Caregivers (family members, friends, health care providers) of individuals with dementia must be supported with resources, education, and respite.

Alzheimer's Disease. Alzheimer's disease (AD) is the most common cause of dementia in older adults, representing 60% to 80% of dementia. Subtypes of AD are defined by age of onset; early-onset AD is used to define onset in age 65 or under, late-onset AD for onset after age 65. It is estimated that currently 4.5 million individuals have AD. Of these 4.5 million individuals, 7% are between ages 65 and 74 years, 53% are between 75 and 84 years, and 40% are over age 85. If population trends hold and no preventive treatment is found, it is estimated that over 13 million people will have AD in 2050 (NIH, 2004). The course of dementia progression varies from individual to individual, but the average duration of the disease is usually about 8 to 10 years after diagnosis. However, AD can sometimes last up to 20 years.

The greatest risk factor for AD is age. Other confirmed risk factors include family history and presence of the apolipoprotein E (ApoE) 4 allele. ApoE, located on chromosome 19, is a serum lipoprotein involved in cholesterol transport. ApoE has three isoforms or alleles, 2, 3, and 4. ApoE 4 is thought to play a role in the deposition of beta-amyloid plaques and is a risk factor for late-onset AD, seen in about 40% of individuals with late-onset AD (NIH, 2004). Presence of ApoE 4 does not mean that an individual will definitely develop AD and is not a recommended guideline to diagnose AD. Lifetime risk of AD for a carrier with at least one copy of the 4 allele (people inherit two) is 29% compared with 9% in the individual without a 4 allele (Cummings & Cole, 2002).

The pathological diagnosis of AD is based on the presence of beta-amyloid plaques, neurofibrillary tangles, and neuronal loss. Although all older adults develop some plaques and tangles as part of the normal aging process, the diagnosis of AD is based on the numbers and location of these plaques and tangles. Neurofibrillary tangles form when the protein that stabilizes the microtubules (the support system of a healthy neuron), tau, changes chemically and threads of tau become tangled and clump together. The microtubules disintegrate, leading to breakdown of the neuron's transport system and communication with other neurons, and ultimately neuron cell death results (NIH, 2003). The cause of the chemical change in tau is not known. Because there is no known way to remove these tangles, there is no treatment therapy that can be directed to this pathological change in AD (DeKosky, 2003). Tau abnormalities are also found in other neurodegenerative diseases, including frontotemporal dementias, corticobasal

degeneration, and supranuclear palsy. Beta-amyloid plaques form when amyloid precursor protein (APP), a protein thought to be important to neuron survival, becomes fragmented and the beta-amyloid fragment clumps together in diffuse plaques. These plaques develop in the hippocampus, which is important to encoding memory, and other areas of the cerebral cortex important to cognition (NIH, 2003). The cause of the fragmentation of APP is unknown. Whether these plaques, and the cascade of events that cause neuronal death, are the cause of AD or the by-product of the disease is also unknown. Research regarding beta-amyloid plaques (how they are toxic to neurons, plaque formation and deposition, and ways to reduce beta-amyloid plaques) is an important focus for potential prevention and treatment mechanisms at this time. Other factors under investigation for a role in the pathology of AD include the inflammatory cascade, oxidative neuronal damage, and neurotransmitter depletion (NIH, 2003).

Most cases of AD are sporadic, but study of rare familial cases of AD has led to greater knowledge of the mechanisms of AD. Findings of specific mutations have led to greater understanding of AD and led to new ideas for possible treatment. Genes identified in the study of these familial cases are outlined in Box 14-10. The mechanisms by which these presenilin mutations cause AD is not fully understood, but data suggest that they influence the concentration of extracellular beta-amyloid and foster beta-amyloid plaque formation (NIH, 2003).

Standard guidelines for the clinical diagnosis of AD were outlined by the American Academy of Neurology (Knopman et al., 2001) and abstracted for use by the American Geriatrics Society (AGS) Clinical Practice Committee (2003). In these criteria, dementia is defined by DSM-III-R criteria, identical to DSM-IV (see Box 14-7, noted earlier). The NINCDS-ADRDA (National Institute of Neurological and Communicative Disorders—Azheimer's Disease and Related Disorders Association) criteria for AD are used to differentiate the cause of dementia. Neuroimaging by CT or MRI is recommended for the initial assessment of dementia to exclude potentially reversible structural causes of dementia, brain

---

BOX 14-10 Genes in Familial Alzheimer's Disease

Chromosome 21 mutation causes production of abnormal amyloid precursor protein

Chromosome 14 mutation produces abnormal protein presenilin 1

Chromosome 1 mutation produces abnormal protein presenilin 2

Data from National Institutes of Health. (2003). *Alzheimer's disease: Unraveling the mystery* (NIH pub. no. 02-3782). Washington, DC: U.S. Government Printing Office.

neoplasm, subdural hematoma, and normal pressure hydrocephalus. The evaluation should include screening for common comorbidities that can cause or worsen cognitive impairment, such as depression, vitamin B_{12} deficiency, and hypothyroidism (Knopman et al., 2001). General screening tools, such as the MMSE, are recommended to detect cognitive change in at-risk groups by the AGS Clinical Practice Committee (2003).

The AGS also recommends neuropsychiatric testing that emphasizes memory as a mechanism to identify at-risk older adults. Cognitive testing reveals problems in memory, category fluency tasks (naming animals), and executive function in AD (Morris, 2005). The literature suggests that informant-based interviews may work as well as cognitive testing when evaluating AD (Knopman et al., 2003; Morris, 2005). An informant can provide information regarding the individual's former level of cognitive and functional abilities, as well as assessing the individual's current level of everyday function, central to the diagnosis of dementia. The informant can provide a thorough history to determine the onset and course of the dementia. The informant-based interview also removes the influence of cultural, educational, and linguistic biases of cognitive testing (Morris, 2005).

Studies such as positron emission tomography (PET), single-photon emission computed tomography (SPECT), electroencephalograms (EEGs), and lumbar puncture for cerebrospinal fluid (CSF) assessment and other invasive procedures are occasionally used to rule out vascular or tissue lesions or infections, but at this time they do not provide definitive proof of the presence of AD and are not recommended in the initial assessment for a diagnosis of AD (Knopman et al., 2001). Currently there are many studies investigating potential biomarkers for AD.

CLINICAL MANIFESTATIONS. The onset of AD is insidious, with gradual progressive decline of cognitive and functional ability. Major symptoms include impaired memory (especially recent memory), disorientation, impaired abstract thinking, impaired judgment and impulse control, and changes in personality and affect. Clinical manifestations and interventions of AD are typically identified by stage of disease, but it is important to realize that there is overlap of these stages. People with AD are individuals, as are their families, and this is important to bear in mind when providing nursing care. The clinical manifestations and key nonpharmacological interventions are presented here by stage of AD.

Very Mild AD. At this stage cognitive change is subtle, and only the individual's immediate family may note any change from prior ability and function. Typically this stage of AD is only detected by dementia specialists because of the very mild nature of the

changes. Individuals may dismiss these very mild changes as normal aging, although individuals with exposure to and personal knowledge of AD may seek evaluation of these very mild changes.

Memory in very mild AD is consistently impaired, and details of recent events are only partially recalled. Although the individual may be fully oriented, there may be difficulty with time relationships, knowing when events happen in relation to one another. The family/individual may note slight impairment in community activities or slight change in interest or participation in hobbies. Complex tasks take longer and errors are evident. For example, in the past an individual handled all the preparations for an annual family gathering but now hosts the event while others share in providing food and organizing the event because of cognitive change. The working individual may continue to work but will require supports to function at the same level or will assume decreased responsibility. For example, the retail shop owner sells her business but continues to work as a consultant and public relations representative for the company with the assistance of a personal assistant. The individual may perform at normal levels on cognitive studies, but in longitudinal studies of cognitive ability individuals with very mild AD will have noted change from their prior performance (Galvin et al., 2005).

Personality changes such as lack of spontaneity and initiative, loss of a previously sharp sense of humor, lack of energy and enthusiasm, or decreased interest in work, family, or recreation may be noted at this very mild stage of AD. Anxiety and depression are not uncommon at this stage and should be treated.

Key interventions involve education and support to maintain autonomy, continue to participate in social activities, and plan for future decision making. The mechanisms to provide support and education for this very mild stage have not yet caught up with the ability to diagnosis AD. At this stage the goal of maintaining a level of independence is attainable. In some areas of the United States there are early-stage AD support groups; for example, the Alzheimer's Association in St. Louis, Missouri, has support groups, Project Esteem, for this group of individuals. They also maintain a telephone support network (a concept developed by an individual with AD) facilitated by volunteers with very mild AD. Long-term planning for future needs must begin now when the individual is most able to make these decisions. Financial and healthcare directives are important to put into place if not already completed. Discussions and exploration of options regarding plans for future living arrangements should begin at this stage. Many people with very mild AD continue to drive, but the ability to drive safely will decline as the disease progresses. A longitudinal on-the-road driving study found that

67% of very mildly demented and 41% of mildly demented drivers were "safe" at baseline assessment but were "unsafe" approximately 2 years later (Duchek et al., 2003). Although not usually reimbursable by healthcare insurers, occupational therapy–based on-the-road drive assessments to establish driving safety should be completed and reassessed at the recommended intervals to help determine when driving is no longer safe.

Mild AD. The individual with mild AD continues to look and act normally to others, and only close family or friends may note any change. There is moderate memory loss, more marked for recent events, that interferes with everyday activities. The individual has difficulty learning and retaining new information. In addition, there may be disorientation in familiar places, difficulty handling complex financial transactions (paying bills, balancing a checkbook), and poor problem solving. Generally the individual functions with assistance in the community and appears independent to the casual observer. The individual is independent in completing usual ADLs but may need prompting to complete the tasks. The ability to participate in complex home repairs and hobbies is reduced; for example, the avid cook no longer experiments in the kitchen but continues to prepare simple meals, relying on recipes for previously well-known dishes. Another example is the skilled handyperson who can no longer complete routine home maintenance or repairs. The individual maintains the semblance of independence with community and family supports, structure, and a daily routine. The neurological examination is generally normal at this stage.

The individual with mild AD may experience personality changes of withdrawal from usual social activities because of fear of others detecting change, lack of confidence in function, or lack of interest in his or her usual activities. Interventions at this stage include those mentioned previously for very mild AD with more attention to assisting the individual and caregiver to adjust to possible role reversal and grief in response to changes caused by AD. At this stage more attention must be given to establishing routines to support cognitive ability, and increased safety monitoring should begin with the goal of maintaining as much independence as is safely possible. Exploration of resources to assist with IADLs and home maintenance to support independence is important, as are measures to support maintenance of social activities and physical health.

Moderate AD. In moderate AD, memory loss is severe, and only highly learned material or established memory is retained while new material is lost rapidly. As the damage of AD spreads in the cerebral cortex, language, reasoning, sensory processing, and conscious thought are impaired. The individual may be confused about the identity and relationships of relatives. The individual becomes increasingly dependent on others and

there is no pretense of independent function at home. Assistance is needed to carry out ADLs. For example, an individual needs assistance setting water temperature in the bath, needs repeated cueing to dress and clothes laid out, and would need prompting to wash hands after toileting. Functional incontinence may become an issue later in this stage. The individual may get lost in familiar settings, has relinquished complex tasks, and even simple tasks of washing dishes or making a bed are completed only with supervision. Language changes are revealed as incomplete sentences and poor comprehension of written and spoken language.

At this stage of AD, disruptive behavioral changes often emerge. Agitation, restlessness (including wandering), sleep disturbances, day-night disorientation, sleep disturbances, verbal or physical aggression, suspiciousness, and hallucinations are common behaviors manifested. Anxiety about separation from a familiar caregiver is seen as the individual seeks to bring meaning to the environment and provide a sense of security. The individual has a decreased tolerance for stress and cannot reliably interpret the environment. Disinhibition, socially inappropriate behaviors, and saying or doing things not usually said or done in public occur at this stage. Manifestation of behavioral changes is highly individualized; not all patients exhibit all these behaviors, though multiple behaviors are common (Monias & Meier, 2003).

Maintaining functional independence for as long as possible, providing a safe environment, and maintaining a sense of person are key issues for the individual with moderate AD. In this stage the safety concerns require greater supervision by others; IADLs are provided and ADLs are supported by others, and increasing behavioral changes require management. AD patients are predisposed to sleep disturbances, weight loss, and dehydration at this stage and require careful monitoring (Monias & Meier, 2003). Social stimulation at this stage is complicated; the patient is unlikely to initiate activity, but can enjoy activity if meaningful, simple, and initiated/supported by others. The coin collector would enjoy sorting coins, the seamstress sorting swatches of fabric by color or texture. Word searches and simple card games are examples of activities appropriate for moderate dementia.

Key interventions for the caregiver are assessing educational and support needs to assist the caregiver role and prevent or intervene in caregiver stress. Problematic behaviors and increasing physical and emotional dependence of the affected individual are a great source of caregiver stress in any setting. Educating the caregiver for providing care, identifying resources to assist in providing care, and providing respite are important nursing interventions. Although this is not an inclusive list, important caregiver resources are the local Alzheimer's

Association, adult day care centers, respite care services, homemaker services, support groups, and geriatric care managers.

Severe AD. At this stage of AD only fragments of memory remain. There may be emotional recognition of family, but names and relationship identification are lost. There is orientation to self only. Language is limited to short phrases and repeated words, and only simple spoken language is understood. The individual may eventually become mute and unable to communicate. There is complete dependence on others for all care, and needs must be anticipated by others. Behavior manifestations disappear, although vocalization (screaming, cursing, or crying) may continue at this stage.

Neurological changes may include parkinsonism (slow, shuffling gait, falls, rigidity, and bradykinesias), occurrence of generalized tonic-clonic seizures, and myoclonus (Morris, 1999). Other clinical changes include weight loss, dysphagia, increased sleeping, and fecal and urinary incontinence. At the end the individual spends most of the time in bed. Death is frequently attributed to complications associated with chronic debilitation: aspiration pneumonia, sepsis, urinary tract infection, pulmonary embolus, or inanition (Cotter, 2002; Morris, 1999; NIH, 2003).

Goals of intervention at this stage are to provide for the physical and emotional needs of the individual, provide comfort, and maximize quality of life. Although this care happens most often in the nursing home setting, it is also provided at home. End-of-life issues regarding treatment interventions of artificial nutrition and hydration, hospitalization or surgery, and cardiopulmonary resuscitation status are important and difficult decisions the caregiver and family must face at this stage. If the individual and family have planned for these issues with advance directives and durable power of attorney to make their wishes known early in the course of AD, the caregiver and family may have less hardship in facing these issues (Monias & Meier, 2003).

TREATMENT. Although there is currently no cure or disease-modifying treatment for AD, there are medications that treat the cognitive and functional symptoms. Four medications—tacrine (Cognex), donepezil (Aricept), rivastigmine (Exelon), and galantamine (Reminyl, soon to be changed to Razadyne)—are cholinesterase inhibitors (ChEIs) that act by stopping or slowing the action of acetylcholinesterase to break down acetylcholine, increasing available acetylcholine. Acetylcholine is thought to be a neurotransmitter important in the neurons of the hippocampus and cerebral cortex for memory (NIH, 2004). Tacrine, the first ChEI approved by the Food and Drug Administration (FDA) in 1993, is no longer marketed because the three new ChEIs (donepezil, FDA approved in 1996; rivastigmine, FDA approved in 2000; and galantamine, FDA approved

in 2001) have improved safety and tolerability profiles and are easier to use (Morris, 2005). These ChEIs provide modest improvement in memory, language, and functional independence in ADLs for a limited period of time, several months to a year. These drugs are not a cure but may slow the progression of symptoms of AD for a period of time. There are ongoing studies to determine if one of these ChEIs is more beneficial, but to date all three are comparable in efficacy. These medications are generally well tolerated; the most common side effects are diarrhea or bowel urgency, nausea, and muscle cramps. Sleep disturbance related to vivid dreams was also noted in a group of individuals and was severe enough to cause medication cessation. Recent studies (Feldman et al., 2003; Trinh, Hoblyn, Mohanty, & Yaffe, 2003) have demonstrated that use of ChEIs may also reduce behavioral symptoms, and manage aggressiveness and agitation, associated with AD.

Memantine (Namenda) was approved by the FDA in 2003 for treatment of symptoms of moderate to severe AD (Morris, 2005). Memantine is thought to work by regulating excess glutamate, another neurotransmitter thought to be important in memory function, which in high levels may damage neurons. Memantine will not reverse or stop AD but in studies demonstrated very modest delay in loss of functional ability in people with moderate to severe AD (Tariot et al., 2004).

Other medications investigated for treatment of AD include estrogen and antiinflammatory agents, antioxidants (vitamins E and C and ginkgo biloba) and statins (cholesterol-lowering agents). The roles of statins and ginkgo biloba are being investigated in clinical trials now. Low estrogen levels were thought to contribute to the development of AD, but several clinical trials of estrogen have failed to demonstrate any benefit of estrogen in the treatment of AD (Kawas, 2003; Morris, 2005). Data recently published from the Women's Health Initiative Memory Study demonstrated that estrogen in combination with progesterone may increase the risk of dementia in women (Kawas, 2003; Morris, 2005). Whereas clinical trials of antiinflammatory agents have not demonstrated treatment benefits for AD, the role of antiinflammatory agents in the prevention of AD is under investigation in clinical trials at present. The American Academy of Neurology's practice parameter for the management of AD provided guidelines for the use of vitamin E to attempt to slow the progression of AD (Doody et al., 2001). This antioxidant is thought to reduce free-radical production and prevent oxidative injury (NIH, 2003). This guideline is based on one randomized control study, and further research is ongoing regarding vitamin E in preventing or postponing the cognitive changes of AD.

Masterman (2003) describes the consequences of the behavioral symptoms of AD as more rapid decline of cognitive ability, increased caregiver burden, earlier institutionalization with attendant increased healthcare costs, and adverse side effects associated with increased use of medications. Treatment of these behaviors can improve the overall quality of life for the person with AD, as well as the caregiver.

Management of behavior problems should always begin with thorough assessment to identify possible medical or environmental causes of the behavior. For example, agitation might be related to fear, pain, constipation, or a urinary tract infection. Correction of the underlying problem can eliminate the behavioral symptom. Nonpharmacological interventions, discussed previously in this chapter, should be the first line of management, and then medication therapy. As with all medication use in older adults, medications should be used cautiously with lower initial doses, longer titration intervals, and lower final dosages. The side effects of certain drugs can produce discomfort and may aggravate the dementia, so the benefits and risks must be weighed. The individual should be observed for drug interactions, keeping in mind that the individual's physical condition affects drug action. Finally, medications should never be used as the only method of treatment but should be used in conjunction with psychological, social, and environmental therapies.

Types of drugs that have been employed for treatment of behavioral symptoms of AD include neuroleptics, antipsychotics, atypical antipsychotics, anticonvulsants, and antidepressants. A recent comprehensive review of randomized clinical trials of medications for treatment of the behavioral symptoms of AD indicates that the atypical antipsychotics, risperidone and olanzapine, demonstrate the most efficacy (Sink, Holden, & Yaffe, 2005). There were no reported studies of the other atypical antipsychotics, clozapine, quetiapine, ziprasidone, and aripiprazole, in the treatment of the behavioral symptoms of AD. There was increased incidence of cerebrovascular events in the treatment arms (risperidone or olanzapine) of these studies compared with the placebo arms, which would warrant discussion with the patient or healthcare decision maker before instituting the use of these atypical antipsychotics. Although the incidence of extrapyramidal symptoms is less with the atypical antipsychotics, the side effect of sedation is still a concern. The neuroleptics, such as haloperidol, thiothixene, thioridazine, chlorpromazine, trifluoperazine, and acetophenazine, have been employed in the treatment of psychotic symptoms, delusions, hallucinations, and agitation. These drugs are not without significant risk, however, because older people with dementia are especially susceptible to adverse effects of neuroleptics, particularly sedation, confusion, and extrapyramidal reactions (Masterman, 2003; Sink et al., 2005). Additionally, recent study reviews show no clear evidence that use of this class of drug was useful in treating the behavioral changes of AD. There have been studies of anticonvulsants to manage behavioral symptoms of AD. These studies have not demonstrated that efficacy outweighs the risk of side effects and so they are not currently recommended based on clinical evidence (Sink et al., 2005). Anxiety disturbances may respond to benzodiazepines, but clinical trials do not demonstrate efficacy in the treatment of agitation or the psychotic symptoms (Masterman, 2003; Sink et al., 2005). Side effects of benzodiazepines include sedation, confusion, and paradoxical disinhibition. Short-acting drugs (oxazepam, lorazepam) are preferred over long-acting drugs (flurazepam, diazepam) to minimize drug accumulation and interactions (Masterman, 2003). Only the antidepressant citalopram has demonstrated efficacy in the treatment of agitation and lability in a 17-day placebo-controlled randomized clinical trial in a specific population. There is an ongoing study, the Clinical Antipsychotic Trials of Intervention Effectiveness (CATIE), designed to evaluate the effectiveness of three atypical antipsychotics (risperidone, olanzapine, and quetiapine) and the antidepressant citalopram in treating the behavioral symptoms of AD (Schneider et al., 2001). The study is expected to publish findings in 2006. Research is also focused on the different presentation of depression in AD and the treatment implications (NIH, 2004).

Other treatments for AD include behavioral interventions, environmental adaptations, and caregiver education. Nonpharmacological management interventions have been discussed earlier in the stages of AD and dementia management.

Vascular Dementia. Vascular dementia is associated with cerebrovascular damage. Many studies report that vascular dementia is the second leading cause of dementia in older adults, representing about 20% of dementia in older adults. The neural systems responsible for cognition are disrupted by ischemia, hemorrhagic brain lesions, or hypoperfusion, resulting in dementia (Morris, 2005; Román, 2003). Rarely does this etiology of dementia exist alone. Increasingly, autopsy studies demonstrate that vascular dementia coexists with other etiologies, usually AD (Knopman et al., 2003; Morris, 2005). Risk factors for vascular dementia include hypertension, cardiac abnormalities, diabetes mellitus, smoking, lipid abnormalities, and autoimmune and infectious vasculitis. The age of onset is usually between 55 and 70 years, and incidence increases with age. This dementia occurs more frequently in men than in women (Neary & Snowden, 2003; Román, 2003).

The pathology of vascular dementia is a result of the cerebrovascular lesion. Primarily this would be hemorrhage or ischemia, with resulting necrosis and cavitation of the involved brain tissue, or evidence of a combination of both. There is also vascular evidence of atherosclerotic disease.

CLINICAL PRESENTATION AND DIAGNOSIS. The presentation of vascular dementia is an abrupt onset of cognitive loss with onset of dementia within 3 months of a symptomatic cerebrovascular accident. The progression of dementia is stepwise, with paroxysmal deterioration of intellectual function that is associated with a clear-cut succession of cerebrovascular insults to the brain. Although initially there may be fluctuating cognitive loss followed by improvement, in vascular dementia a permanent residual disability remains. Focal neurological signs may include limb weakness, asymmetrical reflexes, extensor plantar responses, dysarthria, and gait disturbances (Russell & Burns, 2003). Other clinical features consistent with a diagnosis of vascular dementia based on the NINDS-AIREN (National Institute of Neurological Disorders and Stroke–Association Internationale pour la Recherche et LEnseignement en Neurosciences) diagnostic criteria (Román, 2003) include history of frequent unexplained falls, urinary frequency, urgency or other urinary changes not explained by urological disease, emotional lability, and personality/mood changes.

Cognitive changes of memory loss occur but are not always as prominent as with the presentation of AD. Executive function (the ability to execute complex behavior, sequence information, and problem solve) changes are the more prominent cognitive change of vascular dementia. Other cognitive changes include problems with concentration and comprehension and disturbances in abstract thinking, judgment, and impulse control. Specific changes depend on the areas of the brain affected (Román, 2003).

There are no biomarkers of vascular dementia. Diagnosis is based on the history, physical examination, cognitive assessment, and neuroimaging with MRI or CT. Vascular lesions of a single strategic lacunar stroke, periventricular white matter lesions, or multiple cortical or subcortical strokes are noted on MRI or CT (Knopman et al., 2003; Román, 2003). The Hachinski ischemia score is a useful tool to identify vascular dementias (Table 14-1). A score of 7 or more is compatible with vascular dementia, whereas a score of 4 or less is consistent with AD (Román, 2003).

TREATMENT AND PREVENTION. Treatment of the symptoms of vascular dementia has included vasodilators, calcium channel blockers, and antiplatelet therapy. These are medications aimed at controlling the risks of further stroke. Several recent studies have shown that the cholinesterase inhibitors donepezil, rivastigmine, and galantamine have demonstrated improved cognition and function compared with placebo in patients with vascular dementia (Knopman et al., 2003; Morris, 2005; Román, 2003). This may relate to vascular lesion interruption of the cholinergic pathways.

Table 14-1 *Modified Hachinski Ischemia Score*

Characteristic	Point Score
Abrupt onset	2
Stepwise deterioration	1
Somatic complaints	1
Emotional incontinence	1
History or presence of hypertension	1
History of strokes	2
Focal neurological symptoms	2
Focal neurological signs	2

From Rosen, W. G., Terry, R. D., Fuld, P. A., et al. (1980). Pathological verification of ischemic score in differentiation of dementia. *Annals of Neurology, 7,* 486-488.
NOTE: This tool has been validated on a small number of demented patients by autopsy findings. A score of 4 or more is consistent with vascular dementia.

Treatment of the risk factors of stroke and cardiovascular disease may lower the risk for vascular dementia. Controlling hypertension with diet, exercise, and medications is important because hypertension is the strongest risk factor for stroke (Román, 2003). Other measures include treatment of heart disease, in particular atrial fibrillation; smoking cessation; control of hyperlipidemia with diet and medications; and control of diabetes with diet and medications. Nurses can play an active role in education and support of these possible preventive measures.

Frontotemporal Dementia. Frontotemporal dementia (FTD) is the clinical syndrome of a group of heterogeneous neurodegenerative disorders with predominant frontal and temporal lobe pathological involvement. FTD represents about 5% of the dementias of late life. FTD includes Pick's disease, corticobasal degeneration, progressive supranuclear palsy, primary progressive nonfluent aphasia, and semantic dementia. The Work Group on Frontotemporal Dementia and Pick's Disease (McKhann et al., 2001) suggests that these diverse clinical and pathological entities be collectively called FTD to aid clinical identification. FTDs typically have three neuropathological presentations: abnormal accumulations of tau protein in the neurons and glial cells (tauopathies); tau-negative but ubiquitin protein–positive inclusions in areas of the brain; and FTD with no distinctive pathology (Morris, 2005).

The range of age at onset of FTD is 35 to 75 years, with rare occurrences after age 75. Both men and women are affected equally. Although most cases of FTD are sporadic, familial FTD is reported in up to 40% of cases (McKhann et al., 2001).

CLINICAL PRESENTATION AND DIAGNOSIS. There are two distinct clinical presentations of FTD: behavioral and language. The most common is the behavioral presentation, in which impulsive or inappropriate social conduct is the early change (McKhann et al., 2001; Morris, 2005). The individual becomes disinhibited and impulsive, doing and saying things that are embarrassing. With disease progression, judgment impairment is prominent, there can be a lack of concern regarding personal appearance, and there may also be repetitive or compulsive behavior. Lack of initiative and apathy are also behavioral changes in FTD. Prominent language changes are the early symptom in the language subtype of FTD. The individual has difficulty with expressive language that progresses to difficulty with reading and writing. Language ability/output decreases as the illness progresses so that the individual becomes mute. It is important to note that although the early presentation of symptoms may be either behavioral or language, both behavioral and language changes can occur in FTD as the disease progresses. There is also a subset of FTD in which motor changes occur as the disease progresses. These motor changes include muscle weakness and wasting. FTD with motor disease has a more rapid course, 2 to 3 years on average (Morris, 2005).

Memory changes in FTD are less prominent in the early stages of the disease and worsen as the disease progresses. Other cognitive changes include poor judgment, problem solving, and changes in planning and executing complex tasks (executive function). The individual becomes incapable of handling his or her affairs, cannot work, and social relationships are disrupted (Neary & Snowden, 2003).

Diagnosis is difficult because of the behavioral changes and can be confused with atypical depression in older adults and schizophrenia or antisocial personality disorder in younger adults (McKhann et al., 2001). Individuals with FTD may perform well on memory tasks of cognitive assessment initially but generally will have abnormal scores on executive function. Neuroimaging is helpful in demonstrating prefrontal or temporal atrophy, but atrophy is not always present. There is research investigating possible cognitive assessment batteries to differentiate FTD from AD. There is also ongoing research investigating mutations in the tau gene as a means of improving diagnosis of FTD (Knopman et al., 2003).

TREATMENT. There is no primary treatment for FTD. Nursing interventions aimed at educating the individual and family/caregivers regarding the prominent behavioral changes early in the course of the illness are important. Promoting supervision and safety is crucial in this illness where impulsive or inappropriate social behavior is prominent. There are now resources devoted to promoting understanding FTD available to nurses and family members. The Web site www.ftd-picks.org is just one of these resources.

Dementia Caused by Creutzfeldt-Jakob Disease. Creutzfeldt-Jakob disease (CJD) is a rare, rapidly progressive neurodegenerative disorder that results in dementia and severe neurological impairment. CJD is in the family of diseases called *transmissible spongiform encephalopathies*. CJD is caused by the conversion of normal prion proteins in the brain into abnormally shaped protease-resistant prion proteins. The accumulation of abnormal prions results in neuronal dysfunction and neuronal death. The neuropathological findings of CJD are widespread neuronal loss, gliosis, and spongiform appearance with vacuoles in the sites of abnormal prion accumulation (Will, Alpers, Dormont, & Schonberger, 2004). The human form of this prion disease is different from the new variant CJD (vCJD) that has been a public health focus of interest since 1996 when it was first identified in the United Kingdom. The vCJD is due to the transmission of bovine prions to humans through the consumption of cattle infected with bovine spongiform encephalopathy ("mad cow" disease). The vCJD has clinical and pathological features that are very distinctive from the human prion disease CJD. A striking feature of vCJD is the young age of onset for unclear reasons (Bacchetti, 2003).

Sporadic CJD accounts for about 85% of CJD cases. The cause of sporadic CJD is unknown. One theory is that there is a spontaneous prion protein mutation in a single cell and aberrant mutation causes the conversion of normal prion proteins to the protease-resistant prion protein form (Will et al., 2004). Familial cases of CJD represent about 15% of CJD cases, with 55 mutations and 16 polymorphisms currently identified on the human prion protein gene on chromosome 20 (Pruisner, 2004). Less than 1% of CJD cases are infectious forms (iatrogenic) and have been attributed to improperly decontaminated surgical instruments, corneal transplants, dura mater grafts, and human pituitary extract treatments. Guidelines are now in place to reduce the possibility of infectious CJD; for example, there have been no cases of transmission of CJD via neurosurgical instruments since 1980. There are no well-documented cases of infectious CJD from blood or blood products. The incidence of CJD is 1 in 1 million. The peak age of onset for sporadic CJD is 65 to 79, with a sharp decline in incidence over age 79. The duration of the disease is 2 to 9 months; however, some cases have lasted 2 to 5 years. Familial CJD generally has an earlier age of onset and disease of longer duration compared with the sporadic cases (Will et al., 2004).

The clinical characteristics of CJD are rapidly progressive dementia, ataxia, behavior disturbances, visual-spatial changes, and motor disturbances (including myoclonus). Prodromal symptoms may include fatigue, sleep disturbances, memory disturbances, mild behavioral changes, depression, vertigo, or ataxia (Will et al., 2004). Classic EEG changes, although not specific to

CJD, include generalized slowing or the presence of periodic sharp wave complexes. Serial EEGs have the greatest potential for identifying these EEG changes. Cerebrospinal fluid (CSF) examination may reveal an elevated protein, and some clinicians use the assay for a CSF protein, 14-3-3, to assist in the diagnosis of CJD. This 14-3-3 assay as a tool for diagnosis of CJD is still controversial because of its lack of specificity for CJD, but is an evaluation guideline recommendation of the American Academy of Neurology. At present there is no medical treatment for this devastating illness. Nursing intervention involves supportive assistance and education for the patient and family members. Discussions regarding consideration of autopsy are important, both to establish a definite diagnosis and for public health and epidemiological reasons. The National Prion Disease Pathology Surveillance Center was established in 1997 at Case Western Reserve University to monitor the occurrence of prion disease and can assist in obtaining autopsy. The Web address is www.cjdsurveillance.com.

Dementia with Lewy Bodies. Dementia with Lewy bodies (DLB) is another commonly occurring dementia in older adults, representing 10% to 15% of dementia pathology at autopsy (Knopman et al., 2003). AD pathology (neurofibrillary tangles and senile plaques) is a common concomitant finding in about 66% of DLB cases (Morris, 2005). DLB is a heterogeneous disorder characterized pathologically by neuronal loss and the presence of Lewy bodies in the cerebral cortex. A Lewy body is an inclusion in a neuron and is composed of a protein called alpha-synuclein.

Similar to AD, the incidence of DLB increases with age; the mean age of onset is about 75 years of age. DLB affects men and women equally. The prognosis of DLB is reportedly worse than that of AD, with a faster progression of decline and decreased survival (Knopman et al., 2003).

CLINICAL PRESENTATION AND DIAGNOSIS. A consensus consortium of 1996 outlined the criteria for DLB as a progressive dementia accompanied by at least two of the following: parkinsonian signs, a fluctuating course, and prominent visual hallucinations (McKeith et al., 1996). Other clinical symptoms of DLB include increased sensitivity to neuroleptics, frequent unexplained falls, delusions (misidentification and paranoid delusions), and auditory or olfactory hallucinations (McKeith et al., 1996). Behavioral changes of hallucinations, delusions, depression, apathy, anxiety, and irritability are present in DLB. Despite the diagnostic criteria, the diagnosis of DLB is often difficult (Knopman et al., 2003).

Studies have been conducted to determine if there are specific symptoms that will distinguish DLB from AD (Ferman et al., 2004; Knopman et al., 2003).

Ferman and colleagues (2004) investigated informant-based reports of symptoms of fluctuations and delirium in 200 healthy older adults, 70 individuals with DLB, and 70 individuals with AD. Presence of fluctuations of daytime drowsiness, daytime sleep of 2 hours or more, periods of disorganized speech, flow of ideas, and long periods of staring into space were important in distinguishing DLB from normal aging and AD. Knopman and colleagues (2003) describe REM sleep behavior disorders as occurring in over 50% of DLB individuals and important in distinguishing DLB from AD, Parkinson's disease, and normal aging. Parkinsonism symptoms that are more specific to DLB compared with Parkinson's disease include absence of resting tremor, symmetrical postural tremor, prominent gait and balance disturbance, and little response to levodopa (Knopman et al., 2003). Cognitive changes of DLB include memory loss (similar to AD) and poor executive and visuospatial functions (more than noted in AD).

There are no diagnostic tests specific to DLB. Informant-assisted history to determine the course of dementia and presence and character of motor symptoms, hallucinations, and fluctuations are keys to the diagnosis.

TREATMENT. Management of symptoms is the underlying treatment for DLB. Studies of the use of cholinesterase inhibitors (donepezil and rivastigmine) have demonstrated some benefit in improved cognition and overall function in individuals with DLB (Knopman et al., 2003; Maclean, Collins, & Byrne, 2001). Behavioral symptoms can be very disturbing, and treatment with neuroleptics may worsen the parkinsonism symptoms. Use of the atypical neuroleptics risperidone and olanzapine, which have less binding to dopamine receptors, may prove more beneficial in treating the behavioral symptoms. Quetiapine is an atypical neuroleptic that works within the serotonin system and is also being investigated for potential therapeutic benefits in treating the behavioral manifestations of DLB (AGS Clinical Practice Committee, 2003). Appropriate treatment of depression is an important treatment consideration. Other interventions involve education of caregivers regarding the appropriate management of behaviors and fall risk of individuals with DLB.

Parkinson's Disease

Parkinson's disease (PD) is the most common neurodegenerative movement disorder in older adults. The term *parkinsonian* is often used to describe presence of the cardinal motor features of resting tremor, slowness of voluntary movement (bradykinesia), increased muscle tone or rigidity, postural instability (loss of postural reflexes), and flexed posture or freezing phenomenon (feet "glued to ground") whether or not Parkinson's disease is actually present. PD is in fact the major cause of parkinsonism; however, the administration of major tranquilizers, such as haloperidol and phenothiazines, may produce similar symptoms. Other neurodegenerative illnesses may also have parkinsonian features, such as FTD with motor neuron disease, corticobasal degeneration, DLB, and progressive supranuclear palsy (Fahn, 2003). PD is found worldwide and is estimated to affect 500,000 to 1 million Americans. Onset of symptoms usually occurs between 60 and 69 years of age. About 5% of cases occur before 40 years of age (Burke & Laramie, 2004; Fahn, 2003).

PD is degenerative, involving the basal ganglia and the extrapyramidal nervous system. The basal ganglia contain short anatomical pathways that connect the basal ganglionic structures to the cerebral cortex and to specific cortical and brainstem structures through the thalamus. This interconnecting system has an important role in modifying posture for cortically induced movements. Loss of dopaminergic neurons in the substantia nigra causes a series of changes in the circuitry of the basal ganglia that leads to the motor disturbances of PD. Approximately 90% or more loss of dopamine produces the symptoms of parkinsonism. Symptoms do not usually appear until there is a loss of 70% of the neurons. Pathologically there are spherically shaped intracytoplasmic inclusions, Lewy bodies, present in the remaining neurons of the substantia nigra. Lewy bodies are present in the cerebral cortex in DLB. These Lewy bodies are identified at autopsy microscopically by staining with antibodies against the alpha-synuclein protein. Demyelination of the substantia nigra is visible on gross examination of brain tissue at autopsy.

The etiology of PD is unknown; aging changes, environmental factors, and genetic factors are being investigated. Although PD is primarily sporadic, recent discovery of rare genetic forms of PD may lead to a better understanding of the underlying pathophysiology of PD (Guttman, Kish, & Furukawa, 2003; Meara, 2003).

Symptoms and Clinical Presentation. PD has
an insidious onset with nonspecific complaints of easy fatigability and general malaise initially that often delay diagnosis. Parkinson's disease is characterized by tremor; a slow, progressive rigidity of the limbs and trunk; and decreased voluntary movements. The tremor is typically rapid, rhythmic, and increased by stress. It usually begins unilaterally in the hand and progresses asymmetrically to other parts of the body (Meara, 2003; Rao et al., 2003). There is muscle rigidity, felt as increased resistance of muscle with passive movement by the examiner. A ratchet-like quality of resistance is sometimes called cogwheeling (Meara, 2003).

Bradykinesia (slowness of voluntary movement) or slowing of execution of movement occurs and may become so severe that the person is unable to initiate movements. Freezing ("feet glued to the floor") is present in the later stages of the disease and is noted when stepping onto a different flooring surface, negotiating a curb, or moving in limited spaces. Postural instability manifests as complaints of being unable to turn in bed or get out of a chair without difficulty. Gait may be slow to start, be short-stepped with shuffling, and have decreased arm swing. Gait changes of propulsion (inability to control forward movement) and retropulsion (inability to control backward movement) also occur as the disease progresses (Burke & Laramie, 2004; Fahn, 2003; Meara, 2003). These gait changes, postural instability, and forward-flexed posture place the older adult at risk for falls. Individuals have an expressionless face; whispered, muffled, and monotonous speech; excessive salivation; and reduced blinking. Handwriting becomes progressively smaller until it may be illegible.

Other symptoms frequently seen in PD include depression, anxiety, sleep disorders, constipation, autonomic disturbances, bladder and sexual dysfunction, and sensory complaints (pain, burning, tingling) of the extremities (Burke & Laramie, 2004; Fahn, 2003).

Dementia associated with PD is estimated to occur in about 40% of cases of PD. Pathologically, patients with PD who develop dementia have Lewy bodies present in the cerebral cortex. Risk factors for dementia include increased age and atypical presence of speech changes and axial involvement; severe motor involvement; rapid progression of PD; and presence of depression. Dementia caused by PD typically occurs in the later stages of the disease and is characterized by executive dysfunction, slowed motor and cognitive function, and memory impairment (American Psychiatric Association, 2000; Emre, 2003; Meara, 2003). Cognitive assessment demonstrates executive dysfunction; the inability to organize and plan goal-directed activity is the central feature of dementia caused by PD. The individual benefits from cueing, prompting to problem solve, and prompting to complete tasks. Behavioral and personality changes occur in dementia caused by PD, with increased incidence of depression and visual hallucinations when compared with the behavioral changes of AD (Emre, 2003).

Medications used to treat Parkinson's disease frequently produce side effects of confusion, disorientation, depression, excitement, and hallucinations, a drug-induced psychosis (Guttman et al., 2003; Meara, 2003). Reducing PD medications or using the most efficacious at the lowest doses may help alleviate drug-induced psychosis. Atypical antipsychotics that do not worsen PD symptoms (quetiapine and clozapine) are also used to treat this complication. The potential side effect of leukopenia in clozapine is monitored with frequent blood counts, and both quetiapine and clozapine are given at bedtime because of the side effect of drowsiness (Fahn, 2003; Meara, 2003).

Diagnosis of PD may be difficult in older adults because many of the usual signs and symptoms may be altered or masked. For example, the characteristic tremor may be completely absent, especially when the arms are resting in the person's lap. The flexed posture of the head, shoulders, and thorax; joint rigidity; and bradykinesia may be mistaken for changes associated with aging. In addition, the immobile appearance of the face may be considered a result of depression or deafness rather than Parkinson's disease.

Treatment. Interventions to manage PD should focus on improving the quality of life and maintaining/supporting function. Medication management should treat symptoms (motor and nonmotor) with the least amount of side effects. PD is a long-term illness with many different needs at various stages. A multidisciplinary approach is the most beneficial to meet these interventions. Physical therapy improves muscle tone and strength to enhance function in all stages of PD. Occupational therapy is important to assessing assistive devices for increased function, promotion of independence, and safety, as well as assessing and implementing plans for fall prevention and general safety in all settings. Speech therapy can assist early with communication enhancement and later for swallowing evaluation and safety considerations for diet choices if dysphagia becomes a problem. Social services can assist with increasing social and healthcare supports, as well as education and support for caregivers. Medications provide symptom management only; there is no cure or protective medication for PD. Medication management decisions are based on the level of disability of the individual produced by symptoms, age, and side effects of the medication. Management is an ongoing process with evaluation and adjustments necessary as the disease progresses and the needs of the individual change (Guttman et al., 2003; Meara, 2003).

Anticholinergics are beneficial for tremors in the early stages of the disease; however, they have little effect on rigidity, akinesia (absence of movements), and loss of postural reflexes. Drugs with anticholinergic effects that have been used include trihexyphenidyl (Artane), benztropine (Cogentin), procyclidine (Kemadrin), and antihistamines (Benadryl). Anticholinergics are less suitable for the older adult because of side effects of drowsiness, cognitive impairment, constipation, blurred vision, urinary retention, and aggravation of glaucoma (Guttman et al., 2003).

Amantadine is used in the earlier stages of the disease and has been found to improve akinesia, rigidity, and tremor. It is thought to act by blocking N-methyl-D-aspartate (NMDA) receptors and acetylcholine receptors, promoting release of dopamine from the intact dopaminergic terminals that remain in the basal ganglia. Side effects of the drug are cognitive impairment,

vivid hallucinations, slurred speech, tremor, ataxia, insomnia, depression, ankle edema, and restlessness. In addition, amantadine may exacerbate congestive heart failure (Fahn, 2003; Guttman et al., 2003).

Levodopa is the mainstay of PD therapy and is used by most individuals at some point in the disease. Levodopa increases the level of dopamine in the brain and is highly effective in relieving the symptoms of Parkinson's disease. Levodopa is commonly combined with carbidopa, which prevents the peripheral breakdown of levodopa (Guttman et al., 2003). Levodopa provides rapid improvement in gait, posture, balance, dressing, and handwriting, and productive life expectancy is prolonged to a degree. Initial doses are generally smaller in older people than in the young and are then increased slowly. Side effects of levodopa include nausea and vomiting, cardiac dysrhythmias, postural hypotension, dyskinesias (orofacial movements or choreiform movements involving the head, trunk, or limbs), confusion, and hallucinations. Long-term treatment with levodopa (5 to 7 years) produces fluctuations of effectiveness of the drug, "wearing off" of effects, and an "on-off" syndrome in which the effects intensify or disappear. When the natural dopamine exceeds 90%, levodopa is no longer effective (Fahn, 2003; Guttman et al., 2003, Meara, 2003).

Dopamine agonists are medications that directly stimulate dopamine receptors and are used early in PD to manage symptoms alone or are adjunctive therapy to reduce fluctuations of levodopa in the mild to moderate stages. These medications include bromocriptine (Parlodel), pergolide (Permax), pramipexole (Mirapex), and ropinirol (Requip). Side effects of this class of medications include dyskinesias, confusion, hallucinations, and postural hypotension (Fahn, 2003; Guttman et al., 2003; Meara, 2003).

A recent addition to the drugs available for Parkinson's disease is the catechol O-methyltransferase inhibitors. This class of medications is thought to increase levodopa pharmacokinetics, decreasing fluctuations and producing more "on time," or effectiveness of levodopa. Side effects include exacerbation of levodopa side effects, loose stools, and urine discoloration (Guttman et al., 2003).

Selegiline hydrochloride (Eldepryl), a monoamine oxidase inhibitor, may slow the progression of symptoms by inhibiting dopamine metabolism. It may also be used to boost the effectiveness of levodopa compounds. Side effects frequently include nausea, loose stools, and dizziness. Confusion, hallucinations, and vivid dreams may occur, and the patient may demonstrate signs of CNS depression or overstimulation. Selegiline should not be used in older adults with syncope or falls because of increased incidence of dementia and falls in this group of individuals (Burke & Laramie, 2004; Meara, 2003).

Deep brain stimulation (DBS) of the subthalamic nuclei, globus pallidum, or thalamus is a surgical management of PD. DBS usually improves bradykinesias, rigidity, and drug-induced dyskinesias when used in optimal candidates. These individuals are typically younger, have no cognitive impairments, and have tried all medications without success in controlling symptoms of PD. Transplantation of fetal cells is still investigational (Fahn, 2003; Meara, 2003).

Structural Abnormalities

Normal Pressure Hydrocephalus.
Normal pressure hydrocephalus (NPH) is referred to as a miscellaneous disorder causing dementia in the older adult. NPH is an obstruction of the flow and absorption of CSF that results in a normal high CSF pressure. The ventricles enlarge, exerting a force that compresses cerebral tissue. The etiology of NPH is most often unknown but can be a result of previous head trauma, resolved meningitis, subarachnoid hemorrhage of ruptured aneurysm, or changes in the skull related to Paget's disease (Arciniegas & Dubovsky, 2001; Victor & Ropper, 2001).

Gait changes, dementia, and urinary incontinence are the classic clinical findings of this disorder. The gait changes usually occur first and are a prominent finding. Initially the older adult has leg weakness and an impairment of balance; the unsteadiness is most notable when climbing stairs or stepping off a curb. Gait changes progress to a short-stepped, forward-flexed posture with unexplained falls. Other gait changes characteristic of NPH include walking as though the feet are stuck to the floor ("magnetic gait"). The cognitive changes of NPH have a rapid onset and are characterized as inattention, short-term memory loss, distractibility, poor judgment, lack of initiation, and disinhibition (Arciniegas & Dubovsky, 2001; Victor & Ropper, 2001). Urinary incontinence typically occurs last in the presentation of NPH, with urgency and frequency preceding loss of sphincter control (Victor & Ropper, 2001).

The diagnosis of NPH is based on history, physical changes, and neuroimaging. CT and MRI scans typically reveal ventricular enlargement that is disproportionate to cortical atrophy. Treatment of NPH is the surgical insertion of a ventriculoperitoneal shunt, which produces mixed results with alleviation of symptoms in about 20% of cases as reported by Victor and Ropper (2001). Older adults who have the best response to the shunting procedure are those who have prominent gait changes as the initial feature. Adults with coexisting cerebrovascular disease have lower response rates to shunting. Large-volume CSF drainage by lumbar puncture is a method used to determine if a shunting procedure will relieve the symptoms of NPH. The older adult is assessed with cognitive testing and a comprehensive physical therapy gait assessment before lumbar puncture.

Reassessment is completed several hours later and again after several days to assess for improvement of gait and cognitive changes. Those who have improvement are believed to be better candidates for the shunting procedure. The nurse has the opportunity to provide cognitive assessment and objective behavioral observation of the older adult during this preshunting procedure (Cammermeyer, 2001).

Subdural Hematoma.
A reversible cause of dementia in the older adult is chronic subdural hematoma. Younger adults usually have the clinically relevant acute subdural hematoma, with symptoms evolving over 72 hours. Chronic subdural hematomas are defined as greater than 20 days' duration and have a peak incidence in older adults between 60 and 70. Older persons are predisposed to chronic subdural hematoma because of the increased stress on the bridging cerebral veins with shrinkage of the brain away from the dura. The most common cause of subdural hematoma is trauma, representing about 75% of cases in the older adult. Sometimes the trauma can be so trivial that it is not remembered. Approximately 25% of subdural hematomas have no known etiology and are termed *spontaneous subdural hematomas.* Studies of spontaneous subdural hematomas identify an increased risk associated with the use of anticoagulant and antiplatelet therapy. Risk factors for development of chronic subdural hematoma include age, anticoagulation and antiplatelet therapy, male gender (higher trauma risk), and alcoholism. Alcoholics are at increased risk because of the susceptibility to trauma and the potential underlying liver disease and coagulation abnormalities (Chen & Levy, 2000; Karnath, 2004).

Common symptoms of chronic subdural hematoma include headache, altered mental status, gait changes or ataxia, aphasia, and hemiparesis. The presentation of chronic subdural hematoma mimics other neurological diseases, including dementia, stroke, tumors, and NPH. A history of the onset and time course of symptoms aids in the differentiation of chronic subdural hematoma from these other neurological conditions. Chronic subdural hematoma causes mental status changes that develop over the course of 2 to 6 weeks, may have focal neurological signs, and usually does not have urinary incontinence as an initial feature (NPH). The diagnosis of subdural hematoma is made with neuroimaging of the brain. Brain MRI is the most sensitive diagnostic tool for subdural hematomas of all densities (varies depending on the age of the hematoma); however, CT is more readily available and does not require sedation of the restless patient (Baum et al., 2002; Karnath, 2004).

Surgical intervention to drain the hematoma is the preferred treatment for subdural hematomas. Conservative medical management, hospitalization with serial CT scans, and a trial of steroids can be used in patients who have only mild neurological symptoms (headache without focal deficits or memory changes). The hospital stay can be 1 to 4 weeks for the medical management intervention compared to 1 week with surgical intervention. Risk factors for a poor prognosis include decreased level of consciousness, shorter duration of hematoma (2 to 3 weeks), and age greater than 80. Overall mortality rates are approximately 30% (Karnath, 2004).

Brain Tumors. The overall incidence of brain tumors is increasing, with the highest increase in incidence in adults over age 60 (Flowers, 2000; Hess, Broglio, & Bondy, 2004; Pilkington, 2001). National Cancer Institute statistics reflect a sevenfold increase in incidence of primary brain tumors in people over 70 from 1970 to 1990 (Flowers, 2000). In older adults the most common brain tumors are metastatic tumors, malignant gliomas (particularly glioblastoma multiforme), acoustic neuromas (schwannomas), and meningiomas. Studies report that approximately 25% of cancers metastasize to the brain and surrounding structures. The most common metastatic tumors to the skull and dura originate from breast cancer, prostate cancer, and multiple myeloma. Metastases to the brain originate most commonly from lung cancer, followed by (from most common to least common) breast cancer, melanoma, gastrointestinal tract cancers (colon, rectal), and kidney cancer (Pilkington, 2001; Victor & Ropper, 2001). The most common primary tumor in older adults is malignant glioma (Flowers, 2000; Hess et al., 2004). Factors for the increased incidence of these tumors are not fully understood, but environmental agents such as pesticides and radiation exposure, history of previous head radiation therapy, family history of malignancy, and better diagnostic techniques are being investigated (Flowers, 2000; Pilkington, 2001).

Presentation of brain tumors depends on location and size. Generally, symptoms include headache (persistent and localized), seizures, gait changes, short-term memory loss, and intellectual decline over a short period of time. Diffuse presentations that might resemble a rapid dementia include headache, nervousness, depressed mood, memory changes, and confusion (Victor & Ropper, 2001). Diagnosis of brain tumor in the older adult sometimes is delayed because of these vague presentations. The presentation of acoustic neuromas includes vertigo, sudden unilateral hearing loss, and possible mild facial weakness. MRI and contrast-enhanced CT scans are used most often for neuroimaging diagnosis of brain tumors. Pathological diagnosis is made by examination of the tumor tissue (Victor & Ropper, 2001).

Treatment is determined by tumor type and location, neurological status, and age of the older adult, along with the factor of life expectancy. Coexisting medical conditions and medications are also important factors to consider in the treatment plan (Flowers, 2000). The benign tumors, acoustic neuromas, and meningiomas are managed conservatively depending on symptoms. Gliomas typically are treated aggressively with surgery, radiation therapy, and chemotherapy. Corticosteroid therapy and diuretics are used as needed to control the edema and mass effect of tumors. Age is a factor in survival rates of brain tumors. For example, Flowers (2000) cites Surveillance, Epidemiology and End Results (SEER) data for 1973–1991 to reflect a 5-year survival rate of people over 55 with glioblastoma multiforme to be 1% compared with 10% in people 35 to 54 and 20% in people younger than 35.

Goals of nursing intervention include optimizing the older person's physical performance status, minimizing the side effects of medical treatment, and treating the symptoms of the tumor (Flowers, 2000). Education regarding the treatment choices and quality-of-life issues, ensuring that rehabilitation therapies are in place to optimize physical function, and assessing for reactive depression are important factors in providing nursing care (Flowers, 2000).

NURSING CARE
Assessment

Normal aging changes in mobility, coordination, balance, sensation, and cognitive performance are a consequence of the structural and functional changes in the nervous system. A comprehensive and systematic assessment of the nervous system is critical to distinguish between normal aging and disease in the older adult. Comprehensive neurological assessment and appropriate intervention can have a dramatic impact on the quality of life of older adults. The detection, evaluation, and treatment of vision or hearing loss permit treatment of sensory impairment, thereby increasing quality of life. Gait evaluation can uncover causes of unsteadiness and prevent falls. Early identification of cognitive impairment can lead to earlier treatment options and utilization of social supports to improve quality of life for the older adult with dementia (Kane et al., 2004). This assessment will enable the nurse to do the following:

- Describe the older adult's response to changes in function as a result of the aging process and chronic disease states of the nervous system.
- Formulate tentative nursing diagnostic statements in relation to the functional patterns of health perception–health maintenance, cognition and perception, and activity and rest.
- Refer the patient to other health professionals for further assessment of selected neurological problems, such as gait disturbance, tremor, or cognitive impairment.

The neurological system is complex, and many factors make the neurological assessment of the older adult challenging. First, there are age-related changes to consider. The complaints or symptoms of older adults are often vague and nonspecific. Older adults may attribute change to old age rather than illness and so may underreport or be reluctant to share symptoms or changes. Older adults may need more time to build a trusting relationship than younger persons. Older persons may become fatigued more easily, and, because neuronal functions are associated with a refractory period, fatigue must be considered in the assessment. For example, repetitive testing of a simple reflex over a short period of time, such as pupillary response or deep tendon reflex,

may result in an inaccurate conclusion that the reflex is sluggish when in reality an inadequate refractory period has elapsed. Medication effect is also often an important factor when assessing the neurological function of the older adult. Medications can affect neurological system findings, as well as the functional performance. Careful review with thought to effect of the medication on the neurological system is an important part of nursing assessment.

The unique characteristics of the nervous system also influence the assessment. First, because it is not possible to observe directly neuronal structure or activity, indirect measures of neurological function must be used. Many different methods may be used to assess a particular

---

Box 14-11 Neurological Assessment

Health History
Chief complaint
Family history:
- Any neurological conditions
- Age of onset in the affected individual

Social history:
- Education
- Occupation—retirement and circumstances
- Living arrangements
- Use and availability of social support
- Usual hobbies/community activities—history of changes from usual ability
- Driving status—change from usual ability

Medical history:
- Hospitalizations/surgeries
- Comprehensive review of systems
- Language changes
- Mobility changes
- Cognitive status—baseline and any changes
- Sleep/rest patterns
- Usual weight/weight changes

Medications:
- Prescription
- Over-the-counter
- Nutritional supplements

Personality/behavior:
- Baseline
- Noted changes

Functional assessment:
- ADLs (baseline and noted changes)
- IADLs (baseline and noted changes)

Physical Examination
Level of consciousness
Mental status
Language

Cranial nerves (CNs):
- CN I: Olfactory—sense of smell
- CN II: Optic—visual fields, visual acuity
- CN III: Oculomotor—eyelid movement, pupil responses to light
- CNs III, IV, and VI: Oculomotor, trochlear, abducens—extraocular movements
- CN V: Trigeminal—mastication, facial sensory
- CN VII: Facial—facial motor
- CN VIII: Acoustic—balance and hearing
- CNs IX and X: Glossopharyngeal and vagus—sensory taste, swallow, and gag
- CN XI: Spinal accessory—movement and strength of sternocleidomastoid and trapezius muscles
- CN XII: Hypoglossal—tongue movement

Proprioception and cerebellar function:
- Balance
- Gait
- Fine motor skills

Sensory function
- Superficial touch
- Pain
- Joint position
- Vibratory sense
- Cortical sensory functions
- Stereognosis
- Graphesthesia
- Two-point discrimination

Reflexes
- Deep tendon reflexes
- Plantar reflex (Babinski sign)

Motor function
- Muscle tone
- Muscle strength
- Abnormal motor: tremor, bradykinesia, extrapyramidal

Adapted from Seidel, H. M., Ball, J. W., Dains, J. E., & Benedict, G. W. (1999). *Mosby's guide to physical examination* (4th ed.). St. Louis: Mosby; and Haymore, J. (2004). A neuron in a haystack: Advanced neurologic assessment. *AACN Clinical Issues, 15*(4), 568-581.

domain of function. For example, the simple act of undressing can reveal loss of fine motor function, confusion, visual defects, loss of balance and equilibrium, and stiffness. Second, because neurological functions interrelate with other body system functions, the integrity of the other systems must be considered. Third, the nervous system is characterized by considerable redundancy. Because of this phenomenon, the body often is able to compensate for neuronal loss. Thus a loss of structural integrity does not necessarily lead to a concomitant loss of function. The performance of a functional assessment is an important factor in neurological assessment. Functional assessment is discussed in Chapter 2.

The neurological assessment may have to be prioritized and collected over time. Time constraints may limit data gathering because of slowed responses or limited time allowed during the first encounter. In some cases it is desirable to assess over a period of time and in various locations to validate assessment results or to note the effect of the environment on the assessment situation. Factors influencing the setting of priorities are the prevalence of the problem, the effect of the problem on functional ability, the effect of the problem on patient goals, the ease with which data can be gathered, and the potential for solving the problem.

History. The history information for the neurological assessment should be comprehensive in scope. An important factor when collecting history information for the older adult is the use of a collateral source, particularly when a change in cognitive abilities is suspected. A collateral source is an individual who knows the patient well and can provide information about the patient's usual ability, changes that have occurred in ability, and the time course of the change. Cacchione, Powlishta, Grant, Buckles, and Morris (2003) demonstrated that collateral sources were able to accurately distinguish normal aging from dementia even in the earliest stages of the disease with the use of a semistructured interview. This study demonstrated that the optimal collateral source has a spousal relationship and lives with the individual, but the frequency of contact with the patient was the key factor in accuracy of the collateral source. Another important component in the history is to assess for change in ability from baseline performance. The comprehensive history is outlined in Box 14-11. Important neurological symptoms to investigate include history of sleep patterns, vision or hearing changes, gait changes and fall history, and any focal symptoms.

Physical Assessment. A thorough physical assessment of the neurological system includes examination of level of consciousness, mental status, cranial nerves, language, sensation, movement and coordination, reflexes, functional status, praxis, and potential for rehabilitation. A focused and systematic approach to

---

BOX 14-12 Common Age-Related Changes in the Neurological Physical Assessment of Older Adults

- Decreased sense of smell and taste (sweet and salt diminish first)
- Decreased ability to differentiate colors
- Reduced upward gaze
- Slower adjustment to lighting changes
- Diminished corneal reflex
- Hearing loss in middle- to high-frequency ranges
- Reduced gag reflex
- Gait changes of advanced age: short, uncertain steps; decreased speed and balance; flexion of legs at knees and hips
- Stronger stimuli necessary to detect sensation
- Impaired vibratory and position sense
- Less brisk response of deep tendon reflexes, present in lower extremities before upper extremities
- Absent or difficult to elicit Achilles and plantar reflexes
- Increased incidence of essential tremor
- Impaired fine motor abilities

Data from Seidel, H. M., Ball, J. W., Dains, J. E., & Benedict, G. W. (2006). *Mosby's guide to physical examination* (6th ed.). St. Louis: Mosby.

the neurological examination is important. Box 14-11 illustrates the components of the physical assessment of the neurological system, and Box 14-12 describes the normal age-related changes in the neurological physical assessment of older adults.

Nursing Diagnoses

Nursing diagnoses common to older adults with neurological disorders include the following:

- Communication, impaired verbal, related to aphasia, decreased speech volume, slowness of speech
- Physical mobility, impaired, related to neuromuscular impairment, musculoskeletal impairment, decreased motor agility, and muscle weakness
- Nutrition, altered: less than body requirements, related to chewing or swallowing difficulties, cognitive impairment

---

BOX 14-13 *TOWARD BETTER NEUROLOGICAL HEALTH*

- Protect yourself from excessive stress (e.g., extreme heat or cold, extreme exercise)
- Engage in mentally challenging activities
- Exercise regularly
- Go to bed and get up the same time each day
- Wear glasses and/or hearing aids as needed
- Adhere to prescribed treatments for hypertension, diabetes, and hyperlipidemia

- Self-care deficit: feeding, bathing/hygiene, dressing/grooming, toileting, related to cognitive or neuromuscular impairment
- Sensory-perceptual alterations: kinesthetic, perception, related to neuropathies, immobility

- Sensory perception, disturbed, related to aging process
- Sleep pattern disturbance related to medications (tranquilizers, sedatives, hypnotics), neurological impairments, age-related sleep stage shifts, external factors

Nursing Care Plan: The Older Adult with Sleep Deprivation

Data

An 85-year-old woman who lives alone in her own home. Loss of spouse of 62 years 2 months ago; medical history of stable hypertension, osteoporosis with compression fracture 1 month ago. Medications: Fosamax, Tylenol PM, lisinopril, multivitamin, calcium with vitamin D.

Assessment

Patient reports decreased sleep—increased difficulty in falling asleep, frequent nighttime awakenings, daytime drowsiness, lethargy, and decreased ability to carry out usual daytime activities. She feels sluggish and has difficulty concentrating. She has stopped her usual volunteer activities and bridge participation.

Nursing Diagnoses

Sleep disturbance related to prolonged physical/psychological discomfort.

Goals/Outcomes

The patient will report less nighttime awakening, falling asleep without difficulty, and less daytime fatigue such that she is able to resume her usual daytime activities.

NOC Suggested Outcomes

Rest
Sleep
Mood Equilibrium

NIC Suggested Interventions

Major interventions: Energy Management (0180), Sleep Enhancement (1850), Coping Enhancement (5230)

- Determine causes of fatigue (e.g., treatments, pain, medications).
- Approximate patient's regular sleep-wake cycle in planning care.
- Monitor/record patient's sleep pattern and number of sleep hours.
- Monitor patient for evidence of excess physical and emotional fatigue.
- Monitor patient's sleep pattern, and note physical or psychological circumstances that interrupt sleep.
- Encourage alternate rest and activity periods.
- Adjust environment (light, noise, temperature, mattress, and bed) to promote sleep.

- Monitor participation in fatigue-producing activities during wakefulness to prevent overtiredness.
- Encourage patient to establish a bedtime routine to facilitate transition from wakefulness to sleep.
- Facilitate maintenance of patient's usual bedtime routines (e.g., book to read).
- Assist to eliminate stressful situations before bedtime.
- Instruct patent to avoid bedtime foods and beverages that interfere with sleep.
- Assist patient to limit daytime sleep by providing activity that promotes wakefulness as appropriate.
- Provide calming diversionary activities to promote relaxation.
- Instruct patient how to perform autogenic muscle relaxation or other nonpharmacological forms of sleep inducement.
- Initiate/implement comfort measures of massage, positioning, and affective touch.
- Group care activities to minimize number of awakenings and allow for sleep cycles of at least 90 minutes.
- Adjust medication administration schedule to support patient's sleep-wake cycle.
- Encourage use of sleep medications that do not contain REM sleep suppressors.
- Regulate environmental stimuli to maintain normal day-night cycles.
- Seek to understand the patient's perception of a stressful situation.
- Encourage the use of spiritual resources if desired.
- Explore with the patient previous methods of dealing with life problems.
- Encourage the verbalization of feelings, perceptions, and fears.
- Assist the patient in identifying appropriate short- and long-term goals.
  Other relevant interventions: Anxiety Reduction, Environmental Management: Comfort, Simple Relaxation Therapy, Touch, Grief Work Facilitation, Pain Management.

Evaluation Parameters

Rest: amount of rest, rest pattern, rest quality, physically rested, mentally rested, emotionally rested.

Sleep: hours of sleep (at least 5 hr/24 hr), sleep pattern, sleep quality, sleep efficiency (ratio of sleep time/total time trying), feels rejuvenated after sleep, wakeful at appropriate times.

- Confusion, chronic, related to dementia
- Confusion, acute, related to delirium, dementia
- Falls, risk for, related to impaired physical mobility, impaired balance, proprioceptive deficits, neuropathy, cognitive impairment, medications, environment
- Thermoregulation, ineffective, related to aging process, medications, environment
- Disturbed thought processes related to delirium or dementia

- Violence, risk for self-directed or directed at others, related to inability to control behavior secondary to dementia, delusional thinking
- Environmental interpretation, impaired, related to cognitive impairment
- Wandering related to cognitive impairment
- Health maintenance, ineffective, related to lack of ability to make deliberate and thoughtful judgments, perceptual or cognitive impairment, ineffective family

Nursing Care Plan: The Older Adult with Wandering Behavior

Data

A 78-year-old man with history of Alzheimer's disease for 7 years, now in moderate stage. No other chronic physical illness. Lives at home with spouse of 52 years; they have recently moved to a smaller home. A retired bank executive, he was very social and outgoing. Medications: Aricept, Namenda, multivitamin, Seroquel twice a day, and trazodone at bedtime.

Assessment

Global cognitive impairment and prominent expressive aphasia. MMSE 7, language deficits interfering with testing ability. Functional incontinence. Height, 6 ft; weight, 165 lb, down 15 lb in the last 6 months.

Caregiver history of frequent ambulation from room to room, opening and closing doors that lasts minutes to hours and is repeated at intervals through the day with increasing frequency at meals and bedtime. This behavior is not easily redirected. The caregiver is very concerned about elopement.

Nursing Diagnoses

Wandering related to cognitive impairment

Goals/Outcomes

Patient will be free of falls, have no incidence of elopement, and maintain appropriate body weight. The caregiver will be able to provide a safe environment.

NOC Suggested Outcomes

Caregiver Home Care Readiness
Fall Prevention Behavior
Falls Occurrence

NIC Suggested Interventions

Major interventions: Dementia Management (6460)
- Structure environment such that important destinations are visible and close together.
- Position individuals within visible range of important destinations, such as the bathroom.

- Minimize distractions, especially when they are en route to a desirable destination.
- Interrupt or distract wandering that continues over an extended period or increases anxiety.
- Keep undesired destinations out of sight.
- Provide rest periods.
- Substitute social interaction and structured activities.
- Ascertain and address any underlying problems or concerns.
- Offer comfort and stress-reducing strategies (e.g., music, massage).
- Try signs or labels.
- Substitute repetitive behavior with another (e.g., folding, sorting items, rocking).
- Provide a regularly scheduled and supervised exercise or walking program.
- Modify the environment to protect the patient and prevent elopement.
- Enroll in the Alzheimer's Association's Safe Return Program.
- Develop a plan of action with the caregiver in the event of elopement.
- Teach the caregiver the meaning of wandering behavior.
- Teach the caregiver interventions to manage wandering behavior.
- Refer to occupational therapy for home assessment and environmental adaptations.
- Encourage the caregiver to utilize caregiver support groups and respite services.

Other relevant interventions: Nutrition Management, Urinary Habit Training, Urinary Incontinence Care, Fall Prevention, Caregiver Lifestyle Disruption, Caregiver Stressors, Environmental Management, Surveillance: Safety.

Evaluation Parameters

No elopement, no falls, appropriate weight maintained, physical/psychosocial needs are met, decreased frequency of wandering behavior.

coping, functional dependency, confusion, and immobility
- Home maintenance management, impaired, related to chronic debilitating disease, impaired mental status, unavailable support system, sensory deficits, and immobility
- Family coping: compromised, ineffective, disabling, related to role change, prolonged disease progression that exhausts supportive capacity
- Caregiver role strain, risk for, related to lack of knowledge regarding illness, lack of knowledge regarding resources for support, burden of providing care

Nursing Goals

General goals/outcomes of nursing related to the nursing diagnoses include the following:
- Effective communication
- Mobility (independent, assistive devices, total)
- Self-care: activities of daily living, dressing, grooming, bathing, hygiene, eating, toileting
- Nutritional status: food and fluid intake
- Weight control
- Vision compensation behavior
- Hearing compensation behavior

Nursing Care Plan: The Patient with Parkinson's Disease

Data

A 68-year-old man with history of Parkinson's disease. Lives alone in assisted living setting; admitted to hospital to after repeated falls. Medications: Sinemet, multivitamin.

Assessment

Ambulation is walker assisted. Gait is shuffling, forward flexed with unsteady five-point turn. Slow to rise from chair and uses both arms to "push off" to stand. Arrests ongoing movement when confronted with doorways and floor surface changes. The patient communicates verbally without problem, and no swallowing concerns are noted by the patient or caregivers at present.

Blood pressure (BP) while lying supine, 140/70 mm Hg, heart rate (HR) 72 beats per minute; BP while sitting, 134/70 mm Hg, HR 88 beats per minute; BP while standing, 110/60 mm Hg, HR 90 beats per minute, accompanied by symptoms of dizziness and lightheadedness.

Nursing Diagnoses

Risk for falls related to orthostatic hypotension, impaired mobility, balance, and gait.

Goals/Outcomes

The patient will remain free of falls. The environment will be changed to minimize incidence of falls.

NOC Suggested Outcomes

Fall Prevention Behavior

NIC Suggested Interventions

Major interventions: Fall Prevention (6490); Surveillance Safety (6654)
- Monitor gait, balance, and fatigue level with ambulation.
- Rehabilitation consult referral to evaluate appropriate use and safety of mobility assistance devices.
- Encourage patient to use cane or walker as appropriate.
- Mark doorway thresholds and edges of steps as needed.
- Occupational therapy referral for home assessment and modification recommendations for safety and bathroom.
- Monitor patient for alterations in physical or cognitive function that might lead to unsafe behavior.
- Monitor environment for potential safety hazards.
- Provide appropriate level of supervision/surveillance to monitor patient and to allow for therapeutic actions as needed.
- Place patient in least restrictive environment that allows the necessary level of observation.
- Communicate information about patient's risk to other nursing staff/assisted living facility staff.
- Teach patient interventions to minimize orthostatic hypotension:
  - Increase fluid and salt intake.
  - Have a drink of clear liquid, tea, or coffee before rising and sit on the edge of the bed for 5 to 10 minutes before standing.
  - Remain seated for 20 to 30 minutes after a main meal or dose of medication and for a few minutes after a bowel movement.
  - Sit down to towel off after a hot bath or shower and to urinate (men and women).
  - Stay out of the hot sun.
  - Never stand still (particularly after exercise) to prevent blood pooling in legs.
  - Take medications with food.

Other relevant interventions: Mutual Goal Setting, Self-Responsibility Facilitation.

Evaluation Parameters

Decreased occurrence of falls, increased fall prevention behavior, environmental changes to minimize incidence of falls, patient demonstrates knowledge of methods to prevent falls/injury.

- Rest
- Sleep
- Cognitive orientation
- Distorted thought self-control
- Information processing
- Memory
- Fall prevention behavior
- Safe home environment
- Neurological status: consciousness
- Caregiver home care readiness
- Health-promoting behavior
- Health-seeking behavior
- Caregiver emotional health
- Caregiver performance: direct care, indirect care
- Caregiver physical health
- Role performance
- Family coping
- Leisure participation
- Social support
- Psychosocial safety
- Self-care: instrumental activities of daily living

Nursing Interventions and Evaluation

Nursing interventions for neurological disorders are aimed at promoting safety, maintaining functional independence in the older adult for as long as possible, providing support for family members, and helping caregivers with the management of the symptoms of the neurological diseases. An ongoing evaluation of the neurological status of the individual helps determine whether the condition is acute or reversible and aids in planning and revising interventions to meet the goals of nursing care. Caregivers can be referred to a number of national organizations such as the Alzheimer's Association, Alzheimer's Disease Education and Referral Center (ADEAR), or Parkinson's Association for information on the disease, research findings, and specific strategies for care (Box 14-13).

Evaluation is based on the success with which the older adults are able to safely maintain function and the attainment of social supports for both individuals and families.

SUMMARY

Age-related changes in the nervous system are frequently attributed to disease states, and therefore many people believe that these changes are an inevitable consequence of older age. In fact, the normal changes that take place have little effect on thinking and cognition. Structural changes that occur with normal aging include loss of neurons and brain weight, accumulations of lipofuscin granules in nerve cells, slowed synaptic transmissions, and loss of peripheral nerve function. Functional changes include slowed reaction time, a decline in

proprioceptive capacities, impaired thermoregulation, and altered sleep patterns.

The nervous system is complex, and the common disorders of the nervous system (delirium, dementia, and Parkinson's disease) are challenging. These conditions cause motor impairments, as well as impairments in cognition, reasoning, judgment, and orientation, which in turn cause declines in functional status. As the burden of caregiving falls to the families of these individuals, nursing care must involve provision of support and encouragement to these individuals, as well as the impaired older adult.

REFERENCES

Abrass, I. B. (2003). Disorders of temperature regulation. In W. R. Hazzard, J. P. Blass, J. B. Halter, et al. (Eds.), *Principles of geriatric medicine and gerontology* (5th ed.). New York: McGraw-Hill.

Agostini, J. V., & Inouye, S. K. (2003). Delirium. In W. R. Hazzard, J. P. Blass, J. B. Halter, et al. (Eds.), *Principles of geriatric medicine and gerontology* (5th ed.). New York: McGraw-Hill.

AGS Clinical Practice Committee. (2003). Guidelines abstracted for the American Academy of Neurology's dementia guidelines for early detection, diagnosis, and management of dementia. *Journal of the American Geriatrics Society, 51*(6), 869-873.

American Psychiatric Association (APA). (1994). *Diagnostic and statistical manual of mental disorders* (4th ed.). Washington, DC: American Psychiatric Association.

American Psychiatric Association (APA). (2000). *Diagnostic and statistical manual of mental disorders* (4th ed., text revision). Washington, DC: American Psychiatric Association.

Arciniegas, D. B., & Dubovsky, S. L. (2001). Dementia due to other medical conditions and dementia due to multiple etiologies. In G. O. Gabbard (Ed.), *Treatment of psychiatric disorders* (3rd ed.). Washington, DC: American Psychiatric Press.

Bacchetti, P. (2003, December). Age and variant Creutzfeldt-Jakob disease. *Emering Infectious Diseases.* Retrieved June 5, 2005, from www.cdc.gov/ncidod/EID/vol9no12/03-0361.htm.

Baum, T., Capezuti, E., & Driscoll, G. (2002). Falls. In V. T. Cotter & N. E. Stumpf (Eds.), *Advanced practice nursing with older adults: Clinical guidelines.* New York: McGraw-Hill.

Beck, C. K. (2004, September). Managing behavioral symptoms in persons with dementia. Improving chronic care quality. A National Conference on Transferring Geriatric Research into Practice, University of Missouri, Columbia.

Beck, C. K., & Vogelpohl, T. S. (1999). Problematic vocalizations in institutionalized individuals with dementia. *Journal of Gerontological Nursing, 25*(9), 17-26.

Brotons, M., & Koger, S. M. (2000). The impact of music therapy on language functioning in dementia. *Journal of Music Therapy, 37*(3), 183-195.

Burke, M. M., & Laramie, J. A. (2004). *Primary care of the older adult* (2nd ed.). St. Louis: Mosby.

Cacchione, P. Z., Powlishta, K. K., Grant, E. A., Buckles, V. D., & Morris, J. C. (2003). Accuracy of collateral source reports in very mild to mild dementia of the Alzheimer type. *Journal of the American Geriatrics Society, 51*(6), 819-823.

Cammermeyer, M. (2001). Assessment of cognition. In C. Stewart-Amidei & J. A. Kunkel (Eds.), *AANN's neuroscience nursing: Human responses to neurologic dysfunction* (2nd ed.). Philadelphia: W. B. Saunders.

Chen, J. T., & Levy, M. L. (2000). Causes, epidemiology, and risk factors of chronic subdural hematoma. *Neurosurgery Clinics of North America, 11*(3), 399-406.

Cohen-Mansfield, J. (2001). Nonpharmacologic interventions for inappropriate behaviors in dementia; a review, summary, and critique. *American Journal of Geriatric Psychiatry, 9*(4), 361-381.

Cohen-Zion, M., & Ancoli-Israel, S. (2003). Sleep disorders. In W. R. Hazzard, J. P. Blass, J. B. Halter, et al. (Eds.), *Principles of geriatric medicine and gerontology* (5th ed.). New York: McGraw-Hill.

Cotter, V. T. (2002). Dementia. In V.T. Cotter & N.E. Strumpf (Eds.), *Advanced practice nursing with older adults: Clinical guidelines*. New York: McGraw Hill.

Craft, S., Cholerton, B., & Reger, M. (2003). Aging and cognition: What is normal? In W. R. Hazzard, J. P. Blass, J. B. Halter, et al. (Eds.), *Principles of geriatric medicine and gerontology* (5th ed.). New York: McGraw-Hill.

Cummings, J. L. (1997). The Neuropsychiatric Inventory: Assessing psychopathology in dementia patients. *Neurology, 48*(5 suppl 6), S10-S16.

Cummings, J. L., & Cole, G. (2002). Alzheimer disease. *Journal of the American Medical Association, 287*, 2335-2338.

DeKosky, S. T. (2003). Pathology and pathways of Alzheimer's disease with an update on new developments in treatment. *Journal of the American Geriatrics Society, 51*(5), S314-S320.

Doody, R. S., Stevens, J. C., Beck, C., Dubinsky, R. M., Kaye, J. A., Gwyther, L., et al. (2001). Practice parameter: Management of dementia (an evidence-based review). Report of the Quality Standard Subcommittee of the American Academy of Neurology. *Neurology, 56*(9), 1154-1166.

Duchek, J. M., Carr, D. B., Hunt, L., Roe, C. M., Xiong, C., Shah, K., & Morris, J. C. (2003). Longitudinal driving performance in early-stage dementia of the Alzheimer type. *Journal of the American Geriatrics Society, 51*(10), 1499-1501.

Duckett, S. (2002). The normal human brain. In S. Duckett & J. C. da la Torre (Eds.), *Pathology of the aging human nervous system* (2nd ed.). New York: Oxford University Press.

Emre, M. (2003). Dementia associated with Parkinson's disease. *Lancet, 2*, 229-237.

Fahn, S. (2003). Parkinson's disease and related disorders. In W. R. Hazzard, J. P. Blass, J. B. Halter, et al. (Eds.), *Principles of geriatric medicine and gerontology* (5th ed.). New York: McGraw-Hill.

Feldman, H., Gauthier, S., Hecker, J., Vellas, B., Imir, B., Mastey, V., & Subbiah, P. (2003). Efficacy of donepezil on maintenance of activities of daily living in patients with moderate to severe Alzheimer's disease and the effect on caregiver burden. *Journal of the American Geriatrics Society, 51*(6), 737-744.

Ferman, T. J., Smith, G. E., Boeve, B. F., Ivnik, R. J., Petersen, R. C., Knopman, D., et al. (2004). DLB fluctuations: Specific features that reliably differentiate DLB from AD and normal aging. *Neurology, 62*, 181-187.

Flaherty, J. H., Tariq, S. H., Raghavan, S., Bakshi, S., Moinuddin, A., & Morley, J. E. (2003). A model for managing delirious older inpatients. *Journal of the American Geriatrics Society, 51*(7), 1031-1035.

Flowers, A. (2000). Brain tumors in the older person. *Cancer Control, 7*(6), 523-538.

Folstein, M. F., Folstein, S. E., & McHugh, P. R. (1975). "Mini-Mental State": A practical method for grading the cognitive state of patients for the clinician. *Journal of Psychiatric Research, 12*, 189-198.

Fuzhong, L., Fisher, K. J., Harmer, P., Irbe, D., Tearse, R. G., & Weimer, C. (2004). Tai Chi and self-rated quality of sleep and daytime sleepiness in older adults: A randomized controlled trial. *Journal of the American Geriatrics Society, 52*(6), 892-900.

Galvin, J. E., Powlishta, K. K., Wilkins, K., McKeel, D. W., Xiong, C., Grant, E., et al. (2005). Predictors of preclinical Alzheimer's disease and dementia: A clinicopathologic study. *Archives of Neurology, 62*(5), 758-765.

Guttman, M., Kish, S. J., & Furukawa, Y. (2003). Current concepts in the diagnosis and management of Parkinson's disease. *Canadian Medical Association Journal, 168*(3), 293-301.

Hall, G. R., & Buckwalter, K. C. (1987). Progressively lowered stress threshold: A conceptual mode for care of adults with Alzheimer's disease. *Archives of Psychiatric Nursing, 1*, 399-406.

Hawkins, C., & Shannon, P. (2002). Pathology of the skeletal muscle in aging. In S. Duckett & J. C. da la Torre (Eds.), *Pathology of the aging human nervous system* (2nd ed.). New York: Oxford University Press.

Haymore, J. (2004). A neuron in a haystack: Advanced neurologic assessment. *AACN Clinical Issues, 15*(4), 568-581.

Hess, K. R., Broglio, K. R., & Bondy, M. L. (2004). Adult glioma incidence trends in the United States, 1977-2000. *Cancer, 101*(10), 2293-2299.

Hill, K., & Schwarz, J. (2004). Assessment and management of falls in older people. *Internal Medicine, 34*, 447-564.

Hill-O'Neill, K. A., & Shaughnessy, M. (2002). Dizziness and stroke. In V. T. Cotter & N. E. Strumpf (Eds.), *Advanced practice nursing with older adults: Clinical guidelines*. New York: McGraw-Hill.

Hoffman, S. (2003). Sleep in the older adult: Implications for nurses. *Geriatric Nursing, 24*(4), 210-216.

Hughes, C. P., Berg, L., Danziger, W. L., Coben, L. A., & Martin, R. L. (1982). A new clinical scale for the staging of dementia. *British Journal of Psychiatry, 140*, 566-572.

Hwang, J., Yang, C., Lee, T., & Tsai, S. (2003). The efficacy and safety of olanzapine for the treatment of geriatric psychosis. *Journal of Clinical Psychopharmacology, 23*(2), 113-118.

Inouye, D. K., Bogardus, S. T., Williams, C. S., Leo-Summers, L., & Agostini, J. V. (2003). The role of adherence on the effectiveness of nonpharmacologic interventions. *Archives of Internal Medicine, 163*(4), 958-964.

Inouye, S. K. (2003). Delirium. In C. K. Cassel (Ed.), *Geriatric medicine: An evidence-based approach*. New York: Springer-Verlag.

Inouye, S. K., Foreman, M. D., Mion, L. C., Katz, K. H., & Cooney, L. M. (2001). Nurses' recognition of delirium and its symptoms. *Archives of Internal Medicine, 161*, 2467-2473.

Inouye, S. K., vanDyck, C. H., Alessi, C. A., Balkin, S., Siegel, A. P., & Horwitz, R. I. (1990). Clarifying confusion: The Confusion Assessement Method—a new method for detection of delirium. *Annals of Internal Medicine, 113*, 941-948.

Insel, K. C., & Badger, T. A. (2002). Deciphering the 4 D's. *Journal of Advanced Nursing, 38*(4), 360-368.

Kane, R. L., Ouslander, J. G., & Abrass, I. B. (2004). *Essentials of clinical geriatrics* (5th ed.). New York: McGraw-Hill.

Kapoor, W. N. (2003). Syncope in the elderly. In C. K. Cassel (Ed.), *Geriatric medicine: An evidence-based approach*. New York: Springer-Verlag.

Karnath, B. (2004). Subdural hematoma: Presentation and management in older adults. *Geriatrics, 59*(7), 18-23.

Katzman, R., Brown, T., Fuld, P., Peck, A., Schechter, R., & Schimmel, H. (1983). Validation of a short orientation-memory-concentration test of cognitive impairment. *American Journal of Psychiatry, 140*, 734-739.

Kawas, C. H. (2003). Early Alzheimer's disease. *New England Journal of Medicine, 349*(11), 1056-1063.

Kennedy, G. J. (2003). Dementia. In C. K. Cassel (Ed.), *Geriatric medicine: An evidence-based approach*. New York: Springer-Verlag.

Kenny, R. A. (2003). Syncope. In W. R. Hazzard, J. P. Blass, J. B. Halter, et al. (Eds.), *Principles of geriatric medicine and gerontology* (5th ed.). New York: McGraw-Hill.

Knopman, D. S., Boeve, B. F., & Petersen, R. C. (2003). Essentials of proper diagnoses of mild cognitive impairment, dementia, and major subtypes of dementia. *Mayo Clinic Proceedings, 78*, 1290-1308.

Knopman, D. S., DeKosky, S. T., Cummings, J. L., Chui, H., Corey-Bloom, J., Relkin, N., et al. (2001). Practice parameter: Diagnosis of dementia (and evidence-based review). *Neurology, 56*, 1143-1153.

Kolanowski, A. M. (1999). An overview of the need-driven dementia-compromised behavior model. *Journal of Geronotological Nursing, 25*(9), 7-9.

Kryger, M., Monjan, A., Bliwise, D., & Ancoli-Israel, S. (2004). Sleep, health and aging. *Geriatrics, 59*(1), 24-30.

Kurlowicz, L. H. (2002). Delirium and depression. In V. T. Cotter & N. E. Stumpf (Eds.), *Advanced practice nursing with older adults: Clinical guidelines.* New York: McGraw-Hill.

Lai, H., & Good, M. (2005). Music improves sleep quality in older adults. *Journal of Advanced Nursing, 49*(3), 234.

Laurin, D., Verreault, R., Lindsay, J., MacPherson, K., & Rockwood, K. (2001). Physical activity and risk of cognitive impairment and dementia in elderly persons. *Archives of Neurology, 58*(3), 498-504.

Maclean, L. E., Collins, C. C., & Byrne, E. J. (2001). Dementia with Lewy bodies treated with rivastigmine: Effects on cognition, neuropsychiatric symptoms and sleep. *International Psychogeriatrics, 13*(3), 277-288.

Masdeu, J. C., & Rodriguez-Oroz, M. C. (2003). Abnormalities of posture and movement. In C. K. Cassel (Ed.), *Geriatric medicine: An evidence-based approach.* New York: Springer-Verlag.

Masterman, D. (2003). Treatment of the neuropsychiatric symptoms in Alzheimer's disease. *Journal of the American Medical Directors Association, 4*(6), S146-S154.

Matteson, M. S., Linton, A. D., & Barnes, S. J. (1996). Cognitive developmental approach to dementia. *Image: Journal of Nursing Scholarship, 28*(3), 233-240.

Matteson, M. S., Linton, A. D., Cleary, B. L., Barnes, S. J., & Lichtenstein, M. J. (1997). Management of problematic behavioral symptoms associated with dementia: A cognitive developmental approach. *Aging, 9*(5), 342-355.

Mattson, M. P. (2002). Molecular biology of the aging nervous system. In S. Duckett & J. C. da la Torre (Eds.), *Pathology of the aging human nervous system* (2nd ed.). New York: Oxford University Press.

McKeith, I. G., Galasko, D., Kosaka, K., Perry, E. K., Dickson, D. W., Hansen, L. A., et al. (1996). Consensus guidelines for the clinical and pathologic diagnosis of dementia with Lewy bodies (DLB): Report of the consortium on DLB international workshop. *Neurology, 47*(5), 1113-1124.

McKhann, G. M., Albert, M. S., Grossman, M., Miller, B., Dickson, D., & Trojanowski, J. Q. (2001). Clinical and pathological diagnosis of frontotemporal dementia: Report of the Work Group on Frontotemporal Dementia and Pick's Disease. *Archives of Neurology, 58,* 1803-1809.

McNicoll, L., Pisani, M. A., Zhang, Y., Ely, E. W., Siegel, M. D., & Inouye, S. K. (2003). Delirium in the intensive care unit: Occurrence and clinical course in older adults. *Journal of the American Geriatrics Society, 51*(5), 591-598.

Meara, J. (2003). Parkinsonism and other movement disorders. In R. C. Tallis & H. M. Fillit (Eds.), *Brocklehurst's textbook of geriatric medicine and gerontology* (6th ed.). London: Churchill Livingstone.

Monias, A., & Meier, D. E. (2003). Palliative care in early, moderate, and advanced dementia. In C. K. Cassel (Ed.), *Geriatric medicine: An evidence-based approach.* New York: Springer-Verlag.

Moore, V. (2003). Dementia care mapping. In Hudson, R. (Ed.), *Dementia nursing: A guide to practice.* Melbourne: Ausmed Publications.

Morris, J. C. (1993). The Clinical Dementia Rating (CDR): Current version and scoring rules. *Neurology, 43,* 2412-2414.

Morris, J. C. (1999). Clinical presentation and course of Alzheimer disease. In R. D. Terry, R. Katzman, D. L. Bick, & S. S. Sangram (Eds.), *Alzheimer disease* (2nd ed.). Philadelphia: Lippincott Williams & Wilkins.

Morris, J. C. (2005). *Dementia update 2005.* Unpublished manuscript.

Morris, J. C., Storandt, M., Miller, J. P., McKeel, D. W., Price, J. L, Rubin, E. H., & Berg, L. (2001). Mild cognitive impairment represents early-stage Alzheimer's disease. *Archives of Neurology, 58*(3), 397-405.

Nanda, A., & Besdine, R. W. (2003). Dizziness. In W. R. Hazzard, J. P. Blass, J. B. Halter, et al. (Eds.), *Principles of geriatric medicine and gerontology* (5th ed.). New York: McGraw-Hill.

Nanda, A. & Tinetti, M.E. (2003). Chronic dizziness and vertigo. In C.K. Cassel (Ed.), *Geriatric medicine: An evidence-based approach.* New York: Springer-Verlag.

National Institutes of Health. (2003). *Alzheimer's disease: Unraveling the mystery* (NIH pub. no. 02-3782). Washington, DC: U.S. Government Printing Office.

National Institutes of Health. (2004). *2003 Progress report on Alzheimer's disease: Research advances at NIH* (NIH pub. no. 04-5570). Washington, DC: U.S. Government Printing Office.

Neary, D., & Snowden, J. S. (2003). Classification of the dementias. In R. C. Tallis & H. M. Fillit (Eds.), *Brocklehurst's textbook of geriatric medicine and gerontology* (6th ed.). London: Churchill Livingstone.

Neelon, V. J., Champagne, M. T., Carlson, J. R., & Funk, S. G. (1996). The NEECHAM Confusion Scale: Construction, validation, and clinical testing. *Nursing Research, 45*(6), 324-330.

Petersen, R. C., Smith, G. E., Waring, S. C., Ivnik, R. J., Tangalos, E. G., & Kokman, E. (1999). Mild cognitive impairment: clinical characterization and outcome. *Archives of Neurology, 56*(3), 303-308.

Petersen, R. C., Stevens, J. C., Ganguli, M., Tangalos, E. G., Cummings, J. L. & Dekosky, S. T. (2001). Practice parameter: Early detection of dementia: Mild congitive impairment (an evidence-based review). Report of the Quality Standards Subcommittee of the American Academy of Neurology. *Neurology, 56,* 1133-1142.

Petersen, R. C., Thomas, R. G., Grundman, M., Bennett, D., Doody, R., Ferris, S., et al. (2005). Vitamin E and donepezil for the treatment of mild cognitive impairment. *New England Journal of Medicine, 352*(23), 2379-2388.

Pilkington, G. J. (2001). Brain tumors in the elderly. In S. Duckett & J. C. da la Torre (Eds.), *Pathology of the aging human nervous system* (2nd ed.). New York: Oxford University Press.

Pruisner, S. B. (2004). An introduction to prion biology and diseases. In S. B. Pruisner (Ed.), *Prion biology and disease* (2nd ed.). Cold Spring Harbor, NY: Cold Spring Harbor Laboratory Press.

Rao, G., Fisch, L, Srinivasan, S., D'Amico, F., Okada, T., Eaton, C., & Robbins, C. (2003). Does this patient have Parkinson disease? *Journal of the American Medical Association, 289*(3), 347-353.

Reisberg, B., Ferris, S. H., deLeon, M. J., & Crook, T. (1982). The Global Deterioration Scale for assessment of primary degenerative dementia. *American Journal of Psychiatry, 139,* 1136-1139.

Reisberg, B., Ferris, S. H., deLeon, M. J., & Crook, T. (1988). Global Deterioration Scale (GDS). *Psychopharmacology Bulletin, 24*(4), 661-663.

Roche, V. (2003). Etiology and management of delirium. *American Journal of Medical Science, 325*(1), 20-30.

Román, G. C. (2003). Vascular dementia: Distinguishing characteristics, treatment, and prevention. *Journal of the American Geriatrics Society, 51*(5), S296-S304.

Russell, E. M., & Burns, A. (2003). Presentation and clinical management of dementia. In R. C. Tallis & H. M. Fillit (Eds.), *Brocklehurst's textbook of geriatric medicine and gerontology* (6th ed.). London: Churchill Livingstone.

Schneider, L. S., Tariot, P. N., Lyketsos, C. G., Dagerman, K. S., Davis, K. L., Davis, S., et al. (2001). National Institute of Mental Health Clinical Antipsychotic Trials of Intervention Effectiveness (CATIE): Alzheimer disease trial methodology. *American Journal of Geriatric Psychiatry, 9*(11), 346-360.

Seidel, H. M., Ball, J. W., Dains, J. E., & Benedict, G. W. (1999). *Mosby's guide to physical examination* (4th ed.). St. Louis: Mosby.

Sink, K. M., Holden, K. F., & Yaffe, K. (2005). Pharmacological treatment of neuropsychiatric symptoms of dementia: A review of the evidence. *Journal of the American Medical Association, 293*(5), 596-608.

Smith, M., Gerdner, L. A., Hall, G. R., & Buckwalter, K. C. (2004). History, development, and future of the progressively lowered stress threshold: A conceptual model for dementia care. *Journal of the American Geriatrics Society, 52,* 1755-1760.

Spector, A., Thorgrimsen, L., Woods, B., Royan, L., Davies, S., Butterworth, M., & Orrell, M. (2003). Efficacy of an evidence-based cognitive stimulation therapy programme for people with dementia. *British Journal of Psychiatry, 183,* 248-254.

Tariot, P. N., Farlow, M. R., Grossberg, G. T., Graham, S. M., McDonald, S., & Gergel, I. (2004). Memantine treatment in patients with moderate to severe Alzheimer disease already receiving donepezil: A randomized controlled trial. *Journal of the American Medical Association, 291*(3), 317-324.

Trinh, N. H., Hoblyn, J, Mohanty, S., & Yaffe, K. (2003). Efficacy of cholinesterase inhibitors in the treatment of neuropsychiatric symptoms and functional impairment in Alzheimer disease: A meta-analysis. *Journal of the American Medical Association, 289,* 210-216.

Tullmann, D. F., & Dracup, K. (2000). Creating a healing environment for elders. *AACN Clinical Issues, 11*(1), 34-50.

Verghese, J., Lipton, R. B., Katz, M. J., Hall, C. B., Derby, C. A., Kuslansky, G., et al. (2003). Leisure activities and the risk of dementia in the elderly. *New England Journal of Medicine, 348*(25), 2508-2516.

Victor, M., & Ropper, A. (2001). *Principles of neurology* (7th ed.). New York: McGraw-Hill.

Will, R. G., Alpers, M. P., Dormont, D., & Schonberger, L. B. (2004). Infectious and sporadic prion diseases. In S. B. Pruisner (Ed.), *Prion biology and disease* (2nd ed.). Cold Spring Harbor, NY: Cold Spring Harbor Laboratory Press.

Chapter
15

Gastrointestinal System

Adrianne Dill Linton

Objectives

Describe normal changes in the structure and function of the gastrointestinal system associated with aging.

Describe measures to maintain gastrointestinal health in the older adult.

Explain the cause and treatment of gastrointestinal disorders that are common in older persons.

Describe the components of the gastrointestinal assessment in the older adult.

Formulate nursing diagnoses for older adults with actual or potential gastrointestinal problems.

Develop plans to manage older adults with actual or potential gastrointestinal problems.

The aging digestive tract has been a long-standing topic for humor and a target for numerous commercial products sold as remedies for everything from heartburn to constipation. The major question is, Do older people really have changes in the gastrointestinal system sufficient to cause major problems with digestion and elimination? As with other body systems, it is difficult to determine which changes represent normal aging and which are the result of pathological processes and environmental insults.

CHANGES WITH AGING
Oral Cavity

Changes in the oral cavity can affect appearance, nutrition, and quality of life. Structures that undergo aging changes in the oral cavity are the teeth, soft tissues, jawbones and joints, salivary glands, and taste buds.

Dentition. Some of the changes in the teeth that occur with aging include wearing of tooth surfaces caused by diet, habits, tooth-to-tooth contact, and abrasion. In addition, exposure of the teeth to acids (as in gastric reflux) and frequent intake of acidic foods or

drugs contribute further to erosion. The deposition of cementum on the apical surface of the tooth root maintains its height. Thinning of the enamel on the buccal and lingual surfaces, which may be enhanced by abrasion, reveals the yellowish dentine beneath. This, combined with staining of the enamel, causes the teeth to darken with age. Vertical hairline cracks may develop as a result of shrinkage of dentine with subsequent loss of support for the enamel. The teeth become less sensitive because of a decrease in innervation in the dentine. Apical migration of the gingival margin may eventually expose the entire anatomical crown and part of the cementum-covered root. The more soluble cementum may dissolve and expose the dentine, creating a risk for root caries (Devlin & Ferguson, 2003).

In the United States, the percent of Americans age 65 years and older who are edentulous has declined in recent decades, although the rate varies with geographical area and other factors. In 2002, fewer than half of adults age 65 and older reported having lost six or more teeth (Centers for Disease Control and Prevention [CDC], 2003). A 4-year longitudinal study of African American and non-Hispanic whites in Florida concluded that race and socioeconomic status were strong determinants of tooth loss. African Americans and people of lower socioeconomic status were less likely to obtain dental care, more likely to experience tooth loss, and less likely to report that alternatives to extraction had been presented to them (Gilbert, Duncan, & Shelton, 2003). Similar disparities in tooth retention by socioeconomic and geographical variables have been reported in other countries as diverse as Norway and Australia (Henriksen, Axell, & Laake, 2003; Sanders & Spencer, 2004).

Soft Oral Tissues. The oral mucosa in the older adult becomes thin, smooth, dry, and inelastic. Because of a loss of filiform papillae, the tongue appears smoother as well. Although more fragile, healthy oral tissues retain their healing capacity.

Saliva. Saliva is important for providing protection for all oral tissues. It contains lubricatory factors to keep oral tissues hydrated, pliable, and insulated; buffering acids; and proteins that regulate oral bacterial colonization patterns, thereby modulating dental disease and preventing systemic infections originating from the mouth. It provides for mechanical cleansing of the mouth. Other salivary proteins keep the secretions supersaturated with calcium and phosphate, allowing for remineralization of caries (cavities). Saliva also provides a medium by which the sense of taste is stimulated.

Many older studies reported a decrease of salivary production as a normal aging change. Those findings have since been refuted, and dry mouth is more often attributed to drug side effects, nutritional disturbances, and disease states than to normal aging. Although submandibular flow rates may decrease, parotid salivary flow rates are believed to remain stable so that the total salivary production appears to remain adequate. The large secretory reserve of the major glands probably compensates for changes in the minor glands (Devlin & Ferguson, 2003; Ghezzi & Ship, 2003; Navazesh, 2002).

Jawbone and Joints. With attrition of the molar cusps with aging, the lower jaw slides forward, bringing the incisors into opposition and contributing to attrition of those teeth. Osteoarthritis of the temporomandibular joint is a common radiographic finding in older adults. However, studies of the prevalence of symptomatic joint dysfunction in older adults have had inconsistent results (Devlin & Ferguson, 2003).

Like other bones, the jaws can be affected by osteoporosis. In a study of postmenopausal Asian-American women, Mohammad, Hooper, Vermilyea, Mariotti, and Preshaw (2003) found significant negative correlations between bone mineral density and tooth loss and between bone mineral density and clinical attachment loss. Although tooth loss is not a normal concomitant of aging, it is common and has a profound impact on the jawbone. Following loss of a tooth, the alveolar bone atrophies. When multiple teeth are lost, the atrophy causes a decrease in the height of the face (Devlin & Ferguson, 2003). McCord (2003) asserts that post-extraction bone loss can be reduced by planned retention of roots and/or placement of implants. Loss of posterior teeth permits overclosure of the oral cavity. The muscles of mastication also atrophy, especially with the loss of teeth from the mandible (Devlin & Ferguson, 2003). Tooth loss is an important factor in masticatory performance. Chewing ability can be maintained or improved with appropriate prostheses (Tatematsu et al., 2004). Not only do those without teeth avoid certain foods, they also report experiencing pain and distress and avoid going out (Jones, Orner, Spiro, & Kressin, 2003).

Sense of Taste. Mattes (2003) reviewed the literature regarding the following common assumptions about the chemical senses and nutrition and aging and described the evidence to support or refute those assumptions.

Aging processes result in marked changes of chemosensory function. Multiple studies have demonstrated significant declines of gustatory function in older persons. However, Mattes (2003) questions the practical significance of these findings, noting that the prevalence of chronic chemosensory problems is extremely low even among older adults. Although the number of taste buds and odor identification scores decrease with age, there is no evidence that this translates to a change in taste perception. Also, numerous variables (health disorders, dentures, smoking, oral hygiene, medications) other than age can affect chemosensory function. Once findings are adjusted for confounding variables, it appears that both taste and smell generally are well preserved with age. Compared with young adults, threshold sensitivity is lower in middle-aged adults, but it tends to remain relatively stable thereafter. Mattes (2003) concludes that further study is needed to determine whether the reported changes are simply idiosyncratic or truly part of normal aging, and whether the changes have any practical significance.

Sensory changes associated with aging translate into modifications of food choice and dietary behavior. Studies of individuals with chemosensory complaints have not shown significant changes in weight, body mass index, or specific nutrient deficiencies. Measurable changes in taste have not been predictive of consumption of specific foods. Some data suggest that individuals with olfactory dysfunction tend to reject foods with bitter/sour notes, but once again, there is no evidence that this affects nutritional status (Mattes, 2003). One interesting study sought to determine if residual senses of texture and trigeminal perception in older persons could be compensating for specific losses in taste and smell. The results of the study led Forde, Cantau, Delahunty, and Elsner (2002) to conclude that the selection of preferred textures might help boost food enjoyment. Several sources suggest that sensitivity to sweet and salt is better preserved than sour and bitter tastes (Ikeda, Ikui, & Tomita, 2002; Yamauchi, Endo, & Yoshimura, 2002).

Sensory changes elicit shifts in food selection that increase nutritional risk. Mattes (2003) raises the possibility that chemosensory changes may in fact be beneficial. As energy requirements decline with age, a reduced intake of calories and some specific foods may be a good thing. Also, reduced sensitivity to bitterness, which is characteristic of cruciferous vegetables, may encourage increased intake of these healthy foods.

Age-related declines in chemosensory function increase the risk of food-borne illness in the aging population. There simply is no basis for this statement. Further, Mattes (2003) notes that spores and toxins caused by pathogens in foods usually are tasteless and odorless, so there is no reason to believe that intact senses prevent intake of contaminated or spoiled food.

Esophagus

Esophageal function is essentially preserved with aging. Soergel, Zboralske, and Amberg (1964) coined the term *presbyesophagus* to describe the presence of an abnormal frequency of nonperistaltic contractions and inadequate relaxation of the lower esophageal sphincter, resulting in decreased esophageal motility. This phenomenon was thought to be related to a decrease in esophageal muscle mass, similar to deterioration of the muscle mass in other body organs. This term has since been abandoned, however, because it is now thought that abnormal esophageal motility is more likely to be due to the consequences of the high prevalence of neurological diseases in older people rather than to the process of normal aging.

In the absence of disease, only minor changes in the esophagus have been found in older adults, and these are not considered clinically significant. These changes include decreased amplitude of muscle contractions after swallowing, decreased upper esophageal sphincter pressure and prolonged relaxation of the sphincter, and longer reflux episodes with impaired clearance of refluxed materials (Greenwald & Brandt, 2003; Tepper & Katz, 2003). Therefore individuals who complain of swallowing difficulties should be referred for evaluation and treatment.

Stomach

The major changes in the stomach that commonly are seen in older adults are decreased hydrochloric acid and the delayed emptying of liquids. It has been thought that decreased acid secretion is an age-related change, but that is in question. Current thinking is that chronic infection with *Helicobacter pylori*, which is extremely common, is responsible for the gradual destruction of secretory glands including the parietal cells that produce hydrochloric acid. There is some evidence that older individuals who do not have *H. pylori* actually produce more hydrochloric acid than younger persons (Greenwald & Brandt, 2003). Diminished gastric prostaglandins, bicarbonate, and nonparietal fluid secretion may make the stomach more vulnerable to mucosal damage induced by nonsteroidal antiinflammatory drugs (NSAIDs). In some older adults, gastric emptying time for liquids has been prolonged (Tepper & Katz, 2003).

Small Intestine

The small intestine, with its enormous surface area, has as its major function the absorption of nutrients. The extent to which the small intestine is altered with normal aging has not been well described. A comparative study of older and younger subjects found no difference in small intestine transit rate (Madsen & Graff, 2004). Research has identified some nutrients whose absorption may be altered with age. Jejunal lactase activity declines. Absorption of vitamin D, calcium, and zinc in the small intestine may be reduced with age, whereas absorption of vitamin A increases (Mahan & Escott-Stump, 2000; Tepper & Katz, 2003). Impaired absorption of folate has been reported in some sources, but not others. When evidence of malabsorption exists, it often is associated with achlorhydria, inflammatory bowel disease, bacterial overgrowth, or bowel surgery (Thomas, 2003).

Large Intestine

Histological changes in the colon include increased collagen deposition and atrophy of the muscularis propria (Tepper & Katz, 2003). Experts disagree as to the effects of age on colonic motility and transit rate. Wald (2003) asserts that there are no changes. However, Madsen and Graff (2004) studied transit rate with repetitive gamma camera imaging following ingestion of physiological radiolabeled markers. The procedure was employed with 16 healthy subjects ages 74 to 85 years and 16 healthy subjects ages 20 to 30 years. The colonic transit rate was significantly slower in the older subjects.

Anal sphincter tone and strength diminish with aging, and the rectum becomes less compliant, which may contribute to fecal incontinence (Wald, 2003). Particularly in postmenopausal women, the maximal squeeze pressure declines. The rectum of the older person also accommodates a larger volume before the sensation of a full rectum is recognized (Tepper & Katz, 2003).

Pancreas

Most persons over age 70 have a dilated pancreatic duct. In relation to the exocrine pancreatic function, the flow rate decreases, as does the secretion of bicarbonate and enzymes. With repeated stimulation the flow rate decreases significantly (Tepper & Katz, 2003).

Liver and Biliary Tract

The number and size of hepatocytes decrease with age, resulting in a decrease in organ weight. Hepatic blood flow is reduced, and hepatic regeneration is slower following injury. Phase 1 drug clearance reactions, which include oxidation, hydrolysis, and reduction, are altered. Changes in the liver also affect first-pass metabolism and serum albumin binding capacity (Tepper & Katz, 2003). See Chapter 7 for a more detailed discussion of drug metabolism in the older person.

Some evidence exists that gallbladder contraction in response to stimulation is reduced with age. An increased proportion of phospholipids and cholesterol components in the bile increases the risk of gallstone formation. Because of enlargement of the bile duct, choledocholithiasis also is more common in older persons (Tepper & Katz, 2003). Common changes in the gastrointestinal system of the older adult are summarized in Box 15-1.

Box 15-1 *Age-Related Changes: Gastrointestinal*

Oral Cavity
- Dentition
  - Erosion of tooth surfaces
  - Thinning enamel
  - Staining
  - Decreased sensitivity
- Oral mucosa: thin, smooth, inelastic
- Saliva
  - Submandibular flow rate decreases
  - Parotid flow rate stable
  - Net salivary production adequate
- Jawbone
  - Lower jaw shifts forward
  - Osteoarthritis of joints common
- Taste buds
  - Decreased number
  - Decreased odor identification scores
  - Sensitivity to sweet and salt may be better preserved than other tastes

Esophagus (Effects Measurable but Not Functionally Significant)
- Decreased amplitude of muscle contractions after swallowing
- Decreased upper esophageal sphincter pressure and prolonged relaxation of sphincter
- Longer reflux episodes with impaired clearance of refluxed materials

Stomach
- Decreased hydrochloric acid
- Delayed emptying of liquids

Small Intestine
- Absorption of vitamin A increased
- Absorption of vitamin D, calcium, zinc may be reduced
- Jejunal lactase activity declines

Large Intestine
- Colonic transit rate may be slower
- Atrophy of muscularis propria
- Anal sphincter tone and strength diminish
- Rectum less compliant
- Maximum rectal squeeze pressure declines

Pancreas
- Dilated pancreatic duct
- Flow rate of exocrine secretions declines
- Decreased secretion of bicarbonate and enzymes

Liver and Biliary Tract
- Number and size of hepatocytes decrease
- Hepatic blood flow reduced
- Hepatic regeneration slower
- Phase 1 drug clearance reactions altered
- Reduced gallbladder contraction in response to stimulation
- Increased proportion of phospholipids and cholesterol in bile
- Enlargement of bile duct

COMMON DISORDERS
Disorders of the Oral Cavity

Major problems in the oral cavity that are more common in older age include xerostomia (dry mouth), burning and painful tongue, temporomandibular joint pain, periodontal disease, and oral lesions. Root caries, found almost exclusively in older people, occurs where the tooth root is exposed by receding gingiva (Devlin & Ferguson, 2003). Tooth loss, though less common now than in the past, increases with age.

Xerostomia. Xerostomia is a common complaint with advancing age. Because moisture in the mouth is important for chewing, swallowing, tasting, and speaking, xerostomia can lead to inadequate diet, dental caries, and decreased social interaction. It commonly is attributed to an age-related decrease in salivary production, but more likely causes are certain systemic medications and Sjögren's syndrome (Cassolato & Turnbull, 2003). Major causes of dry mouth are obstructive nasal diseases that promote mouth breathing, drugs, vitamin B complex deficiency, diabetes, dehydration, radiotherapy, anxiety, and fear. Drugs that are often the culprits include anticholinergics, diuretics, some opiates, antidepressants, antipsychotics, tranquilizers, antihistamines, decongestants, antihypertensives, antineoplastics, and antispasmodics (Devlin & Ferguson, 2003). The problem is extremely disturbing to those who experience it; it can result in altered taste sensation, increased vulnerability of the oral mucosa, oral pain, dysphagia, and impaired clearance of the bacteria prominent in causing caries. The oral mucosa appears dry, atrophic, inflamed or pale, and translucent. In addition, sore spots may develop under dentures because of lack of lubrication, interfering with denture retention. The incidence of dental plaque formation and dental caries can increase, especially if sucking on hard candies is used to relieve dry mouth. For the individual with xerostomia, treatment options include salivary substitutes, salivary stimulants, meticulous dental care, and elimination of anticholinergic drugs (Cassolato & Turnbull, 2003). A new drug for xerostomia with Sjögren's syndrome is cevimeline (Evoxac), a muscarinic antagonist similar to bethanechol. The most common side effects of cevimeline are excessive sweating, nausea, rhinitis, and diarrhea. It is contraindicated with narrow-angle glaucoma and uncontrolled asthma and must be used cautiously with cardiac and other obstructive respiratory disorders (Lehne, 2004).

Disorders of the Tongue. Disorders of the tongue may include structural changes, pain (glossodynia), and a burning sensation (glossopyrosis). The tongue is a good indicator of a variety of systemic problems. For example, a red, beefy tongue might indicate the presence of monilial infections or iron deficiency anemia; a flat tongue surface may point to pernicious anemia.

Burning mouth syndrome (BMS) is a common complaint among older adults. It has been associated with allergies to food preservatives or flavoring agents, local denture trauma, nutritional deficiencies, diabetes, and anemia. Three types of BMS have been identified. Type 1 is characterized by increasing discomfort through the waking hours with few symptoms that disrupt sleep. Individuals with type 2 have symptoms on awakening that persist through the day, and those with type 3 have symptom-free periods. Treatment aims to correct the underlying cause. Estrogen replacement therapy may be beneficial in postmenopausal women (Devlin & Ferguson, 2003).

Oral Lesions. The incidence of malignant lesions of the oral cavity rises sharply with age. Most oral malignancies are squamous cell carcinomas. Important risk factors include smoking, use of snuff in the buccal sulcus, and alcohol consumption. Sun exposure is another risk factor for lesions of the lip. The lower lip is the most common site for oral malignancy, followed by the lateral and inferior surfaces of the tongue, then the buccal mucosa and the floor of the mouth. The most important oral cancer detection procedure is careful, regular inspection of the oral mucosa. Lesions commonly are painless and their features variable. Oral malignancies may be manifested as exophytic growths, deep ulcers, swelling of the vermilion border of the lip, or crusty lesions. Cancer of the floor of the mouth is commonly an ulcerated lesion with raised margins near the frenum. Because white patches (leukoplakia) or red patches (erythroplakia) may be premalignant, they should be biopsied (Devlin & Ferguson, 2003).

The prognosis is best when lesions are small and without metastasis, but overall the mortality rate is about 50%. Treatment depends on the location, size, and type of lesion, and usually consists of either surgery or radiation or a combination of the two. Improvements in surgical reconstructive techniques have greatly improved the aesthetic and functional outcomes of surgical intervention (Devlin & Ferguson, 2003).

Oral Malodor

Oral malodor is a common problem in frail, dependent persons. A review by Quirynen, Zhao, and van Steenberghe (2002) concluded that the most effective treatment employed toothbrushing, flossing, tongue cleaning, and use of antimicrobial mouthrinse. The two antiseptic mouthwashes that have American Dental Association (ADA) approval are chlorhexidine (Peridex) and essential oil mouthwash (Listerine) (Santos, 2003).

Periodontal Disease. The major causes of periodontitis are local irritation (including ill-fitting dental work), mouth breathing, food impurities, oral sepsis, malocclusions, malnutrition, endocrine imbalance, diabetes, leukemia, diphenylhydantoin (Dilantin), hypovitaminosis, scurvy, and pellagra. Severe alcoholics are at increased risk of both periodontal disease and tooth loss (Hornecker, Muuss, Ehrenreich, & Mausberg, 2003).

Untreated periodontal disease increases the risk of tooth loss, and when tooth loss is caused by periodontitis, the survival rate of implants declines (Harris, 2003; Karoussis et al., 2003). Advanced periodontitis also can lead to impaired mastication secondary to discomfort and increased tooth mobility, and to gastrointestinal disorders.

The possible relationship between periodontal disease and cardiovascular disease has received considerable attention. The Oral Infections and Vascular Disease Epidemiology Study (INVEST) concluded that tooth loss was associated with periodontitis and with subclinical atherosclerosis (Desvarieux et al., 2003). However, Elter, Champagne, Offenbacher, and Beck (2004) studied more than 8000 individuals ages 52 to 75 and concluded that tooth loss and periodontal disease were associated with prevalent coronary heart disease only in the presence of both. An analysis of periodontal risk profiles in adults with or without a history of myocardial infarction revealed that bone loss was the best individual predictor of individuals with recent acute myocardial infarction (Renvert, Ohlsson, Persson, Lang, & Persson, 2004).

The treatment of periodontal disease depends on the stage of the disease present. When bone loss is present, scaling is done to remove calculus from the sides of tooth roots and the roots are then smoothed to eliminate factors that might cause inflammation of the soft tissues. The goal of treatment at this stage is to maintain existing alveolar bone and to eliminate inflammation. Advanced disease may be treated with gingivectomy, which includes recontouring the alveolar bone and gingival tissues. A newer procedure is the use of bone grafts to replace lost alveolar bone. At any stage, regular home care is essential to prevent the recurrence of active disease.

Research on the effectiveness of oral care products by older adults is limited. Davies (2004) reviewed available literature and concluded that fluoride in the form of toothpaste and other delivery systems may help prevent coronal and root caries in older persons. Further, powered toothbrushes with a rotating oscillating action were found to be more effective than manual toothbrushes in reducing plaque and improving gingival health (Davies, 2004; Heanue et al., 2004; Sicilia, Arregui, Gallego, Cabezas, & Cuesta, 2002). A number of mouthwash preparations have been evaluated for their effects on caries, plaque formation, and gingivitis. A longitudinal study compared the daily use of 0.2% neutral sodium fluoride mouthwash with placebo in long-term care residents. The fluoride solution group had significantly fewer caries and more reversals of carious sites to sound dental surfaces (Wyatt & MacEntee, 2004).

Among the nonsurgical options that have been used to treat periodontal disease are scaling and root planing using manual, sonic, or ultrasonic instrumentation and subgingival debridement with an Er:YAG laser (Cobb, 2002; Sculean et al., 2004). Deep scaling removes calculus from the sides of the roots and is followed by smoothing of the surfaces. The purpose of these procedures is to eliminate the source of inflammation of the gingivae. Eliminating inflammation prevents further bone loss. Advanced periodontitis may require gingivectomy to recontour the alveolar bone and gingival tissues. Following any of these treatments, regular home oral care procedures are essential to prevent recurrence. A longitudinal study of individuals with chronic adult periodontitis who were treated surgically and then followed with maintenance care demonstrated that those who were compliant with their care were far less likely to have tooth loss (Checchi, Montevecchi, Gatto, & Trombelli, 2002). Various types of mouthwashes have been used for both prevention and maintenance care after treatment for periodontal disease; however, the Federation of National Dental Associations (FDI) Commission (2002) notes that they are not equally effective and should be used along with regular tooth cleaning. The use of biological mediators combined with scaffold materials for periodontal and bone regeneration is under study (Oringer, 2002).

Some studies suggest that microbiological identification may be useful in treating periodontal disease, especially for patients who are not responding to standard treatment (Listgarten & Loomer, 2003). Blandino and colleagues (2004) recommend systemic flurithromycin therapy along with scaling and root planing. In a randomized, double-blind trial, persons treated with scaling and root planing followed by oral amoxicillin and metronidazole had significant treatment effects compared with other drug regimens and placebo (Rooney, Wade, Sprague, Newcombe, & Addy, 2002). Loesche, Giordano, Soehren, and Kaciroti (2002) demonstrated that debridement and short-term antibiotic therapy reduced the need for surgery and tooth extraction for individuals with seriously compromised periodontal disease. The effect remained even 5 years after treatment.

Caries and Tooth Loss. Tooth loss may be common with age; however, it is not considered normal or inevitable. According to a report from the Division of Oral Health, Centers for Disease Control and Prevention, dental caries and periodontal disease are the main causes of tooth loss in the United States (Beltran-Aguilar

& Beltran-Neira, 2004). Inflammation produces destruction of the bone that supports the teeth, resulting in a progressive loosening and ultimate shedding of teeth.

The prevalence of oral disease and tooth loss among long-term care residents has been reported in numerous studies. Among Finnish residents, 42% were found to be edentulous. In addition, dental hygiene was judged to be poor in 37%; among denture wearers, 25% had stomatitis and 28% had angular cheilitis. Of those with teeth, 37% needed restorations, 51% needed periodontal treatment, and 42% needed extractions (Peltola, Vehkalahti, & Wuolijoki-Saaristo, 2004). A study of 866 subjects in Swedish long-term care found that 61% needed evaluation and some treatment (Isaksson, Soderfeldt, & Nederfors, 2003).

Smoking has emerged as a strong predictor of periodontal bone loss and tooth loss. For nonsmokers, predictors of tooth loss include number of teeth, mean alveolar bone level, percent of periodontally healthy approximal sites, and educational level (Paulander, Wennstrom Axelsson, & Lindhe, 2004; Ylostalo, Sakki, Laitinen, Jarvelin, & Knuuttila, 2004). With cessation of smoking, the accelerated loss of periodontal bone height has been shown to slow to the rate of nonsmokers (Bergstrom, 2004). During a 10-year longitudinal study in Finland, 52% of the subjects lost one tooth or more, with the most common reason for extraction being root caries (Fure, 2003).

Whereas most studies have focused on periodontal disease and heart disease, Frisk, Hakeberg, Ahlqwist, and Bengtsson (2003) assessed the relationship of coronary heart disease (CHD) with endodontic variables (number of root filled teeth, number of teeth with periapical radiolucencies). Their conclusion was that there was no significant association between endodontically treated teeth and CHD, nor between teeth with periapical disease and CHD. In contrast, the work of Hung, Willett, Merchant, and colleagues (2003) found that cumulative tooth loss was associated with peripheral arterial disease, especially in men with periodontal disease. Based on their findings that total tooth loss was associated with low citrus intake and low plasma vitamin C, Lowe and colleagues (2003) proposed that inadequate vitamin C deficiency could contribute to low-grade inflammation and thrombosis.

Tooth loss can have important implications for nutrition, body image, and quality of life. A relationship has been shown between a declining number of teeth and dietary alterations. Loss of teeth requires adjustments in food choices that may affect nutrition, including reduced intake of fiber, whole fruits, and raw vegetables (Daly, Elsner, Allen, & Burke, 2003; Hung, Willett, Ascherio, et al., 2003). The work of Marcenes, Steele, Sheiham, and Walls (2003) in Great Britain demonstrated that the likelihood of having an acceptable body mass index correlated with having 21 or more teeth.

The impact of tooth loss on quality of life has been explored from several perspectives. Steele and colleagues (2004) found that oral health–related quality of life was related to age, number of teeth, and cultural background in the United Kingdom and Australia. The importance of culture in relation to quality of life was illustrated in a study of Saudi elders. Investigators explored the sentiments about tooth loss in edentulous people, and the themes that emerged included unqualified acceptance and inevitability with age. The subjects in this study gave no outward indications of bereavement (Omar, Tashkandi, Abduljabbar, Abdullah, & Akeel, 2003). In another Saudi study, 82% of those with missing teeth expressed a need for replacement. However, only 42% thought tooth loss negatively affected their appearance. About 63% said tooth loss affected their chewing (Akeel, 2003). In a U.S. study, patients who had lost teeth or wore dentures reported a need to avoid certain foods. Other reported consequences included pain and distress and reluctance to go out (Jones et al., 2003).

Other factors that may play a role in tooth loss in older persons include diet, genetics, and early life circumstances. Among subjects in the Baltimore Study on Aging, age was the only significant predictor of tooth loss over a 10-year period. However, in a cohort from the Veterans Administration (VA) Dental Longitudinal Study, predictors were baseline percent of teeth with restorations, mean probing pocket depth score, age, tobacco use, alcohol consumption, number of teeth present, and male sex (Copeland, Krall, Brown, Garcia, & Streckfus, 2004). Pearce, Steele, Mason, Walls, and Parker (2004) studied the impact of early life factors on eventual tooth loss and found that those factors (e.g., childhood socioeconomic status) explained very little variation in tooth retention in middle age.

Genetic factors, including the vitamin D receptor gene and the matrix Gla protein gene, have been implicated in natural tooth loss; however, the research in this field is just beginning (Hirano et al., 2003; Inagaki, Krall, Fleet, & Garcia, 2003).

Oral disease and tooth loss are especially problematic in the nursing home population. Residents may be unable to perform oral hygiene independently, may resist oral care by others, and may have less access to professional dental services. Several studies have revealed that dental problems (poor oral hygiene, oral disease, decreased use of dentures, increased denture-related oral lesions, increased plaque, increased coronal and root caries, increased decayed retained tooth roots) are more prevalent in cognitively impaired individuals and those with impaired functional abilities (Avlund, Holm-Pedersen, Morse, Viitanen, & Winblad, 2004;

Chalmers, Carter, & Spencer, 2003; Shimazaki, Soh, Koga, Miyazaki, & Takehara, 2003).

Oral Candidiasis. *Candida albicans* is part of the normal gastrointestinal flora that manifests as candidiasis only when the other flora is disrupted or the immune function is disturbed. Common reasons for mucosal candidiasis in older adults are antibiotic therapy and immunosuppressive cancer chemotherapy. Candidiasis appears as soft white plaques that can be readily scraped from the mucosa, exposing a raw mucosal surface. This is in contrast to leukoplakia, in which the lesions cannot be stripped (Greenwald & Brandt, 2003).

Treatment of oral candidiasis depends in part on the cause. When antibiotics are implicated, the condition is likely to resolve when drug therapy is discontinued and normal flora returns. For chemotherapy patients, oral nystatin suspension or troches often are effective. The oral antifungal agent fluconazole may be needed in some cases. Topical anesthetics can be used if discomfort is severe (Greenwald & Brandt, 2003).

Stomatitis and candidiasis may develop in denture wearers, particularly with poorly fitting dentures and poor oral hygiene. Treatment includes education in denture hygiene and replacement or repair of dentures. Miconazole oral gel may be applied to the denture four times daily. Instruct the patient to remove and clean the dentures each night. Chronic candidiasis may be accompanied by angular cheilitis (painful fissures at the corners of the mouth) (Devlin & Ferguson, 2003).

Disorders of the Esophagus

Three esophageal disorders that are more common among older people are dysphagia, hiatus hernia, and carcinoma. Esophageal dysfunction usually is secondary to diseases of the nervous system that cause neuromuscular incoordination, such as Parkinson's disease, amyotrophic lateral sclerosis, pseudobulbar palsy, peripheral neuropathy, diabetes mellitus, and stroke.

Dysphagia. Dysphagia is a symptom of an esophageal problem rather than a specific disease entity. It is experienced immediately after deglutition when the passage of food through the esophagus is impaired. The patient typically reports that food is "stuck in the throat." However, symptoms are perceived as being at a higher level than the actual site of the obstruction because sensation is referred proximally in the esophagus (Greenwald & Brandt, 2003).

The two basic causes of dysphagia are esophageal motility disorders and obstruction. A precise history can assist the care provider in determining the cause. Intermittent symptoms are associated with motility disorders, whereas steadily progressive worsening of symptoms is more characteristic of a neoplasm or peptic stricture. The type of foods that are difficult to swallow also is a clue to the underlying cause. Primary neuromuscular abnormalities and disordered motility create problems swallowing both liquids and solids. When a mechanical obstruction is present, the individual may be able to swallow liquids but not solids (Greenwald & Brandt, 2003). Some patients with dysphagia are able to handle solids and thick liquids better than thin liquids. Thickening agents can be used to improve the intake of fluids in these patients.

Among the conditions that can contribute to secondary esophageal motility disorders are diabetes mellitus, myxedema, connective tissue diseases, and amyloidosis. Despite typical changes in esophageal motility, most people with diabetes do not have significant dysphagia.

Achalasia is characterized by the absence of esophageal peristalsis, usually with increased resting lower esophageal sphincter pressure and the lack of sphincter relaxation to allow contents to exit the esophagus. Food accumulates in the esophagus, which may become dilated. Typically the patient complains of progressive dysphagia and coughing and aspiration when reclining. Chest pain may occur, though older adults usually have less pain than younger persons. Whereas the dysfunction is fairly localized with achalasia, some patients have diffuse spasms with segmental contractions (Cohen & Parkman, 2000).

When possible, dysphagia is treated by reversing the underlying cause. Drugs that may be used to treat primary motility disorders despite limited evidence of efficacy are nitrates, anticholinergics, calcium channel blockers, nifedipine, and sedatives. Dilation may be indicated for achalasia; however, it carries about a 5% risk of perforation (Cohen & Parkman, 2000; Greenwald & Brandt, 2003). If conservative management fails, surgical treatment is myotomy, which is the surgical division of the muscle of the lower esophageal sphincter. To prevent postoperative reflux, a fundoplication may be done as well. A controversial treatment for achalasia is the endoscopic injection of botulinum toxin, which relaxes the sphincter and relieves symptoms for several months (Cohen & Parkman, 2000). Speech therapists are experts in swallowing disorders and are helpful in recommending or implementing interventions. Prolonged enteral feedings are sometimes necessary. For stroke patients with severe dysphagia, percutaneous endoscopic gastrostomy may be recommended.

Gastroesophageal Reflux Disease. Gastroesophageal reflux disease (GERD) is the reflux of gastric contents through the lower esophageal sphincter (LES) into the esophagus or oropharynx. The classic symptoms of this chronic condition are heartburn and acid regurgitation. The cause is not fully understood but is thought to be related to abnormal LES pressure with transient relaxations that permit reflux (Kahrilas, 2003a). Current anatomical and histological studies of the normal esophagus are producing new understandings that may elucidate the pathophysiology of GERD (Chandrasoma, 2003; Melciades, Costa, & Pires-Neto, 2004). Evidence exists to support a genetic role in the development of various manifestations of GERD (Quigley, 2003). The relationship between *H. pylori* and GERD is a topic of controversy, with most studies to date having identified a negative association between the two (Massey, 2004). One study assessed the prevalence of individuals with symptomatic GERD compared with control subjects. Among those with symptomatic erosive esophagitis, 34.7% had *H. pylori* compared with 64.9% of the controls (Wu, Wu, Huang, & Lin, 2004). Most patients who have GERD also have hiatus hernia (Manes et al., 2003). Nonreducible hiatus hernia is associated with severe GERD (Mattioli, Lugaresi, Pierluigi, DiSimone, & D'Ovidio, 2003). Individuals with GERD may or may not have increased gastric acid secretion; in fact, it actually is decreased in some individuals (Shimatani et al., 2004). Complications of GERD include esophageal stricture and stenosis and bleeding.

Some sources recommend that GERD be categorized into three distinct diagnoses: nonerosive esophageal reflux disease (NERD), erosive esophagitis, and Barrett's esophagus. Others argue that these conditions represent a single disease that can progress from a mild nonerosive form to metaplasia and then to neoplasia (Pace & Porro, 2004). Individuals with NERD have symptoms typical of GERD but do not have esophagitis. However, long-term follow-up has demonstrated that most of these patients eventually developed reflux esophagitis (Pace, Bollani, Molteni, & Bianchi Porro, 2004).

Among older adults, approximately 8% of men and 15% of women report having symptoms of GERD on a daily basis. Substernal burning that is worse in a reclining position is the most common complaint. Those individuals who have erosive or complicated esophagitis are more likely to report dysphagia; respiratory symptoms such as chronic cough, hoarseness, or wheezing; and vomiting (Koretz & Reuben, 2003). Older adults experience complications of GERD more often than younger persons. This may be due in part to diminished sensitivity of the esophagus, which allows the inflammation to become severe before the patient seeks medical care (Byrne, Mulligan, O'Riordan, Keeling, & Reynolds, 2003). Patients who have chest pain must be carefully evaluated to differentiate GERD from angina. Older adults who have recurrent pneumonia or exacerbations of other chronic respiratory disease may be aspirating refluxed gastric contents. Endoscopy should be done promptly when GERD is suspected to confirm the diagnosis and to detect premalignant changes or malignant lesions. This examination is especially important if the patient has more ominous symptoms such as dysphagia, bleeding, weight loss, or odynophagia (Kahrilas, 2003b). Manometry and pH-metry are recommended in patients with atypical symptoms (Bresadola et al., 2003).

The impact of GERD on quality of life was assessed using the Gastrointestinal Quality of Life Index (GIQLI) before and after laparoscopic antireflux surgery. The results showed that GERD symptoms had a negative effect on quality of life that was reversed by surgical treatment (Kamolz, Granderath, & Pointner, 2003).

The specific anatomical and functional abnormalities that underlie GERD must be determined in order to select the most appropriate treatment (Mattioli, D'Ovidio, et al., 2003). Initial treatment is started and then adjusted to determine the lowest effective dosing regimen. A stepped care approach uses antacids and over-the-counter histamine-2 blockers (step 1), prescription histamine-2 blockers (step 2), and proton pump inhibitors (step 3). The practitioner may start with step 1 and move upward as needed, or start with step 3 and adjust downward as tolerated (Heitkemper, 2004). Proton pump inhibitors are believed to be most effective in suppressing acid secretion, thereby controlling reflux symptoms and permitting healing of erosions (Moss et al., 2003). Kahrilas (2003b) advises keeping the patient on that regimen for at least 8 weeks. If symptoms continue, additional evaluation is recommended. If symptoms resolve, the prescribed drugs should be discontinued on a trial basis to assess the need for maintenance therapy. Continuous therapy usually is needed if symptoms recur within 3 months, whereas individuals who remain in remission for 3 months or longer can be managed intermittently. Persons with NERD respond poorly to proton pump inhibitors and are not good candidates for surgery (Quigley, 2003).

Management of GERD in older persons is essentially the same as for younger persons except that the older individuals often require more acid suppression for the inflamed esophagus to heal (Tepper & Katz, 2003). Nonpharmacological measures that can improve LES resting pressure are weight loss; low-fat, low-glucose, high-protein diet; and avoidance of mint, chocolate, alcohol, and tobacco (Todd, Corsnitz, Ray, & Nassar, 2002).

Surgical options include several versions of fundoplication, a procedure that involves wrapping the gastric fundus around the lower esophagus to improve LES pressure. Usually performed laparoscopically, these procedures prevent movement of the junction and increase LES resting and postglutition relaxation pressures (Chrysos et al., 2004). Nissen fundoplicaton can be disrupted, most often by weight lifting and vomiting (Kakarlapudi et al., 2002).

A newer procedure is the endoscopic introduction of a catheter that delivers radiofrequency energy to the smooth muscle at the gastroesophageal junction, causing contraction of collagen and creating a barrier to reflux (Heitkemper, 2004). Esophageal lengthening procedures have been done along with antireflux surgery. However, the work of Lin, Swafford, Chadalavada, Ramshaw, and Smith (2004) questions the value of this procedure. Further, Madan, Frantzides, and Patsavas (2004) present data that bring into question the "myth of the short esophagus."

Hiatal Hernia. The incidence of hiatus hernia rises progressively from about 10% at age 40 to approximately 70% of persons over age 70. A study of more than 11,000 patients over a 10-year period revealed a steady increase in the incidence. The incidence was greater in men than in women. Hiatal hernia was present in 79% to 88% of those individuals with active reflux esophagitis (Loffeld & van der Putten, 2003). Hiatus hernia has been associated with Barrett's metaplasia (Rajendra, Kutty, & Karim, 2004). Iron deficiency anemia that occurs even in the absence of bleeding from erosions may be found in individuals with hiatal hernia (Panzuto et al., 2004).

Some investigators believe that *H. pylori* protects against GERD in patients with hiatal hernia, especially the elderly (Manes et al., 2003). Others contend that the presence of *H. pylori* and hiatal hernia in people with reflux has no effect on the risk for severe esophagitis (Awad & Camacho, 2002).

Paraesophageal hernia is an uncommon type of hiatal hernia that occurs most often in persons age 60 to 70. It is important because it causes only vague symptoms unless it becomes entrapped, leading to gangrene, perforation, and hemorrhage. Therefore surgical correction of paraesophageal hernia is recommended despite relatively minor symptoms (Greenwald & Brandt, 2003; Leeder, Smith, & Dehn, 2003). Laparoscopic surgery is an option that has been reported to be safe and effective (Anduhar et al., 2004; Leeder et al., 2003; Migliori, 2004). One study reports a relatively high incidence of recurrent hiatal hernias while noting that few require reoperation (Diaz, Brunt, Klingensmith, Frisella, & Soper, 2003). Opinions vary as to whether primary repair or the use of a mesh prosthesis is superior. An alternative that is being evaluated is the use of small intestine submucosa instead of synthetic mesh (Oelschlager, Barreca, Chang, Oleynikov, & Pelligrini, 2003a; Strange, 2003).

Although many older people with hiatal hernia are asymptomatic, they may report regurgitation, flatulence, and acid vomiting. Heartburn more commonly is reported by younger than older persons (Greenwald & Brandt, 2003). Bending over or lying down may aggravate the symptoms. If reflux esophagitis becomes severe enough, peptic ulceration or stricture may occur, and occult bleeding may lead to iron deficiency anemia.

Medical therapy is similar to that for GERD. In addition, drugs that lower LES pressure such as anticholinergics and calcium antagonists should be avoided. Surgical options may be advised in selected circumstances. The advent of laparoscopic surgery has made such procedures less risky for older adults who might previously have been denied corrective treatment.

Individuals with hiatal hernias are advised to decrease intraabdominal pressure that can result from wearing restrictive clothing, avoid lifting or straining, and elevate the head of their bed 4 to 6 inches. In addition, they should lose weight if obese; eat small, frequent meals; and avoid eating before going to bed. Smoking and alcohol consumption are discouraged because they promote reflux and impair healing.

Barrett's Esophagus. Barrett's esophagus, also called Barrett's metaplasia, is a condition in which the normal stratified squamous cell epithelium in the lower esophagus is replaced by specialized columnar cells. This change in the esophageal lining is believed to represent a response to trauma caused by the reflux of gastric contents into the esophagus. Barrett's esophagus is age related, and it is more common in patients with hiatal hernia and antral intestinal metaplasia who have a long duration of symptoms (Toruner et al., 2004). It is less common in women, possibly because they have more severe GERD symptoms (specifically heartburn, regurgitation, belching, and nocturnal symptoms) and may seek treatment earlier than men (Lin, Gerson, Lascar, Davila, & Triadafilopoulos, 2004).

The significance of Barrett's metaplasia is the increased risk of strictures and neoplasia. Screening and periodic biopsies are indicated in an effort to detect early malignant changes while resection still is possible (Greenwald & Brandt, 2003). Symptoms may be improved with reflux therapy. Thermal ablation of the abnormal tissue may be done, but recurrence is possible. Laparoscopic antireflux surgery (LARS) can effectively treat symptoms. At least one study has reported regression of intestinal metaplasia in patients with Barrett's esophagus following LARS (Oelschlager, Barreca, Chang, Oleynikov, & Pellegrini, 2003b).

Esophageal Carcinoma. Most cancers of the esophagus and gastric cardia are squamous cell carcinomas (SCCs) or adenocarcinomas. In recent decades a marked increase in the incidence of adenocarcinomas in developed countries has been noted. The reason for this increase remains elusive. The incidence of esophageal carcinoma increases with age, with three times as many men affected as women in the United States. The main risk factors for SCC are alcohol and tobacco use, older age, and previously treated head and neck cancer. The primary risk factors for adenocarcinoma are long-standing gastroesophageal reflux disease, obesity, older age, and male sex (Tytgat et al., 2004). After controlling for demographics, smoking, and body size, Wu, Tseng, and Bernstein (2003) also found that hiatal hernia remained as an independent risk factor for esophageal carcinoma. Among subjects with both hiatal hernia and reflux symptoms, the risk for adenocarcinoma was increased eightfold. Greenwald and Brandt (2003) cite evidence of esophageal stasis, achalasia, poor oral hygiene, thermal irritation, lye stricture, and previous gastric surgery as additional risk factors. Esophageal cancer always should be suspected when an older adult has symptoms such as achalasia and marked weight loss. By the time the patient has dysphagia, the disease is usually quite advanced (Greenwald & Brandt, 2003).

Efforts to identify tumor markers for esophageal cancer are ongoing. The increasing sophistication of imaging procedures (computed tomography [CT], magnetic resonance imaging [MRI], positron emission tomography) permits more accurate staging, which can guide treatment decisions. Diagnostic laparoscopy and thorascopy provide additional valuable data, though they are expensive and carry a risk of serious complications (Tytgat et al., 2004). The value of endoscopic ultrasound combined with fine-needle aspiration biopsy has been reported to yield highly accurate data for tumor and lymph node staging, which can be used to guide treatment decisions (Chang, Soetikno, Bastas, Tu, & Nguyen, 2003; Vazquez-Sequeiros et al., 2003).

Treatment options for esophageal cancer include surgery, radiotherapy, and (less commonly) chemotherapy. Although surgery offers the best long-term prognosis, fewer than half of all esophageal tumors are resectable. The traditional surgical approach has been resection of the tumor and surrounding tissue with adjacent lymph nodes by way of thoracotomy and laparotomy. This procedure carries significant mortality and morbidity rates and offers poor long-term survival. A variety of less invasive surgical procedures are under study. The role of chemotherapy in esophageal cancer is the focus of much research. A large, recently completed study concluded that preoperative chemotherapy with cisplatin and 5-fluorouracil (5-FU) demonstrated a modest but significant survival advantage over surgery alone (Tytgat et al., 2004). The gastrointestinal toxicity of cisplatin/5-FU regimens has prompted the study of alternative agents, including paclitaxel/cisplatin and irinotecan/cisplatin for combination therapy. Investigators at Sloan-Kettering are now assessing the use of these alternative agents in combination with radiation (Anderson, Minsky, Bains, Kelsen, & Ilson, 2003). The use of neoadjuvant chemoradiotherapy can be relatively toxic and currently is considered investigational (Brenner, Ilson, & Minsky, 2004; Donington et al., 2004; Tytgat et al., 2004; Zacherel et al., 2003). Several studies have reported encouraging responses to combined modalities

(Goldberg et al., 2003). A study that compared patients treated with neoadjuvant chemoradiation with patients treated with surgery alone reported similar rates of complications in the two groups (Kelley, Coppola, & Karl, 2004). A study of pathology specimens revealed that multimodal therapy, compared with surgery alone, reduced margin involvement and provided a significant survival advantage (Mulligan, Dunne, Griffin, Keeling, & Reynolds, 2004). A review of neoadjuvant therapy for adenocarcinoma by Zacherel and colleagues (2003) provides a good overview of the current state of the science. Other approaches under study include molecularly targeted agents and gene therapy.

Various studies have reported 5-year survival rates ranging from 5% to 29% (Tytgat et al., 2004). A Finnish study reported an overall rate of 12.5% with the highest survival rate (50%) with esophagectomy with two-field lymphadenectomy (Sihvo, Luostarinen, & Salo, 2004). Palliative care aims to improve the quality of life by controlling symptoms with esophageal dilation, tumor debulking, endoscopically placed stents, lasers, external beam radiation, brachytherapy, and photodynamic therapy (Greenwald & Brandt, 2003; Tytgat et al., 2004). Patients with advanced disease may tolerate brachytherapy better than external radiotherapy. Chemotherapy in advanced esophageal cancer may extend survival and reduce dysphagia (Tytgat et al., 2004).

Because of the known relationship between acid reflux and esophageal cancer, management of reflux is one preventive strategy. However, the best way to manage reflux is a topic of current research. It appears that antireflux surgery is somewhat more effective than proton pump inhibitors in reducing the risk of Barrett's esophagus and, subsequently, esophageal malignancy. Some evidence exists that a high intake of fruits and vegetables and nutritional fibers decreases the risk of esophageal cancer. In addition, *H. pylori* infection may confer a protective effect against adenocarcinoma (Tytgat et al., 2004). Evidence that invasive tumors of the stomach and esophagus demonstrate increased COX-2 expression has sparked interest as a potential target for chemopreventive agents. This approach is supported by the established reduction in risk in individuals who use aspirin regularly.

Disorders of the Stomach

Common stomach disorders in older persons are gastritis, peptic ulcer disease, and carcinoma.

Gastritis and Peptic Ulcer Disease. The most common cause of gastritis is *Helicobacter pylori* infection of the gastric mucosa, which causes inflammation, alterations in cell function, metaplasia, and cell death.

H. pylori infection usually is acquired in childhood. It sometimes causes transient symptoms and resolves, but more often persists as chronic gastritis. The infection is more common among older adults in the United States because they grew up during a time when sanitary standards were less rigid (Greenwald & Brandt, 2003). Whereas the antrum is affected initially, the infection spreads into the body and fundus over time and invades deeper layers of tissue that contain the gastric secretory cells. Gradually metaplastic glands or atropic mucosa replace normal glands, a condition that predisposes to gastric cancer (Kuipers et al., 2004). Submucosal hemorrhage, edema, epithelial erosion, and peptic ulcers may occur with chronic active gastritis. The severity of *H. pylori* gastritis has been associated with profound suppression of gastric acid (Kuipers et al., 2004).

Symptoms associated with active gastritis and gastric mucosal atrophy include intermittent dyspepsia, abdominal pain, distention, and nausea and vomiting; however, these conditions often are asymptomatic. The presence of *H. pylori* can be assessed with biopsy specimens of the stomach (obtained endoscopically), serum antibody studies, stool assay, and a urea breath test.

Treatment of *H. pylori* infection consists of a combination of several drugs, typically a proton pump inhibitor with various combinations of metronidazole, a tetracycline, a macrolide, a fluoroquinolone, a beta lactam, or a bismuth preparation. An antisecretory agent also is recommended in the presence of active ulcers to facilitate healing. The effectiveness of the drug therapy should be evaluated with a urea breath test 4 weeks after completion of the course of therapy (Greenwald & Brandt, 2004). In a small study ($n = 17$) of individuals with a clarithromycin-resistant strain of *H. pylori*, the subjects were effectively treated with a 2-week course of rabeprozole and amoxicillin (Furuta et al., 2004).

After *H. pylori* infection, NSAID ingestion is the most common cause of peptic ulcer disease. NSAIDs inhibit the synthesis of prostaglandins, which normally protect the stomach by stimulating the production of bicarbonate and mucus and increasing mucosal blood flow. The use of NSAIDs by older adults is startling. In the United States, 1.2% of the population takes at least one NSAID each day, and the number increases with age. One study in the United Kingdom revealed that for every 1000 women over age 64, 1400 prescriptions for NSAIDs were written in 1 year. It is estimated that 12% to 30% of chronic NSAID users develop gastric ulcers and 2% to 19% develop duodenal ulcers (Greenwald & Brandt, 2003). Until recently, COX-2 inhibitors appeared to be a good alternative to other NSAIDs because of fewer gastrointestinal effects. However, an increase in myocardial infarctions and strokes among individuals taking Vioxx resulted in its withdrawal from the market. Therefore the use of the COX-2 inhibitors is being reexamined.

Misoprostol and famotidine (in high doses) have been used with NSAIDs to prevent ulcers. Misoprostol is a synthetic prostaglandin analog that has been shown to reduce the incidence of both duodenal and gastric ulcers in people on NSAID therapy. Side effects of misoprostol that have limited its usefulness include diarrhea, abdominal cramping, and flatulence.

Older persons with peptic ulcer disease are at greater risk for complications and death than their younger counterparts. Duodenal ulcers are more common, but gastric ulcers are more often associated with death. The complication rate for individuals age 75 to 79 is 76%. Although bleeding or perforation may be the first sign of ulcer disease, the clinical manifestations in the older adult may be subtle. If chronic blood loss occurs, the chief complaint may be fatigue and cardiac symptoms. When ulcers develop high in the cardia, symptoms may be mistaken for cardiac or esophageal problems. In addition to bleeding and perforation, complications of peptic ulcer disease in older persons include gastric outlet obstruction. In some cases the disease is not discovered until major complications occur (e.g., acute upper gastrointestinal hemorrhage, perforation, or pyloric stenosis).

Giant ulcers may occur in the stomach and in the duodenum. The duodenal version is most commonly found in men over age 70 and is typically manifested by abdominal pain that radiates to the back or right upper quadrant. Giant gastric ulcers are more common after age 65 and have high morbidity and mortality rates associated with hemorrhage. Pain with giant gastric ulcers is more likely to radiate to the chest, umbilicus, or lower abdomen. Giant ulcers in both locations usually can be treated effectively with histamine antagonists, proton pump inhibitors, and antibiotics (if *H. pylori* is present).

Although antiulcer drugs often are effective, some precautions must be mentioned when prescribed for older persons (Greenwald & Brandt, 2003):

- Depending on the type, antacids can cause diarrhea, constipation, and/or fluid retention.
- Antacids interfere with the absorption of many other drugs.
- Histamine antagonists interfere with the metabolism of other drugs.
- Cimetidine interferes with the elimination of other drugs, including warfarin, and can cause confusion when given intravenously.
- Ranitidine and famotidine can cause headache.
- Sucralfate can cause constipation.

Hematemesis is more common than melena in older persons with upper gastrointestinal bleeding. Surgical intervention should not be withheld on the basis of age alone; however, the mortality and complication rates are higher among older individuals. They are especially at risk for cardiac, neurological, and renal disease; sepsis;

and reactions to medications and transfusions (Greenwald & Brandt, 2003).

ATROPHIC GASTRITIS AND PERNICIOUS ANEMIA. Type A gastritis is associated with an autoimmune process, in contrast to type B, which is associated with *H. pylori*. Parietal cells eventually are destroyed, and the production of hydrochloric acid and intrinsic factor falls. Without adequate intrinsic factor, vitamin B_{12}, which is required for the growth and maturation of red blood cells, is not absorbed. Affected individuals develop pernicious anemia and neurological complications (Heitkemper, 2004). Vitamin B_{12} deficiency is treated with regular injections of the vitamin.

Gastric Adenocarcinoma. The incidence of adenocarcinoma of the proximal stomach has been increasing, whereas the incidence of distal gastric carcinoma is declining (Crew & Neugut, 2004). Gastric cancer is most likely to occur after 60 years of age, and the incidence rate is considerably higher among men than among women. Dietary factors and *H. pylori* have been implicated in the pathogenesis of gastric adenocarcinoma (Crew & Neugut, 2004; Huang & Hunt, 2003; Rautelin & Kosunen, 2004). Early symptoms typically are vague and include early satiety, anorexia, epigastric discomfort, and weight loss. Enlarged left axillary and supraclavicular lymph nodes, an umbilical node, or a firm left hepatic lobe may be palpable. Though uncommon, some patients suddenly develop multiple skin lesions referred to as the sign of Leser-Trelat. At this time, complete tumor resection is believed to be the only curative option (Macdonald, 2004; Yeh & Cheng, 2004). Unfortunately, gastric cancer often is inoperable by the time it is diagnosed, and the 5-year survival rate is reported to be only 5% to 15%. A combination of chemotherapy and radiotherapy may also be employed (Greenwald & Brandt, 2003). Among the treatment strategies being explored are preoperative neoadjuvant chemoradiation, growth receptor antagonists, antiangiogenesis agents, postoperative chemoradiotherapy, and intraperitoneal chemotherapy (Macdonald, 2004; Sakar et al., 2004; Sugarbaker, Yu, & Yonemura, 2003). One study at the M. D. Anderson Cancer Center employed a three-step treatment strategy consisting of induction chemotherapy, followed by a combination of chemotherapy and radiation, and then surgery. The investigators concluded that the strategy increased survival time in individuals with potentially resectable carcinomas (Ajani et al., 2004). In a Japanese study, palliative resection was demonstrated to significantly prolong survival in individuals with incurable gastric cancer with distant metastases (Moriwaki et al., 2004). However, surgical intervention carries a significant risk. The in-hospital mortality rate following gastric resection in the United States is 7.4%, a figure that had remained constant over 13 years (Wainess,

Dimick, Upchurch, Cowan, & Mulholland, 2003). Measures that may help prevent gastric cancer are dietary modifications and treatment of *H. pylori* infections (Plummer, Franceschi, & Munoz, 2004).

Disorders of the Small Intestine

In general, age alone is not thought to cause significant changes in small intestine structure or function. One disorder of the small intestine sometimes encountered in the older patient is malabsorption.

Malabsorptive Disorders. The prevalence of malabsorption in older adults is uncertain, with estimates ranging from 7% to 30%. Most cases of malabsorption result from bacterial overgrowth syndrome, chronic pancreatitis, or celiac disease (Rodrigues, 2003). Symptoms of malabsorption in the older person may differ from those in younger persons. For example, older persons with fat malabsorption are unlikely to have steatorrhea, probably because of slow bowel transit time and lower fat intake. With carbohydrate malabsorption, the bacterial action on carbohydrates in the colon causes watery diarrhea, abdominal distention, borborygmi, and flatulence. Other clinical manifestations might include nausea, fatigue, poor mobility, anorexia, anemia, weight loss, and confusion. Deficiencies of specific nutrients account for other manifestations. For example, hypoproteinemia can result in peripheral edema; osteomalacia can cause muscle weakness and generalized aches; and bruising, petechiae, and bleeding may represent vitamin K deficiency. Abdominal pain is not common with malabsorption, but may be present with chronic pancreatitis, inflammatory bowel disease, strictures, or chronic mesenteric ischemia.

Because of the atypical presentation, malabsorption should be suspected in the older person with evidence of malnutrition even if there are no gastrointestinal symptoms. A dietary assessment is essential to rule out inadequate nutrient intake. The history should document factors that may be associated with malabsorption, such as gastric surgery, intestinal bypass procedures, and small bowel resection. Blood studies should include blood cell counts, ferritin, vitamin B_{12}, red cell folate level, alkaline phosphatase, calcium and phosphorus, international normalized ratio (INR), and protein. Absorption tests are available but inconvenient and relatively insensitive. Bacterial overgrowth can be determined with analysis of small bowel fluid obtained during endoscopy or through one of several breath tests and a urine test. Small bowel enteroscopy and CT and MRI scanning may yield additional data. Capsule endoscopy is a relatively new diagnostic procedure that is proving to be especially valuable in the study of the small bowel (Rodrigues, 2003).

Effective treatment of malabsorption depends on accurate diagnosis and may employ drug and diet therapy, nutritional supplementation, and enzyme replacement. If bacterial overgrowth is the precipitating factor in malabsorptive disorders, treatment is accomplished with antibiotics.

Some other small bowel disorders seen in older adults are summarized in Table 15-1.

Disorders of the Large Intestine

Important disorders of the large intestine that are more common in older persons are diverticular disease, cancer, ischemic colitis, vascular ectasias, fecal incontinence, constipation, and antibiotic-associated diarrhea and colitis (Wald, 2003).

Diverticular Disease. Diverticular disease, including diverticulitis and diverticulosis, is extremely common among older persons, affecting about two thirds by age 80. A colonic diverticulum is a herniation of the colonic mucosa through the otherwise normal colonic wall, with weakness or abnormalities (or both) of intracolonic pressure. There is also a pronounced thickening of the longitudinal and circular muscle layers (Figure 15-1). The major factors leading to diverticula formation are thought to be weakness of the colonic muscle and insufficient dietary fiber. Most diverticula

Table 15-1 *Small Bowel Disorders in the Older Adult*

Disorder	Characteristics	Manifestations	Management
Bacterial overgrowth syndrome	Malabsorption related to increased population of anaerobes in the small bowel. Usually associated with disordered motility.	Nonspecific signs of malabsorption. History of gastroparesis, irritable bowel syndrome, chronic pancreatitis.	Antibiotics: co-metronidazole with a cephalosporin; co-amoxyclav; norfloxacin. Cyclic courses may be needed every 4-6 months. Prokinetic agents. Avoid antacids.
Crohn's disease	Segmental inflammation and ulceration. Relapsing. Isolated small bowel involvement more common in older persons.	Diarrhea, weight loss, fever, right iliac fossa pain (may be absent in older persons). Signs and symptoms of obstruction or perforation in some cases.	Antimicrobials. For small bowel involvement, need mesalazine preparations that release the drug in the small bowel. Corticosteroids. Immunosuppressive agents. Nutritional supplementation. Surgery for complications.
Acute small bowel ischemia	Caused by embolism, thrombus, or nonocclusive ischemia of superior mesenteric artery. High mortality rate.	Acute: severe abdominal pain. May have abdominal distention, gastrointestinal bleeding, leukocytosis, metabolic acidosis. Hypotension, vomiting, fever with peritonitis.	Acute: fluids, inotropics, broad-spectrum antibiotics. Papaverine to dilate mesenteric arteries. Thrombolytics in selected cases. Emergency surgery for infarction. Postoperative anticoagulation for thrombus.
Chronic small bowel ischemia	Caused by atherosclerosis of blood vessels. Mesenteric blood vessels cannot meet demands after meals.	Upper abdominal pain begins 30 minutes after a meal, increases in intensity, lasting several hours. Lying prone or squatting may bring relief. May have constipation or diarrhea.	Surgical revascularization.
Malignant small bowel tumors	Incidence peaks in sixth and seventh decades	Abdominal pain, bleeding, intestinal obstruction, weight loss.	Surgical resection for adenocarcinomas and leiomyosarcomas. Surgery and drug therapy (serotonin antagonists, octreotide, chemotherapy, interferon-A) for carcinoid tumors.

Data from Rodrigues, C. A. (2003). The small bowel. In R. C. Tallis & H. M. Fillit (Eds.), *Brocklehurst's textbook of geriatric medicine and gerontology* (6th ed.). London: Churchill Livingstone.

are asymptomatic. Individuals with painful diverticular disease experience crampy lower left abdominal discomfort and tenderness, often associated with diarrhea or constipation. The symptoms are similar to irritable bowel disease except for the absence of fever, leukocytosis, and rebound tenderness (Wald, 2003).

As many as a quarter of individuals with diverticulosis develop diverticulitis. The inflamed diverticulum becomes obstructed, leading to microperforations and macroperforations that usually are localized but can result in abscesses, fibrosis and bowel obstruction, fistula formation, and perforation with peritonitis. It can be difficult to distinguish painful diverticular disease from diverticulitis because the older person may not have fever, leukocytosis, or rebound tenderness even with inflammation (Wald, 2003). CT scanning and ultrasonic imaging are useful for initial evaluation, with barium enema performed after inflammation has diminished.

The medical treatments of painful diverticulosis and diverticulitis are detailed in Table 15-2. When bleeding occurs, a colonoscopy permits identification of the source. A bleeding scan or selective mesenteric angiography is indicated with brisk bleeding. A vasopressor can be administered through the angiography catheter to control bleeding. Bowel resection is indicated for those who do not respond to medical therapy or who develop specific complications. A one-step procedure is preferred, but sometimes a two-step process with a temporary colostomy may be necessitated by peritonitis or perforation with abscess or high-grade obstruction (Wald, 2003).

Cancer

Colorectal cancers are the third most common type of new cancers and cause of cancer deaths in the United States. More than 90% are diagnosed in individuals age 50 and older. In addition to age, risk factors include smoking, alcohol consumption, obesity, physical inactivity, high-fat and/or low-fiber diet, inadequate intake of fruits and vegetables, and a family history of colorectal cancer, polyps, or inflammatory bowel disease. The 5-year survival rate is 90% when detected while still localized; however, only about one third of colorectal cancers are detected at that stage. The 5-year survival rate drops to 65% with regional involvement and 9% with distant metastasis (American Cancer Society, 2004).

The absence of symptoms during the early stage explains why these cancers are seldom detected early. When symptoms do occur, they may include rectal bleeding, blood in the stool, change in bowel function, and cramping in the lower abdomen. Informative diagnostic procedures include colonoscopy, abdominal imaging studies, and (to stage rectal cancers) rectal

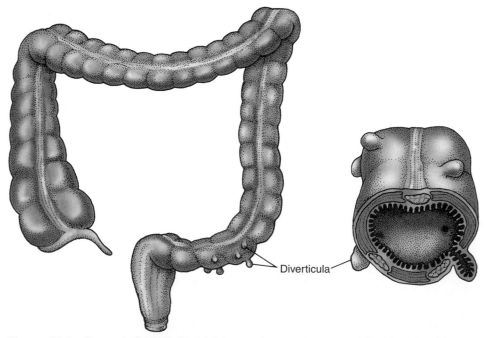

Diverticula

Figure 15-1 Several *diverticula,* which are abnormal outpouchings, or herniations, in the wall of the intestine. These can occur anywhere in the small or large intestine but are found most often in the sigmoid, as shown in this figure. Diverticulitis is the inflammation of a diverticulum that occurs when undigested food or bacteria become trapped in the diverticulum. (From Ignatavicius, D. D., & Workman, M. L. [2006]. *Medical-surgical nursing: Critical thinking for collaborative care* [5th ed.]. Philadelphia: Saunders.)

Table 15-2 *Medical Treatment of Diverticular Disease*

Measure	Painful Diverticulosis	Diverticulitis
Diet	Increase fiber	Reduce fiber (or nothing by mouth [NPO])
Bulk laxatives	Sometimes effective	Not indicated
Analgesics	Avoid opioids	Avoid morphine; meperidine is best
Antispasmodics	Propantheline bromide Dicyclomine hydrochloride Hyoscyamine sulfate	Not indicated
Antibiotics	Not indicated	Oral: amoxicillin/clavulanate K Parenteral: gentamycin or tobramycin plus clindamycin; cefoxitin; ampicillin/ sulbactam sodium

Modified from Wald, A. (2003). The large bowel. In R. C. Tallis & H. M. Fillit (Eds.), *Brocklehurst's textbook of geriatric medicine and gerontology* (6th ed.). London: Churchill Livingstone.

endosonography. Surgical resection is the primary treatment. Adjuvant chemotherapy has been shown to prolong survival in individuals with colon cancer who have regional lymph node metastasis and those with tumor penetration through the muscularis propria or through the serosa into pericolic fat. For rectal cancer, survival is improved by adjuvant combined chemotherapy and radiotherapy (Wald, 2003).

For early detection, the American Cancer Society (2004) recommends the following beginning at age 50 for individuals who are at average risk for colorectal cancer:

■ Annual fecal occult blood test *or* flexible sigmoidoscopy every 5 years *or* both every 5 years (preferred)
■ Colonoscopy every 10 years if normal *or* double-contrast barium enema every 5 years if normal
■ Digital rectal examination at same time as endoscopy or barium enema

Changes in Bowel Habits. Normal adult bowel function is the result of a complex interplay of the central nervous system, the peripheral nerves, the autonomic nervous system, the endocrine system, the gastrointestinal tract, and the musculoskeletal system, as outlined in Table 15-3. This chart can be used to illustrate how various factors contribute to the development of constipation and fecal incontinence by affecting these essential components of bowel function. Changes in bowel habits actually are symptoms rather than disease states, but they are listed as separate entities because they are so bothersome to older adults.

DIARRHEA. *Diarrhea* is defined by the North American Nursing Diagnosis Association (NANDA) as "the passage of loose, unformed stools" (NANDA

Table 15-3 *Components of Normal Bowel Function*

Component	Function
Food and water	Nothing in—nothing out; fiber produces bulk in the stool
Central nervous system	Judgment: to take in sufficient quantities of food and fluid Control of motor functions: inhibits defecation until socially appropriate time
Intestines	Where nutrients are absorbed and feces are formed (in large intestine or colon); feces propelled by peristaltic action of intestines
Muscles	Propel fecal matter along intestinal tract Allow one to walk to toilet and get on the commode Abdominal muscles assist peristaltic action Sphincter muscles hold feces in rectum until time to defecate
Nerves	Carry messages to the central nervous system about need to defecate; carry messages to the muscles (sphincters) to relax and defecate
Rectum	Holding area for feces until place to defecate is found

From Snow, T. L., & McConnell, E. S. (1985). Bowel and bladder management training program. Unpublished educational aid.

International, 2003, p. 60). Defining characteristics are a minimum of three loose liquid stools per day, hyperactive bowel sounds, urgency, abdominal pain, and cramping. Consequences of untreated diarrhea include fluid and electrolyte disturbance, predisposition to fecal incontinence, pain, impaired skin integrity, and low self-image.

Acute diarrhea persists for less than 3 weeks and most often is caused by infection. In the United States, the death rate associated with acute diarrhea is 15 per 100,000 for individuals age 75 and older. Chronic diarrhea can be classified as prolonged infectious, fat malabsorptive, watery, secretory, or inflammatory. Conditions associated with watery diarrhea include ingestion of nonabsorbable solutes, carbohydrate malabsorption, high bile salt level, and irritable bowel syndrome. True secretory disorders are related to endocrine tumors, nonendocrine malignancies, alcoholism, or diabetes. In addition, factitious diarrhea sometimes is seen, in which the patient surreptitiously ingests laxatives or diuretics to induce diarrhea. Several conditions may cause inflammatory diarrhea, including Crohn's disease, ulcerative colitis, food intolerance or allergy, and pelvic radiation.

Diagnosis is based on the duration of the condition, the presence of blood in the stool, a recent history of constipation, a medical and drug history, and recent changes in dietary habits. Patients should be assessed for signs and symptoms of volume depletion, such as tachycardia, postural hypotension, poor skin turgor, absence of axillary sweat, and an increase in the hematocrit or blood urea nitrogen level, as well as changes in serum potassium. Radiography, endoscopy, biopsy, and laboratory testing of blood, stool, and urine all may be needed to determine the specific cause.

Many older adults enjoy traveling in other countries, which places them at risk for traveler's diarrhea (TD). One large study found incidence rates between 5.4% and 31.5% with considerable variations between countries visited. The investigators noted that travelers tended not to heed warning about consuming potentially dangerous food items (Steffen et al., 2004). Measures to reduce the risk of TD include meticulous handwashing, drinking bottled water where recommended, and avoidance of foods known to be dangerous.

Contributing Factors. In addition to infection, diarrhea in older persons may be caused by fecal impactions, food intolerance, dietary indiscretions (too much fruit, especially bananas; caffeine), misuse of laxatives, improper hyperosmolar tube feedings, side effects of radiation therapy to the abdomen, autonomic neuropathy, inflammatory bowel disease, anxiety, malignancy, malabsorption syndromes, and protein-calorie malnutrition. Among the drugs that increase motility in the small and large intestine are laxatives, diuretics, cholinergics, angiotensin-converting enzyme (ACE) inhibitors,

antidepressants, H-2 blockers, prokinetic agents (metoclopromide), and prostaglandins (Powell, 2000).

An especially serious drug effect is pseudomembranous colitis, a *Clostridium difficile* superinfection that is associated with antibiotics. "C. diff," as it commonly is called, is most likely with cephalosporins, ampicillin, clindamycin, and combination therapy. Diarrhea and colitis associated with *C. difficile* is common in nursing homes, where as many as 30% of residents with a history of antibiotic therapy may be asymptomatic carriers (Fekety, 2000). The onset of symptoms may be as soon as the first week of antibiotic therapy or as long as 6 weeks after therapy has been completed. Diarrhea is profuse, with cramping, fever, and leukocytosis, but usually without blood or mucus. In severe cases, hypoalbuminemia develops because of protein-losing enteropathy. Treatment is with oral metronidazole or vancomycin. Relapses are not uncommon, but usually respond to standard treatment. *C. difficile* is commonly found in the environment, but the best prevention is good hygiene to prevent spread among individuals (Fekety, 2000). An evidence-based nursing review concluded that the coadministration of probiotics such as lactobacillus reduces the incidence of antibiotic-associated diarrhea (Gagan, 2003). Diarrhea associated with chemotherapy or radiotherapy is treated with loperamide and NSAIDs in addition to symptom management.

Several factors have been implicated in diarrhea associated with enteral feedings, including lack of fiber, high fat content in the presence of fat malabsorption, bacterial contamination, and rapid advancement in the rate of administration. Formula hyperosmolarity has been blamed, but this has not been demonstrated in controlled studies. Lactose also has been blamed for causing diarrhea; however, it is absent from almost all enteral feeding formulas (Rombeau, 2000).

Treatment. Treatment is aimed at providing support, relieving symptoms, and treating the underlying condition. The patient is supported by replacing fluid and electrolyte losses, and symptomatic relief is provided by giving antidiarrheals to decrease the number of bowel movements or to improve the consistency of the stool. The underlying condition may be treated medically or surgically. Depending on the condition, drug therapy may include antimicrobials, corticosteroids, and enzyme preparations.

Treatment of acute diarrhea depends on the cause and the individual's general condition. In the absence of dehydration, fluid/electrolyte replacement and antidiarrheals may suffice. Intravenous therapy may be needed until the oral intake is sufficient. For infectious bacterial diarrhea, bismuth subsalicylate is safe and efficacious. Opiates and anticholinergics are contraindicated with infectious diarrhea because they prolong microorganism excretion time. Loperamide, especially in combination with appropriate antibiotics, may be helpful.

Fluoroquinolones are the treatment of choice while awaiting stool culture results. Diarrhea associated with chemotherapy or radiotherapy is treated with loperamide and NSAIDs in addition to symptom management (Powell, 2000).

As with acute diarrhea, the treatment of chronic diarrhea depends on the cause. Drugs that often are used include those that decrease secretory activity, slow peristalsis, decrease inflammation, or increase sphincter tone. With severe inflammatory disease, opiates and anticholinergics are contraindicated because of the risk of toxic megacolon (Powell, 2000).

CONSTIPATION. NANDA defines *constipation* as a "decrease in normal frequency of defecation accompanied by difficult or incomplete passage of stool and/or passage of excessively hard, dry stool" (NANDA International, 2003, p. 40). In the United States, over 2 million physician visits each year are related to constipation, causing a significant burden for the health care system. In addition, over $1 billion is spent each year on laxatives (Merli & Graham, 2003). An extensive review of the literature sought to document the prevalence of constipation in North America. A fundamental problem in compiling results was the variation in the definition of constipation that was used in various studies. Studies that relied on self-report claimed higher prevalence rates than those that used objective criteria such as the Rome II criteria. Older adults who reported constipation typically defined it as "straining" or "hard stools" regardless of the frequency of bowel movements. However, when the Rome II criteria were applied, the rate ranged from 12% to 19%. Box 15-2 lists criteria for constipation.

An increasing incidence of constipation with advancing age was demonstrated in several large national databases included in the review. The prevalence also was higher among women, individuals with less formal education, and non-whites (Higgins & Johanson, 2004). In a survey of a large sample of Taiwanese women, 32.4% of women over age 65 reported constipation, but that figure fell to 8.3% when medical criteria for constipation were applied (Chen, Hu, Chen, Lin, & Lin, 2003).

The pathophysiological basis for constipation may include alterations in innervation, smooth muscle activity, or neuroendocrine function that increase colonic transit time and create difficulty in defecation and changes in anal rectal sensation (Potter, 2003). One system classifies constipation as either functional constipation or rectal outlet delay constipation. The two types of functional constipation are slow transit constipation and dyssynergic defecation. Older adults with constipation have been found to have a total gut transit time of 4 to 9 days compared with a normal rate of less than 3 days. The delay has been attributed to segmental dysmotility with predominant slowing in the left colon. Transit time may be as long as 14 days in institutionalized, bedridden individuals. The slower transit time allows for greater reabsorption of water from the feces, creating a smaller fecal mass and subsequently less intraluminal pressure to stimulate travel through the colon. Other factors that can slow transit time are dilation of the colon and reduced sigmoid response to stimuli (Harari, 2003). Individuals with slow-transit idiopathic constipation have been found to have decreased colonic motor activity that leads to reduced propulsion of colon contents (Hagger, Kumar, Benson, & Grundy, 2003).

Anorectal dysfunctions are classified as rectal dyschezia, pelvic dyssynergia, pelvic floor descent, or irritable bowel syndrome. Rectal dyschezia is characterized by impaired rectal sensation of distention, reduced rectal tone, increased rectal compliance, and impaired rectal sensitivity. It may be caused by suppression of defecation. Patients may have leakage of liquid stool and mucus around a fecal impaction. With pelvic dyssynergy, the puborectalis and external anal sphincter muscles contract rather than relaxing with attempted defecation, causing the individual to strain. Pelvic floor descent is more common among women who have given birth, resulting in a loss of pelvic muscle strength. Following a long history of constipation, some patients develop irritable bowel syndrome with increased rectal tone and decreased compliance. They pass small fecal pellets with difficulty, and experience abdominal pain and distention that is relieved by defecation (Harari, 2003). Defocography was used to evaluate 52 women with a mean age of 78 who complained of constipation. Abnormalities, including perineal descent, rectocele, intussusception, and enterocele, were detected in 77% of the women (Savoye-Collet, Savoye, Koning, Leroi, & Dacher, 2003). Figure 15-2 provides an algorithm for evaluating constipation in older persons.

BOX 15-2 Rome II Criteria for Constipation

Twelve or more weeks of two or more of the following:

- Fewer than three stools per week
- Hard or lumpy stools with at least 25% of bowel movements
- Straining with at least 25% of bowel movements
- A sense of incomplete evacuation in at least 25% of bowel movements
- Manual maneuvers required for at least 25% of bowel movements
- Sense of anorectal obstruction with at least 25% of bowel movements

From Drossman, D. A., Talley, N. J., Thompson, W. G., et al. (1999). Rome II: A multinational consensus document on functional gastrointestinal disorders. *Gut, 45*(suppl 2), 1-81.

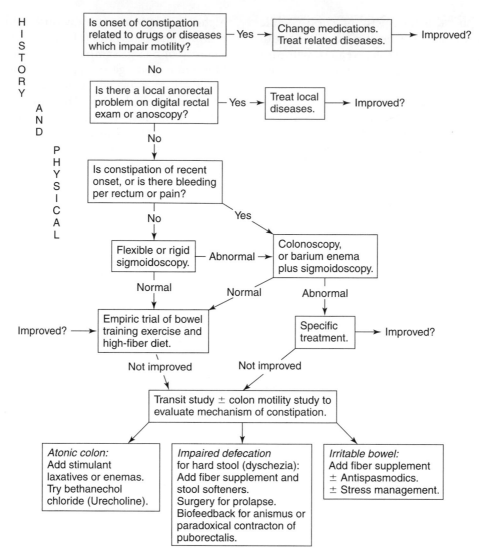

Figure 15-2 Evaluation of constipation in older persons. (From Cheskin, L. J., & Schuster, M. M. [1994]. Constipation. In W. R. Hazzard, E. L. Bierman, J. P. Blass, et al. [Eds.], *Principles of geriatric medicine and gerontology* [3rd ed.]. New York: McGraw-Hill, p. 1270. Copyright 1994. Reproduced with permission of McGraw-Hill, Inc.)

Risk Factors. Risk factors for functional constipation in the older adult include specific disease states, medications, immobility, dehydration, low dietary fiber, metabolic disturbances, and mechanical obstruction. Rectal outlet delay and self-reported constipation are associated with different factors as listed in Box 15-3 (Harari, 2003).

DISEASE STATES. People with dementing disorders, such as Alzheimer's disease, multi-infarct dementia, and Parkinson's disease, often experience constipation and fecal incontinence. The impairments of judgment, memory, and problem solving associated with dementia can result in an individual who is unable independently to take in proper amounts of fiber and fluid. Inability to find a toilet when the urge to defecate is sensed also contributes to constipation and fecal incontinence.

Motor dysfunction and incoordination that may accompany progressive dementing disorders also make independent toileting difficult.

Endocrine disorders, such as hypothyroidism and hypercalcemia, can result in constipation, as can depression. Neurological disorders, including demyelinating diseases, autonomic neuropathy, spinal cord injuries, and cerebrovascular accidents, may interfere with the sensation of the urge to defecate or the ability to defecate on command. If a regular toileting regimen is not established, constipation ensues because too much water is reabsorbed in the large intestine, resulting in feces that are hard and difficult to pass. Musculoskeletal disorders, such as severe arthritis, muscular dystrophies, and fractures resulting in prolonged immobility, all may lead to constipation. In these cases, immobility results

BOX 15-3 Pharmacological Treatment of Constipation in Older People

Functional Constipation

- Bulk laxative one to three times daily with fluids in ambulant elderly persons
- In less mobile individuals, those with questionable fluid intake, or those intolerant of bulk laxatives, give lactulose 30 mL daily titrating upward to achieve regular (three or more times per week) and comfortable evacuation
- In high-risk patients (e.g., immobile nursing home residents, patients with Parkinson's disease, etc.) or those with persistent constipation, add senna 1 to 3 tablets at bedtime

Rectal Outlet Delay

- Manual disimpaction where necessary, followed by enema for initial clearance
- Glycerin suppository once daily after breakfast for 2 weeks, then use as required to relieve symptoms; for recurrent rectal impaction or overflow fecal incontinence, use bisacodyl suppositories instead
- If stool is hard, add daily bulk laxative or lactulose

Colonic Transit Impaction

- Daily arachis oil retention enema, or phosphate or enema with extension nozzle
- When obstruction resolves, give senna 3 tablets at bedtime and lactulose 30 mL two times daily with daily enemas until no further washout result
- Polyethylene glycol* (Movicol) ½ to 1 sachet daily with fluids may be given instead of lactulose for rapid disimpaction (e.g., in hospital) or where stool retention is persistent; provisions must be taken to manage the likely side effect of fecal incontinence
- When impaction resolves, return to maintenance regimen for functional constipation

From Harari, D. (2003). Constipation and fecal incontinence in old age. In R. C. Tallis & H. M. Fillit (Eds.), *Brocklehurst's textbook of geriatric medicine and gerontology* (6th ed.). London: Churchill Livingstone.
*If not available, an alternative to Movicol is Miralax.

in diminished activity, which produces decreased peristalsis because voluntary muscles do not assist peristalsis. Tumors in either the colon, peritoneal cavity, or rectum may interfere with the peristaltic action required to move fecal material through the colon and out the anus. Hemorrhoids and fistulas may result in pain on defecation that inhibits the normal urge to defecate.

DRUGS. Many drugs contribute to constipation. Key offenders are anticholinergic drugs, including many antipsychotics and antidepressants; opioids; antacids containing aluminum, bismuth, or calcium; bulk-forming laxatives taken without sufficient fluids; stimulant laxatives taken on a regular basis; and some less frequently thought of drugs, such as diuretics and calcium channel blockers.

INADEQUATE DIETARY FIBER INTAKE. Feces are composed of food that is not absorbed in the stomach or small intestine. A diet of highly refined foods and few fruits or vegetables predisposes to constipation, because there is insufficient bulk to stimulate peristaltic movement.

INADEQUATE FLUID INTAKE. The large intestine is part of the body's system for maintaining fluid and electrolyte balance. If a person is poorly hydrated, more water will be absorbed in the large intestine in an attempt to maintain homeostasis. This results in dry feces that become hardened and more difficult to pass.

ENVIRONMENTAL FACTORS. Defecation is a complex process involving the autonomic nervous system and the use of voluntary muscles. Both spinal reflexes and cortical control are involved. The process involves simultaneous contraction of some muscles and relaxation of others. Inadequate privacy may result in habitual and inappropriate inhibition of the urge to defecate, resulting in constipation.

When older adults were interviewed about problems with constipation, their first concern was to preserve their dignity (Potter, 2003). Creating an environment for toileting that respects privacy and dignity is especially problematic in nursing homes and hospitals. Bedside commodes often are provided because of the distance to the bathroom, and privacy is limited to a flimsy curtain pulled around the individual. Persons who cannot get to the toilet independently must wait for assistance and risk incontinence if the wait is excessive.

Complications. Chronic constipation is not just an inconvenience; it can have serious complications, including overflow incontinence, fecal impaction, perforation of the colon, sigmoid volvulus, and urinary retention (Harari, 2003). In addition, frequent use of laxatives and enemas to treat actual or perceived constipation can create new problems.

Constipation contributes to incontinence when the patient never completely evacuates the rectum, resulting in frequent, small stools, or the patient oozes liquid stool around an impaction. Other major contributing factors to fecal incontinence are summarized in Table 15-4. A fecal impaction is a hard mass of feces lodged in the colon or rectal vault. This severe form of constipation may result in two major problems: (1) soiling, which may be incorrectly diagnosed as diarrhea, and (2) stercoral ulceration, a pressure necrosis of the large intestine.

Management. An abundance of advice on the prevention and management of constipation exists, but surprisingly there is limited evidence of best practices. Meta-analyses and systematic reviews are stymied by inconsistent definitions and methodological weaknesses (Potter, 2003). From 2000 to 2004 the Cochrane Database of Systematic Reviews and the EBM Reviews—Cochrane Central Register of Controlled Trials contained

Table 15-4 *Techniques for Patients with Fecal Incontinence*

Etiology	Identifying Characteristics	Intervention
CENTRAL NERVOUS SYSTEM		
Disorientation		
Alzheimer's/dementia	Can't find the right place (early disease)	Establish toileting schedule
Coma	Can't figure out how to get undressed, defecate, and get dressed again	Staff must take initiative to prevent "accidents"
Stroke		
Advanced Parkinson's	Can't ask for help	
Acute confusion		
No control over spinal reflexes	Can't control the urge to defecate (late disease)	Establish toileting regimen using patient's habit pattern as a guide
	Can't sense the urge to defecate	
		Behavior modification:
No social awareness	Doesn't care where defecation occurs "I'm not worth it"	• Obtain street clothes for patient
		• Explore patient's decreased feeling of self-worth
	Never taught that it matters where one defecates	• Determine rewards for correct toilet use, explain to patient and implement
		Staff development/behavior modification:
Negative self-image	No one else cares where defecation occurs	• Assess caregivers' actions toward patient
Low energy		
Too much trouble	"The slows"—it's just too much trouble	• Assess for physiological problems and treat accordingly
Depressed		• Provide structure, reinforce good performance
Chronically ill		
Anemia		• Modify the environment to facilitate function and equipment
METABOLIC ABNORMALITIES		
Endocrine disorders	Abnormal lab values—diagnosis of hypercalcemia, hyperthyroidism, hypokalemia	Medical diagnosis and treatment of etiologic disorder:
		• During evaluation, resolve constipation, using medications if necessary
PSYCHOLOGICAL		
Depression . . . which leads to constipation . . . which leads to impaction . . . which leads to fecal incontinence	Marked sadness, loss of interest and pleasure in daily activities	Drug therapy, antidepressants
		Psychotherapy, cognitive-behavioral therapy
Inappropriate expression of anger	Attention getter—"He's just doing that to get attention"	Supportive counseling/behavior modification:
		• Positive reinforcement of "good" bowel habits
Misinformed about "normal" bowel habits	"I need to go once a day"	• Look at other ways of giving attention
	"I've got to have a bowel movement every day"	Counsel and teach:
	"I drink too much"	• Teach and support new knowledge regarding bowel habits
LACK OF PRIVACY		
Lack of private/comfortable place to defecate	"Habit constipation"	Provision of adequate privacy
	Ignoring/suppressing the urge to defecate	Attend to proper equipment and positioning
	Bedpans	
GASTROINTESTINAL SYSTEM		
Reduced peristalsis	Immobility	Start exercise program
	Drug-induced: anticholinergics, narcotics	Consider whether change in drugs is possible
	Chronic laxative abuse	Stop laxatives
	Low-fiber diet	Increase bulk and fluid
No assistance of peristalsis with voluntary muscles	Muscle inactivity: bedbound/chairbound, cord injury	Start exercise program to increase use of abdominal muscles

Table 15-4 *Techniques for Patients with Fecal Incontinence—cont'd*

Etiology	Identifying Characteristics	Intervention
GASTROINTESTINAL SYSTEM—CONT'D		
Diarrhea in individuals with reduced mobility	Soiling on clothes— "I couldn't get there in time"	Treat diarrhea with medications or diet Protective padding until diarrhea resolved
Not eating fresh vegetables or any fiber	Oral problems: dentures not fitting, edentulous	Refit dentures, or use bulk-forming laxatives
INTAKE PROBLEMS: FLUID AND FIBER		
Not enough intake to form bulk or stimulate peristalsis	Poor appetite Low-fiber diet	Increase bulk and water
Too much bulk for amount of water	Decreased skin tugor Tongue dry/fissured Intake <2000 ml/day	More water—offer small amounts frequently
MUSCULOSKELETAL SYSTEM		
No assist from voluntary muscle action	Neurological disease Muscular dystrophy ALS Cord injury Inability to sit up in bed voluntarily	ROM—passive sit-ups Assist patients to get upright and sustain upright position while defecating
Reduced assist from voluntary muscles	Neurological disease leading to decreased activity CVA Alzheimer's	Teach active exercises Support in doing exercises
	Other problems leading to decreased activity Hip fracture with traction Terminal illness	Teach isometric exercises to strengthen abdominal muscles
Can't get to the bathroom	Problems as above	Bedside commode Toileting schedule
Lack of dexterity to wipe and redress	Stroke with hemiplegia, rheumatoid arthritis	Adaptive equipment
PERIPHERAL NERVOUS SYSTEM		
Sphincter dysfunction	Surgical trauma Anorectal disease	Surgical repair
Dysfunction of nerves to the gut	Diabetic neuropathy Tertiary syphilis "I can't use a bedpan"	Enemas
Positioning problems	"I can't sit on the toilet—I'm afraid I'll fall"	Arrange for bedside commode or toilet use Arrange for SAFE and comfortable restraint system Either stay with the patient or use vest restraint

11 reviews on constipation and 5 on fecal incontinence. In addition to general reviews of studies on management of constipation, the limited findings focused on laxatives in palliative care (Goodman & Wilkinson, 2004), bowel programs for persons with central neurological diseases (Coggrave, Wiesel, Norton, & Brazzelli, 2005), acupuncture for chronic constipation (Zhao, Liu, Liu, & Peng, 2004), and colonic pacing for colonic inertia (Shafik, Shafik, El-Sibai, & Ahmed, 2003). The review of bowel care programs for individuals with central neurological diseases concluded that well-designed controlled trials with adequate numbers of subjects and clinically relevant outcome measures are needed (Coggrave et al., 2005).

A psychophysiological approach to bowel problems generally is recommended. This approach integrates understanding of the principles of normal bowel function, psychological influences on bowel function, the effects of specific pathological states, and cultural beliefs about excretion and bowel habits. A study of the effects of exercise and scheduled toileting on appetite and constipation in nursing home residents found no change in daily food intake or in frequency of bowel movements. The investigators concluded that these interventions alone were not sufficient to produce the desired outcomes (Simmons & Schnelle, 2004). Simren (2002) notes that a relationship between constipation and inactivity is accepted, but the value of physical exercise in chronic constipation has not been clearly demonstrated. Japanese investigators who used self-report data to study the relationship of defecation and lifestyle factors concluded that high fiber intake (in the form of rice) and walking (only in men) appeared to prevent constipation (Nakaji et al., 2002).

When nonpharmacological interventions fail, laxatives sometimes are necessary and appropriate. The types of laxatives available are summarized in Table 15-5.

The most important consideration in using a laxative is ensuring that a program to prevent future episodes of constipation is implemented. If a good faith effort to prevent further episodes of constipation is established, the laxative of choice can be either a bulk-forming,

saline, hyperosmotic, or stimulant laxative. The choice depends on the patient's other medical problems and preference. In general, bulk-forming laxatives are preferred to other types because of their better side effect profile. Bulk laxatives often are recommended for prevention of constipation; however, many people find them to be unpleasant. In addition, these drugs can harden in the intestines if the individual does not take in adequate fluids. One study found a methylcellulose caplet to be effective and more acceptable than suspensions (Smith, Hellebusch, & Mandel, 2003). Some sources question the effectiveness of surfactant laxatives such as docusate sodium and claim that it is most appropriately used to prevent straining at stool (Harari, 2003). It commonly is believed that chronic use of stimulant or saline cathartics may result in an atonic colon, sometimes referred to as "cathartic colon," characterized by bloating, cramping, and inability to defecate without a cathartic or an enema. However, Lembo and Camilleri (2003) contend that data do not support this theory that stimulants are to blame. Overuse of saline cathartics may result in fluid and electrolyte imbalances.

Table 15-5 *Pharmacological Management of Constipation*

Class	Examples	Mechanism of Action	Comments
Bulk forming	Methylcellulose (Citrucel) Psyllium (Metamucil, etc.)	Soften fecal mass and increase bulk by forming viscous solution or gel. Distends intestinal wall, which stimulates peristalsis.	Take with full glass of water or juice to reduce risk of esophageal or intestinal obstruction. Contraindicated with narrowed intestinal lumen.
Surfactant	Docusate sodium (Colace, etc.) Docusate calcium	Soften stool by lowering surface tension, which allows water to penetrate feces. May have some stimulant action.	Take with full glass of water. Requires 1-3 days for therapeutic response.
Stimulant	Bisacodyl (Dulcolax, etc.) Senna (Senokot, etc.)	Increases secretion of water/ electrolytes into intestinal lumen. Decreases absorption of water and electrolytes from intestines. Simulates peristalsis.	Widely abused. Senna can cause harmless yellow-brown or pink color to urine.
Osmotic	Milk of magnesia Polyethylene glycol (Miralax)	Draw water into intestinal lumen, which softens fecal mass, distends intestines, and stimulates peristalsis.	Magnesium salts are contraindicated with renal dysfunction.
Other	Mineral oil Lactulose Glycerin suppository	Mineral oil is a lubricant. Lactulose is not absorbed and draws water into the feces. Therapeutic effect may take up to 3 days. Glycerin suppositories have osmotic effect that softens and lubricates feces, and may stimulate rectal peristalsis.	Mineral oil is not recommended for older persons. Can cause lipid pneumonia if aspirated. Can cause anal leakage. Excessive use decreases absorption of fat-soluble vitamins. Lactulose is expensive; often causes flatulence and cramping. Glycerin suppositories may help restore normal pattern of evacuation following period of laxative abuse.

Data from Lehne, R. A. (2004). *Pharmacology for nursing care* (5th ed.). Philadelphia: Saunders.

Mineral oil, another emollient laxative, is contraindicated in debilitated people or those with dysphagia because of the risk of lipid aspiration. Further, frequent use of mineral oil may interfere with the absorption of fat-soluble vitamins. Saline and hyperosmotic laxatives are inappropriate for dehydrated persons because of the increased fluid loss.

Several trials have studied lactulose and polyethylene glycol (PEG) 4000. Zhang, Zhang, Zhang, and Fu (2003) compared PEG and lactulose in 85 older persons with functional constipation. After 4 weeks of treatment, 69% of those in the PEG group had complete remission of constipation compared with 42.1% percent of those taking lactulose. Chaussade and Minic (2003) compared various doses of Forlax and Transipeg in ambulatory persons with idiopathic chronic constipation. The standard-dose Transipeg (5.9 grams) induced the most normal stool consistency in that sample. Lactulose is more expensive than bulk-forming laxatives, and commonly causes flatulence and abdominal cramping (Lehne, 2004).

The use of opioids may be especially problematic for older persons who already have multiple risk factors for constipation. Some sources recommend that laxative therapy be started concurrently with opioid therapy. However, a study of prescribing patterns for community-dwelling persons in the Netherlands found that only 31% of individuals who were prescribed opioids started taking laxatives within 5 days (Bouvy, Buurma, & Egberts, 2002). An intervention by pharmacists increased the rate of concurrent laxative prescribing to 42%.

Swedish investigators studied the effect of laxative use on plasma homocysteine in individuals ages 82 and older. They determined that the subjects who were using laxatives had lower plasma folate and higher homocysteine levels than those who were not using laxatives (Nilsson et al., 2004).

Other treatments for constipation that are under investigation are colonic pacing, resection rectopexy, and biofeedback. Colonic pacing uses electrodes placed in the colon with a stimulator embedded in the inguinal area to induce rectal evacuation in patients with total colonic inertia. In one study, the procedure was successful in six out of nine subjects ages 39 to 52 (Shafik, Shafik, El-Sibai, & Ahmed, 2004). A second study that included normal subjects and individuals with total colonic inertia also concluded that pacing effectively produced electrical activity. All subjects in this study were younger than age 50 (Shafik, Shafik, El-Sibai, & Ahmed, 2003). In 22 patients with internal rectal intussusception, Norwegian physicians reported improvement in constipation following rectopexy with sigmoid resection (Johnsson, Carlsen, Mjaland, & Drolsum, 2003). Biofeedback and electrical stimulation were found to be equally effective in constipated patients with impaired rectal sensation (Chang et al., 2003).

According to Rao (2003), biofeedback is the preferred therapy for dyssynergia at this time. Abdominal massage effectively relieved constipation in some participants in a small sample of hospice patients in the United Kingdom. The author suggested formal study of this technique to better assess its usefulness (Preece, 2002).

Fecal Incontinence. *Fecal incontinence* is the involuntary passage of feces. Fecal incontinence can be classified as overflow, functional, dementia related, comorbidity related, and anorectal. These types are described in Table 15-6. The prevalence of fecal incontinence in community-dwelling older adults in the United States has been estimated at 11% in men and 15% in women, with the greatest number being age 85 and older. For acutely ill hospitalized older adults, the prevalence has been reported as 14% to 22%, and for individuals residing in nursing homes, approximately 54% (Harari, 2003). Among the factors implicated in fecal incontinence are internal anal sphincter dysfunction, childbirth trauma, pudendal neuropathy, and stool impaction. In addition, other physical and cognitive disorders may interfere with normal toileting.

The adverse consequences of fecal incontinence are many, including increased predisposition to skin ulceration and bacteriuria. Additionally, it is a degrading condition. When associated with constipation, efforts to manage incontinence and impaction are unlikely to succeed until the constipation is addressed.

Assessment of the person with fecal incontinence should include a bowel history, a general neurological assessment (including cognition), medication history, and ability to access and use a toilet. Failure of providers to ask and failure of patients to report this problem mean that it often goes untreated even when reversible. One study in a primary care setting revealed that only half of those persons with fecal incontinence had reported it to their care provider. The physical examination should include digital assessment of basal and squeeze tone, observation of pelvic floor descent, and assessment of sacral reflexes (Harari, 2003).

Treatment of fecal incontinence varies with the cause and includes conservative interventions (biofeedback, pelvic floor muscle training, dietary manipulation, and drug therapy) and surgical interventions, including sphincter repair, postanal repair, and placement of a neosphincter (Cheetham, Brazzelli, Norton, & Glazener, 2004). Studies of antidiarrheal drugs and drugs intended to improve sphincter tone have generally been of short duration with small samples, and most addressed diarrhea-related incontinence with limited evidence of effectiveness. Larger comparative studies are needed to guide pharmacological interventions (Cheetham et al., 2004). Surgical intervention may be appropriate when the basic problem is a structural or functional defect in the pelvic floor muscles or the anal

Table 15-6 *Types of Fecal Incontinence*

Type	Characteristics	Contributing Factors	Interventions
Overflow	Fecal impaction present with leakage of liquid stool around obstruction	Immobility, medication side effects Low fluid and fiber intake	Acute: enemas until no further response, then lactulose. Prevention: may require ongoing use of laxatives, suppositories, and enemas.
Functional	Physical impairments prevent timely access to the toilet	Poor mobility Poor vision Poor dexterity	Modification of physical environment and clothing to facilitate self-toileting.
Dementia related	Neurologically disinhibited rectum; rectum empties with mass peristaltic movement	Failure to recognize or respond to urge to defecate; failure to inhibit defecation until appropriate time and place	Prompted or scheduled toileting (with or without suppositories). Controlled evacuation (e.g., daily codeine phosphate or loperamide with twice-weekly enemas or suppositories).
Comorbidity related		Stroke Long-term incontinence may be due to medication effects and functional problems Diabetes mellitus: may be related to multilevel anorectal dysfunction and/or nocturnal diarrhea caused by bacterial overgrowth in sluggish gut	
Anorectal		Age-related and neurogenic anal sphincter dysfunction	Loperamide unless constipated. Biofeedback and exercises to strengthen sphincter and pelvic floor muscle have been recommended, but may have limited value with older persons. Surgical correction of rectal prolapse or external sphincter damage. Estrogen replacement therapy may help older women.
Loose stools	Incontinence occurs with diarrhea	Excessive use of laxatives Lactose malabsorption Antibiotic-related diarrhea	Evaluate laxative use; institute other measures for constipation Dietary adaptation Restore normal flora

sphincter. A Cochrane Database of Systematic Reviews could not determine clinically important differences among the various surgical procedures (Bachoo, Brazzelli, & Grant, 2004). Likewise, reviews of studies of bowel management in people with neurological disease failed to yield empirical evidence of the most appropriate approaches (Coggrave et al., 2006).

Disorders of the Pancreas

Important pancreatic diseases that affect older persons include acute and chronic pancreatitis and pancreatic carcinoma. Diabetes mellitus is addressed with other endocrine disorders. $\mathcal{S}$

Pancreatitis. Age is not a risk factor for acute pancreatitis; however, it typically is more severe in older people. This acute inflammatory condition is initiated by some trigger that results in blockage of the secretion of pancreatic enzymes while enzyme production continues. Autodigestion occurs as proteolytic enzymes are activated. Cell injury releases additional enzymes, resulting in progressive destruction of the pancreas and surrounding tissues. The great majority of acute episodes are triggered by alcohol or gallstones, with gallstone disease being the most common cause in older persons. Pancreatic ischemia associated with vascular surgery (e.g., coronary artery bypass grafts), vasculitis, drug therapy, atypical infections, and endoscopic retrograde cholangiopancreatography (ERCP) are other risk factors in the older adult. Among the medications that have been implicated in acute pancreatitis are immunosuppressants, corticosteroids, some antibiotics and diuretics, ACE inhibitors, and estrogens.

The classic symptom of acute pancreatitis is steady, boring pain in the upper abdomen that radiates through to the back, often accompanied by nausea and vomiting. However, pain is absent in some older persons in whom acute confusion progressing to coma may be the first manifestation. Because serum amylase rises soon after the onset of the attack, it is an important diagnostic tool.

The prognosis is related to the severity of the inflammation. The mortality and complication rates are low for mild acute pancreatitis. It usually responds to intravenous therapy, nothing by mouth, and opioid analgesics. The mortality rate for severe acute pancreatitis is 10% to 20%. Intravenous fluid therapy is especially important because of intravascular fluid loss; however, close monitoring is vital to prevent pulmonary and peripheral edema. Antibiotics that penetrate the pancreas (third-generation cephalosporins, fluoroquinolones, metronidazole, piperacillin, and imipenem) have been shown to reduce mortality rates related to infection (Kaushik & Makin, 2003). Complications of acute pancreatitis include necrosis, infection, hypotension, acute tubular necrosis, hypoxia and lung injury, pseudocyst, and pancreatic duct leak.

The pathogenesis of chronic pancreatitis is not fully understood. A hereditary form related to a protein defect manifests mostly in young people, and alcohol-related inflammation peaks in males ages 35 to 40 years. Anecdotal evidence suggests that chronic pancreatitis follows repeated acute episodes. Researchers are exploring factors that initiate the process that leads to irreversible destruction of pancreatic tissue. Among the current leads are evidence of reduced ductal bicarbonate secretion, a possible autoimmune process, a protein defect that prevents dilution and alkalinization of pancreatic juices, and obstruction of the pancreatic duct caused by scarring, tumor, pseudocyst, or congenital abnormalities. Chronic pancreatitis is called *idiopathic* when the cause is unknown. The incidence of this form peaks twice, once among 15- to 30-year-olds and again among 50- to 70-year-olds.

The typical symptom of chronic pancreatitis is persistent epigastric pain that radiates through to the back and is exacerbated by eating. Nausea and vomiting may occur. Acute intermittent episodes of pain usually become continuous. If pancreatic lipase secretion falls below 10% of normal, the individual will be unable to absorb complex foods, resulting in steatorrhea and bloating. Protein malnutrition and weight loss ensue in the absence of proteolytic enzymes. As the disease progresses, glucose intolerance and eventually diabetes

require treatment. Because the cells that produce glucagon are damaged along with the insulin-producing cells, the risk for treatment-related hypoglycemia exists.

Pain management is a treatment priority. NSAIDs should be tried first for chronic pain; if ineffective, opioids are required. Smoking cessation and avoidance of alcohol are advised and may reduce the frequency and severity of intermittent attacks.

Proton pump inhibitors, histamine-2 receptor antagonists, and pancreatic enzymes have been tried, with mixed results. Unrelieved pain may be treated with pancreatic sphincterotomy. Stents placed in the pancreatic duct temporarily relieve obstruction but should only be placed in expert endoscopy centers. When pancreatic stones obstruct the duct, endoscopic extraction and extracorporeal shock wave lithotripsy may be effective. Should all conservative measures fail and severe pain persist, surgical intervention is an option. Procedures include longitudinal pancreaticojejunostomy and pancreatic resection.

Nutrition management is different for acute and chronic pancreatitis. Depending on the severity of an acute attack, a low-fat, clear-liquid diet may be provided or oral feedings may be withheld and fluids provided intravenously. The diet is gradually progressed to small, low-fat meals as tolerated. Total parenteral nutrition sometimes is necessary because of the hypermetabolic and catabolic state. Lipid emulsions may or may not be given, depending on the patient situation. Jejunal feedings are another option. For chronic pancreatitis, advise the patient to avoid large, high-fat meals and alcohol. However, fat is needed as tolerated to maintain weight or promote weight gain. Supplements of vitamin B complex and vitamins A, D, E, and K often are required. Supplemental pancreatic enzymes help reduce pancreatic stimulation, thereby reducing pain. When pancreatic function falls to 10%, enzyme replacement is essential. As insulin secretion declines, glucose intolerance develops and must be managed similar to diabetes mellitus (Mahan & Escott-Stump, 2000).

Complications of chronic pancreatitis include pseudocyst, pancreatic ascites, pseudoaneurysm, common bile duct and duodenal obstruction, and pancreatic cancer. A pseudocyst forms when a pool of pancreatic secretions is walled off, creating a risk for infection, rupture, hemorrhage, and obstruction. Several procedures can be employed to drain pseudocysts.

Pancreatic Cancer. Pancreatic cancer, most often adenocarcinoma in the head of the gland, usually appears in persons over age 65. Risk factors in addition to age are male gender; black race; cigarette smoking; diet high in fat, meat, and fish and low in fruits and vegetables; alcoholism; chronic pancreatitis; familial predisposition; and exposure to industrial toxins.

The initial symptoms are vague and nonspecific, so that diagnosis is frequently made in the advanced stages of the disease. The classic presentation includes weight loss, painless obstructive jaundice, and a palpable gallbladder; however, few cases are classic. Epigastric pain radiating to the back may be worse after eating and when reclining. The recent onset of diabetes in an older person may signal the presence of pancreatic cancer. Also, depression has been reported as a common symptom in older persons with pancreatic cancer. Because the disease is generally inoperable when it is diagnosed, the 5-year survival rate is 2% to 5% (Kaushik & Makin, 2003). Several diagnostic procedures commonly are used to confirm the diagnosis and to stage the cancer. A transabdominal ultrasound scan may be used for initial evaluation. Dual-phase contrast-enhanced helical (spiral) CT is considered the best means of determining the diagnosis and resectability. Other useful procedures are measures of the tumor marker CA_{19-9}, ERCP, and endoscopic ultrasound.

If the tumor is located in the head of the pancreas and judged to be resectable, pancreaticoduodenectomy is the usual procedure. For people over age 70, the morbidity and mortality rates are 39.1% and 4.3%, respectively. Tumors in the body or tail of the pancreas are treated with distal pancreatectomy. Postoperative neoadjuvant chemoradiation using external-beam radiation combined with 5-FU has been shown to increase survival by 4 to 6 months over surgery alone.

When the tumor is not considered to be resectable, surgery may be performed only to bypass the obstructed common duct to promote drainage and relieve jaundice and pruritus. This bypass may be done during ERCP or by percutaneous transhepatic cholangiography, thereby sparing the patient major abdominal surgery (Kaushik & Makin, 2003). Survival may be prolonged with chemotherapy or radiotherapy, individually or in combination. Other new therapies being investigated in the treatment of pancreatic cancer are immunotherapy and monoclonal antibodies. To manage symptoms and effects of pancreatic cancer, the patient also requires analgesics, insulin, pancreatic enzyme supplements, and enteral nutritional supplements. Pruritus may require antihistamines, cholestyramine, or ursodeoxycholic acid. If analgesics do not relieve pain, a thoracic splanchnicectomy or celiac plexus block may be performed (Kaushik & Makin, 2003).

Disorders of the Liver

Although alcoholic liver disease is most highly associated with older age, viral hepatitis also is mentioned here because it is increasing in this population.

Hepatitis. There are four types of viral hepatitis: A, B, C, and D. Acute hepatitis A virus (HAV) infection is rare in older persons; however, those individuals are at greater risk for serious complications than younger persons. The incidence of HAV among older persons is predicted to rise because fewer older adults now have acquired immunity to the virus (James, 2003). Hepatitis B virus (HBV) is decreasing mostly because of routine screening of donated blood. Although older persons with chronic HBV are generally not infective, replication may be reactivated by cancer chemotherapy. Hepatitis C virus (HCV) is the most common hepatitis virus; over 80% of individuals who acquire acute HCV become chronic carriers. Although studies of older persons with HCV are limited, it appears that they progress more rapidly toward cirrhosis. HCV probably accounts for most posttransfusion hepatitis (James, 2003). The hepatitis D virus can replicate only in the presence of HBV, and it increases the severity of HBV infection.

The aims of treatment for hepatitis are adequate nutrition, relief of symptoms, and avoidance of further liver injury by inappropriate drugs. Any hepatotoxic drugs are discontinued. Pharmacological therapy for hepatitis is evolving, with research using antivirals and interferon; however, questions about their efficacy, tolerability, and cost-effectiveness in older persons have not been answered (James, 2003).

Alcoholic Liver Disease and Cirrhosis. Alcoholic liver disease (ALD) represents the toxic effects of alcohol on the liver. Once thought to be uncommon in older persons, data from the United States and Europe have found that 20% to 28% of individuals treated for the first time with ALD were older than 60 years. James (2003) reports that older individuals with ALD have a higher proportion of clinical manifestations of severe liver disease when first seen. Also, mortality rates of older persons with ALD are around 75% at 1 year and 90% at 3 years, figures much higher than those of persons below age 60.

The spectrum of liver disease is described as stages that include steatosis ("fatty liver"), alcoholic hepatitis, and alcoholic cirrhosis. Even though the three stages are marked by specific histological changes, stages overlap. In older persons, alcoholic hepatitis usually progresses to cirrhosis and typically is present with cirrhosis. Cirrhosis is a chronic condition marked by degeneration and destruction of hepatic parenchymal cells. The course is progressive, ultimately resulting in severe liver failure and death. Manifestations of compensated ALD include telangiectasia, parotid enlargement, spider nevi, loss of body hair, gynecomastia, vertebral and rib fractures, liver palms, clubbing with leukonychia, muscle wasting, and testicular atrophy. Liver and spleen enlargement may or may not be present. Evidence of decompensation includes encephalopathy, alcohol withdrawal symptoms, jaundice, fetor hepaticus, ascites, dilated abdominal veins, asterixis, and peripheral edema. At this stage, the prognosis is poor (James, 2003).

The most important treatment of ALD is abstinence from alcohol. Abstinence is believed to contribute to reversal of steatosis and to improve the 5-year survival rate. It should be noted that some addiction specialists view alcoholism as a chronic disease marked by relapses that is more realistically managed by efforts to control drinking behavior rather than requiring strict abstinence (Tome & Lucey, 2004).

Symptoms of acute alcohol withdrawal can be treated with a benzodiazepine (chlordiazepoxide) and a beta blocker (atenolol). Among the types of drugs that have been studied for treatment of ALD are corticosteroids, anabolic-androgenic steroids (Rambaldi, Iaquinto, & Gluud, 2003), oxpentifylline, infliximab, antioxidants such as silymarin, membrane stabilizers such as S-adenosyl methionine (Purohit & Russo, 2002), propylthiouracil (Rambaldi & Gluud, 2002), colchicine, and phosphatidylcholine (Lieber, 2004; Lieber, Weiss, Groszmann, Paronetto, & Schenker, 2003). For most of these, evidence of benefits is limited or conflicting results have been reported. Corticosteroids are absolutely contraindicated in the presence of infection or variceal bleeding (Tome & Lucey, 2004). Although evidence is limited at this time, oxpentifylline appears to decrease the risk of hepatorenal syndrome, which is a common cause of death in individuals with acute alcoholic hepatitis. Liver transplantation in individuals with end-stage ALD has survival rates similar to those of individuals transplanted for other reasons. From 10% to 15% of transplant recipients resume heavy alcohol consumption (Tome & Lucey, 2004; Young, Neuberger, Longworth, Ratcliffe, & Buxton, 2003).

Nutritional support with intravenous glucose and vitamins is recommended. A high-protein diet is advised for long-term nutrition. Some sources claim that correction of protein-energy malnutrition may improve survival, whereas others contend that the benefits of enteral and parenteral nutrition have not been demonstrated (James, 2003; Stickel, Hoehn, Schuppan, & Seitz, 2003). The best nutritional management of persons with ALD remains unresolved.

Disorders of the Gallbladder

Cholelithiasis (gallstones) is common in older adults, affecting as many as half of persons over 80 years of age (Raimondo & Burroughs, 2003). Biliary pain is the most common manifestation. Typically, biliary pain is located in the epigastrium and right hypocondrium, some-times radiating around to the interscapular region and accompanied by jaundice and fever. When a gallstone obstructs the gallbladder outlet or lodges in the cystic duct, inflammation results and can progress (rarely) to gangrene and perforation. Symptoms usually are severe. However, older individuals with diabetes and diabetic neuropathy may have an atypical presentation with only mild abdominal complaints, low fever, and no leukocytosis (Raimondo & Burroughs, 2003). Older persons with cholecystitis frequently have common bile duct stones. Acute cholangitis may occur with bile duct obstruction or following ERCP. Clinical manifestations of cholangitis include fever, upper abdominal pain, and jaundice. Gram-negative septicemia may be present in older persons.

The most appropriate diagnostic procedures are magnetic resonance cholangiopancreatography (MRCP), ERCP, and percutaneous cholangiography (PTC). The primary advantage of MRCP is that it is noninvasive. ERCP and PTC both are invasive, but also permit therapeutic intervention during the procedure (Raimondo & Burroughs, 2003).

When the older adult is suspected of having acute cholecystitis or cholangitis, initial care is supportive, with replacement of fluids and electrolytes, pain management, correction of metabolic imbalances, and antimicrobial therapy. Cholecystectomy is the treatment of choice for symptomatic gallstones. The laparoscopic procedure is generally preferred for older persons because of the low mortality and complication rates, as well as the short hospitalization required. An alternative to surgery is endoscopic sphincterotomy and stone extraction. When stones cannot be removed, a stent may be placed to bypass the obstruction in the common bile duct.

NURSING CARE
Nursing Assessment

A thorough assessment of the gastrointestinal system includes an accurate history of oral hygiene and dietary and elimination habits. Physical assessment includes inspection and palpation of the oral cavity and inspection, auscultation, percussion, and palpation of the upper and lower abdomen. (Note the deviation from the usual order of inspection, palpation, percussion, and auscultation.) The nutritional assessment is addressed separately in Chapter 8.

Health History. Individuals who are seeking care because of gastrointestinal problems may be experiencing a variety of symptoms such as pain, dysphagia, dyspepsia, nausea, vomiting, changes in stool characteristics, and gastrointestinal bleeding. Many symptoms, including anorexia and weight loss, can be related to nutritional problems. Obtain a detailed description of symptoms. With gastrointestinal complaints, timing in relation to eating may be significant.

Significant past health problems include GERD, peptic ulcer disease, cancer, hepatitis, gallstones, and diabetes mellitus. Document any surgical procedures involving the gastrointestinal system. Note all current medications because many affect the gastrointestinal tract: anticholinergics, laxatives, calcium channel blockers, aspirin and other NSAIDs, calcium- and aluminum-based antacids, opioids, and most antiemetics.

In the review of systems, ask whether the older adult has had a recent weight change. Inquire about oral problems, including lesions, pain, and bleeding; prostheses used; and daily oral care practices. If the person has dentures, ask when they are worn and whether they cause any problems (pain, slipping). Document appetite; food intolerance; heartburn; indigestion; pain; nausea; vomiting; flatulence; usual bowel pattern and changes; use of laxatives, stool softeners, suppositories, or enemas; ability to control bowel movements; stool characteristics; rectal bleeding or pain; and hemorrhoids. When the individual reports constipation, it is helpful to assess beliefs about normal bowel function and how that person defines constipation. Record the date and results of the last sigmoidoscopy or colonoscopy, if done. The nutritional assessment is relevant, and covered in detail elsewhere. If a person is unable to give a reliable history, these data may be obtained from family and other caregivers.

Physical Examination. The physical examination of the individual with gastrointestinal complaints focuses on the oral cavity, the abdomen, and the rectum. The process is the same as for other adults, but areas of special interest with the older adult will be noted.

ORAL CAVITY. Inspect the palate and lips for lesions, particularly looking for cracks at the corners of the mouth. Note the condition of the natural teeth and gums. If the individual wears dentures, the mouth should be inspected with the dentures in place and again when removed. Be alert for clicking or whistling sounds when the person talks, which may indicate poorly fitting dentures. Note whether the oral mucosa is moist or dry.

ABDOMEN. The appearance of the abdomen may be rounded even in thin older persons because of decreased muscle tone. Also, peristalsis may be visible because of thinning of the musculature. Jaundice and ascites may be present with liver disease. Bowel sounds and vascular sounds should be normal. The fluid wave test will be positive in the presence of a large amount of ascitic fluid. Findings on palpation are unchanged in a healthy older person. It may actually be easier to palpate the liver and kidneys. Even with acute abdominal conditions, the older person may complain of only mild pain and the abdomen may not be rigid.

ANUS AND RECTUM. For assessment of the anus and rectum, consider the older person's ability to stand or to assume a lithotomy position. The side-lying position may be more comfortable. With the Valsalva maneuver, the perineal musculature and rectal sphincter may relax (Jarvis, 2004).

ASSESSMENT OF CONSTIPATION. Assessment of the individual suspected of having constipation is designed to (1) determine whether the person truly has constipation, (2) identify risk factors for development of constipation, and (3) isolate factors in the individual that contribute to the constipation or high-risk status. Most of the areas for assessment that are relevant to constipation already have been discussed. To summarize, they are

- Activity level
- Usual bowel pattern, history of bowel disease
- Characteristics of constipation
- Medications, including pattern of laxative use
- Findings on rectal ination
- Bowel sounds
- Hydration status
- Diet: amount of fiber; special diet
- Beliefs about normal bowel function

Other variables that may affect the individual's ability to follow through with a bowel management program include sensory acuity, motor function, short-term memory, judgment, and problem-solving ability. Toileting can be complex for the person with cognitive impairment, poor vision, and poor coordination.

The rectal examination is an important part of the gastrointestinal assessment. Inspect the perianal area for scars, fistulas, fissures, and hemorrhoids. With the patient in the left lateral position, observe the perineum at rest, and then ask the patient to bear down while observing for perineal descent (normally 1 to 3.5 cm). If descent is reduced, the patient may be unable to relax the pelvic floor muscles for defecation. Increased descent is associated with laxity of the perineum as may occur with many years of straining because of constipation. Over many years, excessive descent may damage sacral nerves, causing a loss of rectal sensation and possibly incontinence. The digital examination is useful in detecting fecal impaction, anal stricture, and rectal masses.

Typically, multiple factors contribute to constipation; therefore it is helpful to summarize baseline and ongoing assessment data in a central place. This method aids in evaluating the effectiveness of various interventions. A flow sheet to record this information, developed for use in institutions, is shown in Figure 15-3.

**ASSESSMENT—BASELINE
CIRCLE APPROPRIATE ANSWERS**

1. **History**
   Stool Pattern Previously:
   >1 time/day
   1 time/day
   1 time/3 days
   1 time/day
   Time of Day of Stool:
   early AM   late PM
   late AM   at night
   early PM   variable
2. **Laxative Use**
   Frequency:
   never   occasionally
   sometimes   weekly   daily
   Type of laxative:
   juice   diet   laxative
   enema   suppos.   other
3. **Medical Diagnoses**
   CVA
   Diabetes
   Diverticulitis
   Metastatic disease
   Colon cancer
   Parkinson's disease
   Severe arthritis
4. **Physical Findings**
   Fecal impaction   yes/no
   Abdominal mass   yes/no
   Bowel sounds:
   Hypoactive
   Normal
   Hyperactive
5. **Activity Status**
   a) bedridden
   b) bed-to-chair
   c) wheelchair-bound
   d) exercises
   e) wheelchair-mobile
   f) walks <25 feet/day
   g) walks >25 feet/day
   h) in P.T.
6. **Medications**
   C) constipating drugs
   opiates
   antidiarrheals
   psychotropics
   iron supplements
   antacids
   high-dose aspirin
   L) laxative-like drugs
   stool softeners
   antacids
7. **Fluid Intake**
   a) unknown
   b) inadequate (<1000 ml)
   c) marginal (1000-2000)
   d) adequate (>2000 ml)
8. **Diet**
   a) no solid intake
   b) no roughage
   c) high-fiber diet

KEY TO ABBREVIATIONS:

Y/N = toileted
X = MEDS—PRN, or Meds—REG
     administered
* = episode of incontinence or
     accidental bowel movement
† = bowel movement in correct
     location
SUPP = suppository administered
EN = enema administered
LAX = laxative administered

	Day 1			Day 2			Day 3			Day 4			Day 5			Day 6			Day 7		
	D	E	N	D	E	N	D	E	N	D	E	N	D	E	N	D	E	N	D	E	N
Week 1																					
Bowel Movmnt																					
Toileted																					
Diet																					
Fluid Intake	\} Use codes from baseline assessment on the left, items 5–8																				
Activities																					
LAX SUPP EN																					
Meds—REG																					
Meds—PRN																					
Week 2																					
Bowel Movmnt																					
Toileted																					
Diet																					
Fluid Intake																					
Activities																					
LAX SUPP EN																					
Meds—REG																					
Meds—PRN																					
Week 3																					
Bowel Movmnt																					
Toileted																					
Diet																					
Fluid Intake																					
Activities																					
LAX SUPP EN																					
Meds—REG																					
Meds—PRN																					
Week 4																					
Bowel Movmnt																					
Toileted																					
Diet																					
Fluid Intake																					
Activities																					
LAX SUPP EN																					
Meds—REG																					
Meds—PRN																					
Week 5																					
Bowel Movmnt																					
Toileted																					
Diet																					
Fluid Intake																					
Activities																					
LAX SUPP EN																					
Meds—REG																					
Meds—PRN																					
Week 6																					
Bowel Movmnt																					
Toileted																					
Diet																					
Fluid Intake																					
Activities																					
LAX SUPP EN																					
Meds—REG																					
Meds—PRN																					

Figure 15-3 Assessment form to record alteration in bowel elimination. (From Snow, T., & McConnell, E. S. [1985]. Bowel and bladder management training program. Unpublished educational aid.)

ASSESSMENT OF DIARRHEA. When a person has diarrhea, the nursing assessment should include stool count, observation of stool consistency, and digital rectal and abdominal examinations for fecal impaction. Fecal impaction and infectious causes must be ruled out before drugs are administered for diarrhea. The person's usual bowel elimination pattern should be determined, along with the current pattern. Diarrhea that occurs only during the day suggests a functional rather than an organic cause. Obtain a drug and diet history, placing particular emphasis on recent changes in medications or dietary habits. Medicines in elixir form may contain sorbitol, which may act as an osmotic laxative. Ask specifically about patterns of laxative use. Diarrhea that is accompanied by bloating and cramps after ingesting milk products likely is caused by lactose intolerance, which is common in older persons. Diarrhea that persists over a 5-day period, diarrhea characterized by bloody stools, or widespread diarrhea in an institutional setting calls for laboratory examination of stool, including Gram stain, presence of fecal leukocytes, culture for ova and parasites, and examination for the presence of the toxin produced by *Clostridium difficile. C. difficile* often is the culprit among older women and nursing home residents (Harari, 2003). Persistent diarrhea requires extensive medical evaluation to determine the cause and definitive treatment.

Assessment of the impact of diarrhea on other aspects of the individual's function also is important. The patient's emotional reaction to the diarrhea and ability to maintain continence, adequate hydration, and skin integrity should be assessed.

Box 15-4 Gastrointestinal Assessment

History

Oral Cavity, Mouth, Pharynx, and Larynx

Complaints of disturbances in the sense of taste
Pain or bleeding of the tongue, lips, or gums
Abnormalities of salivation
Dental problems
Dentures
  Ability to chew
Last dental examination
Difficult or painful swallowing of liquids or solids (or both)
Sore throat
Hoarseness
Lump in throat

Upper and Lower Gastrointestinal Tract

Diet, especially liquids
Appetite; anorexia; weight loss; appetite changes
Intolerance to certain foods
Nausea (circumstances, time of day, relation to meals)
Vomiting (type, color, quantity, relation to meals)
Heartburn, epigastric pain
Pain (type, location, intensity, duration)
Jaundice
Bowel habits; use of laxatives
Flatulence; tarry stools; bloody stools

Physical Assessment

Oral Cavity, Mouth, Larynx, and Pharynx

Face (anterior and side view)
  Observe for asymmetry, pigmentations, masses, ulcers, inflammatory lesions, lacerations
  Describe location, size, and depth of deviations
Lymph nodes
  Palpate cervical chain of lymph nodes, starting with the posterior cervical region through the submandibular, sublingual, and anterior cervical areas

Lips
  Observe for normal and abnormal changes
  Compress lips gently to palpate for masses
Teeth
  Observe caries, missing teeth, dentures
Buccal mucosa
  Observe color, masses, or inflammatory lesions
  Examine alveolar ridges in edentulous patients, palpating for any unusual lumps or bumps
Tongue
  Examine ventral and dorsal aspects of tongue
  Grasp tongue with a 2-by-2 gauze pad and examine the lateral borders and base of the tongue and the floor of the mouth
Palate
  Observe for lesions or masses
  Observe uvula for deviation
Throat
  Note condition, color, vascularity, and evidence of postnasal drip

Upper and Lower Gastrointestinal Tract

Inspection
  Observe for scars, striae, dilated veins, lesions, masses, color changes, increased pigment, tautness
  Note contour, especially symmetry, herniations along midline, swelling
  Check movement and rigidity; look for arterial pulsations, peristalsis
Auscultation
  Listen for bowel sounds, vascular bruits, and rubs
Percussion
  Check for tympany (normal abdominal sounds) and dullness (solid viscera)
Palpation
  Assess for rebound tenderness or pain, organomegaly

A summary of the gastrointestinal assessment is shown in Box 15-4.

Nursing Diagnoses

Numerous nursing diagnoses may apply to persons with gastrointestinal disorders. Examples include the following:

- Chronic or acute pain related to oral lesions, gastrointestinal disorders, malignancy
- Constipation related to neuromuscular impairment, intestinal obstruction, megacolon, painful defecation, drug side effects, immobility, inadequate intake of fluids and fiber, metabolic problems
- Perceived constipation related to inappropriate use of aids to elimination based on custom or lack of information
- Risk for constipation related to inadequate fluid and fiber intake, inactivity
- Diarrhea related to gastrointestinal disorders, infectious processes, adverse effects of laxatives or other drugs
- Bowel incontinence related to neuromuscular impairment, diarrhea, fecal impaction, cognitive impairment, inability to access toilet
- Deficient fluid volume related to abdominal cancer, hemorrhage, diarrhea
- Risk for deficient fluid volume related to decreased fluid intake, drug effects, inability to obtain fluids because of immobility, abnormal loss of fluid through diarrhea or vomiting
- Knowledge deficit of oral hygiene and dental care, diet, nutrition, self-medication
- Altered nutrition, less than body requirements, related to chewing difficulties, anorexia, difficulty in procuring or preparing food

Nursing Goals

The goals of nursing care related to alterations in the older adult's gastrointestinal function include (1) maintenance or restoration of regular bowel elimination, (2) prevention of complications of bowel incontinence, and (3) prevention of complications of diarrhea. Nursing interventions to maintain or improve nutritional status are addressed in Chapter 8. They include (1) maintenance or restoration of normal fluid volume, (2) establishment of regular oral hygiene and dental care practices, and (3) maintenance or restoration of appropriate intake of nutrients.

Nursing Interventions

Interventions to Promote Regular Bowel Elimination. Older adults may need education about normal bowel function and what actually defines

constipation. The cycle of repeated laxative use leading to dependence begins with lack of understanding of normal bowel function. Well-established laxative dependence may not be reversible, requiring continued regular laxative therapy. When constipation has been confirmed, treatment should begin with nonpharmacological interventions (Harari, 2003) (Box 15-5).

Although it can be difficult with frail elders, make every effort to provide for comfort and privacy for toileting. Encourage efforts to defecate within half an hour after breakfast to coincide with the gastrocolic reflex. A toilet chair with arms may allow the individual to safely use the toilet in private.

The natural position for defecation allows the assistance of gravity in evacuating the rectum. Attempts to use a bedpan may result in discomfort and less than optimal benefit from the forces of gravity. Discomfort may also lead to the inhibition of the urge to defecate. If at all possible, provide a bedside commode or access to a bathroom toilet. Have the patient bend over from the waist, or press firmly on the lower abdomen. Allow a reasonable amount of time—5 to 10 minutes or longer if patient preference dictates—to facilitate relaxation. For persons whose legs do not reach the floor, provide a footstool to allow hip flexion. The footstool also may be helpful for individuals with muscle weakness and those who strain. Individuals with limited hip flexion may be more comfortable with a raised toilet seat.

To prevent constipation, the time-honored nonpharmacological interventions are generally recommended. These include adequate fluid intake, appropriate activity level, daily dietary fiber, and regularly scheduled toileting. If the patient depends on family or professional caregivers, include them in education and other interventions designed to prevent constipation. Increased dietary fiber long has been recommended to prevent constipation. Interestingly, limited high-level evidence of

---

BOX 15-5 *TOWARD BETTER GASTROINTESTINAL HEALTH*

- Practice good oral hygiene; have regular dental care.
- Salivary substitutes are available for dry mouth.
- Seek treatment promptly for lesions in the mouth.
- Use a powered toothbrush with a rotating oscillating action.
- Avoid smoking.
- Dietary fiber, fluids, and physical activity may reduce the risk of constipation.
- Bulk laxatives generally are preferred, but must be taken with adequate fluids.
- Many prescription and over-the-counter drugs can cause diarrhea or constipation, and dry mouth.

the efficacy of this intervention exists. Nevertheless, the demonstrated value of fiber in lowering serum cholesterol and improving glycemic control has provided adequate support to continue recommending a high-fiber diet (James, Muir, Curtis, & Gibson, 2003). To increase dietary fiber, encourage ambulatory community-dwelling individuals to consume whole-grain bread products, fresh fruits, vegetables, and seeded berries. Coarse bran is effective in softening the stool, but it is not very palatable, and it can significantly reduce absorption of calcium and iron. Unless contraindicated, a fluid intake of 1500 mL/day is recommended. However, evidence is lacking that increased fluids are helpful except in individuals who are dehydrated. Also, this can be difficult to achieve with frail disabled persons. Encourage and assist older adults to exercise within their limitations. Although these time-honored interventions are widely accepted, Annells and Koch (2003) contend that little scientific evidence exists to explain the relationships, if any, between constipation and fiber, exercise, and fluid intake. An analysis of self-report data from the Nurses Health Study found that women ages 36 to 61 with higher activity levels and those with higher dietary fiber intake had lower prevalence rates of constipation (Dukas, Willett, & Giovannucci, 2003). Even if laxatives become necessary, the nonpharmacological measures should be continued.

Recent nursing intervention studies on the management of constipation are limited. One successful quality improvement project designed to reduce constipation and fecal impaction on a vascular surgery ward used a combination of dietary modification, positioning, and abdominal strengthening exercises to reduce the occurrence of constipation and fecal impaction. The protocol included 4.2 to 5.2 grams of fiber delivered in cookies or muffins, fluid intake of between 1500 and 2000 mL per day, and daily toileting in the upright position with privacy. The prevalence of constipation on this unit dropped from 59% to 9%, the prevalence of fecal impaction dropped from 36% to 0%, and requests for enemas or laxatives declined from 59% to 8% (Hall, Karstens, Rakel, Swanson, & Davidson, 1995).

Interventions to Prevent and Treat Fecal Impaction.

The wisest approach to fecal impaction is prevention. Patients at risk for impaction should be identified and a preventive bowel regimen established. High-risk individuals are those with a previous history of impaction, immobilized patients, and those taking doses of medicines with constipating properties, such as opioids and drugs with anticholinergic properties. Unfortunately, many patients develop fecal impaction before a bowel management program is implemented.

Most approaches to the management of fecal impaction use some combination of enemas and manual disimpaction. Oil retention enemas often are given first to soften the stool, followed by disimpaction. Another approach is to manually disimpact and then administer a tap water cleansing enema (Harari, 2003). The protocols for pharmacological treatment of constipation and fecal impaction recommended by Harari (2003) appear in Table 15-7. No rigorous evaluations of treatment for fecal impaction are reported in the literature.

Interventions to Treat Fecal Incontinence.

A key element in the management of overflow fecal incontinence is ongoing monitoring of bowel elimination,

Table 15-7 *Causes of Constipation in Older People*	
Functional constipation	*Medications*
	Anticholinergic drugs (tricyclics, antipsychotics, antihistamines, antiemetics, drugs for detrusor hyperactivity)
	Opiates
	Iron supplements
	Calcium channel antagonists
	Calcium supplements
	Nonsteroidal antiinflammatory drugs
	Immobility
	Neurological conditions
	Parkinson's disease
	Diabetes mellitus
	Stroke
	Spinal cord injury or disease
	Dehydration
	Low dietary fiber
	Metabolic disturbances
	Hypothyroidism
	Hypercalcemia
	Hypokalemia
	Mechanical obstruction (e.g., tumor)
Rectal outlet delay	Dementia
	Depression
	Lack of privacy or comfort
	Anorectal disease or prior surgery
	Weak pelvic and abdominal muscles
	Rectal dyschezia
Self-reported constipation	Misperceptions regarding normal bowel habits
	Anxiety/depression

From Harari, D. (2003). Constipation and fecal incontinence in old age. In R. C. Tallis & H. M. Fillit (Eds.), *Brocklehurst's textbook of geriatric medicine and gerontology* (6th ed.). London: Churchill Livingstone.

including rectal examinations. One effective treatment is enemas until no further response occurs, followed by lactulose. If incontinence is functional, the basic problem (mobility, dexterity, communication) must be identified and a plan designed to consider the basic problem. Dementia-related fecal incontinence is common among nursing home residents. The initial intervention to be used is prompted toileting. If this is not successful, try scheduled toileting with daily suppositories. The last measure, if others fail, is controlled bowel evacuation. Controlled evacuation includes regular loperamide to control spontaneous evacuation and periodic suppositories or enemas to promote evacuation (Harari, 2003). In addition to measures to control bowel evacuation, persons with fecal impaction and their families need guidance on skin care, odor control, and incontinence products.

Interventions to Prevent Complications of Fecal Incontinence and Diarrhea. After each episode of diarrhea, provide meticulous perineal hygiene to frail individuals. Use emollient creams following cleansing to help protect the skin against the caustic effects of fecal material. Fecal collection bags may protect the skin of individuals who have incontinence with diarrhea. Socially active patients who experience incontinence secondary to diarrhea may also find these devices useful while the diarrhea is being evaluated. Temporary use of a bedside commode for people with immobility problems may prevent diarrhea-induced fecal incontinence.

Employ standard precautions for handling all body fluids, regardless of whether diarrhea is present. However, if an infectious diarrhea outbreak in a long-term care facility is suspected, additional steps should be taken. Consider instituting gastroenteritis outbreak management procedures if greater than 3% of all patients in a facility, or more than three patients on one ward, develop diarrhea (Edmond, 1994). Follow guidelines related to notification of health department and attending physicians. Food service employees should be interviewed regarding recent gastrointestinal illness, and ill employees should be excused from work. If a bacterial pathogen is isolated, stool specimens for culture should be obtained from food service employees, and asymptomatic infected workers should be reassigned until stool cultures are negative. Use contact precautions for infected patients, reminding paraprofessional staff or family caregivers about the rationale for extra precautions. Observe strict handwashing between all patients. In some instance, isolation of patients until infection is resolved is recommended. In addition, if an infectious cause for the diarrhea is suspected, preventing transmission to other people is a high priority.

Evaluation

The outcomes of nursing management include comfort level, bowel elimination, hydration, symptom control, health beliefs, toileting self-care, electrolyte and acid/base balance, fluid balance, symptom severity, bowel continence, and tissue integrity of skin and mucous membranes; knowledge of diet and disease process, health behaviors, illness care, prescribed activity, and treatment regimen; and nutritional status.

Indicators of goal achievement for individuals with gastrointestinal disorders include the following:

- The patient reports that pain control is effective.
- The patient's stools are soft and formed and passed easily and without discomfort.
- The patient acknowledges the ability to improve control of health outcomes related to perceived constipation.
- The patient responds to the urge to have a bowel movement in a timely manner.
- The patient's serum electrolytes and pH are within normal limits.
- The patient's fluid intake and output are approximately equal and mucous membranes are moist.
- The patient maintains a predictable pattern of stool evacuation and maintains control of stool passage.
- The patient accurately describes health behaviors to promote normal gastrointestinal function, and explains disease process, illness care, and treatment regimen.
- The patient's nutritional intake is sufficient to maintain appropriate body weight.

A protocol for developing a bowel management program is detailed in Box 15-6.

SUMMARY

Studies have shown that normal age-related changes in the gastrointestinal system are difficult to differentiate from pathological states. Some age-related changes that probably occur in the gastrointestinal system include decreases in the blood flow to the organs, the size of the organs, and motility.

Pathological problems most commonly found in the gastrointestinal system in older age include periodontal disease of the mouth, malignant lesions, dysphagia, hiatus hernia, gastritis, peptic ulcer disease, malabsorption syndromes, diverticular disease, pancreatitis, hepatitis, cirrhosis, cholelithiasis, and cholecystitis. These disease states produce problems with nutrition and elimination, resulting in pain, discomfort, anorexia, constipation, and diarrhea. The nurse should provide measures to relieve these problems through direct interventions and patient teaching to promote the highest level of functioning.

BOX 15-6 Protocol for Development of a Bowel Management Program

Dos and Don'ts

Do

1. Make sure the person is well hydrated.
2. Start with the technique that has the fewest side effects.
3. Move to a new technique only after the first approach has had 2 weeks of documented application.
4. Make sure everyone involved in the patient's care (patient, family, volunteers, dietary staff, AND THE NIGHT SHIFT!) knows the goals of the bowel management program, the plan, the reasons for the plan, and when the plan will be re-evaluated.
5. Remember to document your interventions.

Don't

1. Use negative reinforcement—ever!
2. Do anything before assessing the patient thoroughly.
3. Use medicines when nursing care will work better.
4. Underestimate the power of lifelong habits, both good and bad.

First: Look Before You Leap—Assessment

1. Check for fecal impaction.
   If there is an impaction, GO TO IMPACTION PROTOCOL.
   If there is NO impaction, continue to step 2.
2. Check for diarrhea.
   If there is diarrhea WITHOUT an impaction, GO TO DIARRHEA PROTOCOL.
   If there is NO diarrhea, continue to step 3.
3. Record intake and output for 1 week.
4. Identify preadmission and preillness bowel habits.
   Frequency
   Time of day
   Surrounding events: cup of coffee, commode vs. toilet vs. bedpan
   Laxative use
5. Activity patterns
   (Good, fair, and poor is not enough—need to specify type of activity)
6. Diet
   Amount of bulk
   Prune juice?
7. Medications

Second: Start by Doing What Comes Naturally

1. Up, in the bathroom, on the toilet
2. At their usual time
3. With enough privacy
4. Feeling secure
5. For long enough time

Third: Look at the Things You Can Do That Won't Hurt

1. Exercise to increase or assist peristalsis.
2. Increase fluid intake.
3. Increase fiber content of diet.
4. Counsel regarding "need" for daily bowel movement.

The vast majority of your patient's bowel problems will be resolved using these three steps. However . . . If you have done these things, given patients sufficient time, and believed in their ability to do the job, with no success, then and only then should you turn to medications or enemas for treating constipation.

Warning

Medications and Enemas

All have side effects that may be harmful to your patients and may create new and more difficult problems for you and them!

BOX 15-6 Protocol for Development of a Bowel Management Program—cont'd

If these things don't work, then look again at your assessments to diagnose the problem.
1. Medications
2. Undiagnosed medical illness: hypothyroidism, hypokalemia, hypercalcemia
3. Complication of already-diagnosed illness:
   End-stage diabetes mellitus w/neuropathy
   End-stage demyelinating diseases
   Anorectal disease
4. Psychological problems—adjustment reaction, depression

Impaction Protocol
First: Assessment
1. Perform digital examination.
   If hard stool is present, manual disimpaction is indicated.
   If large amount of soft stool, use either glycerin suppository, oil enema, or hyperosmolar enema.

Second: Intervention
1. Provide privacy.
2. Explain procedure (either manual disimpaction or enema).
3. Ask patient to breathe deeply, slowly, and quietly throughout procedure to promote relaxation.
4. Stop manual disimpaction if patient complains of excessive pain.
5. Do not manipulate impaction beyond the fatigue tolerance of the patient. Allow for a rest period during and following the disimpaction.
6. Follow manual disimpaction with hyperosmotic laxative or enema.

Third: Evaluation
1. Note results of laxative or enema.
2. Check for impaction.
3. Has a bowel management program to prevent recurrent impaction been implemented?

Diarrhea Protocol
First: Look Before You Leap—Assessment
1. Check for impaction. If impacted, GO TO IMPACTION PROTOCOL.
2. Begin intake and output, including stool count. Older patients are at high risk for dehydration and electrolyte imbalance if diarrhea goes untreated.
3. If patient is tube fed, consider possibility of tube feeding as the culprit. Tube feedings administered too fast or hyperosmotic feedings may cause diarrhea.
4. Review medications, especially if a new medication has recently been started. Many drugs have the potential to cause diarrhea as a side effect. Consult with pharmacist.
5. Get diet history. Excessive intake of high-fiber foods may result in diarrhea in some patients.
6. Consider infection (either viral or bacterial) as source of diarrhea. Consult with physician or nurse practitioner.

Second: Intervene
1. Make sure toilet is close by and notify staff of patient's diarrhea and high risk for incontinence. People with diarrhea have a shorter time to respond to the urge to defecate.
2. Match the treatment to the suspected cause of the diarrhea. Bowel rest may be all that is necessary.
3. Remember that antidiarrheals are all strong medications with potential for adverse side effects and drug-drug interactions.

Third: Evaluate
1. If a diet modification or drug is prescribed to treat the diarrhea, make sure you establish agreement with the physician or nurse practitioner on criteria to discontinue treatment.
2. Set criteria for discontinuing stool counts and intake and output.
3. If fecal incontinence is prevented or resolved, pat yourself on the back!

From Snow, T. L., & McConnell, E. S. (1985). *Bowel and bladder management training program.* Unpublished educational aid.

Nursing Care Plan: The Older Adult with Constipation

Data

Mr. Martin, age 81, had a stroke 9 years ago that left him with left hemiplegia. He is able to walk with considerable effort using a cane. He lives at home with his 78-year-old wife. Most of his time is spent in a chair in his bedroom, where he watches television. He rarely ventures from home because of the difficulty getting into and out of the car. He is able to use the toilet with a raised seat and also has a bedside commode in his room that he uses at night. He reports having a good appetite, and his weight has been stable for several years. His wife keeps a glass of fresh water next to him at all times. Before his stroke, he had a daily bowel movement with only occasional constipation. He now has frequent episodes of constipation, which he describes as hard stools that are difficult to pass. He says if he does not have a stool for 2 days, he takes milk of magnesia. In a typical week, he takes milk of magnesia three to four times. The laxative sometimes causes diarrhea and urgency, making it difficult to reach the toilet in time. He would like to find a better way to manage his constipation.

Nursing Diagnoses

Constipation related to insufficient physical activity
Perceived constipation related to faulty appraisal

NOC Suggested Outcomes

Bowel Elimination (0501), Symptom Control (1608), Health Beliefs (1700), Health Beliefs: Perceived Threat (1704).

NIC Suggested Interventions

Major interventions: Bowel Management (0430), Constipation Management (0450), Individual Teaching (5606).

- Establish rapport.
- Determine the patient's learning needs.
- Appraise the patient's current level of knowledge and understanding of content, educational level, and abilities/disabilities.
- Determine the patient's ability and motivation to learn specific information.
- Set mutual, realistic learning goals with the patient.
- Tailor the content to the patient's cognitive, psychomotor, and affective abilities/disabilities.
- Select appropriate teaching methods/strategies.
- Provide an environment that is conducive to learning.
- Instruct the patient when appropriate.
- Evaluate the patient's achievement of stated objectives.
- Instruct patient/wife to record color, volume, frequency, and consistency of stools.
- Teach patient (and wife) about foods that assist in promoting bowel regularity.
- Encourage patient to drink warm liquids after meals.
- Evaluate medication profile for gastrointestinal side effects.
- Identify factors that may cause or contribute to constipation.
- Institute a toileting schedule as appropriate.
- Instruct patient/wife on appropriate use of laxatives.
- Suggest use of laxative/stool softener as appropriate.
- Teach patient and wife about normal digestive processes.

Evaluation Parameters

Bowel elimination: elimination pattern, control of bowel movements, stool amount for diet, stool soft and formed, ease of stool passage, comfort of stool passage, constipation

Symptom control: monitors symptom persistence, uses preventive measures, uses relief measures, reports symptoms controlled

Health beliefs: perceived benefits of action, perceived control of health outcome, perceived ability to perform action

Health beliefs: perceived impact on current lifestyle (perceived threat to current lifestyle habits)

REFERENCES

Ajani, J. A., Mansfield, P. F., Janjan, N., Morris, J., Pisters, P. W., Lynch, P. M., et al. (2004). Multi-institutional trial of preoperative chemoradiotherapy in patients with potentially resectable gastric carcinoma. *Journal of Clinical Oncology, 22*(14), 2774-2780.

Akeel, R. (2003). Attitudes of Saudi male patients toward the replacement of teeth. *Journal of Prosthetic Dentistry, 90*(6), 571-577.

American Cancer Society. (2004). Cancer facts and figures—2003. Retrieved November 15, 2004, from www.cancer.org.

Anderson, S. E., Minsky, B. D., Bains, M., Kelsen, D. P., & Ilson, D. H. (2003). Combined modality therapy in esophageal cancer: The Memorial experience. *Seminars in Surgical Oncology, 21*(4), 228-232.

Andujar, J. J., Papasavas, P. K., Birdas, T., Robke, J., Raftopoulos, Y., Gagne, D. J., et al. (2004). Laparoscopic repair of large paraesophageal hernia is associated with a low incidence of recurrence and reoperation. *Surgical Endoscopy, 18*(3), 444-447.

Annells, M., & Koch, T. (2003). Constipation and the preached trio: Diet, fluid intake, exercise. *International Journal of Nursing Studies, 40*(8), 843-852.

Avlund, K., Holm-Pedersen, P., Morse, D. E., Viitanen, M., & Winblad, B. (2004). Tooth loss and caries prevalence in very old Swedish people: The relationship to cognitive function and functional ability. *Gerodontology, 21*(1), 17-26.

Awad, R. A., & Camacho, S. (2002). *Helicobacter pylori* infection and hiatal hernia do not affect acid reflux and esophageal motility in patients with gastroesophageal reflux. *Journal of Gastroenterology, 37*(4), 247-254.

Bachoo, P., Brazzelli, M., & Grant, A. (2004). Surgery for fecal incontinence in adults. *Cochrane Database of Systematic Reviews, 4.*

Beltran-Aguilar, E. D., & Beltran-Neira, R. J. (2004). Oral diseases and conditions throughout the lifespan. 1. Diseases and conditions directly associated with tooth loss. *General Dentistry, 52*(1), 21-27.

Bergstrom, J. (2004). Influence of tobacco smoking on periodontal bone height: Long term observations and a hypothesis. *Journal of Clinical Periodontology, 31*(4), 260-266.

Blandino, G., Lo Bue, A. M., Milazzo, I., Nicolosi, D. V., Cali, G., Cannavo, V., & Rossetti, B. (2004). Comparison of systemic flurithromycin therapy and clinical procedures in the treatment of periodontal disease. *Journal of Chemotherapy, 16*(2), 151-155.

Bouvy, M. L., Buurma, H., & Egberts, T. C. G. (2002). Laxative prescribing in relation to opioid use and the influence of pharmacy-based intervention. *Journal of Clinical Pharmacy and Therapeutics, 27*(2), 107-110.

Brenner, B., Ilson, D. H., & Minsky, B. D. (2004). Treatment of localized esophageal cancer. *Seminars in Oncology, 31*(4), 554-565.

Bresadola, V., Dado, G., Terrosu, G., Alessandrini, V., Marcellino, M. G., & Bresadola, F. (2003). Role of manometry and pH-metry in patients with symptoms and signs of gastroesophageal reflux disease. *Chirugia Italiana, 55*(6), 785-590.

Byrne, P. J., Mulligan, E. D., O'Riordan, J., Keeling, P. W., & Reynolds, J. V. (2003). Impaired visceral sensitivity to acid reflux in patients with Barrett's esophagus. The role of esophageal motility. *Diseases of the Esophagus, 16*(3), 199-203.

Cassolato, S. F., & Turnbull, R. S., (2003). Xerostomia: Clinical aspects and treatment. *Gerodontology, 20*(2), 64-67

Centers for Disease Control and Prevention. (2003). Public health and aging: Retention of natural teeth among older adults—United States, 2002. *MMWR Morbidity and Mortality Weekly Report, 52*(50), 1226-1229.

Chalmers, J. M., Carter, K. D., & Spencer, A. J. (2003). Oral diseases and conditions in community-living older adults with and without dementia. *Special Care in Dentistry, 23*(1), 7-17.

Chandrasoma, P. (2003). Pathological basis of gastroesophageal reflux disease. *World Journal of Surgery, 27*, 986-993.

Chang, H. S., Myung, S. J., Yang, S. K., Jung, H. Y., Kim, T. H., Yoon, I. J., et al. (2003). Effect of electrical stimulation in constipated patients with impaired rectal sensation. *International Journal of Colorectal Disease, 18*(5), 433-438.

Chang, K. J., Soetikno, R. M., Bastas, D., Tu, C., & Nguyen, P. T. (2003). Impact of endoscopic ultrasound combined with fine-needle aspiration biopsy in the management of esophageal cancer. *Endoscopy, 35*(11), 962-966.

Chaussade, S., & Minic, M. (2003). Comparison of efficacy and safety of two doses of two different polyethylene glycol–based laxatives in the treatment of constipation. *Alimentary Pharmacology and Therapeutics, 17*(1), 165-172.

Checchi, L., Montevecchi, M., Gatto, M. R., & Trombelli, L. (2002). Retrospective study of tooth loss in 92 treated periodontal patients. *Journal of Clinical Periodontology, 29*(7), 651-656.

Cheetham, M., Brazzelli, M., Norton, C., & Glazener, C. M. A. (2004). Drug treatment for faecal incontinence in adults. *Cochrane Database of Systematic Reviews, 4.*

Chen, G. D., Hu, S. W., Chen, Y. C., Lin, T. L., & Lin, L. Y. (2003). Prevalence and correlations of anal incontinence and constipation in Taiwanese women. *Neurourology and Urodynamics, 22*(7), 664-669.

Chrysos, E., Athanasakis, E., Pechlivanides, G., Tzortzinis, A., Mantides, A., & Xynos, E. (2004). The effect of total and anterior

partial fundoplication on antireflux mechanisms of the gastroesophageal junction. *American Journal of Surgery, 188*(1), 39-44.

Cobb, C. M. (2002). Clinical significance of non-surgical periodontal therapy: An evidence-based perspective of scaling and root planning. *Journal of Clinical Periodontology, 29*(suppl 2), 6-16.

Coggrave, M., Wiesel, P. H., Norton, C., & Brazzelli, M. (2006). Management of fecal incontinence and constipation in adults with central neurological diseases. *Cochrane Database of Systematic Reviews, 4.*

Cohen, S., & Parkman, H. P. (2000). Diseases of the esophagus. In L. Goldman & J. C. Bennett (Eds.), *Cecil textbook of medicine* (21st ed.). Philadelphia: Saunders.

Copeland, L. B., Krall, E. A., Brown, L. J., Garcia, R. I., & Streckfus, C. F. (2004). Predictors of tooth loss in two U.S. adult populations. *Journal of Public Health Dentistry, 64*(1), 31-37.

Crew, K. D., & Neugut, A. I. (2004). Epidemiology of upper gastrointestinal malignancies. *Seminars in Oncology, 31*(4), 450-464.

Daly, R. M., Elsner, R. J., Allen, P. F., & Burke, F. M. (2003). Associations between self-reported dental status and diet. *Journal of Oral Rehabilitation, 30*(10), 964-970.

Davies, R. M. (2004). The rational use of oral care products in the elderly. *Clinical Oral Investigation, 8*, 2-5.

Desvarieux, M., Demmer, R. T., Rundek, T., Boden-Albala, B., Jacobs, D. R., Jr., Papaanou, P. N., & Sacco, R. I. (2003). Relationship between periodontal disease, tooth loss, and carotid artery plaque: The Oral Infection and Vascular Disease Epidemiology Study (INVEST). *Stroke, 34*(9), 2120-2125.

Devlin, H., & Ferguson, M. W. J. (2003). Aging and the orofacial tissues. In R. C. Tallis & H. M. Fillit (Eds.), *Brocklehurst's textbook of geriatric medicine and gerontology* (6th ed.). London: Churchill Livingstone.

Diaz, S., Brunt, L. M., Klingensmith, M. E., Frisella, P. M., & Soper, N. J. (2003). Laparoscopic paraesophageal hernia repair, a challenging operation: Medium-term outcome of 116 patients. *Journal of Gastrointestinal Surgery, 7*(1), 59-66.

Donington, J. S., Miller, D. L., Deschamps, C., Nichols, F. C., 3rd, & Pairolero, P. C. (2004). Preoperative chemoradiation therapy does not improve early survival after esophagectomy for patients with clinical stage III adenocarcinoma of the esophagus. *Annals of Thoracic Surgery, 77*(4), 1193-1198.

Dukas, L., Willett, W. C., & Giovannucci, E. L. (2003). Association between physical activity, fiber intake, and other lifestyle variables and constipation in a study of women. *American Journal of Gastroenterology, 98*(8), 1790-1796.

Edmond, M. (1994). Enteric infections in the nursing home. Paper presented at 17th Midwestern Conference on Health Care in the Elderly. University of Iowa, Iowa City.

Elter, J. R., Champagne, C. M., Offenbacher, S., & Beck, J. D. (2004). Relationship of periodontal disease and tooth loss to prevalence of coronary heart disease. *Journal of Periodontology, 75*(6), 782-790.

FDI Commission. (2002). Mouthrinses and periodontal disease. *International Dental Journal, 52*(5), 346-352.

Fekety, R. (2000). Pseudomonas colitis. In L. Goldman & J. C. Bennett (Eds.), *Cecil textbook of medicine* (21st ed.). Philadelphia: W. B. Saunders.

Forde, C. G., Cantau, B., Delahunty, C. M., & Elsner, R. J. (2002). Interactions between texture and trigeminal stimulus in a liquid food system: Effects on elderly consumers' preferences. *Journal of Nutrition, Health, and Aging, 6*(2), 130-133.

Frisk, F., Hakeberg, M., Ahlqwist, M., & Bengtsson, C. (2003). Endodontic variables and coronary heart disease. *Acta Odontologica Scandinavica, 61*(5), 257-262.

Fure, S. (2003). Ten-year incidence of tooth loss and dental caries in elderly Swedish individuals. *Caries Research, 37*(6), 462-469.

Furuta, T., Shirai, N., Xiao, F., Takashita, M., Sugimoto, M., Kajimura, M., et al. (2004). High-dose rabeprazole/amoxicillin therapy as the second-line regimen after failure to eradicate *H. pylori* by triple therapy with the usual doses of a proton pump inhibitor, clarithromycin, and amoxicillin. *Hepato-Gastroenterology, 50*(54), 2274-2278.

Gagan, M. J. (2003). Review: Probiotics are effective in preventing antibiotic associated diarrhea. *Evidence-Based Nursing, 6*(1), 16.

Ghezzi, E. M., & Ship, J. A. (2003). Aging and sensory reserve capacity of major salivary glands. *Journal of Dental Research, 82*(2), 844-848.

Gilbert, G. H., Duncan, R. P., & Shelton, B. J. (2003). Social determinants of tooth loss. *Health Services Research, 38*(6 pt 2), 1843-1862.

Goldberg, M., Farma, J., Lampert, C., Colarusso, P., Coia, L., Frucht, H., et al. (2003). Survival following intensive preoperative combined modality therapy with paclitaxel, cisplatin, 5-fluorouracil, and radiation in resectable esophageal carcinoma: A phase 1 report. *Journal of Thoracic and Cardiovascular Surgery, 126*(4), 1168-1173.

Goodman, M. L., & Wilkinson, S. (2004). Laxatives for the management of constipation in palliative care. *Cochrane Database of Systematic Reviews, 4.*

Greenwald, D. A., & Brandt, L. J. (2003). The upper gastrointestinal tract. In R. C. Tallis & H. M. Fillit (Eds.), *Brocklehurst's textbook of geriatric medicine and gerontology* (6th ed.). London: Churchill Livingstone.

Hagger, R., Kumar, D., Benson, M., & Grundy, A. (2003). Colonic motor activity in slow-transit idiopathic constipation as identified by 24 hr pancolonic ambulatory manometry. *Neurogastroenterology and Motility, 15*(5), 515-522.

Hall, G. R., Karstens, M., Rakel, B., Swanson, E., & Davidson, A. (1995). Managing constipation using a research based protocol. *MEDSURG Nursing, 4*(1), 11-20.

Harari, D. (2003). Constipation and fecal incontinence in old age. In R. C. Tallis & H. M. Fillit (Eds.), *Brocklehurst's textbook of geriatric medicine and gerontology* (6th ed.). London: Churchill Livingstone.

Harris, R. J. (2003). Untreated periodontal disease: A followup on 30 cases. *Journal of Periodontology, 74*(5), 672-678.

Heanue, M., Deacon, S. A., Deery, C., Robinson, P. G., Walmsley, A. D., Worthington, H. V., & Shaw, W. C. (2004). Manual versus powered toothbrushing for oral health. *Cochrane Database of Systemic Reviews, 3.*

Heitkemper, M. M. (2004). Nursing management: Upper gastrointestinal problems. In S. M. Lewis, M. M. Heitkemper, & S. R. Dirksen (Eds.), *Medical-surgical nursing* (6th ed.). St. Louis: Mosby.

Henriksen, B. M., Axell, T., & Laake, K. (2003). Geographic differences in tooth loss and denture wearing among the elderly in Norway. *Community Dentistry and Oral Epidemiology, 31*(6), 403-411.

Higgins, P. D. R., & Johanson, J. F. (2004). Epidemiology of constipation in North America: A systematic review. *American Journal of Gastroenterology, 99,* 750-759.

Hirano, H., Ezura, Y., Ishiyama, N., Yamaguchi, M., Nasu, I., Yoshida, H., et al. (2003). Association of natural tooth loss with genetic variation at the human matrix G1a protein locus in elderly women. *Journal of Human Genetics, 48*(6), 288-292.

Hornecker, E., Muuss, T., Ehrenreich, H., & Mausberg, R. F. (2003). A pilot study on the oral conditions of severely alcoholic persons. *Journal of Contemporary Dental Practice, 4*(2), 51-59. Retrieved February 1, 2006, from www.thejcdp.com/issue014/hornecker/index.htm.

Huang, J. Q., & Hunt, R. H. (2003). The evolving epidemiology of *Helicobacter pylori* infection and gastric cancer. *Canadian Journal of Gastroenterology, 17*(suppl B), 18B-20B.

Hung, H. C., Willett, W., Ascherio, A., Rosner, B. A., Rimm, E., & Joshipura, K. J. (2003). Tooth loss and dietary intake. *Journal of the American Dental Association, 134*(9), 1185-1192.

Hung, H. C., Willett., W., Merchant, A., Rosner, B. A., Ascherio, A., & Joshipura, K. J. (2003). Oral health and peripheral arterial disease. *Circulation, 107*(8), 1152-1157.

Ikeda, M., Ikui, A., & Tomita, H. (2002). Gustatory function of the soft palate. *Acta Oto-Laryngologica Supplement, 546,* 69-73.

Inagaki, K., Krall, E. A., Fleet, J. C., & Garcia, R. I. (2003). Vitamin D receptor alleles, periodontal disease progression, and tooth loss in the VA dental longitudinal study. *Journal of Periodontology, 74*(2), 161-167.

Isaksson, R., Soderfeldt, B., & Nederfors, T. (2003). Oral treatment need and oral treatment intention in a population enrolled in long-term care in nursing homes and home care. *Acta Odontologica Scandinavica, 61*(1), 11-18.

James, O. F. W. (2003). The liver. In R. C. Tallis & H. M. Fillit (Eds.), *Brocklehurst's textbook of geriatric medicine and gerontology* (6th ed.). London: Churchill Livingstone.

James, S. L., Muir, J. G., Curtis, S. L., & Gibson, P. R. (2003). Dietary fibre: A roughage study. *Internal Medicine Journal, 33*(7), 291-296.

Jarvis, C. (2004). *Physical examination and health assessment* (4th ed.). Philadelphia: W. B. Saunders.

Johnsson, E., Carlsen, E., Mjaland, O., & Drolsum, A. (2003). Resection rectopexy for internal rectal intussusception reduces constipation and incomplete evacuation of stool. *European Journal of Surgery, Acta Chirurgica, Supplement, 588,* 51-56.

Jones, J. A., Orner, M. B., Spiro, A., 3rd, & Kressin, N. R. (2003). Tooth loss and dentures: Patients' perspectives. *International Dental Journal, 53*(5 suppl), 327-334.

Kahrilas, P. J. (2003a). GERD pathogenesis, pathophysiology, and clinical manifestations. *Cleveland Clinic Journal of Medicine, 70*(suppl 5), S4-S19.

Kahrilas, P. J. (2003b). GERD pathophysiology: The importance of acid control. *Revista de Gastroenterologia de Mexico, 68*(suppl 3), 14-19.

Kakarlapudi, G. V., Awad, Z. T., Haynatzki, G., Sampson, T., Stroup, G., & Filipi, C. J. (2002). The effect of diaphragmatic stressors on recurrent hiatal hernia. *Hernia, 6*(4), 163-166.

Kamolz, T., Granderath, F., & Pointner, R. (2003). Laparoscopic antireflux surgery: Disease-related quality of life assessment before and after surgery in GERD patients with and without Barrett's esophagus. *Surgical Endoscopy, 17*(6), 880-885.

Karoussis, I. K., Salvi, G. E., Heitz-Mayfield, L. J., Bragger, U., Hammerle, C. H., & Lang, N. P. (2003). Long-term implant prognosis in patients with and without a history of chronic periodontitis: A 10-year prospective cohort study of the ITI Dental Implant System. *Clinical Oral Implants Research, 14*(3), 329-339.

Kaushik, V., & Makin, A. (2003). The pancreas. In R. C. Tallis & H. M. Fillit (Eds.), *Brocklehurst's textbook of geriatric medicine and gerontology* (6th ed.). London: Churchill Livingstone.

Kelley, S. T., Coppola, D., & Karl, R. C. (2004). Neoadjuvant chemoradiotherapy is not associated with a higher complication rate vs. surgery alone in patients undergoing esophagectomy. *Journal of Gastrointestinal Surgery, 8*(3), 227-231.

Koretz, B., & Reuben, D. B. (2003). Presentation of disease in old age. In R. C. Tallis & H. M. Fillit (Eds.), *Brocklehurst's textbook of geriatric medicine and gerontology* (6th ed.). London: Churchill Livingstone.

Kuipers, E. J., Nelis, G. F., Klinkenberg-Knol, E. C., Snel, P., Goldfain, D., Kolkman, J. J., et al. (2004). Cure of *Helicobacter pylori* infection in patients with reflux oesophagitis treated with long term omeprazole reverses gastritis without exacerbation of reflux disease: Results of a randomized controlled trial. *Gut, 53*(1), 12-20.

Leeder, P. C., Smith, G., & Dehn, T. C. (2003). Laparoscopic management of large paraesophageal hiatal hernia. *Surgical Endoscopy, 17*(9), 1372-1375.

Lehne, R. A. (2004). *Pharmacology for nursing care* (5th ed.). Philadelphia: Saunders.

Lembo, A., & Camilleri, M. (2003). Chronic constipation. *New England Journal of Medicine, 349*(14), 1360-1368.

Lieber, C. S. (2004). New concepts of the pathogenesis of alcoholic liver disease lead to novel treatments. *Current Gastroenterology Reports, 6*(1), 60-65.

Lieber, C. S., Weiss, D. G., Groszmann, R., Paronetto, F., & Schenker, S. (2003). Veterans Affairs Cooperative Study of polyenylphosphatidylcholine in alcoholic liver disease. *Alcoholism: Clinical and Experimental Research, 27*(11), 1765-1772.

Lin, E., Swafford, V., Chadalavada, R., Ramshaw, B. J., & Smith, C. D. (2004). Disparity between symptomatic and physiologic outcomes following esophageal lengthening procedures for antireflux surgery. *Journal of Gastrointestinal Surgery, 8*(1), 31-39.

Lin, M., Gerson, L. B., Lascar, R., Davila, M., & Triadafilopoulos, G. (2004). Features of gastroesophageal reflux disease in women. *American Journal of Gastroenterology, 99*(8), 1442-1447.

Listgarten, M. A., & Loomer, P. M. (2003). Microbial identification in the management of periodontal disease: A systematic review. *Annals of Periodontology, 8*(1), 182-192.

Loesche, W. J., Giordano, J. R., Soehren, S., & Kaciroti, N. (2002). The nonsurgical treatment of patients with periodontal disease: Results after five years. *Journal of the American Dental Association, 133*(3), 311-320.

Loffeld, R. J., & van der Putten, A. B. (2003). Rising incidence of reflux oesophagitis in patients undergoing upper gastrointestinal endoscopy. *Digestion, 68*(2-3), 141-144.

Lowe, G., Woodward, M., Rumley, A., Morrison, C., Tunstall-Pedoe, H., & Stephen, K. (2003). Total tooth loss and prevalent cardiovascular disease in men and women: Possible roles of citrus fruit consumption, vitamin C, and inflammatory and thrombotic variables. *Journal of Clinical Epidemiology, 56*(7), 694-700.

Macdonald, J. S. (2004). Treatment of localized gastric cancer. *Seminars in Oncology, 31*(4), 566-573.

Madan, A. K., Frantzides, C. T., & Patsavas, K. L. (2004). The myth of the short esophagus. *Surgical Endoscopy, 18*(1), 31-34.

Madsen, J. L., & Graff, J. (2004). Effects of ageing on gastrointestinal motor function. *Age and Ageing, 33*, 154-159.

Mahan, L. K., & Escott-Stump, S. (2000). *Krause's food, nutrition, and diet therapy* (10th ed.). Philadelphia: W. B. Saunders.

Manes, G., Pieramico, O., Uomo, G., Mosca, S., de Nucci, C., & Balzano, A. (2003). Relationship of sliding hiatus hernia to gastroesophageal reflux disease: A possible role for *Helicobacter pylori* infection. *Digestive Diseases and Sciences, 48*(2), 303-307.

Marcenes, W., Steele, J. G., Sheiham, A., & Walls, A. W. (2003). The relationship between dental status, food selection, nutrient intake, nutritional status, and body mass index in older people. *Cadernos de Saude Publica, 19*(3), 809-816.

Massey, B. T. (2004). The implications of *Helicobacter pylori* infection for gastroesophageal reflux disease: Studies presented at Digestive Disease Week 2003. *Current Gastroenterology Reports, 6*(3), 191-195.

Mattes, R. D. (2003, February). The chemical senses and nutrition in aging: Challenging old assumptions. *Journal of the American Dietetic Association, 102*(2), 192-196.

Mattioli, S., D'Ovidio, F., Pilotti, V., DiSimone, M. P., Lugaresi, M. L., Bassi, F., & Brusori, S. (2003). Hiatus hernia and intrathoracic migration of esophagogastric junction in gastroesophageal reflux disease. *Digestive Diseases and Sciences, 48*(9), 1823-1831.

Mattioli, S., Lugaresi, M. L., Pierluigi, M., DiSimone, M. P., & D'Ovidio, F. (2003). Review article: Indications for anti-reflux surgery in gastroesophageal reflux disease. *Alimentary Pharmacology and Therapeutics, 17*(suppl 2), 60-67.

McCord, R. (2003). Understanding prosthodontics—where did it all go wrong? *International Dental Journal, 53*(5 suppl), 335-339.

Melciades, M., Costa, B., & Pires-Neto, M. A. (2004). Anatomical investigation of the esophageal and aortic hiatuses: Physiologic, clinical, and surgical considerations. *Anatomical Science International, 79*, 21-31.

Merli, G. J., & Graham, M. G. (2003, June). Three steps to better management of constipation. *Patient Care for the Nurse Practitioner, 6*.

Migliori, S. J. (2004). The surgical management of gastroesophageal reflux disease. *Medicine and Health, Rhode Island, 87*(2), 33-35.

Mohammad, A. R., Hooper, D. A., Vermilyea, S. G., Mariotti, A., & Preshaw, P. M. (2003). An investigation of the relationship between systemic bone density and clinical periodontal status in postmenopausal Asian-American women. *International Dental Journal, 53*(3), 121-125.

Moriwaki, Y., Kunisaki, C., Kobayashi, S., Harada, H., Imai, S., & Kasaoka, C. (2004). Does the surgical stress associated with palliative resection for patients with incurable gastric cancer with distant metastasis shorten their survival? *Hepato-Gastroenterology, 51*(57), 872-875.

Moss, S. F., Armstrong, D., Arnold, R., Ferenci, P., Fock, K. M., Holtman, G., et al. (2003). GERD 2003—a consensus on the way ahead. *Digestion, 67*(3), 111-117.

Mulligan, E. D., Dunne, B., Griffin, M., Keeling, N., & Reynolds, J. V. (2004). Margin involvement and outcome in oesophageal carcinoma: A 10-year experience in a specialist unit. *European Journal of Surgical Oncology, 30*(3), 313-317.

Nakaji, S., Tokunaga, S., Sakamoto, J., Todate, M., Shimoyama, T., Umeda, T., & Sugawara, K. (2002). Relationship between lifestyle factors and defecation in a Japanese population. *European Journal of Nutrition, 41*(6), 244-248.

NANDA International. (2003). *Nursing diagnoses: Definitions and classification 2003-2004*. Philadelphia: NANDA International.

Navezesh, M. (2002). Dry mouth: Aging and oral health. *Compendium of Continuing Education in Dentistry, 23*(10 suppl), 41-48.

Nilsson, S. E., Takkinen, S., Johansson, B., Dotevall, G., Melander, A., Berg, S., & McClearn, G. (2004). Laxative treatment elevates plasma homocysteine: A study of a population based Swedish sample of old people. *European Journal of Clinical Pharmacology, 60*(1), 45-49.

Oelschlager, B. K., Barreca, M., Chang, L., Oleynikov, D., & Pellegrini, C. A. (2003a). The use of small intestine submucosa in the repair of paraesophageal hernias: Initial observations of a new technique. *American Journal of Surgery, 186*(1), 4-8.

Oelschlager, B. K., Barreca, M., Chang, L., Oleynikov, D., & Pellegrini, C. A. (2003b). Clinical and pathologic response of Barrett's esophagus to laparoscopic antireflux surgery. *Annals of Surgery, 238*(4), 458-464.

Omar, R., Tashkandi, E., Abduljabbar, T., Abdullah, M. A., & Akeel, R. F. (2003). Sentiments expressed in relation to tooth loss: A qualitative study among edentulous Saudis. *International Journal of Prosthodontics, 16*(5), 515-520.

Oringer, R. J. (2002). Biological mediators for periodontal and bone regeneration. *Compendium of Continuing Education in Dentistry, 23*(6), 501-504.

Pace, F., Bollani, S., Molteni, P., & Bianchi Porro, G. (2004). Natural history of gastro-esophageal reflux disease without esophagitis (NERD)—a reappraisal 10 years on. *Digestive and Liver Disease, 36*(2), 111-115.

Pace, F., & Porro, B. (2004). Gastroesophageal reflux disease: A typical spectrum disease (a new conceptual framework is not needed). *American Journal of Gastroenterology* [Electronic version]. Retrieved October 1, 2004, via OVID.

Panzuto, F., DiGiulio, E., Capurso, G., Baccini, F., D'Ambra, G., Delle Fave, G., & Annibale, B. (2004). Large hiatal hernia in patients with iron deficiency anemia: A prospective study of prevalence and treatment. *Alimentary Pharmacology and Therapeutics, 19*(6), 663-670.

Paulander, J., Wennstrom, J. L., Axelsson, P., & Lindhe, J. (2004). Some risk factors for periodontal bone loss in 50-year-old individuals: A 10 year cohort study. *Journal of Clinical Periodontology, 31*(7), 489-496.

Pearce, M. S., Steele, J. G., Mason, J., Walls, A. W., & Parker, L. (2004). Do circumstances in early life contribute to tooth retention in middle age? *Journal of Dental Research, 83*(7), 562-566.

Peltola, P., Vehkalahti, M. M., & Wuolijoki-Saaristo, K. (2004). Oral health and treatment needs of the long-term hospitalized elderly. *Gerodontology, 21*(2), 93-99.

Plummer, M., Franceschi, S., & Munoz, N. (2004). Epidemiology of gastric cancer. *IARC Scientific Publications, 157*, 311-326.

Potter, J. (2003). Bowel care in older people. *Clinical Medicine, 3*(1), 48-51.

Powell, D. W. (2000). Approach to the patient with diarrhea. In L. Goldman & J. C. Bennett (Eds.), *Cecil textbook of medicine* (21st ed.). Philadelphia: W. B. Saunders.

Preece, J. (2002). Introducing abdominal massage in palliative care for the relief of constipation. *Complementary Therapies in Nursing and Midwifery, 8*(2), 101-105.

Purohit, V., & Russo, D. (2002). Role of S-adenosyl-L-methionine in the treatment of alcoholic liver disease: Introduction and summary of the symposium. *Alcohol, 27*(3), 151-154.

Quigley, E. M. (2003). New developments in the pathophysiology of gastroesophageal reflux disease (GERD): Implications for patient management. *Alimentary Pharmacology and Therapeutics, 17*(suppl 2), 43-51.

Quirynen, M., Zhao, H., & van Steenberghe, D. (2002). Review of the treatment strategies for oral malodor. *Clinical Oral Investigations, 6*(1), 1-10.

Raimondo, M. L., & Burroughs, A. (2003). Biliary tract disease. In R. C. Tallis & H. M. Fillit (Eds.), *Brocklehurst's textbook of geriatric medicine and gerontology* (6th ed.). London: Churchill Livingstone.

Rajendra, S., Kutty, K., & Karim, N. (2004). Ethnic differences in the prevalence of endoscopic esophagitis and Barrett's esophagus: The long and short of it all. *Digestive Diseases and Sciences, 49*(2), 237-242.

Rambaldi, A., & Gluud, C. (2002). Propylthiouracil for alcoholic liver disease. *Cochrane Database of Systematic Reviews, 2*, CD002800.

Rambaldi, A., Iaquinto, G., & Gluud, C. (2003). Anabolic-androgenic steroids for alcoholic liver disease. *Cochrane Database of Systematic Reviews, 1*, CD003045.

Rao, S. S. (2003). Constipation: Evaluation and treatment. *Gastroenterology Clinics of North America, 32*(2), 659-683.

Rautelin, H., & Kosunen, T. U. (2004). *Helicobacter pylori* infection in Finland. *Annals of Medicine, 36*(2), 82-88.

Renvert, S., Ohlsson, O., Persson, S., Lang, N. P., & Persson, G. R. (2004). Analysis of periodontal risk profiles in adults with or without a history of myocardial infarction. *Journal of Clinical Periodontology, 31*(1), 19-24.

Rodrigues, C. A. (2003). The small bowel. In R. C. Tallis & H. M. Fillit (Eds.), *Brocklehurst's textbook of geriatric medicine and gerontology* (6th ed.). London: Churchill Livingstone.

Rombeau, J. L. (2000). Enteral nutrition. In L. Goldman & J. C. Bennett (Eds.), *Cecil textbook of medicine* (21st ed.). Philadelphia: Saunders.

Rooney, J., Wade, W. G., Sprague, S. V., Newcombe, R. G., & Addy, M. (2002). Adjunctive effects to non-surgical periodontal therapy of systemic metronidazole and amoxicillin alone and combined. *Journal of Clinical Periodontology, 29*(4), 342-350.

Sakar, B., Karagol, H., Gumus, M., Basaran, M., Kaytan, E., Argon, A., et al. (2004). Timing of death from tumor recurrence after curative gastrectomy for gastric cancer. *American Journal of Clinical Oncology, 27*(2), 205-209.

Sanders, A. E., & Spencer, A. J. (2004). Social inequality in perceived oral health among adults in Australia. *Australian and New Zealand Journal of Public Health, 28*(2), 159-166.

Santos, A. (2003). Evidence-based control of plaque and gingivitis. *Journal of Clinical Periodontology, 30*(suppl 5), 13-16.

Savoye-Collet, C., Savoye, G., Koning, E., Leroi, A. M., & Dacher, J. N. (2003). Defecography in symptomatic older women living at home. *Age and Ageing, 32*(3), 347-350.

Sculean, A., Schwartz, F., Berakdar, M., Romanos, G. E., Arweiler, N. B., & Beeker, J. (2004). Periodontal treatment with an Er:YAG laser compared to ultrasonic instrumentation: A pilot study. *Journal of Periodontology, 75*(7), 966-973.

Shafik, A., Shafik, A. A., El-Sibai, O., & Ahmed, I. (2003). Colonic pacing in patients with constipation due to colonic inertia. *Medical Science Monitor, 9*(5), CR191-196.

Shafik, A., Shafik, A. A., El-Sibai, O., & Ahmed, I. (2004). Colonic pacing: A therapeutic option for the treatment of constipation due to total colonic inertia. *Archives of Surgery, 139*(7), 775-779.

Shimatani, T., Inoue, M., Harada, N., Horikawa, Y., Nakamura, M., & Tazuma, S. (2004). Gastric acid normosecretion is not essential in the pathogenesis of mild erosive gastroesophageal reflux disease in relation to *Helicobacter pylori*. *Digestive Diseases and Sciences, 49*(5), 787-794.

Shimazaki, Y., Soh, I., Koga, T., Miyazaki, H., & Takehara, T. (2003). Risk factors for tooth loss in the institutionalized elderly: A six-year cohort study. *Community Dental Health, 20*(2), 123-127.

Sicilia, A., Arregui, I., Gallego, M., Cabezas, B., & Cuesta, S. (2002). A systematic review of powered vs manual toothbrushes in periodontal cause-related therapy. *Journal of Clinical Periodontology, 29*(suppl 3), 39-54.

Sihvo, E. I., Luostarinen, M. E., & Salo, J. A. (2004). Fate of patients with adenocarcinoma of the esophagus and the esophagogastric junction: A population-based analysis. *American Journal of Gastroenterology, 99*(3), 419-424.

Simmons, S. F., & Schnelle, J. F. (2004). Effects of an exercise and scheduled-toileting intervention on appetite and constipation in nursing home residents. *EBM Reviews—Cochrane Central Register of Controlled Trials.*

Simren, M. (2002). Physical activity and the gastrointestinal tract. *European Journal of Gastroenterology and Hepatology, 14*(10), 1053-1056.

Smith, C., Hellebusch, S. J., & Mandel, K. G. (2003). Patient and physician evaluation of a new bulk fiber laxative tablet. *Gastroenterology Nursing, 26*(1), 31-37.

Soergel, K. H., Zboralske, F. E., & Amberg, J. R. (1964). Presbyesophagus: Esophageal motility in nonagenarians. *Journal of Clinical Investigations, 43*, 1472.

Steele, J. G., Sanders, A. E., Slade, G. D., Allen, P. F., Lahti, S., Nuttall, N., & Spencer, A. J. (2004). How do age and tooth loss affect oral health impacts and quality of life? A study comparing two national samples. *Community Dentistry and Oral Epidemiology, 32*(2), 107-114.

Steffen, R., Tornieporth, N., Clemens, S. C., Chatterjee, S., Cavalcanti, A., Collard, F., et al. (2004). Epidemiology of travelers' diarrhea: Details of a global survey. *Journal of Travel Medicine, 11*(4), 231-238.

Stickel, F., Hoehn, B., Schuppan, D., & Seitz, H. K. (2003). Review article: Nutritional therapy in alcoholic liver disease. *Alimentary Pharmacology and Therapeutics, 18*(4), 357-373.

Strange, P. S. (2003). Small intestinal submucosa for laparoscopic repair of large paraesophageal hiatal hernia: A preliminary report. *Surgical Technologies International, 11*, 141-143.

Sugarbaker, P. H., Yu, W., & Yonemura, Y. (2003). Gastrectomy, peritonectomy, and perioperative intraperitoneal chemotherapy: The evolution of treatment strategies for advanced gastric cancer. *Seminars in Surgical Oncology, 21*(4), 233-248.

Tatematsu, M., Mori, T., Kawaguchi, T., Takeuchi, K., Hattori, M., Morita, I., et al. (2004). Masticatory performance in 80 year old individuals. *Gerodontology, 21*(2), 112-119.

Tepper, R. F., & Katz, S. (2003). Geriatric gastroenterology: Overview. In R. C. Tallis & H. M. Fillit (Eds.), *Brocklehurst's textbook of geriatric medicine and gerontology* (6th ed.). London: Churchill Livingstone.

Thomas, A. J. (2003). Nutrition. In R. C. Tallis & H. M. Fillit (Eds.), *Brocklehurst's textbook of geriatric medicine and gerontology* (6th ed.). London: Churchill Livingstone.

Todd, S., Corsnitz, D., Ray, S., & Nassar, J. (2002). Outpatient laparoscopic Nissen fundoplication. *AORN Journal, 75*(5), 955-956.

Tome, S., & Lucey, M. R. (2004). Review article: Current management of alcoholic liver disease. *Alimentary Pharmacology and Therapeutics, 19*, 707-714.

Toruner, M., Soykan, I., Ensari, A., Kuzu, I., Yurdaydin, C., & Ozden, A. (2004). Barrett's esophagus: Prevalence and its relationship with dyspeptic symptoms. *Journal of Gastroenterology and Hepatology, 19*(5), 535-540.

Tytgat, G. N. J., Bartelink, H., Bernards, R., Giaccope, G., van Lanschot, J. J. B., Offerhaus, G. J. A., & Peters, G. J. (2004). Cancer of the esophagus and gastric cardia: Recent advances. *Diseases of the Esophagus, 17*, 10-26.

Vazquez-Sequeiros, E., Wiersema, M. J., Clain, J. E., Norton, I. D., Levy, M. J., Romero, Y., et al. (2003). Impact of lymph node staging on therapy of esophageal carcinoma. *Gastroenterology, 125*(6), 1626-1635.

Wainess, R. M., Dimick, J. B., Upchurch, G. R., Jr., Cowan, J. A., & Mulholland, M. W. (2003). Epidemiology of surgically treated gastric cancer in the United States. *Journal of Gastrointestinal Surgery, 7*(7), 879-883.

Wald, A. (2003). The large bowel. In R. C. Tallis & H. M. Fillit (Eds.), *Brocklehurst's textbook of geriatric medicine and gerontology* (6th ed.). London: Churchill Livingstone.

Wu, A. H., Tseng, C. C., & Bernstein, L. (2003). Hiatal hernia, reflux symptoms, body size, and risk of esophageal and gastric adenocarcinoma. *Cancer, 98*(5), 940-948.

Wu, C. H., Wu, M. S., Huang, S. P., & Lin, J. T. (2004). Relationship between *Helicobacter pylori* infection and erosive gastroesophageal reflux disease. *Journal of the Formosan Medical Association, 103*(3), 186-190.

Wyatt, C. C., & MacEntee, M. I. (2004). Caries management for institutionalized elders using fluoride and chlorhexidine mouthrinses. *Community Dentistry and Oral Epidemiology, 32*(5), 322-328.

Yamauchi, Y., Endo, S., & Yoshimura, I. (2002). A new whole mouth gustatory test procedure. II. Effects of aging, gender and smoking. *Acta Oto-Laryngologica Supplement, 546*, 49-56.

Yeh, K. H., & Cheng, A. L. (2004). Recent advances in therapy for gastric cancer. *Journal of the Formosan Medical Association, 103*(3), 171-185.

Ylostalo, P., Sakki, T., Laitinen, J., Jarvelin, M. R., & Knuuttila, M. (2004). The relation of tobacco smoking to tooth loss among young adults. *European Journal of Oral Sciences, 112*(2), 121-126.

Young, T. A., Neuberger, J., Longworth, L., Ratcliffe, J., & Buxton, M. J. (2003). Survival gain after liver transplantation for patients with alcoholic liver disease: A comparison across models and centers. *Transplantation, 76*(10), 1479-1486.

Zacherel, J., Sendler, A., Stein, H. J., Ott, K., Feith, M., Jakesz, R., et al. (2003). Current status of neoadjuvant therapy for adenocarcinoma of the distal esophagus. *World Journal of Surgery, 27*(9), 1067-1074.

Zhang, C. Q., Zhang, G. W., Zhang, K. L., & Fu, Y. Q. (2003). Clinical evaluation of polyethylene glycol 4000 in treatment of functional constipation in elderly patients. *World Chinese Journal of Digestology, 11*(9), 1399-1401. In *EBM Reviews—Cochrane Central Register of Controlled Trials.*

Zhao, H., Liu, J. P., Liu, Z. S., & Peng, W. N. (2004). Acupuncture for chronic constipation. *CochraneDatabase of Systematic Reviews, 4.*

16 Genitourinary System

Adrianne Dill Linton

Objectives

Describe the normal changes in the genitourinary system associated with aging.

Describe measures to maintain genitourinary health in the older adult.

Explain the cause and treatment of genitourinary disorders that are common in older persons.

Describe the components of the genitourinary assessment in the older adult.

Formulate nursing diagnoses for older adults with actual or potential genitourinary problems.

Develop plans to manage older adults with actual or potential genitourinary problems.

The changes in the genitourinary system, particularly changes related to urinary elimination, present problems to older people and challenges to nurses. Part of the challenge to health care providers is to dispel the myth that dysfunction is inevitable and not amenable to treatment.

NORMAL STRUCTURE AND FUNCTION

The genitourinary system functions to eliminate bodily wastes formed in the kidneys and, in men, to provide a pathway for sperm in the reproductive process. The normal functioning of this system depends on the interrelated activities of the circulatory, endocrine, and nervous systems.

The system components are the kidneys, ureters, urinary bladder, and urethra (Figure 16-1). Each kidney comprises approximately 1 million nephrons, which in turn are made up of a vascular component (the glomerulus) and a tubular component. The glomerulus protrudes into one side of Bowman's capsule, a blind sac lined with epithelial cells. On the other side, the tubule originates from Bowman's capsule and consists of the proximal convoluted tubule, Henle's loop, the distal convoluted tubule, and the collecting duct (Figure 16-2).

The kidneys excrete end products of metabolism and foreign substances, including drugs, and regulate fluid and electrolyte balance by selectively conserving or excreting molecules based on serum levels, pH, and hormonal influences. The kidneys produce renin, various prostaglandins, erythropoietin, and active forms of vitamin D. The process of urine formation takes place in the nephrons and includes glomerular filtration, solute reabsorption and secretion, urine concentration and dilution, and urinary acidification and alkalinization. The urine is collected in the renal pelvis before it flows through the ureter into the bladder, from which it is eliminated via the urethra.

The organs of the male reproductive system are the testes, ducts, and external genitalia. The female reproductive organs are the ovaries, ducts, uterus, vagina, sex glands, and external genitalia.

NORMAL CHANGES IN GENITOURINARY STRUCTURE AND FUNCTION
Kidney

Whereas aging itself does not cause renal disease, the risk increases with age as a result of the increased prevalence of atherosclerosis, hypertension, heart failure, diabetes, obstructive nephropathy and prostatic disease, infection, immune insult, and exposure to nephrotoxins. Among the anatomical changes in the kidneys that occur with aging are decreases in weight, total renal area, cortical area, and number of glomeruli (Lamb, O'Riordan, & Delaney, 2003). It is significant that kidney size alone, as determined by ultrasound, is not predictive of renal function in older persons (Burkhardt, Hahn, & Gladisch, 2003). Although adaptive capacity decreases, sufficient reserve capacity exists to permit the aging kidney to maintain homeostasis under stable conditions. When pathological changes are superimposed on the age-related changes, however, the older person is more vulnerable because of lessened reserve (Jassal & Oreopolous, 2003).

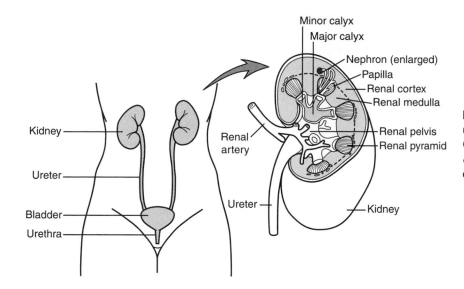

Figure 16-1 General organization of the urinary system and the kidney. (From Guyton, A. C., & Hall, J. E. [2006]. *Textbook of medical physiology* [11th ed.]. Philadelphia: Saunders, p. 309.)

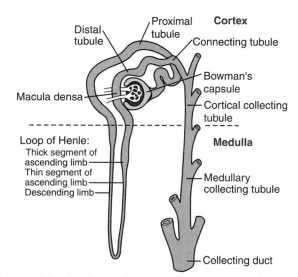

Figure 16-2 Basic tubular segments of the nephron. The relative lengths of the different tubular segments are not drawn to scale. (From Guyton, A. C., & Hall, J. E. [2006]. *Textbook of medical physiology* [11th ed.]. Philadelphia: Saunders, p. 310.)

Nephron. Anatomical changes in the nephron include a decrease in the number and size of nephrons in the cortex; increased interstitial connective tissue; fewer identifiable glomeruli, and a greater percentage of sclerotic glomeruli. The effective filtering surface is diminished by glomerular sclerosis and loss of lobulation of the glomerular tuft. To compensate, remaining healthy glomeruli enlarge and begin to hyperfilter. The number of mesangial cells progressively increases while the number of epithelial cells decreases. The glomerular basement membrane is thickened by the deposition of thrombospondin, an extracellular glycoprotein. An increasing number of diverticuli appear in the distal convoluted tubules. These diverticuli may contribute to the

increased prevalence of recurrent urinary tract infections in older persons and may be the origin of simple retention cysts (Jassal & Oreopoulos, 2003; Lamb, O'Riordan, & Delaney, 2003).

The large renal blood vessels show sclerotic changes that are more prominent in hypertensive individuals. Changes in small blood vessels are minimal in normotensive people. Arteriolar-glomerular alterations revealed in microangiographical and histological studies include hyalinization and collapse of the glomerular tuft and obliteration of the lumen of the preglomerular arteriole, resulting in diminished blood flow. Another change is the development of connections between the afferent and efferent arterioles, which allows blood to bypass the sclerosed glomeruli. Blood flow to the medullary area is maintained via the vasa recta (Jassal & Oreopolous, 2003; Lamb, O'Riordan, & Delaney, 2003). Among persons with newly diagnosed vascular disease, atherosclerosis has been found to accelerate the decline in size of the kidneys and the increase in serum creatinine (Bax et al., 2003).

As renal vascular resistance increases, plasma flow progressively declines about 10% for each decade from young adulthood to age 80 (Jassal & Oreopolous, 2003; Lamb, O'Riordan, & Delaney, 2003). Sources disagree as to whether the decrease in total renal blood flow alters the filtration fraction; some indicate that it increases (Lamb, O'Riordan, & Delaney, 2003; Melk, 2003) whereas others report that it is unaffected (Jassal & Oreopoulos, 2003). Most filtration occurs in the juxtamedullary nephrons where medullary plasma flow is preserved rather than the cortex where vasculature is lost.

A decline in the glomerular filtration rate (GFR) is typical, but not universal with aging. Even when the GFR is decreased, serum creatinine normally remains stable. This is possible because muscle mass, from which creatinine is derived, also declines with age. Poor nutrition may be a factor in some individuals. Therefore GFR may be overestimated if based on serum creatinine. On the other hand, when creatinine clearance is used, GFR may be underestimated.

The accurate assessment of GFR is important because early recognition of chronic kidney disease permits treatment that could slow the progress of the disease. Early detection can also allow for dosage adjustments thereby reducing the risk of nephrotoxicity, and complications of chronic kidney disease can be assessed and treated (Lamb, O'Riordan, & Delaney, 2003). Numerous formulas have been devised using serum creatinine to estimate GFR. Two of these are the Cockcroft and Gault formula and the Modification of Diet in Renal Disease (MDRD) formula. The Cockcroft and Gault formula may be the most widely used:

Estimated creatinine clearance =
$$\frac{(140 - \text{Age in years}) \times (\text{Weight in kg})}{72 \times (\text{Serum creatinine in mg/dL})}$$

For women, multiply the figure obtained by 85.

Criticisms of this formula are that it was derived in a younger population that was 96% male, the method used to assess serum creatinine is different from the methods now used, and it initially was validated against measured creatinine clearance. Despite these validity issues, Lamb and colleagues concluded that the Cockcroft and Gault formula "was unlikely to misclassify patients with mild renal failure as having GFR >50 mL min^{-1}/1.73 m^{2}" (Lamb, O'Riordan, & Delaney, 2003, p. 28).

The MDRD formula was developed based on data from 1628 adults, mostly middle aged. A later, abbreviated formula has been published. Neither has been tested in older people. The MDRD formulas have been found more likely to miscategorize individuals than the Cockcroft formula (Lamb, O'Riordan, & Delaney, 2003). A study was conducted that compared serum and urinary urea and creatinine in hospitalized octogenarians who had indwelling urinary catheters. Seventy percent of the participants had normal serum creatinine; however, half of those had abnormally low urinary creatinine clearance. When the Cockcroft formula was applied, only 9% fell within (plus or minus) 10% of their measured creatinine clearance. With the MDRD formula, 17% fell within (plus or minus) 10% of their measured creatinine clearance. These investigators recommended simply avoiding nephrotoxic drugs and drugs excreted mainly by the kidneys as a practical way to address the dilemma of which formula to use (Rimon et al., 2004). Another study compared the use of the Jelliffe, Cockcroft-Gault, and Wright formulas in persons over age 70 years who had recent GFR measurements. In this sample, the Wright formula was found to be the most accurate, most precise, and least biased for older persons with a GFR greater than 50 mL/min (Marx et al., 2004).

It is hardly surprising that formulas based on serum creatinine are imperfect given that serum creatinine is a poor indicator of GFR in older persons. Therefore some investigators recommend timed urine collections of short duration to more accurately assess creatinine clearance (Jassal & Oreopolous, 2003).

Cystatin C is a protein whose serum concentration is mainly determined by the GFR. The utility of serum measurements of this protein as a marker of GFR has been the subject of several studies. A study of 1246 older persons in Finland demonstrated considerable variability in estimates of renal function using formulas based on serum creatinine, and the authors proposed cystatin C as a promising alternative (Wasen et al., 2004). Lamb, O'Riordan, and Delaney (2003) report that an elevated serum cystatin C suggests moderately reduced GFR; however, they contend that insufficient data on cystatin C in older persons are available for this test to be recommended at this time.

The endocrine functions of the kidneys change with age. In older persons, baseline levels of renin, angiotensin II, and aldosterone are reduced by about 50%. Renin release in response to stimuli is reduced. Renal arterioles regulate renal blood flow and the GFR in response to circulating and local mediators. In general, "an overall picture of increased vasoconstriction and decreased vasodilator reserve of the renal vascular bed is seen with age" (Jassal & Oreopoulos, 2003, p. 1082). The vasoconstrictor response is not affected by age, but there may be changes in the vasodilating system.

Tubules. Tubular function declines with aging as a result of tubulointerstitial fibrosis, loss of tubular mass, and shortening of the proximal tubules (Lamb, O'Riordan, & Delaney, 2003). Under normal circumstances, function is adequate to maintain electrolyte and acid-base balance. However, the older person adapts more slowly to changes in water and sodium balance. With the reduction in aldosterone and renin secretion, sodium conservation and excretion both are impaired, which contributes to nocturnal polyuria. In contrast with declining renin and aldosterone, plasma natriuretic peptide rises (Richardson et al., 2004). Despite a rising antidiuretic hormone level, the maximal urine osmolarity progressively falls. As with sodium and water, potassium and phosphate balance is impaired in the older adult when stressed. Because of the propensity for potassium loss and a 20% decrease in total body potassium, Jassal and Oreopoulos (2003) advise that the older person is at risk for hypokalemia. However, data from 18,723 noninstitutionalized persons in the National Health and Nutrition Examination Survey (NHANES) III study demonstrated a progressive rise in serum potassium from ages 30 to 90 and older. Males consistently had higher levels than females (Wysowski, Kornegay, Nourjah, & Trontell, 2003).

The urinary excretion of albumin rises with aging. Factors that contribute to microalbuminemia are diabetes, hypertension, and cardiovascular disease. In older persons who do not have diabetes, microalbuminemia is a predictor of increased mortality rate (Lamb, O'Riordan, & Delaney, 2003).

Several theories have been proposed to explain the progressive glomerulosclerosis that occurs in the aging kidney. One such theory is hyperfiltration, which proposes that the loss of glomeruli increases the capillary blood flow through the remaining glomeruli with a resultant increase in intracapillary pressure. Elevated pressure damages endothelial cells, which sets in motion a sequence of events that results in glomerular injury. The elevated pressure also disrupts ion exchange and alters cell membrane voltage and protein transcription within endothelial cells.

Much support exists for the hyperfiltration theory; however, it is thought that other mechanisms probably are relevant as well. The genetic theory assumes that cells have a predetermined number of replications so that older persons are at increasing risk for injury to the genetic code and cellular malfunction. The toxin-mediated theory proposes that progressive kidney damage occurs because of exposure to by-products of normal metabolism. It is possible that all three of these theories work together to bring about the changes observed in the aging kidney (Jassal & Oreopoulos, 2003).

A study designed to determine the relative contribution of genetic and environmental factors to kidney changes in older persons assessed 688 older twins in Denmark. Biochemical kidney markers selected for comparison included serum urea, creatinine, urate, and sodium. Genetic factors were found to account for one third to one half of the variation in these markers, except creatinine in males. Furthermore, all four markers were shown to affect survival. Individuals with values that deviated from reference intervals were at increased risk for death (Bathum, Fagnani, Christiansen, & Christensen, 2004).

Ureters

The major defects in the ureters are related to the vesicoureteral junction and the possible reflux of urine into the ureter and subsequently into the renal pelvis. Bilateral obstruction of the ureters can occur when the uterus is prolapsed, causing pressure on the ureters.

Bladder

Age-related changes in the bladder include replacement of smooth muscle and elastic tissue with fibrous connective tissue, and the formation of trabeculae, diverticula, and pseudodiverticulosis. The bladder muscles weaken, the force of the urine stream decreases, and incomplete emptying may occur. Bladder capacity decreases, and frequency of urination increases. The ability to postpone voiding declines. Beta-adrenergic responsiveness declines with age, and this may be a factor in the reduced bladder compliance in older persons (Li, Li, Li, & Wang, 2003). Bladder outlet changes may cause obstruction or incontinence, and overstretching of the bladder wall may occur with urinary retention. The risk of bladder tumors increases with age.

Micturition Cycle. The phases of the micturition cycle are as follows: (1) the bladder fills until the need to void is perceived, (2) urination is voluntarily postponed, and (3) the bladder is emptied voluntarily at the appropriate time and place. Common aging changes combined with pathological states can affect each of these phases, creating problems with urinary retention or incontinence. Interference in the urination process may arise from alterations in the sphincter muscle, neural controls, outlet size, muscle strength, or sensation of need to void. Defects in peripheral innervation may occur with prostatic surgery, alcoholism, and diabetes mellitus. Uninhibited bladder contractions may occur. Incontinence may occur as a result of neurogenic disease, overflow in the absence of a lesion, impaired mobility, cognitive impairment, or drug side effects.

Urethra

There may be difficulty in opening or closing the bladder outlet. An inverse relationship exists between age and maximum urethral closure pressure (Schick, Tessier, Bertrand, Dupont, & Jolivet-Tremblay, 2003). Decreased closing pressure may be caused by loss of striated muscle that makes up the external sphincter. Both men and women may experience difficulty in starting the urinary stream. In men the problem may be related to benign prostatic hypertrophy. In women the problem commonly is related to weakened pelvic musculature caused by childbirth, surgery, or urethral stenosis. Diminished estrogen secretion affects all tissues of the perineal area, including the urethra.

Prostate

The major change in the prostate that occurs with aging is hyperplasia that is most prominent in the periurethral zone. Hyperplasia may be a factor in obstruction and urinary symptoms; however, those symptoms also can be attributed to vesicourethral dysfunction. Some men with significant prostate enlargement report no related symptoms. The interdependence of hyperplasia, obstruction, and lower urinary tract symptoms is represented by the interlocking circles in Figure 16-3. Understanding these relationships is important because it illustrates why treatment focused only on the prostate

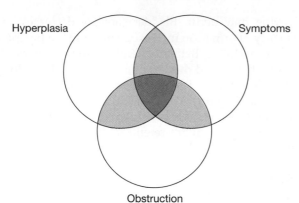

Hyperplasia   Symptoms

Obstruction

Figure 16-3 Interlocking diagram demonstrating the interdependence of lower urinary tract symptoms, out-flow tract obstruction, and hyperplastic tissue when considering symptoms of patients with "prostatism." Significant volumes of hyperplasia may not necessarily be associated either with obstruction or symptoms, whereas all three may be present in some cases. (From George, N. J. R. [2003]. The prostate gland. In R. C. Tallis & H. M. Fillit [Eds.], *Brocklehurst's textbook of geriatric medicine and gerontology* [6th ed.]. London: Churchill Livingstone, p. 1123. Adapted from Hald with permission. Hald, T. [1989]. Urodynamics in benign prostatic hypertrophy: A survey. *The Prostate* [suppl 2], 69-77. Reprinted with permission of Wiley-Liss, Inc., a subsidiary of John Wiley & Sons, Inc.)

gland will not necessarily resolve the symptoms (George, 2003).

The enlarging prostate can create problems in both the filling and voiding phases of micturition. Bladder instability is a condition in which abnormal intrinsic detrusor pressure waves occur during the filling phase of the micturition cycle. The patient experiences frequency, urgency, nocturia, and sometimes urge incontinence. Although bladder instability may be related to benign prostatic hyperplasia, it also can be caused by neurological disorders, in which case it is labeled *detrusor hyper-reflexia*. Prostatectomy effectively treats bladder instability in only about two thirds of cases. Two types of dysfunction in the voiding phase that are associated with prostate enlargement are high-pressure obstructed voiding and low-pressure underactive detrusor function. High-pressure obstructed voiding is the effect of mechanical obstruction and is manifested by hesitancy, poor stream, and increasing frequency. Low-pressure underactive bladder also is manifested by frequency and poor stream. The two dysfunctions can only be differentiated by invasive urodynamic testing. Symptoms related to high pressure are more likely to be resolved by prostatectomy than those related to low pressure (George, 2003).

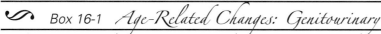

∽ Box 16-1 *Age-Related Changes: Genitourinary*

Kidneys
- Decreased weight
- Decreased total renal area, cortical area
- Decreased adaptive capacity

Nephrons
- Decreased number and size
- Increased interstitial connective tissue
- Fewer identifiable glomeruli
- Greater percentage of sclerosed glomeruli
- Reduced filtering surface
- Healthy glomeruli enlarge and hyperfiltrate
- Thickened glomerular basement membrane
- Increased diverticuli in distal convoluted tubules
- Large renal blood vessels: sclerosis
- Small renal blood vessels: diminished cortical blood flow
- Decline in glomerular filtration rate
- Reduced baseline levels of renin, angiotensin II, and aldosterone
- Decreased erythropoietin

Tubules
- Decreased tubular function
- Shortening of proximal tubules
- Slowed response to changes in water and sodium balance
- Maximal urine osmolarity declines
- Increased urinary excretion of albumin
- Ureters: increased risk of reflux of urine into ureters

External Genitalia

Changes in the male external genitalia include thinning of pubic hair and testicular atrophy. Changes in the female include labial atrophy, vaginal atrophy, and thinning of the vaginal walls associated with estrogen deficiency. Secretions diminish; vaginal pH rises; the normal flora is altered; and the lining is thinner, drier, less elastic, and more easily traumatized. The length and width of the vagina diminish. The outcome frequently is painful intercourse, pruritus, and increased risk for vaginal and bladder infections.

Sexual Response

In both men and women, the production of sex hormones declines, affecting all phases of sexual response. Menopause marks the end of a woman's reproductive capacity, whereas a healthy man can remain fertile throughout life (Butler & Lewis, 2003). The concept of a male menopause is a topic of interest, but it is not universally accepted. Effects of aging changes in the male include increased time needed to achieve an erection, greater difficulty maintaining an erection, delayed ejaculation, decreased volume of semen, and prolonged refractory period. Psychic stimulation is less effective so that more direct stimulation of the penis is required. Erections are less firm, and the expulsion of seminal fluid is less forceful (Brown & Cooper, 2003). Sexual function in men may be affected by altered blood flow to the penis, physical discomforts of chronic illnesses, depression, and the effects of drugs, including alcohol.

Changes in sexuality in older women appear to be influenced most by the changes in estrogen and androgen rather than by age per se (Box 16-1). A significant reduction in sexual interest and activity has been reported in women between 50 and 60 years of age, a time period that coincides with the average menopause. In older

---

 Box 16-1 *Age-Related Changes: Genitourinary — cont'd*

Bladder
- Increased fibrous connective tissue
- Formation of trabeculae, diverticula, and pseudodiverticulosis
- Bladder muscle weakens
- Ability to postpone voiding declines

Urethra
- Opening and closing of bladder outlet may be impaired
- Maximum urethral closure pressure declines

Prostate
- Hyperplasia

External Genitalia
Male
- Thin pubic hair
- Testicular atrophy

Female
- Labial atrophy
- Vaginal atrophy
- Thin, inelastic vaginal walls
- Diminished secretions
- Increased vaginal pH
- Reduced length and width of vagina

Sexual Response
Male
- Increased time to achieve erection
- Greater difficulty maintaining erection
- Delayed ejaculation
- Decreased semen volume
- Prolonged refractory period

Female
- Delayed arousal phase
- Reduced vaginal secretions and expansion
- Orgasm shorter; contractions lessened and sometimes painful

women, the arousal phase is marked by delayed and diminished vaginal secretions and expansion, which may result in dyspareunia (painful intercourse). Vaginal stenosis may occur, especially in women who are not sexually active. Studies of orgasmic capacity in older women have yielded conflicting results, with some reports of diminished capacity and other reports of no change (Brown & Cooper, 2003). The orgasm is shorter and the strength of the contractions is lessened; painful uterine contractions sometimes are experienced.

IMPLICATIONS OF GENITOURINARY CHANGES WITH AGE

Changes in the urinary system can significantly affect the older person's ability to maintain fluid and electrolyte and acid-base balance. Despite these challenges, the older adult usually can maintain homeostasis under stable conditions. However, when the adaptive capacity is tested, the risk for imbalances is increased. There is less compensatory renal hypertrophy in the aging kidney, and therefore the kidney is less able to compensate for function lost after a unilateral nephrectomy.

Other changes in renal function can affect other body systems or structures. The conversion of 1-OH-cholecalciferol to 1-25-(OH)$_2$-cholecalciferol is decreased. This may be a factor in the decrease in intestinal absorption of calcium seen in normal subjects and subjects with osteoporosis. A decrease in erythropoietin may contribute to anemia.

The social impact of problems with urinary elimination can be profound. Control over elimination, like many other self-care tasks, is achieved early in life and is an essential aspect of self-concept as an adult. Difficulties with urination are not typically discussed in ordinary social conversation. The subject is in many ways taboo. Changes in urinary elimination patterns may be worrisome to people of all ages because of the threat of eventual loss of control, resulting in social ostracism. The fearfulness is compounded by the fact that little information is available for the lay public about the normal and abnormal changes in patterns of urinary elimination that occur with age, and the meanings of those changes.

Despite the normal changes in the reproductive system, the healthy older person usually remains capable of satisfying sexual activity. It now is generally accepted that sexual function and interest persist throughout life, although the mode of expression may change. Whereas younger people tend to relate intimacy to sexual intercourse, older persons may define intimacy more broadly. Reasons for changing sexual expression in older persons may be related to common aging changes, various health deviations, social expectations, and lack of a sexual partner.

Fluid and pH Balance

Various changes affect the ability of the older adult to maintain fluid and electrolyte balance. In addition to decreased urinary concentrating ability and limitations in excretion of water, sodium, potassium, and acid, the older person may have impaired thirst perception (Luckey & Parsa, 2003).

The transport maximum declines at a rate parallel to the decline in GFR. This change results in a higher renal threshold for glucose. An older person may have an elevated blood glucose level but no evidence of glycosuria. The change in tubular transport is also reflected in the specific gravity and maximum osmolarity of the urine, the ability to dilute the urine, and the ability to handle acid-base loads.

Water balance is affected by the diminished ability of the loop of Henle, the distal convoluted tubule, and the collecting ducts to concentrate the urine, which is compounded by an age-related decrease in response to antidiuretic hormone (ADH). These factors are important when water intake is limited (overnight dehydration before tests) and when water losses are increased (fever, vomiting, diarrhea). In the presence of dehydration, contrast agents with high osmolarity may lead to acute renal failure. Individuals with decreased GFR are at even greater risk for injury from such agents or hypotension caused by hypovolemia.

An aged person responds more slowly to decreased salt intake. A salt-losing tendency in illness is compounded by inadequate salt intake and may result in impaired cardiac, renal, and mental function. Careful administration of salt-containing fluids is required in older persons who are volume depleted.

Dehydration can cause an acute confusional state. Although reduced thirst sensation has been documented in older persons, dehydration problems more commonly arise from physical difficulty in obtaining and drinking fluids. Altered mental status can contribute to decreased water intake. Also, people who are incontinent may restrict their fluid intake in an attempt to avoid the problem.

Excessive salt intake without an appropriate increase in water may result in dehydration with hyperosmolarity. If an excess of sodium is ingested, resulting in volume overload, the kidney is less able to handle the problem if the GFR is decreased. Problems occur when the older person increases salt in the diet or receives it in intravenous fluids, medications, or sodium-containing contrast agents.

Water intoxication may result in hyponatremia. This may occur because of the decreased ability to excrete water related to decreased renal blood flow. Although the response to ADH may be blunted, excess secretion of ADH further contributes to the problem. Medications that increase ADH secretion (e.g., chlorpropamide, carbamazepine, aspirin, acetaminophen) should be used with caution.

The normal excretion of potassium and retention of sodium is altered. An excess of potassium may occur because of decreased renin and aldosterone levels and decreased GFR. Other factors that may contribute to hyperkalemia are gastrointestinal bleeding, intravenous administration of potassium-containing salts, acidosis, and potassium-sparing diuretics such as spironolactone.

Problems in acid excretion by the kidney are probably associated with defects in the tubular and collecting ducts that impair the excretion of ammonium. They do not appear to be related to decreased GFR.

Pharmacokinetics

A low protein intake may result in low serum albumin levels with less binding of drug molecules, thereby making more free drug molecules available.

Changes in renal function with aging slow the elimination of many drugs, possibly resulting in accumulation of drugs and their toxic metabolites (Turnheim, 2003). A decrease in clearance means an increase in the half-life for drugs that are excreted primarily by the kidneys. Therefore, the dosage should be reduced while the dosing interval remains constant, or the dosage should remain constant while the dosing interval is increased. Dosages of nephrotoxic drugs and those with a narrow therapeutic range (e.g., digitalis, aminoglycosides, and other antibiotics) should be calculated using the creatinine clearance. Though imperfect, these formulas provide some estimate of renal function.

Surgery

Noting that acute renal failure following cardiac surgery is more common in older than younger persons, German researchers assessed kidney-specific proteins in persons younger than 60 years and older than 70 years who did not have known preoperative renal dysfunction. Urine specimens were obtained during the perioperative period and on the first and second postoperative days. In older persons, all of the proteins measured higher, suggesting transient alterations in kidney integrity that were not detected with measures of creatinine (Boldt, Brenner, Lang, Kumle, & Isgro, 2003).

COMMON DISORDERS

Disorders of the kidney in aging usually are caused by atherosclerosis, infection, and simultaneously age-induced changes (Jassal & Oreopoulos, 2003). Eleven percent of persons in the United States over age 65 have renal disease, not including individuals with diabetes or

hypertension. The most common underlying cause of renal dysfunction in older persons is glomerular disease. Zheng and colleagues (2003) studied aging mice to determine the etiology of age-related renal dysfunction. They concluded that progressive glomerular enlargement and scarring is characterized by phenotypic changes in mesangial (glomerular smooth muscle) cell progenitors and is an entity distinct from all other causes of renal disease (Zheng et al., 2003).

This section discusses some of the most common genitourinary problems of older adults. Each part includes a brief description with prevalence, pathophysiology, clinical presentation, methods of diagnosis and treatment, and prognosis. Of note is that the clinical presentation of renal disease in older persons often is confounded by multisystem disease. The following are some of the common manifestations of renal disease in older persons (Jassal, Fillit, & Oreopoulos, 2003):
- Deterioration in renal function, acute or gradual
- Proteinuria
- Hypertension and renal vascular disease
- Systemic disease with renal involvement
- Urinary tract infection

Acute Renal Failure

Acute renal failure (ARF) is a sudden decrease in GFR caused by disease of the blood vessels, glomeruli, tubules, or interstitial tissue. The resulting decrease in function may or may not be reversible. ARF may be caused by prerenal, intrarenal, or postrenal problems (Guyton & Hall, 2000). Prerenal acute kidney failure occurs secondary to decreased renal blood flow as might occur with dehydration, hypotension, heart failure, sepsis, and severe hemorrhage. Intrarenal failure is the result of abnormalities in the renal blood vessels, glomeruli, or tubules. Such abnormalities may be associated with diabetes mellitus; multiple myeloma; atherosclerosis; and exposure to nephrotoxic agents such as contrast media, nonsteroidal antiinflammatory drugs, and antibiotics (e.g., aminoglycosides, penicillins, and cephalosporins) (Jassal, Fillit, & Oreopoulos, 2003). Postrenal causes of ARF include urinary tract obstruction from tumors, prostatism, calculi, papillary necrosis, and blood clots. Older persons are particularly at risk for ARF because of the combination of age-related renal changes and the increased frequency of common inciting events.

The signs and symptoms seen most frequently are azotemia, oliguria, hypotension or hypertension, hyperkalemia, acidosis, and altered mental status. Nonoliguric failure may occur and is manifested by elevated serum blood urea nitrogen (BUN) and creatinine without oliguria for several days after a brief hypotensive episode or exposure to nephrotoxic agents. Renal function normally improves gradually.

Diagnostic studies include renal function tests. The decrease in urine output expected with ARF is less common in older persons, a factor that may cause ARF to be overlooked. A history of exposure to contrast media or renal insufficiency is important. It is especially important to detect contributing factors such as diabetes mellitus, urinary obstruction, strictures of renal blood vessels, or nephrotoxic exposure.

Reversible causes such as obstruction are addressed promptly, and antibiotics are ordered if infection is present. Treatment options for ARF include intermittent or continuous hemodialysis and peritoneal dialysis with cautious monitoring of fluid balance. A loss of about 0.5 kg of body mass per day is expected because of increased catabolism. During the recovery period, the older person must be protected from nephrotoxic substances and volume depletion. Serum BUN and creatinine are used to monitor renal function (Jassal, Fillit, & Oreopoulos, 2003).

The aged kidney can recover from episodes of transient and reversible ARF. Although age, per se, does not predict the prognosis with ARF, the mortality rate has been reported as 40% to 60%, with the higher rates for persons with hepatic failure, shock, renal parenchymal disease, and renovascular disease. Other factors associated with a high death rate are hypophosphatemia and hypokalemia. Most persons who survive recover complete or adequate renal function; only about 3% require long-term dialysis (Jassal, Fillit, & Oreopoulos, 2003).

Glomerular Diseases

The incidence of glomerular disease in older adults is about equal to that in younger persons. Hallmark features are proteinuria and hematuria, with or without hypertension and renal dysfunction. Some of the systemic diseases associated with glomerular disease are diabetes, myeloma, and systemic lupus erythematosus. Renal biopsy is the gold standard for diagnosis; however, interpretation is complicated by arteriosclerosis and global sclerosis related to aging.

Glomerular diseases can be classified as nephrotic syndromes, proliferative syndromes, and systemic disorders causing glomerular disease. Nephrotic syndrome is characterized by a predominantly proteinuric manifestation, and proliferative syndrome by hematuria and proteinuria, often with cellular casts. It most often is caused by membranous nephropathy, but may also be associated with minimal change disease, amyloidosis, and myeloma. On initial examination, 40% of older persons with membranous nephropathy have hypertension, 30% to 90% have hematuria, and 15% have renal impairment. Corticosteroid therapy alone has produced poor results. The condition is best treated with low-dose chlorambucil over a 3- to 6-month period with or without low-dose corticosteroid therapy. Compared with younger patients, older adults on this therapy have a higher incidence of severe side effects and a longer time to remission (Jassal, Fillit, & Oreopoulos, 2003).

Older individuals with minimal change nephropathy (MCN) initially have a much higher incidence of microscopic hematuria, hypertension, and renal impairment than younger persons. When MCN is caused by nonsteroidal antiinflammatory drugs, discontinuation of those drugs may induce remission. Otherwise, corticosteroid therapy for as long as 16 weeks may be required. If corticosteroids fail, chlorambucil, cyclophosphamide, or cyclosporine A may be needed; however, these drugs pose a risk of bone marrow depression.

Chronic Renal Failure and End-Stage Renal Disease

Chronic renal failure (CRF) is a permanent loss of renal function. The classic picture of CRF may include azotemia, oliguria, hypertension, nausea and vomiting, edema, itching and dry skin, fatigue, malaise, weakness, cognitive and personality changes, and infection. However, older persons with CRF have decompensation of preexisting medical conditions rather than symptoms of uremia. The serum creatinine level does not rise in proportion to the loss of renal function.

The cause of CRF in the older person most often is nephrosclerosis, diabetes, or renal disease of unknown etiology. Although tubulointerstitial disease, glomerulonephritis, and polycystic kidney disease can culminate in CRF, they more often are factors among younger persons than older ones. Determining the etiology is important so that any reversible contributors can be treated. For example, obstruction should be relieved and infection treated.

Predialysis Management. Early referral to a nephrologist is strongly advised so that measures can be implemented to slow the rate of renal deterioration, control uremic complications, prepare the older person and family for dialysis, and commence dialysis at the most appropriate time. The rate of deterioration can be slowed by maintaining strict control of blood pressure, preventing hyperglycemia, and moderately restricting dietary protein. Creatinine clearance must be monitored because of the poor correlation between serum creatinine and GFR. Fluid balance also requires careful monitoring to prevent dehydration or fluid volume overload. High-dose loop diuretics usually are effective in managing fluid overload. Constipation, which may be severe, can contribute to hyperkalemia because persons in CRF lose more potassium through the gastrointestinal system (Jassal, Fillit, & Oreopoulos, 2003). Nutrition is another problem for the older person with chronic renal failure. Severe restriction of protein and sodium usually is not necessary for older persons in the predialysis stage. Protein restriction of less than 0.86 g/kg of body weight in older persons is controversial because of increased risk for malnutrition. As the serum phosphate level rises, serum calcium falls, placing the person at risk for renal osteodystrophy. Calcium carbonate, given with meals, helps restore balance by reducing phosphate absorption. Persistent hypocalcemia is treated with vitamin D or one of its active metabolites. Potassium restriction is implemented if indicated by serum levels. The tendency toward dry skin makes the older person particularly prone to pruritus. Skin moisteners and ultraviolet light may relieve symptoms. Antihistamines are not recommended because of limited efficacy and adverse neurological effects (Jassal, Fillit, & Oreopoulos, 2003). In older persons with known renal impairment, angiotensin-converting enzyme (ACE) inhibitors, angiotensin receptor blockers, and protein restriction may decrease angiotensin II and reduce glomerular capillary pressure (Jassal & Oreopoulos, 2003).

Prevention and treatment of anemia can greatly improve activity tolerance, quality of life, sleep quality, and even cognition, in addition to reducing the risk of heart failure. Human recombinant erythropoietin is recommended for symptoms of anemia in persons with a GFR less than 15 mL/min. Transferrin saturation and ferritin should be assessed to detect iron deficiency because red blood cell indices are not reliable indicators. If needed, oral or parenteral iron supplements are ordered. Individuals who do not respond to erythropoietin may require blood transfusions. To reduce the risk of acute pulmonary edema, packed red cells are preferred over whole blood. The target for hemoglobin is 11 to 12 g/dL.

Chronic Dialysis Therapy. The use of renal replacement therapy in older persons is becoming increasingly common. Options include hemodialysis at home or in a special outpatient setting and peritoneal dialysis, which can be done on a continuous or an intermittent basis (Table 16-1). The mortality rate in the first 90 days of dialysis is 11% for persons age 65 to 69 years and rises progressively to 26% for persons age 85 years and older. Excluding these early deaths, the survival rate is 70% to 75% at 1 year and 20% to 25% at 5 years. The best survival predictors are low comorbidity, good nutritional state, and high functional state before dialysis. Predictors of poor outcomes include diabetes, cardiac disease, and underdialysis. Research has not shown clearly a consistent advantage of one type of dialysis over the other.

Wound healing in older persons is poor after vascular access surgery. Therefore access surgery should be done as early as possible so the fistula or graft will have time to heal and mature. Establishing access commonly is advised when the GFR reaches less than 25 mL/min. In older persons, it also is recommended if the plasma creatinine concentration exceeds 354 μmol/L or if function is deteriorating rapidly. Potential problems related to vascular access include high-output cardiac failure and, in persons with severe peripheral vascular disease, steal syndrome.

Complications of hemodialysis that are of special concern with older persons are hypotension, hypoxemia, and cardiac dysrhythmias. Measures to reduce the risk of hypotension during dialysis are avoidance of rapid ultrafiltration, avoidance of antihypertensive drugs before dialysis, and not eating immediately before

Table 16-1 *Hemodialysis versus Peritoneal Dialysis*

Type of Dialysis	Advantages	Disadvantages
Hemodialysis In-center hemodialysis (ICD) Home hemodialysis	May have slight survival advantage for older persons. May have better outcomes for older women with diabetes. Better cardiovascular stability, reduced dialysis-induced dysrhythmias, easier control of hypertension, and preservation of residual renal function.	Requires venous access, which is sometimes more difficult to establish and maintain in older persons. Arteriovenous fistula survival rates are commonly less than 1 year. More than half of prosthetic grafts survive over 2 years.
Peritoneal dialysis Continuous ambulatory peritoneal dialysis (CAPD) Intermittent peritoneal dialysis (IPD) Continuous cycling peritoneal dialysis (CCPD)	Avoids vascular access difficulties.	Requires good family support to assist with exchanges. Abdominal wall herniation and catheter leaks are more common related to poor tissue turgor and wound healing. Greater protein loss may contribute to malnutrition, reduced immune function, and abnormal bone mineralization. CCPD: more flexibility; performed at night

or during dialysis. Hypoxemia is not common, but can be avoided by the use of biocompatible membranes and bicarbonate-buffered dialysate. Excessive protein loss is a concern with peritoneal dialysis that contributes to malnutrition, hypoalbuminemia, and hyperlipidemia. The recommended nutritional intake for energy expenditure is greater than 35 kcal/kg/day and 1 to 1.2 g/kg/day for protein. Fluids traditionally have been restricted to limit weight gain between dialysis treatments to 5%; however, recent research has reported improved nutritional state with additional weight gain. Because water-soluble vitamins are lost during dialysis, supplements are needed. Various interventions to improve nutrition during dialysis are under investigation, including the use of human growth hormone, parenteral nutrition, and anabolic steroids. For older adults beginning renal replacement therapy, functional independence is a strong predictor of both mortality and morbidity. The prevalence of disability in terms of activities of daily living increases with age among persons with end-stage renal disease. A comparison of older and younger persons on dialysis has shown that older persons have a more positive outlook and life satisfaction despite having more disability. However, when objective measures of quality of life are used, life satisfaction scores are lower among older persons.

Complications of dialysis, including gastric bleeding, hyperparathyroidism, rapidly progressing cardiac disease, left ventricular hypertrophy, and falls, occur in all age-groups, but may be especially threatening in older persons. The use of heparin during hemodialysis increases the risk of subdural hematoma with falls and injuries.

Transplantation. Generally, kidney transplantation is safe for older persons and enhances life expectancy (Baid-Agrawal, Reinke, Schindler, Tullius, & Frei, 2004). Two issues arise in relation to organ transplantation and older persons. First, the scarcity of kidneys available for transplantation has presented an ethical question: should age be a criterion in deciding who should receive donated organs? Second, is the older person equally likely to benefit from transplantation? Older kidneys accepted for transplantation must meet the same criteria as those obtained from younger donors. Graft survival and function of kidneys obtained from donors ages 65 and older have been found to be the same as for kidneys obtained from donors ages 55 to 64 (Jassal, Fillit, & Oreopoulos, 2003).

At one time, transplantation was not considered an option for individuals over age 55. Since the advent of cyclosporine, the procedure has become more common for older persons. The risk of death after transplantation is higher among older persons, usually as the result of infection or cardiac disease. However, the acute rejection rate is lower, probably because of declining immunocompetence in the older person. Because the older individual is more sensitive to immunosuppressants, some sources recommend lower drug dosages (Jassal, Fillit, & Oreopoulos, 2003). Others question whether this is indeed the best course, citing accelerated chronic graft deterioration associated with recipient age-dependent immune responses (Pascher, Pratschke, Neuhaus, & Tullius, 2004). Compared with older individuals treated with dialysis, older persons treated with transplantation generally have lower mortality rates. A major benefit in terms of quality of life is the freedom afforded by transplantation (Jassal, Fillit, & Oreopoulos, 2003). One complication is erectile dysfunction which is common after renal transplantation (El-Bahnasawy et al., 2004).

Bertoni and colleagues (2004) compared outcomes in 101 persons over age 55 who received single kidneys from donors over age 50 with 263 younger persons who received kidneys from younger donors. No significant differences were found for delayed graft function or acute rejections. For the older recipients, the 5-year recipient survival rate and the 5-year graft survival rate were lower. However, when adjustments were made for death with a functioning kidney, the difference among age-groups was not significant. The investigators concluded that excellent outcomes (higher than 80%) were possible for old persons using single cadaveric kidneys (Bertoni et al., 2004). Although some evidence suggests that allograft survival is improved by matching older kidneys with older recipients, not all studies support this conclusion (Baid-Agrawal et al., 2004).

A study of compliance with diet, medications, and routine physician visits among renal transplant recipients found that compliance was related to smoking and alcohol intake, but not to age. Also, interestingly, compliance was not related to mortality rate (Yavuz et al., 2004).

Lower Urinary Tract Symptoms

The term *lower urinary tract symptoms* (LUTS) is used to describe problems with storage or voiding and postmicturition symptoms. They commonly are encountered in many older men, but may occur in women as well (Andersson, 2003). These problems include urinary frequency, urgency, nocturia, and slow stream. Although these symptoms have been attributed to prostatic enlargement, about one third of men continue to have the symptoms after obstruction is relieved. Detrusor overactivity or excessive urine output can contribute to symptoms whether obstruction is present or not. Muscarinic receptors and central nervous system changes are hypothesized to play a role in LUTS. It is likely that multiple, overlapping factors are involved, which explains why some individuals respond to certain treatments while others do not (Andersson, 2003). Other contributing factors may be constipation and alterations in mobility or fluid balance. Pharmacological options for LUTS include antispasmodics, alpha antagonists, and 5-alpha reductase inhibitors (Hsieh, Taylor, & Albertsen, 2003). Whereas obstructive symptoms in men most commonly are associated with benign prostatic disease, in women they usually are related to prior antiincontinence surgery or to pelvic organ prolapse (Ellerkmann & McBride, 2003).

Benign Prostatic Hyperplasia

Benign prostatic hyperplasia (BPH) occurs in more than half of men over age 60 years and in nearly 90% of 85-year-old men. It is characterized by increased prostate size and increased prostate smooth muscle tone that is governed by alpha1-adrenergic receptors (Schwinn, Price, & Narayan, 2004). When BPH causes partial outlet obstruction, bladder dysfunction, notably loss of compliance of bladder smooth muscle, may develop (Levin & Hudson, 2004). A relationship between prostate enlargement and LUTS has been presumed because of improved LUTS following relief of obstruction. The finding that LUTS is equally distributed in males and females has redirected attention to the bladder as the basis for LUTS. It is hypothesized that chronic bladder outflow obstruction causes bladder decompensation with possible permanent bladder damage. Current research is focused on the attenuation of mitochondrial energy production that occurs with outlet obstruction and may underlie the loss of compliance of the bladder smooth muscle (Levin & Hudson, 2004).

Clinical Manifestations. Most often BPH is asymptomatic, although enlargement of the intracapsular tissue may obstruct the bladder outlet. When this occurs, patients may have urinary tract infections, incontinence, difficulty in starting urine flow, retention of urine, dysuria, posturination dribbling, decreased force and size of urine stream, frequency, nocturia, and urgency. These last three symptoms may not be related to the severity of the disease. Over time, obstruction can lead to bladder decompensation, overflow incontinence, hydronephrosis, and renal failure.

Diagnosis. Investigations of symptoms that may be related to prostate enlargement may begin with having the person maintain a chart of voiding frequency and volume. This record may suggest causes of the symptoms that are not related to the prostate. Urine studies should include microscopy and culture. The physical examination should include abdominal palpation for bladder distention and a rectal examination. Diagnostic measures include a plain abdominal radiograph and an independent flow rate test. If the residual urine volume exceeds 300 mL, an upper urinary tract ultrasound is advised to assess the renal anatomy (George, 2003). Blood studies include serum creatinine and prostate-specific antigen (PSA). Several tools are available to assess the presence and severity of symptoms. These provide a baseline against which to evaluate treatment response. Cystoscopic examination is not routine but may be done for further evaluation when surgery is contemplated and to exclude bladder tumors (Partin, 2000).

Management. The management of persons with BPH varies according to the types of dysfunction experienced. Persons with hesitancy, poor stream, frequency, and nocturia, but not incontinence or urgency, may choose to undergo treatment or adapt to their symptoms. Decisions often are based on the extent to which the symptoms pose a problem for the individual on a routine basis. The most common interventions are drug therapy and surgical intervention. Alpha-adrenergic antagonists are useful because they relax the muscle tone of the urinary sphincter and the bladder neck, thereby reducing urethral resistance (Schwinn, Price, & Narayan, 2004). Furthermore, preliminary experimental evidence indicates that alpha1-adrenergic antagonists may actually reduce the damage to the bladder caused by obstruction (Tubaro et al, 2003). Alpha reductase inhibitors improve voiding by decreasing prostate size. Therapeutic effects of alpha antagonists may take a month, whereas it may be as long as 3 months for the reductase inhibitors.

The types of prostatectomy used to treat BPH symptoms are transurethral resection (TUR), suprapubic prostatectomy, retropubic prostatectomy, and perineal prostatectomy. Transurethral prostatectomy (TUR) is the gold standard for treatment of severe obstructive symptoms. Age alone does not contraindicate surgical intervention. Some newer options include prostate incision, laser therapy, thermotherapy, and stent therapy. The effectiveness of these interventions compared with TUR remains to be seen (George, 2003). A review of trials comparing transurethral microwave thermotherapy (TUMT) with TUR in men with BPH concluded that the treatments were equally effective in the short term, but that TUR resulted in greater symptom improvement and fewer needs for subsequent treatment. TUMT was associated with fewer complications, required shorter hospitalization, and could be used on an outpatient basis (Hoffman, MacDonald, Monga, & Wilt, 2004). When the effects of TUR and neodymium laser prostatectomy on sexual function were compared, the only significant difference was a higher incidence of decreased or absent ejaculate after TUR (Tuhkanen, Heino, Aaltoma, & Ala-Opas, 2004). A systematic review of studies of laser prostatectomy reported the pooled percentage improvements in urinary symptoms as 59% to 68% with the laser and 63% to 77% with TUR. Individuals who had the laser procedure were less likely to require transfusions or develop strictures and had shorter hospitalizations. However, they also were more likely to require reoperation. The preferred type of laser could not be determined in this review (Hoffman, MacDonald, Monga, & Wilt, 2005).

Complications of TUR include blood loss (requiring transfusion), catheter clot obstruction, infections, strictures, sexual dysfunction, urinary incontinence, and urinary retention (Hoffman et al., 2004). Furthermore, symptoms are not relieved in about one third of persons treated surgically. Persons with urinary incontinence as a complication of radical prostatectomy or TUR may be managed conservatively with pelvic floor muscle training, biofeedback, electrical stimulation, penile clamps, lifestyle changes, or extracorporeal magnetic innervation. A systematic review of these options found some research support only for early pelvic floor muscle training with biofeedback. Regardless of the intervention, most men's symptoms gradually improve (Hunter, Moore, Cody, & Glazener, 2005).

Underactive detrusor function is best treated pharmacologically, reserving TUR for those who do not respond well or cannot tolerate drug therapy. If there is weakness of the detrusor muscle and a hypotonic bladder, surgery will not improve the urine flow rate. For persons with bladder instability, a trial of drug therapy with an antimuscarinic agent often is recommended. Unfortunately, treatment often is ineffective (George, 2003).

Spigt, van Schayck, van Kerrebroeck, van Mastrigt, and Knottnerus (2004) proposed that male voiding dysfunction commonly attributed to prostate enlargement is actually caused by functional behavior of the bladder. In animal studies, increased urine output stimulated improved bladder function, forming the basis for the authors' hypothesis that increased fluid intake could improve bladder function by increasing urine output (Spigt et al., 2004).

Prostate Cancer

Among men in the United States, cancer of the prostate was predicted to be the most common type of cancer and the second most frequent cause of cancer deaths in 2004 (American Cancer Society, 2005). Epidemiological studies reveal the incidence to be much lower in the Far East, Japan, and China. The difference is attributed to lifestyle because of the increased rate among persons who migrate from low-risk regions (George, 2003). The incidence of prostate cancer increases with age, but tumors appearing in younger men are more lethal. The etiology is not clear. It once was thought that some prostate tumors were inactive or latent, but newer studies indicate that almost all continue to grow, though some may be very slow. Italian investigators found an increased risk of prostate cancer among men

with a family history of prostate cancer, especially those with two or more affected relatives or a brother who was affected. The risk also was increased with a family history of ovarian, bladder, or kidney cancer (Negri et al., 2005).

Localized tumors most often are found in the peripheral zone of the gland, an advantage because they may be detected by palpation. Tumors may be confined to the prostate, invade the capsule, or metastasize to nearby tissues: nodes, liver, lung, and bone. Metastases spread by local growth or by hematogenous or lymphatic routes.

There are no early symptoms of prostate cancer; however, persons with more advanced disease may have obstructive symptoms or hematuria. Elevated PSA screening results or lower urinary tract symptoms may prompt a person to seek medical evaluation. A firm mass or nodule may be found on rectal examination. Suspicious findings on examination warrant biopsy per transurethral ultrasound or TUR. If the PSA level is less than 20 ng/mL, bony metastasis is unlikely and some sources say that a bone scan is unnecessary (George, 2003). Staging is done to guide the selection of appropriate therapy. A variety of staging systems are used. Tests and procedures used to stage the cancer may include chest radiographs, bone scans, excretory urography, computed tomography, magnetic resonance imaging, PSA and prostatic acid phosphatase (PAP) measurements, and transurethral ultrasonography. Pelvic lymph nodes should be examined.

Treatment depends on the stage, the patient's age, and the patient's preference. The four approaches to localized prostate cancer for older men are watchful waiting, conventional radiotherapy, brachytherapy, and radical surgery. Watchful waiting is based on the assumption that tumor growth is slow and that older persons may succumb to something else before prostate cancer advances to become a serious threat. When watchful waiting and radical surgery are not appropriate options, intensity-modulated conformal radiotherapy may be an acceptable method of treatment with minimal toxicity to surrounding structures. Brachytherapy is relatively simple and imposes comparatively minimal disruption of lifestyle; however, the outcome of this therapy compared with other approaches remains under study.

Radical prostatectomy commonly is the first treatment choice for prostate cancer in the United States, especially for younger men. Incontinence and erectile dysfunction are important complications of radical surgery. Age is a consideration in the choice of therapy, with men over age 70 more likely to be offered conservative management. With PSA screenings becoming routine, extensive local disease is more frequently found than in the past. This involves advanced local disease without evidence of bone metastasis. Because radical surgery is not curative at this stage, hormone therapy or orchidectomy may be offered. Some studies have shown improvement when hormone therapy is used in combination with radiotherapy. The nonsteroidal antiandrogen bicalutamide has been found to be equally as effective as castration in persons with locally advanced prostate cancer.

Various new approaches to prostatectomy are reported in the literature. Minimally invasive radical prostatectomy uses laparoscopic techniques and robot-assisted technology, which are not available in all settings. As surgical experience increases, outcomes are improving. Data comparing minimally invasive robotic radical prostatectomy (MIRP) with conventional open prostatectomy in the treatment of cancer still are limited, but seem to demonstrate comparable operative, oncological, and functional results (Trabulsi & Guillonneau, 2005). Advantages to these less invasive approaches appear to be lower operative blood loss, reduced need for transfusions, and less postoperative pain (Humphreys, Gettman, Chow, Zincke, & Blute, 2004). In one study of persons who had laparoscopic prostatectomy, 10% required blood transfusion, one patient had clot retention that required manual bladder irrigation, and 83% were continent after 6 months (Wilson, Kennett, & Gilling, 2004). Although retropubic transvesical prostatectomy reportedly has a low incidence of complications, patients may have bleeding, permanent incontinence, urinary tract infection, and secondary wound healing (Adam et al., 2004). Lepor and Kaci (2004), who assessed the outcomes of radical open prostatectomy in 500 men, determined that LUTS improved significantly (40% decrease in symptom score) and that most men regained continence within 24 months. A study of nearly 3000 men treated for stage T1 or T2 localized prostate cancer found similar relapse-free survival rates with radical prostatectomy, permanent seed implantation, external beam radiotherapy, high-dose external beam radiotherapy (72 Gy or greater), and combination treatment with seeds and external beam radiotherapy. The outcomes for low-dose external beam radiotherapy (less than 72 Gy) were significantly worse than for other treatments (Kupelian et al., 2004). A review of studies comparing radical prostatectomy and brachytherapy for localized prostate cancer concluded that no evidence existed to support one treatment over the other with low-risk and intermediate-risk disease. Neither treatment achieved biochemical control rates above 50% in persons with high-risk disease (Quaranta, Marks, & Anscher, 2004).

Once bone metastases are present, the 5-year survival rate drops to less than 15%. Medical or surgical androgen deprivation typically induces remission that lasts 9 to 12 months. Flutamide and bicalutamide are nonsteroidal antiandrogens that block testosterone action peripherally with fewer side effects than traditional agents used for hormone manipulation. Some controversy exists over the timing of initial therapy if the person has bone metastasis without symptoms. Whereas some sources recommend delaying treatment until symptoms appear, research in the United Kingdom clearly has demonstrated increased morbidity with delayed treatment (George, 2003). The management of bone pain is yet to be mastered.

Erectile dysfunction is a potential complication of radical prostate surgery, external beam radiation therapy, and hormonal therapy. Before nerve-sparing techniques were available, the incidence of erectile dysfunction with radical prostatectomy was very high. New surgical techniques have greatly decreased this complication. In addition, a number of treatment options are available for older patients who experience posttreatment dysfunction. Interventions recommended for erectile rehabilitation during the first few postoperative months include intracavernosal injections or a vacuum device. After the initial recovery period, an oral phosphodiesterase 5 inhibitor may be effective for individuals who are able to achieve a partial erection (Gontero & Kirby, 2004).

A German study compared quality of life following permanent brachytherapy and radical prostatectomy. After 1 year, the percentage of individuals with urinary incontinence was similar for both treatments. Fecal soiling was more common after brachytherapy. Sexual activity was more impaired after nerve-sparing radical prostatectomy than after brachytherapy (Borchers et al., 2004).

Bladder Cancer

Bladder cancer is the fourth most common malignancy in the United States and the fifth most common in Europe. The incidence increases with age and peaks in the fifth to the seventh decade. It is about four times higher in men than women, and higher in whites than African Americans. It tends to recur, requiring repeated cystoscopies and resections (American Cancer Society, 2005; Sengupta, Siddiqui, & Mumtaz, 2004). The great majority of bladder tumors are urothelial (transitional cell carcinoma [TCC]); the others are mesenchymal or epithelial tumors (squamous cell carcinoma, adenocarcinoma, small cell/neuroendocrine carcinoma) of other histological types. Nonepithelial types are sarcoma, lymphoepithelioma-like carcinoma, pheochromocytoma, and melanoma (Manunta, Vincendeau, Kiriakou, Lobel, & Guille, 2005).

Risk Factors. Among the known risk factors for bladder cancer are smoking and industrial exposure to dye, rubber, and leather (American Cancer Society, 2005; Rosenman & Reilly, 2004). In terms of occupation, increased risk also has been identified in male truck drivers, male molding/casting machine operators, female sales workers, and female health service workers (Colt et al., 2004). Additional risk factors identified in a Canadian study were asbestos and mineral, cutting, and lubricating oils (Ugnat, Luo, Semenciw, & Mao, 2004). Radium treatments appear to increase the risk of cancers of several organs, including the kidney and bladder (Ron, 2003). Personal hair dye products and, in women, aspirin use also have been implicated in bladder cancer (Huncharek & Kupelnick, 2005; Ratnasinghe et al., 2004). Although arsenic has been suspected, an analysis of arsenic content in drinking water and data on bladder cancer over 30 years revealed no increase in bladder cancer when the level of arsenic in water ranged from 3 to 60 mcg/L (Lamm et al., 2004). Whether alcohol consumption is a risk factor for bladder cancer is controversial. Data from over 10,000 Framingham Heart Study participants revealed no significant relationship between alcohol consumption and bladder cancer (Djousse et al., 2004).

Diagnosis. Painless gross hematuria is the most common symptom; however, the patient may have signs of bladder irritation or asymptomatic pyuria. Bleeding with clot formation may cause urinary retention. Multiple diagnostic methods are commonly employed because no single procedure, including endoscopy, detects all bladder malignancies (Grossman et al., 2005). The diagnostic potential of various tumor markers for bladder cancer is under study. The role of positron emission tomography (PET) in relation to prostate, bladder, and renal cancer is evolving; it may prove to be most valuable in disease staging and in monitoring response to therapy. At this time, the use of PET for prostate cancer has received more attention than its use for other genitourinary cancers (Schoder & Larson, 2004).

Management. The most common treatment is surgery alone or with other treatments. Intravesical immunotherapy or chemotherapy may be used for superficial, localized cancers. Chemotherapy with or without radiation may be done before cystectomy (American Cancer Society, 2005). Survival varies with the stage of urethral TCC, with the median being 28 months after diagnosis (Clark et al., 2005). Urethral transitional cell carcinoma sometimes occurs after radical cystectomy for TCC.

In an effort to conserve the bladder, transurethral resection may be used in combination with radiotherapy and brachytherapy for solitary bladder tumors 5 cm or less in diameter. The instillation of chemotherapy immediately following transurethral resection of stage Ta T1 bladder cancers has been shown to reduce the risk of recurrence (Sylvester, Oosterlinck, & van der Meijden, 2005). In the Netherlands, this procedure resulted in 5- and 10-year disease-specific survival rates of 73% and 67%, respectively. The investigators noted that 90% of

the long-term survivors had their native bladders (Pos, Horenblas, Dom, Moonen, & Bartelink, 2005). A tumor-free bladder preservation rate of 75% has been reported for another bladder-sparing approach that uses intraarterial cisplatin and abdominal radiotherapy (Eapen, Stewart, Collins, & Peterson, 2004). The new gold standard for definitive surgical therapy for muscle-invasive bladder cancer is the neobladder (Beitz, 2004).

A review of National Cancer Institute cancer registry data on 3311 individuals age 80 years and older with bladder cancer revealed patterns of treatment. Seven percent were treated with watchful waiting, 1% with radiotherapy alone, 12% with full or partial cystectomy, and 79% with transurethral resection. Cystectomy was chosen more often for younger persons than their older counterparts. However, radical or partial cystectomy was related to the greatest reduction in risk for death from bladder cancer in the older group. The investigators concluded that more aggressive therapy for bladder cancer, with good risk evaluation, might improve survival rates among older persons (Hollenbeck et al., 2004).

A meta-analysis of comparative studies on the progression of bladder cancer found no significant difference in persons treated with intravesical bacille Calmette-Guérin (BCG) and those treated with mitomycin C. However, when the subgroup that received BCG maintenance therapy was examined, the results were superior to mitomycin C (Bohle & Bock, 2004).

European Association of Urology guidelines on the diagnosis and treatment of superficial bladder tumors are as follows:

- For low- and intermediate-risk tumors, TUR followed by an immediate chemotherapy instillation is believed to prevent recurrence but not progression. Long-term therapy is not considered useful.
- Tumors at high risk for recurrence should be treated with BCG including maintenance therapy.
- Cystectomy is indicated if the tumor is still present after two cycles of BCG.
- Possible preventive measures include vitamins E and A, *Lactobacillus casei*, and smoking cessation.
- Follow-up cystoscopy should be done at 3 months and repeated as indicated.

Low-risk tumors require follow-up for 5 years; high-risk tumors require lifelong follow-up (Oosterlinck, 2004). A study of survival rates among 1054 persons following radical cystectomy for transitional cell carcinoma of the bladder showed rates by age as follows: less than 60 years of age, 72%; 60 to 69 years, 58%; 70 to 79 years, 54%; and 80 years and older, 33%. (The investigators noted that older persons were more likely to have extravesical TCC and less likely to receive adjuvant chemotherapy than younger persons (Clark et al., 2005). The American Cancer Society (2005) reports the 5-year survival rate by tumor stage: localized (94%), regional (48%), and distant (6%). Clark and colleagues

(2005) compared survival rates following radical cystectomy in relation to age. Pathological features were similar among the age-groups; however, more older persons had advanced disease. Older persons also were less likely to have received adjuvant chemotherapy—26% of those under age 70 compared with 6% of those 80 and older (Clark et al., 2005).

Prevention. Although results of epidemiological studies have been contradictory, some evidence exists that dietary carotenoids reduce the risk of bladder cancer (Schabath et al., 2004). The possible value of nonsteroidal antiinflammatory drugs in the prevention and treatment of genitourinary cancers also is a topic of research (Sabichi & Lippman, 2004).

Urinary Tract Infections

Urinary tract infections (UTIs) can be classified as uncomplicated or complicated. An uncomplicated UTI is one that occurs in persons who are basically healthy and have normal voiding mechanisms. Typically, uncomplicated UTIs occur in women, are caused by *Escherichia coli*, respond well to antibiotics, and seldom cause permanent renal damage. In contrast, complicated UTIs occur with structural or functional abnormalities in the voiding mechanism; resist treatment; pose a risk of severe renal damage, bacteremia, and sepsis; and increase mortality risk (Kunin, 2000).

In most populations, about 80% of all UTIs occur in women, the exception being nursing homes, where the rates are similar for both genders (Griebling, 2005). The incidence of UTI in men dramatically increases with aging. This may be explained by the bladder outlet obstruction associated with BPH. It also may be associated with invasive procedures that often are performed related to LUTS, including cystoscopy, prostate needle biopsy, and transrectal ultrasonography.

UTIs are common health problems in older people. Up to 20% of persons over age 65 have significant bacteriuria. In institutions, the incidence increases to 43% in noncatheterized persons and 50% in those who have intermittent catheterization. Risk factors for UTI in older persons include urinary stasis (decrease in fluid intake, less frequent washout of bladder and urethra), increase in urine pH, institutionalization, concomitant disease, obstruction to the outflow of urine, sexual activity (postmenopausal changes increase the susceptibility of women), immunosuppression, and catheterization or other instrumentation. Causes of obstruction include prostatic hypertrophy and carcinoma, changes in the bladder neck, malformations, nephrolithiasis and ureterolithiasis, and vaginal or uterine prolapse. Neurological causes may be related to stroke, diabetes, Parkinson's disease, motor neuron disease, and spinal injury.

Organisms most often identified in uncomplicated UTIs are *E. coli, Klebsiella, Staphylococcus saprophyticus, Enterococcus,* and *Proteus.* The prognosis for uncomplicated UTI is good, although recurrence is common.

Diagnosis. Diagnostic procedures include microscopic and dipstick methods to assess the presence and number of organisms and leukocytes, leukocyte esterase, and nitrites; culture and sensitivity; and urological and radiological investigations such as renal ultrasonography with bladder studies to assess for structural defects. Ultrasonography has greatly reduced the need for more invasive procedures (Kunin, 2000). Wang, Chang, Yang, Lin, and Huang (2003) recommended ultrasonography only in individuals with a history of urolithiasis or a fever lasting 3 days or more. When UTI is suspected in a person with a catheter, the urine culture results will be more accurate if the sample for culture is collected after changing the catheter (Trautner & Darouiche, 2004).

Management. The goals of treatment for UTIs are to eradicate microorganisms that invade the renal parenchyma and blood and to prevent chronic infection and scarring. Various studies have advised courses of treatment for UTIs ranging from 3 to 14 days (Jassal, Fillit, & Oreopoulos, 2003; Kunin, 2000). Several studies of once-daily dosing have reported outcomes equivalent to multiple daily doses (Talan et al., 2004). Uncomplicated infections can be treated with cotrimoxazole or amoxicillin; a 3-day course of treatment usually is sufficient. Complicated infections require 7 to 10 days or more of treatment (Kunin, 2000; Ooi, Frazee, & Gardner, 2004). The ideal treatment duration has not been determined (Lutters & Vogt, 2005). Long-term therapy for UTIs is recommended only for individuals with distressing symptoms and a high rate of recurrence (Williams & Schaeffer, 2004). As noted earlier, asymptomatic bacteriuria in older persons need not be treated.

Drug therapy for complicated infections should be based on culture and sensitivity testing, and often requires aminoglycosides, beta-lactam/beta-lactamase inhibitors, imipenem, or advanced-generation cephalosporins or fluoroquinolones (Carson & Naber, 2004). The risk of *Pseudomonas* infection is higher with catheter-related infection; therefore treatment requires penicillin with an aminoglycoside, or a quinolone.

Factors that may account for failure of therapy are reinfection with a new pathogen, bacterial resistance, and inadequate duration of therapy. In both the United States and Europe, regional differences in antimicrobial resistance exist (Grabe, 2004; Sannes, Kuskowski, & Johnson, 2004). Drug selection should consider local resistance patterns (Williams & Schaeffer, 2004).

Prevention. Catheter-associated UTI is the result of biofilm formation by uropathogens on the catheter itself. Biofilm is composed of microorganisms, their extracellular products, and host components that adhere to the catheter. At this time no measures to prevent biofilm formation are adequate (Trautner, Hull, & Darouiche, 2005). However, antibiotic therapy may be more effective if the catheter is changed because it removes the biofilm that likely serves as a nidus for reinfection (Trautner & Darouiche, 2004). When indwelling urinary catheters are used for less than 2 weeks, the risk for infection may be decreased by use of silver-impregnated or antibiotic-impregnated catheters. Because UTIs may occur following catheter removal, a short course of antibiotics at the time of removal has been proposed. A survey of British health care providers who managed persons with urinary catheters revealed that 60% favored antibiotics after catheter removal. The specific antibiotic and duration of therapy varied (Wazait, van der Meulen, et al., 2004). However, one clinical trial found no difference in infection rate among persons treated with a 48-hour course of ciprofloxacin and those treated with placebo. All infections that occurred in the ciprofloxacin group were found to be resistant to ciprofloxacin (Wazait, Patel, et al., 2004). If the antibiotics have no real advantage, the cost and risk of resistant strains should be considered. This is a topic that merits further study.

A two-chamber urine collection device has been designed that is intended to reduce the rate of UTI associated with ascending bacteria. In a randomized study of 311 persons comparing a traditional urinary drainage collection device with the two-chamber device, there was no difference in the rate of acquisition of bacteriuria (Leone et al., 2003).

A multicenter study compared nitrofurantoin with placebo to prevent UTIs in persons having surgery for pelvic organ prolapse and/or stress incontinence with suprapubic catheterization. The nitrofurantoin significantly decreased postoperative positive urine cultures and symptomatic UTIs (Rogers et al., 2004). Another study found oral nitrofurantoin superior to estriol-containing vaginal pessaries in postmenopausal women (Raz et al., 2003).

On occasion, infection-suppressive agents such as methenamine mandelate (Mandelamine) are used. Methenamine is a second-line agent that is recommended only for chronic infection. It is not effective in the treatment of upper urinary tract infection or in the prevention of catheter-related infections. Methenamine is contraindicated with sulfonamides because the combination poses a risk for crystalluria (Lehne, 2004). There is evidence that continuous antimicrobial therapy reduces the rate of UTI in women with recurrent UTI (defined as three or more episodes in a 12-month period).

However, many women experience side effects, some severe, of continuous therapy (Schoof & Hill, 2005). Vaginal estrogen has been found to reduce recurrent infections in postmenopausal women. The benefit of estrogen appears to be negated if progesterone is given concurrently (McCully & Jackson, 2004).

A review article in a European journal reported that probiotic lactobacilli, taken orally, were delivered to the vagina and inhibited pathogens including *E. coli*. *Lactobacillus rhamnosus* GR-1 was specifically identified as colonizing and protecting the urogenital tract against infection (Marelli, Papaleo, & Ferrari, 2004). One study recommended the inclusion of *L. acidophilus* CRL 1259 in probiotic products that could be used for vaginal application to prevent UTI (Juarez Tomas, Ocana, Wiese, & Nader-Macias, 2003).

Asymptomatic Bacteriuria. Asymptomatic bacteriuria, defined as 100,000 or more colony-forming units per milliliter of urine on two or more consecutive occasions, is increasingly common with age. In the absence of symptoms such as incontinence or frequency, routine screening for asymptomatic bacteriuria is not justified because treatment provides no improvement in mortality rate and increases the risk of resistant organisms. Exceptions are individuals with a history of symptomatic UTI, structural abnormalities, diabetes, and renal transplantation. Treatment also is indicated for 2 weeks before urological interventions (Jassal, Fillit, & Oreopoulos, 2003; Kunin, 2000). Because antibiotics usually are ineffective with indwelling catheters, they are recommended only if the patient is septic (Kunin, 2000).

Pyelonephritis. Acute pyelonephritis is an infection of the renal parenchyma. Most persons are asymptomatic, but some have fever, vomiting, hematuria, or the classic signs of UTI: frequency, dysuria, and urgency. Foul urine odor may be detected, but this sometimes occurs in the absence of bacteriuria. The picture may not be the same as that seen in a younger person (fever, chills, flank pain). This is a medical emergency because septicemia may develop.

Chronic pyelonephritis is the result of chronic infection that has caused cortical scarring, tubulointerstitial damage, and calyx deformity. It is described as *active* if infection still is present, or *inactive* if infection no longer is present (Kunin, 2000). Pyelonephritis most commonly is the result of ascending infection in which bacteria enter through the urethra and ascend the urinary tract, causing bacteremia. Also, septicemia can cause pyelonephritis. Even after bacteria are no longer detected, endotoxins and immunological mechanisms can induce prolonged damage to the renal interstitium. Because the course of the disease commonly is asymptomatic in older persons, it often goes undetected until an advanced stage of uremia. Studies of autopsy specimens have placed the rate of chronic pyelonephritis at 20% to 28%. In the United States, pyelonephritis accounts for more than 100,000 hospitalizations each year, with *E. coli* as the most common causative organism (Ramakrishnan & Scheid, 2005).

RISK FACTORS. Diabetes and incontinence are two risk factors for pyelonephritis that may be particularly relevant to older persons. Among women of reproductive age, the risk increases with frequency of sexual intercourse, recent UTI, and new sexual partner in the previous year (Scholes et al., 2005).

DIAGNOSIS. Diagnosis may be delayed because of the absence of classic symptoms. A clean-catch urine specimen may reveal bacteriuria and pyuria; however, the significance of bacteriuria in elderly people is in question, as discussed earlier. The combination of the leukocyte esterase test and the nitrite test has good sensitivity and specificity; a diagnosis of UTI is made if either is positive. Despite being highly specific, the nitrite test is sensitive only when the first morning specimen is tested (Kunin, 2000). Ninety percent of persons with pyelonephritis will have a positive urine culture (Ramakrishnan & Scheid, 2005). Shen and Brown (2004) recommend routine renal ultrasound for persons hospitalized for pyelonephritis based on their discovery that abnormalities (e.g., urinary tract obstruction) have been found in 16% of these individuals.

MANAGEMENT. Antibiotic therapy is the mainstay of treatment for pyelonephritis, with a recommended course of 7 to 14 days. An oral fluoroquinolone usually is effective in outpatients with mild uncomplicated pyelonephritis. Other choices are extended-spectrum penicillins, amoxicillin-clavulanate potassium, cephalosporins, and trimethoprim-sulfamethoxazole. Ampicillin and amoxicillin without beta-lactamase inhibitors are not recommended because of the high frequency of resistance to those drugs (Kunin, 2000). Hospitalization is indicated for complicated infections, sepsis, persistent vomiting, failed outpatient treatment, or age extremes. Complicated cases typically require intravenous antibiotic therapy with a fluoroquinolone, an aminoglycoside with or without ampicillin, or a third-generation cephalosporin (Ramakrishnan & Scheid, 2005).

A Canadian study compared treatment outcomes of community-acquired acute pyelonephritis with trimethoprim-sulfamethoxazole or fluoroquinolones. Young women responded better to fluoroquinolones, whereas there were no differences in outcomes in women over age 60. Notably, this study also showed that a treatment duration of less than 10 days increased the risk of treatment failure (Carrie, Metge, Collins, Harding,

& Zhanel, 2004). Regional pathogen susceptibility must be considered when choosing antibiotics. A study of antimicrobial agents and 165 *E. coli* isolates from women with pyelonephritis showed that resistance to ampicillin, trimethoprim, and trimethoprim-sulfamethoxazole was most common in the eastern United States and least common in the western United States (Sannes, Kuskowski, & Johnson, 2004). In an Australian study, 46% of the *E. coli* cultured was resistant to ampicillin, but not to ampicillin-clavulanate (Shen & Brown, 2004).

Follow-up is imperative because treatment failure can occur due to resistant organisms, underlying renal abnormalities, or immunosuppression. A urine culture is recommended 1 to 2 weeks after completing antibiotic therapy. Continued infection warrants blood culture and imaging studies if structural abnormalities are suspected (Ramakrishnan & Scheid, 2005).

Urinary Retention

Urinary retention may be an acute problem that develops rapidly or a more chronic one that develops over time. Acute urinary retention (AUR), characterized by the sudden inability to pass urine accompanied by lower abdominal pain, is a urological emergency. Mechanisms that may be responsible for AUR include increased resistance to urine flow created by mechanical or dynamic means, interrupted sensory or motor innervation of the detrusor, and bladder overdistention. Mechanical obstruction may result from BPH, stricture, or increased muscle tone. Neurological impairment can be caused by diabetic neuropathy, spinal cord lesions, or stroke. Risk factors for overdistention include general anesthesia, large fluid challenge, and drug therapy with opioids and anticholinergics (Table 16-2). Studies of risk factors for AUR in men have found age to be significant, as well as a prostate volume exceeding 30 mL, a single peak flow rate measure of less than 12 mL, and moderate or severe lower urinary tract symptoms (Thomas, Chow, & Kirby, 2004).

During the postoperative period, the risk of retention increases with older age, anorectal procedures, and use of spinal anesthesia (Lau & Lam, 2004). When ultrasound was used to assess bladder contents in persons in the surgical recovery room, 44% had a volume greater than 500 mL. Half of those had no symptoms of bladder distention and were not able to void within 30 minutes. Risk factors for urinary retention in this sample were age over 60 years, spinal anesthesia, and surgical duration greater than 120 minutes (Lamonerie et al., 2004).

Diagnosis. Diagnostic procedures for urinary retention include catheterization, cystoscopy, and excretory urography. The onset, duration, and precipitating factors should be identified.

Table 16-2 *Drugs That May Cause Varying Degrees of Urinary Retention or Obstructive Symptoms*

CENTRAL NERVOUS SYSTEM
Antiepileptic agents
Opioids
Baclofen

BLADDER
Anticholinergic agents
Antihistamines
Antiparkinsonism drugs
  Benztropine
  Biperiden
  Levodopa
  Procyclidine
  Trihexyphenidyl
  Selegiline
Beta-adrenergic agonists (not common)
Calcium antagonists: nifedipine
Diuretics
Ganglionic blocking agents
Skeletal muscle relaxants: diazepam
Prostaglandin inhibitors
Phenothiazine
Tricyclic antidepressants
Other
  Bromocriptine
  Hydralazine
  Isoniazid
  Theophylline

BLADDER OUTLET
Alpha-adrenergic agonists
Beta-adrenergic antagonists
Estrogen combinations
Others
  Levodopa
  Tricyclic antidepressants

Modified from Bissade, N. K., & Finkbeiner, A. E. (1988). Urologic manifestations of drug therapy. *Urology Clinics of North America, 15*, 725.

Management. The immediate goal of treatment is prompt relief of retention and pain. Urethral catheterization is the most common intervention, although suprapubic catheterization is an option. Some studies have reported a significantly lower incidence of UTIs and stricture with the suprapubic route. Lower infection rates also have been reported with clean intermittent self-catheterization. The ideal duration for leaving a catheter in place after an AUR episode has not been determined. Men over age 75 years are less likely than younger men to void successfully during a trial without a catheter (Thomas, Chow, & Kirby, 2004). A comparison of intermittent and 24-hour indwelling catheterization for postoperative AUR found no difference in infection rates

(Lau & Lam, 2004). If retention has been prolonged and azotemia has developed, postobstructive diuresis may occur. The fluid lost should be monitored and replaced. The retained urea, salt, and water are excreted.

Long-term management may employ pharmacological therapy with alpha-adrenergic antagonists and/or 5-alpha reductase inhibitors to prevent AUR when it is caused by prostatic obstruction. Alpha antagonists such as terazosin and alfuzosin decrease resistance to urinary flow by relaxing the smooth muscle in the bladder neck and prostate. In a placebo-controlled study, persons with AUR related to BPH were started on daily alfuzosin or placebo after emergency catheterization. Even among persons over age 65 and those with a drained volume exceeding 1000 mL, those receiving alfuzosin had significantly better rates of successful trials without catheters than those on placebo (McNeill & Hargreave, 2005). 5-Alpha reductase inhibitors, including finasteride and dutasteride, reduce the size of the prostate by inhibiting the conversion of testosterone to dihydrotestosterone. Both of these drugs have demonstrated efficacy in reducing the risk of AUR and the need for prostate surgery (Brown & Nuttall, 2003; Roehrborn et al., 2004). In an Italian study of 4500 men with BPH or LUTS suggesting BPH, individuals treated with 5-alpha reductase inhibitors had a significantly lower incidence of complications and surgical intervention than those treated with alpha antagonists (Boyle et al., 2004). Combination therapy has been the topic of several studies with conflicting results. The development of effective drug therapy has greatly reduced the popularity of surgery, which once was the only option available (Chapple, 2004) (Table 16-3).

Surgical intervention (TUR) including various new technological approaches significantly reduces the risk of AUR. It must be noted that TUR does not prevent AUR in all cases. Preoperative factors that predict failure of surgical intervention include residual volume greater than 1500 mL, lack of detrusor instability, detrusor pressure at maximum fill of less than 9 cm water, and maximal detrusor pressure less than 28 cm water. Urethral stents are relatively new and success rates have been inconsistent (Thomas, Chow, & Kirby, 2004). An evaluation of the Urolume wall stent in 60 men over a 12-year period reported that almost half were removed because of stent malposition or migration, symptom progression, or poor case selection. Nevertheless, the investigators concluded that the device provides a safe alternative to other minimally invasive treatments for men with BPH (Masood, Djaladat, Kouriefs, Keen, & Palmer, 2004). A small study that evaluated the use of prostate stents in persons with severe overactive bladder combined with bladder outlet obstruction found that individuals who had improvement of symptoms and did not leak with the stent were more likely to have a good outcome of TUR (Knutson, 2004).

Table 16-3 *Drugs Used to Treat Urinary Retention*

Action	Classification	Examples
Increase bladder contractility	Cholinergics Prostaglandins (bladder instillation) Alpha-adrenergic antagonists	Bethanecol (Urecholine) Prostaglandin E_2 Phenoxybenzamine (Dibenzyline) Prazosin (Minipres) Terazosin (Hytrin)
Decrease bladder outlet resistance	Alpha-adrenergic antagonists	Phenoxybenzamine (Dibenzyline) Prazosin (Minipres) Terazosin (Hytrin)

For urethral stricture, urethroplasty using one of several procedures may be helpful. A multiinstitutional study of urethroplasty in men older than 65 years found a success rate of 91%, which was lower than younger men but not statistically significant. Few perioperative complications developed (Santucci et al., 2004).

Various strategies have been employed to manage retention in women, which sometimes is caused by anterior vaginal wall prolapse. One study reported a 79% cure rate with surgical intervention for prolapse. A retrospective study of participant data revealed that relief of urinary retention with a pessary during a trial before surgery was a good predictor of a successful surgical outcome (Lazarou, Scotti, Mikhail, Zhou, & Powers, 2004). In women with sphincter overactivity, sacral neuromodulation may restore voiding by increasing detrusor pressure (DasGupta & Fowler, 2004). A urethral prosthesis that uses a magnetic control unit to activate the device and to achieve micturition was rated satisfactory by half of the women with chronic urinary retention who tested it. Reasons for discontinuation included bladder migration, urinary leakage, cystitis, and spontaneous expulsion (Mazouni, Karsenty, Bladou, & Serment, 2004).

The impact of AUR on quality of life has received little attention. Some studies have reported that persons with indwelling catheters had high complication rates and levels of dissatisfaction, whereas others found little disruption of their daily lives (Thomas, Chow, & Kirby, 2004).

Urinary Incontinence

Urinary incontinence is a condition in which involuntary losses of urine occur, causing a social or hygienic problem. The prevalence of urinary incontinence is probably much higher than documented reports because many people fail to report it. The prevalence among nursing home residents is estimated at 50%.

Unquestioning acceptance of incontinence in the aged is inappropriate. It is not an expected, permanent outcome of aging, but age-related factors increase the risk of variables that can lead to incontinence. These factors are weakened pelvic floor, BPH, increased incidence of UTIs, fecal incontinence, and impaired mobility. Many drugs commonly prescribed for older persons affect voiding. Assessment of urinary incontinence should include mobility, cognition, and fluid balance (LaSala & Kuchel, 2003).

One study of lower urinary tract symptoms in women demonstrated a significant correlation between age, parity, and urethral mobility and uroflow rates (Yang & Huang, 2003). In another study, 1253 Chinese women were interviewed using the Bristol Female Urinary Tract Symptoms Questionnaire. The frequency of dysfunctions of storage (frequency, urgency, nocturia, urge incontinence) and voiding (incomplete emptying, discontinuous urine flow, dribbling) increased after menopause and with aging (Chen, Chen, Hu, Lin, & Lin, 2003). Another study compared ultrastructural changes in detrusor biopsies from normal and underactive bladders. Bladder dysfunction was associated with an increased number of disrupted cells in the specimens; however, the number was not correlated with age. The investigators concluded that underactive detrusor activity was not part of the aging process per se (Brierly, Hindley, McLarty, Harding, & Thomas, 2003). Using intraurethral sonography to assess the function of the rhabdosphincter in women with stress incontinence, Klauser and colleagues (2004) found that sphincter muscle thickness and urethral closure pressure decreased with age.

In a survey of women with bladder control disorders, two distinct groups emerged. One group comprised those who thought their symptoms were age related and did not feel embarrassed about discussing it with their physician. The other group did not feel comfortable discussing the problem and were reluctant to seek professional help. The second group especially reported the negative effect of incontinence on their daily life. Both groups wanted their health care providers to initiate discussion on incontinence and to provide information about its management (Newman, 2004a).

Types of Urinary Incontinence. A variety of overlapping categories of incontinence are described in the literature. The International Continence Society defines four types:

- *Stress incontinence:* Involuntary loss of urine that occurs with increased abdominal pressure but in the absence of a detrusor contraction or an overdistended bladder (International Continence Society, 1990)
- *Urge incontinence:* Involuntary loss of urine associated with an abrupt and strong desire to void (Urinary Incontinence Guideline Panel, 1992)
- *Overflow incontinence:* Involuntary loss of urine when the intravesical pressure exceeds the maximum urethral pressure associated with bladder distention but in the absence of detrusor activity (Urinary Incontinence Guideline Panel, 1992)
- *Reflex incontinence:* Involuntary loss of urine caused by abnormal activity in the spinal cord in the absence of sensation usually associated with the desire to micturate

Additional categories of interest to gerontological nurses include the following:

- *Mixed incontinence:* Involuntary loss of urine due to a combination of the aforementioned factors
- *Functional incontinence:* Involuntary loss of urine because of a functional limitation of either neurological, musculoskeletal, or psychiatric origin
- *Total incontinence:* Continuous, unpredictable loss of urine associated with neuropathy, spinal cord disorder, neurological dysfunction, or independent contraction of detrusor reflex caused by surgery (North American Nursing Diagnosis Association [NANDA], 2005)

Categories specified by NANDA International (2005) are functional, reflex, stress, total, and urge urinary incontinence. In addition to the terms just defined, urinary incontinence is often classified as either "transient" or "established." The term *transient incontinence* is generally reserved for incontinence of abrupt onset, generally associated with a specific precipitant, such as delirium, a drug side effect, or presence of infection. Whether transient or established, urinary incontinence should be considered remediable until proved otherwise. Causes of transient incontinence include infection, atrophic vaginitis and urethritis, fecal impaction, immobility, drug therapy, hyperglycemia, delirium, and depression (Tables 16-4 and 16-5).

Established incontinence is basically due to one of two problems: failure to empty the bladder or failure to store urine. The bladder may not empty owing to decreased bladder contractility (as with diabetic neuropathy) or increased bladder outlet resistance (as in prostate hypertrophy). Failure to empty leads to urinary retention and overflow. Failure to store urine, as in stress incontinence and detrusor instability, can be attributed to increased bladder pressure, decreased bladder outlet resistance, or both. The most common cause of urinary incontinence is detrusor instability manifested by abnormal bladder contractions of uncertain etiology. The term *functional incontinence* is used to describe the situation in which the bladder functions normally but the patient voids inappropriately. Factors that contribute to established urinary incontinence in older persons are listed in Table 16-6.

Management of Urinary Incontinence. Identification and treatment of the underlying problem should relieve transient incontinence, but some people have multiple contributing factors, some of which may lead to established incontinence. Treatments for

Table 16-4 *Factors That Contribute to Transient Urinary Incontinence*

Potential Causes	Comment
Delirium (confusional state)	In the delirious patient, incontinence is usually an associated symptom that will abate with proper diagnosis and treatment of the underlying cause of confusion.
Infection (symptomatic urinary tract infection)	Dysuria and urgency from symptomatic infection may defeat the older person's ability to reach the toilet in time. Asymptomatic infection, although more common than symptomatic infection, is rarely a cause of incontinence.
Atrophic urethritis or vaginitis	Atrophic urethritis or vaginitis may cause dysuria, dyspareunia, burning on urination, urgency, agitation (in demented patients), and occasionally incontinence. Both disorders are readily treated by conjugated estrogen administered either orally (0.3-1.25 mg/day) or locally (2 mg or fraction/day).
Pharmaceuticals (e.g., sedatives-hypnotics)	Benzodiazepines, especially long-acting agents such as flurazepam and diazepam, may accumulate in elderly patients and cause confusion and secondary incontinence. Alcohol, frequently used as a sedative, can cloud the sensorium, impair mobility, and induce a diuresis, resulting in incontinence.

Table 16-5 *Drugs That May Cause Urinary Incontinence or Reduce Bladder Storage Function*

Bladder level
  Alpha-adrenergic agonists
    (minimal effect)
  Anticholinesterases
    Distigmine
    Neostigmine
  Beta-adrenergic blocking
    agents
  Direct smooth muscle
    stimulants
    Angiotensin
    Bradykinin
    Ergotamine
    Histamine
    5-Hydroxytryptamine
    Oxytocin
    Prostaglandins
    Vasopressin
  Ganglionic stimulants
    Lobeline
    Nicotine
    Tetramethylammonium
  Opioid antagonists
    (methadone)
  Parasypathomimetics
    Arecholine
    Bethanechol
    Carbachol
    Dehydromuscarone
    Furtrethonium
    Methacholine
    Muscarine
    Mecarone
  Prostaglandins
  Others
    Digitalis
    Furrosemide
    Metoclopramide
    Metronidazole

  Testosterone
  Thioridazine (nocturnal
    enuresis)
  Valproic acid

Bladder outlet level
  Alpha-adrenergic
    blocking agents
    Alpha-methyldopa
    Clonidine
    Guanethidine
    Phenoxybenzamine
    Phentolamine
    Prazosin
    Reserpine
  Beta-adrenergic agonists
    Isoproterenol
    Terbutaline
  Smooth-muscle relaxants
    Chlordiazepoxide
    Diazepam
    Methocarbamol
    Orphenadrine
  Striated-muscle relaxants
    Baclofen (Lioresal)
    Dantrolene
    Hydramitrazine
      (Lisidonil)
  Others
    Bromocriptine
    Bupivacaine
    Demecarium
    Isoflurophate
    Ketanserin
    Levodopa
    Lithium
    Pheothiazines
    Phenytoin
    Progesterone

From Bissada, N. K., & Finkbeiner, A. E. (1988). Urologic manifestations of drug therapy. *Urologic Clinics of North American, 15*, 725.

established incontinence may include drug therapy, surgery, catheterization, and behavioral therapy (LaSala & Kuchel, 2003; Madigan & Neff, 2003).

DRUG THERAPY. A review of drugs used to treat urge incontinence concluded that only the anticholinergics oxybutynin and tolterodine have adequate efficacy and tolerability data to support their use. Transdermal and controlled-release oral preparations may promote better adherence than other forms because they require less frequent administration and are more tolerable

(Guay, 2003). However, a placebo-controlled study of low-dose intravaginal estriol demonstrated improvement in urogenital symptoms, including incontinence, in 68% of postmenopausal women (Dessole et al., 2004). A review of 15 trials comparing estrogen with placebo concluded that about 50% of women taking estrogen claimed cure or improvement, with the most impressive results for those with urge incontinence. The results of one large study showed better response to placebo than to combination estrogen/progesterone therapy (Moehrer, Hextall, & Jackson, 2005). When randomized trials comparing adrenergic agonists and placebo were reviewed, the authors concluded that weak evidence existed that the adrenergic agonists were better than placebo (Alhasso, Glazener, Pickard, & N'Dow, 2005).

Stress incontinence may respond to a dual serotonin and norepinephrine reuptake inhibitor such as duloxetine. Duloxetine may be even more effective when combined with pelvic floor muscle training (McCormack & Keating, 2004). In women with urge-predominant mixed urinary incontinence, extended-release tolterodine has proved to be effective (Khullar et al., 2004).

SURGICAL INTERVENTION. Several surgical approaches to urinary incontinence are in use. A Cochrane Review of surgical approaches to management of pelvic organ prolapse in women concluded that the rate of recurrent prolapse was lower with abdominal sacrocolpopexy than with vaginal sacrospinous colpopexy. The review also noted that a polyglactin mesh overlay could reduce the risk of recurrent cystocele with anterior vaginal wall repair (Maher, Baessler, Glazener, Adams, & Hagen, 2005). A review that looked specifically at open retropubic colposuspension reported this procedure to be the most effective treatment for stress incontinence based on the available data. Following this procedure, 85% to 90% of individuals treated were continent; 5 years later, 70% remained continent. The reviewers concede that new, less invasive procedures may prove to be equally effective, but their effectiveness is not yet known (Lapitan, Cody, & Grant, 2005; Moehrer, Ellis, Carey, & Wilson, 2005). A retrospective study of women who had undergone colposuspension found that 69% were objectively cured and 48% were subjectively cured of stress incontinence. Among those who were cured, there was an increase in opening detrusor pressure. Younger women had a higher cure rate than older women (Dolan, Smith, & Hosker, 2004).

Suburethral slings use a variety of materials to treat stress or mixed incontinence; comparative data are lacking at this time (Bezerra, Bruschini, & Cody, 2005). A review of trials in which bladder neck needle suspension was used for stress incontinence showed that needle suspension had a higher failure rate (29%) than open abdominal retropubic suspension (16%). The failure rates

Table 16-6 *Factors That Contribute to Established Urinary Incontinence in Older Persons*

	Impact on Continence
CNS disturbance—e.g., delirium, dementia, CVA	Difficulty finding the toilet Inability to inhibit detrusor action Inability to sense urge to void Apraxia, resulting in difficulty with transfer, dressing, and hygiene tasks associated with toileting Loss of social inhibitions that make toileting important
Depression	Loss of self-esteem, combined with fatigue, makes maintaining continence too costly
Drugs	CNS depressants may interfere with ability to sense the urge to void or to act on the sensation Anticholinergic drugs may induce urinary retention, resulting in overflow incontinence

Psychological impairments
  Learned helplessness
  Inappropriate
    expression of anger
  Attention-getting device
	Reduced motivation to use toilet to urinate

Vision impairment	Difficulty finding the toilet
Fluid	Dehydration predisposes to fecal impaction and urinary tract infection: both contribute to incontinence by obstructing bladder outlet and serving as irritants to detrusor, respectively
Hormones: Estrogen	Influences function of external urinary sphincter in women
Kidneys	Diuretics stimulate increased production of urine, which may overwhelm patient's usual routines for maintaining continence
Bladder	Hyperreflexia produces urge incontinence—hyperreflexia, or detrusor instability, is precipitated by foreign bodies in bladder, such as catheter balloons, stones, and tumors
Nerves	Loss of bladder innervation because of spinal cord lesions, autonomic neuropathies, or demyelinating neurological disorders results in inability to sense urge to void or inability to adequately contract detrusor, resulting in overflow incontinence
Musculoskeletal system	Pain or limited mobility may limit patient's ability to get to the toilet in a timely manner or to perform associated dressing and hygiene tasks
Sphincters	Weak sphincter muscles result in reduced ability to resist detrusor hyperreflexia or dribbling from distended bladder

From Snow, T., & McConnell, E. (1985). *Bowel and bladder management training program.* Unpublished educational aid.

for needle suspension and anterior vaginal repair were similar (Glazener & Cooper, 2005).

The periurethral injection of bulking agents may be used to treat stress urinary incontinence in women. Available data suggest that the procedure has resulted in improved symptoms on a short-term basis when manufactured bulking agents were used. The effects do not appear to be superior to those obtained with surgery. Long-term effects are not known at this time (Pickard et al., 2005).

MECHANICAL AND ELECTRICAL DEVICES. Although mechanical devices such as pessaries have been used for pelvic organ prolapse, no randomized trials

have been reported that compare them with other treatments (Adams, Thomson, Maher, & Hagen, 2005). A decision to recommend a pessary must consider the ability of the individual to provide proper care.

Electrical stimulation of the pelvic viscera, muscles, or nerves has also been used with varying degrees of success in different types of urinary incontinence. Stimulation of afferent nerve fibers is thought to facilitate storage of urine, and stimulation of efferent fibers is believed to facilitate emptying. Electrical stimulation has been associated with pain and discomfort. Evaluation of it is made difficult by the variability in protocols, including differences in type and placement of electrodes and differences in methods of delivering the electricity.

CATHETERIZATION. Individuals with overflow incontinence for whom medical therapies and surgical intervention are not possible must receive some form of regular bladder drainage, either in the form of intermittent or indwelling catheterization. Clean intermittent catheterization (CIC) is the preferred treatment for those with overflow incontinence caused by inoperable obstruction, underactive detrusors, or detrusor hyperreflexia with sphincter dyssynergia. Complications of CIC include urethritis, UTI, difficulty with inserting the catheter, urethral stricture, epididymitis, and bladder stones. Nevertheless, the incidence of complications with CIC is generally lower than that of indwelling catheterization.

The use of an indwelling catheter may be considered when treatment of reversible contributing factors and noninvasive approaches have failed, and when skin integrity is compromised. However, long-term catheterization may cause more problems than it solves. Complications commonly associated with long-term urinary catheters include bacteriuria, encrustation, and blockage. As previously noted, the risk for bacteriuria increases with age and female gender; however, bacteremia and renal disease occur less often in older persons. The best indicator of urinary tract infection is the presence of white blood cells in the urine. Nursing interventions are detailed later in this chapter.

Overactive Bladder

Overactive bladder (OAB) is characterized by a sudden intense desire to pass urine that is difficult to defer. Related manifestations may include urge incontinence, nocturia, and frequent micturition. Incontinence with OAB is more common in women than in men (Newman, 2004b).

Normal bladder contractions result from the activation of muscarinic receptors by acetylcholine. The symptoms of OAB may be related to decreased cholinergic neurotransmission, increased purinergic neurotransmission, and increased ATP. These findings may explain the effectiveness of antimuscarinic agents in the treatment of OAB (Yoshida, Miyamae, Iwashita, Otani, & Inadome, 2004). At the usual dosage, however, antimuscarinics act mainly by reducing bladder tone during the bladder storage phase; they have little effect on voiding contractions. Stretching the bladder muscle increases acetylcholine release thereby contributing to detrusor overactivity and OAB (Andersson & Yoshida, 2003). Anticholinergics have demonstrated effectiveness in the management of OAB (Hay-Smith, Herbison, Ellis, & Moore, 2005). Oxybutynin and tolterodine are anticholinergics commonly used for OAB. Although they are effective, their nonselectivity causes common adverse effects, including dry mouth and constipation. Extended-release formulations of these drugs generally have fewer side effects and were deemed cost effective in a British study (Hughes & Dubois, 2004). Likewise, the transdermal route provides good symptom control with fewer systemic side effects (Abramov & Sand, 2004). Small studies of intravesical oxybutynin have demonstrated good symptom response, but this route requires additional evaluation (Abramov & Sand, 2004; Saito et al., 2004). Selective M3 muscarinic receptor antagonists (e.g., darifenacin, solifenacin) have demonstrated usefulness in the management of OAB with fewer incontinent episodes; improved voiding frequency, bladder capacity, frequency of urgency, and severity of urgency; and improved quality of life (Kelleher, Cardozo, Chapple, Haab, & Ridder, 2005; Steers, Corcos, Foote, & Kralidis, 2005). Several studies of selective muscarinic antagonists have reported no adverse effects on cognitive function in healthy older persons (Croom & Keating, 2004). Tropsium chloride, a newly approved antimuscarinic drug in the United States, is another option for OAB, as well as reflex neurogenic bladder, postoperative bladder irritation, and radiation-induced cystitis (Rovner, 2004). Urologists generally are reluctant to prescribe anticholinergics in persons with glaucoma; however, Kato and colleagues contend that these drugs can be safely used in individuals with open-angle glaucoma or angle-closure glaucoma that has been treated by laser iridotomy (Kato, Yoshida, Suzuki, Murase, & Gotoh, 2005).

Lee, Kim, and colleagues (2004) studied the use of doxazosin alone and in combination with tolterodine in men with symptomatic bladder outlet obstruction. Whereas doxazosin improved symptoms in about 75% of men with bladder outlet obstruction alone, only a third of those with bladder outlet obstruction and OAB benefited (Lee, Kim, et al., 2004).

Some studies report effective use of botulinum toxin for idiopathic and neurogenic detrusor overactivity, urinary retention, and prostatic conditions (Rackley & Abdelmalak, 2004). Behavioral treatments, including Kegel exercises, bladder stretching, and fluid regulation, may be useful independently or in combination with drug therapy (Herschorn, Becker, Miller, Thompson, & Forte, 2004).

Sexual Dysfunction

Pathological conditions that are common with advancing age often contribute to sexual dysfunction. Disorders such as stroke or arthritis may make intercourse difficult or painful. The person with chronic pulmonary disease may be affected by dyspnea and activity intolerance. Diabetic neuropathy, chronic renal disease, Parkinson's disease, and atherosclerosis can cause erectile dysfunction. Individuals who have cardiac disease may avoid sexual activity out of fear. Drugs that can affect sexual desire and function adversely include many antihypertensive agents, antidepressants, psychotropics, antipsychotics, antianxiety agents, diuretics, alcohol, and tobacco. In addition to the many physical causes, sexual dysfunction can have a psychological origin such as performance anxiety, stress, and depression. After loss of a partner, some people experience guilt, grief, and depression that interfere with engaging new sexual partners (Butler & Lewis, 2003).

Treatment varies with the cause. When possible, underlying physical problems should be treated or corrected. Drug therapy can be changed to an agent with less negative impact on function. For example, ACE inhibitors seem to have fewer sexual side effects than many other types of antihypertensives. When the cause is psychological, psychotherapy, marital counseling, group therapy, or sex therapy may be helpful.

Options for the treatment of persistent erectile dysfunction include drug therapy, penile implants, and vacuum devices. Surgical intervention to improve blood flow to the penis is experimental. The advent of sildenafil marked a turning point in the public recognition of erectile dysfunction, and made seeking treatment acceptable. Sildenafil is an oral drug that dilates penile blood vessels sufficient to produce an erection within an hour, but only when a man is stimulated. Because of its vasodilating effect, it is contraindicated in persons taking nitrates for angina. The combination could cause serious hypotension. Another type of drug therapy is the intracavernosal injection of vasoactive agents. The patient is taught self-injection. The effects should occur within 10 minutes and persist for about 30 minutes. A potential adverse effect of these drugs, including sildenafil, is *priapism*, which is defined as tumescence of more than 4 hours' duration that can damage the penis. Another option is alprostadil, which is administered transurethrally (Butler & Lewis, 2003).

Penile implants are either inflatable or noninflatable. The inflatable devices have a pump that is placed in the penis or the scrotum. A reservoir that is implanted in the scrotum is compressed to fill the cylinder, resulting in an erection. Noninflatable implants are semirigid or positionable rods. Implant complications are infection, penile fibrosis, and mechanical failure of the pump (Butler & Lewis, 2003).

Vacuum therapy uses a cylinder that is placed over the flaccid penis. Air is extracted from the cylinder, which draws blood into the penis, producing an erection. A wide band then is placed at the base of the penis to maintain the erection when the cylinder is removed. This device is contraindicated in men on anticoagulant therapy and those with low platelet counts (Butler & Lewis, 2003).

Effective treatment of sexual dysfunction may enhance relationships, but that is not always the case. If the sexual partner is not interested in or able to resume sexual intercourse, it may become a source of conflict. It is crucial that the health care provider explore the older

person's views and expectations before initiating therapy for erectile dysfunction.

Vaginitis

Inflammation of the vaginal tissues is associated with the age-related changes known as atrophic or senile vaginitis. Such changes increase the susceptibility to trauma and infection. The vaginal walls are thin and easily traumatized, thus permitting the introduction of microorganisms. Pruritus may lead to areas of excoriation. Coitus or douching may cause injury. All elderly women are at risk unless they are receiving estrogen replacement therapy.

Patients complain of vaginal bleeding, pruritus, and dyspareunia. A vaginal examination will help rule out other problems. Estrogen cream applied nightly for 3 to 4 months is the usual treatment. If there is a concurrent infection, an antibacterial or antifungal cream is used also.

Diabetic Cystopathy

Diabetic cystopathy is a complication of diabetes that is manifested as decreased bladder sensation, increased bladder capacity, and impaired detrusor contractility. Increased postvoid residual poses increased risk for UTI. Although little research exists to guide management of diabetic cystopathy, current approaches emphasize glycemic control, voiding strategies, catheterization (intermittent preferred), and management of nocturnal polyuria. Specific voiding strategies are scheduled toileting, double voiding, and bladder expression if no vesicoureteral reflux. Nocturnal polyuria is managed by taking most fluids during the day and voiding before going to bed. Various drugs are under study for treatment of diabetic cystopathy.

Nocturia

Nocturia is so common among older people that it is not considered a symptom of underlying urinary pathology. Some sources indicate that less than three nighttime voiding episodes requires no intervention or investigation. Among the factors that can cause or contribute to nocturia are nocturnal polyuria, reduced bladder capacity, or a combination of the two. Conditions that can cause nocturnal polyuria are diabetes insipidus, diabetes mellitus, heart failure, and sleep apnea. Nocturnal polyuria syndrome (NPS) is a disturbance of the vasopressin system that causes diuresis to shift from daytime to night. NPS affects about 3% of older persons and affects men and women equally. Treatment includes oral desmopressin at bedtime, limited fluids before bedtime, and taking diuretics in the afternoon rather than in the morning. Nocturia can profoundly influence general health and quality of life. Sleep deterioration can be associated with daytime sleepiness, loss of energy, and falls (Asplund, 2004).

An interesting study compared community-dwelling older persons with and without nocturia. Participants recorded the time and volume of each void, as well as their bedtime and time of awakening. Those with nocturia had a higher nocturnal urine production and lower volume per void compared with individuals who did not have nocturia. The investigators concluded that nocturia resulted from a mismatch between nocturnal urine volume and the largest volume voided rather than abnormal values of either (Rembratt, Norgaard, & Andersson, 2003).

Table 16-7 summarizes the various types of drugs used for urinary symptoms in older adults.

Table 16-7 *Drug Therapy for Urinary Symptoms in Older Persons*

Class	Examples	Action and Use	Comments
Anticholinergics (muscarinic antagonists)	Oxybutynin (Ditropan, Ditropan XL)	Decreases bladder muscle tone by blocking receptors for acetylcholine	Anticholinergic side effects common. Risk of confusion in older persons.
	Tolterodine (Detrol, Detrol LA)	Used for overactive bladder and urge incontinence	Less dry mouth with tolterodine and with extended-release preparations.
			Numerous contraindications.
	Tropsium chloride		M3 selective antagonists do not appear to affect cognition in older persons (Lipton, Kolodner, & Wesnes, 2005).
	M3 selective antagonists: darifenacin, solifenacin, trospium, duloxetine		Symptoms of excessive muscarinic blockade: hallucinations, delirium, hyperthermia, hot dry skin, dry mouth, blurred vision, and respiratory depression (Lehne, 2004).
Anticholinergics (muscarinic agonists)	Bethanechol (Urecholine)	Stimulates contraction of detrusor muscle and relaxation of sphincter Used to treat postoperative nonobstructive urinary retention and neurogenic bladder atony	Contraindicated with obstruction.
Cholinesterase inhibitors	Neostigmine	Indirectly increases acetylcholine by inhibiting enzyme that breaks acetylcholine	
Estrogen replacement therapy	Intravaginal cream Estradiol ring, tablets	Improves urogenital symptoms caused by atrophic vaginitis	Dose is insufficient to treat systemic symptoms of hormone deficiency.
Alpha-adrenergic agonists		Increases bladder sphincter tone	Can raise blood pressure.
Alpha-adrenergic antagonists	Terazosin, prazosin, doxazosin	Decreases tone of sphincter and bladder neck Used to decrease outflow obstruction in men with mild obstruction	Lowers blood pressure.
5-Alpha reductase inhibitors	Finasteride (Proscar)	Improves voiding by decreasing prostate size	Most common side effect (3.7% of subjects) is sexual dysfunction. Usually well tolerated.
Tricyclic antidepressants	Imipramine, doxepine, desipramine, nortriptyline		Not recommended in older adults.

Tests Of Urinary Function

A variety of specialized tests may be used to assess genitourinary disorders or dysfunction, in order to more precisely guide treatment. Laboratory studies include hemoglobin or hematocrit; blood urea nitrogen or serum creatinine, or both; and urinalysis for albumin, glucose, and pH, with microscopic examination and screening for bacteria. Urinalysis is performed to detect the presence of conditions contributing to urinary incontinence, such as hematuria, pyuria, bacteriuria, glycosuria, and proteinuria. Positive findings mandate referral for further evaluation and management of the associated medical conditions. Simply obtaining a clean urine specimen can be a challenge with impaired older adults. Catheterization should be a last resort because of the risk of introducing bacteria into the bladder.

The microscopic examination of urinary sediment in the older person commonly reveals increased leukocytes and epithelial cells. A leukocyte count greater than 10 per milliliter is not necessarily a sign of infection in older individuals. Bacterial screening tests, including dipstick testing for urinary nitrites, leukocyte esterase, and urine microscopy for urinary leukocytes, generally lack sensitivity and specificity. Therefore multiple tests may be done to increase the certainty of the results. The presence of casts, dysmorphic red cells, and high levels of proteinuria and hematuria warrants further study because it may represent glomerular disease or vasculitis. The urine of older adults commonly has increased leukocytes, even without infection, and epithelial cells. Mixed infections sometimes occur in persons with indwelling catheters. However, bacteriological evidence of a mixed infection more often means the specimen has been contaminated (Jassal, Fillit, & Oreopoulos, 2003).

Uroflowmetry measures the urine flow rate and may help in detecting abnormal voiding patterns, although it is not helpful in distinguishing among various types of urinary incontinence in women and cannot differentiate bladder outlet obstruction from detrusor weakness. *Cystometry* allows the testing of detrusor function. Simple cystometry may be performed at the bedside by using a sterile catheter and filling the bladder with sterile saline. Bladder sensation and capacity can be assessed, along with the presence and strength of involuntary detrusor contractions. More sophisticated cystometrograms can be obtained using pressure transducers to allow measurement of intraabdominal pressures and intravesicular pressure, but they must be done in specialized clinics. Cystometry results can be affected by patient cooperation and therefore must be interpreted within the context of the patient's behavior during the test. Both false-positive and false-negative results can occur. Bacteriuria is increasingly common with age. Among women, about 20% of those ages 65 to 70, and 50% of those over age 80, have bacteriuria. For men, the

percentages are 3% and 20%, respectively, for the two age-groups (Malone-Lee, 2003).

The urodynamic study assesses lower urinary tract function. It includes measurement of urine flow rate, postvoid residual, and detrusor pressure, and it allows the examiner to determine the presence of unstable bladder versus detrusor hyperreflexia (Malone-Lee, 2003).

Cystoscopy is used to help identify bladder lesions and foreign bodies, as well as urethral diverticula, fistulas, strictures, and intrinsic urethral sphincter deficiency caused by radiation injury, trauma, or congenital malformations.

The prostate assessment consists of digital rectal examination, measurement of serum markers, and various imaging procedures, including plain abdominal radiographs, intravenous urogram, transrectal ultrasound (TRUS), computed tomography, and magnetic resonance imaging. The digital examination provides information only about the posterior aspect of the peripheral zone of the prostate. TRUS is most informative when cancer is suspected.

The primary serum markers of prostate disease include PSA and acid phosphatase (George, 2003). PSA has largely replaced acid phosphatase. Contrary to popular belief, PSA is not specific to cancer, but reflects prostatic epithelial activity. It may be elevated with cancer, inflammation, or benign hyperplasia. About one third of men with PSA levels of 4 to 10 ng/mL, and two thirds of those with a level over 10 ng/mL, have neoplastic change. Among persons with a PSA greater than 50 ng/mL, most will have skeletal metastases (George, 2003).

NURSING CARE

Control over elimination, like many other self-care tasks, is achieved early in life and is an essential aspect of self-concept as an adult. Difficulties with urination are not typically discussed in ordinary social conversation. The subject is in many ways taboo. Changes in urinary elimination patterns may be worrisome to people of all ages because of the threat of eventual loss of control, resulting in social ostracism. The fearfulness is compounded by the fact that little information is generally available for the lay public about the normal and abnormal changes in patterns of urinary elimination that occur with age, and the meanings of those changes. In addition to social withdrawal and emotional reactions to urinary incontinence, economic costs can also be documented. The annual direct costs of urinary incontinence care in the United States are estimated to exceed $10 billion. Many nursing interventions are available to correct or manage problems associated with urinary elimination.

Renal disease can easily be overlooked in the older person because of comorbidity. Therefore routine assessments should include hemoglobin and hematocrit; BUN or serum creatinine (or both); urine albumin, glucose, and pH; microscopic examination of urinary sediment; and screening for bacteriuria (Jassal, Fillit, & Oreopoulos, 2003). Obtaining a clean urine specimen can be a special challenge in the older person, especially when the individual is cognitively impaired or physically disabled. A clean-catch specimen obtained in the morning is preferred. It may be necessary to obtain a specimen by catheterization; however, this method may introduce bacteria. Bladder puncture and suprapubic aspiration are difficult in the older person and should be reserved as a last resort (Jassal, Fillit, & Oreopoulos, 2003).

Nursing Assessment

Initial assessment for alterations in urinary elimination patterns includes the following:

- History of urinary symptoms: nocturia, dysuria, frequency, urgency, incontinence. Ask specifically about urine leakage or wetting, otherwise this important symptom may be minimized or overlooked.
- Physical examination: observation for smell of urine on clothes, evidence of poor perineal hygiene, ability to urinate on demand, difficulty starting or stopping a stream of urine, palpable or percussable bladder after voiding; rectal examination for size of prostate, presence of fecal impaction; vaginal examination for atrophic vaginitis, cystocele, or rectocele.
- Laboratory: urinalysis is advised if symptoms of urinary tract infection are present (e.g., dysuria, frequency, urgency, incontinence).

This assessment protocol is sufficient to identify alterations and likely causes and provides a base for counseling older patients about age-related changes in their urinary elimination patterns. Patients with urinary retention, prostate abnormalities, or symptoms of urinary tract infection should be referred for medical evaluation and treatment. Individuals who show signs of incontinence require more detailed assessment to determine the type of incontinence and likely contributors. When symptoms of overactive bladder are reported, the assessment should include not only the medical history, physical examination, and urinalysis, but also determination of postvoid residual (Maloney-Monaghan & Cafiero, 2004). The in-depth assessment is described next. Before beginning the evaluation, assessment of mental function and mobility is worthwhile, because these domains of function may influence the individual's ability to cooperate with some aspects of urinary incontinence evaluation and may themselves be contributors to urinary incontinence.

Health History. Individuals seeking care because of genitourinary problems may be experiencing a variety of symptoms such as changes in energy level, urinary function or patterns of urine elimination, urinary retention or incontinence, pain, fluid retention, confusion, and changes in urine characteristics. Ask specifically about frequency, urgency, nocturia, hesitancy or straining, narrowed stream, and loss of urinary control when laughing, coughing, or sneezing. If pain is reported, the location is important because pain associated with urinary tract disorders typically is experienced in the suprapubic region, flank, groin, or lower back. Ask about fluid intake and dietary habits, including intake of dairy products and alcohol.

PAST HEALTH HISTORY. Significant past health problems include hypertension, diabetes mellitus, gout, connective tissue disorders, uterine prolapse, prostatic hyperplasia, and urinary cancer, infection, and calculi. Inquire about surgery or instrumentation of the urinary tract. As always, document all current medications, including regular and as needed, prescription, and over-the-counter drugs. Types of drugs relevant to the genitourinary system include diuretics, antibiotics, corticosteroids, cholinergics and anticholinergics, anticoagulants, antidepressants, and calcium channel blockers. Among the many nephrotoxic drugs are streptomycin, vancomycin, cephalosporins, contrast medium, heavy metals, nonsteroidal antiinflammatory drugs, and large quantities of salicylates (Gray, 2004).

REVIEW OF SYSTEMS. Ask specifically about pain in the flank, back, costovertebral angle, abdomen, pelvis, or scrotum. Describe any symptoms directly related to the urinary pattern: any changes in frequency, amount, timing, sensation, control, and appearance of the urine. For the male patient, inquire about penile pain, sores, or discharge; testicular pain or lumps; and hernia. Document whether testicular self-examination is done and, if so, whether any changes have been detected. For female patients, record menstrual status, including age at menopause, menopausal symptoms, and postmenopausal bleeding. Also inquire about vaginal discharge and pruritus. Note the last gynecological examination and Papanicolaou (Pap) smear results. In relation to sexual function, note whether the person is sexually active and whether sexual function is satisfactory. Note any known exposure to or history of sexually transmitted disease, and "safe sex" practices if not in a monogamous relationship. The review of other systems may yield important data. For example, independent toileting requires mobility, manual skills, normal sensory perception, and cognitive abilities.

Assessment of Incontinence. The purpose of documenting incontinence is to determine the pattern in terms of frequency and amount and to determine the environmental circumstances surrounding episodes of incontinence. Describing incontinence over time requires the use of some form of diary. Checklists such as the one in Figure 16-4 are very helpful. However, the tool must be tailored to the abilities of the individual completing the record. If the older person is too impaired cognitively to keep a diary, enlist the aid of a family member, friend, or caregiver.

Stress incontinence often is characterized by dribbling of urine associated with increases in intraabdominal pressure. Urge and reflex incontinence is suggested by a pattern of periodic "floods" of urine, often en route to the toilet. Overflow incontinence is also characterized by dribbling, but a large postvoid residual is typically found on physical examination, allowing differentiation from stress incontinence. Mixed incontinence is likely to produce a pattern of both dribbling and flooding. No particular pattern is associated with functional incontinence, because the underlying contributors are not urological but cognitive, musculoskeletal, or psychological. However, the record may still provide cues about possible interventions.

INCONTINENCE MONITORING RECORD

INSTRUCTIONS: EACH TIME THE PATIENT IS CHECKED:
1) Mark *one* of the circles in the BLADDER section at the hour closest to the time the patient is checked.
2) Make an X in the BOWEL section if the patient has had an incontinent or normal bowel movement.

● = Incontinent, small amount ∅ = Dry X = Incontinent BOWEL
● = Incontinent, large amount △ = Voided correctly X = Normal BOWEL

PATIENT NAME ______________________ ROOM # ________ DATE ________

	BLADDER			BOWEL			
	INCONTINENT OF URINE	DRY	VOIDED CORRECTLY	INCONTINENT X	NORMAL X	INITIALS	COMMENTS
12 AM	● ●	○	△ cc ____				
1	● ●	○	△ cc ____				
2	● ●	○	△ cc ____				
3	● ●	○	△ cc ____				
4	● ●	○	△ cc ____				
5	● ●	○	△ cc ____				
6	● ●	○	△ cc ____				
7	● ●	○	△ cc ____				
8	● ●	○	△ cc ____				
9	● ●	○	△ cc ____				
10	● ●	○	△ cc ____				
11	● ●	○	△ cc ____				
12 PM	● ●	○	△ cc ____				
1	● ●	○	△ cc ____				
2	● ●	○	△ cc ____				
3	● ●	○	△ cc ____				
4	● ●	○	△ cc ____				
5	● ●	○	△ cc ____				
6	● ●	○	△ cc ____				
7	● ●	○	△ cc ____				
8	● ●	○	△ cc ____				
9	● ●	○	△ cc ____				
10	● ●	○	△ cc ____				
11	● ●	○	△ cc ____				
TOTALS:							

Figure 16-4 Form for monitoring incontinence. (From Greengold, G. A., & Ouslander, J. [1986]. Bladder retraining. *Journal of Gerontological Nursing, 12*[6], 31-35.)

In relation to incontinence, the history should include information about the onset, duration, and characteristics. Based on that information, a medical history should be obtained and reviewed for possible causes of transient incontinence with an emphasis on medications, recent functional and cognitive changes, and other contributing medical problems such as diabetes or cardiac disease. In addition, information about the individual's fluid intake, caffeine use, bowel habits, sexual function, use of pads or briefs, and other attempts to treat the urinary incontinence should be elicited.

FUNCTIONAL ASSESSMENT. Various tools are available to assess the impact of genitourinary symptoms or disorders on daily life, self-concept, and self-esteem. Inquire about the symptom effects on socialization, occupation, and relationships. Because of known risk factors for some genitourinary cancers, occupation and environmental exposure to carcinogens should be noted, as should smoking history.

Ask about usual dietary and fluid intake, including types of fluids, amounts, and intake pattern. Specifically record intake of dairy products and alcohol. Patterns of activity and rest help establish the extent to which symptoms are disruptive. Nocturia is common among older persons, and one to three episodes per night is considered acceptable (Gray, 2004).

Mental status testing includes evaluation of cognitive function, presence of delusions or hallucinations, and affect. The ability to follow simple instructions is basic to participating in any continence treatment plan.

Elements of the assessment of mobility include the ability to transfer out of chairs of various heights, ability to transfer on and off the toilet, ability to dress and undress, and length of time required to travel to the toilet in customary settings. For men who are wheelchair bound, the ability to manipulate buttons, zippers, and underclothes and the ability to place a urinal are important aspects of performance to observe directly. For women, toileting is dependent not only on transferring on and off a toilet, but also on sufficient standing balance to arrange clothing before toileting.

Physical Examination. The physical examination of the older person with genitourinary complaints begins with a general inspection and focuses on the abdomen and the external genitalia. The process is the same as for other adults, but areas of special interest with the older person will be stressed. Assess the weight and vital signs and compare with previous measures.

Inspect and palpate the skin for turgor, color, and scratches that might indicate pruritus. Consider signs of either fluid volume excess or deficit. With renal disease, skin color may be pale or yellow-gray. The oral examination should include assessment for stomatitis and the odor of ammonia on the breath. Inspect and palpate for generalized and dependent edema. Observe the suprapubic area for distention. Palpate for kidney enlargement and bladder distention. Normally the kidneys are not palpable. A full bladder sounds dull when percussed. Percuss for costovertebral angle tenderness, which is indicative of kidney infection or polycystic kidney disease. Blood flow to the kidneys can be assessed by auscultating over both kidneys.

Genital examination in men should focus on identifying abnormalities of the foreskin, penis, scrotum, and perineal skin. The digital rectal examination permits assessment of the size of the prostate and the presence of lumps. Pelvic examination in women may reveal atrophic vaginitis, pelvic prolapse, or mass. Experienced clinicians may be able to assess for urethral and bladder neck hypermobility. Rectal examination is performed to assess for perineal sensation, sphincter tone, and the bulbocavernosus reflex, and to determine whether fecal impaction or rectal mass is present. If vaginal or urethral discharge is present, obtain a specimen for examination.

Other assessments of bladder function are also commonly recommended. Postvoid residual volume may be estimated using palpation and percussion during physical examination; it can be determined more accurately by urinary catheterization or ultrasound. Care must be taken in interpreting the postvoid residual volume, because it may be influenced by situational factors, such as inability of the patient to void on request. Provocative stress testing is also commonly recommended. The patient is asked to cough vigorously while being observed for urine loss. Urine loss that occurs immediately after coughing is considered indicative of stress incontinence. If urine loss is delayed or persists after the cough, urge incontinence is the more likely diagnosis. Box 16-2 summarizes the nursing assessment of the genitourinary system.

Nursing Diagnoses

Numerous nursing diagnoses may apply to persons with genitourinary disorders. Examples include the following:

- Acute pain related to pruritus, vaginitis, urinary tract infection
- Deficient fluid volume related to excessive fluid losses, decreased fluid intake
- Excess fluid volume related to compromised regulatory mechanism, excess sodium intake
- Toileting self-care deficit related to environmental barriers, weakness, impaired mobility status, perceptual or cognitive impairment, neuromuscular impairment
- Sexual dysfunction related to altered body structure or function, lack of significant other
- Ineffective sexuality pattern related to knowledge deficit about alternative responses to health-related

Box 16-2 Genitourinary Assessment

Health History
- **General:** fatigue, confusion
- **Personal or family history** of genitourinary disease
- **Recent surgery or instrumentation**
- **Review of systems:**
- **Chronic illnesses:** Hypertension, diabetes mellitus, cardiac disease
- **Medications:** antidepressants, antipsychotics, diuretics, antibiotics, corticosteroids, cholinergics and anticholinergics, anticoagulants, calcium channel blockers, NSAIDs
- **Symptoms:**
  Urine characteristics: color, amount
  Urination: frequency, urgency, nocturia, dysuria, dribbling, loss of control, inability to empty the bladder, hesitancy, straining
  Bladder: feeling of fullness, distention
  Pain: suprapubic, flank, lower back, groin
  Sexual dysfunction: lack of interest, erectile dysfunction, satisfaction with current function, known exposure to STDs, safe sex practices
  Male genitalia: penile pain, sores, discharge, testicular pain or lumps, hernia, whether testicular self-examination is done
  Female genitalia: menstrual status, menopausal symptoms, postmenopausal bleeding, vaginal discharge, pruritus, last gynecological exam and Pap smear results.
- **Functional assessment:** occupational history, exposure to carcinogens, smoking history, usual fluid intake, dietary patterns, mental status, mobility

Physical Examination
- **Weight and vital signs:** usual, current
- **Skin:** turgor, color, abrasions
- **Oral cavity:** stomatitis, odor
- **Extremities:** edema
- **Thorax and abdomen:** bladder distention, kidney enlargement, CVA tenderness, bruits over kidneys
- **Male genitalia:** abnormalities of foreskin, penis, scrotum, perineal skin, penile discharge, digital examination for palpation of prostate
- **Female genitalia:** atrophic vaginitis, pelvic prolapse, masses, vaginal discharge

transitions, altered body function or structure, illness, or medical treatment
- Ineffective tissue perfusion related to hypervolemia secondary to acute renal failure
- Impaired urinary elimination related to urinary tract infection, anatomical obstruction, sensorimotor impairment, multiple causality
- Urinary retention related to blockage, weak detrusor

Nursing Goals

The goals of nursing care related to alterations in the older adult's genitourinary function include the following: (1) maintenance or restoration of continence, (2) prevention of complications of urinary incontinence, (3) prevention or elimination of urinary tract infection and related complications, (4) relief of urinary retention, (5) maintenance or restoration of satisfying sexual relationships, and (6) maintenance or restoration of normal fluid balance.

Nursing Interventions

Interventions to Reduce or Eliminate Incontinent Episodes. Urinary incontinence has many causes—physiological, psychological, and environmental—and nursing interventions must be geared toward the cause. If problems with toileting occur, determine the factors that interfere with self-care and remove any barriers that exist. These may include clearing pathways, providing assistance in ambulating, providing adequate lighting, allowing privacy, and providing sufficient space in toilet areas. Commodes and urine-containment devices at the bedside also are useful.

Nursing care includes assessment of the patient, which often includes maintenance of voiding records, implementation of prescribed therapy, and evaluation of outcomes. The nurse is the key person in planning and implementing strategies to deal with functional incontinence. Before interventions can be implemented, it may be necessary to convince the patient and family that improvement probably is possible.

The first step in the management of urinary incontinence is to identify factors that may be causing or contributing to it, such as UTI, fecal impaction, atrophic vaginitis, poorly controlled diabetes mellitus, drug therapy, motor disorder, inconvenient toileting facilities, or cognitive impairment. Correction of underlying problems, alterations in drug regimens, or environmental modifications may restore continence. If incontinence remains a problem, the intervention depends on the type of incontinence diagnosed. The interventions suggested for various alterations in urinary elimination are summarized in Table 16-8.

Various behavioral interventions have been developed and evaluated to varying extents. These include prompted voiding, habit training, and scheduled voiding. Prompted voiding commonly is recommended for nursing home patients, including those with substantial cognitive impairments. It requires the staff to attempt to teach the incontinent person to become more aware of the incontinent status and to ask for help from caregivers. The staff asks patients at established intervals if the patients are wet or dry. Patients then are asked to try to use the toilet. Patients are praised for trying to use the

Table 16-8 *Treatment Approaches for Alterations in Urinary Elimination in Older Persons*

Alteration	Approaches
Nocturia	Explain that this pattern is normal in older persons. Explore whether the patient experiences associated difficulties, such as difficulty falling asleep
Dysuria	Evaluate for urinary tract infection and other causes and treat as indicated If no cause is evident or the cause is not remediable, consider pyridium as a urinary tract anesthetic
Urinary frequency	Evaluate for urinary tract infection or atrophic vaginitis in women and obtain treatment as indicated Obtain postvoid residual: if present, evaluate for possible causes of urinary retention and treat. If not treatable, teach patient Credé maneuver or bending over from waist while on toilet to see if more urine can be expelled Obtain record of toileting frequency and amount over 3 days Try a toileting schedule, based on previous records of voiding frequency and amount, setting goal of an increase in intervals by 30 minutes progressively, until q 2-3 hr voiding pattern is reached. Document toileting pattern, including amounts voided at each toileting Teach relaxation exercises as a form of distraction and anxiety alleviation, which may decrease the sense of urgency Teach Kegel exercises to raise patient's confidence in competence of urinary sphincter
Hesitancy	Evaluate for obstructive process: e.g., prostatic hypertrophy, fecal impaction, and treat as indicated Teach deep breathing and relaxation exercises, to assist in relaxation of sphincters during urination
Urinary retention	Obtain postvoid residual Determine cause of retention: anatomical obstruction, side effect of drug therapy, autonomic neuropathy, and treat as indicated
Stress incontinence	Kegel exercises Biofeedback Medications: anticholinergics, estrogen replacement (if atrophic vaginitis diagnosed) Padding Surgery
Overflow incontinence	Toileting schedule Positioning and Credé maneuver Medications: parasympathomimetics, such as bethanechol Catheterization: intermittent, clean self-catheterization; indwelling
Urge incontinence (detrusor instability; reflex bladder)	Toilet schedule Biofeedback Medications: anticholinergics and adrenergic antagonists
Functional incontinence 　Mobility problems	Toilet schedule Bedside commode to reduce distance to toilet Kegel exercises Intervene to optimize mobility
Learned helplessness	Help patient resume control over decisions in life in small ways (e.g., choice of clothing, food), then set expectations that patient control bodily functions and positively reinforce expected outcomes
Inappropriate expression of and anger	Explore anger with patient. Help find more appropriate means of expressing anger
Attention-getting maneuver	Respond to incontinent episodes with as little attention or fuss as possible. Find positive behaviors in patient; pay attention, reward those behaviors

toilet, and for times when monitoring shows them to be dry.

Habit training, or adapting toileting schedules to a patient's natural voiding pattern, has also been shown to be effective. It can be contrasted with a technique called bladder training, in which scheduled voiding, distraction techniques, and positive reinforcement are combined as a therapy for urge or stress incontinence. The general goal is to reduce the number of incontinent episodes and to increase the time between scheduled voids.

When a reversible cause such as UTI is identified, correction may resolve the problem. However, older persons often have multiple predisposing factors, making it difficult to predict the impact of treatment on incontinence. Numerous other approaches to management of incontinence are commonly recommended. Considering the scope of the problem of urinary incontinence and the variety of time-honored interventions, surprisingly limited research evidence exists to guide best practices. The major intervention modalities most commonly employed for urinary incontinence in older persons and conclusions of relevant Cochrane Reviews are summarized in Table 16-9.

Some individuals who have episodes of inappropriate voiding are able to control urination, but they may have motor or sensory deficits, problems with coordination, physical barriers, or cognitive impairment. In that case, interventions are individualized for the situation. When environmental barriers exist, consider a bedside commode, nightlights to the bathroom, or moving the person to a location that is more bathroom accessible. The person with impaired motor function might benefit from a raised toilet seat and simplified clothing. Velcro closures and elastic waistbands can greatly facilitate toileting. For persons with dementia, the management will vary with the stage of the disease. For those with mild to moderate dementia, simple clothing, a convenient bathroom, and periodic reminders may be all that is needed to maintain dryness most of the time. More impaired persons should be taken to the toilet at intervals, and environmental cues should be used (e.g., a picture of a toilet on the bathroom door). As dementia progresses, incontinence becomes more common. When the aforementioned strategies no longer work, incontinence briefs or pads will be needed. As long as good skin integrity can be maintained, indwelling catheters should be avoided.

Interventions to Prevent or Eliminate Urinary Tract Infections.
In persons with indwelling catheters, the most important way to prevent UTI is to encourage removal as soon as possible. One study involved simply providing daily reminders to physicians to remove unnecessary catheters after they had been in place for 5 days. The rate of catheter-associated infection was significantly reduced over a 12-month intervention (Huang et al., 2004).

Intermittent catheterization is a commonly used procedure for community-dwelling persons with urinary retention. In some situations, it is necessary to reuse catheters. Disinfection can be achieved by immersing the catheter in a 70% alcohol solution for a minimum of 5 minutes. The catheter should not be rinsed, but placed in a resealable plastic bag (Bogaert et al., 2004).

To reduce the risk of infection, daily rinsing of the urine collection bag with 1:10 solution of diluted bleach is recommended. Antibiotic ointment applied to the urinary meatus has not been proven effective (Madigan & Neff, 2003). When urinary catheters are used, nurses should pay particular attention to infection control procedures, so that other patients are not infected from the colonized patient. Vigilant handwashing between emptying catheter bags and taping of the catheter to prevent traction are recommended. Table 16-10 lists the various containment options in incontinence, along with the advantages and disadvantages of each type.

Cranberry juice has been touted as a product that might reduce the risk of UTI by acidifying the urine or preventing the adherence of E. coli to uroepithelial cells in the urinary tract. Following a review of controlled trials of cranberry products in the prevention of UTIs, Jepson, Mihaljevic, and Craig (2004) concluded that there was some evidence that products decreased the number of symptomatic UTIs in women. Their review identified no difference in the effects of juice versus capsules; however, another study did not demonstrate the same benefit when cranberry capsules were used. A prospective, double-blinded, placebo-controlled, crossover study comparing cranberry tablets with placebo in persons with neurogenic bladders found no differences in urine pH, bacterial count, urinary white blood cell count, and UTIs (Linsenmeyer et al., 2005). The ideal dosage and dosage form have not been determined.

Because UTIs commonly are caused by fecal bacteria, Finnish investigators sought to determine whether dietary habits were associated with the infections. The data indicated a decreased risk of recurrent UTI in women who frequently consumed fresh fruit juices (especially berry juices) and who consumed fermented milk products three or more times each week (Kontiokari et al., 2003).

Interventions to Relieve Urinary Retention.
The best strategy for removal of a catheter from a person with a short-term indwelling urethral catheter was the subject of a Cochrane Review. Although the data were inconclusive, there was evidence to suggest a benefit to midnight removal of the catheter. In eight randomly controlled trials involving 1020 participants, midnight catheter removal (compared with daytime removal) was associated with larger urine volume at first void, longer

Table 16-9 *Evidence Supporting Common Interventions for Urinary Incontinence*

Intervention	Type of Incontinence	Research Evidence
Individualized toileting schedules, habit training	Functional, possibly urge	Possible short-term benefit of prompted voiding; insufficient evidence to draw conclusions about effectiveness.[3] Lack of quality studies of outcomes of habit training in older persons.[6] Limited evidence that bladder training may improve continence.[9]
Pelvic floor muscle training (PFMT) and biofeedback	Urge, stress	Vaginal cones better than no treatment for stress incontinence; may be similar in effectiveness to PFMT and electrostimulation.[1] Insufficient evidence that PFMT before prostate surgery decreased occurrence of postoperative urinary incontinence.[4] PFMT appears to benefit women with stress or mixed incontinence. Benefits with urge incontinence uncertain. Limited evidence of additive effectiveness of other therapies with PFMT. Most research on premenopausal women.[5] PFMT with biofeedback soon after catheter removal following prostatectomy may promote return to continence.[7]
Drug therapy	Urge, stress, overflow	Estrogen improves or cures stress, urge, and mixed incontinence in approximately half the women treated.[11] Anticholinergics decrease symptoms of overactive bladder syndrome.[12] Limited evidence of adrenergic agonist benefits.[13]
Catheterization	Overflow, other forms if refractory to other treatments, skin integrity is threatened	Insufficient evidence to guide use of indwelling or sheath catheters in adults with neurogenic bladder.[8]
Absorbent products: incontinence garments or underpads		Limited data suggest that disposable products may be more effective and associated with fewer skin problems.[10]
Timed voiding	Functional	Insufficient data to draw conclusions about effectiveness.[2]

[1]Herbison, P., Plevnik, S., & Mantle, J. (2005). Weighted vaginal cones for urinary incontinence. *Cochrane Database of Systematic Reviews, 2.*

[2]Ostaszkiewicz, J., Johnston, L., & Roe, B. (2005). Timed voiding for the management of urinary incontinence in adults. *Cochrane Database of Systematic Reviews, 2.*

[3]Eustice, S., Roe, B., & Paterson, J. (2005). Prompted voiding for the management of urinary incontinence in adults. *Cochrane Database of Systematic Reviews, 2.*

[4]Hay-Smith, J., Herbison, P., & Morkved, S. (2005). Physical therapies for prevention of urinary and faecal incontinence in adults. *Cochrane Database of Systematic Reviews, 2.*

[5]Hay-Smith, E. J. C., Bo, K., Berghmans, L. C. M., Hendriks, H. J. M., de Bie, R. A., & van Waalwijk van Doorn, E. S. C. (2005). Pelvic floor muscle training for urinary incontinence in women. *Cochrane Database of Systematic Reviews, 2.*

[6]Ostaszkiewicz, J., Johnston, L., & Roe, B. (2005). Habit retraining for the management of urinary incontinence in adults. *Cochrane Database of Systematic Reviews, 2.*

[7]Hunter, K. F., Moore, K. N., Cody, D. J., & Glazener, C. M. A. (2005). Conservative management for postprostatectomy urinary incontinence. *Cochrane Database of Systematic Reviews, 2.*

[8]Jamison, J., Maguire, S., & McCann, J. (2005). Catheter policies for management of long term voiding problems in adults with neurogenic bladder disorders. *Cochrane Database of Systematic Reviews, 2.*

[9]Wallace, S. A., Roe, B., Williams, K., & Palmer, M. (2005). Bladder training for urinary incontinence in adults. *Cochrane Database of Systematic Reviews, 2.*

[10]Brazzelli, M., Shirran, E., & Vale, L. (2005). Absorbent products for containing urinary and/or faecal incontinence in adults. *Cochrane Database of Systematic Reviews, 2.*

[11]Moehrer, B., Hextall, A., & Jackson, S. (2005). Oestrogens for urinary incontinence in women. *Cochrane Database of Systematic Reviews, 2.*

[12]Hay-Smith, J., Herbison, P., Ellis, G., & Moore, K. (2005). Anticholinergic drugs versus placebo for overactive bladder syndrome in adults. *Cochrane Database of Systematic Reviews, 2.*

[13]Alhasso, A., Glazener, C. M. A., Pickard, R., & N'Dow, J. (2005). Adrenergic drugs for urinary incontinence in adults. *Cochrane Database of Systematic Reviews, 2.*

Table 16-10 *Advantages and Disadvantages of Various Forms of Management of Urinary Incontinence*

Method of Management	Advantages	Disadvantages
Incontinence pads	Nonintrusive Can be managed easily by patients and caregivers Removable for toileting Not visible under most clothing	Cost ($6-$8/dozen) "Diapers" Odor Medicare does not pay as medical supply
Condom catheters	Nonintrusive Easier to manage than indwelling Leg bags are available Covered as a medical expense	Not available for women Risk of infections Adhesives irritate genitals Need frequent replacements
Intermittent catheterization	Limited intrusion Self-done/private Limited expense Lower infection risk than Foley	Some skill needed to do task Scheduling necessary for effectiveness Not thought of for OLD patients
Indwelling catheterization	Limited leakage No retention Covered as a medical supply Entitles patient to RN home health	Risk of infection greater Less independent mobility Risk of trauma greater Risk of skin breakdown greater Need for more medical supervision greater

Adapted from Giduz, B. H., et al. (1986). *A geriatric first aid kit.* Chapel Hill, NC: University of North Carolina School of Medicine, p. 24.

time until first void, and shorter hospitalization. Advantages of catheter clamping, if any, are unknown (Griffiths & Fernandez, 2005).

Interventions to Maintain or Restore Normal Fluid Balance.

Insufficient fluid intake is a problem for many older people for multiple reasons. Individuals who may be dependent on others to provide adequate fluids include those with poor mobility or dexterity and those with cognitive impairment. Persons with urinary incontinence sometimes severely limit fluid intake in an effort to reduce incontinent events. These problems are compounded by the diminished thirst sensation and decreased ability of the kidneys to respond to fluid volume deficits.

Older persons with renal failure may need assistance to manage their medications. It is especially important to avoid nephrotoxic drugs. Monitor the serum levels of K^+ and Ca^{++} and report abnormalities. Explain the reason for any dietary and fluid restrictions. For persons with cognitive impairment, intake will require supervision by caregivers. Provide emotional support and teaching to enable older patients and their families to adapt to the management of acute and chronic renal failure. These include dialysis, renal transplantation (if an option), self-monitoring skills, and sexual dysfunction related to renal disease.

Interventions to Address Sexual Dysfunction.

Nurses and other health care providers may be uncomfortable with the subject of sexual dysfunction and avoid bringing it up, which is a missed opportunity. One reason for this is the often incorrect assumption that older persons, particularly those without a partner, are unlikely to be interested in sexual activity. Sexual dysfunction can result from age-related changes, psychological factors, pathology affecting the sex organs, or other disorders (e.g., renal failure, diabetes mellitus, arthritis, pulmonary disease, stroke). Older patients and their partners may need information about the normal changes of aging and expected alterations in sexual

---

BOX 16-3 *TOWARD BETTER GENITOURINARY HEALTH*

- Measures to discourage smoking may reduce the risk of bladder and cervical cancer.
- The American Cancer Society recommends a diet with plenty of fruits and vegetables and limited foods that are high in saturated fats.
- Maintaining ideal body weight may reduce the risk of genitourinary cancers.
- All sexually active people, regardless of age, need to understand the risk for sexually transmitted diseases and the use of preventive measures.
- Renal function should be monitored in persons taking nephrotoxic drugs.
- Regular screenings with Pap smears and PSA measurements may detect cancer in an early stage when it is most likely curable.

functioning. Some older patients benefit from referral to a professional counselor.

Various additional interventions to promote genitourinary health are discussed in Box 16-3.

Evaluation

NOC outcomes of nursing management include comfort level, pain control, pain level, electrolyte and acid-base balance, fluid balance, hydration, nutritional status: food and fluid intake, self-care: activities of daily living, self-care: hygiene, self-care: toileting, physical aging status, sexual functioning, circulation status, urinary elimination, urinary continence, and tissue integrity: skin and mucous membranes.

Indicators of goal achievement for individuals with genitourinary disorders include the following:

- The patient reports that pain has been eliminated or is controlled.
- The patient's fluid balance is normal as evidenced by acceptable pulse, blood pressure, and hemodynamic measures; balanced intake and output; stable body weight; normal urine specific gravity; and normal serum electrolytes.

Nursing Care Plan: The Older Adult with Urinary Incontinence

Data

Maria Martinez, age 83, has resided in an assisted living facility for 1 year. She decided to move here after she fell in her yard and could not attract help for 6 hours. She says she manages pretty well despite rheumatoid arthritis that affects her hands and feet. During a recent visit, Mrs. Martinez asks the nurse where she can get some of those waterproof briefs for adults that she has seen advertised on television. She goes on to tell the nurse that sometimes she just cannot get to the toilet quickly enough to avoid leaking urine. This has been a problem for about 6 months. She says, "I guess that just happens when you get old." Mrs. Martinez has been using feminine hygiene pads to stay dry, and says she has some perineal irritation from the damp pads. A urine specimen was obtained; the urinalysis results were normal.

Nursing Diagnoses (NANDA International, 2005)

Knowledge deficit of normal aging and management of functional urinary incontinence

Functional urinary incontinence related to neuromuscular limitations, weakened supporting pelvic structures, altered environmental factors

NOC Suggested Outcomes (Moorhead, Johnson, & Maas, 2004)

Knowledge: Disease Process (1803)
Urinary Continence (0502)
Urinary Elimination (0503)
Self-Care: Toileting (0310).

NIC Suggested Interventions (Dochterman & Bulechek, 2004)

Major interventions: Teaching: Disease Process (5602), Urinary Incontinence Care (0610), Urinary Bladder Training (0570), Environmental Management (6480).

- Identify multifactorial causes of incontinence (impaired mobility and dexterity, environmental barriers).
- Explain etiology of problem and rationale for (suggested) actions.
- Place furniture in room in an appropriate arrangement that best accommodates patient disabilities.
- Assist to select appropriate incontinence garment/pad for short-term management while more definitive treatment is designed.
- Instruct patient to respond immediately to urge to void.
- Ask patient to keep record of urinary output and pattern.
- Assist patient to identify patterns of incontinence.
- Establish interval of initial prompted voiding schedule based on voiding pattern.
- Establish interval for toileting of not less than 1 hour and preferably not less than 2 hours.
- Reduce toileting interval by one-half hour if there are more than three incontinence episodes in 24 hours.
- Maintain toileting interval if there are three or fewer incontinence episodes in 24 hours.
- Increase toileting interval by one-half hour if patient is unable to void at two or more scheduled toileting times.
- Increase toileting interval by 1 hour if patient has no incontinence episodes for 3 days until optimal 4-hour interval is achieved.
- Express confidence that continence can be improved.
- Teach patient to consciously hold urine until the scheduled toileting time.
- Discuss daily record of continence with patient to provide reinforcement.
- Provide positive feedback for any decrease in episodes of incontinence.

- The patient responds to full bladder in a timely manner, gets to and from the toilet, removes clothing, empties bladder, wipes self after urinating, and adjusts clothing after toileting.
- The patient cleans perineal area and washes hands after toileting.
- The patient consumes oral fluids.
- The patient expresses sexual interest, attains sexual arousal, sustains arousal through orgasm, adapts sexual technique as needed, performs sexually with assistive device as needed, expresses comfort with sexual expression, and expresses knowledge of sexual capabilities of self and partner.
- The patient recognizes the urge to void, responds to urge to void in a timely manner, voids in appropriate receptacle, voids greater than 150 mL each time, and toilets independently.
- The patient's perineal skin remains intact.

SUMMARY

Normal anatomical and physiological changes include loss of nephrons and renal mass, sclerotic changes in the renal blood vessels and diminished renal blood flow, decreased creatinine clearance, and a decline in the endocrine functions of the kidney. Bladder changes include replacement of the smooth muscle and elastic tissue with fibrous connective tissue and reduction in bladder capacity. In women, the external genitalia and vagina may atrophy and become less elastic. In men, alterations in hormones combined with various pathological states and drug effects may lead to erectile dysfunction.

Common disorders associated with the genitourinary system in older age are acute and chronic renal failure, benign prostatic hyperplasia, cancer of the prostate and bladder, urinary tract infections, urinary retention and incontinence, and vaginitis. Treatment and nursing care are geared toward maintaining continence, functional independence, and self-care. Multiple factors place the older person at risk for disorders of the genitourinary system. Although not a normal effect of aging, urinary incontinence is common and presents challenging problems to nurses, older patients, and their families. These problems can be embarrassing, isolating, and debilitating.

REFERENCES

Abramov, Y., & Sand, P. K. (2004). Oxybutynin for treatment of urge urinary incontinence and overactive bladder: An updated review. *Expert Opinion on Pharmacotherapy, 5*(11), 2351-2359.

Adam, C., Hofstetter, A., Deubner, J., Zaak, D., Weitkunat, R., Seitz, M., & Schneede, P. (2004). Retropubic transvesical prostatectomy for significant prostatic enlargement must remain a standard part of urology training. *Scandinavian Journal of Urology and Nephrology, 38*(6), 472-476.

Adams, E., Thomson, A., Maher, C., & Hagen, S. (2005). Mechanical devices for pelvic organ prolapse in women. *Cochrane Database of Systematic Reviews, 2.*

Alhasso, A., Glazener, C. M. A., Pickard, R., & N'Dow, J. (2005). Adrenergic drugs for urinary incontinence in adults. *Cochrane Database of Systematic Reviews, 2.*

American Cancer Society. (2005). Cancer facts and figures 2004. Retrieved April 20, 2005, from www.cancer.org.

Andersson, K. E. (2003). Storage and voiding symptoms: Pathophysiologic aspects. *Urology, 62*(5; suppl 2), 3-10.

Andersson, K. E., & Yoshida, M. (2003). Antimuscarinics and the overactive bladder—which is the main mechanism of action? *European Urology, 43*(1), 1-5.

Asplund, R. (2004). Nocturia, nocturnal polyuria, and sleep quality in the elderly. *Journal of Psychosomatic Research, 56*(5), 517-525.

Baid-Agrawal, S., Reinke, P., Schindler, R., Tullius, S., & Frei, U. (2004). WCN 2003 Satellite Symposium on Kidney Transplantation in the Elderly, Weimar, Germany, June 12-14, 2003. *Nephrology, Dialysis, Transplantation, 19*, 43-46.

Bathum, L., Fagnani, C., Christiansen, L., & Christensen, K. (2004). Heritability of biochemical kidney markers and relation to survival in the elderly—results from a Danish population-based twin study. *Clinica Chimica Acta, 349*(1-2), 143-150.

Bax, L., van der Graaf, Y., Rabelink, A. J., Algra, A., Beutler, J. J., & Mali, W. P. (2003). Influence of atherosclerosis on age-related changes in renal size and function. *European Journal of Clinical Investigation, 33*(1), 34-40.

Beitz, J. M. (2004). Continent diversions: The new gold standards of ileoanal reservoir and neobladder. *Ostomy Wound Management, 50*(9), 26-35.

Bertoni, E., Rosati, A., Zanazzi, M., Di Maria, L., Becherelli, P., Gallo, M., & Salvadori, M. (2004). Excellent outcome of renal transplantation using single old kidneys in old recipients. *Annals of Transplantation, 9*(2), 25-26.

Bezerra, C. A., Bruschini, H., & Cody, D. J. (2005). Suburethral sling operation for urinary incontinence in women. *Cochrane Database of Systematic Reviews, 2.*

Bogaert, G. A., Goeman, L., de Ridder, D., Wevers, M., Ivens, J., & Schuermans A. (2004). The physical and antimicrobial effects of microwave heating and alcohol immersion on catheters that are reused for clean intermittent catheterization. *European Urology, 46*(5), 641-646.

Bohle, A., & Bock, P. R. (2004). Intravesical bacilli Calmette-Guerin versus mitomycin C in superficial bladder cancer: Formal meta-analysis of comparative studies on tumor progression. *Urology, 63*(4), 682-686.

Boldt, J., Brenner, T., Lang, J., Kumle, B., & Isgro, F. (2003). Kidney-specific proteins in elderly patients undergoing cardiac surgery with cardiopulmonary bypass. *Anesthesia and Analgesia, 97*(6), 1582-1589.

Borchers, H., Kirschner-Hermanns, R., Brehmer, B., Tietze, L., Reineke, T., Pinkawa, M., et al. (2004). Permanent ^{125}I-seed brachytherapy or radical prostatectomy: A prospective comparison considering oncological and quality of life results. *BJU International, 94*(6), 805-811.

Boyle, P., Roehrborn, C., Harkaway, R., Logie, J., de la Rosette, J., & Emberton, M. (2004). 5-Alpha reductase inhibition provides superior benefits to alpha blockade by preventing AUR and BPH-related surgery. *European Urology, 45*(5), 620-626.

Brierly, R. D., Hindley, R. G., McLarty, E., Harding, D. M., & Thomas, P. J. (2003). A prospective controlled quantitative study of ultrastructural changes in the underactive detrusor. *Journal of Urology, 169*(4), 1374-1378.

Brown, A. D. G., & Cooper, T. K. (2003). Gynecological disorders. In R. C. Tallis & H. M. Fillit (Eds.), *Brocklehurst's textbook of geriatric medicine and gerontology* (6th ed.). London: Churchill Livingstone.

Brown, C. T., & Nuttall, M. C. (2003). Dutasteride: A new 5-alpha reductase inhibitor for men with lower urinary tract symptoms secondary to benign prostatic hyperplasia. *International Journal of Clinical Practice, 57*(8), 705-709.

Burkhardt, H., Hahn, T., & Gladisch, R. (2003). Is kidney size a useful predictor of renal function in the elderly? *Clinical Nephrology, 59*(6), 415-422.

Butler, R. N., & Lewis, M. I. (2003). Sexuality in old age. In R. C. Tallis & H. M. Fillit (Eds.), *Brocklehurst's textbook of geriatric medicine and gerontology* (6th ed.). London: Churchill Livingstone.

Carrie, A. G., Metge, C. J., Collins, D. M., Harding, G. K., & Zhanel, G. G. (2004). Use of administrative healthcare claims to examine the effectiveness of trimethoprim-sulfamethoxazole versus fluoroquinolones in the treatment of community-acquired acute pyelonephritis in women. *Journal of Antimicrobial Chemotherapy, 53*(3), 512-517.

Carson, C., & Naber, K. G. (2004). Role of fluoroquinolones in the treatment of serious bacterial urinary tract infections. *Drugs, 64*(12), 1359-1373.

Chapple, C. R. (2004). Pharmacological therapy of benign prostatic hyperplasia/lower urinary tract symptoms: An overview for the practicing clinician. *BJU International, 94*(9), 738-744.

Chen, Y. C., Chen, G. D., Hu, S. W., Lin, T. L., & Lin, L. Y. (2003). Is the occurrence of storage and voiding dysfunction affected by menopausal transition or associated with the normal aging process? *Menopause, 10*(3), 191-192.

Clark, P. E., Stein, J. P., Groshen, S. G., Cai, J., Miranda, G., Lieskovsky, G., & Skinner, D. G. (2005). Radical cystectomy in the elderly: Comparison of survival between younger and older patients. *Cancer, 103*(3), 546-552.

Colt, J. S., Baris, D., Stewart, P., Schned, A. R., Heaney, J. A., Mott, L. A., et al. (2004). Occupation and bladder cancer risk in a population-based case-control study in New Hampshire. *Cancer Causes and Control, 15*(8), 759-769.

Croom, K. F., & Keating, G. M. (2004). Darifenacin: In the treatment of overactive bladder. *Drugs and Aging, 21*(13), 885-892.

DasGupta, R., & Fowler, C. J. (2004). Urodynamic study of women in urinary retention treated with sacral neuromodulation. *Journal of Urology, 171*(3), 1161-1164.

Dessole, S., Rubattu, G., Ambrosini, G., Gallo, O., Capobianco, G., Cherchi, P. L., et al. (2004). Efficacy of low-dose intravaginal estriol on urogenital aging in postmenopausal women. *Menopause, 11*(1), 49-56.

Djousse, L., Schatzkin, A., Chibnik, L. B., D'Agostino, R. B., Kreger, B. E., & Ellison, R. C. (2004). Alcohol consumption and the risk of bladder cancer in the Framingham Heart Study. *Journal of the National Cancer Institute, 96*(18), 1397-1400.

Dochterman, J. M., & Bulechek, G. M. (Eds.). (2004). *Nursing interventions classification (NIC)* (4th ed.). St. Louis: Mosby.

Dolan, L. M., Smith, A. R., & Hosker, G. L. (2004). Opening detrusor pressure and the influence of age on success following colposuspension. *Neurology and Urodynamics, 23*(1), 10-15.

Eapen, L., Stewart, D., Collins, J., & Peterson, R. (2004). Effective bladder sparing therapy with intra-arterial cisplatin and radiotherapy for localized bladder cancer. *Journal of Urology, 172*(4 pt 1), 1276-1280.

El-Bahnasawy, M. S., El-Assmy, E., Ali-El Dein, B., Shehab, E. A. B., Refaie, A., & El-Hammady, S. (2004). Critical evaluation of the factors influencing erectile dysfunction after renal transplantation. *International Journal of Impotence Research, 16*(6), 521-526.

Ellerkmann, R. M., & McBride, A. (2003). Management of obstructive voiding dysfunction. *Drugs of Today, 39*(7), 513-540.

George, N. J. R. (2003). The prostate gland. In R. C. Tallis & H. M. Fillit (Eds.), *Brocklehurst's textbook of geriatric medicine and gerontology* (6th ed.). London: Churchill Livingstone.

Glazener, C. M. A., & Cooper, K. (2005). Bladder neck needle suspension for urinary incontinence in women. *Cochrane Database of Systematic Reviews, 2.*

Gontero, P., & Kirby, R. (2004). Proerectile pharmacological prophylaxis following nerve-sparing radical prostatectomy. *Prostate Cancer and Prostatic Diseases, 7*(3), 223-226.

Grabe, M. (2004). Controversies in antibiotic prophylaxis in urology. *International Journal of Antimicrobial Agents, 23*(suppl 1), S17-S23.

Gray, M. (2004). Nursing assessment: The urinary system. In S. M. Lewis, M. M. Heitkemper, & S. R. Dirksen (Eds.), *Medical-surgical nursing: Assessment and management of clinical problems* (6th ed.). St. Louis: Mosby.

Griebling, T. (2005). Urologic diseases in America project: Trends in resource use for urinary tract infections in men. *Journal of Urology, 173*, 1288-1294.

Griffiths, R., & Fernandez, R. (2005). Policies for the removal of short-term indwelling urethral catheters. *Cochrane Database of Systematic Reviews, 2.*

Grossman, H. B., Messing, E., Soloway, M., Tomera, K., Katz, G., Berger, Y., & Shen, Y. (2005). Detection of bladder cancer using a point-of-care proteomic assay. *Journal of the American Medical Association, 293*(7), 810-816.

Guay, D. R. (2003). Clinical pharmacokinetics of drugs used to treat urge incontinence. *Clinical Pharmacokinetics, 42*(14), 1243-1285.

Guyton, A. C., & Hall, J. E. (2000). *Textbook of medical physiology* (10th ed.). Philadephia: Saunders.

Hay-Smith, J., Herbison, P., Ellis, G., & Moore, K. (2005). Anticholinergic drugs versus placebo for overactive bladder syndrome in adults. *Cochrane Database of Systematic Reviews, 2.*

Herschorn, S., Becker, D., Miller, E., Thompson, M., & Forte, L. (2004). Impact of health education intervention in overactive bladder patients. *Canadian Journal of Urology, 11*(6), 2430-2437.

Hoffman, R. M., MacDonald, R., Monga, M., & Wilt, T. J. (2004). Transurethral microwave thermotherapy vs transurethral resection for treating benign prostatic hyperplasia: A systematic review. *BJU International, 94*(7), 1031-1036.

Hoffman, R. M., MacDonald, R., Monga, M., & Wilt, T. J. (2005). Laser prostatectomy for benign prostatic obstruction. *Cochrane Database of Systematic Reviews, 1*, CD001987.

Hollenbeck, B. K., Miller, D. C., Taub, D., Dunn, R. L., Underwood, W., 3rd, Montie, J. E., & Wei, J. T. (2004). Aggressive treatment for bladder cancer is associated with improved overall survival among patients 80 years old or older. *Urology, 64*(2), 292-297.

Hsieh, K., Taylor, J. A., & Albertsen, P. C. (2003). Lower urinary tract symptoms in the older male. *Connecticut Medicine, 67*(8), 487-490.

Huang, W. C., Wann, S. R., Lin, S. L., Kunin, C. M., Lin, C. H., Hsu, C. W., et al. (2004). Catheter-associated urinary tract infections in intensive care units can be reduced by prompting physicians to remove unnecessary catheters. *Infection Control and Hospital Epidemiology, 25*(11), 974-978.

Hughes, D. A., & Dubois, D. (2004). Cost-effectiveness analysis of extended-release formulations of oxybutynin and tolterodine for the management of urge incontinence. *Pharmacoeconomics, 22*(16), 1047-1059.

Humphreys, M. R., Gettman, M. T., Chow, G. K., Zincke, H., & Blute, M. L. (2004). Minimally invasive radical prostatectomy. *Mayo Clinic Proceedings, 79*(9), 1169-1180.

Huncharek, M., & Kupelnick, B. (2005). Personal use of hair dyes and the risk of bladder cancer: Results of a meta-analysis. *Public Health Reports, 120*(1), 31-38.

Hunter, K. F., Moore, K. N., Cody, D. J., & Glazener, C. M. A. (2005). Conservative management for postprostatectomy urinary incontinence. *Cochrane Database of Systematic Reviews, 2.*

International Continence Society. (1990). Report of the Committee for Standardization of Terminology of Lower Urinary Tract Function. *British Journal of Obstetrics and Gynecology, 6*(suppl), 1-16.

Jassal, S. V., Fillit, H. M., & Oreopolous, D. G. (2003). Diseases of the aging kidney. In R. C. Tallis & H. M. Fillit (Eds.), *Brocklehurst's textbook of geriatric medicine and gerontology* (6th ed.). London: Churchill Livingstone.

Jassal, S. V., & Oreopoulos, D. G. (2003). Aging of the urinary tract. In R. C. Tallis & H. M. Fillit (Eds.), *Brocklehurst's textbook of geriatric medicine and gerontology* (6th ed.). London: Churchill Livingstone.

Jepson, R. G., Mihaljevic, L., & Craig, J. (2004). Cranberries for preventing urinary tract infections. *Cochrane Database of Systematic Reviews, 2*, CD001321.

Johnson, M., Bulechek, G., Dochterman, J. M., Maas, M., & Moorhead, S. (Eds.). (2001). *Nursing diagnoses, outcomes, and interventions: NANDA, NOC, and NIC linkages.* St. Louis: Mosby.

Juarez Tomas, M. S., Ocana, V. S., Wiese, B., & Nader-Macias, M. E. (2003). Growth and lactic acid production by vaginal *Lactobacillus acidophilus* CRL 1259, and inhibition of uropathogenic *Escherichia coli. Journal of Medical Microbiology, 52*(pt 12), 1117-1124.

Kato, K., Yoshida, K., Suzuki, K., Murase, T., & Gotoh, M. (2005). Managing patients with an overactive bladder and glaucoma: A questionnaire survey of Japanese urologists on the use of anticholinergics. *BJU International, 95*(1), 98-101.

Kelleher, C. J., Cardozo, L., Chapple, C. R., Haab, F., & Ridder, A. M. (2005). Improved quality of life in patients with overactive bladder symptoms treated with solifenacin. *BJU International, 95*(1), 81-85.

Khullar, V., Hill, S., Laval, K. U., Schiotz, H. A., Jonas, U., & Versi, E. (2004). Treatment of urge-predominant mixed urinary incontinence with tolterodine extended release: A randomized placebo-controlled trial. *Urology, 64*(2), 269-274.

Klauser, A., Frauscher, F., Strasser, H., Helweg, G., Kolle, D., Strohmeyer, D., et al. (2004). Age-related rhabdosphincter function in female urinary stress incontinence: Assessment of intraurethral sonography. *Journal of Ultrasound in Medicine, 23*(5), 631-637.

Knutson, T. (2004). Can prostate stents be used to predict the outcome of transurethral resection of the prostate in the difficult cases? *Current Opinion in Urology, 14*(1), 35-39.

Kontiokari, T., Laitinen, J., Jarvi, L., Pokka, T., Sundqvist, K., & Uhari, M. (2003). Dietary factors protecting women from urinary tract infection. *American Journal of Clinical Nutrition, 77*(3), 600-604.

Kunin, C. M. (2000). Urinary tract infection and pyelonephritis. In L. Goldman & J. C. Bennett (Eds.), *Cecil textbook of medicine* (21st ed.). Philadelphia: W. B. Saunders.

Kupelian, P. A., Potters, L., Khuntia, D., Ciezki, J. P., Reddy, C. A., Reuther, A. M., et al. (2004). Radical prostatectomy, external beam radiotherapy <72 Gy, external beam radiotherapy = or >72 Gy, permanent seed implantation, or combined seeds/external beam radiotherapy for stage T1-T2 prostate cancer. *International Journal of Radiation Oncology, Biology, Physics, 58*(1), 25-33.

Lamb, E. J., O'Riordan, S. E., & Delaney, M. P. (2003). Kidney function in older people: Pathology, assessment, and management. *Clinical Chimica Acta, 334*(1-2), 25-40.

Lamm, S. H., Engel, A., Kruse, M. B., Feinleib, M., Boyd, D. M., Lai, S., & Wilson, R. (2004). Arsenic in drinking water and bladder cancer mortality in the United States: An analysis based on 133 U.S. counties and 30 years of observation. *Journal of Occupational and Environmental Medicine, 46*(3), 298-306.

Lamonerie, L., Marret, E., Deleuze, A., Lembert, N., Dupont, M., & Bonnet, F. (2004). Prevalence of postoperative bladder distention and urinary retention detected by ultrasound measurement. *British Journal of Anaesthesia, 92*(4), 544-546.

Lapitan, M. C., Cody, D. J., & Grant, A. M. (2005). Open retropubic colposuspension for urinary incontinence in women. *Cochrane Database of Systematic Reviews, 2*.

LaSala, C. A., & Kuchel, G. A. (2003). Evaluation and management of urinary incontinence in elderly women. *Connecticut Medicine, 67*(8), 491-495.

Lau, H., & Lam, B. (2004). Management of postoperative urinary retention: A randomized trial of in-out versus overnight catheterization. *Australian and New Zealand Journal of Surgery, 74*(8), 658-661.

Lazarou, G., Scotti, R. J., Mikhail, M. S., Zhou, H. S., & Powers, K. (2004). Pessary reduction and postoperative cure of retention in women with anterior vaginal wall prolapse. *International Urogynecology Journal, 15*(3), 175-178.

Lee, J. Y., Kim, H. W., Lee, S. J., Koh, J. S., Suh, H. J., & Chancellor, M. B. (2004). Comparison of doxazosin with or without tolterodine in men with symptomatic bladder outlet obstruction and an overactive bladder. *BJU International, 94*(6), 817-820.

Lehne, R. A. (2004). *Pharmacology for nursing care* (5th ed.). Philadelphia: Saunders.

Leone, M., Garnier, F., Antonini, F., Bimar, M. C., Albanese, J., & Martin, C. (2003). Comparison of effectiveness of two urinary drainage systems in intensive care unit: A prospective, randomized clinical trial. *Intensive Care Medicine, 29*(3), 410-413.

Lepor, H., & Kaci, L. (2004). The impact of open radical retropubic prostatectomy on continence and lower urinary tract symptoms: A prospective assessment using validated self-administered outcome instruments. *Journal of Urology, 171*(3), 1216-1219.

Levin, R. M., & Hudson, A. P. (2004). The molecular genetic basis of mitochondrial malfunction in bladder tissue following outlet obstruction. *Journal of Urology, 172*(2), 438-447.

Li, G., Li, K., Li, Z., & Wang, P. (2003). Age-dependent changes in beta-adrenergic function in human detrusors and possible mechanisms. *Chinese Medical Journal, 116*(10), 1511-1514.

Linsenmeyer, T. A., Harrison, B., Oakley, A., Kirshblum, S., Stock, J. A., & Millis, S. R. (2005). Evaluation of cranberry supplement for reduction of urinary tract infections in individuals with neurogenic bladders secondary to spinal cord injury. A prospective, double-blinded, placebo-controlled, crossover study. *Scientific Nursing, 22*(1), 20-25.

Lipton, R. B., Kolodner, K., & Wesnes, K. (2005). Assessment of cognitive function in the elderly population: Effects of darifenacin. *Journal of Urology, 173*(2), 493-498.

Luckey, A. E., & Parsa, C. J. (2003). Fluid and electrolytes in the aged. *Archives of Surgery, 138*(10), 1055-1060.

Lutters, M., & Vogt, N. (2005). Antibiotic duration for treating uncomplicated, symptomatic lower urinary tract infections in elderly women. *Cochrane Database of Systematic Reviews, 2*.

Madigan, E., & Neff, D. F. (2003). Care of patients with long-term indwelling urinary catheters. *Online Journal of Issues in Nursing, 8*(3), 7.

Maher, C., Baessler, K., Glazener, C. M. A., Adams, E. J., & Hagen, S. (2005). Surgical management of pelvic organ prolapse in women. *Cochrane Database of Systematic Reviews, 2*.

Malone-Lee, J. (2003). Urinary incontinence. In R. C. Tallis & H. M. Fillit (Eds.), *Brocklehurst's textbook of geriatric medicine and gerontology* (6th ed.). London: Churchill Livingstone.

Maloney-Monaghan, C., & Cafiero, M. (2004). Male bladder control problems: A guide to assessment. *Ostomy Wound Management, 50*(12), 42-48.

Manunta, A., Vincendeau, S., Kiriakou, G., Lobel, B., & Guille, F. (2005). Non-transitional cell bladder carcinomas. *BJU International, 95*, 497-502.

Marelli, G., Papaleo, E., & Ferrari, A. (2004). Lactobacilli for prevention of urogenital infections: A review. *European Review for Medical and Pharmacological Sciences, 8*(2), 87-95.

Marx, G. M., Blake, G. M., Galani, E., Steer, C. B., Harper, S. E., Adamson, K. L., et al. (2004). Evaluation of the Cockcroft-Gault, Jelliffe and Wright formulae in estimating renal function in elderly cancer patients. *Annals of Oncology, 15*(2), 291-295.

Masood, S., Djaladat, H., Kouriefs, C., Keen, M., & Palmer, J. H. (2004). The 12-year outcome analysis of an endourethral wallstent for treating benign prostatic hyperplasia. *BJU International, 94*(9), 1271-1274.

Mazouni, C., Karsenty, G., Bladou, F., & Serment, G. (2004). Urethral device in women with chronic urinary retention: An alternative to self-catheterization. *European Journal of Obstetrics, Gynecology, and Reproductive Biology, 115*(1), 80-84.

McCormack, P. L., & Keating, G. M. (2004). Duloxetine: In stress urinary incontinence. *Drugs, 64*(22), 2567-2573.

McCully, K. S., & Jackson, S. (2004). Hormone replacement therapy and the bladder. *Journal of the British Menopause Society, 10*(1), 30-32.

McNeill, S. A., & Hargreave, T. B. (2005). Alfuzosin once daily facilitates return to voiding in patients in acute urinary retention. *Journal of Urology, 171*(6; pt 1), 2316-2320.

Melk, A. (2003). Senescence of renal cells: Molecular basis and clinical implications. *Nephrology, Dialysis, Transplant, 18*(12), 2474-2478.

Moehrer, B., Ellis, G., Carey, M., & Wilson, P. D. (2005). Laparoscopic colposuspension for urinary incontinence in women. *Cochrane Database of Systematic Reviews, 2,* CD001405.

Moehrer, B., Hextall, A., & Jackson, S. (2005). Oestrogens for urinary incontinence in women. *Cochrane Database of Systematic Reviews, 2.*

Moorhead, S., Johnson, M., & Maas, M. (Eds.). (2004). *Nursing outcomes classification (NOC)* (3rd ed.). St. Louis: Mosby.

NANDA International. (2005). *Nursing diagnoses: Definitions and classification 2005-2006.* Philadelphia: NANDA International.

Negri, E., Pelucchi, C., Talamini, R., Montella, M., Gallus, S., Bosetti, C., et al. (2005). Family history of cancer and the risk of prostate cancer and benign prostatic hyperplasia. *International Journal of Cancer, 114*(4), 648-652.

Newman, D. K. (2004a). Report of a mail survey of women with bladder control disorders. *Urologic Nursing, 24*(6), 499-507.

Newman, D. K. (2004b). Stating the case for overactive bladder: A nurse practitioner's perspective. *Journal of the American Academy of Nurse Practitioners, 16*(10; suppl), 1-3.

Ooi, S. T., Frazee, L. A., & Gardner, W. G. (2004). Management of asymptomatic bacteriuria in patients with diabetes mellitus. *Annals of Pharmacotherapy, 38*(3), 490-493.

Oosterlinck, W. (2004). Guidelines on diagnosis and treatment of superficial bladder cancer. *Minerva Urologica e Nefrologia, 56*(1), 65-72.

Partin, A. W. (2000). Diseases of the prostate. In L. Goldman & J. C. Bennett (Eds.), *Cecil textbook of medicine* (21st ed.). Philadelphia: W. B. Saunders.

Pascher, A., Pratschke, J., Neuhaus, P., & Tullius, S. G. (2004). Modifications of immune regulations with increasing donor and recipient age. *Annals of Transplantation, 9*(1), 72-73.

Pickard, R., Reaper, J., Wyness, L., Cody, D. J., McClinton, S., & N'Dow, J. (2005). Periurethral injection therapy for urinary incontinence in women. *Cochrane Database of Systematic Reviews, 2.*

Pos, F., Horenblas, S., Dom, P., Moonen, L., & Bartelink, H. (2005). Organ preservation in invasive bladder cancer: Brachytherapy, an alternative to cystectomy and combined modality treatment? *International Journal of Radiation Oncology, Biology, Physics, 61*(3), 678-686.

Quaranta, B. P., Marks, L. B., & Anscher, M. S. (2004). Comparing radical prostatectomy and brachytherapy for localized prostate cancer. *Oncology (Huntington), 18*(10), 1289-1302.

Rackley, R., & Abdelmalak, J. (2004). Urologic applications of botulinum toxin therapy for voiding dysfunction. *Current Urology Reports, 5*(5), 381-388.

Ramakrishnan, K., & Scheid, D. C. (2005). Diagnosis and management of acute pyelonephritis in adults. *American Family Physician, 71*(5), 933-942.

Ratnasinghe, L. D., Graubard, B. I., Kahle, L., Tangrea, J. A., Taylor, P. R., & Hawk, E. (2004). Aspirin use and mortality from cancer in a prospective cohort study. *Anticancer Research, 24*(5B), 3177-3184.

Raz, R., Colodner, R., Rohana, Y., Battino, S., Rottensterich, E., Wasser, I., & Stamm, W. (2003). Effectiveness of estriol-containing vaginal pessaries and nitrofurantoin macrocrystal therapy in the prevention of recurrent urinary tract infection in postmenopausal women. *Clinical Infectious Diseases, 36*(11), 1362-1368.

Rembratt, A., Norgaard, J. P., & Andersson, K. E. (2003). Differences between nocturics and non-nocturics in voiding patterns: An analysis of frequency-volume charts from community dwelling elderly. *BJU International, 91*(1), 45-50.

Richardson, J. D., Cocanour, C. S., Kern, J. A., Garrison, R. N., Kirton, O. C., Cofer, J. B., et al. (2004). Perioperative risk assessment in elderly and high-risk patients. *Journal of the American College of Surgeons, 199*(1), 133-146.

Rimon, E., Kagansky, N., Cojocaru, L., Gindin, J., Shattner, A., & Levy, S. (2004). Can creatinine clearance be accurately predicted by formulae in octogenarian in-patients? *Quarterly Journal of Medicine, 97*(5), 281-287.

Roehrborn, C. G., Bruskewitz, R., Nickel, J. C., McConnell, J. D., Saltzman, B., Gittelman, M. C., et al. (2004). Sustained decrease in incidence of acute urinary retention and surgery with finasteride for 6 years in men with benign prostatic hyperplasia. *Journal of Urology, 17*(3), 1194-1198.

Rogers, R. G., Kammerer-Doak, D., Olsen, A., Thompson, P. K., Walters, M. D., Lukacz, E. S., & Qualls, C. (2004). A randomized, double-blind, placebo-controlled comparison of the effect of nitrofurantoin monohydrate macrocrystals on the development of urinary tract infections after surgery for pelvic organ prolapse and/or stress urinary incontinence with suprapubic catheterization. *American Journal of Obstetrics and Gynecology, 191*(1), 182-187.

Ron, E. (2003). Cancer risks from medical radiation. *Health Physics, 85*(1), 47-59.

Rosenman, K. D., & Reilly, M. J. (2004). Cancer mortality and incidence among a cohort of benzidine and dichlorbenzidine dye manufacturing workers. *American Journal of Industrial Medicine, 46*(5), 505-512.

Rovner, E. S. (2004). Trospium chloride in the management of overactive bladder. *Drugs, 64*(21), 2433-2446.

Sabichi, A. L., & Lippman, S. M. (2004). COX-2 inhibitors and other nonsteroidal anti-inflammatory drugs in genitourinary cancer. *Seminars in Oncology, 31*(2 suppl 7), 36-44.

Saito, M., Watanabe, T., Tabuchi, F., Otsubo, K., Satoh, K., & Miyagawa, I. (2004). Urodynamic effects and safety of modified intravesical oxybutynin chloride in patients with neurogenic detrusor overactivity: 3 years experience. *International Journal of Urology, 11*(8), 592-596.

Sannes, M. R., Kuskowski, M. A., & Johnson, J. R. (2004). Geographical distribution of antimicrobial resistance among *Escherichia coli* causing acute uncomplicated pyelonephritis in the United States. *FEMS Immunology and Medical Microbiology, 42*(2), 213-218.

Santucci, R. A., McAninch, J. W., Mario, L. A., Rajpurkar, A., Chopra, A. K., Miller, K. S., et al. (2004). Urethroplasty in patients older than 65 years: Indications, results, outcomes, and suggested treatment modifications. *Journal of Urology, 172*(1), 201-203.

Schabath, M. B., Grossman, H. B., Delclos, G. L., Hernandez, L. M., Day, R. S., Davis, B. R., et al. (2004). Dietary carotenoids and genetic instability modify bladder cancer risk. *Journal of Nutrition, 134*(12), 3362-3369.

Schick, E., Tessier, J., Bertrand, P. E., Dupont, C., & Jolivet-Tremblay, M. (2003). Observations on the function of the female urethra: I: Relation between maximum urethral closure pressure at rest and urethral hypermobility. *Neurourology and Urodynamics, 22*(7), 643-647.

Schoder, H., & Larson, S. M. (2004). Positron emission tomography for prostate, bladder, and renal cancer. *Seminars in Nuclear Medicine, 34*(4), 274-292.

Scholes, D., Hooton, T. M., Roberts, P. L., Gupta, K., Stapleton, A. E., & Stamm, W. E. (2005). Risk factors associated with acute pyelonephritis in healthy women. *Annals of Internal Medicine, 142*(1), 20-27.

Schoof, M., & Hill, K. (2005). Antibiotics for recurrent urinary tract infection. *American Family Physician, 71*(7), 1301-1302.

Schwinn, D. A., Price, D. T., & Narayan, P. (2004). Alpha-1 adrenoceptor subtype selectivity and lower urinary tract symptoms. *Mayo Clinic Proceedings, 79*(11), 1423-1434.

Sengupta, N., Siddiqui, E., & Mumtaz, F. H. (2004). Cancers of the bladder. *Journal of the Royal Society of Health, 124*(5), 228-229.

Shen, Y., & Brown, M. A. (2004). Renal imaging in pyelonephritis. *Nephrology, 9*(1), 22-25.

Spigt, M. G., van Schayck, C. P., van Kerrebroeck, P. E., van Mastrigt, R., & Knottnerus, J. A. (2004). Pathophysiological aspects of bladder dysfunction: A new hypothesis for the prevention of "prostatic" symptoms. _Medical Hypothesis, 62_(3), 448-452.

Steers, W., Corcos, J., Foote, J., & Kralidis, G. (2005). An investigation of dose titration with darifenacin, an M3 selective receptor antagonist. _BJU International, 95_(4), 580-586.

Sylvester, R. J., Oosterlinck, W., & van der Meijden, A. P. (2005). A single immediate postoperative instillation of chemotherapy decreases the risk of recurrence in patients with stage Ta T1 bladder cancer: A meta-analysis of published results of randomized clinical trials. _Journal of Urology, 171_(6 pt 1), 2186-2190.

Talan, D. A., Klimberg, I. W., Nicolle, L. E., Song, J., Kowalsky, S. F., & Church, D. A. (2004). Once daily, extended release ciprofloxacin for complicated urinary tract infections and acute uncomplicated pyelonephritis. _Journal of Urology, 171_(2 pt 1), 734-739.

Thomas, K., Chow, K., & Kirby, R. S. (2004). Acute urinary retention: A review of the aetiology and management. _Prostate Cancer and Prostatic Diseases, 7_(1), 32-37.

Trabulsi, E. J., & Guillonneau, B. (2005). Laparoscopic radical prostatectomy. _Journal of Urology, 173_(4), 1072-1079.

Trautner, B. W., & Darouiche, R. O. (2004). Role of biofilm in catheter-associated urinary tract infection. _American Journal of Infection Control, 32_(3), 177-183.

Trautner, B. W., Hull, R. A., & Darouiche, R. O. (2005). Prevention of catheter-associated urinary tract infection. _Current Opinion in Infectious Diseases, 18_(1), 37-41.

Tubaro, A., Carter, S., Trucchi, A., Punzo, G., Petta, S., & Miano, L. (2003). Early treatment of benign prostatic hyperplasia: Implications for reducing the risk of permanent bladder damage. _Drugs and Aging, 20_(3), 185-195.

Tuhkanen, K., Heino, A., Aaltoma, S., & Ala-Opas, M. (2004). Sexual function of LUTS patients before and after neodymium laser prostatectomy and transurethral resection of prostate. A prospective, randomized trial. _Urologia Internationalis, 73_(2), 137-142.

Turnheim, K. (2003). When drug therapy gets old: Pharmacokinetics and pharmacodynamics in the elderly. _Experimental Gerontology, 38_(8), 843-853.

Ugnat, A. M., Luo, W., Semenciw, R., & Mao, Y., (2004). Occupational exposure to chemical and petrochemical industries and bladder cancer in four western Canadian provinces. _Chronic Diseases in Canada, 25_(2), 7-15.

Urinary Incontinence Guideline Panel. (1992). _Urinary incontinence in adults: Clinical practice guideline._ AHCPR pub. no. 92-0038. Rockville MD: Agency for Health Care Policy and Research, Public Health Service, U. S. Department of Health and Human Services.

Wang, I. K., Chang, F. R., Yang, B. Y., Lin, C. L., & Huang, C. C. (2003). The use of ultrasonography in evaluating adults with febrile urinary tract infection. _Renal Failure, 25_(6), 981-987.

Wasen, E., Isoaho, R., Mattila, K., Vahlberg, T., Kivela, S. L., & Irjala, K. (2004). Estimation of glomerular filtration rate in the elderly: A comparison of creatinine-based formulas with serum cystatin C. _Journal of Internal Medicine, 256_(1), 70-78.

Wazait, H. D., Patel, H. R., van der Meulen, J. H., Ghei, M., Al-Buheissi, S., Kelsey, M., et al. (2004). A pilot randomized double-blind placebo-controlled trial on the use of antibiotics on urinary catheter removal to reduce the rate of urinary tract infection: The pitfalls of ciprofloxacin. _BJU International, 94_(7), 1048-1050.

Wazait, H. D., van der Meulen, J. H., Patel, H. R., Brown, C. T., Gadgil, S., Miller, R. A., et al. (2004). Antibiotics on urethral catheter withdrawal: A hit and miss affair. _Journal of Hospital Infection, 58_(4), 297-302.

Williams, D. H., & Schaeffer, A. J. (2004). Current concepts in urinary tract infections. _Minerva Urologica e Nefrologica, 56_(1), 15-31.

Wilson, L. C., Kennett, K. M., & Gilling, P. J. (2004). Laparoscopic radical prostatectomy: Early safety and efficacy. _Australian and New Zealand Journal of Surgery, 74_(12), 1065-1068.

Wysowsky, D. K., Kornegay, C., Nourjah, P., & Trontell, A. (2003). Technical briefs: Sex and age differences in serum potassium in the United States. _Clinical Chemistry, 49_(1), 190-192.

Yang, J. M., & Huang, W. C. (2003). Factors associated with voiding function in women with lower urinary tract symptoms: A mathematic model explanation. _Neurology and Urodynamics, 22_(6), 574-581.

Yavuz, A., Tuncer, M., Erdogan, O., Gurkan, A., Cetinkaya, R., Akbas, S. H., et al. (2004). Is there any effect of compliance on clinical parameters of renal transplant recipients? _Transplantation Proceedings, 36_(1), 120-121.

Yoshida, M., Miyamae, K., Iwashita, H., Otani, M., & Inadome, A. (2004). Management of detrusor dysfunction in the elderly: Changes in acetylcholine and adenosine triphosphate release during aging. _Urology, 63_(3 suppl 1), 17-23.

Zheng, F., Plati, A. R., Banerjee, A., Elliot, S., Striker, L. J., & Striker, G. E. (2003, July 23). The molecular basis of age-related kidney disease. _Science of Aging Knowledge Environment, 2003_(29), PE20.

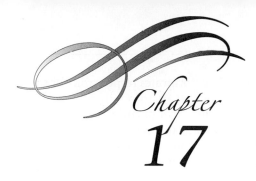

Chapter 17

Endocrine System

Adrianne Dill Linton § Lisa J. Hooter §
Coleen R. Elmers

Objectives

Discuss normal changes in the structure and function of the endocrine system associated with aging.

Describe measures to maintain endocrine health in the older adult.

Explain the cause and treatment of endocrine disorders that are common in older persons.

Describe the components of the endocrine assessment in the older adult.

Formulate nursing diagnoses for older adults with endocrine disorders.

Develop plans to manage older adults with actual or potential endocrine problems.

ORGANIZATION OF THE ENDOCRINE SYSTEM

The endocrine system consists of various tissues and glands whose function is to produce and secrete hormones into the bloodstream. The major hormone-secreting glands are the pituitary gland, thyroid gland, parathyroid glands, pancreatic islets, pineal gland, ovaries, testes, and adrenal glands (Figure 17-1). Hormones are released in low concentrations and are transported to other parts of the body, where they exert regulatory effects on cellular processes. Their purpose is to coordinate body activities, control growth and development, and maintain homeostasis. The endocrine system also acts with the nervous system to instigate various responses to changes in the external and internal environment. Overactivity of most hormones is controlled by negative feedback mechanisms. An exception is leutinizing hormone (LH), which stimulates estrogen secretion that in turn stimulates the secretion of additional LH. Hormones are cleared from the blood by metabolic destruction, tissue binding, excretion by the liver into the bile, or excretion by the kidneys. The endocrine glands and their secretions are listed in Table 17-1.

Pituitary Gland

The pituitary gland, or hypophysis, consists of an anterior and a posterior segment. It is about 1 cm in diameter, weighs 0.5 to 1 gram, and lies in a bony cavity at the base of the brain called the sella turcica. The posterior pituitary gland does not actually produce any hormones, but it stores the hormones oxytocin and antidiuretic hormone (ADH), whose release is governed by nerve impulses from the hypothalamus. The major function of ADH is to regulate the concentration of water in body fluids by controlling the rate of water excretion into the urine. The primary action of oxytocin (pitocin) is to influence the lactating breast to release milk from the glandular cells into the ducts. Oxytocin also may play a role in delivery at the end of gestation (Guyton & Hall, 2006).

The anterior pituitary gland produces human growth hormone (GH, somatotropin), thyroid-stimulating hormone (TSH), prolactin, adrenocorticotropin (ACTH), and two gonadotrophic hormones: follicle-stimulating hormone (FSH) and leutinizing hormone (LH). Growth hormone affects protein formation, cell multiplication, and cell differentiation in almost all tissues throughout the body. The activity of GH is mediated by insulin-like growth factors I and II (IGF-I and IGF-II). IGF-I in the plasma is increased by GH, whereas IGF-II is less affected. The steps in the regulation of circulating growth hormone are as follows (Davies, 2003):

1. Growth hormone–releasing hormone (GHRH) is produced in the hypothalamus.
2. GHRH stimulates somatotrophs in the anterior pituitary to release growth hormone (GH).
3. GH stimulates the liver to produce IGF-I.
4. IGF-I stimulates the release of somatostatin in the hypothalamus.
5. Somatostatin causes somatotrophs to reduce GH release.

The other pituitary hormones control the activities of their target glands—the thyroid gland, mammary glands, adrenal cortex, ovaries, and testes. Hypothalamic

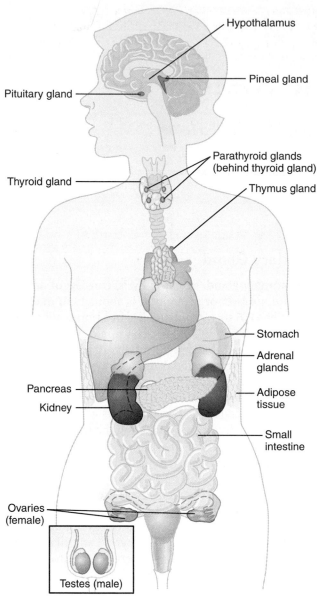

Figure 17-1 Anatomical location of principal endocrine glands and tissues of the body. (Used with permission from Guyton, A. C., & Hall, J. E. [2006]. *Textbook of medical physiology* [11th ed.]. Philadelphia: Saunders.)

surface of the trachea. The hormones responsible for the major functions of the thyroid are triiodothyronine (T_3) and thyroxine (T_4). Calcitonin, a hormone that participates in calcium metabolism, also is secreted by the thyroid. TSH, secreted by the anterior pituitary, stimulates iodine uptake by the thyroid gland as well as the synthesis and ultimate release of T_3 and T_4. Most T_4 is converted into T_3 in the tissues. The actions of T_3 and T_4 are to raise the basal metabolic rate, develop the central nervous system, stimulate all aspects of glucose and fat metabolism, increase the demand for vitamins, increase the rates of secretion of other endocrine glands, and enhance normal sexual functioning. Among the many effects of thyroid activity are enhanced glycolysis and gluconeogenesis; increased insulin secretion; increased fatty acid levels in the plasma; decreased cholesterol, phospholipid, and triglyceride levels in the plasma; increased blood flow and cardiac output; increased rate and strength of the heartbeat; increased systolic blood pressure; increased secretion of digestive juices; and increased intestinal motility. A 2- to 3-month supply of thyroid hormones is stored in thyroglobulin molecules in the gland (Guyton & Hall, 2006).

Parathyroid Glands

The parathyroid glands usually are located behind the thyroid gland. Typically there are four of the glands although sometimes more are found. These glands secrete parathyroid hormone (PTH), which helps to regulate calcium and phosphate concentrations in body fluids by controlling intestinal reabsorption, renal excretion, and movement of these ions between the bones and the extracellular fluid. Parathyroid secretion is primarily regulated by the serum calcium concentration through negative feedback. A decrease in extracellular calcium concentration produces a prompt increase in PTH secretion, whereas excess calcium concentration suppresses the secretion of PTH (Guyton & Hall, 2006).

Adrenal Cortex

The adrenal cortex is the outer layer of the two adrenal glands, which rest on top of the kidneys. The major types of hormones secreted by the adrenal cortex are the corticosteroids: mineralocorticoids, glucocorticoids, and small amounts of androgens. Aldosterone, the principal mineralocorticoid, regulates the fluid and electrolyte balance by increasing the reabsorption of sodium and decreasing the reabsorption of potassium by the kidneys. Cortisol, the principal glucocorticoid, influences the metabolism of glucose, protein, and fat, is required for a normal response to stress, and exerts antiinflammatory and antiallergic actions. The androgenic hormones have the same effects as testosterone.

releasing and inhibitory hormones secreted within the hypothalamus control the release of anterior pituitary hormones. Major releasing and inhibiting hormones include TSH-releasing hormone, corticotropin-releasing hormone, growth hormone-releasing hormone, growth hormone inhibitory hormone, gonadotropin-releasing hormone, and prolactin inhibitory factor (Guyton & Hall, 2006) (Figure 17-2).

Thyroid Gland

The thyroid gland is composed of two lobes lying on either side of the trachea that are connected at the midline by a thin isthmus extending over the anterior

Table 17-1 *Endocrine Glands and Their Secretions*

Gland/Tissue	Hormones	Major Functions	Chemical Structure
Hypothalamus	Thyrotropin-releasing hormone (TRH)	Stimulates secretion of TSH and prolactin	Peptide
	Corticotropin-releasing hormone (CRH)	Causes release of ACTH	Peptide
	Growth hormone–releasing hormone (GHRH)	Causes release of growth hormone	Peptide
	Growth hormone inhibitory hormone (GHIH) (somatostatin)	Inhibits release of growth hormone	Peptide
	Gonadotropin-releasing hormone (GnRH)	Causes release of LH and FSH	
	Dopamine or prolactin-inhibiting factor (PIF)	Inhibits release of prolactin	Amine
Anterior pituitary	Growth hormone	Stimulates protein synthesis and overall growth of most cells and tissues	Peptide
	Thyroid-stimulating hormone (TSH)	Stimulates synthesis and secretion of thyroid hormones (thyroxine and triiodothyronine)	Peptide
	Adrenocorticotropic hormone (ACTH)	Stimulates synthesis and secretion of adrenocortical hormones (cortisol, androgens, and aldosterone)	Peptide
	Prolactin	Promotes development of female breasts and secretion of milk	Peptide
	Follicle-stimulating hormone (FSH)	Causes growth of follicles in ovaries and sperm maturation in Sertoli cells of testes	Peptide
	Luteinizing hormone (LH)	Stimulates testosterone synthesis in Leydig cells of testes; stimulates ovulation, formation of corpus luteum, and estrogen and progesterone synthesis in ovaries	Peptide
Posterior pituitary	Antidiuretic hormone (ADH) (also called vasopressin)	Increases water reabsorption by kidneys and causes vasoconstriction and increased blood pressure	Peptide
	Oxytocin	Stimulates milk injection from breasts and uterine contractions	Peptide
Thyroid	Thyroxine (T_4) and triiodothyronine (T_3)	Increases rates of chemical reactions in most cells, thus increasing body metabolic rate	Amine
	Calcitonin	Promotes deposition of calcium in bones and decreases extracellular fluid calcium ion concentration	Peptide
Adrenal cortex	Cortisol	Has multiple metabolic functions for controlling metabolism of proteins, carbohydrates, and fats; also has antiinflammatory effects	Steroid
	Aldosterone	Increases renal sodium reabsorption, potassium secretion, and hydrogen ion secretion	Steroid
Adrenal medulla	Norepinephrine, epinephrine	Same effects as sympathetic stimulation	Amine
Pancreas	Insulin (beta cells)	Promotes glucose entry in many cells, and in this way controls carbohydrate metabolism	Peptide
	Glucagon (alpha cells)	Increases synthesis and release of glucose from liver into body fluids	Peptide
Parathyroid	Parathyroid hormone (PTH)	Controls serum calcium ion concentration by increasing calcium absorption by gut and kidneys and releasing calcium from bones	Peptide
Testes	Testosterone	Promotes development of male reproductive system and male secondary sexual characteristics	Steroid

Continued

Table 17-1 *Endocrine Glands and Their Secretions—cont'd*

Gland/Tissue	Hormones	Major Functions	Chemical Structure
Ovaries	Estrogens	Promotes growth and development of female reproductive system, female breasts, and female secondary sexual characteristics	Steroid
	Progesterone	Stimulates secretion of "uterine milk" by uterine endometrial glands and promotes development of secretory apparatus of breasts	Steroid
Placenta	Human chorionic gonadotropin (HCG)	Promotes growth of corpus luteum and secretion of estrogens and progesterone by corpus luteum	Peptide
	Human somatomammotropin	Probably helps promote development of some fetal tissues as well as mother's breasts	Peptide
	Estrogens	See actions of estrogens from ovaries	Steroid
	Progesterone	See actions of progesterone from ovaries	Steroid
Kidney	Renin	Catalyzes conversion of angiotensinogen to angiotensin I (acts as enzyme)	Peptide
	1,25-Dihydroxycholecalciferol	Increases intestinal absorption of calcium and bone mineralization	Steroid
	Erythropoietin	Increases erythrocyte production	Peptide
Heart	Atrial natriuretic peptide (ANP)	Increases sodium excretion by kidneys, reduces blood pressure	Peptide
Stomach	Gastrin	Stimulates HCl secretion by parietal cells	Peptide
Small intestine	Secretin	Stimulates pancreatic acinar cells to release bicarbonate and water	Peptide
	Cholecystokinin (CCK)	Stimulates gallbladder contraction and release of pancreatic enzymes	Peptide
Adipocytes	Leptin	Inhibits appetite, stimulates thermogenesis	Peptide

From Guyton, A. C., & Hall, J. E. (2006). *Textbook of medical physiology* (11th ed.). Philadelphia: Saunders, p. 907.

The stress response occurs in the hypothalamic-pituitary-adrenal (HPA) axis. When the body is stressed, the neural and hormonal input into the hypothalamus increases. Corticotropin-releasing factor is then secreted into the hypothalamic-hypophyseal portal tract and transmitted to the anterior pituitary gland. ACTH release is stimulated, causing a twofold to sevenfold increase in plasma cortisol concentration, which in turn regulates the metabolic response of the stressed person.

Gonads

The gonads serve two basic functions: they secrete sex steroids (predominantly testosterone from the testes and estradiol and progesterone from the ovaries) and they produce gametes (sperm and ova). In general, production of the sex steroids from the gonads is stimulated by the secretion of LH from the pituitary, and production of gametes is stimulated by FSH, also secreted from the pituitary. Growth hormone is essential for normal

spermatogenesis. Sex steroids are responsible for the establishment and maintenance of secondary sex characteristics, whereas gametes are responsible for reproduction (Guyton & Hall, 2006).

Pancreas

The two major types of tissue that make up the pancreas are the acini and the islets of Langerhans. Acini secrete digestive juices into the duodenum. About 2% of the glandular tissue of the pancreas consists of the islets of Langerhans, which are scattered throughout. The islets secrete two polypeptide hormones—insulin and glucagon. Alpha, beta, delta, PP, and D1 cells are found in the islets. The alpha cells form glucagon, and the beta cells form insulin. The delta cells produce somatostatin, which is thought to inhibit the secretion of glucagon and insulin (Guyton & Hall, 2006). PP cells secrete pancreatic polypeptide, which inhibits gallbladder contraction and the release of pancreatic enzymes, but further

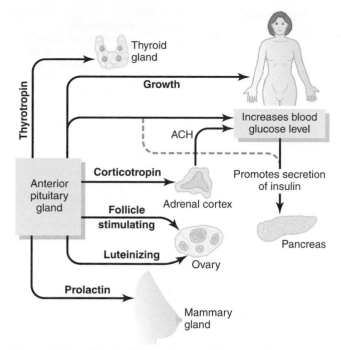

Figure 17-2 Metabolic functions of the anterior pituitary hormones. *ACH*, Adrenal corticosteroid hormones. (Used with permission from Guyton, A. C., & Hall, J. E. [2006]. *Textbook of medical physiology* [11th ed.]. Philadelphia: Saunders.)

biological function is not clear (Vinik, 2004). Little is known about D1 cells.

Pineal Gland

The pineal gland once was considered a vestigial organ (Zahid, 2003). We now understand that it produces melatonin—a hormone that plays an important role in the regulation of circadian rhythms (Wu & Swaab, 2005). Interest in the pineal gland has led to studies linking it to circadian rhythm, sleep disorders, immunocompetence, antioxidant protection, and specific age-related neurodegenerative disorders (Karasek, 2004).

NORMAL CHANGES IN STRUCTURE AND FUNCTION

The study of neuroendocrine aging, like that of other systems, is complicated by confounding factors. The complex interdependence of neural and hormonal factors has been the focus of considerable study aimed at understanding why and how aging occurs.

Pituitary Gland

The pituitary gland reaches maximum size during middle age and then gradually diminishes. There is a decrease in cell mass and weight because of atrophy,

fibrosis, and decreased vascularity. The secretion of growth hormone declines by about 15% per decade after age 30. The decrease in GH may be related to increased hypothalamic somatostatin release or decreased GHRH secretion. It also is possible that somatotrophs are less responsive to GHRH because of decreased receptors or declining signal transduction mechanisms. Circulating levels of insulin-like growth factor (IGF), which is a peripheral mediator of the somatic effects of GH, also decline. The effects of growth hormone deficiency include decreased lean body mass, decreased bone density, and increased fat mass. Because these changes are commonly seen in "normal" aging, there is interest in the potential for growth hormone as an anti-aging agent. At this time, GH therapy is recommended only for persons with pituitary disease who have a clear GH deficiency (Belchetz & Hammond, 2003; Davies, 2003).

In humans, circulating IGF-I peaks in mid-adolescence and then gradually decreases through the remaining years. The mean basal concentration of IGF-I is similar among young and older men although the total GH peak area and the amplitude of the peaks are lower in older men. Notably, the plasma concentrations of IGF-I are lower in older men and women than in younger persons. This may indicate older persons do not achieve the threshold concentration of GH needed to stimulate IGF-I release. There also is some evidence that the sensitivity of somatotrophs to GHRH stimulation declines with age (Davies, 2003). The regulation of the GH/IGF-I pathway and changes with age are depicted in Figure 17-3.

The prevalence of pituitary tumors decreases with age with a few exceptions. Lesions that occur more often in older persons are nonfunctioning adenomas, pituitary metastases, and pituitary incidentalomas (small adenomas without clinical sequelae) that usually are found incidentally and require no intervention (Belchetz & Hammond, 2003).

Thyroid Gland

It once was believed that the thyroid gland mass declined considerably with aging. However, newer data based on ultrasounds in healthy older persons have revealed little change in the size of the gland. Changes that commonly are found but are not universal are progressive fibrosis, the appearance of lymphocytes, and reduced amount of colloid. Even in the presence of these changes, thyroid function appears not to change significantly. Possibly because of age-related changes in the mechanisms that control TSH release, the serum concentration of TSH shows less circadian variation in older men than younger men. The release of T_3 and T_4 after TSH stimulation appears to be normal. Whereas the young adult produces 80 micrograms of T_4 and 30

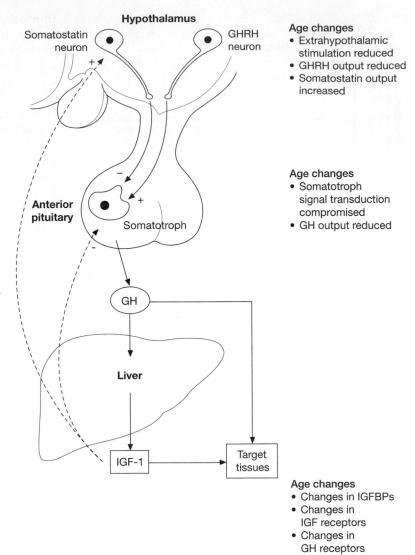

Hypothalamus

Somatostatin neuron

GHRH neuron

Age changes
- Extrahypothalamic stimulation reduced
- GHRH output reduced
- Somatostatin output increased

Anterior pituitary

Somatotroph

Age changes
- Somatotroph signal transduction compromised
- GH output reduced

GH

Liver

IGF-1

Target tissues

Age changes
- Changes in IGFBPs
- Changes in IGF receptors
- Changes in GH receptors

Figure 17-3 Regulation of the GH/IGF-I pathway. (Used with permission from Tallis, R. C., & Fillit, H. M. [Eds.] [2003]. *Brocklehurst's textbook of geriatric medicine and gerontology* [6th ed.]. Edinburgh: Churchill Livingstone.)

micrograms of T_3 daily, the older person produces 60 micrograms and 20 micrograms, respectively. Thyroid binding globulin, the primary thyroid hormone transport protein, appears unaffected by age. The circulating levels of T_3 and T_4 should remain constant with aging. Studies of centenarians have shown no difference in serum-free T_4 levels, but a reduction in TSH and serum-free T_3 concentrations (Miller, 2005).

Parathyroid Glands

With age, the serum concentration of PTH increases by about 30%, a change that coincides with a decline in vitamin D levels in the serum. Inadequate vitamin D, which is believed to be common among older adults, triggers a secondary increase in PTH concentration that stimulates bone resorption, possibly leading to osteoporosis (Hammond & Belchetz, 2003; Simon, Leboff, Wright, & Glowacki, 2002).

Numerous studies are adding to our understanding of parathyroid activity and calcium homeostasis in older persons. In a study of institutionalized older adults, Deplas and colleagues found vitamin D deficiency and low calcium intake to be common. Secondary hyperparathyroidism was present in the individuals with the lowest bone mineral density values (Deplas, Debiais, Alcalay, Bontoux, & Thomas, 2004). The 2004 study of Dawson-Hughes of the relationships among PTH levels, bone mineral density, and serum vitamin D levels found that higher PTH levels were associated with lower bone mineral density, and higher serum levels of vitamin D were associated with lower levels of parathyroid hormone. When the serum concentration of vitamin D increased to 75 to 80 nmol/L, the PTH concentration declined, the rate of bone loss decreased, and fracture rates declined. Another study determined that serum PTH concentration began to increase when serum 25-hydroxyvitamin D concentration fell below

80 nmol/L. Body weight and age had a positive relationship to PTH, and in turn PTH had a negative relationship to serum-ionized calcium (Need, O'Loughlin, Morris, Horowitz, & Nordin, 2004). Campbell, Fleet, Hall, & Carnell (2004) assessed the effects of short-term (12 to 14 days) low-protein diets on serum PTH concentration. Although urinary total nitrogen excretion and BUN levels fell progressively as the protein intake decreased, PTH hormone did not increase.

Russo de Boland (2004) found that the response of intestinal cells to PTH was impaired because of changes in parathyroid binding sites. Although most studies have examined bone mass in women, the MINOS study (Szulc, Munoz, Marchand, Chapuy, & Delmas, 2003) looked at the role of vitamin D and PTH in the regulation of bone turnover and bone mass in men aged 19 to 85 years. In this sample, "elderly" men (>55 years) demonstrated seasonal variation: PTH levels and bone resorption markers were highest in winter when the vitamin D level was lowest. Both 25-hydroxyvitamin D and PTH were predictive of bone mineral content and cortical thickness of the femoral neck. Not surprisingly, men with vertebral deformities were found to have lower vitamin D levels, higher PTH levels, and slightly elevated markers of bone resorption (Szulc et al., 2003). However, another study failed to demonstrate an increase in a bone resorption marker in response to suppression of PTH (Kennel, Riggs, Achenbach, Oberg, & Khosla, 2003). As part of the Longitudinal Aging Study Amsterdam, investigators examined the relationships between vitamin D and PTH levels and sarcopenia (loss of muscle mass) in persons aged 65 and older. Individuals with baseline levels of vitamin D below 25 nmol/L and those with elevated PTH levels were significantly more likely to experience sarcopenia (Visser, Deeg, & Lips, 2003).

An interesting study compared the relationships between 25-hydroxyvitamin D and PTH concentrations in individuals aged 19 to 97 years. The mean PTH concentration increased after age 70 although older persons with vitamin D concentrations greater than 100 nmol/L had PTH levels similar to those of younger persons with vitamin D levels of 70 nmol/L. Creatinine concentration correlated with PTH concentration only in older persons. The investigators concluded that older adults need more vitamin D to yield the 25-hydroxyvitamin levels necessary to overcome the hyperparathyroidism associated with their declining renal function (Vieth, Ladak, & Walfish, 2003).

A study to determine the effects of age on calcium absorption in postmenopausal women confirmed that absorption in women older than 75 years was 28% lower than in younger women. The investigators noted that the decline could be due to a decrease in active calcium transport or diffusion (Nordin, Need, Morris, O'Loughlin, & Horowitz, 2004).

Adrenal Glands

Sufficient evidence exists that basal, circadian, and stimulated cortisol secretion is intact in the older adult. The catabolism of cortisol decreases, but is balanced by a reduction in cortisol production. Immunosenescence has been compared with the effects of chronic stress or glucocorticoid (GC) therapy. Compared with younger persons, healthy older adults have been found to be more stressed and show activation of the HPA axis. It has been noted that immunosenescence may be related to both psychological distress and stress hormones, and that older persons are at particular risk of stress-related pathology because of altered GC-immune signaling. The neuroendocrine hypothesis of immunosenescence attributes the immunological changes to an increase in the cortisol/DHEA ratio (Bauer, 2005). A study of stress hormones and human memory function across the life span determined that long-term exposure to high endogenous levels of glucocorticoids was associated with memory impairment in older adults (Lupien et al., 2005). Using dexamethasone suppression tests, researchers found that frail institutionalized older persons had a deficient feedback regulation of the HPA axis when compared with the responses of independent community-dwelling older persons (Carvalhaes-Neto, Huayllas, Ramos, Cendoroglo, & Kater, 2003). In lab studies, peripheral lymphocytes from older persons responded poorly to glucocorticoid treatment (Bauer, 2005).

Androgen synthesis by the adrenal cortex begins around age 7 and declines through the adult years. The exact function of these androgens other than affecting body hair is uncertain. It is possible that one of these hormones (dehydroepiandrosterone [DHEA]) has an immunomodulatory and antioncogenic action (Belchetz & Hammond, 2003). A decline in adrenal androgens has been found to coincide with diminution of the zona reticularis of the adrenal cortex. The plasma levels of the adrenal steroids DHEA and DHEA-S decline markedly with aging. Researchers are studying the role of these steroids for possible beneficial antiaging effects including immune system stimulation and antidiabetes, antiatherosclerosis, antidementia, antiobesity, and antiosteoporosis effects (Dharia & Parker, 2004; Nawata et al., 2004). In one study, DHEA replacement in older adults increased natural killer cell cytotoxicity and reportedly dramatically improved the sense of physical and psychological well-being (Morales, Nolan, Nelson, & Yen, 1994, cited in Belchetz & Hammond, 2003).

Aldosterone secretion appears to be well preserved in older age (Belchetz & Hammond, 2003). The renin-angiotensin system (RAS) is the primary regulator of aldosterone. Angiotensin II stimulates the secretion of aldosterone from the adrenal cortex, which results in the renal conservation of sodium and loss of potassium.

Some investigators believe the RAS has a significant protective effect on the function and structure of the cardiovascular system, kidneys, and brain. This conclusion is based on animal studies in which chronic long-term inhibition of the RAS prevented the common harmful effects of aging in these structures in rats and mice (Basso et al., 2005; Ferder, Inserra, & Basso, 2002). RAS inhibition was achieved with either an angiotensin converting enzyme inhibitor or an angiotensin II receptor antagonist. The benefits were attributed not only to lowered arterial blood pressure but also to antioxidant effects that preserved mitochondrial function (de Cavanagh, Piotrkowski, & Fraga, 2004).

Pancreas

Histological changes in the pancreas of the older adult are minimal. Ultrasonography commonly reveals high echogenicity. The pancreatic duct often appears dilated in persons over age 70. The flow rate of pancreatic enzymes and bicarbonate slows (Tepper & Katz, 2003).

The prevalence of glucose intolerance and type 2 diabetes increases with age. Insulin resistance may accompany age-related glucose intolerance. Defects in insulin secretion have been demonstrated even after controlling for insulin sensitivity (Chang & Halter, 2003; Yates & Laing, 2002). In glucose-tolerant non-Hispanic whites, non-Hispanic blacks, and Hispanics, beta cell function has been found to decline about 1% each year. This is believed to account for the positive correlation between age and glycosylated hemoglobin (HbAIC) and fasting glucose concentrations, and the negative correlation between age and beta cell function (Chiu, Martinez, & Chu, 2005). In a review of the literature, Elahi and colleagues concluded that the age-related decline in insulin production remains even after adjustments for differences in adiposity, fat distribution, and physical activity (Elahi et al., 2002). A study of the impact of intraabdominal fat and age on insulin sensitivity and beta cell function revealed a relationship between insulin sensitivity and intraabdominal fat, but not age. Both intraabdominal fat and age were correlated with the index used to assess beta call function (Utzschneider et al., 2004). Animal studies of beta cell regeneration showed that the only source of new beta cells was replication of beta cells. No new cells were contributed by stem cells or other non-beta cells (Bock, 2004).

Pineal Gland

Like many other hormones, melatonin production declines through the adult years. Despite a decline in melatonin levels and altered circadian profile, studies of pineal size, weight, volume, and density have not revealed age-related changes (Golan, Torres, Staskiewicz, Opielak, & Maciejewski, 2002). Comparisons of plasma melatonin levels in healthy young, healthy old, and demented old persons demonstrated a flattened circadian profile in all older persons. However, the decline in circadian amplitude was especially pronounced in older persons with dementia (Magri et al., 2004; Skene & Swaab, 2003). The production of melatonin has been found to be disrupted with aging, which may account for the increasing prevalence of sleep disturbances. Investigators also believe melatonin acts as an antioxidant and a neuroprotector. For that reason, its relationship to Alzheimer's disease is under study (Karasek, 2004). Melatonin has been promoted as a rejuvenating agent; however, sufficient data do not exist proving that it has a role in extending normal longevity (Karasek, 2004).

Changes in the Female Reproductive System

Menopause (the cessation of menses) is just one facet of the larger climacteric, which is the long transition phase extending many years before and after the last menstrual event. The climacteric encompasses endocrine, somatic, and psychological changes and involves an intricate relationship between the ovarian and hypothalamic-pituitary factors. It begins at approximately age 40 with gradually decreasing ovarian sensitivity to gonadotropins and reduced estrogen production. The circulating level of FSH rises gradually followed by an increase in LH concentration and a decline in estradiol concentration. Eventually, the amount of estradiol produced is insufficient to stimulate the endometrium and amenorrhea ensues. FSH and LH levels continue to rise until they peak 3 to 5 years after menopause, and then gradually decline. Whereas ovarian production of estradiol and progesterone decreases after menopause, the ovaries continue to produce androstenedione and testosterone. Estrone is produced from androstenedione and is subsequently converted to estradiol. The bulk of androstenedione is produced by the adrenal cortex. Estradiol continues to play an important role in maintaining hormone-dependent tissues (Brown & Cooper, 2003; Hall, 2004).

The estrogen deficiency that accompanies menopause produces changes in the vulva, vagina, cervix, uterus, fallopian tubes, ovaries, and pelvic and supportive ligaments and tissue. After menopause, the ovary and myometrium shrink and become sclerotic. The size of the uterus is greatly reduced, and the cervix is more even with the vaginal vault. Recession of the squamocolumnar junction can cause stenosis of the external os. Atrophy of subcutaneous fat, epithelium, and associated glands and loss of elasticity occur in the entire pelvic region. Pelvic floor weakness is related to diminished collagen and nerve damage associated with parturition and prolapse. Atrophy of the vaginal epithelium causes the vaginal walls to thin, and vaginal secretions become more alkaline. These changes make the vaginal tissues more vulnerable to infections. Genital sensation declines, indicating deterioration of neurological function (Brown & Cooper, 2003; Connell et al., 2005).

Neurodegenerative changes with aging are hypothesized to result from dysregulation of the hypothalamic-pituitary-gonadal axis that occurs with menopause and andropause (Atwood et al., 2005). Weiss and colleagues also examined the relationship between the hypothalamic-pituitary response to estrogen feedback and the onset of menopause. Study findings provided evidence of hypothalamic-pituitary insensitivity to estrogen in aging perimenopausal women (Weiss, Skurnick, Goldsmith, Santoro, & Park, 2004).

Some research has suggested that replacement of sex hormones might prevent Alzheimer's disease. Bhavnani (2003) claims that the neurotoxic effects of oxidized low-density lipoprotein (LDL) and glutamate can be inhibited by estrogens, particularly the ring B unsaturated estrogens, which are among the types found in conjugated equine estrogens. In a longitudinal study of menopause and cognitive decline, nulliparous women and women who experienced menopause later in life had significantly less cognitive decline (McLay, Maki, & Lyketsos, 2003).

Breast tissue becomes involuted, accompanied by a decrease in the number of mammary ducts and a disappearance of the alveoli. Atrophy of the urogenital tract can lead to excessive dryness, bleeding, inflammation and infections, and atrophic and hypertrophic lesions. These may be treated with estrogen, antimicrobials, corticosteroids, and antipruritics (Barzel, 1989; Brown & Cooper, 2003).

The inhibin hypothesis proposes that the menopausal transition is initiated by the loss of inhibin negative feedback on FSH as a result of diminished follicular reserve (Santoro et al., 2004).

Systemic Effects of Menopause. Numerous systemic effects have been attributed to menopause. Hormonal fluctuations during the menopausal transition may account for vasomotor symptoms, vaginal dryness, breast tenderness, sleep disturbances, and premenstrual dysphoria. Signs of the menopausal transition are abnormal uterine bleeding, diminishing bone mineral density, increased body mass index, increased central adiposity, and worsening lipid profile (Guthrie et al., 2004; Zapantis & Santoro, 2003). The skin is affected significantly by menopause. Diminished estrogen levels influence dermal cellular metabolism, which leads to changes in collagen content, water content, and altered concentration of glycosaminoglycans. The result of these changes is loss of elasticity and skin strength that leads to wrinkling. Hair loss sometimes occurs at the beginning of menopause (Raine-Fenning, Brincat, &

Muscat-Baron, 2003). Perimenopausal mood disorders may be triggered in vulnerable women by loss of the modulating effects of estrogen and progesterone (Steiner, Dunn, & Born, 2003). Sleep disorders in the perimenopausal period may be related to hot flashes, mood disorders, and an increase in sleep-disordered breathing (Moline, Broch, Zak, & Gross, 2003).

Research on the topic of menopausal symptoms is abundant. The Menopause Symptom List (MSL) classifies symptoms as psychological, somatic-sensory, somatic-sleep, and vasomotor (Kalpakjian, Toussaint, Quint, & Reame, 2005). In addition to the common vasomotor symptoms, mood and sleep disturbances, and bone demineralization, investigators have studied possible relationships between menopause and oral dryness, nocturia, and effects on tears and intraocular pressure. Among Swedish women in the menopausal transition, 17.8% reported oral dryness at baseline. This figure increased steadily to 34.5% 10 years or more postmenopause and was independent of drug therapy. Nocturia was an independent correlate of oral dryness (Asplund & Aberg, 2005). Chinese investigators sought to determine whether the increased prevalence of nocturia in older women is age-related or a symptom of the menopausal transition. Whereas nocturia was significantly higher in older age-groups, it was not related to perimenopausal stage (Lin, Ng, Chen, Hu, & Chen, 2005). The structure and function of the larynx are affected by the sex hormones (Amir & Biron-Shental, 2004). Compared with healthy age-matched women who still are menstruating, menopausal women have been found to have decreased tear volume and quality, increased intraocular pressure (IOP), and increased ocular blood flow. In one study, the initiation of hormone replacement therapy (HRT) was accompanied by increased tear volume and quality, decreased IOP, and decreased peak systolic velocity and resistivity index in some retrobulbar arteries (Altintas, Caglar, Yuksel, Demirci, & Karabas, 2004).

A 9-year study of women initially aged 45 to 55 years described the natural history of the menopausal transition. Increased body weight accompanied by increased free testosterone concentration and decreased estradiol concentration was associated with increased risk for cardiovascular disease (CVD). Symptoms and stressors during this period increased depression (Guthrie et al., 2004). The low prevalence of cardiovascular disease in premenopausal women suggests that endogenous estrogens protect the cardiovascular system. However, two large, randomized clinical trials have failed to demonstrate the same benefit from exogenous estrogen in older women (Dubey, Imthurn, Barton, & Jackson, 2005).

HOT FLASHES. Hot flashes, the most common symptom of menopause, are characterized by increased perspiration, increased skin blood flow or vasodilation, and a 10% to 15% increase in pulse rate. They may be triggered by acute estrogen withdrawal, surges in LH levels, small increases in core body temperature in a narrowed thermoneutral zone, or increased central noradrenergic activation (Freedman, 2005). The velocity of capillary blood flow is reduced, and profound vasodilation in the dermal papillae accounts for flushing. About one third of women experience hot flashes before they become aware of any changes in their menstrual cycles and before serum estrogen levels change. In general, hot flashes persist from 6 months to 2 years, although they are more persistent is some individuals. Most women can identify a recurring pattern. The frequency typically peaks in the early evening, which follows a peak in core body temperature (North American Menopause Society, 2004). Differences in the incidence of hot flashes have been found among racial and ethnic groups in the United States, with the highest rates among African Americans (45.6%) and the lowest among Japanese Americans (17.6%) (North American Menopause Society, 2004). Women who experience bilateral oophorectomy may have more acute symptoms; however, they resolve over about the same period of time as women undergoing natural menopause (North American Menopause Society, 2004).

Hot flashes have been the focus of numerous studies. Based on a study of thermoregulatory parameters in symptomatic and asymptomatic women, Freedman and Subramanian (2005) concluded that women with postmenopausal hot flashes had lower sweating thresholds and higher sweat rates. Smoking is a known risk for hot flashes; hormone levels, body size, tubal ligation, surgical menopause, and race/ethnicity also have been found in some studies to increase risk (Whiteman, Staropoli, Benedict, Borgeest, & Flaws, 2003). Survey data from Asian American women revealed their most common menopausal symptoms as worrying about the body, aches in the back of the neck and skull, and weight gain. Most of these women attributed their symptoms to aging, and elected not to pursue treatment (Im & Chee, 2005).

Variables Affecting the Menopausal Experience.
Data from the SWAN study revealed differences in menstrual cycle alterations in the early menopausal transition based on body size and ethnicity. Women with a body mass index (BMI) less than 25 kg/m^2 had shorter menstrual cycles and higher total-cycle LH, FSH, and pregnanediol glucuronide levels than heavier women. Also, women of Chinese and Japanese ethnicity had lower total-cycle estradiol levels (Santoro et al., 2004). It appears that high body mass index and low socioeconomic status increase the burden of morbidity during the menopausal transition (Santoro & Chervenak, 2004). This is contrary to long-held beliefs that thin women are most likely to experience

significant symptoms. A large study of health functioning during the menopausal transition found that women who reported the most severe menopausal symptoms were those who experienced the greatest declines in functioning (Kumari, Stafford, & Marmot, 2005).

Quality of Life.
In a 2-year study of women (mean age 46), factors that reportedly reduced quality of life included body pain, emotional role limits, physical function role limits, social role function, and vitality. Other symptoms that were reported during the study period were genitourinary symptoms, psychological symptoms, vasomotor symptoms, and poor sleep quality (Bair et al., 2005). Another study that also used the SF-36 (a 36-item, short-form health survey) to assess quality of life found a strong relationship between all aspects of health functioning and menopausal symptoms (Kumari, Stafford, & Marmot, 2005).

Osteoporosis.
An evaluation of bone-related biochemical variables at menopause reported a rise in calculated serum ionized calcium levels without a decrease in PTH levels, which reflects a change in the PTH setpoint. The intestinal absorption of calcium declines as does the reabsorption in the renal tubules, both attributed to the effects of estrogen deficiency on receptor sites in the intestines and the kidneys (Nordin et al., 2004). A study of elite runners compared bone mineral density (BMD) in the hip and spine before, during, and after menopause. Those who remained estrogenized throughout the study had no bone loss at any site. Postmenopausal runners who were not taking HRT had a decline in BMD from the femoral neck and spine at the expected rate. The rate of BMD loss in the femoral trochanter was less than average; calcaneus measures were close to those of young women (Tomkinson, Gibson, Lunt, Harries, & Reeve, 2003).

It has been hypothesized that the duration of the fertile period of a woman's life might predict menopausal changes in bone density. However, when Gerdhem & Obrant (2004) assessed bone mineral density among women age 75 or older, no relationship was found between BMD and the age at menarche, age at menopause, or the length of the fertile period.

The increased bone remodeling rate following menopause contributes to the increased risk for fractures (Recker, Lappe, Davies, & Heaney, 2004). Osteoporosis also has been related to oral health; therefore women presenting with oral disease should be evaluated for osteoporosis (Chohayeb, 2004).

The use of HRT appears to protect menopausal women against osteoporosis. Recent reports that the health risks posed by HRT may outweigh the benefits have resulted in many women discontinuing HRT. Researchers are seeking to determine whether lower HRT dosage might relieve menopausal symptoms and protect bone without other significant risks (Mirza & Prestwood, 2004). For a more comprehensive discussion of osteoporosis, see Chapter 11.

Female Sexual Functioning.

Components of female sexual function are desire, arousal, lubrication, and orgasm. Although some women do report changes in libido, menopause is most likely not the cause. Changes associated with menopause that may affect sexuality include diminished vaginal lubrication; changes in the vascular and urogenital systems; alterations in mood, sleep, and cognitive function; changes in health status; medications; changes in the partner relationship, social status, and cultural attitudes toward older women. Physical conditions that may affect sexual function include cardiac disease, stroke, diabetes mellitus, arthritis, recurrent cystitis and urethritis, Parkinson's disease, and pulmonary disease. In addition, women who have had traumatic injuries or surgical procedures, such as hysterectomies, mastectomies, and ostomies, may have changes in body image that affect sexual interest and enjoyment. Problems related to estrogen deficiency can be improved with estrogen supplementation, vaginal lubricants, and moisturizers (Bachmann & Leiblum, 2004). Medical conditions and interventions that can affect sexual dysfunction are listed in Tables 17-2 and 17-3.

The postmenopausal woman is capable of full sexual performance and pleasure with regular exposure to effective stimulation (Masters & Johnson, 1966). Many women have heightened sexual interest because of the lessened fear of pregnancy, more leisure time, and fewer distractions—such as children—at home. Although the testosterone level does not rise, its effect is probably less mitigated by estrogen than in the premenopausal period. Masters & Johnson (1966) assembled baseline data in their classic work. They found that sexual responses in older women, as in older men, are characterized by a gradual decrease in the duration and intensity of the response. However, continuation of sexual activity throughout the climacteric may delay and prevent some of the atrophic vaginal changes associated with aging, including decreased lubrication and accompanying discomfort. Table 17-4 summarizes the changes in sexual response in aging women.

Survey data from Colombian-born pre- and postmenopausal women aged 40 to 62 revealed sexual dysfunction to be most commonly related to desire or arousal. When the pre- and postmenopausal groups were compared, menopause was associated only with changes in lubrication and pain. Postmenopausal women on HRT reported a higher level of sexual satisfaction than those not taking HRT. However, HRT did not improve desire or arousal (Gonzalez, Viafara, Caba, & Molina, 2004). When premenopausal, perimenopausal, and postmenopausal women were compared, investigators in one study found no differences in depression and

Table 17-2 Effects of Surgery on Sexuality

Surgical Procedure	Effect on Sexuality
Hysterectomy	Need to refrain from sexual activity during healing (6-8 weeks after surgery); depression; possible reduction in sensation during orgasm
Mastectomy	Emotional reactions such as depression; loss of sexual desire caused by emotional reactions of patient and partner
Prostatectomy	Need to refrain from sexual activity during healing (6 weeks); possible impotence because of surgery (nerve-sparing techniques help avoid this effect in some cases); possible psychogenic impotence
Orchiectomy	Impotence is common
Colostomy and ileostomy	Emotional reactions that can affect desire and potency (participation in ostomy clubs is recommended)
Rectal cancer surgery	Impotence is common

From Butler, R. N., & Lewis, M. I. (2003). Sexuality. In R. C. Tallis & H. M. Fillit (Eds.), *Brocklehurst's textbook of geriatric medicine and gerontology* (6th ed.). Edinburgh: Churchill Livingstone, pp. 1407-1412.

anxiety among the three groups. However, high scores on measures of depression and anxiety were related to sexuality. Women with high depression scores reported the lowest frequency of sexual intercourse. Painful intercourse was more common among those with high anxiety scores, and there was a decline in frequency of sexual intercourse, sexual desire, and orgasm (Danaci, Oruc, Adiguzel, Yildirim, & Aydemir, 2003).

Symptom Management.

Only 20% to 30% of all older women seek medical attention for symptoms associated with menopause. This may be explained by variations in levels of endogenous estrogens or by the perceptions of many women that menopausal symptoms are expected and do not require medical intervention.

At this time, only HRT (hormone replacement therapy with both estrogen and progesterone) has been approved by the FDA for treatment of menopausal symptoms. The lowest effective dose for the shortest duration is recommended (Sikon & Thacker, 2004). For many years estrogen therapy was routinely prescribed to relieve menopausal symptoms including hot flashes and atrophic vaginitis, to maintain bone density, and (it was believed)

Table 17-3 *Effects of Medical Conditions on Sexuality*

Medical Condition	Effect on Sexuality	Treatment
Arthritis	Sexual desire usually unaffected, but disability resulting from osteoarthritis and rheumatoid arthritis may interfere with performance	Trying sexual positions that do not aggravate joint pain; planning sexual activity for times of day when pain and stiffness are diminished
Chronic emphysema and bronchitis	Shortness of breath hinders physical activity, including sex	Rest; supplemental oxygen
Chronic prostatitis	Pain may diminish sexual desire	Antibiotics; warm sitz baths, prostatic massage; Kegel exercises
Chronic renal disease	Impotence, possibly with anxiety and depression	Dialysis; psychotherapy for underlying emotional problems; kidney transplantation may restore sexual capacity
Diabetes mellitus	Impotence is common	Very tight control of diabetes may restore potency
HEART AND VASCULAR DISEASE		
Myocardial infarction	8-14-week recuperation period recommended before resuming sexual intercourse; depression and anti-depressant drugs may reduce libido and capacity; fear of causing another heart attack if patient resumes sexual activity	Reassurance from doctor about safety of sexual activity; exercise programs to improve cardiac function
Heart failure	Sexual dysfunction because of physical symptoms or medications; 2-3-week recovery period advised before resuming sex in cases of pulmonary edema	Reassurance from doctor about safety of sexual activity for patients with effectively managed heart failure; exercise programs to improve cardiac function
Coronary bypass surgery	4 weeks or more of abstinence recommended before resuming sexual intercourse	Alternatives such as self-stimulation or masturbation can usually be started earlier in recovery period; exercise programs to improve cardiac function
Pelvic steal syndrome	Example of vascular impotence—male loses erection as soon as he enters his partner and begins pelvic thrusting (as a result of gravity's redirecting blood supply away from pelvis)	Changing position may help (man should lie on his back or side)
Hypertension	Incidence of impotence in untreated male hypertensive patients is about 15%; effects on women not established	Choose hypertensive drugs that do not impair sexual response
Parkinson's disease	Lack of sexual desire in both men and women; impotence in men	Levodopa can improve sex drive and performance in some men for a limited period
Peyronie's disease	Intercourse is painful for many men with disease; penetration may be difficult or impossible when penis is angled too sharply	Psychotherapy to help patient adjust to changes in enis; symptoms occasionally disappear spontaneously; surgery helps in some cases
Stress incontinence	Sexual dysfunction has been reported in up to 50% of women with this condition	Solving underlying problem may help; Kegel exercises to strengthen muscles supporting bladder; estrogen taken orally or locally to increase firmness of vaginal lining; biofeedback training
Stroke	Sexual desire may not be impaired, but sexual performance likely to be affected (e.g., male erectile dysfunction because of either physical or psychological reasons, anesthetic areas, and/or physical limitations because of paralysis)	Mechanical adjustments to assist positioning necessary for sexual activities; treatments for impotence

From Butler, R. N., & Lewis, M. I. (2003). Sexuality. In R. C. Tallis & H. M. Fillit (Eds.), *Brocklehurst's textbook of geriatric medicine and gerontology* (6th ed.). Edinburgh: Churchill Livingstone, pp. 1407-1412.

Table 17-4 *Phase-Specific Changes in the Sexual Response Cycle of Aging Women*

Target Tissue	Excitement	Plateau	Orgasm	Resolution
	Phase of Sexual Response			
Breast	Vasocongestive increase in size less pronounced, especially in more pendulous breasts	Engorgement of areola less intense	—	Loss of nipple erection slowed
Skin	Sex flush does not occur as frequently	Sex flush does not occur as frequently	—	—
Muscle	Degree of myotonia decreases with age	Degree of myotonia decreases with age	—	—
Urethra and urinary bladder	—	—	Minimal distention of meatus*	—
Rectum	—	—	Contraction of rectal sphincter only with severe tension levels	—
Clitoris	—	—	—	Retracts rapidly; tumescence lost rapidly
Labia majora	No women past age 51 demonstrates flattening, separation, and elevation of labia majora	—	—	—
Labia minora	Vasocongestion reduced	Labial color change (sex skin) usually pathognomonic of orgasm decreases in frequency among women ≥61 years of age	—	—
Bartholin's glands	—	Reduction in amount of secretions and activity, especially among postmenopausal women	—	—
Vagina	Rate and amount of vaginal lubrication decreased; lubrication occurs 1 to 3 minutes after stimulation; vaginal expansion in breadth and width decreases	Inner two thirds of vagina may still be expanding during this phase; vasocongestion of orgasmic platform reduced in intensity	Postmenopausal orgasmic platform contracts 3 to 5 times versus 5 to 10 times in younger women	Rapid involution and loss of vasocongestion
Cervix	—	—	—	Dilation of cervix not noted
Uterus	Uterine elevation and tenting of transcervical vagina develop more slowly and are less marked	Uterine elevation and tenting of transcervical vagina develop more slowly and are less marked	Some women report painful contractions with orgasm	—

Summary of findings from Masters, W., & Johnson, V. (1966). The aging female. In *Human sexual response.* Boston: Little, Brown, pp. 233-247.
Adapted from Woods, N. F. (1978). Human sexuality and the healthy elderly. In M. Brown (Ed.), *Readings in gerontology* (2nd ed.). St. Louis: Mosby, pp. 69-87.
*Mechanical irritation of urethra and bladder may occur as a result of thinning of vagina, which minimizes protection of these structures during thrusting.

to protect against cardiovascular disease. For women whose uteruses were intact, combination estrogen-progestin therapy was recommended because the unopposed estrogen increased the risk of uterine cancer.

In 2001 and 2002, two important studies found that not only did hormone therapy not protect against heart disease, it could actually be harmful to women with existing risk factors for heart disease. A primary criticism of these conclusions was that the average ages of study participants were more than 60 years at baseline. The critics contend that these studies really did not assess the benefits of estrogen therapy for primary prevention in perimenopausal women (Smith, 2005). Nevertheless, estrogen therapy is not advised for any woman with cardiovascular disease. The Women's Health Initiative found a modest increase in the risk for breast cancer among women on combined hormone therapy, but no increase in risk for those on estrogen alone. A significant reduction in colon cancer also was found for women on combination therapy in this study (Smith, 2005).

Estrogen can be effectively administered by the oral, topical (vaginal), and transdermal routes. Although vaginal administration provides some relief from vaginitis, effective systemic absorption via this route is questionable. Among the many adverse effects of estrogen replacement therapy (ERT) are headache, nausea, mastalgia, slight impairment of glucose tolerance, hypertension, increased risk of thromboembolism, increased risk of gallbladder disease, edema, weight gain, and dermatitis. Estrogen also causes endometrial hyperplasia and contributes to the development of endometrial adenocarcinoma. Because of its inhibitory effect on the development of estrogen-induced endometrial hyperplasia, progestin should be added to the regimen for the woman who retains her uterus and who is receiving long-term ERT. Side effects of progestin therapy are mood swings, breast tenderness, and uterine bleeding (Smith, 2005). Among the contraindications to ERT are breast or genital cancer (or a family history of either), undiagnosed vaginal or uterine bleeding, active or chronic liver disease, uterine leiomyomata, history of cerebrovascular disease, thromboembolic disorders, coronary artery disease, and hypertension. Note that sometimes estrogen therapy is specifically employed for the treatment of metastatic cancer (Abrams, 2004).

Although we can reassure patients that hot flashes almost always resolve over time, the symptoms may be distressing to the individual. The severity of hot flashes is considered in selecting management strategies. Mild symptoms are treated primarily with lifestyle changes, whereas more severe symptoms may also require nonhormonal prescription drugs or hormonal drugs. The risks associated with estrogen therapy are well documented and must be taken into consideration (North American Menopause Society, 2004). A summary of The North American Menopause Society position statement on the treatment of menopause-associated vasomotor symptoms is presented in Table 17-5.

Psychosocial Considerations. Both the Heart and Estrogen/Progestin Replacement Study (HERS) and the Women's Health Initiative (WHI) found that quality of life among postmenopausal women did not improve after starting hormone therapy. The mean age of study

Table 17-5 *Management of Hot Flashes: Recommendations from the North American Menopause Society Position Statement*

Symptom Severity	Management Strategies Supported by Research	Management Strategies with Limited or No Evidence of Effectiveness
Mild	**Lifestyle-related strategies:** keep core body temperature cool, regular exercise, relaxation techniques (specifically slow, controlled diaphragmatic breathing at onset of hot flash)	**Lifestyle-related strategies:** Losing excess weight, smoking cessation **Nonallopathic therapies with some/limited evidence of effectiveness:** isoflavone found in soy and red clover; black cohosh, vitamin E, topical progesterone **Nonallopathic therapies that have not been shown to be effective:** dong quai, evening primrose oil, ginseng, acupuncture, magnet therapy
Moderate to severe	**Pharmacological therapy with evidence of significant effectiveness:** estrogen (ET), combined estrogen and progestogen (EPT), estrogen-progestin oral contraceptive **Nonhormonal prescription drugs:** Antidepressants: venlafaxine, paroxetine, fluoxetine Anticonvulsant: gabapentin Antihypertensives: clonidine and methyldopa	

Data from *Menopause: The Journal of the North American Menopause Society, 11*(1), 11-33.

participants might have been a factor in these findings (Smith, 2005).

Views of menopause are culturally influenced. A study of the knowledge and attitudes of older Pakistani women towards menopause found a range of views. Most consider menopause a normal transition rather than a medical condition requiring treatment. About 75% knew about menopause and associated symptoms, and were satisfied with the cessation of menstruation. However, only 46% were satisfied with their present sexual relations. There was a general interest in learning more about menopause (Mazhar & Gul-e-Erum, 2003).

Complementary and Alternative Therapies.

Longitudinal data from the Study of Women's Health Across the Nation (SWAN) indicated that women who used complementary and alternative therapies (CAM) also had more conventional health care contact than women who did not use CAM. The types of CAM used were classified as nutritional remedies, herbal remedies, psychological remedies, or folk medicine. At baseline, 51.4% used some type of CAM; 2 years later, the number had increased to 57.7% (Bair et al., 2005).

Breasts

Without sufficient hormonal influence, the glandular tissue of the breasts atrophies and is replaced with fibrous connective tissue. Atrophy of the fat envelope that begins in middle age is pronounced by the eighth decade. Decreasing size and elasticity cause the breasts to sag. Tissue atrophy makes palpation of lumps easier. The lactiferous ducts around the nipple feel firm and stringy. Some males develop gynecomastia because of decreased testosterone concentration (Jarvis, 2000).

Changes in the Male Reproductive System

The male reproductive system undergoes significant changes with aging. Testicular volume decreases, there is some sclerosis of the tubules, and the number of testosterone-producing Leydig and Sertoli cells decline. Spermatogenesis is somewhat impaired, so there is a decrease in the number of spermatozoa, but reproduction can take place even into very old age. Degenerative and atrophic changes occur in the epididymis, seminal vesicles, and prostate gland, with loss of epithelial cells. An increase in estrogen values increases the ratio of estrogen to testosterone. Beginning in the late third or early fourth decade, the total testosterone level declines steadily while the sex hormone binding globulin (SHBG) level rises (Allan & McLachlan, 2004; Veldhuis, Veldhuis, Keenan, & Iranmanesh, 2005). These changes result in a decrease in calculated free testosterone of 2% to 3% each year. Related factors may be relative failure of gonadotropin-releasing hormone, luteinizing hormone, and/or gonadal testosterone secretion (Veldhuis et al., 2005). There are increases in both LH and FSH, which suggests that the decline in testicular function is related to changes in the testicle rather than in regulatory structures (Allen & McLachlan, 2004; Dakouane et al., 2005; Mahmoud et al., 2003). Age-related changes in the hypothalamic-pituitary-testicular (HPT) axis are not fully understood (Allan & McLachlan, 2004). Results of numerous studies suggest that the neuroendocrine control mechanisms within the HPT axis may be altered with age. This is illustrated by the failure of aging men to respond to falling testosterone levels with a compensatory LH response (Figure 17-4).

Sexual responses normally become slower and less intense with aging. For example, erection may take longer

Figure 17-4 The different stages of male sexual function as reflected by average plasma testosterone concentrations (solid line) and sperm production (broken line) at different ages. (Modified from Griffin, J. F., & Wilson, J. D. [2006]. The testis. In P. K. Bondy & L. E. Rosenberg [Eds.], *Metabolic control and disease* [8th ed.]. Philadelphia: Saunders. From Guyton, A. C., & Hall, J. E. [2006]. *Textbook of medical physiology* [11th ed.]. Philadelphia: Saunders.)

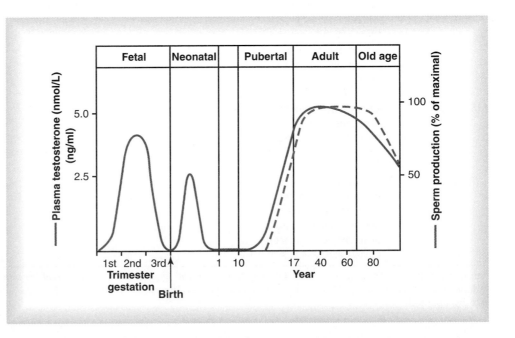

to achieve and may be less full than in younger men. Erection can be maintained for extended periods without ejaculation; however, if erection is lost without ejaculation, a secondary refractory period may result. The ejaculatory force is decreased, along with the volume of the semen. The refractory period lasts for an extended amount of time, and there is rapid loss of the erection (Table 17-6) (Brown & Cooper, 2003; Butler & Lewis, 2003).

Some sources have referred to declining testosterone production as *male menopause* or *andropause*. Others prefer that this change be referred to as *partial androgen deficiency in aging men (PADAM)* or *partial endocrine deficiency in aging men (PEDAM)*. Androgen deficiency has been linked with sleep disorders, irritability, mood change, memory loss, and a decrease in sexual interest and libido (Segal, 2003).

The prevalence of androgen deficiency in aging males is difficult to determine because of the great variety of populations studied, methods used, and lack of consistency in defining biochemical hypogonadism. To illustrate, in one study, 30% of institutionalized men ages

Table 17-6 *Phase-Specific Changes in the Sexual Response Cycle of Aging Men*

Target Tissue	Excitement	Plateau	Orgasm	Resolution
	Phase of Sexual Response			
Breast	Nipple erection less discernible	—	—	Nipple erection lost more slowly
Skin	Sex flush does not occur as frequently	Sex flush does not occur as frequently	—	—
Muscle	Degree of myotonia decreased	Degree of myotonia decreased	—	—
Rectum	—	—	Rectal sphincter contractions decreased in frequency	—
Penis	Erection may be less full; time required to achieve erection 2 to 3 times that of younger males; erection can be maintained for extended periods without ejaculation; if erection is lost without ejaculation, there may be a secondary refractory period (rare in men under 50 years)	Color change at coronal ridge not observed in men over 60 years of age	Ejaculatory force is decreased (expulsion of semen 6-12 inches versus 12-14 inches in younger men); volume of semen decreases; fewer contractions with orgasm	Refractory period lasts for extended period of time; rapid loss of erection
Scrotum	Decreased evidence of vasocongestion; less tensing of scrotal sac evident	—	—	Slow involution of vasocongestion
Testes	Testes do not elevate fully to perineum; less contractile tone of cremasteric musculature observed; rare vasocongestive increase in size	—	—	Testicular descent extremely rapid

Summary of findings from Masters, W., & Johnson, V. (1966). The aging male. In *Human sexual response.* Boston: Little, Brown, pp. 248-270. Adapted from Woods, N. F. (1978). Human sexuality and the healthy elderly. In M. Brown (Ed.), *Readings in gerontology* (2nd ed.). St. Louis: Mosby, pp. 69-87.

46 to 89 years were classified testosterone-deficient. Another study of ambulant healthy men aged 60 and older reported deficiency in only 20%. For the most accurate assessment of serum testosterone levels, blood samples should be drawn in the morning. At least two samples should be analyzed because of the variability over weeks or months. A diagnosis of hypoandrogenism is supported by an elevated LH level. However, the LH level may be within normal range when the serum testosterone concentration is borderline. The possibility of actual LH deficiency related to possible pituitary tumors or hemochromatosis should not be overlooked (Allan & McLachlan, 2004).

Decreased testosterone level has been linked with numerous variables including chronic illness, drug therapy, and obesity. Medical conditions that have been implicated are lung disease and diabetes. Serum testosterone level has been found to drop during acute illness, but returns to baseline upon recovery. Opioids and anticonvulsants also lower serum levels. Over time, it appears that obesity has the greatest impact on serum testosterone and SHBG levels. Studies assessing the effects of smoking have yielded contradictory or inconclusive results, as have studies of the effects of exercise patterns. Alcohol consumption is interesting because it initially lowers testosterone production. However, with sustained stable intake, the level does not appear to be affected (Allan & McLachlan, 2004).

Unlike the female menopause that is commonly marked by specific symptoms, symptoms of androgen deficiency tend to be nonspecific. Among the variables that have been studied are sexual and physical performance, mood/behavior, and quality of life. However, no tools yet exist that predict testosterone level based on these types of symptoms (Allan & McLachlan, 2004).

Testosterone Therapy. Testosterone replacement/supplementation therapy is being prescribed more frequently. Testosterone is available in numerous formulations including oral, buccal, transdermal, and intramuscular and subdermal implants. Special considerations for each of these are detailed in Table 17-7. The aims of drug therapy are to increase muscle mass and strength, and improve bone strength. The studies that have been conducted to evaluate the drug effects have used a variety of dosages and formulations for various durations in cohorts with a wide range of baseline testosterone levels, making generalizations difficult. The question of adverse effects of treatment also must be addressed. The cardiovascular benefits and risks are currently under study. In the male skeleton, it is likely that androgens and estradiol have independent roles in the maintenance of bone mass. One study demonstrated that estrogen prevented an increase in bone resorption markers whereas both estrogen and testosterone played a role in bone formation (Allan & McLachlan, 2004). Although large, long-term studies are needed for conclusive results, it appears that testosterone replacement therapy may decrease total fat mass and increase lean body mass. Improved sexual function appears to be limited to improved libido in men with the lowest baseline testosterone levels. Usefulness for erectile dysfunction (ED) has not been demonstrated although one study found that the response to sildenafil improved when men were also treated with transdermal testosterone (Allan & McLachlan, 2004). Cognitive benefits also require additional study. The increasing use of testosterone supplementation mandates well-designed, large, controlled studies regarding the benefits and adverse effects of testosterone therapy in older men (Morley & Perry, 2003).

Table 17-7 *Options for Testosterone Therapy*

Formulation	Comments
Oral	Testosterone undecanoate NOT recommended for first-line therapy because of inadequate androgenic effect, frequent administration, and GI side effects
Buccal	Well tolerated in young hypogonadal men; not yet evaluated in older men
Transdermal	Therapy of choice for older men Types: gel, transscrotal patches, nonscrotal patches—reservoir and nonreservoir Gel least irritating to skin; should avoid transfer to female partners Well absorbed through scrotal skin, but requires shaving skin at application site Nonscrotal reservoir may cause skin irritation that can be reduced by applying topical corticosteroid cream first (note: cream, not ointment, because it will impair absorption)
Intramuscular	Contraindicated with anticoagulant therapy
Implants	Duration of action: 6 months; caution with older men; possible coincidental diagnosis of prostate cancer

Data from Allan, C. A., & McLachlan, R. I. (2004). Age-related changes in testosterone and the role of replacement therapy in older men. *Clinical Endocrinology, 60,* 653-670.

Like any drug, exogenous testosterone has side effects that must be considered. Testosterone does stimulate the prostate, especially when supraphysiological blood levels are attained. Prostate-specific antigen (PSA), hemoglobin, and hematocrit have been found to increase, whereas both LDL and high-density lipoprotein (HDL) cholesterol decrease. Some studies have reported exacerbation of sleep apnea when the patient uses supraphysiological doses. Testosterone therapy is contraindicated in men with prostate and breast cancer (Tenover, 2003).

Erectile Dysfunction. ED, which is defined as failure in sexual encounters in at least one fourth of all attempts, may occur at any age but is more common in older men. This disorder is discussed later in this chapter.

The age-related changes in the endocrine system are summarized in Box 17-1.

 Box 17-1 *Age-Related Changes: Endocrine*

Pituitary Gland
- Atrophy, fibrosis, decreased vascularity
- Decreased secretion of growth hormone
- Decreased circulating IGF-I level

Thyroid Gland
- Adequate function even with progressive fibrosis
- Less circadian variation of serum TSH level
- Thyroid binding globulin unchanged

Parathyroid Glands
- Increased serum PTH level
- Impaired response of intestinal cells to PTH

Adrenal Glands
- Basal, circadian, and stimulated cortisol secretion intact
- Decreased cortisol catabolism balanced by reduced cortisol production
- Diminished synthesis of adrenal androgens
- Aldosterone secretion well preserved

Pancreas
- Pancreatic duct dilated
- Flow rate of pancreatic enzymes and bicarbonate slows
- Decline in insulin production

Pineal Gland
- Melatonin production declines

Female Sex Hormones
- Ovarian sensitivity to gonadotropins decreases
- Reduced estrogen production
- FSH and LH rise, then decline 3 to 5 years after menopause
- Decline in ovarian production of estradiol and progesterone
- Ovarian production of androstenedione and testosterone continues
- Ovary and myometrium shrink and become sclerotic
- Size of uterus reduced

Male Sex Hormones
- Decreased testicular volume
- Sclerosis of testicular tubules
- Decline in Leydig and Sertoli cells
- Degeneration and atrophy in epididymus, seminal vesicles, prostate
- Decrease in number of spermatozoa
- Ratio of estrogen to testosterone increases
- Increased LH and FSH levels
- Decline in testosterone level
- Rise in SHBG level
- Neuroendocrine control within hypothalamo-pituitary-testicular axis may be altered

PATHOLOGICAL CHANGES AND COMMON DISORDERS
Diabetes Mellitus (Type 2)

The American Diabetes Association (ADA) defines diabetes mellitus as a group of metabolic diseases characterized by hyperglycemia resulting from defects in insulin production, insulin action, or a combination of both. The pathogenesis of diabetes can be a result of destruction of pancreatic cells or can be caused by changes in the metabolism of glucose, fat, and protein. Until 1997 diabetes was classified according to treatment modalities under the National Diabetes Data Group (NDDG) system developed in the late 1970s. In 1995 an international committee of experts began meeting to develop a new classification system based on more recent research findings and disease etiology. The new classification system was announced in 1997. Type 1 diabetes mellitus (formerly known as insulin-dependent diabetes mellitus [IDDM] or juvenile diabetes) is defined as beta cell destruction usually resulting in absolute insulin deficiency. Type 2 diabetes mellitus (formerly known as non–insulin-dependent diabetes mellitus [NIDDM] or adult-onset diabetes) is defined as hyperglycemia resulting from one or more of the following: insulin resistance, altered hepatic glucose production, or decreased insulin secretion. Reference to age in both type 1 and type 2 diabetes was removed because of the fact that both types of diabetes can occur at any age. The third classification of diabetes is other specified types and includes causes for hyperglycemia such as pancreatitis, carcinoma, and drug-induced diabetes. The fourth classification is gestational diabetes mellitus (GDM). Impaired glucose tolerance (IGT) and impaired fasting glucose (IFG) were added to the classification system to recognize the condition where glucose levels are above normal but not within the diagnostic criteria for diabetes. IGT and IGF were previously called borderline diabetes or attributed to normal aging, but now are referred to as prediabetes (American Diabetes Association, 1997, 2005a). In 2002 the Centers for Disease Control (CDC) estimated that approximately 6.3% of persons in the United States (18.2 million) have diabetes. Most alarming is the increase in the older adult population. Current estimates of diabetes incidence among persons 65 years and older are 40% to 42% (CDC, 2005) with projections as high as 53% by 2025 and 58% by 2050 (Boyle et al., 2001; King, Aubert, & Herman, 1998). These increases can be attributed to the overall aging of the population, increased prevalence of diabetes in all age-groups, and changes in the diagnostic criteria for diabetes (Engelgau et al., 2004; Gregg, Engelgau, & Narayan, 2002). Another important statistic shows that the highest prevalence increase in the older population occurred in minority groups, especially Hispanic and Asians (McBean, Gilbertson, Li, &

Collins, 2004). The estimated direct and indirect medical expenditures attributable to diabetes reached $132 billion in 2002 with over 51.8% of direct medical expenditures being incurred by people 65 years and older (ADA, 2003).

The increased prevalence of diabetes in the older adult population can be attributed to genetic predisposition, lifestyle, and age-related changes in metabolism. Obesity and sedentary lifestyles increase the risk for developing diabetes. Diets high in fat and simple sugars also contribute to changes in carbohydrate metabolism. The Framingham cohort study reported 30% to 40% of participants 65 years and older exhibited some degree of glucose intolerance (Kannel, 2001). Age-related changes in carbohydrate metabolism are due to a combination of increased hepatic glucose production, decreased glucose-mediated insulin response, and insulin resistance. It now is thought that the actual mechanism for glucose intolerance more closely correlates to body mass. Lean older individuals with type 2 diabetes show relatively normal rates of hepatic glucose production and insulin-mediated glucose disposal but have impaired insulin release in response to elevated glucose production. On the other hand, obese older persons with type 2 diabetes show marked insulin resistance but relatively normal insulin secretion in response to elevated glucose levels (Chau & Edelman, 2001; Chau, Shumaker & Plodkowski, 2003; Meneilly & Tessier, 2001).

Diagnosis and Symptoms. The diagnostic criteria for diabetes mellitus are presented in Box 17-2.

Diagnosis of type 2 diabetes mellitus becomes difficult in older persons because the usual symptoms of polyuria, polydipsia, and polyphagia may be absent or

---

BOX 17-2 Diagnostic Criteria for Diabetes Mellitus (Excluding GDM)

Casual plasma glucose concentration ≥200 mg/dl (11.1 mmol/L) with symptoms on two occasions

Or

Fasting plasma glucose concentration ≥126 mg/dl (7.0 mmol/L) on two occasions

Or

Two-hour postprandial glucose concentration ≥200 mg/dl after a 75-g glucose load

Impaired Fasting Glucose (IFG)
Fasting plasma glucose concentration ≥100 mg/dl (6.1 mmol/L) and <126 mg/dl (11.1 mmol/L)

Impaired Glucose Tolerance (IGT)
Two-hour postprandial glucose concentration ≥140 mg/dl (7.8 mmol/L) and <200 mg/dl (11.1 mmol/L)

seen as normal age-related changes. Decreased fluid intake and altered thirst perception are common age-related changes and decrease the presence of polydipsia. Because of age-related changes in the renal threshold, glucosuria is not seen until glucose levels are very elevated. The clinical presentation of diabetes mellitus in the older person is often atypical and may include non-specific problems, such as fatigue, weight loss, confusion, incontinence, and recurrent infections. It is not uncommon for a diagnosis of diabetes to be made only after an older person is treated for complications that are associated with diabetes, such as nephropathy, peripheral vascular disease, stroke, and myocardial infarction. Nonketotic hyperosmolar coma may also be the first sign of diabetes in the very old and frail person (Chau et al., 2003; Meneilly & Tessier, 2001).

It has been believed for some time that early detection and good management of hyperglycemia could delay or prevent some of the complications of diabetes. Therefore general health screenings usually include some measure of blood glucose level. According to the Diabetes Epidemiology and Collaborative Analysis of Diagnostic Criteria in Europe (DECODE) trials, fasting plasma glucose levels are normal in over 30% of older persons with abnormal 2-hour glucose tolerance test, and these individuals are at increased risk in all-cause mortality (Chau et al., 2003). Because of this, many practitioners are evaluating fasting plasma glucose levels and 2-hour glucose tolerance tests in older patients.

Prevention of Complications.

Historically, chronic complications of diabetes have been categorized as macrovascular disease (cardiovascular, cerebrovascular, and peripheral vascular disease) and microvascular disease (retinopathy, nephropathy, and neuropathy). These complications have been well documented in the literature and affect persons with diabetes across the age-span. Other unique complications related to diabetes in older persons include neuropathic cachexia, amyotrophy, malignant otitis externa, papillary necrosis, and hypothermia (Meneilly & Tessier, 2001). According to 2002 data, diabetes is the seventh leading cause of death in the United States for persons 65 years and older. It is generally accepted that this statistic is understated because diabetes is a contributing factor for deaths attributed to cardiovascular disease and cerebrovascular disease. Older persons with diabetes have twice the death rate related to cardiovascular disease as older persons without diabetes. Diabetes increases the risk of cardiovascular disease events twofold in men and fourfold in women (Sowers, 2004). Classic studies, such as the Diabetes Control and Complications Trial (DCCT, 1998) and the UK Prospective Diabetes Study (UKPDS, 1998), clearly document the benefits of improved glycemic control.

Studies of the aging diabetes population show that diabetes is associated with declining cognitive functioning, increased falls, and impaired physical mobility. More recent clinical trials document an association between diabetes and the increased risk for developing dementia (Fontbonne, Berr, Ducimetiere, & Alperovitch, 2001; Luchsinger, Tang, Stern, Shea, & Mayeux, 2001). Diabetes also is associated with increased risk for impaired mobility and a decline in activities of daily living, such as housework, preparing meals, and managing money (Gregg et al., 2002; Schwartz et al., 2001). These added complications in older persons have a direct impact on quality of life, which in turn affects both independence of the person with diabetes as well as demands on the caregiver. In the long run, age-related complications of diabetes may become more concerning than the macrovascular and microvascular complications (Chau et al., 2003; Gregg, Engelgau, & Narayan, 2002; Knopman et al., 2001).

Management.

The goals of management for persons with diabetes mellitus are to relieve symptoms, control hyperglycemia, and prevent acute and chronic complications while maintaining quality of life and independence. The treatment is essentially the same for all age-groups: meal planning, exercise, self-monitoring, and medications when necessary. With an increasing life expectancy, prevention of complications should be the goal of treatment, and appropriate treatment goals should be individualized to include coexisting health problems. Because of treatment challenges in the older population, achieving glucose levels within normal values may not be realistic but maintaining fasting glucose levels below 126 mg/dl and 2-hour postprandial glucose levels below 200 mg/dl is possible. Although hypoglycemia is a concern and should be a consideration when treatment goals are identified, only those with a marked risk for hypoglycemia (dementia, kidney or liver damage, poor nutritional status) need higher glucose level targets (Chau & Edelman, 2001; Meneilly & Tessier, 2001).

MEAL PLANNING. Obesity is highly associated with the onset of diabetes, and weight reduction has an extremely positive effect on reducing symptoms, eliminating or reducing the need for medications, and maintaining control of diabetes. Many older persons with diabetes are overweight and would benefit from maintaining a normal weight. There also is a large population of older adults with diabetes that are malnourished, especially in long-term care facilities. This fact underscores the role a dietitian plays in establishing individualized medical nutrition therapy (Oiknine & Mooradian, 2003). Development of a proper meal plan should begin with a careful diet history and include input from the client. A meal plan must be individualized based on eating habits, motivation, and therapeutic goals. This promotes modification of eating habits without making drastic changes in the meal plan that make adherence more difficult.

The ADA still recommends a meal plan consisting of 50% to 60% calories from carbohydrates, 10% to 20% calories from protein, and less then 30% calories from fat (Franz et al., 2002). Media attention in recent years that has focused on carbohydrate types (simple or complex), glycemic index of foods, and protein levels has been confusing and controversial. Basic principles regarding carbohydrate portion control, increasing fiber intake, limiting simple sugars, and increasing intake of leafy vegetables may be more effective in controlling glucose levels. Protein intake of 0.8 g/kg of weight usually is sufficient for the healthy older adult. Some chronic disease states (such as malabsorption) may require increased protein intake while other disease states (such as renal failure) may require decreased protein intake. A majority of fat should be obtained from monounsaturated fats. In the older population, goals for medical nutrition therapy should be individualized and as simple as possible. Dramatic changes and heavy restrictions are less likely to be followed.

EXERCISE. Physical activity has been shown to be beneficial for all individuals with diabetes because exercise increases insulin sensitivity, increases glucose uptake in peripheral tissue, decreases plasma lipid levels, decreases blood pressure, and increases bone density (ADA, 2003). Maintaining a physically active lifestyle in the older adult also improves quality of life and decreases the risk for falls. Even exercise programs performed from a sitting position can improve strength, improve the ability to perform activities of daily living, and reduce the signs of depression (Perry, 2001). Realistic activity goals should be set after evaluating coexisting medical problems. All older persons with diabetes should be cautioned to obtain approval from their primary care provider before beginning an exercise program. Choosing an enjoyable activity may increase the likelihood that individuals adhere to an exercise program. Non–weight-bearing activities, such as swimming or cycling, may be beneficial for persons with arthritis, neuropathy, and obesity because of the decreased stress on joints. Blood glucose levels should be checked before exercising to avoid hypoglycemia. Exercise should also be avoided during times of peak action for medications and when the risk for hypoglycemia is high, such as immediately before a meal.

SELF-MONITORING. It is imperative that older persons with diabetes self-monitor blood glucose levels in order to control the disease and prevent complications. Blood glucose testing is simple and has become relatively painless. Medicare and supplemental insurances cover most of the cost associated with blood glucose monitoring. Most people can learn blood glucose testing, although motor and visual impairments must be considered in the older individual. A certified diabetes educator (CDE) can be useful in identifying a glucose meter to fit individual needs. Self-monitoring of glucose levels provides immediate feedback regarding the effects of diet, exercise, and medication on glucose levels. The benefits of improved glucose control include an improved sense of well-being, decreased lethargy, less blurring of vision, fewer symptoms of hyperglycemia, improved lipid levels, improved fluid and electrolyte balance, and possibly a decrease in long-term complications.

DRUG THERAPY. If diet and exercise do not control hyperglycemia, drug therapy is indicated. Drugs do not replace diet and exercise but are used in conjunction with them. There are six classes of oral agents currently used to treat diabetes. Care must be taken when considering an agent to use with the older diabetic population. Considerations should include the medication action, metabolism, safety profile, and cost (Oiknine & Mooradian, 2003). Unfortunately, cost often is not considered by practitioners, and this factor directly affects adherence to prescribed treatment plans. The presence of coexisting diseases, the high cost of medications, and the lack of supplemental coverage make following medical advice difficult for the older person. Often they must choose between taking certain medications or taking less than the prescribed amount in order to make their supply last longer.

Sulfonylureas are the oldest and, until recently, have been the most commonly used oral drugs for diabetes. The oral sulfonylureas act by directly stimulating insulin production with a secondary effect of decreasing tissue resistance to insulin. They are ineffective in the absence of functioning beta cells. The first-generation sulfonylureas (tolbutamide, acetohexamide, tolazamide, and chlorpropamide) should not be used because of the increased risk for side effects, especially hypoglycemia and hyponatremia. Second-generation sulfonylureas are preferred for the older patient because the risk of adverse effects is lower, especially when the shorter acting agents are used. Second-generation sulfonylureas include glyburide (Micronase, DiaBeta, Glynase) and glipizide (Glucotrol). Glipizide may be advantageous in the older person because it metabolizes in the liver into inactive metabolites, thus reducing the risk for hypoglycemia (Oiknine & Mooradian, 2003). As a result of increased insulin production, sulfonylureas can cause weight gain and hypoglycemia and may be more effective on lean older persons with diabetes (Meneilly & Tessier, 2001).

Biguanides reduce hepatic gluconeogenesis, decrease hepatic glucose production, and have an indirect effect on glucose utilization by peripheral tissue. Currently, metformin (Glucophage) is the only biguanide on the market in the United States. It is used most effectively in obese persons with insulin resistance (Oiknine & Mooradian, 2003). Biguanides do not cause hypoglycemia when used as monotherapy, but common side effects include nausea, bloating, and loose stools. These side effects are usually dose-related and can be diminished if metformin is started at lower doses with a gradual increase to a therapeutic dosage. Because of the risk of lactic acidosis, metformin should not be used in individuals over age 80, in men with serum creatinine levels >1.5 mg/dl, or in women with serum creatinine levels >1.4 mg/dl. If the older person with diabetes has a low muscle mass, a creatinine clearance <60 mg/dl would also contraindicate use of metformin (Chau & Edelman, 2001). Other contraindications include alcohol abuse, hepatic dysfunction, congestive heart failure, sepsis, and dehydration. Metformin must be held for 48 hours after administration of IV contrast media in order to prevent acute renal failure.

Thiazolidinediones (TZDs) such as rosiglitazone (Avandia) and pioglitazone (Actos) enhance glucose uptake and improve insulin resistance, especially in skeletal muscle. TZDs are well tolerated, have the added benefit of improving HDL cholesterol levels, and do not cause hypoglycemia when used as monotherapy. TZDs can also be used in combination with insulin, metformin, and sulfonylureas. TZDs are metabolized in the liver and eliminated by the biliary route, so dosages do not need to be adjusted in renal insufficiency (Oiknine & Mooradian, 2003). However, weight gain secondary to fluid retention and stimulation of adipogenesis are common side effects of TZDs, and they are contraindicated for use in older persons with heart failure and hepatic disease (Mooradian, Chehade, & Thurman, 2002). Earlier formulations of drugs in this category were removed from the market because of hepatic toxicity; therefore liver functions should be monitored before initiating therapy and periodically during therapy with TZDs (Meneilly & Tessier, 2001). TZDs are expensive; thus cost may be a factor when considering this medication.

α-Glucosidase inhibitors inhibit the brush border enzymes of the proximal small intestine, which in turn delays carbohydrate absorption and blunts postprandial glucose elevations usually seen in persons with diabetes. Medications in this classification include acarbose (Precose) and miglitol (Glyset). α-Glucosidase inhibitors are most effective in patients with a high-carbohydrate diet. They can be used as monotherapy to treat modest elevations in fasting plasma glucose levels

or in combination with other oral agents or insulin. Hypoglycemia can occur when α-glucosidase inhibitors are used in combination therapy and should be treated with glucose rather than sucrose (Oiknine & Mooradian, 2003). Gastrointestinal side effects (mainly diarrhea and flatulence) may limit the use of α-glucosidase inhibitors, but the side effects may be useful if constipation is a problem. Multiple premeal dosing and cost may also limit the usefulness of medication in this class (Chau & Edelman, 2001).

Meglitinides are insulin secretagogues that target different binding sites on pancreatic beta cells, triggering insulin release and targeting postprandial hyperglycemia. Meglitinides such as repaglinide (Prandin) and nateglinide (Starlix) are shorter acting than traditional sulfonylureas, resulting in less hypoglycemia. Insulin secretagogues should be avoided in the presence of hepatic and renal disease. Meglitinides can result in weight gain and hypoglycemia, making it more effective on lean older persons with diabetes. Dosing with each meal increases effectiveness but may affect compliance (Oiknine & Mooradian, 2003).

In 2005, two new injectable medications were approved by the FDA. Pramlintide (Symlin) is a synthetic form of the hormone amylin, which plays a role in glucose homeostasis. Pramlintide, used to treat type 1 and type 2 diabetes, increases the risk for hypoglycemia and gastrointestinal side effects. Exenatide (Byetta), which is classified as an incretin mimetic, has been shown to lower blood glucose levels by increasing insulin secretion. Exenatide is used only with type 2 diabetes and works only in the presence of elevated glucose levels, so there is no increased risk of hypoglycemia unless the patient is also on sulfonylureas. Most individuals on this medication experience decreased appetite and weight loss. Both of these new medications have complex dosing regimens and require injections before each meal. They are also very costly and are not covered by many insurance companies, so use in the older population may be limited (Brunk, 2005; Hussar, 2005).

Oral medications usually are started at the lowest possible dose and then increased at 1- to 2-week intervals until the desired clinical response is attained. Failure of oral drug therapy may be associated with disease progression, acute illness, lack of adherence to dietary and exercise prescriptions, or weight gain. Another often overlooked reason for failure of oral drug therapy is the cost of medications, especially for older persons with comorbid disease. Efforts should be made to improve glycemic control through diet and exercise before insulin therapy is initiated because of the increased risk of hypoglycemia with insulin therapy, especially during the night. Insulin therapy has been demonstrated to improve glycemic control and lower very low-density lipoprotein levels on a long-term basis after secondary failure of oral agents. A variety of regimens are being studied

Table 17-8 *Insulin Types*

Insulin	Appearance	Onset	Peak	Duration
Lispro, aspart	Clear	<15 minutes	1-2 hours	3-4 hours
Regular	Clear	0.5-1 hour	2-3 hours	3-6 hours
NPH	Cloudy	2-4 hours	4-10 hours	10-16 hours
Glargine	Clear	2-4 hours	Does not peak	20-24 hours

Copyright 2005 by American Diabetes Association. (2005, January). *Diabetes Forecast, 58*(1), RG10-15. Reprinted with permission from the American Diabetes Association.

that include insulin therapy alone and combinations of oral sulfonylureas and insulin. Combination therapy may pose special disadvantages for older patients, who often already have problems with polypharmacy.

The major concern with insulin therapy is the risk of hypoglycemia, which can lead to cardiac dysrhythmias. It is important to consider the onset, peak, and duration of insulin action (Table 17-8). Other problems associated with insulin therapy in the older person are delayed excretion, hyperinsulinemia, weight gain, and possibly sodium and fluid retention. Other factors that must be considered with insulin therapy are the ability of the older person to prepare and self-administer insulin and the willingness of the person to accept insulin therapy. When patients are taking insulin, they need to be able to monitor blood glucose levels. Periodic measurements of glycosylated hemoglobin level should be obtained to evaluate blood glucose control over time. Because of the wide variation in absorption from injection sites, the patient is advised to rotate sites in the same anatomical region. Absorption is best from the abdomen. Unless the patient is thin, the medication can be injected at a 90-degree angle. Various devices are available to facilitate self-injection for people with visual or motor impairments (Box 17-3).

Special Problems in Managing Older Persons with Diabetes. In planning the care and treatment of older persons with diabetes, it is important to consider the normal and pathological changes associated with aging (Box 17-4). Dietary planning must account for changes in the perceptions of taste and smell, as well as any difficulties in preparing food and eating. Social and economic factors may also influence the nutrition of older patients, especially those who are poor and living alone. Other diseases, including chronic diseases, neoplasms, and infections, may have an impact on the control of diabetes in older adults. The prevalence of chronic disease increases with age, especially hypertension, atherosclerosis, and arthritis. A high proportion of the older population with diabetes also has hypertension, which can aggravate the microvascular and macrovascular complications.

In older people, drugs cleared through the kidneys may accumulate so that serum concentrations of these drugs may rise, producing increased pharmacological effects. In addition, insulin degradation, which occurs largely in the liver, diminishes with age, reflecting a decrease in hepatic function. Many drugs commonly used by older people interact with hyperglycemic agents. Beta blockers that are used as antihypertensives and antidysrhythmics are particularly problematic. They inhibit insulin secretion, but they also lower serum glucose levels, prolong recovery from hypoglycemia, and inhibit the tachycardia that is normally a sign of hypoglycemia. Therefore people with diabetes who take beta blockers may experience hypoglycemia without the usual symptoms and may delay seeking appropriate treatment. These effects occur even with ophthalmic beta blockers. If systemic beta blockers are indicated, selective $beta_1$ blockers like atenolol are recommended because they have less impact on serum glucose level. Other drugs that enhance the hypoglycemic effects of drugs used to

BOX 17-3 Insulin Injection Aids

Syringe Magnifiers
- Insul-eze
- Magni-Guide
- Syringe magnifier

Dose Gauges
- Andros IDM
- Click-Count Syringe
- Count-a-dose
- Dos-Aid
- Insulgauge

Needle and Vial Holders
- Dos-Aid
- Holdease
- Inject-Aid
- Insul-eze
- Load-Matic
- Insulin Needle Guide
- Magni-Guide
- Vial Center Aid

Insulin Pens
- Autopen
- Novo pen
- Novolin pen

BOX 17-4 Factors That May Interfere with or Alter Control of Diabetes in the Older Adult

Alterations in the Senses
- Diminished vision
- Diminished smell
- Altered taste perception

Difficulties in Preparing Food and Eating
- Tremor
- Arthritis
- Poor dentition
- Alterations in gastrointestinal function

Altered Renal and Hepatic Function

Diminished Exercise and Mobility

Effects of Other Diseases
- Other chronic diseases
- Neoplasms
- Infection

Neuropsychiatric Problems
- Depression
- Cognitive impairment

Social Factors
- Lack of education
- Poor dietary habits
- Living alone
- Poverty

Drugs
- Other medications
- Alcoholism

From Lipson, L. G. (1985). *Diabetes mellitus in the elderly: Special problems, special approaches.* New York: Pfizer Pharmaceuticals, p. 9.

treat diabetes include nonsteroidal antiinflammatory drugs, sulfonamides, ethanol, ranitidine, cimetidine, and chloramphenicol. A number of other drugs counteract the hypoglycemic effects of drugs used to treat diabetes. They include calcium channel blockers, combination oral contraceptives, glucocorticoids, phenothiazines, and thiazide diuretics. The fact that so many drugs affect serum glucose levels poses a challenge to the health care provider in managing osteoarthritis, hypertension, infections, and cancer. Special care must be taken to teach older clients about drug interactions and side effects (Amella, 2004; Wooten & Galavis, 2005).

Cognitive factors, such as dementia or depression, can interfere with eating habits and proper management of diabetes. Confused older people may eat sporadically, paying little attention to proper diet. They may not be able to manage their medications or be able to prevent complications such as infection. Infections and abnormal serum glucose level may produce more confusion, further exacerbating the problem. Older persons who are depressed also may have a poor appetite and lack motivation to follow the prescribed diet. If their medications are not adjusted, hypoglycemia may result. Social factors, such as lack of education, poor dietary habits, isolation, and poverty, may influence the older person's ability to cope with diabetes. Care must be taken with teaching and management of the symptoms of the disease, so that interventions are tailored to the special needs of the individual. A patient's motivation to modify lifestyle and adhere to the diabetic regimen is of the utmost importance and must be assessed and encouraged. One approach to managing diabetes in older adults is presented in Figure 17-5.

Thyroid Disease

Thyroid gland dysfunction is common among older adults and is associated with significant morbidity if left untreated (Rehman, Cope, Senseney, & Brzezinski, 2005). Because thyroid dysfunction in older adults often goes unnoticed, routine screening for both hyperthyroidism and hypothyroidism has been recommended for this age-group (Gussekloo et al., 2004). Diagnosis of thyroid disease in the older patient is often difficult. The clinical presentation frequently differs significantly from those of younger patients, making diagnosis challenging. Some of the classic clinical features seen in younger patients are completely absent in the geriatric patient (Beers, Jones, Berkwits, Kaplan, & Porter, 2000; Mohandas & Lal Gupta, 2003; Rehman et al., 2005). Often these symptoms that are subtle or absent become easily confused with coexisting illnesses or are attributed to normal aging.

Hyperthyroidism. The incidence of hyperthyroidism in persons older than 60 years ranges from 0.2% to 2.3% depending on the study (Beers et al., 2000; Mohandas & Lal Gupta, 2003; Rehman et al., 2005). Rehman et al. (2005) estimate that 10% to 15% of patients with hyperthyroidism are older than 60 years of age. The condition typically affects women in greater proportions than men.

Hyperthyroidism in the older adult is a great masquerader, even more so than hypothyroidism. In general the classic signs and symptoms of hyperthyroidism that are often striking in younger patients (hyperactive reflexes, increased sweating, heat intolerance, tremor, nervousness, polydypsia, and increased appetite) are muted in the older person (Hall, 1997; Mohandas & Lal Gupta, 2003). In these patients even severe, life-threatening hyperthyroidism can easily be missed, leading to potentially significant morbidity (Rehman et al., 2005).

Older patients typically have fewer signs and symptoms and a different complex of symptoms than younger patients. Many age-specific differences in symptoms are

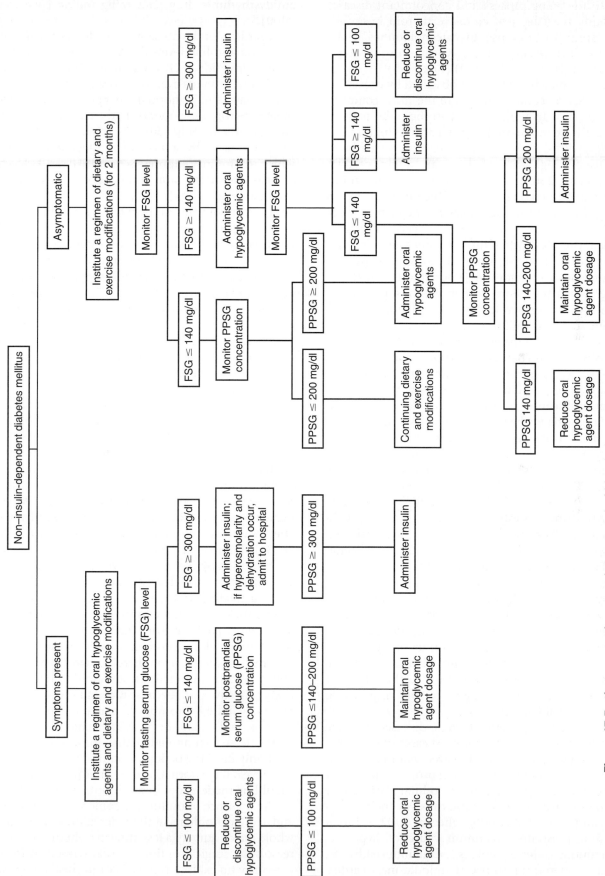

Figure 17-5 A suggested approach to control of blood glucose levels of older adults with type 2 diabetes mellitus.

related to the aging process and concomitant diseases that modify the effects of excessive thyroid hormone. For example, the response to catecholamines is decreased in older persons. This may explain some atypical symptoms (Beers et al., 2000) (Box 17-5).

Symptoms may be subtle and obscured by coexisting diseases. Cardiac complications are the most common manifestation of hyperthyroidism in the older patient. They usually are manifested as atrial arrhythmias (atrial fibrillation with slow ventricular rates), congestive heart failure (usually high-output failure), and angina pectoris (Rehman et al., 2005). The hyperthyroid condition imposes a great burden on the heart of the older person. An excess of thyroid hormone makes the heart beat more forcefully and increases the muscle's need for oxygen. Chest pain can result when the coronary arteries cannot carry the extra blood the heart demands, as is the case with acute coronary syndrome (Anonymous, 2002).

Congestive heart failure is often the most prominent symptom of hyperthyroidism in the older patient. Symptoms of heart failure and angina may dominate the clinical picture to the exclusion of the usual features of hyperthyroidism (Beers et al., 2000; Felicetta, 2002). Atrial fibrillation, the most common complication in older patients, is found in 27% of patients at the time of presentation (Beers et al., 2000; Mohandas & Lal Gupta, 2003). Prognosis for heart failure and early death is increased if atrial fibrillation does not convert to normal sinus rhythm when a normal thyroid state is achieved. Atrial fibrillation also carries a high risk of embolic stroke in this age-group (Beers et al., 2000).

One common clinical presentation—"apathetic hyperthyroidism"—is estimated to occur in 10% to 15% of older adults. The predominant features are weakness, lethargy, and depression (Beers et al., 2000; Felicetta, 2002; Fisher, 2002; Mohandas & Lal Gupta, 2003; Rehman et al., 2005). In a study of clinical features of hyperthyroidism in older persons (Trivalle et al., 1996), apathy was present in 41% and depression in 24% of the individuals studied. Although the precise etiology of apathetic hyperthyroidism remains unclear, age-related attenuation of adrenergic tone and altered autonomic nervous system and tissue resistance to the effects of thyroid hormone are thought to be responsible (Mohandas & Lal Gupta, 2003).

As with younger patients, Graves' disease and toxic multinodular goiter account for most cases of hyperthyroidism in older patients. However, compared with younger patients, a somewhat higher proportion of older hyperthyroid patients have multinodular toxic goiter rather than Graves' disease as the cause of their hyperthyroidism (Beers et al., 2000; Felicetta, 2002; Rehman et al., 2005). Another common cause of hyperthyroidism among older patients is iodine-induced hyperthyroidism, often from the use of amiodarone, a cardiac antidysrhythmic drug containing iodine (Beers et al., 2000).

Regardless of the cause, elevated levels of total or free thyroxine and low levels of TSH confirm the diagnosis of hyperthyroidism (Rehman et al., 2005). In a minority of older patients even with low TSH levels, thyroxine levels may remain normal. In approximately 10% of older hyperthyroid patients, T_3 toxicosis occurs, causing an elevation in only serum T_3 level. This condition is usually caused by a nodule producing excessive T_3, which in turn may suppress serum TSH and T_4 levels because of the suppression of the rest of the thyroid gland (Rehman et al., 2005).

Hyperthyroidism can be a life-threatening disease in the older person and requires prompt attention. There are three treatment strategies for hyperthyroidism: medication to suppress the gland, surgery to remove the hyperfunctioning tissue, and radioactive iodine (RAI) to destroy the gland (Rehman et al., 2005). Radioactive iodine has been the preferred treatment in the older person for many reasons, including ease of administration, higher age-related surgery risks, and the polypharmacy often present in the older patient (Beers et al., 2000; Felicetta, 2002; Rehman et al., 2005).

Older patients, especially those with coronary artery disease, should be treated with antithyroid drugs to achieve normal or near-normal T_4 levels before undergoing radioablation (Mohandas & Lal Gupta, 2003). One drawback of RAI therapy is that hyperthyroidism is gradually reversed over weeks to months, and cardiac problems must be aggressively managed until the thyrotoxic state is reversed (Rehman et al., 2005). Many patients treated with RAI therapy develop hypothyroidism after treatment (Felicetta, 2002; Mohandas & Lal Gupta, 2003; Rehman et al., 2005).

Drug therapy is very effective, but the potential for side effects and a high recurrence rate make this an unpopular treatment of choice. Because antithyroid drugs (propylthiouracil or methimazole) work very quickly, they are reserved for those individuals with special circumstances, whose unstable conditions warrant rapid suppression of the hyperthyroid state (Rehman et al., 2005). Antithyroid medications should be given at the lowest effective dose because they can cause serious side effects including thrombocytopenia, anemia, hepatitis, arthritis, and agranulocytosis (Mohandas & Lal Gupta, 2003). It is recommended that these medications be used only until the patient's condition is stable and thyroid levels have normalized. At that point the decision should be made about definitive treatment.

The presence of multiple chronic medical conditions and cardiac problems in the older adult population as a whole makes surgery a less attractive alternative. For that reason the surgical option is usually reserved for older patients who exhibit dysphagia or tracheal compression

BOX 17-5 Clinical Features of Hyperthyroidism in the Older Patient

SYMPTOM	FREQUENCY (%)
Hyperhidrosis	38
Heat intolerance	63
Weight loss	69
Palpitation	63
Angina pectoris	20
Respiratory symptoms consistent with congestive heart failure	66
Polyphagia	11
Anorexia	36
Increased stool frequency	12
Constipation	26
Tremor/nervousness	55

SIGN	FREQUENCY (%)
Hyperkinesis	25
Apathy	16
Cachexia/chronically ill appearance	39
Classical skin changes (warm, fine, moist)	81
Proptosis	8
Lid lag	35
Extraocular muscle palsy	22
Impalpable or normal-sized thyroid gland	37
Multinodular thyroid gland	20
Solitary thyroid nodule	21
Diffuse thyroid enlargement	22
Atrial fibrillation (AF)	39
Supraventricular tachycardia (rate >120 beats/min)	11
Brisk deep tendon reflexes, shortened relaxation phase	26

From Davis, P. J., & Davis, F. B. (1992). Endocrine diseases. In E. Calkins, A. B. Ford, & P. R. Katz (Eds.), *Practice of geriatrics* (2nd ed.). Philadelphia: Saunders, p. 485.

or if there is a high suspicion of malignant tumor (Fisher, 2002; Rehman et al., 2005).

Hypothyroidism. Hypothyroidism, which is common in older persons, is often difficult to recognize because the symptoms bear such a close resemblance to the process of aging. The incidence of hypothyroidism in patients over 60 years of age is estimated to be between 2% and 10% depending on the study (Beers et al., 2000; Mohandas & Lal Gupta, 2003; Rehman et al., 2005). The prevalence increases with age and is much higher in women than in men at all ages. By age 75 the incidence of hypothyroidism increases to about 17.4% of women and 3.5% of men exhibiting signs and symptoms of the disease (Felicetta, 2002).

The causes of primary hypothyroidism in older persons include thyroid autoimmune disease, neck irradiation, previous surgical or medical treatment of hyperthyroidism, and administration of drugs such as lithium or amiodarone (Beers et al., 2000; Rehman et al., 2005).

Classic signs and symptoms of hypothyroidism in the younger patient—cold intolerance, weight gain, dry skin, constipation, and mental and physical slowing—can easily be mistaken for the normal aging process (Mohandas & Lal Gupta, 2003; Rehman et al., 2005). These factors along with the fact that hypothyroidism often has an insidious onset and affects multiple organs can lead to considerable delays in treatment. Side effects of medications can further mask the symptoms of hypothyroidism (Mohandas & Lal Gupta, 2003; Rehman et al., 2005) (Box 17-6).

Clinical manifestations of hypothyroidism in the older patient include unexplained elevations in plasma cholesterol or triglyceride levels, congestive heart failure (especially in patients with restrictive cardiomyopathy), fecal impaction, macrocytic anemia, vague arthritic complaints, and mild psychiatric disturbances, especially depression (Beers et al., 2000; Felicetta, 2002; Rehman et al., 2005). Diagnosis is based on the presence of symptoms and on laboratory findings, including a marked elevation in serum TSH and decreased free T_4 levels (Beers et al., 2000; Rehman et al., 2005).

Proper treatment of hypothyroidism completely corrects the metabolic condition in most older patients. The mantra for treating the older patients with hypothyroidism is "start low and go slow." Conservative dosing for hypothyroidism in the older patient is very appropriate. With the increased prevalence of coronary artery disease with advancing age, significant cardiac disease is more likely in the older hypothyroid patient than the younger one. This means that great caution must be exercised when treating an older hypothyroid patient. Prescribing a too vigorous schedule for replacing thyroid hormone can precipitate angina pectoris, rhythm disturbances, or even myocardial infarction

BOX 17-6 Features of Hypothyroidism in the Older Patient*

- General: unexplained medical deterioration, insidious onset, reversible sleep apnea syndrome Constipation and weight gain may be present
- Nervous system: mental slowing, fatigue, excessive sleepiness, acute decline in mental status with physiological stress, delayed reflex relaxation stage, hyporeflexia, cold intolerance, decreased sweating, hypothermia
- Integument: dry skin, facial puffiness, periorbital edema, skin yellowing, hair coarse and thin
- Cardiovascular: hypertension, bradycardia, narrowed pulse pressure
- Musculoskeletal: slow movement, weakness, gait disorders
- Renal: decreased glomerular filtration rate with sodium and water retention
- Laboratory findings: elevated TSH, low serum T_4, hyponatremia, hyperuricemia, elevated serum antithyroid antibody titer
- Electrocardiogram: low voltage QRS, flat or inverted T wave, ventricular dysrhythmias
- Radiographs: asymmetrical hypertrophy of myocardial ventricular septum
- Other: voice coarse, speech slow and slurred, hearing impairment

Data from Davis, P.J., & Davis, F. B. (1998). Endocrine disorders. In E. H. Duthie & P. R. Katz (Eds.), *Practice of geriatrics* (3rd ed.). Philadelphia: Saunders, pp. 563-578; and Miller, M. (2003). Disorders of the thyroid. In R. C. Tallis and H. M. Fillit (Eds.), *Brocklehurst's textbook of geriatric medicine and gerontology* (6th ed.). London: Churchill-Livingstone, pp. 1165-1183. *The clinical presentation of hypothyroidism in the older person is easily missed. The above may or may not be present in an individual.

(Felicetta, 2002; Mohandas & Lal Gupta, 2003; Rehman et al., 2005). The daily starting dose of levothyroxine in the older person is 25 mcg; however, if there is any uncertainty regarding the cardiac status, start with 12.5 mcg daily. The geriatric patient's hypothyroid state has developed over a prolonged period, and correction should be made slowly over a period of months. Levothyroxine doses should be increased by small increments of 12.5 to 25 mcg every 2 to 4 weeks until the dosage is therapeutic and the serum TSH and T_4 levels normalize. It is important to monitor for tachycardia and reduce the dose if necessary (Rehman et al., 2005). The physiological dose in the older adult is approximately 75 mcg daily. Occasionally, when an older patient has severe coronary artery disease, only partial replacement is possible because severe angina develops. Unfortunately, these patients will exhibit a modest degree of hypothyroidism and may still be at risk for accelerated coronary artery disease related to elevated cholesterol levels (Rehman et al., 2005).

Subclinical Thyroid Disorders. Subclinical hypothyroidism and hyperthyroidism represent the earliest stages of thyroid dysfunction and are relatively common in older persons. Population surveys have identified a subset of older persons with either high or suppressed levels of thyroid-stimulating hormone (TSH) despite having normal levels of circulating thyroxine (T_4, free T_3, and free T_3) (Col, Surks, & Daniels, 2004; Cooper, 2004; Diez & Iglesias, 2004; Hall, 2005; Miller, 2005; Surks et al., 2004). Geriatric patients experiencing elevated serum TSH levels have subclinical hypothyroidism while those with suppressed serum TSH levels are considered to have subclinical hyperthyroidism.

The incidence of subclinical hypothyroidism in the older persons is estimated at between 4% and 20% depending on the study cited (Col, Surks, & Daniels, 2004; Cooper, 2004; Miller, 2005; Surks et al., 2004). There appears to be a relationship between the degree of elevation of TSH level and the long-term risk of developing overt hypothyroidism especially when the TSH concentration is higher than 12 milliunits/L, resulting in a 77% incidence of overt hypothyroidism by the 10-year follow-up (Miller, 2005). Adverse effects associated with subclinical hypothyroidism include symptoms of mild hypothyroidism, dyslipidemia, altered left ventricular function, coronary artery disease, peripheral vascular disease, and cognitive impairment (Miller, 2005).

Subclinical hyperthyroidism is much less common than subclinical hypothyroidism. The incidence of subclinical hyperthyroidism in the older population is between 2.1% and 6.3% depending on the study cited (Miller, 2005; Surks et al., 2004). Untreated subclinical hyperthyroidism with suppressed TSH levels <0.1 milliunit/L carries the potential risks of atrial fibrillation, cardiovascular mortality, and osteoporosis (Kumeda et al., 2000; Mohandas & Lal Gupta, 2003; Parle, Maisonneuve, Sheppard, Boyle, & Franklyn, 2001; Surks et al., 2004). The risk of developing osteoporosis is greatest in postmenopausal women.

Considerable controversy surrounds the issue of treating subclinical thyroid disease. For this very reason a panel made up of experts from the American Association of Clinical Endocrinologists, the American Thyroid Association, and the Endocrine Society came to a consensus and released recommendations after completing a review of the literature on this subject. These statements were published in 2004 and made the following recommendations (Col, Surks, & Daniels, 2004; Surks et al., 2004). The panel stated treatment was reasonable for subclinical hypothyroidism for patients with TSH levels above 10 milliunits/L. The decision was based on the projected rate of progression to overt hypothyroidism. It also considered the positive effects of treatment on symptoms of depression, lipid profiles, and cardiac function. Treatment for subclinical hyperthyroidism also was recommended for those patients with complete

TSH suppression of lower than 0.1 milliunit/L. This decision was based on the higher cardiovascular and all-cause death rates in older persons with complete TSH suppression (Miller, 2005).

Thyroid Carcinoma. Thyroid cancer is relatively rare, representing only 5% to 10% of all thyroid nodules. The majority of thyroid carcinomas are slower growing papillary or follicular carcinomas (Beers et al., 2000; Mandel, 2004; Simon & Jabbour, 2005). In all age-groups, papillary carcinoma is the most common type of thyroid cancer, accounting for approximately 80% of all thyroid carcinomas. In older patients, papillary carcinoma is more aggressive (Felicetta, 2002; Gambert, 2005; Simon & Jabbour, 2005). In one study the 10-year survival rate among patients older than 50 was only 60%, compared to 90% among those younger than 50 (Felicetta, 2002).

Follicular cancer is the second most common cancer of the thyroid gland. It is responsible for approximately 12% of all thyroid cancer and accounts for only a small number of thyroid cancer deaths. It generally affects individuals between the ages of 20 and 60 years and affects more women than men. Follicular carcinoma has a greater tendency to metastasize, invading neighboring blood vessels and more distant sites (Gambert, 2005).

Less common than either papillary or follicular cancer, medullary carcinoma of the thyroid gland most commonly affects women in their fifties. Medullary carcinoma accounts for only 3% to 4% of thyroid cancers and has an 80% survival rate (Gambert, 2005). The most serious and life-threatening form of thyroid cancer is anaplastic carcinoma. Anaplastic carcinoma of the thyroid for the most part affects older persons, women only slightly more than men, and is responsible for 90% of the deaths from thyroid cancer. It has a dismal 1-year survival rate of approximately 10% and 5-year survival rate of only 5%. This is a very rapidly growing carcinoma that is difficult to treat and frequently metastasizes to distant sites (Gambert, 2005).

Most thyroid nodules are benign. However, if there is a history of therapeutic irradiation of the head, neck, or upper chest, there is an increased risk of both benign and malignant thyroid nodules. Diagnosis is made through needle biopsy. Thyroid scans, ultrasound study, and soft tissue radiography may also be employed in evaluating thyroid nodules (Simon & Jabbour, 2005). Symptoms of thyroid carcinoma include a new, rapidly enlarging, solitary mass or nodule; pain; hoarseness; dysphasia; and hemoptysis. Anaplastic carcinoma often has features that clearly suggest malignancy—a large, growing, stony hard thyroid mass that is irregular, immobile, and fixed to other tissues (Beers et al., 2000).

Surgery is the treatment choice when fine-needle aspiration indicates evidence of malignancy unless the older patient's comorbidities create an absolute contraindication (Beers et al., 2000; Mandel, 2004). If the cytological exam is not determinant, meaning the pathologist cannot identify whether the nodule is benign or malignant, a better treatment choice may be levothyroxine sodium to suppress TSH to a subnormal but not hyperthyroid state. A repeat fine-needle aspiration should be completed in 6 to 12 months (Beers et al., 2000). The use of thyroxine suppressive therapy in euthyroid patients to suppress thyroid nodule growth remains controversial. There is conflicting evidence regarding the value of suppressive therapy in shrinking most nodules. Suppressive therapy is not without risks and may cause osteoporosis and increased atrial fibrillation in some older patients (Simon & Jabbour, 2005).

Cancer of the Female Reproductive System

The prevalence of malignant female reproductive system tumors increases with age. Breast cancer is the most frequently diagnosed malignancy of the reproductive system (American Cancer Society [ACS], 2005b). Additional sites of postmenopausal primary cancers are the endometrium, vulva, vagina, uterine cervix, and ovaries.

Breast Cancer. In the United States, the breast is the most common site of cancer and the second leading cause of cancer deaths in adult women (ACS, 2005a; Gosney, 2003).

INCIDENCE. The probability of developing invasive breast cancer before age 40 is 1 in 270. For women aged 40 to 59, the probability is 1 in 24, and for those aged 60 to 79, it is 1 in 13 (ACS, 2005a). Among participants in the NHS Screening Programme in the United Kingdom, the mammography detection rate among women over age 65 was 13.1 per 1000 compared with 5.9 per 1000 in younger women (Mansel, 2003). UK statistics further reflect increasing incidence of breast cancer from 1971 to 1999 in women younger than age 65, but static rates for women age 65 and older (Johnson & Shekhdar, 2005). Analysis of age-specific incidence of in situ breast carcinomas from 1980 to 2001 revealed a 7.2-fold increase in ductal carcinoma in situ and a 2.6-fold increase in lobular carcinoma in situ (Li, Daling, & Malone, 2005). Analysis of data from the Geneva Cancer Registry (Switzerland) revealed that age was not related to 5-year survival/mortality from breast cancer (Rapiti et al., 2005). In the United States, the prevalence of breast cancer is higher in white women, but the mortality is higher in black women (Harris, Miller, & Davis, 2003).

Worldwide, breast cancer is the most common cause of cancer death among women. The incidence rates are highest in North American and northern European countries and lowest in Eastern Europe, South and Latin America, and Asia. Differences in incidence and death rates among developed and developing countries are attributed to differential use of screening mammography, and differences in lifestyle and hereditary factors (Althuis, Dozier, Anderson, Devesa, & Brinton, 2005). Not surprisingly, in the United States, the percent of breast cancers detected in situ correlates with the number of mammography facilities per 10,000 women (Marchick & Henson, 2005).

RISK FACTORS. The most important risk factors for breast cancer are increasing age and female gender. Other known risks are recent oral contraceptive use, long-term postmenopausal hormone replacement therapy, previous therapeutic radiation exposure, and benign proliferative breast disease such as hyperplasia and papillomas. A small proportion of breast cancers are attributed to inherited mutations of the BRCA1 and BRCA2 genes (Dell, 2005).

Older women tend to have estrogen receptor positive tumors (Mansel, 2003). Because about two thirds of breast cancers are stimulated by estrogen, it has been thought that early menarche and later menopause increase the risk because of the longer exposure to unopposed estrogen. The role of hormone replacement therapy (HRT) for menopausal symptoms has been subject to scrutiny, particularly since the publication of data from the Women's Health Initiative that found estrogen and estrogen-progestin therapy increased the risk of stroke, deep vein thrombosis, and dementia, and that estrogen-progestin therapy increased the risk of breast cancer (Barrett-Connor, Grady, & Stefanick, 2005). A Danish cohort study confirmed the increased risk of breast cancer in HRT users who were aged 50 or older. The risk increased with the duration of use (Ewertz et al., 2005). In an editorial in the *Archives of Women's Mental Health*, Birkhaeuser (2005) questioned the application of findings from the Women's Health Initiative (WHI) to symptomatic perimenopausal and early postmenopausal women because the WHI participants were older, more obese, and less healthy than the typical woman on hormone replacement therapy.

Research continues efforts to improve our understanding of risk factors. Among participants in the Long Island Breast Cancer Study Project, women who gained more than 33 lb after age 20 and those who gained more than 24 lb in the perimenopausal and postmenopausal years were at a 1.6-fold increased risk of breast cancer compared with their counterparts whose weight remained stable (Eng et al., 2005). The relationship between exposure to low-frequency electromagnetic fields (EMF) and breast tumors in older women was explored by Beniashvili, Avinoach, Baazov, & Zusman (2005). EMF exposure was measured by the frequency of use of personal computers, mobile telephones, television sets, air conditioners, and other household appliances known to generate EMF. Those women who were regularly exposed to EMF for at least 3 hours a day had a significantly higher incidence of epithelial mammary tumors, particularly invasive ductal carcinomas.

Some studies have shown an inverse relationship between long-term regular use of NSAIDs (aspirin and ibuprofen) and the risk of breast cancer, particularly in premenopausal women (Zhang, Coogan, Palmer, Strom, & Rosenberg, 2005). After examining aspirin frequency and duration of use, Swede, Mirand, Menezes, & Moysich (2005) concluded that both regular and occasional aspirin users had reduced risks of breast cancer. On the contrary, analysis of data from the California Teachers Study cohort failed to show a relationship between long-term daily NSAID use and breast cancer risk. Furthermore, this study reported that use of ibuprofen was associated with increased risk of breast cancer (Marshall et al., 2005). Obviously, no firm conclusions can be drawn at this time.

Attempts to relate specific foods and breast cancer also have yielded inconsistent results. One study examined the dietary patterns of women with post-menopausal breast cancer. The two major patterns in this sample were the Western diet—characterized by a higher intake of red and processed meat, refined grains, sweets and desserts, and high-fat dairy products—and the "prudent" diet—which included more fruits, vegetables, whole grains, low-fat dairy products, fish, and poultry. No relationship was found between risk for postmenopausal breast cancer and dietary pattern. However, there was some evidence that the combination of smoking and a Western dietary pattern elevated risk. There was also an inverse relationship between the prudent pattern and estrogen receptor-negative cancer (Fung et al., 2005).

MANIFESTATIONS. Breast cancer should be suspected any time an older woman has a discrete breast mass. Other less common signs are nipple discharge (which is present in about 30% of older women with carcinoma), persistent localized pain or tenderness, and an eczema-like eruption on the nipple (even without a palpable mass). Older women are more likely than younger women to present with locally advanced, neglected tumors (Mansel, 2003).

DIAGNOSTIC METHODS. A number of diagnostic methods may be employed to detect, diagnose, or stage breast cancer. Among the diagnostic procedures are fine-needle aspiration cytology, needle biopsy, and imaging with mammography, ultrasound, positron emission tomography, and magnetic resonance imaging (Dell, 2005; Mansel, 2003). Mammography screening is thought to advance the time of diagnosis, which is one factor that can decrease mortality (Moller et al., 2005).

Core needle biopsy (with a 14-gauge needle) with ultrasound guidance is the preferred diagnostic method (Mansel, 2003). The search for breast cancer biochemical markers is underway. Among the markers being studied are CEA, CA 15-3, and CA 125 in breast aspiration fluid, and APC and cyclin D2 gene promoter hypermethylation (Lee et al., 2004). After the diagnosis of breast cancer is confirmed by biopsy, the tumor is staged by the tumor-nodes-metastases system (Table 17-9).

MANAGEMENT. TNM Classification of Breast Cancer guides the treatment options. Initial treatment is primarily surgical, with the extent of surgery and additional treatment dependent on many factors: stage and type of the cancer, age and physical status of the patient, and judgment of the physician. Surgical options for early (stage 1 or 2) breast cancer are simple total mastectomy, modified radical mastectomy, and local excision alone or with radiotherapy or tamoxifen. Sentinel node biopsy may be performed to detect malignancy in axillary nodes, in which case dissection of the nodes may be done. In some cases tamoxifen alone is used. In the UK, older women with hormone-responsive disease typically are treated with tamoxifen, but the treatment of women with non–hormone-responsive cancer is less definitive (Leonard & Malinovszky, 2005). After potentially curative treatment is completed, adjuvant chemotherapy with cytotoxic agents or endocrine therapy may be used. Endocrine therapy includes tamoxifen, aromatase inhibitors that suppress the peripheral synthesis of estrogens, an estrogen-receptor antagonist (fulvestrant), and mesestrol acetate. Examples of aromatase inhibitors are formestane, anastrozole, letrozole, and exemestane (Mansel, 2003). Preliminary results from clinical trials using aromatase inhibitors in adjuvant therapy are showing improved disease-free survival rates and decreased contralateral breast cancer when given alone for 5 years or for 2 to 5 years after tamoxifen. Noting that tamoxifen remains the standard adjuvant for low-risk primary breast cancer, Sulkes (2005) recommends that an aromatase inhibitor also should be offered to postmenopausal women with higher risk hormone-positive primary breast cancer. An encouraging development in the treatment of HER2-positive breast cancers is the use of the monoclonal antibody Herceptin (trastuzumab). HER2 is a protein that is present in 15% to 25% of breast cancers (ACS, 2005a). Issues still under study are whether to use Herceptin with adjuvant chemotherapy or afterwards. An important adverse effect of Herceptin therapy is congestive heart failure, which occurred in 2.9% to 4.1% of study participants (ACS, 2005b).

The aims of treatment for stage III (locally advanced) breast cancer are to control both the primary disease and the systemic disease. Unless the tumor is firmly attached to the chest wall or involves a wide area of skin,

Table 17-9 TNM Classification of Breast Cancer

PRIMARY TUMOR (T)

T_0 No evidence of primary tumor
T_{is} Carcinoma in situ
T_1 Tumor <2 cm
T_2 Tumor 2-5 cm
T_3 Tumor >5 cm
T_4 Extension to chest wall, inflammation

REGIONAL LYMPH NODES (N)

N_0 No tumor in regional lymph nodes
N_1 Metastasis to movable ipsilateral nodes
N_2 Metastasis to matted or fixed ipsilateral nodes
N_3 Metastasis to ipsilateral internal mammary nodes

DISTANT METASTASIS (M)

M_0 No distant metastasis
M_1 Distant metastasis (includes spread to ipsilateral supraclavicular nodes)

STAGE GROUPING

Stage 0	T_{is}	N_0	M_0
Stage I	T_1	N_0	M_0
Stage IIA	T_0	N_1	M_0
	T_1	N_1	M_0
	T_2	N_0	M_0
Stage IIB	T_2	N_1	M_0
	T_3	N_0	M_0
Stage IIIA	T_0	N_2	M_0
	T_1	N_2	M_0
	T_2	N_2	M_0
	T_3	N_1, N_2	M_0
Stage IIIB	T_4	Any N	M_0
	Any T	N_3	M_0
Stage IV	Any T	Any N	M_1

From Lewis, S. M., Heitkemper, M. M., & Dirksen, S. R. (2004). *Medical-surgical nursing* (6th ed.). St. Louis: Mosby, p. 1370.

surgical treatment may be effective. Radiotherapy is an option for tumors that cannot be resected. With stage III, relapse is common regardless of the type of treatment. Hormone therapy has been shown to reduce the rate of both relapse and mortality (Mansel, 2003). The goal of treatment for stage IV (metastatic) breast cancer is palliation. Treatment may employ radiotherapy and endocrine therapy. A phase I trial was conducted to determine dosage ranges for capecitabine and vinorelbine in the treatment of older persons with metastatic breast cancer. The drugs were tolerated well; however, persons with bone involvement experienced toxicity at a lower dosage level than individuals with no bone involvement (Hess et al., 2004).

Neoadjuvant chemotherapy may be used in an effort to downstage the disease before surgical intervention.

One study that compared neoadjuvant chemotherapy with conventional therapy in stage III breast cancer patients saw no survival benefit to the neoadjuvant therapy, though the investigators noted that the data hinted at improved disease-free survival in those women who had neoadjuvant therapy (Alassas et al., 2005).

SPECIAL CONSIDERATIONS WITH OLDER BREAST CANCER PATIENTS. Even among older women, surgical treatment of breast cancer has become less extensive. Depending on the status of axillary lymph nodes and the patient's "fitness" for anesthesia, simple mastectomy is sometimes the treatment of choice. For women over age 80, the risk of death from other causes is greater than the risk of recurrence when axillary nodes are retained. Axillary node dissection sometimes is omitted in older women based on the belief that it is unlikely to alter the treatment recommendations.

The burgeoning older population has made us confront the lack of clinical guidelines for the oldest old. Practitioners are forced to individualize treatment as much as possible using data extrapolated from studies of other populations (Mano et al., 2005). Some of the studies relevant to care of older persons with breast cancer are presented here. Older patients may not tolerate chemotherapy well, and it may offer little benefit over hormone therapy (Mansel, 2003). Data on chemotherapy in women over age 69 are limited (Leonard & Malinovszky, 2005). It has been found that older women with breast cancer are less likely to be referred to a medical oncologist. Those who were seen by a medical oncologist were more likely to have been informed about tamoxifen, and to have been prescribed the drug (Thwin, Fink, Lash, & Silliman, 2005). Noting that 20% to 30% of older persons experience toxic effects from docetaxel, investigators tested the response to a modified weekly dosage schedule in patients with metastatic disease. The response rate was 33%, with only mild toxicity reported (Maisano et al., 2005).

Various aspects of breast cancer prevention, diagnosis, and treatment are under study. Using small-size tin colloids for sentinel lymph node (SLN) biopsy, Japanese investigators found no differences among subjects of varying ages in relation to successful mapping rates and false-negative rates (Jinno et al., 2005). After performing SNL biopsy on 241 women over age 70, Italian researchers reported an SNL identification rate of 100%. Among the 151 patients with negative sentinel nodes, there were no axillary recurrences over the follow-up period of 3 to 87 months (Gennari, Rotmensz, Perego, dos Santos, & Veronesi, 2004). In addition, a review of a prospectively collected breast cancer sentinel lymph node mapping database demonstrated that SNL mapping and biopsy had a significant influence on treatment decisions (McMahon, Gray, & Pockaj, 2005).

Women being treated for breast cancer are at risk for lymphedema, a complication that can affect function, relationships, self-image, and self-esteem. Furthermore, it can eventually result in lymphangitis and cellulitis. It is quite possible that age-related changes in tissue density, skin, immune function, fluid balance, and comorbid conditions affect the older patient's risk for lymphedema (Armer & Heckathorn, 2005). Recommendations to reduce the risk of lymphedema are summarized in Box 17-7. Even though there is some evidence that women under age 60 have more prevalent symptoms of lymphedema (numbness, tenderness, aching) than older women, even older women must be considered at risk (Armer & Fu, 2005).

COPING AND ADAPTATION. Older women with newly diagnosed breast cancer reported that partners and adult children were important sources of support. Perceived support from these sources and their adjustment were associated with less patient depression and anxiety. In this sample, only 15% reported that their physicians asked support persons how they were coping, and only 3% made referrals to support groups (Maly et al., 2005).

RECONSTRUCTION AND BREAST IMPLANTS. If reconstruction is desired, it should be discussed before treatment is initiated because reconstruction and some therapies are incompatible (Dell, 2005). Reconstruction

---

BOX 17-7 18 Steps to Prevention Revised: Lymphedema Risk-Reduction Practices

I. Skin Care—Avoid Trauma/Injury and Reduce Infection Risk
1. Keep extremity clean and dry.
2. Apply moisturizer daily to prevent chapping/chafing of skin.
3. Pay attention to nail care; do not cut cuticles.
4. Protect exposed skin with sunscreen and insect repellent.
5. Use care with razors to avoid nicks and skin irritation.
6. If possible, avoid punctures such as injections and blood draws.
7. Wear gloves while performing activities that may cause skin injury (i.e., gardening, working with tools, using chemicals such as detergent).
8. If scratches/punctures to skin occur, wash with soap and water, apply antibiotics, and observe for signs of infection (i.e., redness).
9. If rash, itching, redness, pain, increased skin temperature, fever or flulike symptoms occur, contact your physician immediately.

II. Activity/Lifestyle
1. Gradually increase the duration and intensity of any activity or exercise.
2. Take frequent rest periods during activity to allow for limb recovery.
3. Monitor the extremity during and after activity for any change in size, shape, tissue, texture, soreness, heaviness, or firmness.
4. Maintain optimal body weight.

III. Avoid Limb Constriction
1. If possible, avoid having blood pressure measurement taken on the at-risk arm.
2. Wear loose-fitting jewelry and clothing.

IV. Compression Garments
1. Ensure garment fits properly.
2. Support the at-risk limb with a compression garment for strenuous activity (i.e., weight lifting, prolonged standing, running).
3. Wear a well-fitting compression garment for air travel.

V. Extremes of Temperature
1. Avoid exposure to extreme cold, which can be associated with rebound swelling, or chapping of skin.
2. Avoid prolonged (>15 minutes) exposure to heat, particularly hot tubs and saunas.
3. Avoid immersing limb in water temperatures above 102° F.

VI. Additional Practices Specific to Lower Extremity Lymphedema
1. Avoid prolonged standing or sitting.
2. When possible, avoid crossing legs.
3. Wear proper, well-fitting footwear.

employs implants (usually saline filled) or uses the patient's own tissue.

The popularity of breast implants has raised questions about whether prostheses interfere with breast cancer detection. The review of the literature by Smalley (2003) on this topic concluded that implants might facilitate breast self-examination (BSE) and clinical breast examination (CBE), but challenge mammography interpretation. Concerns that this might delay diagnosis or be related to a poor prognosis were not supported in this review.

EARLY DETECTION AND PREVENTION. Screening mammography and proper breast examinations can reduce mortality from breast cancer (Humphrey, Helfand, Chan, & Woolf, 2002; Vahabi, 2003). The ACS recommends periodic screening for breast cancer. A clinical breast examination should be performed as part of an annual health examination beginning at age 40. Annual mammography also is recommended beginning at age 40 along with education about mammography. Additional screening, such as more frequent mammography and the addition of MRI or ultrasound, may be recommended for women with increased risk for breast cancer (ACS, 2003).

Various educational strategies have been tested to encourage older women to have mammograms or to practice breast self-examination (BSE). Wood & Duffy (2004) used educational kits intended to increase breast cancer screening in older black and white women. Although knowledge increased and technique and proficiency in detecting lumps in simulation models improved, the kits were not associated with increased mammogram compliance. The Witness Project was an educational offering designed to improve mammography rates among African American women. The program, which was delivered by African American women, incorporated repetition, modeling, building comprehension, reinforcement, hands-on learning, a social story on breast health for African American women, and role playing about breast and cervical health and support. Investigators reported a 79% increase in the number of women who mastered the didactic material when these strategies were employed (Hurd, Muti, Erwin, & Womack, 2003). In contrast, an intervention program delivered by lay health educators in the apartments of participants did not significantly affect CBE or mammogram rates (Zhu et al., 2002). One study of low-income African American and Hispanic women age 40 and older found that physician recommendations for BSE and mammography were significant predictors of patient compliance with these practices. Another predictor was health insurance, with those covered being more likely to have had a mammogram and/or to perform BSE (Bazargan, Bazargan, Calderon, Husaini, &

Baker, 2003). In a Canadian study, variables associated with mammography screening included annual clinical breast examinations, compliance with cervical screening, and physician suggestion (Miedema & Tatemichi, 2003). Even when screening is available, some women do not access it because of fear or embarrassment (Garbers, Jessop, Foti, Uribelarrea, & Chaisson, 2003). An interesting study looked at the influence of perceived barriers and health conception on BSE performance. Women who had a clinical conception of health practiced BSE less often. Women who identified barriers such as worry about breast cancer or embarrassment were less thorough when they performed BSE (Gasalberti, 2002). In a follow-up survey of women who had participated in a formal teaching program in Denmark and a matched control group, participants reported a significantly greater frequency of BSE, and more correct technique (Sorensen, Hertz, & Gudex, 2005).

One population that may be overlooked for screening comprises persons in long-term care facilities. A study that was confined to a single state determined that health screening practices, including BSE, were not being implemented in rural long-term care facilities (Bassett & Smyer, 2003).

The impact of BSE on breast cancer mortality has been a subject of debate in recent years. A meta-analysis of the effect of regular BSE on breast cancer mortality did not find BSE to be an effective method of reducing mortality from breast cancer (Hackshaw & Paul, 2003).

Evidence exists that the risk of breast cancer is reduced by physical activity, particularly in postmenopausal women (Friedenreich, 2004). Fortunately, many risks can be mitigated by maintenance of a healthy body weight and regular, moderate to vigorous exercise (Dell, 2005; Friedenreich, 2004). Preventive behaviors advised by the American Cancer Society (ACS, 2003) include performing at least 30 minutes of physical activity a minimum of 5 days a week, achieving and maintaining a healthy weight, and limiting alcohol intake to one drink per day.

FACTORS RELATED TO SCREENING BEHAVIORS. Numerous studies have explored screening behaviors among women of varying cultures, races, and nationalities. Interviews of women ages 50 and older about BSE technique revealed that African American women relied more on visual examination whereas Caucasian women relied more on tactile examination (Mitchell, Mathews, & Mayne, 2005). The degree of acculturation of African American women was found to be related to adherence to BSE frequency guidelines (Guevarra et al., 2005).

Interviews of Canadian women demonstrated differences among various ethnocultural groups in knowledge, attitudes, beliefs, and practices regarding breast and cervical cancer screening. Compared with other groups, Ojibwa and Oji-Cree women generally were less likely to have practiced BSE or to have received information about breast examination. They also were more likely to have refused a clinical breast examination or mammogram (Steven et al., 2004). Predictors of breast and cervical screening in Vietnamese women in Harris County, Houston, Texas, were found to be married status, high educational level, older age, lack of barriers, family history of cancer, and increased perception of seriousness (Ho et al., 2005). In a study of Latinas in a U.S. city, women with poor functional health literacy were less likely to use mammography (Guerra, Krumholz, & Shea, 2005).

Bowen and colleagues explored the relationship between affect (general anxiety, perceived risk, cancer worry, general depression) and health behaviors. Significant predictors of BSE were general anxiety and breast cancer worry. None of the variables predicted mammography use (Bowen, Alfano, McGregor, & Anderson, 2004). Data from the Canadian National Population Health Survey found that regular BSE did not predict mammography use. The investigators concluded that not recommending BSE was unlikely to influence mammography participation (Jelinski, Maxwell, Onysko, & Bancej, 2005).

Although it should not replace other screening methods, all women should be taught to perform breast self-examination by the circular, vertical strip, or wedge method (Figure 17-6). It is easier to palpate the breasts of postmenopausal women than those of premenopausal women because of the older woman's progressive atrophy of breast tissue and the lack of confusing findings related to pregnancy and to the menstrual cycle. Nevertheless, because older women may be less able to detect lumps, it is important to assess her ability to accurately palpate her breasts. The patient needs to understand that failure to find any lumps does not mean that mammography and regular examination by a professional health care provider can be omitted.

Cancer of the Vulva, Cervix, Uterus, and Ovary.
Not only does the prevalence of gynecological cancers rise with aging, but the cancers often are detected at a more advanced stage. Cervical cancer is the most common whereas ovarian cancer is the most lethal (Brown & Cooper, 2003).

CANCER OF THE VULVA. Vulval cancer occurs most often in women aged 60 to 70 years. Pruritus and a symptomatic lump are early signs; however, it often is diagnosed in a later stage when bleeding or an offensive discharge is noted. The treatment of choice is radical vulvectomy with bilateral groin node dissection. Wide dissection sometimes requires closure with a myocutaneous flap. Perhaps surprisingly, older women usually tolerate

these surgical procedures well. Surgical treatment may be followed by pelvic radiotherapy and/or topical chemotherapy (Brown & Cooper, 2003).

VAGINAL CANCER. Vaginal cancers, which are rare and confined almost exclusively to older women, usually are metastatic lesions. Bleeding and offensive discharge are common presenting symptoms. Treatment may include radiotherapy and vaginectomy. Urinary diversion may be necessary for fistula formation (Brown & Cooper, 2003).

UTERINE CANCER. Factors associated with cervical cancer are early age of coitus, multiple sexual partners, a history of a sexually transmitted disease, and human papilloma virus types 16 and 18. Offensive vaginal discharge and postmenopausal or postcoital bleeding are the most common symptoms though some patients present with obstructive renal failure resulting from advanced disease. When a tumor is confined to the cervix, it is treated with radical hysterectomy and pelvic node dissection or radiotherapy. Radiotherapy is more often used in older women; however, otherwise healthy older women will usually tolerate the surgical procedure well (Brown & Cooper, 2003).

CANCER OF THE CORPUS UTERI. Factors associated with endometrial cancer are celibacy, nulliparity, late menopause, obesity, unopposed estrogen therapy, hypertension, and diabetes mellitus. The usual symptom is postmenopausal bleeding. Early stage cancers may be cured with total abdominal hysterectomy and bilateral salpingo-oophorectomy. Depending on the extent of myometrial invasion, a combination of vaginal and external radiotherapy may be given postoperatively. Progestational agents may be used as adjunctive therapy to control vaginal bleeding and reduce pain (Brown & Cooper, 2003).

OVARIAN CANCER. Almost 50% of ovarian cancers occur in women aged 65 and older. Unfortunately, the disease is more likely to be advanced in these women, and they are less likely to be offered radical surgery and chemotherapy. Symptoms generally are vague, such as abdominal discomfort and swelling, malaise, and weight loss. Ascites is a late sign. The tumor marker CA125 is elevated in about 90% of ovarian carcinomas. Surgical treatment entails tumor debulking with bilateral salpingo-oophorectomy, total hysterectomy, and omentectomy. Except in patients with stage 1 disease, postoperative chemotherapy commonly is used. If first line treatment fails, the outlook usually is poor. Ascites becomes a persistent problem requiring repeated paracentesis. Spironolactone may help control fluid retention.

Breast self-examination (BSE) should be done once a month so that you become familiar with the usual appearance and feel of your breasts. Familiarity makes it easier to notice any changes in the breast from one month to another. Early discovery of a change from what is baseline is the main idea behind BSE.

If you menstruate, the best time to do BSE is 2 or 3 days after your period ends, when your breasts are least likely to be tender or swollen. If you no longer menstruate, pick a day, such as the first day of the month, to remind yourself it is time to do BSE.

Here is how to do BSE:

1. Stand before a mirror. Inspect both breasts for anything unusual, such as any discharge form the nipples, puckering, dimpling, or scaling of the skin.

The next two steps are designed to emphasize any change in the shape or contour of your breasts. As you do them, you should be able to feel your chest muscles tighten.

2. Watching closely in the mirror, clasp hands behind your head and press hands forward.
3. Next, press hands firmly on hips and bow slightly toward your mirror as you pull your shoulders and elbows forward.

Some women do the next part of the examination in the shower. Fingers glide over soapy skin, making it easy to appreciate the texture underneath.

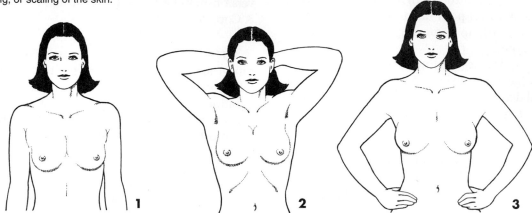

4. Raise your left arm. Use three of four fingers of your right hand to explore your left breast firmly, carefully, and thoroughly. Beginning at the outer edge, press the flat part of your fingers in small circles, moving the circles slowly around the breast. Gradually work toward nipple. Be sure to cover the entire breast and the armpit, including the armpit itself. Feel for any unusual lump or mass under the skin.

5. Gently squeeze the nipple and look for a discharge. Repeat the examination on your right breast.
6. Steps 4 and 5 should be repeated lying down. Lie flat on your back, left arm over your head and a pillow or folded towel under your left shoulder. This position flattens the breast and makes it easier to examine. Use the same circular motion described earlier.
7. Repeat on your right breast.

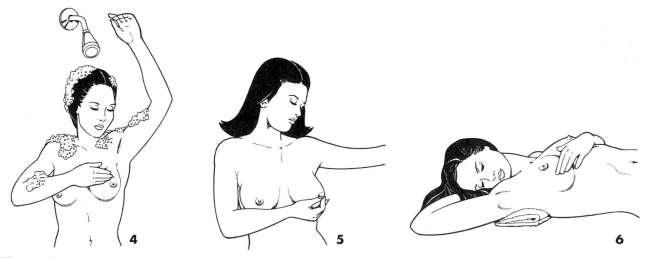

Figure 17-6 Technique for breast self-examination. (From U.S. Department of Health and Human Services.)

Radiotherapy may be used for palliation in individuals with unresectable tumors (Brown & Cooper, 2003).

SCREENING RECOMMENDATIONS. ACS (2005c) recommendations for the early detection of cervical cancer include:

■ Pap tests should begin about 3 years after the beginning of vaginal intercourse, but no later than 21 years of age.
■ Screening should be done annually with regular Pap tests or every other year using the liquid-based Pap test.

- After age 30, a woman who has had three consecutive normal tests can decrease screening frequency to every 2 to 3 years depending on the type of test performed (Pap, liquid Pap, HPV DNA test plus Pap).
- Yearly testing still is advised for women with poor immune function and those whose mothers took diethylstilbestrol (DES) during pregnancy.
- Screening may be discontinued at age 70 if a woman has had no abnormal results for 10 years and normal results for 3 or more years.
- A woman who has had a total hysterectomy including removal of the cervix does not require screening unless she has been treated for cervical cancer or precancer.
- A woman who has had a hysterectomy without removal of the cervix should continue screening at least until age 70.

Erectile Dysfunction

A diagnosis of ED is based on failure in sexual encounters in at least one fourth of all attempts (Butler & Lewis, 2003). ED may occur at any age, but it is more likely in older men. The great majority of cases of ED are attributed to physical causes, including vascular, neurological, and endocrine disorders. Only about 4% of men have low testosterone levels. Psychological causes such as depression, performance anxiety, and stress account for about 10% of ED cases (see Tables 17-2 and 17-3). Drugs frequently inhibit sexual responses in older males. Sex is more likely if there is a willing partner available and if there has been no interruption in sexual activity during the middle years. Because ED may be an early sign of heart disease, hypertension, or diabetes, practitioners should perform a careful evaluation before recommending a treatment.

A healthy lifestyle including a balanced diet, weight management, exercise, avoidance of tobacco, and only moderate alcohol consumption may help to prevent sexual dysfunction. Underlying causes such as hypertension or depression should be treated. Psychotherapy, marital therapy, or sex therapy may be helpful even when a physical cause exists because ED commonly evokes emotional distress in the patient and his/her partner (Butler & Lewis, 2003). Other options are drugs, vacuum therapy, implants, and surgery. Pharmacological agents for ED are summarized in Box 17-8. As noted earlier, testosterone supplementation may enhance the response to sildenafil by improving the response to phosphodiesterase inhibitor type 5 in hypogonadal persons (Frajese & Pozzi, 2005).

Vacuum therapy uses a cylinder that is placed over the flaccid penis. As air is drawn out of the cylinder, blood is drawn into the penis. A wide band is placed around the base of the penis to maintain the erection. This treatment, which is effective for about one third of men, is contraindicated in men with low platelet counts or receiving anticoagulant therapy. Inflatable and non-inflatable penile implants are permanent prostheses that may be used when other approaches fail. Implants are contraindicated in men with psychosis and men with untreated depression. Revascularization surgery is considered experimental at this time (Butler & Lewis, 2003).

Prostate Disorders. Benign prostatic hypertrophy and prostate cancer are addressed in Chapter 16.

BOX 17-8 Pharmacotherapy for Erectile Dysfunction

DRUG	COMMENTS
Phosphodiesterase inhibitors: sildenafil, tadalafil	Taken orally 1 hour before sexual encounter Dilates penile blood vessels Produces erection only in presence of sexual stimulation Contraindicated with nitrates Side effects: headache, upset stomach, bluish vision, nasal congestion, and (rarely) priapism
Phentolamine, atropine, prostaglandin E	Vasodilating drugs injected into corpus cavernosum Erection occurs within 10 minutes and lasts approximately 30 minutes Contraindicated with sickle cell anemia, multiple myeloma, leukemia, anatomical deformities, penile implants
Transurethral alprostadil	Vasodilating drug administered into urethra with applicator

Data from Butler, R. N., & Lewis, M. I. (2003). Sexuality. In R. C. Tallis & H. M. Fillit (Eds.), *Brocklehurst's textbook of geriatric medicine and gerontology* (6th ed.). Edinburgh: Churchill Livingstone, pp. 1407-1412.

NURSING CARE: PERSON WITH ENDOCRINE DYSFUNCTION
Nursing Assessment

Nursing assessment of the endocrine system is centered mainly on the conditions that commonly occur—diabetes mellitus, thyroid disorders, and breast cancer. Information regarding sexuality, menstruation and childbearing, and menopause is also elicited.

History

DIABETES MELLITUS. Ask if the patient has a recent history of fatigue, generalized weakness, excessive appetite and thirst, and rapid weight loss, which may indicate type 1 or type 2 diabetes mellitus. Obesity may be associated with type 2 diabetes mellitus.

THYROID DISORDERS. Inquire about a history of thyroid problems and treatment received, which might include drug therapy, surgery, and/or radiation. Assess for intolerance of heat or cold, fatigue, weakness, nervousness, depression, and unexplained weight changes.

Hypothyroidism. Symptoms suggestive of hypothyroidism include decreased tolerance to cold, lethargy, and constipation. Patients' responses may be slowed and inappropriate. Patients may also complain about muscle weakness, pain, stiffness, and loss of sense of smell or nasal stuffiness.

Hyperthyroidism. There may be a history of cardiovascular symptoms, such as angina pectoris or atrial fibrillation. Other symptoms to assess include confusion, depression, emotional lability, weakness, fatigue, weight loss, increased cold tolerance, and decreased heat tolerance.

BREAST CANCER. Ask if the patient has noticed changes in the appearance of the breasts or the presence of a mass, tenderness, or discharge. Record whether the patient performs breast self-examinations and has periodic mammograms. Note a positive family history of breast cancer.

SEXUALITY. Information regarding sexual activity should include the availability of a partner, interest, and ease of intercourse. Men should be questioned about erectile dysfunction.

Menstruation, Childbearing, and Menopause. The general medical history for the female patient should document blood clots, hypertension, stroke, cancer, uterine fibroids, endometriosis, migraine headaches, diabetes, liver disorders, and fractures. Significant data from the family history include osteoporosis, heart disease before age 50, breast cancer among first-degree relatives, diabetes, and mental illness. Lifestyle information should include dietary patterns, particularly calcium and fat intake, caffeine and alcohol consumption, recreational drug use, tobacco history, and exercise and sleep patterns. Introduce the topic of sexuality by asking about marital status, sexual activity, and changes that may have affected sexual activity (Smith, 2005).

The specific menstrual and pregnancy history records pregnancy, age at menarche, age at full-term pregnancy, and any relevant surgical history. Information about menopause includes age of onset and symptoms such as hot flashes, chills, sweating, and palpitations. Other complaints that may be relevant include headaches, irritability, mood swings, loss of libido, depression, and changes in well-being, sleeping, or management of daily activities. Also inquire about routine gynecological examinations, Pap smears, and bone density studies. In relation to the breasts, note any abnormal mammograms or breast biopsies. If hormone therapy has been used at any time, note the type and duration of the therapy. A standardized rating scale for menopause symptoms can be very useful. However, these tools should be used cautiously with women with physical disabilities (Kalpakjian et al., 2005).

Physical Assessment

MENOPAUSE. The physical examination of the menopausal woman is comprehensive and should assess cardiovascular, skeletal, genitourinary, and neuroendocrine function. Common findings on the gynecological examination include sparse pubic hair, and atrophy of the fat pad on the mons pubis, the labia, the clitoris, and the uterus. The vaginal epithelium may appear dry, irritated, or inflamed. The atrophied ovaries are no longer palpable. Relaxation of the sacral ligaments and the pelvic musculature allows the uterus to descend, sometimes into the vagina (Jarvis, 2000).

A blood sample may be drawn to determine FSH and estradiol levels. Hormonal medications should be discontinued 1 to 2 weeks before obtaining the sample. Test sensitivity will be best if the sample is drawn on day 3 to 6 of the menstrual cycle (Smith, 2005). Tests for TSH level, fasting blood glucose level, lipid profile, and liver enzymes may be ordered as appropriate based on the patient assessment and risk factors (Smith, 2005).

DIABETES MELLITUS. Older persons with diabetes mellitus may appear chronically ill and fatigued. There may be thinning of the skin and subcutaneous tissue in the lower extremities with plantar redness of the feet. Skin infections and foot ulcers may be present. An examination of the eye may reveal cataracts or retinopathy. Neuropathy can result in diminished patellar and Achilles tendon reflexes as well as decreased temperature sensation.

THYROID DISORDERS. Inspect the neck for any swelling. The thyroid gland can be palpated with the examiner standing in front of or behind the patient with the hand positioned on either side of the trachea. The examiner feels for lobe enlargement and nodules as the patient swallows. Auscultate the thyroid gland for a bruit if the gland is enlarged.

Hypothyroidism. Observe for coarse, dry, thickened skin and hair that is dry and lifeless. The lips and nostrils may appear prominent, and the eyebrows sparse with loss of the outer third of the margin. The voice often is husky and weak. There may be evidence of an enlarged heart or congestive heart failure.

Hyperthyroidism. In the presence of hyperthyroidism, the skin often is smooth, warm, and damp with perspiration. The eyes may have the bulging appearance of exophthalmia or may appear to be staring. Tremors may be observed in the tongue when it is extended from the mouth, or in the hands when the arms and fingers are extended. Tachycardia or atrial fibrillation also occurs with hyperthyroidism. Turbulent blood flow heard on auscultation is characteristic of hyperthyroidism.

EXAMINATION OF THE BREASTS. Older women may have large, pendulous breasts that make examination difficult. The nurse should observe for symmetry, changes in contour, swelling, dimpling of the skin, and changes in the nipple. The nurse should also palpate for lumps, thickening, and hard knots. Self-breast examination should be taught to all older women.

Assessment of the patient with an endocrine disorder is outlined in Box 17-9

NANDA Nursing Diagnoses (NANDA International, 2005)

Nursing diagnoses common to multiple endocrine disorders include the following:

- Effective therapeutic regimen management
- Deficient Knowledge (breast examination, diabetes self-care; sexuality in the aged) related to lack of exposure, cognitive limitation, unfamiliarity with information resources
- Anxiety related to threat to self concept (erectile dysfunction, mastectomy, symptoms of menopause)

Box 17-9 Endocrine Assessment

Health History
Family history of diabetes mellitus, thyroid disease, or cancer

Symptoms
- Diabetes mellitus: fatigue, generalized weakness, excessive appetite, thirst, rapid weight loss, obesity
- Hypothyroidism: decreased tolerance to cold, lethargy, constipation, muscle weakness, pain, stiffness, loss of sense of smell or nasal stuffiness, answers questions slowly and inappropriately
- Hyperthyroidism: angina, confusion, emotional lability, weakness, fatigue, weight loss, increased cold tolerance, decreased heat tolerance
- Breast cancer: changes in appearance of breast, tenderness, mass, discharge

Sexual history and functioning
- Availability of a partner
- Interest
- Ease of intercourse

Menstruation, childbearing, and menopause
- Gynecological care
- Menstruation history
- Number of pregnancies
- Menopause
  - Age of onset
  - Symptoms: "hot flashes," chills, sweating, palpitations, headaches, irritability, and depression

Physical Assessment
Diabetes mellitus
- Thinning of skin and subcutaneous tissue in lower extremities
- Skin infections, foot ulcers
- Decreased temperature sensation
- Cataracts: diabetic retinopathy
- Diminished patellar and Achilles reflexes
  Hypothyroidism:
- Lifeless, dry hair
- Coarse, dry, and thickened skin
- Prominent lips and nostrils
- Sparse eyebrows with loss of outer one-third margin
- Enlarged heart and congestive heart failure
- Husky and weak voice

Hyperthyroidism
- Skin warm, damp, fine, and smooth
- Exophthalmia or staring eyes
- Tremors of tongue or hands
- Tachycardia or atrial fibrillation
  Breast examination:
- Symmetry, contour, swelling, dimpling, and changes in nipples
- Lumps, thickening, and hard knots

Other nursing diagnoses that are more specific to a particular diagnosis include:

- Death anxiety related to diagnosis of cancer
- Disturbed body image related to surgery, illness treatment, erectile dysfunction
- Sexual Dysfunction related to altered body structure or function, lack of significant other, misinformation or lack of knowledge
- Imbalanced Nutrition: Less Than Body Requirements related to symptoms of diabetes, hyperthyroidism
- Risk for constipation related to decreased motility of the gastrointestinal tract
- Risk for impaired skin integrity related to altered sensation, altered circulation secondary to diabetes mellitus
- Risk for imbalanced body temperature related to altered metabolic rate

NOC Nursing Goals/Outcomes (Moorhead, Johnson, & Maas, 2004)

The outcomes of nursing care for the person with an endocrine disorder might include adherence behavior, participation in health care decisions, and family participation in professional care; knowledge: diabetes care, illness care, medication, sexual functioning, and treatment regimen; and decreased indicators of anxiety.

NIC Nursing Interventions

Because of the diverse nature of nursing care for the disorders addressed in this chapter, specifics are addressed with each disorder. This section will summarize only topics general to the care of persons with endocrine disorders. Common interventions are directed toward enabling patients to manage their therapeutic regimens effectively and reducing anxiety associated with medical diagnoses that might be life-threatening or require changes in lifestyle.

Interventions to Foster Effective Therapeutic Regimen Management.

Although many older persons are capable of managing their own therapeutic regimens, an assessment of functional and cognitive abilities is vital. Educational interventions should be designed to accommodate the specific needs of the older person. For example, reading material should use larger font, content should be broken into manageable units, and reading level should be appropriate for the target audience. Individuals with hearing deficits may have difficulty in a large group setting. Some individuals may prefer videos or even computer-assisted instruction. Drug management such as the preparation and administration of insulin is often difficult for older persons with sensory and motor deficits. These same patients may need assistance to perform self blood glucose monitoring. When the patient is not able to manage independently, family members or community nurses must be involved in the preparation of medications to be sure that proper doses and schedules are maintained.

Interventions to Manage Anxiety.

Counseling may be necessary to help older patients to adjust to changes in lifestyle, such as diet modification and exercise. Older people are willing to modify their diets and to engage in exercise programs if they are able and see the need to do so. Dietary changes and exercise regimens should be developed based on individual preferences and abilities, cultural background, and previously held attitudes and beliefs. Unfortunately, health care providers often have limited time to elicit concerns and provide support. Some older patients are reluctant to impose on the care provider's time. Patient education and community support groups conducted by health professionals or volunteers provide a venue to express concerns, to problem-solve, and to receive support.

Diagnosis of a new disease can be a source of anxiety. The older adult may not be aware of the range of treatment options available. Even with potentially life-threatening diagnoses, protocols often are available that can be customized to the older person.

Older people may have difficulty in discussing intimate matters related to sexuality. Thoughtful discussion may reveal attitudes and beliefs that may be untrue and that interfere with satisfactory sexual functioning. For example, they may assume that sexual dysfunction is a normal and inevitable consequence of aging. This perception may have changed with the availability of sildenafil. Although it is not effective or appropriate in all situations, it has fostered the idea that ED often can be treated. Nurses must also examine their own attitudes toward sexuality in older persons and must be aware that sexuality is a normal part of life at any age.

Evaluation

Evaluation is based on the amount of compliance and ability to carry out drug, dietary, and exercise regimens. In addition, older clients should be able to express satisfaction with their sexual outlets.

SUMMARY

The endocrine system consists of tissues and glands whose function is to produce and secrete hormones into the bloodstream. Age-related changes occur in both the reception and the production of hormones and affect the functioning of the pituitary and thyroid glands, adrenal cortex, gonads, parathyroid glands, and pancreas. Major changes occurring in the older male include decreases in testicular volume and spermatogenesis;

Nursing Care Plan: The Older Patient with Type 2 Diabetes Mellitus

Assessment Data

78 y.o. white female, widowed, lives alone, 2 adult children live in the same community. Is a homemaker who worked as a file clerk. Height 5'4", weight 170 lbs. Diagnosed with type 2 DM 1 year ago. She attended diabetes education classes and lost 10 pounds initially but has since regained the lost weight. She has been walking for half an hour "most days." Efforts to maintain blood glucose control with lifestyle changes have not been effective. Patient states "I know I should eat right, but I don't think my diabetes is really that bad, is it?" Health is good except for hypertension and osteoarthritis. Medications: calcium channel blocker (Norvasc 5 mg qd) ; OTC NSAIDs prn for joint pain. The provider has ordered glipizide (Glucotrol).

Nursing Diagnoses (Johnson, Bulechek, Dochterman, Maas, & Moorhead, 2001)

Knowledge deficit related to management of type 2 DM

Ineffective denial related to need to alter lifestyle to cope with type 2 DM

Noncompliance related to motivational factors

Goals/Outcomes

- The patient will correctly describe dietary, activity, and pharmacological measures to maintain blood glucose with acceptable range.
- The patient will explain the complications of poorly controlled diabetes.
- The patient will acknowledge the diagnosis of diabetes mellitus and the need to make lifestyle changes to manage it.
- The patient will adhere to guidelines for diet and activity to manage her diabetes.

NOC Suggested Outcomes (Moorhead, Johnson, & Maas, 2004)

Diabetes self-management (1619): patient accepts health care provider's diagnosis, performs treatment regimen as prescribed, monitors blood glucose level, follows recommended diet, follows recommended activity level, uses effective weight control strategies, and uses medications as prescribed

Acceptance: *Health status:* recognizes reality of health situation, adjusts to changes in health status, pursues information about health status, makes decisions about health, performs self care tasks

Health beliefs: perceived threat: Perceived vulnerability to progressive health problems, concern regarding potential complications

Health seeking behavior: performs self-screening when indicated, adheres to self described strategies to eliminate unhealthy behavior

NIC Nursing Interventions (Dochterman & Bulechek, 2004)

Major interventions: Teaching: Disease Process (5206), Coping Enhancement (5230), Counseling (5240)

- Review patient's knowledge about condition.
- Describe possible chronic complications as appropriate.
- Discuss lifestyle changes that may be required to prevent future complications and/or control the disease process.
- Discuss therapy/treatment options.
- Describe rationale behind management/therapy/ treatment recommendations.
- Instruct the patient on measures to control/minimize symptoms as appropriate.
- Help patient to identify the information she is most interested in obtaining.
- Support the use of appropriate defense mechanisms.
- Encourage verbalization of feelings, perceptions, and fears.
- Assist the patient in breaking down complex goals into small, manageable steps.
- Assist patient to list and prioritize all possible alternatives to a problem.
- Identify any differences between patient's view of the situation and the view of the health care team.

Evaluation Parameters

Knowledge: disease process, knowledge: diabetes management, patient knowledge of condition, complications, treatment, measures to manage symptoms: patient expression of intent to make lifestyle changes; patient verbalization of feelings, perceptions, fears; patient acknowledgement of actions to move toward goal achievement; patient acknowledges how her views differ from those of health care team.

BOX 17-10 *TOWARD BETTER ENDOCRINE HEALTH*

- Ensure adequate vitamin D levels by regular exposure to sunlight.
- Ensure adequate intake of calcium through diet or supplements.
- Attain and maintain weight within a healthy range.
- Exercise on a regular basis.
- Discuss benefits and risks of postmenopausal estrogen replacement therapy with health care provider.
- Have periodic health screenings to detect endocrine dysfunction.
- Have periodic health screenings to detect malignancies (breast, prostate) at an early stage.

however, serum testosterone levels remain constant. Females experience menopause, decreased serum estrogen levels, and atrophy of the subcutaneous tissues of the breast and external genitalia. Sexual responses tend to become slower and are less intense in both men and women in older age.

Pathological changes in the endocrine system that commonly occur with older age include type 2 diabetes mellitus, thyroid disorders, and cancer of the breast and reproductive organs. Treatment is aimed toward proper management of medications, diet and exercise, and sexual counseling (Box 17-10).

REFERENCES

Abrams, A. C. (2004). *Clinical drug therapy* (7th ed.). Philadelphia: Lippincott.

Alassas, M., Chu, Q., Burton, G., Ampil, F., Mizell, J., & Li, B. D. (2005). Neoadjuvant chemotherapy in stage III breast cancer. *American Surgeon, 71*(6), 487-492.

Allan, C. A., & McLachlan, R. I. (2004). Age-related changes in testosterone and the role of replacement therapy in older men. *Clinical Endocrinology, 60,* 653-670.

Althuis, M. D., Dozier, J. M., Anderson, W. F., Devesa, S. S., & Brinton, L. A. (2005). Global trends in breast cancer incidence and mortality 1973-1997. *International Journal of Epidemiology, 34*(2), 405-412.

Altintas, O., Caglar, Y., Yuksel, N., Demirci, A., & Karabas, L. (2004). The effects of menopause and hormone replacement therapy on quality and quantity of tear, intraocular pressure and ocular blood flow. *Ophthalmologica, 218*(2), 120-129.

Amella, E. (2004). Presentation of illness in older adults. *AJN, 104*(10), 40-51.

American Cancer Society (ACS). (2003). Cancer facts for women, 2003. Retrieved October 28. 2005 from www.cancer.org.

American Cancer Society (ACS). (2005a). Herceptin "revolutionary" for breast cancer. Retrieved October 28, 2005, from www.cancer.org.

American Cancer Society (ACS). (2005b). Leading sites of new cancer cases and deaths—2005 estimates. Retrieved October 28, 2005, from www.cancer.org.

American Cancer Society (ACS). (2005c). New cervical cancer early detection guidelines released. Retrieved October 28, 2005, from www.cancer.org.

American Cancer Society (ACS). (2005d). Probability of developing invasive cancers over selected age intervals, by sex, U. S., 1999-2001. Retrieved October 28, 2005, from www.cancer.org.

American Diabetes Association. (1997). Report on the expert committee on the diagnosis and classification of diabetes mellitus. *Diabetes Care, 20*(suppl), 1183-1197.

American Diabetes Association. (2002). Economic costs of diabetes in the U.S. *Diabetes Care, 26*(3), 917-932.

American Diabetes Association. (2003). Physical activity/exercise and diabetes mellitus. *Diabetes Care, 26*(suppl 1), S73-S77.

American Diabetes Association. (2005a). Diagnosis and classification of diabetes mellitus. *Diabetes Care, 28,* S37-S42.

American Diabetes Association. (2005b). Insulin: There are many different insulins for many different situations and lifestyles. *Diabetes Forecast, 59*(1), RG 10-15.

Amir, O., & Biron-Shental, T. (2004). The impact of hormonal fluctuations on female vocal folds. *Current Opinion in Otolaryngology & Head & Neck Surgery, 12*(3), 180-184.

Anonymous. (2002, November). The heart can ail when the thyroid gland fails. *Harvard Heart Letter, 13*(3), 4-5.

Armer, J. A., & Fu, M. R. (2005). Age differences in post-breast cancer lymphedema signs and symptoms. *Cancer Nursing, 28*(3), 200-207.

Armer, J. M., & Heckathorn, P. W. (2005). Post-breast cancer lymphedema in aging women: Self management and implications for nursing. *Journal of Gerontological Nursing, 31*(5), 29-39.

Asplund, R., & Aberg, H. E. (2005). Oral dryness, nocturia, and the menopause. *Maturitas, 50*(2), 86-90.

Atwood, C. S., Meethal, S. V., Liu, T., Wilson, A. C., Gallego, M., Smith, M. A., & Bowen, R. L. (2005). Dysregulation of the hypothalamic-pituitary-gonadal axis with menopause and andropause promotes neurodegenerative senescence. *Journal of Neuropathology & Experimental Neurology, 64*(2), 93-103.

Bachmann, G. A., & Leiblum, S. R. (2004). The impact of hormones on menopausal sexuality: A literature review. *Menopause, 11*(1), 120-130.

Bair, Y. A., Gold, E. B., Azari, R. A., Greendale, G., Sternfeld, B., Harkey, M. R., & Kravitz, R. L. (2005). Use of conventional and complementary health care during the transition to menopause: Longitudinal results from the Study of Women's Health Across the Nation (SWAN). *Menopause: The Journal of the North American Menopause Society, 12*(1), 31-39.

Barrett-Connor, E., Grady, D., & Stefanick, M. L. (2005). The rise and fall of menopausal hormone therapy. *Annual Review of Public Health, 26,* 115-140.

Barzel, U. S. (1989). Endocrinology and aging. In Reichel, W., (Ed.). *Clinical aspects of aging* (3rd.ed.). Baltimore: Williams & Wilkins, pp. 373-381.

Bassett, S. D., & Smyer, T. (2003). Health screening practices in rural long-term care facilities. *Journal of Gerontological Nursing, 29*(4), 42-49.

Basso, N., Paglia, N., Stella, I., de Cavanagh, E. M. V., Ferder, L., Arnaiz, M.D. L., & Inserra, F. (2005). Protective effect of the inhibition of the renin-angiotensin system on aging. *Regulatory Peptides, 128,* 247-252.

Bauer, M. E. (2005). Stress, glucocorticoids, and aging of the immune system. *Stress, 8*(1), 69-83.

Bazargan, M., Bazargan, S. H., Calderon, J. L., Husaini, B. A., & Baker, R. S. (2003). Mammography screening and breast self-examination among minority women in public housing projects: The impact of physician recommendation. *Cellular and Molecular Biology, 49*(8), 1213-1218.

Beers M., Jones, T., Berkwits, M., Kaplan, J., & Porter, R. (Eds). (2000). Metobolic and endocrine disorders. Chapter 65: Thyroid disorders, *The Merck maual of geriatrics.* Rahway, NJ: Merck (online edition).

Belchetz, P., & Hammond, P. (2003). Adrenal and pituitary disorders. In R. C. Tallis & H. M. Fillit (Eds.), *Brocklehurst's textbook of geriatric medicine and gerontology* (6th ed.). Edinburgh: Churchill Livingstone, pp. 1157-1164.

Beniashvili, D., Avinoach, I., Baazov, D., & Zusman, I. (2005). Household electromagnetic fields and breast cancer in elderly women. *In Vivo, 19*(3), 563-566.

Bhavnani, B. R. (2003). Estrogens and menopause: Pharmacology of conjugated equine estrogens and their potential role in the prevention of neurodegenerative diseases such as Alzheimer's. *Journal of Steroid Biochemistry & Molecular Biology, 85*(2-5), 473-482.

Birkhaeuser, M. H. (2005). The Women's Health Initiative conundrum. *Archives of Women's Mental Health, 8*(1), 7-14.

Bock, T. (2004). The source(s) for new pancreatic beta cells in adult life. *Bioessays, 26*(11), 1156-1159.

Bowen, D. J., Alfano, C. M., McGregor, B. A., & Anderson, M. R. (2004). The relationship between perceived risk, affect, and health behaviors. *Cancer Detection & Prevention, 28*(6), 409-417.

Boyle, J. P., Honeycutt, A. A., Narayan, V., Hoerger, T. J., Geiss, L. S., Chen, H., and Thompson, T. J. (2001). Projection of diabetes burden through 2050. *Diabetes Care, 24*(11), 1936-1940.

Bressler, R., & Katz, M. D. (1993). *Geriatric pharmacology*. New York: McGraw-Hill, p. 420.

Brown, A. D. G., & Cooper, T. K. (2003). Gynecological disorders. In R. C. Tallis & H. M. Fillit (Eds.), *Brocklehurst's textbook of geriatric medicine and gerontology* (6th ed.). Edinburgh: Churchill Livingstone, pp. 1136-1144.

Brunk, D. (2005). Byetta approved as first in new class of medications to treat type 2 diabetes. *Family Practice News, 35*(11), 2-3.

Butler, R. N., & Lewis, M. I. (2003). Sexuality. In R. C. Tallis & H. M. Fillit (Eds.), *Brocklehurst's textbook of geriatric medicine and gerontology* (6th ed.). Edinburgh: Churchill Livingstone, pp. 1407-1412.

Campbell, W. W., Fleet, J. C., Hall, R. T., & Carnell, N. S. (2004). Short-term low-protein intake does not increase serum parathyroid hormone concentration in humans. *Journal of Nutrition, 134*(8), 1900-1904.

Carvalhaes-Neto, N., Huayllas, M. K., Ramos, L. R., Cendoroglo, M. S., & Kater, C. E. (2003). Cortisol, DHEAS and aging: Resistance to cortisol suppression in frail institutionalized elderly. *Journal of Endocrinological Investigation, 26*(1), 17-22.

Centers for Disease Control and Prevention. (2005). Diabetes surveillance system. Atlanta: U.S. Department of Health and Human Services. Accessed October 21, 2005, at www.cdc.gov/diabetes/statistics/index.htm.

Centers for Disease Control and Prevention. (2005). Leading causes of death and number of deaths according to age: U.S. 1980-2002. Atlanta: U.S. Department of Health and Human Services, pp. 178-179. Accessed October 21, 2005, at www.cdc.gov/nchs/hus.htm.

Chang, A. M., & Halter, J. B. (2003). Aging and insulin secretion. *American Journal of Physiology—Endocrinology & Metabolism, 284*(1), E7-E12.

Chau, D., and Edelman, S. (2001). Clinical management of diabetes in the elderly. *Clinical Diabetes, 19*(4), 172-174.

Chau, D., Shumaker, N., & Plodkowski, R. (2003). Complications of type 2 diabetes in the elderly. *Geriatric Times, 4*(2), 11.

Chiu, K. C., Martinez, D. S., & Chu, A. (2005). Comparison of the relationship of age and beta cell function in three ethnic groups. *Clinical Endocrinology, 62*(3), 296-302.

Chohayeb, A. A. (2004). Influence of osteoporosis on the oral health of menopausal women. *General Dentistry, 52*(3), 258-261.

Col, N., Surks, M., & Daniels, G. (2004). Subclinical thyroid disease, clinical applications. *Journal of the American Medical Association, 291*(2), 239-243.

Connell, K., Guess, M. K., Bleustein, C. B., Powers, K., Lazarou, G., Mikhail, M., & Melman, A. (2005). Effects of age, menopause, and comorbidities on neurological function of the female genitalia. *International Journal of Impotence Research, 17*(1), 63-70.

Cooper, D. (2004). Thyroid disease in the oldest old, the exception to the rule. *Journal of the American Medical Association, 292*(21), 2651-2654.

Dakouane, M., Bicchieray, L., Bergere, M., Albert, M., Vialanr, F., & Selva, J. (2005). A histomorphic and cytogenetic study of testis from men 29-102 years old. *Fertility and Sterility, 83*(4), 923-928.

Danaci, A. E., Oruc, S., Adiguzel, H., Yildirim, Y., & Aydemir, O. (2003). Relationship of sexuality with psychological and hormonal features in the menopausal period. *West Indian Medical Journal, 52*(1), 27-30.

Davies, L. (2003). Aging and the endocrine system. In R. C. Tallis & H. M. Fillit (Eds.), *Brocklehurst's textbook of geriatric medicine and gerontology* (6th ed.). Edinburgh: Churchill Livingstone, pp. 1149-1156.

Davis, P. J., & Davis, F. B. (1992). Endocrine diseases. In E. Calkins, A. B. Ford, & P. R. Katz (Eds.), *Practice of geriatrics* (2nd ed.). Philadelphia: Saunders, p. 485.

Davis, S. R., & Burger, H. G. (2003). The role of androgen therapy. *Best Practice & Research. Clinical Endocrinology & Metabolism, 17*(1), 165-175.

Dawson-Hughes, B. (2004). Racial/ethnic considerations in making recommendations for vitamin D for adult and elderly men and women. *American Journal of Clinical Nutrition, 80*(6; suppl), 1763S-1766S.

de Cavanagh, E. M. V., Piotrkowski, B., & Fraga, C. G. (2004). Concerted action of the renin-angiotensin system, mitochondria, and antioxidant defenses in aging. *Molecular Aspects of Medicine, 25*, 27-36.

DECODE Study Group. (1999). Is fasting glucose sufficient to define diabetes? *Diabetologia, 42*(6), 647-654.

Dell, D. D. (2005). Breast cancer. *Nursing 2005, 35*(10), 56-64.

Deplas, A., Debiais, F., Alcalay, M., Bontoux, D., & Thomas, P. (2004). Bone density, parathyroid hormone, calcium and vitamin D nutritional status of institutionalized elderly subjects. *Journal of Nutrition, Health, & Aging, 8*(5), 400-404.

Dharia, S., & Parker, C. R., Jr. (2004). Adrenal androgens and aging. *Seminars in Reproductive Medicine, 22*(4), 361-368.

Diabetes Control and Complications Trial Research Group. (1998). The effect of intensive treatment of diabetes on the development and progression of long-term complications in insulin-dependent diabetes mellitus. *New England Journal of Medicine, 329*, 837-853.

Dick, I. M., Devine, A., Beilby, J., & Prince, R. L. (2005). Effects of endogenous estrogen on renal calcium and phosphate handling in elderly women. *American Journal of Physiology—Endocrinology & Metabolism, 288*(2), E430-E435.

Diez, J., & Iglesias, P. (2004). Spontaneous subclinical hypothyroidism in patients older than 55 years: An analysis of the natural course and risk factors for the development of overt thyroid failure. *Journal of Clinical Endocrinology and Metabolism, 89*(10), online October 2004.

Dochterman, J. M., & Bulechek, G. M. (Eds.). (2004). *Nursing interventions classification (NIC)* (4th ed.). St. Louis: Mosby.

Dubey, R. K., Imthurn, B., Barton, M., & Jackson, E. K. (2005). Vascular consequences of menopause and hormone therapy: Importance of timing of treatment and type of estrogen. *Cardiovascular Research, 66*(2), 295-306.

Elahi, D., Muller, D. C., Egan, J. M., Andres, R., Veldhuist, J., & Meneilly, G. S. (2002). Glucose tolerance, glucose utilization and insulin secretion in ageing. *Novartis Foundation Symposium, 242*, 222-242.

Eng, S. M., Gammon, M. D., Terry, M. B., Kushi, L. H., Teitelbaum, S., Britton, J. A., & Neugut, A. I. (2005). Body size changes in relation to postmenopausal breast cancer among women on Long Island, New York. *American Journal of Epidemiology, 162*(3), 229-237.

Engelgau, M.M., Geiss, L. S., Saaddine, J. B., Boyle, J. P., Benjamin, S. M., Gregg, E. W., et al. (2004). The evolving diabetes burden in the United States. *Annals of Internal Medicine, 140*(11), 945-950.

Ewertz, M., Mellemkjaer, L., Poulsen, A. H., Friis, S., Sorensen, H. T., Pedersen, L., et al. (2005). Hormone use for menopausal symptoms and risk of breast cancer. A Danish cohort study. *British Journal of Cancer, 92*(7), 1293-1297.

Felicetta, J. (2002). Thyroid disease in the elderly, when to suspect, when to treat. *Consultant, 42*(13), 1597-1599, 1603-1606.

Ferder, L. F., Inserra, F., & Basso, N. (2002). Advances in our understanding of aging: Role of the renin-angiotensin system. *Current Opinion in Pharmacology, 2*, 189-194.

Fisher, J. (2002). Management of thyrotoxicosis. *Southern Medical Journal, 95*(5), 493-505.

Fontbonne, A., Berr, C., Ducimetiere, P., & Alperovitch, A. (2001). Changes in cognitive abilities over a 4-year period are unfavorably affected in elderly diabetic subjects. *Diabetes Care, 24*(2), 366-370.

Frajese, G. V., & Pozzi, F. (2005). New achievement and novel therapeutic applications of PSE5 inhibitors in older males. *Journal of Endocrinological Investigation, 28*(3 Suppl), 45-50.

Franz, M. J., Bantle, J. P., Beebe, J. D., Burnzell, J. L., Jean-Louis Chiasson, A., Garg, A., et al. (2002). Technical review: Evidence-based nutrition principles and recommendations for the treatment and prevention of diabetes and related complications. *Diabetes Care, 25*(1), 148-198.

Freedman, R. R. (2005). Pathophysiology and treatment of menopausal hot flashes. *Seminars in Reproductive Medicine, 23*(2), 117-125.

Freedman, R. R., & Subramanian, M. (2005). Effects of symptomatic status and the menstrual cycle on hot flash-related thermoregulatory parameters. *Menopause, 12*(2), 156-159.

Friedenreich, C. M. (2004). Physical activity and breast cancer risk: The effects of menopausal status. *Exercise & Sport Sciences Review, 32*(4), 180-184.

Fung, T. T., Hu, F. B., Holmes, M. D., Rosner, B. A., Hunter, D. J., Colditz, G. A., et al. (2005). Dietary patterns and the risk of post-menopausal breast cancer. *International Journal of Cancer, 116*(1), 116-121.

Gambert, S. (2005). The difficult problem of timely diagnosis. *Clinical Geriatrics, 13*(2), 10.

Garbers, S., Jessop, D. J., Foti, H., Uribelarrea, M., & Chiasson, M. A. (2003). Barriers to breast cancer screening for low income Mexican and Dominican women in New York City. *Journal of Urban Health, 80*(1), 81-91.

Gasalberti, D. (2002). Early detection of breast cancer by self-examination: The influence of perceived barriers and health conception. *Oncology Nursing Forum. Online, 29*(9), 1341-1347.

Gennari, R., Rotmensz, N., Perego, E., dos Santos, G., & Veronesi, U. (2004). Sentinel node biopsy in elderly breast cancer patients. *Surgical Oncology, 13*(4), 193-196.

George, N. J. R. (2003). The prostate gland. In R. C. Tallis & H. M. Fillit (Eds.), *Brocklehurst's textbook of geriatric medicine and gerontology* (6th ed.). Edinburgh: Churchill Livingstone, pp. 1119-1133.

Gerdhem, P., & Obrant, K. J. (2004). Bone mineral density in old age: The influence of age at menarche and menopause. *Journal of Bone & Mineral Metabolism, 22*(4), 372-375.

Golan, J., Torres, K., Staskiewicz, G. J., Opielak, G., & Maciejewski, R. (2002). Morphometric parameters of the human pineal gland in relation to age, body weight, and height. *Folia Morphologica (Warszawa), 61*(2), 111-113.

Gonzalez, M., Viafara, G., Caba, F., & Molina, E. (2004). Sexual function, menopause and hormone replacement. *Maturitas, 48*(4), 411-420.

Gosney, M. (2003). Geriatric oncology. In R. C. Tallis and H. M. Fillit (Eds.), *Brocklehurst's textbook of geriatric medicine and gerontology* (6th ed.). London: Churchill-Livingstone, pp. 1297-1309.

Gregerman, R. I., & Katz, M. S. (1994). Thyroid diseases. In W. R. Hazzard, E. L. Bierman, J. P. Blass, W. H. Etinger, J. B. Halter, J. G. Ouslander, et al. (Eds.), *Principles of geriatric medicine and gerontology* (3rd ed.). New York: McGraw-Hill, pp. 807-824.

Gregg, E. W., & Brown, A. (2003). Cognitive and physical disabilities and aging-related complications of diabetes. *Clinical Diabetes, 21*(1), 113-118.

Gregg, E. W., Engelgau, M. E., & Narayan, V. (2002). Complications of diabetes in elderly people: Underappreciated problems include cognitive decline and physical disability. *BMJ, 325*(7370), 916-917.

Gregg, E. W., Mangione, C. M., Cauley, J. A., Thompson, T. J., Schwartz, A. V., Ensrud, K. E., et al. (2002). Diabetes and incidence of functional disability in older women. *Diabetes Care, 25*(1), 61-68.

Griffin, J. E., & Wilson, J. D. (2006). The testis. In P. K. Bondy & L. E. Rosenberg (Eds.), *Metabolic control and disease* (8th ed.). Philadelphia: Saunders.

Guerra, C. E., Krumholz, M., & Shea, J. A. (2005). Literacy and knowledge, attitudes and behavior about mammography in Latinas. *Journal of Health Care for the Poor and Underserved, 16*(1), 152-166.

Guevarra, J. S., Kwate, N. O., Tang, T. S., Valdimarsdottir, H. B., Freeman, H. P., & Bovbjerg, D. H. (2005). Acculturation and its relationship to smoking and breast self-examination frequency in African American women. *Journal of Behavioral Medicine, 28*(2), 191-199.

Gussekloo, J., van Exel, E., de Craen, A., Meinders, A., Frolich, M., & Westendorp, R. (2004). Thyroid status, disabiilty and cognitive function, and survival in old age. *Journal of the American Medical Association, 292*(21), 2591-2599.

Guthrie, J. R., Dennerstein, L., Taffe, J. R., Lehert, P., & Burger, H. G. (2004). The menopausal transition: A 9-year prospective population-based study. The Melbourne Women's Midlife Health Project. *Climacteric, 7*(4), 375-389.

Guyton, A. C., & Hall, J. E. (2000). *Textbook of medical physiology* (10th ed.). Philadelphia: Saunders.

Guyton, A. C., & Hall, J. E. (2006). *Textbook of medical physiology* (11th ed.). Philadelphia: Saunders.

Hackshaw, A. K., & Paul, E. A. (2003). Breast self-examination and death from breast cancer: A meta analysis. *British Journal of Cancer, 88*(7), 1047-1053.

Hall, J. E. (2004). Neuroendocrine physiology of the early and late menopause. *Endocrinology & Metabolism Clinics of North America, 33*(4), 637-659.

Hall, R. (2005). How should we manage sub-clinical thyroid disease? *Internal Medicine Alert*, March 29, 2005.

Hall, W. (1997). Update in geriatrics; hyperthyroidism presented like hypothyroidism. *Annals of Internal Medicine, 127*(7), 557-559.

Hammond, P., & Belchetz, P. (2003). Disorders of the parathyroids. In R. C. Tallis & H. M. Fillit (Eds.), *Brocklehurst's textbook of geriatric medicine and gerontology* (6th ed.). Edinburgh: Churchill Livingstone, pp. 1185-1191.

Harris, D. M., Miller, J. E., & Davis, D. M. (2003). Racial differences in breast cancer screening, knowledge and compliance. *Journal of the National Medical Association, 95*(8), 693-701.

Hess, D., Thurlimann, B., Pagani, O., Aebi, S., Rauch, D., Ballabeni, P., et al. (2004). Capecitabine and vinorelbine in elderly patints (> or = 65 years) with metastatic breast cancer: A phase I trial (SAKK 25/99). *Annals of Oncology, 15*(12), 1760-1765.

Ho, V., Yamal, J. M., Atkinson, E. N., Basen-Engquist, K., Tortolero-Luna, G., & Follen, M. (2005). Predictors of breast and cervical screening in Vietnamese women in Harris County, Houston, Texas. *Cancer Nursing, 28*(2), 119-129.

Humphrey, L. L., Helfand, M., Chan, B. K., & Woolf, S. H. (2002). Breast cancer screening: A summary of the evidence for the U.S. Preventive Services Task Force. *Annals of Internal Medicine, 137*(5 Part 1), 347-360.

Hurd, T. C., Muti, P., Erwin, D. O., & Womack, S. (2003). An evaluation of the integration of non-tradtional learning tools into a community based breast and cervical cancer education program: The Witness Project of Buffalo. *BMC Cancer, 3*(1), 18.

Hussar, D. A. (2005). New drugs: Exenatide, pramlintide acetate and micafungin sodium. *Journal of the American Pharmacological Association, 45*(4), 524-527.

Im, E. O., & Chee, W. (2005). A descriptive Internet survey on menopausal symptoms: Five ethnic groups of Asian-American university faculty and staff. *Journal of Transcultural Nursing, 16*(2), 126-135.

Jarvis, C. (2000). *Physical examination and health assessment* (4th ed.). Philadelphia: Saunders.

Jelinski, S. E., Maxwell, C. J., Onysko, J., & Bancej, C. M. (2005). The influence of breast self-examination on subsequent mammography. *American Journal of Public Health, 95*(3), 506-511.

Jen, K. L., Buison, A., Darga, L., & Nelson, D. (2005). The relationship between blood leptin level and bone density is specific to ethnicity and menopausal status. *Journal of Laboratory and Clinical Medicine, 146*(1), 18-24.

Jinno, H., Ikedo, T., Asaga, S., Muto, T., Kitagawa, Y., Fujii, H., et al. (2005). Increasing age does not affect efficacy of sentinel lymph node biopsy using smaller-sized technetium-99m tin colloids for breast cancer patients. *American Journal of Surgery, 190*(1), 51-54.

Johnson, A., & Shekhdar, J. (2005). Breast cancer incidence: What do the figures mean? *Journal of Evaluation in Clinical Practice, 11*(1), 27-31.

Johnson, M., Bulechek, G., Dochterman, J. M., Maas, M., & Moorhead, S. (Eds.). (2001). *Nursing diagnoses, outcomes, and interventions: NANDA, NOC, and NIC linkages.* St. Louis: Mosby.

Kalpakjian, C. Z., Toussaint, L. L., Quint, E. H., & Reame, N. K. (2005). Use of a standardized menopause symptom rating scale in a sample of women with physical disabilities. *Menopause, 12*(1), 78-87.

Kannel, W. B. (2001). Risk factors for cardiovascular disease in woman. *Cardiology Review, 18*(3), 11-15.

Karasek, M. (2004). Melatonin, human aging, and age-related diseases. *Experimental Gerontology, 39*, 1723-1729.

Kaushik, V., & Makin, A., (2003). The pancreas. In R. C. Tallis & H. M. Fillit (Eds.), *Brocklehurst's textbook of geriatric medicine and gerontology* (6th ed.). Edinburgh: Churchill Livingstone, pp. 987-1000.

Kennel, K. A., Riggs, B. L., Achenbach, S. J., Oberg, A. L., & Khosla, S. (2003). Role of parathyroid hormone in mediating age-related changes in bone resorption in men. *Osteoporosis International, 14*(8), 631-636.

King, H., Aubert, R. E., & Herman, W. H. (1998). Global burden of diabetes 1995-2025: Prevalence, numerical estimates and projections. *Diabetes Care, 21*, 1414-1431.

Knopman, D., Boland, L. L., Mosley, T., Howard, G., Liao, D., Szklo, M., et al. (2001). Cardiovascular risk factors and cognitive decline in middle-aged adults. *Neurology, 56*(1), 42-48.

Kumari, M., Stafford, M., & Marmot, M. (2005). The menopausal transition was associated in a prospective study with decreased health functioning in women who report menopausal symptoms. *Journal of Clinical Epidemiology, 58*, 719-727.

Kumeda, Y., Inaba, M., Tahara, H., Kurioka, Y., Ishikawa, T., Morii, H., et al. (2000). Persistent increase in bone turnover in Graves' patients with subclinical hyperthyroidism. *Journal of Clinical Endocrinology & Metabolism, 85*, 4157-4161.

Lee, A., Kin, Y., Han, K., Kang, C. S., Jeon, H. M., & Shim, S. I. (2004). Detection of tumor markers including carcinoembryonic antigen, APC, and cyclin D2 in fine-needle aspiration of fluid of breast. *Archives of Pathology & Laboratory Medicine, 128*(11), 1251-1256.

Leonard, R. C., & Malinovszky, K. M. (2005). Chemotherapy for older women with early breast cancer. *Clinical Oncology, 17*(4), 244-248.

Lewis, S. M., Hietkemper, M. M., & Dirksen, S. R. (2004). *Medical surgical nursing* (6th ed.). St. Louis: Mosby, p. 1370.

Li, C. I., Daling, J. R., & Malone, K. E. (2005). Age-specific incidence rates of in situ breast carcinoma by histologic type, 1980-2001. *Cancer Epidemiology, Biomarkers & Preventions, 14*(4), 1008-1011.

Lin, T. L., Ng, S. C., Chen, Y. C., Hu, S. W., & Chen, G. D. (2005). What affects the occurrence of nocturia more: Menopause or age? *Maturitas, 50*(2), 71-77.

Lipson, L. G. (1985). *Diabetes mellitus in the elderly: Special problems, special approaches.* New York: Pfizer Pharmaceuticals, p. 9.

Luchsinger, J. A., Tang, M., Stern, Y., Shea, S., & Mayeux, R. (2001). Diabetes mellitus and risk of Alzheimer's disease and dementia with stroke in a multiethnic cohort. *American Journal of Epidemiology, 154*(7), 635-641.

Lupien, S. J., Fiocco, A., Wan, N., Maheu, F., Lord, C., Schramek, T., & Tu, M. T. (2005). Stress hormones and human memory function across the lifespan. *Psychoneuroendocrinology, 30*(3), 225-242.

Magri, F., Sarra, S., Cinchetti, W., Guazzoni, V., Fioravanti, M., Cravello, L., & Ferrari, E. (2004). *Journal of Pineal Research, 36*(4), 256-261.

Mahmoud, A. M., Goemaere, S., El-Garem, Y., Van Pottelbergh, I., Comhaire, F. H., & Kaufman, J. M. (2003)). Testicular volume in relation to hormonal indices of gonadal function in community-dwelling elderly men. *Journal of Clinical Endocrinology & Metabolism, 88*(1), 179-184.

Maisano, R., Mare, M., Caristi, N., Chiofalo, G., Picciotto, M., Carboni, R., et al. (2005). A modified weekly docetaxel schedule as first-line chemotherapy in elderly metastatic breast cancer: A safety study. *Journal of Chemotherapy, 17*(2), 242-246.

Maly, R. C., Leake, B., & Silliman, R. A. (2004). Breast cancer treatment in older women: Impact of the patient-physician interaction. *Journal of the American Geriatrics Society, 52*(7), 1138-1145.

Maly, R. C., Umezawa, Y., Leake, B., & Silliman, R. A. (2005). Mental health outcomes in older women with breast cancer: Impact of perceived family support and adjustment. *Psycho-Oncology, 14*(7), 535-545.

Mandel, S. (2004). A 64 year-old woman with a thyroid nodule. *JAMA, 282*(21), 2632-2642.

Mano, M., Fraser, G., McIlroy, P., Stirling, L., MacKay, H., Ritchie, D., & Canney, P. (2005). Locally advanced breast cancer in octogenarian women. *Breast Cancer Research & Treatment, 89*(1), 81-90.

Mansel, R. E. (2003). Carcinoma of the breast. In R. C. Tallis & H. M. Fillit (Eds.), *Brocklehurst's textbook of geriatric medicine and gerontology* (6th ed.). London: Churchill-Livingstone, pp. 1145-1148.

Marchick, J., & Henson, D. E. (2005). Correlations between access to mammography and breast cancer stage at diagnosis. *Cancer, 103*(8), 1571-1580.

Marshall, S. F., Bernstein, L., Anton-Culver, H., Deapen, D., Horn-Ross, P. L., Mohrenweiser, H., et al. (2005). Nonsteroidal anti-inflammatory drug use and breast cancer risk by stage and hormone receptor status. *Journal of the National Cancer Institute, 97*(11), 805-812.

Masters, W., & Johnson, V. (1966). *Human sexual response.* Boston: Little, Brown, pp. 233-247.

Mazhar, S. B., & Gul-e-Erum (2003). Knowledge and attitude of older women towards menopause. *Journal of the College of Physicians and Surgeons—Pakistan, 13*(11), 621-624.

McBean, A. M., Gilbertson, D. T., Li, S., & Collins, A. J. (2004). Difference in diabetes prevalence, incidence, and mortality among the elderly of four racial/ethnic groups. *Diabetes Care, 27*(10), 2317-2324.

McLay, R. N., Maki, P. M., & Lyketsos, C. G. (2003). Nulliparity and late menopause are associated with decreased cognitive decline. *Journal of Neuropsychiatry and Clinical Neurosciences, 15*(2), 161-167.

McMahon, L. E., Gray, R. J., & Pockaj, B. A. (2005). Is breast cancer sentinel lymph node mapping valuable for patients in their seventies and beyond? *American Journal of Surgery, 190*(3), 366-370.

Meneilly, G. S., & Tessier, D. (2001). Diabetes in elderly adults. *The Journals of Gerontology. Series A, Biological Sciences and Medical Sciences, 56*(A), M5-M13.

Miedema, B. B., & Tatemichi, S. (2003). Breast and cervical cancer screening for women between 50 and 69 years of age: What prompts women to screen? *Womens Health Issues, 13*(5), 180-184.

Miller, M. (2005). Subclinical thyroid disorders. *Clinical Geriatrics, 13*(8), 38-45.

Mirza, F. S., & Prestwood, K. M. (2004). Bone health and aging: Implications for menopause. *Endocrinology & Metabolism Clinics of North America, 33*(4), 741-759.

Mitchell, J., Mathews, H. F., & Mayne, L. (2005). Differences in breast self-examination techniques between Caucasian and African American elderly women. *Journal of Women's Health, 14*(6), 476-484.

Mohandas, R., & Lal Gupta, K. (2003). Managing thyroid dysfunction in the elderly; answers to seven common questions. *Postgraduate Medicine, 113*(5), 54-57.

Moline, M. L., Broch, L., Zak, R., & Gross, V. (2003). Sleep in women across the life cycle from adulthood through menopause. *Sleep Medicine Reviews, 7*(2), 155-177.

Moller, B., Weedon-Fekkaer, H., Hakulinen, T., Tryggvadottir, L., Storm, H. H., Talback, M., & Haldorsen, T. (2005). The influence of mammographic screening on national trends in breast cancer incidence. *European Journal of Cancer Prevention, 14*(2), 117-128.

Mooradian, A. D., Chehade, J. M., & Thurman, J. E. (2002). The role of thiazolidinediones in the treatment of patients with type 2 diabetes mellitus. *Treatments in Endocrinology, 1,* 13-20.

Moorhead, S., Johnson, M., & Maas, M. (2004). *Nursing outcomes classification (NOC).* St. Louis: Mosby.

Morley, J. E., & Perry, H. M., III (2003). Androgen treatment of male hypogonadism in older males. *Journal of Steroid Biochemistry & Molecular Biology, 85*(2-5), 367-373.

NANDA International. (2005). *Nursing diagnoses: Definitions and classification 2005-2006.* Philadelphia: NANDA International.

Nawata, H., Yanase, T., Goto, K., Okabe, T., Nomura, M., Ashida, K., & Watanabe, T. (2004). Adrenopause. *Hormone Research, 62*(3; suppl), 110-114.

Need, A. G., O'Loughlin, P. D., Morris, H. A., Horowitz, M., & Nordin, B. E. (2004). The effects of age and other variables on serum parathyroid hormone in postmenopausal women attending an osteoporosis center. *Journal of Clinical Endocrinology & Metabolism, 89*(4), 1646-1649.

Nordin, B. E., Need, A. G., Morris, H. A., O'Loughlin, P. D., & Horowitz, M. (2004). Effect of age on calcium absorption in postmenopausal women. *American Journal of Clinical Nutrition, 80*(4), 998-1002.

Nordin, B. E., Wishart, J. M., Clifton, P. M., McArthur, R., Scopacasa, F., Need, A. G., et al. (2004). A longitudinal study of bone-related biochemical changes at the menopause. *Clinical Endocrinology, 61*(1), 123-130.

North American Menopause Society (2004). Treatment of menopause-associated vasomotor symptoms: Position statement of The North American Menopause Society. *2004 North American Menopause Society, 11*(1), 11-33.

Oiknine, R., & Mooradian, A. D. (2003). Drug therapy of diabetes in the elderly. *Biomedicine & Pharmacotherapy, 57*(5-6), 231-239.

Parle, J. V., Maisonneuve, P., Sheppard, M. C., Boyle, P., & Franklyn, J. A. (2001). Prediction of all-cause and cardiovascular mortality in elderly people from one low serum thyrotropin result: A 10-year cohort study. *Lancet, 358,* (9285) 861-865.

Perry, M. (2001). Diabetes in the elderly. *Practice Nurse, 20*(10), 30-33.

Raine-Fenning, N. J., Brincat, M. P., & Muscat-Baron, Y. (2003). Skin aging and menopause: Implications for treatment. *American Journal of Clinical Dermatology, 4*(6), 371-378.

Rapiti, E., Fioretta, G., Verkooijen, H. M., Vlastos, G., Schafer, P., Sappino, A. P., et al. (2005). Survival of young and older breast cancer patients in Geneva from 1990 to 2001. *European Journal of Cancer, 41*(10), 1446-1452.

Recker, R., Lappe, J., Davies, K. M., & Heaney, R. (2004). Bone remodeling increases substantially in the years after menopause and remains increased in older osteoporosis patients. *Journal of Bone and Mineral Research, 19*(10), 1628-1633.

Rehman, S., Cope, D., Senseney, A., & Brzezinski, W. (2005). Thyroid disorders in elderly patients. *Southern Medical Journal, 98*(5), 543-549.

Russo de Boland, A. (2004). Age-related changes in the response of intestinal cells to parathyroid hormone. *Mechanisms of Ageing and Development, 125*(12), 877-888.

Santoro, N., & Chervenak, J. L. (2004). The menopause transition. *Endocrinology & Metabolism Clinics of North America, 33*(4), 627-636.

Santoro, N., Lasley, B., McConnell, D., Allsworth, J., Crawford, S., Gold, E. B., et al. (2004). Body size and ethnicity are associated with menstrual cycle alterations in women in the early menopausal transition: The Study of Women's Health across the Nation (SWAN) Daily Hormone Study. *Journal of Clinical Endocrinology & Metabolism, 89*(6), 2622-2631.

Saskia, R. J., & Thiadens, R. N. (2005). 18 Steps to prevention revised: Lymphedema risk-reduction practices. Retrieved November 13, 2005, from http://lymphnet.org.

Schwartz, A. V., Sellmeyer, D. E., Ensrud, K. E., Cauley, J. A., Tabor, H. K., Schreiner, P. J., et al. (2001). Older women with diabetes have an increased risk of fracture: A prospective study. *Journal of Clinical Endocrinology & Metabolism, 86*(1), 32-38.

Segal, S. J. (2003). The aging gonad. *Molecular and Cellular Endocrinology, 202,* 1-3.

Sikon, A., & Thacker, H. L. (2004). Treatment options for menopausal hot flashes. *Cleveland Clinic Journal of Medicine, 71*(7), 578-582.

Simon, B., & Jabbour, S. (2005). Working up the thyroid nodule. *Patient Care; Best Practices for Today's Physicians,* online January 1, 2005.

Simon, J., Leboff, M., Wright, J., & Glowacki, J. (2002). Fractures in the elderly and vitamin D. *Journal of Nutrition, Health, & Aging, 6*(6), 406-412.

Skene, D. J., & Swaab, D. F. (2003). Melatonin rhythmicity: Effect of age and Alzheimer's disease. *Experimental Gerontology, 38*(1), 199-206.

Smalley, S. M. (2003). Breast implants and breast cancer screening. *Journal of Midwifery & Women's Health, 48*(5), 329-337.

Smith, P. E. (2005). Menopause assessment, treatment, and patient education. *Nurse Practitioner, 30*(2), 32-43.

Sorensen, J., Hertz, A., & Gudex, C. (2005). Evaluation of a Danish teaching program in breast self-examination. *Cancer Nursing, 28*(2), 141-147.

Sowers, J. R. (2004). Diabetes in the elderly and in women: Cardiovascular risks. *Cardiology Clinic, 22*(4), 541-551.

Steiner, M., Dunn, E., & Born, L. (2003). Hormones and mood: From menarche to menopause and beyond. *Journal of Affective Disorders, 74*(1), 67-83.

Steven, D., Fitch, M., Dhaliwal, H., Kirk-Gardner, R., Sevean, P., Jamieson, J., & Woodbeck, H. (2004). Knowledge, attitudes, beliefs, and practices regarding breast and cervical cancer screening in selected ethnocultural groups in Northwestern Ontario. *Oncology Nursing Forum Online, 31*(2), 305-311.

Sulkes, A. (2005). The emerging role of the new aromatase inhibitors in the treatment of breast cancer. *Israel Medical Association Journal, 7*(4), 257-261.

Surks, M., Ortiz, E., Daniels, G., Sawin, C., Col, N. F., Cobin, R. H., et al. (2004). Subclinical thyroid disease, scientific review and guidelines for diagnosis and management. *Journal of the American Medical Association, 291*(2), 228-238.

Swede, H., Mirand, A. L., Menezes, R. J., & Moysich, K. B. (2005). Association of regular aspirin use and breast cancer risk. *Oncology, 68*(1), 40-47.

Szulc, P., Munoz, F., Marchand, F., Chapuy, M. C., & Delmas, P. D. (2003). Role of vitamin D and parathyroid hormone in the regulation of bone turnover and bone mass in men: The MINOS study. *Calcified Tissue International, 73*(6), 520-530.

Tenover, J. S. (2003). Declining testicular function in aging men. *International Journal of Impotence Research, 15*(4; suppl), S3-S8.

Tepper, R. E., & Katz, S. (2003). Geriatric gastroenterology: Overview. In R. C. Tallis & H. M. Fillit (Eds.), *Brocklehurst's textbook of geriatric medicine and gerontology* (6th ed.). Edinburgh: Churchill Livingstone, pp. 943-950.

Thwin, S. S., Fink, A. K., Lash, T. L., & Silliman, R. A. (2005). Predictors and outcomes of surgeons' referral of older breast cancer patients to medical oncologists. *Cancer, 104*(5), 936-942.

Tomkinson, A., Gibson, J. H., Lunt, M., Harries, M., & Reeve, J. (2003). Changes in bone mineral density in the hip and spine before, during, and after the menopause in elite runners. *Osteoporosis International, 14*(6), 462-468.

Trivalle, C., Doucet, J., Chassagne, P., Landrin, I., Kadri, N., Menard, J. F., et al. (1996). Differences in the signs and symptoms of hyperthyroidism in older and younger patients. *Journal of the American Geriatric Society, 44*(1), 50-53.

UK Prospective Diabetes Study Group. (1998). Intensive blood-glucose control with sulfonylureas or insulin compared with conventional treatment and risk of complications in patients with type 2 diabetes (UKPDS 33). *Lancet, 352*(9131)837-853.

Utzschneider, K. M., Carr, D. B., Hull, R. L., Kodama, K., Shofer, J. B., Retzlaff, B. M., et al. (2004). Impact of intra-abdominal fat and age on insulin sensitivity and beta-cell function. *Diabetes, 53*(11), 2867-2872.

Vahabi, M. (2003). Breast cancer screening methods: A review of the evidence. *Health Care for Women International, 24*(9), 773-779.

Veldhuis, J. D., Veldhuis, N. J., Keenan, D. M., & Iranmanesh, A. (2005). Age diminishes the testicular steroidogenic response to repeated intravenous pulses of recombinant human LH during acute GnRH-receptor blockade in healthy men. *American Journal of Physiology—Endocrinology & Metabolism, 288*(4), E775-E781.

Vieth, R., Ladak, Y., & Walfish, P. G. (2003). Age-related changes in the 25-hydroxyvitamin D versus parathyroid hormone relationship suggest a different reason why older adults require more vitamin D. *Journal of Clinical Endocrinology & Metabolism, 88*(1), 185-191.

Vinik, A. (2004). Pancreatic polypeptide ppoma. Accessed October 21, 2005, at www.endotext.com/guthormones/guthormone9/guthormoneframe9.htm.

Visser, M., Deeg, D. J., & Lips, P. (2003). Low vitamin D and high parathyroid hormone levels as determinants of loss of muscle strength and muscle mass (sarcopenia): The Longitudinal Aging Study Amsterdam. *Journal of Clinical Endocrinology & Metabolism, 88*(12), 5766-5772.

Weiss, G., Skurnick, J. H., Goldsmith, L. T., Santoro, N. F., & Park, S. J. (2004). Menopause and hypothalamic-pituitary sensitivity to estrogen. *Journal of the American Medical Association, 292*(24), 2991-2996.

Whiteman, M. K., Staropoli, C. A., Benedict, J. C., Borgeest, C., & Flaws, J. A. (2003). Risk factors for hot flashes in midlife women. *Journal of Women's Health, 12*(5), 459-472.

Wood, R. Y., & Duffy, M. E. (2004). Video breast health kits: Testing a cancer education innovation I older high-risk populations. *Journal of Cancer Education, 19*(2), 98-104.

Woods, N. F. (1978). Human sexuality and the healthy elderly. In M Brown (Ed.), *Readings in gerontology* (2nd ed.). St. Louis: Mosby, pp. 69-87.

Wooten, J., & Galavis, J. (2005). Polypharmacy: Keeping the elderly safe. *RN 68*(8), 44-48.

Wu, Y. H., & Swaab, D. F. (2005). The human pineal gland and melatonin in aging and Alzheimer's disease. *Journal of Pineal Research, 38*(3), 145-152.

Yates, A. P., & Laing, I. (2002). Age-related increase in haemoglobin A1c and fasting plasma glucose is accompanied by a decrease in beta cell function without change in insulin sensitivity: Evidence from a cross-sectional study of hospital personnel. *Diabetic Medicine, 19*(3), 254-258.

Zahid, A. (2003). Unravelling the role of the pineal gland. *Journal of the College of Physicians and Surgeons—Pakistan, 13*(10), 611-615.

Zapantis, G., & Santoro, N. (2003). The menopausal transition: Characteristics and management. *Best Practice & Research. Clinical Endocrinology & Metabolism, 17*(1), 33-52.

Zhang, Y., Coogan, P. F., Palmer, J. R., Strom, B. L., & Rosenberg, L. (2005). Use of nonsteroidal anti-inflammatory drugs and risk of breast cancer: The Case-Control Surveillance Study revisited. *American Journal of Epidemiology, 162*(2), 165-170.

Zhu, K., Hunter, S., Bernard, L. J., Payne-Wilks, K., Roland, C. L., Elam, L. C., Feng, Z., & Levine, R. S. (2002). An intervention study on screening for breast cancer among single African American women aged 65 and older. *Preventive Medicine, 34*(5), 536-545.

Chapter 18

Immune System

Adrianne Dill Linton

Objectives

Describe the normal age-related changes in the structure of the immunological system.

Discuss the normal age-related changes in immunological function including responses to tissue injury and to vaccines.

Describe measures to maintain immunological health in the older adult.

Explain the cause and treatment of immunological disorders that are common in older persons, including autoimmune disorders and acquired immune deficiency.

Describe the components of the immunological assessment of the older adult.

Formulate nursing diagnoses for older adults with immunological disorders.

Develop management plans for older adults with actual or potential immunological problems.

The immune system and aging are so closely related that one theory explains many aspects of the aging process as the outcome of changes in the immune system. As science unfolds the mysteries of the immune system, we increasingly appreciate its complexity and importance in relation to health and aging.

The functions of the immune system include defense, homeostasis, and surveillance. The defense function involves protection against invading pathogens and foreign antigens. The digestion and removal of damaged cellular substances serves to maintain homeostasis. Surveillance refers to the continual monitoring for and subsequent destruction of foreign cells (Lewis & Kang, 2004). An essential characteristic of the immune system is the ability to distinguish between the host tissues and foreign antigens. The immune system should be tolerant of host tissues while capable of rejecting foreign tissues and pathogens (Rote, 2000a).

NORMAL ANATOMY AND PHYSIOLOGY
Structures

The lymphoid system comprises central lymphoid organs (bone marrow and thymus) and peripheral lymphoid organs, which are the tonsils, lymph nodes, spleen, and lymphoid tissues in the gut, genitals, bronchi, and skin (Lewis & Kang, 2004).

Bone Marrow. The bone marrow is the site where immunological cell lines originate and mature. Most cell production occurs in the vertebrae, ribs, skull, pelvis, and proximal epiphyses of the femur and humerus.

Thymus. The thymus is a lymphoid organ in the mediastinum that grows rapidly during fetal development and during the first 2 years of life. Lymphocytes that are released from the bones migrate to the thymus, mature into T cells, and then are released into the circulation. After puberty, the long-lived T cell population is maximized and the thymus slowly involutes.

Lymph System. As blood flows through the capillaries, some plasma and blood components shift between the capillary beds and the tissues. The lymph system is a network of vessels that picks up the plasma and leukocytes that remain in the tissues, filters the fluid, and returns it to the circulation. Lymph fluid comprises plasma, leukocytes, enzymes, and antibodies. The lymph system is dependent on skeletal muscle contraction to move the fluid through the system toward the right lymphatic and thoracic ducts, which drain into the subclavian veins. Scattered along the lymphatic channels are the lymph nodes, which are patches of tissue that filter microorganisms from the lymph fluid. Lymph nodes can become enlarged as a result of infection or malignancy. When infection is present, white blood cells can accumulate in the nodes that serve the affected area, causing them to swell.

Spleen. The spleen, which is located in the upper left abdominal quadrant, removes damaged and non-functioning red blood cells. It also filters antigens from the blood. The spleen is comprised of white pulp that contains B and T lymphocytes, and red pulp that contains erythrocytes (Lewis & Kang, 2004).

Immune System Components

The components of the immune system are stem cells, white blood cells, complement, cytokines, and eicosanoids.

Stem Cells. All bone marrow cell lines are derived from pluripotent stem cells. Pluripotency refers to the "ability to develop in any one of several different ways, or to affect more than one organ or tissue" (O'Toole, 2003). This characteristic explains the current interest in stem cells for the regeneration of various types of tissue.

White Blood Cells (WBCs). The role of WBCs is to detect and destroy bacteria, viruses, fungi, parasites, and other foreign proteins. WBCs primarily mature in the bone marrow. After being released into the circulation, the average life span is 12 hours. The major types of WBCs are granulocytes and lymphocytes.

GRANULOCYTES. Granulocytes include neutrophils, monocytes and macrophages, eosinophils, basophils, and mast cells. Neutrophils, which may be referred to as "segs," "PMNs," "polys," "neuts," or "grans," comprise the greatest number of WBCs. Although they are capable of migrating through endothelial cells to reach areas of pathogenic invasion, they often are destroyed by phagocytosis. Cellular debris from microorganisms and damaged neutrophils accumulates as "pus."

Monocytes mature after they are released into the circulation, and they become phagocytic macrophages after entering the body tissues. Some macrophages remain in specific tissues whereas others circulate throughout the body. Stationary macrophages are located in the liver, skin, alveoli, kidney, and central nervous system. The life span of macrophages can be months to years.

Eosinophils respond to multicellular parasitic infections, allergic reactions, and other inflammatory processes. Unlike monocytes, neutrophils, and eosinophils, basophils are not phagocytic. Rather, they attract immunoglobulin E (IgE) to their cell membranes. Subsequently, the IgE binds with antigens, which triggers the release of histamine and initiates the inflammatory response. Mast cells, which reside in body tissue, also attract IgE antibodies and trigger the inflammatory response. Mast cells may survive for several months, compared with basophils, which have a life span of several days.

LYMPHOCYTES. Lymphocytes include B cells, T cells, and natural killer (NK) cells.

B Cells. B cells manufacture immunoglobulins, which are proteins that bind with antigens on the B cell membranes, thereby inducing the cell to differentiate into plasma cells and memory B cells. Plasma cells manufacture antibodies that bind with the antigen; memory B cells are inactive until reactivated by future exposure to the same antigen. The major types of antibodies are immunoglobulin M (IgM), immunoglobulin G (IgG), immunoglobulin A (IgA), and immunoglobulin E (IgE). When an antigen is encountered, IgM is the first immunoglobulin to be secreted in the primary immune response. IgG, which is secreted in the secondary immune response, has more antigen specificity. IgA is found in mucus, breast milk, and other secretions. As mentioned earlier, IgE triggers the release of histamine when an antigen is encountered.

T Cells. T cells are lymphocytes that migrate from the bone marrow to the thymus where they differentiate into T lymphocytes. Of circulating lymphocytes, 70% to 80% are comprised of T cells. They primarily are responsible for immunity to viruses, tumor cells, and fungi. Their life span may be as short as a few months, or they may survive for the life of the individual (Lewis & Kang, 2004).

T lymphocytes can be classified as cytotoxic, helper, or suppressor cells. T cytotoxic cells destroy pathogens by attacking foreign antigens and releasing substances that lyse the pathogen. T cytotoxic cells are sensitized by exposure to an antigen and are specific to that antigen. Following sensitization, some T cells become memory cells, causing a cell-mediated immune response if a second exposure occurs. T helper and T suppressor cells regulate cell-mediated immunity and humoral antibody response. In autoimmune disorders, T suppressors commonly are decreased in relation to T helper cells. As a result, the immune response is overaggressive. In persons with HIV, the virus invades and destroys T helper cells, leaving the infected individual susceptible to infection and malignancy (Lewis & Kang, 2004) (Figure 18-1).

When T helper cells recognize a particular type of foreign antigen-cell membrane protein complex, they secrete cytokines, which activate other immune components. T helper cells also are called CD4 cells because of the type of antigen on the cell membranes. T cytotoxic cells recognize a different type of complex and respond by secreting a substance that directly destroys the cell.

Natural Killer Cells. Natural killer cells are not T or B lymphocytes, and they do not express antigen-binding receptors. They are, however, cytotoxic against tumor cells and cells infected with bacteria and viruses.

Complement. Complement is not a single substance, but a group of proteins that act sequentially to lyse microorganisms and infected cells.

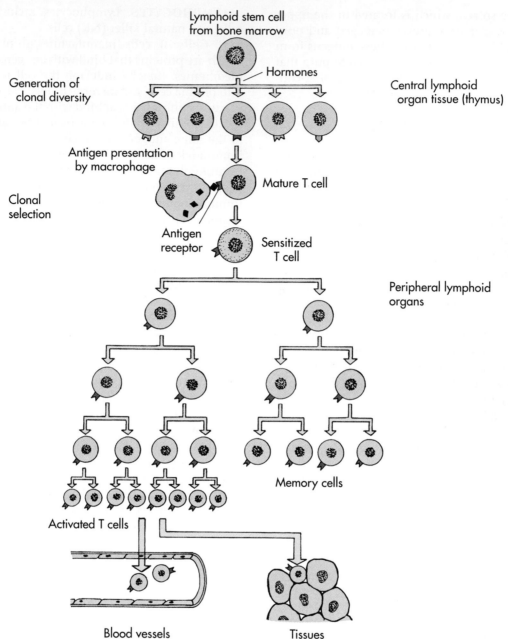

Lymphoid stem cell
from bone marrow

Hormones

Generation of
clonal diversity

Central lymphoid
organ tissue (thymus)

Antigen presentation
by macrophage

Clonal
selection

Mature T cell

Antigen
receptor

Sensitized
T cell

Peripheral lymphoid
organs

Memory cells

Activated T cells

Blood vessels

Tissues

Figure 18-1 T cell production: Generation of clones of antigen-reactive T lymphocytes. Under the control of hormones and without antigen, T lymphocyte precursors undergo cellular division in the central lymphoid organ (the thymus) and generate receptors against all possible antigens that may be encountered in the host's adult life. Later, antigen encountered in the peripheral lymphoid organs reacts with the clones of cells expressing appropriate receptors on their surfaces, causing those cells to proliferate and produce functional T lymphocytes. (From Rote, N. S. [2004]. Immunity. In S. E. Huether & K. L. McCance [Eds.], *Understanding pathophysiology* [3rd ed.]. St. Louis: Mosby.)

Cytokines. Cytokines serve as messengers among macrophages and various lymphocytes. They are secreted by cells that participate in the immune response. They bind to specific receptors on neighboring cells that they instruct to respond in a particular fashion (e.g., increase production of proteins to serve as receptors' complement or antibodies; initiate cell proliferation and differentiation in hemopoietic blood cells). Cytokines include a variety of interleukins, interferons, tumor necrosis factors, colony-stimulating factors, and transforming growth factor. Interleukins are produced by macrophages or leukocytes and enhance the response of leukocytes to foreign substances. Interferon helps to protect the body against viruses and tumor cell growth (Rote, 2000a).

Eicosanoids. Eicosanoids include prostaglandins, thromboxanes, and leukotrienes. They regulate various processes by signaling cells in a local area. For example, prostaglandins play a role in temperature elevation, antiplatelet aggregation, and the inflammatory response.

FUNCTION
Innate Immunity

The term "innate immunity" is used to describe the immunity a person has to a specific antigen without ever having been exposed to that antigen. This response is nonspecific and employs primarily neutrophils and monocytes. Innate immunity is not an outcome of the immune response described above.

Lines of Defense. Anatomical barriers, the skin and mucous membranes, present the first line of defense against harmful substances and pathogens. Not only do they create a physical barrier but also they provide biochemical barriers such as antibacterial fatty acids and lactic acid. When the anatomical barriers are penetrated or bypassed, the body may use mechanical means such as vomiting or diarrhea to clear the offending agents from the body. The normal bacterial flora also plays a role in inhibiting the growth of invading pathogens (Rote, 2000a).

The next line of defense is the inflammatory response that occurs when pathogens, harmful chemicals, or foreign bodies penetrate cells and tissues. The inflammatory process brings cells and fluids into the affected tissue to isolate, remove, and destroy the unwelcome substance. Anatomical barriers, mechanical clearance mechanisms, and inflammation are all nonspecific lines of defense, meaning they respond to all invaders in essentially the same, generalized manner (Rote, 2000a).

The third line of defense is the immune response, which occurs more slowly but is specific in that it forms antibodies against particular organisms. Immunity refers to a state of responsiveness to foreign substances (antigens), and is classified as innate or adaptive (acquired). In response to an antigen, two types of lymphocytes, B cells and T cells, are activated. B cells produce antibodies that attack the antigen whereas T cells attack the antigen directly. B cells and T cells are specific, meaning they recognize or respond to only one antigen. Once these cells have been activated by a particular antigen, some of them become memory cells. They are able to respond quickly if the antigen should reappear (Rote, 2000a). Box 18-1 summarizes the lines of defense.

Inflammation

Inflammation is an immediate response to cellular injury or dead cells. The response to cellular injury engages cells, platelets, complement, clotting, and kinin systems and immunoglobulins. Immediately following an injury, local arterioles constrict briefly and then dilate. Capillary permeability increases, allowing the flow of plasma and blood cells into the tissues. Junctions between cells in the vascular epithelium widen, permitting leukocytes to squeeze out. Phagocytic leukocytes arrive first to ingest bacteria, dead cells, and cellular debris; they are followed by monocytes and monophages that act in a similar manner but remain present longer. The inflammatory process is protective but if prolonged may cause damage to host structures.

Mast Cells. Mast cells are bags of granules located close to blood vessels that play a vital role in the inflammatory response. In response to physical or chemical injury or immunological processes, these cells release their contents and synthesize mediators that respond to specific stimuli. Biochemical mediators (histamine, neutrophil chemotactic factor [NCF], and eosinophil chemotactic factor of anaphylaxis [ECF -A]) are released and cause dilation of postcapillary venules and increased capillary permeability. Chemotactic factors attract blood cells to the area. To prevent local inflammation from becoming generalized, eosinophils provide enzymes that degrade the vasoactive amines.

Mast cells also synthesize leukotrienes and prostaglandins. The effects of leukotrienes are similar to those of histamine, but the action is slower and more prolonged. Prostaglandins also increase vascular permeability and NCF and cause pain. Nonsteroidal antiinflammatory drugs act by blocking prostaglandin synthesis (Rote, 2000b). The sequence of events in acute inflammation is depicted in Figure 18-2.

Phagocytosis

The most important phagocytes are neutrophils and macrophages (the mature form of monocytes) although eosinophils, basophils, and monocytes also are capable of phagocytosis. When inflammation occurs, neutrophils and macrophages that are circulating in the blood migrate to the affected area and pass through vessel walls into the tissue. Neutrophils arrive first, but macrophages remain active for a longer period of time. The cells become entrapped in a meshwork of fibrinous exudates where they ingest (phagocytose) foreign and dead cells for the remainder of their life span. As phagocytes die, they break down and become part of the exudate (pus) that is removed through the epithelium or the lymphatic system (Figure 18-3).

BOX 18-1 Lines of Defense

TYPE OF DEFENSE	SPECIFIC MECHANISM
Surface defenses	Physical barriers: skin, conjunctivae, mucous membranes Mechanical removal: desquamation of skin, tears, mucus, ciliary action, coughing, salivation, swallowing, urination, defecation Normal bacterial flora: antibacterial factors Chemical inhibitors: gastric acid, lactic acid, fatty acids, spermine, lactoperoxidase, bile salts Antimicrobial substances: lysozyme, secretory IgA
Nonspecific resistance factors	Fevers, interferons, complement, lysozyme, C-reactive protein (reacts with bacterial surface polysaccharides and activates complement), lactoferrin (binds and removes iron as a bacterial nutrient), α_1-antitrypsin (inhibits bacterial enzymes)

Inflammation	Soluble factors
	    Clotting system: Hageman factor (factor XII)
	    Complement systems: chemotactic factors, anaphylatoxins
	    Kinin system: bradykinin
	Phagocytes
	    Circulating neutrophils, eosinophils, monocytes, macrophages
	    Fixed cells (of mononuclear phagocyte system) in alveoli, spleen, liver, bone marrow

Immune response	Humoral immune response: B cells, plasma cells, immunoglobulins Cell-mediated immune response: T cells, lymphokines

From Rote, N. S. (2004). Immunity. In S. E. Huether & K. L. McCance (Eds.), *Understanding pathophysiology* (3rd ed.). St. Louis: Mosby, pp. 127-152.

Complement System

The complement system is one of the plasma protein systems that mediate inflammation. Because the proteins of the complement are nonspecific, they are powerful defenders against bacterial invasion. Antigen-antibody complexes, by-products of invading bacteria, and components of other plasma protein systems can activate the complement system (Rote, 2000a).

Acquired (Adaptive) Immunity

Acquired or adaptive immunity develops as a result of exposure to an antigen or administration of antibodies. It may be either active acquired or passive acquired immunity. A person who develops antibodies as a result of exposure to an antigen either naturally or by immunization is said to have active acquired immunity. If preformed antibodies are administered as an immune

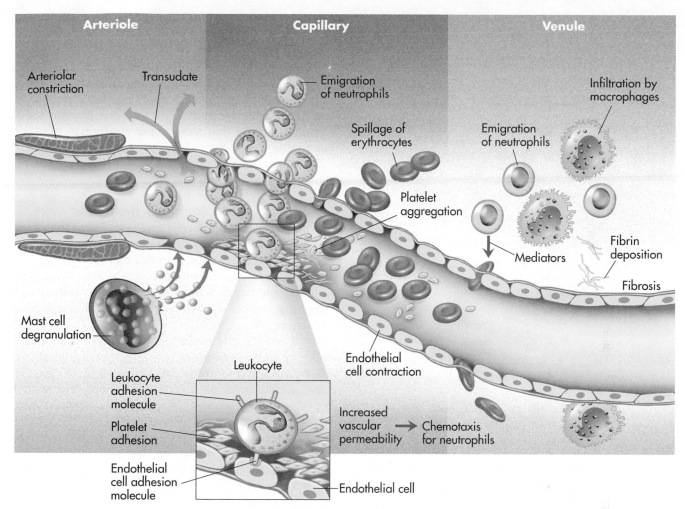

Figure 18-2   The sequence of events in the process of inflammation. (From Rote, N. S. [2004]. Inflammation. In S. E. Huether & K. L. McCance [Eds.], *Understanding pathophysiology* [3rd ed.]. St. Louis: Mosby.)

serum, the individual is said to have passive acquired immunity. Passive immunity is temporary (Rote, 2000a).

Lymphocyte precursors known as stem cells form in the liver, spleen, and bone marrow. They mature as they migrate through lymphoid tissues throughout the body and emerge as either B cells (B lymphocytes) or T cells (T lymphocytes). B cells are responsible for humoral immunity and T cells for cell-mediated immunity (Rote, 2000a). B lymphocytes are the cells that migrate to the bone marrow, where they are preprocessed. T lymphocytes migrate to the thymus, where they are preprocessed.

Antibody-Mediated (Humoral) Immunity

Antibody production is a two-step process. In the first step, B cells migrate through lymphoid tissue where they acquire the capacity to react with antigens and generate antibodies of the IgM and IgD classes. In the second step, an initial encounter with an antigen stimulates the

proliferation of the immunocompetent B cells whose antibody receptors match the specific antigen. Thereafter, these B cells (which now are called plasma cells) can be found in various parts of the body. T cells become sensitized to specific antigens, which they then recognize and attack directly. With this mechanism in place, a subsequent encounter with the same antigen initiates the immune response. The antigen binds and interacts with antibody receptors on the surface of the mature B cell. Through a sequence of proliferation and differentiation, immunoglobulin-secreting plasma cells and long-lived memory cells are produced (Rote, 2000a).

The process of antibody production inside the body is governed by the systemic immune system. Another system, called the secretory (or mucosal) immune system, provides protection of the external body structures. Antibodies found in body secretions (tears, sweat, saliva, mucus, and breast milk) also are produced by B cells but the maturation process is different. In the secretory immune system, B cells leaving the bone marrow migrate through the lacrimal and salivary glands

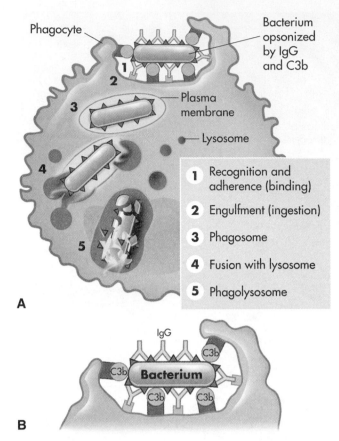

Figure 18-3 Phases of phagocytosis. **A,** Opsonized microorganisms (1) bind to the surface of a phagocyte and (2) are ingested into a phagocyte vacuole, or phagosome (3). Lysosomes fuse with the phagosome (4), releasing their digestive enzymes into the vacuole. This results in the formation of a phagolysosome (5), within which the microorganism is killed and digested. **B,** Enlargement showing bacterium opsonization. *IgG,* Immunoglobulin G; *C3b,* complement component. (From Rote, N. S. [2004]. Inflammation. In S. E. Huether & K. L. McCance [Eds.], *Understanding pathophysiology* [3rd ed.]. St. Louis: Mosby.)

and the lymphoid tissue in the breast, bronchi, intestines, and genitourinary tract (Rote, 2000a).

IMMUNOGLOBULINS. Serum glycoproteins that are produced by plasma cells in response to antigens are called immunoglobulins. Those immunoglobulins that are specific for a particular antigen are called antibodies. Based on their antigenic, structural, and functional characteristics, immunoglobulins are classified as IgG, IgA, IgM, IgE, and IgD with subclasses for each of these (Rote, 2000a).

ANTIBODIES. The specificity of an antibody is determined by its exact amino acid sequence. Antibodies protect the host by several mechanisms that include neutralization of bacterial toxins and viruses, phagocytosis

(opsonization) of bacteria, and activation of components of the inflammatory response. The process of antibody production is illustrated in Figure 18-4.

Monoclonal Antibodies. In the body various B lymphocytes that respond to the same antigen produce antibodies with slight variations in structure. Monoclonal antibodies that are produced in the laboratory are identical antibodies that have many advantages over conventional antibody-containing sera. They are showing promise in cancer treatment and early diagnosis of viral infections (Rote, 2000a).

Cell-Mediated Immune Response. After maturing in the thymus, T cells produce plasma membrane receptors that stimulate proliferation when bound to an antigen. All cells produced in this manner recognize the same antigen. Not all antigens can induce the B cell immune response; they must first interact with intermediary cells. Each of the five types of T cells has a different function:

- **T-lymphocyte memory cells:** induce the secretory immune response
- **Lymphokine-producing cells:**
  secrete proteins that activate other cells such as macrophages
  transfer delayed hypersensitivity
- **Cytotoxic cells:**
  directly attack antigens
  destroy cells bearing foreign antigens
- **Helper T cells:** control cell-mediated and humoral processes
- **Suppressor T cells:** control cell-mediated and humoral processes

The cell-mediated immune response is illustrated in Figure 18-5.

ANTIGEN PROCESSING, PRESENTATION, AND RECOGNITION. Depending on the route by which an antigen enters the body, it may be filtered by the spleen or ingested by phagocytes in the lymph nodes. The antigen is degraded and then a portion is expressed and "presented" to T or B cells to initiate the immune response (Figure 18-6).

Hypersensitivity

Hypersensitivity is defined as "an altered immunologic reaction to an antigen that results in a pathologic immune response after reexposure" (Rote, Huether, & McCance, 2000, p. 181). Three types of hypersensitivity are autoimmunity, alloimmunity, and allergy. In autoimmunity, the immune response is misdirected against the host's own tissues. Alloimmunity is the immune response directed against antigens on foreign tissues that are intended to be beneficial, such as transfused blood or transplanted tissue. An allergic reaction

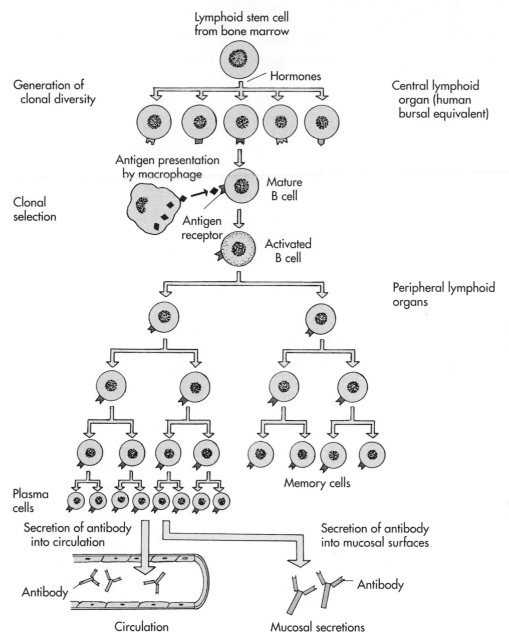

Figure 18-4 Antibody production: Generation of clones of B cells. Under the control of hormones and without antigen, B lymphocyte precursors undergo cellular division in the central lymphoid organs (bursal equivalent tissues, probably bone marrow) and generate receptors against all possible antigens that may be encountered in the host's adult life. Later, primarily in the peripheral lymphoid organs (spleen, lymph nodes), antigen, either directly or presented by macrophages (phagocytic cells of inflammation), reacts with the clones of B cells having appropriate receptors on their surfaces, causing those cells to proliferate and produce antibody. (From Rote, N. S. [2004]. Immunity. In S. E. Huether & K. L. McCance [Eds.], *Understanding pathophysiology* [3rd ed.]. St. Louis: Mosby.)

is an exaggerated response to an environmental antigen. Anaphylaxis is an immediate, life-threatening hypersensitivity reaction.

The four types of hypersensitivity reactions are classified as type I, type II, type III, or type IV. A type I reaction, which is IgE-mediated, occurs as a result of the release of

inflammatory substances including histamine. A type II reaction is tissue-specific and may be caused by complement-mediated lysis, opsonization and phagocytosis, antibody-dependent cell-mediated cytotoxicity, or modulation of cellular function. A type III reaction results from the formation of immune complexes that are

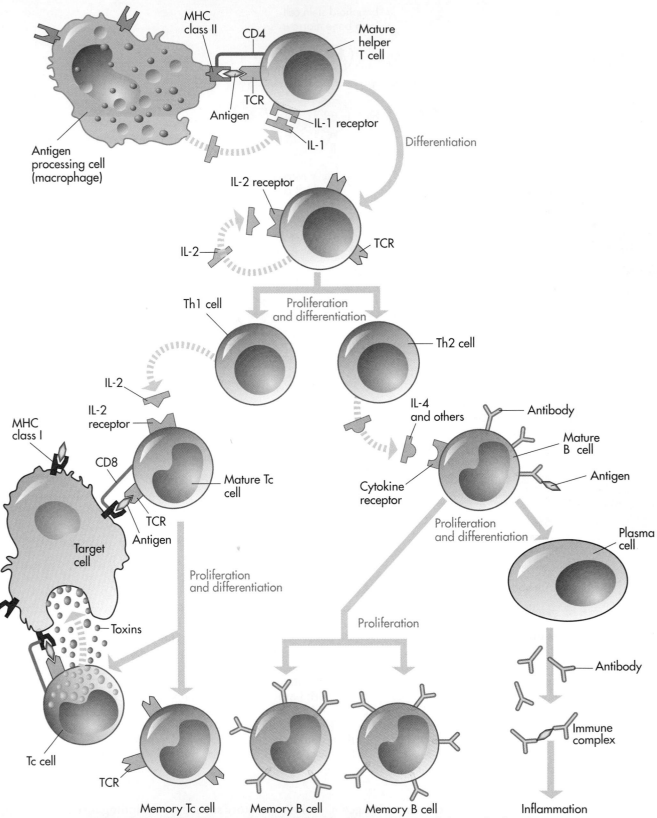

Figure 18-5 Cellular interactions and the immune response. Schematic showing activation and differentiation of T and B cell immune responses. Solid arrows indicate differentiation steps. Hatched arrows indicate indirect effects through cytokine. (From Rote, N. S. [2004]. Immunity. In S. E. Huether & K. L. McCance [Eds.], *Understanding pathophysiology* [3rd ed.]. St. Louis: Mosby.)

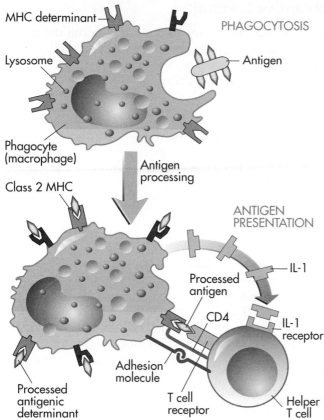

Figure 18-6 Antigen processing and presentation. Circulating antigen is phagocytosed by macrophages. Remnants of the digested antigen are expressed on the membrane of the phagocyte and, in conjunction with MHC molecules, are presented to lymphocytes to initiate the immune response. The macrophage and T cell are also held together by adhesion molecules, and the macrophage produces interleukin-1 (IL-1) that helps the T cell respond to the antigen. (From Rote, N. S. [2004]. Immunity. In S. E. Huether & K. L. McCance [Eds.], *Understanding pathophysiology* [3rd ed.]. St. Louis: Mosby.)

deposited in target tissues and activate the complement cascade that attracts neutrophils. A type IV reaction, caused by specifically sensitized T cells, destroys antigens either directly or by using macrophages (Rote, Huether, & McCance, 2000).

NORMAL AGING CHANGES

Compared with other major body systems, research on the immune system and aging has been limited. Much of the research on aging and immunity has been in animals (Gravenstein, Fillit, & Ershler, 2003). Like studies on aging in general, the use of cross-sectional data and participants along the entire health-illness continuum makes it difficult to determine what changes truly are age-related.

The term immunosenescence refers to the changes that occur in the immune system with advancing age,

including serious alterations in critical B cell and T cell subpopulations, elevations in proinflammatory cytokines, and remodeling of innate immunity (Hakim, Flomerfelt, Boyiadzis, & Gress, 2004; Mishto et al., 2003). Some experts prefer the term remodeling of the immune system over immunosenescence because of the profound structural changes that modify immune function with age (Bonafe, Valensin, Gianni, Marigliano, & Franceschi, 2001). The changes in the immune system are associated with marked reduction in immune responsiveness (Effros, Cai, & Linton, 2003). Immunosenescence comprises changes in both natural (innate) and acquired (adaptive) components of the immune system. Despite progressive involution, the thymus continues to function at some level throughout life. However, the function eventually fails to supply sufficient naïve T cells to replace those lost daily from the periphery (Hakim et al., 2004). Changes in the T cell population include fewer naïve cells, increased memory cells with resultant increased cytokine production, and an accumulation of activated effector cells that occupy T cell space but have limited T cell repertoire. Because proinflammatory cytokines are overexpressed, the synthesis of enzymes that control the expression of inflammatory lipid mediators and reactive oxygen species increases (Daynes, Enioutina, & Jones, 2003).

Age-related changes in the innate immune system have been considered less significant in relation to immunosenescence, but this thinking is changing. We now know that innate immunity interacts with the adaptive immune system at several levels to ensure optimal immune response (Provinciali & Smorlesi, 2005). The innate system plays a key role in stimulating adaptive immunity such that changes in innate immunity have the potential to affect adaptive immunity (Mocchegiani & Malavolta, 2004).

The absolute number of NK cells increases with advancing age as does the number of NK cells expressing NK receptors. Nevertheless, cytotoxicity and the production of cytokines and chemokines by activated NK cells are impaired (Mocchegiani & Malavolta, 2004). In relation to cell humoral immunity, there is an increase in autoantibodies even though vaccine responses diminish.

Clearly, apoptosis (cell death) is involved in many aspects of immunosenescence including thymic involution, alteration of T cell repertoire, the accumulation of memory/effector cells, and autoimmunity. Age-related changes in activation-induced apoptosis and damage-induced apoptosis could lead to disease (Ginaldi, DeMartinis, Monti, & Franceschi, 2004). Disequilibrium between cell survival/proliferation and programmed cell death in the immune system may explain various pathological consequences (Ginaldi et al., 2000). Immunosenescence normally is counterbalanced by continuous adaptation.

Innate Immunity

Aging changes can affect the body's first line of defense, which includes mucocutaneous barriers, phagocytosis, and complement.

Mucocutaneous Barriers. Changes in the skin and mucous membranes are discussed in detail in Chapter 10. In relation to the immune system, the most important changes in the skin are decreased amounts of circulating thymus-derived lymphocytes, cytokines, and epidermal Langerhans cells (the cells responsible for immunosurveillance). In addition to reduced protection against invasion of pathogens, older persons have slower and less dramatic hypersensitivity reactions. This may explain the decreased incidence of allergic contact dermatitis in older adults (Brooke & Griffiths, 2003).

Phagocytosis. Variables affecting the efficiency of phagocytosis include the number of neutrophils, macrophages, and monocytes; endothelial adherence and chemotaxis; and phagocytosis with subsequent digestion of invading organisms (Gravenstein et al., 2003). With age, the following changes have been reported:

- The effectiveness of chemotaxis may decline in less vascular areas such as the skin. In vitro studies of neutrophil function show no significant changes with age; however, when skin abrasion sites of older persons were studied, fewer neutrophils had reached the sites (Gravenstein et al., 2003).
- The number of local T cells activated in response to infection declines, and the homing markers that normally attract additional T cells from peripheral blood are defective (Gravenstein et al., 2003).
- The capacity to focus mediator cells and the additional cytokines they may express at sites of infection is impaired (Gravenstein et al., 2003).
- Changes in the number of circulating monocytes and polymorphonuclear leukocytes occur. Cell adhesion is the first-line response in acute inflammation. The presence of an increased proportion of CD62L-negative leukocytes in older persons impairs cell adhesion, which likely makes them more susceptible to acute infection (De Martinis, Modesti, & Ginaldi, 2004).
- Altered intracellular signaling renders aged macrophages and neutrophils less able to destroy bacteria. Neutrophils are less able to respond to "rescue from apoptosis" (Gravenstein et al., 2003).

Cell Lysis

The complement system, natural killer cell activity, and neutrophil activity mediate cell lysis. In animal studies, only natural killer cell activity has been found to decline with age (Gravenstein et al., 2003).

Adaptive Immunity

Both cellular immunity and humoral immunity are altered with aging. Because the thymus normally involutes during adolescence, few thymic peptides are present in peripheral blood after age 60 (Gravenstein et al., 2003).

Cell-Mediated Immunity. Changes in cellular immunity include:

- "Equivocal changes in the ratio of helper cells to suppressor cells (T4/T8) occur in normal aging" (Gravenstein et al., 2003, p. 114).
- Memory cells increase.
- Cell-mediated immunity declines, particularly in relation to T cell function, which coincides with increased autoantibody frequency (Boren & Gershwin, 2004).
- Antigen-specific declines to specific viruses are seen in T cells. Although the number and affinity of mitogen receptors on T cells do not change with age, the number of T lymphocytes that are capable of dividing in response to mitogens is reduced. Further, the T cells that are activated do not undergo as many divisions.
- The predominance of helper T cell responses shifts from type I to type II. Type I cells predominantly mediate cell-mediated immune and inflammatory responses; type II cells produce factors that enhance antibody-mediated immunity (Gravenstein et al., 2003).
- In human lymph nodes, the relative number of $CD8^+$ T cells decreases with age, but the relative number of $CD4^+$ T cells does not. Naïve T cells are depleted (Lazuardi et al., 2005).
- The reduced proliferative capacity of T cells may be influenced by the accumulation of virus-specific memory T cells. It is thought that cytomegalovirus (CMV) may be detrimental to the immunocompetent host because it may suppress heterologous virus-specific immunity in aging (Khan et al., 2004).
- Across a lifetime, CD8 T cells reach an end stage of replicative senescence. These changes may exert negative effects on both immune and nonimmune organ systems during aging (Effros, 2004).
- Delayed type skin hypersensitivity reactions decline, possibly because of reduced lymphocyte proliferation.
- The ability of dendritic cells to stimulate T and B cells declines with age. The altered T cell stimulation results from changes in human leukocyte antigen expression and cytokine production. Lower B cell stimulation results from changes in dendritic cell-immune complex binding (Plackett, Boehmer, Faunce, & Kovacs, 2004).

- Natural killer cells from older persons are less capable of destroying tumor cells (Plackett et al., 2004).

Importantly, certain aspects of immune function remain stable with aging. The total number of peripheral blood cells is unchanged, and the percentages of B and T lymphocyte populations usually are stable, though some chronically ill persons have a decline in total T cell numbers (Gravenstein et al., 2003).

Antibody-Mediated Immunity. The number of peripheral blood B cells is unchanged with age. Antibodies increase; total serum immunoglobulin G (IgG) and IgA levels tend to be higher while IgM levels remain stable. Research in this area has demonstrated that physically active men ages 60 to 69 years of age responded to novel antigenic challenge in a more robust manner than their sedentary counterparts (Smith, Kennedy, & Fleshner, 2004). Another study assessed organ-specific and non–organ-specific autoantibodies in relation to disability and comorbidity among Danish centenarians. Although organ-specific autoantibodies were high, they did not reflect an equally high level of overt autoimmune disease. However, less disabled subjects with low comorbidity had significantly fewer autoantibodies than subjects with organ-specific autoantibodies. Non–organ-specific autoantibodies were distributed equally among individuals with varying degrees of disability and comorbidity (Andersen-Ranberg, Hoier-Madsen, Wiik, Jeune, & Hegedus, 2004).

Cytokine Dysregulation. Proinflammatory cytokines (particularly interleukin-6 [IL-6]) increase with aging. Serum levels of IL-6 normally are undetectable until menopause because sex hormones regulate IL-6 concentration. It has been proposed that chronic exposure to proinflammatory signals may contribute to the metabolic changes of frailty. The finding that elevated IL-6 levels correlate with functional decline and mortality in community-dwelling older persons provides support for this relationship (Gravenstein et al., 2003; van den Biggelaar et al., 2004). In addition to increased IL-6 production by peripheral blood mononuclear cells (PBMC), frail older adults also have been found to have decreased lipopolysaccharide (LPS)-induced proliferation (Leng, Yang, & Walston, 2004). Overexpression of IL-10 may reduce cardiac cellular proliferation after myocardial injury (Dotson, Horak, Alwardt, & Larson, 2004). Box 18-2 summarizes the common changes in the immune system in older adults.

S Box 18-2 *Age-Related Changes: Immune*

Mucocutaneous Barriers (Skin and Mucous Membranes)
- Decreased circulating thymus-derived lymphocytes, cytokines, and epidermal Langerhans cells
- Slower, less dramatic hypersensitivity reactions

Phagocytosis
- Decline in effectiveness of chemotaxis in less vascular areas
- Fewer local T cells activated in response to infection
- Markers that normally attract peripheral T cells are defective
- Impaired capacity to focus mediator cells and the cytokines they express
- Impaired cell adhesion
- Macrophages and neutrophils less effective against bacteria

Cell Lysis
- Natural killer cell activity declines

Cell-Mediated Immunity
- Equivocal changes in ratio of helper cells to suppressor cells
- Increased memory cells
- Decline in T-cell function and proliferative capacity in response to mitogens
- Predominance of helper T cell responses shifts from type 1 to type 2
- Depletion of naïve T cells
- Decreased relative number of CD8 (+) T cells
- Aged dendrites less able to stimulate T and B cells
- Percentages of B and T lymphocytes stable

Antibody-Mediated Immunity
- Total number of peripheral blood cells is stable
- Increased autoantibody frequency
- Increased serum IgG and IgA

Cytokine Dysregulation
- Proinflammatory cytokines (particularly IL-6) increase

IMPACT OF CHANGES IN THE IMMUNE SYSTEM

The impact of changes in the immune system with aging may be profound. Not only is the response to vaccines altered, but immune aging also may be related to increased autoimmune phenomena, neoplasia, and predisposition to infection (Gravenstein et al., 2003; Ramos-Casals, Brito-Zeron, Lopez-Soto, & Font, 2004). Some changes may be adaptive, as in the case of increased NK cells in very old persons that may compensate for decreases in other immune functions (Leng et al., 2004).

Many avenues of study are seeking strategies to improve immune function in older persons. According to the free radical theory of aging, accumulated oxygen-derived free radicals cause cellular damage. It is proposed that dietary antioxidants can protect the body, including the immune system, by supporting the inactivation of the free radicals and by decreasing oxidative stress (De la Fuente, 2002). Noting the relationship between thymic atrophy and immunosenescence, and the importance of IL-7 in the early stages of thymocyte development, investigators are exploring the use of IL-7 to boost immune function (Henson, Pido-Lopez, & Aspinall, 2004). Some antidepressants have been found to stimulate the production of IL-6 in adults (mean age 50.6 years). Specifically, imipramine, venlafaxine, 5-hydroxytryptophan (5-HTP), and a combination of 5-HTP and fluoxetine all increased IL-6 production in this age-group sample (Kubera et al., 2004).

Vaccination in Older Persons

The response of older persons to vaccine is a good representation of immune changes. In older individuals, many sources report that primary and secondary responses to vaccination are altered. Peak antibody titers are lower, the peak titer occurs 2 to 6 weeks after vaccination (compared with 2 to 3 weeks in younger persons), and the titers decline more rapidly. However, in the work of Kang and colleagues the response of healthy elderly persons to vaccination was like that of younger persons, except the older persons failed to maintain or expand the responses (Kang et al., 2004).

Vaccine researchers continue to seek methods to induce better immunity in older persons. Strategies under exploration include the use of immunomodulators as adjuvant therapy with vaccines, mucosal delivery of vaccines, and DNA vaccination (Katz et al., 2004). Prevaccination NK has been found to affect vaccination response, with higher postvaccination titers occurring in individuals with high prevaccination NK. Those persons with higher titers also had better health status and a lower incidence of respiratory tract infections.

Influenza Vaccination. Older persons with influenza are at higher risk for morbidity than younger persons, presumably because of reduced antibody responsiveness and influenza-specific cell-mediated immunity (Gravenstein et al., 2003). Therefore much emphasis is placed on vaccination as a means of reducing the risk for influenza in older persons. Influenza vaccine has been shown to augment NK activity (Mysliwska et al., 2004). Just how effective is the influenza vaccine in preventing influenza in this population? A meta-analysis of studies of influenza vaccine efficacy in healthy adults obtained an efficacy estimate of 22% for the prevention of clinically diagnosed cases and 63% for the prevention of laboratory confirmed cases. The efficacy decreased significantly with increasing age (Villari, Manzoli, & Boccia, 2004). Despite diminished response to vaccine in older persons, vaccination has been shown to be highly effective in decreasing the incidence and severity of influenza. In a healthy, unvaccinated population, the duration of illness from influenza is twice as long in older persons as in younger persons. Among older persons who contract the infection despite vaccination, the duration is like that of younger patients (Gravenstein et al., 2003). An interesting study assessed the feasibility of using reduced dosages of influenza vaccine administered intradermally (half of the usual intramuscular dose) because of a vaccine shortage. The antibody response was similar to the usual dose response in persons under age 60, but not for those over age 60 (Belshe et al., 2004).

Cancer and Immunosenescence

Advancing age is a risk factor for many kinds of cancer, predominantly carcinomas. Denduluri and Ershler (2004) point out that normal aging and the development of cancer have much in common. Autopsy data show the greatest prevalence of metastatic disease between ages 75 and 90, followed by a decline in the tenth decade. The increase in natural killer cells, increased production of cytokines, and progressive acquisition of T cells with phenotypes that are intermediate between T lymphocytes and NK cells may actually serve to slow the growth and spread of tumors in the oldest old (Bonafe et al., 2001; Provinciali & Smorlesi, 2005).

The relationship between immunosenescence and cancer is not completely understood. Factors thought to play a role in the development of cancer include lymphocyte proliferative disorders, defective immune surveillance, and an imbalance between immune-restraining and growth-enhancing effects on tumors. Unknown mechanisms may trigger spontaneous tumor growth to which the aging antitumoral immune defenses are unable to respond adequately. Immunosenescence also might provide avenues that enable cancer cells to escape immune clearance. For example, many tumors produce immunosuppressive cytokines that suppress inflammatory T cell responses and cell-mediated immunity (Provinciali & Smorlesi, 2005). By comparing persons who had cancer with others who did not, Motta and colleagues (2003) concluded that alterations in immunocompetent cells, particularly of the T cell pool, may play a role in carcinogenesis in older persons (Motta et al., 2003).

In a discussion of prostate cancer, Leibovitz, Baumoehl, & Segal (2004) note that the inability of the gland to eradicate emergent malignant cells in the older person may be related to the age-related decline in immune surveillance of the already immune-privileged prostate.

Infection and Immunosenescence

The number and severity of infections increase with age, a fact attributed to numerous factors including immunosenescence. Changes in cellular immunity may help to explain reactivation of infections such as tuberculosis and shingles (Gravenstein et al., 2003).

Manifestations of infection in older persons commonly are atypical. Classic signs (high fever, leukocytosis, prominent inflammatory infiltrates on chest x-ray with pneumonia, rebound tenderness with acute conditions in the abdomen) may be absent. Temperature change relevant to the individual's usual temperature may be more significant than the same reading in a younger person. Older persons, particularly the oldest old, may present with infections caused by unusual organisms, recurrent infections with the same pathogen, or reactivation of quiescent diseases such as those caused by tuberculosis and herpes zoster virus. They also may not respond as well to therapy for infection (Gravenstein et al., 2003).

Patch Test Reactivity

A study of patch test reactivity in 1444 persons over age 65 with suspected allergic contact dermatitis demonstrated a decline in overall patch test reactions. However, the test subjects also demonstrated a higher sensitization rate to some allergens that commonly are used in topical products. Because the allergic response tended to be delayed, the investigators recommended an additional reading after 7 days. They also recommended that even weak reactions should be considered positive patch test reactions (Piaserico et al., 2004).

COMMON DISORDERS
Infectious Disease

Diminished immune function alone is sufficient to explain the increased incidence and severity of infection in older persons. Older adults who are debilitated and poorly nourished are at even greater risk for infections with serious consequences. Two infectious diseases that are more commonly seen in older persons are pneumococcus and varicella (herpes zoster).

Pneumococcal Disease. The incidence of pneumococcal disease in adults younger than 70 years of age is estimated at 5/100,000. After age 70, it increases to 70/100,000. Infections associated with *Streptococcus pneumoniae* include pneumonia, otitis media, sinusitis, meningitis, septic arthritis, pericarditis, endocarditis, peritonitis, cellulitis, glomerulonephritis, and sepsis. Factors found to increase the risk of pneumococcal disease are chronic obstructive pulmonary disease (COPD) and swallowing disorders as might occur with dementia, stupor, stroke, alcoholism, seizure disorders, and foreign bodies in the esophagus. Pneumococcal vaccines are recommended, especially in long-term care facilities, even though their effectiveness is debated. Currently efforts are underway to develop a more effective vaccine. Revaccination is recommended for individuals 65 and older who were vaccinated 5 or more years in the past and before the age of 65 (Gravenstein et al., 2003).

Varicella (Herpes Zoster) Viral Disease. The incidence and severity of herpes zoster infection (shingles) increase with age. Complications include postherpetic neuralgia and cranial nerve zoster, which commonly affects the ophthalmic nerve. Cranial nerve zoster can also cause severe conjunctivitis with possible corneal scarring. Correlates of postherpetic neuralgia are sleep disturbance, depression, Bell's palsy, and Meniere's disease. Immune suppression is a risk factor for varicella zoster infection.

Chickenpox, caused by this organism, is generally thought of as a childhood disease, and many older persons have acquired immunity as a result of exposure as a child. However, any person who has never had chickenpox or has not been vaccinated for it should avoid contact with persons with herpes zoster infection because it is communicable.

Autoimmune Disorders and Immunosenescence

An increase in autoantibodies has been implicated in the increasing incidence of vascular disease and autoimmune disorders (e.g., rheumatoid arthritis, temporal arteritis, thyroiditis, pernicious anemia). Rheumatoid arthritis and temporal arteritis are addressed in Chapter 11. Aspects of the various types of thyroiditis are summarized in Table 18-1.

Pernicious Anemia. Pernicious anemia is an autoimmune disease in which antibodies destroy gastric parietal cells and intrinsic factor (IF). It most often affects persons over 60 years of age, occurs equally in men and women, is found in all racial and ethnic groups, and is more common in people with other autoimmune conditions. The basic problem is a deficiency of intrinsic factor, which interferes with the absorption of

Table 18-1 Types of Thyroiditis

Type of Thyroiditis	Etiology	Features	Management
Acute (suppurative)	Bacterial, fungal, or other infectious agent	Tenderness, swelling; fever and leukocytosis common	Fine-needle aspiration to identify organism; antibiotics; abscess drainage if needed
Subacute painful (granulomatous)	Inflammatory: thyroid antibodies secondary to thyroid damage caused by viral infection	Most common in women ages 40 to 50 years; most frequent cause of severe thyroid pain and tenderness; gland enlarged; T_4 elevated initially; may have temporary hypothyroidism after acute phase	Mild analgesics usually sufficient; prednisone if symptoms severe, tapered over 4 weeks; beta blockers if thyrotoxic in early phase
Subacute painless (lymphocytic)	Probably autoimmune and unrelated to viral infection	Most common in women ages 30 to 40 years; abrupt thyrotoxicosis initially, then hypothyroid; may have small, firm, painless goiter; no signs of Graves' disease; biopsy shows lymphocyte infiltration	Beta blockers for symptoms of thyrotoxicosis; thyroid replacement for hypofunction only until normal function regained
Chronic lymphocytic (Hashimoto's thyroiditis)	Most common autoimmune thyroid disease; most common cause of thyroid failure in older persons	Most common in women ages 20 to 40 years; genetic propensity; very high level of thyroid antibodies; anti-TSH receptor blockers may be present; usually goitrous but may be atrophic; some individuals have initial hypothyroidism; some people have symptoms of Graves' disease, transient hyperthyroidism; other autoimmune diseases commonly present	Thyroxine replacement if T_4 low and TSH high; marginal hypothyroidism treated to prevent further thyroid enlargement; surgery if obstructing trachea; beta blockers for symptoms of transient hyperthyroidism
Fibrous (Riedel's thyroiditis)	Inflammation	Gland very hard	Aspiration to rule out cancer; surgery if obstructs trachea; thyroid replacement if hypothyroid

Data from Dillman, W. H. (2003). The thyroid. In L. Goldman & J. C. Bennett (Eds.), *Cecil textbook of medicine* (21st ed.). Philadephia: Saunders, pp. 1231-1250; Miller, M. (2003). Disorders of the thyroid. In R. C. Tallis & H. M. Fillit (Eds.), *Brocklehurst's textbook of geriatric medicine and gerontology* (6th ed.). London: Churchill Livingstone, pp. 1164-1184.

cobalamin (vitamin B_{12}). Whereas some persons present with only fatigue, others have the classic signs of glossitis, mild jaundice, lemon-yellow skin color, and neurological manifestations such as paresthesias, abnormal position and vibration sensation, gait ataxia, personality changes, and even dementia. Laboratory studies reveal macrocytosis and hypersegmented polymorphonuclear leukocytes on the peripheral blood smear, elevated serum bilirubin and LDH levels, and decreased serum vitamin B_{12} levels. Platelets and white blood cell counts also may be low. Because the dementia of pernicious anemia resembles Alzheimer's disease, persons presenting with neuropsychiatric symptoms

should be evaluated promptly for vitamin B_{12} deficiency (Nierodzik, Sutin, & Freedman, 2003).

Absorption of oral vitamin B_{12} can be improved with intrinsic factor. However, persons with long-standing pernicious anemia may have intestinal malabsorption usually requiring lifelong treatment with parenteral vitamin B_{12}. Vitamin B_{12} 1000 mcg may be given daily for the first week, weekly for 4 doses, and monthly thereafter. During initial therapy, the patient should be monitored for hypokalemia and hypophosphatemia, and supplementation should be provided as needed. If a transfusion is needed, the risk of circulatory overload demands careful monitoring of the older person.

Treatment does not always reverse all neurological symptoms (Nierodzik et al., 2003).

It should be mentioned that older persons sometimes have signs of vitamin B_{12} deficiency that are not caused by pernicious anemia. For example, gastric HCl and pepsin are necessary to free vitamin B_{12} from dietary proteins. Other causes of B_{12} deficiency are bacterial overgrowth in the stomach, ileal disease, gastric surgery, and use of the gastric acid inhibitor omeprazole. When the deficiency is caused by a lack of HCl, it can be treated with oral vitamin B_{12} administered on an empty stomach (Nierodzik et al., 2003).

Acquired Immune Deficiency

Factors other than aging that can diminish immune function in older persons include malnutrition, polypharmacy, HIV infection, and psychosocial factors such as social isolation, depression, and stress. Malnutrition can have a profound effect on the immune system. Resistance to infection is diminished by deficiencies of protein, calories, vitamins, and elemental substances such as zinc. Among the many drugs that can suppress the inflammatory immune response are analgesics, NSAIDs, steroids, antithyroid drugs, antibiotics, antipsychotics, antidepressants, hypnotics/sedatives, anticonvulsants, antihypertensives, diuretics, H_2 blockers, and hypoglycemics. In addition, some drugs can cause neutropenia and lymphocytopenia. Because T lymphocytes have calcium channels and cholinergic, histaminic, and adrenergic receptors, they are subject to various drug effects (Gravenstein et al., 2003, p. 118).

HIV/AIDS IN OLDER PERSONS. Although "older adult" commonly is defined as age 65 and older, the Centers for Disease Control and Prevention (CDC) classifies persons with HIV as "older" after age 49. HIV/AIDS commonly is perceived as a disease of young and middle-aged persons; however, the mean age at diagnosis of HIV infection and AIDS has been progressively increasing. Persons aged 50 and older comprise 10% to 15% of new HIV cases, and individuals 65 and older comprise 2%. In addition to shifts in age at diagnosis, the mode of transmission has shifted from IV drug use and contaminated blood products to heterosexual and homosexual activity. Also, the proportion of females has been increasing (Manfredi, 2003).

Compared with their younger counterparts, older persons with HIV/AIDS are more likely to be diagnosed late in disease, experience a more rapid immunological decline, progress more rapidly from known date of seroconversion to AIDS, and have a shorter survival time after the diagnosis of AIDS (Valcour, Shikuma, Watters, & Sacktor, 2004). Older persons also tend to have more comorbidities and treatment sensitivity that can complicate the disease process and its management, resulting in increased morbidity and premature mortality (Dolder, Patterson, & Jeste, 2004). One factor that may explain the late diagnoses in this population is that they are less likely to perceive themselves at risk for HIV infection (Goodroad, 2003).

PREVALENCE. About 11% of people with AIDS are age 50 and over; as noted 10% of all new cases of AIDS are in people older than 50 (Becker, Lopez, Dew, & Aizenstein, 2004; Gravenstein et al., 2003). The CDC estimates of new AIDS cases diagnosed in the United States in 2003 were as follows: ages 45 to 54 = 10,051; ages 55 to 64 = 2888; and ages 65+ = 886 (CDC Division of HIV/AIDS Prevention, 2005). There now are more than 60,000 persons age 50 and older living with AIDS in the United States (Mack & Ory, 2003). The expanding number of older persons with AIDS is largely due to prolonged survival, and can be expected to continue. With the advent of highly active antiretroviral therapy (HAART), more people diagnosed during young adulthood survive to middle and older age. Racial and ethnic minorities are disproportionately represented among persons with HIV/AIDS. By race/ethnicity, the greatest number of cases in 2003 were in black non-Hispanics (21,304), followed by white non-Hispanics (12,222), Hispanics (8757), Asian/Pacific Islanders (497), and American Indian/Alaska natives (196) (CDC Division of HIV/AIDS Prevention, 2005). Like their younger counterparts, older men who have sex with men comprise the largest group of individuals in the United States affected by HIV. This pattern is different from other parts of the world where heterosexual transmission is more common. Education and prevention need to consider the increasing representation of ethnic and racial minorities. Men who are minorities and have sex with men are at special risk (Levy, Ory, & Crystal, 2003).

An integrative review of research on transmission risks of HIV in older adults identified inadequate HIV transmission education, poor awareness of risk, and insufficient communication between patients and health care providers about HIV transmission (Savasta, 2004). Additional risk factors that were identified in urban senior housing were intravenous drug use and contact with commercial sex workers. It was assumed that individuals would be reluctant to admit to these behaviors (Radda, Schensul, Disch, Levy, & Reyes, 2003). Interestingly, Kwiatkowski and Booth (2003) found older IV drug users to be less likely to use previously used needles or to share drug paraphernalia. Research has given less attention to older women, who have their own set of risk factors. They may be less likely to use barrier contraceptives, and age-related changes in the vagina may enhance susceptibility to disease. Women who find themselves newly single in the middle or later years may be less well informed about the risks of HIV and safe sex

(Levy et al., 2003). Global travel and tourism may be a factor in the spread of HIV. Older travelers may engage in risky behavior when removed from the home environment. The Internet presents opportunities for sexual encounters.

FEATURES. Although clinical manifestations of HIV are similar regardless of age, older persons typically report fewer symptoms (Levy et al., 2003). However, the older adult is more likely to have comorbidity that might modify the clinical expression. Symptoms such as fatigue, anorexia, cognitive disorders, weight loss, chronic pain, rash, and itching could easily be attributed to other, more common, conditions or even to drug therapy. The presentation of Kaposi's sarcoma may be atypical (Manfredi, 2003). Older persons have been found to have lower plasma viral loads than younger persons with HIV (Goodkin et al., 2004). The reason for the shorter survival times for older adults is not completely understood. Proposed explanations include more advanced disease at diagnosis and immunosenescence (Levy et al., 2003).

Neurological symptoms are varied and may include cognitive, behavioral, and psychomotor disturbances. Neurological disturbances require careful evaluation because they could be related to vascular or degenerative conditions (some treatable) instead of HIV/AIDS (Manfredi, 2003). Symptoms similar to Parkinson's disease may develop with psychomotor declines (Vance, 2004). Despite generally lower viral loads in older individuals, viral burden and age are significant predictors of neuropsychological impairment. Older persons with detectable virus in the CSF are much more likely to have neurological impairment (Cherner et al., 2004). Alcohol abuse also has been identified as a risk factor for neurocognitive disorders with HIV (Becker et al., 2004). A study of persons with HIV showed that older persons had longer reaction times that significantly correlated with higher viral loads and lower CD4 cell counts. Learning and memory retrieval deficits were found in all age-groups (Wilkie et al., 2003).

HIV-associated dementia (HAD) and minor cognitive and motor disorders (MCMD) are thought to be more prevalent among older HIV-seropositive persons perhaps because the aging brain may be at increased risk of injury in HIV (Valcour, Shikuma, Watters, & Sacktor, 2004). Indeed, some patients with AIDS present with dementia. HIV-related neurocognitive disorders are characterized by acquired deficits affecting motor function, behavior, and cognition. Impairment is greater in HAD than in MCMD (Valcour, Shikuma, Watters, & Sacktor, 2004). Some similarities have been noted in the immune system changes in both HAD and Alzheimer's disease. In addition to immune changes, comorbid neurodegenerative disorders, vascular co-pathology, and astrocytic function may also contribute

to the pathogenesis of neurocognitive dysfunction. An association has been found between APOE4 and dementia among older but not among younger HIV-1 infected individuals (Valcour, Shikuma, Shiramizu, Watters, Poff, et al., 2004). Not only are older persons with HIV at risk for central nervous system effects, but they also are at increased risk for symptomatic distal sensory polyneuropathy characterized by vibratory loss and increased severity of pinprick loss. Correlates are dementia and low nadir CD4 in HIV-positive patients aged 50 and older (Watters et al., 2004).

SPECIAL CONCERNS. Providers sometimes fail to assess risk factors for HIV infection in older persons with immunodeficiency, an omission that can have serious consequences for direct care providers (Gravenstein et al., 2003). Late diagnosis, which is common among older persons with HIV, reduces the likelihood of a good response to HAART therapy (slowed disease progression, immune recovery, delay of opportunistic complications) (Manfredi, 2003). Earlier detection needs to be a priority to improve outcomes for older individuals.

Psychosocial issues facing individuals with HIV/AIDS include the following: facing morbidity and mortality, social isolation, loss and grieving, decline in physical function, and pathological changes in multiple organ systems (Ress, 2003). Studies of quality of life among older persons with HIV have revealed reactive depression, emotional stress, and distress related to awareness of a transmissible and life-threatening illness (Manfredi, 2003). Unfortunately, many older persons with HIV lack psychological support networks, and others choose not to use them. Many have experienced multiple AIDS-related deaths. Schrimshaw and Siegel (2003), who studied social support among persons with HIV/AIDS, found adults age 50 and over with HIV to be more socially isolated than their younger counterparts. Of the persons interviewed, 42% said they did not receive adequate emotional support, and 27% percent expressed the need for more practical support. Identified barriers to meeting their support needs included nondisclosure of HIV status, others' fear of HIV/AIDS, desire to be self-reliant and independent, not wanting to be a burden, family unavailability, death of friends to AIDS, and ageism. Building social support groups is an important intervention (Levy et al., 2003).

Comorbidity. As noted above, care of the older person with HIV/AIDS is complicated by the increased prevalence of comorbid conditions. Not only do the multiple conditions require management, but multiple drugs also increase the risk of adverse drug effects. For example, prolonged HAART treatment is associated with metabolic disturbances such as dyslipidemia and diabetes mellitus, and peripheral neuropathies (Manfredi, 2003). Consider the implications for older persons who

Table 18-2 *Organ Toxicity of Antiretroviral Drugs*

Drug Class	Organ/Tissue							
	Liver	Pancreas	Kidney	Bone Marrow	Skin and Soft Tissues	GI Tract	Eye	Peripheral Nervous System
Nucleoside analogues	X	X	X	X	X	X	X	X
Protease inhibitors	X	X	X		X	X		
Nonnucleoside reverse transcriptase inhibitors	X	X			X			

Data from Manfredi, R. (2003). HIV infection and advanced age: Emerging epidemiological, clinical, and management issues. *Ageing Research Reviews, 3,* 31-54.

also have cardiovascular disease or diabetes mellitus. Data from the Hawaii Aging with HIV cohort revealed a relationship between dementia and diabetes that was not fully explained by covariates including age. Even among individuals who did not have diabetes, fasting glucose levels were elevated (Valcour, Shikuma, Shiramizu, Williams, Watters, et al., 2005). Forty-three percent of HIV-positive patients in the Veterans Aging 3-Site Cohort Study also were infected with hepatitis C (Fultz et al., 2003).

Treatment Considerations. Since the first antiretroviral drug was introduced in 1986, 4 different classes and 17 specific drugs have been developed. Because of major problems with resistance and toxicity, numerous combinations have been used. Current recommendations are to select at least three drugs from different classes with specific selections tailored to the individual on the basis of clinical manifestations, CD4 and lymphocyte count, and plasma viral load thresholds (Manfredi, 2003). The cost of lifelong drug therapy is considerable ($15,000 to $20,000 per year), but still less expensive than the repeated hospitalizations that occur without therapy.

The goal of HAART is improved immunological function, a response that may be slow and incomplete in the older person (Manfredi, 2003). The major obstacle to efficacy is emerging resistance. Variables associated with more effective treatment are lower baseline viremia, limited resistance profile, possibility of using drugs from novel classes, and elevated patient adherence and motivation. Genotypic and phenotypic assays are very useful during HAART. The most common sequence of events leading to resistance is believed to be reduced compliance, which permits a rapid spread of viral resistance and accelerated virological failure (Manfredi, 2003). After HAART is initiated, the decrease in viral load is similar regardless of age; however, some studies found delayed or a less favorable response in CD4 lymphocytes. The magnitude of the increase is usually less in older persons possibly because of the age-related changes in the thymus (Valcour et al., 2004).

Antiretroviral drugs have multiple adverse effects that may require changes from one combination of drugs to another. Among the adverse effects are disorders of lipid and glucose metabolism, accelerated atherosclerosis, and hypertension that predispose to cardiovascular and cerebrovascular events; other adverse effects are fat redistribution syndrome (similar to that seen in corticosteroid therapy), avascular osteonecrosis, early osteopenia and osteoporosis, muscle damage, hepatic steatosis, pancreatitis, peripheral neuropathy, gynecomastia, lactic acidosis, and hyperlactatemia (Table 18-2). Suggested interventions for these adverse effects are low-fat, low-glucoside diet, increased physical exercise, and lipid-lowering drugs. Adjustments are necessary when individuals have concurrent liver or kidney failure, but no detailed recommendations are available (Manfredi, 2003).

Like most other conditions that require long-term drug therapy, issues of adherence mandate efforts to select programs that are easy to self-administer. No standardized recommendations have been designed specifically for treatment of the older person with HIV, probably because controlled data on this population are lacking (Manfredi, 2003). Some strategies to improve compliance with therapy are listed in Box 18-3.

BOX 18-3 Strategies to Improve Adherence with HAART

- Consider patient characteristics and lifestyle when selecting drugs.
- Use technology (phone, email) to maintain daily communication with health care personnel.
- Select drug formulations and combinations that reduce the number and frequency of drugs taken daily.

Data from Manfredi, R. (2003). HIV infection and advanced age: Emerging epidemiological, clinical, and management issues. *Ageing Research Reviews, 3,* 31-54.

Drug selection is more complicated in the older person who has comorbidities and drug therapy for other purposes (Manfredi, 2003). One study found that 81% of persons with HIV were taking non-HIV medications, most commonly inhaled β_2 agonists, calcium channel blockers, and NSAIDs (Shah et al., 2002, cited in Manfredi, 2003). Of special concern is the potential for serious drug interactions if antiretroviral drugs are taken concurrently with antitubercular drugs, antimycobacterial drugs, some antimicrobials and antifungals, various antihistamines, estrogen-progesterone preparations, methadone, theophylline, sildenafil, hypolipemic drugs, calcium channel blockers, and some psychotropic drugs. The effects of the interactions may be to increase the serum level of the antiretroviral, thereby increasing the risk of toxicity, or decreasing the serum level, causing reduced drug activity (Manfredi, 2003).

NURSING CARE
Assessment of the Immune System

The assessment of the immunological system actually incorporates multiple systems because immunological problems are manifested in many ways.

Health History. Important clues to immunological dysfunction are complaints of recent, recurrent, or chronic infections. Relevant data include a past history of cancer, liver, or kidney disorders, HIV infection, or malabsorption. Also significant are reports of delayed healing, prolonged bleeding, blood transfusions, splenectomy, and placement of a prosthetic heart valve or an indwelling venous access device.

The review of systems assesses general well-being, noting fatigue, fever, chills, and night sweats. Inquire about skin lesions, pruritus, and bruising or bleeding. Document any complaints of headache, sore throat, or enlarged lymph nodes. Note respiratory symptoms such as dyspnea, cough, or hemoptysis and cardiovascular symptoms including palpitations and dizziness with position changes. Determine if the patient has had changes in appetite or weight, dysphagia, nausea, vomiting, hematemesis, melena, painful defecation, or a change in bowel habits. Genitourinary symptoms that may be significant are hematuria, dysuria, and menorrhagia. Joint pain or swelling and bone pain should be assessed.

Significant data from the family history include cancer and blood or immune system disorders. Within the social history, chemical exposure, heavy alcohol consumption, and sexual preference and patterns are important. Factors that may indicate increased risk include the number of sexual partners, a history of STDs, and safe sex practices. There is no justification for omitting the sexual history when assessing an older patient. Based on survey results of older patients, Ress (2003)

found that less than 10% of the patients said they would be unwilling to answer a physician's questions about their sexual behavior.

MEDICATION. The drug history is important because many drugs are used to treat immunological symptoms, and others can affect the immunological function. Some drugs are used specifically as immunosuppressants. Others, including corticosteroids, nonsteroidal antiinflammatory drugs, antineoplastics, and some antibiotics, also suppress immune function.

Physical Examination. Begin the physical examination by taking vital signs. Note temperature elevation, tachycardia, hypotension, or tachypnea. Inspect the skin and the mucous membranes for lesions, pallor, purpura, ecchymoses, hematomas, and rashes. Inspect the tongue for the glossy appearance characteristic of pernicious anemia. Document how long any lesions have been present. Immunocompromised patients including those with HIV are at risk for Kaposi's sarcoma, which is manifested by bluish-red cutaneous nodules that appear first on the lower extremities and spread proximally. Inspect and palpate the joints for swelling and tenderness. Palpate for enlarged lymph nodes, liver, and spleen. Auscultate heart rate and breath sounds. The nursing assessment of the person with an immune disorder is summarized in Box 18-4

Diagnostic Tests. Diagnostic tests that are useful in assessing immunological function include blood studies, radiologic procedures, and invasive procedures.

BLOOD STUDIES. Laboratory tests to assess the humoral immune system are serum protein electrophoresis, immunoelectrophoresis, quantitation of Ig levels, and specific antibody titers (e.g., isoagglutinins). To assess the cellular immune system, obtain blood leukocyte count, absolute lymphocyte counts, delayed skin test hypersensitivity with at least six antigens, and in vitro testing "such as measurements of suppressor and helper lymphocyte ratios (T4/T8), and the ability of lymphocytes to proliferate in response to mitogens and specific antigens" (Gravenstein et al., 2003, p. 119).

The differential measures the proportions of each type of white blood cell (monocytes, neutrophils, basophils, eosinophils, and lymphocytes). When only a small proportion of the WBCs are neutrophils, the blood sample is said to reflect a "shift to the right." The patient with a low neutrophil count is at risk for infection. When a large proportion of WBCs are neutrophils, the patient is said to have a "shift to the left," a finding that usually indicates that a severe infection has stimulated the bone marrow to produce more neutrophils (Young-McCaughan & Jennings, 1998).

Box 18-4 Immune System Assessment

Health History
- **Chief complaint:** Recent, recurrent, or chronic infections; delayed healing, prolonged bleeding
- **Past medical history:** Cancer, liver, or kidney disorders, HIV infection, malabsorption, blood transfusions, spleenectomy, prosthetic heart valve, indwelling venous access device
- **Review of systems:**
  - **General:** Fatigue, fever, chills, night sweats, headache
  - **Integument:** Lesions of skin and mucous membranes, pruritus, bruising or bleeding
  - **Respiratory:** Sore throat, dyspnea, cough, hemoptysis
  - **Cardiovascular:** Palpitations, dizziness with position changes
  - **Gastrointestinal:** Change in appetite or weight, dysphagia, nausea, vomiting, hematemesis, melena, painful defecation, change in bowel habits
  - **Genitourinary:** Hematuria, dysuria, menorrhagia
  - **Musculoskeletal:** Joint pain, swelling, bone pain
  - **Family history:** Cancer, blood or immune system disorders
- **Social history:** Chemical exposure, heavy alcohol consumption, sexual preference and patterns, number of sexual partners, history of STDs, safe sex practices
- **Medications:** Particularly immunosuppressants, corticosteroids, nonsteroidal antiinflammatory drugs, antineoplastics, antibiotics

Physical Examination
- **Vital signs:** Fever, tachycardia, hypotension, tachypnea
- **Cardiopulmonary:** Heart rate, breath sounds
- **Integument:** Lesions, pallor, purpura, ecchymoses, hematomas, rash
- **Oral cavity:** Appearance of tongue
- **Musculoskeletal:** Joint swelling, tenderness
- **Lymph nodes, liver, and spleen:** Enlargement

Other diagnostic laboratory tests and their findings that may be relevant to immunological function are the T cell counts, serum electrophoresis, and HIV antibody tests (enzyme-linked immunosorbent assay [ELISA] and Western blot). Serum electrophoresis determines protein levels in the serum, particularly immunoglobulins. HIV antibody tests (ELISA and Western blot) detect antibodies to HIV. The Western blot is considered more sensitive.

RADIOLOGIC PROCEDURES. Ultrasonography is used to estimate the size of the spleen. A radioactive tracer can be used in a liver-spleen scan to provide information about the size and function of both organs. The gallium scan, which also uses a radioactive tracer, is useful in detecting malignancies in lymphoid and other tissues. To visualize the lymph system, a lymphangiogram with contrast dye is helpful.

INVASIVE PROCEDURES. Lymph nodes sometimes are removed and submitted for pathological examination. Skin tests may be used to assess immune functioning by judging the response to specific antigens.

Nursing Diagnoses
- Risk for infection related to suppressed immune response, inadequate secondary defenses
- Ineffective coping related to uncertainty, high degree of threat, inadequate social support created by characteristics of relationships
- Interrupted family processes related to shift in health status of a family member, situational crisis
- Fatigue related to anxiety, depression, disease state, drug side effects
- Grieving related to change in health status, risk for life-threatening complications
- Ineffective health maintenance related to perceptual/cognitive impairment, lack of material resources, ineffective individual coping
- Imbalanced nutrition: less than body requirements related to anorexia
- Deficient knowledge related to lack of exposure, cognitive limitation
- Social isolation related to altered state of wellness
- Ineffective therapeutic regimen management related to perceived barriers, social support deficit, complexity of therapeutic regimen
- Disturbed thought processes related to disease process

Interventions

Common interventions for the patient with altered immune function include measures to improve immune function, manage symptoms of HIV and adverse effects of treatments, reduce the risk of infection, promote effective self-care, and provide support.

Measures to Improve Immune Function.
Efforts to improve immune function that are within the nurse's purview focus on nutrition and exercise. Nutrition is viewed as one approach because of the recognized relationship between good nutrition and immunity. Also, it is hypothesized that antioxidants help to maintain the health of the immune system by breaking

down free radicals. Because nutrient deficiencies may be related to impaired immunity in older persons, some investigators are exploring the benefits of nutritional supplements. Vitamins C and E are two antioxidants that have drawn much attention. Zinc and vitamin E have been shown to improve selected immune responses, but not to reduce morbidity related to infection. A multinutrient with essential trace elements and vitamins may enhance immune function and reduce infections (Chandra, 2004).

Exercise has been studied as an intervention to restore immune function in older individuals. A review of the research investigating this hypothesis suggests that exercise, particularly long term, may indeed restore the immune response. However, current data are limited and leave many questions unanswered (Kohut & Senchina, 2004). Moderate exercise (65% to 75% heart rate reserve, 25″ to 30″, 3 times per week for 10 months) has been found to enhance the antibody response to influenza vaccine (Kohut et al., 2004). Smith et al. (2004) studied the response of physically active and sedentary men to a novel protein antigen. Not surprisingly, the responses were better in younger men than the older participants. However among the older participants measures of the primary antibody and T cell responses were significantly higher in those who were physically active with the exception of IgG2.

Measures to Manage Symptoms of HIV and Adverse Effects of Treatments.

The symptoms experienced by persons with HIV can have a negative effect on quality of life and can be related to the disease itself or to side effects of treatment. The most frequently reported symptoms are fatigue, joint pain or stiffness, muscle aches, diarrhea, neuropathy, and depression. Weight loss; diarrhea; white patches in the mouth; pain, numbness, and tingling in the hands and feet; and cough with fever and/or dyspnea also have been reported. Symptoms attributed to HIV disease include tender lymph nodes, night sweats, weight loss, fever, and weakness. Side effects of treatment include upset stomach, nausea/vomiting, constipation, and changes in the sense of taste (Asch et al., 2004; Johnson, Stallworth, & Neilands, 2003; Lorenz, Shapiro, Asch, Bozzette, & Hays, 2001; Nicholas, Kirksey, Corless, & Kemppainen, 2005).

Some studies that have examined the effects of antiretroviral therapy on mental health have concluded that the therapy resulted in improved mental health (Chan et al., 2003; Rabkin, Ferrando, Lin, Sewell, & McElhiney, 2000). In the study by Rabkin et al. (2000), physical symptoms were more strongly related to psychological distress than to CD4 cell count. Studies of medication adherence (compliance) determined that good adherence was predicted by having emotional support, being employed, and having higher levels of HIV symptoms (Cox, 2002).

Testosterone treatments have been found to reduce the loss of lean body and muscle mass. When administered to persons with HIV, testosterone reportedly improves mood and libido in women and increases bone density in men (Dobs, 2003).

Kilbourne and colleagues (2002) hypothesized that vulnerable populations were less likely to receive the same care for HIV symptoms as other groups. They were surprised to find that the only group that was less likely to receive care were those who had private, non-HMO insurance.

Measures to Reduce the Risk of Infection.

Health care acquired infections continue to contribute significantly to morbidity and mortality. In one large United States city with a higher than average rate of malpractice claims, hospital-acquired infections most commonly involved surgical sites, specifically the knees, back, sternum, and harvest site. Methicillin-resistant *Staphylococcus aureus* (MRSA) was responsible for about one third of the infections (Guinan, McGuckin, Shubin, & Tighe, 2005). Hospitals with a low volume of a specific surgical procedure have been found to have higher rates of surgical site infection (Geubbels et al., 2005). Despite guidelines for procedures that pose an infection hazard, many practitioners fail to exercise proper precautions (Rubinson, Wu, Haponik, & Diette, 2005). A study of adults admitted to intensive care units found higher morbidity and mortality among older persons. Independent risk factors for mortality for persons 75 years and older included infection on admission, impaired level of consciousness, ICU-acquired infection, and severity of illness score (Vosylius, Sipylaite, & Ivaskevicius, 2005).

Prevention of infection depends on basic nursing techniques—including handwashing, aseptic technique, and oral care. Technology has introduced new vectors for transmission including bedside and office computers and personal digital assistants (PDAs). Several studies have reported colonization on these articles (Braddy & Blair, 2005; Waghorn et al., 2005). Oropharyngeal colonization has been implicated in nosocomial pneumonia. Strategies to reduce respiratory infection associated with microaspiration of oropharyngeal secretions include oropharyngeal decontamination with topical antibiotics, application of antimicrobial chlorhexidine gluconate, and tooth brushing with dental prophylaxis. Oral care for intensive care patients may employ a toothbrush and toothpaste, antibacterial mouth rinses, and lubricants for the lips. Toothbrushes generally are superior to foam swabs for persons with their natural teeth (Brinkley, Furr, Carrico, & McCurren, 2004).

One strategy intended to reduce catheter-related urinary tract infection is the administration of an antibiotic when the catheter is removed. A survey of this practice in the UK found that about half of the practitioners followed it despite the lack of clinical trials to confirm its effectiveness (Wazait et al., 2004).

Gastrointestinal infections can be especially dangerous for older persons who adapt less readily to changes in fluid balance. Noroviruses have been implicated in outbreaks of gastroenteritis in long-term care facilities. A study of the features of norovirus identified prodromal excretion at least 24 hours before the onset of symptoms and continued fecal excretion for as long as 15 days even after stool became formed (Goller,

Dimitriadis, Tan, Kelly, & Marshall, 2004). These findings are important reminders that measures to prevent the spread of infection from patient to patient are important even when both are asymptomatic.

An individual who has a defect in the immunological system is said to be immunosuppressed. Sometimes immune suppression is intentional, as after organ transplantation. One type of immunosuppression is neutropenia. The patient with abnormally low neutrophils is particularly at increased risk for pneumonia, septicemia,

---

BOX 18-5   Nursing Actions for the Patient at Risk for Injury from Infection: Compromised Host Precautions

1. The patient should have a private room, though it does not have to be an isolation room. The door may be left open. A "Compromised Host Precaution" sign should be posted on the door.
2. All persons entering the patient's room must wash hands before touching the patient for any reason. This is the most important way to prevent infection. The patient and family should be encouraged to remind all staff and visitors to wash their hands before touching the patient.
3. Monitor vital signs every 2 to 4 hours. Notify physician immediately of a temperature greater than 101° F to consider the need for an infectious fever workup and initiation or change of antibiotics. An infectious fever workup usually includes two sets of blood cultures, a chest radiograph, sputum culture, urine culture, wound culture, and cultures of other sites suggestive of infection. Patients with a central line or permanent, indwelling venous access device usually have one set of specimens for culture drawn from the line and one set drawn from a peripheral site. Mark the culture bottles clearly regarding where the specimen was obtained to assist with localization of the infection. Blood cultures are more likely to yield the offending organism if the blood is drawn as the patient's temperature is rising instead of after the patient's temperature has peaked.
4. Invasive procedures should be kept to a minimum. Invasive devices such as catheters and tubes should be removed as soon as the patient's medical condition permits.
5. Careful attention to aseptic technique must be observed, especially when performing phlebotomy, handling intravenous lines, or performing other invasive procedures.
6. Designate a particular stethoscope and thermometer to be used exclusively in caring for the patient.
7. Masks are not required; they are actually discouraged. Staff with upper respiratory tract or other infections should not care for the patient.
8. Clean table tops, equipment, and the floor frequently with hospital-approved disinfectant, clean cloths, and clean mops.
9. The patient should be taught to wash his or her hands before and after eating, using the toilet, and doing any self-care procedure. If possible, the patient should shower every day. Liquid soap instead of bar soap should be used.
10. Encourage the patient to cough and deep breathe every 4 hours. Mobility should be encouraged. Smoking should be discouraged.
11. Only canned or cooked foods should be served. Raw fruits, raw vegetables, and milk products are not served because of the risk of *Escherichia coli, Pseudomonas aeruginosa,* and *Klebsiella* species bacteria on or in these food items. The patient should be encouraged to choose appropriate foods from the menu. The diet roster should be annotated "Compromised Host Precautions" so that the nutrition care staff can verify that appropriate choices are being made.
12. Tests, scans, and appointments away from the patient's room should be coordinated in advance to eliminate or minimize waiting time in common waiting areas.
13. The patient should wear a clean mask when outside the room, especially in heavily traveled public areas such as corridors, elevators, and waiting rooms. The mask may be removed when the patient is in less public areas. A new mask should be used for each trip out of the room.
14. Some hospitals allow flowers and plants in the patient's room; however, they should not be handled by the patient because of the possibility of *Escherichia coli* contamination of the water and dirt.
15. No humidifiers with standing water should be used in the patient's room. If a wall humidifier is needed, the water should be changed every day.
16. Teach the patient and family about the underlying pathophysiology that puts the patient at risk for infection and about precautions to minimize the risk of infection.

From Young-McCauhgan, S. (In press). Immunologic disorders. In A. D. Linton (Ed.). *Introduction to medical-surgical nursing* (4th ed.). Philadelphia: Saunders.

and infections of the skin, urinary tract, and gastrointestinal tract. Fever may be the only sign of infection because the neutropenic patient is unable to launch a full immunological response. Therefore fever in these individuals is treated with a broad-spectrum antibiotic even when the source of infection has not been identified. Failure to respond to antibiotics within 5 days suggests a fungal or viral infection (Young-McCaughan & Jennings, 1998). Box 18-5 lists nursing actions for the patient who is neutropenic.

Antimicrobial therapy is used to treat and sometimes to prevent infection. HIV infection is treated with combinations of antiretrovirals. Prophylactic agents such as trimethoprim-sulfamethoxazole or aerosolized pentamidine may be ordered also to prevent opportunistic infections. Prophylactic antibiotic therapy for respiratory tract infections and mortality in adult intensive care patients was the subject of a Cochrane review. The reviewers concluded that a combination of systemic and topical antibiotics reduces not only respiratory tract infection rates but also mortality. Notably, topical prophylaxis alone reduces infection but not mortality (Liberati, D'Amico, Pifferi, Torri, & Brazzi, 2005). In all cases, the choice of antibiotics should consider not only organism sensitivity but also comorbidities and concurrent drug therapy in the older patient.

Investigators in the UK have recommended that immunocompromised patients be given drinking water that is filtered with commercial devices (Hall, Hodgson, & Kerr, 2004).

Measures to Promote Effective Self-Care.
For the individual with a disorder of the immune system, education for self-care should include hygiene measures, avoidance of exposure, general health promotion activities, and information about vaccinations as appropriate (Box 18-6). It is especially important that prevention and treatment strategies consider cultural characteristics, family relationships, and language differences (Montoya & Whitsett, 2003). A challenge with HIV prevention is that some older adults perceive themselves to be at low risk. Furthermore, practitioners who assume older persons do not engage in risky behaviors may fail to provide education about self protection. Persons at special risk may be those who lost a spouse after being monogamous for years, and are now ready to develop new relationships. They may never have been educated in "safe sex." In addition to sexual activity, intravenous drug use remains an important mode of HIV transmission. Interviews with older American drug users revealed that they were less likely to have had sex in the month before the interview. However, older individuals generally reported risky sex-related behavior equal to their younger counterparts (Kwiatkowski & Booth, 2003).

BOX 18-6 *TOWARD BETTER IMMUNE HEALTH*

- Take care of your skin; treat minor injuries promptly.
- Practice good oral hygiene; have regular dental care.
- Protect yourself from others with infectious diseases.
- Take recommended immunizations.
- Eat a balanced diet, ensuring an adequate intake of protein, calories, vitamins, and zinc.
- Practice safe sex; do not assume that older persons do not have HIV infection.
- Engage in stress-reducing activities.

Older persons with disorders, including HIV, that affect the immune system require special attention because of the prevalence of the other chronic conditions. Drug interactions and adverse effects of drugs used for one condition may aggravate another condition. Research related to effective educational strategies has not often targeted older adults. More commonly, implications for the older individuals are determined on the basis of smaller subsets. This is an area where nursing research could make an important contribution.

Measures to Provide Support.
Support can come in many forms including support groups, educational opportunities, assistance with meeting basic needs, individual and family counseling, and mental health care. HIV social workers and other health care providers need to be knowledgeable about resources for older persons (Emlet & Poindexter, 2004). Some model programs and strategies have been reported. The Senior HIV Intervention Project (SHIP) in South Florida implements early intervention activities, as well as HIV testing and counseling. A network of trained staff and volunteers helps HIV-positive seniors access needed services and treatment (Agate, Mullins, Prudent, & Liberti, 2003).

Another approach is a weekly telephone support and education group for persons aged 50 and older with HIV. Groups of one to five clients "met" with a registered nurse and a social worker for approximately an hour each week over a 10-week period. Issues that were addressed included staying healthy, symptom management, other chronic illnesses, diagnostic tests, strategies for interacting with health care providers, antiretroviral drug therapy, new developments in HIV treatment, coping with losses, and finding commonalities. The authors also noted the need to explore ineffective treatments (Nokes, Chew, & Altman, 2003).

Spiritual support can be a significant comfort to the patient and many even play a role in immune function.

Nursing Care Plan: The Older Patient with HIV

Assessment Data

Alice Moore, age 68, tested positive for HIV 2 years ago. She is a widow with two adult children. She is a retired teacher with a modest income who owns her own home and cares for her 2 grandchildren twice a week. Her current medications are:

- Saquinavir
- AZT and Epivir
- Dactrim DS
- Fluconazole
  Results of her most recent blood studies include:
- CD4 100 cells/mm^3
- HIV RNA 35,000 copies/mL

She reports increasing fatigue that has required her to give up some of her social activities. She has confided her diagnosis only to her daughter.

Nursing Diagnoses (Johnson, Bulechek, Dochterman, Maas, & Moorhead, 2001)

Risk for infection related to suppressed immune response, inadequate secondary defenses
Ineffective coping related to high degree of threat
Altered family processes related to shift in health status of a family member
Fatigue related to disease state, drug side effects
Grieving related to change in health status, risk for life-threatening complications
Deficient knowledge related to lack of education
Social isolation related to altered state of wellness
Ineffective therapeutic regimen management related to complexity of therapeutic regimen

Goals/Outcomes

- The patient will remain afebrile and free of other signs of infection.
- The patient will adopt effective coping mechanisms to handle condition and treatment.
- The family unit will reorganize responsibilities to assist and support the patient.
- The patient will report using strategies to conserve energy and diminish fatigue.
- The patient will express her feelings about her diagnosis.
- The patient will describe her self-care regimen and measures to prevent transmission to others.
- The patient will seek opportunities to establish or restore social relationships.
- The patient will take her medications as prescribed and keep follow-up appointments.

NOC Suggested Outcomes (Moorhead, Johnson, & Maas, 2004)

Knowledge: Infection control
Coping
Decision Making
Information Processing
Role Performance
Social Support
Family Coping
Energy Conservation
Psychomotor Energy
Psychosocial Adjustment: Life change
Knowledge Deficit (disease process, treatment, health behaviors)
Leisure Participation
Adherence Behavior
Knowledge: Treatment regimen
Risk Control: Sexually transmitted disease

NOC Suggested Interventions (Dochterman & Bulechek, 2004)

Major interventions: Infection Control (6540), Infection Protection (6550), Coping Enhancement (5320), Mutual Goal Setting (4410), Decision Making Support (5250), Learning Readiness Enhancement (5540), Health Education (5510), Teaching: Disease Process (5602), Teaching: Prescribed Medication (5616), Role Enhancement (5370), Support System Enhancement (5440), Family Support (7140), Energy Management (0180), Health System Guidance (7400), Recreation Therapy (5360)

- Instruct patient to take antibiotics and antiretrovirals as prescribed.
- Teach patient and family about signs and symptoms of infection, when to report them to the health care provider, and how to avoid infection.
- Monitor for systemic and localized signs and symptoms of infection.
- Administer an immunizing agent as appropriate.
- Appraise the impact of the patient's life situation on roles and relationships and the patient's current level of knowledge related to specific disease process.
- Explain the pathophysiology of the disease and how it relates to anatomy and physiology as appropriate.
- Describe common signs and symptoms of the disease as appropriate, the disease process as appropriate, and the rationale behind management/therapy/treatment recommendations.

Continued

Nursing Care Plan: The Older Patient with HIV—cont'd

- Identify possible etiologies as appropriate.
- Discuss lifestyle changes that may be required to prevent future complications and/or control the disease process, as well as therapy/treatment options.
- Instruct the patient on measures to prevent/minimize side effects of treatment for the disease, measures to control/minimize symptoms, and which signs and symptoms to report to health care provider, all as is appropriate.
- Explore possible resources/support as appropriate.
- Refer the patient to local community agencies/support groups as appropriate.
- Use a calm, reassuring approach.
- Provide an atmosphere of acceptance.
- Establish a learning environment with patient as early as possible.
- Help patient to identify information she is most interested in obtaining.
- Provide factual information concerning diagnosis, treatment, and prognosis, as well as a time for the patient to ask questions and discuss concerns.
- Assist the patient to realize the severity of the illness, realize that treatment options exist, and realize susceptibility to complications, all as is appropriate.
- Encourage an attitude of realistic hope as a way of dealing with feelings of helplessness, social and community activities; the use of spiritual resources if desired; verbalizations of feelings, perceptions, and fears; and the patient's ability to identify own strengths and abilities.
- Evaluate the patient's decision-making ability.
- Support the use of appropriate defense mechanisms.
- Assist the patient in identifying appropriate short-term and long-term goals, solving problems in a constructive manner, breaking down complex goals into small, manageable steps, examining available resources to meet the goals, prioritizing (weighting) identified goals, and developing a plan to meet the goals.
- Coordinate periodic review dates with the patient for assessment of progress toward goals.
- Determine whether there are differences between the patient's view of own condition and the view of health care providers.
- Inform patient of alternative views or solutions.
- Identify internal or external factors that may enhance or reduce motivation for health behavior.
- Determine current health knowledge and lifestyle behaviors of the individual.
- Review patient's knowledge of medications.

- Instruct the patient on the proper administration of each medication; the dosage, route, and duration of each medication; specific precautions to observe when taking the medication(s) as appropriate; possible side effects of medication(s); how to relieve and/or prevent certain side effects as appropriate; and carrying documentation of her prescribed medication regimen.
- Inform the patient what to do if a dose is missed, of consequences of not taking or abruptly discontinuing medication(s) as appropriate, and of possible drug-food interactions as appropriate.
- Assist the patient to develop a written medication schedule.
- Provide information on cost savings programs/organizations to obtain medications and devices as appropriate.
- Assist patient to identify usual role in family, specific role changes required because of illness or disability, and positive strategies for managing role changes.
- Facilitate discussion of role adaptations of family to compensate for ill member's role changes.
- Assess psychological response to situation and availability of support system.
- Determine adequacy of existing social networks.
- Identify degree of family support.
- Appraise family's emotional reaction to patient's condition.
- Determine psychological burden of prognosis for family.
- Listen to family concerns, feelings, and questions.
- Facilitate communication of concerns/feelings between patient and family or between family members.
- Respect and support adaptive coping mechanisms used by family.
- Encourage alternate rest and activity periods.
- Assist patient to schedule rest periods.
- Assist the patient to understand energy conservation principles.
- Assist the patient to identify tasks that family and friends can perform in the home to prevent/relieve fatigue.
- Assist patient to identify preferences for activity.
- Assist patient or family to coordinate health care and communication.
- Inform patient of appropriate community resources and contact persons.
- Coordinate referrals to relevant health care providers as appropriate.
- Assist to explore the personal meaning of favorite recreational activities.

Nursing Care Plan: The Older Patient with HIV—cont'd

- Assist patient to choose recreational activities consistent with physical, psychological, and social capabilities.
- Monitor emotional, physical, and social responses to recreational activity.

Evaluation Parameters

Patient description of disease process, mode of transmission, symptoms, complications, treatment, and prognosis; coping patterns; adaptation to life changes; symptoms of stress; rest/activity balance; emotional assistance provided by others; supportive social contacts; patient description of prescribed drug actions, side effects, proper administration; patient adherence to medication regimen; use of methods to control STD transmission

---

In one study, attendance at religious services more than twice weekly predicted lower subsequent 12-year mortality and elevated IL-6 levels. The investigators concluded that IL-6 plays a role in mediating the relationship between religious attendance and mortality (Lutgendorf, Russell, Ullrich, Harris, & Wallace, 2004).

SUMMARY

One major theory of aging proposes that it is primarily the result of immunosenescence. Changes in the immune system that are common in older adults increase the risk for infections, neoplasms, and autoimmune phenomena. Researchers are seeking interventions to bolster immune function in older persons. Care of the older adult in any setting should consider measures that can be implemented to compensate for the reduced defenses of the aging immune system.

REFERENCES

Agate, L. L., Mullins, J. M., Prudent, E. S., & Liberti, T. M. (2003, June 1). Strategies for reaching retirement communities and aging social networks: HIV/AIDS prevention activities among seniors in South Florida. *Journal of Acquired Immune Deficiency Syndromes: JAIDS, 33*(suppl 2), S238-S242.

Andersen-Ranberg, K., Hoier-Madsen, M., Wiik, A., Jeune, B., & Hegedus, L. (2004). High prevalence of autoantibodies among Danish centenarians. *Clinical & Experimental Immunology, 138*(1), 158-163.

Asch, S. M., Fremont, A. M., Turner, B. J., Gifford, A., McCutchan, J. A., Mathews, W. M., et al. (2004). Symptom-based framework for assessing quality of HIV care. *International Journal for Quality in Health Care, 16*(1), 41-50.

Becker, J. T., Lopez, O. L., Dew, M. A., & Aizenstein, H. J. (2004). Prevalence of cognitive disorders differs as a function of age in HIV virus infection. *AIDS, 18*(1; suppl), S11-S18.

Belshe, R. B., Newman, F. K., Cannon, J., Duane, C., Treanor, J., VanHoecke, C., et al. (2004). Serum antibody responses after intradermal vaccination against influenza. *New England Journal of Medicine, 351*(22), 2286-2294.

Bonafe, M., Valensin, S., Gianni, W., Marigliano, V., & Franceschi, C. (2001). The unexpected contribution of immunosenescence to the leveling off of cancer incidence and mortality in the oldest old. *Critical Reviews in Oncology-Hematology, 39*(3), 227-233.

Boren, E., & Gershwin, M. E. (2004). Inflamm-aging: Autoimmunity, and the immune-risk phenotype. *Autoimmunity Review, 3*(5), 401-406.

Braddy, C. M., & Blair, J. E. (2005). Colonization of personal digital assistants used in a health care setting. *American Journal of Infection Control, 33*(4), 230-232.

Brinkley, C., Furr, L. A., Carrico, R., & McCurren, C. (2004). Survey of oral care practices in US intensive care units. *American Journal of Infection Control, 32*(3), 162-169.

Brooke, R. C. C., & Griffiths, C. E. M. (2003). Aging of the skin. In R. C. Tallis & H. M. Fillit (Eds.), *Brocklehurst's textbook of geriatric medicine and gerontology* (6th ed.). London: Churchill Livingstone, pp. 1135-1144.

Centers for Disease Control and Prevention (CDC) Division of HIV/AIDS Prevention. (2005). Basic statistics. Retrieved March 17, 2005, from www.cdc.gov/hiv/stats.htm.

Chan, K. S., Orlando, M., Joyce, G., Gifford, A. L., Burnam, M. A., Tucker, J. S., & Sherbourne, C. D. (2003). Combination antiretroviral therapy and improvements in mental health: Results from a nationally representative sample of persons undergoing care for HIV in the United States. *Journal of Acquired Immune Deficiency Syndromes, 33*(1), 104-111.

Chandra, R. K. (2004). Impact of nutritional status and nutrient supplements on immune responses and incidence of infection in older individuals. *Ageing Research Reviews, 3*(1), 91-104.

Cherner, M., Ellis, R. J., Lazzaretto, D., Young, C., Mindt, M. R., Atkinson, J. H., et al. (2004). Effects of HIV-1 infection and aging on neurobehavioral functioning, preliminary findings. *AIDS, 18*(1; suppl), S27-S34.

Cox, L. E. (2002). Social support, medication compliance and HIV/AIDs. *Social Work in Health Care, 35*(1-2), 425-460.

Daynes, R. A., Enioutina, E. Y., & Jones, D. C. (2003). Role of redox imbalance in the molecular mechanisms responsible for immunosenescence. *Antioxidants & Redox Signaling, 5*(5), 537-548.

De la Fuente, M. (2002). Effects of antioxidants on immune system ageing. *European Journal of Clinical Nutrition, 56*(3; suppl), S5-S8.

De Martinis, M., Modesti, M., & Ginaldi, L. (2004). Phenotypic and functional changes of circulating monocytes and polymorphonuclear leucocytes from elderly persons. *Immunology & Cell Biology, 82*(4), 415-420.

Denduluri, N., & Ershler, W. B. (2004). Aging biology and cancer. *Seminars in Oncology, 31*(2), 137-148.

Dennett, N. S., Barcia, R. N., & McLeod, J. D. (2002). Age associated decline in CD25 and CD 28 expression correlate with an increased susceptibility to CD95 mediated apoptosis in T cells. *Experimental Gerontology, 37*(2-3), 271-283.

Dillman, W. H. (2003). The thyroid. In L. Goldman & J. C. Bennett (Eds.), *Cecil textbook of medicine* (21st ed.). Philadephia: Saunders, pp. 1231-1250.

Dion, M. L., Poulin, J. F., Bordi, R., Sylvestre, M., Corsini, R., Kettaf, N., et al. (2004). HIV infection rapidly induces and maintains a substantial suppression of thymocyte proliferation. *Immunity, 21*(6), 757-768.

Dobs, A. (2003, August). Role of testosterone in maintaining lean body mass and bone density in HIV infected patients. *International Journal of Impotence Research, 15*(4; suppl), S21-S25.

Dochterman, J. M., & Bulechek, G. M. (2004). *Nursing interventions classification* (4th ed.). St. Louis: Mosby.

Dolder, C. R., Patterson, T. L., & Jeste, D. V. (2004). HIV, psychosis and aging: Past, present, and future. *AIDS, 18*(1; suppl), S35-S42.

Dotson, V., Horak, K., Alwardt, A., & Larson, D. F. (2004). Relationship of aging and cardiac IL-10. *Journal of Extracorporeal Technology, 36*(2), 197-201.

Effros, R. B. (2004). Replicative senescence of CD8 T cells: Effect on human aging. *Experimental Gerontology, 39*(4), 517-524.

Effros, R. B., Cai, Z., & Linton, P. J. (2003). CD8 T cells and aging. *Critical Reviews in Immunology, 23*(1-2), 45-64.

Emlet, C. A., & Poindexter, C. C. (2004). Unserved, unseen, and unheard: Integrating programs for HIV-infected and HIV-affected older adults. *Health and Social Work, 29*(2), 86-96.

Fultz, S. L., Justice, A. C., Butt, A. A., Rabeneck, L., Weissman, S., & Rodriguez-Barradas, M. (2003). Testing, referral, and treatment patterns for hepatitis C virus coinfection in a cohort of veterans with human immunodeficiency virus infection. *Clinical Infectious Diseases, 36*(8), 1039-1046.

Geubbels, E. L. P., Willie, J. C., Nagelkerke, N. J. D., Vandenbrouchke-Grauls, C. M. J., Grobbee, D. E., & de Boer, A. S. (2005). Hospital-related determinants for surgical-site infection following hip arthroplasty. *Infection Control and Epidemiology, 26*(5), 435-441.

Ginaldi, L., DeMartinis, M., D'Ostilio, A., Marini, L., Loreto, M. F., Corsi, M. P., & Quaglino, D. (2000). Cell proliferation and apoptosis in the immune system in the elderly. *Immunologic Research, 21*(1), 31-38.

Ginaldi, L., DeMartinis, M., Monti, D., & Franceschi, C. (2004). The immune system in the elderly: Activation-induced and damage-induced apoptosis. *Immunologic Research, 30*(1), 81-94.

Goller, J. L., Dimitriadis, A., Tan, A., Kelly, H., & Marshall, J. A. (2004). Long-term features of norovirus gastroenteritis in the elderly. *Journal of Hospital Infection, 58*(4), 286-291.

Goodkin, K., Shapshak, P., Asthana, D., Zheng, W., Concha, M., Wilkie, F. L., et al. (2004). Older age and plasma viral load in HIV-1 infection. *AIDS, 18*(1; suppl), S87-S98.

Goodroad, B. K. (2003). HIV and AIDS in people older than 50. A continuing concern. *Journal of Gerontological Nursing, 29*(4), 18-24.

Gravenstein, S., Fillit, S. M., & Ershler, W. B. (2003). Clinical immunology of aging. In R. C. Tallis & H. M. Fillit (Eds.), *Brocklehurst's textbook of geriatric medicine and gerontology* (6th ed.). London: Churchill Livingstone, pp. 113-124.

Guinan, J. L., McGuckin, M., Shubin, A., & Tighe, J. (2005). A descriptive review of malpractice claims for health care acquired infections in Philadelphia. *American Journal of Infecton Control, 33*(5), 310-312.

Hakim, F. T., Flomerfelt, F. A., Boyiadzis, M., & Gress, R. E. (2004). Aging, immunity, and cancer. *Current Opinion in Immunology, 16*, 151-156.

Hall, J., Hodgson, G., & Kerr, K. G. (2004). Provision of safe portable water for immunocompromised patients in hospital. *Journal of Hospital Infection, 58*(2), 155-158.

Henson, S. M., Pido-Lopez, J., & Aspinall, R. (2004). Reversal of thymic atrophy. *Experimental Gerontology, 39*(4), 673-678.

Johnson, M., Bulechek, G., Dochterman, J. M., Maas, M., & Moorhead, S. (2001). *Nursing diagnoses, outcomes, & interventions.* St. Louis: Mosby.

Johnson, M. O., Stallworth, T., & Neilands, T. B. (2003). The drugs or the disease? Causal attributions of symptoms held by HIV-positive adults on HAART. *AIDS and Behavior, 7*(2), 109-117.

Kang, I, Hong, M. S., Nolasco, H., Park, S. H., Dan, J. M., Choi, J. Y., & Craft, K. (2004). Age associated change in the frequency of memory CD4+ T cells impairs long term CD4+ T cell responses to influenza vaccine. *Journal of Immunology, 173*(1), 673-681.

Katz, J. M., Plowden, J., Renshaw-Hoelscher, M., Lu, X., Tumpey, T. M., & Sambhara, S. (2004). Immunity to influenza: The challenges of protecting an aging population. *Immunologic Research, 29*(1-3), 113-124.

Khan, N., Hislop, A., Gudgeon, N., Cobbold, M., Khanna, R., Nayak, L., et al. (2004). Herpesvirus-specific CD8 T cell immunity in old age: Cytomegalovirus impairs the response to a coresident EBV infection. *Journal of Immunology, 173*(12), 7481-7489.

Kilbourne, A. M., Andersen, R. M., Asch, S., Nakazono, T., Crystal, S., Stein, M., et al. (2002). Response to symptoms among a U. S. nations probability sample of adults infected with human immunodeficiency virus. *Medical Care Research & Review, 59*(1), 36-58.

Kohut, M. L., Arntson, B. A., Lee, W., Rozeboom, K., Yoon, K. J., Cunnick, J. E., & McElhaney, J. (2004). Moderate exercise improved antibody response to influenza immunization in older adults. *Vaccine, 22*, 17-18.

Kohut, M. L., & Senchina, D. S. (2004). Reversing age-associated immunosenescence via exercise. *Exercise Immunology Review, 10*, 6-41.

Kubera, M., Kenis, G., Bosmans, E., Kajta, M., Basta-Kaim, A., Scharpe, S., et al. (2004). Stimulatory effect of antidepressants on the reduction of IL-6. *International Immunopharmacology, 4*(2), 185-192.

Kwiatkowski, C. F., & Booth, R. E. (2003). HIV risk behaviors among older American drug users. *Journal of Acquired Immune Deficiency Syndromes, 33*(2; suppl), S131-S137.

Lazuardi, L., Jenewein, B., Wolf, A. M., Pfister, G., Tzankov, A., & Grubeck-Loebenstein, B. (2005). Age related loss of naïve T cells and dysregulation of T-cell/B-cell interactions in human lymph nodes. *Immunology, 114*(1), 37-43.

Leibovitz, A., Baumoehl, Y., & Segal, R. (2004). Increased incidence of pathological and clinical prostate cancer with age: Age-related alterations of local immune surveillance. *Journal of Urology, 172*(2), 435-437.

Leng, S. X., Yang, H., & Walston, J. D. (2004). Decreased cell proliferation and altered cytokine production in frail older adults. *Aging—Clinical & Experimental Research, 16*(3), 249-252.

Levy, J. A., Ory, M. G., & Crystal, S. (2003). HIV/AIDS interventions for midlife and older adults: Current status and challenges. *Journal of Acquired Immune Deficiency Syndromes, 33*, S59-S67.

Lewis, S. M., & Kang, D. (2004). Genetics and altered immune responses. In S. M. Lewis, M. M. Heitkemper, & S. R. Dirksen (Eds.), *Medical-surgical nursing: Assessment and management of clinical problems* (6th ed.). St. Louis: Mosby, pp. 234-263.

Liberati, A., D'Amico, R., Pifferi, Torri, V., & Brazzi, L. (2005). Antibiotic prophylaxis to reduce respiratory tract infections and mortality in adults receiving intensive care. *The Cochrane Library*, CD000022.

Lorenz, K. A., Shapiro, M. F., Asch, S. M., Bozzette, S. A., & Hays, R. D. (2001). Associations of symptoms and health-related quality of life: Findings from a national study of persons with HIV infection. *Annals of Internal Medicine, 134*(9; part 2), 854-860.

Lutgendorf, S. K., Russell, D., Ullrich, P., Harris, T. B., & Wallace, R. (2004). Religious participation, interleukin-6, and mortality in older adults. *Health Psychology, 23*(5), 465-475.

Mack, K. A., & Ory, M. G. (2003, June 1). AIDS and older Americans at the end of the Twentieth century. *Journal of Acquired Immune Deficiency Syndromes, 33*(2; suppl), S68-S75.

Manfredi, R. (2003). HIV infection and advanced age: Emerging epidemiological, clinical, and management issues. *Ageing Research Reviews, 3*, 152-173.

Miller, M. (2003). Disorders of the thyroid. In R. C. Tallis & H. M. Fillit (Eds.), *Brocklehurst's textbook of geriatric medicine and gerontology* (6th ed.). London: Churchill Livingstone, pp. 1164-1184.

Mishto, M., Santoro, A., Bellavista, E., Bonafe, M., Monti, D., & Frencheschi, C. (2003). Immunoproteasomes and immunosenescence. *Ageing Research Reviews, 2*(4), 419-432.

Mocchegiani, E., & Malavolta, M. (2004). NK and NKT cell functions in immunosenescence. *Aging Cell,* 177-184.

Montoya, I. D., & Whitsett, D. D. (2003). New frontiers and challenges in HIV research among older minority populations. *Journal of Acquired Immune Deficiency Syndromes, 33*(2; suppl), S218-S221.

Moorhead, S., Johnson, M., & Maas, M. (2004). *Nursing outcomes classification (NOC)* (3rd ed.). St. Louis: Mosby.

Motta, M., Ferlito, L., Malaguarnera, L., Vinci, E., Bosco, S., Maugeri, D., & Malaguarnera, M. (2003). Alterations of the lymphocytic set-up in elderly patients with cancer. *Archives of Gerontology and Geriatrics, 36*(1), 7-14.

Mysliwska, J., Trzonkowski, P., Szmit, E., Brydak, L. B., Machala, M., & Mysliwski, A. (2004). Immunomodulating effect of influenza vaccination in the elderly differing in health status. *Experimental Gerontology, 39*(10), 1447-1458.

North American Nursing Diagnosis Association (NANDA). (2005). *Nursing diagnoses: Definitions & classification 2005-2006.* Philadelphia: NANDA International.

Nicholas, P. K., Kirksey, K. M., Corless, I. B., & Kemppainen, J. (2005). Lipodystrophy and quality of life in HIV: Symptom management issues. *Applied Nursing Research, 18*(1), 55-58.

Nierodzik, M. L. R., Sutin, D., & Freedman, M. L. (2003). Blood disorders and their management in old age. In R. C. Tallis & H. M. Fillit (Eds.), *Brocklehurst's textbook of geriatric medicine and gerontology* (6th ed.). London: Churchill Livingstone, pp. 1229-1268.

Nokes, K. M., Chew, L., & Altman, C. (2003). Using a telephone support group for HIV positive persons aged 50+ to increase social support and health related knowledge. *AIDS Patient Care and Standards, 17*(7), 345-351.

O'Toole, M. T. (2003). *Encyclopedia and dictionary of medicine, nursing, and allied health* (7th ed.). Philadelphia: Saunders.

Pedersen, M., Steensberg, A., Keller, C., Osada, T., Zacho, M., Saltin, B., et al. (2004). Does the aging skeletal muscle maintain its endocrine function? *Exercise Immunology Review, 10,* 42-55.

Piaserico, S., Larese, F., Recchia, G. P., Corradin, M. T., Scardigli, F., Carriere, C., et al. (2004). Allergic contact sensitivity in elderly patients. *Aging—Clinical & Experiment Research, 16*(3), 221-223.

Plackett, T. P., Boehmer, E. D., Faunce, D. E., & Kovacs, E. J. (2004). Aging and innate immune cells. *Journal of Leukocyte Biology, 76*(2), 291-299.

Provinciali, M., & Smorlesi, A. (2005). Immunoprevention and immunotherapy of cancer in ageing. *Cancer, Immunology, Immunotherapy, 54,* 93-106.

Rabkin, J. G., Ferrando, S. J., Lin, S. H., Sewell, M., & McElhiney, M. (2000). Psychological effects of HAART: A 2-year study. *Psychomatic Medicine, 62*(3), 413-422.

Radda, K. E., Schensul, J. J., Disch, W. B., Levy, J. A., & Reyes, C. Y. (2003). Assessing human immunodeficiency virus (HIV) risk among older urban adults. *Family Community Health, 26*(3), 203-213.

Ramos-Casals, M., Brito-Zeron, P., Lopez-Soto, A., & Font, J. (2004). Systemic autoimmune diseases in elderly patients: Atypical presentation and association with neoplasia. *Autoimmunity Reviews, 3*(5), 376-382.

Ress, B. (2003). HIV disease and aging: The hidden epidemic. *Critical Care Nurse, 23*(5), 38-42.

Rote, N. S. (2000a). Immunity. In S. E. Huether & K. L. McCance (Eds.), *Understanding pathophysiology* (2nd ed.). St. Louis: Mosby, pp. 125-152.

Rote, N. S. (2000b). Inflammation. In S. E. Huether & K. L. McCance (Eds.), *Understanding pathophysiology* (2nd ed.). St. Louis: Mosby, pp. 153-180.

Rote, N. S., Huether, S. E., & McCance, K. L. (2000). Hypersensitivities, infection, and immunodeficiencies. In S. E. Huether & K. L. McCance (Eds.), *Understanding pathophysiology* (2nd ed.). St. Louis: Mosby, pp. 180-220.

Rubinson, L., Wu, A. W., Haponik, E. E., & Diette, G. B. (2005). Why is it that internists do not follow guidelines for preventing intravascular catheter infections? *Infection Control Hospital and Epidemiology, 26*(6), 525-533.

Sainz, R. M., Mayo, J. C., Reiter, R. J., Tan, D. X., & Rodriguez, C. (2003). Apoptosis in primary lymphoid organs with aging. *Microscopy Research & Technique, 62*(6), 524-539.

Savasta, A. M. (2004). HIV: Associated transmission risks in older adults—an integrative review of the literature. *Journal of the Association of Nurses in AIDS Care, 15*(1), 50-59.

Schrimshaw, E. W., & Siegel, K. (2003). Perceived barriers to social support from family and friends among older adults with HIV/AIDS. *Journal of Health Psychology, 8*(6), 738-752.

Shah, S. S., McGowan, J. P., Smith, S., Blum, S., & Klein, R. S. (2002). Comorbid conditions, treatment, and health maintenance in older persons with human immunodeficiency virus infection in New York City. *Clinical Infectious Disease, 35,* 1243-1248.

Smith, T. P., Kennedy, S. L., & Fleshner, M. (2004). Influence of age and phsyical activity on the primary in vivo antibody and T cell mediated responses in men. *Journal of Applied Physiology, 97*(2), 491-498.

Valcour, V. G., Shikuma, C., Shiramizu, B., Watters, M., Poff, P. Selnes, O. A., et al. (2004). Age, apolipoprotein E4, and the risk of HIV dementia: The Hawaii Aging with HIV Cohort. *Journal of Neuroimmunology, 157,* 197-202.

Valcour, V. G., Shikuma, C. M., Shiramizu, B. T., Williams, A. E., Watters, M. R., Poff, P. W., et al. (2005). Diabetes, insulin resistance, and dementia among HIV-1 infected patients. *Journal of Acquired Immune Deficiency Syndrome, 38*(1), 31-36.

Valcour, V. G., Shikuma, C. M., Watters, M. R., & Sacktor, N. C. (2004). Cognitive impairment in older HIV-1-seropositive individuals: Prevalence and potential mechanisms. *AIDS 2004, 18*(1; suppl): S79-S86.

Vance, D. E. (2004). Cortical and subcortical dynamics of aging with HIV infection. *Perceptual and Motor Skills, 98*(2), 647-655.

van den Biggelaar, A. H., Huizinga, T. W., de Craen, A. J., Gussekloo, J., Heijmans, B. T., Frolich, M., & Westendorp, R. G. (2004). Impaired innate immunity predicts frailty in old age. The Leiden 85-plus study. *Experimental Gerontology, 39*(9), 1407-1414.

Villari, P., Manzoli, L., & Boccia, A. (2004). Methodological quality of studies and patient age were major sources of variation in efficacy estimates of influenza vaccination in healthy adults: A meta analysis. *Vaccine, 22*(25-26), 3475-3486.

Vosylius, S., Sipylaite, J., & Ivaskevicius, J. (2005). Determinants of outcome in elderly patients admitted to the intensive care unit. *Age and Ageing, 34*(2), 157-162.

Waghorn, D. J., Wan, W. Y., Greaves, C., Whittome, N., Bosley, H. C., & Cantrill, S. (2005). Contamination of computer keyboards in clinical areas: Potential reservoir for nosocomial spread of organisms. *British Journal of Infection Control, 6*(3), 22-24.

Watters, M. R., Poff, P. W., Shiramizu, B. T., Holck, P. S., Fast, K. M. S., Shikuma, C. M., & Valcour, V. G. (2004). Symptomatic distal sensory polyneuropathy in HIV after age 50. *Neurology, 62,* 1378-1383.

Wazait, H., van der Meullen, J., Patel, H. R. H., Brown, C. T., Gadgil, S., Miller, R. A., et al. (2004). Antibiotics on urethral catheter withdrawal: A hit and miss affair. *Journal of Hospital Infection, 58*(4), 297-302l.

Wilkie, F. L., Goodkin, K., Khamis, I., van Zuilen, M. H., Lee, D., Lecusay, R., et al. (2003). Cognitive functioning in younger and older HIV-1 infected adults. *Journal of Acquired Immune Deficiency Syndromes, 33*(2; suppl), S93-S105.

Young-McCaughan, S., & Jennings, B. M. (1998). Hematologic and immunologic systems. In J. G. Alspach (Ed.), *AACN core curriculum for critical care nursing* (5th ed.). Philadelphia: Saunders, pp. 601-646.

Chapter 19

Age-Related Changes in the Special Senses

Adrianne Dill Linton

Objectives

Discuss normal changes in vision, hearing, taste, smell, and touch associated with aging.

Describe measures to maintain sensory health in the older adult.

Explain the cause and treatment of sensory disorders that are common to older persons including cataracts, glaucoma, senile macular degeneration, diabetic retinopathy, and senile entropion and ectropion, as well as sensorineural, conductive, and central hearing loss.

Describe the components of the sensory assessment in the older adult.

Formulate nursing diagnoses for older adults with sensory disorders.

Develop plans to manage older adults with actual or potential sensory disorders.

Sensory changes can have a great impact on the lifestyle of older persons, substantially altering the quality of life and independence they once took for granted. Visual and hearing impairments may interfere with written and verbal communication, enjoyment of previously meaningful activities, and important social interactions. Older persons may become socially isolated because they are unable to endure the strain of attempting to hear a muted or indistinguishable conversation or because they cannot see well enough to provide their own transportation to social activities. Changes in the senses of taste and smell can affect the enjoyment of food and present a safety hazard. It is important to understand the sensory changes associated with aging to help older adults adjust and function at their highest possible level.

People of all ages require a minimum of stimulation of sense organs to evoke any sensory experience. The minimum physical energy needed to activate a particular sensory system is known as the absolute threshold. It is determined by finding a range of intensities over which the physical energy moves from having no effect to having a complete effect. The absolute threshold is generally considered to be the value at which the stimulus is perceived 50% of the time. The threshold varies among individuals and also within an individual from time to time, depending on physical condition, motivational state, and the conditions under which the observations are made (Rich, 1990). With advanced aging, it is generally thought that greater sensory inputs are required to evoke responses. Thus the absolute threshold is higher for the older person than it is for the younger person.

Sensory decrements, like absolute threshold levels, vary among and within individuals. The senses of vision, hearing, taste, smell, and touch may all be affected by the changes of aging, but vision and hearing changes are the most dramatic and have the greatest impact.

THE VISUAL SYSTEM

The external structures of the eye consist of the orbital cavity, extrinsic ocular muscles, eyebrows, eyelids, eyelashes, conjunctiva, cornea, sclera, and lacrimal apparatus. Every sense organ responds to a particular type of physical energy. The eye is sensitive to light—a portion of electromagnetic energy that travels in waves through space. The colors that are perceived by the eye travel at varying wavelengths (the distance from the crest of one wave to the crest of the next) that are related to the colors of the rainbow. The red end of the rainbow is produced by longer wavelengths and the violet end by shorter wavelengths. Light enters the eye through the transparent cornea and is focused on the retina by the lens. The pupil regulates the amount of light entering the visual system and is controlled by the autonomic nervous system.

The internal structures of the eye are the sclera (fibrous protective coat), cornea (transparent tissue serving as refractive surface), choroid (vascular pigmented middle layer), ciliary body, iris, pupil, lens, and retina (inner layer containing visual receptor cells). The eyeball is divided into two cavities: (1) the anterior cavity, which consists of anterior and posterior chambers, located in front of the lens; and (2) the posterior cavity, located behind the lens. The anterior cavity contains a fluid called the aqueous humor, and the posterior cavity contains a soft, jellylike material called the vitreous humor. The ciliary body is an anterior continuation of the choroid lining of the sclera. It contains the ciliary muscle, which governs the convexity of the lens, and the ciliary processes, which produce the aqueous humor.

The retina is composed of (1) rods and cones, which convert light energy into nerve impulses; (2) the bipolar cells, which make synaptic connections with the rods and cones; and (3) the ganglion cells, which contain the fibers forming the optic nerve. The fovea, located on the retina, is the most sensitive portion of the eye and plays a major role in visual perception (Rich, 1990) (Figure 19-1).

Age-Related Changes in the Visual System

Structural Changes. Changes occurring in the orbital areas are similar to those that occur with aging in other parts of the body. There is a graying of the eyebrows and eyelashes and a wrinkling and loosening of the skin around the eyelids, which is due to loss of tonus and decreased elasticity of the eyelid muscle. The muscle that supports the upper eyelid may atrophy so that the opened lid partially covers the pupil. Loss of orbital fat causes the eyes to sink deeper into the orbit and limits upward gaze. Orbital fat may herniate into the lower lid tissue, producing baggy lids. Tear secretions may diminish, producing a condition known as "dry eyes." This phenomenon may cause discomfort and irritation for older people and can be relieved by the use of eyedrops or "artificial tears" (Brodie, 2003).

Age-related changes in the cornea produce a decrease in the number of endothelial cells. Corneal sensitivity is often diminished, so that the older adult may be less aware of injury or infection. The corneal reflex also may be diminished or absent in relatively healthy older individuals. Another phenomenon characteristic of aging is the arcus senilis (Figure 19-2), which is found on the periphery of the cornea. It is a grayish-yellow ring surrounding the iris and is thought to be caused by an accumulation of lipids.

With aging, the ciliary body secretes less aqueous humor; however, because there is generally less outflow of fluid from the anterior and posterior chambers, intraocular pressure remains relatively stable. The length of the ciliary muscle tends to decrease because of atrophy, and the lost muscle tissue is replaced with connective tissue. Because ciliary muscle action is responsible for the changing curvature of the lens, the focusing ability of the

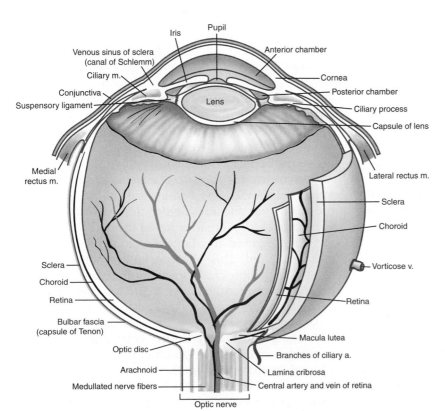

Figure 19-1 Midsaggital section through the eyeball, showing layers of retina and blood supply. (From Drain, C. B. D. [2003]. *Perianesthesia nursing: A critical care approach* [4th ed.]. St. Louis: Saunders.)

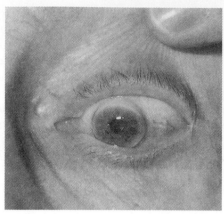

Figure 19-2 Arcus senilis. (From Schwartz, M. H. [2006]. *Textbook of physical diagnosis* [5th ed.]. Philadelphia: Saunders.)

lens is compromised when deterioration of the muscle takes place. The process of focusing the image on the retina is known as accommodation, and the inability to focus properly is called presbyopia (Brodie, 2003).

Accommodation is also difficult because the lens becomes less elastic, larger, and more dense as a result of continued production of new cells and accumulation of old and dead cells within the lens capsule. Increased density of the lens, together with the accumulation of loosened, degenerated cells on the iris, cornea, and lens capsule, causes increased scattering of light and sensitivity to glare. The lens also becomes progressively yellowed and opaque, probably as a result of absorption of ultraviolet light over the years. Although there is diminished discrimination at all ages for blues and greens than for reds and yellows, the aged have particular difficulty in this respect. This phenomenon is thought to be related to the fact that the effect of age is greatest on short wavelengths of light (violet, blue, green), which are filtered by the yellowed lenses (Corso, 1971). The generous use of warm (yellow, orange, red) contrasting colors can greatly increase the ease with which older persons maneuver in their environments and carry out activities of daily living. It must be noted, however, that although older people do have difficulty with blue-green discrimination, general color vision defects either are of genetic origin or are indicative of a pathological process (Kline, Ikeda, & Schieber, 1982; Mashiah, 1978).

The iris, which is a diaphragm containing the pupil, loses its pigment with age, so that most older people appear to have grayish or light blue eyes. The pupil becomes progressively smaller with advancing age; by age 60, it is one third of the size it was at age 20. Decreased pupil size results in a smaller amount of light reaching the retina, and the light must pass through the densest, most opaque area of the lens.

In the posterior cavity, the vitreous gel begins to liquefy and collapse. Bits of condensation and debris may become visible as "floaters," a common occurrence with aging. Although the condition is not pathologically significant nor does it impair vision, it may be a source of annoyance to older people. The retina also begins to degenerate because of local ischemia and loss of neurons.

Functional Changes. Major visual changes with aging include decreased visual acuity, decreased tolerance of glare, decreased ability to adapt to dark and light, and decreased peripheral vision. The major refractive change is an increase in myopia or a decrease in hyperopia. As this shift occurs, some individuals have a temporary improvement in acuity that allows reading without glasses—a phenomenon referred to as second sight (Brodie, 2003). All of these changes in visual function are related to changes in eye structure that affect the quality and intensity of the light reaching the retina (Rich, 1990).

Because of a general decline in visual acuity, almost everyone over age 55 needs eyeglasses for either reading or distance vision. However, failure of visual function is not inevitable with older age, and some older people retain excellent visual acuity.

Glare is a particular problem for older people and is one of the major reasons, along with poor adjustment to dark and light, that older adults frequently give up night driving. Oncoming lights produce light scattering in the cornea and lens, rendering the older person virtually blind at times. Sunlit rooms in which window light reflects on shiny floors are equally difficult to negotiate. Rooms should be well lighted with soft, incandescent rather than fluorescent lighting to minimize glare. Sheer curtains and rugs can be used to reduce window glare.

Because dark and light adaptation take longer with advancing age, older adults are at greater risk for falls and injuries. Entering and leaving a theater, going to the bathroom at night, and moving from a well-lighted room to a dark room can therefore be most dangerous for older people. Interestingly, the dark-adapted eye makes use of the rods rather than the cones and is much more sensitive to blue-green wavelengths than to the longer red wavelengths. Because red light stimulates the cones but not the rods, older persons may see well enough by red light to function in the dark. In addition, the time required for dark adaptation in red light is greatly reduced. This phenomenon is noteworthy because older people can be encouraged to keep a red light on in darkened rooms at all times to improve the rate of dark adaptation and to increase visibility at night.

Loss of peripheral vision is a common occurrence with aging and greatly limits social interactions and physical activities. Older persons may not communicate with others sitting next to them because they are out of their range of vision. At the dining table, they may spill food and drinks located on their visual periphery, or they may not be able to find objects placed out of visual range. Driving also can be hazardous because of their inability to see oncoming motorists. In a study of 397 volunteers from the Baltimore Longitudinal Study of Aging, Kline and colleagues, Kline, Fozard, Kosnki, Schieber, & Sekuler (1992) found that visual problems of driving increased with age along five dimensions: (1) unexpected vehicles, (2) vehicle speed, (3) dimly lit displays, (4) windshield problems, and (5) sign reading. It is important that older drivers be made aware of these limitations so that they can compensate for them.

Common Disorders and Diseases

Prevalent disorders of the visual system with older age are cataracts, glaucoma, senile macular degeneration, and diabetic retinopathy. These conditions are the major causes of blindness in developed countries. Corneal scarring also is a common cause of blindness in Third World countries. In the United States, the prevalence of blindness and poor vision increases gradually through the adult years. Among persons ages 80 and older, 7% are blind and 16.7% have poor vision (NEI, 2004) (Table 19-1).

Cataracts. Cataracts are the most common age-related eye disease, accounting for about half of the cases of vision loss in whites, Hispanics, and African Americans. They are somewhat more prevalent among women than men. Compared with white males, African American males are more likely to be blind from cataracts (Gohdes, Balamurugan, Larsen, & Maylahn, 2005). Most cataracts develop bilaterally in persons older than 50 years; by the ninth decade of life 68.3% of individuals have cataracts (NEI, 2004). Various mechanical or metabolic insults can result in cataracts (Brodie, 2003). The three types of cataracts are nuclear, cortical, and posterior subcapsular, which can be present alone or in combination. Nuclear sclerosis is slowly progressive and may be associated with "second sight," loss of color discrimination, and loss of far vision.

Cortical opacities may be discrete and cause no visual disturbance unless they involve the visual axis. Posterior subcapsular cataracts are granular opacities that occur mainly in the central posterior cortex. They are associated with glare and tend to affect near vision (Asbell et al., 2005). Blurred vision associated with cataracts has been shown to increase postural instability in older persons, placing them at risk for falls (Anand, Buckley, Scally, & Elliott, 2003).

Risk factors for cataracts include age, exposure to sunlight, and possibly family history, obesity, hypertension, diabetes, and certain iris colors. Some risk factors are associated with one or more specific types of cataract. For example, data from the Framingham study identified a relationship between hypertriglyceridemia and posterior subcapsular cataract, but not nuclear or cortical cataract (Hiller, Sperduto, Reed, D'Agostino, & Wilson, 2003). Systemic corticosteroids have been clearly linked to cataracts; however, the evidence for inhaled corticosteroids has not been conclusive (Asbell et al., 2005). A slightly higher prevalence among women has raised questions as to whether hormonal influences are a factor. Smoking is widely believed to be a risk factor for cataracts; however, evidence is not sufficient to conclude that the risk is decreased by smoking cessation (Gohdes et al., 2005). Other risk factors are low socioeconomic status and heavy alcohol use (Asbell et al., 2005).

The disorder is characterized by a clouding or opacity of the normally clear, crystalline lens. Structural changes in the proteins of the lens cause liquefication and swelling within the lens capsule. In rare cases, the hypermature cataract leaks lens protein, causing uveitis or obstructing the trabecular meshwork, which causes glaucoma (Fay & Jakobiec, 2000). There is a gradual painless loss of vision in one or both eyes. Some patients complain of glare, general darkening of vision, change in refraction, and loss of contrast sensitivity. Ophthalmoscopic examination reveals a haziness of the lens, an inability to see the fundus in detail, and a reduced red reflex (Lichtenstein, 1992). Even when a

Table 19-1 *Prevalence of Cataract, Age-Related Macular Degeneration, and Open-Angle Glaucoma Among Adults 40 Years and Older in the United States*

Age (Years)	Cataract Persons	Cataract Percent	Advanced AMD Persons	Advanced AMD Percent	Intermediate AMD Persons	Intermediate AMD Percent	Glaucoma Persons	Glaucoma Percent
40-49	1,046,000	2.5	20,000	0.1	851,000	2.0	290,000	0.7
50-59	2,123,000	6.8	113,000	0.4	1,053,000	3.4	318,000	1.0
60-69	4,061,000	20.0	147,000	0.7	1,294,000	6.4	369,000	1.8
70-79	6,973,000	42.8	388,000	2.4	1,949,000	12.0	530,000	3.9
≥80	6,272,000	68.3	1,081,000	11.8	2,164,000	23.6	711,000	7.7
Total	20,475,000	17.2	1,749,000	1.5	7,311,000	6.1	2,218,000	1.9

From National Eye Institute. Retrieved December 4, 2005, from www.nei.nih.gov/eyedata/pbd_tables.asp.

cataract is evident, a thorough eye examination should be performed to prevent overlooking other causes of reduced vision such as glaucoma or macular degeneration (Asbell et al., 2005).

There is no medical treatment for cataract. Approaches under investigation include drug therapy, nutritional supplements, and antioxidants. Surgical removal of the cataract is the treatment of choice. The location of the cataract, the degree of visual impairment, and the effect on the individual's ability to carry out activities of daily living all influence the decision to perform surgery. Because postoperative visual acuity of 20/40 or better is expected, surgery usually is delayed until acuity has fallen to 20/50 or worse. However, surgery is almost always performed before a cataract becomes "ripe," that is, when water is drawn into the lens with resultant swelling. Visual improvement after surgical intervention usually is excellent in the absence of concomitant eye disease (Fay & Jakobiec, 2000).

Two types of surgical procedures can be used to remove cataracts: (1) intracapsular extraction and (2) extracapsular extraction. Intracapsular extraction involves removal of the lens intact in its capsule through a wide incision in the cornea. In developed countries, it is generally reserved for difficult or complicated cases (Asbell et al., 2005). In an extracapsular extraction, the contents of the lens are aspirated, leaving the capsule intact. The intact capsule serves as a barrier between the anterior and posterior chambers and may reduce complications. Current techniques include minimally invasive surgery in which a rapidly vibrating needle liquefies the cataract (phacoemulsion) so that it can be aspirated through a small, self-sealing incision in the cornea (Brodie, 2003). Anesthesia requirements have lessened with the advent of newer surgical procedures. Whereas retrobulbar anesthesia was once the standard in most cases, topical agents and anesthesia delivered to the anterior chamber often suffice now (Asbell et al., 2005).

The condition in which the lens is absent from the eye is known as aphakia. Because removal of the lens' contents or capsule deprives the eye of focusing power, some type of replacement is necessary. There are three ways to provide focusing power for the visual system. The first is an intraocular lens—a surgically implanted lens positioned in place of the natural lens. The intraocular lens implant is highly desirable because it is most like a natural lens. The posterior-chamber lens, which is placed in the intact lens capsule, is used most often. If the patient's eyes lack the integrity of the posterior capsule to support a posterior lens, an anterior chamber lens can be implanted anterior to the iris (Asbell et al., 2005). Contact lenses are the second type of lens replacement and are the next best treatment for aphakia. They are particularly appropriate and safe for younger persons. Hard or soft lenses may be used; the long-wearing type are best because they require care

only once a month. Eyeglasses are the third and least effective means of treating aphakia, although they are the simplest, safest, and most proven method. Persons using aphakic eyeglasses may have difficulty with depth perception and peripheral vision. Individuals who require surgery in only one eye often have great difficulty with eyeglasses because of optical distortion caused by the unequal perceived image size in the two eyes (Brodie, 2003).

The most common late postoperative complication after cataract extraction is posterior capsular calcification, which occurs in about 25% of persons within 5 years of the surgery. It can be treated with laser capsulotomy on an outpatient basis. Although retinal detachment is not common, the risk is increased with extracapsular extraction, severe myopia, younger age, and male gender (Asbell et al., 2005).

Research related to cataract focuses on risk factors, etiology, and treatment. Particularly interesting is the relationship that some studies have found between age-related eye disease and mortality. Investigators in the Rotterdam Study found that age-related maculopathy (ARM) and cataract were predictors of shorter survival. However, once adjusted for known risk factors (e.g., smoking status, body mass index, cardiovascular disease), ARM and cataract were not significantly associated with mortality (Borger et al., 2003). The Age-Related Eye Disease Study (AREDS) found an increased death rate for individuals with age-related macular degeneration (AMD) and cataracts. The investigators concluded that this relationship may signify that these vision disorders are part of a systemic process rather than just a local process (Clemons, Kurinij, & Sperduto, 2004). Nutritional status as a contributing factor has been another topic of study. A 4-year prospective, randomized study found that treatment with daily 500 international units of vitamin E did not reduce the incidence or rate of progression of age-related cataracts (McNeil et al., 2004). A study that measured plasma levels of vitamins A, C, and E and β-carotene concluded that higher levels of vitamin C were associated with reduced prevalence of nuclear and posterior subcapsular cataracts. A randomized trial of β-carotene supplementation over a period of 12 years indicated no overall benefit in terms of the incidence of cataract. An exception was a subgroup of smokers in whom the excess risk of cataract appeared to be reduced by about one fourth (Christen et al., 2003). Surprisingly, in this sample, higher levels of vitamin E were associated with increased prevalence of nuclear and posterior subcapsular cataract (Ferrigno, Aldigeri, Rosmini, Sperduto, & Maraini, 2005). Shichi (2004) cautions that we do not yet have clear evidence that antioxidants delay or prevent cataracts. Several studies of the risk of cataracts in women suggested that high fruit and vegetable intake may have a modest protective effect (Christen, Liu, Schaumberg, & Buring, 2005;

Moeller et al., 2004). Data from the Nurses Health Study showed that carbohydrate quantity, but not quality, was associated with early cortical opacities but not with nuclear opacities (Chiu et al., 2005). Among the drugs under study for the treatment of cataracts is *N*-acetylcarnosine in the form of Can-C (Babizhayev, Deyev, Yermakova, Brikman, & Bours, 2004).

Glaucoma. Among adults ages 40 and older, almost 2% have open-angle glaucoma. The prevalence is greatest after age 70 (NEI, 2004). In addition to age, risk factors for glaucoma are family history, diabetes, and African American ancestry (Gohdes et al., 2005). Characterized by progressive atrophy of the optic nerve, glaucoma often is associated with increased intraocular pressure. Glaucoma is classified according to the cause of the obstruction of the aqueous outflow. These causes are classified as follows:

1. Primary or secondary (primary is genetic in origin; secondary is caused by other ocular disorders—tumor, inflammation, trauma—that obstruct aqueous outflow)
2. Open-angle or closed-angle (angle is the point in the anterior chamber where the iris inserts into the corneoscleral junction)
3. Congenital or developmental (disease develops during gestation or the first year of life, but signs and symptoms may not appear until adulthood)

Primary open-angle glaucoma (POAG) is the most common form in the United States. It is an insidious, chronic condition that has been characterized as a "thief in the night" because it robs its victims of vision without any noticeable symptoms. The condition is related to changes in the trabecular meshwork that impede the outflow of aqueous humor, causing intraocular pressure (IOP) to rise. As many as 40% of the optic nerve fibers must be destroyed before losses in the visual fields are detectable. The damage to the visual fields begins in the periphery and progresses so slowly that the patient typically is unaware of the loss.

Drug therapy is the cornerstone of treatment of POAG. First-line drugs are beta-adrenergic antagonists, alpha$_2$-adrenergic agonists, and prostaglandin analogs (Lehne, 2004) (Table 19-2). Initial treatment commonly is medical and is intended to lower IOP with parasympathomimetic miotics, anticholinesterase miotics, sympathomimetics, beta-adrenergic blockers, carbonic anhydrase inhibitors, and prostaglandin analogs. Another option, or one that may be used if drug therapy fails, is laser treatment of the trabecular meshwork.

Angle-closure glaucoma occurs with sudden obstruction of the trabecular meshwork that causes acute elevation of IOP. Age-related enlargement of the lens predisposes the older adult to this condition. Unlike open-angle glaucoma, the symptoms are dramatic with severe pain, blurred vision, a perception of colored

Table 19-2 *Drugs Used to Treat Glaucoma*	
Beta Blockers	**Prostaglandin Analogs**
Betaxolol (Betoptic)	Latanoprost (Xalatan)
Levobetaxolol (Betaxon)	Travoprost (Travatan)
Carteolol (Ocupress)	Bimatoprost (Lumigan)
Levobunolol (Betagan Liquifilm, AKBeta)	Unoprostone (Rescula)
Metipranolol (Optipranolol)	
Timolol (Timoptic, Betimol)	

Data from Lehne, R. A. (2004). *Pharmacology for nursing care* (5th ed.). St. Louis: Saunders.

haloes around lights, nausea, and vomiting. If not corrected, permanent damage to the optic nerve may occur within weeks. Treatment is directed toward lowering intraocular pressure, and may employ miotic eyedrops, carbonic anhydrase inhibitors, topical beta-adrenergic antagonists, and systemic osmotic agents (Lehne, 2004). Analgesics are also given for pain. Peripheral iridectomy may be performed to permit aqueous humor to pass from the posterior to the anterior chamber, which helps to prevent recurrence (Brodie, 2003).

The patient with normal-tension glaucoma develops optic atrophy and loss of visual fields in the presence of normal IOP (Brodie, 2003).

Age-Related Macular Degeneration. The macula, located on the retina, is functionally the most important part of the eye. It is the area that contains the fovea—the central focusing point for the optic system of the eye. Forms of age-related macular degeneration (AMD) include exudative AMD and atrophic AMD. Exudative ("wet") AMD, which causes central vision loss, is characterized by abnormal vascularization under the retina. The growth of abnormal blood vessels causes irreversible damage to the macula and vision loss. Degenerative changes of the macula usually are bilateral and increase significantly with age. Because the loss is central, reading and recognition of objects are impaired, whereas side vision and mobility remain intact. Eyeglasses are not effective in improving vision. Laser treatment sometimes arrests the growth of the abnormal tissue and seals off the damaged vessels, preventing bleeding, fluid leakage, scar tissue formation, and destruction of nerve tissue. Photodynamic therapy attempts to treat the vessels with an intravenous infusion of a sensitizing agent followed by treatment of the affected area with a low-power ultraviolet laser. A surgical procedure aims to separate and then reattach the affected area of the retina over a healthier patch of choroids. These treatments at best arrest the progression and preserve existing vision (Brodie, 2003).

Research efforts focus on early diagnosis and the development of effective treatments. Drusen are pale white dots commonly seen on the retinas of older persons. They appear to predispose the individual to exudative AMD. Efforts to prevent or delay AMD in these persons with nutritional therapy (vitamins C and E, β-carotene, zinc) have shown some promise (Brodie, 2003).

The atrophic ("dry") form, for which no treatment exists, is characterized by degeneration of the retinal pigment epithelium and choriocapillaris underlying the macula. Among persons aged 80 and older, as many as 16% of white women and 12% of white men have advanced AMD. AMD accounts for approximately half of cases of blindness in white Americans, affecting males and females equally. It is less prevalent among African Americans than whites (Gohdes et al., 2005).

One study has shown that high doses of vitamins C and E, β-carotene, and zinc slowed the rate of progressive vision loss. Some forms of wet AMD respond to laser therapy and photodynamic therapy. The injection of antivascular endothelial growth factor slowed the loss of vision with wet AMD in a randomized trial. Laser photocoagulation is being studied for treatment of dry AMD (Gohdes et al., 2005).

Diabetic Retinopathy.

Approximately 3.4% of all persons with diabetes have diabetic retinopathy, with the highest prevalence among those 65 to 74 years of age (5.8%) (NEI, 2004). The duration of hyperglycemia is more important than age in the development of diabetic retinopathy. It is rare for serious visual complications to occur before 10 to 15 years after the onset of diabetes. The major symptom of diabetic retinopathy is central visual impairment; complete blindness is rare. Visual deterioration is more rapid in older patients with diabetes, as evidenced by the fact that 3% of patients younger than 60 and 20% of those older than 60 with diabetic retinopathy are legally blind. Blindness may be avoided with early diagnosis and treatment, which includes aggressive control of blood glucose levels and blood pressure. The goal of treatment is to delay or retard visual impairment (Brodie, 2003).

The first observable sign of diabetic retinopathy is innocuous microaneurysms. Eventually fluid begins to leak from the retinal capillaries, causing edema and the precipitation of exudates into the retina that impair visual acuity. Laser treatment at this stage may reduce the visual loss. The late stage is characterized by localized retinal infarctions that create "cotton wool spots" visible on ophthalmoscopic examination. Remaining capillaries become dilated, leaky, and irregular. New blood vessels that form may grow along the surface of the retina. Fibroblastic membranes exert traction on the retina that may further diminish vision. In severe cases, the fibrovascular membrane obstructs the trabecular meshwork, causing refractory neovascular glaucoma. Treatment may include laser photocoagulation to arrest

the proliferative retinopathy and pars plana vitrectomy to remove blood and fibrovascular membranes. Some evidence exists that good glucose level control in the period following the onset of diabetes may delay the onset of retinopathy. However, there does not appear to be improvement when tight control is instituted after onset of the condition (Brodie, 2003).

Senile Entropion and Ectropion.

Two other disorders that are not necessarily threatening to visual integrity but are most troublesome and uncomfortable for older people are senile entropion and senile ectropion. Entropion, a complete inversion of the lower lid, is caused by a general weakening and wasting of the muscles, fat, and skin surrounding the orbit of the eye, resulting in decreased support of the lower lid against the globe. The eye may become irritable, watery, and prone to conjunctivitis, or it may develop keratitis or corneal ulceration from the constant rubbing of the eyelashes against the eyeball. Temporary relief can be obtained by strapping the lid outward with a short strip of adhesive. For permanent correction, surgery or cautery is the treatment of choice.

Senile ectropion, also called involutional, atonic, relaxation, or senescent ectropion, is an outward turning of the eyelid margin from its position of contact with the globe. It may occur as a result of facial nerve paralysis; however, with increasing age, it may simply be the result of atrophy of eyelid tissues. The position of the lid may prevent the tears from flowing into the lacrimal sac, resulting in persistent tearing. Ectropion is due to relaxation and loss of muscle tone, which results in laxity of the lid. The lid is in a good position but no longer has any snap and can easily be pulled away from the globe. The lid becomes elongated, leading to conjunctival hypertrophy and keratonization. Ectropion may also result from mechanical weighting of the lids from growths or lesions. Surgical treatment is aimed toward shortening the lid to produce better tone (Brodie, 2003).

HEARING

The ear has two functions: hearing and maintenance of balance. Hearing is achieved through the vibration of sounds transmitted through the tympanic membrane, or eardrum. The vibrations are then conveyed to the inner ear and are transformed into tiny nerve impulses to the brain. Equilibrium is controlled through the hairs located in the inner ear that innervate fibers of the vestibular branch of the eighth cranial, or acoustic, nerve.

The three parts of the ear are (1) the external ear, (2) the middle ear, and (3) the inner ear (Figure 19-3). The external ear, consisting of the auricle and the external

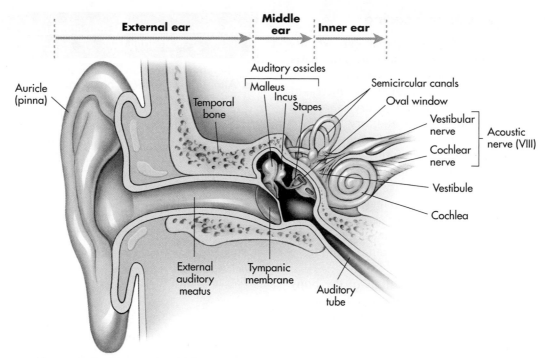

Figure 19-3 External, middle, and inner ear. (From Lewis, S. M., Heitkemper, M. M. & Dirksen, S. R. [2004]. *Medical-surgical nursing: Assessment and management of clinical problems* [6th ed.]. St. Louis: Mosby.)

auditory canal, conducts sound to the tympanic membrane (eardrum) and protects the deeper parts of the ear. The middle ear consists mainly of an air space in the temporal bone, which is bounded laterally by the tympanic membrane. This space contains three bones—the malleus, the incus, and the stapes—that are responsible for transmitting sound vibrations from the tympanic membrane to the middle ear and for reducing the amplitude of large vibrations. The inner ear is made up of the osseous (bony) labyrinth, which contains the semicircular canals, the vestibule, and the cochlea, and the membranous labyrinth, which contains the semicircular ducts, the utricle, the saccule, and the cochlear duct. The organ of Corti with its sensitive hair cells lies at the base of the cochlear duct. The cochlea is the essential organ of the auditory system.

The ear is sensitive to mechanical energy or pressure changes among the molecules in the atmosphere. The vibration of molecules produces sound waves, which are the stimuli for hearing. Sound waves have two main characteristics—frequency and amplitude. Frequency is measured by the number of vibrations or cycles per second; amplitude is the amount of compression and expansion of the sound waves. Frequency is related to the pitch of a sound, so that the higher the vibration frequency, the higher the perceived pitch. Hertz (Hz) is used to denote cycles per second. Amplitude is related to the loudness of a sound, so that the greater the intensity with which the sound pressure strikes the

eardrum, the louder the tone. Intensity of sound is measured in decibels (dB). Table 19-3 shows the relative intensities of some common sounds. Sound waves differ from light waves in that light waves are specified in terms of length of the wave, whereas sound waves are specified on the basis of the number of waves per unit of time. When dimensions of light and color are compared with sound and tone, hue can be likened to pitch and brightness can be equated with loudness.

Table 19-3 *Decibel Levels for Normal Sounds*	
Decibel Level at 1000 Hz	
160	Bursting of eardrum
140	Severe pain
120	Pain threshold; thunder
100	Damage to hearing after prolonged exposure; average factory, loudest passages of orchestra for close listener
80	Class lecture, loud radio
60	Conversational speech
40	Very soft music, typical living room
20	Very quiet room
0	Threshold of hearing

Adapted from Nave, C. R., & Nave, B. C. (1985). *Physics for the health sciences* (3rd ed.), Philadelphia: WB Saunders; Goodhill, V. (1992). Evaluation of the aging ear. *Emergency Medicine, 24*(15), 165-166.

Age-Related Changes in Hearing

Structural Changes. The external ear exhibits changes with aging similar to those seen in other parts of the body. The skin of the auricle often becomes dry and lax with increased wrinkling. There is also increased itching and dryness in the external auditory canal. The tragi (hairs on the lateral external auditory canal) of adult males become longer, coarser, and more noticeable beginning during the third and fourth decades. The ceruminal glands, which are modified apocrine sweat glands, decrease in number and activity, producing drier cerumen (earwax). The dried cerumen may result in impactions within the external auditory canal, especially in older men, whose large tragi become imbedded in the accumulated wax and prevent the natural dislodging of the cerumen.

In the middle ear, some degeneration of the bony joints may take place, but there is no apparent effect on sound transmission. The eardrum thickens, and there may be scarring accumulated over the years from infections, injuries, or other disorders.

The most important age-related changes occur in the inner ear and the auditory nerve. Significant atrophy and degeneration of hair cells, supporting cells, and stria vascularis occur in addition to a reduction in the number of functional spiral ganglia and nerve fibers that make up the auditory portion of the eighth cranial nerve. Though not common to all older persons, changes in the central auditory nervous system can significantly affect the understanding of speech in noisy conditions and also can limit hearing aid benefit (Weinstein, 2003).

Functional Changes. In the United States, an estimated 28 million people have hearing loss. Thirty-one percent of persons over the age of 65 and 40% to 50% of those age 75 and older have hearing loss (NIDCD, 2004). Furthermore, it is estimated that 70% to 80% of all nursing home residents have a sensorineural hearing impairment. The prevalence is believed to be even higher among persons with dementia (Weinstein, 2003). In the UK, 41.7% of persons over age 50 and 71.1% of persons over age 70 reportedly have some kind of hearing loss (RNID, 2005). The psychosocial consequences of hearing impairment for the older person are listed in Box 19-1. Hearing loss can be classified as conductive, sensorineural, or central. Some persons have mixed loss, which means they have conductive loss superimposed on sensorineural loss.

Conductive Hearing Loss. Conductive hearing loss results from any interference with the normal movement of sound vibrations through the external and middle ears. This type of mechanical hearing loss may be caused by impacted cerumen, otitis media, otosclerosis,

> **BOX 19-1 Psychosocial Consequences of Hearing Loss**
>
> - Negative impact on communicative behavior
> - Altered psychosocial behavior
> - Strained family relations
> - Limited enjoyment of daily activities
> - Threat to physical well-being
> - Threat to ability to live independently and safely
> - Difficult telephone communication
> - Interference with medical diagnosis, treatment, and management
> - Nonadherence to drug regimens
> - Interference with therapeutic interventions
>
> From Weinstein, B. E. (2003). Disorders of hearing. In R. C. Tallis & H. M. Fillit (Eds.), *Brocklehurst's textbook of geriatric medicine and gerontology* (6th ed.). London: Churchill Livingstone, pp. 749-761.

trauma, congenital malformations of the external or middle ear, and glomus body tumor (Baloh, 2000).

A person with conductive hearing loss has equal loss at all frequencies, and can hear speech better in a noisy setting than a quiet one. Once the threshold for hearing is exceeded, these individuals have well-preserved speech discrimination. Individuals with conductive hearing loss may speak more softly than normal hearing persons because the sound of their voice to themselves is enhanced by the conductive blockage.

Sensorineural Hearing Loss. Sensorineural loss involves damage to the cochlea and/or the auditory division of the eighth cranial nerve. Numerous factors can cause sensorineural hearing loss: bacterial or viral infection, head trauma, vascular occlusion, acoustic trauma caused by noise, presbycusis, drugs, heredity, acoustic nerve tumors, and postinflammatory reactions. Drugs including salicylates, furosemide, and ethacrynic acid can cause reversible bilateral sensorineural hearing loss when taken in high doses. Other drugs that may be even more toxic to the cochlea are aminoglycosides and some antineoplastics, especially cisplatin (Baloh, 2000b). A perilymphatic fistula, which may be congenital or may occur after stapes surgery or head trauma, can account for sudden unilateral hearing loss. Persons with sensorineural hearing loss hear low-frequency tones better than high-frequency tones. Background noise increases this person's difficulty hearing speech.

Meniere's syndrome is characterized by fluctuating hearing loss and tinnitus, episodes of vertigo, and a feeling of fullness in the ear. The acute episodes are attributed to recurrent endolymphatic hypertension. Over time the endolymphatic sac dilates, the hair cells become atrophic, and deafness, which is reversible in the early stages, eventually becomes permanent.

PRESBYCUSIS. Presbycusis is the term used to describe the most common sensorineural hearing loss associated with age. It may be associated with loss of hair cells at the basal turn, degeneration of the spiral ganglion, atrophy of the stria vascularis, or loss of elasticity of the basement membrane.

Presbycusis is characterized by a decline in pure-tone hearing sensitivity that usually is bilateral and symmetrical. Adults with normal hearing can perceive sound at a frequency range of 300 to 3500 Hz. With aging, loss begins to affect hearing of sound in the higher frequency ranges (1500 to 4000 Hz) and gradually affects the hearing of lower frequencies (500 to 1500 Hz) (Figure 19-4). Noise trauma initially affects the ability to hear sound at frequencies of around 4000 Hz, and with continued exposure, the lower frequencies are affected. The loss is greater with louder noise and longer exposure (Goodhill, 1992; Voeks et al., 1993).

Individuals with presbycusis commonly complain that they can hear other people talking but cannot understand what they are saying, particularly in noisy settings. Loud sounds may become uncomfortably loud, a process called recruitment, and this may limit the effectiveness of amplification or the use of hearing aids. Speech discrimination and comprehension are affected by reduced speech perception and high-tone hearing loss. Reduced speech perception results from the increase in time required to process information in the higher auditory centers. Thus accelerated speech (increase in word rate per minute) is more difficult for the old to understand than it is for the young. High-tone hearing loss, which results from impaired hearing of high-frequency sounds, causes poor discrimination of consonants such as "s," "t," "f," and "g," which have high frequencies. Older persons with presbycusis have difficulty discriminating among phonetically similar words and find it difficult to follow a normal conversation. Background noise exaggerates the problem because the noise tends to mask the weaker speech sounds of the consonants. Table 19-4 reveals difficulties encountered in specific listening situations.

Central Hearing Loss. Central hearing disorders are the results of lesions of the central auditory pathways. Depending on the site of the damage, it can be unilateral or bilateral. In the absence of background noise, the person with a central hearing disorder can understand clearly-spoken speech (Baloh, 2000).

INTERVENTIONS. The treatment of hearing loss depends on the basic etiology. Stapedectomy may be effective for persons with otosclerosis. A perilymph fistula may be surgically closed. Treatment of otitis media with antibiotics and decongestants may prevent permanent hearing loss. In some cases, a low-salt diet and diuretics bring relief from acute episodes of Meniere's syndrome (Baloh, 2000).

As noted, cerumen impaction is a common cause of conductive hearing loss. Research related to prevention of cerumen impaction showed that the topical emollient

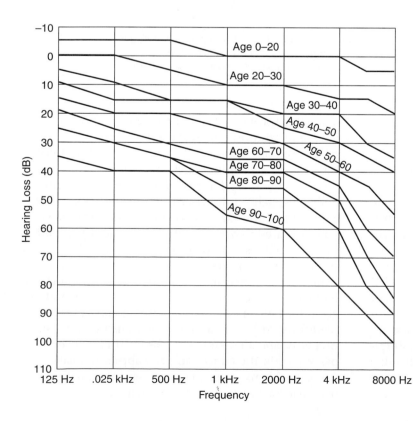

Figure 19-4 This decade audiogram shows the normal aging patterns in an urban environment. (From Goodhill, V. [1992]. Evaluation of the aging ear. *Emergency Medicine, 24*(5), 166.)

Table 19-4 Residents' Responses to Questions Regarding Difficulty in Specific Listening Situations According to Hearing Status and Sensitivity for Each Question

| "Do you have difficulty hearing when . . ." | Answer* | Hearing Status Based on Audiometry | | Sensitivity |
		Normal, % ($n = 91$)	Impaired, % ($n = 107$)	
Talking with several people	No	64	26	73.8
	Equivocal	7	16	
	Yes	30	58	
Watching TV	No	64	38	61.7
	Equivocal	27	31	
	Yes	9	31	
On the telephone	No	64	40	59.8
	Equivocal	27	32	
	Yes	9	28	
There are no facial cues	No	75	42	57.9
	Equivocal	7	8	
	Yes	19	50	
In the dining room	No	64	50	49.5
	Equivocal	30	31	
	Yes	7	19	
Talking one-to-one	No	92	78	21.5
	Equivocal	3	7	
	Yes	4	15	
There are facial cues	No	96	78	21.5
	Equivocal	3	10	
	Yes	1	11	

From Voeks, S. K., Gallagher, C. M., Langer, E. H., & Drinka, P. J. (1993). Self-reported hearing difficulty and audiometric thresholds in nursing home residents. *Journal of Family Practice, 36*(1), 54-58.
*Equivocal and "Yes" responses were both considered positive indicators. "No" responses were considered negative indicators.

Ceridal lipolotion instilled in the ear canal once a week significantly decreased the formation of impacted earwax (Saloranta & Westermarck, 2005). Another study compared the number of irrigations needed to clear the ear of occlusive wax with and without first instilling water into the canal for 15 minutes. After instilling water, an average of 7.5 attempts were needed to clear the canal compared with an average of 25.4 attempts without initial water instillation (Pavlidis & Pickering, 2005). Reviews of studies on the management of earwax have concluded that further large trials are needed (Burton & Doree, 2003; Guest, Greener, Robinson, & Smith, 2004; Hand & Harvey, 2004).

Hearing aids are essentially amplifiers that are intended to make speech intelligible. Simple amplification will suffice for the person with conductive hearing loss. Individuals with sensorineural loss often need frequency-selective amplification. An optimal hearing aid makes speech audible without being uncomfortably loud and restores the normal loudness relations for speech and other sounds (Baloh, 2000). The technological options are summarized in Box 19-2.

There are several types of hearing aids, including body aids, behind-the-ear (postauricular) aids, eyeglass aids, and in-the-ear aids (Figure 19-5). Hearing aids may be placed in one or both ears (binaural), according to individual losses and needs. Binaural aids help to improve the speech reception threshold and speech discrimination (especially in a noisy environment) and provide better localization of sound. A trained audiologist is the person best qualified to test and fit older people for hearing aids. A period of adjustment is usually necessary, and all members of the health care team must participate in the education and support of hearing aid users. Problems most frequently encountered include nervousness because of the sudden increase in noise,

BOX 19-2 Technological Options for Hearing Loss

For mild, moderate, moderately severe, severe sensorineural hearing loss, and speech recognition difficulties in quiet and noise:
- Hearing Aids (Analog, Digitally Programmable Analog, Digital)
  - Behind the ear
  - In the ear
  - In the canal
  - Completely in the canal

For postlingual profound sensorineural hearing loss with extreme difficulty understanding speech using hearing aids:
- Cochlear implants

For mild, moderate, moderately severe, severe sensorineural hearing loss, and speech recognition difficulties in noise—needs unmet by hearing aids:
- Assistive Hearing Devices
  - Personal listening system (e.g., remote microphone FM system)
  - TV listening system (e.g., infrared system)
  - Telephone devices (e.g., TDD, telephone amplifiers)
  - Interactive pagers
  - Fax machines, e-mail
  - Altering devices
  - Auditorium-type assistive listening systems

From Weinstein, B. E. (2003). Disorders of hearing. In R.C. Tallis & H. M. Fillit (Eds.), *Brocklehurst's textbook of geriatric medicine and gerontology* (6th ed.). London: Churchill Livingstone, pp. 749-761.

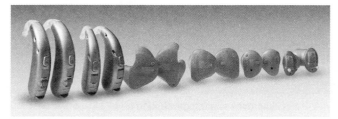

Figure 19-5 A family of hearing instruments that redefines what is possible in a hearing system. Pictured from left to right are a set of ACURIS P BTEs (Behind-the-Ear), ACURIS S BTEs, ACURIS ITEs (In-the-Ear), ACURIS ITCs (In-the-Canal), ACURIS MCs (Mini-Canal), and ACURIS Micro-CICs (Completely-in-the-Canal). (Courtesy of Siemens Hearing Instruments, Piscataway, New Jersey.)

BOX 19-3 Guidelines for Hearing Aid Users

1. Practice inserting and removing the hearing aid until you can do these things easily. Put the aid on when relaxed. If you are unable to handle the aid, make sure that your relative or friend can help you.
2. Wear the hearing aid 4 to 5 hours at first. Wear it for a longer period of time the next day. After a week, it should be worn all day.
3. Remove the hearing aid before going to bed, bathing, or showering.
4. Make sure the battery is inserted correctly. Follow + sign for placement of + side of battery. If there is no on-off switch, open the battery case at night to shut the aid off; this will conserve the battery power. If there is an M-T-O (microphone-telephone-off) switch on the aid, turn to O for off at night. Do not forget to turn back to M in the morning to turn the aid on. Store unused batteries in a cool, dry place.
5. Clean the ear mold daily with a damp cloth. Once a week wipe the mold with a cloth dampened with mild soapy water. Do not immerse the mold in water. If the ear mold gets plugged with wax, clean it out with a toothpick or bent paper clip or wax-removing tool—carefully!
6. Change the batteries every 10 days to 2 weeks. If a whistle (feedback) is not heard when the volume control is fully on, change the battery, and the whistle should then be heard. If no whistle is heard despite a new battery, then the problem is in the aid itself.
7. Remember, the aid is a mechanical instrument. Sounds and voices are made louder, not clearer. Expectations should be realistic.
8. Extraneous noises may annoy you at first. Identify the sounds and then forget them. You will get used to hearing background sounds in a short period of time.
9. If the problem persists, the aid should be tested by an audiologist or hearing aid dealer.

Adapted from Margolis, E. M., Levy, B., & Sherman, F. T. (1981). Hearing disorders. In L. S. Libow & F. T. Sherman (Eds.), *The core of geriatric medicine*. St. Louis: CV Mosby, p. 20; Beltone Electronics (1987). *The better hearing book*. Chicago: Beltone.

embarrassment from appearing with the hearing aid in public, forgetting to turn off or change the batteries in the hearing aid because of poor memory, and difficulty in manipulating the parts of the hearing aid because of poor vision or lack of manual dexterity. Guidelines for hearing aid users are listed in Box 19-3.

Evaluation for a hearing aid is a complex process, requiring a sensitive audiologist who must consider not only the older person's audiologic profile but also the finances, motivation, manual dexterity, and ability to learn the skill of using a hearing aid. If a hearing aid is obtained, the older person may need considerable support and encouragement in using it, for there are disadvantages to the increased volume, such as increased background noise, new problems with speech discrimination, and new tasks to learn.

Even though hearing aids are effective for various kinds of hearing losses, many older people do not use

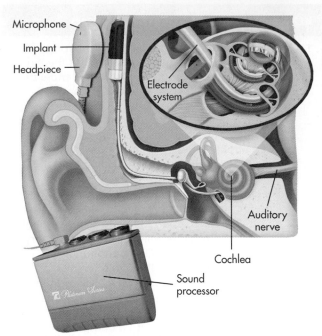

Figure 19-6   Cochlear implant. (From Lemmi, F. D., & Lemmi, C. A. E. [2000]. *Physical assessment findings CD-ROM.* Philadelphia: Saunders.)

them. Thinking that deafness is normal and inevitable with aging, they may withdraw from social interaction, rendering hearing aid use less necessary. Thus many elderly people postpone audiological evaluation until after it is too late for a hearing aid to be effective. Older people may also deny that they have a hearing problem, thereby avoiding any association with older age. The

negative social stigma attached to hearing aid users may be another deterrent. The cost of a hearing aid may be prohibitive for many older people on fixed incomes, especially because there is no Medicare reimbursement for this expense. Hearing aid molds also may cause irritation to the external ear manifested as contact dermatitis and itching. In addition, increased humidity in the external auditory canal can cause infection, a condition known as otitis externa.

Technological developments have provided a variety of options in addition to hearing aids for hearing-impaired persons. Cochlear implants are options for adults with severe to profound bilateral sensorineural hearing loss who are unable to benefit from conventional amplification (Figure 19-6). Candidates must be able to undergo general anesthesia, and have no anatomical deformities that would prevent implantation of the device. As the technology continues to develop, outcomes are progressively improving. Benefits include improved ability to detect sound at lower intensities than with hearing aids and improved lipreading. Many adults who were deafened postlinguistically have significantly improved word recognition; more than half are able to converse to some degree on the telephone. The level of speech perception is predicted by duration of deafness, duration of implant use, and hearing ability before implantation. Adults who were deafened prelinguistically have poorer speech scores but still report improved quality of life and communication abilities (Koch, Staller, Jaax, & Martin, 2005). Bioengineering solutions for hearing impairment are summarized in Table 19-5. Predictions of future developments

Table 19-5 *Bioengineering Solutions for Hearing Loss*

Device	Features	Outcomes
Electro-acoustic (hybrid) cochlear implants	Used with hearing aid; provides high-frequency speech cues electrically in combination with low-frequency speech cues acoustically	Improves speech perception
Auditory brainstem implants	Used for patients with neurofibromatosis type 2 who become deaf when auditory nerve is severed during surgery to remove tumors on nerve	Permits detection of sound and lipreading; speech perception abilities are poor
Middle ear implants	Uses electromagnetic or piezoelectric transducers to mechanically drive middle ear ossicles; designed to overcome disadvantages of acoustic hearing aids (canal occlusion, acoustic feedback, sound distortion, cosmesis); for adults with moderate-severe hearing loss with normal middle ear function, good aided speech perception, and prior experience with conventional amplification	Compared with conventional hearing aids, word recognition is similar; less acoustic feedback, occlusion effect, and distortion; increased satisfaction
Bone-anchored hearing aids	Delivers acoustic information to inner ear through direct bone conduction	May be useful for all types of hearing loss in selected persons; improved speech perception in noise

Data from Koch, D. B., Staller, S., Jaax, K., & Martin, E. (2005). Bioengineering solutions for hearing loss and related disorders [electronic version]. *Otolaryngologic Clinics of North America, 38*(2).

include fully implantable cochlear devices, improved delivery of signals to the auditory nerve, and the use of drugs to preserve neural tissue or induce neural growth (Koch et al., 2005).

Tinnitus. Tinnitus is the perception of sound in the absence of an apparent acoustic stimulus (Ahmad & Seidman, 2004, p. 297). It is thought to result from spontaneous and aberrant neural activity at any level along the auditory axis. This disturbing concomitant of both conductive and sensorineural hearing loss affects approximately 50 million Americans, with adults aged 40 to 70 most often affected (Noell & Meyerhoff, 2003; Seidman & Babu, 2003). Fortunately, for most persons, it is not disturbing. Tinnitus may be characterized as objective or subjective. Subjective tinnitus is apparent only to the patient. It is characterized by hissing, buzzing, or ringing. The sound is generally high pitched with sensorineural loss and low pitched with conductive loss; however, tinnitus may be present with or without hearing loss. The intensity is so low that the sound is heard only during quiet times and is masked by extraneous environmental noises. Objective tinnitus, which is rare, can be heard by both the patient and an examiner (usually with auscultation). It usually is associated with vascular or muscular causes. Tinnitus does not usually awaken afflicted persons, nor does it interfere with pleasurable activity.

Factors leading to tinnitus are otological, neurological, traumatic, and pharmacological. Otological causes include infection, neoplasms, labyrinthine disorders such as Meniere's disease, otosclerosis, and impacted cerumen. Neurological causes include multiple sclerosis, migraine, seizure disorders, and stress. Traumatic causes include head injury, ossicular discontinuity, tympanic membrane perforation, and neck injuries. Ototoxic drugs include aspirin, NSAIDs, loop diuretics, and aminoglycosides. Tinnitus also has been associated with temporomandibular joint disorders, nutritional deficiencies, metabolic disorders (e.g., hyperlipidemia), and dietary intake (for example, salt, caffeine, alcohol, simple sugars, monosodium glutamate) (Ahmad & Seidman, 2004).

Although there is no cure for tinnitus, treatment may improve symptoms and quality of life. Box 19-4 summarizes the treatment options for mild to severe tinnitus. Among the options are counseling, stress reduction programs, biofeedback, dietary modification, hearing aids, masking devices, tinnitus retraining therapy (TRT), and drug therapy. Masking devices produce sounds such as ocean waves (called "white noise") that may reduce the annoyance of tinnitus. Some devices include a hearing aid and a masker in the same case. TRT induces habituation to tinnitus by exposing the patient to low-level noise that is just below the patient's perceived

---

BOX 19-4 Management of Tinnitus Based on Severity

Mild
- Reassurance and counseling
- Dietary modifications: reduction in sodium, alcohol, caffeine, sweets, nicotine

Moderate to Moderately Severe
- Hearing aid
- Masking device
- Habituation therapy (tinnitus retraining therapy)

Moderately Severe to Severe
Drug Therapy
- Antidepressants
- Antiepileptics
- Antianxiety agents
- Antihistamines
- Diuretics
- Vasoactive drugs
- Herbs
- Vitamins and minerals
- Intratympanic corticosteroids or gentamicin

Severe Intractable
- Transcochlear cochleovestibular neurectomy (CVN)
- Translabyrinthine CVN
- Microvascular decompression

Data from Ahmad, N., & Seidman, M. (2004). Tinnitus in the older adult. *Drugs Aging, 21*(5), 297-305; Dodson, K. M., & Sismanis, A. (2004). Intratympanic perfusion for the treatment of tinnitus. *Otolaryngologic Clinics of North America, 37*(5), 991-1000; and Smith, P. F., Zheng, Y., & Darlington, C. L. (2005). Ginkgo biloba extracts for tinnitus: More hype than hope? *Journal of Ethnopharmacology, 100*(1), 95-99.

---

tinnitus sound (Ahmad & Seidman, 2004). Surgical options are reserved for severe, intractable tinnitus. The success rates for various procedures range from 29% to 67% (Ahmad & Seidman, 2004). Various drugs have been used to treat tinnitus. Lidocaine has been used in the past, but has generally been abandoned. Several reviews of studies of ginkgo biloba concluded that there was limited evidence of effectiveness (Hilton & Stuart, 2004; Smith et al., 2005). Current technological efforts are focusing on tinnitus suppression devices that apply electrical stimulation in a variety of manners. The Bion microstimulator is a miniature, self-contained, rechargeable neurostimulator that was developed to stimulate nerves and muscles. It is controlled by a remote handheld device. The goal of using the Bion with tinnitus is to chronically suppress tinnitus by implanting it behind the ear with an electrode running to the middle ear. The patient could use the remote control to provide continuous or intermittent stimulation as needed (Koch et al., 2005).

TASTE AND SMELL

The senses of taste and smell are intertwined in a person's appreciation of food, and they provide sensitive responses to the environment. The safety of the environment as well as its pleasantness or unpleasantness can be detected by these senses. The smell of smoke can warn of a dangerous fire, and the scent of a light perfume can provide a delightful background for a romantic interlude. The taste of tainted food or drink can be nauseating, whereas a sip of fine wine can provide a rosy glow to an evening with friends. Changes in the senses of taste and smell with aging are not definitively known, but there is some evidence that they are diminished. If so, this decrease certainly has an effect on the quality of life and on the ability of older people to react safely to the environment.

Taste

The sense of taste is perceived through approximately 9000 taste buds located on the edges and toward the back of the human tongue, the soft palate, the pharynx, and the larynx. The primary taste qualities of sweet, sour, salt, and bitter are associated with particular taste receptors distributed in various parts of the tongue. Generally, sensitivity to sweet taste is located at the tip of the tongue, sourness at the sides, bitterness at the back, and saltiness at the tip and sides of the tongue. Each of the taste buds has 15 to 20 taste cells arranged in a budlike form on its tip. The taste cells, which have a life span of 10 to 101 days, are constantly replacing themselves. However, turnover may be slower in older persons. Because the taste signal pathway is complicated, errors can occur at many different points. For example, saliva is critical for normal taste perception because it is essential for the transport of water-soluble tastants. Therefore xerostomia is associated with alterations in taste.

In general, the chemical senses peak in the third or fourth decade of life, and then decline. Older persons experience changes in taste-detection and taste-recognition. A decreased sense of taste often is noticed around age 60; severe loss is typical after age 70 (Seiberling & Conley, 2004). It has been assumed that these changes are caused by a loss of taste buds; however, some studies have reported gradual diminution in the number of taste buds whereas other studies report no loss. Some investigators attribute the decline in taste to changes in the taste cell membranes rather than a loss of taste buds (Seiberling & Conley, 2004). Because changes in taste are more prevalent in older persons, they have been labeled as normal age-related changes. However, many other factors that are more common among older people may be responsible for change. These include disease states, medications, surgery, head trauma, malnutrition,

and cumulative exposure to toxins (Doty & Bromley, 2004; Sieberling & Conley, 2004) (Box 19-5).

Research on taste commonly uses a variety of substances representing salt, sweet, bitter, and sour to assess the patient's ability to recognize the substance. Results typically are measured in terms of two types of thresholds: (1) detection threshold—the lowest concentration of a substance that can be distinguished from water; (2) recognition threshold—the lowest concentration of a substance that can be recognized by taste. Both detection and recognition thresholds are elevated in older adults. Medical conditions and drug therapy can

---

BOX 19-5 Partial List of Factors That Alter the Senses of Taste and Smell

Medical Conditions
- Nervous system disorders: Alzheimer's disease, head trauma, Parkinson's disease
- Nutritional disorders: cancer; chronic renal failure; liver disease; deficiencies of zinc, vitamin B_{12}, or vitamin B_3
- Endocrine disorders: diabetes mellitus, hypothyroidism
- Local disorders: allergic rhinitis, bronchial asthma, sinusitis, xerostomia
- Viral infections: influenza-like infections

Medications
- Lipid-lowering drugs
- Antihistamines
- Antimicrobials
- Antineoplastics
- Antiinflammatory drugs
- Asthma drugs including bronchodilators
- Antihypertensive drugs
- Cardiac medications
- Muscle relaxants
- Antiparkinsonian drugs
- Antidepressants
- Anticonvulsants
- Vasodilators

Oral Sources of Smell and Taste Disorders
- Oral trauma
- Removable prosthodontic appliances
- Dental caries
- Periodontal disease
- Drugs in saliva
- Salivary dysfunction
- Chemotherapy
- Head and neck radiotherapy
- Tooth loss
- Impaired chewing

Data from Seiberling, K. A., & Conley, D. B. (2004). Aging and olfactory and taste function. *Otolaryngologic Clinics of North America, 37,* 1209-1228.

significantly raise the thresholds even more. Of the five tastes, sucrose (sweet) remains the most robust over the years. Citric acid (sour) and quinine (bitter) are most likely to decline (Seiberling & Conley, 2004).

Smell

The sense of smell is perceived through a series of receptors—bipolar nerve cells—located in the mucous membranes high in the nasal cavity. Impulses are relayed to the olfactory bulbs of the brain, which lie just below the frontal lobes, and then to the temporal lobes, the primary olfactory areas of the cortex. The olfactory area comprises both olfactory and respiratory epithelium. The thickness of the olfactory epithelium depends on the number of neuronal cells. One type of cell in this layer is the ciliated olfactory receptor neurons (ORNs) that transmit the stimulus signal from the molecules of odorants. Basal cells in the olfactory epithelium are the stem cell population that differentiate and replace lost ORNs, which have a life span of 3 to 7 weeks. Normally, the production of new ORNs (olfactory neurogenesis) replaces lost neurons to maintain consistent thickness of the olfactory epithelium (Seiberling & Conley, 2004).

Like the sense of taste, the sense of smell peaks in the third or fourth decade and declines thereafter. In the sixth and seventh decades, olfactory identification declines sharply. Histologic studies of the olfactory epithelium in older persons reveal an increase in respiratory cells in relation to the olfactory cells. This change is believed to reflect loss of ORNs with age, and is a major explanation for the age-related changes in the sense of smell (Seiberling & Conley, 2004). Factors that may contribute to these changes are summarized in Box 19-5. Among persons aged 65 to 80, about half have olfactory dysfunction; 75% of those over age 80 have marked olfactory dysfunction. In healthy older adults, the threshold for odors has been found to be 2 to 15 times that of younger persons. Older persons also have deficits in odor recognition memory, odor recall, odor discrimination, and the ability to track increases in odor concentration. Among persons with Alzheimer's disease, the primary change is impaired odor identification (Seiberling & Conley, 2004).

The implications of olfactory dysfunction for the older person are significant as it may affect food intake, including the social aspects of food preparation and mealtime. Olfactory dysfunction also has been associated with diminished quality of life, decreased ability to perform some activities of daily living, and safety hazards such as the inability to detect spoiled food, smoke, or gas. Individuals who are concerned that they will not recognize body or breath odor sometimes overuse scented products.

Conclusions from the results of studies of chemosensory function must be tempered by the fact that there is often considerable bias (older people respond more slowly and carefully to psychomotor testing) in the testing process and that sample sizes are generally small.

TOUCH, VIBRATION, AND PAIN SENSITIVITY

The sensory apparatus of the human body consists of a series of sensory receptors that send signals through the spinal cord, brainstem, thalamus, and cerebral cortex to evoke various types of motor and sensory responses. Sensory receptors are located in the skin, muscles, tendons, joints, and viscera. Receptors in the skin, called exteroceptors, record information about the external environment of the body; specialized receptors, such as Meissner's or Ruffini's corpuscles, detect sensations of touch, heat, or pain. These specialized receptors are distributed throughout the body, but some areas are more sensitive to particular stimuli than others. In addition, different sensory fibers conduct impulses at different rates, so that various sensory modalities (heat, pain, touch) may be perceived differently.

Most somatic sensations evoke affective responses that determine whether the sensation received is pleasant (warmth), unpleasant (pain, excess heat or cold), or neutral (touch). Drugs, brain surgery, or brain lesions may decrease or abolish the affective response while leaving intact the ability to recognize sensory modalities. Thus individuals can feel and recognize pain, but it no longer bothers them. This phenomenon can be important in the care of older clients with delirium or dementia in whom assessment of pain, heat, or cold is extremely difficult.

Proprioceptors are located in muscles, tendons, joints, and visceral organs. They transmit information regarding the position and condition of these deeper organs, although this information does not enter conscious thinking. Many of the responses to proprioceptive stimuli are related to reflex activity that is mediated through the spinal cord or cerebellar areas where posture and movement are controlled.

Changes in Structure and Function

Touch and Vibration. The sense of touch declines with age, perhaps beginning as early as adolescence. Even in healthy older persons, detection of a vibratory stimulus declines. Studies have consistently shown a loss of sensitivity to vibration in a significant proportion of aged subjects who were apparently free of disease or detectable neuropathy. Studies using a variety of stimulators and quantitative measurements have shown that it is sensitivity to high frequencies that declines, while no change is found at low frequencies. It should be noted that vibratory sense may be affected by diabetes, alcohol, vitamin B_{12} deficiency, and neurotoxic drugs (Assal & Cummings, 2003).

A study of healthy individuals aged 85 and older revealed a decline in balance testing, a diminished sense of touch, especially with neurologically demanding tasks, some decline in proprioception, and diminished two-point discrimination. However, the most significant declines were in stereognosis and vibratory sensation (Kaye et al., 1994, cited in Nusbaum, 1999).

Pain. Pain is a complicated phenomenon that is difficult to measure. Data regarding measurement of pain sensitivity are inconsistent and are confounded by variables in the test situation such as the subjects, investigators, and environmental conditions. In healthy older persons, the ability to perceive painful stimuli appears to remain relatively intact (Nusbaum, 1999).

Clinical observations that about one half of older persons suffering a myocardial infarction or peritonitis do not report the classic pain normally found with those conditions have contributed to a common belief that older persons perceive pain differently than younger persons. Some studies have reported that they also appear to have less postoperative pain than younger persons. However, the stereotypical stoic, uncomplaining older person may in fact be reluctant to label a stimulus as painful or may fear addiction to pain medication (Barkin, Barkin, & Barkin, 2005; Katz & Helme, 2003).

Schuler and colleagues studied the clinical characteristics of acute and chronic pain in older persons with and without cognitive impairment in acute and rehabilitiation facilities. In this sample, individuals with chronic pain described more pain sites, used more pain descriptors, used more analgesics at discharge, and reported less pain reduction with therapy than persons with acute pain (Schuler, Njoo, Hestermann, Oster, & Hauer, 2004). A study of the pattern of pain occurrence revealed that pain that interfered with daily activities increased incrementally with age. One other finding was a decline with aging in the prevalence of regional pains except for the lower extremities (Thomas, Peat, Harris, Wilkie, & Croft, 2004).

Reports of the prevalence of pain in older persons are varied. Studies have consistently reported a prevalence rate of chronic pain of about 30% in older community-dwelling individuals, and 66% to 80% in residential care settings (Katz & Helme, 2003). The pain prevalence in a stratified random sampling of older nursing home residents in Taiwan was 65.3%. The average number of pain sites was 3.24 (Tsai, Tsai, Lai, & Chu, 2004). Pain affecting the joints, feet, and legs increases with aging whereas head, abdominal, and chest pain decreases.

Multiple studies around the world have documented gender differences in the pain experience. In general, the prevalence of pain is higher in women for all age-groups (Katz & Helme, 2003). Some studies also report more widespread pain in older women than in older men (Leveille, Zhang, McMullen, Kelly-Hayes, & Felson, 2005). Not only is the prevalence of chronic pain higher in women, but also they rate the pain at higher levels of intensity than men (Donald & Foy, 2004; Gerdle, Bjork, Henriksson, & Bengtsson, 2004; Rustoen et al., 2004; Thomas et al., 2004). Despite a progressive increase in prevalence rates for pain in older adults, Zarit, Griffiths, & Berg (2004) demonstrated in a sample ages 86 to 92 years that pain worsened in some individuals over 1 year whereas it improved in others. These findings suggest that intervention can be beneficial in even the oldest patients.

Swedish investigators described the stress of musculoskeletal pain in primary care patients of various ages. Compared with younger patients, the older patients were found to have had pain of longer duration and greater frequency, and they felt more disabled. They consumed more analgesics, sedatives, and other medications, had more health problems, and were more likely to use passive coping for pain (Soares, Sundin, & Grossi, 2004).

The impact of pain on older persons is significant. It is associated with decreased quality of life, functional limitations, fatigue, sleeping problems, and depression (Jakobsson, Klevsgard, Westergren, & Hallberg, 2003).

Age-related changes of the special senses are summarized in Box 19-6.

NURSING CARE
Assessment

Assessment of the special senses in the older adult is one of the most important parts of a generalized health assessment, because inability to accurately receive and process sensory information seriously impedes any assessment maneuver that requires interpretation of patient responses to questions or directions. For example, the results of a mental status examination are unreliable and invalid if the patient cannot hear the questions being asked. Similarly, historical information about a specific complaint is not very reliable if the patient has poor comprehension of the examiner's questions but is eager to please. Choice of interventions is also influenced by the person's sensory abilities. If the individual is severely impaired, the amount of patient education that can be conducted without a significant other present is quite limited. The elements of the nursing assessment of the senses are outlined in Box 19-7.

History. Inquire about visual disturbances—such as diplopia (double vision), inability to focus on far or near objects, tunnel vision, and transient blindness—and note the onset, duration, and circumstances under which they occur. Also record complaints of intermittent or persistent discomfort related to vision, such as

Box 19-6 _Age-Related Changes: Special Senses_

General Sensory Response
- Greater absolute threshold for sensory stimuli

Visual System
Eyebrows and Eyelashes
- Gray

Eyelids
- Wrinkling and loosening of skin
- Decrease in muscle tone and elasticity
- Herniation of fat into lower lids

Orbit
- Loss of fat

Tears
- Secretion may diminish

Cornea
- Decrease in number of endothelial cells
- Diminished sensitivity
- Diminished corneal reflex
- Arcus senilis (grayish ring around iris)

Ciliary Body
- Decreased secretion of aqueous humor
- Atrophy of ciliary muscle
- Decreased ability to focus (presbyopia)
- Decreased visual acuity

Lens
- Enlargement, yellowing
- Loss of elasticity
- Increased density
- Decreased tolerance of glare
- Decreased ability to adapt to dark and light
- Increased myopia or decreased hyperopia

Iris
- Loss of pigment

Pupil
- Smaller
- Decreased peripheral vision

Vitreous Gel
- Liquefies and collapses
- Condensation and debris common as "floaters"

Retina
- Local ischemia
- Loss of neurons

Hearing
External Ear
- Skin of auricle dry and wrinkled
- Itching and dryness of external auditory canal
- Tragi longer, coarser, more noticeable
- Ceruminal glands decrease in number and activity
- Cerumen drier

Middle Ear
- Degeneration of bony joints
- Eardrum thickens

Continued

◇ Box 19-6 *Age-Related Changes: Special Senses—cont'd*

Hearing—cont'd

Inner Ear

■ Atrophy and degeneration of hair cells, supporting cells, and stria vascularis
■ Decrease in number of functional spiral ganglia and nerve fibers

Taste

■ Slower turnover of taste buds; may decrease in number
■ Elevated thresholds for taste detection and recognition
■ Detection of sour and bitter tastes declines most

Smell

■ Elevated thresholds for smell detection and recognition
■ Number of olfactory cells in epithelium declines in relation to respiratory cells
■ Loss of olfactory receptor neurons

Touch, Vibration, and Pain

■ Decline in sense of touch
■ Decline in sensitivity to high-frequency vibration
■ Some decline in proprioception
■ Decline in two-point discrimination
■ Decline in balance testing
■ Ability to perceive painful stimuli remains relatively intact in healthy older persons

---

headaches, eye fatigue, or eye pain. Older clients usually wear bifocal, trifocal, or progressive lens glasses, so it is important to know the date of the most recent eye examination and the name of the examiner.

Investigate reports of hearing loss, whether sudden or gradual, bilateral or unilateral. Document related complaints such as tinnitus, vertigo, drainage from the ears, and pain. Because family members may be more cognizant of the hearing loss than older clients, their input is useful. The American Speech and Hearing Association (1996) advocates the use of the screening version of the "Hearing Handicap Inventory" (Ventry & Weinstein, 1982) or the Self Assessment of Communication (Schow & Nerbonne, 1982) to identify the impact of a hearing loss on the patient's function. Determine whether the individual has ever used a hearing aid in the past and what that experience was like. Behaviors that mask the impact of the hearing loss should be noted. For example, many people are embarrassed by having to ask a speaker to repeat—instead they will simply smile and nod as if they understood. Ask questions that test comprehension, to ensure that the message has been understood despite a hearing impairment.

Complaints of diminished taste and smell are unusual, partly because many individuals are unaware of the loss (Seiberling & Conley, 2004). However, these sensations may be blunted in the presence of colds or allergies. Therefore record any changes that have been noted in these senses. The impact of sensory losses on activities of daily living should also be explored. Consider the effects on communication, mobility, nutrition,

social activities, work, and relationships. Changes in somatic sensations should be investigated, especially the occurrence of acute or chronic pain. The impact of any sensory deficits may be determined by asking the patient to describe a typical day. Explore any problems with activities of daily living, instrumental activities of daily living, employment, relationships, and social activities.

Physical Assessment. In addition to the standard physical assessment, imaging procedures may be helpful in evaluating problems related to the special senses. For example, functional MRI may demonstrate olfactory loss with early neurodegenerative disease (Seiberling & Conley, 2004).

EYE AND VISION. Inspect the external eye, including the lids and lacrimal ducts, for deviations from normal, particularly the presence of excess tearing, discharge, ectropion, entropion, or swelling. The conjunctiva and sclera should be free from lesions or redness. The cornea may have some opacity or abnormal curvature, and an arcus senilis may be seen on the iris surrounding the cornea. Inspect the pupils for size, shape, and equality.

Perform a fundoscopic examination to detect abnormalities of the optic disc (optic atrophy, papilledema, glaucoma), hemorrhages, exudates, and vascular abnormalities. Various types of tonometers can be used to measure intraocular pressure (Figure 19-7). Normal intraocular pressure is 10 to 21 mm Hg.

Box 19-7 Assessment: Sensory Function

History
- History of cataracts, glaucoma, diabetes

Symptoms
- Visual problems: diplopia (double vision), inability to focus, tunnel vision, transient blindness, discomfort, headaches, eye fatigue, eye pain
- Hearing loss (sudden or gradual, bilateral or unilateral), ringing in the ears or tinnitus, dizziness, vertigo, pain
- Diminished taste, smell, or touch

Use of aids
- Eyeglasses, hearing aids

Physical Assessment
Eye/vision
Inspection
- External eye, lids, and lacrimal ducts for excess tearing, discharge, ectropion, entropion, swelling
- Conjunctiva and sclera for lesions, redness
- Cornea for opacity, curvature
- Pupils for size, shape, equality, reaction to light

Funduscopic examination of internal eye
- Optic disc (optic atrophy, papilledema, glaucoma), hemorrhages, exudates, vascular abnormalities
- Intraocular pressure test for glaucoma

Vision
- Snellen's chart
- Acuity, color, depth perception, peripheral vision, light and dark adaptation, glare, halos

Ear/hearing
Inspection
- External ear for lesions, dryness, exudates
- Ear canal for cerumen, scarring, infections

Measure air and bone conduction
- Weber's test
- Rinne test

Hearing
- Tone, frequency, speech discrimination

Smell, taste, and touch
- Identification of odors, food tastes (sweet, sour, bitter, salty), and objects
- Somatic sensations (pinprick, cotton, temperature)

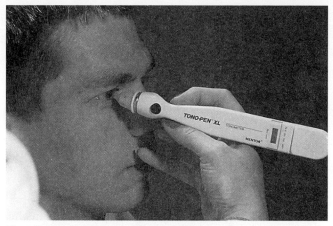

Figure 19-7 Tono-pen tonometry. (Courtesy of Eye Institute, Department of Ophthalmology and Visual Sciences, University of Iowa Health Care, Iowa City, Iowa.)

identify colors in the environment. Peripheral vision, glare, depth perception, and light and dark adaptation should also be tested. Vision should be assessed with and without glasses. Ask about behavioral changes such as bumping into objects, straining to read or watch television, or social withdrawal that could be related to sensory losses.

An approximation of the ability to function in the environment should be obtained. Can the older person find a number in the telephone directory? Can the person read medicine labels and differentiate pills based on color and shape? Does the older person appear clumsy and bump into furniture? In institutional settings, can the menu or patient education materials be read? Is the person bothered by the visual impairments experienced? The Activities of Daily Vision Scale is a questionnaire that measures the amount of functional deficit associated with vision loss (Mangione et al., 1992). High reliability and good validity have been demonstrated in elderly patients before and after cataract surgery; however, its use in other populations has not been reported. The instrument is composed of 20 visual activities, representing the following 5 areas of visual function: distance vision, near vision, glare disability, night driving, and daytime driving. Each subscale is rated from 0 to 100, ranging from inability to perform an activity because of visual difficulty to no visual difficulty. Individuals with significant deficits but without an explanatory medical diagnosis should be referred to an ophthalmologist for further evaluation.

EAR AND HEARING. Inspect the external ear for lesions, dryness, or exudate. The ear canal should be examined for cerumen, scarring, and signs of infections. Assessment of hearing loss can be carried out through sophisticated audiometric testing or through cursory

Visual acuity traditionally is measured by using the Snellen chart. If this is not available, ask the older adult to read a newspaper aloud, starting with the larger headlines and ending with the finest, smallest print. This provides a gross measure of near vision. Colors can be distinguished with color charts or by asking patients to

examinations in the clinical setting. Some clues to hearing loss may be detected during a conversation with the older person. Be alert to discrepancies between questions and answers and to remarks such as, "Would you repeat the question," or "Stop mumbling," or "Please speak louder." Many older persons are embarrassed, sensitive, or unaware of hearing loss and may not acknowledge a hearing difficulty. Some will simply answer "yes" or smile in reply to questions. If you suspect the patient is responding without understanding, stand out of the patient's field of vision and ask questions that require answers other than "yes" or "no."

Pure-tone air and bone conduction tests (the Weber and Rinne tuning fork tests) may be performed in the clinical setting. Air conduction is the measured level of sound transmitted through the ear canal and middle ear ossicles to the inner ear. Bone conduction is measured by placing a vibrator on the mastoid bone behind the auricle, which directly stimulates the inner ear. If air conduction is greater than bone conduction, there is sensorineural loss; if bone conduction is greater than air conduction, there is conductive loss.

Older people who do not "pass" screening measures or who report that they have difficulty following conversations or are unable to hear extraneous environmental noises, such as birds singing or the wind blowing, may be referred to an audiologist to determine the nature and extent of their hearing loss. The audiologist may use an array of screening techniques, including self-estimates of hearing loss by the individual, pure-tone audiometry, and speech perception tests, to facilitate the selection of proper rehabilitative techniques if needed.

If the patient has a hearing aid, assess knowledge of the use and care of the device. Observe for difficulties with manual dexterity as the person manipulates the aid, during battery changing or insertion.

SMELL AND TASTE. Smell and taste can be assessed by asking the older patient to identify odors and flavors. Spices can be used for tests of the sense of smell, and foods that are sour, sweet, bitter, and salty may be used to test for the sense of taste. A more sophisticated test of olfactory function is the University of Pennsylvania Smell Identification Test that uses 40 microencapsulated odorants that are released when rubbed with an eraser (Seiberling & Conley, 2004). Aspects of the physical examination that are relevant to smell and taste include inspection of the nasal and oral cavities and the neurological examination. Because some neurological conditions such as Alzheimer's disease and Parkinson's disease are associated with chemosensory changes, mental status is important as well (Seiberling & Conley, 2004).

TOUCH AND VIBRATION. The person's ability to accurately report light touch, pinprick, deep pressure, vibration, hot and cold, and proprioception of distal portions of the extremities should be assessed, using standard sensory testing methods. Small objects placed in a paper bag can be used to test the sense of touch; the client can reach in and try to identify the object. Somatic sensations can be measured by using pinpricks or by brushing cotton lightly on the skin. Such information guides development of individualized self-care programs, such as regular foot inspection for injury and use of appropriate footwear, and testing of bathwater with a thermometer instead of relying on inadequate temperature sensitivity to prevent accidental burns. Vibratory sense is determined by placing a tuning fork on the area to be measured and looking at the frequency threshold.

KINESTHESIA. The sense of where the body is in space requires information from the vestibular apparatus, proprioceptors, and the visual system. Minimal testing of kinesthesia involves observation of the person's ability to maintain a sitting and standing balance, the ability to recover from a disequilibrating force, such as a gentle shove on one shoulder, and observation for nystagmus. During the testing, attention should be paid to the patient's emotional response and complaints of symptoms. For example, an impaired kinesthetic sense may underlie the older person's fear of falling. This fear or diffuse anxiety may be elicited during the testing, and the nurse should be prepared to provide reassurance by describing the safety precautions incorporated into the testing procedures.

PAIN. A special problem is the assessment of pain in older persons who are cognitively impaired. A small study ($n = 55$) concluded that older patients with cognitive impairments were less precise in describing their pain than less impaired patients (Schuler et al., 2004). Particularly for community-dwelling individuals, the caregiver may be relied upon to recognize behaviors indicative of pain. A study of pain reports of dementia patients and their caregivers found a "fair" degree of congruence between the reports of the two. Interestingly, these patients also reported less pain than dementia patients in nursing homes (Shega, Hougham, Stocking, Cox-Hayley, & Sachs, 2004).

Nursing Diagnoses

Among the many possible nursing diagnoses for the individual with sensory impairment are the following:
- Impaired Adjustment related to limited resources to cope with sensory losses
- Disturbed Body Image related to impact of altered sensory function on view of self
- Impaired Verbal Communication related to hearing or visual disorder

- Confusion related to inability to receive or interpret sensory input
- Deficient Diversional Activity related to loss of ability to perform usual or favorite activities secondary to sensory losses
- Impaired Home Maintenance related to sensory losses
- Risk for Injury related to sensory losses
- Impaired Physical Mobility related to sensory losses
- Imbalanced Nutrition: Less than body requirements related to altered sense of taste, smell
- Self-Care Deficit: Bathing/Hygiene, Dressing/Grooming, Feeding, Toileting, related to sensory losses
- Sensory-Perceptual Alterations: Visual, Auditory, Kinesthetic, Gustatory, Tactile, Olfactory related to aging processes
- Impaired Social Interactions related to sensory losses
- Disturbed Thought Processes related to inability to evaluate reality secondary to sensory losses
- Disturbed Sensory Perception related to sensory losses
- Grieving related to sensory losses
- Deficient Knowledge related to sensory-perceptual alterations

Goals/Outcomes

The following goals apply to individuals with alterations in the special senses:
- The patient will retain or regain maximum possible independence.
- The patient will use adaptive devices or other strategies to communicate effectively.
- The patient will employ strategies to prevent injury related to sensory losses.
- The patient will resolve psychosocial difficulties associated with sensory losses.

Nursing Interventions

Nursing interventions for older persons with any type of sensory deficit aim toward maintaining the highest possible level of functioning and teaching patients and families strategies for maximizing sensory function.

Phillips (1981) proposes a useful model of sensory alteration in the aged. It is based upon theories of sensoristasis, which state that individuals have a basic drive to maintain "an optimal range and variety of external stimulation to maintain awareness" (p. 173) and that individual differences exist in the optimal level of stimulation. At the neurological level, Phillips contends the reticular activating system is programmed with expectations about acceptable levels of stimuli. The reticular

activating system is stimulated by both internal and external sources; if stimulation from either source becomes excessive, disturbances of awareness and attention result. Under conditions of external stimulus deprivation, uncontrolled input from internal stimuli may produce cognitive disturbances.

Sensory distortion results from both overload and deprivation. Sensory deprivation occurs as the result of too little intensity or variation in the patterning or complexity of sensory stimulation while the relevance of stimuli is also low. Sensory overload occurs when the intensity or variation of patterns and complexity of stimuli is high and the relevance is low.

Interventions to Promote Adaptation to Sensory Losses. Referral for evaluation of treatable disorders that cause sensory impairment is essential. Support groups for persons with vision and hearing impairments can be helpful resources. A nationally affiliated hearing-impaired support group called "Shh," which is located in many communities, is an avenue of support for the person learning to cope with hearing impairment. Nonprofit organizations exist for most sensory disorders and can be a source of information and, in some cases, can facilitate access to services and adaptive devices.

Interventions for Sensory-Perceptual Alterations. Disturbed sensory-perception is defined as "change in the amount or patterning of incoming stimuli accompanied by a diminished, exaggerated, distorted, or impaired response to such stimuli" (North American Nursing Diagnosis Association [NANDA], 2005, p. 172) Sensory-perceptual alterations include sensory deprivation, sensory overload, and sensory distortion.

Difficulty in accurately processing sensory stimuli is further compounded if the patient is cared for in a place where environmental stimulation is minimal, because hypostimulation may lead to further deterioration of central processing abilities. Hospital and nursing home environments contain many unfamiliar sensory experiences for the older patient. Odors, noises, sights, textures, routines, and activity patterns are all different from those experienced at home. This applies especially to persons with preexisting dementia or perceptual deficits, who have increased difficulty interpreting new stimuli. There is great potential for reduced relevance of stimulation, predisposing to disturbed sensory-perception In addition, the intensity of stimulation in hospitals is typically quite high: many caregivers, around-the-clock noise, many questions and procedures, and disruptions in habit patterns, resulting in a high likelihood of sensory overload and associated adverse outcomes. In the nursing home and at home, sensory deprivation is more likely to be the predominant problem.

The pace of activity is slower and more routine, and stimulation may be less varied, producing monotony. All predispose to sensory deprivation.

Disturbances in one sensory modality also may affect function of other modalities. For example, vision plays a role in kinesthesia because of central connections between the visual apparatus and the vestibular system. In visual impairment, the sense of balance and position in space is affected, and adaptations must be made for safe locomotion to take place. Older people are at high risk for both sensory deprivation and distortion because of the high prevalence of disorders that influence sensory function in old age.

Interventions for Chemosensory Loss (Taste, Smell).

Taste and smells can be enhanced through the liberal use of spices and condiments, attractive food preparation, and food served at the appropriate temperature. Attention to oral health can remove some factors that influence taste. Good oral hygiene and regular dental care are recommended. Artificial saliva preparations are helpful with xerostomia. Chlorhexidine mouthwash reduces salty or bitter dysgeusia (Doty & Bromley, 2004). Persons with olfactory dysfunction who live independently should have smoke alarms. Leftover food should be discarded if not eaten within a few days so the older person does not consume spoiled food.

Social interactions can include varied scents, such as cosmetic-sharing parties, thematic food tastings, flower arranging, and wheelchair gardening. The clinician or volunteer should draw attention to the scent or taste during the activity. Varying the smells and tastes available in both institutional settings and home care settings should be a conscious effort. Although much of the sensory stimulation literature emphasizes group intervention, nurses have many opportunities to focus an older patient's attention on a taste or smell that may help stimulate further sensory exploration or reminiscence. For example, when serving a cognitively impaired patient medication with juice, the conversation might touch on the flavor of the juice and whether the taste evokes any special memories.

When chemosensory loss is attributed to drug therapy, discontinuing the offending drug may solve the problem. In some cases, however, the drug effects may linger for months after the drug is stopped. Also, the problem may be caused by the condition for which the patient is receiving a drug, in which case stopping the drug may actually worsen the symptom. Based on the hypothesis that some medications deplete tissue-bound zinc, supplemental zinc and multivitamins may produce some improvement. Avoidance of environmental toxins including cigarette smoke may be helpful (Doty & Bromley, 2004).

Interventions for Vision Loss.

Early identification of vision disorders provides the best chance for optimal treatment results. It is important, therefore, that older people have ready access to eye care professionals to obtain routine assessment for glaucoma, cataracts, and the diverse other eye diseases that affect older persons. Teaching older people and their family members about the possibilities for treatment of visual disorders is an important nursing function, along with coordinating referrals. Unfortunately, reimbursement for routine eye examinations and refraction to fit eyeglasses is not currently available under Medicare. However, treatment for diseases of the eye is reimbursed under Medicare; therefore treatment of pathological conditions is affordable by many.

For the visually impaired, visual aids and environmental adaptations can be extremely helpful. Eyeglasses and contact lenses can provide dramatic improvements in visual acuity, particularly for aphakic patients. However, they are of no use unless they are worn as prescribed. Unfortunately, it is commonplace to find eyeglasses in the bedside tables of older patients in hospitals and nursing homes. Nurses should know which patients require eyeglasses and be vigilant in making sure they are regularly cleaned and used.

Contact lenses are being used more often in people of all ages. Nurses should know how to insert, remove, and care for contact lenses, so that if the patient lacks the manual dexterity or mental ability to care for the lenses properly the problem can be identified and a compensatory system developed. Good handwashing is essential before handling the lenses. Follow the specific instructions for lens removal, insertion, cleaning, and disinfection recommended by the patient's eye care professional. Eye prostheses usually require removal once each day to cleanse the eye socket and then can be replaced immediately. Nurses should be prepared to function in an advocacy role for demented individuals. The fact that an older person has a cognitive impairment should not preclude treatment of visual disturbance. Sensory-perceptual disturbances are likely to exacerbate the patient's confusion and therefore should be treated as aggressively as in any other patient.

Modification of the environment requires creativity and familiarity with available resources (for example, the *Lighthouse International* catalogue, available at www.thelighthousecatalog.com). Two basic principles facilitate visual perception for all people and should be incorporated when possible into the physical environments of older people: use of adequate lighting intensity and use of color. People over age 60 years require twice the illumination for close tasks as people aged 20 years. However, with increasing lighting intensity the problem of glare should be considered. Glare occurs when the peripheral field is much darker than the central field, or when the eyes pass from a darkened area to a greatly illuminated area. Factors that create glare include lighting that is not diffuse and shiny surfaces, such as floors, magazine paper, and walls with glossy paint. Older people and health care administrators should be counseled on the need for bright, indirect environmental lighting.

Color contrast can be used quite effectively to provide cues for people with poor vision and to reduce the monotony of the environment. Monochromatic color schemes are to be avoided, such as white plates on a white placemat or gray chairs on gray carpeting, as the older person may have difficulty discriminating the borders of the plate or the chair, leading to embarrassment or injury. Use of black borders or of contrasting colors, such as red and yellow, will enhance the visual capacity of the older person.

For individuals with some intact visual function, large-print materials—books, periodicals, patient education materials, clocks, calendars, and telephone dials —are examples of useful environmental modifications. Safety considerations, including sufficient time to adapt, night lights, color borders on steps, increased caution or even a decrease in night driving, and medication assessment, are also important. Regardless of the extent of the visual impairment, caregivers should be cautioned not to move objects in the visually impaired person's environment without warning; to do so impairs the older person's independent function and may precipitate an accident. Individuals who are completely without vision should have the opportunity to receive the services of specialists in visual rehabilitation. Sometimes blind people will need to develop a relationship with others who can assist with tasks such as grocery shopping, bill paying, and transportation. If the individual has disabilities in addition to blindness and demonstrates difficulty in managing simple self-care tasks, use of a paid companion or institutionalization may be warranted.

Interventions for Hearing Loss. For talking with hearing-impaired people, the rate of speech should be moderate, and the volume should be even throughout each sentence. Take care to articulate words clearly, especially consonants. Do not shout but try to lower the pitch of your voice. Loudness can be irritating because it induces recruitment of sound. Face the individual so that your lip movements and facial expressions can be seen. Many people read lips without realizing it. The use of gestures and body language gives visual clues to the conversation. If the older person expresses difficulty in understanding a sentence, try rephrasing it rather than repeating the same words. Rephrase content and verbal cues when changing subjects.

If a hearing aid is used, be certain that it is in place, turned on, and in working order. In addition to hearing aids, handheld assistive hearing devices can be used for many patients within a facility or a clinic.

Where available, a stethoscope can be a handy amplifier. Place the earpieces in the patient's ears and speak into the diaphragm. Visual cues may be used as substitutes for auditory cues, such as lights that signal the telephone ringing or someone at the door. Trained assist dogs are taught to respond to certain auditory cues, and in turn alert the hearing-impaired person.

Modify the environment to promote hearing ability in those with presbycusis or other hearing impairments. Eliminate background noise as much as possible before trying to communicate. Focus on the most common sources, such as the television set, radio, air conditioners, fans, people talking in the next room, or rattling of cutlery at a meal. It may be necessary to go to a different room if background noise cannot be adjusted. Some people have such severe hearing impairments that verbal communication becomes nearly impossible. Written communication may be the only alternative.

Residential facilities where hearing-imparied persons live should have light-signal devices for fire alarms, smoke detectors, room doorbells, telephones, and alarm clocks. Closed captioning for the television is helpful. A communication board for basic needs or a staff member fluent in American Sign Language for interpretation of more complex information is also indicated.

Impacted cerumen is common among nursing home residents. Older people should be taught or assisted to clean the ear canal correctly to remove wax accumulations. The ear canal should never be gouged with cotton swabs, bobby pins, or other objects that can harm the external auditory canal or the tympanic membrane. Over-the-counter eardrops, such as Cerumenex or Debrox, can be used as directed, followed by lavage to remove the cerumen and the medication (prolonged instillation of the drugs can cause severe external otitis). Another safe and easy method is instillation of mineral oil into the ear canal for 24 hours, followed by gentle lavage with one part hydrogen peroxide to three parts water at room temperature.

INTERVENTIONS FOR KINESTHETIC DISTURBANCES. Immobilized patients are at most risk from kinesthetic deprivation and distortion. Regular exercise that carries the body parts through various planes stimulates proprioceptive and vestibular function. People who have been immobile for long periods of time may find such activity very anxiety provoking, because their position sense is impaired and they fear injury. Therefore, introduce exercise gradually, explain the rationale for the exercise, and reassure the patient about the safety measures being employed during the exercise session.

Interventions to Manage Pain. Numerous studies of pain prevalence and management in various settings report that therapy often is inadequate (Strohbuecker, Mayer, Evers, & Sabatowski, 2005; Visentin, Zanolin, Trentin, Sartori, & de Marco, 2005). This may be especially true with older persons. Interventions may be guided by misperceptions, such as older persons being less sensitive to pain, at increased risk for addiction to opioids, and unable to take opioid analgesics safely. Another problem is that some older people believe that pain is inevitable with aging and is meant to be endured. An important nursing intervention is to

Nursing Care Plan: The Older Adult with Vision Loss

Data

Mrs. Marion is a 75-year-old female with a diagnosis of atrophic macular degeneration. Her vision loss has progressed so that she is no longer able to read. She is proud of her ability to manage activities of daily living in the home where she has resided for 25 years with some help from her husband. When her husband was hospitalized after a stroke, Mrs. Marion's daughter invited her parents to stay in her home until both were able to manage in their own home. The home health nurse who visits Mr. Marion notices that Mrs. Marion sits quietly in a chair in front of the television. She answers only briefly when the nurse attempts to engage her in conversation. Her daughter frequently cautions her against doing anything that could lead to injury. She also reports that Mrs. Marion seems confused at times about time and place, and has to be prompted to initiate self-care activities. The daughter is concerned that her parents will never again be able to live independently in their own home.

Nursing Diagnoses (Johnson, Bulechek, Dochterman, Maas, & Moorhead, 2001)

Impaired adjustment related to vision impairment, relocation to unfamiliar setting, stress of husband's illness
Acute confusion related to sensory loss, unfamiliar environment, stress
Fear related to unfamiliar environment, sensory impairment

Goals/Outcomes

The patient will adapt to vision impairment in new environment as evidenced by resuming usual social and self-care activities.
The patient will remain oriented to person, place, and time in her new environment.
The patient will express increased confidence in her ability to manage in her new setting.

NOC Suggested Outcomes (Moorhead, Johnson, & Maas, 2004)

Coping
Motivation
Psychosocial adjustment: Life change
Cognitive orientation
Fear level

NIC Suggested Interventions (Dochterman & Bulechek, 2004)

Major interventions: Coping Enhancement (5230), Cognitive Stimulation (4720), Anxiety Reduction (5820), Environmental Management (6480)
- Create an atmosphere to facilitate trust.
- Orient to time and place.
- Talk to patient.
- Provide planned sensory stimulation.
- Assist the patient in developing an objective appraisal of the event.
- Provide the patient with factual information about diagnosis, treatment, and prognosis.
- Seek to understand the patient's perception of a stressful situation.
- Encourage gradual mastery of the situation.
- Encourage social and community activities.
- Arrange situations that encourage the patient's autonomy.
- Explore with the patient previous methods of dealing with life problems.
- Encourage verbalization of feelings, perceptions, and fears.
- Assist the patient in identifying appropriate short- and long-term goals.
- Assist the patient to grieve and work through the losses of chronic illness and/or disability.
- Remove environmental hazards.
- Place furniture in room in an appropriate arrangement that best accommodates patient disabilities.
- Place frequently used objects within reach.
- Bring familiar objects from home.

Evaluation Parameters

Adapts to life changes, identifies multiple coping strategies, verbalizes sense of control, reports decrease in stress, identifies current place, identifies correct day, plans for the future, develops an action plan, expresses belief in ability to perform action, maintains positive self-esteem, sets realistic goals, verbalizes optimism about present, uses effective coping strategies, expresses satisfaction with living arrangements (Moorhead, Johnson, & Maas, 2004)

educate the patient about the benefits of good pain control and the safe and appropriate use of analgesics. Opioids can be used safely by starting with low doses and gradually increasing them to achieve good pain control without excessive side effects.

Evaluation Parameters

Evaluation is made by ongoing measurement of the ability to carry out activities of daily living independently. This provides a good measure of visual and hearing capacity and adaptation to deficits. Other useful evaluation data include the effectiveness of communication and the use of safety measures. Successful adaptation to sensory losses also requires resolution of grief and formulation of a new, healthy body image.

SUMMARY

Sensory changes greatly affect the life of older people and can substantially alter the quality of life and independence once taken for granted. Normal age-related changes in vision include decreases in visual acuity, tolerance to glare, ability to adapt to dark and light, and decrease in peripheral vision. Presbyopia, the inability to accommodate for far and near vision, also is common. Disorders of the eye that occur frequently in older age include cataracts, glaucoma, senile macular degeneration, diabetic retinopathy, and senile entropion and ectropion.

Hearing loss is highly associated with aging. The three types of hearing loss are conductive, sensorineural, and central. Hearing loss for high frequencies is especially common, and older people often have difficulty distinguishing words spoken too fast. Presbycusis, which is frequently found in older age, produces bilateral loss of hearing acuity, and poor discrimination and comprehension. Tinnitus may occur with many different types of hearing disorders.

The senses of taste, smell, and touch are thought to diminish with older age; however, more studies are needed in these areas.

Nursing assessment and interventions are geared toward maximizing the ability to see, hear, taste, smell, and touch. Older people and their families should be taught to use more effective methods of communication and to use aids for communication, such as hearing aids and eyeglasses. These measures help to promote functional independence and well-being in older clients (Box 19-8).

BOX 19-8 *TOWARD BETTER SENSORY HEALTH*

Vision
- Protect eyes from sunlight.
- Keep hypertension and diabetes under control.
- Avoid smoking.
- Have annual eye examinations.
- Report changes in sensory function to care provider.
- Use medications for glaucoma as prescribed.

Hearing
- Protect the ears from extremely loud noise.
- Do not use an instrument to remove cerumen deep in the ear canal.
- Use drops to soften earwax followed by irrigation as prescribed.

REFERENCES

Ahmad, N., & Seidman, M. (2004). Tinnitus in the older adult. *Drugs Aging, 21*(5), 297-305.

American Speech and Hearing Association. (1996). Screening for hearing disorders—adults. Retrieved December 5, 2005, from www.asha.org.

American Speech-Language-Hearing Association. (1997-2005). The prevalence and incidence of hearing loss in adults. Retrieved December 4, 2005, from www.asha.org.

Anand, V., Buckley, J. G., Scally, A., & Elliott, D. B. (2003). Postural stability changes in the elderly with cataract simulation and refractive blur. *Investigative Ophthalmology & Visual Science, 44*(11), 4670-4675.

Asbell, P. A., Dualan, I., Mindel, J., Brocks, D., Ahmad, M., & Epstein, S. (2005). Age-related cataract. *Lancet, 365,* 599-609.

Assal, F., & Cummings, J. L. (2003). Neurological signs in old age. In R. C. Tallis & H. M. Fillit (Eds.), *Brocklehurst's textbook of geriatric medicine and gerontology* (6th ed.). London: Churchill Livingstone, pp. 541-548.

Babizhayev, M. A., Deyev, A. I., Yermakova, V. N., Brikman, I. V., & Bours, J. (2004). Lipid peroxidation and cataracts: *N*-Acetylcarnosine as a therapeutic tool to manage age-related cataracts in human and in canine eyes. *Drugs in R & D, 5*(3), 125-139.

Baloh, R. W. (2000). Hearing and equilibrium. In L. Goldman & J. C. Bennett (Eds.), *Cecil textbook of medicine* (21st ed.). Philadelphia: Saunders, 2250-2257.

Barkin, R. L., Barkin, S. J., & Barkin, D. S. (2005). Perception, assessment, treatment, and management of pain in the elderly (electronic version). *Clinics in Geriatric Medicine, 21*(3), 465-490.

Beltone Electronics. (1987). *The better hearing book.* Chicago: Beltone.

Borger, P. H., van Leeuwen, R., Hulsman, C. A., Wolfs, R. C., van der Kuip, D. A., Hofman, A., & de Jong, P. T. (2003). Is there a direct association between age-related eye diseases and mortality? The Rotterdam Study. *Ophthalmology, 110*(7), 1292-1296.

Brodie, S. E. (2003). Aging and disorders of the eye. In R. C. Tallis & H. M. Fillit (Eds.), *Brocklehurst's textbook of geriatric medicine and gerontology* (6th ed.). London: Churchill Livingstone, pp. 735-747.

Burton, M. J., & Doree, C. J. (2003). Ear drops for the removal of ear wax. *Cochrane Database of Systematic Reviews, 3,* CD004400.

Chiu, C. J., Morris, M. S., Rogers, G., Jacques, P. F., Chylack, L. T., Jr., Tung, W., et al. (2005). Carbohydrate intake and glycemic index in relation to the odds of early cortical and nuclear lens opacities. *American Journal of Clinical Nutrition, 81*(6), 1411-1416.

Christen, W. G., Liu, S., Schaumberg, D. A., & Buring, J. E. (2005). Fruit and vegetable intake and the risk of cataract in women. *American Journal of Clinical Nutrition, 81*(6), 1417-1422.

Christen, W. G., Manson, J. E., Glynn, R. J., Gaziano, J. M., Sperduto, R. D., & Buring, J. E. (2003). A randomized trial of beta carotene and age-related cataract in U.S. physicians. *Archives of Ophthalmology, 121*(3), 372-378.

Clemons, T. E., Kurinij, N., & Sperduto, R. D. (2004). Associations of mortality with ocular disorders and an intervention of high-dose antioxidants and zinc in the Age-Related Eye Disease Study: AREDS Report No. 13. *Archives of Ophthalmology, 122*(5), 716-726.

Congdon, N., Broman, K. W., Lai, H., Munoz, B., Bowie, H., Gilbert, D., et al. (2005). Cortical, but not posterior subcapsular, cataract shows significant familial aggregation in an older population after adjustment for possible shared environmental factors. *Ophthalmology, 1112*(1), 73-77.

Corso, J. F. (1971). Sensory processes and age effects in normal adults. *Journal of Gerontology, 26*(1), 90-105.

Dochterman, J. C., & Bulechek, G. B. (Eds.) (2004). *Nursing interventions classification (NIC)* (4th ed.). St. Louis: Mosby.

Dodson, K. M., & Sismanis, A. (2004). Intratympanic perfusion for the treatment of tinnitus. *Otolaryngologic Clinics of North America, 37*(5), 991-1000.

Donald, I. P., & Foy, C. (2004). A longitudinal study of joint pain in older people. *Rheumatology, 43*(10), 1256-1260.

Doty, R. L., & Bromley, S. M. (2004). Effects of drugs on olfaction and taste. *Otolaryngologic Clinics of North America, 37*, 1229-1254.

Drain, C. B. D. (2003). *Perianesthesia nursing: A critical care approach* (4th ed.). St. Louis: Saunders.

Fay, A., & Jakobiec, F. A. (2000). Diseases of the visual system. In L. Goldman & J. C. Bennett (Eds.), *Cecil textbook of medicine* (21st ed.). Philadelphia: Saunders, pp. 2224-2235.

Ferrigno, L., Aldigeri, R., Rosmini, F., Sperduto, R. D., & Maraini, G. (2005). Associations between plasma levels of vitamins and cataract in the Italian-American Clinical Trial of Nutritional Supplements and Age-Related Cataract (CTNS): CTNS Report #2. *Ophthalmic Epidemiology, 12*(2), 71-80.

Gerdle, B., Bjork, J., Henriksson, C., & Bengtsson, A. (2004). Prevalence of current and chronic pain and their influences upon work and healthcare-seeking: A population study. *Journal of Rheumatology, 31*(7), 1399-1406.

Gohdes, D. M., Balamurugan, A., Larsen, B. A., & Maylahn, C. (2005, July). Age-related eye diseases: An emerging challenge for public health professionals. *Preventing Chronic Disease: Public Health Research, Practice, and Policy, 2*(3), A17.

Goodhill, V. (1992). Evaluation of the aging ear. *Emergency Medicine, 24*(15), 165-166.

Guest, J. F., Greener, M. J., Robinson, A. C., & Smith, A. F. (2004). Impacted cerumen: Composition, production, epidemiology, and management. *QJM, 97*(8), 477-488.

Hand, C., & Harvey, I. (2004). The effectiveness of topical preparations for the treatment of earwax: A systematic review. *British Journal of General Practice, 54*(508), 862-867.

Hiller, R., Sperduto, R. D., Reed, G. F., D'Agostino, R. B., & Wilson, P. W. (2003). Serum lipids and age-related lens opacities: A longitudinal investigation: The Framingham Studies. *Ophthalmology, 110*(3), 578-583.

Hilton, M., & Stuart, E. (2004). Ginkgo biloba for tinnitus. *Cochrane Database of Systematic Reviews, 2*, CD003852.

Iliff, C. E., Iliff, W. J., & Iliff, N. T. (1979). *Oculoplastic surgery.* Philadelphia: Saunders, pp. 128, 136.

Jakobsson, U., Klevsgard, R., Westergren, A., & Hallberg, I. R. (2003). Old people in pain: A comparative study. *Journal of Pain and Symptom Management, 26*(1), 625-636.

Johnson, M., Bulechek, G., Dochterman, J. M., Maas, M., & Moorhead, S. (2001). *Nursing diagnoses, outcomes, & interventions.* St. Louis: Mosby.

Katz, B., & Helme, R. D. (2003). Pain in old age. In R. C. Tallis & H. M. Fillit (Eds.), *Brocklehurst's textbook of geriatric medicine and gerontology* (6th ed.). London: Churchill Livingstone, pp. 1392-1398.

Kline, D. W., Ikeda, D. M., & Schieber, F. J. (1982). Age and temporal resolution in color vision: When do red and green make yellow? *Journal of Gerontology, 37*, 705-709.

Kline, D. W., Kline, T. J., Fozard, J. L., Kosnik, W., Schieber, F., Sekuler, R., et al. (1992). Vision, aging, and driving: The problems of older drivers. *Journal of Gerontology, 47*, 27-34.

Koch, D. B., Staller, S., Jaax, K., & Martin, E. (2005). Bioengineering solution for hearing loss and related disorders (electronic version). *Otolaryngologic Clinics of North America, 38*(2).

Kuang, T. M., Tsai, S. Y., Hsu, W. M., Cheng, C. Y., Liu, J. H., & Chou, P. (2005). Body mass index and age-related cataract: The Shihpai Eye Study. *Archives of Ophthalmology, 123*(8), 1109-1114.

Lehne, R. A. (2004). *Pharmacology for nursing care* (5th ed.). St. Louis: Mosby.

Leveille, S. G., Zhang, Y., McMullen, W., Kelly-Hayes, M., & Felson, D. T. (2005). Sex differences in musculoskeletal pain in older adults. *Pain, 116*(3), 332-338.

Lichtenstein, M. J. (1992). Hearing and vision impairments. *Clinics in Geriatric Medicine, 8*(1), 173-182.

Malmstrom, J. (2005). Gerontologic nurse practitioner care guidelines: Assessing managing hearing deficits in the older adult. *Geriatric Nursing, 26*(1), 57-59.

Mangione, C. M., Phillips, R. S., Seddon, J. M., Lawrence, M. G., Cook. E. F., Dailey, R., et al. (1992). Development of the "Activities of Daily Vision Scale": A measure of visual functional status. *Medical Care, 30*(12), 1111-1126.

Margolis, E. M., Levy, B., & Sherman, F. T. (1981). Hearing disorders. In L. S. Libow & F. T. Sherman (Eds.), *The core of geriatric medicine.* St. Louis: Mosby, p. 20.

Mashiah, T. (1978). The effect of ageing on colour vision in females. *Age & Ageing, 7*, 114-115.

McNeil, J. J., Robman, L., Tikellis, G., Sinclair, M. I., McCarty, C. A., & Taylor, H. R. (2004). Vitamin E supplementation and cataract: Randomized controlled trial. *Ophthalmology, 111*(1), 75-84.

Moeller, S. M., Taylor, A., Tucker, K. L., McCullough, M. L., Chylack, L. T., Jr., Hankinson, S. E., et al. (2004). Overall adherence to the dietary guidelines for Americans is associated with reduced prevalence of early age-related nuclear lens opacities in women. *Journal of Nutrition, 134*(7), 1812-1819.

Moorhead, S., Johnson, M., & Maas, M. (2004). *Nursing outcomes classification (NOC)* (3rd ed.). St. Louis: Mosby.

National Academy on an Aging Society. (n.d.). Hearing loss: A growing problem that affects quality of life. Retrieved December 4, 2005, from www.agingsociety.org.

National Eye Institute. (2004). Statistics and data: Prevalence of blindness data. Retrieved November 15, 2005, from http://www.nei.nih.gov/eyedata/pbd_tables.asp.

National Institute on Deafness and Other Communication Disorders (NIDCD). (2004). Statistics about hearing disorders, ear infections, and deafness. Retrieved November 19, 2005, from www.nidcd.nih.gov/health/statistics/hearing/asp.

Nave, C. R., & Nave, B. C. (1985). *Physics for the health sciences* (3rd ed.). Philadelphia: Saunders.

Noell, C. A., & Meyerhoff, W. L. (2003). Tinnitus. Diagnosis and treatment of this elusive symptom. *Geriatrics, 58*(2), 28-34.

North American Nursing Diagnosis Association (NANDA). (2005). *Nursing diagnoses: Definitions and classification 2005-2006.* Philadelphia: NANDA International.

Nusbaum, N. J. (1999). Aging and sensory senescence. *Southern Medical Journal, 92*(3), 267-275.

Pavlidis, C., & Pickering, J. A. (2005). Water as a fast acting wax softening agent before ear syringing. *Australian Family Physician, 34*(4), 303-304.

Phillips, L. R. F. (1981). Care of the client with sensoriperceptual problems. In M. O. Wolanin & L. R. F. Phillips. *Confusion: Prevention and care.* St. Louis: Mosby.

Rich, L. F. (1990). Ophthalmology. In C. K. Cassel, D. E. Riesenberg, L. B. Sorensen, & J. R. Walsh (Eds.), *Geriatric medicine* (2nd ed.). New York: Springer-Verlag, pp. 394-404.

Royal National Institute for Deaf People (RNID). (2005). RNID: For deaf and hard of hearing people. Retrieved November 19, 2005, from www.rnid.org.uk/information_resources/aboutdeafness/statistics.

Rustoen, T., Wahl, A. K., Hanestad, B. R., Lerdal, A., Paul, S., & Miaskowski, C. (2004). Gender differences in chronic pain—findings from a population-based study of Norwegian adults. *Pain Management Nursing, 5*(3), 105-117.

Saloranta, K., & Westermarck, T. (2005). Prevention of cerumen impaction by treatment of ear canal skin. A pilot randomized controlled study. *Clinical Otolaryngology, 30*(2), 112-114.

Schele, H. G., & Albert, D. M. (1977). *Textbook of ophthalmology* (9th ed.). Philadelphia: Saunders.

Schow, R. L., & Nerbonne, M. A. (1982). Communication screening profile: Use with elderly clients. *Ear and Hearing, 3*, 135-147.

Schuler, M., Njoo, N., Hestermann, M., Oster, P., & Hauer, K. (2004). Acute and chronic pain in geriatrics: Clinical characteristics of pain and the influence of cognition. *Pain Medicine, 5*(3), 253-262.

Seiberling, K. A., & Conley, D. B. (2004). Aging and olfactory and taste function. *Otolaryngologic Clinics of North America, 37*, 1209-1228.

Seidman, M. D., & Babu, S. (2003). Alternative medications and other treatments for tinnitus: Facts from fiction. *Otolaryngologic Clinics of North America, 36*(2), 359-381.

Shega, J. W., Hougham, G. W., Stocking, C. B., Cox-Hayley, D., & Sachs, G. A. (2004). Pain in community-dwelling persons with dementia: Frequency, intensity, and congruence between patient and caregiver report. *Journal of Pain and Symptom Management, 28*(60), 585-592.

Shichi, H. (2004). Cataract formation and prevention. *Expert Opinion on Investigational Drugs, 13*(6), 691-701.

Smith, P. F., Zheng, Y., & Darlington, C. L. (2005). Ginkgo biloba extracts for tinnitus: More hype than hope? *Journal of Ethnopharmacology, 100*(1), 95-99.

Soares, J. J., Sundin, O., & Grossi, G. (2004). The stress of musculoskeletal pain: A comparison between primary care patients of various ages. *Journal of Psychosomatic Research, 56*(3), 297-305.

Strohbuecker, B., Mayer, H., Evers, G. C., & Sabatowski, R. (2005). Pain prevalence in hospitalized patients in a German university teaching hospital. *Journal of Pain and Symptom Management, 29*(5), 498-506.

Tallis, R. C., & Fillit, H. M. (Eds.), *Brocklehurst's textbook of geriatric medicine and gerontology* (6th ed.). London: Churchill Livingstone.

Thomas, E., Peat, G., Harris, L., Wilkie, R., & Croft, P. R. (2004). The prevalence of pain and pain interference in a general population of older adults: Cross sectional findings from the North Staffordshire Osteoarthritis Project (NorStOP). *Pain, 110*(1-2), 361-368.

Truscott, R. J. (2005). Age-related nuclear cataract—oxidation is the key. *Experimental Eye Research, 80*(5), 709-725.

Tsai, Y. F., Tsai, H. H., Lai, Y. H., & Chu, T. L. (2004). Pain prevalence, experiences and management strategies among the elderly in Taiwanese nursing homes. *Journal of Pain and Symptom Management, 28*(6), 579-584.

Ventry, I. M., & Weinstein, B. E. (1982). The Hearing Handicap Inventory for the Elderly: A new tool. *Ear and Hearing, 3*, 128-134.

Vernon, J. A., & Meikle, M. B. (2003). Masking devices and alprazolam treatment for tinnitus. *Otolaryngologic Clinics of North America, 36*(2), 307-320.

Visentin, M., Zanolin, E., Trentin, L., Sartori, S., & de Marco, R. (2005). Prevalence and treatment of pain in adults admitted to Italian hospitals. *European Journal of Pain, 9*(1), 61-67.

Voeks, S. K., Gallagher, C. M., Langer, E. H., & Drinka, P. J. (1993). Self-reported hearing difficulty and audiometric thresholds in nursing home residents. *Journal of Family Practice, 36*(1), 54-58.

Weinstein, B. E. (2003). Disorders of hearing. In R. C. Tallis & H. M. Fillit (Eds.), *Brocklehurst's textbook of geriatric medicine and gerontology* (6th ed.). London: Churchill Livingstone, pp. 749-761.

Zarit, S. H., Griffiths, P. C., & Berg, S. (2004). Pain perceptions of the oldest old: A longitudinal study. *Gerontologist, 44*(4), 459-468.

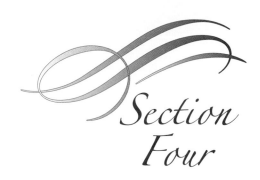

Section Four

Psychosocial Aging

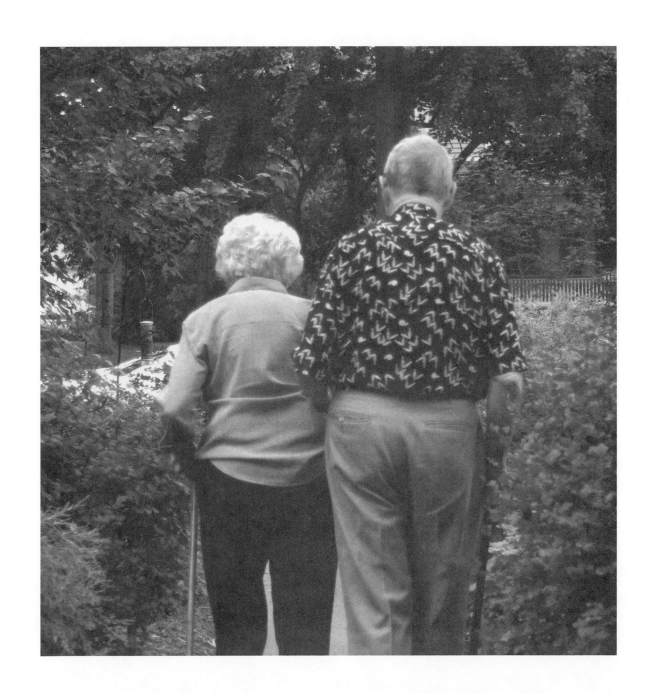

Chapter 20

Age-Related Psychological Changes

David W. Carroll & Adrianne Dill Linton

Objectives

Describe the normal psychological changes associated with aging.

Describe measures to maintain psychological health.

Explain the cause and management of psychological problems that are common in older persons.

Describe the components of the psychological assessment of the older adult.

Formulate nursing diagnoses for older persons with actual or potential psychological problems.

Develop plans to manage older adults with actual or potential psychological problems.

The separation of physical, social, and psychological dimensions of human beings is artificial, but it is useful as a framework for study. While focusing on the mind and mental processes, psychology helps us to understand many aspects of the human experience. This chapter provides an overview of psychological functioning in older persons by addressing personality, cognition, and attitudes. Mental disorders among older adults are discussed with emphasis on the special considerations in caring for older persons.

NORMAL AGING CHANGES

Refer to Box 20-1 for age-related psychological changes.

Personality

"Personality is the pattern of thoughts, feelings, and behaviors that shape an individual's interface with the world, distinguish one person from another, and manifest across time and situations. It is impacted by biological, cognitive, and environmental determinants" (Allen, Welsh, Willis, & Schale, 2003, p. 151). Models of personality development generally can be classified as "stage models," "trait models," or "social-cognitive approaches." The once popular developmental approach is less favored now than in the past.

Stage Models. Stage models or theories explain the growth of the personality as the individual moves through stages in a specific sequence. Among the stage model theorists are Freud, Jung, Loevinger, and Erikson. Several measurement issues have hampered the development and validation of the stage models. Like much other aging research, cross-sectional samples commonly are studied, making it difficult to separate the impact of aging from external influences on various cohorts. This field of study has limited standardized tools, lacks specification of change mechanisms, and challenges investigators to derive precise, testable hypotheses. Furthermore, studies of personality and growth and development have used mostly very select subjects so that older adults from diverse cultural and racial groups have not been well represented. Therefore the universality and generalizability of many findings are in question (Allen, Welsh, Willis, & Schale, 2003).

FREUDIAN THEORY. Freudian theory uses a psychoanalytical approach to personality development. It has limited application to personality in the older adult because Freud believed that personality development was complete by adolescence.

POST-FREUDIAN THEORISTS. Among the post-Freudian theorists whose work is more valuable in the study of older adults are Carl Jung, Jane Loevinger, and Erik Erikson. Jung proposed that adults gradually achieve balance between their masculine and feminine characteristics as they age. Loevinger identified six stages of personality development in adults: conformist, conscientious-conformist, conscientious, individualistic, autonomous, and integrated. Factors that she believes influence development are character, interpersonal style, and conscious preoccupation. Erikson's stages of development progress from infancy to old age. For each stage, he defines specific tasks that the

---

$\curlyeqprec$ Box 20-1 *Age-Related Changes: Psychological*

Personality
- Balance between masculine and feminine characteristics (Jung)
- Moves toward being more conscientious, individualistic, autonomous, and integrated (Loevinger)
- Strive to achieve ego integrity versus despair (Erikson)
- Uses life review to define meaning of one's life
- Variability in stability of personality traits
- More present-orientation; decreased range of activities (Carstensen)
- Relatively stable self-concept
- Morale and emotional stability related to well-being
- Life satisfaction related to well-being, activity, independence, and adaptation

Cognition
- Stable locus of control
- Fluid intelligence thought to decline; crystallized intelligence to remain stable
- Intelligence scores correlate with educational level
- Diminished short-term memory; remote memory may be stable
- Less efficient processing, storage, and encoding of information

Learning
- Less able to attend to multiple tasks
- Distracted by extraneous stimuli

Wisdom, Creativity, and Attention
- Lower scores on tests of creativity
- Decreases output of creative work for many
- Sustained attention retained; selective and divided attention diminish
- Executive function decreases for abstract testing but is retained for real-life problem-solving
- Intact executive skills when assessed with real-life problems

Attitudes
- Most attitudes stable
- Paid work is valued
- Increasing acceptance of cohabitation without marriage
- Death
  - Death thoughts are relatively rare
  - Think of death as a process rather than a moment in time
- Religion and spirituality
  - Both religiousness and spirituality relate positively to well-being
  - Persons who are religious may have lower levels of depression
  - Religious activities provide spiritual and social support
- Health
  - Believe physical activity is beneficial
  - Enjoy leisure activities and volunteer work
  - General acceptance of physician authority
  - Satisfied with nonphysician primary care providers
  - Less likely to perceive need for mental health care
  - Generally positive about nutrition education
  - Perception of function health varies among cultures
- Attitudes toward sex highly variable

---

individual strives to achieve. According to Erikson, the adult from ages 25 to 65 years focuses on *generativity versus stagnation*. Individuals who resolve the tasks of this stage achieve generativity. They care about the next generation as demonstrated by sharing knowledge and talents in a generous way. Failure to resolve the tasks of this stage can lead to *stagnation*—a state of self-absorption. The developmental task after age 65 is *ego integrity versus despair*. This stage continues until death. Individuals who achieve ego integrity recognize the increasing nearness of death. They examine their lives and are able to find meaning in it. Failure to achieve ego integrity results in a sense of meaninglessness and despair (Allen, Welsh, Willis, & Schale, 2003).

LIFE REVIEW. *Life review* is a systematic cognitive-emotional process in which the older "individual thinks back across his or her life experiences and integrates disparate events into general themes" (Allen, Welsh, Willis, & Schale, 2003, p. 144). It may be that the physical, social, and other changes of old age activate life review. Life review is more than just storytelling; sifting through memories allows older persons to gain new understanding of their life experiences that helps to define the meaning of their lives (Silver, 2002). The concept of life review has been the subject of numerous studies. Whereas some investigators have uncovered themes of generativity and ego integrity, others have not.

LIFE SPAN APPROACH. Whitbourne and Connolly's life span approach, which emphasizes identity and the sense of self, is applicable to older persons. *Identity* refers to the developing sense of self, which serves as a schema for interpreting life experiences. Physical functioning, cognition, social relationships, and environmental experiences all are dimensions of identity. Underlying identity are the constructs of *scenario* (expectations for one's future life path) and *life story* (personal history). Incompatibilities between the scenario and the life story must be resolved by the individual. The development of identity occurs in the context of family relationships, work experiences, and life/cohort experiences. Whitbourne and Connolly (1999; cited in Allen, Welsh, Willis, & Schale, 2003) conclude that older adults respond to aging changes by cognitive reinterpretation of experiences that are at odds with their identity and by making behavioral changes in their identity. These adaptations allow the older person to age in a healthy manner.

The "possible selves" model also has a life span perspective. Possible selves are defined as aspects of the self that represent what a person could or would like to become, and what the individual fears becoming. They are believed to motivate and direct future behavior (Allen, Welsh, Willis, & Schale, 2003).

Trait Models. Trait approaches provide the basis for most of the current instruments designed to measure personality. Despite the use of various instruments, the results have been remarkably consistent in the identification of five "big" traits: neuroticism, extroversion, openness to experience, agreeableness, and conscientiousness. The Big Five Model describes personality in terms of individual differences in relation to those traits. Factor analysis of data obtained from self-report and peer or observer ratings have yielded the five broad domains of personality characteristics (Box 20-2).

The traditional belief that personality traits stabilize by age 30 does not have universal support. A

BOX 20-2 The Big Five Personality Traits

- Emotional stability versus neuroticism: anxiety, depression, emotional instability, self-consciousness, hostility, and impulsiveness versus relaxation, poise, and steadiness
- Extroversion or surgency: gregariousness, assertiveness, activity level, and positive emotions versus silence, passivity, and reserve
- Culture/intellect or openness to experience: imagination, curiosity versus shallowness, imperceptiveness, and stupidity
- Agreeableness or pleasantness: attributes such as kindness, trust, and warmth that are considered pleasant and attractive to others versus hostility, selfishness, and distrust.
- Conscientiousness or dependability: encompasses organization, responsibility, ambition, perseverance, and hard work versus carelessness, negligence, and unreliability

Adapted from Goldberg, L. R. (1993). The structure of phenotypic personality traits. *The American Psychologist, 48,* 26-34. Copyright 1993 by the American Psychological Association. Adapted with permission.

---

meta-analysis of data from 152 longitudinal studies did find increasing rank order trait consistency from childhood to age 30. However, when rank order trait consistency was measured at standard intervals of 6.7 years, it plateaued between ages 50 and 70 (Roberts & Delvecchio, 2000). Evidence is building that personality traits do not stop changing at a specific point in life.

An interesting study conducted by Igier and Mullet (2003) assessed how five age-groups described personality traits of people by age. Given a list of 300 different adjectives, subjects indicated which they perceived applied to people of various ages. In this sample, participants perceived that conscientiousness increased linearly with age and openness decreased with age beginning in young adulthood; neuroticism was highest for adolescents and neutral for adults, the pattern for introversion scores was U shaped, and middle-aged adults scored lower than all others on agreeableness (Igier & Mullet, 2003).

Like other models, the trait model is plagued by measurement issues such as a predominance of cross-sectional studies. The personality traits of individuals over age 74 have received little attention. In addition, the impact of biological and environmental variables and social, historical, and life span-related influences on personality stability and change have not been fully explored (Allen, Welsh, Willis, & Schale, 2003).

Social-Cognitive Models. The social-cognitive approaches focus on the development of a sense of self through the interaction of internal and external factors.

The need for adaptive personality adjustments in response to maturational and cohort changes is stressed. The applicability of social-cognitive approaches to diverse cultural and racial/ethnic groups has not been studied adequately. Findings may be different among some groups, particularly those that have a more present time orientation. Some evidence exists that perceived limitation of remaining time may not be restricted to the end of life. It also may be related to important anticipated sociocultural changes (Allen, Welsh, Willis, & Schale, 2003).

Using data from the Berlin Aging Study, Lang, Rieckmann, and Baltes (2002) assessed the impact of sensorimotor-cognitive and social-personality resources on functioning in everyday life. Older persons who were rich in social-personality resources used more selection, compensation, and optimization in everyday function than those who were considered resource poor.

"AINTEGRATION". Lomranz (1998; cited in Allen, Welsh, Willis, & Schale, 2003, p. 149) takes a different approach with the concept of *aintegration,* which is described as "intra-individual differences in the need for personal consistency." Lomranz contends that the integration of various biopsychosocial levels is not essential to well-being. This notion is significant to gerontologists because the concept of aintegration may be linked to resiliency, a trait that is seen as a strength in aging.

SOCIO-EMOTIONAL SELECTIVITY. Carstensen's socio-emotional selectivity theory is especially relevant to older adults. According to this theory, social motives are directed either toward knowledge acquisition or the regulation of affect (Carstensen, Isaacowitz, & Charles, 1999; cited in Allen, Welsh, Willis, & Schale, 2003). Which of these takes priority depends on the individual's perceived time left in life. The healthy younger person perceives much time ahead and therefore prioritizes activities that lead to knowledge acquisition. Older persons and individuals who face a shortened life span perceive a shortened time of life and prefer to optimize their social networks. They may decrease their range of interests and activities, let go of casual acquaintances, and invest in the social relationships that they believe will be reciprocal and have positive affective outcomes. Carstensen's theory is consistent with findings that older adults tend to be more present oriented than young adults.

Stability of Personality. It long was thought that personality traits become stable by age 30. Stereotypical views of personality and aging are reflected in comments such as "older people are rigid and grouchy." It sometimes is said that personality traits just become exaggerated as a person ages. In an effort to confirm or disprove this perception, numerous studies have addressed

stability of personality. Based on three cross-sectional studies, Caprara, Caprara, and Steca (2003) concluded that personality functioning does not necessarily decline in late adulthood, although a greater decline was seen in men than in women, particularly for emotional stability and self-efficacy beliefs.

The Victoria Longitudinal Study provided data on personality traits in 223 adults ages 55 to 85 years. Findings confirmed significant stability over a 6-year period, as well as unique evidence of significant individual differences in late adulthood (Small, Hertzog, Hultsch, & Dixon, 2003). The Normative Aging Study extended over 12 years and studied personality trait trajectories for extroversion and neuroticism in adults. Considerable variability was found in personality trajectories, with extroversion defined by a linear model and neuroticism by a quadratic decline in age. Variables that predicted individual differences included birth cohort, marriage or remarriage, death of a spouse, and memory complaints (Mroczek & Spiro, 2003).

The impact of major changes in health and life circumstances in later life was assessed in a longitudinal study of personality stability in older women (mean age 80 years). Data analysis revealed moderate stability in neuroticism, extroversion, and openness; however, negative occurrences influenced trait stability. Increased neuroticism was associated with decreased social support and increased unmet needs. Extroversion decreased with poorer health and greater psychosocial needs. Openness was affected least by life circumstances. The investigators reconciled their findings with other data supportive of trait stability by viewing personality development within an interaction framework (Maiden, 2003).

The California Psychological Inventory was administered multiple times between ages 21 and 75 to assess normative personality change in two cohorts over 40 years. The results showed much quadratic change and much individual variability. Both period of life and social climate were identified as factors in change. For example, during the peak years of the culture of individualism, scores for responsibility were low. During the middle years, scores on dominance and independence peaked. These findings were inconsistent with beliefs that personality changes little after age 30 (Ravenna, Jones, & Kwan, 2002).

Personality development was assessed over a 30-year period in 78 women. From young to middle adulthood, subjects increased in dominance. Femininity/masculinity increased, and then decreased. Changes in both dominance and femininity/masculinity were associated with life events such as divorce and paid employment (Roberts, Helson, & Klohnen, 2002).

As the time of life after the middle years increases, it is useful to consider that "old age" encompasses several substages. A study that assessed personality traits (e.g., sensitivity, radicalism) and states (e.g., fatigue, depression) of German centenarians, octogenarians, and sexagenarians found differences among the age-groups. Centenarians scored higher than the other groups in suspiciousness but lower in intelligence and stress. Sexagenarians scored higher than octogenarians in arousal, intelligence, dominance, and conscientiousness, and lower on regression. In a follow-up study, centenarians were the least stable of the age-groups, with lower scores for sensitivity but higher scores for radicalism, fatigue, and depression. Changes in the younger groups were increased sensitivity and suspiciousness (Martin, Long, & Poon, 2002).

Personality and Self-Concept. Self-concept is a component of personality that can be viewed as an attitude toward the self. Personality type appears to influence self-concept and adaptation to role transitions such as widowhood or retirement. Research supports the notion of a relatively stable self-concept through the life span, with life events more than the aging process itself affecting self-concept. Research related to personality traits and self-concept indicates that individuals can maintain continuity and coherence in the course of adult life. People who are happy and well adjusted in early adulthood are likely to remain so in later life.

Holahan (2003) investigated stability and change in self-appraisal from 1960 to 1996 among subjects in the Terman Study of the Gifted. At the final data collection point, the average age of participants was 85 years. In general, the two ratings were similar, and the net change reflected a positive view of aging. Positive self-appraisals were associated with better education, better self-rated health in midlife, higher-level occupations, and greater satisfaction with achievements in early aging. Current life satisfaction was related to self-appraisal in later life.

Personality and Health. Various aspects of the relationship between personality and health have been explored. The work of Gerend, Aiken, and West (2004) examined personality factors and perceived susceptibility to diseases of aging in women ages 40 to 86 years. General perceived susceptibility was predicted by affect-related personality traits (neuroticism, extroversion, optimism, worry, and self-deceptive enhancement) and internal and chance locus of control. The investigators concluded that the link between personality traits and perceived risk may be mediated by cognitive heuristics, specifically the perceived similarity to those who contracted specific diseases.

Negative emotions and stressful experiences can stimulate the production of proinflammatory cytokines, which have been linked to a variety of conditions, including cardiovascular disease, osteoporosis, arthritis, type 2 diabetes mellitus, Alzheimer's disease, periodontal disease, frailty, functional decline, prolonged

infection, and delayed wound healing (Kiecolt-Glaser, McGuire, Robles, & Glaser, 2002). This has powerful implications for nursing because of the opportunity to decrease health risks by stress management and interventions to reduce negative emotions.

Personality and Intelligence. The Wechsler Adult Intelligence Scale—Revised (WAIS-R) and Revised Personality Inventory was administered to 100 individuals 75 years and older. From the personality inventory, openness to experience was a weak, but the best, predictor of intelligence scores. Additional study is required to confirm these findings (Saggino & Balsamo, 2003).

Personality and Quality of Life. Life satisfaction is an attitude toward one's own life; it may be defined as a reflection of feelings about the past, present, and future. Life satisfaction and morale are closely related to well-being. Evidence exists that various personality characteristics are related to various dimensions of quality of life. The work of Swedish investigators Hagberg, Hagberg, and Saveman (2002) found that vigor alone predicted current quality of life. Emotional stability was associated with psychological well-being and satisfaction with significant relationships. Optimism and the absence of psychosomatic symptoms were associated with ascendancy and the ability to maintain personal relationships. Psychosomatic symptoms increased with original thinking and sociability. A negative correlation was found between sociability and satisfaction with personal relationships.

Cognition

Cognition is the process by which sensory input is transformed, reduced, elaborated, stored, and retrieved. Memory, learning, and attention all are aspects of cognition that have complex relationships. Memory is essential to cognition; it involves the mental processes of retaining information for later use and retrieving such information. *Learning* is defined as the acquisition of information, skills, and knowledge measured by an improvement in some overt response. Learning depends on memory, and both memory and learning depend on attention. *Attention* is defined as the mechanisms by which we prepare to process stimuli, focus on what to process, and determine how far it will be processed and whether it should call us to action. Deficits in attention may affect learning and memory (Birren and Schaie, 1990; Sugar & McDowd, 1992; Whitbourne & Sperbeck, 1981). Cognition, learning, memory, and attention all can be affected by age-associated changes.

The extent to which cognitive changes occur because of age alone versus physiological or psychosocial variables is a topic of debate. Using data from the Victoria Longitudinal Study, investigators derived a biological age for older adults based on visual and auditory acuity, peak expiratory flow rate, blood pressure, grip strength, and body mass index. Cognitive domains, including verbal processing speed, working memory, reasoning, episodic memory, and semantic memory, were assessed at 3-year intervals over 12 years. Changes were examined in relation to both chronological and biological age. Biological age was found to be an independent predictor of actual cognitive change in older adults, thus suggesting that cognitive decline is likely due to causal factors other than chronological aging (MacDonald, Dixon, Cohen, & Hazlitt, 2004).

Survey data from the National Longitudinal Study of Older Men were used to assess the associations between psychosocial experience over the life course and cognitive function. Among the findings were that locus of control is highly stable over time, unlike affect, which fluctuates between positive and negative. Cognitive function had an inverse relationship with external locus of control, enduring negative affect, and the absence of positive affect. Level of education was a moderating factor, with low educational attainment appearing to enhance the risk for poor cognitive function (Wight, Aneshensel, Seeman, & Seeman, 2003). A study of brain aging in normal Egyptians had produced similar findings. Advancing age and lower levels of education emerged as risk factors for cognitive decline in normal aging (Elwan et al., 2003).

Perhaps not surprisingly, cognitive decline has been associated with the loss of relationships with friends and neighbors. The number of potential supporters has been shown to increase when a person's physical status declines; in contrast, the number is more likely to decrease when a person has cognitive decline (Aartsen, van Tilburg, Smits, & Knipscheer, 2004).

Intelligence. Wechsler (1971) defined *intelligence* as the "ability to perceive relationships between things, regardless of substance; to recognize and recall what has been perceived, to think logically and to plan." Cattel (1963) further defined intelligence as either fluid or crystallized. *Fluid intelligence* is the integration of neuroanatomical functioning that is used to solve novel problems for which no previous knowledge provides the solution; it has been correlated with performance subtests on the WAIS-R. *Crystallized intelligence*, which is the assimilation of learning and experience, has been associated with verbal subtests. It is determined on the basis of acquired knowledge and cannot be "figured out."

Studies of aging and intelligence have described a classic aging curve, which represents rising intelligence test scores through childhood that peak in the late teens, plateau, and decline in the sixties. This pattern has been consistent over many years of study, the only real difference being that earlier studies indicated that

the decline began in the late twenties or early thirties. Stuart-Hamilton (2003) contends that the classic aging curve is an overly simplistic description of aging and intelligence for three reasons. First, the curve applies only to the number of questions answered correctly (raw score). The raw score needed for a specific intelligence quotient (IQ) score varies for different ages. An IQ score is derived by measuring a person's cognitive status in relation to the rest of her or his age group. Although the mean score may decline with age, the extent of change is quite variable. A person's IQ score generally remains about the same throughout life. A person who is in the upper or lower percentile likely will remain in that same percentile. Stuart-Hamilton's (2003) second point is that many studies of cognitive aging look at performance (the end result of cognitive function) on standardized intelligence tests whereas others focus on the *process* of cognitive functioning with no concern for performance. His third, and last, point is that most intelligence tests assess aptitude rather than knowledge. Because much of what the older person knows is based on experience and education, a relatively large component of the older adult's mental life and abilities will be discounted. The history of today's older adults compared with that of today's young persons, who have had more educational opportunities, more access to information, better health care, and so on, should also be considered before deciding that the older cohort is less intelligent. Consideration of cohort effects, though difficult to accomplish, generally mitigates age differences (Stuart-Hamilton, 2003).

Many issues revolve around the measurement of intelligence, particularly in older adults. The validity of intelligence test scores may be questioned because of the nature and content of the instruments used. For example, the WAIS test originally was developed as an aid in placing children in appropriate academic settings and measuring skills emphasized in educational settings (Watson, 1982). The items on the test are not relevant to the everyday functioning of average older adults and therefore have little value in predicting the success with which they can manipulate their environment. Demming and Pressey (1957) attempted to overcome this validity problem by measuring intellectual functioning according to the ease of using telephone directories, understanding common paralegal concepts, and securing essential social services. It was found that middle-aged and older adults scored higher on tests measuring everyday tasks but continued to score lower on standard IQ tests. When tests are relevant to everyday functioning of older adults, some studies have shown that intelligence does not decrease with age.

Intelligence tests generally do not allow for physical conditions that might affect the outcome. Health status can play an important role in influencing IQ test scores. Many older persons have visual, hearing, or motor problems that affect their ability to read adequately and respond appropriately to the test items. Older people with one or more chronic illnesses may tire easily or not feel well on the testing day, so that one set of test scores may be unreliable. In addition, health problems that affect cognitive functioning may affect test scores.

Another factor that complicates interpretation of intelligence scores is that intelligence tests may be measuring fluid intelligence, crystallized intelligence, or both. Older persons typically demonstrate a decline in fluid intelligence; however, crystallized intelligence generally is preserved or improved (Hagberg, Bauer Alfredson, Poon, & Homma, 2001; Stuart-Hamilton, 2003). Numerous factors might account for this difference. Fluid, but not crystallized, intelligence has been found to correlate positively with physical health. Interpretation of these findings must consider that fluid tests often are timed and may require manual dexterity, putting the older person with motor or visual problems at a disadvantage. Tasks that require rapid responses commonly are more difficult for older persons.

One interesting finding in longitudinal studies has been a phenomenon referred to as *terminal drop* in which a rather abrupt decline in abilities predicted an individual's death within a few months after the last testing session (Stuart-Hamilton, 2003).

Another concern in assessing changes in intelligence with aging is the fact that most studies rely on cross-sectional data, which can be colored by cohort effects. Because the reported changes in measures of intelligence occur so gradually, a longitudinal study would seem to be the answer. However, measuring changing intelligence over multiple decades would be very expensive and fraught with practical problems. Even longitudinal studies would not resolve the problem of cohort effect because it cannot be said that a different group of individuals would demonstrate the same pattern of change. The solution would be an overlapping longitudinal study in which several age-groups are followed longitudinally. It was this kind of study that revealed that appreciable cognitive decline typically occurs in the midsixties, rather than the twenties to thirties as previously thought (Stuart-Hamilton, 2003). One other consideration is that subjects in longitudinal studies frequently are relatively healthy volunteers who are most able to participate in the studies over a long period of time.

Because most older persons have had less education than the young, and studies have shown that educational levels are positively correlated with intelligence test scores, the comparisons among scores by age-group are not valid. Also, the types of tests used today are quite different from those that older adults have been accustomed to. Finally, testing procedures and extraneous influences can affect the outcome of IQ tests. The increase in reaction time, ubiquitous in the normal aging process, can have a profound influence on the performance test and timed test scores.

The issue of flaws in the measurement of intelligence aside, what might explain apparent age-related declines in intelligence in some people? The two primary factors that have been implicated are the general slowing hypothesis and the disuse theory. The general slowing hypothesis proposes that basic processes of intellectual activity are impaired by declining physiological functioning, including neural transmission. The slowed reaction time is used to illustrate this effect. Changes in the frontal lobes, which are involved in planning, memory, and sequential activity, also are implicated. The disuse theory applies the "use it or lose it" way of thinking. Evidence to support these theories is equivocal. It is likely that both play a role in explaining changes in intelligence. One additional factor that might be an influence in some individuals is the loss of interest in cognitively demanding activities (Stuart-Hamilton, 2003).

Memory. Change in memory attributed to aging is a topic of concern, conversation, and humor. It commonly is said that a patient can describe the time he won a race in the fourth grade, but cannot recall what he had for breakfast. To what extent does the stereotype conform to reality? Like most other age-related changes, memory does decline, but to varying degrees among individuals. Also, memory is multidimensional, and some types are affected more than others. One classification describes the types of memory as short term or long term (Stuart-Hamilton, 2003).

SHORT-TERM MEMORY. Short-term memory, which is used to recall information that will need to be retained briefly (e.g., dialing a phone number that was just located in a directory), typically declines with age. This mental activity requires efficient information processing that is best accomplished without distractions. According to the working memory model developed by Baddeley and Hitch (1974), incoming information is processed by one mechanism for visuospatial material and another for verbal material. The information is forwarded from the working memory to long-term memory where a permanent memory trace can be formed with sufficient rehearsal. Factors that may contribute to diminished short-term memory in older persons include difficulty organizing incoming material, ineffective storage, and poor retrieval (Stuart-Hamilton, 2003).

LONG-TERM MEMORY. Long-term memory, which actually encompasses a set of skills concerned with various types of subject matter, is used to store material for longer periods of time. Long-term memory can be classified as autobiographical (life events), remote, semantic, implicit, or prospective. Regardless of age, when asked to produce a memory of some event, most adults report something that occurred in the past 10 years. When older memories are elicited, they most often are drawn from the period when the individual was 10 to 30 years of age ("reminiscence peak"). Autobiographical memory may remain intact; however, the quality of recall of such memories may decline. The accuracy of these old memories of personal experiences correlates with intelligence measures. One problem in assessing long-term memory is that there often is no one to corroborate the accuracy (Stuart-Hamilton, 2003).

A second type of long-term memory is remote memory, which covers events that occurred during a person's lifetime but were not part of the individual's personal history. To test remote memory, patients are asked if they recall specific "briefly famous" names or events from some point in their life. Although persons of all ages have better recall of more recent events, older persons typically perform as well as or better than younger persons in more remote material.

Older persons often perform well on tests of semantic memory and implicit memory tasks. Semantic memory is used to describe facts retained in memory that are independent of experience. No significant difference has been found in the quantity of facts retained, although the older person's retention and retrieval of newly learned material is less effective. Implicit memory is tested by asking a person to recall something presented earlier without prior notification that the information needed to be remembered. As long as the task is simple, there are no differences in results on the basis of age.

Prospective memory is used to maintain a memory of something that will or should occur in the future, such as a medical appointment or medication schedule.

Many older persons may demonstrate good prospective memory because their generation was taught to be punctual, or because their schedules are less full than those of younger persons. Interestingly, young people do perform better if the task is do something just a few minutes in the future, possibly because of the increased time required for the older person to process the information. Older persons' prospective memory also is negatively affected when the complexity of the tasks increases (Stuart-Hamilton, 2003).

Table 20-1 summarizes the components of memory and what is known about changes in older persons.

The decreased efficiency with which older persons process, store, and encode information probably results from multiple contributing factors. If memory stores can be thought of as physical space, that space is smaller. Material may be processed and stored incompletely, and retrieval may be slower and less accurate. These changes all can be explained by the general slowing of the nervous system. Memory traces may fade before storage occurs because of delays in processing and loss of neurons.

Memory complaints in older persons without manifest cognitive decline have been associated with physical health problems, depressive and anxiety symptoms, low feelings of mastery, low perceived self-efficacy, and high neuroticism. Based on these findings, it has been recommended that these individuals be assessed for psychoaffective and health problems (Comijs, Deeg, Dik, Twisk, & Jonker, 2002). In a study of anxiety disorder and subjective memory loss in older persons, Sinoff and Werner (2003) found both direct and indirect effects of anxiety on the prediction of future cognitive decline.

Table 20-1 *Changes in Memory with Aging*

Categories of Memory Skills	Changes with Age	Implications
TEMPORAL		
Short term: recall within 30 seconds	Small but significant decline; decline is greater when complexity of task increases Performance better on recognition tasks than recall tasks	Eliminate extraneous stimuli. Concentrate on one task at a time. Use notes, lists, mnemonics, etc. Method of loci strategy: picture a familiar scene and imaging objects representing ideas to be remembered placed prominently in the scene. Chunking: arrange items in small groups rather than long lists.
Long term	Autobiographical memory: may remain intact although the quality of those memories may decline Remote memory: remains intact Semantic memory: intact for quantity but may decline in retention and ease of retrieval Implicit memory: same for older and younger persons if task is simple Prospective memory: generally intact unless the task is complex	Distant personal events may be reported accurately; difficult to validate historical data. Long-term memory less accurate for more complex tasks. To promote retention of information, break into small steps. Simplify.

Further, path analysis revealed that the effect of memory loss on cognitive decline was via anxiety.

In another longitudinal study that examined memory loss of older persons, the investigators concluded that much memory loss may be attributed to the progression of preclinical dementia and other nonnormative processes rather than chronological age. No subjects were demented at the beginning of the study; however, 25% of the sample developed dementia during the course of the study. In the dementia group, virtually all of the memory loss was attributed to disease progression (Sliwinski, Hofer, Hall, Buschke, & Lipton, 2003).

Wisdom, Creativity, and Attention. Some important intellectual skills may not be assessed by usual measures of intelligence. These include wisdom, creativity, and attention. Wisdom, which refers to a pragmatic approach to problem solving, is not unique to older persons. Creativity is a type of divergent thinking that enables a person to devise novel and appropriate solutions. In contrast, intelligence tests measure convergent thinking that requires selection of a single "correct" answer. Older persons typically score lower than young persons on tests of creativity. The output of creative work decreases for most individuals when they reach their sixties. Certainly, this is not universal, and many older individuals remain creative throughout life. The differences may be explained by cohort differences in educational experiences. In decades past, education emphasized knowledge acquisition over creativity.

Attention is the ability to concentrate despite distractions. Attention can be further described as sustained, selective, or divided. Sustained attention is used by a radar observer who watches a screen for specific targets. Selective attention is required to seek a specific target in the midst of multiple distractors. Divided attention requires attending to more than one stimulus simultaneously. Sustained attention generally is retained by older persons, whereas selective attention (for both visual and auditory stimuli) and divided attention diminish.

Learning. In light of the cognitive changes that commonly occur with aging, what is known about the older person and learning? Not only is the older learner affected by the previously described changes, but the perception of information also can be affected by environmental influences, age-related sensoriperceptual changes, and pacing of instruction. Older people may be less motivated to learn and more threatened in a setting in which declining cognitive abilities may be publicly demonstrated. They may have difficulty attending to more than one task or topic at a time and may be distracted by extraneous stimuli. Impairments in vision and hearing can pose major barriers in the teaching-learning situation. Common visual problems in older adults include presbyopia (inability to focus the lens at various

distances), altered color perception (difficulty in distinguishing blues and greens because of a yellowing of the lens), diminished depth perception, decreased peripheral vision, slowed adaptation to dark and light, and poor tolerance for glare. Sensorineural hearing loss (presbycusis) affects mainly high frequencies and is often a barrier to communication in the elderly. Problems hearing consonants or high-pitched voices are a special concern, especially when unfamiliar material is presented. Background noises also interfere with hearing in a group setting, so that perception and processing of information are virtually impossible.

Interventions to Preserve Cognitive Function with Age. Interest is high in identifying variables that have a protective effect on cognitive function during aging. Among the variables that are being studied are literacy level, physical exercise, hormones, and nutrition. Some evidence exists that literacy skills have a protective effect against memory decline in nondemented older persons. In a longitudinal study of literacy level and cognitive skills in an ethnically diverse sample of older adults, the individuals with low literacy levels had a steeper decline in immediate and delayed word recall (Manly, Touradji, Tang, & Stern, 2003). However, a study of 3263 persons in the United Kingdom reflected that vocabulary scores did not change, whereas measures of fluid intelligence declined from age 49 to 92 years. The rate of age-related decline did not vary with gender, level of ability, or socioeconomic status (Rabbitt, Chetwynd, & McInnes, 2003).

The cognitive benefits of physical exercise among older persons have been shown to be domain specific. In the work of Woo and Sharps (2003), older adults who engaged in relatively high levels of exercise had better recall of verbal but not pictorial stimuli. Another study showed that individuals who were more physically active performed better on a test of fluid intelligence. However, when the data were entered into the hierarchical regression equation, 16% of the unique variance in intelligence test scores was explained by openness to experience (Lochbaum, Karoly, & Landers, 2002).

Despite high hopes, the Women's Health Initiative Memory Study failed to demonstrate that hormone therapy protected postmenopausal women against cognitive decline. In fact, the risk of cognitive decline actually increased in women over age 64 taking conjugated equine estrogens (Craig, Maki, & Murphy, 2005).

The benefits of good nutrition on both cognitive and physical function are apparent. Malnourished older persons have been found to have more impairment in cognition, function, and general well-being (Odlund, Koochek, Ljungqvist, & Cederholm, 2005). Attention now has turned to dietary patterns and specific nutrients that may play a role in enhancing brain function and reducing the risk of dementia. The Dietary

Approaches to Stop Hypertension (DASH) diet, which is rich in fruits, vegetables, and low-fat dairy products and low in saturated fat and sodium, may lessen the risk of vascular dementia by decreasing the risk of stroke. Indeed, a high dietary intake of saturated or trans-unsaturated fats and a low intake of nonhydrogenated unsaturated fats have been related to cognitive decline (Morris, Evans, Bienias, Tangney, & Wilson, 2004). Among the nutrients now being evaluated for their impact on cognitive function are the antioxidants vitamin C and E, ginkgo biloba, folate, beta carotene, selenium, and omega-3 polyunsaturated fatty acids. Additional clinical trials are needed for definitive answers about the cognitive benefits of these nutrients. Researchers at Rush Institute compared various forms of tocopherol for their protective effects against Alzheimer's disease. The rate of cognitive decline in the older participants was lowest in those who obtained tocopherol from multiple sources (Morris et al., 2005). The best recommendation at this time is a healthy diet with plenty of vitamins and minerals and appropriate calorie intake (Whalley, Starr, & Deary, 2004; Yen, 2003). U.S. Army researchers are interested in the effects on cognitive function of caffeine, carbohydrates, and the amino acids tryptophan and tyrosine. Whereas their motivation is to identify military applications, any other useful outcomes remain to be seen (Lieberman, 2003). Many questions remain unanswered in relation to diet and cognition function. If specific nutrients preserve or restore function, what form, source, and dose are optimal? If cognitive impairment is present at baseline, can nutritional therapy improve cognition?

Executive Function. Executive function enables a person to plan and execute activities. Pathological states such as Alzheimer's disease that impair executive function have significant impact on all aspects of daily life. Normal aging is associated with decreased executive skills as assessed by abstract neuropsychological tests. However, when presented with real-life-type problems, the problem-solving skills of older and younger individuals are comparable (Crawford & Channon, 2002). To determine the relationship between affect and executive function, executive function was assessed after a neutral, positive, or negative mood induction procedure. In this study, the older subjects were more impaired in planning than younger persons in both the negative and positive mood conditions (Phillips, Smith, & Gilhooly, 2002).

Developmental Tasks

The life span developmental theory is based somewhat on Erikson's psychosocial stage model of ego development. Erikson defined the task of older adulthood as ego integrity versus despair. The characteristics of ego integrity, which is not well defined, might include emotional integration, acceptance of the reality of death without fear, adaptation to changes in capacities, and ongoing meaningful connections with others (Glass, 2003). Developmental tasks of older persons are included in the earlier discussion of personality.

Life Satisfaction and Morale

Life satisfaction is an attitude toward one's own life; it may be defined as a reflection of feelings about the past, present, and future. Life satisfaction and morale are closely related to well-being. According to George (1991), life satisfaction is the cognitive assessment of well-being, and happiness is the affective assessment. The two major components of well-being—affect (happiness) and satisfaction (realized expectations)—may reflect a changing balance with age. Thus age-related declines in positive affect may be countered by increases in the sense of satisfaction with life accomplishments (Maddox, 1962).

Research has explored many variables in relation to life satisfaction. In one study, 15 individuals ages 80 to 94 were interviewed during and after a period of rehabilitation to obtain their perceptions of factors that affected their life satisfaction. The three major themes that emerged as important for life satisfaction from the interview data were activity, independence, and adaptation (Aberg, Sidenvall, Hepworth, O'Reilly, & Lithell, 2005). These same themes emerged from a survey of older whites and Japanese-Americans when Phelan, Anderson, LaCroix, and Larson (2004) assessed participant perceptions of successful aging. Responses were obtained from 717 Japanese Americans and 1173 whites with an average age of 80 years. The 13 most highly rated attributes were shared by the two groups (Box 20-3).

Some relationships between personality characteristics, well-being, and quality of life have been identified. A positive life orientation is associated with satisfaction with life, zest for life, having plans for the future, feeling needed, and seldom feeling lonely or depressed (Pitkala, Laakkonen, Strandberg, & Tilvis, 2004).

ATTITUDES

Attitudes are important determinants of behavior. It is thought that most attitudes are remarkably stable over the course of adulthood, and the older the individual, the more firmly attitudes are held. Attitudes are related to other psychological variables. For example, lowered mood is associated with a pessimistic attitude toward life, as well as cognitive impairment and impaired survival (Pitkala, Kahonen-Vare, Valvanne, Strandberg, & Tilvis, 2003).

Studies have shown that older and younger Americans share many attitudes and stereotypes about

BOX 20-3 Perceptions of Older White and Japanese American Adults Regarding Successful Aging: Items Rated Most Important for Successful Aging by 75% or More of Participants

- Remaining in good health until close to death
- Being able to take care of myself until close to the time of my death
- Remaining free of chronic disease
- Being able to cope with the challenges of my later years
- Being able to make choices about things that affect how I age, such as my diet, exercise, and smoking
- Having friends and family who are there for me
- Being able to meet all of my needs and some of my wants
- Being able to act according to my own inner standards and values
- Feeling good about myself
- Adjusting to changes that are related to aging
- Not feeling lonely or isolated
- Staying involved with the world and people around me
- Feeling satisfied with my life the majority of the time

Data from Phelan, E. A., Anderson, L. A., LaCroix, A. Z., & Larson, E. B. (2004). Older adults' views of "successful aging"—how do they compare with researchers' definitions? *Journal of the American Geriatrics Society, 52,* 211-216.

old age. In addition, many older people maintain attitudes about other "old people" that they do not apply to themselves. Many of the problems commonly associated with old age, such as loneliness, shrinking job opportunities, boredom, and lack of adequate medical care, actually occur in the same proportions in younger people as in older people. Two exceptions are poor health and fear of crime, which are more evident in the aged.

Much of the literature related to attitudes and older people is concerned with how younger people, health care providers, or society in general view aging. An encouraging study of psychologists' perceptions of older patients revealed slightly more positive attitudes about older patients than younger ones. Furthermore, the participants in this study were knowledgeable about aging and mental health issues of older adults. Younger psychologists were less likely than their older counterparts to make negative or discriminatory comments about older persons (Treadwell, 2003). A study of 1250 Swedes between ages 20 and 85 revealed generally positive attitudes toward physical aging and older persons, with equally positive views toward both older men and women (Oberg & Tornstam, 2003). Other studies have explored how older persons view aging. A large cohort of older Canadians was asked to define successful aging

and whether they thought they had aged successfully. The most frequent themes from their definitions of successful aging were related to health and disease (Tate, Lah, & Cuddy, 2003).

Work and Retirement

Ample evidence suggests that older people work in a competent manner, despite the prevailing stereotype that older workers are less competent. Past research has shown that the performance of older workers depends on the nature of the work being undertaken (Welford, 1984). In jobs with low physical demand, such as clerical work, older workers are more accurate and have steadier work output patterns; however, productivity can decline when jobs require significant physical exertion, such as manufacturing positions (Kelleher & Quirk, 1973). A study of hotel employees in Thailand sought to determine whether age and tenure are individual determinants of job satisfaction. The employee's age was not significantly associated with satisfaction, but tenure was. Tenure and facets of job satisfaction such as pay and fringe benefits were related; however, the effect of tenure on satisfaction was modified by age (Sarker, Crossman, & Chinmeteepituck, 2003).

By age 65, 16% to 18% of all men and 9.4% of all women remain in the labor force, either working or actively seeking work. A qualitative approach was used to explore the meaning that older women make of their work life. Fifty-three ethnically and economically diverse women ages 55 to 84 years made up the sample. The majority was Caucasian; others were Hispanics, African Americans, and Asians. Participants strongly valued their paid work for a number of reasons. Two themes that emerged were independence from men and lost dreams and regrets. Lost dreams and regrets were reflected in comments made by some who had not pursued their career goals because of cultural and family pressure into marriage. Some who came from poor and working-class families had not seen options other than marriage and motherhood for themselves when they were younger. Specific regrets voiced by some included having any or too many children and quitting school. Participants commonly reported pride in having instilled in their daughters the importance of preparing for a meaningful career. In the work world, these women's experiences varied, with some having experienced perceived discrimination on the basis of age and gender, and some being perceived and treated as a mother figure (positive in some cases; negative in others). It was clear that most of these women believed they worked above and beyond the call of duty (Altschuler, 2004).

Retirement from work is a relatively modern concept. Various patterns of retirement have been observed, with many individuals choosing to withdraw from the work world gradually or substituting volunteer activities as a source of fulfillment. Attitudes toward retirement and adjustment to retirement are influenced by preretirement lifestyles and values. Contrary to stereotypes, older retirees often are financially secure, satisfied with life, and claim good health (Hyde, Ferrie, Higgs, Mein, & Nazroo, 2004). However, many of today's older persons have worked almost all of their lives and it is an important part of their identity. When work is gone, some of them experience a profound sense of loss.

Table 20-2 summarizes historical events affecting work and retirement in the elderly.

Some employers offer retirement planning to assist individuals to make the transition to retirement. After the introduction of such a program for bank employees in Nigeria, their attitudes toward both retirement and preretirement education were assessed. The respondents anticipated retirement positively and cited advantages to preretirement education (Ogunbameru & Bamiwuye, 2004). In another study, persons in professional managerial positions who planned for retirement were compared with those who did not. Planning was found not to be related to depression and quality of life (Earl, 2005).

Relationships

Retirement affects not only the retiree, but also the significant other. Personal relationships may be realigned. Data pooled from Waves 1 to 4 of the Health and Retirement Surveys suggested that retirement transitions that enhance the partner's influence in the relationship reduce the satisfaction of married retirees. Retirees were found to be least satisfied when their spouses continued

employment and assumed greater responsibility in decisions (Szinovacz & Davey, 2005). The importance of the dyadic relationship is reinforced by the work of Schwarzer (2003), who found that positive dyadic coping of the partner predicted coping efforts and emotions of the retiree after 1 year.

A social phenomenon that seems to be increasingly common is cohabitation—residing together without marriage. Cohabitating older persons tend to view their relationships as an alternative to marriage, whereas younger couples more often see it as a trial period preceding marriage. Compared with younger cohabitants, older cohabitants report better quality and stability of relationships (King & Scott, 2005).

Death

Studies of attitudes about death reveal a complex, multidimensional concept. It is assumed that older persons, because they are closer to the end of life, think about death more often than younger people. It also is assumed that human beings fear death. How individuals view death probably varies with age because of differences in understanding and experience. "For many elderly individuals death is a process rather than a moment in time, resting on a need for balance between the technology of science and the transcendence of spirituality" (Proulx & Jacelon, 2004, p. 116). Some may be surprised to learn that death thoughts among mentally healthy older adults are relatively rare (DeLeo & Spathonis, 2003). Terror management theory asserts that the fear of death is buffered by self-esteem and beliefs about literal and symbolic immortality (Cicirelli, 2002).

Attitudes toward death are difficult to measure, because some people are reluctant to discuss their thoughts and fears about death and because different methods of measuring the concept can uncover different dimensions. Two tools that assess attitudes toward death are the Death Attitudes Profile—Revised (DAP-R) and the Multidimensional Fear of Death Scale (MFDS). The DAP-R and the MFDS illustrate the different concepts that tools might measure. The subscales on the DAP-R are Fear of Death, Death Avoidance, Approach Acceptance, Escape Acceptance, and Neutral Acceptance (Clements & Rooda, 2000; Gesser, Wong, & Reker, 1987). The MFDS has subscales such as Fear of the Unknown, Fear of the Dying Process, Fear of Conscious Death, and Fear for the Body after Death. It was used to explore death anxiety and attitudes in a group of 197 older men and women. Differences were found on some subscales on the basis of gender and race. Women's scores were higher on Fear of the Dead. Caucasians scored higher than African Americans on Fear of the Dying Process, and African Americans scored higher on Fear of the Unknown, Fear of Conscious Death, and Fear for the Body after Death (Depaola, Griffin, Young,

Table 20-2 Historical Events Shaping Attitudes toward Retirement and Work

Year	Event	Impact
1889	Germany: Old Age and Survivors Benefits Act	First nationalized pension plan, set 65 as retirement age
1908	Great Britain: similar	Set pensionable age at 70
1935	United States: Social Security Act	First nationalized pension system in the United States, pensionable age at 65
1967	Age Discrimination in Employment Act	Made age discrimination in places of employment illegal
1978	Amendments to Age Discrimination in Employment Act	Mandatory retirement age raised to 70

& Neimeyer, 2003). Individuals who expressed personal anxieties about aging and death were found to hold more negative attitudes toward other older adults. Cultural and ethnic differences in attitudes about death might be anticipated. However, when the MFDS was used to assess death attitudes among older whites and African Americans, Cicirelli (2000) found the two ethnic groups to be similar in relation to their strongest and weakest death fears. The sociocultural context of thoughts about death was illustrated in an ethnographic study of older Korean women who identified the following meanings attached to death: end of pain, dispersion of existence, moving to the next life by transcending the boundary, returning to the original place, and escalating into the world of the men's group (Shin, Cho, & Kim, 2005).

Communication about end-of-life preferences between older persons and their health care providers still needs improvement, as evidenced by the finding of investigators in the United Kingdom. Eighty persons over age 64 with acute heart failure were interviewed about their preferences when facing the last stages of their disease. Although only two individuals previously had expressed their wishes in regard to cardiopulmonary resuscitation (CPR), 40% did not wish to have CPR. In addition, only 41% expressed a desire for spiritual support (Formiga et al., 2004). Some similarities were found in a study of older terminally ill Finns who indicated they wanted active treatment and more conversations with their physicians about active care. They were reluctant to "trouble" caregivers with their needs because of the caregivers' heavy workload (Laakkonen, Pitkala, & Strandberg, 2004). When older people in the United Kingdom were queried about their preferred location for end of life, home was identified as the ideal location, but perhaps not the most appropriate. Participants cited concerns about the burden placed on family caregivers, questioned the quality of care that could be provided at home, and did not want intimate care to be provided by their children. Some saw the nurse in the home setting as intrusive (Gott, Seymour, Bellamy, Clark, & Ahmedzai, 2004). These findings emphasize the importance of determining, rather than assuming, the patient's wishes.

The expression "a good death" often is reported as a goal. The literature lists six themes of a good death: pain and symptom management, clear decision making, preparation for death, completion, contribution to others, and affirmation of the whole person (Bosek, Lowry, Lindeman, Burck, & Gwyther, 2003). A survey of seriously ill patients, recently bereaved families, physicians, and other health care providers sought to determine the factors that they considered important at end of life (Steinhauser et al., 2000). Box 20-4 lists the factors that

---

BOX 20-4 Factors Considered Important at End of Life

RATED IMPORTANT BY PATIENTS, FAMILIES, AND HEALTH CARE PROVIDERS	RATED MORE IMPORTANT BY PATIENTS THAN BY PHYSICIANS	INCONSISTENT RATINGS WITHIN AND AMONG PATIENTS, FAMILIES, AND HEALTH CARE PROVIDERS
Pain and symptom management	Being mentally aware	Using all available treatments regardless of chance of recovery
Preparation for death	Having funeral arrangement planned	Not being connected to machines
Achieving a sense of completion	Not being a burden	Dying at home
Decisions about treatment preferences	Helping others	Being with one's pets
Being treated as a "whole person"	Coming to peace with God	Talking about the meaning of death
		Knowing the timing of death
		Meeting with a clergy member
		Discussing spiritual beliefs with physician
		Controlling the time and place of one's death
		Discussing personal fears

Data from Steinhauser, K. E., Christakis, N. A., Clipp, E. C., McNeilly, M., McIntyre, L., & Tulsky, J. A. (2000). Factors considered important at end of life by patients, family, physicians, and other care providers. _Journal of the American Medical Association, 284_(19), 2476-2482.

consistently were rated as important by all groups of participants, those rated more important by patients than by physicians, and those factors that had broad variation within and among groups. The factors that received inconsistent ratings remind us that we must not assume that we know our patients' wishes. For example, only 35% of seriously ill patients in this sample thought it was important to die at home.

Religion

Religion is a multidimensional and complex phenomenon. Some dimensions of religion include the ritualistic (praying, attending services), the ideological (religious beliefs), the intellectual (knowledge of scriptures, creeds), the experiential (religious feelings, sensations, emotions), and the consequential (effects of the other four dimensions on daily life) (Glock, 1962). Religiousness may include institutional religious participation or an individual religion or personal faith. All of these concepts overlap with one another in complex combinations, so that it is difficult to characterize an individual as simply "religious" or "nonreligious." Spirituality and religiosity can be considered distinct but overlapping traits. Spirituality often is defined as a universal connection to the transcendent and a search for meaning in life. It may or may not center around a divinity (McClain-Jacobson et al., 2004). An analysis of the relationships among religiousness, spirituality, and domains of psychosocial function (i.e., sources of well-being, involvement in everyday life, generativity, and wisdom) in older adults revealed that both religiousness and spirituality related positively to well-being, but the sources of well-being differed. With religiousness, well-being came from positive relations with others, involvement in social and community tasks, and generativity, whereas well-being associated with spirituality came from personal growth, involvement in creative and knowledge-building life tasks, and wisdom (Wink & Dillon, 2003). Spirituality was one of themes that emerged when Hispanic and African American elders were asked how they defined health (Collins, Decker, & Esquibel, 2004).

Historically, older persons have made up the cohort that is most involved in organized religion. This involvement is thought to have several important benefits. Not only is it associated with general well-being, but it provides an opportunity for active contributions by older persons (Hepburn, 2003). Community-dwelling older persons have identified spirituality and reflection as a restorative activity (i.e., one that refreshes, brings peace and feelings of greater mental energy) (Jansen & von Sadovszky, 2004). One study of older persons residing in the rural United States revealed that religiousness/spirituality was associated with subjective well-being among whites, African Americans, and Native Americans (Yoon & Lee, 2004). Data from the Assets and

Health Dynamics among the Oldest Old Survey found that more frequent attendance at religious activities was associated with fewer functional limitations; salience of religion was associated with more functional limitations (Benjamins, 2004). Data from a large, ethnically diverse sample of community-dwelling older persons were used to examine the relations between ethnicity and patterns of socioemotional adaptation. Profiles derived from the data were then related to physical resiliency. Among the findings were that religious beliefs played a greater role in adaptation to aging among resilient participants of African American descent, but not among resilient whites (Consedine, Magai, & Conway, 2004). Magai, Consedine, King, and Gillespie (2003) found that patterns of adaptation characterized by religiosity were associated with greater physical hardiness in a large sample of older adults.

Numerous studies have addressed the relationships between religiosity and various other psychosocial variables, particularly depression. In a study of older persons in the southern United States, persons who scored high on all three dimensions of religiosity (organized, nonorganized, and intrinsic) reported better mental health and fewer symptoms of depression than persons who scored low on the three dimensions (Parker et al., 2003). Similarly, interviews with 1000 older adults in the southern United States found lower levels of depression in highly religious persons (Roff et al., 2004). Among Asian Indian immigrants age 50 and older in the southeastern United States, religiosity was one factor that predicted less negative affect (Diwan, Jonnalagadda, & Balaswamy, 2004). Likewise, church attendance was negatively associated with depressive symptoms in older Dutch citizens (Braam et al., 2004). Citing high rates of depression among older persons and Hispanics in the northeastern United States, Robison and colleagues (2003) assessed relationships between depression and social stressors, social support, and religiosity. In a sample of older Puerto Ricans in the United States, no relationship was found between religiosity and religious participation and depression (Robison et al., 2003). The relationship of religiosity to health and illness also has been studied.

Religiosity may be one factor that influences the type of supports that persons need. It has been suggested that persons who are more religious are more likely to benefit from a strong social network, whereas persons who are more spiritual are more likely to benefit from psychotherapy (Payman, 2005). African Americans often identify religious resources for coping whereas Jewish Americans are more likely to cite personal resources (Nelson-Becker, 2004). In a study of African American women with breast cancer, the participants indicated that they relied more on God than on the support of family and friends (Henderson & Fogel, 2003). When facing declining health, some older persons withdraw from religious involvement, and some substitute religious media for attendance (Benjamins, Musick, Gold, & George, 2003).

Among the proposed explanations for increased religiosity among older persons are the following: more religious training in early life; different life experiences, such as the world wars or the Great Depression; more free time to devote to religion; and a need to resolve the existential fear of death (Moberg, 1990). It also may be that more religious people tend to have healthier habits. Religious participation can fill both spiritual and social needs for older persons. Many churches offer transportation, recreation, counseling, support, education, and even material assistance in crisis situations.

Despite the mutual benefits of religiosity for older persons and for organized religions, various barriers exist to continued participation in institutional religion for some older individuals. Although access to public buildings has improved greatly in recent years, many older facilities may not be very accommodating for persons with physical limitations. Young clergy may not understand the needs and concerns of older members.

Physical Activity

After retirement, many individuals do not engage in sufficient activity to compensate for activity previously performed in the work setting (Berger, Der, Mutrie, & Hannah, 2005). Understanding the attitudes of older persons about physical activity may guide the development of exercise programs. This area has been the focus of numerous studies. In a Canadian sample of adults ages 26 to 95, attitudes related to physical exercise were assessed. Subjects in each of four age-groups were classified as sedentary, modest exercisers, or high exercisers. Sedentary persons identified barriers to exercise as negative exercise attitudes, attributions of negative bodily changes to aging, and low levels of exercise motivation and self-efficacy. Both modest and high exercisers reported positive exercise attitudes (O'Connor, Rousseau, & Maki, 2004). When Americans of various ages were asked about reasons for exercising, older persons were more likely to cite health benefits whereas younger persons cited interpersonal attraction outcomes (Trujillo, Brougham, & Walsh, 2004).

When independent older adults in Scotland were surveyed about leisure time physical activity, 95% indicated that they believed that physical activity was beneficial. Most believed that they engaged in sufficient physical activity to remain healthy despite the fact that 36% of them engaged in no leisure time physical activity, and another 17% did less than 2 hours a week. Lack of interest was the most powerful identified deterrent (Crombie et al., 2004). A study of older persons in Finland, Sweden, and Denmark revealed no change in attitudes toward physical activity between ages 75 and 80 despite a decrease in the actual amount of free time physical activity (Pedersen, Rothenberg, & Maria, 2002).

Leisure Pursuits and Volunteerism

Evidence of increasing interest of older persons in hobbies and leisure pursuits is found in the expansion of the elder hostel movement, a growing number of community-based activities directed toward older persons, and growth of a travel industry that focuses on older customers (Hepburn, 2003). Leisure activities are largely related to education and financial status (Weagley & Huh, 2004). Among the leisure activities most popular with older persons are travel and the creative arts such as needlework, painting, music, pottery or ceramics, writing, and dancing.

As work occupies less of the older person's time and energy, volunteer activities provide an avenue for continued involvement in the community. Individuals who participate in volunteer activities in midlife commonly continue that involvement into later life. Older persons have been described as "the backbone of the U.S. volunteer network" (Hepburn, 2003, p. 187). According to the U.S. Bureau of Labor, 22.7% of persons age 65 and older engaged in volunteer activities in 2002; about half of those volunteered for religious organizations. The median number of volunteer hours per year was approximately 88 hours, the highest of all age-groups. Whites and college graduates were the most likely to report volunteer work. The most common volunteer activities involved fund raising; coaching, tutoring, teaching (mostly parents of children under age 18); collecting, preparing, distributing, or serving food; providing information; and engaging in general labor (U.S. Department of Labor, Bureau of Labor Statistics, 2002).

Sex

The importance of sex among older persons has been found to vary with the availability of a sexual partner. In a study in the United Kingdom, those who reported sex as unimportant were without a current partner and did not anticipate having a future sexual partner. Among participants with a current sexual partner, all reported sex to be of some importance. Factors reported to diminish the importance of sex included health problems and widowhood. Some individuals described decreasing sexual desire with age, and found that being in a long-term relationship made it easier to cope with declining desire (Gott & Hinchliff, 2003).

Health and Health Care

Attitudes toward health care encompass beliefs about health and illness, care during illness, the health care system, health care providers, and the roles of sick persons and their families. Older people today were born before the advent of many of the miracles of modern health care, such as antibiotics, vaccines, and coronary bypass operations. Older persons appear to have a greater acceptance of physician authority than the young; however, this generalization is dependent on factors such as previous experiences with the health care world and general attitudes toward authority. Future cohorts of older persons are likely to be similar to the population at large regarding questioning the authority of physicians and other health professionals. The apparent acceptance of physician authority by older persons should not be construed to mean that they are not accepting of health care provided by other disciplines. Research to evaluate the impact of nonphysician primary care providers on the health care of older persons and their satisfaction with care received has shown health outcomes to be good and satisfaction to be high. Mezey's (2004) review of the literature between 1966 and 2004 provided evidence that nurse practitioners (NPs) in nursing homes were cost-effective, had clinical outcomes equivalent to those of physicians, and had patients with fewer hospital admissions and fewer visits to emergency departments. Furthermore, NPs spent more time with nursing home patients and had higher levels of family satisfaction. A study that compared nursing home care by NP-physician teams versus care by only physicians concluded that the teams provided additional access to care without additional costs (Kluger, 2004). Other studies comparing various types of practitioners (NPs, physician assistants, physicians) have reported higher levels of patient satisfaction with NPs (Edwards, Oppewal, & Logan, 2003; Mark, Byers, & Mays, 2001; Roblin, Becker, Adams, Howard, & Roberts, 2004). Medical directors of long-term care facilities also have credited NPs with maintaining physician, family, and resident satisfaction (Rosenfeld, Kobayashi, Barber, & Mezey, 2004).

Martin and colleagues (2005) assessed gender differences in patients' attributions for myocardial infarction. Attributions to diet and exercise were more common among men than women. Three months later, men were more likely to report attempts to improve their diet and increase their exercise. The investigators concluded that gender differences in causal attributions for myocardial infarction may contribute to subsequent differences in health-related behaviors (Martin et al., 2005).

Using data from over 9000 telephone surveys, Klap, Unroe, and Unutzer (2003) determined that older adults who met diagnostic criteria for mental disorders were less likely than younger persons to perceive the need for mental health care, receive specialty mental health care, or be referred to mental health care by a primary provider. Investigators implemented an individualized early intervention to address the attitudes of older patients about depression and mental health treatment.

Individuals who participated in the intervention along with standard treatment reported greater improvement in symptoms and continued treatment longer than persons who received only standard treatment (Sirey, Bruce, & Alexopoulos, 2005).

Jang, Poon, and Martin (2004) examined the role of age and subjective perception of health in the relationship between disease and disability and depressive symptoms in older adults. Participants were divided into age categories of 60s, 80s, and 100s. In the oldest group, which had more health problems, the effects on their perceptions of health and depressive symptoms were less than in younger persons with less disability.

A longitudinal study of health behaviors and attitudes among older persons in Nordic countries revealed that 60% to 70% believed their own efforts were important in maintaining health—a belief that did not change across the 5-year study period. The proportion of subjects who tried to improve their health decreased between ages 75 and 80 (Pedersen, Rothenberg, & Maria, 2002). When focus groups were used to assess the attitudes of older adults toward nutrition education, the investigators found that the participants were generally positive about nutrition education, viewed food as "good or bad," and thought of nutrition guidelines as "rules" or "orders" (Patacca, Rosenbloom, Kicklighter, & Ball, 2004). Differences between adherent and nonadherent older participants in the dietary modification arm of the Women's Health Initiative aimed at reducing fat intake were examined. Adherence was related to assertiveness, long-time commitment to reducing dietary fat, satisfaction with lifestyle changes, and necessary knowledge and skill. Nonadherence was related to difficulty resisting negative emotions in addition to prior food preferences and habits (Kearney, Rosal, Ockene, & Churchill, 2002). It is important to remember that perceptions of functional health may vary from one culture to another. To illustrate, McCarthy, Ruiz, Gale, Karam, and Moore (2004) found vastly different views when they interviewed Anglo and Latina older women. The use of alternative therapies among older adults in the United States has not been discerned. A survey of 145 persons ages 65 to 74 revealed use of alternative therapies by 43.3% of the sample. The most common therapies used were spiritual practices, exercise/movement therapy, special diets, chiropractic, and meditation (McMahan & Lutz, 2004).

Aging and Old Age

Despite the frequent challenges commonly encountered in late life, it also is a time with the potential for continued development and growth. The attitude of older persons toward their own aging has received minimal attention, which is unfortunate because their attitudes can significantly affect the way late life is experienced and managed (O'Hanlon & Coleman, 2004). A study in the United Kingdom explored the worries that persons might have about their future old age. The investigators found that the older participants generally were not overwhelmed with worry and were coping adequately with their daily challenges. The highest worry scores were among middle-aged persons (Neikrug, 2003). How older individuals view aging may be especially important for those with chronic and disabling conditions.

Some research has focused on persons with specific health deviations. For example, women with spinal cord injuries expressed concern about declining health, increasing dependency, and financial stresses. For successful aging, they identified the need for better environmental accessibility, assistive devices, household help/support, access to recreational and fitness facilities, peer support, and psychological support. These women perceived a lack of sensitivity of health care providers to their unique issues (Pentland et al., 2002).

AFFECT

A study of stress reactivity across the age continuum revealed that the association between daily stress and negative affect was stronger for older adults than for young adults. The investigators suggested that reactivity to stressors was heightened in older adulthood (Mroczek & Almeida, 2004). Isaacowitz and Smith (2003) used data from the Berlin Aging Study to examine the relationship between age and affect in very old individuals. After controlling for demographic, personality, and health and cognitive functioning variables, no unique effects of age were found. The strongest predictors of positive and negative affect were personality and general intelligence. Comparisons by age and gender found minimal differences in predictor patterns. The investigators concluded that much of the variance in affect remains unexplained (Isaacowitz & Smith, 2003).

BOX 20-5 *TOWARD BETTER PSYCHOLOGICAL HEALTH*

- Use relaxation techniques such as progressive muscle relaxation, guided imagery, hypnosis, massage, meditation, biofeedback, or exercise to reduce anxiety.
- Participate in meaningful activities.
- Music can restore the spirit and enhance quality of life.
- Develop strategies to deal with changes in health status or functional abilities.
- Express specific fears and make realistic plans to deal with them.
- Take control of fearful situations by learning all you can about it.

A longitudinal study assessed the impact of positive life orientation in older adults on mortality rate and institutionalization at 5 and 10 years. Those who did not have a positive orientation had significantly higher mortality rates and greater risk for permanent institutionalization (Pitkala et al., 2004) (Box 20-5).

COMMON MENTAL DISORDERS

The elder population of the United States is expected to double between 2000 and 2030. Mental health problems in older persons are significant in their frequency, impact on mental status, and influence on the course of physical illness in later life. It has been estimated that 20% of people age 55 and older exhibit signs and symptoms of significant mental illness at any given time (U.S. Department of Health and Human Services, 1999). The problems occur in both community and institutional settings. The number of people in nursing homes continues to rise, and although psychiatric admissions to state hospitals have declined in past years, admissions to private psychiatric and general hospitals have increased. The statistics may be skewed by closure of state hospital beds nationwide.

Attempts to estimate the prevalence of mental illness in the older population are complicated by the tendency of older persons to underutilize mental health services and to underreport psychiatric symptoms. A study of the needs for support services among aging families of adults with severe mental illness found very low use of services despite high perceived needs for services. Specific needs that were not being met were related to social/recreational programs, behavior management, and planning for the future (Smith, 2003a). Other factors include transportation issues, financial constraints, and the stigma of using mental health services.

Many mental disorders are amenable to treatment with pharmacotherapy, psychotherapy, environmental manipulation, or family therapy (Bartels et al., 2003). However, access to services has been hampered by the stereotypical views of care providers toward older persons and their ability to be treated and by the suspicions with which older adults view the service providers (Lagana & Shanks, 2002). A small shift in the attitudes of older persons toward mental health services was detected in a longitudinal study in rural New York. From 1987 to 1994, the percentage of older persons who expressed willingness to use mental health services increased from 5% to 18%. Unfortunately, participants judged to be in the greatest need of such services were the least likely to use them (Maiden & Peterson, 2002).

The most common mental disorders in persons 65 and older are anxiety disorders and severe cognitive impairment (Hybels & Blazer, 2003). Lehmann (2003) reports that women are at greater risk than men for late-onset depressive disorders, schizophrenia, and mood disorders. Gonadal steroids affect mood, cognition, and behavior, and gender differences have been observed in the prevalence, course, and treatment response of schizophrenia and mood disorders, so the role of hormones in these disorders is under study (Ozcan & Banoglu, 2003). One avenue of study is the relationship between estrogen and the dopaminergic system. The researchers believe that postmenopausal estrogen deficiency may contribute to gender differences in the prevalence of late-onset neuropsychiatric disorders, including schizophrenia and Parkinson's disease (Craig et al., 2004). Although some researchers believe that estrogen actually has a protective effect against schizophrenia, studies of age of menarche and the age of onset of schizophrenia have yielded conflicting results (Hochman & Lewine, 2004).

It should be noted that older persons often are caregivers for offspring or spouses with mental illness. Older caregivers have the same concerns as other aging adults but also must face questions such as who will care for the person if the caregiver becomes disabled or dies. The nurse should encourage consideration of this issue including involvement of other family members (Smith, 2003b).

Mood Disorders

The Depression and Bipolar Support Alliance is the largest patient-directed, illness-specific organization in the United States. In 2001, the organization convened a consensus panel including experts in mood disorders and mental health and aging to draft a statement "defining the crisis in late life mental health care" and providing recommendations (Charney et al., 2003, p. 665). Major conclusions in the consensus statement were as follows:

- Safe and efficacious treatments for mood disorders in older persons exist.
- Mood disorders pose a significant health care issue for older persons.
- Mood disorders in older persons are associated with disability, functional decline, diminished quality of life, and death from comorbid medical conditions or suicide.
- Mood disorders in older persons increase demands on caregivers and the utilization of services.
- Coverage and reimbursement policies for mental health care are discriminatory.
- Older persons lack adequate access to mental health services, a situation that is complicated by poor coordination of services.

Depression. Depression in late life is not a normal part of aging. Dysthymic disorder occurs in about 1.8% of persons 65 or older, followed by major depressive

disorder at about 0.7%. In both disorders, women are afflicted at over twice the rate of men. The reasons for this disparity may be due to various psychosocial and biological factors. Women are more likely to report depression and seek treatment than their male counterparts. Gender roles, societal expectations, past trauma, and social status may also play a role (Sloan, 2003). The hormonal changes that take place during and after menopause may also put women at particular risk for depression. Estrogen levels are linked by complex mechanisms to serotonin, norepinephrine, and dopamine with regard to serum levels and receptor site function (Marcus, 1995). Declining estrogen levels may precipitate mood changes, as well as other physical symptoms such as migraine, hot flashes, sleep disturbance, and joint pain (Warnock, 2004). Male depression has been associated with different factors than depression in women. For example, some men with depression have benefited from testosterone augmentation (Orengo, Fullerton, & Tan, 2004). Although the incidence of depression is generally lower than that found in the younger population (25 to 44 years), the prevalence of depressive disorders dramatically increases in those older persons in home health care, nursing homes, hospitals, and primary care (Hybels & Blazer, 2003).

The physiological basis for late-life depression is multifactorial. The consideration of a genetic etiology for depression has attracted great attention for decades. The use of twin and family studies consistently has shown strong evidence for the heritability of depression (Johansson et al., 2001). However, genetics may not play as significant a role in late-life depression as it does in younger people. As individuals age, genetic influences may be tempered by numerous factors, including past lifestyle, exercise, diet, substance use, levels of stress, and comorbid medical illnesses such as heart disease and stroke (Burke & Wengel, 2003). The assumption that the brain loses neurons as it ages has been challenged by new findings from animal studies that show the brain to be remarkably stable over time. Although there may not be a frank loss of neurons, loss of dendritic spines can occur (Li, 2002). In addition, there may be decreases in the rate of metabolism of neurotransmitters or changes in the number of receptors or receptor sites (Yew, Li, Webb, Lai, & Zhang, 1999). Serotonin and norepinephrine both are strongly associated with the neurobiology of mood and emotion. Age-related decreases in serotonin levels have been shown to occur in both animal and human neuroimaging studies (Goldberg et al., 2004). Monoamine oxidase B, an enzyme responsible for breaking down serotonin and dopamine, seems to increase with age and further contributes to decreased serotonin levels in the aging brain (Rehman & Masson, 2001). The hypothalamic-pituitary-adrenal (HPA) axis plays a crucial role in mood regulation and is probably related to elevated levels of glucocorticoids and their effects within the brain. The glucocorticoids, especially cortisol, are crucial in our body's adaptation to stress. However, depression is a common symptom of both iatrogenic administration of cortisol and metabolic disorders that elevate cortisol levels in the body (Alesci, De Martino, Ilias, Gold, & Chrousos, 2005). Prolonged elevated levels of cortisol can damage neurons, especially those within the hippocampus, a key mood-related structure in the limbic system. The effects of aging on the HPA axis are unclear at this time. This may be due to the great variability of individuals in their genetic makeup, ability to cope with stress, and life experience. We do know that the system endures a certain level of "wear" over time that has been shown to affect obesity, hypertension, hyperlipidemia, and insulin resistance, as well as cardiovascular disease, diabetes, and atherosclerosis, all commonly associated with aging. The literature remains conflicted as to whether the HPA reactivity is increased or decreased with aging (Traustidottir, Bosch, & Matt, 2005). Depression may be related to hormonal dysregulation as well. Growth hormone production declines in both frequency and amount in older men and women (Horani & Morley, 2004) and is associated with depression. Hypothyroidism, commonly associated with aging, may initially manifest as depressive symptoms in older persons (Joffe, Brasch, & MacQueen, 2003). Depression as a result of cerebrovascular disease and its deleterious impact on pathways between the prefrontal cortex and the basal ganglia has been identified as a depressive subtype. Depression after stroke occurs in 25% to 50% of cases, with some data suggesting increased rates when the damage occurs in the left anterior pole of the cerebral cortex or left basal ganglia (Burke & Wengel, 2003). White matter hyperintensities have been seen on magnetic resonance imaging studies of older depressed patients, suggesting ischemic lesions in the dorsolateral prefrontal cortex as a contributing factor (Thomas, 2002).

Social factors are an important consideration in late-life depression. The older patient is susceptible to multiple life stressors, which include decline in function; disability; social isolation; lack of social support; death of spouse, friends, and relatives; economic stresses; medical illness; and injury (Bruce, 2002).

The disorder is characterized by marked sadness and loss of interest and pleasure in daily activities. Affected individuals may experience weight change, sleep disturbance, difficulty concentrating, feelings of guilt, fatigue, disinterest in personal hygiene, psychomotor retardation, and suicidal ideation (Friedlander, Friedlander, Gallas, & Velasco, 2003; Pier, Halstijn, & Sabbe, 2004).

One factor that cannot be overlooked when discussing depression is the possible influence of drug therapy. Data on medications used by 2646 community-dwelling older adults were obtained from the Longi-

tudinal Aging Study in Amsterdam. After controlling for other known risk factors for depression, 22 individual medications and 9 groups of medications remained uniquely associated with depression. This study highlights the importance of considering iatrogenic causes of depression in older persons (Dhondt, Beekman, Deeg, & Van Tilburg, 2002). Van Ness and Larson (2002) reviewed studies of the relationships between religion, senescence, and mental health in people near the end of life. Fairly consistent inverse relationships were found between religiousness and rates of suicide and depression. The writers concluded that religion generally had a protective, though modest, effect on mental health. An important challenge for the practitioner is to differentiate depression from dementia. Approximately one third of those referred for evaluation for dementia are found to be suffering from depression. Maynard (2003) suggests a six-step process to making an accurate diagnosis (Box 20-6).

Treatment of depression generally falls into two categories: nonpharmacological and pharmacological. Nonpharmacological methods involve psychotherapy and electroconvulsive therapy (ECT). Cognitive-behavioral therapy is a form of therapy that helps people change behavior by changing the way that they think about, or perceive, events in their life. Behaviorally, the individual is encouraged by the therapist to engage in one or more interventions such as keeping thought/feeling/behavior logs, graded assignments, and workbook exercises. Cognitively, the individual attempts to restructure his or her automatic or negative thoughts, as well as challenge irrational, stress-inducing thoughts. Cognitive-behavioral therapy has the greatest empirical support for effectiveness in the treatment of geriatric depression. Other psychosocial interventions are likely to be efficacious in older adults, including problem-solving therapy, interpersonal therapy, brief psychodynamic therapy, and reminiscence therapy. A common finding suggests that the combination of pharmacological and psychosocial interventions is more effective than either intervention alone in preventing major depression from recurring (Bartels et al., 2003).

ECT has been used in the treatment of depression since its inception in the 1930s. Its mechanism of action is unclear, although human and animal studies have demonstrated that it causes changes at the neurotransmitter and receptors site levels. It has been shown to "downregulate" noradrenergic receptors, similar to the longer-term effects of antidepressant medications, as well as exerting effects on serotonin and acetylcholine levels in the brain and cerebrospinal fluid (Kamat, Lefevre, & Grossberg, 2003). ECT is safe and effective for the treatment of psychiatric disorders in the elderly. It is an especially attractive option for those older patients who have not responded to or cannot tolerate higher doses of psychotropic drug treatment. It is also

---

BOX 20-6 Steps to Differentiate Depression and Dementia

1. Assess Personal Assumptions
Avoid jumping to a diagnosis of dementia because you expect it in older persons.

2. Rule Out Normal Aging
Occasionally forgetting names of acquaintances, occasionally misplacing items, and somewhat slowed learning are normal. Forgetting names of family members, getting lost in familiar locales, and progressive, disabling cognitive changes are not normal.

3. Know the Characteristics of Depression
Persons with dementia commonly cannot express when they feel depressed. Manifestations of depression can include a variety of somatic, cognitive, and affective complaints, as well as self-neglect, especially in the absence of objective evidence to explain the symptoms.

4. Understand Dementia
The onset of dementia typically is insidious and the course progressive. The *Diagnostic and Statistical Manual of Mental Disorders* (fourth edition) defines the criteria for a diagnosis of dementia as multiple cognitive deficits including memory impairment and apraxia, aphasia, or agnosia; and disturbed executive function. Changes must be sufficient to interfere with daily function and represent a decline from usual level of functioning.

5. Perform a Thorough Assessment
Interview the patient first, then family members separately. A thorough history and physical examination should include screening tools for depression and cognitive impairment (e.g., MMSE, Draw a Clock, 7-Minute Screen).

6. Differentiate the Diagnosis
Rule out various causes of the symptoms by assessing vitamin B_{12} and folate levels, thyroid function, metabolic disorders, blood dyscrasias, malignancy, small blood vessel disease, cardiac and pulmonary disorders, infections, and other neurological disorders.

Data from Maynard, C. K. (2003). Differentiate depression from dementia. *Nurse Practitioner, 28*(3), 18-27.

---

an alternative in the case of those patients taking multiple medications when the addition of one or more psychotropic agents becomes impractical. ECT can be used safely in elderly patients, even those with multiple comorbid illnesses (Tomac, Rummans, Pileggi, & Li, 1997).

Antidepressants work just as well for older persons as they do for other populations. Geriatric patients may take longer than the 4 weeks generally considered as the

benchmark for response in the younger patient. One study comparing sertraline versus nortriptyline suggested that up to 12 weeks of observation may be required to adequately assess the efficacy of an antidepressant in an older patient (Bondareff et al., 2000). Starting low and going slow can lead to prolonged symptoms, making psychotherapy a valuable adjunct to treatment. Efficacy seems to be equal among all the classes of antidepressants (Williams et al., 2000). However, as a class, the tricyclic antidepressants (TCAs) present a more problematic set of side effects that can be dangerous in the older person. These include their ability to cause cardiac conduction delays and lethality in overdose. The tertiary amine tricyclics, amitriptyline, imipramine, doxepin, and clomipramine, are more prone to causing hypotension and anticholinergic side effects such as dry mouth, blurred vision, and constipation. They can aggravate narrow-angle glaucoma and prostatic hyperplasia and cause delirium in susceptible patients. The secondary amine tricyclics, nortriptyline and desipramine, are less commonly associated with these side effects. However, the tricyclics are valuable in that sometimes the anticholinergic side effects can be advantageous, such as in patients with bladder leakage along with depression (Potter, Manji & Rudorfer, 2001).

The selective serotonin reuptake inhibitors (SSRIs) present their own set of concerns, as well, although overall they are much safer. They have been associated with the syndrome of inappropriate antidiuretic hormone in older persons (Desai, 2003). They sometimes are more difficult to tolerate from a gastrointestinal perspective (Papakostas et al., 2003), along with hemostatic dysfunction and prolonged bleeding (Tassini et al., 2002). They also can cause sexual side effects, such as impotence, anorgasmia, and lack of sexual desire, all problems sometimes overlooked in older individuals (Lenahan & Willwood, 2004). Fluoxetine and paroxetine are potent inhibitors of the cytochrome P450 2D6 isoenzyme and have many drug interactions. Paroxetine also is anticholinergic, although less so than the TCAs, and is associated with a discontinuation syndrome when abruptly stopped. This syndrome is characterized by dizziness, anxiety, and flulike symptoms lasting 1 to 3 days after stopping the medication (Shatzberg et al., 1997). The best choice of an SSRI in the older individual is one that has few drug interactions and a short half-life. Sertraline, citalopram, and escitalopram are drugs that fit this profile. Fluvoxamine generally is used for obsessive-compulsive disorder in children. Venlafaxine, although effective for the treatment of depression and anxiety, should be used with caution in older persons with uncontrolled hypertension because of its propensity to increase blood pressure (Tollefson & Rosenbaum, 2001). It also is associated with a discontinuation syndrome when abruptly discontinued. Mirtazapine, with its lack of cardiotoxicity, few drug interactions, and potential to stimulate appetite and cause weight gain, is an attractive choice for the older patient (Gray, 2004). It is also beneficial for inducing sleep because of its antihistaminic properties at low doses. As doses increase, it becomes more noradrenergic and therefore more stimulating. Bupropion is generally well tolerated by older persons because of its availability in generic form and lack of sedation, cardiotoxicity, and sexual side effects. It should generally be avoided in patients with a history of seizures or stroke because of the possibility of seizures at doses greater than 400 mg per day. Trazodone is mainly used for its sedative properties. It can cause orthostatic hypotension and can oversedate older patients at higher doses (Golden, Dawkins, Nicholas, & Bebchuk, 2001). Duloxetine is a newer antidepressant with both serotonergic and noradrenergic properties. A British research study into its effects and tolerability in older persons indicated that it is generally well tolerated (Cowen, 2005).

There are several special situations that the practitioner should be aware of in treating depression in the older patient. The first involves using caution with antidepressants in bipolar I and II patients because of their ability to induce mania and hypomania. They have been known to increase the number of manic and depressive episodes, and induce rapid cycling, defined as more than four episodes per year (Mackin & Young, 2004; Stoll et al., 1994). Depression and heart disease are frequently comorbid conditions. TCAs should be avoided in individuals with any history of cardiac problems. SSRIs are a safer alternative and have the added benefit of decreasing platelet adhesiveness and may decrease coronary artery vasospasms. In patients with swallowing difficulties, several medications are available in easy-to-swallow preparations. These include liquid solutions for fluoxetine and citalopram, venlafaxine extended-release sprinkles, and rapidly dissolving mirtazapine orally disintegrating wafers. Sexual dysfunction

caused by SSRIs can be treated in several ways, including decreasing the dose of the offending medication, switching to bupropion or mirtazapine, or treating male erectile symptoms with sildenafil, tadalafil, or vardenafil (Abels, 2003). Monoamine oxidase inhibitors, as always, are a last-resort agent for the treatment of depression because of drug and food interactions and hypotension (Table 20-3).

Bipolar Disorder. Bipolar disorder can be classified as early or late onset depending on the age of the individual at first contact. Studies comparing the two types have not provided consistent answers. An Australian study found only small differences in the two and attributed those to illness duration (Almeida & Fenner, 2002). Another study comparing the two concluded that persons with late-onset bipolar disorder are more likely to have less severe illness, a negative family history, a better treatment response, and a better prognosis (Engstrom, Brandstrom, Sigvardsson, Cloninger, & Nylander, 2003). According to Burke and Wengel (2003), older adults tend to experience more "mixed episodes," or those manifesting both depressive and manic symptoms simultaneously, than younger persons with bipolar disorder. They may be irritable and grumbling or complaining, as opposed to their younger counterparts' agitation and euphoria. Diagnosis and treatment of the older bipolar patient presents unique challenges because of the number of comorbid medical problems that can mimic symptoms of depression and mania, including hyperthyroidism, hypothyroidism, cerebrovascular pathology, dementia, and delirium. Treatment must be tempered by consideration of drug interactions and sensitivity to medication side effects.

Lithium remains a first-line drug for bipolar disorder. Despite its narrow therapeutic index of 0.6 to 1.2 mEq/L, it can be safely used in the older person. However, these individuals generally respond to lower serum levels of

Table 20-3 *Antidepressant Use in the Elderly*

Antidepressant	Normal Dosage (mg/day)	Medically Ill Elderly (mg/day)	Possible Side Effects
Fluoxetine	20-80	10-20	Restlessness, insomnia, sexual side effects
Paroxetine	20-60	10-20	Sedation, weight gain, sexual side effects
Paroxetine (controlled release)	12.5-75	12.5-25	Sedation, weight gain, sexual side effects
Sertraline	25-200	12.5-50	Nausea, vomiting, dry mouth, sexual side effects
Citalopram	20-60	10-20	Nausea, diarrhea
Escitalopram	10-20	5-10	Nausea, diarrhea
Venlafaxine (extended release)	37.5-225	37.5-75	Hypertension, nausea, insomnia, sexual side effects
Mirtazapine	15-45	7.5-15	Fatigue, sedation, weight gain
Bupropion	75-300	75-150	Restlessness, insomnia, tremor, anorexia
Duloxetine	20-60	20-40	Nausea, dry mouth, insomnia

lithium, specifically, 0.2 to 0.4 mEq/L. Patients not showing a therapeutic response at these lower levels should be increased very slowly until symptoms resolve. It should be started at 75 to 150 mg per day. The clinician must remember that lithium is not metabolized by the liver, but excreted by the kidney, making effective renal function a must (Holroyd, 2004). Hyponatremia, dehydration, diuretics, and angiotensin-converting enzyme inhibitors can reduce lithium clearance and increase serum levels (Desan, 2004). Increased levels can lead to toxicity, with symptoms ranging from upset stomach to confusion, tremor, and death (Mokhlesi, Leikin, Murray, & Corbridge, 2003). Older patients are particularly susceptible to its side effects of polydipsia, polyuria, hand tremor, dry mouth, and fatigue. Lithium can induce hypothyroidism in some patients (Hanna & LaFranchi, 2002) and can result in flattened or even inverted T waves on electrocardiogram in 20% to 30% of patients. It can cause sinus node dysfunction and first-degree heart block in a small number of patients (Van Mieghem, Sabbe, & Knockaert, 2004). It is available in pill and liquid forms. Long-term therapy demands periodic renal function studies. Even with normal creatinine levels, toxicity can occur because the loss of lean body mass with age makes serum creatinine levels a poor indicator of creatinine clearance (Williams, 2002).

Valproate is becoming a first-line treatment for bipolar disorder in older persons because it is better tolerated than lithium. Valproate can be titrated faster than lithium, making it more effective in the treatment of acute mania. It is started at 125 to 250 mg per day and can be increased by the same amount every 3 to 5 days as tolerated by the patient (Desai, 2003). It is measurable in the blood and is therapeutic at levels of 50 to 100 mcg/L. It is available in oral, extended-release, sprinkle form, suppository, and intravenous forms, making it easy to use—an advantage in older persons who have difficulty with medications. The divalproex extended-release form may require higher doses than the immediate-release form (Birnbaum et al., 2004). It can cause weight gain and sleepiness. Other side effects include gastrointestinal upset, ataxia, and tremor, and it can lead to elevated liver enzymes, hepatitis, and life-threatening pancreatitis (Shneker & Fountain, 2003). Carbamazepine can be used for bipolar disorder, but with caution in the older patient because of its ability to induce liver enzyme production, which may decrease the effects of other drugs. Clearance of carbamazepine is reduced in older persons, making lower doses necessary. There also is an increased risk of hyponatremia and conduction delays in the older patient on the drug. All this combines to make carbamazepine a second- or even third-line choice in older people. Even though lamotrigine generally is better tolerated in older patients and has few side effects (Bergey, 2004), it should be titrated very slowly to avoid Stevens-Johnson syndrome. It is safely prescribed at 25 mg per day for 2 weeks, then 50 mg per day for 2 weeks, then 100 mg per day for 1 week, and then 200 mg per day as a maintenance dose. The lamotrigine dose should be lowered if taken with valproate because it slows the elimination of lamotrigine (Singh, Muzina, & Calabrese, 2005). Oxcarbazepine and topiramate are other anticonvulsants used off label for bipolar disorder.

Anxiety

Anxiety disorders are the most prevalent disorders among older adults, with prevalence rates ranging from 10.2% to 15% (Lauderdale & Sheikh, 2003). Although the reasons are unclear, many factors contribute to anxiety among older persons. As people age, they begin to develop concerns about a multitude of issues, including their physical health, finances, social support systems, cognition, and death. The character of anxiety varies across the life span. In one study comparing worry in younger and older adults, both groups were found to worry equally in general; however, the subject of the worry, as well as methods of coping, varied between the groups. The older sample tended to worry more about health, world issues, and family concerns (Hunt, Wisocki, & Yanko, 2003).

Phobias are high in prevalence among older adults. Fear of specific things or situations occurs in about 3% to 12% of elders. They tend to fear flying, heights, and lightning more so than younger people. This may be a function of life experience and the probability that earlier phobias continue into late life (Lauderdale & Sheikh, 2003).

Generalized anxiety disorder is the second most common anxiety disorder among older adults. Although point prevalence ranges from 0.7% to 7.1%, these rates are actually lower than younger subjects and may represent lifelong problems with anxiety (Beyer, 2004). Panic disorder is relatively uncommon in older persons, with a prevalence rate of 0.1% (Hybels & Blazer, 2003). These figures may reflect underreporting because of decreased ability to recall anxiety symptoms (Beyer, 2004).

Late-life onset of obsessive-compulsive disorder (OCD) is uncommon. Prevalence rates up to 1.5% have been reported in persons age 65 and older. Obsessions and compulsions in older persons are marked by an elevated focus on somatic preoccupations and may reflect continuation of OCD symptoms from younger life or even organic neurological events in late life (Carmin, Wiegartz, Yunus, & Gillock, 2002).

Posttraumatic stress disorder (PTSD) can occur at any age. Trauma research with older adults has tended to focus on veterans of war; however, the elder population is vulnerable to ongoing trauma associated with aging. The loss of friends and loved ones, relocation, isolation, and financial problems can be viewed as traumatic. In addition, the need for time to work through and integrate traumatic experiences into one's life presents challenges for older adults in view of perceptual, memory, and expressive difficulties. Stress reactions can follow trauma quickly or be delayed for many years and surface in old age (Busutill, 2004).

Nonpharmacological treatment includes cognitive-behavioral therapy, as discussed earlier. Cognitive-behavioral therapy has proven its usefulness in panic disorder and generalized anxiety disorder. However, little research exists into its efficacy for PTSD and OCD (Lauderdale & Sheikh, 2003).

Benzodiazepines are the mainstay of treatment for anxiety. However, they pose a danger because older individuals are more sensitive to their effects. Declining liver function with decreased ability to clear the drug from the body and increased receptor site sensitivity in the older brain can lead to untoward effects from benzodiazepines (Bogunovic & Greenfield, 2004). Chronic use is associated with drowsiness, ataxia, fatigue, confusion, cognitive impairment, depression, disinhibition, paranoia, hallucinations, delirium, and aggressiveness. They have been shown to be a cause of falls in nursing homes (Tamblyn, Abrahamowicz, du Berger, McLeod, & Bartlett, 2005). When benzodiazepines are discontinued in nursing home patients with dementia, their cognition has been shown to improve. Benzodiazepines are also associated with withdrawal potential after long-term use. Short-acting benzodiazepines such as lorazepam and alprazolam can be used if concerns arise about accumulation caused by their hydrophilic properties (Bogunovic & Greenfield, 2004). Both are available in pill and liquid form, with lorazepam also available in parenteral form. Clonazepam is a longer-acting benzodiazepine that is also available in a rapidly dissolving wafer, as well as the standard pill form. Diazepam and chlordiazepoxide are longer-acting agents that are stored in fat. Although they have less potential for withdrawal after short-term use because of autotapering, their side effects can remain constant over time and should be a consideration. Buspirone, a 5HT1A receptor partial agonist, has been shown to be effective as an antianxiety agent in older persons (Majercsik & Haller, 2004). Its advantages are the lack of physical dependence potential, safety in overdose, and cost efficiency over the benzodiazepines.

Antihistamines are sometimes used for treating anxiety because of their sedating effects. Nevertheless, their use in older adults should be limited because of their anticholinergic side effects and propensity to precipitate delirium in some individuals (Gurwitz et al., 2005). The SSRIs are particularly effective in the treatment of anxiety disorders in older persons and are preferable to the benzodiazepines, tricyclics, and antihistamines. As discussed earlier in this chapter, they are well tolerated among elders. They are efficacious in the treatment of panic disorder, generalized anxiety disorder, OCD, social phobia, and PTSD. Given the high comorbidities of depression and anxiety, they are an attractive choice for the older patient to treat both simultaneously with a single agent (Spalleta, Pasini, & Caltagirone, 2002).

Stress, Defense Mechanisms, and Coping Strategies

A study of stressful life events among community-dwelling older persons found that similar events could have either negative or positive consequences for individuals. The investigators attributed the differences to differing degrees of resilience. Interestingly, the stressful event reported by the greatest number of participants was death of a family member or friend, followed by illness of family member or friend, a personal illness, and a nonmedical event (Hardy, Concato, & Gill, 2002).

Whitty (2003) studied age-group differences in coping strategies and defense mechanisms. The youngest group used immature defense mechanisms compared with the middle and oldest groups, which both used more mature mechanisms. Coping strategies used were similar across all age-groups. Boerner (2004) used the model of assimilative and accommodative coping to study the effects of coping and disability on mental health among middle-aged and older adults who experienced age-related vision loss. Accommodative coping was found to play a critical role in adaptation. In this sample, dealing with disability posed a greater threat to mental health among middle-aged adults than older persons.

Data from the Berlin Aging Study (Lang et al., 2002) examined strategies used to adapt to aging losses in relation to everyday functioning and personal resources. Individuals who were richer in sensorimotor-cognitive and social-personality resources had a higher survivor rate, invested more social time with their families, reduced the diversity of their leisure activities, slept more during the daytime, and increased the variety of time investments across activities. Better-functioning, resource-rich older persons used more selection, compensation, and optimization to adapt to aging losses.

Personality Disorders

An empirical study of the prevalence of personality disorders in groups of individuals from adolescence to old age detected a specific effect for aging. Community-dwelling older persons demonstrated more schizoid and obsessive-compulsive characteristics. Compared with younger groups, the older mental health patients had more schizoid disorder characteristics and fewer high-energy disorder characteristics (Engels, Duijsens, Haringsma, & van Puttern, 2003).

Schizophrenia

Schimming and Harvey's (2004) review of the literature on older adults with schizophrenia addressed several common beliefs about this population. The first of these beliefs is that people with schizophrenia "burn out" with age, meaning that severe positive symptoms decrease and are replaced with more negative symptoms. Cross-sectional studies have reported significant positive symptoms in later life. A small number of longitudinal studies (up to 6 years) have failed to detect improvement in positive symptoms in individuals. One subgroup that does appear to have a reduction in the severity of positive symptoms comprises community-dwelling persons who have never required extended institutionalization. In relation to negative symptoms, existing data do not support an increase, particularly among community-dwelling individuals with better functional outcomes.

Second, the belief that cognitive function deteriorates throughout the course of the illness has not been supported across the range of outcomes (Hijman, Pol, Sitskoorn, & Kahn, 2003; Jeste et al., 2003; Kondel, Mortimer, Leeson, Laws, & Hirsch, 2003; Schimming & Harvey, 2004). Although some cross-sectional studies have demonstrated a trend toward declining cognitive and functional status, this pattern is more prevalent in individuals with lifelong poor functional status and chronic institutionalization than in those with good outcomes. Schimming and Harvey (2004) point out that the comorbidities of aging persons should be taken into consideration in the interpretation of these data. Examination of autopsy brain specimens from a small group of individuals with late-onset schizophrenia and individuals with no known neuropsychiatric pathology found no evidence that schizophrenia is a risk factor for Alzheimer's disease (Bozikas, Kovari, Bouras, & Karavatos, 2002).

The third issue is whether early-onset and late-onset schizophrenia represent the same or different entities. Depending on the age of onset, schizophrenia can be classified as early onset (up to age 40), late onset (ages 40 to 59), and very late onset (age 60 or older). It is not clear how these differ other than the age of onset. Some researchers believe that onset of very late schizophrenia-like psychosis represents a different entity with a different symptom profile and risk factors (Howard & Reeves, 2003). Late-onset schizophrenia is associated with better social and occupational function, as well as more schizoid symptoms before the onset of illness (Schimming & Harvey, 2004). To illustrate, in a sample of community-dwelling subjects with a mean age of 59 years, 30% had been employed at least half time following the onset of schizophrenia, 73% were living in a house or an apartment and meeting their own daily needs, and 43% were driving (Palmer et al., 2002). A

study in the United Kingdom compared social functioning in healthy older adults, depressed older adults, and older adults with schizophrenia. Those with schizophrenia were the most isolated and had the fewest private leisure activities (Graham, Arthur, & Howard, 2002).

Schimming and Harvey (2004) also examined the treatment of older persons with schizophrenia. Importantly, typical antipsychotics were deemed to have debilitating side effects, treatment resistance, and risk for toxicity. Anticholinergic drugs that have been used to manage extrapyramidal side effects have been shown to worsen cognitive performance. New antipsychotic drugs improve both negative and positive symptoms with less risk of extrapyramidal side effects and tardive dyskinesia. Cognitive improvements have even been reported in older persons taking risperidone and olanzapine. On the other hand, the newer drugs are associated with weight gain and the induction of diabetes mellitus.

Heterogeneity in cognitive function also was apparent in a study designed to assess the ability of persons with schizophrenia to understand information presented to obtain informed consent for treatment. Though persons with schizophrenia generally had poorer understanding than healthy controls, the variability was wide (Palmer, Dunn, Appelbaum, & Jeste, 2004).

Hasset (2003) described a stress-vulnerability model to explain the late-life onset of schizophrenia-like psychosis in persons without a primary diagnosis of affective disturbance or dementia.

Reportedly, suicide attempts are frequent among individuals with schizophrenia. A study of 1066 persons age 60 and over with schizophrenia revealed 49 suicide attempts by 30 individuals. No risk factors for suicide attempt could be determined from this study (Barak, Knobler, & Aizenberg, 2004).

A review of health service usage by age revealed that older persons with schizophrenia had fewer psychiatric hospitalizations but longer lengths of stay, fewer outpatient psychiatric visits, and more medical outpatient visits and hospitalizations (Barry, Blow, Dornfeld, & Valenstein, 2002).

Treatment of Psychosis in Older Persons

The risks and benefits of antipsychotic drug use in older persons is a topic of debate. In general, antipsychotic drugs are the medications of choice for older persons with psychosis. However, the practitioner must consider the fact that older persons are more sensitive to both the therapeutic and toxic effects. Although data currently are limited, it appears that the second-generation or atypical antipsychotics are equally as effective as the first-generation antipsychotics but better tolerated. Adverse effects of the first-generation antipsychotics that are of special concern for older persons are sedation, anticholinergic effects, cardiovascular effects, and extrapyramidal symptoms (EPS), including tardive dyskinesia (Sable & Jeste, 2003). Although generally more tolerable, the atypical antipsychotics are not without their own problems. Various agents are associated with weight gain, diabetes, metabolic syndrome, and hyperprolactinemia. Recent placebo-controlled studies have demonstrated an increased risk of cardiac events or infectious processes with the use of the atypical antipsychotics in elderly patients with dementia-related psychosis (U.S. Food and Drug Administration, 2005). However, despite the fact that all antipsychotics pose some treatment risk, the clinician must help the patient decide the best choice of treatment in light of the patient's symptoms and side effect tolerability. The goal is overall improvement of the patient's quality of life, and the patient must sometimes choose between side effects and the debilitating effects of his or her illness. Thorough patient education and baseline evaluations such as body mass index, weight, fasting glucose, complete blood count, and lipid profile can help the clinician and patient alike make the appropriate choices for treatment (McKinley, 2005).

Despite their side effects, the older drugs do still hold a place in our drug armamentarium. Haloperidol remains a first-line drug for psychiatric emergencies in patients of all ages. It is available in oral, intramuscular, and intravenous forms, and it acts rapidly and effectively, making it the mainstay of many emergency departments and inpatient units (Kapur & Seeman, 2001). When used intravenously, it produces less risk of EPS (Riker, Fraser, & Richen, 1997). This implies short-term use only, with most practitioners transitioning to a newer agent for longer-term maintenance. Several situations arise that make first-generation antipsychotics more acceptable in the older patient. These include patients who have responded to these drugs on a long-term basis and tolerate them, those who require a long-term injectable decanoate form, and those for whom only this class will control symptoms (Desai, 2003).

Clozapine, the prototype second-generation antipsychotic, is highly effective in refractory psychosis and psychosis associated with Parkinson's disease (Fernandez, Treischmann, & Okun, 2004). However, it is associated with agranulocytosis and delirium in older patients. Its impact on adrenergic, histaminic, cholinergic, and serotonergic receptors makes it more likely to cause tachycardia, hypotension, and a host of anticholinergic side effects (Finkel, 2004). It should be used with caution, if at all, in elderly patients and avoided in the very frail and medically ill geriatric patient.

Olanzapine, chemically similar to clozapine, is generally well tolerated in older adults. Nevertheless, like clozapine, it is strongly associated with weight gain, hyperglycemia, and dyslipidemia (Wirshing, Pierre, Erhart, & Boyd, 2003). However, olanzapine is associated with

lower weight gain in the elderly (Street et al., 2000). It does have anticholinergic properties that can be troublesome in patients prone to delirium. Along with most of the other newer antipsychotics, it also is indicated for treatment of bipolar disorder. It is available in pill form, as a rapidly dissolving disk, and in intramuscular form.

Risperidone is well studied in the elderly. It works well for delirium, and improves psychotic, positive, negative, and cognitive symptoms of schizophrenia in older patients. It has been shown to be useful in controlling the athetoid movements and psychotic symptoms of Huntington's disease (Sharma & Standaert, 2002). It is available in an oral solution, a rapidly dissolving tablet, and a long-acting intramuscular form with a unique delivery system that allows about 2 weeks between injections. Risperidone is associated with increased prolactin levels (Volavka et al., 2004) that can lead to galactorrhea, gynecomastia, impotence, and a possible role in osteoporosis (Leung & Pacaud, 2004). This can be problematic in patients with prolactin-secreting pituitary tumors or breast cancer.

Ziprasidone has been shown to be weight neutral (Wiegle, 2003) and less sedating than prior antipsychotics (Mendelowitz, 2004). It can, however, cause QT complex (QTc) prolongation and should not be used in cardiac patients. Although most of the antipsychotics can lead to QTc prolongation, ziprasidone and an older agent, thioridazine, are more associated with cardiac effects than the others (Harrigan et al., 2004). It is available in pill, intramuscular, and intravenous formulations (Young & Lujan, 2004).

Quetiapine is a highly effective antipsychotic and possesses an attractive feature of being one of the least tightly bound to the dopamine 2 receptor site of all the antipsychotics along with clozapine (Kapur & Seeman, 2001). This makes it useful in patients with Parkinson's disease and other neurological problems (Jankovic, 2002). It is sedating and can cause hypotension. Nevertheless, it has less incidence of weight gain, dyslipidemias (Wirshing et al., 2003), EPS (Sajatovic, Mullen, & Sweitzer, 2002; Zimmet, 2005), and diabetes. Aripiprazole is the newest of the antipsychotics with unique properties as a dopamine agonist/antagonist. It is not associated with elevated prolactin levels, EPS, weight gain, or QTc prolongation. It is, however, activating in some patients and can cause insomnia, anxiety, and restlessness (Desai, 2003).

Neuroleptic malignant syndrome is a potentially fatal reaction to the dopamine blockade of the antipsychotics that can occur with a single dose of the medication. Although more commonly associated with the older agents, the second-generation antipsychotics can cause it as well. Symptoms include hypertension, mental status changes, fever, and muscle ridigity. Treatment involves intensive care monitoring with cooling blankets and muscle relaxants (Chandran, Mikler, & Keegan, 2003).

Table 20-4 *Antipsychotic Use in the Elderly*

Antipsychotic	Available Route	Healthy Elderly (mg/day)	Medically Ill Elderly (mg/day)	Possible Side Effects
Clozapine	PO, RDT	50-75	6.25-50	Agranulocytosis, weight gain, hyperglycemia, hypotension
Olanzapine	PO, RDT, IM	5-20	1.25-5	Weight gain, hyperglycemia, hyperprolactinemia
Risperidone	PO, RDT, LAI	0.5-6	0.25-1	Hypotension, sedation, extrapyramidal symptoms, weight gain, hyperprolactinemia
Quetiapine	PO	25-200	25-100	Hypotension, sedation
Ziprasidone	PO, IM, IV	20-160	20-80	QTc prolongation, rash, hypertension
Aripiprazole	PO	5-30	5-15	Headache, insomnia, agitation
Haloperidol	PO, IM, IV, LAI	1-15	0.5-6	Extrapyramidal symptoms, hypotension

IM, Intramuscular; *IV,* intravenous; *LAI,* long-acting injection; *PO,* oral; *RDT,* rapidly dissolving tablet.

One concern about psychotropics is the possibility of negative effects on memory in older persons. Data from the Eugeria longitudinal study compared cognitive abilities of older individuals taking psychotropics ("consumers") on a chronic basis with those who were not taking them ("nonconsumers"). Among consumers, a significant positive effect of antidepressants was found for both verbal and visual recall; benzodiazepines had no effect (Llard, Artero, & Ritchie, 2003).

Table 20-4 outlines antipsychotic use in older adults.

Suicide

Over the past few decades, suicide rates increased in Asian and Latin countries while declining in Anglo-Saxon countries (DeLeo & Spathonis, 2003).

Although older adults have the highest suicide rate of all age-groups, the prevalence of late-life suicide still is low. In a prospective study of 14,456 community-dwelling individuals, 21 suicides occurred over a 10-year period. Factors that predicted suicide in this sample were depressive symptoms, perceived health status, sleep quality, and absence of a confidant (Turvey et al., 2002).

Compared with younger persons, older adults are more likely to use highly lethal methods and to complete suicide. Factors that may contribute to suicide in older adults are listed in Box 20-7. In cases of assisted suicide and euthanasia, the older adult commonly seeks to escape chronic physical pain and suffering associated with a terminal illness. It also may be a response to profound mental anguish, feelings of hopelessness, depression, and being extremely tired of living (DeLeo & Spathonis, 2003). Among the personality traits that have been correlated with suicide are hostility, hopelessness, and the inability to verbally express psychological pain. Other factors are dependency on others, recent life events, and losses.

Mentally healthy older persons report that death thoughts and suicidal ideation are relatively rare (DeLeo & Spathonis, 2003). A German study that assessed the wish to die among persons age 70 and older determined

BOX 20-7 Factors That May Contribute to Suicide in Older Adults

- Mental disorders (especially depression)
- Physical illness
- Personality traits such as hostility
- Hopelessness
- The inability to verbally express psychological pain and dependency on others
- Recent life events and losses

Data from DeLeo, D., & Spathonis, K. (2003). Suicide and euthanasia in later life. *Aging: Clinical and Experimental Research, 15*(2), 99-110.

that death wishes were associated strongly with mental illness, particularly major depression. Older age, female gender, perceived physical health, and negative living conditions were only moderately related (Barnow, Linden, & Freyberger, 2004).

Among older persons who attempt suicide, a high risk of repeated attempts exists. Italian investigators followed 63 individuals age 60 and over who had attempted suicide. Over a 1-year period, 12.7% took their own life and another 11.1% attempted suicide again. One interesting difference found between repeaters and nonrepeaters was that repeaters were more likely to have experienced death of their father during childhood (DeLeo et al., 2002). In addition to the usual sense of loss, bereaved relatives and friends of an older person who commits suicide may also experience stigma, shame, and a sense of rejection in bereavement (Harwood, Hawton, Hope, & Jacoby, 2002).

NURSING CARE RELATED TO PSYCHOSOCIAL NEEDS

Nursing Assessment

Because there is considerable overlap in the assessment of sociological and psychological factors, this section addresses both. The purpose of the psychosocial assessment is to characterize the patient's functioning in a particular social environment. As with other assessments of older persons, the clinician should consider pace, patient fatigue, trust, validation of information with other sources, and the purposes for which the assessment is being made when selecting assessment techniques. In addition, knowledge of the most prevalent psychosocial problems encountered by older persons and their families, as well as knowledge of typical potential areas for growth, should guide the assessment.

Elements of a Psychosocial Assessment.
Psychosocial assessment should include the individual, the family, and the community, with consideration for the cultural environment. Essential content in assessment of the *individual* includes:

- Perception of current life situation
- Current roles and recent role changes
- Lifestyle
- Cultural background
- Location/residence
- Financial resources
- Mental status
- Goals and plans for the future

Essential content in the assessment of *family and significant others* includes:

- Perception of the family or caregiver of the patient's life situation and goals
- Family structure
- Family patterns of functioning
- Roles of the patient's significant others

Essential content in the assessment of the patient's *community* includes:

- Special resources in the current environment/ community
- Special demands of the current environment/ community

These elements of assessment are discussed in the context of three different types of assessment: screening, comprehensive assessment, and problem-specific assessment.

SCREENING. The purpose of screening is to identify potential patient, family, or community attributes that may signify a need for either preventive action or treatment. Screening may be problem oriented, or it may identify potential for growth in some area of function. The emphasis on particular psychosocial screening techniques varies with the expectations of the health care setting, the perspective from which the nurse practices, and the purpose for the screening examination. In all health care settings, a wellness focus can be maintained, along with an illness perspective.

During the screening process, it is important to determine whether an individual has certain prevalent problems related to aging, such as depression, substance abuse, and elder abuse. Because the current population of older adults matured in an era when psychological problems were not openly discussed or acknowledged, it is sometimes difficult to detect whether they exist. However, simple screening maneuvers such as drug and alcohol histories; depression questionnaires; and observation of appearance, hygiene, and dress are useful.

Psychological or social barriers may exist that interfere with achieving nursing care goals. These should be assessed during the screening process. These barriers may be economic, attitudinal, or cultural. Examples of economic barriers are insufficient funds with which to purchase medicines, equipment, food, or transportation to medical facilities; inability to pay for medical or nursing care; and lack of financial coverage for rehabilitation. Attitudinal barriers are related to health beliefs that interfere with prescribed medical or health care regimens, family issues that prevent rehabilitative measures because of the need to maintain dependence in the older member, or beliefs about services provided that may be viewed as "charity." Cultural barriers are related to religious, racial, or ethnic issues. Beliefs of older persons of particular racial or ethnic groups regarding the medical and health care system or its providers may lead to what appears to be "lack of compliance." Religious beliefs may also interfere with the carrying out of various medical and self-care regimens.

Mechanics of Screening and Assessment.
At a screening level, the interview/assessment is necessarily superficial. In many cases, information may be gained through a social, conversational manner to put older patients at ease. An informal format usually is preferable to a structured interview, especially with older people, who may be uncomfortable discussing psychological or social issues.

The interview should begin with open-ended questions and should focus on matters of primary importance to the patient. This allows the patient the opportunity to discuss issues of greatest concern and reinforces the impression that the nurse truly is concerned with the major problems. The following data are particularly helpful in eliciting psychosocial data:

1. In a clinical setting with a high proportion of low-income elderly, ask whether *income* is sufficient to provide needed groceries, drugs, and medical supplies.
2. If the individual lives alone and volunteers no information about family or friends, determine whether the person has a close friend or family member who acts as a *confidant*. A confidant increases life satisfaction.
3. If the older person has obvious dependencies, note on the first encounter who is *assisting with care* and who else in the family or friendship network is available to provide assistance.

4. Identify any *major life changes* that have occurred within the past year and chart the dates of key life events, such as retirement, widowhood, death of close friends, and anniversaries.

5. By asking an older person to *describe a typical day,* it is possible to gain insight into role-relationship patterns, self-concept, and demands of daily living.

6. Because many values and beliefs regarding health, illness, aging, and dying are culturally determined, it is beneficial to note the *racial and ethnic background* of an individual. Older persons are closer to their culture of origin than the young, and membership in a particular cultural group may influence health beliefs or self-care practices.

7. Find out the *religious background* of the older person to assist in determining whether spiritual distress is being experienced. National survey data have shown that members of the current cohort of old people are more likely to be a part of organized religion than younger persons. Religious organizations may also provide an important source of informal support.

8. *Note recent losses,* because a high number of losses in a short amount of time can predispose to illness, including depression, in all ages.

9. Ask *what the patient does for pleasure.* This information is helpful in indicating whether depression is present. An inability to enjoy life is one of the cardinal symptoms of depression, and the individual who is unable to describe any pleasurable activity should be assessed further.

10. Assess *employment status* and *work history,* including year of retirement, if applicable. This helps prevent inaccurate stereotyping of older people as universally retired and also identifies current roles that may be affected by an illness status.

After a screening, in-depth data gathering may be indicated. The nurse should judge the timing and depth of further assessment. Generally, primary care or continuing care nurses should prepare a comprehensive database for their patients. Nurses in acute care settings will probably do so only if psychosocial problems affect the handling of an acute problem or result in discharge difficulties.

COMPREHENSIVE PSYCHOSOCIAL ASSESSMENT. The major areas to be addressed in a comprehensive psychosocial assessment are financial status, role-relationship patterns, sexuality, coping and stress tolerance, health perception, and value-belief patterns. The data may be gathered in a conversational style; sometimes structured questioning of the individual or a significant other may be necessary. The geriatric psychiatric assessment is detailed separately.

Financial Status. For older individuals, especially those in need of long-term care, assessment of financial status is essential. Most people who are retired are faced with diminished income and, at the same time, may encounter markedly increased expenditures for medical care. Long-term care services are costly and frequently not covered by insurance or Medicare. Failure to acknowledge economic realities impedes planning of resource allocation and may result in impoverishment without the patient's goals being met.

The following story illustrates the importance of the financial assessment. Mr. J. had always said that he would "sooner die than go to a nursing home." When he experienced inoperable lung cancer and became weak secondary to radiation therapy and the progress of his disease, his family assumed that home care would be prohibitively expensive. They arranged for admission to a skilled nursing home. He died 2 weeks later. Had his financial status been assessed, adequate financial resources to purchase 24-hour daily help for 9 months would have been found. Failure to assess his financial status thus resulted in Mr. J.'s not meeting an important goal despite adequate resources.

Role-Relationship Patterns. Assessment of role-relationship patterns provides information regarding self-concept and sources of social support. One method of determining the pattern of role relationships is to obtain detailed information about the day's activities. If the patient is vague, this may indicate a paucity of social roles or lack of integration into the larger community. Vague responses may also indicate the presence of cognitive impairment or other mental disorders.

Sexuality. Barriers to assessment of the sexual patterns of older adults include generational barriers, myths about sexuality in old age, and perceived taboos about discussion of sexual concerns. Nurses typically belong to a younger age cohort than their older patients, which may make discussion of sexual matters more uncomfortable. In addition, most older persons grew up during a time when sexual mores were more restrictive and there was less explicit discussion of sexual matters. The myths that older persons are uninterested in sex, are unable to enjoy it, or are sexually inactive further complicate the issue, from the standpoint of both the nurse and the older person.

Assessment of sexual patterns requires a nonjudgmental, matter-of-fact manner. Older patients should be asked whether they are sexually active or whether there have been recent changes in sexual patterns. If concerns about sexual function are expressed, provide an opportunity for further exploration. In-depth assessment need not be pursued unless there is evidence of sexual dysfunction or the patient is at risk for alterations in sexual function.

Anxiety, Coping, and Stress Tolerance. Inquire about specific stressors or situations that cause anxiety. Understanding an older individual's lifetime patterns of coping can greatly facilitate the planning of nursing care. Explore how major problems were handled in the past and how these techniques could be used to handle present and future problems. One way to elicit information about past coping strategies is to ask the patient to focus on memories of past stressful situations that were successfully resolved. If the patient has relied on family members or friends for support, are these individuals still living and in good health? How does the patient typically cope with pain, uncertainty, or new situations? Does the patient use alcohol or drugs to cope with stressful situations? How much does the patient value religion as a means of coping with life's problems? The answers to these and similar questions affect the approach to patient teaching and counseling and indicate areas of potential lifestyle modifications and growth.

Health Perception. The following question may provide a picture of the older person's health perception: How do you rate your overall health—excellent, good, fair, or poor? Self-perception of health is significantly correlated with objective measures of health and longevity. In addition, responses to this question may give the nurse important insight into the individual's self-concept, need for knowledge, and motivation for change. Many older individuals perceive their health as "good," despite long lists of chronic diseases; this may reflect excellent coping abilities or denial of illness. Follow up by asking about personal goals for health and practices that the patient believes to be important in maintaining health. Understanding the patient's goals can reduce frustration for patients and nurses alike. Older people do not necessarily have experience in formulating goals with their health care providers, so nurses should be prepared to explain the importance of the patient's involvement in the management and prevention of chronic disease.

Value-Belief Pattern. Maintaining certain beliefs and adhering to values may become more important as older people grow closer to death. Often, decisions about priorities in health care for dependent older people must be made; knowledge of the individual's values and beliefs is central to making these decisions in an ethical manner. Religious beliefs, concerns about dependency and control, and prolongation of life if severe functional impairment exists should be discussed with the older person and involved family members to plan thoughtfully for nursing and health care.

Geriatric Psychiatric Assessment. Geriatric psychiatric assessments can take place in a variety of settings. These include the home, outpatient health care facilities, inpatient units, skilled nursing facilities, and hospices. The complexity of geriatric care demands comprehensive assessment, which is best accomplished by a team approach. The core team usually is made up of the physician, nurse, and social worker. The extended care

team varies with the needs of the patient and may include the pharmacist, psychiatrist or psychiatric nurse practitioner, dentist, psychologist, occupational therapist, physical therapist, or dietitian (Elon, Phillips, Loome, Denman, & Woods, 2000).

The psychiatric interview is the most essential tool the psychiatric clinician possesses. It elicits the information needed to establish a diagnosis and treatment plan. The psychiatric interview is strikingly different than a standard medical interview. In most cases, the clinician will have more time set aside for an initial interview because of the scope of the information necessary for diagnosis and treatment. Most clinicians consider 1 to 1.5 hours as sufficient. The psychiatric interview delves much deeper and covers areas such as social background and family psychiatric history that usually affect a visit for a cough or fever. The longer time serves another, more personal purpose. It allows the clinician and patient time to establish a rapport and begin the therapeutic alliance. Clinicians should always keep in mind that they are being assessed as closely as they are assessing the patient. The patient will be forming an opinion on how well the clinician interacts, speaks, and, most importantly, listens.

The interview begins rather generally and delves deeper as it progresses. It provides a logical sequence that allows the patient to describe symptoms and the thoughts and feelings that go along with them before moving to more historical data. We begin with the identifying demographic data. It is important to remember that the interviewer will probably not be the only person reading the report. This demographic data allows the reader or listener to at least form something of an image of the person, considering cultural characteristics, as well as age-related factors.

The chief complaint is what drives the interview. It should be in the patient's own words and is brief. The chief complaint may come from a family member or friend if the patient is having difficulty with self-expression or does not speak your language. There may be times when the patient is too demented, psychotic, or delirious to respond.

The largest portion of the interview is usually the history of present illness. This portion allows the patient to do the talking. You may need to prompt or redirect the person, but the purpose is to learn the patient's perception of his or her chief complaint. Allow or assist the patient to essentially paint you a picture of the problem and its symptoms. Key areas to assess are the patient's responses to his or her symptoms. What appears to be the patient's psychological makeup? In other words, how does the patient define the problem? How well is the patient coping and what are his or her defense mechanisms? What has the patient done to alleviate the problem and how well has it worked? What brought the patient to seek your help? What strengths and weakness does the patient bring to the situation? How has the health problem affected the person's life? Meanwhile, you will be gathering even more data about the patient as you listen and observe. Do consistent themes or schemas emerge? What does the nonverbal communication imply? How well does the patient communicate verbally? How organized is the patient's thinking? In other words, the clinician has already begun the mental status examination.

When a sufficient picture of the patient emerges, it is time to delve into the patient's history, which more times than not will reveal other problems or situations that need to be addressed in the care plan or that may affect the diagnosis.

The past psychiatric history is a crucial component of the interview. The data gathered, at a minimum, should include any past diagnoses, therapy or counseling, past psychiatric admissions, any psychotropic medications taken in the past, and their effect. Finally, you must assess past suicidal behaviors, be they gestures or attempts.

It is essential to obtain the past medical history. It provides clues about the patient that will affect your choice of treatments and can yield a great deal of information about the patient's past behavior. The patient's sexual history may be relevant, and the medical history may serve as a safe, clinical mechanism for discussing such a sensitive topic. The detail considered in the medical history is based on clinical judgment. There may be cases where the medical history is a major component, as in a patient with somatization disorder or pain disorder.

Substance abuse history should include tobacco, alcohol, recreational drugs, prescription drug abuse, and any intravenous drug abuse. Past family psychiatric history is another important source of information, especially considering the strong genetic component of many substance use and psychiatric disorders. It is important to go back at least two generations of blood relatives. Using a genogram can be helpful in diagramming the family history (Bennet, 2004). Asking about psychiatric medications that family members have taken in the past and their effect may elicit valuable data that can help in choosing a medication for the patient. Queries about family history of suicide are also valuable in assessing for safety.

The importance of knowing all the medications that the patient is currently taking cannot be overstated. Given the high incidence of drug interactions with many psychotropic medications, patient safety demands it. This includes all herbals, supplements, and any complementary or alternative therapies the patient might be using at the time. It is estimated that over 2.5 million adults use homeopathic modalities (D'Huyvetter & Corhssen, 2002). It is always a good idea to have patients keep a list of current medications with them or bring their prescriptions to the appointment. Although allergies to psychotropic medications are infrequent, it is still important to assess allergies. Many patients consider side effects as allergies, so it is important to document what the reaction was and educate the patient properly.

The social history can be time consuming, especially in the older patient, but it is an important tool. Determine where the person was born and raised, as well as where the person falls in the birth order of the family. A brief description of a person's childhood can yield valuable cues to explore abuse and abandonment issues or childhood/adolescent psychiatric problems that may not have been elucidated in the psychiatric history. Assessing school life gives a good idea of the patient's level of intelligence and early social relationships. Essential facts include the last grade completed, academic performance, and relationships. It is important to ask about military service because of its major impact on people's lives. Assessing job history tells you about the ability to maintain routines, be responsible, and interact with others. Marital status includes the number of marriages, how long they lasted, and what caused any relationship to end. It is important not to ignore sexuality in the elderly patient, especially when it may have a bearing on the health problem. If a thorough assessment is indicated, it is important to ask about sexual history, which can include any history of sexually transmitted diseases, childhood sexuality, experience in puberty, current sexual activity, and any history of conflict or dysfunction. It is a matter of clinical judgment based on the case as to whether to ask about sexual orientation. The number of children the patient has or has fathered and their status is important. Again, clinical judgment is used in assessing any marital infidelity and its relevance to the case.

Assessing spirituality is valuable in identifying support systems and affiliations with others. Knowing in what conditions the patient is living is important. Is the patient homeless? Does the patient live with a friend or with his or her children? Is the patient's living situation, especially for patients in nursing homes, stressful? Financial stress also is important, as well as any current or past legal problems that might factor into current symptoms. Asking about abuse requires discretion and a nonjudgmental attitude. It is important to ask about any physical, sexual, or emotional abuse or neglect. National estimates of 550,000 elders over age 60 suffering abuse or neglect in a 1998 study make it imperative to ask about current or past abuse or neglect (National Center on Elder Abuse, 1998). The mental status examination is the description of all the areas of the patient's mental functioning. The AMSIT framework is a useful mnemonic for structuring the examination (Brackley, 1997) (Table 20-5).

Appearance encompasses several aspects of the patient visible to the interviewer. Is appearance congruent with stated age? Is dress appropriate given the situation and weather? Keep in mind that some older patients

Table 20-5 *AMSIT Framework for Mental Status Assessment*

Category	Components	Abnormal Findings
Appearance	Stated age vs. apparent age	Older/younger appearance
	Dress and hygiene	Unkempt, unusual color combinations, body odor
	Posture	Slumped or rigid
	Behavior	Hostile, suspicious, dramatic, seductive
	Psychomotor activity	Agitated or retarded, echopraxia, stereotypical movements
	Speech	Pressured, echolalia, mute
	Gait	Ataxia, steppage, shuffling
Mood and affect	Mood: patient's subjective emotional state	Expansive, euphoric, depressed, dysphoric
	Affect: outward expression of emotional state	Incongruent, flat, inappropriate laughing/crying
Sensorium	Level of consciousness	Lethargic, obtunded, stupor, coma
	Orientation	Disorientation to time, person, place, situation
	Memory	Poor short- or long-term recall
	Calculation abilities	Inability to perform simple calculations
	Attention	Short attention span
	Concentration	Inability to focus on a simple task
Intellectual function	General fund of knowledge	Inability to produce basic knowledge
	Executive function	Inability to plan, sequence, or organize
Thought	Thought processes	Illogical, tangential, circumstantial, loose thought associations
	Thought content	Suicidal/homicidal ideations, delusions
	Abstracting ability	Inability to interpret proverbs or make logical connections between things
	Insight and judgment	Lack of logical response to a given situation
	Perceptions	Hallucinations

Courtesy of David S. Fuller, San Antonio, Texas, 2006.

wear more clothes than the younger person because of increased sensitivity to cold with decreased body fat. Patients with dementia frequently mismatch clothes. Note the patient's behavior in the interview, observing for hostility, seductiveness, anger, fear, or other signs of distress. Is the patient exhibiting psychomotor agitation or retardation? Posture can provide clues about neurological status, such as the stooped posture characteristic of parkinsonism, which could be pathological, idiopathic, or iatrogenic as a side effect of antipsychotic medications. Gait is another important neurological aspect that is easily assessed in the ambulatory patient. Shuffling or a "freezing" gait is indicative of parkinsonism. A rigid gait is suggestive of progressive supranuclear palsy. Steppage is a gait characterized by completely lifting the foot off the floor with each step, a symptom of paralysis of the frontal muscles of the legs caused by stroke, multiple sclerosis, neuropathies, or drug toxicities.

The clinician must assess speech as well, focusing on rate, rhythm, and inflection, and looking for any pressured speech, muteness, or odd speechlike neologisms or clanging. Mood is the subjective description of the patient's emotional state. It is most accurately described using the patient's own words. Affect, or outward expression of the mood, is up to the clinician's observation and falls along a continuum from full ranged to a flat, emotionless expression. Also important to note is the appropriateness of the affect to the stated mood. If the patient laughs while stating that he or she is depressed, this can be a sign of mania or psychosis. A flattened affect in the presence of a stated good mood can be a sign of depression or the masklike facies of parkinsonism.

Sensorium involves the patient's level of consciousness and orientation to person, place, time, and situation. The clinician also might assess the patient's ability to concentrate based on the ability to perform simple calculations, spell the word "world" backwards, or repeat the days of the week in reverse. Attention is easily assessed by having the patient tap a finger every time the clinician says the letter "A" while reciting a series of letters with "A" interspersed at random intervals in the sequence.

Intellectual function is assessed by simple questions such as "What states border ours?" and "Who are the president and vice president?" Use of language also is a component of the assessment of intellect. Executive function, the ability to utilize intact connections from the frontal lobes to the rest of the brain, can be assessed in many different ways; for example, have the patient complete a sequence such as the following: 1A, 2B, 3C, 4, and so on; have the patient name as many things that start with a particular letter as he or she can; or have the patient complete a "go/no go" sequence ("If I touch my ear, you touch your ear and if I touch my nose, you touch your nose"; then switch the sequence to "If I touch my ear, you touch your nose, and if I touch my nose, you touch your ear"). A formal test of executive functioning is discussed later in this section.

The dimensions of thought to assess include thought content, thought processes, ability to abstract, and judgment and insight. Thought content involves assessing for delusions or suicidal or homicidal ideations. Delusions may be of various types, including persecutory, somatic, jealous, erotomanic, or grandiose. In older patients, delusions frequently are persecutory in nature, such as beliefs that they are being stolen from or poisoned. They may believe that someone else is living in their house or that their relatives have been replaced by duplicates (known as Capgras' syndrome) (Moore & Jefferson, 2005). Thought process is the flow of thought, which may be logical and linear, tangential, or without any discernable connections. Confabulation, which is making up information, occurs in many neurological disorders, and is especially common in Alzheimer's disease (Geldmacher, 2004) and Wernicke-Korsakoff syndrome. Perseveration, the repetition of words or tasks, is common in dementia (Kertesz & Munoz, 2002). An example can be seen when the patient is asked to perform a repetitive task, such as writing "X" and "O" repeatedly across a single line on a page, and does not stop, but resumes the writing on the next line despite instructions to the contrary. Asking the patient to interpret a proverb is a good way to assess the patient's ability to abstract. Always keep in mind the culture of the patient when asking for proverb interpretation. Judgment and insight can be assessed by reviewing the patient's recent behavior. If that is not possible, asking a simple question that requires reasoning (e.g., "If you found a letter on the street with an address and stamp, what would you do with it?") gives an idea of the patient's judgment. The patient's understanding of his or her illness also gives clues as to the patient's insight. Hallucinations are most commonly auditory or visual, but they can be olfactory, gustatory, or tactile as well. They are indicative of psychosis, whether from schizophrenia, mania, Alzheimer's disease, Lewy body dementia, or delirium, as well as brain tumors and alcohol withdrawal.

Rating scales and standardized tests are useful tools that not only assist with initial diagnosis of various mental disorders, but also are effective for ongoing assessment of the patient. Some of the more common instruments used in the geriatric population are reviewed.

Structured interviews for diagnostic purposes are available. The most widely used instrument is the Scheduled Clinical Interview for DSM IV-TR (SCID). Although not specifically geared toward older persons, it provides a useful structure and flexibility for a diagnostic interview. However, it can take 2.5 to 3 hours to administer, making it difficult for some older adults. The Geriatric Mental State Schedule is a semistructured interview that allows the interviewer to explore symptoms commonly associated with psychiatric disorders. The instrument requires training and computer interpretation (Blazer, 2004).

One of the most widely used instruments for assessing cognition is the Folstein Mini-Mental State Examination (MMSE). It is divided into sections covering orientation, registration, attention and calculation, recall, and language. The maximum score is 30; the lower the score, the lower the cognitive functioning. Older adults with depression and cognitive impairment score higher than those with dementias and tend to improve their own scores with treatment of the depression, whereas the demented individual's scores do not improve (Gallo, Fulmer, Paveza, & Reichel, 2000). Another brief cognitive screen is the Short Portable Mental Status Questionnaire (SPMSQ). It is a 10-item tool designed to assess orientation, memory, general fund of knowledge, and calculation ability. Intact cognitive functioning is indicated by two or fewer errors. Progressive errors imply a decreasing level of functioning consciousness (Blazer, 2004). The Executive Interview (EXIT) is a comprehensive 25-item test administered by the interviewer. It tests the frontal lobes' capacity for reasoning, number/letter sequencing, memory, word and design fluency, and primitive reflexes, among other items (Royall, Mahurin, & Gray, 1992).

Several scales are useful for the assessment of depression in the older person. The first is the Center for Epidemiological Studies Depression Scale (CES-D). It consists of 20 basic questions on mood and behavior administered by the interviewer with rating scales for each item (e.g., 0 for rarely or never to 3 for most or all of the time) (Osterweil, Brummel-Smith, & Beck, 2000). The Geriatric Depression Scale (GDS) is a simple, 30-item scale covering symptoms such as cognitive complaints, self-image, and losses in a format of "present" or "not present" responses. The Beck Depression Inventory (BDI) is a 21-item self-report questionnaire that assesses depressive symptoms and attitudes on a scale of 0 to 3. The Hamilton Rating Scale for Depression (HAM-D) is probably the most commonly used scale. It is a 25-item scale administered by the interviewer on a number of symptoms from mood, insomnia, and psychomotor activity to sex drive and hypochondriasis (Blazer, 2004).

The Confusion Assessment Method—ICU can be a valuable contribution to the assessment of delirium for clinical and research purposes, with its optimal target population limited to intensive care unit (ICU) patients (McNicoll et al., 2005). The scale uses *Diagnostic and Statistical Manual of Mental Disorders* criteria for confusion and incorporates them into nine domains, including acute onset, course, inattention, disorganized thinking, and altered level of consciousness (Blazer, 2004).

Assessing alcohol abuse in the elderly can be made easier with the use of one of several instruments. The first and easiest to use is the CAGE test, a quick, four-item test in which the clinician asks about the perceived need to *cut down* on drinking, feeling *annoyed* by others' criticism of drinking, *guilt* over drinking, and using morning *"eye openers"* of alcohol to control withdrawal symptoms. Two or more positive responses can indicate problem drinking. The Michigan Alcoholism Screening Test—Geriatric (MAST-G) is a 24-item instrument that assesses a multitude of different physiological, social, and psychological aspects of drinking. It takes a few minutes to complete and score. The Alcohol Use Disorders Identification Test (AUDIT) is a 10-item scale used to assess current drinking patterns that can indicate alcohol abuse, alcohol dependence, and hazardous drinking (O'Connell et al., 2004). All three tests are available from multiple sources with no copyright restrictions.

It often is necessary to assess an older person's decision-making *capacity* in order to ascertain the person's ability to give informed consent for procedures. This differs from *competency*, a legal determination assessed by a judge in a formal hearing (Kassutto & Vaught, 2003). Physicians and advanced practice nurses with training are capable of determining capacity. The clinician assesses the patient's mental status and ability to communicate, the patient's level of understanding of the procedure or drug, and the patient's insight and judgment into his or her decisions. Low-risk procedures infer a lower threshold for capacity than high-risk, low-yield tests, procedures, or treatments. If the patient is determined not to have capacity, a surrogate decision maker must be obtained as needed.

Testing and evaluating the older adult can be a challenge because of a number of factors, including visual and hearing impairment, memory, fatigability issues, and distrust of psychiatric personnel. Older patients often need special attention during the interview. The pace of the interview may need to be slower. Hearing-impaired or visually impaired patients may need to sit closer to, and directly in front of, the interviewer. It is important to speak clearly and at a volume the patient does not find distorted. You may need to offer more physical assistance than with a younger patient. Necessarily, the interview will take longer because of a longer history and probably more medications that must be assessed for drug interactions.

If the patient is exhibiting psychotic symptoms or the interview seems to be agitating the patient, it may need to be abbreviated. In all, flexibility is important, especially in emergency situations such as having to admit the patient with suicidal ideations. The most important aspect of setting is privacy. This is sometimes difficult when seeing patients in the hospital, when other patients may be only a few feet away and nursing staff members are frequently in and out of the room. The clinician should feel free to ask visitors to step out for a while, perhaps to eat or have a snack. If the patient's medical condition allows, you may opt to see the patient in another area. The physical layout of the setting should be comfortable for the patient. In any setting, it is wise to position yourself between the patient and the door, making rapid egress possible if safety is a concern. If collateral data are needed, the patient must give permission for the clinician to interview others, unless the patient lacks the capacity to make his or her own medical decisions.

Note taking is a bone of contention for many patients. Some patients may object to the clinician writing during the interview; others may be concerned that the interviewer will not remember everything the patient says if the interviewer does not take notes. It is important at the start of the interview to ask whether the patient minds note taking. A simple statement can be made, such as "I'd like to take some notes at times in our interview so that I make sure I have all the important information I need. If it bothers you, just let me know and I'll stop." Interruptions are something to be dealt with as best as possible. In the office setting, support personnel are aware that the time the clinician is with the patient is protected time. Placing a "do not disturb" sign on the door is important. In addition, turning off cell phones or muting them, as well as pagers, is important so that the patient can see that the clinician takes his or her problem seriously. Any measures taken to decrease interruptions are important.

The patient may want a family member or friend in the room during the interview. This is the patient's prerogative as long as he or she understands that very personal issues may be discussed. Additionally, there may be times when the clinician will want someone else in the room, as in the case of some patients of the opposite sex or severely disordered patients who pose a threat either physically or legally. This is usually dealt with based on the clinician's own clinical judgment and the rules of the agency or practice.

There are several specific situations that make the psychiatric interview challenging. The first is the delusional patient, who often has been brought to the interview by a third party. It is important to remain neutral about the delusion, but discussing it can yield information about stressors in the patient's life and underlying psychodynamic issues. Reassuring the patient that you are there only to help may set the patient at ease. As the patient begins to express doubts about the delusion, the clinician can begin to doubt it as well. Most patients do not see their delusion as a clinical problem, and in that case it is usually best to work on other issues for which they want help. As the overall clinical condition improves, they will usually stop talking about the delusion, and it is up to the clinician how much the delusional content is revisited.

One of the more challenging interviews is the somatic patient. These patients will have probably been referred by their primary physician when the medical complaints are not consistent with the physical findings. A referral to a mental health clinician alone will probably create some defensiveness on the part of patients. They will probably feel that their doctor has given up on them or thinks that they are "crazy." Communication with the referring clinician can help the clinician prepare for the interview by knowing how the patient was prepared for the referral. It is imperative for the clinician to reassure these patients that the clinician does not doubt their complaints, but wants to understand the stress that it has caused for them. This neutral stance is sometimes reassuring and allows the clinician to explore the stress that may be contributing to the patient's symptoms. Several visits may be necessary before the patient even approaches the notion of the stress-causing symptoms.

Violent patients are most likely to be seen in the emergency department. The patient may be physically restrained by handcuffs or other restraints. Whether you have them removed or have a law enforcement officer in the room is based on clinical judgment and the law. Logically, a quiet environment with decreased stimuli should be arranged.

By using basic principles of interviewing combined with recognized tests and measurements or collateral information, a comprehensive assessment of the older person is possible. It is essential in this vulnerable population to obtain the most accurate data possible in order to ensure accurate diagnosis, develop a comprehensive care plan, and continually reassess the patient and your treatment.

All instruments should be considered copyright protected unless otherwise indicated.

For additional assessment information, refer to Box 20-8.

Nursing Diagnoses

Among the many nursing diagnoses that might be made related to the older person's psychological status are the following (North American Nursing Diagnosis Association [NANDA], 2005):

- Impaired adjustment related to negative attitudes toward health behavior, multiple stressors, absence of social support for changed beliefs and practices,

---

Box 20-8 Psychiatric Assessment

History
- Identifying data
- Chief compaint
- History of present illness
  - Perception of problem and symptoms
  - Response to symptoms
  - Coping strategies
  - Reason for seeking help
  - Strengths and weaknesses
  - Impact of problem/symptoms on life
- Past history
  - Psychiatric:
    Past diagnoses and treatment
    Past and current medications
    Suicidal behavior
    Substance abuse history
    Family psychiatric history
  - Medical
- Social history
  - Place of birth, birth order
  - Description of childhood
  - Education, academic performance
  - Relationships
  - Military service
  - Job history
  - Marital history and current status
  - Sexual history
  - Children
  - Spirituality
  - Current or past abuse or neglect
  - Economic, attitudinal, and cultural barriers to achieving goals

Physical Examination
- General appearance
  - Appropriateness of dress
  - Congruence of appearance with age
  - Behavior
  - Psychomotor function
  - Posture and gait
  - Speech rate, rhythm, inflection
- Mood and affect
- Sensorium
- Intellectual function
  - Language
  - Executive function
  - Thought content, processes, ability to abstract
  - Judgment and insight
  - Suicidal or homicidal ideations
  - Cognition
  - Decision making

disability or change in health status, low state of optimism

■ Anxiety related to unmet needs; change in health status, environment, role function, interaction status, economic status; threat of death, threat to self-concept

■ Disturbed body image related to developmental changes, trauma, illness, illness treatment

■ Decisional conflict related to support system deficit, perceived threat to value system, lack of relevant information, multiple or divergent sources of information

■ Ineffective coping related to uncertainty, inadequate resources available, high degree of threat, inability to conserve adaptive energies, inadequate level of confidence in ability to cope

■ Fear related to separation from support system in potentially stressful situation, sensory impairment

■ Dysfunctional grieving related to actual or perceived object loss

■ Hopelessness related to prolonged activity restriction creating isolation, long-term stress, abandonment, lost belief in transcendent values/God, failing or deteriorating physiological condition

■ Risk for loneliness related to affectional deprivation, social isolation, physical isolation

■ Impaired memory related to neurological disturbances, fluid and electrolyte imbalance, anemia, acute or chronic hypoxia, decreased cardiac output

■ Noncompliance related to health care plan cost, complexity; personal abilities, knowledge and skills relevant to regimen behavior, credibility of providers, relationship with provider

■ Powerlessness related to health care environment, illness-related regimen, interpersonal interaction, lifestyle

■ Ineffective role performance related to physical illness, cognitive deficits, mental illness, health alterations, fatigue, depression, low self-esteem

■ Situational low self-esteem related to disturbed body image, functional impairment, social role change, failures/rejections

■ Spiritual distress related to loneliness/social alienation, death and dying of self and others, life change, chronic illness of self or others

■ Risk for suicide related to behavioral, verbal, situational, psychological, demographic, physical, or social factors (specify)

Nursing Goals

The general goals of nursing care for individuals with needs related to psychological status are to (1) reduce anxiety, fear; (2) improve coping, adjustment/adaptation to aging and pathological states; (3) maintain cognitive function; (4) promote learning; (5) improve self-esteem, confidence in abilities; (6) facilitate grief work; and (7) foster feelings of hope and spiritual well-being.

Nursing Interventions

Interventions to Reduce Anxiety. The specific techniques used to reduce anxiety are highly variable, because they depend not only on the individual's current level of function but also on coping strategies developed over a lifetime. Capitalize on coping mechanisms and habit patterns that have been successful in the past. Using familiar strategies may serve to heighten the patient's sense of mastery over the situation, which itself contributes to anxiety reduction. Interventions may focus on the immediate reduction of anxiety or on better management of anxiety and stress over time.

Useful techniques to reduce the current level of anxiety and to prevent further severe anxiety states include the following:

■ Use consistent caregivers (i.e., do not change patient care assignments capriciously).

■ Use short, simple explanations for procedures.

■ Be predictable. Follow through on promises, especially regarding time.

■ Provide companionship in small, regular, frequent doses. During this time, gentle, firm touch may be useful rather than conversation. Spend quiet time with the patient.

■ Consider the patient's pace. It is likely to be slower than yours! A calm, unhurried manner is transmitted to the patient.

■ Coach the patient in deep breathing.

■ Inform all persons involved in the patient's care of factors that cause anxiety.

■ Useful techniques to prevent severe anxiety episodes in the future include the following:

■ Explore life events that contribute to anxiety.

■ Assess antecedents of anxiety. The use of a diary may be helpful.

■ Document responses to environmental stimuli, and to drugs if they are used.

■ Document the effectiveness of interventions used in the short term.

■ Model or describe to caregivers behaviors that successfully reduce anxiety and praise their successes in reducing or preventing anxiety in the patient.

■ Explore the need for referral for psychotherapy to deal with the anxiety problem on a long-term basis.

In addition to these guidelines for reducing or preventing anxiety in the older patient, general treatment approaches include environmental manipulation, behavioral therapies, pharmacotherapy, and psychotherapy. Drug therapy and psychotherapy were discussed earlier. The purpose of *environmental manipulation* is to alleviate the fears associated with the older person's feelings of dependency. Environmental manipulation can be applied to either the physical environment or the family and social support system. A more structured, safe, and protective physical environment and in some cases relocation to a group home, assisted living, or institutional setting may be required to alleviate symptoms of severe anxiety. Strengthening support systems can be accomplished by helping family and friends understand factors underlying anxiety such as increasing dependency and fears of dependency. Support persons who understand the causes of anxiety are better prepared to offer support.

Behavioral therapies may include systematic desensitization, progressive muscle relaxation, hypnosis, biofeedback, massage, meditation, and exercise. Research in behavioral therapies has been plagued with methodological problems, making generalizations difficult (Canter, 2003). Also, many studies have focused on specific groups such as persons with pain, cancer, headache, or irritable bowel syndrome, and individuals undergoing chemotherapy. Nevertheless, nursing literature commonly recommends reassurance, relaxation techniques, and diversional strategies for anxiety reduction.

Truthful reassurance, providing information, and providing clear explanations certainly are appropriate. Evidence exists to support the use of relaxation techniques for panic disorder, generalized anxiety disorders, and OCD. One outcome of relaxation therapy is that patients learn that they have the ability to reduce some of their own anxiety. However, it should be noted that effective relaxation training typically requires 8 to 12 treatment sessions. Also, this therapy is not without risk because some individuals experience relaxation-induced anxiety or even panic (Short, Kitchiner, & Curran, 2004).

Guided imagery also is often recommended to reduce anxiety. Various mechanisms that have been proposed to explain possible benefits of this strategy include refocusing attention, reduced autonomic responses, and blocking of painful stimuli (Baird & Sands, 2004). Much of the research on guided imagery has focused on pain reduction and has employed combinations of strategies (often progressive relaxation with guided imagery). Many studies include multiple outcomes such as anxiety and depression. Benefits have been demonstrated in various samples, including cardiac bypass patients (Rose, 2004) and older persons having joint replacement surgery (Antall & Kresevic, 2004). Sloman's (2002) study of relaxation and imagery in patients with advanced cancer found no improvement in anxiety, but significant positive changes in depression and quality of life. A meta-analysis of the effect of guided imagery practice on outcomes showed that the effect size increased over the first 5 to 7 weeks, and decreased at 18 weeks (Van Kuiken, 2004). Although cognitive-behavioral

therapy and relaxation therapy have been found effective for generalized anxiety disorder, drug therapy may be needed as well (Culpepper, 2002). Music often is used alone or in combination with other strategies to reduce anxiety (Cooke, Chaboyer, & Hiratos, 2005; Lai, 2004; West, 2003).

Psychotherapy for anxiety should be based on a supportive relationship rather than on the development of insight. The older person should be reassured that the anxiety symptoms are emotionally related and are not signals of impending physical breakdown. Regular, frequent meetings help provide assurance that a caring, supportive person is available. The meetings may be gradually tapered off as the level of anxiety lowers. Therapy should aim at returning to patients a sense of control over their own lives (Stetter, Walter, Zimmernann, Zahress, & Straube, 1994).

INTERPERSONAL TECHNIQUES KEYED TO SPECIFIC CONTRIBUTING FACTORS. Interpersonal interventions are best when individualized to address factors that contribute to the individual's anxiety. These interventions are powerful and, unlike drugs, have no dangerous side effects. An additional benefit is their potential for addressing the cause of the anxiety rather than simply alleviating the symptoms.

Figure 20-1 is an algorithm that helps simplify the assessment of factors that contribute to anxiety. A variety of ways to elicit the data are needed to follow the algorithm, but the cornerstone is careful history taking and observation of patient responses. Differentiating one contributing factor from another may require noting the individual's response to several different interventions. Remember that multiple factors may be contributing to the anxiety simultaneously.

Common factors contributing to anxiety are unconscious conflicts related to essential values or goals, threat to self-concept, threat of death, and change in health status. Each of these is discussed next along with specific intervention techniques.

Unconscious Conflict Related to Essential Values or Goals. Life review therapy may enable the individual to work through unresolved conflict. This may take place in a group or individually. Family members, interested volunteers, and paraprofessional workers can be taught the principles and techniques applicable to facilitating an individual's life review.

Threat to Self-Concept. When a threat to the self-concept is the basis of anxiety, explore the patient's feelings about self at present and in the past. Assist patients to identify ways in which they are important despite changes in roles. Help them to identify meaningful activities at which they can succeed. Teach new skills as indicated, or help the individual search for new meaning in previously learned skills.

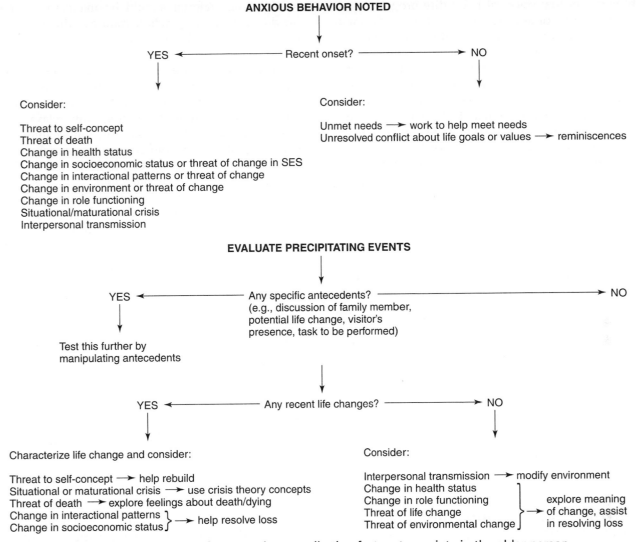

Figure 20-1   Algorithm for assessing contributing factors to anxiety in the older person.

Threat of Death. Responding to a patient's anxiety based on fear of death considers whether the patient is terminally ill or not. When the patient is not terminally ill, clarify the patient's prognosis and explain available treatment options. Experiencing death anxiety may motivate nonterminally ill people to pay more attention to their health. After a life-threatening exacerbation of a chronic disease such as diabetes mellitus, people who previously used denial as their main coping mechanism may become motivated to learn and practice better techniques of disease management. Likewise, individuals in the early recovery phase of a myocardial infarction may be motivated to learn about lifestyle modification to reduce their risk of a second infarction.

When the patient is terminally ill, nurses first must explore their own feelings about dying and achieve some comfort in viewing dying as a part of living to avoid transmitting their anxieties to the patient. Dying is a highly emotionally charged issue. Give patients the opportunity to share feelings, fears, and concerns about

the process of dying. Use active listening techniques to encourage them to express their concerns. Although older people generally talk about death more easily and express less fear, some do experience death anxiety. Some older patients are more comfortable talking with someone of their own chronological age or cultural background. Be sensitive to the patient's ability and willingness to discuss dying, which may change over the course of the terminal illness. Several sources report the value of music as a creative outlet (Hogan, 2003) that can restore the spirit and enhance quality of life in a person with a terminal illness (Halstead & Roscoe, 2002). Initiate contact with other health team members such as the chaplain, social worker, or hospice team, as indicated by patient wishes, stress level, and proximity of death.

CHANGE IN HEALTH STATUS. When anxiety stems from a change in health status, interventions must include information, support, and guidance. Many diseases such as cancer that once carried a dire prognosis now often are curable or at least treatable, but patients may not know this. Teach them about their diagnoses and current treatment options and prognoses. All health care team members should communicate to ensure that the patient is given consistent information. The anxiety that accompanies a new diagnosis interferes with comprehension and memory of details. Therefore reinforcement, "take home" educational materials, and resources (e.g., American Diabetes Association) are essential. Some changes in health status result in changes in role relationships, which represent a potential threat to self-concept. Assist individuals and their significant others to explore potential changes in roles, and guide them in developing strategies to adapt to those changes.

Some individuals experience health anxiety characterized by catastrophic interpretations of their symptoms. They tend to constantly seek reassurance, but are satisfied with responses for only a short period of time. Their behavior has been compared to that of an addict who seeks a substance (in this case, reassurance) that provides short-term relief of anxiety. Soon the anxiety resurfaces, and the person again seeks another "dose" of reassurance. Once reasonable investigation of the symptoms has revealed no cause for alarm, this cycle can exhaust the patience of health care providers and significant others. To break the cycle of dependence on reassurance, consistent responses from all involved parties (e.g., "We all have agreed not to answer those kinds of questions") may be effective (Short, Kitchiner, & Curran, 2004).

NEUROBIOLOGICAL ETIOLOGIES. Anxiety disorders tend to run in families, therefore inferring a genetic link and biological etiology in some patients. Twin studies have shown increased rates of panic disorder in monozygotic twins over their dizygotic counterparts. Studies suggest that panic disorder could result from abnormalities in the firing of neurons within the amygdala, the principle structure in formulating emotional reactions, primarily fear. Neuroimaging studies have shown increased blood flow in the hippocampus, a related structure within the limbic system, in patients with panic disorder even when not having panic attacks. Similar increased amygdaloid activity occurs in PTSD. OCD can also have neurological roots as manifested by an inability to "turn off" a signal that continues to loop through a well-defined pathway from the cerebral cortex to the thalamus, thus leading to the inability to stop repetitive behaviors or ruminating thoughts (Pliszka, 2003).

EVALUATION. The number and duration of extreme anxiety states are two critical outcome variables. These parameters can be monitored using a simple flow sheet (Figure 20-2). If anxiety persists despite nursing

interventions, referral should be made to other care providers, such as psychotherapists, who can follow through with treatment.

Interventions to Reduce Fear. Interventions to reduce fear in older persons generally involve increasing the patient's knowledge, competence, or awareness of the feared situation or object. Progressive relaxation and guided imagery are two stress reduction techniques that may be applicable to older persons experiencing fear. Possible interventions for common sources of fear in older people include the following:

- *Fear of pain:* Tell patients what sensations to expect during procedures. Use premedication and deep breathing, systematic relaxation techniques, distraction, or imagery for painful procedures. Remain with the older person during the procedure, if possible. Consider whether the patient is a candidate for self-management of pain medication and offer the option if feasible.

- *Fear of nursing home placement:* Encourage the patient to express fantasies about nursing home life. Then enlist the assistance of family or friends to obtain firsthand information about local nursing homes regarding the feared attributes. If the fantasized fears are based in reality, try anticipatory problem solving to allow the patient opportunity to exert some control over the situation. Consider shopping for a nursing home that has the least number of feared characteristics. If at all possible, the patient should be able to visit facilities and participate in making a choice.

- *Fear of falling:* Assess the patient's previous fall patterns and risk factors for fall-related injury. Fears may be based on an experience in which situational elements were quite different—for example, the patient's sister died after a fall, but the patient's risk of fall-related injury is not high. Explain the risks of inactivity and the benefits of ambulation. Implement a plan to reduce the risk for fall-related injury, and include the patient in establishing goals and evaluation criteria. Discuss environmental modifications and ambulatory aids as appropriate.

- *Fear of crime:* Contact the local police department for information about neighborhood watch programs, and other resources for frail, isolated individuals. Some religious institutions have programs to assist older persons. Senior companion programs may assist with shopping or accompany older persons on outings. Encourage the patient to express specific fears about crime and facilitate reality testing and problem solving.

- *Fear of incontinence:* Explore meanings and fears of incontinence with the individual. This may be the first opportunity offered to the patient to discuss the social and psychological aspects of incontinence. Knowledge deficits about incontinence may be revealed, which in

DATE/TIME	Anxiety State	Activities Since Last Assessment	Coping Strategies Used During Assessment Period (Client Perception)	Medications

Figure 20-2   Flow sheet for anxiety documentation.

turn may suggest some strategies for intervention. For example, if a woman no longer goes to church because she fears the embarrassment associated with an episode of stress incontinence, she could be counseled about the options available to treat or manage this problem.

EVALUATION. Effectiveness of interventions for those with fears can be judged by the extent to which the patient states that fear has been resolved, and alleviation of the signs of dysfunction or restricted activity associated with the fear(s). It is reasonable to assume that the more complex the intervention required, the more time will be required for resolution.

Case Example. A. N. was an 86-year-old woman admitted to the hospital because of a septic knee and uncompensated heart failure. Before the hospitalization she was functionally independent in all domains and lived alone. She had not been hospitalized in the past 50 years. The knee inflammation caused her to have considerable pain on motion. As a result, she limited her mobility to such an extent that she performed no activities of daily living independently because she was afraid of inducing more pain. She became increasingly weak and developed a grade II sacral pressure sore.

To reverse this declining function secondary to fear of pain, the nurse began giving the patient regular doses of analgesia rather than administering pain medication only on an "as requested" basis. The nurse also instructed A. N. on the relationship between immobility and decreased strength and ability. Finally, the nurse stayed with the patient and assisted her in performing activities within her functional capacity, such as sitting on the bedside commode and bathing and grooming activities. Increased activity helped reduce the edema associated with the infection. The experience of increased activity without an increase in knee pain served to resolve the patient's fear of pain with increased activity.

Interventions to Promote Effective Individual Coping. Providing support is the most important immediate intervention. Initially the patient may require what the self-care model terms a *wholly compensatory mode* in which the nurse makes the majority of decisions, moving next through a partially compensatory care system, and finally achieving a supportive educative system, in which the older patient has the primary decision-making role. Immediate interventions for ineffective coping include increasing the support available to the older person through use of formal agencies and informal support networks. Formal agencies include home health agencies, social service agencies, clinics, and hospitals; informal support networks involve church groups, extended family, and volunteers.

Efforts then can shift to identify the care system that will enable the individual to cope with life demands more effectively. This usually involves a combination of helping the individual enhance coping skills and increasing the available social and environmental support. Care should be offered in the least restrictive environment possible; however, institutional care may be needed on a short-term or long-term basis.

Specific interventions depend to a great degree on the specific factors contributing to the coping difficulty and on the resources available for support in a given setting. Factors that may contribute to ineffective coping are clouded perception of life events, reduced social support, knowledge deficit, massive functional disability, and environmental change.

CLOUDED PERCEPTION OF LIFE EVENTS. Physical dysfunction, physiological imbalance, and drug adverse effects should be considered as possible contributors to ineffective coping in the older adult. Any disorder that impairs tissue oxygenation, cellular metabolism, sensory perception and interpretation, or mobility could affect the individual's ability to cope. The intervention of choice is correction of the underlying disturbance; when drug adverse effects are implicated, a medication adjustment is warranted.

It is important to distinguish ineffective coping related to acute, reversible causes from that related to chronic impairments. Those with a chronic impairment in mentation that affects coping require some form of surrogate to provide ongoing support. Those with temporary and reversible coping difficulties require transient support but will later be able to resume former coping patterns.

REDUCED SOCIAL SUPPORT. Older persons often experience a gradual or sudden diminution of social supports as they age. Loss of a spouse, friendly neighbor, or confidant may affect the ability to maintain independent living. In determining the appropriate intervention, assess the roles performed by the lost member of the support network. Some losses can be compensated, particularly in the case of instrumental support services. Even in the case of loss of affective support, new, emotionally satisfying relationships can be formed, although this may require an extended period of time. In the interim, the individual may require transient instrumental support to prevent deterioration of health status.

KNOWLEDGE DEFICIT. Information is a key coping resource. Some older persons may be at a disadvantage in acquiring new knowledge because of slowed responses, memory impairment, and sensory impairment. Sometimes information is not provided to older persons because of the stereotype that they cannot, or will not, learn. There is every indication that older persons benefit from new knowledge if it is presented appropriately. For a more detailed discussion of teaching methods available to enhance the knowledge of older persons, refer to the section on learning in this chapter.

MASSIVE FUNCTIONAL DISABILITY. Although humans have an enormous capacity for adaptation, at some point the number or nature of stressors in comparison to a person's coping resources and situational support can become overwhelming. This may occur on a transient or chronic basis. For example, the individual who sustains bilateral cerebral infarctions with a total loss of function initially will be overwhelmed, even with excellent coping resources and social support. Although it is possible for such a person to adapt eventually, nursing action usually is required to compensate for overwhelmed psychological defenses. The key to intervention lies in maximizing the individual's remaining abilities, facilitating the grief process of the patient and family, and helping the individual clarify on an ongoing basis both progress and prognosis. The patient's perception is most important because the patient and family often do not understand the powerful impact of skillful rehabilitation in helping individuals compensate for lost function. It is essential that patient and family be included in goal setting and prioritization.

ENVIRONMENTAL CHANGE. Nurses should have a high index of suspicion for environmental change as a factor that precipitates ineffective coping in older persons because they are sensitive to such changes. Those with sensory impairments or mobility impairments are particularly vulnerable. It is vital to determine the older person's functional level before the environmental change took place in order to ascertain whether the functional disability has been induced merely by a change in the environment. For example, older persons who are continent at home may become incontinent in the hospital. This change may be inaccurately perceived by family or patient as an inevitable part of aging and a signal that the older person is losing the ability to cope independently. The true etiology of the functional impairment should be determined (in this case, for example, a new diuretic, lack of privacy, activity restriction, reduced mobility, inaccessible toilet, or urinary tract infection), and both the causes and their treatment should be discussed with the patient and family. Failure to do so may well contribute to a downward spiral leading to increased dependency and reduced coping capacity.

Evaluation. Criteria for evaluation of nursing care for patients with ineffective coping should reflect expected outcomes of the desired health state of a patient and specify indicators addressing the extent of achievement of the patient goal. The critical outcome variable for the patient with ineffective coping is developing an adequate response repertoire. This may be demonstrated by the patient verbalizing or demonstrating cognitive knowledge learned, skills achieved, and new behaviors acquired, and by the patient using the new knowledge, behavior, and skill in daily life activities. Additional outcomes might include meeting daily physical needs, realistic cognitive/perceptual domains, and a functional kin/social support network. Questions that might be relevant in evaluating the support network include the following: What is the nature of the social support available to the patient? Does the patient have a confidant? Has the patient identified a surrogate to act in his or her behalf should ineffective coping again be a problem? Have these support persons been included in plans for the patient's care? Will the patient receive support from any formal agencies? If the nature of this help is time limited, is there a mechanism to reevaluate the need for support when these services are terminated?

Interventions to Maintain Cognitive Function.

"Learning slows down specific aspects of aging and its side effects" (Schneider, 2003, p. 809). This statement represents the view of many who believe that frequent, stimulating activity helps preserve cognitive function in older age. Wilson (2003) demonstrated the relationship between lifetime participation in cognitively stimulating activities and cognitive reserve. After controlling for age, sex, and education, he found that individuals with more frequent stimulating activity had better perceptual speed, visuospatial ability, and semantic memory.

Interventions to Promote Learning.

How the older learner perceives the information can be affected by environmental influences, age-related sensoriperceptual changes, and pacing of instruction. Adaptations that assist the older learner include the following:

- Implement learning experiences in familiar settings whenever possible. For group instruction, churches or senior centers may be more attractive to older persons than schools or health care facilities.
- Relate learning experiences to real life.
- Direct the learner's attention to only one topic or task at a time; eliminate extraneous stimuli.
- Be sure patients have glasses and hearing aids if normally worn.

- Consider the needs of persons with poor vision. Use large-print, written materials. Dark letters on a light yellow paper or background is recommended. Avoid excessively "busy" designs. Avoid dim lighting and glare.
- For persons with poor hearing, provide written material, repeat as needed, and use amplifier if needed. Moderate rate of speech. Validate understanding.
- Provide written material that the person can refer to after the learning experience.
- Adapt instruction to the pace of the learner. Break content into small blocks.
- Persons with chronic illness, physical impairment, or poor nutrition may tire quickly. Slower pacing helps when fatigue is a factor.
- Adapt pace to accommodate slower reaction time and information processing.

Interventions to Improve Self-Esteem.

Almost any situation that involves loss places individuals at risk for situational low self-esteem. Nurses have numerous opportunities to implement or foster the development of strategies to enhance self-esteem in the older adult. A primary goal of nurses who work with individuals who are faced with disease-related assaults is to help the individual compensate for losses and make sense of those losses. Nurses can have a powerful influence on how people view themselves when their lives are altered by disability, chronic illness, or major role changes.

Many interventions have been successfully applied to the problem of disturbances in self-concept and self-perception. Individual counseling, group approaches, network interventions, exercise, and environmental modification all have a place in the nurse's armamentarium. Individual counseling is aimed at helping the individual resolve losses by facilitating the grief process. This intervention is particularly useful for those who are experiencing disturbances in role performance, personal identity, and body image (Norris, 1992). For those with disturbances in self-esteem, the focus of individual therapy is helping the individual identify strengths and lower unrealistic expectations (Figure 20-3). Reminiscence may help achieve both objectives. Individual counseling need not take place only in an office setting or with an explicitly formulated contract for counseling. Nurses have numerous opportunities at the bedside or chairside to provide the active listening, guided reminiscence, gentle confrontation, and support needed by an older person who is grieving or working to reduce unrealistic expectations of self.

Reminiscence groups are another form of intervention for self-concept disturbance (Stevens-Ratchford, 1993). In addition to the general advantages of group treatment, reminiscence groups have the added

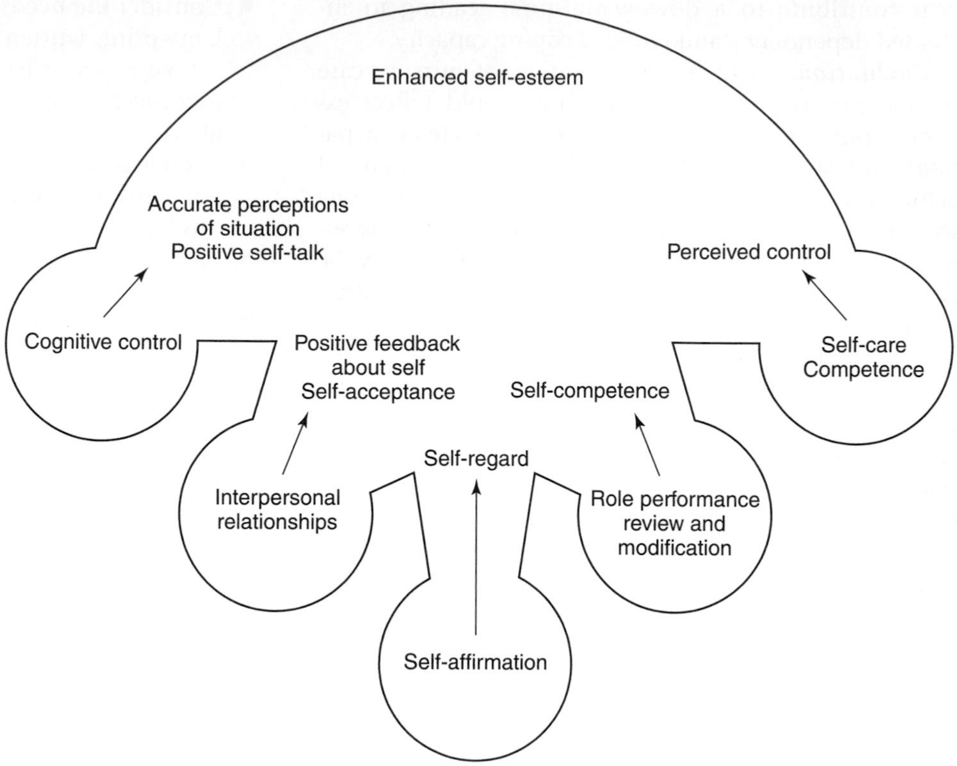

Figure 20-3 Interventions for altered self-esteem. (From Miller, J. F. [1992]. *Coping with chronic illness: Overcoming powerlessness* [2nd ed.]. Philadelphia: FA Davis.)

advantage of providing the experiences of many people to stimulate reminiscence, increasing the possibility of empathic responses by group members of a similar life station and birth cohort. Points to consider in organizing these groups include the following:

A. Minimum skill requirements for a reminiscence therapist (Butler, 1960, 1968; quoted in Blum & Tross, 1980)
  1. Someone who can serve as an active listener, helping the individual summarize the reflections stimulated
  2. Someone knowledgeable about techniques that stimulate reminiscence
B. Therapist's attitudes
  1. Empathy for the older person's frame of reference
  2. Tolerance for defensive distortion of memories
  3. Positive concern for the patient's emotional struggle and progress in that struggle
  4. Sense of professional purpose and the ability to persevere
C. Considerations in group reminiscence therapy (Ebersole, 1984)
  1. Keep group size small, no more than five or six people, with men and women participants
  2. The group should meet at the same time and place on a regular basis
  3. Groups may be short term or long term
  4. Props, such as food, pictures, or objects, are excellent stimuli for discussion and reminiscence

  5. Relaxation exercises at the beginning of the group meeting stimulate awareness and facilitate discussion

Nurses who establish reminiscing groups should review an authoritative reference on group process and therapy with the aged.

Exercise groups are used successfully in all settings of care for the elderly. The many benefits of exercise are addressed in Chapters 11 and 27. In relation to self-esteem, exercise may improve both self-perception and self-image. Setting realistic goals and individualizing the exercise program are important because an overly ambitious or inappropriate program will only serve to reinforce feelings of inadequacy. Increased strength, endurance, and coordination enhances the individual's competence, which in turn favorably influences self-esteem and increases the person's ability to assume new roles. A greater variety of role opportunities may thus become available. Personal identity is enhanced by the successful fulfillment of roles. Participants should be allowed to follow their own pace. Music can be a useful adjunct. Individual participants may require extra attention from the group leader to maintain participation or to receive accurate directions about exercises.

The purpose of network interventions is to increase the role opportunities available to older persons, thus affecting personal identity, self-esteem, and role performance. Ehrlich (1979) reports that the development of mutual support networks in residential neighborhoods provides older persons with meaningful work and social and service roles and enhances both the level of informal support in the community and individual morale.

Network interventions are applicable to both community and institutional care settings. They are a form of primary prevention for self-concept disturbance but can also be used therapeutically in communities where there is a high prevalence of self-concept disturbance, for example, in nursing homes or age-segregated communities.

Some of the advantages of group approaches to self-concept disturbance include efficient use of the nurse's or therapist's time, increased social contact for participants, the realization that human responses to aging are shared by others, and opportunities to see how others resolve problems.

ENVIRONMENTAL MODIFICATION. Environmental modifications encompass a variety of interventions that have the potential for significant impact on a person's self-concept. Self-esteem is enhanced in an environment that allows individuals to function at their highest possible level. The attitudes and nonverbal behaviors of others in the older person's environment can significantly affect self-concept. If others think old people are just like children, it is difficult for the older person to maintain a positive adult self-image. Nurses must educate caregivers about the importance of treating older persons as adults to prevent deterioration of self-image.

Touch also can be used to enhance self-esteem by conveying warmth and acceptance. However, the social background of the individual influences how touch is perceived. Nurses are in a key position to influence the use of touch with older persons because lay and paraprofessional caregivers often look to professionals for guidance. Modeling therapeutic use of touch and teaching this to caregivers modifies the interpersonal environment of the older person in a manner that should promote increased self-esteem.

Respecting personal space and territory and promoting privacy are environmental interventions that preserve the self-concept. Territory is the area that an individual lays claim to and that can be seen, whereas personal space is an invisible boundary around the individual that varies with relationship, situation, and culture (Potter & Perry, 2005). In hospital and nursing home settings, needs for space are difficult to meet and are often belittled or ignored. The older person's insistence on fixed seating arrangements in the dining room is an attempt to establish and protect a territory—a very normal human response. The distress of nursing home residents at other residents rummaging through their drawers is understandable as a response to violated territory. It is important for staff to make every attempt not to violate territory and personal space. It is risky for a patient to become upset with staff members, yet the insult to self-concept is just as real. A reasonable alternative is to request permission before entering established territory or personal space. Personal possessions are another aspect of the environment. Retaining and respecting personal possessions may be one way to help the older person maintain self-identity. Possessions also can be helpful tools in facilitating reminiscence.

EVALUATION. Self-care behaviors, eye contact, posture, statements about self, and extent of role repertoire are all measurable behaviors that may be used when evaluating the effectiveness of nursing care for those with self-concept disturbances.

Interventions to Facilitate Grief Work. The primary nursing goals for persons experiencing anticipatory grief are to facilitate the grieving process and to assist the bereaved person to focus on the here-and-now aspects of life. Promoting the individual's ability to function in the present is important because the dying individual needs support from family and friends, and "unfinished business" may remain. Resolution of such matters reduces feelings of ambivalence about the death, which in turn reduces the likelihood of dysfunctional grieving for survivors.

For individuals who are dealing with a loss, the primary nursing goal is to facilitate the grief process. A secondary goal is to identify the ways in which the grieving process interferes with other goals or tasks of the older person, such as rehabilitation or strengthening of social networks.

Gerontological nurses and other health care professionals have important roles in caring for the bereaved. The specific interventions of individual health professionals for the bereaved depends on the care setting; the religious, psychosocial, and cultural characteristics of the bereaved; the characteristics, interest, competence, accessibility, and availability of the gerontological nurse; and the nature of the relationship with the bereaved. Although the exact nature of patient interventions may vary, several professional tasks following bereavement are well documented (Caserta & Lund, 1992; Cleirin, 1993; Osterweis, Solomon, & Green, 1984) and include the following:

- Information and education, with sensitivity to what significant others want to know
- Emotional support
- Clinical recognition of dysfunctional grieving
- Management and appropriate referral to mental health resources
- Legitimization of the occurrence of death, so that the bereaved are assured that all appropriate measures were attempted

In planning specific interventions to assist patients and accomplish these professional tasks, the nurse will be prepared to do the following (Ackley & Ladwig, 1993; NANDA, 1994):

- Observe cause/contributing factors of potential loss.
- Monitor the stage of grief (anger, denial, bargaining, depression, acceptance).
- Use open, facilitative communications to aid emotional support and sharing.
- Use silence, use touch with permission, or sit and make eye contact if appropriate to the situation.
- Review past experiences, role changes, coping skills, and strengths.
- Permit expressions of anger and fear free from judgment, but be cautious that all members of the bereaved party may not feel the same and may be in conflict with some emotional states.
- Be honest in all responses; trust is usually enhanced and communication paths opened; do not give false reassurances.
- Identify and discuss problems of eating, activity, sexual desire, sleep, finances, and so on.
- Identify other social supports: friends, family, religious leaders, mental health support services, and self-help groups.
- Provide clear explanations of the cause of death that may prevent misconceptions and self-blame by the bereaved.

Other resources that may help facilitate grief work include mutual self-help groups, hospice, psychotherapy, and drug therapy. The gerontological nurse may be involved to some degree in each. The bereaved may avail themselves of one or more of these interventions sequentially or simultaneously. Bereavement groups aim to help resolve the conflicts of separation, facilitate grief tasks, provide social support, and grant permission to mourn (Gray, Zide, & Wilker, 2000). A meta-analysis of group bereavement intervention studies concluded that participants improved (usually in relation to depression) compared with persons who did not participate in the groups (Sharpnack, 2001). Benefits of cognitive-behavioral group interventions have been demonstrated for coping with acquired immunodeficiency syndrome (AIDS) bereavement (Sikkema, Hansen, Meade, Kochman, & Lee, 2005) and grief related to suicide (Constantino, Sekula, & Rubinstein, 2001). Group therapy provides opportunities for participants to learn more about themselves, their behavior, and their relationships with others (Douglas, 2004). Based on his work with bereavement groups with older persons, Cohen (2000) identified the following factors derived from participation: hope, acceptance, less social isolation, new identity and meaning in life, support, catharsis, amelioration of fears, education, help in processing and dealing with painful or intense feelings, and an opportunity to help others. An intervention study based on the symbolic interactional model found that social worker-facilitated grief work helped bereaved persons to regain the number and types of social connections they had before their loss (Forte, Barrett, & Campbell, 1996).

Hospices also serve as excellent resources for bereaved persons. The National Hospice and Palliative Care Organization (NHPCO) (2005) defines *hospice* as "a philosophy of care that accepts dying as a natural part of life." The Hospice Foundation of America (HFA) (2005) further describes it as "a special concept of care designed to provide comfort and support to patients and their families when a life-limiting illness no longer responds to cure-oriented treatments." Hospice serves not only the patient, but also the family, with bereavement and counseling services before and after the patient's death (HFA, 2005). Because hospice care is covered by Medicare, Medicaid, and most private insurance plans and managed care organizations, it is accessible by most individuals and their families. There are at least five predominant models of hospice: freestanding, hospital affiliated, hospital based, within a nursing facility, and the home care program. The nurse might assist the patient and family by educating them about hospice and the types of hospice care available. Surprisingly, an NHPCO (2005) survey revealed that 75% of Americans were unaware that hospice home care was available and that it can be covered fully by Medicare.

For individuals who feel overwhelmed by the pain and sad emotions attributable to grief or who are experiencing dysfunctional grief, psychotherapeutic intervention may be warranted. The gerontological nurse might refer patients to a psychiatric clinical nurse specialist for short-term crisis intervention or to other mental health professionals for longer treatments. Psychotherapeutic intervention should be offered to individuals, families, or groups of similarly bereaved persons.

Medications may be used alone or in combination with other interventions. The medications most often used to assist the bereaved are antianxiety agents, hypnotics, and antidepressants. The value of psychopharmacological agents for bereaved patients is unsubstantiated. Some researchers argue that the use of medications interferes with the "normal" process of grief and causes delays that may have detrimental consequences. As with all medications and issues of polypharmacy with older adults, drugs must be carefully selected and outcomes closely monitored.

EVALUATION. Evaluative criteria that suggest successful resolution of both anticipatory grieving and dysfunctional grieving include observations that the grieving individual

1. Performs activities of daily living and instrumental activities of daily living at functional baseline
2. Has the ability to appropriately express feelings of anxiety and sadness

3. Has developed new plans, habits, and relationships with others that acknowledge that life goes on despite the lost object
4. Has the ability to approach life one day at a time

Interventions to Combat Powerlessness.

The NANDA (2005) definition of *powerlessness* is "perception that one's own action will not significantly affect an outcome: a perceived lack of control over a current situation or immediate happening." In the most severe state, defining characteristics might include apathy and verbal expressions of not having control over one's self-care and no influence over one's situation and the outcome. Factors related to powerlessness are health care environment, illness-related regimen, interpersonal interaction, or lifestyle of helplessness (NANDA, 2005).

Successful intervention with an individual who experiences powerlessness requires a team effort. The team membership may be patient and nurse, or it may span a much larger group, including family, staff members in a clinic, several community agencies, or staff in an institution such as a hospital or nursing home. Planning is important because powerlessness is predominantly a socially constructed experience. Its resolution, therefore, depends to a large extent on social solutions. If the team is composed of a patient and a nurse only, an explicit contract with the patient may be useful. A contract specifying nurse and patient responsibilities and privileges immediately restructures the nurse-patient relationship on a more egalitarian basis, returning some power to the individual. If the patient refuses to agree to the contract or is unable to do so because of physical or emotional impairment, develop a written plan of approach with other team members to enhance consistency.

Enhancing the older person's self-esteem is essential to reducing powerlessness. Avoid the temptation to assume the older person cannot make independent decisions about his or her life and health care. Patients may need help to recognize their strengths and accomplishments. Encourage independence within the patient's limitations. Focus on the patient's abilities, rather than losses and disabilities. Give feedback, but avoid negative criticism. Support the patient in establishing realistic goals and priorities consistent with personal values and beliefs. Help patients to identify options, encourage them to make decisions, and respect their decisions (NANDA, 2005). Facilitate responsibility for self by providing information needed for the patient to make good decisions. Patients need to know not only what is recommended for self-care, but also the consequences of not assuming responsibility for self. Once the care plan has been implemented, evaluate goal attainment with the patient, and consider alternative actions if needed.

One situation that may precipitate feelings of powerlessness is relocation, especially when it occurs suddenly or when a major change has occurred. Whenever possible, the patient should participate in relocation plans. Family and caregivers must recognize that relocation, especially if it is likely to be permanent, evokes a grief response because of "loss" of the home, neighbors, and familiar objects. The patient should be encouraged to make personal decisions within the new setting.

Many older persons, especially older women, have never learned to assert themselves. They may be especially reticent in the health care setting. Encouraging them to express both negative and positive feelings is a first step. When older persons are intimidated by health care providers, help them formulate their questions in advance and practice how to make their needs and views known. Cognitive restructuring may enable the patient to achieve a more realistic view of self. It can help assist the patient to verbalize feelings of powerlessness or helplessness and to identify factors that create that feeling. The nurse or therapist may challenge the patient's faulty beliefs and suggest alternative ways of perceiving a situation in which the person feels powerless. For example, the patient may assume that the physician will not answer questions because "she is always so busy." With coaching, the patient may find that the physician is quite willing to answer questions when asked.

EVALUATION. Patient responses indicating successful resolution of powerlessness might include (1) verbalizing feelings of increased control over the situation, (2) making more active choices about life situation or care regimen, (3) expressing hope, and (4) participating in health care decisions.

Powerlessness is not a state of being that develops quickly; therefore it is unrealistic to expect that it will be easily remedied. However, focusing on the day-by-day activities of the patient's world and setting day-by-day goals for increasing frequency of choice provides ample opportunity to measure progress toward enhancing the individual's control.

Interventions to Instill Hope and Spiritual Well-Being.

The NANDA classification system defines *hopelessness* as a "subjective state in which an individual sees limited or no alternatives or personal choices available and is unable to mobilize energy on own behalf" (NANDA, 2005, p. 93).

Among the defining characteristics are passivity, withdrawal, verbal cues such as "I can't," increased or decreased sleep, and lack of initiative. A sense of hopelessness in the older person may occur in response to isolation, declining physical condition, or lost belief in transcendent values (NANDA, 2005). In planning interventions to assist the older adult during periods of hopelessness, the patient care goal should focus on uncovering and highlighting the older adult's multiple internal and external resources and the focus of his or her hope. To instill hope is to facilitate "the development of a positive outlook in a given situation" (Dochterman & Bulechek, 2004, p. 420). The planning is highly individualized. A basic step is to determine how accurately the patient perceives the situation. A person may assume that a diagnosis of cancer is hopeless, when in fact treatment with the possibility of cure or remission is possible. Selected interventions to enable hope and prevent hopelessness need to be recorded in the health care record. Specified outcomes and evaluation methods must be delineated.

EVALUATION. The nurse needs to create an atmosphere that fosters the expression and sharing of hopes, fears, questions, and expectations. Older adults may need to be reminded that both hope and hopelessness may coexist in a situation. For example, the older adult newly admitted to a nursing home may feel hopeless about the potential for independent living but may be hopeful about being in a safe, caring, and supportive environment. It is important for the integrity of the older adult to be protected even in the face of despair. A perspective that acknowledges hopelessness may be

Nursing Care Plan: The Older Adult with Dysfunctional Grief

Data

Rudolph Bernard is a 78-year-old resident of Boston whose wife of 55 years died suddenly 6 months ago. He has two grown sons; one lives in a Boston suburb and the other lives in California. His sons communicate frequently, but they visit only twice a month because "they are very busy with their jobs and families." Mr. Bernard lives in a neighborhood of older single-family homes. He is friendly with one couple who live next door. He and his wife used to visit with other couples, but they rarely call since her death. He depends on the bus for transportation. Most basic services are accessible on the bus line. Mr. Bernard is seeing a nurse practitioner in a clinic. He complains that he has little appetite, has no energy, and sleeps poorly. He has not been to church since his wife's death, although they used to attend services irregularly. He says he keeps dreaming about his wife in her casket and that she is reaching out for him. He wonders if she might still be alive if he had recognized that she was ill earlier. He tells the nurse, "I really don't have anything to live for. I am just waiting for my time to go."

Assessment

Other than a 10-pound weight loss, the physical examination is normal for a person of his age.

Nursing Diagnoses (NANDA, 2005)

Dysfunctional grieving related to major life event (death of wife) as manifested by prolonged difficulty coping, loss-associated sense of despair, intrusive images, and self-criticism.

Goals/Outcomes (Moorhead, Johnson, & Maas, 2004)

Mr. Bernard will progress toward resolving his dysfunctional grief as evidenced by verbalizing acceptance of his loss, discussing unresolved conflicts, reporting fewer somatic complaints, and resuming involvement in social activities.

NIC Suggested Interventions (Dochterman & Bulechek, 2004)

Major interventions: Coping Enhancement (5230), Grief Work Facilitation (5290)
- Encourage expression of feelings about the loss.
- Encourage the patient to verbalize memories of the loss, both past and current.
- Make empathetic statements about grief.
- Instruct in phases of the grieving process.
- Identify sources of community support.
- Encourage the patient to implement cultural, religious, and social customs associated with the loss.
- Support progression through personal grieving stages.
- Appraise impact of situation on roles and relationships.
- Provide atmosphere of acceptance.
- Encourage gradual mastery of the situation.
- Encourage relationships with persons who have common interests and goals.
- Encourage social and community activities.
- Explore reasons for the patient's self-criticism.
- Explore previous coping methods.
- Introduce the patient to person (or groups) who have successfully undergone the same experience.
- Encourage the patient to identify own strengths and abilities.
- Assist the patient to identify appropriate short-term and long-term goals.
- Encourage family involvement as appropriate.

Evaluation Parameters (Moorhead, Johnson, & Maas, 2004)

Outcomes may include coping, family coping, appetite, sleep, and grief resolution

balanced by presenting options for thinking, feeling, and behaving.

Strategies for enhancing hope include providing physical and emotional comfort and encouraging the person to verbalize why and how hope is significant in his or her life. The nurse may assist the older adult to identify and express feelings to determine if there is a sense of entrapment. Sometimes the use of a diary (written or tape recorded) can facilitate the discovery process and relieve some of the emotional discomfort associated with hopelessness. Life review or reminiscence may enable the older adult to relive and savor past achievements and experiences.

Some older adults feel abandoned and need to feel connected to someone or something. Nurses might attempt to create conditions that foster a caring relationship among peers, family members, professional caregivers, and pets. Use of community resources, including religious groups, may be helpful in restoring a sense of hope when few family members or significant others are available.

Although energy-conserving measures may be necessary initially, progressive physical activity may enhance energy and promote cognitive and emotional well-being. Guided imagery and relaxation techniques may be used to promote positive thought processes and reenergize individuals who feel hopeless.

Control and autonomy are significant factors in restoring hope. The older adult should be respected as a competent decision maker and involved in obtaining information and making rational decisions.

Counseling by psychiatric nurses is available in most acute care settings. Unfortunately, community resources may be scant. The nurse should refer to psychiatric counseling older adults with suicidal ideation or threatening behaviors to self or others. Emergency services may be needed to help stabilize and restore some sense of hope for the older adult with dysphoria.

These clinical strategies must be documented and evaluated for effectiveness in sustaining hope and preventing hopelessness. Documentation is needed to determine which strategies work best with particular populations. Evaluation must also consider specific dose requirements. What frequency of pet visitation offers the best prospect for health promotion and hopefulness? Future investigations also need to address wellness response to treatment and quality of life.

Evaluation

The outcomes of nursing management of psychological disturbances include the following: anxiety control, fear control, coping, perceived ability to perform, grief resolution, body image, decision making, hope, self-esteem, psychological adjustment, life changes, and spiritual well-being.

REFERENCES

Aartsen, M. J., van Tilburg, T., Smits, C., & Knipscheer, K. (2004). A longitudinal study of the impact of physical and cognitive decline on the personal network in old age. *Journal of Social and Personal Relationships, 21*(2), 249-266.

Abels, A. Z. (2003). Antidepressants: An update on new agents and indications. *American Family Physician, 67*(3), 547-554.

Aberg, A. C., Sidenvall, B., Hepworth, M., O'Reilly, K., & Lithell, H. (2005). On loss of activity and independence, adaptation improves life satisfaction in old age: A qualitative study. *Quality of Life Research, 14*(4), 1111-1125.

Ackley B. J., & Ladwig, G. B. (1993). *Nursing diagnosis handbook: A guide to planning care.* St. Louis: Mosby.

Alesci, S., De Martino, M. U., Ilias, I., Gold, P. W., & Chrousos, G. P. (2005). Major depression is associated with significant diurnal elevations in plasma interleukin-6 levels, a shift of its circadian rhythm, and loss of physiological complexity in its secretion: Clinical implications. *Journal of Clinical Endocrinology and Metabolism, 90*(5), 2522-2530.

Allen, R. S., Welsh, D. L., Willis, S. L., & Schale, K. W. (2003). The aging personality and self: Diversity and health issues. In R. C. Tallis & H. M. Fillit (Eds.), *Geriatric medicine and gerontology* (6th ed.). London: Churchill Livingstone.

Almeida, O. P., & Fenner, S. (2002) Bipolar disorder: Similarities and differences between patients with illness onset before and after 65 years of age. *International Psychogeriatrics, 14*(3), 311-322.

Altschuler, J. (2004). Beyond money and survival: The meaning of paid work among older women. *International Journal of Aging and Human Development, 58*(3), 223-239.

American Psychiatric Association (APA). (2002). The diagnostic and statistical manual of mental disorders (4th ed.) (text revision). Washington, DC: The Association.

Antall, G. F., & Kresevic, D. (2004). The use of guided imagery to manage pain in an elderly orthopaedic population. *Orthopaedic Nursing, 23*(5), 335-340.

Baddeley, A. D., & Hitch, G. J. (1974). Working memory. In G. H. Brown (Ed.), *The psychology of learning and motivation.* New York: Academic Press.

Baird, C. L., & Sands, L. (2004). A pilot study of the effectiveness of guided imagery with progressive muscle relaxation to reduce chronic pain and mobility difficulties of osteoarthritis. *Pain Management Nursing, 5*(3), 97-104.

Barak, S., Knobler, C. Y., & Aizenberg, D. (2004). Suicide attempts amongst elderly schizophrenia patients: A 10-year case control study. *Schizophrenia Research, 71*(1), 77-81.

Barnow, S., Linden, M., & Freyberger, H. J. (2004). The relation between suicidal feelings and mental disorders in the elderly: Results from the Berlin Aging Study. *Psychological Medicine, 34*(4), 741-746.

Barry, K. L., Blow, F. C., Dornfeld, M., & Valenstein, M. (2002). Aging and schizophrenia: Current health services research and recommendations. *Journal of Geriatric Psychiatry and Neurology, 15*(3), 121-127.

Bartels, S. J., Dums, A. R., Oxman, T. E., Schneider, L. S., Arean, P. A., Alexopoulos, G. S., & Jeste, D. V. (2003). Evidence-based practices in geriatric mental health care: An overview of systematic reviews and meta-analyses. *Psychiatric Clinics of North America, 26*(4), 971-990.

Benjamins, M. R. (2004). Religion and functional health among the elderly: Is there a relationship and is it constant? *Journal of Aging and Health, 16*(3), 355-374.

Benjamins, M. R., Musick, M. A., Gold, D. T., & George, L. K. (2003). Age-related declines in activity level: The relationship between chronic illness and religious activities. *Journals of Gerontology Series B: Psychological Sciences and Social Sciences, 58*(6), S377-S385.

Bennett, R. L. (2004). The family medical history. *Primary Care: Clinics in Office Practice, 31*(3), 479-495.

Berger, U., Der, G., Mutrie, N., & Hannah, M. K. (2005). The impact of retirement on physical activity. *Ageing and Society, 25*(2), 181-195.

Bergey, G. K. (2004). Initial treatment of epilepsy: Special issues in treating the elderly. *Neurology, 63*(10 suppl 4), S40-S48.

Beyer, J. L. (2004). Anxiety and panic disorders. In D. G. Blazer, D. C. Steffens, & E. W. Busse (Eds.), *The American Psychiatric Publishing textbook of geriatric psychiatry* (3rd ed.). Washington, DC: American Psychiatric Publishing.

Birnbaum, A. K., Hardie, N. A., Conway, J. M., Bowers, S. E., Lackner, T. E., Graves, N. M., & Leppik, I. E. (2004). Valproic acid doses, concentrations, and clearances in elderly nursing home residents. *Epilepsy Research, 62*(2-3), 157-162.

Birren, J., & Schaie, K. (1990). *Handbook of the psychology of aging* (3rd ed.). San Diego: Academic Press.

Blazer, D. G. (2004). The psychiatric interview of older adults. In D. G. Blazer, D. C. Steffens, & E. W. Busse (Eds.), *Textbook of geriatric psychiatry*. Washington, DC: American Psychiatric Publishing.

Blum, J. E., & Tross, S. (1980). Psychodynamic treatment of the elderly: A review of issues in theory and practice. In C Eisdorfer (Ed.), *Annual Review of Gerontology and Geriatrics, 1,* 204-234.

Boerner, K. (2004). Adaptation to disability among middle-aged and older adults: The role of assimilative and accommodative coping. *Journals of Gerontology Series B: Psychological Sciences and Social Sciences, 59B*(1), P35-P42.

Bogunovic, O. J., & Greenfield, S. F. (2004). Practical geriatrics: Use of benzodiazepines among elderly patients. *Psychiatric Services, 55,* 233-235.

Bondareff, W., Alpert, M., Friedhoff, A. J., Richter, E. M., Clary, C. M., & Balzar, E. (2000). Comparison of sertraline and nortriptyline in the treatment of major depressive disorder in late life. *American Journal of Psychiatry, 157,* 729-736.

Bosek, M. S. D., Lowry, E., Lindeman, D. A., Burck, R., & Gwyther, L. P. (2003). Promoting a good death for persons with dementia in nursing facilities: Family caregivers' perspectives. *JONA's Healthcare, Law, Ethics, and Regulations, 5*(2), 34-41.

Bozikas, V. P., Kovari, E., Bouras, C., & Karavatos, A. (2002). Neurofibrillary tangles in elderly patients with late onset schizophrenia. *Neuroscience Letters, 342*(2), 109-112.

Braam, A. W., Hein, E., Deeg, D. J. H., Twisk, J. W. R., Beekman, A. T. F., & Van Tilburg, W. (2004). Religious involvement and 6-year course of depressive symptoms in older Dutch citizens. *Journal of Aging and Health, 16*(4), 467-489.

Brackley, M. (1997). Mental health assessment/mental status examination. *Nurse Practitioner Forum, 8*(3), 105-113.

Bruce, M. (2002). Psychosocial risk factors for depressive disorders in late life. *Biological Psychiatry, 52,* 175-184.

Burke, W. J., & Wengel, S. P. (2003). Late-life mood disorders. *Clinics in Geriatric Medicine, 19*(4), 777-797.

Busutill, W. (2004). Presentation and management of post traumatic stress disorder and the elderly: A need for investigation. *International Journal of Geriatric Psychiatry, 19,* 429-439.

Butler, R N. (1960). Intensive psychotherapy for the hospitalized patient. *Geriatrics, 15,* 653-664.

Butler, R. N. (1968). Toward a psychiatry of the life-cycle: Implications of socio-psychologic studies of the aging process for the psychotherapeutic situation. *Psychiatic Research Report, 23,* 233-248.

Canter, P. H. (2003). The therapeutic effects of meditation. *BMJ, 326*(7398), 1049-1050.

Caprara, G. V., Caprara, M., & Steca, T. (2003). Personality correlates of adult development and aging. *European Psychologist, 8*(3), 131-147.

Carmin, C. N., Wiegartz, P. S., Yunus, U., & Gillock, K. L. (2002). Treatment of late onset OCD following basal ganglia infarct. *Depression and Anxiety, 15*(2), 87-90.

Carstensen, L. L., Isaacowitz, D. M., & Charles, S. T. (1999). Taking time seriously: A theory of socioemotional selectivity. *American Psychologist, 54*(3), 165-181.

Caserta, M., & Lund, D. (1992). Bereavement stress and coping among older adults: Expectations versus the actual experience. *Omega, 25*(1), 33-45.

Cattel, R. B. (1963). Theory of fluid and crystallized intelligence: A critical experiment. *Journal of Educational Psychology, 54,* 1-22.

Chandran, G. J., Mikler, J. R., & Keegan, D. L. (2003). Neuroleptic malignant syndrome: A case report and discussion. *Canadian Medical Association Journal, 169*(5), 439-442.

Charney, D. S., Reynolds, C. F., Lewis, L., Lebowitz, B. D., Sunderland, T., Alexopoulos, G. S., et al. (2003). Depression and bipolar support alliance consensus statement on the unmet needs in diagnosis and treatment of mood disorders in late life. *Archives of General Psychiatry, 60,* 664-672.

Cicirelli, V. G. (2000). Older adults ethnicity, fear of death, and end-of-life decisions. In A. Tomer (Ed.), *Death attitudes and the older adult: Theories, concepts, and applications. Series in death, dying, and bereavement.* New York: Brunner-Routledge.

Cicirelli, V. G. (2002). Fear of death in older adults: Predictions from terror management theory. *Journals of Gerontology Series B: Psychological Sciences and Social Sciences, 57B*(4), P358-P366.

Cleirin, M. (1993). *Bereavement and adaptation: A comparative study of the aftermath of death.* Washington, DC: Hemisphere.

Clements, R., & Rooda, L. A. (2000). Factor structure, reliability, and validity of the Death Attitude Profile—Revised. *Journal of Death and Dying, 40*(3), 453-463.

Cohen, M. A. (2000). Bereavement groups with the elderly. *Journal of Psychotherapy in Independent Practice, 1*(2), 33-41.

Collins, C. A., Decker, S. I., & Esquibel, K. A. (2004). Definitions of health: Comparison of Hispanic and African-American elders. *Journal of Multicultural Nursing and Health, 10*(3), 13-18.

Comijs, H. C., Deeg, D. J., Dik, M. G., Twisk, J. W., & Jonker, C. (2002). Memory complaints: The association with psycho-affective and health problems and the role of personality characteristics. *Journal of Affective Disorders, 72*(2), 157-165.

Consedine, N. S., Magai, C., & Conway, F. (2004). Predicting ethnic variation in adaptation to later life: Styles of socioemotional functioning and constrained heterotypy. *Journal of Cross-Cultural Gerontology, 19*(2), 97-131.

Constantino, R. E., Sekula, L. K., & Rubinstein, E. N. (2001). Group intervention for widowed survivors of suicide. *Suicide and Life-Threatening Behavior, 31*(4), 428-441.

Cooke, M. Chaboyer, W., & Hiratos, M. A. (2005). Music and its effects on anxiety in short waiting periods: A critical appraisal. *Journal of Clinical Nursing, 14*(2), 145-155.

Cowen, P. J. (2005). Efficacy, safety, and tolerability of duloxetine 60 mg once daily in major depression. *Current Medical Research and Opinion, 21*(3), 345-356.

Craig, M. C., Cutter, W. J., Wickham, H., van Amelsvoort, T. A., Rymer, J., Whitehead, M., & Murphy, D. G. (2004). Effect of long-term estrogen therapy on dopaminergic responsivity in post-menopausal women—a preliminary study. *Psychoneuroendocrinology, 29*(10), 1309-1316.

Craig, M. C., Maki, P. M., & Murphy, D. G. (2005). The Women's Health Initiative Memory Study: Findings and implications. *Lancet Neurology, 4*(3), 190-194.

Crawford, S., & Channon, S. (2002). Dissociation between performance on abstract tests of executive function and problem solving in real-life-type situations in normal aging. *Aging and Mental Health, 6*(1), 12-21.

Crombie, I. K., Irvine, L., Williams, B., McGinnis, A. R., Slane, P. W., Alder, E. M., & McMurdo, M. E. (2004). Why older people do not participate in leisure time physical activity: A survey of activity levels. *Age and Ageing, 33*(3), 287-292.

Culpepper, L. (2002). Generalized anxiety disorder in primary care: Emerging issues in management and treatment. *Journal of Clinical Psychiatry, 63*(8 suppl), 35-42.

DeLeo, D., Padoani, W., Lonnqvist, J., Kerkhof, A. J., Bille-Brahe, U., Michel, K., et al. (2002). Repetition of suicidal behaviour in elderly Europeans: A prospective longitudinal study. *Journal of Affective Disorders, 72*(3), 291-295.

DeLeo, D., & Spathonis, K. (2003). Suicide and euthanasia in late life. *Aging—Clinical and Experimental Research, 15*(2), 99-110.

Demming, J. A., & Pressey, S. L. (1957). Tests "indigenous" to the adult and older years. *Journal of Counseling Psychology, 4,* 144-148.

Depaola, S. J., Griffin, M., Young, J. R., & Neimeyer, R. A. (2003). Death anxiety and attitudes toward the elderly among older adults: The role of gender and ethnicity. *Death Studies, 27*(4), 335-354.

Desai, A. K. (2003). Use of psychopharmacologic agents in the elderly. *Clinics in Geriatric Medicine, 19*(4), 697-719.

Desan, P. H. (2004). Assessment and management of patients with psychiatric disorders. *Critical Care Medicine, 32*(4 suppl), 166-173.

Dhondt, T. D., Beekman, A. T., Deeg, D. J., & Van Tilburg, W. (2002). Iatrogenic depression in the elderly. Results from a community-based study in the Netherlands. *Social Psychiatry and Psychiatric Epidemiology, 37*(8), 393-398.

D'Huyvetter, K., & Corhssen, A., (2002). Homeopathy. *Primary Care: Clinics in Office Practice, 29*(2), 407-418.

Diwan, S., Jonnalagadda, S. S., & Balaswamy, S. (2004). Resources predicting positive and negative affect during the experience of stress: A study of older Asian Indian Immigrants in the United States. *Gerontologist, 44*(5), 605-614.

Dochterman, J. M., & Bulechek, G. M. (2004). *Nursing interventions classification.* St. Louis: Mosby.

Douglas, D. H. (2004). The lived experience of loss: A phenomenological study. *Journal of the American Psychiatric Nurses Association, 10*(1), 24-32.

Earl, B. T. (2005). Effects of pre-retirement preparation on depression and quality of life in retirement for professional managerial males. *Dissertation Abstracts International Section B: The Sciences and Engineering, 65*(8-B).

Ebersole, P. P. (1984). Establishing reminiscing groups. In I. Burnside (Ed.), *Working with the elderly: Group process and techniques* (2nd ed.). North Scituate, MA: Duxbury Press.

Edwards, J. B., Oppewal, S., & Logan, C. L. (2003). Nurse-managed primary care: Outcomes of a faculty practice network. *Journal of the American Academy of Nurse Practitioners, 15*(12), 563-569.

Ehrlich, P. (1979). *Mutual help for community elderly: Mutual help model.* Carbondale, IL: Southern Illinois University.

Elon, R., Phillips, C., Loome, J. F., Denman, S., & Woods, A. (2000). General issues and comprehensive approach to assessment of elders. In D. Osterweil, K. Brummel-Smith, & J. C. Beck (Eds.), *Comprehensive geriatric assessment.* New York: McGraw-Hill.

Elwan, O., Madkour, O., Elwan, F., Mostafa, M., Abbas Helmy, A., Abdel-Naseer, M., et al. (2003). Brain aging in normal Egyptians: Cognition, education, personality, genetic and immunological study. *Journal of the Neurological Sciences, 211*(1-2), 15-22.

Engels, G. I., Duijsens, I. J., Haringsma, R., & van Puttern, C. M. (2003). Personality disorders in the elderly compared to four younger age groups: A cross sectional study of community residents and mental health patients. *Journal of Personality Disorders, 17*(5), 447-459.

Engstrom, C., Brandstrom, S., Sigvardsson, S., Cloninger, R., & Nylander, P. O. (2003). Bipolar disorder II: Personality and age of onset. *Bipolar Disorders, 5*(5), 340-348.

Fernandez, H. H., Treischmann, M. E., & Okun, M. S. (2004). Rebound psychosis: Effect of discontinuation of antipsychotics in Parkinson's disease. *Movement Disorders, 20*(1), 104-105.

Finkel, S. (2004). Pharmacology of antipsychotics in the elderly: A focus on the atypicals. *Journal of the American Geriatrics Society, 52*(s12), 258.

Formiga, F., Chivite, D., Ortega, C., Casas, S., Ramon, J. M., & Pujol, R. (2004). End of life preferences in elderly persons admitted for heart failure. *QJM: An International Journal of Medicine, 97*(12), 803-808.

Forte, J. A., Barret, A. V., & Campbell, M. H. (1996). Patterns of social connectedness and shared grief work: A symbolic interactionist perspective. *Social Work with Groups, 19*(1), 29-51.

Friedlander, A. H., Friedlander, I. K., Gallas, M., & Velasco, E. (2003). Late-life depression: Its oral health significance. *International Dental Journal, 53*(1), 41-50.

Gallo, J. J., Fulmer, T., Paveza, G. J., & Reichel, W. (2000). *Handbook of geriatric assessment* (3rd ed.). Gaithersburg, MD: Aspen.

Geldmacher, D. S. (2004). Differential diagnosis of dementia syndromes. *Clinics in Geriatric Medicine, 20*(1), 27-43.

George, L. K. (1991). Social factors and depression in late life. Paper presented for the NIH Consensus Development Conference on the Diagnosis and Treatment of Depression in Late Life. November 4-6, 1991. Bethesda, MD.

Gerend, M. A., Aiken, L. S., & West, S. G. (2004). Personality factors in older women's perceived susceptibility to diseases of aging. *Journal of Personality, 72*(2), 243-270.

Gesser, G., Wong, P. T. P., & Reker, G. T. (1987). Death attitudes across the life-span: The development and validation of the Death Attitude Profile (DAP). *Journal of Death and Dying, 18*(2), 125-133.

Glass, T. A. (2003). Successful aging. In R. C. Tallis & H. M. Fillit (Eds.), *Geriatric medicine and gerontology* (6th ed.). London: Churchill Livingstone.

Glock, C. Y. (1962). On the study of religious commitment. *Religious Education, 57*(res suppl), S98-S110.

Goldberg, S., Smith, G. S., Barnes, A., Ma, Y., Kramer, E., Robeson, K., et al. (2004). Serotonin modulation of cerebral glucose metabolism in normal aging. *Neurobiology of Aging, 25*(2), 167-174.

Golden, R. N., Dawkins, K., Nicholas, L., & Bebchuk, J. M. (2001). Trazodone, nefazodone, buproprion, and mirtazapine. In A. F. Schatzberg & C. B. Nemeroff (Eds.), *Essentials of clinical psychopharmacology.* Washington, DC: American Psychiatric Publishing.

Gott, M., & Hinchliff, S. (2003). How important is sex in later life? The views of older people. *Social Sciences and Medicine, 56*(8), 1617-1628.

Gott, M., Seymour, J., Bellamy, G., Clark, D., & Ahmedzai, S. (2004). Older people's views about home as a place of care at the end of life. *Palliative Medicine, 18*(5), 460-467.

Graham, C., Arthur, A., & Howard, R. (2002). The social functioning of older adults with schizophrenia. *Aging and Mental Health, 6*(2), 149-152.

Gray, K. F. (2004). Managing agitation and difficult behavior in dementia. *Clinics in Geriatric Medicine, 20*(1), 69-82.

Gray, S. W., Zide, M. R., & Wilker, H. (2000). Using the solution focused brief therapy model with bereavement groups in rural communities: Resiliency at its best. *Hospice Journal, 15*(3), 13-30.

Gurwitz, J. H., Field, T. S., Judge, J., Rochon, P., Harrold, L. R., Cadoret, C., et al. (2005). The incidence of adverse drug events in two large academic long-term care facilities. *American Journal of Medicine, 118*(3), 251-258.

Hagberg, B., Bauer Alfredson,B., Poon, L. W., & Homma, A. (2001). Cognitive functioning in centenarians: a coordinated analysis of results from three countries. *Journals of Gerontology Series B: Psychological Sciences and Social Sciences, 56,* P141-P151.

Hagberg, M., Hagberg, B., & Saveman, B. I. (2002). The significance of personality factors for various dimensions of life quality among older people. *Aging and Mental Health, 6*(2), 178-185.

Halstead, M. T., & Roscoe, S. T. (2002). Restoring the spirit at the end of life: Music as an intervention for oncology nurses. *Clinical Journal of Oncology Nursing, 6*(6), 332-336.

Hanna, C. E., & LaFranchi, S. H. (2002). Adolescent thyroid disorders. *Adolescent Medicine, 13*(1), 13-35.

Hardy, S. E., Concato, J., & Gill, T. M. (2002). Stressful life events among community-living older persons. *Journal of General Internal Medicine, 17*(11), 832-838.

Harrigan, E. P., Miceli, J. J., Anziano, R., Watsky, E., Reeves, K. R., Cutler, N. R., et al. (2004). A randomized evaluation of the effects of six antipsychotic agents on QTc, in the absence and presence of metabolic inhibition. *Journal of Clinical Psychopharmacology, 24*(1), 62-69.

Harwood, D., Hawton, K., Hope, T., & Jacoby, R. (2002). The grief experiences and needs of bereaved relatives and friends of older people dying through suicide: A descriptive and case-control study. *Journal of Affective Disorders, 72*(2), 185-194.

Hasset, A. (2003). Psychosis and schizophrenia disorders in the elderly: An exploration of psychosocial factors which may influence emergence in late life. *Journal of Nutrition, Health, and Aging, 7*(6), 401-408.

Henderson, P. D., & Fogel, J. (2003). Support networks used by African American breast cancer support group participants. *ABNF Journal, 14*(5), 95-98.

Hepburn, K. W.. (2003). Social gerontology. In R. C. Tallis & H. M. Fillit (Eds.), *Brocklehurst's textbook of geriatric medicine and gerontology* (6th ed.). London: Churchill-Livingstone, pp. 183-191.

Hijman, R., Pol, H. E. H., Sitskoorn, M. M., & Kahn, R. S. (2003). Global intellectual impairment does not accelerate with age in patients with schizophrenia: A cross sectional analysis. *Schizophrenia Bulletin, 29*(3), 509-517.

Hochman, K. M., & Lewine, R. R. (2004). Age of menarche and schizophrenia onset in women. *Schizophrenia Research, 69*(2-3), 183-188.

Hogan, B. E. (2003). Soul music in the twilight years: Music therapy and the dying process. *Topics in Geriatric Rehabilitation, 19*(4), 275-281.

Holahan, C. K. (2003). Stability and change in positive self-appraisal from midlife to later aging. *International Journal of Aging and Human Development, 56*(3), 247-267.

Holroyd, S. (2004). Managing dementia in long-term settings. *Clinics in Geriatric Medicine, 20*(1), 83-92.

Horani, M. H., & Morley, J. E. (2004). Hormonal fountains of youth. *Clinics in Geriatric Medicine, 20*(2), 275-292.

Hospice Foundation of America. (2005). What is hospice? Retrieved July 20, 2005, from www.hospicefoundation.org.

Howard, R., & Reeves, S. (2003). Psychosis and schizophrenia-like psychosis in the elderly. *Journal of Nutrition, Health, and Aging, 7*(6), 410-411.

Hunt, S., Wisocki, P., & Yanko, J. (2003). Worry and use of coping strategies among older and younger adults. *Journal of Anxiety Disorders, 17*(5), 547-560.

Hybels, C. F., & Blazer, D. G. (2003). Epidemiology of late-life mental disorders. *Clinics in Geriatric Medicine, 19*(4), 663-696.

Hyde, M., Ferrie, J., Higgs, P., Mein, G., & Nazroo, J. (2004). The effects of pre-retirement factors and retirement route on circumstances in retirement: Findings from the Whitehall II study. *Ageing and Society, 24*(2), 279-296.

Igier, V., & Mullet, E. (2003). Application of the five-factor model of personality to intergenerational perception. *Journals of Gerontology Series B: Psychological Sciences and Social Sciences, 58*(3), P177-P186.

Isaacowitz, D. M., & Smith, J. (2003). Positive and negative affect in very old age. *Journals of Gerontology Series B: Psychological Sciences and Social Sciences, 58*(3), P143-P152.

Jang, Y., Poon, L. W., & Martin, P. (2004). Individual differences in the effect of disease and disability on depressive symptoms: The role of age and subjective health. *International Journal of Aging and Human Development, 59*(2), 125-137.

Jankovic, J. (2002). Levodopa strengths and weaknesses. *Neurology, 58*(4 suppl 1), S19-S32.

Jansen, D. A., & von Sadovszky, V. (2004). Restorative activities of community-dwelling elders. *Western Journal of Nursing Research, 26*(4), 381-404.

Jeste, D. V., Twamley, E. W., Eyler Zorrilla, L. T., Golshan, S., Patterson, T. L., & Palmer, B. W. (2003). Aging and outcome in schizophrenia. *Acta Psychiatrica Scandinavia, 107*(5), 336-343.

Joffe, R. T., Brasch, J. S., & MacQueen, J. M. (2003). Psychiatric aspects of endocrine disorders in women. *Psychiatric Clinics of North America, 26*(3), 683-691.

Johansson, C. M., Jansson, M., Linner, L., Yuan, Q. P., Pedersen, N. L., Blackwood, D., et al. (2001). Genetics of affective disorders. *European Neuropsychopharmacology, 11*(6), 385-394.

Kamat, S. M., Lefevre, P. J., & Grossberg, G. T. (2003). Electroconvulsive therapy in the elderly. *Clinics in Geriatric Medicine, 19*(4), 825-839.

Kapur, S., & Seeman, P. (2001). Does fast dissociation from dopamine D2 receptor explain the action of atypical antipsychotics? A new hypothesis. *American Journal of Psychiatry, 158*(3), 360-369.

Kassutto, Z., & Vaught, W. (2003). Informed decision making and refusal of treatment. *Clinical Pediatric Emergency Medicine, 4*(4), 285.

Kearney, M. H., Rosal, M. C., Ockene, J. K., & Churchill, L. C. (2002). Influences on older women's adherence to a low-fat diet in the Women's Health Initiative. *Psychosomatic Medicine, 64*(3), 450-457.

Kelleher, C. H., & Quirk, D. A. (1973, Fall). Age, functional capacity, and work: An annotated bibliography. *Industrial Gerontology, 19*, 80-98.

Kertesz, A., & Munoz, D. G. (2002). Frontotemporal dementia. *Medical Clinics of North America, 86*(3), 501-518.

Kiecolt-Glaser, J. K., McGuire, L., Robles, T. F., & Glaser, R. (2002). Emotions, morbidity: New perspectives from psychoneuroimmunology. *Annual Review of Psychology, 53*, 83-107.

King, V., & Scott, M. E. (2005). A comparison of cohabiting relationships among older and younger adults. *Journal of Marriage and Family, 67*(2), 271-285.

Klap, R., Unroe, K. T., & Unutzer, J. (2003). Caring for mental illness in the United States: A focus on older adults. *American Journal of Geriatric Psychiatry, 11*(5), 517-524.

Kluger, M. (2004). Research brief: Physicians and NPs in nursing homes. *American Journal of Nursing, 104*(9), 72.

Kondel, T. K., Mortimer, A. M., Leeson, V. C., Laws, K. R., & Hirsch, S. R. (2003). Intellectual differences between schizophrenic patients and normal controls across the adult lifespan. *Journal of Clinical and Experimental Neuropsychology, 25*(8), 1045-1056.

Laakkonen, M., Pitkala, K. H., & Strandberg, T. E. (2004). Terminally ill elderly patient's experiences, attitudes, and needs: A qualitative study. *Omega: Journal of Death and Dying, 49*(2), 117-129.

Lagana, L., & Shanks, S. (2002). Mutual biases underlying the problematic relationship between older adults and mental health providers: Any solutions in sight? *International Journal of Aging and Human Development, 55*(3), 271-295.

Lai, H. (2004). Music preference and relaxation in Taiwanese elderly people. *Geriatric Nursing, 25*(5), 286-291.

Lang, F. R., Rieckmann, N., & Baltes, M. M. (2002). Adapting to aging losses: Do resources facilitate strategies of selection, compensation, and optimization in everyday functioning? *Journal of Gerontology Series B: Psychological Sciences and Social Sciences, 57*(6), P501-P509.

Lauderdale, S. A., & Sheikh, J. I. (2003). Anxiety disorders in older adults. *Clinics in Geriatric Medicine, 19*(4), 721-741.

Lehmann, S. W. (2003). Psychiatric disorders in older women. *International Review of Psychiatry, 15*(3), 269-279.

Lenahan, P. M., & Willwood, A. L. (2004). Sexual health and aging. *Clinics in Family Practice, 6*(4), 917-939.

Leung, A. K., & Pacaud, D. (2004). Diagnosis and management of galactorrhea. *American Family Physician, 70*(3), 543-550.

Li, S. C. (2002). Aging of the brain, sensorimotor, and cognitive processes. *Neuroscience and Biobehavioral Reviews, 26*(7), 729-732.

Lieberman, H. R. (2003). Nutrition, brain function, and cognitive performance. *Appetite, 40*, 245-254.

Llard, J., Artero, S., & Ritchie, K. (2003). Consumption of psychotropic medication in the elderly: A re-evaluation of its effects on cognitive performance. *International Journal of Geriatric Psychiatry, 18*(10), 874-878.

Lochbaum, M. R., Karoly, P., & Landers, D. M. (2002). Evidence for the importance of openness to experience on performance of a fluid intelligence task by physically active and inactive participants. *Research Quarterly for Exercise and Sport, 73*(4), 437-444.

Lomranz, J. (1998). An image of aging and the concept of aintegration: Coping and mental health implications. In J. Lomranz (Ed.), *Handbook of aging and mental health: An integrative approach. The Plenum series in adult developing and aging.* New York: Plenum Press.

MacDonald, S. W. S., Dixon, R., Cohen, A., & Hazlitt, J. E. (2004). Biological age and 12 year cognitive change in older adults: Findings from the Victoria Longitudinal Study. *Gerontology, 50*(2), 64-81.

Mackin, P., & Young, A. H. (2004). Rapid cycling bipolar disorder: Historical overview and focus on emerging treatments. *Bipolar Disorders, 6*(6), 523-529.

Maddox, G. L. (1962). Some correlates of differences in self-assessments of health status among the elderly. *Journal of Gerontology, 17,* 180-185.

Magai, C., Consedine, N. S., King, A. R., & Gillespie, M. (2003). Physical hardiness and styles of socioemotional functioning in later life. *Journals of Gerontology Series B: Psychological Sciences and Social Sciences, 58*(5), P269-P279.

Maiden, R. J. (2003). Personality changes in the old-old. *Journal of Adult Development, 10*(1), 31-39.

Maiden, R. J., & Peterson, S. A. (2002). Use of mental health services by the rural aged: Longitudinal study. *Journal of Geriatric Psychiatry and Neurology, 15*(1), 1-6.

Majercsik, E., & Haller, J. (2004). Interactions between anxiety, social support, health status, and buspirone efficacy in elderly patients. *Progress in Neuropsychopharmacology and Biological Psychiatry, 28*(7), 1161-1169.

Manly, J. J., Touradji, P., Tang, M., & Stern, Y. (2003). Literacy and memory decline among ethnically diverse elders. *Journal of Clinical and Experimental Neuropsychology, 25*(5), 680-690.

Marcus, D. A. (1995). Interrelationships of neurochemicals, estrogen, and recurring headache. *Pain, 62*(2), 129-139.

Mark, D. D., Byers, V. L., & Mays, M. Z. (2001). Primary care outcomes and provider practice styles. *Military Medicine, 166*(10), 875-880.

Martin, P., Long, M. V., & Poon, L. W. (2002). Age changes and differences in personality traits and states of the old and very old. *Journals of Gerontology Series B: Psychological Sciences and Social Sciences, 57*(2), P144-P152.

Martin, R., Johnsen, E. L., Bunde, J., Bellman, S. B., Rothrock, N. E., Weinrib, A., & Lemos, K. (2005). Gender differences in patients' attributions for myocardial infarction: Implications for adaptive health behaviors. *International Journal of Behavioral Medicine, 12*(1), 39-45.

Maynard, C. K. (2003). Differentiate depression from dementia. *Nurse Practitioner, 28*(3), 18-27.

McCarthy, M. C., Ruiz, E., Gale, B. J., Karam, C., & Moore, N. (2004). The meaning of health: Perspectives of Anglo and Latino older women. *Health Care for Women International, 25*(10), 950-969.

McClain-Jacobson, C., Rosenfeld, B., Kosinski, A., Pessin, H., Cimino, J. E., & Breitbart, W. (2004). Belief in an afterlife, spiritual well-being, and end of life despair in patients with advanced cancer. *General Hospital Psychiatry, 26*(6), 484-486.

McDonald, W. M., Salzman, C., & Schatzberg, A. F. (2002). Depression in the elderly. *Psychopharmacological Bulletin, 36*(suppl 2), 112-122.

McKinley, E. (2005). Protecting the atypical antipsychotic-medicated patient. *Psyched Up: Psychopharmacology Educational Update, 1*(3), 5.

McMahan, S., & Lutz, R. (2004). Alternative therapy use among the young-old (ages 65-74): An evaluation of the MIDUS database. *Journal of Applied Gerontology, 23*(2), 91-103.

McNicoll, L., Pisani, M. A., Ely, E., Gifford, D., & Inouye, S. K. (2005). Detection of delirium in the intensive care unit: Comparison of confusion assessment method for the intensive care unit with confusion assessment method ratings. *Journal of the American Geriatrics Society, 53*(3), 495-500.

Mendelowitz, A. J. (2004). The utility of intramuscular ziprasidone in the management of acute psychotic agitation. *Annals of Clinical Psychiatry, 16*(3), 145-154.

Mezey, M. (2004). NPs in nursing homes: An issue of quality. *American Journal of Nursing, 104*(9), 71.

Moberg, D. (1990). Religion and aging. In K. Ferraro (Ed.), *Gerontology: Perspective and Issues.* New York: Springer.

Mokhlesi, B., Leikin, J. B., Murray, P., & Corbridge, T. C. (2003). Adult toxicology in critical care: Part 2: Specific poisonings. *Chest, 123*(3), 897-922.

Moore, D. P., & Jefferson, J. W. (2005). *Handbook of medical psychiatry* (2nd ed.). St Louis: Elsevier Mosby.

Moorhead, S., Johnson, J., & Maas, M. (2004). *Nursing outcomes classification (NOC)* (3rd ed.). St. Louis: Mosby.

Morris, M. C., Evans, D. A., Bienias, J. L., Tangney, C. C., & Wilson, R. S. (2004). Dietary fat intake and 6 year cognitive change in an older biracial community population. *Neurology, 62*(9), 1573-1579.

Morris, M. C., Evans, D. A., Tangney, C. C., Bienias, J. L., Wilson, R. S., Aggarwal, N. T., & Scherr, P. A. (2005). Relation of the tocopherol forms to incident Alzheimer disease and to cognitive change. *American Journal of Clinical Nutrition, 81*(2), 508-514.

Mroczek, D. K., & Almeida, D. M. (2004). The effect of daily stress, personality, and age on daily negative affect. *Journal of Personality, 72*(2), 355-378.

Mroczek, D. K., & Spiro, A., 3rd. (2003). Modeling intraindividual change in personality traits: Findings from the Normative Aging Study. *Journals of Gerontology Series B: Psychological Sciences and Social Sciences, 58*(3), P153-P165.

National Center on Elder Abuse. (1998). *The National Elder Abuse Incidence Study.* Washington, DC: American Public Human Services Association.

National Hospice and Palliative Care Organization. (2005). What is hospice and palliative care? Retrieved July 20, 2005, from www.nhpco.org.

Neikrug, S. M. (2003). Worrying about a frightening old age. *Aging and Mental Health, 7*(5), 326-333.

Nelson-Becker, H. B. (2004). Meeting life challenges: A hierarchy of coping styles in African American and Jewish American older adults. *Journal of Human Behavior in the Social Environment, 10*(1), 155-174.

Norris, J. (1992). Nursing interventions for self-esteem disturbance. *Nursing Diagnoses, 3*(2), 48-53.

North American Nursing Diagnosis Association. (1994). *Nursing diagnoses: Definitions and classifications 1994-1995.* Philadelphia: NANDA International.

North American Nursing Diagnosis Association. (2003). *Nursing diagnoses: Definitions and classifications 2003-2004.* Philadelphia: NANDA International.

North American Nursing Diagnosis Association. (2005). *Nursing diagnoses: Definitions and classifications 2005-2006.* Philadelphia: NANDA International.

Oberg, P., & Tornstam, L. (2003). Attitudes toward embodied old age among Swedes. *International Journal of Aging and Human Development, 56*(2), 133-153.

O'Connell, H., Ai-vyrn, C., Hamilton, F., Cunningham, C., Walsh, J. B., Davis, C., & Lawlor, B. A. (2004). A systematic review of the utility of self-report alcohol screening instruments in the elderly. *International Journal of Geriatric Psychiatry, 19,* 1074-1086.

O'Connor, B. P., Rousseau, F. L., & Maki, S. A. (2004). Physical exercise and experienced bodily changes: The emergence of benefits and limits on benefits. *International Journal of Aging and Human Development, 59*(3), 177-203.

Odlund, O. A., Koochek, A., Ljungqvist, O., & Cederholm, T. (2005). Nutritional status, well-being and functional ability in frail elderly service flat residents. *European Journal of Clinical Nutrition, 59*(2), 263-270.

Ogunbameru, O., & Bamiwuye, S. (2004). Attitudes toward retirement and preretirement education among Nigerian bank workers. *Educational Gerontology, 30*(5), 391-401.

O'Hanlon, A., & Coleman, P. (2004). Attitudes toward aging: Adaptation, development, and growth into later years. In Pennsylvania State University, *Handbook of communication and aging research* (2nd ed.). Mahway, NJ: Lawrence Erlbaum Associates.

Orengo, C. A., Fullerton, G., & Tan, R. (2004). Male depression: A review of gender concerns and testosterone therapy. *Geriatrics, 59*(10), 24-30.

Osterweil, D., Brummel-Smith, K., & Beck, J. C. (Eds.). (2000). *Comprehensive geriatric assessment* (pp. 737-738). New York: McGraw-Hill.

Osterweis, M., Solomon, F., & Green, M. (1984). *Bereavement: Reactions, consequences, and care.* Washington, DC: National Academy Press.

Ozcan, M. E., & Banoglu, R. (2003). Gonadal hormones in schizophrenia and mood disorders. *European Archives of Psychiatry and Clinical Neuroscience, 253*(4), 193-196.

Palmer, B. W., Dunn, L. B., Appelbaum, P. S., & Jeste, D. V. (2004). Correlates of treatment-related decision-making capacity among middle-aged and older patients with schizophrenia. *Archives of General Psychiatry, 61*(3), 230-236.

Palmer, B. W., Heaton, R. K., Gladsjo, J. A., Evans, J. D., Patterson, T. L., Golshan, S., & Jeste, D. V. (2002). Heterogeneity in functional status among older outpatients with schizophrenia: Employment history, living situation, and driving. *Schizophrenia Research, 55*(3), 205-215.

Papakostas, G. I., Petersen, T., Denninger, J. W., Montoya, H. D., Nierenberg, A. A., Alpert, J. E., & Fava, M. (2003). Treatment-related adverse events and outcome in a clinical trial of fluoxetine for major depressive disorder. *Annals of Clinical Psychiatry, 15*(3/4), 187-192.

Parker, M., Roff, L. L., Klemmack, D. L., Koenig, H. G., Baker, P., & Allman, R. M. (2003). Religiosity and mental health in southern, community-dwelling older adults. *Aging and Mental Health, 7*(5), 390-397.

Patacca, D., Rosenbloom, C. A., Kicklighter, J. R., & Ball, M. (2004). Using a focus group approach to determine older adults' opinions and attitudes toward a nutrition education program. *Journal of Nutrition for the Elderly, 23*(3), 55-72.

Payman, V. (2005). Book review: *New directions in the study of late life religiousness and spirituality* by S. H. McFadden, M. Brennan, & J. H. Patrick (Eds.). *International Psychogeriatrics, 17*(1), 136-138.

Pedersen, A. N., Rothenberg, E., & Maria, A. (2002). Health behaviors in elderly people. A 5 year follow-up of 75 year old people living in three Nordic localities. Smoking, physical activity, alcohol consumption, and healthy eating, and attitudes to their importance. *Aging: Clinical and Experimental Research, 14*(3 suppl), 75-82.

Pentland, W., Walker, J., Minnes, P., Tremblay, M., Brouwer, B., & Gould, M. (2002). Women with spinal cord injury and the impact of aging. *Spinal Cord, 40*(8), 374-387.

Phelan, E. A., Anderson, L. A., LaCroix, A. Z., & Larson, E. B. (2004). Older adults' views of "successful aging"—how do they compare with researchers' definitions? *Journal of the American Geriatrics Society, 52,* 211-216.

Phillips, L. H., Smith, L., & Gilhooly, K. J. (2002). The effects of adult aging and induced positive and negative mood on planning. *Emotion, 2*(3), 263-272.

Pier, M. P., Halstijn, W., & Sabbe, B. G. (2004). Psychomotor retardation in elderly depressed persons. *Journal of Affective Disorders, 81*(1), 73-77.

Pitkala, K., Kahonen-Vare, M., Valvanne, J., Strandberg, T. E., & Tilvis, R. S. (2003). Long-term changes in mood of an aged population: Repeated Zung-tests during a 10 year follow-up. *Archives of Gerontology and Geriatrics, 36*(2), 185-195.

Pitkala, K. H., Laakkonen, M. L., Strandberg, T. E., & Tilvis, R. S. (2004). Positive life orientation as a predictor of 10-year outcome in an aged population. *Journal of Clinical Epidemiology, 57*(4), 409-414.

Pliszka, S. R. (2003). *Neuroscience for the mental health clinician* (pp. 216-220). New York: Guilford Press.

Potter, P. A., & Perry, A. G. (2005). *Fundamentals of nursing* (6th ed.). St. Louis: Mosby.

Potter, W. Z., Manji, H. K., & Rudorfer, M. V. (2001). Tricyclics and tetracyclics. In A. F. Schatzberg & C. B. Nemeroff (Eds.), *Essentials of clinical psychopharmacology.* Washington, DC: American Psychiatric Publishing.

Proulx, K., & Jacelon, C. (2004). Dying with dignity: The good patient versus the good death. *American Journal of Hospice and Palliative Care, 21*(2), 116-120.

Rabbitt, P., Chetwynd, A., & McInnes, L. (2003). Do clever brains age more slowly? Further exploration of a nun result. *British Journal of Psychology, 94*(pt 1), 63-71.

Ravenna, H., Jones, C., & Kwan, V. S. (2002). Personality change over 40 years of adulthood: Hierarchical linear modeling analyses of two longitudinal samples. *Journal of Personality and Social Psychology, 83*(3), 752-766.

Rehman, H. U., & Masson, E. A. (2001). Neuroendocrinology of aging. *Age and Ageing, 30,* 279-287.

Riker, R. R., Fraser, G. L., & Richen, P. (1997). Movement disorders associated with withdrawal from high dose intravenous haloperidol therapy in delirious ICU patients. *Chest, 111*(6), 1778-1781.

Roberts, B. W., & Delvecchio, W. F. (2000). The rank order consistency of personality traits from adulthood to old age: Continuity or change? *Psychological Bulletin, 126,* 3-25.

Roberts, B. W., Helson, R., & Klohnen, E. C. (2002). Personality development and growth in women across 30 years: Three perspectives. *Journal of Pesonality, 70*(1), 79-102.

Robison, J., Curry, L., Cruman, C., Covington, T., Gaztambide, S., & Blank, K. (2003). Depression in late life Puerto Rican primary care patients: The role of illness, stress, social integration, and religiosity. *International Psychogeriatrics, 15*(3), 239-251.

Roblin, D. W., Becker, E. R., Adams, E. K., Howard, D. H., & Roberts, M. H. (2004). Patient satisfaction with primary care: Does type of practitioner matter? *Medical Care, 42*(6), 579-590.

Roff, L. L., Klemmack, D. L., Parker, M., Koenig, H. G., Crowther, M., Baker, P. S., & Allman, R. M. (2004). Depression and religiosity in African American and white community-dwelling older adults. *Journal of Human Behavior in the Social Environment, 10*(1), 175-189.

Rose, S. R. (2004). The psychological effects of anxiolytic music/imagery on anxiety and depression following cardiac surgery (doctoral dissertation, research). Walden University, AN 2005094456.

Rosenfeld, P., Kobayashi, M., Barber, P., & Mezey, M. (2004). Utilization of nurse practitioners in long term care: Findings and implications of a national survey. *Journal of the American Medical Directors Association, 5*(1), 9-15.

Royall, D. R., Mahurin, R. K., & Gray, K. F. (1992). Bedside assessment of executive cognitive impairment: The Executive Interview. *Journal of the American Geriatrics Society, 40,* 1221-1226.

Sable, J. A., & Jeste, D. V. (2003). Pharmacologic management of psychosis in the elderly. *Journal of Nutrition, Health and Aging, 7*(6), 421-427.

Saggino, A., & Balsamo, M. (2003). Relationship between WAIS-R intelligence and the five factor model of personality in a normal elderly sample. *Psychological Reports, 92*(3, pt 2), 1151-1161.

Sajatovic, M., Mullen, J. A., & Sweitzer, D. E. (2002). Efficacy of quetiapine and risperidone against depressive symptoms in outpatients with psychosis. *Journal of Clinical Psychiatry, 63*(12), 1156-1163.

Sarker, S. J., Crossman, A., & Chinmeteepituck, P. (2003). The relationship of age and length of service with job satisfaction: An examination of hotel employees in Thailand. *Journal of Managerial Psychology, 18*(7), 745-758.

Schimming, C., & Harvey, P. D. (2004). Disability reduction in elderly patients with schizophrenia. *Journal of Psychiatric Practice, 10*(5), 283-295.

Schneider, K. (2003). The significance of learning for aging. *Educational Gerontology, 29*(10), 809-823.

Schwarzer, C. (2003). Social support and emotions in the elderly. *Ansieded y Estres, 9*(2-3), 191-202.

Sharma, N., & Standaert, D. G. (2002). Inherited movement disorders. *Neurologic Clinics, 20*(3), 759-778.

Sharpnack, J. D. (2001). The efficacy of group bereavement interventions: An integrative review of the research literature. *Dissertation Abstracts International: Section B: The Sciences and Engineering, 61*(12-B).

Shatzberg, A. F., Haddad, P., Kaplan, E. M., Lejoyeux, M., Rosenbaum, J. F., Young, A. H., & Zajecka, J. (1997). Serotonin reuptake discontinuation syndrome: A hypothetical definition. *Journal of Clinical Psychiatry, 58*(suppl 7), S5-S10.

Shin, K. R., Cho, M. O., & Kim, J. S. (2005). The meaning of death as experienced by elderly women of a Korean clan. *Qualitative Health Research, 15*(1), 5-18.

Shneker, B. F., & Fountain, N. B. (2003). Epilepsy. *Disease a Month, 49*(7), 426-478.

Short, N. P., Kitchiner, N. J., & Curran, J. (2004). Unreliable evidence. *Journal of Psychiatric and Mental Health Nursing, 11*(1), 106.

Sikkema, K. J., Hansen, N. B., Meade, C. S., Kochman, A., & Lee, R. S. (2005). Improvements in health-related quality of life following a group intervention for coping with AIDS bereavement among HIV-infected men and women. *Quality of Life Research, 14*(4), 991-1005.

Silver, M. H. (2002). The significance of life review in old age. *Journal of Geriatric Psychiatry, 35*(1), 11-23.

Singh, V., Muzina, D. J., & Calabrese, J. R. (2005). Anticonvulsants in bipolar disorder. *Psychiatric Clinics of North America, 28*(20), 301-323.

Sinoff, G., & Werner, P. (2003). Anxiety disorder and accompanying subjective memory loss in the elderly as a predictor of future cognitive decline. *International Journal of Geriatric Psychiatry, 18*(10), 951-959.

Sirey, J. A., Bruce, M., & Alexopoulos, G. S. (2005). The treatment initiation program: An intervention to improve depression outcomes in older adults. *American Journal of Psychiatry, 162*(1), 184-186.

Sliwinski, M. J., Hofer, S. M., Hall, C., Buschke, H., & Lipton, R. B. (2003). Modeling memory decline in older adults: The importance of preclinical dementia, attrition, and chronological age. *Psychology and Aging, 18*(4), 658-671.

Sloan, D. M. (2003). Gender differences in depression and response to antidepressant treatment. *Psychiatric Clinics of North America, 26*(3), 581-594.

Sloman, R. (2002). Relaxation and imagery for anxiety and depression control in community patients with advanced cancer. *Cancer Nursing, 25*(6), 432-435.

Small, B. J., Hertzog, C., Hultsch, D. F., & Dixon, R. A. (2003). Stability and change in adult personality over 6 years: Findings from the Victoria Longitudinal Study. *Journals of Gerontology Series B: Psychological and Social Sciences, 58*(3), P166-P176.

Smith, G. C. (2003a). Patterns and predictors of service use and unmet needs among aging families of adults with severe mental illness. *Psychiatric Services, 54*(6), 871-877.

Smith, G. C. (2003b). Predictors of the stage of residential planning among aging families of adults with severe mental illness. *Psychiatric Services, 55*(7), 804-810.

Spalleta, G., Pasini, A., & Caltagirone, C. (2002). Fluoxetine alone in the treatment of first episode anxious-depression: An open clinical trial. *Journal of Clinical Psychopharmacology, 22*(3), 263-266.

Steinhauser, K. E., Christakis, N. A., Clipp, E. C., McNeilly, M., McIntyre, L., & Tulsky, J. A. (2000). Factors considered important at end of life by patients, family, physicians, and other care providers. *Journal of the American Medical Association, 284*(19), 2476-2482.

Stetter, F., Walter, G., Zimmernann, A., Zahress S., & Straube E. R., (1994). Ambulatory short-term therapy of anxiety patients with autogenic training and hypnosis. Results of treatment and 3 months follow-up. *Psychotherapie, Psychosomatik, Medizinische Psychologie, 44*(7), 226-234.

Stevens-Ratchford, R. (1993). The effect of life review activities on depression and self-esteem in older adults. *American Journal of Occupational Therapy, 47*(5), 413-420.

Stoll, A. L., Mayer, P. V., Kolbrener, M., Goldstein, E., Suplit, B., Lucier, J., et al. (1994). Antidepressant-associated mania: A controlled comparison with spontaneous mania. *American Journal of Psychiatry, 151*, 1642-1645.

Street, J. S., Tollefson, G. D., Tohen, M., Sanger, T. M., Clark, S., Gannon, K. S., & Wei, H. (2000). Olanzapine for psychotic conditions in the elderly. *Psychiatric Annals, 30*(3), 191-196.

Stuart-Hamilton, I. A. (2003). Normal cognitive aging. In R. C. Tallis & H. M. Fillit (Eds.), *Geriatric medicine and gerontology* (6th ed.). London: Churchill Livingstone.

Sugar, J. A., & McDowd, J. M. (1992). Memory, learning, and attention. In J. E. Birren, R. B. Sloane, & G. D. Cohen (Eds.), *Handbook of mental health and aging* (2nd ed.). New York: Academic Press, pp. 307-337.

Szinovacz, M. E., & Davey, A. (2005). Retirement and marital decision making: Effects on retirement satisfaction. *Journal of Marriage and Family, 67*(2), 387-398.

Tamblyn, R., Abrahamowicz, M., du Berger, R., McLeod, P., & Bartlett, G. (2005). A 5-year prospective assessment of the risk associated with individual benzodiazepines and doses in new elderly users. *Journal of the American Geriatrics Society, 53*(2), 233-241.

Tassini, M., Vivi, A., Gaggelli, E., Valensin, G., Pasini, F. L., Puccetti, L., & Di Perri, T. (2002). Effects of fluoxetine treatment on carbohydrate metabolism in human blood platelets: A 1H-NMR study. *Archives of Biochemistry and Biophysics, 404*(1), 163-165.

Tate, R. B., Lah, L., & Cuddy, T. E. (2003). Definition of successful aging by elderly Canadian males: The Manitoba follow-up study. *Gerontologist, 43*(5), 735-744.

Thomas, A. (2002). Ischemic basis for deep white matter hyperintensities in major depression: A neuropathological study. *Archives of General Psychiatry, 59*, 785-792.

Tollefson, G. D., & Rosenbaum, J. F. (2001). Selective serotonin reuptake inhibitors. In A. F. Schatzberg & C. B. Nemeroff (Eds.), *Essentials of clinical psychopharmacology.* Washington, DC: American Psychiatric Publishing.

Tomac, T. A., Rummans, T. A., Pileggi, T. S., & Li, H. (1997). Safety and efficacy of electroconvulsive therapy in patients over age 85. *American Journal of Geriatric Psychiatry, 5*(2), 126-130.

Traustidottir, T., Bosch, P. R., & Matt, K. S. (2005). The HPA axis response to stress in women: Effects of aging and fitness. *Psychoneuroendocrinology, 30*(4), 392-402.

Treadwell, B. E. (2003). Psychologists' perception of older clients: The effect of age, gender, knowledge, and experience. *Dissertation Abstracts International Section A: Humanities and Social Sciences, 63*(12-A).

Trujillo, K. M., Brougham, R. R., & Walsh, D. A. (2004). Age differences in reasons for exercising. *Current Psychology: Developmental, Learning, Personality, Social, 22*(22), 348-365.

Turvey, C. L., Conwell, Y., Jones, M. P., Phillips, C., Simonsick, E., Pearson, J. L., & Wallace, R. (2002). Risk factors for late-life suicide: A prospective, community-based study. *American Journal of Geriatric Psychiatry, 10*(4), 398-406.

U.S. Department of Health and Human Services. (1999). *Mental health: A report of the Surgeon General—executive summary.* Rockville, MD: U.S. Department of Health and Human Services, Substance Abuse and Mental Health Services Administration, Center for Mental Health Services, National Institutes of Health, National Institute of Mental Health.

U.S. Department of Labor, Bureau of Labor Statistics. (2002). Retrieved June 18, 2005, from www.bls.gov.

U.S. Food and Drug Administration. (2005, April). FDA issues public health advisory for antipsychotic drugs used for treatment of behavioral disorders in elderly patients. U.S. FDS Talk Paper Online. Retrieved July 24, 2005, from www.fda.gov.bbs/topics/answers/2005/ANSO1350.html.

Van Kuiken, D. (2004). A meta-analysis of the effect of guided imagery practice on outcomes. *Journal of Holistic Nursing, 22*(2), 164-179.

Van Mieghem, C., Sabbe, M., & Knockaert, D. (2004). The clinical value of the EKG in noncardiac conditions. *Chest, 125*(4), 1561-1576.

Van Ness, P. H., & Larson, D. B. (2002). Religion, senescence, and mental health: The end of life is not the end of hope. *American Journal of Geriatric Psychiatry, 10*(4), 386-397.

Volavka, J., Czobor, P., Cooper, T. B., Sheitman, B., Lindenmayer, J. P., Citrome, L., et al. (2004). Prolactin levels in schizophrenia and schizoaffective disorder patients treated with clozapine, olanzapine, risperidone, or haloperidol. *Journal of Clinical Psychiatry, 65*(1), 57-61.

Warnock, J. K. (2004). Major depression in women: Unique issues (monograph). *University of Virginia School of Medicine Reports on Psychiatric Disorders, 1*(1). Newtown, PA: Associates in Medical Marketing Co., Inc.

Watson, W. (1982). *Aging and social behavior.* Monterey, CA: Wadsworth Health Sciences Division.

Weagley, R. O., & Huh, E. (2004). The impact of retirement on household leisure expenditures. *Journal of Consumer Affairs, 38*(2), 262-281.

Wechsler, D. (1971). Intelligence: Definition, the IQ. In R. Caucio (Ed.), *Intelligence: Genetic and environmental influence.* New York: Grune and Stratton, pp. 50-55.

Welford, A. T. (1984). Psychomotor performance. *Annual Review of Gerontology and Geriatrics, 4,* 237-274.

West, T. M. (2003). The effects of music attention and music imagery on mood and salivary cortisol following a speech stress task. Doctoral dissertation. University of Miami.

Whalley, L. J., Starr, J. M., & Deary, I. J. (2004). Diet and dementia. *Journal of the British Menopause Society, 10*(3), 113-117.

Whitbourne, S. K. & Connolly, L. A. (1999). The developing self in midlife. In S. L. Willis & J. D. Reid (Eds.), Life in the middle: The psychological and social developments of middle age. San Diego: Academic Press, pp. 25-45.

Whitbourne, S. K. & Sperbeck, D. J. (1981). Dependency in the institutional setting: A behavioral training program for geriatric staff. *Gerontologist, 21,* 268-275.

Whitty, M. T. (2003). Coping and defending: Age differences in maturity of defense mechanisms and coping strategies. *Aging and Mental Health, 7*(2), 123-132.

Wiegle, D. S. (2003). Pharmacological therapy of obesity: Past, present and future. *Journal of Clinical Endrocrinology and Metabolism, 88*(6), 2462-2469.

Wight, R. G., Aneshensel, C. S., Seeman, M., & Seeman, T. E. (2003). Late life cognition among men: A life course perspective on psychosocial experience. *Archives of Gerontology and Geriatrics, 37*(2), 173-193.

Williams, C. M. (2002). Using medications appropriately in older adults. *American Family Physician, 66*(10), 1917-1924.

Williams, J. W., Jr., Mulrow, C. D., Chiquette, E., Noel, P. H., Aguilar, C., & Cornell, J. (2000). A systematic review of newer pharmacotherapies for depression in adults: Evidence report summary. *Annals of Internal Medicine, 132*(9), 743-756.

Wilson, R. S. (2003). Assessment of lifetime participation in cognitively stimulating activities. *Journal of Clinical and Experimental Neuropsychology, 25*(5), 634-642.

Wink, P., & Dillon, M. (2003). Religiousness, spirituality, and psychosocial functioning in late adulthood: Findings from a longitudinal study. *Psychology and Aging, 18*(4), 916-924.

Wirshing, D. A., Pierre, J. M., Erhart, S. M., & Boyd, J. A. (2003). Understanding the new and evolving profile of adverse drug effects in schizophrenia. *Psychiatric Clinics of North America, 26*(1), 165-190.

Woo, E., & Sharps, M. J. (2003). Cognitive aging and physical exercise. *Educational Gerontology, 29*(4), 327-337.

Yen, P. K. (2003). Maintaining cognitive function with diet. *Geriatric Nursing, 24*(1), 62-63.

Yoon, D. P., & Lee, E. O. (2004). Religiousness/spirituality and subjective well-being among rural elderly whites, African Americans, and Native Americans. *Journal of Human Behavior in the Social Environment, 10*(1), 191-211.

Young, C. C., & Lujan, E. (2004). Intravenous ziprasidone for treatment of delirium in the intensive care unit. *Anesthesiology, 101*(3), 794-795.

Yew, D. T., Li, W. P., Webb, S. E., Lai, H. W., & Zhang, L. (1999). Neurotransmitters, peptides, and neural cell adhesion molecules in the cortices of normal elderly humans and Alzheimer patients: A comparison. *Experimental Gerontology, 34*(1), 117-133.

Zimmet, P. (2005). Epidemiology of diabetes mellitus and associated cardiovascular risk factors: Focus on human immunodeficiency virus and psychiatric disorders. *American Journal of Medicine, 118*(2; suppl), S3-S8.

Chapter 21

Age-Related Sociological Changes

Cheryl Lyn Zukerberg § Adrianne Dill Linton

THEORETICAL APPROACH TO SOCIOLOGICAL ISSUES

Two theories are viewed as particularly important in guiding nurses as they work with older adults. The first theory is Symbolic Interaction Theory, which enables nurses to understand their older adult patients. The second theory is the Theory of Caring. Effective integration of the Theory of Caring by nurses is essential for patient well-being. It also is an important positive motivator of nursing actions (Benner & Wrubel, 1989).

Symbolic Interaction Theory

Symbolic Interaction Theory is used throughout this chapter in considering sociological and sociocultural issues related to aging. This theory, developed by George Herbert Mead, was used by Herbert Blumer (1969) to describe the ways people develop and interact with one another. Three premises from this theory are particularly useful to nurses working with older adults.

The first premise is that people act toward things, other people, or events based on the symbolic meanings these have for them. Life experiences, which vary for each person, influence the meanings each person develops (Blumer, 1969). It is important for nurses to determine how their older patients are interpreting their experiences rather than providing care based on the nurses' perceptions of what they think older patients need. To ensure meaningful communication and appropriate responses, nurses must develop skill in observing, interpreting, and responding to their patients based on their patients' understandings.

The second premise is that meanings are developed in social contexts in the process of interacting with others (Blumer, 1969). Therefore it is important that nurses consider the social and cultural environment of each older adult. A complete assessment includes examining the interaction patterns in the older adult's social world and recognizing how these patterns are changing over time. Nurses have the potential to help older adults redefine their experiences in more satisfying ways that can enhance the quality of their older patients' lives and social worlds.

The third premise is that people behave in ways that are consistent with the meanings they have developed over time (Blumer, 1969). Understanding an older adult's behavior requires the nurse to carefully identify the meanings this behavior has for the patient. Concerns that may seem relatively unimportant to the nurse may be very serious for the older person. This may result in behavior that to the nurse seems strange or out of proportion to the situation. The nurse who understands and uses Symbolic Interaction Theory effectively will not make the mistake of minimizing the patient's concerns. Instead the nurse will identify how those concerns are interpreted by the older adult and will appropriately intervene with sensitivity to the patient's needs.

685

Theory of Caring

The Theory of Caring has been used extensively in nursing since the days of Florence Nightingale; however, it is only recently that nurse theorists have begun to describe some of its major components. Benner and Wrubel (1989) indicated that a caring relationship sets up the conditions of trust necessary for the person receiving care to perceive that care as helpful. Leininger (1984) suggested that the meanings and patterns of caring are culturally derived and best understood in a cultural context. Watson's Theory of Caring examined the kinds of relationships and interactions necessary between the caregiver and the care receiver in order to promote and protect the care recipient's humanity and well-being (Watson, 1988). She particularly emphasized the importance of the psychological, emotional, and spiritual dimensions of care. Wolf, Giardino, Osborne, and Ambrose (1994) proposed five dimensions of caring for nurses: (1) respectful deference to others; (2) assurance of human presence; (3) positive connectedness; (4) professional knowledge and skill; and (5) attentiveness to the experiences of others. Morse, Solberg, Neander, Bottorff, and Johnson (1990) identified the following attributes of caring: compassion, competence, confidence, character, and commitment.

The nurse must exhibit each of the characteristics of caring in ways that the older adult can perceive if a trusting relationship is to be developed. Even skillful use of interaction theory will not meet the patient's needs if the patient does not see the nurse as compassionate and caring. Older adults need to feel that nurses are competent and have confidence in their own abilities, as well as confidence in their patients. To work effectively with their older patients, nurses must demonstrate that they are trustworthy in character and that they are committed to their patients' well-being.

AGE CATEGORIES
Gerontologists' View of Aging

Several views exist on the age categories of older adults. Most gerontologists consider old age to start at 65 years, with subsequent stages of life divided into three categories: *young-old*, 65 to 74 years; *old-old*, 75 to 84 years; and *very old*, 85 years and older. Because the older adult population is living longer, some gerontologists have modified the categories to include another upper age category for those 100 years old and older. They define the *old-old* as 85 to 100 years, and those over 100 years are defined as the *elite-old* (Eliopoulos, 2005, p. 5). The National Institute on Aging (see www.nia.nih.gov/) refers to adults 100 years old and older as *centenarians*. Gosline (2003) refers to those over 85 years old as *frail elders*. These older adults have "increased multiple losses associated with aging, increased effects from chronic diseases, greater vulnerability to illness, and a higher incidence of cognitive impairment" (Gosline, 2003, p. 286).

Sociologists' View of Aging

Sociologists divide older adult years into two categories: *young-old*, 55 to 75 years, as long as the older adult is independent; and *old-old*, which includes those 76 years and older or any age if an older adult becomes dependent.

U.S. Government's View of Aging

In the United States, the federal government has set the beginning of "old age" as the time when full Social Security benefits begin. For older adults born before 1943, this point in time will be age 65. For those born in 1943 and later, the beginning of old age has been raised to age 66 plus a certain number of months. The retirement age depends on the year of birth and increases as the birth year increases (Social Security Administration, 2004).

Older Adults' View of Aging

Regardless of which point of view is deemed the "correct" one by society, older adults have their own view of aging and age categories. Thompson, Itzin, and Abendstern (1990) extensively interviewed adults over 80 years of age and found that these individuals did not perceive themselves as old. Being old is how adults over 80 are perceived by young people and adults in midlife. The younger person equates age with "being old," not the 80-year-old (Thompson, Itzin, & Abendstern, 1990, pp. 111–113). According to Cunningham (2004, p. 278), the individual's perception that "old age" has happened comes with a stroke or any illness that strikes suddenly and significantly affects the ability to speak, walk, or carry out any activities of daily living (ADLs) or instrumental activities of daily living (IADLs). One major factor in helping the older adult perceive and feel younger is laughter, "generous, wholehearted, spontaneous laughter" and the bonding with another human being that occurs when this type of laughter is shared (Cunningham, 2004, p. 280).

For changes related to aging, see Box 21-1.

CULTURAL AND SOCIOLOGICAL CHANGES

According to the 2000 U.S. Census, the older adult population, which doubled from 1970 to 2000, was 35 million persons, or 12.4% of the population. Of the 12.4%, 8.1% were minorities. By 2030, the older adult population will increase to 70 million (20%), with a projection of 24% minorities (Heitkemper, 2004, p. 58). Falk and Falk's (2002) research found that adults ages 65 and

⌐ *Box 21-1* *Age-Related Changes:*
Sociological

- View of personal aging changes and differs from society's view of aging.

- Experiences change in family roles.

- Reflects on life purposes (including unaccomplished goals).

- Family relationships increase in importance and provide emotional and material support when available.

- Religious activities provide spiritual and social support.

- Experiences diminished social network and support as friends age and mobility decreases.

- Experiences financial difficulty related to fixed income, with decreased ability to work and increase income.

- Experiences diminished physical ability and energy level; unable to maintain independence through upkeep of home and activities of daily living (ADLs).

- Has an increased need for formal networks (e.g., senior nutrition sites, senior transportation).

older are the most diverse group of older adults in U.S. history. Based on the growing numbers of older adults, it becomes critical for all nurses to have a solid understanding and working knowledge of the impact of normal age-related cultural and sociological changes.

Relationships

Family. For most older adults, family relationships and continued care are the cornerstone of their social support networks. They often provide material support and usually serve as an important source of socialization within each culture (Spector, 2004). In the last 10 to 15 years, the family structure has changed in that there are fewer family members per generation, yet often there are four or five generations within a family. It is through these family ties that specific cultural behavioral patterns, beliefs, and values are passed from generation to generation (Santrock, 2004).

Fewer children in the family and longer life spans have increased the time individuals spend within the intergenerational family. Older adults may spend up to 50 years with their children, as compared with 20 or 30 years in the 1880s. This may change with the current trend to delay childbearing into the thirties and forties.

Grandparenthood also has become an expanded and more delineated role that is separate from parenthood. People who become grandparents at the median age of 45 to 50 years old and who live to the current life expectancy of 75 to 80 years can expect to be a grandparent for nearly half of their lives (Falk & Falk, 2002).

Most older adults have a small immediate family but are likely to belong to an extended kin network. Thus children often have the opportunity to interact on a regular basis with older adults in their families, with the result that many older adults continue to have the potential to form a viable role in the kinship network. For the majority of older adults, aging serves to reduce the size of the household but increases the number and complexity of role relationships within the extended kinship network, as subsequent generations produce more extended family members.

The Intimate Dyad Relationship. Over half of all persons age 65 to 74 years and older are married, with 78% of men married as compared with 56% of women. As adults age, the proportion who marry is lower for both genders; however, the percentage of men who marry at any age is higher than women (Federal Interagency Forum on Aging-Related Statistics, 2004). Couples who have been married for many years find that their marriage is different from that in their earlier years. Marital satisfaction in these older marriages is strongly related to the individual's emotional and economic well-being. This sense of well-being is affected by the type and amount of care during illness, household management, living arrangements, and emotional gratification (Federal Interagency Forum on Aging-Related Statistics, 2000).

Parent-Child Relationship. For most adults, the parent-child bond persists throughout life and does not weaken appreciably over the years. The relationship is based on affection and is characterized by closeness and caring. Aging parents and adult children become closer in many cases, and the two households often develop a strong spirit of shared responsibility and mutual support. Often it is the parent generation that prefers the separate living arrangement (Family and Consumer Sciences, 2005).

The number of white non-Hispanic older women (9%) living with adult children is higher when compared with older men (5%) living with adult children. The percentage of Asian American men (31%) living with adult children is lower than Asian American women (36%). More black older women (13%) live with their adult children as compared with men (6%), and 25% of older Hispanic women live with adult children as compared with 15% of men (Federal Interagency Forum on Aging-Related Statistics, 2004). The relationship between older parents and their children appears to be healthier when there is some distance between them. However, the attachment between parent and adult child in midlife and later life is influenced by the relationship before birth and as a young child (Family and Consumer Sciences, 2005). Into the upper years, parents continue to maintain the role of advisor to children in later life. Most advising occurs when older parents are vigorous and healthy. However, the role of advisor often shifts to the adult children and adult grandchildren when parents or grandparents become frail or needy (Falk & Falk, 2002).

As the role of global communication, transportation, and computer technology increases, job opportunities and military conflicts will continue to spread adult children over a wider radius as compared with previous years. With diverse mobility, the explosion of health-related knowledge, and medical advances, older adults will live longer and experience the loss of their adult children through death. The death of a child of any age affects the parent because it is an event that occurs out of sequence. The parent, regardless of age, is supposed to die first. It has been estimated that 10% of parents age 60 and older have experienced the loss of one of their adult children (Moss, 2002). For the older adult, sudden death of an adult child may have wider implications than the death of a nonadult child. The adult child may have been the one who carried out instrumental activities that were vital to older parents' ability to stay in their home: grocery shopping, transportation, financial supplements, and performance of household tasks. With the loss of this particular helping relationship, older adult parents may not be able to replace the services that are necessary for them to remain in their home, and the result will be a dramatic change in lifestyle. Brubaker's (1985) model of pertinent factors for determining the possibility of lifestyle change is centered on the formal and informal support systems in place at the time of the adult child's death and the older adult's feelings about death, his or her religious beliefs, and his or her previous experiences with death. With the death of an adult child and the loss of the parent-child relationship, it is common for the older adult to become immersed in social isolation and loss of independence. These are the major causes of lifestyle change for older adults whose adult children were a large part of their formal and informal support systems.

Grandparent Relationship. Older adult grandparents also may serve as caregivers to their grandchildren, transmitting family culture and values. Grandparenting is frequently a joyous reward in older age. Neugarten and Weinstein (1964) developed a typology of five grandparenting styles:

1. Formal: in which the grandparents have rigid role expectations for themselves and their grandchildren, with interaction being somewhat constrained and characterized as fairly authoritarian.
2. Fun seekers: in which the grandparents tend to interact with grandchildren around pleasurable, leisure activities.
3. Surrogate parents: in which the grandparents assume caregiving responsibilities for the grandchildren on a frequent and regular basis.
4. Reservoirs of family wisdom: in which the primary role is to pass down information about family culture and heritage.
5. Distant: in which interactions are infrequent and limited to holidays.

These styles tend to change according to the age of the grandchild and also change according to the age of the grandparent. Baydar and Brooks-Gunn (1991) presented four different categories of grandmothers. (1) The "homemaker" group consisted of grandmothers who were the most apt to take care of any family member needing care. Most of the women in this group were under 65. Most of their time was spent doing household chores, such as baking cookies. (2) The "young and connected" grandmothers were mainly under 55 years of age, had higher education, and had good jobs. They were active and provided care to grandchildren on a regular basis. (3) The "remote" group lived away from their grandchildren and did not provide any care. (4) The "frail" grandmothers had diminished physical or mental health. Most in this group were over 65 years of age. Falk and Falk (2002) also found that grandparents were actively contributing to the life of the grandchild.

Access to grandchildren often depends on factors related to the parents. Grandchildren who come from single or divorced homes or live in the inner city seem to rely on grandparents more than those grandchildren who have both father and mother and live in a more urban area (Falk & Falk, 2002).

Most people view the grandparent role as having vital meaning in their life. Grandparents are valued and loved for just "being there" and are looked on as a stabilizing force in the family. In a time of crisis, they often step in to keep the family afloat and provide emotional support and other types of help. They also can be family mediators or "kin-keepers" who help keep the family connected.

Sibling Relationships. The relationship between older adult siblings can be significant, meaningful, and enriching. It is often the longest lasting relationship in the life of an older adult. If the sibling was in the same cohort they often were first friends and shared each other's history. Many times social losses caused by retirement, relocation, and death can be better supplemented by siblings, because of their peer status, than by adult children. Older adults who maintained frequent contact with their siblings had a greater sense of control in life than adults with infrequent interaction. It has also been found that the loss of a sibling or lack of sibling interaction contributes to loneliness, less life satisfaction, and depression among older persons. Sibling ties are particularly close and active in women and in older adult siblings who are single, divorced, widowed, or childless (Price, 2002a, 2002b; White, 2001).

Intergenerational Family Relationships.

Support within families flows in multiple directions, so that chronological age is not useful in distinguishing support providers from recipients. Intergenerational support takes many forms, including the giving and receiving of money and material resources, care, household assistance, companionship, and advice. The configuration of the family has a significant effect on family support. For example, it is not uncommon to find siblings caring for one another if no spouses or children are present. Another growing phenomenon is the younger-old, who, in their late sixties, may be caring for older-old relatives in their eighties or nineties. This may occur in mother-daughter relationships or some other kin combinations. The cooperation, interaction, and exchange between intergenerational family members who share resources benefit all (Generations United, 2005).

Older adults often serve as standard bearers of family values. They provide emotional support to children and grandchildren, and they care for dependents, including their children, or their dependent elders. These activities assist older adults in coping with age-related losses. It also helps intergenerational family members to recognize the uniqueness of each generation within the family. Intergenerational relationships between older parents and their adult children are important to both parties. Although adult children provide a sense of satisfaction and well-being to older parents, contact with friends and neighbors appears to be more closely associated with well-being in social activities. Close relationships between an adult child and grandchildren are more important for many active older adults when those older adults are dependent for basic needs on family. Other findings emphasize the influence of past experiences on intergenerational interactions and expectations. Lawson and Brossart (2004) found that experiences that occurred in one generation often were repeated in some degree by members from other generations in the same family. Women often have greater intergenerational family roles than men if there are adult children of both genders. Female-linked intergenerational networks usually have greater interaction, more emotional exchanges, and more frequent patterns of mutual aid. However, Lawson and Brossart (2004) determined that there was a difference in contact with the older parent related to the number of female adult children in the family; the number of phone calls and contact with the older parent decreased when there were several female adult children to interact with and care for the parent.

Cohort Relationships.

With the normal aging process, older adults experience loss of friends though death or relocation. Friends of the older adult are usually from the same age, class, race, and ethnic cohort, with friendships based on shared interests, experiences, and concerns. Today's older adult cohort, over age 75, lived through the Depression Era, World War II, the Cold War, the Korean Conflict, the Vietnam War, and the Middle East crises. Out of these experiences came shared interests and similar concerns that formed the older adults' perceptions of the world, country, and home. Older adults usually share attitudes that are similar, such as work ethic, patriotism, productivity in society, and legacy to future generations (Brokaw, 1998).

Lifelong friends are significant and often are considered as part of the family or as an extension of themselves. Lifelong friends supply companionship, stimulation, physical support, ego support, and intimacy. Often these friends are chosen by the older adult to meet intimacy needs for self-disclosure and sharing of private thoughts. Older adult women often have emotionally closer friends than men. As the adult moves into the upper age categories, most friendships are with people of the same gender.

As the cohort grows older and friends die or relocate out of reach, their loss may be profound and affect well-being both emotionally and physically. This may result in symptoms of disease and the inability to meet one's health care needs. The older adult may experience increased depression and a loss of motivation. In the social realm, the older adult may experience increased isolation and may lack the support to be able to live independently at home (Price, 2002b).

Today's young older adult cohort, ages 65 to 75, is more diverse because of world events and social events in the United States during the late 1950s and the 1960s. Those older adults who were "hippies" in the 1960s and opposed the Vietnam War have different perceptions of aging than same-age older adults who supported or fought in the Vietnam War. Perceptions among this young older adult cohort also differ because of the media explosion and faster global communication. One example of the differences within the younger cohort is that even though "these older adults will be more demanding and sophisticated users of information, their ability to access the information and act on it differs" (Kirsch & Jeffery, 2003, p. 4). According to the research by Kirsch and Jeffery (2003), some of the differences that will make a change in public policy as the boomer generation approaches the older adult years include the following: (1) how acute and chronic health issues are dealt with; (2) a changed definition of aging to include "active and productive older life"; (3) creation of more health-focused communities and more support groups for age-related transitions; (4) personal health choices that include going outside "the system"; (5) creation of easy access to health care delivery systems that address mental health issues of older adults; (6) increased choices to spend monies on nonessential health care, including cosmetic surgery and alternative care; (7) changed attitudes and role expectations of women who work and may be unavailable to provide care for aging parents, dependent adult children, and grandchildren; and (8) personal retirement issues such as leisure activities and ongoing financial stability during the older years.

Pets. For older adults, another significant loss is often that of the family pet. Pets can make up a large portion of the older adult's informal support system by providing comfort and by awakening the human desire to respond and love (Schoen, Proctor, & Winter, 2003). Research has shown many benefits when older adults own pets or have regular contact with pets while hospitalized. These benefits include the following: lower blood pressure; decreased anxiety reaction to stress; increased interest in mobility and increased activity levels; significant improvement in emotional and psychosocial well-being; increased feelings of comfort and security; better coping with the consequences of aging; decreased use of the health care delivery system; and decreased loneliness (Keil & Barba, 1995; Lavoie-Vaughn & Vaughn, 2003; Raina, Waltner-Toews, Bonnett, Woodward, & Abernathy, 1999; Rogers & Hart, 1993).

Role Changes

Overall Role Changes. For many older adults, role transitions that occur during the passage into the older years, such as widowhood, retirement, institutionalization, and dying, are considered normal and met without much difficulty. However, as some older adults give up roles, voluntarily or involuntarily, leading to a socially unstructured life in which there are few responsibilities, expectations, or standards by which to judge themselves, depression may occur. With each involuntary surrendering of a role, Ritchie (2003) found that the older adult perceives this as an assault on the human spirit. Role change at any age is generally considered to be stressful, but role change for older adults may be particularly difficult because of diminished socialization opportunities. Older adults need lifestyle management skills, which include daily socialization and meaningful activities within the cultural context (Ritchie, 2003).

Impact on Caregiving Roles within the Context of Family. Cultural factors undoubtedly influence the experience of aging and giving care to older adults within the family. Changes that have occurred over the past 50 years at times have created cultural barriers that subtly create misunderstandings and tensions between family members (Spector, 2004, p. 18). Spector (2004, pp. 19-21) brings up other variables that add to cultural and generational conflicts in families, such as decade of birth; number of generations born in the United States; social class; main language spoken and degree of accent; level of education; and physical problems, such as hearing loss. Any of these may affect the caregiving roles within the family. The role of women in the family changed from the early 1900s, when the mother or adult female children stayed home and helped with family responsibilities, to the late 1900s, when women, because of economic necessity, became a strong economic force in the workplace. However, the tensions between the woman as wage earner and the need for the woman to be family caregiver to young children or older parents continues to create conflict within women and within the family setting (Cuellar, Lundy, & Callahan, 2001, pp. 732-733).

Widowhood. Loss of a spouse is a highly significant life event that can have negative implications for the survivor; however, most widows and widowers cope remarkably well. The grieving process depends on many variables, including spiritual beliefs, life experiences, type of loss, relationship with the deceased, type of death (sudden, suicide, or prolonged illness), and individual coping styles. There is no orderly step-by-step process of getting through the loss of one's spouse. Many factors may affect the depth of bereavement and the ease of recovery, including (1) antecedent factors, such as the nature of the marital relationship and cause of death; (2) concurrent factors, such as health, gender, and age; and (3) subsequent factors, such as social support or secondary stressors.

Relationships, Roles, and Ethnicity. American culture is highly pluralistic, meaning that it is composed of many subcultures. The traditional predominating cultural values include (1) an emphasis on self-reliance and independence, (2) an appreciation for accomplishments and productivity over longevity, and (3) a higher value placed on "new and improved" rather than "old and trusted." Older adults often experience difficulties in a culture that has values differing from theirs on aging. Some of these differences include decreased role opportunities because work for the young is valued over work for the old, and decreased access to health care because economic factors many times weigh heavier than health factors. For the nurse working with the older adult's aging issues and chronic illnesses, relationships and role are wrapped in culture. Because of the tremendous diversity within American culture, the

Box 21-2 Sociological Assessment

Health History

- Identifying data
- Chief complaint
- History of present illnesses (including perceived functional deficit)
  - Perception of social/mobility problems and symptoms (including perceptions of degrees of social isolation)
  - Responses to symptoms
  - Evaluation of past coping strategies (e.g., strategies that worked or did not work)
  - Reason for seeking help
  - Strengths that promote and weaknesses that inhibit socialization
  - Impact of problem/symptoms on life (including social lifestyle)
- Past history
  - Medical: chronic illnesses/exacerbations/medications/review of systems including gastrointestinal/genitourinary causes that may interfere with times of socialization (lactose intolerance, ileostomy, colostomy, urinary incontinence)
  - Functional assessment for activities of daily living (ADLs) and instrumental activities of daily living (IADLs)
  - Social history:
    Past social history (include activities from younger years, hobbies, clubs)
    Current social contacts (formal and informal senior activities)
    Past and current job history (paid and volunteer)
    Effect of medical regime on social activities
    Educational attainment
    Current adult school or community classes
    Current goals

Relationships within family and extended kin network
Relationships outside of family
Relationships with negative consequences (current or past abuse, coercion, or neglect; including current and failed marriages)
Spirituality (formal and informal religious activities)
Economic, attitudinal, and cultural barriers to achieving goals

Physical Examination

- General appearance
  - Appropriateness of dress
  - Congruence of appearance with age
  - Behavior (including spontaneity and congruence of verbals and nonverbals)
  - Mood and affect (rate, rhythm, inflection), depression, reaction to loses, suicidal or homicidal ideations
  - Cognition (including high brain function: orientation, alertness, language, memory, thought content, processes, ability to abstract, judgment, insight, decision-making, critical thinking ability)
- Review of systems
  - HEENT
  - Respiratory
  - Cardio/peripheral vascular
  - Abdomen (genitourinary/gastrointestinal)
  - Musculoskeletal (including ADL and IADL functional ability)
  - Neurological (including cranial nerve testing; posture, gait, and use of assistive devices; coordination)

---

nurse must take many variables into consideration. These include the following: (1) older adult patients' traditional methods of maintaining, protecting, and restoring their health; (2) which spiritual practices and rituals are necessary and important for healing or coping with the illness; and (3) which allopathic, homeopathic, folk, or alternative medications/treatments are preferred. The key to working with older adult patients from diverse backgrounds is to be culturally competent in the setting of mutual health goals to ensure compliance with treatment regimens. In 2003, non-Hispanic whites accounted for 83% of the U.S. population (Federal Interagency Forum on Aging-Related Statistics, 2004, p. 4). As the population ages, immigration from other countries will lend itself to more intercultural marriages. The nurse will need to increase the depth of interviewing and listening skills in order to be culturally competent to make care plans and do case management.

For more information on assessment, see Box 21-2.

SOCIAL NETWORKS AND SUCCESSFUL AGING

Normal changes that come with aging may cause physical or cognitive alterations in older adults' abilities to continue certain roles and social interactions. The age-related changes compounded by changes brought on by disease processes may require specialized assistance for the older adult in order to maintain the desired quality of life. Therefore, as individuals age, support resources that were not necessary for independence and continuance of roles and activities at an earlier stage now become a necessary part of life because the lack of social support is linked to physical and mental health problems (Yeh & Lo, 2004). Depending on the physical or cognitive impairments, the required resources or social networks may range from an occasional card or weekly phone call to extensive daily involvement. The resources may involve informal networks, such as family, friends, and neighbors; formal networks, such as religious or voluntary organizations; and professional organizations in order to provide the needed physical or financial assistance (Allender & Spradley, 2005).

Social Networks

Social networks are defined as relationships between individuals or groups that provide guidance, increase coping skills, offer feedback, and foster independence by promoting a sense of control for individuals with life transitions caused by short-term crises or long-term problem situations (Litwin, 2001).

Successful Aging

Successful aging occurs when the older adult experiences active engagement with life, has a strong connection with at least one other person, and maintains a positive attitude accompanied by a sense of humor about life. These positive attitudes integrate the past with the present and provide a feeling of security for the future (Crowther, Parker, Achenbaum, Larimore, & Koenig, 2002; Easley & Schaller, 2003). Building on the concept of active engagement with life, Easley and Schaller (2003) point out that despite having multiple health problems, older adults who age successfully build a structure in their lives that gives them a sense of control over the consequences of their health problems.

For more information, see Box 21-3.

Most older adults receive support from more than one source. The type and amount of assistance received is partly determined by family availability and its willingness to help. Many times alternative support systems are pulled in to help older adults because family is not available or family members do not have the physical, cognitive, emotional, or financial ability to help.

Support networks are important to the elderly in helping individuals (1) maintain physical and psychological health, (2) maintain self-concept, and (3) obtain material assistance with mental or physical impairments. It is important for the nurse to consider which networks are most effective in providing support for older adults.

One characteristic of old age for most adults is increased dependence on others because of decreasing physical strength, mobility, and economic resources. This may result in conflicts between personal needs and the Western cultural values of self-reliance and

---

BOX 21-3 *TOWARD BETTER SOCIOLOGICAL HEALTH*

- Work with health care providers to stabilize physical and psychosocial issues.
- Utilize positive coping mechanisms (include appropriate use of assertiveness skills to articulate needs).
- Develop balance between needs of dependent family members and own needs.
- Participate in activities that nurture meaningful relationships.
- Participate in activities that provide cognitive and physical stimulation; exercise; music; and humor and spontaneous laughter.
- Develop strategies to deal with changes in health status or functional abilities (e.g., become more mobile with use of assistive devices and public transportation for seniors [such as Dial-a-Ride]).
- Participate in family get-togethers and engage in intergenerational activities, including use of technical equipment (computers and the Internet) to maintain contact.
- Define (or redefine) life purpose and include new goals.
- Continue hobbies and find new activities of interest to increase expressions of self (e.g., art, creative writing, music, folk dancing).
- Identify resources older adults can utilize to increase socialization (e.g., senior centers, church groups, telephone partners, groups around organized games, pets).
- Evaluate own feelings about aging.
- Evaluate and appropriately deal with society's view of aging (for example, by joining senior support/advocacy group such as AARP and the Gray Panthers).

---

independence in adulthood. The use of informal networks, such as family, neighbors, and friends, may reduce the psychological damage of dependency because older people tend to view members of informal support networks as extensions of themselves. However, informal support systems are not always sufficient to meet the needs of older people, particularly the frail elderly. Older adults most often turn for assistance to family first, followed by friends, neighbors, and lay organizations. Older adults and their families typically engage the formal networks last.

Major Types of Social Support Systems

These systems can be viewed as three concentric circles, going from the smaller, inner circle to the largest, outer circle with the older adult in the center (Figure 21-1). The circle closest to the older adult is the informal support system.

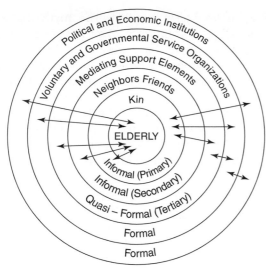

Figure 21-1 The circle closest to the older adult is the informal support system. (From Cantor, M. [1977]. Neighbors and friends: An overlooked resource in the informal support system. Paper presented at the 30th Annual Meeting of the Gerontological Society, San Francisco. Reprinted in Cantor, M., & Little, V. [1985]. Aging and social care. In R. Binstock & E. Shanas [Eds.], *Handbook of aging and the social sciences* [2nd ed.]. New York: Van Nostrand Reinhold, p. 748.)

Informal Support Network. The informal network is made up of the primary support group, which consists of family members and close friends who are considered as family. McIntosh, Sykes, and Kubena (2002) conducted a literature review and found that older adults with regular attendance at religious services believed that relationships inside their religious organizations were the most important feature of their networks. For many older adults, these groups are their cornerstone of social support. Older adults tend to view members of the informal support network as extensions of themselves, including specially trained service pets. The use of this informal support system, for older adults, is related to several well-being outcomes. These include (1) a reduction of the psychological damage of dependency, (2) an increase in morale, (3) improved self-esteem, and (4) an increase in effective problem solving (Kim & Nesselroade, 2003; Litwin, 2001). In the informal network there is a greater likelihood that the individual's lifestyle and preferences will be respected. Pets often are a significant part of the older adult's informal support system.

Semiformal Support Network. The secondary support system is the semiformal network. It is made up of neighbors, religious organizations, and service groups, such as Alcoholics Anonymous, Salvation Army, grief groups for widows/widowers, homeowners' groups, fraternal organizations (e.g., Shriners, Masons), groups

for those with chronic diseases or impairments (e.g., ostomy clubs, cancer support groups), and hobby or special interest groups (including senior citizen clubs). In some of these organizations specific services are provided. For example, many churches, synagogues, temples, and mosques have programs of visitation. They may have congregational or parish nurses who provide care for homebound older adults with chronic problems or care for older adults with temporary problems, such as newly discharged postoperative patients. The services provided vary in different organizations. They often are individualized and diverse, depending on the person's need. Semiformal networks usually attempt to provide services that will ensure that the older adult's lifestyle and preferences are respected.

Formal Support Network. The tertiary support system is usually a part of a formal network. These professional organizations often are bureaucracies sponsored by the local, state, or federal government. They offer certain services for those who are frail and living alone. The services are delivered in a uniform manner to all participants, based on efficiency and rationality. An example of this is the Postal Carrier Alert Program provided by the U.S. Postal Service. The external environments of older adults who enroll in this program are assessed by the letter carrier on his or her delivery route. If there is a buildup of delivered mail or newspapers in the yard, the letter carrier attempts to determine if anyone is home. It there is no response, the letter carrier contacts the route supervisor, who in turn notifies the police department. The police then follow up to determine if the older adult has fallen or is injured. Families often are mediators in securing support for older adults from bureaucratic organizations.

Informal support networks are an important part of older adults' physical, emotional, cognitive, and spiritual well-being. They advocate for older adults with health care delivery systems and provide close relationships that semiformal and formal networks do not. Older adults who lose their primary informal support network through relocation, death of significant person, or illness may experience increased exacerbations of chronic illnesses, feelings of aloneness, loneliness secondary to lack of socialization, depression, or lack of motivation to comply with medical regimen (Yeh & Lo, 2004).

There are times when the informal and semiformal support systems can no longer handle the complexity of the older adult's needs, and the older adult must turn to a formal support network for the assistance of professionals (Beerman & Rappaport-Musson, 2002). The nurse is key in promoting communication and collaboration between informal and formal networks to establish mutually set goals. This is especially true when a coordinated effort is needed among agencies and health care professionals to better meet the needs of older adults. With the increase in technology in Western society and the increasing proportion of dependent older adults with decreased economic power, formal support networks will become increasingly important to meet the daily needs of older adults (see further discussion in the section on public policy later in this chapter). To find specific informal and formal networks for older adults, contact the city hall information center in the patient's city of residence.

AGING AND AGEISM

Positive Aging

Aging is a gift that brings many positive things into the older adult's life. The word "gift" is used because certain characteristics come only with the aging process and these have the potential to change an individual, a family, a community, and society as a whole. Positive aging is based on the definition of aging that is incorporated into the older adult's being. This definition must include the older adult's perspective of wholeness, how the older individual sees himself or herself as fitting into the history of family and time in his or her life space, regardless of the chronological factor.

To be effective, the health care professional also must integrate a definition of aging with the positive components. It is important that the health care professional equate health with aging rather than equating illness with aging. Health is a feeling of satisfaction or well-being about one's physical conditions. This well-being involves a balance between the internal and external environments (the physical, emotional, spiritual, social, and cultural processes of life). For society to change the current negative view of aging it now holds, the health care professional's thinking regarding the aging process must change.

Aging is not static but a moving, natural, and normal process on a continuum. There are no discrete lines of demarcation between adolescence, young adulthood, middle adulthood, and old age. With older adults, most age changes are so gradual that many people develop successful coping skills and accept the changes as a normal part of life. For example, when eyesight begins to change and visual acuity diminishes, the individual goes to the ophthalmologist or optometrist for glasses. Normal aging does not happen all of a sudden. Any change that occurs suddenly is the result of pathology.

Older adults are a heterogeneous group. Adolescents and young adults have only 10 to 20 years of life experience. Older adults have lived three to four times longer and have more life experiences. They have (1) more varied experiences; (2) lived through a variety of problems and environmental conditions for decades; (3) triumphed over years; and (4) coped from day to day,

resulting in long-term survival. The myth that older adults are all alike is not true. Over the years of life experience, older adults have developed increased wisdom, better judgment, a broader perspective of situations, and a wider range of coping mechanisms because they have lived so long.

Despite all of the positive aspects of aging, America tends to be a youth-oriented society where physical beauty, strength, and productivity are prized above characteristics that only come with years of life experience. The term for this is *ageism*. Butler (1975) defined *ageism* as systematic discrimination toward a group of people based on chronological age. He explored this attitude of society and concluded that "ageism allows the younger generation to see older people as different from themselves thus they subtly cease to identify with their elders as human beings" (Butler, 1975, p. 12). Binstock (1983) described society's attitude of ageism as combining a diverse group of people with different characteristics, status, goals, and interests into a single group. Society then views these older adults as "artificially homogenized," packaged, and labeled, to be marketed as "the aged" (Binstock, 1983, p. 136).

Ageism

With ageism, there often is a subtle relationship between society's attitude and its behavior. An individual, or a society, may say that there is no attitude of ageism, but many times behavior speaks louder than words. For example, many older adults are on fixed incomes, which requires them to purchase generic or less expensive items. Often grocery stores place those items on the highest or lowest shelves while catering to the younger populations by placing higher-priced items on shelves that are at eye level and easy to reach. In order to buy the more inexpensive items, many older adults, with less agility and flexibility, have to do more stooping down or reaching high; the younger person, who has more flexibility and agility and is able to purchase more expensive items, only has to reach to eye level. Similar problems occur in department stores. Items for the younger generations are found near the store entrance. Older adults must walk further from the entrance to find the departments they want.

Many communities exhibit ageism in subtle ways, such as the timing of "walk/don't walk" signs on street corners. With normal aging, reflexes slow and ability to move quickly decreases. The timing on the street signs assumes that people can cross the street quickly. It is not unusual to see older adults trapped in the middle of the street when the light changes and traffic begins to move. Ageism also is manifested when cities use small street signs and poorly lit signs. Maps and map books that use small print are not geared for the visual problems of older adults, which also may be a form of ageism.

Stereotypical attitudes of ageism are held by many health care professionals. One can look at the behavior of nurses and acknowledge that older adults are treated like children, such as being called "sweetie" or "honey." These are examples of the use of *elderspeak*. Williams, Kemper, and Hummert (2004) use this term to describe the way that health care workers give older adults communication messages that are patronizing, reinforce dependency, and cause the older adult to feel incompetent and inadequate. Elderspeak communicates a lack of respect for older adults and reinforces the view that American society is a "culture of disrespect" (Lueckenotte, 2004, p. 2).

Another common example of ageism from health care professionals often occurs in the acute facility and is passed along to staff in the long-term care facility, with the use of the word "diapers." Table 21-1 compares behaviors used by health care workers with children and older adults.

Society is more tolerant of young children than of older adults. Both very young children and very old adults are at high risk for health care problems, but there is a major difference between the way society treats a young child and the older adult. Children should be treated with dignity because they are human, and society feels that they have potential and are worthy. However, that same sentiment does not always extend to older adults, especially those over 75 years of age. These older adults have been contributing members of society; built communities; and invented new methods of transportation, such as intercontinental freeway

Table 21-1 *Behaviors of Health Care Workers toward Children and Older Adults*

Behaviors toward Children	Behaviors toward Older Adults
Use diapers for incontinence	Use briefs (incontinence pads) but referred to as "diapers"
Dependent but will have gains	Increasingly dependent
Smelly (do not have the development to take care of themselves)	Smelly older people do not realize they need to wash; with decreases in hearing, smell, and sphincter control, cannot tell when they let out flatus
Use of "baby talk" to communicate endearing feelings to child	Use of "elderspeak" communicates dependence and incompetence

systems, trains, air travel, and space travel. They created the inventions that made our lives easier: telephones, cell phones, and wireless communication. They sacrificed their well-being and lives in World War I, World War II, and the Korean Conflict to give us the freedom to live as we want and make our own choices.

According to Weir (2004), the impact of ageism on health care outcomes may be caused by unresolved fears of the health professional's own aging process, thoughts of his or her own death, and, in some degree, a sense of impotence in treating the chronic health problems that can accompany aging. This form of ageism is subtle; it gives the older adult a sense of being unimportant, yet allows the health care professional to remain detached from the personal implications of the aging process.

Consequences of Ageism: Social Breakdown Syndrome.
Scapegoating is a predecessor of the social breakdown syndrome. Scapegoating is placing the blame for problems on older adults for taking up resources that could be used for other, more valued, groups. One example occurs when a younger driver who causes an accident while speeding and weaving in and out of traffic blames an older adult who was driving the posted speed limit and remaining in one lane.

Ageism has devastating consequences for older adults and can lead to the downward spiral of the social breakdown syndrome (SBS). This downward spiral is caused by society's attitudes and behavior toward older adults and results in a breakdown of the social system for older adults in America. This breakdown affects the well-being of older adults and occurs because society tends to place older adults into a homogeneous, stereotyped group and begins to discriminate against them (Kuypers & Bengtson, 1973). The SBS spiral is usually precipitated by retirement, loss of spouse, or a health crisis resulting in some disability. This precipitating event causes the older adult to become vulnerable.

The first step downward, *vulnerability*, means the older adult is at risk to lose capacity to perform certain roles, adapt to new skills, or have the power to control events or change circumstances. At this stage, the abilities of the older adult are questioned by family, employers, and others in the community.

The second step downward is *dependence*. At this point many older adults doubt their ability to cope with what society demands, and they turn to external sources for help, such as formal networks. This leads to the third step downward, *labeling*. In many areas of society, there is social labeling of older adults as incompetent and incapable of caring for themselves. The older adult is made to feel helpless and inadequate. The fourth step in the downward spiral is *induced dependency*. In this step others force themselves on older adults to take over the caregiving role for them. Often when older adults are placed in institutions for illness or because some help is needed, they are bathed and told when to get out of bed, go to the bathroom, and eat, whether or not this level of care is required. Often they are put into a "sick role" and made more dependent. This step is easily reinforced by families, who, through love, want to do things for older adults that they could do for themselves.

Once the older adult is forced into a dependent role, the fifth downward step is *learned helplessness and atrophy of present skills.* Older adults once competent in self-care skills are viewed as unable to do for themselves and are treated as if they were totally helpless. The sixth and last stage is *internalization.* This occurs when older adults internalize the sick role and perceive themselves as inadequate and unable to care for themselves.

As an older adult enters and continues down the SBS spiral, society assumes the attitude that results in *infantilization.* This is the treatment of the older adult as a child instead of as a mature adult suffering from ill health or in the natural process of aging. In the concept of infantilization, society communicates to the older adult that he or she is not capable. Infantilization is an interpersonal issue. The person involved in the infantilization process can be a family member, friend, health care worker, or anyone else with whom the older adult comes in contact. That person is the problem, not the older adult. Often the infantilization is done out of love because people want to take care of the older adult. However, if the older adult is capable of doing something on his or her own but the caregiver is not letting the older adult perform this task, that is infantilization. Unfortunately, American society is very good at infantilization of the older adult. Infantilization of the older adult is exhibited in many ways: using the older adult's first name or a pet name if it is not requested; patting the older adult on the head; referring to an older adult as a little old boy or a cute little old lady; patronizing the older adult with phrases such as, "Good girl, you ate all of your breakfast"; speaking in other childish terms or the use of baby talk; little or no inclusion of the older adult in decision making about his or her own care; or combing older women's hair into pigtails and attaching bows. Infantilization leads to depersonalization and increased disability. Infantilization is considered as a form of psychological abuse that is not necessarily less damaging than actual physical abuse (Yan & Tang, 2004, p. 270).

It is important to note that this downward spiral of the SBS does not occur with all older adults. When crisis situations arise, older adults often become vulnerable. However, many individuals are able to cope, adapt, and maintain competence and mastery over the circumstances and do not move further down the spiral.

Many health care professionals hold negative attitudes toward care of older adults. They may believe that older adults are dependent, that older adults require considerable physical care, and that there is little professional skill in providing such care. Older adults have a narrow range of homeostasis in body systems. Because of decreased reserves in the different organ systems, the older adult patient is considered "fragile," with a precarious balance. For this reason, nurses need a higher level of assessment skills and knowledge of older adults' issues. Research has shown that many negative attitudes about older adults come from nurses who take care of older adults in the gerontological nursing settings. Nursing outcomes often are not congruent with the nursing goal of promoting maximum independence in older adult patients (Williams, Kemper, & Hummert, 2004, p. 19).

Competent Gerontological Nursing Practice

In the early 1980s the boards of registered nursing recognized the need for a specialized body of gerontological knowledge as part of minimal nursing educational preparation that is necessary for basic competence for the beginning registered nurse. The American Nurses Association (ANA) built on this and set minimal gerontological nursing standards for every nurse (see the ANA Web site at www.ana.org). The National Gerontological Nursing Association (NGNA) added practice details required for certification (see http://ngna.org). The American Nurses Credentialing Center (ANCC) set the criteria for testing eligibility, developed, and administered the national tests for certification (see www.ancc.org).

In addition, two major organizations, the American Association of Colleges of Nursing (AACN; see www.aacn.org) and the John A. Hartford Foundation Institute for Geriatric Nursing (see www.hartfordign.org) also are trying to change these negative stereotypical attitudes of health care providers through provision of grant monies, awards to improve curriculum in schools of nursing, and continuing education activities. Their goals include increasing knowledge related to the physical, psychological, and social aspects of aging throughout the life span and resultant impact on the individual and family. Recommended content includes the following: (1) assessment of the functional status of older adults; (2) signs and symptoms of atypical manifestation of diseases in older adults; (3) pathophysiology, epidemiology, and treatment of chronic diseases; (4) altered pharmacology of drugs used by older adults; and (5) planning and providing appropriate nursing interventions and other health care services. The acquisition of this content will enable the health care worker to provide care for older adults that will maximize functional ability, prevent and minimize disabilities, maintain life with dignity, and provide comfort until death.

Social Responses to Growth in the Older Adult Population

With the current increasing numbers of older adults and even larger increases predicted in the next 10 to 15 years, society is becoming more aware of the older adult's needs. This is exhibited in the following: (1) increased local, state, and federal services to deal with rapidly increasing numbers of dependent older adults; (2) changes in attitudes toward balance of work and leisure; (3) increased recognition of the pressure on women as demands build for their time and energies from their nuclear family, the workplace, and dependent older adults in their extended family; and (4) development of special interest groups to advocate on behalf of older adults (Federal Interagency Forum on Aging-Related Statistics, 2004).

The increasing population of older adults has occurred at a time when Americans have increasingly turned to government for assistance with social problems. Additionally, because American families have never had a legal responsibility to care for their elders, only a moral one, there has been an increased need for solutions generated by formal network organizations. These two factors have contributed to a plethora of bureaucratic "solutions" to some of the problems associated with aging. The Social Security system is perhaps the largest and most visible example. Others include the Medicaid program (which funds approximately 75% of nursing home care in the United States), various programs sponsored under the Older Americans Act, and local bureaucracies established to disburse private sector philanthropy. The nature of the problems of older adults has not basically changed over the past century, but the numbers of older adults who need care have increased; however, the mechanisms for addressing those needs have not increased sufficiently to meet the needs.

Special Interest Groups. Older adults and professionals in the field of gerontology are organized into several key special interest groups, which have gained recognition as powerful forces for social change. Some of the groups are the American Association of Retired Persons (AARP; see www.aarp.org), the National Council on the Aging (NCOA; see www.ncoa.org), the Gray Panthers Network (see www.graypanthers.org), and the Gerontological Society of America (GSA; see www.geron.org). These groups have been in the forefront of lobbying for maintaining services currently available to older adults, increasing community-based options for long-term care, and improving access to specialized training in gerontology and geriatrics for health care providers. These special interest groups have been actively working to change society's stereotypes of older adults and change public policy through demonstration projects, research, public education, and lobbying efforts. Some examples of the specific activities of these special interest groups are as follows. AARP is the largest organization for older adults in the United States. Among other activities, it produces a variety of widely read publications for older adults; operates an economical, high-volume pharmaceutical service; and does extensive lobbying at the federal level. It also sponsors small-scale research projects designed to enhance the quality of life for the aged (see www.aarp.org).

The NCOA is involved in such diverse projects as (1) developing standards for senior centers and adult day care, (2) stimulating medical student interest in geriatrics through funding of small-scale predoctoral fellowships, (3) producing publications for individuals working in the field of gerontology, and (4) sponsoring national meetings to provide a communications network for service innovations that contribute to well-being in old age (see www.ncoa.org).

The Gray Panthers Network is an intergenerational group that focuses on local issues, where strong networks are in place. The organization is interested in a fairly broad social agenda that includes concerns of older adults (see www.graypanthers.org).

The GSA is a multidisciplinary professional and scientific organization for those working in the field of gerontology. It produces research publications, holds scientific meetings, publishes compilations of relevant research, and is a resource for experts in the field of gerontology. Annual scientific meetings are held to enhance communication among researchers and practitioners. The GSA also sponsors a postdoctoral fellowship program in applied gerontology to help link academics with practical problems of aging service delivery or policy formulation (see www.geron.org).

Ageism and Nursing

Ageism is strong in American society. The nurse's behavior and attitudes toward older adults must be examined before trying to educate colleagues and society (Wells, Foreman, Gething, & Petralia, 2004). Box 21-4 presents a few questions for self-examination.

The nurse's goal for society in promoting change from ageism to advocacy is through interventions that empower both the nurse and the older adult. Society can be empowered with knowledge through health education and by increases in financial and social resources. Table 21-2 lists several examples of ageism against older adults and effective advocacy to change them.

The principles noted in Box 21-5 are important in order to raise awareness and combat ageism as a health care professional.

Nursing Diagnosis. Social isolation related to ageism manifested by feelings of loneliness.

BOX 21-4 Self-Assessment of Attitudes toward Older Adults

ASK: What are some losses associated with aging (e.g., strength, vision)?

ASK: What are some gains associated with aging (e.g., wisdom, insight with life experience)?

ASK: What are some changes you have already noticed in your body?

ASK: What are some gains you have now that you did not have at age 15?

DEFINING CHARACTERISTICS. Sample subjective data include the following:

- Expresses feelings of aloneness because of other people or circumstances
- Expresses feelings of being unable to meet expectations of others
- Expresses feelings of being different from others or being treated as different
- Expresses feelings of being rejected or not accepted by others
- Expresses feelings of anger or hostility toward caregivers, family, or friends
- Expresses feelings of being abandoned by God, family, or friends
  Sample objective data include the following:
- Lives alone or in extended care facility
- Recent change in living arrangements
- Limited access to transportation
- Limited contact with family, friends, neighbors, or socialization activities
- Unable to maintain usual social activities
- Limited knowledge of resources for transportation or socialization
- Impaired mobility, sensory deficits, or limited energy level
- Lacks perception of a significant purpose for life
- Limited spiritual resources
- Affect appears sad, dull, bored, or withdrawn

Outcomes. The older adult will demonstrate increased social involvement within 1 month as evidenced by the following indicators:

- Verbally identifies reasons for feelings of isolation
- Verbally identifies four ways of increasing meaningful relationships and activities
- Reports a satisfying individual social interaction with at least one person each day for a minimum of 15 minutes
- Reports participation in and enjoyment of at least one weekly group social activity
- Verbally identifies at least one resource that will assist in decreasing feelings of isolation
- Reports feeling an increase in social support (e.g., person to contact when feeling lonely or isolated)

Interventions
COMPLEX RELATIONSHIP BUILDING (5000)
- Establish rapport and a trusting relationship with patient

Table 21-2 Examples of Ageism and Effective Advocacy

Daily Events	Examples	What Actions to Take
Financial	Being refused interest-free credit, a new credit card, or car insurance because of age.	File complaints through the customer services manager and always try to speak, or write, to the most senior person who deals with complaints.
Social care	Finding that an organization's attitude toward older people results in older adults receiving a lower quality of service.	File complaints through local authority complaints procedure. If unsuccessful, contact the local government ombudsman. Inform and encourage others to take similar action.
Health service	Age limits on benefits such as disability living allowance. Physician deciding not to refer older adults to a consultant because of age. Being denied travel insurance.	File complaints. Discuss with physician, registered nurse, or case manager. Use the insurance company's official complaints procedure.
Career	Receiving less or unfair training and development than other staff. Coerced to retire early or losing job based solely on age.	Let employer know that younger staff only stay for 2 years on average after receiving training.

Data from Age Concern England. (2002). Ageism exists. Have you seen the signs? Retrieved January 10, 2005, from www.ageconcern.org.uk/AgeConcern/media/ace_week_booklet.pdf; and Levy, B. (2001). Eradication of ageism requires addressing the enemy within. *Gerontologist, 41*(5), 578-580.

1. Compliment people on an inner quality rather than on how young they look.
2. Promote intergenerational job sharing, full or part time.
3. Use a single standard of behavior. (Do not blame old age for fatigue, disorganization, or forgetfulness. As with young persons, they could be due to poor planning or lack of sleep.)
4. Contact local news media when a headline or cartoon is offensive.
5. When selecting a birthday card, keep your sense of humor. (Recognize the difference between laughing *with* and laughing *at* someone.)
6. Educate on implications of ageism on older adults.

Adapted from National Gray Panthers, Washington, DC.

COPING ENHANCEMENT (5230)

- Encourage patient verbalization of feelings of isolation
- Identify variables patient views as contributing to feelings of isolation

FAMILY INTEGRITY PROMOTION (7100)

- Promote family cohesion and unity

FAMILY INVOLVEMENT PROMOTION (7110)

- Facilitate family participation in emotional or physical care of the patient

SUPPORT SYSTEM ENHANCEMENT (5440)

- Decrease barriers to social interactions (e.g., transportation, finances, special equipment needs)
- Identify resources patient can use to increase socialization and initiate referrals as indicated (e.g., senior centers, religious/church groups, day care centers for elderly, retirement communities, house sharing, college classes for older adults, telephone partners, pets)

SOCIALIZATION ENHANCEMENT (5100)

- Facilitation of patient's ability to interact with others (Carpenito, 2002; Dochterman & Bulechek, 2000; Wilkinson, 2005)

ELDER MISTREATMENT
Definition and Scope of the Problem

Definition of Elder Mistreatment. Elder mistreatment (EM) is a broad construct that encompasses categories of defined behavior toward older adults that violate their individual rights by infliction of pain, injury, debilitating mental anguish, physical or emotional isolation, or deprivation of services. EM is a serious, underreported, and often undetected situation that affects thousands of older adults.

Elder abuse, an international problem, is increasing in many countries (Litwin & Zoabi, 2004). In the United States, it has been estimated that approximately 2 million older adults are abused or neglected yearly, yet the full extent of abuse is not known because many cases are not recognized by health care providers. This lack of recognition of EM perhaps is due to lack of education in assessment techniques, lack of assessment tools, the misinterpretation of assessment data as signs and symptoms of many common chronic medical conditions found in older adults, or misinterpretation of findings as normal age-related changes (Fulner, 2002; MacNeill & MacNeill, 2004; National Center on Elder Abuse, 2000; Pavlik, Hyman, Festa, & Dyer, 2001). EM occurs in varied settings, including board and care facilities, long-term care facilities, acute care hospitals, and at home. It has been found that persons most likely to mistreat older adults are family members who are direct caregivers and who are experiencing increased stress under the burden of caregiving (Litwin & Zoabi, 2004; MacNeill & MacNeill, 2004). Hospitals and police are the most frequent reporters of EM, followed by friends and neighbors (National Center on Elder Abuse, 1998).

Adult children are the most frequent abusers (47.3%); next are spouses (19.3%), siblings and other relatives (8.8%), and grandchildren (8.6%). Nonfamily abusers include friends, neighbors, and service providers (12.4%). The highest incidence of abuse is reported in older adults having some degree of confusion and depression. The incidence of all types of EM increases with advancing age. Two to three times more dependent elders over 80 years suffered EM as compared with those from ages 65 to 79. The reports of EM include more women and whites. Hispanic and black older adults were underrepresented in the national statistics (Administration on Aging, 2005; National Center on Elder Abuse, 1998).

Concept Clarification

The term *elder mistreatment* is synonymous with the term *abuse*. EM continues to be difficult to define, categorize, and recognize. Victims of EM may demonstrate signs and symptoms similar to the signs and symptoms of many common chronic medical conditions found in older adults, such as bruising, weight loss, and fractures. According to Litwin and Zoabi (2004), this is a major reason EM is not recognized. Another reason it is difficult to define and categorize types of EM is the lack of standardization in reporting. In a study that surveyed reports of abuse to adult protective services (APS) in the United States, it was indicated that approximately 52% of the states did not maintain a central abuse registry and only 39% of the states reported maintaining registries on the abusers (National Center on Elder Abuse, 2000). According to the report, *A Response to the Abuse of Vulnerable Adults,* APS determined that of the substantiated reports, 42.5% occurred in domestic settings, 8.3% occurred in institutional settings, and 2.4% occurred in mental health settings. The other 42.1% of substantiated reports were not tracked by specific settings; therefore the reports were put under the category of "all settings." A third reason for lack of congruity in reporting abuse is that many investigated reports of EM have been unsubstantiated and many cases simply are unreported (National Center on Elder Abuse, 2000; Pavlik, Hyman, Festa, & Dyer, 2001).

Ethical Issues

Ethical difficulties related to defining and describing EM exist. These difficulties stem from differences among individuals and cultural groups in defining quality of life, survival needs, and well-being. Moon (2000) found that there were significant group differences in perceptions of abuse among African Americans, Hispanics, non-Hispanic whites, Koreans, Korean Americans, Japanese Americans, and Native Americans. Verbal abuse by adult children was tolerated more in the Japanese American and non-Hispanic white groups. Psychological neglect and abuse was considered as hurtful as physical abuse among the Hispanic and European American groups. Use of medication to calm the older adult or to leave the bedridden older parent alone occasionally was seen as acceptable by many in the Hispanic and Korean groups. Korean and Korean American older adults and their adult children share a sense of co-ownership of parents' wealth and property. The adult children in these two ethnic groups agree that it is acceptable not to repay the parents. Native Americans disapprove of adult children using elderly parents' money without reimbursement (Moon, 2000). All of the groups would use formal and informal sources of help for EM differently. Moon (2000) determined that the type of intervention sought was predicted by the identification and tolerance of EM in specific cultural groups.

Many gaps exist in the knowledge about EM. It is unlikely that there will be one definition of EM that is accepted by everyone. Thus nurses must continue to integrate their clinical experience and social skills to recognize the problem and provide appropriate intervention. Nurses must also be aware of the values that underlie each definition of abuse and be prepared to use principles of ethical decision making as guides to intervention (see Chapter 9).

Risk Factors for Elder Mistreatment

Theoretical Bases. Several theories have been proposed to explain EM, yet no single theory explains the dynamic. The four major theories are (1) Social Learning or Transgenerational Violence Theory, (2) Psychopathology of the Abuser Theory, (3) Stressed Caregiver Theory, and (4) Dependency Theory (Krouse, 2004).

According to Transgenerational Violence Theory, family violence is a learned behavior that is passed down from one generation to another. Children who are abused tend to grow up to abuse their own children and abuse their older parents as well. Most cases of EM involve family members in which there have been longstanding conflicts. According to a literature review by Wolf (2000), there was an increased incidence of elder abuse victims when there was evidence of depression or psychological distress. Unfortunately, there was no way to know if the depression or psychological distress was present before the abuse or occurred as a consequence. Wolf (2000, pp. 8-9) emphasizes that "some studies on the relationships between caregiver stress, Alzheimer's disease, and elder abuse suggest that the long-term or preabuse nature of the relationship between the caregiver and the care recipient may be the important factor in predicting instances of mistreatment." In many instances abuse of the older adult adds a high risk for death. Factors that may increase the risk for elder abuse resulting in death are age, gender, income, functional status, cognitive status, diagnosis, social supports, and possibly extreme interpersonal stress (Wolf, 2000).

Psychopathology of the Abuser Theory asserts that nonnormal personality characteristics of the abuser result in abuse. These abusers are typically primary caregivers who are unemployable due to mental retardation, dementia, or personality disorders.

Stressed Caregiver Theory suggests that pressures of direct caregiving plus stresses outside the home build up in the caregiver and culminate in behavioral expressions of anger (Krouse, 2004). Ramsey-Klawsnik (2000) refers to this theory as a *typology of abuser,* which is discussed in more detail later in the chapter. Numerous stressors are placed on primary caregivers of older adults. Caregivers may have unrealistic perceptions of their abilities to care for older adults without resources. Plowfield, Raymond, and Blevins (2000) found that caregivers' lack of knowledge and time often led to frustration and exhaustion as the older adult's needs increased. "A situation once thought to be tolerable may become impossible" (Plowfield, Raymond, & Blevins, 2000, p. 53). Most caregivers also have family responsibilities, and as the patient care needs increase, the caregiver feels that there is not enough time in the day to do everything required. "In-home caregiving can be perceived as disruptive to the family's lifestyle and privacy" (Plowfield, Raymond, & Blevins, 2000, p. 54). Older adults with chronic illnesses may have times of exacerbations of one or more illnesses. Conditions such as congestive heart failure or chronic obstructive pulmonary disease may have acute illness episodes because of intrapersonal or environmental factors. Acute episodes

Irresponsibility	Assertiveness	Nurturance	Hyperresponsibility
No true guilt Passive elder abuse	Needs of caregiver	Needs of care recipient	Much false guilt Active abuse/burnout

Figure 21-2   Caregiver continuum. (From Watson, J. [1990]. Someone in the family is sick. In T. Smick, J. Duncan, J. P. Moreland, & J. Watson (Eds.), *Eldercare for the Christian family: What to do when a loved one becomes dependent.* Dallas: Word Publishing.)

will require more of the caregiver's finances and more of the caregiver's time and energy. Employment needed to ensure financial stability may not be feasible because of the time commitment needed to give care and coordinate health care services. Many adult children and siblings of older adults who are not directly involved with caregiving may experience guilt and frustration because they do not want the responsibility and their lives are not as affected as the caregiver's life (Plowfield, Raymond, & Blevins, 2000).

Nurses who work with caregivers and family members should remind these support people that they are in a marathon, not a sprint. The loved one's needs are great, but so are the caregivers' needs (Watson, 1990). Watson (1990) put the caregiver's role on a continuum starting with *irresponsibility,* followed by *assertiveness,* then *nurturance,* and ending with *hyperresponsibility* (Figure 21-2).

When the caregiver is obsessed with his or her own needs, irresponsibility is manifested by neglect of the older adult or abandonment. When the caregiver is overcommitted to the patient's needs, hyperresponsibility is manifested by caregiver burnout, breakdown, or active abuse. To remain healthy, the caregiver needs to balance the needs of the caregiver and the needs of the dependent older adult between assertiveness and nurturance (Watson, 1990).

Smick (1990) formulated some key questions that are useful for assessing overload in the primary caregiver (Box 21-6). Nursing interventions that must be included in any care plan are based on empowerment of the caregiver.

Dependency Theory implies that functional frailty and medical illness of the victim lead to abuse. However, recent studies show no direct correlation between patient frailty and abuse. Krouse (2004) suggests that dependency causes vulnerability in the older adult and that leads to abuse.

Ramsey-Klawsnik (2000) identified five types of abusers of older adults: (1) overwhelmed, (2) impaired, (3) narcissistic, (4) domineering or bullying, and (5) sadistic abusers. The overwhelmed abusers are qualified, have good intentions, and give adequate care. However, when the amount of care that is needed is more than the overwhelmed individual can provide, verbal or physical abuse occurs. Caregiver factors that

BOX 21-6 Questions to Assess Primary Caregiver Overload

Is the patient's condition worsening despite the primary caregiver's best efforts?

Does the primary caregiver feel that no matter what he or she does for the patient, it is never enough?

Does the primary caregiver have time for respite?

Does the primary caregiver have other responsibilities in addition to the direct care of the patient?

Are family relationships breaking down because of the caregiving pressures?

Do the caregiving duties interfere with the primary caregiver's work and social activities to an unacceptable degree?

Does the primary caregiver refuse to think of herself or himself because that would be "selfish"?

Is the primary caregiver using destructive coping methods such as overeating, undereating, abusing alcohol, or abusing drugs?

Is the primary caregiver's voice tone or language harsh, bitter, rushed, or sharp?

Are the primary caregiver's physical actions forceful toward the family member?

Does the primary caregiver express loss of happy times?

From Smick, T. (1990). The sandwiched generation. In T. Smick, J. Duncan, J. P. Moreland, & J. Watson, *Eldercare for the Christian family: What to do when a loved one becomes dependent.* Dallas: Word Publishing.

play into abusive situations include lack of sleep, inadequate food intake, insufficient respite time, or conflict with a family member. Care recipient factors that are present in abusive situations occur when the older adults are impatient, critical, uncooperative, or demanding (Ramsey-Klawsnik, 2000). Ramsey-Klawsnik (2000) found that some environmental factors influence occurrences of abuse, including lack of supplies, equipment, financial resources, or assistance with care.

The impaired abuser also is a well-meaning care provider; however, the presence of some type of physical, mental, or developmental impairment limits the ability to adequately provide care for the older adult (Ramsey-Klawsnik, 2000). Problems such as drug addiction may make the impaired abuser particularly dangerous to the patient.

The primary reason a narcissistic abuser becomes a caregiver is not out of the desire to help the older adult but for personal gain. This individual uses the older adult's resources to get what he or she wants. Ramsey-Klawsnik (2000) refers to the narcissistic behavior toward the older adult as a means to an end. This behavior is used to obtain the person's financial assets, such as Social Security or pension checks or inheriting the older adult's home.

The domineering or bullying abuser perceives himself or herself as having power and authority over the older adult, which leads to coercion and demanding verbal behavior. This type of abuser also is high risk to engage in sexual abuse with the older adult (Ramsey-Klawsnik, 2000).

The sadistic abuser uses behavior to humiliate and terrify the older adult. This gives the abuser feelings of power and control. This abuser takes great pleasure in producing fear in the victim by using torture or manipulation. This abuser is very dangerous because threats of harm or death are made to the victim about family members or pets, and these can be carried out. The older adult does everything possible to please the abuser and is too fearful to seek or accept outside assistance (Ramsey-Klawsnik, 2000).

Major Categories of Elder Mistreatment

Different names are used for EM in the literature. However, forms of elder abuse are comparable to those that occur in the abuse of children. In elder abuse, as in child abuse, it is common to identify the coexistence of several types of abuse in a single older adult (Marshall, Benton, & Braizer, 2000). The five major categories of EM are physical (includes sexual abuse), psychological, financial (exploitation, undue influence), neglect (includes self-neglect), and abandonment (MacNeill & MacNeill, 2004).

Physical Abuse (Including Sexual Abuse).
Physical abuse is an act of assault or battery. It includes infliction of physical pain, abrasions, lacerations, burns, sprains, dislocations, whiplash, fractures, burns, and bruises. It includes behaviors such as hitting, beating, pushing, shoving, kicking, and pinching. This category of abuse contains the largest number of substantiated reports. Coerced sexual intercourse or nonconsensual sexual contact with an older adult is usually classified as physical abuse but may be categorized separately. Sexual abuse also includes unwanted touching, rape, molestation, and sexually explicit photographing (National Center on Elder Abuse, 2005).

Psychological Abuse.
Psychological abuse, also called emotional abuse, is the use of words with an aggressive, coercive tone toward the older adult. It may be manifested by insults, threats, intimidations, humiliation, harassment, and withdrawal of acts of affection. Emotional abuse also includes infantilization and enforced social isolation.

Financial Abuse.
Financial abuse, also called exploitation, carries coercive undertones toward the older adult. It refers to behavior geared to take advantage of the older adult for financial benefits, such as forging the older adult's signature on legal documents, cashing checks without authorization, misusing an older adult's money or possessions, or improper use of power of attorney. Older adults are easy prey for financial frauds, such as buying property that looks wonderful in brochures but does not exist as advertised or is not available for sale. Another scam is the inclusion of an additional name on the older adult's bank signature card (National Center on Elder Abuse, 2005).

Another type of financial abuse is *undue influence* (UI). Quinn (2002) used UI to denote intense psychological pressure rather than persuasion. It involves an individual using "his or her role and power to exploit the trust, dependency, or fear to gain psychologic control over the older adult's decision-making for financial gain" (Quinn, 2002, p. 11). UI is a combination of financial abuse and psychological abuse. The process of UI is deliberate and involves trusting relationships. As the trusting relationship deepens, the abuser isolates, monitors, and manipulates the older adult's contact with other people. During the process, the older adult is made to believe that only the abuser cares for the elder and can keep him or her safe. The older adult is made to feel powerless and totally dependent on the abuser for food, medications, care, and psychological and financial well-being. Ultimately the older adult forms a strong bond with the abuser and gives financial control of assets to the abuser (Quinn, 2002). For the older adult victim, financial abuse often results in poverty, depression, and ultimately the loss of ability to sustain oneself financially.

Neglect.
Neglect can be active or passive. Active neglect refers to withholding goods or services necessary for the older adult's physical or mental health, including food, water, clothing, shelter, or medical attention. Neglect may involve inappropriate clothing, resulting in hypothermia, hyperthermia, or frostbite; poor hygiene; lack of medical attention; contractures from lack of position change; dehydration; malnutrition; pressure sores; and burns of the perineum and anal areas caused by inadequate cleansing after urination or defecation. Passive neglect refers to the legitimate inability of the caregiver to perform caregiving activities, such as bathing, dressing, or caring for an incontinent older person.

Self-neglect occurs when older adults make decisions to refuse medical care or services that are necessary for their quality of life. Self-neglect also occurs when the older adult is too weak to meet his or her own needs with ADLs and IADLs. This type of abuse is very difficult for the nurse to deal with because the older adult has the right to refuse medical care and the benefits of health care (O'Keefe, 2001).

Abandonment (Geriatric Orphan).

Abandonment refers to desertion or the purposeful withdrawal of care with no provision for alternative care; the term used is *geriatric orphan*. This is commonly seen when the older adult is dropped off at a hospital emergency department. The caregiver or family member leaves the older adult and assumes no further responsibility for care. According to a study by the National Center on Elder Abuse (1998), abandonment occurs most often to older, black men; approximately 96% of these abandoned men are in the $5000 to $9000 income bracket.

Nurses' Care: Elder Mistreatment

With the population growth of older adults, it is expected that nurses will see an increase in elder mistreatment cases and an increase in the number of substantiated mistreatment reports. The problem of EM and its causes have important implications for nurses working with older adults, families, and caregivers. Because older adults are at risk for mistreatment by any family member, peer, paid caregiver, or agencies designed to help them, nurses have the opportunity and responsibility to alter the abuse course for the older adult and reduce the consequences of any type of EM. While working with older adults, whether in the acute hospital, long-term care facility, clinic, or home setting, nurses should always be alert for signs and symptoms of all types of EM. Elder abuse occurs mainly in the home setting, with the most likely abusers being spouses, children, siblings, relatives, or paid caregivers (Marshall, Benton, & Braizer, 2000). Because of their intimate contact with older adults and their assessment skills, nurses may be able to identify abuse, observe the effects of EM, and identify high-risk families. Nursing assessment is the key in prevention and treatment of abuse (Table 21-3).

Case Study.

Mr. R. is an 88-year-old physically dependent man who lives with his daughter, Maggi, and her family. Maggi works full time as a stock clerk in a department store. She has four grown children. Maggi's youngest son and 15-year-old grandson live with her. Maggi cannot afford caregivers for Mr. R. so he is home alone while she works. Her son and grandson are usually not home until late evening. Sometimes Mr. R. is home alone for 12 to 15 hours without food and water.

In the mornings, Maggi bathes and feeds her father. When she comes home in the evenings, she cleans and feeds him again. Maggi gets angry over the situation and yells at Mr. R. whenever he complains. Maggi says she feels guilty about having to leave him alone so long but does not feel she has a choice. Mr. R. has one stage 1 and three stage 2 pressure areas over both hips and coccygeal areas. Maggi says she has no life of her own and is tired all the time.

NURSING DIAGNOSIS. Ineffective family coping: disabling, related to caregiver role strain and manifested by elder abuse.

Defining Characteristics. Sample subjective data include the following:

- Older adult patient complains that caregiver leaves patient alone with no access to any means of communication for long periods of time; is rough when assisting with personal care; refuses to leave room when visitors are present; shouts at patient, using abusive and demeaning language; and threatens to put patient in a long-term care facility.
- Older adult expresses ambivalent feelings of appreciation for the caregiver but also fear, anger, and hostility about the caregiver.
- Older adult expresses helplessness and fear of being abandoned.
- Caregiver expresses feelings of being overwhelmed by the responsibilities of providing care for the older adult patient.
- Caregiver expresses feelings of being unable physically and financially to meet the needs of the older adult patient.
- Caregiver expresses feelings of anger and frustration toward the patient and states that the patient complains about everything the caregiver does.
- Caregiver expresses feelings of guilt and incompetence about the care provided for the patient.

Sample objective data include the following:

- Older adult has significant self-care deficits of 6 months' duration related to stroke. These are not expected to improve.
- Limited finances on fixed income.
- Limited contact with family, friends, and neighbors.
- Caregiver is unable to maintain usual recreational activities.
- Caregiver has limited knowledge of resources for assistance in caregiver responsibilities.
- Caregiver is experiencing fatigue and claims to have limited energy level.

Suggested alternative diagnoses include the following:

- Caregiver role strain (actual or risk for)
- Management of therapeutic regimen: families/individual, ineffective
- Violence: directed at others, risk for

Table 21-3 *Categories of Elder Mistreatment, Manifestations, Signs, and Symptoms*

	Physical	Psychological	Financial	Neglect	Abandonment
Definition	Use of physical force that results in bodily injury, physical pain, or impairment.	Infliction of emotional pain or distress through verbal or nonverbal acts.	Illegal or improper use of older adult's monies, property, or assets.	Refusal or failure to fulfill any part of obligations or duties to older adult.	Purposeful withdrawal of care with no provision for alternative care.
Manifesting behaviors	Strike, hit, beat, push, shove, shake, slap, kick, pinch, and burn.	Verbal assaults, insults, threats, intimidation, humiliation, and harassment.	Cashing checks without permission, forging signature for financial gain, misusing older adult's money or possessions, and improper use of power of attorney.	Failure of a person who has fiduciary responsibilities to provide care, including food, water, clothing, shelter, and medical attention.	Caregiver or family member with responsibility for care, leaving older adult alone.
Signs and symptoms	Multiple fractures in various stages of healing. Bruises clustered together and located in unusual places. Burns located in or around the soles, palms, or buttocks. Sprains or dislocations of joints. Listen for key words on admission, such as older adult is "accident prone" or "clumsy."	Upset or agitated. Unusual behavior usually attributed to dementia (sucking, biting, and rocking). Paranoia. Fear of family or friends. Exhibits fear in own environment. Unusual quietness when caregiver is present. Low self-esteem. Hunger for attention and socialization.	Unexplained loss of pension/Social Security checks, lack of adequate food and medications. Little knowledge about financial status.	Dehydration. Malnutrition. Pressure ulcers. Odor on body or clothing, poor personal hygiene, bug bites, lice, maggots, scabies, and urine or stool excoriations.	Leaving older adult alone, without basic care, for long periods of time or without intention of returning.

OUTCOMES

Caregiver Emotional Health

- The caregiver will demonstrate increased emotional well-being within 1 month as evidenced by the following indicators:
  - The caregiver verbally identifies reasons for feelings of anger and frustration.
  - The caregiver verbally identifies four constructive ways of handling anger and frustrations with the patient.
  - The caregiver verbally states improved ability to care for the patient.

Caregiver-Patient Relationship

- Caregiver and patient verbalize an increased satisfaction with their interactions and a reduction in negative interactions.

Caregiver Well-Being

- Caregiver reports feeling more comfortable in caregiver role.
- Caregiver uses appropriate resources to handle stress.

INTERVENTIONS

Complex Relationship Building (5000)

- Establish rapport and a trusting relationship with patient and caregiver.

Coping Enhancement (5230)

- Encourage verbalization of feelings.
- Identify variables contributing to feelings of frustration.
- Encourage caregiver to problem solve about alternatives and use assistance of others.

Family Involvement Promotion (7110)

- Facilitate participation by the adult children in emotional care for the patient and caregiver.

Support System Enhancement (5440)

- Identify resources caregiver can use to decrease role strain and fatigue; initiate referrals as indicated (e.g., senior centers, day care centers/respite care for elderly, and services for the elderly by churches/religious organizations) (Carpenito, 2002; Dochterman & Bulechek, 2000; Wilkinson, 2005).

Mandatory Reporting

Many incidents of elder abuse have gone unreported in the past. All 50 states have enacted reporting laws and have instituted protective service programs. In 42 states, reporting is mandatory for all health care professionals. Eight states have mandated reporting by specified health care professionals: Colorado, Illinois, Wisconsin, New York, Pennsylvania, North Dakota, South Dakota, and New Jersey. States that require mandatory reporting have implemented fines, imprisonment, or license revocation if reporting is not completed within the required time frame following the recognition of abuse. All states provide immunity for the reporter, even if the abuse is not substantiated (Marshall, Benton, & Braizer, 2000). EM has been increasingly recognized as a social problem. Unfortunately, both professionals and the public continue to underreport cases of abuse. Reasons cited for underreporting include lack of knowledge of identifying signs and symptoms, denial, concern about appearing in court to testify against the abuser, reluctance to report abuse, and lack of awareness of abuse laws. For more information on reporting in individual states, the following Web sites provide helpful information: the American Bar Association (www.abanet.org), the Politics and Policy News, State By State (www.stateline.org), and the National Center for State Courts/NCSC (www.ncsconline.org) (Table 21-4).

ECONOMIC AND PUBLIC POLICY ISSUES

Economic Issues

Poverty is measured by a family's annual income and their risk level for being unable to meet their basic needs such as adequate food, housing, clothing, and health care. The poverty level varies by family size and composition. Older adults, with fewer people living in the home and lower incomes, may easily fall into the poverty category. The poverty level for adults age 65 and older has declined in the last 40 years from 35% to 11%. However, for Americans ages 85 and older, the poverty level rises to around 14%. The highest group of adults experiencing poverty are those 65 and older who are nonmarried, female, and minority. As reported by the Federal Interagency Forum on Aging-Related Statistics (2004), among minorities, there is a 47% poverty rate for divorced black women ages 65 to 74, as compared with the same age of non-Hispanic white females.

Table 21-4 *Interventions for Elder Abuse*

Interventions	Resources
ONE-ON-ONE INTERVIEW Interview the patient privately. Document the interview accurately and be as objective as possible. Avoid confrontation. Remember, the less you talk, the more information you will get. Be alert for inconsistencies between answers and related physical evidence.	**NATIONAL CENTER ON ELDER ABUSE** Provides information on all aspects of elder abuse and a list of state hotline numbers. Phone: 202-898-2586 Web site: www.elderabusecenter.org
DOCUMENT SUSPECTED ABUSE Gather all data of your assessment. Include specifically what the patient said about his or her injuries. Identify each speaker and exact words with quotations. Document any discrepancies in the patient's and caregiver's stories.	**ADULT PROTECTIVE SERVICES** Offers help for vulnerable and frail older adults. Web site: www.elderabusecenter.org/default.cfm?p=apsstate.cfm
REPORT ABUSE Always provide the patient with access numbers to report abuse. Reassure the patient that abuse is not normal and that it is not a result of something the patient has done.	**THE NATIONAL LONG TERM CARE OMBUDSMAN RESOURCE CENTER** Provides advocacy for rights of residents of long-term care facilities. Phone: 202-332-2275 Web site: www.ltcombudsman.org **NATIONAL ORGANIZATION FOR VICTIM ASSISTANCE** Phone: 1-800-TRY-NOVA, 202-232-6682

Education has a strong influence on socioeconomic status in the 65- to 74-year-old age category differentiated by ethnic and racial groups. In 1998, 22% of Asian and Pacific Islander Americans had bachelor's or higher degrees compared with 16% of non-Hispanic white, 7% of black, and 5% of Hispanic Americans (Federal Interagency Forum on Aging-Related Statistics, 2004).

Another factor that is included with higher education and better jobs is earning ability and the establishment of a preretirement savings plan. Older middle-class adults who were forced to retire early and live on an inadequate pension years before they qualified for Social Security usually have drained their savings or have not planned for the cost of inflation necessary to maintain their preretirement lifestyle. A major concern that comes with retirement and affects finances is the cost of a postretirement health care plan with affordable copayments, which includes long-term care insurance, coverage for catastrophic illnesses, a health promotion focus, and an adequate medication program for both common brand names and generic drugs. As adults age, the need for health care increases, and older adults often find that the greatest threat to their economic security is the out-of-pocket expense for health costs. Because the total budget of older adults is smaller and health is more fragile, the amount spent on health care, including medications, usually is substantially higher than the amount spent on health care by younger people (U.S. Food and Drug Administration, 2003).

Many older adults experience the economic crunch when they can no longer help younger family members with financial needs; are unable to maintain the upkeep on a home, an automobile, and car insurance; or are unable to participate in desired socialization and leisure activities because of fixed income. Living on a fixed income and having reduced financial earning power created by the death of the working spouse; loss of the spouse's Social Security funds; or inability to work even at low-paying jobs because of diminished hearing, vision, cognitive, and mobility deficits may put the older adult at or below the poverty level. It is common for older adults in these situations to scale down their living conditions by finding a safe and affordable place to live or finding another person with whom to share living expenses. However, these solutions may cause other problems for many older adults. Older adults who depend on a housemate for financial reasons or help with dependence needs are vulnerable to fraud or theft. Major concerns are use of credit cards or the slow, subtle pilfering of finances by the housemate. Older adults have a deep need for financial security and peace about having enough money in their "golden years." This is increased for those who lived during the Great Depression, which began with the financial crash of the stock market in 1929 and ended in 1941 when the United States entered World War II. Many experienced up to 12 years of deprivation and concerns about how they could survive. The economic impact of the Depression Era on older adults and their adult children was reinforced on September 11, 2001, with the acts of terrorism in New York, Washington, D.C., and Pennsylvania and the subsequent loss in value of stocks and bonds that were the source of income for retirement. After September 11, 2001, with the unexpected demise of some companies, foreign trade deficits, and a plunge in value of stocks and bonds, some adults who were ready to retire were thrust back into the job market. They were suddenly in a competitive market for skills found in younger employees for less salary.

Prevention of Late-Life Poverty

Although the prospects for preventing poverty in old age for those who have always been economically disadvantaged are not good, there may be some potential for preventing late-life impoverishment. Although no easy solutions exist, it is clear that those who plan carefully for their retirement years will probably fare better than those who do not. Taking economic needs in retirement seriously as a young adult is an important factor in having adequate income in retirement.

An important step in preretirement planning is to plan retirement in phases instead of suddenly stopping one lifestyle schedule and trying to start another. "Phased retirement" begins with years of preretirement planning and includes a self-structuring of slowly changing from one lifestyle schedule to another. One way older adults successfully begin to retire is to cut down on the number of working hours and by going to some degree of part-time work instead of ending employment. It has been reported that older workers expect their retirement to include some form of work, but with different criteria, such as flexible hours so that time can be taken to care for relatives or other high-priority activities; a compressed work week; or time off with pay after having worked extra hours (see www.aarp.org). Senior centers in most cities have classes on retirement, postretirement job opportunities, and volunteer positions. The AARP Web site has numerous articles with suggestions on how to make retirement pleasurable and productive (see www.aarp.org/Articles/a2004-10-18-retiring-happy/tools/printable). This Web site also has links to numerous books on successful retirement.

Preretirement planning also includes evaluating life goals and setting new ones. Hershey, Jacobs-Lawson, and Neukam (2002, p. 163) assert that "having clear goals for retirement is a critical determinant of life satisfaction and adjustment during the post-employment transition period." Some of the best predictors of "late life satisfaction and adjustment in retirement involve having positive, concrete, and stable goals upon which to rely" (Hershey, Jacobs-Lawson, & Neukam, 2002,

p. 164). Preretirement not only involves economic planning but also making goals for hobbies and leisure activities.

Public Policy and the Impact on Older Adults

The local, state, and federal levels of the U.S. government have a history of changing economic policies related to older adults. The making of public policy, which includes the depth of support for older Americans, depends on the balance of power of the two major political parties. The political climate influences the amount of funding available and length of time for suggested formal support network programs. The major attempts to increase support to older adults have helped but not solved their economic concerns.

Supplemental Security Income. Since 1972, older adults with the lowest incomes have been eligible for a monthly check from Social Security under the Supplemental Security Income (SSI) program. This program for people 65 years and older (as well as blind and disabled persons) was designed to supplement the income of those who do not qualify for standard Social Security benefits or whose Social Security benefits are not adequate for subsistence. Eligibility is determined by a means test based on income and assets of the individual. As of January 1, 2005, the federal benefit rate for an individual was $579 per month. However, in order to qualify for SSI, the individual must sell his or her resources so that only $2000 is left that could be turned into cash for food and shelter. Although SSI has resulted in a guaranteed source of income for many older persons, some have criticized the program because the benefit levels still leave many older people below the poverty level. Because benefits may change yearly, the health care professional should obtain the latest information from the nearest Social Security office or access the Social Security Web site at www.ssa.gov.

Although SSI is tied into the Medicaid program, many people do not realize that being under SSI entitles them to gain health care benefits under Medicaid. Because of the high degree of unfamiliarity with and confusion about the SSI program, nurses may encounter older persons who are eligible for this type of assistance but not receiving it.

Older Americans Act Programs. The Older Americans Act (OAA) was first enacted in 1965. The mission of the OAA is "to foster maximum independence by providing a wide array of social and community services to those older persons in greatest economic and social need. The key philosophy of the program has been to help maintain and support older persons in their homes and communities to avoid unnecessary and costly institutionalization" (U.S. Senate, 1993, p. 313). Designed to address a number of the problems of older persons without regard to income, its programs have nonetheless addressed some of the problems of economically disadvantaged older adults. Three specific programs are worthy of note: nutrition programs, senior employment programs, and transportation programs.

Nutrition programs offered under the auspices of the OAA include both home-delivered meals and congregate meal programs. Both provide one third of the minimum daily requirements for anyone age 60 or older regardless of income. This partially addresses the problem of inadequate nutrition related to poverty, without the embarrassment or ordeal of a means test or eligibility determination. These programs have been helpful in averting institutionalization by providing meals to the homebound who are unable or unwilling to prepare meals for themselves and a source of socialization as well as nutrition for those who are able to get out of the house.

Senior employment services under OAA are designed to help develop employment opportunities for those age 55 or older who wish to work. These services include job training, job placement, and demonstration of the effectiveness of older workers. Workers are placed in part-time minimum wage positions in community service organizations. This type of service helps the economically disadvantaged minority older adults who are capable of employment.

Transportation programs are also aimed at resolving one of the problems associated with poverty. Although older adults who are not impoverished cite transportation as a major problem, it is clear that without adequate income to purchase or maintain a car or to pay cab or bus fare, transportation is a serious problem. OAA funds have been used in diverse ways to address this problem, from funding "dial-a-ride"–type services using volunteers to providing bus or van transportation for grocery shopping or medical appointments.

OAA funds also have been applied to the development of senior centers, which, in many communities, serve as an important source for information about available services, as well as a place where diverse services may be obtained. OAA monies have additionally been applied to the development of health-related services such as adult day care and in-home health care.

The 2000 amendments to the OAA continue to target provisions for low-income minorities, older individuals residing in rural areas, and in-home and legal services. The amendments also included extending the program for 5 years to allow time for changes to be implemented, results to be tracked, and reports to get back to Congress before the new date for further decision making. The 2000 amendments consolidated 3 of the original 10 objectives from the 1992 amendment. Two strong positives that came out of the 2000 amendments were the creation of the National Family Caregiver Support Program and a caregiver support program for Native American elders. Therefore, with the amendments, state and local agencies on aging will have more flexibility in developing comprehensive and coordinated service systems (see www.aoa.dhhs.gov/about/legbudb/oaa/legbudg_oaa.asp). When working with older adults who are seeking current information, the health care professional can use online sources to stay current.

Title XX of the Social Security Act. Title XX of the Social Security Act is a "block grant" to the states that provides funding for a wide array of social services to low-income people. Although this money is not specifically targeted for the elderly, services such as homemakers for disabled older people, home-delivered meals, and adult day care are provided through this funding in some communities. Decisions about allocation of these scarce dollars are made at the local level, so the services available to older persons vary from community to community. The eligibility guidelines for recipients of these services are much less stringent than those for Medicaid. The problem most communities face is a greater need among potential recipients than can be met through available funding. This results in long waiting lists for services in many communities.

Medicare. Medicare is the national health insurance program that provides coverage to approximately 40 million Americans. Those who qualify are adults age 65 or older, some people under age 65 with disabilities, and people with end-stage renal disease (ESRD). For the latest out-of-pocket costs and benefits, the nurse can call the nearest Medicare office or get the information from the Centers for Medicare and Medicaid Services Web site (www.cms.hhs.gov/medicaid).

Beginning January 2005, the Medicare Modernization Act, signed into law in December 2003, enlarged the benefits to Medicare recipients. These benefits include prescription drug coverage, expanded health plan options, improved health care access for rural Americans, and preventive care services, such as flu shots and mammograms.

Medicaid. Medicaid is a program that funds medical care for economically disadvantaged older persons, disabled people, and families with dependent children. The program deserves special mention because of the major role it plays in the financing of nursing home care. Medicaid is a federal program that is administered at the state level. Its financing is a combination of federal, state, and local funds. For this reason, there is considerable variability from state to state as to the type of services provided under Medicaid. Criteria and procedures for eligibility also vary by state. Medicaid is designed so

that those who cannot afford to pay for medical care will not be denied this care regardless of their living arrangement. Owing to the complexities of eligibility and coverage, the reality is that the majority of elderly Medicaid recipients are in nursing homes, although Medicaid will pay for some non–institution-based services. Three fourths of nursing home care is paid for by Medicaid.

Eligibility for Medicaid benefits requires the older person to exhaust nearly all savings and income on medical expenses. Stiff penalties exist for those who try to defraud the system by giving away property or other assets in an attempt to become eligible for Medicaid. Determination of eligibility is a long and somewhat laborious process, generally carried out through a local department of social services. The process involves extensive financial disclosure and repeated recertification. For those without other means to pay for medical care, it is an important resource. Some older adults are reluctant to apply for Medicaid for a variety of reasons, including pride or refusal to accept charity, fear of losing their home, assumption that they would not qualify for welfare, and inability to withstand or understand complex bureaucratic processes. It takes considerable sensitivity to help older adults and their families understand the benefits to which they may be entitled. Assistance may be needed in going through the necessary bureaucratic processes to obtain such benefits. Like other public programs, the funding, qualifications, and benefits change frequently. For the latest information on Medicaid, call the nearest Medicaid office or access the Centers for Medicare and Medicaid Services Web site (www.cms.hhs.gov/medicaid).

Senior Citizen Discount Programs. One example of a public sector–private sector joint initiative in reducing the economic burden on older people is the existence of senior citizen discount programs for goods and services, including hot meals, retail merchandise, hotels, and transportation. One of the problems with this type of program is that there is no consistency in the definition of "senior citizen" among agencies. Some programs start at age 50, whereas others do not give discounts until age 65.

Nurse's Role of Advocacy

Perhaps the most important role for nurses caring for older adults is the advocacy role. Box 21-7 shows many of the activities involved in the effective performance of this role.

Case Study. Mrs. L., a 67-year-old woman, is facing retirement in a year. She has worked for 20 years as a medical office assistant and has been able to save a little over the years. Even with income from Social

Box 21-7 Nurses' Advocacy Role

Facilitate the establishment of social support networks to enable older adults to live as independently as possible.

Educate on different health care insurance plans and what types of services are necessary to maintain the health of older adults.

Refer to resources to assist in the application process; refer the older adult to reputable, formal resources for unbiased, knowledgeable financial advice.

Talk with legislators on pending bills regarding public policy issues.

Encourage older adults to become active participants in their homeowners' association.

Encourage older adults and nurses to attend city council meetings to give voice on local issues.

Lobby for senior discounts in businesses older adults frequent.

Write articles on issues affecting older adults, such as quality of life, ageism, and financial well-being after retirement.

Security supplemented with her savings, Mrs. L. is anxious about being able to sustain her current lifestyle with the anticipated drop in income after she retires. She has difficulty getting to sleep and staying asleep at night, trying to problem solve where to relocate, the type of health insurance needed, how to afford the maintenance on her car, and how to provide some of her grandson's finances for college. Mrs. L. has been the family matriarch for the past 8 years, guiding her siblings and immediate family without difficulty problem solving. For the first time she feels completely overwhelmed by the future.

NURSING DIAGNOSIS. Ineffective individual coping related to multiple stressful events, including retirement, change in financial status, and change in residence, manifested by verbalization of inability to cope, anxiety, and difficulty problem solving.

Defining Characteristics. Sample subjective data include the following:

- Expresses feelings of anxiety
- Expresses feelings of incompetence related to making good decisions
- Expresses feelings of being overwhelmed by all the changes that need to be made
  Sample objective data include the following:
- Recent change in living arrangements and financial resources
- Decreased contact with support system
- Difficulty structuring time
- Inadequate problem solving

- Difficulty sleeping for several weeks
- Decreased confidence in ability to cope with changes
  Suggested alternative diagnoses include the following:
- Adjustment, impaired
- Anxiety
- Denial, ineffective
- Fear
- Violence, risk for: self-directed or directed at others

OUTCOMES. The older adult will demonstrate effective coping within 1 month as evidenced by the following indicators:

- Verbally identifies effective and ineffective coping strategies
- Identifies and uses at least two effective coping strategies
- Reports feeling an increased ability to cope with life changes
- Reports a decrease in anxious feelings
- Reports improved ability to sleep
- Verbally identifies at least one resource that will assist in coping with life changes
- Verbalizes and uses effective problem-solving strategies in making appropriate decisions about finances, living arrangements, and postretirement activities

INTERVENTIONS
Coping Enhancement (5230)
- Encourage patient verbalization of feelings of being overwhelmed.
- Identify patient views as contributing to difficulty coping with changes.
Decision-Making Support (5250)
- Provide information, resources, and support for patient related to retirement, finances, and residential changes.
Family Involvement Promotion (7110)
- Facilitate family participation in emotional support for patient's adjustment to life changes.
Learning Facilitation (5520)
- Promote patient's ability to process and comprehend information related to life changes.
Support System Enhancement (5440)
- Identify resources patient can use to assist in information acquisition and decision making.
- Initiate referrals as indicated (e.g., senior centers, legal aid resources, religious groups) (Carpenito, 2002; Dochterman & Bulechek, 2000; Wilkinson, 2005).

REFERENCES

Administration on Aging. (2005). Elder abuse. Retrieved March 1, 2005, from www.aoa.gov/eldfam/Elder_Rights/Elder_Abuse/Elder_Abuse.asp.

Age Concern England. (2002). Ageism exists. Have you seen the signs? Retrieved January 10, 2005, from www.ageconcern.org.uk/AgeConcern/media/ace_week_booklet.pdf.

Allender, J., & Spradley, B. (2005). *Community health nursing: Promoting and protecting the public's health* (6th ed.). Philadelphia: Lippincott Williams & Wilkins.

Baydar, N., & Brooks-Gunn, J. (1991). *Profiles of America's grandmothers: Those who provide care for their grandchildren and those who do not.* Seattle, WA: University of Washington Battelle.

Beerman, S., & Rappaport-Musson, J. (2002). *Eldercare 911.* New York: Prometheus.

Benner, P., & Wrubel, J. (1989). *The primacy of caring: Stress and coping in health and illness.* Menlo Park, CA: Addison Wesley.

Binstock, R. H. (1983). The aged as scapegoat. *Gerontologist, 23*(2), 136-143.

Blumer, H. (1969). *Symbolic interaction: Perspective and method.* Englewood Cliffs, NJ: Prentice Hall.

Brokaw, T. (1998). *The greatest generation.* New York: Random House.

Brubaker, E. (1985). Older parents' reactions to the death of adult children: Implications for practice. *Journal of Gerontological Social Work, 9*(1), 35-48.

Butler, R. N. (1975). *Why survive? Being old in America.* New York: Harper & Row.

Carpenito, L. (2002). *Nursing diagnoses: Application to clinical practice* (9th ed.). Philadelphia: Lippincott.

Crowther, M., Parker, M., Achenbaum, W., Larimore, W., & Koenig, H. (2002). Rowe and Kahn's model of successful aging revisited: Positive spirituality—the forgotten factor. *Gerontologist, 42*(5), 612-620.

Cuellar, N., Lundy, K., & Callahan, V. (2001). Women's health. In K. Lundy & S. Janes, *Community health nursing: Caring for the public's health.* Boston: Jones & Bartlett.

Cunningham, M. (2004). Old is a three-letter word. *Geriatric Nursing, 25*(5), 277-280.

Dochterman, J. M., & Bulechek, G. M. (2000). *Nursing intervention classification* (NIC) (4th ed.). St. Louis: Mosby.

Easley, C., & Schaller, J. (2003). The experience of being old-old: Life after 85. *Geriatric Nursing, 24*(5), 273-277.

Eliopoulos, C. (2005). *Gerontological nursing* (6th ed.). Philadelphia: Lippincott Williams & Wilkins.

Falk, U., & Falk, G. (2002). *Grandparents: A new look at the supporting generation.* New York: Prometheus.

Family and Consumer Sciences. (2005). Texas cooperative extension. Texas A&M University System. Retrieved February 23, 2005, from http://fca.tamu.edu/families/aging/elder_care/building_positive_relationships.php.

Federal Interagency Forum on Aging-Related Statistics. (2000). *Older Americans 2000: Key indicators of well-being.* Washington, DC: U.S. Government Printing Office.

Federal Interagency Forum on Aging-Related Statistics. (2004). *Older Americans 2004: Key indicators of well-being.* Washington, DC: U.S. Government Printing Office.

Fulner, T. (2002). *Try this: Best practices in nursing care to older adults.* New York: Hartford Institute for Geriatric Nursing.

Generations United. (2005). People of all ages. Retrieved January 5, 2005, from www.pbs.org/americanfamily/gap/people.html.

Gosline, M. B. (2003). Client participation to enhance socialization for frail elders. *Geriatric Nursing, 24*(5), 286-289.

Heitkemper, M. (2004). Older adults. In S. Lewis, M. Heitkemper, & J. Dirksen, *Shannon's medical-surgical nursing: Assessment and management of clinical problems* (6th ed.). St. Louis: Mosby.

Hershey, D., Jacobs-Lawson, J., & Neukam, K. (2002). Influences of age and gender on workers' goals for retirement. *International Journal of Aging and Human Development, 55*(2), 163-179.

Keil, C., Barba, B. (1995, September 6-9). *The relationship of loneliness and stress to human-animal attachment in the elderly.* Paper presented at the 7th International Conference on Human-Animal Interactions, Animals, Health and Quality of Life, Geneva, Switzerland.

Kim, J., & Nesselroade, J. (2003). Relationships among social support, self-concept, and well-being of older adults: A study of process using dynamic factor models. *International Journal of Behavioral Development, 27*(1), 49-65.

Kirsch, S., & Jeffery, L. (2003). *Boomers in transition: The future of aging and health.* Palo Alto, CA: Institute for the Future.

Krouse, L. (2004, August 18). Elder abuse. Retrieved March 24, 2005, from www.emedicine.com/emerg/topic160.htm.

Kuypers, J. A., & Bengtson, V. (1973). Social breakdown and social competence. *Human Development, 16*(3), 181-201.

Lavoie-Vaughn, N., & Vaughn, D. (2003, April). Pet project: Four-legged caregivers benefit patients and staff. *Networks, Nursing Spectrum Western Edition, 4*(4), 8-10.

Lawson, D., & Brossart, D. (2004). The association between current intergenerational family relationships and sibling structure. *Journal of Counseling and Development, 82*(4), 472-482.

Leininger, M. (1984). *Care: The essence of nursing and health.* Thorofare, NJ: Slack.

Levy, B. (2001). Eradication of ageism requires addressing the enemy within. *Gerontologist, 41*(5), 578-580.

Litwin, H. (2001). Social network type and morale in old age. *Gerontologist, 41*(4), 516-524.

Litwin, H., & Zoabi, S. (2004). A multivariate examination of explanations for the occurrence of elder abuse. *Social Work Research, 28*(3), 133-142.

Lueckenotte, A. (2004). Editorial on safety and straight talk. *Supporting Innovations in Gerontological Nursing, 11*(5), 2. National Gerontological Nursing Association.

MacNeill, M., & MacNeill, A. (2004). Ten signs that elder abuse is occurring at an LTC facility. *Long-Term Care Interface, 5*(4), 27-28.

Marshall, C. E., Benton, S., & Braizer, J. M. (2000). Using clinical tools to identify clues of mistreatment. *Geriatrics, 55*(2), 42-53.

McIntosh, W. A., Sykes, D., & Kubena, K. S. (2002). Religion and community among the elderly: The relationship between the religious and secular characteristics of their social networks. *Review of Religious Research, 44*(2), 109-125.

Moon, A. (2000). Perceptions of elder abuse among various cultural groups: Similarities and differences. *Generations, 24*(2), 75-80.

Morse, J., Solberg, S., Neander, W., Bottorff, J., & Johnson, J. (1990). Concepts of caring and caring as a concept. *Advances in Nursing Science, 13*(1), 1-14.

Moss, M. (2002). Living with grief: Loss in later life. Retrieved March 10, 2005, from www.hospicefoundation.org/teleconference/2002/moss.asp.

National Center on Elder Abuse. (1998). *The national elder abuse incidence study.* Washington, DC: American Public Health Services Association.

National Center on Elder Abuse. (2000). *A response to the abuse of vulnerable adults: The 2000 survey of state adult protective services.* Washington, DC: American Public Health Services Association.

National Center on Elder Abuse. (2005). The basics. Retrieved March 2, 2005, from www.elderabusecenter.org/default.cmf?p=basics.cfm.

National Gray Panthers. (1995, September/October). *Network, 1*(2), 14. Retrieved January 10, 2005, from www.graypanthersmetrodetroit.org/Ageism.html.

Neugarten, B. L. & Weinstein, K. K. (1964). The changing American grandparent. *Journal of Marriage and the Family, 26*(2), 199-204.

O'Keefe, M. (2001). *Nursing practice and the law: Avoiding malpractice and other legal risks.* Philadelphia: F.A. Davis.

Pavlik, V., Hyman, D., Festa, N., & Dyer, C. (2001). Quantifying the problem of abuse and neglect in adults—analysis of a statewide database. *Journal of the American Geriatrics Society, 49*(1), 45-48.

Plowfield, L., Raymond, J., & Blevins, C. (2000). Wholism for aging families: Meeting needs of caregivers. *Holistic Nursing Practice, 14*(4), 51-59.

Price, C. (2002a). Siblings are forever. Senior Series 180-01. Retrieved January 3, 2005, from http://ohioline.osu.edu/ss-fact/0180.html.

Price, C. (2002b). Sibling relations in later life. Aging Families—Senior Series Bulletin #1. Retrieved January 3, 2005, from www.hec.ohio-state.edu/famlife/aging/PDFs/Siblings %20Bulletin.final.pdf.

Quinn, M. J. (2002). Undue influence and elder abuse: Recognition and intervention strategies. *Geriatric Nursing, 23*(1), 11-16.

Raina, P., Waltner-Toews, D., Bonnett, B., Woodward, C., & Abernathy, T. (1999). Influence of companion animals on the physical and psychological health of older people: An analysis of a one-year longitudinal study. *Journal of American Geriatric Society, 47*(3), 323-329.

Ramsey-Klawsnik, H. (2000). Elder abuse offenders: A typology. *Generations, 24*(2), 17-22.

Ritchie, L. (2003). Adult day care: Northern perspectives. *Public Health Nursing, 20*(2), 120-131.

Rogers, J., & Hart, L. A. (1993). Retrieved February 10, 2005, from www.deltasociety.org.

Santrock, J. (2004). *Peer and the sociocultural word. A topical approach to life-span development.* Columbus, OH: McGraw-Hill.

Schoen, A., Proctor, P., & Winter, N., of Therapy Dogs International Inc. (2003). Retrieved January 10, 2005, from www.tdi-dog.org.

Smick, T. (1990). The sandwiched generation. In T. Smick, J. Duncan, J. P. Moreland, & J. Watson, *Eldercare for the Christian family: What to do when a loved one becomes dependent.* Dallas: Word Publishing.

Social Security Administration. (2004). Retrieved January 10, 2005, from www.ssa.gov.retire2/retirechart.htm.

Spector, R. (2004). *Cultural diversity in health and illness* (6th ed). Englewood Cliffs, NJ: Prentice Hall.

Thompson, P., Itzin, C., & Abendstern, M. (1990). *I don't feel old: The experience of later life.* New York: Oxford University Press.

U.S. Food and Drug Administration. (2003). Medications and older people. *FDA Consumer,* FDA03-1315C. Retrieved March 29, 2005, from www.fda.gov.

U.S. Senate. (1993). *Developments in aging: 1992* (volume 1). Washington, DC: U.S. Government Printing Office.

Watson, J. (1988). *Nursing: Human science and human care: A theory of nursing.* New York: National League for Nursing.

Watson, J. (1990). Someone in the family is sick. In T. Smick, J. Duncan, J. P. Moreland, & J. Watson (Eds.), *Eldercare for the Christian family: What to do when a loved one becomes dependent.* Dallas: Word Publishing.

Weir, E. C. (2004). Identifying and preventing ageism among healthcare professionals. *International Journal of Therapy and Rehabilitation, 11*(2), 56-63.

Wells, Y., Foreman, P., Gething, L., & Petralia, W. (2004). Nurses' attitudes toward aging and older adults. *Journal of Gerontological Nursing, 30*(9), 5-13.

White, L. K. (2001). Sibling relationships over the life course: A panel analysis. *Journal of Marriage and Family, 63*(2), 555-568.

Wilkinson, J. (2005). *Prentice Hall nursing diagnoses handbook with NIC interventions and NOC outcomes.* Englewood Cliffs, NJ: Prentice Hall.

Williams, K., Kemper, S., & Hummert, M. L. (2004). Enhancing communication with older adults: Overcoming elderspeak. *Journal of Gerontological Nursing, 30*(10), 17-25.

Wolf, R. (2000). The nature and scope of elder abuse. *Generations, 24*(2), 6-12.

Wolf, Z., Giardino, E., Osborne, P., & Ambrose, M. (1994). Dimensions of nurse caring. *Image: Journal of Nursing Scholarship, 26*(2), 107-111.

Yan, C., & Tang, S. (2004). Elder abuse by caregivers: A study of prevalence and risk factors in Hong Kong Chinese families. *Journal of Family Violence, 19*(5), 269-277.

Yeh, S., & Lo, S. (2004). Living alone, social support, and feeling lonely among the elderly. *Social Behavior and Personality, 32*(2), 129-138.

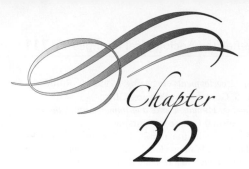

Chapter 22

End of Life Care of the Older Adult

Pamela Z. Cacchione & Patrick J. Cacchione

DEFINING END OF LIFE

A chapter on end of life care should begin with a definition of "end of life" so there is agreement as to when this type of care commences. Lamont (2002) describes it as "the time period preceding an individual's natural death from a process that is unlikely to be arrested by medical care." The term commonly refers to the interval when the prognosis is poor, the chance of dying soon is near, and treatments intended to cure or prolong life are likely to be rejected (Finucane, 2004). This period of life is important because the type of medical care often shifts from invasive intervention aimed at prolonging life to supportive intervention that focuses on control of symptoms. From an insurance and hospice point of view, the end of life stage begins 6 months before death. The major problem with this definition is the difficulty in predicting the period of patient survival. Physicians are likely to overestimate survival time, which probably is one reason that the average patient lives only 24 days after being admitted to hospice (Christakis & Lamont, 2000).

HISTORICAL PERSPECTIVE

Whether we like it or not we are a death-denying society. It is deep in our nature to resist dying. This is apparent in our society's investment into life-saving and life-prolonging treatments and technology. It also may be a factor in the large number of persons who decline to make advance directives, and who reach for every option that offers a chance of prolonged survival. Technological advances have changed the way we live and die. People used to die at home, surrounded by family and friends, after a short illness. Now over one half of all deaths in the United States occur in hospitals. It has taken several pioneers and significant investments by foundations and the federal government to focus attention on improving care at the end of life. Nurses have played pivotal roles in this transition. Some of the early leaders in the movement to improve care at the end of life include Dame Cicely Saunders and Florence Wald, PhD, RN. Dame Cicely Saunders trained first as a nurse, then as a social worker, and finally as a physician. She is known as the crusader of the Hospice Movement, which she initiated in 1964. In 1967, she opened St. Christopher's In-patient Hospice in the United Kingdom. There she pioneered a new approach to end of life care. Dame Saunders described the concept of "Total Pain" as pain that incorporates the physical, social, emotional, and spiritual realms. Basic to Dame Saunders' principles of hospice care are the patient's acceptance of death, interdisciplinary team managed care, management of symptoms (especially pain), recognition of the patient and family as one unit, home care for the dying, and bereavement care for the family following the patient's death (Sheehan & Forman, 1996).

Florence Wald, PhD, RN, is recognized as the leader of the hospice movement in the United States. While Dean of the School of Nursing at Yale University she heard Dame Cicely Saunders speak on the subject of end of life care, which inspired her to visit St.

Christopher's Hospice in the late 1960s. She brought the movement to the United States in the early 1970s and with a multidisciplinary team opened "Hospice Incorporated" in Branford, Connecticut, in 1974 (Krisman-Scott, 2003; Lentz, 2004).

After only 30 years, some type of hospice care exists in almost every community in the United States. There are approximately 2200 Medicare-funded hospices and another 200 volunteer hospice programs (NAHC, 2002). Federal agencies including the Institute of Medicine and the National Institutes of Health have become involved by helping set the agenda to study end of life care. The impact of funding from the Robert Wood Johnson Foundation (RWJF) has been far-reaching. Numerous organizations dedicated to improving end of life care exist through initial funding from the RWJF. These include the following: Last Acts, Rallying Points, Circle of Life, Supportive Care of the Dying, and the End of Life Nursing Education Consortium. Other foundations that have invested in improving care at the end of life care are the Henry J. Kaiser Foundation, National Hospice Foundation, and the Soros Foundation. These organizations have helped push the public policy agenda to improve care at the end of life.

In the United States, hospice care is financed through private insurance, Medicare part A, and Medicaid. Conditions that qualify a person for care include end-stage cardiovascular or pulmonary disease, cancer, HIV-related illness, unspecified debility, end-stage dementia, and multiple system organ failure. The patient should have a life expectancy of no more than 6 months; however, recertification is possible if the person survives beyond 6 months. When a primary care provider determines that a person meets the criteria for hospice services, a referral is made.

The advanced practice nurse (APN) can help patients and families negotiate the layers of the care continuum and maximize continuity of care. APNs not only are respected by patients and their families but also are highly valued by their clinical colleagues and administrators (Emmet, Byock, & Sheils Twohig, 2002). APNs have been a powerful force in helping to reshape the way care at the end of life is managed regardless of the setting.

MODELS OF CARE AT END OF LIFE: HOSPICE AND PALLIATIVE CARE
Hospice Care

Hospice is an interdisciplinary model of care that surrounds and supports the patient, the family, and significant others through the final phase of a life-threatening illness. Hospice care is a model for quality end of life care focusing on the last phase of an illness, the dying process, and the bereavement period. Whereas the home once was the only setting for hospice, it now is available as inpatient and long-term care settings.

Unfortunately, hospice care is not well understood and sometimes is feared by the general population. One common misconception about hospice is that it is only for individuals with cancer. Depending on the severity of the illness, many conditions common to older persons qualify a person for hospice care. In addition to cancer, these include Alzheimer's dementia, end-stage congestive heart failure, recurrent cerebral vascular accidents, Parkinson's disease, end-stage renal disease, and failure to thrive. End of life coalitions such as Last Acts and Supportive Care of the Dying encourage primary care providers to ask if they would be surprised if the older adult was still alive in a year. If the answer is yes, it is time to refer to hospice. Criteria for hospice include a prognosis of 6 months or less based on the clinical judgment of two physicians—the primary care physician and the medical director of the hospice. Hospices use guidelines for identifying patients with non–cancer diagnoses as appropriate for hospice. One common method is the Karnofsky scale, also known as the Karnofsky performance index (Karnofsky, et al., 1948) (Box 22-1). An individual with a score of 70 and below with a life-threatening diagnosis will qualify for hospice care.

Palliative Care

In the 1990s the hospice movement and baby boomer generation spawned a philosophy of care for individuals with life-threatening illnesses. Called **palliative care,** this movement built on the hospice model but was not limited to the 6-month window commonly used to define the period of hospice care. Palliative care can include potentially curative treatments as well as the supportive interventions of hospice care.

Palliative care is both a philosophy of care and a highly structured system for delivery of care. The World Health Organization (WHO) defines it as an approach that improves the quality of life of patients facing life-threatening illness and their families through the prevention, assessment, and treatment of pain and other physical, psychosocial, and spiritual problems (WHO, 2002). The intent, as described by WHO, is that palliative care is gradually integrated as needs change from the time of diagnosis to death (Higginson, 2004). Key elements of palliative care identified by the clinical practice guidelines for quality palliative care are listed in Box 22-2. Palliative care can be delivered in any setting including an intensive care unit and typically segues into hospice care as the disease progresses to the final phase. Figure 22-1 depicts the trajectory of illness and a place for palliative care and hospice.

Palliative Care in Long-Term Care. End of life care in nursing homes and other long-term care settings has special challenges including high staff/patient ratios,

BOX 22-1 Karnofsky Performance Scale

SCORE	FUNCTIONAL DESCRIPTION
100	Able to work; normal: no complaints; no evidence of disease
90	Able to work; able to carry on normal activity; minor symptoms
80	Able to work; normal activity with effort; some symptoms
70*	Independent; not able to work; cares for self; unable to carry on normal activity
60	Disabled; dependent; requires occasional assistance; cares for most needs
50	Moderately disabled; dependent; requires considerable assistance
40	Severely disabled; dependent; requires special care and assistance
30	Severely disabled; hospitalized, death not imminent
20	Very sick; active supportive treatment needed
10	Moribund; fatal process rapidly progressing

From Karnofsky, D. A., & Burchenal, J. H. (1949). The clinical evaluation of chemotherapeutic agents in cancer. In C. M. MacLeod (Ed.), *Evaluation of chemotherapeutic agents.* New York: Columbia University Press, p. 196.
*Scores of 70 or below may qualify for hospice depending upon the disease or condition.

high staff turnover, poor communication between care institutions, primary care providers who do not know the patients or their families, resistance from community pharmacies that serve nursing homes, and resistance from physicians and nurses (Rochon & Heller, 2002). Some sources report that older persons in nursing homes reportedly have the worst pain and receive the least effective treatment (Merrick, cited in Hall, 1999).

Rochon and Heller (2002) describe a nurse practitioner palliative care consult service for nursing homes in the United States. The innovative service was designed by a family nurse practitioner to provide palliative care for nursing home residents who are ineligible for the Medicare Hospice Benefit or have chosen not to use it. Current policies discourage nursing home residents from switching from the skilled nursing benefit to the hospice benefit because Medicare will not pay for skilled nursing care in a long-term care facility at the same time the patient is receiving a per diem for hospice care. If the patient switches to the hospice benefit, he or she will be charged $250 per day for skilled nursing home care. However, a person receiving skilled nursing care is eligible for consultation services. The nurse practitioner was able to be paid through Medicare or private insurance by billing as an independent consultant. This arrangement also meant that the nurse practitioner did not interfere with the practice of the primary care provider (Rochon & Heller, 2002).

VALUES HISTORY

To provide individualized care to patients and their families at the end of life, it is important to understand the patient's core values because those values will play a large role in the decisions patients make in directing their end of life care. The values history is an important tool to identify those values. It can take the form of a written questionnaire or an interview. The questions in the values' history are related to quality of life versus quantity of life. These questions may stimulate reflections and questions between patients and their loved ones as well as their health care providers. By expressing their wishes and desires for the quality of their life, patients can guide their families and health care providers to provide care consistent with the patient's wishes when they can no longer speak for themselves. Common questions included in a values history are provided in Box 22-3.

ADVANCE DIRECTIVES

The Patient Self Determination Act (PSDA, Public Law 101-508) was passed in 1990 and became effective December 1, 1991. The purpose of the PSDA was to encourage people to make and document their choices and decisions about the types and extent of medical care they want to accept or refuse should they become unable to make their wishes known. The Patient Self Determination Act was a response to the complex health care issues faced by families of persons who were in persistent vegetative states and had not put in writing their wishes regarding life-prolonging measures. APNs can help families avoid having to make agonizing choices about what their loved one might have wanted by encouraging discussion about advance directives.

The PSDA imposed specific requirements on all health care agencies (hospitals, long-term care facilities, and home health agencies) that receive Medicare or Medicaid reimbursement. When treating adult patients, this law requires agencies to:

- Assess and document whether patients have advance directives.

BOX 22-2 Core Elements of Palliative Care

CORE ELEMENT	DESCRIPTION
1. Patient population	Refers to patients of all ages experiencing debilitating, chronic, or life-threatening illness, condition, or injury.
2. Patient- and family-centered care	Patient and family (where patient defines family) are respected. Care plan is determined by goals and preferences of patient and family with guidance of health care team.
3. Timing of palliative care	Ideally starts with diagnosis of life-threatening disease or injury and continues through to cure or until death occurs, and then into family's bereavement period.
4. Comprehensive care	Multidimensional assessments identify and relieve suffering through prevention or alleviation of physical, psychological, social, and spiritual distress. Palliative care requires regular, formal, clinical process of patient-appropriate assessment, diagnosis, planning, interventions, monitoring, and follow-up.
5. Interdisciplinary team	Involves core group of professionals from medicine, nursing, social work, and combination of volunteer coordinators: chaplains, psychologists, pharmacists, nursing assistants, dietitions, therapists, case managers, and trained volunteers.
6. Relief of suffering	Goal of palliative care is to prevent and relieve burdens brought on by diseases and their treatments, including pain and other symptoms of distress.
7. Communication	Includes developmentally appropriate and effective sharing of information, active listening, determination of goals and preferences, assistance with medical decision making, and effective communication with all individuals involved in care of patients and their families.
8. Care of dying and bereaved	Knowledgeable teams are involved in prognostication, signs and symptoms of imminent death, and associated care and support needs of patients and their families before and after death.
9. Continuity of care across settings	Palliative care team collaborates with professional and informal caregivers in each setting (hospital, emergency department, nursing home, assisted living, and outpatient facility) to ensure coordination, communication, and continuity of palliative care across institutional and home care settings, as well as prevention of crises and unnecessary transfers.
10. Equitable access	Palliative care teams work toward equitable access to palliative care across all ages and patient populations regardless of race, ethnicity, sexual preference, or ability to pay.
11. Address regulatory barriers	Palliative care professionals collaborate with policymakers, law enforcement, and regulators to achieve balanced and positive environment for pain management and palliative care.
12. Quality improvement	Attention paid at all times to safety and systems of care that reduce error and are timely, patient- and family-centered, beneficial, and effective. Care should also be accessible and equitable, evidence-based, and efficient.

From National Consensus Project for Quality Palliative Care. (2004). *Clinical practice guidelines for quality palliative care.* National Hospice and Palliative Care Organization. Accessed online at www.nhpco.org.

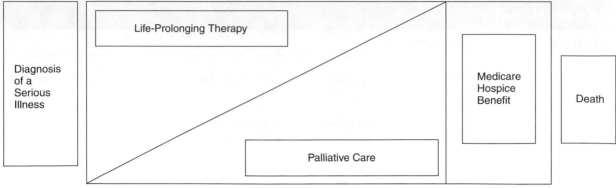

Figure 22-1 Trajectory of illness and a place for palliative care and hospice. (From National Consensus Project for Quality Palliative Care [2004]. *Clinical practice guidelines for quality palliative care.* National Hospice and Palliative Care Organization. Accessed online at www.nhpco.org.)

- Provide a copy of the agency policies related to the patient's rights to make decisions, formulate advance directives, and refuse treatment.
- Provide an opportunity for patients to complete advance directives.
- Provide care regardless of whether or not the patient has an advance directives.
- Recognize the living will and power of attorney for health care as advance directives.

BOX 22-3 Common Value History Questions

1. How important are independence and self-sufficiency in your life?
2. If you experience a decrease in your physical functioning and your mental abilities, how would that affect your attitude toward independence and self-sufficiency?
3. What activities do you enjoy?
4. Are you happy to be alive?
5. Do you feel that life is worth living?
6. What do you fear most?
7. What goals do you have for the future?
8. What will be important to you when you are dying?
9. Where would you prefer to die?
10. What is your attitude toward death?
11. How do you feel about the use of life-sustaining measures in the face of:
    - terminal illness?
    - permanent coma?
    - irreversible chronic illness?
12. How do your religious beliefs affect your attitude toward serious or terminal illness?
13. Does your attitude towards death find support in your religion?

Data from Center for Health and Law Ethics, Institute of Public Law, University of New Mexico, Albuquerque, New Mexico.

- Comply with state laws related to advance directives.
- Provide education about living wills and durable powers of attorney.

The main criticism of the PSDA is that hospitals, long-term care facilities, and home health agencies are the wrong places to have this dialog. Rather, these conversations should occur in the community and primary care settings before a crisis or long-term health concern. The SUPPORT Study (the Study to Understand Prognoses and Preferences for Outcomes and Risks of Treatments) was designed to assess end of life care in patients with serious illnesses and to test an intervention to improve the process of end of life decision making (SUPPORT Principal Investigators, 1995). This study identified that pain was poorly managed at end of life, and that do not resuscitate (DNR) orders were written only 2 days prior to death. Only 47% of the physicians knew that the patient's wish was to avoid CPR. The SUPPORT investigators identified that even if patients have advance directives, they often are not adhered to and rarely discussed with the patients or their families.

An issue that sometimes is overlooked in relation to advance directives is that some cultures and some individuals do not agree that planning for life-threatening possibilities is a good thing. Health care providers must respect the rights of persons who choose not to express their wishes. For some persons, being presented with information about advance directives when being admitted for surgery, for example, is anxiety-producing.

Durable Powers for Health Care, Living Wills, and Five Wishes

Various mechanisms can be used to convey a person's preferences in case he or she becomes incapacitated. Most health care providers will recommend an advance directive that designates someone who can make decisions for an individual if that person becomes incapacitated in any way. Directives for health care are documents that allow individuals to put in writing their wishes regarding health care including the use of certain medical treatments and procedures. Durable power of attorney for health care is a document that is executed by competent individuals to describe their desires regarding death-delaying procedures. It also designates another person as the individual's "agent" or "designee" to make health care decisions on their behalf if they are not able to make decisions for themselves. It is essential that the individual named as agent is someone who knows the patient's values and is trusted to act in accordance with the patient's wishes. An important aspect of the durable power of attorney for health care is that it becomes effective only if the principal becomes unable to make decisions. Also, it is more comprehensive than a living will because it grants the agent authorization to make decisions not only about life-sustaining treatment but also about other issues such as medications and surgical consent (Rain, 1999).

A living will is a document in which individuals can stipulate what their wishes are regarding life-prolonging treatments or procedures if they develop a terminal condition. Like the durable health care power of attorney, it must be executed while the patient is fully capable of understanding the implications. This document can free the physician from liability if treatment is discontinued according to the patient's expressed wishes. Because most states do not define terminal illness, it is subject to various interpretations. One solution to this problem is for the person drafting the document to specify conditions under which further treatment is not desired. Some states require notarization of living wills and specify certain parties that may not serve as witnesses. There are some advantages to having both a living will and a durable health care power of attorney. An attorney can advise the individual as to the most appropriate options in that person's situation.

Another form of advance directive is the "Five Wishes" document, which is unique in the broad range of issues it addresses. It is honored in more than 40 states as a legal document. This document not only provides information, such as choosing a health care agent, but also asks questions to elicit the person's values and wishes. Common statements can be endorsed or marked out, and space is provided for other personal comments. The amount of detail elicited can be extremely helpful to families in planning care not only during the patient's life but afterwards as well. The document provides an opportunity for a person to record his or her wish for:

- "The person I want to make care decisions for me when I can't"
- "The kind of medical treatment I want or don't want"
- "How comfortable I want to be"
- "How I want people to treat me"
- "What I want my loved ones to know"

After the Five Wishes document is completed, the patient should sign and date it. Two witness signatures are required, and some states require notarization. The patient is encouraged to provide copies to family members and physicians and to discuss it with them. The original should be retained in an accessible place where the patient resides, and a copy taken with the patient when hospitalized or admitted to a long-term care facility. A wallet card is provided to alert medical personnel to the document. A copy of the Five Wishes document can be obtained for a fee by calling 1-888-594-7437 or online at www.agingwithdignity.org.

COMMUNICATING ABOUT DEATH AND DYING

The SUPPORT study highlighted the problem with communication about life-threatening illness and death and dying. APNs have the opportunity to promote open communication about end of life decisions between patients and their families. When patients and their families are informed that cure is no longer likely, the APN often is in a position to facilitate communication. To deliver such information requires great sensitivity. The APN should prepare and practice before embarking on sharing such news with patients and families. It is important for APNs to reflect on their own feelings about the patient and to be prepared for a variety of patient and family reactions that might range from disbelief, anger, or extreme sadness to denial.

Baile and colleagues (2000) developed a six-step protocol for delivering bad news in a patient-centered approach (Radziewicz & Baile, 2001). The protocol uses the acronym SPIKES. The six steps include the following: S for Setting, P for Perception, I for Invitation, K for Knowledge, E for Emotion, and S for Summary. In relation to the **setting,** the location should provide for comfort and privacy with all the appropriate people present. Sufficient time for questions should be reserved. **Perception** refers to what the patient and family understand about the illness. Obtaining their perceptions allows the APN to build on that understanding so they will be able to comprehend the new information they are about to receive. By **inviting** the patient and family to share how much information they are ready to receive, the nurse is asking permission to provide them with more information. Patients and their families usually are very clear about how much information they are ready to hear. APNs are particularly skilled at providing the **knowledge** needed and wanted by patients and families. Baile and colleagues (2000) suggest warning the patient and family before delivering unfavorable news and then moving forward with information as needed, pausing to assess its effect. The nurse should avoid being blunt, giving incomplete information, or offering false hope. When the patient and family react emotionally, respond to their **emotions** empathetically rather than proceeding with the information. Pause to clarify, discuss, and validate the feelings of the patient and family. Last, provide a **summary** of the new direction of care. Answer questions, discuss options further, and provide appropriate referrals. Identify a time to meet again to answer any questions that may arise in 1 or 2 days. In this situation, much that is said may not be comprehended or recalled later. With practice the SPIKES six-step protocol will serve as a useful framework to support patients and families when receiving bad news.

SYMPTOM MANAGEMENT

Both palliative and hospice care aim to provide the highest quality of care in order to improve the quality of the life for the patient who has a life-threatening illness or has entered the final phase of an illness. To achieve the highest quality of care at the end of life, troubling symptoms must be managed. Consistent with both palliative and hospice care is the precept that patients are living until they die. Good symptom management allows the patient to continue to function at the highest level possible during each remaining day. Therefore it is essential for nurses and APNs to be skilled in symptom management at end of life. The End of Life Nursing Education Consortium (ELNEC) has developed an extensive "train the trainer" program to improve nursing care of patients at the end of life. This program has developed multiple resources and educational materials for nurses (ELNEC, 2000).

The most common symptoms experienced by patients in palliative and hospice care are pain, nausea, dyspnea, cough, anxiety, gastrointestinal (GI) distress, delirium, depression, and spiritual distress. Although pain has become a central focus in end of life care, patients commonly require management of multiple symptoms.

Pain

Pain now is recognized as the fifth vital sign in all care settings, but the assessment and management are particularly important in end of life care. Many common progressive, potentially life-limiting illnesses including cancer, heart disease, and stroke have painful symptoms. As many as 4 out of 10 dying patients report having severe pain most of the time (Hall, 1999). Persons who cannot communicate are at increased risk for undertreated pain (Hospice and Palliative Care Nurses Association [HPNA], 2003c). The two main types of pain are nociceptive, which includes somatic or visceral

pain, and neuropathic pain. Nociceptive pain occurs as a result of direction stimulation of intact afferent nerve endings. It typically is described as dull, sharp, aching, or a combination of these terms. Nociceptive pain usually responds to analgesics, and can be relieved if the cause can be removed or treated (Texas Cancer Council, 2003). The organ most commonly associated with nociceptive pain is the bowel (Miller et al., 2001). Neuropathic pain is due to nervous system dysfunction and is experienced as burning, tingling, shooting, or electrical sensations (ELNEC, 2000). Examples of neuropathic pain are nerve damage caused by tumors or the effects of chemotherapy, acute herpes zoster and postherpetic neuralgia, and phantom limb pain. It may be characterized by a delayed onset after an injury, and is sometimes accompanied by sympathetic nervous system dysfunction (e.g., complex regional pain syndrome). Drug therapy for neuropathic pain is more complex and may require treatment by a pain specialist. Table 22-1 describes each type of pain and suggested pharmacological management. In addition to pain directly related to the diagnosis or treatment, patients at end of life are at risk for pressure ulcers, joint contractures, bowel obstruction, and other complications that may cause or contribute to discomfort. Untreated pain consumes energy, interferes with function, affects quality of life and social interactions, and contributes to sleep disturbances, hopelessness, and loss of control (American Pain Foundation, 2005; HPNA, 2003c). Therefore pain management is a priority in end of life care.

Assessment. An outdated belief is that older persons are less sensitive to pain. However, it has been found that they have a tendency to underreport their pain. A thorough pain assessment is essential to guide the most appropriate interventions for the patient's pain. If the patient reports pain, the nurse is obligated to accept that report (HPNA, 2003c). When pain is reported, determine the location and radiation, character, and intensity. The quantitative assessment uses various approaches to determine pain intensity. Intensity scales are useful only as a gauge of change over time, making it important to use the same scale each time an individual is assessed. There are no norms for these scales as there is no way to know how different people are "defining" a pain level of 5. However, the rating allows us to determine whether the patient perceives the pain as unchanged, better, or worse. The qualitative assessment determines the character of the pain and can be helpful in recognizing its origin and directing treatment.

With increasing cultural diversity, nurses are encountering more and more persons of backgrounds different from their own. Responses to pain and expectations for management vary among cultures. Understanding the patient's viewpoint will help the nurse to provide sensitive and appropriate care. In terms of assessment, two

Table 22-1 *Pain Descriptions with Suggested Treatments*

Pain Syndrome	Description	Management
Nociceptive pain	Actual or potential tissue damage	
Somatic	Skin or musculoskeletal pain Aching, throbbing	NSAIDs first NSAIDs and corticosteriods for bone pain May need palliative radiation
Visceral	Organ related, most common organ is bowel Squeezing, cramping	Limit to clear liquids Antiemetics Refractory pain may require scopolamine, Sandostatin, and/or corticosteroids
Neuropathic pain	Pain associated with peripheral nervous system	
Continuous dysesthesias	Continuous burning, or paresthesias	Tricyclic antidepressants Local anesthetics Transdermal clonidine Opioids often not sufficient
Lancinating or paroxysmal	Lancinating pain that is sharp, stabbing, shooting, with a sudden onset	Anticonvulsants are first choice: carbamazepine or gabapentin Topical capsaicin Tricyclics and clonidine may also be helpful

Data from Miller, K. E., Miller, M. M., & Jolley, M. R. (2001). Challenges in pain management at the end of life. *American Family Physician, 64,* 1227-1234.

patients with similar pain may demonstrate very different behavioral responses, with one crying out and thrashing and the other lying perfectly still. One may be satisfied with reducing the pain to a tolerable level whereas the other may want to be completely pain-free even if it means sleeping most of the time.

Other appropriate questions for the pain assessment might include the following: "Are there any other symptoms associated with the pain?" "How long have you been having this pain?" "Does anything make the pain better?" "Does anything make the pain worse?" "Are you currently taking any medications for the pain (including over the counter and herbal)?" The medication history is especially important because patients may be using prescription and/or over the counter drugs, herbal products, or even illegal substances that may affect the response to conventional therapy. A nonjudgmental approach to this topic is critical; otherwise the patient may not disclose all pertinent information. Once a treatment plan is initiated, ongoing assessment is vital. As a disease progresses and tolerance to drugs develops, drug changes and dosage adjustments are necessary. Also, remember to monitor for side effects and adverse effects of drugs and take measures to manage them.

Persons who cannot speak for themselves are at particular risk for undertreatment of pain (HPNA, 2003c). Individuals with cognitive impairment fall into this

category. Pain assessment in cognitively impaired patients often relies on nonverbal presentations of pain, which is not necessarily valid. Sometimes family members are able to recognize behavioral clues that a patient is in pain; this information should be shared. Several pain assessment tools are available including the Pain Assessment Tool in Confused Older Adults (PATCOA) (Decker & Perry, 2003) and the Check List of Nonverbal Pain Indicators (CNPI) (Feldt, Ryden, & Miles, 1998). The PATCOA is a nine-item ordinal scale used to evaluate nonverbal cues in order to assess pain in acutely confused older adults. This tool has a high degree of interrater reliability, internal consistency, reliability, and construct validity (Decker & Perry, 2003). The CNPI (Feldt et al., 1998) also evaluates nonverbal and vocal signs of pain in confused elders. This instrument has very good interrater reliability (93%) and good face validity (Feldt et al., 1998). Depending on the level of cognitive impairment, some persons may be able to use the FACES scale or a pain intensity scale. Some sources recommend a 5-point rather than a 10-point scale as being easier for the person with dementia to use.

Management. Once pain is recognized, the challenge is to bring it under control in a manner that is consistent with the patient's values, beliefs, and culture. According to the American Pain Foundation (2005)

"... close to 98 percent of all pain problems can be relieved or reduced." However, treatment must consider the level of comfort desired by the patient. Some persons want their pain relieved as much as possible without sedation whereas others may want pain relief regardless of the amount of sedation needed. The first-line treatment for unrelieved pain is drug therapy, starting with nonopioids. If pain persists, opioids alone or in combination with nonopioids are the next choice. Specific guidelines for drug choice and dosage are available from the American Pain Society, American Geriatrics Society, and the National Comprehensive Cancer Network. As tolerance develops, patients may require increasing dosages to achieve pain relief. With gradually increased opioid dosage, the risk of significant respiratory depression is low although constipation and miosis will persist. Prevention is the best way to manage constipation with opioid therapy. A combination of senna and a stool softener commonly is recommended when opioid therapy is initiated. The dosage is adjusted to maintain regular, comfortable bowel movements at least every other day. Some symptoms such as nausea and sedation usually resolve as tolerance to opioids develops. Until then, antiemetics may be needed for nausea. Sedation is expected when opioids are begun, but this typically improves over a few days without a reduction in dosage. The temptation to reduce the dosage may result in the return of poorly controlled pain. Particularly in older males, urinary retention may be a side effect of opioid therapy. Noninvasive interventions should be tried, followed by intermittent catheterization if needed. If this effect persists after several catheterizations, an alternate analgesic should be tested (Texas Cancer Council, 2003).

A major challenge for palliative care nurses is to overcome the reluctance of many physicians and nurses to use opioids, especially for frail older persons. Many fear that opioid doses high enough to relieve pain could hasten death, although there is no convincing scientific evidence that this is true (HPNA, 2004). Concerns about addiction are unwarranted in persons at end of life. Educating other care providers about the benefits of opioids and the management of side effects is an important nursing role.

Although nonopioid and/or opioid analgesics usually are required to manage pain at end of life, nonpharmacological interventions may be effective alone or as complementary therapies. Interventions that are effective for some patients are massage, biofeedback, distraction, music therapy, and relaxation therapy (HPNA, 2003c). Some patients choose to use complementary and alternative therapies to treat their symptoms. These therapies are classified by the National Center for Complementary and Alternative Medicine (NCCAM) as alternative medical systems, mind-body interventions, biologically-based therapies, manipulative and body-based methods, and energy therapies. Nurses in hospice and palliative care settings need to be familiar with these therapies and the implications for their use. Before rejecting a therapy just because it is unfamiliar, think about the complementary therapies in common use such as massage, relaxation therapy, aromatherapy, and guided imagery. HPNA (2003b) suggests the following

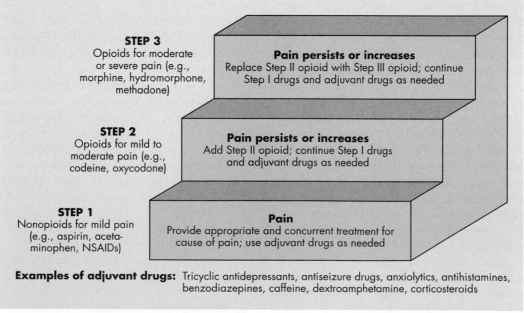

Figure 22-2 World Health Organization's step-care approach. (From World Health Organization, Geneva.)

questions to assist patients in making decisions about the types of therapies they might be considering:

- What are the specific goals of therapy (i.e., cure, palliation, reduction of drug side effects)?
- Is there scientific evidence that the therapy can achieve the goal?
- What benefits are expected?
- What risks are incurred?
- What side effects might occur?
- What are the effects on other therapy?
- What are the costs? Are they covered by insurance?
- What are the practitioner's qualifications?
- Is the therapy part of an approved clinical trial?

Three principles guide pain control at the end of life:

- Pain can be controlled in most patients by following the WHO's step-care approach (Figure 22-2).
- Acute or escalating pain is a medical emergency that requires prompt attention. Delaying treatment for pain makes it more difficult to control.
- Addiction is not an issue in patients with a terminal illness (Miller et al., 2001).

An important ethical principle, the principle of double effect, applies to pain relief at end of life. This principle differentiates between providing pain medications with the intent to relieve pain that might inadvertently hasten death and providing medications to intentionally cause death. The difference in the two actions is the intent. The American Nurses' Association (ANA) supports, as ethically acceptable, the provision of pain medications intended to relieve pain (ELNEC, 2000).

Dyspnea

Dyspnea is the next most troubling symptom following pain. Dyspnea is defined as distressing shortness of breath. It may be related to pulmonary, cardiac, neuromuscular, or metabolic disorders, or to other causes including obesity, anxiety, and spiritual distress (Dudgeon, 2001). Of concern to families in particular is the gurgling sound, often described as the "death rattle," that occurs close to the end of life. Alleviating dyspnea and congestion as much as possible can contribute much to the patient's comfort. An acronym for the evaluation of a patient with shortness of breath is BREATHES (ELNEC, 2000; Box 22-4).

Interventions for dyspnea may address only the symptom or may aim to correct the underlying cause (Sherman, Matzo, Coyne, Ferrell, & Penn 2004). Providing oxygen and elevating the head of the bed often help. Some patients, especially those with chronic obstructive pulmonary disease (COPD), breathe more easily when leaning slightly forward and resting the elbows on a table. A fan gently blowing on the patient may help to relieve the sensation of air hunger. Depending on the cause of dyspnea, medical interventions

---

BOX 22-4 BREATHES Program for Management of Dyspnea in the Elderly Palliative Care Patient

- B—Bronchospasm. Consider nebulized albuterol and/or steroids.
- R—Rales/crackles. If present, reduce fluid intake. If patient is receiving IV hydration, reduce fluid intake or discontinue. Consider gentle diuresis with Lasix 20-40 mg daily and/or spirolactone daily.
- E—Effusion. Determine if effusion is present by physical examination or chest x-ray. Consider thoracentesis or chest tube if appropriate.
- A—Airway obstruction. If patient is at risk or has had aspiration from food, puree solid food, avoid thin liquids, and keep the patient upright during and after meals for at least 1 hour.
- T—Tachypnea and breathlessness. Opioids reduce respiratory rate and feelings of breathlessness as well as anxiety. Assess daily. If patient is opioid naive, begin with morphine sulfate 5-10 mg by mouth every 4 hours and titrate opioids 25% to 50% daily to every other day as needed. Consider nebulized morphine and an anxiolytic such as Ativan 0.5-2 mg twice daily by mouth. Use of a fan may reduce feelings of breathlessness.
- H—Hemoglobin low. Consider a blood transfusion if anemia is contributing to dyspnea.
- E—Educate and support the patient and family during this highly stressful period.
- S—Secretions. If secretions are copious, consider a trial of scopolamine patch every 72 hours, atropine 0.3-0.5 mg subcutaneously every 4 hours as needed, or Rubinol (glycopyrrolate) 0.1-0.4 mg intramuscularly or subcutaneously every 4-12 hours as needed.

From Storey, P. (1994). Symptom control in advanced cancer. *Seminars in Oncology, 21*(6), 748-753.

---

might include drug therapy, blood transfusions for anemia, thoracentesis or paracentesis to remove accumulated fluid, or stent placement to prevent airway collapse (Dudgeon, 2001). Classes of drugs that may be employed to decrease dyspnea and increase comfort are:

- Opioids: relieve pain that may precipitate dyspnea; also relieve wheezing by relaxing bronchial smooth muscles; decrease anxiety
- Diuretics: improve breathing by decreasing fluid in the lungs
- Benzodiazepines: reduce anxiety and relax skeletal muscles; useful if the individual is tachypneic or anxious
- Steroids: decrease inflammation around a tumor, or manage the inflammation or bronchospasm occurring because of a tumor or exacerbation of COPD

- Antibiotics: treat respiratory tract infections
- Anticoagulants: treat or prevent pulmonary emboli
- Anticholinergics: reduce pulmonary secretions that cause the "death rattle" and the need for suctioning

Intense shortness of breath, sometimes called "air hunger," can cause both patients and their families to panic. Sometimes patients who had indicated they did not wish to have mechanical ventilation change their minds in the face of air hunger. It is hoped that timely use of medications (morphine and anxiolytics), positioning, and measures to relieve anxiety will avoid this type of crisis. It is especially important that the patient and family not feel abandoned at this time. Patients who fear suffocation may be comforted to know that they can choose sedation to relieve their suffering (Tarzian, 2000).

Anxiety

Anxiety is described as a subjective feeling of apprehension, tension, insecurity, and uneasiness ranging in intensity from mild to severe (Pasacreta, Minarik, & Nield-Anderson, 2001). At end of life, anxiety may be associated with various physical and emotional factors including dyspnea, a lifelong pattern of responding to stress, or a preexisting anxiety disorder. Whatever the reason for the anxiety, it is essential to bring it under control to allow the patient some peace.

When anxiety progresses, the physical signs and symptoms also increase. Anxiety can manifest as sweating, tachycardia, hyperventilation, trembling, agitation, chest pain, and muscular tension (Sherman et al., 2004). A two-pronged approach to managing anxiety begins with nonpharmacological interventions followed by pharmacological agents as needed. Nonpharmacological interventions include relaxation techniques such as visual imagery and music therapy, empathetic listening, reassurance, and reinforcement of previously successful anxiety-reducing strategies (Sherman et al., 2004). When these interventions are not effective, pharmacological management may be necessary. Options include selective serotonin reuptake inhibitors (SSRIs), benzodiazepines, and nonbenzodiazepines. The SSRIs, which increase the level of serotonin in the brain, are most commonly used for their antidepressant effect, but paroxetine (Paxil) has also been used effectively to treat anxiety. Benzodiazepines produce an anxiolytic effect by acting on the limbic-thalamic-hypothalamic areas of the central nervous system (Sherman et al., 2004). Nonbenzodiazepines that may be useful are Desyrel and buspirone. Desyrel is an atypical antidepressant used mostly for sleep or adjunctive therapy with another antidepressant. Buspirone is an anxiolytic that also may be helpful in mixed anxiety and depressive symptoms; however, it typically takes up to 3 weeks to take effect.

The APN should confirm whether the prescription of benzodiazepines is within the scope of practice.

Gastrointestinal Symptoms

Gastrointestinal (GI) symptoms can take many forms including nausea, vomiting, gastritis, constipation, and diarrhea. If not controlled, they can negatively impact the patient's comfort and quality of life.

Nausea and Vomiting. Nausea is an unpleasant sensation that often signals the onset of vomiting. It is caused by excitation of an area of the medulla that is either part of the vomiting center or located nearby. Vomiting may be initiated by several mechanisms including gastrointestinal irritation or overdistention, stimulation of the chemoreceptor trigger zone in the medulla by motion sickness or drugs such as morphine, or by psychic stimuli that elicit cerebral excitation (Guyton & Hall, 2000).

The principles of managing nausea include blocking the responses of the gut and the central nervous systems to stimuli. Although this is best accomplished with drug therapy, nonpharmacological measures such as distraction, music therapy, guided imagery, and acupuncture can enhance drug effects. Types of drugs used to relieve nausea include antihistamines, dopa-antagonists, serotonergic antagonists, and pro-motility agents. A diet of clear liquids or small, frequent meals also may be helpful.

Constipation. Constipation can be caused by a disease process such as colon cancer, end-stage diabetes, or Parkinson's disease; drug side effects; metabolic disturbances; and other neurogenic and systemic disease states. Among the medications that can contribute to constipation in older adults at the end of life are opiates, anticholinergics, calcium channel blockers, antiparkinsonian drugs, diuretics, calcium supplements, and iron supplements. At the end of life, inactivity and poor diet and fluid intake also increase the risk of constipation.

The principles of managing constipation at end of life emphasize prevention first, followed by establishing a normal pattern for the patient. Measures to accomplish this include regular toileting and adequate fluids as long as possible, and laxatives or cathartics as needed. A laxative of some kind should be prescribed routinely whenever opioid analgesics are used. Some sources recommend a combination of a stimulant and a stool softener with doses titrated to achieve the desired effect (Welsh, Fallon, & Kelley, 2003). Table 22-2 summarizes the pharmacological options for constipation. A "rescue enema" may be required if constipation persists (Economou, 2001).

Table 22-2 *Pharmacological Treatment for Constipation*

Class of Drug	Examples	Mechanism of Action	Comments
Stimulant	Senna	Stimulates bowel	Use with caution in patients with liver disease
Bulk laxatives	Psyllium	Increases intestinal transit time	Not recommended in patients with decreased fluid intake or if impending bowel obstruction
Detergent softener	Docusate	Softens stool; may stimulate colon	
Osmotic	Sorbitol, lactulose	Combines mild stimulant with softener	Often used with opiate use and chronic constipation
Magnesium salts	Milk of magnesia	Osmotic	Prolonged use can cause electrolyte disturbances Avoid in end-stage renal patients

From End of Life Nursing Education Consortium (ELNEC). (2000). *ELNEC course syllabus.* Washington, DC: American Association of Colleges of Nursing and the City of Hope National Medical Center.

Diarrhea. Diarrhea, like constipation, can be multifactorial (Sherman et al., 2004). Contributing factors are chemotherapy, radiation, partial bowel obstructions, malabsorption, excessive dietary fiber, laxative abuse, parasitic or bacterial infections, and superinfections associated with antibiotic therapy (e.g., *Clostridium difficile*). Good management of diarrhea is vital for the individual's comfort and quality of life.

Management of diarrhea includes identification and treatment of the underlying cause, dietary modification such as a low residue or clear liquid diet, hydration as appropriate, and use of pharmacological agents. Common treatments for diarrhea include opioids such as loperamide hydrochloride, bulk-forming agents to promote absorption of fluid from the bowel, antibiotics for infectious diarrhea, and steroids to decrease inflammation of the gut. Somatostatin may be used to slow transit time by decreasing GI secretions (ELNEC, 2000).

Anorexia and Cachexia

Anorexia and cachexia frequently are associated with advanced terminal illness. Cachexia is distressing to patients and their families because of the muscle wasting and altered appearance that result. Anorexia and cachexia also are multifactorial with causes including alterations in oral mucosa and taste, pathological changes, drug effects, chronic nausea/vomiting, metabolic disturbances, diarrhea, sedation, and depression.

Anorexia and cachexia should be managed in accordance with the goals of the patient and the family. For the patient who wants to eat, the enjoyment of pleasure foods is more important than adhering to a therapeutic diet. Some appetite stimulants can be used safely in older adults. Dexamethasone and Marinol may be used short term to improve appetite (ELNEC, 2000). Megesterol

acetate also has been used short term in older adults but usually is avoided in individuals with vascular disease because of the increased risk of deep vein thrombosis and stroke. This is a good example of an ethical dilemma where risks and benefits must be weighed. At a certain point in the process of dying, patients commonly lose the will to eat. This is thought to be a normal part of the process that culminates in death. The body not only requires less nourishment but also is less able to process nutrients. Although artificial feeding has not been shown to reverse the wasting process, the patient's wishes should be respected. Decisions about artificial feedings are best made before the final stage of life and documented in advance directives.

Evidence exists that dehydration actually improves the quality of life in the last few days by reducing respiratory and gastrointestinal secretions, edema, and ascites (Critchlow & Bauer-Wu, 2002; Seery, 2004). The Hospice and Palliative Care Coalition (HPCC) is an organization comprised of the American Academy of Hospice and Palliative Medicine, the Hospice and Palliative Nurses Association, and the National Hospice and Palliative Care Organization. The following is an excerpt from a statement issued by the HPCC (2005) in response to public concerns surrounding the death of Terri Schiavo:

One of the most important aims of hospice and palliative care is to minimize suffering and discomfort. Many patients, families, and other caregivers fear that undernourished patients may experience hunger. They may also believe that forgoing artificial nutrition results in troublesome symptoms such as thirst, dry mouth, headache, delirium, nausea, vomiting, and abdominal cramps. Contrary to expectations, however, studies show that most patients with complex medical conditions nearing the end of their lives do not experience hunger even if they have inadequate caloric intake. Dry mouth is the most common symptom but it can easily be alleviated with conscientious mouth care.

These points echo the HPNA (Hospice and Palliative Nurses Association) Position Statement on Artificial Nutrition and Hydration in End of Life Care (HPNA, 2003a) that cites the lack of empirical evidence that artificial nutrition and hydration (ANH) prolong life, prevent aspiration, maintain independence and function, or decrease suffering and discomfort at the end of life. The HPNA statement further lists the complications of ANH. Vascular access may require repeated venipunctures and presents a portal for infection. Fluid therapy may worsen peripheral and peritumor edema, heart failure, and pulmonary congestion. Problems associated with tube-feedings include infection, fluid overload, skin excoriation, nausea and vomiting, diarrhea, and throat and nose pain. In addition, it is likely that physical restraint will be needed to maintain venous lines or enteral tubes (Critchlow & Bauer-Wu, 2002; HPNA, 2003a).

Various theories have been offered to explain the apparent benefits of what is called terminal dehydration (TD). One theory is that electrolyte imbalances and ketosis resulting from inadequate fluid and food intake account for partial loss of sensation through either a local or a central mechanism. Rat studies have demonstrated an increase in β-endorphin and dynorphin levels, which are natural opiates. Another avenue of study has looked at the consequence of hydration in the terminal phase. When patients already were in a state of TD, the administration of intravenous fluids and glucose reversed ketonemia and discomfort increased.

Despite the body of evidence supporting TD as beneficial, nurses' beliefs vary. A survey assessing the perceptions and attitudes of nurses in long-term care toward TD revealed considerable variation. For reactions to statements such as "Dehydration provides relief from distressing symptoms" and "Dehydration can be beneficial to the dying patient," responses were almost evenly distributed along the continuum from "strongly disagree" to "strongly agree." RNs were much more likely than LPNs to strongly agree with these two statements. A positive correlation existed between nurse age and positive perception of TD (Critchlow & Bauer-Wu, 2002). The best approach may be to examine each case on an individual basis to determine what action is most likely to promote patient comfort (Dunphy, Finlay, Rathbone, Gilbert, & Hicks, 1995). As long as they are able, patients should be allowed to make their own decisions about whether to accept food and fluids.

Psychiatric Symptoms

Psychiatric symptoms are very common at end of life. Depression rates among individuals with advanced illness have been reported as 25% to 77% (Chochinov,

Wilson, Enns, & Lander, 1998). Delirium also is quite common in older adults nearing the end of life. Unfortunately, both depression and delirium may remain untreated if clinicians attribute the symptoms to normal aging or dementia. It is important to recognize symptoms of depression and delirium because these conditions can rob individuals nearing death of the quality of life and quality of care they deserve.

Depression. Depression is defined as a continuum with reactive depression at one end, the middle occupied by an adjustment disorder, and depressed mood to major depressive disorder at the other end. It is realistic to expect most individuals with a terminal diagnosis to have some level of reactive depression. Unfortunately, many of the symptoms of depression (weight loss, fatigue, decreased ability to concentrate) mimic symptoms of many disease processes (Gullate, Kaplow, & Heidrich, 2005). A diagnosis of a major depressive disorder requires at least five of the following symptoms to be present most of the day, or almost every day for at least 2 weeks: depressed mood; markedly decreased interest or pleasure in all or almost all activities; significant weight loss; insomnia or hypersomnia; psychomotor agitation or retardation; fatigue or loss of energy; feelings of worthlessness or excessive or inappropriate guilt; diminished ability to think or concentrate or indecisiveness; and current thoughts of death, recurrent suicidal ideation, or suicide attempt (APA, 2000). Tools to assess for depression include the Yesavage Geriatric Depression Scale, the Hamilton Depression Rating Scale, and the Cornell Depression Scale in dementia patients.

Depression is best managed by a combination of psychotherapy and medications (APA, 2000). The mainstay of medication management is the selective serotonin reuptake inhibitor (SSRI), an effective class of antidepressants that takes about 2 weeks to take effect. Mirtazapine, an atypical sedating antidepressant that has been found to help with appetite, commonly is used in end of life care. The long-acting tricyclic antidepressants have significant anticholinergic activity that can increase an individual's risk of falling because of orthostatic hypotension, exacerbate constipation, and cause delirium in older adults. Psychostimulants such as methylphenidate may be used to "jump start" the treatment of depression. Knowledge of the side effect profile of the many available antidepressants will aid in the choice of drugs.

Major depression may lead to suicidal ideations. APNs should monitor individuals closely for suicidal thoughts or expressions. Feelings of worthlessness and hopelessness and thoughts of harming oneself are clear indications an individual is at risk for suicide. A family history of suicide and a history of substance abuse also are risk factors for suicide. The following questions should be asked if there is concern about suicidal ideation: (a) Have you ever thought of harming yourself? (b) Are you thinking about it now? (c) Have you ever thought about how you might harm yourself? (d) Do you have the means and a time frame to harm yourself? (Gullate et al., 2005).

The individual who has a plan, means, and time frame should have a psychiatric evaluation immediately. Exploration of the patient's feelings may reveal unrelenting suffering and a lack of hope for relief. The palliative care nurse should explore options to improve the patient's comfort and sense of well-being.

Delirium. Delirium is common toward the end of life. It is characterized by the acute onset of confusion that fluctuates over hours to days and inattention that may be accompanied by disorganized thinking and hallucinations (APA, 1994). The three subtypes of delirium are *hyperactive* (associated with restlessness and agitation), *hypoactive* (associated with lethargy), and *mixed* (a combination of both hyperactive and hypoactive) (Liptzin & Levkoff, 1992). This section will address delirium specifically in regard to end of life care. For a full discussion of delirium including assessment tools such as the CAM and the NEECHAM, see Chapters 2 and 14.

ETIOLOGY. The causes of delirium at end of life include many of the same etiologies as in non–terminally ill patients such as dehydration, hypoxia, and sepsis (Wakefield & Johnson, 2001). Risk factors for delirium often are related to progression of the disease process. Although terminal illness often is equated with a diagnosis of cancer, other common causes in older adults are congestive heart failure, kidney disease, pulmonary disease, or neurological conditions including end-stage dementia. Some general risk factors for delirium include:

- Infections of the bladder, respiratory tract, gastrointestinal tract, or skin
- Medications: newly started or abruptly stopped; side effects
- Fluid and electrolyte or metabolic disturbances, such as abnormal serum sodium, potassium, or calcium levels; atypical BUN/creatinine ratios; abnormal glucose levels; or thyroid or liver dysfunction
- Pain syndromes (probably most important)

MANAGEMENT. Delirium at end of life may increase the distress of both the older adult and the family. If it is attributed to a medication, a decision must be made regarding the drug's benefits versus its adverse effect. Perhaps an alternate drug could be tried. In general, comfort and quality of life take priority and potentially delirium-inducing drugs may be necessary. It also may not be possible to prevent symptoms related to the progression of the disease process.

Delirium may be resolved if the cause can be identified and is reversible. Consider the possibility of bladder infection, dehydration, poorly managed pain, constipation, bladder distention, and hypoxemia. Determine whether the onset of symptoms coincided with starting a new drug (e.g., an anticholinergic) or with the withdrawal of a drug (Sherman et al., 2004). A focused physical examination may enable the nurse to identify possible causes or contributing factors. If the patient is too agitated for the examination, it may be necessary to administer a sedative. Preferred sedatives are low-dose neuroleptics such as haloperidol or an intermediate-acting benzodiazepine such as lorazepam. These medications should be used only if agitation disturbs the patient or endangers the patient or others. Analgesics may have a calming effect if the basic problem is pain.

Nonpharmacological management of delirium includes low-level lighting, a quiet room, or soft music playing. If family members provide a calming presence, encourage them to be present as much as possible. When family is unavailable, a sitter at the bedside can reassure the patient and prevent injury. Assist with regular toileting and fluid intake if appropriate. To maintain sensory function, be sure the patient's hearing aids and eyeglasses are worn. Be sure hearing aids are turned on and in working order.

Because the etiology of delirium may be multifactorial, more than one intervention may be necessary. Addressing potential causes one at a time may enable you to identify the major cause and contributing factors. Making too many changes at once can exacerbate the delirium rather than improve it.

Delirium often is an ominous sign that the individual is declining, particularly if a precipitating cause is not obvious and the patient is not responsive to treatment. In this case, the patient's family should be notified of the change in the patient's condition. Every effort, pharmacological and nonpharmacological, should be made to enable the patient to be peaceful at the end of life.

SPIRITUAL CARE

Spirituality is recognized by both professionals and patients as an important element at the end of life. Spirituality is a broad concept that encompasses the search for meaning in life experiences and relationships with others. Religion is that aspect of spirituality that is associated with a sense of connectedness to a personal deity. Both spirituality and religion help to create a sense of purpose and meaning that makes life worthwhile. To ascribe meaning to life means that a person believes he or she is fulfilling a unique role and purpose, that life is a gift that comes with responsibility for striving to fulfill one's potential, and that finding meaning brings peace and transcendence by connecting with a greater power (Chochinov, 2004).

Spiritual distress is defined as "impaired ability to experience and integrate meaning and purpose in life through a person's connectedness with self, others, art, music, literature, nature, or a power greater than oneself" (NANDA, 2005). Among the factors that may be related to spiritual distress are death and dying, pain, anxiety, life change, and chronic illness of self or others. The first step in helping persons with spiritual distress is to recognize this state of mind. Clues to spiritual distress might include expressions of lack of meaning and purpose in life, refusing interactions with others who offer support, loss of interest in creative expression, and a sense of having been abandoned by God (NANDA, 2005).

An acronym that can be used to guide the assessment of spiritual well-being is FICA (Puchalski & Romer, 2000). The components of this guide and examples of related questions follow.

- F—Faith: Faith and Belief
  "Do you consider yourself spiritual or religious?" "Do you have spiritual beliefs that help you cope with stress?" If the patient responds "No" the clinican might ask, "What gives your life meaning?" Sometimes patients respond with answers such as family, career, or nature.
- I—Importance
  "What importance does your faith or belief have in your life?" "Have your beliefs influenced how you take care of yourself in this illness?" "What role do your beliefs play in regaining your health?"
- C—Community
  "Are you part of a spiritual or religious community?" "Is this a source of support to you; if so, how?" "Is there a group of people you really love or who are important to you?" Communities such as churches, temples, and mosques, or a group of like-minded friends can serve as strong support systems for some patients.
- A—Address in Care
  "How would you like me, your health care provider, to address these issues in your health care?" The patient should be given the opportunity to express spiritual concerns although some will choose not to discuss these issues with a physician or nurse.

Opening a dialogue about spiritual concerns can be therapeutic in itself. Various therapeutic approaches seek to reduce spiritual suffering by focusing on meaning and dignity.

LIMITATIONS ON TREATMENT

When care is provided in a hospice or palliative care environment, the focus is on quality of life and symptom management. However, 20% of all deaths in the United States take place in critical care settings where the focus traditionally is on cure or sustaining life (Angus, et al., 2004). Some studies have shown that ethics or palliative care consultations may improve end of life care in the intensive care unit or shorten the stay in that setting (Curtis, 2004). Inherent in this discussion is the decision to discontinue or withhold life-sustaining treatment. Some protocols for withdrawing life support have been designed. For example, one protocol has four sections: (1) discontinuing routine laboratory and x-ray studies, (2) guidelines for analgesia and sedation, (3) a ventilator withdrawal protocol, and (4) principles of life support withdrawal (Treece et al., 2004).

Of course, decisions about limited treatment are faced outside the intensive care unit as well. For example, a significant number of persons who die from end-stage renal disease do so following withdrawal of hemodialysis. Therefore the American Society of Nephrology and Renal Physicians Association have published guidelines for the withdrawal process. The guidelines address numerous issues including shared decision making between the patient and the physician, and symptom control issues (Galla, 2000). Research relating to care when treatment is withdrawn is greatly needed to improve quality of care in this and other life-threatening situations.

FAMILY CAREGIVING

For many persons at end of life, family caregivers play a vital role. Caregivers may do everything from assisting with ADLs to giving medications and managing medical equipment and treatments. Furthermore, the family caregiver often is the person who serves as a go-between for the patient and health care providers. Although caregivers may find great satisfaction in their role, they often experience stress and diminished physical health. Some caregivers take on more than they can reasonably manage out of a sense of duty or because of cultural or family pressure. Interventions to assist family caregivers have focused primarily on education and support, and outcomes have been inconsistent (McMillan, 2004). Few studies have focused specifically on care giving during the end of life period and palliative care. Clearly, this is an area where more nursing research is needed.

SIGNS OF DYING

No one can predict exactly when death actually will occur, but there are common signs and symptoms that suggest that it is near. Klinkenberg and colleagues (2004) used retrospective data collected from relatives to study symptom burden in older persons in the last week of life. Most commonly reported were fatigue (83%), pain (48%), and shortness of breath (50%). Others that were important but affected fewer than 40% of the individuals were confusion, anxiety, depression,

---

BOX 22-5 Signs of Dying

The following signs are common 1 to 2 weeks before death (Seery, 2004):

- Weakness, lethargy
- Increased sleeping or restlessness
- Progressive disorientation
- Short attention span
- Withdrawal
- Less interest in food and fluids
- Dysphagia
- Incontinence

The following signs may be evident 2 to 3 days before death:

- Decreased level of awareness
- Glassy eyes, unfocused pupils
- Loss of interest in food and fluids
- Abnormal breathing pattern
- Faint blood pressure and pulse rate
- Unexpected energy surges
- Progressive cooling and mottling of extremities

From Seery, D. H. (2004). Shifting gears: From cure to comfort. *RN, 67*(11), 52-57. *RN* is a copyrighted publication of Advanstar Communications. All rights reserved.

---

and nausea and/or vomiting. Patients with cancer were the most likely to have pain, and those with COPD were most likely to have shortness of breath. Symptoms that patients were more likely to discuss with relatives included pain, nausea, vomiting, and fatigue; symptoms discussed least were confusion, anxiety, depression, and shortness of breath. Compared with individuals with normal cognition, persons with cognitive impairment had higher scores on confusion, depression, anxiety, fatigue, and nausea and vomiting. Their scores for pain were consistent with the scores of patients who did not have cognitive impairment (Klinkenberg, Willems, van der Wal, & Deeg, 2004). Another study monitored physical changes in terminally ill cancer patients. In this sample, the onset of the death rattle preceded death by a mean of 57 hours, cyanosis on extremities by a mean of 5.1 hours, and absence of radial pulse by a mean of 2.6 hours (Morita, Ichiki, Tsunoda, Inoue, & Chihara, 1998). One week before death, none of the patients was comatose. That number rose to 50% in the last 6 hours. Common signs of dying are summarized in Box 22-5.

DEALING WITH GRIEF: SURVIVOR BEREAVEMENT

One of the most important points to remember when working with people who have experienced a loss is that this experience is very deep and personal. Although bereavement is a normal and natural process that resolves in most cases, it has been associated with mental and physical illness for some. In fact, following the loss

through death of a significant person, the survivor is at increased risk for death (Stroebe, 2004).

Several models have been constructed to explain how people grieve and go through bereavement, yet the experiences of many individuals do not fit any of these models. Good communication is essential to understand the experience of someone who has recently lost a loved one and to be able to be therapeutic and supportive. Important theorists regarding the grieving process include Freud (1957), Lindeman (1994), Kubler-Ross (1969), Parkes (1972), Bowlby (1980), Rando (1986), Worden (1991), and Copp (1990). Table 22-3 briefly describes their views. Common elements of these models are the concept of mourning, and grief and bereavement as processes with stages through which individuals move back and forth. Other common features of these models are that each person goes through these stages at his or her own pace and that not everyone moves in and out of these stages without complications.

Normal responses to grief are physical, psychological, cognitive, and/or spiritual (Potter, 2001). Cowles (1996) describes uncomplicated grief as a dynamic, pervasive, highly individualized process. The term **complicated grief** is used to describe persistent maladaptive behaviors that occur following loss. Complicated grief is defined as the intensification of grief to the level where the individual is overwhelmed, develops maladaptive behavior, or remains interminably in the state of grief without progression through the mourning process to completion (Worden, 1991). The diagnostic criteria for complicated grief include the persistence of the following symptoms for more than 1 year after a loss: the current experience of intensive intrusive thoughts, pangs of severe emotion, distressing yearnings, feeling excessively alone and empty, excessively avoiding tasks reminiscent of the deceased, unusual sleep disturbances, and maladaptive loss of interest in personal activities (Horowitz et al., 1997, p. 904).

The majority of individuals who experience a loss progress through their bereavement process with informal social support systems. Social support systems include friendly visitors, provision of meals, support from friends who have had the experience of bereavement, lay support groups, friendly listeners, and even exercise groups (Corless, 2001). The nature of the nurse-client relationship places nurses and APNs in a position to help identify and manage complicated grief. However, it is important for nurses or APNs to know their limitations. The National Council for Hospice and Specialist Palliative Care Services (1993) identifies the need for generalists to refer persons with complicated grief to the right provider, such as a bereavement counselor. Professional care for the bereaved includes clergy visiting and/or counseling, health professional counseling, professionally led support groups, and professional

Table 22-3 *Models and Theories of Grief and Bereavement*

Freud (1957)	Lindemann (1994)	Kubler-Ross (1969)	Bowlby (1980)	Rando (1986)	Worden (1991)	Copp (1990)
Mourning and Melancholia (1917): Mourning is reaction to loss of loved person, or to loss of one's country, liberty, and ideal, meaning that grieving is response to loss, not just to loss from death. Mourning takes time and once work of mourning is completed, ego is free to be uninhibited again.	Lindemann described three stages of grief: (1) shock and disbelief (2) acute mourning (3) resolution of grief process Three tasks involved: (1) emancipation from bondage of deceased (2) readjustment to environment without deceased (3) formation of new relationships	Stages of death and dying: (1) denial (2) anger (3) bargaining (4) depression (5) acceptance This is not a linear process. Individuals and families go through stages at various rates and sequences.	Uses attachment theory to describe four phases of mourning: (1) phase of numbness (2) yearning and searching (3) disorganization and despair (4) reorganization	Mourning has a sociocultural dimension with religious beliefs and values. Grief is response to perception of loss and is transitional process of mourning. Mourning is intrapsychic process initiated by loss. Bereavement is state of suffering a loss.	Four essential tasks of mourning: (1) to accept reality of loss (2) to work through pain of grief (3) to adjust to environment in which deceased is gone (4) to relocate deceased emotionally and move on with living	Personal acceptance of imminent death and physical condition determined readiness to die. States of readiness: (1) person ready, body not ready (2) person ready, body ready (3) person not ready, body ready (4) person not ready, body not ready The dying experience impacts everyone who is involved with dying patient.

bereavement programs (Corless, 2001). Hospice and palliative care programs provide professional bereavement services for the immediate family of the deceased. Research on the effectiveness of bereavement interventions has provided no justification for routine intervention. However, intervention has been found to be effective in persons suffering complicated or pathological grief. Stroebe (2004) notes that the need for additional research in the identification of risk factors for complicated grief and the application of guidelines for grief intervention. As nurses, we can guide patients who express a need for help or seem to be especially vulnerable to find appropriate services. When the death of a loved one is sudden, it is especially important to assess for complicated grief and to connect the individual or family to appropriate professional care as needed.

ETHICAL CONSIDERATIONS IN END OF LIFE CARE AND RESEARCH

Nurses in end of life care are dealing constantly with situations that require ethical decision making. Various professional organizations, including the ANA, have published ethical guidelines, both general and specific, to end of life issues. Of particular interest, the American Society for Pain Management Nursing (ASPMN) (2003) lists the following ethical tenets relevant to pain management at end of life:

- The nurse who provides pain management uses personal and professional codes of ethics to guide pain management practice that is characterized by respect for human dignity (ASPMN, 1996).

- Beneficence is the ethical principle of 'commitment to do good and avoid harm' (Thompson, 1994).
- Nurses individually and collectively have an obligation to provide comprehensive and compassionate end of life care, which includes the promotion of comfort and the relief of pain, and, at times, forgoing life-sustaining treatments (ANA, 1998).
- "The duty to benefit through relief of pain is by itself adequate to support the use of increasing doses (of opioids) to alleviate pain, even if there might be life shortening and expected side effects" (Cain & Hannes, 1994, p. 161).
- There is an ethical obligation to provide relief that is based on the pain report and mutually agreed upon goals as defined by the patient in collaboration with the health care team (AHCPR, 1994).

Admittedly, there are many gaps in our understanding of the process of dying and the care that is most appropriate at that time. Considerable efforts have gone into defining the problems and ethical dilemmas at end of life (e.g., allocation of scarce resource, withholding treatment, termination of life support). However, advancing the science of end of life care requires research and that raises other ethical issues. Casarett (2004) identified the following ways to examine the ethics of research with persons nearing the end of life:

- Determine whether a planned project is research or quality improvement
- Consider potential benefits for future patients in terms of validity and value
- Consider potential benefits to subjects
- Consider risks for subjects
- Consider the decision-making capacity of subjects
- Ensure that there is no coercion, and that patients can withdraw if they wish

The American Academy of Hospice and Palliative Medicine (2002a, 2002b) affirms that research in palliative care is ethical as long as risks are assessed, the patient's decision-making capacity and the role of the surrogate are considered, participation is voluntary, placebo use is appropriate, and suffering is considered. As with all clinical research, the concepts of minimal risk and informed consent must be honored.

ASSISTED SUICIDE

Few topics generate emotional response as strongly as euthanasia and assisted suicide. Whereas suicide is the taking of one's own life, assisted suicide is the provision of a means for a person to take his or her own life while aware of that person's intent (ANA, 2002). The term euthanasia is used when a person deliberately and actively administers the means (e.g., medication) to end a person's life. Nurses who work with patients at end of life may confront this issue when a patient who is suffering

asks for help to die. The position of most professional bodies is that every effort must be made to relieve the suffering, but not to deliberately cause death. The principles that must be weighed in this situation are autonomy, beneficence, and nonmaleficence. The dilemma is in weighing which principle takes priority (AAHPM, 1997).

In a position statement on assisted suicide, the HPNA (2001) published the following:

It is the position of the HPNA Board of Directors to:

- Oppose the legalization of assisted suicide
- Affirm the value of end of life care, which includes aggressive and comprehensive symptom management
- Affirm that nurses must be vigilant advocates for humane and ethical care for the alleviation of suffering and for the non-abandonment of patients (ANA, 1994)
- Support public policy that ensures access to hospice and palliative care for persons facing the end of life
- Direct those nurses practicing in states where assisted suicide is legal that they may choose to continue to provide care or may withdraw from the situation after transferring responsibility for care to a nursing colleague (Oncology Nursing Society [ONS], 2001)

In the United States at this time, physician-assisted suicide is legal only in Oregon; however, nurses must

---

BOX 22-6 Web Resources Relevant to End of Life Nursing Care

- Americans for Better Care of the Dying: www.abcd-caring.org
- Center for Advance Palliative Care: www.capcmssm.org
- Center to Improve Care of the Dying: www.gwu.edu/~cicd
- Community-State Partnerships to Improve End-of Life Care: www.midbio.org
- Hospice and Palliative Care Nurses Association: www.hpna.org
- Innovations in End-of-Life Care: www.edc.org/lastacts
- National Hospice and Palliative Care Organization: www.nhpco.org
- Partnership for Caring: www.partnershipforcaring.org
- Supportive Care of the Dying: www.careofdying.org
- Toolkit Nurturing Excellence in End of Life Transitions: www.tneel.uic.edu/tneel.asp
- www.palliativecarenursing.net/
- www.stronghealth.com/services/palliative/nursingeducation.cfm
- www.dyingwell.com/PE.htm

Source: www.promotingexcellence.org/.

Nursing Care Plan: The Older Patient at the End of Life

Data

Maria is a 74-year-old widow and retired school teacher. She was first diagnosed with breast cancer 10 years ago that was treated with a right radical mastectomy and followed with chemotherapy. Five years later, a lump in her left breast proved to be malignant. Once again she had surgery, chemotherapy, and radiation therapy. Six months ago, she began having headaches and blurred vision. She was hospitalized after a grand mal seizure. A thorough medical evaluation revealed extensive metastatic cancer, including brain lesions that were considered inoperable. Maria was advised of this by her physician. She was discharged in stable condition on anticonvulsant therapy. She sought comfort from her priest and her neighbor, who had been her friend for 30 years. She called her daughter and son who lived in nearby communities and informed them of her diagnosis. Maria felt she was being strong when she listened to her physician with a growing sense of sadness but maintained control over her emotions. However, when telling her children of her illness, she was overcome with emotions that fluctuated between anger and sadness.

Most days she felt pretty good, but she began to notice some weakness in her right arm and sometimes it was hard to write. One time she stumbled and fell while walking in the yard. These incidents made her realize that she would continue to have changes in her ability to care for herself and needed to plan for the future. She made an appointment with an attorney to review her will and make some minor revisions. At that time, she completed an advance directive and filled out a Five Wishes form to share with her family how she wanted to live the rest of her life. At night she often lay awake thinking about her life, her family, her accomplishments, and her disappointments. In accord with her religious faith, she believed that she would enter a state of peace and joy after her death and would be reunited with her beloved parents and brother. She felt regret that she would not see her grandchildren grow up. Prompted by her daughter, she called her older sister to whom she had not spoken since a disagreement 2 years ago. Her greatest fear about dying was that she would be in pain. Her father had died of lung cancer many years before, but she remembered his painful death, gasping for breath in a hospital bed. Maria hoped that she would be able to stay in her own home until she died, but she did not know if that was realistic.

Over a period of months, Maria had several hospitalizations—one hospitalization for a pleural effusion that caused shortness of breath and another time because of progressive neurological deficits. Maria's daughter or teenaged granddaughter has been staying with Maria in her own home at nights. Following the latest hospitalization after a fall, Maria and her daughter agreed that it was not safe for her to be alone at home all day. Following a conference with Maria's physician, a referral was initiated for hospice care. The hospice nurse visited Maria in the hospital and talked to Maria alone and in the presence of her daughter. Based on a series of assessment interviews, the following was decided upon:

- Maria would move into an inpatient hospice setting.
- Maria would receive both pharmacological and nonpharmacological treatments to manage her pain.
- Maria wanted pain control even if it meant that she slept much of the time.
- Maria wanted sedation and opioids as needed to control shortness of breath; but not mechanical ventilation.
- Maria did not want to have artificial feedings when she could no longer take oral nourishment.
- Maria wanted visits from family, friends, and her priest.

Maria arrived at the hospice in a wheelchair accompanied by her daughter. She was wearing her own clothing. Despite right-sided weakness, she was able to assist in transferring out of the wheelchair into a chair in her room. She was alert and oriented. She stated she felt fine except for a dull headache. During the admission process, she tired quickly and asked to be allowed to rest. Later that day she had an episode of urinary incontinence when she was unable to get to the bathroom unassisted.

Assessment

As the weeks pass, Maria's pain escalates, requiring increasing amounts of opioids. She is given laxatives and stool softeners to prevent constipation. She now spends most of her day in bed and has very little oral intake—small amounts of sherbet and tea. She now has an indwelling catheter, and her urine is dark with a total output of 600 to 800 ml/day. She has oxygen per cannula when needed, and becomes dyspneic if flat in bed. The distant breath sounds on her left side suggest that the pleural effusion has recurred. She has had one episode of acute air hunger that resolved with morphine and lorazepam. She sleeps much of the time, and has been slightly confused on occasion, once thinking the nursing assistant was her sister. Her family and friends are attentive, visiting in shifts so that she is never alone.

Nursing Diagnoses (NANDA, 2005)

At this stage of Maria's life, appropriate nursing diagnoses might include:

- Acute confusion related to delirium

Nursing Care Plan: The Older Patient at the End of Life—cont'd

- Acute pain related to disease process—metastatic cancer
- Death anxiety related to fear of pain, breathlessness at end of life
- Impaired bed mobility related to weakness, incoordination, confusion, sedation
- Impaired gas exchange related to ventilation/perfusion imbalance
- Imbalanced nutrition: Less than body requirements related to inability to ingest foods and fluids
- Impaired oral mucous membranes related to mouth breathing, dehydration, malnutrition
- Ineffective protection related to inadequate nutrition, effects of cancer
- Risk for deficient fluid volume related to inadequate intake
- Self-care deficit
- Risk for impaired skin integrity related to weight loss, pressure, immobilization
- Readiness for enhanced spiritual well-being
In addition, the following diagnoses may apply to Maria's family:
- Interrupted family processes related to shift in health status of a family member
- Readiness for enhanced coping
- Anticipatory grieving

Goals/Outcomes

The goals of nursing care for the patient at this phase of the end of life include achieving the best comfort level attainable, minimal anxiety, prevention of complications of immobility, and a sense of spiritual well-being. These goals should be consistent with the wishes of the patient. The nursing goal for the family is for them to feel supported and to know that the best care possible was provided.

NOC Suggested Outcomes (Moorhead, Johnson, & Maas, 2004)

Comfort Level, Anxiety Control, Immobility Consequences: Physiological, Spiritual Well-Being, Family Coping, Grief Resolution

NIC Suggested Interventions (Dochterman & Bulechek, 2004)

Major interventions: Comfort level: Medication management (2380), Pain management (1400)
Observe for nonverbal cues of discomfort, especially in those unable to communicate effectively.
Determine the needed frequency of making an assessment of patient comfort and implement monitoring plan.
Control environmental factors that may influence the patient's response to discomfort.

Reduce or eliminate factors that precipitate the pain experience.
Administer analgesics around the clock to prevent peaks and troughs of analgesia.
Consider use of continuous infusion, either alone or in conjunction with bolus opioids, to maintain serum levels.
Institute safety precautions as appropriate.
Correct misconceptions/myths patient or family members may hold regarding analgesics, particularly opioids.
Document response to analgesics and any untoward effects.
Implement actions to decrease untoward effects of analgesics.
Collaborate with the physician if drug, dose, route of administration, or interval changes are indicated, making specific recommendations based on equianalgesic principles.
Major interventions: Anxiety control: Anxiety reduction (5820)
- Observe for verbal and nonverbal signs of anxiety.
- Use a calm, reassuring approach.
- Explain all procedures, including sensations likely to be experienced during the procedure.
- Encourage family to stay with patient as appropriate.
- Administer backrub, neckrub as appropriate.
- Control stimuli as appropriate for patient needs.
- Administer medications to reduce anxiety as appropriate.
Major interventions: Immobility consequences: Physiological: Positioning (0840), Bed rest care (0740)
- Place on an appropriate therapeutic mattress/bed.
- Position in proper body alignment.
- Keep bed linen clean, dry, and wrinkle free.
- Use devices on the bed (e.g., sheepskin) to protect the patient.
- Raise siderails as appropriate.
- Turn, as indicated by skin condition.
- Monitor skin condition.
- Assist with hygiene measures.
- Position to alleviate dyspnea (e.g., semi-Fowler's position) as appropriate.
- Position to facilitate ventilation/perfusion matching ("good lung down") as appropriate.
- Minimize friction and shearing forces when positioning and turning the patient.
- Prop with a backrest as appropriate.
- Develop a written schedule for repositioning as appropriate.
- Turn the immobilized patient at least every 2 hours, according to a specific schedule, as appropriate.
Major interventions: Spiritual well-being: Spiritual support (5420)
- Treat individual with dignity and respect.

Nursing Care Plan: The Older Patient at the End of Life—cont'd

- Pray with the individual.
- Assure individual that nurse will be available to support individual in times of suffering.
- Be available to listen to individual's feelings.
- Be open to individual's feelings about illness and death.
- Encourage individual to review past life and focus on events and relationships that provided spiritual strength and support.
- Facilitate individual's use of meditation, prayer, and other religious traditions and rituals.

Major interventions: Family coping: Family support (7140)

- Assure family that best care possible is being given to patient.
- Appraise family's emotional reaction to patient's condition.
- Determine the psychological burden of prognosis for family.
- Listen to family concerns, feelings, and questions.
- Facilitate communication of concerns/feelings between patient and family or between family members.
- Promote trusting relationship with family.
- Accept the family's values in a nonjudgmental manner.
- Answer all questions of family members or assist them to get answers.
- Identify nature of spiritual support for family.
- Respect and support adaptive coping mechanisms used by family.
- Provide feedback for family regarding coping.
- Provide spiritual resources for family as appropriate.

- Provide family with information about patient's progress frequently, according to patient preferences.
- Provide necessary knowledge of options to family that will assist them to make decisions about patient care.
- Include family members with patient in decision making about care when appropriate.
- Advocate for family as appropriate.
- Provide opportunities for visitation by extended family members as appropriate.
- Assist family members through the death and grief process as appropriate.

Major interventions: Grief resolution: Grief work facilitation (5290)

- Encourage expression of feelings about the loss.
- Listen to expressions of grief.
- Make empathetic statements about grief.
- Encourage identification of greatest fears about the loss.
- Encourage patient to implement cultural, religious, and social customs associated with the loss.
- Support efforts to resolve previous conflicts as appropriate.

Evaluation Parameters

Relaxed appearance; no verbalization of pain, other discomfort, or anxiety; skin intact, absence of persistent signs of pressure; expressions of peace, acceptance; family members supportive of patient and one another, accept approaching death (Box 22-7); family expresses satisfaction with care provided.

BOX 22-7 Defining a "Good Death": Patient, Family, Provider Views

- Pain and symptom management
- Clear decision making that reduces fears
- Preparation for death—that is, knowing what to expect; planning events, and so on
- Completion, including life review, dealing with issues of faith, resolution of conflicts, saying goodbye, sharing time with family and friends
- Contributing to others by sharing gifts, time, knowledge
- Affirmation of the whole person by recognition of the uniqueness of the individual

From Stajduhar, K. (2001). Patients, family members, and providers identified 6 components of a "good death." *Evidence-Based Nursing, 4*(1), 32.

continue the discussion about the ethics of this practice, what safeguards must be in place, and what role, if any, a nurse might assume.

Palliative Sedation

Palliative sedation is the use of drugs to decrease the level of consciousness in order to decrease suffering, but not with the goal of ending life. When suffering is "unrelenting and unendurable" in imminently dying patients, palliative sedation is justified on the principles of dignity, autonomy, beneficence, fidelity, nonmaleficence, and the rule of double effect. This stance is supported even if the use of sedation should hasten death (HPNA, 2003d). The position of the AAHPM is similar, and further notes that the decision to use palliative sedation is separate from decisions to withhold treatments (AAHPM, 2002a).

NURSING CARE AT END OF LIFE

As the needs of the patient evolve toward the end of life, the nurse monitors how the person is doing physically, emotionally, and spiritually and adapts care as needed. When a terminal diagnosis is made or the futility of curative interventions is recognized, the nurse anticipates a kaleidoscope of emotions that come and go in unique patterns. Patients face practical questions about their future and existential questions about their place in the universe. If older adults have not already done so, most want to be certain their legal affairs are in order. There may be a need to repair relationships, or lifetime dreams to be fulfilled. During the time when the patient may still be physically able, the nurse might encourage continued physical activity and socialization to maintain connections. Some people set about creating a legacy by which they hope to be remembered.

As symptoms become more troubling and function declines, the patient's world begins to shrink. Activities that are less valued or require too much energy are discarded. Physical needs consume more time, but are no more important than the continuing emotional and spiritual needs. For an illustration of the events leading up to the final days of life, see the Nursing Care Plan. Also, for various Web resources related to end of life nursing care, see Box 22-6.

SUMMARY

The role of the nurse is to promote the highest possible quality of life from birth to death. When the end of life approaches, the nurse strives to preserve the dignity and comfort of the patient, to assure that the patient's directives are followed, and to provide support to the patient and the family. Connecting older adults and their families at the end of life with the services they require is also a role of the health care team. It is essential that nurses themselves are healthy if they are to provide appropriate support and care to those who are at or near the end of life. Nurses who care for patients at the end of life must recognize that they also experience a loss when a patient dies. To continue to be supportive of patients and families, nurses must take care of themselves as well, whether it is through the use of friends and lay support or the use of professional services. Nurse researchers have much work to do in terms of end of life care. Lorenz (2004) studied the evidence available to support the use of various interventions at end of life. He identified thousands of articles on the topic, but noted that most were exploratory, leaving the following questions to be addressed:

- What services are needed at end of life?
- What is the ideal time before death to implement those services?
- What are the aims of those services?

In a state of the science paper on end of life research, George (2002) points out the lack of rigorous testing of accepted approaches such as use of the WHO ladder of analgesics or the merits of palliative care.

REFERENCES

Agency for Health Care Policy and Research (AHCPR). (1994). *Guidelines for management of pain*. Bethesda, MD: National Institutes of Health.

American Academy of Colleges of Nursing. (2001). Peaceful death: Recommended competencies and curricular requirements for quality end of life care. Retrieved May 10, 2006, from www.aacn.nche.edu/Publications/deathfin.htm.

American Academy of Hospice and Palliative Medicine. (1997). Comprehensive end of life care and physician assisted suicide. Retrieved August 21, 2005, from www.aahpm.org.

American Academy of Hospice and Palliative Medicine. (2002a). Statement on sedation at the end of life. Retrieved August 21, 2005, from www.aahpm.org.

American Academy of Hospice and Palliative Medicine. (2002b). Statement on the ethics of palliative care research. Retrieved August 21, 2005, from www.aahpm.org.

American Nurses Association (ANA). (2002). *Position statement: Assisted suicide*. Washington, DC: The Association.

American Nurses Association (ANA). (1998). *Position statement: Assisted suicide*. Washington, DC: The Association.

American Nurses Association (ANA). (1994). Position statement: Assisted suicide: Retrieved March 25, 2002, from http://nursingworld.org/redroom/position/ethics/etsuic.htm.

American Pain Foundation. (2005). Pain management for end of life. Retrieved August 24, 2005, from www.painfoundation.org.

American Psychiatric Association (APA). (2000). *Practice guidelines for the treatment of patients with major depression* (2nd ed.). Washington, DC: American Psychiatric Publishing.

American Psychiatric Association (APA). (1994). *Diagnostic and statistical manual of mental disorders IV*. Washington, DC: The Association.

American Society for Pain Management Nursing (ASPMN). (2003). ASPMN position statement: Pain management at the end of life. Retrieved August 24, 2005, from www.aspmn.org.

American Society for Pain Management Nursing (ASPMN). (1996). Position statement: Pain management at the end of life. Retrieved August 24, 2005, from www.aspmn.org.

Angus, D. C., Barnato, A. E., Linde-Zwirble, W. T., Weissfeld L. A., Watson R. S., Richert T., Rubenfeld G. D., & Robert Wood Johnson Foundation ICU End-Of-Life Peer Group. (2004). Use of intensive care at the end of life in the United States: an epidemiological study. *Critical Care Medicine, 32(3)*, 638-643.

Baile, W. F., Buckman, R., Lenzi, R., Glober, G., Beale, E. A., & Kudelka, A. P. (2000). SPIKES—A six-step protocol for delivering bad news: Application to the patient with cancer. *The Oncologist, 5*, 302-311.

Ballard, D. (2000). Legal and ethical issues. In A. G. Lueckenotte (Ed.), *Gerontological nursing*. St. Louis: Mosby, pp. 34-62.

Baggs, J. G. (2002). End of life care for older adults in ICUs. *Annual Review of Nursing Research, 32*, 181-229.

Bowlby, J. (1980). *Attachment and loss: Loss, sadness and depression* (Vol. 3). New York: Basic Books.

Bruera, E., & Neumann, C. M. (1998). Management of specific symptom complexes in patients receiving palliative care. *Canadian Medical Association Journal, 158*, 1717-1726.

Cain, J. M., and Hannes, B. L. (1994). Ethics and pain mangement: Respecting patient wishes. *Journal of Pain and Symptom Management, 9*, 160-165.

Casarett, D. (2004, December 6-8). Ethical considerations in end-of-life care and research. NIH State-of-the-Science Conference on Improving End-of-Life Care, Bethesda, MD.

Chochinov, H., Wilson, K., Enns, M., & Lander, S. (1998). Depression, hopelessness and suicidal ideation in the terminally ill. *Psychosomatics, 39*, 366-370.

Chochinov, H. M. (2004, December 6-8). Interventions to enhance the spiritual aspects of dying. NIH State-of-the-Science Conference on Improving End-of-Life Care, Bethesda, MD.

Christakis, N. A., & Lamont, E. B. (2000). The extent and determinants of error in physicians' prognoses for terminally ill patients. *British Medical Journal, 320*(7233), 469-473.

Copp, L. A. (1990). The spectrum of grief suffering. *American Journal of Nursing, 90*, 35-39.

Corless, I. B. (2001). Bereavement. In B. R. Ferrell & N. Coyle (Eds.), *Textbook of palliative nursing.* New York: Oxford University Press, pp. 352-362.

Costello, J. (2001). Nursing older dying patients: Findings from an ethnographic study of death and dying in elderly care wards. *Journal of Advanced Nursing, 35*(1), 59-68.

Council on Scientific Affairs. (1996). Good care of the dying patient. *Journal of the American Medical Association, 275*, 474-478.

Cowles, K. V. (1996). Cultural perspectives of grief: An expanded concept analysis. *Journal of Advanced Nursing, 23*, 287-294.

Critchlow, J., & Bauer-Wu, S. M. (2002). Dehydration in terminally ill patients. *Journal of Gerontological Nursing, 28*(12), 31-39.

Curtis, J. R. (2004, December 6-8). Interventions to facilitate withdrawal of life-sustaining treatments. NIH State-of-the-Science Conference on Improving End-of-Life Care, Bethesda, MD.

Decker, S. A., & Perry, S. A. (2003). The development and testing of the PATCOA to assess pain in confused older adults. *Pain Management Nursing, 4*(2), 77-86.

Derby, S., & O'Mahony, S. (2005). Elderly patients. In B. R. Ferrell & N. Coyle (Eds.), *Textbook of palliative nursing.* New York: Oxford University Press, pp. 635-660.

Desbiens, N. A., Wu, A. W., Broste, S. K., Wenger, N. S., Connors, A. F., Lynn, J., et al. (1996). Pain and satisfaction with pain control in seriously ill hospitalized adults: Findings from the SUPPORT research investigations. *Critical Care Medicine, 24*, 1953-1961.

Dochterman, J. M., & Bulechek, G. M. (2004). *Nursing interventions classification (NIC)* (4th ed.). St. Louis: Mosby.

Dudgeon, D. (2001). Dyspnea, death rattle and cough. In B. R. Ferrell & N. Coyle (Eds.), *Textbook of palliative nursing.* New York: Oxford University Press, pp. 164-174.

Dunphy, K., Finlay, I., Rathbone, G., Gilbert, J., & Hicks, F. (1995). Rehydration in palliative and terminal care: if not—why not? *Palliative Medicine, 9*(3), 221-228.

Economou, D. C. (2001). Bowel management: Constipation, diarrhea, obstruction, and ascites. In B. R. Ferrell & N. Coyle (Eds.), *Textbook of palliative nursing.* New York: Oxford University Press, pp. 139-155.

End of Life Nursing Education Consortium (ELNEC). (2000). *ELNEC course syllabus.* Washington, DC: American Association of Colleges of Nursing and City of Hope National Medical Center.

Emmet, J., Byock, I., & Sheils Twohig, J. (2002). Advanced practice nursing: Pioneering practices in palliative care. *Promoting excellence in end-of-life care.* New York: The Robert Wood Johnson Foundation.

Feldt, K. S. (2000). The Checklist of Nonverbal Pain Indicators (CNPI). *Pain Management Nursing, 1*, 13-21.

Feldt, K. S., Ryden, M. B., & Miles, S. (1998). Treatment of pain in cognitively impaired compared with cognitively intact older patients with hip-fracture. *Journal of the American Geriatrics Society, 46*, 1079-1085.

Finucane, T. (2004, December 6-8). Preferences and changes in the goals of care. NIH State-of-the-Science Conference on Improving End-of-Life Care, Bethesda, MD.

Freud, S. (1957). *General psychological theory.* London: Thunderbolt Books.

Galla, J. H. (2000). Clinical practice guideline on shared decision-making in the appropriate initiation of and withdrawal from dialysis. The Renal Physicians Association and the American Society of Nephrology. *Journal of the American Society of Nephrology, 11*, 1340-1342.

George, L. K. (2002). Research design in end of life research: State of science. *Gerontologist, 42*(3), 86-98.

Gullate, M. M., Kaplow, R., & Heidrich, D. E. (2005). Oncology. In K. K. Kuebler, M. P. Davis, & C. D. Moore (Eds.), *Palliative practices: An interdisciplinary approach.* St. Louis: Elsevier, pp. 197-245.

Guyton, A. C., & Hall, J. E. (2000). *Textbook of medical physiology* (10th ed.). Philadelphia: Saunders.

Hall, C. T. (1999). In search of a good death. *San Francisco Chronicle.* Retrieved August 4, 2005, from www.sfgate.com.

Higginson, I. J. (2004, December 6-8). Lessons from other nations. NIH State-of-the-Science Conference on Improving End-of-Life Care, Bethesda, MD.

Horowitz, M. J., Siegel, B., Holen, A., Bonanno, G. A., Milbrath, C., & Stinson, C. H. (1997). Diagnostic criteria for complicated grief disorder. *American Journal of Psychiatry, 154*, 904-910.

Hospice and Palliative Care Nurses Association (HPNA). (2001). HPNA Position Statement: Legalization of assisted suicide. Retrieved August 21, 2005, from www.HPNA.org.

Hospice and Palliative Care Nurses Association (HPNA). (2003a). HPNA Position Statement: Artificial nutrition and hydration in end of life care. Retrieved August 21, 2005, from www.HPNA.org.

Hospice and Palliative Care Nurses Association (HPNA). (2003b). HPNA Position Statement: Complementary therapies. Retrieved August 21, 2005, from www.HPNA.org.

Hospice and Palliative Care Nurses Association (HPNA). (2003c). HPNA Position Statement: Pain. Retrieved August 21, 2005, from www.HPNA.org.

Hospice and Palliative Care Nurses Association (HPNA). (2003d). HPNA Position Statement: Palliative sedation at end of life. Retrieved August 21, 2005, from www.HPNA.org.

Hospice and Palliative Care Nurses Association (HPNA). (2004). HPNA Position Statement: Providing opioids at the end of life. Retrieved August 21, 2005, from www.HPNA.org.

Hospice and Palliative Care Coalition (HPCC). (2005). HPCC responds to misleading information regarding forgoing artificial nutrition and hydration. Retrieved August 21, 2005, from www.aahpm.org/positions.

Karlawish, J. H., Quill, T., & Meier, D. E. (1999). A consensus based approach to providing palliative care to patients who lack decision-making capacity. *Annals of Internal Medicine, 130*, 835-840.

Karnofsky, D. A., & Burchenal, J. H. (1949). The clinical evaluation of chemotherapeutic agents in cancer. In C. M. MacLeod (Ed.), *Evaluation of chemotherapeutic agents.* New York: Columbia University Press, p. 196.

Karnofsky, D. A., Abelmann, W. H., Craver, L. F., et al. (1948). The use of the nitrogen mustards in the palliative treatment of carcinoma. *Cancer, 1*, 634-656.

Kazanowski, M. (2001). Symptom management in palliative care. In M. Matzo & W. Sherman (Eds.), *Palliative care nursing: Quality care to the end of life.* New York: Springer-Verlag, pp. 327-361.

Klinkenberg, M., Willems, D. L., van der Wal, G., & Deeg, D. J. H. (2004). Symptom burden in the last week of life. *Journal of Pain and Symptom Management, 27*(1), 5-13.

Krisman-Scott, M. A. (2003). Origins of hospice in the United States: The care of the dying 1945-1975. *Journal of Hospice & Palliative Nursing, 5*(4), 205-210.

Kubler-Ross, E. (1969). *On death and dying.* New York: Macmillan.

Lamont, E. (2002, December 6-8). A demographic and prognostic approach to defining the end of life. NIH State-of-the-Science Conference on Improving End-of-Life Care, Bethesda, MD.

Leland, J. Y. (2000). Death and dying management of patients with end-stage disease. *Clinics in Geriatric Medicine, 16*(4), 875-890.

Lentz, J. (2004). A conversation with Florence Wald. *Journal of Hospice & Palliative Nursing, 6*(1), 9-10.

Lewis, M., Pearson, V., Corcoran-Perry, S., & Narayan, S. (1997). Decision making by elderly patients with cancer and their caregivers. *Cancer Nursing, 20,* 389-397.

Lindemann, E. (1994). Symptomatology and management of acute grief. 1944. *American Journal of Psychiatry, 151*(6; suppl), 155-160.

Liptzin, B., & Levkoff, S. E. (1992). An empirical study of delirium subtypes. *British Journal of Psychiatry, 161,* 843-845.

Lorenz, K. (2004, December 6-8). Evidence-based practice center presentation: Interventions to improve outcomes for patients and families. NIH State-of-the-Science Conference on Improving End-of-Life Care, Bethesda, MD.

Mallison, R. K. (1999). Griefwork of HIV-positive persons and their survivors. *Nursing Clinics of North America, 34*(1), 163-177.

Marshall, P. L. (2001). End of life care symptom management, *Kansas Nurse, 76*(7), 1-3.

McMillan, S. C. (2004, December 6-8). Interventions to facilitate family caregiving. NIH State-of-the-Science Conference on Improving End-of-Life Care, Bethesda, MD.

Miller, K. E., Miller, M. M., & Jolley, M. R. (2001). Challenges in pain management at the end of life. *American Family Physician, 64,* 1227-1234.

Moorhead, S., Johnson, M., & Maas, M. (2004). *Nursing outcomes classification (NOC)* (3rd ed.). St. Louis: Mosby.

Morita, T., Ichiki, T., Tsunoda, J., Inoue, S., & Chihara, S. (1998). A prospective study on the dying process in terminally ill cancer patients. *American Journal of Hospice and Palliative Care, 15*(4), 217-222.

NANDA International. (2005). *Nursing diagnoses: Definitions and classification 2005-2006.* Philadelphia: NANDA International.

National Association of Hospice Care. (2002). *Hospice facts & statistics.* Retrieved March 28, 2005, from www.nahc.org/Consumer/hpstats.html.

National Consensus Project for Quality Palliative Care. (2004). *Clinical practice guidelines for quality palliative care.* National Hospice and Palliative Care Organization. Accessed online at www.nhpco.org.

National Council for Hospice and Specialist Palliative Care Services (NCHSPCS). (1993). In I. Higginson (Ed.), *Matching services to individual needs.* London: NCHSPC.

Oncology Nurses Society (ONS). (2001). The nurse's responsibility to the patient requesting assisted suicide. *Oncology Nursing Forum. 28*(3), 442.

Pantilat, S. Z., & Steimle, A. E. (2004). Palliative care for patients with heart failure. *Journal of the American Medical Association, 291,* 2476-2482.

Parkes, C. P. (1972). *Bereavement studies of grief in adult life.* London: Pelican.

Pasacreta, J., Minarik, P., & Nield-Anderson, L. (2001). In B. R. Ferrell & N. Coyle (Eds.), *Textbook of palliative nursing.* New York: Oxford University Press, pp. 269-289.

Potter, M. L. (2001). Loss, suffering, bereavement, and grief. In M. L. Matzo & D. W. Sherman (Eds.), *Palliative care nursing: Quality care to the end of life.* New York: Springer, pp. 275-321.

Puchalski, C. (1999). Promoting excellence: HIV care: An agenda for change: Appendix B. FICA: Taking a spiritual history. Retrieved April 30, 2005, from www.promotingexcellence.org/tools/index.

Puchalski, C. & Romer, A. L. (2000). Taking a spiritual history allows clinicians to understand patients. *Journal of Palliative Medicine, 3,* 129-137.

Radziewicz, R., & Baile, W. F. (2001). Communication skills: breaking bad news in the clinical setting. *Oncology Nursing Forum, 28,* 951-953.

Rain, R. (1999). Alternatives to guardianship. In L. A. Polk (Ed.), *Aging and the law.* Philadelphia: Temple University Press, pp. 285-294.

Rando, T. (1986). *Loss and anticipatory grief.* Lexington, MA: Lexington Books.

Roberts, K. F., & Berry, P. H. (2002). In K. K. Kuebler, P. H. Berry, & D. E. Heidrich (Eds.), *End of life care, Clinical practice guidelines.* Philadelphia: Saunders, pp. 53-63.

Rochon, T., & Heller, K. S. (2002). A nurse practitioner palliative care consult service for nursing homes. *Innovations in End of Life Care, 4*(2). Retrieved August 24, 2005, from www2.edc.org/lastacts/archivesMarch02/promprac.asp.

Seery, D. H. (2004). Shifting gears: from cure to comfort. *RN, 67*(11), 52-57.

Sheehan, D., & Forman, W (1996). *Hospice & palliative care: Concepts & practice.* Boston: Jones & Bartlett.

Sherman, D. W. (1999). End of life care: Challenges and opportunities for health professionals. *The Hospice Journal, 14,* 109-121.

Sherman, D. W., Matzo, M. L., Coyne, P., Ferrell, B. R., & Penn, B. K. (2004). Teaching symptom management in end of life care: The didactic content and teaching strategies based on the end of life nursing education curriculum. *Journal for Nurses in Staff Development, 20*(3), 103-115.

Shotton, L. (2000). Can nurses contribute to better end-of life care? *Nursing Ethics, 7*(2), 134-139.

Singer, P. A., Martin, D. K., & Kelner, M. (1999). Quality end of life care: Patients' perspectives. *Journal of the American Medical Association, 281,* 163-168.

Stajduhar, K. (2001). Patients, family members, and providers identified 6 components of a "good death." *Evidence-Based Nursing, 4*(1), 32.

Stroebe, M. (2004). *Interventions to enhance grief resolution.* NIH State of the Science Conference on Improving End of Life Care. Bethesda, MD: National Institutes of Health.

SUPPORT Principal Investigators. (1995). A controlled trial to improve care for seriously ill hospitalized patients. The study to understand prognosis and preferences for outcomes and risks of treatment. *Journal of the American Medical Association, 274,* 1591-1598.

Tarzian, A. J. (2000). Caring for dying patients who have air hunger. *Journal of Nursing Scholarship, 32*(2), 137-143.

Texas Cancer Council. (2003). *Guidelines for treatment of cancer pain.* Austin, TX: Texas Cancer Council.

Thompson, M. H. (1994). Ethics committees: Their share in the advocacy role. *Seminars in Perioperative Nursing, 5,* 62-67.

Treece, P. D., Engelberg, R. A., Crowley, L., Chan, J. D., Rubenfeld G. D., Steinberg K.P., & Curtis J. R. (2004). Evaluation of a standardized order form for the withdrawal of life support in the intensive care unit. *Critical Care Medicine, 32,* 1141-1148.

Virani, R., & Sofer, D. (2003). Improving the quality of end of life care: Making changes at every level. *American Journal of Nursing, 103*(5), 52-60.

Wakefield, B., & Johnson, J. A. (2001). Acute confusion in terminally ill hospitalized patients. *Journal of Gerontological Nursing, 27*(4), 49-55.

Welsh, J., Fallon, M., & Kelley, P. W. (2003). Palliative care. In R. C. Tallis & H. M. Fillit (Eds.), *Brocklehurst's textbook of geriatric medicine and gerontology* (6th ed.). London: Churchill Livingstone, pp. 257-271.

World Health Organization (WHO). (2002).

Worden J. W. (1991). *Grief counseling and grief therapy: A handbook for the mental health practitioner* (2nd ed.). New York: Springer.

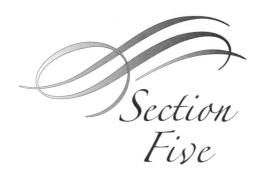

Section Five

Competencies and Roles in Gerontological Nursing

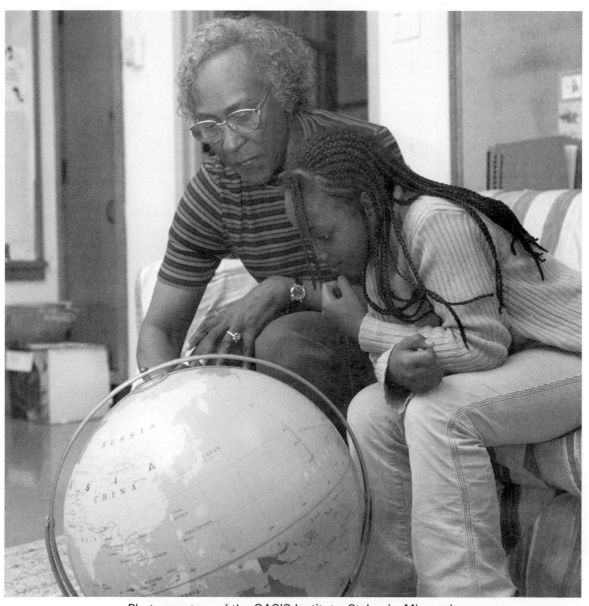

Photo courtesy of the OASIS Institute, St. Louis, Missouri.

Chapter 23

Leadership Skills

Nina Tumosa & Helen W. Lach

Objectives

Identify core competencies associated with leadership.
Discuss traits associated with gerontological nursing for each core competency.
Describe the importance of change management to gerontological nurses.
Identify traits the nurse should cultivate in different settings to be effective agents of change.

Leadership is an important tool for the gerontological nurse, especially in this new age of rapid health care changes that have been instigated to reduce the costs of health care. As in any time of change, there are many opportunities to influence how health care is delivered. As the primary patient advocate, nurses have a responsibility to seize every opportunity to better serve the patient. This is more easily accomplished by being a leader, by being in a position of authority to affect outcomes, and by influencing systems to change to the advantage of the patient. However, some misguided assumptions about leadership may hinder nurses' perceptions or applications of leadership skills.

First, many assume that leadership roles are held solely by those in administrative positions. In fact, the interdisciplinary nature of clinical geriatrics and gerontology means that clinical leaders are also needed to inform others of the best patient outcomes and the best paths for achieving positive outcomes. As a result, gerontological nurses need to develop leadership competencies so that they can fill either formal leadership roles as administrators or informal leadership roles as clinical leaders to help improve the health care system for older patients. They may serve on interdisciplinary teams or in quality improvement projects; as patient advocates, teachers, or role models; and in many other applications of leadership. Advance practice nurses are likely to be in many situations in which they can assume leadership roles and influence change.

Another misconception of leadership is that leaders have innate abilities rather than skills that can be learned and developed. Some leaders have more natural charisma than others, which is a helpful quality. However, most people are not born leaders; they have worked to develop and hone their skills over time. McConnell (2003) states that "the fundamental difference between the leader and the non-leader is often marked by no more than the extent to which the individual has succeeded in learning about leadership and putting what has been learned into practice" (p. 361). Unfortunately, nurses often receive little formal leadership training (Tourangeau, 2003), and so may not have the opportunities to learn and develop skills needed in this time of growing shortages of nurses and nurse educators.

Great leaders are often created by a crisis. Everyone can think of great leaders who took charge and did whatever was needed to avert or ameliorate a crisis. We all have heroes whom we admire for their ability to "do the right thing" against impossible odds or against usual expectations. Florence Nightingale and Clara Barton are but two nurses that are heroes not only of other nurses but also for many people in health careers today.

Leadership, however, need not be quite so dramatic. Some people quietly do their jobs, identifying and solving problems, taking advantage of opportunities, and generally leaving the world a better place than they found it. These people are also effective leaders. It is to these prospective leaders that this chapter is addressed. This chapter is designed to provide an overview of competencies that every gerontological nurse can develop, through self-assessment, reflection, and acquisition of the knowledge and skills that will ultimately improve the care for our older patients.

Another issue that affects leadership in gerontological nursing is the small number of nurses trained in the care of older adults. As a result, each of us who is so trained has an obligation to develop and use leadership competencies and skills, even if we apply them to only one unit in one facility. In addition, because staff come and go, they will take what they learn to other units or facilities. Thus gerontological nurses can have an influence that reaches far beyond the traditional vision. The following sections will describe the core competencies of leadership, leadership styles, and issues related to leading through change.

CORE COMPETENCIES OF LEADERSHIP

Leadership is often defined as a process of influencing people to accomplish goals (Huber et al., 2000). Many qualified people have published papers on models of leadership styles and characteristics of great leaders (Deming, 1993; Roberts, 1987; Senge, 1994). For the purposes of this chapter, we will use a set of competencies of leadership developed by Flannery et al. (1996) and adapted by the Veteran's Administration (American College of Hospital Administration, 1997). They include personal mastery, organizational stewardship, systems thinking, customer service, creative thinking, flexibility/adaptability, technical expertise, and interpersonal effectiveness (Table 23-1). These core competencies all

Table 23-1 *Core Competencies of Leadership*	
Personal mastery	Develops both personally and professionally
Organizational stewardship	Supports the mission and values of the organization, especially when there is change
Systems thinking	Sees the big picture and knows how individual components interact
Customer service	Integrates all stakeholders to provide successful services that are of high quality and also cost effective
Creative thinking	Solves problems creatively
Flexibility/adaptability	Embraces change
Technical expertise	Maintains up-to-date skills and knowledge
Interpersonal effectiveness	Builds and sustains collaborative working relationships, resolves conflict, and communicates and negotiates effectively

have unique qualifiers that can be adapted to nursing paradigms.

Each of these qualifiers is briefly described below for each of the core competencies. Also included are examples and resources to help increase the gerontological nurse's knowledge and skills in these competencies. This discussion is accompanied by the reflections of one of the important leaders in gerontological nursing today—Dr. May Wykle, who is the Dean of the Frances Payne Bolton School of Nursing at Case Western Reserve University (Box 23-1). She is gracious in sharing information about how her career developed. We have many exceptional leaders in gerontological nursing today, and readers should take advantage of the opportunity to hear and learn from these leaders through readings and national conferences. These leaders have much to share to help shape gerontological nursing in the future.

Personal Mastery

Personal mastery requires that a leader invest in himself or herself. As stated in the introduction, knowledge and skills about leadership can be developed through a variety of learning methods (Grossman & Valiga, 2000). In addition, nurses should strive for a balanced life, taking a holistic approach to themselves much as they do with their patients. By working to develop as healthy human beings, nurses will develop a strong base from which to grow as a leader.

The leader should develop short-term and long-term goals and demonstrate a passion for excellence in every aspect of his or her life and career. In order to do that, a leader must:

- Assume responsibility for personal development toward career goals
- Find a balance between personal and career demands
- Learn from personal failures as well as from personal successes
- Safeguard physical, mental, and emotional health
- Continuously improve skills, knowledge, and behavior
- Understand how he/she is perceived by others

Good leaders are aware of how their personal and emotional states impact others around them, a feature known as emotional intelligence (Goleman, 1998). Leaders reflect and manage emotionally charged issues by attending to their own responses as well as the responses of others. The leader develops empathy by listening and attempting to understand others' positions and feelings and using appropriate leadership styles for specific situations and groups. Porter-O'Grady (2003a) concurs that emotional intelligence is an important attribute the nurse leader needs to develop.

Currently, there is a shortage of leaders who understand the challenges of caring for older people, who can articulate how special gerontological nursing is, and who will help us continue to build this important specialty. We have a great need for gerontological nurses, faculty, curriculum, and resources to educate practitioners about geriatric issues and the challenge of improving the quality of life for seniors. The leadership competencies outlined in this chapter describe skills that are developed through experience, education, reflection, self-appraisal, and exchange with others. Leadership in gerontological nursing is a continual process of "becoming" that addresses these competencies.

My many nursing experiences have contributed immensely to my development as a leader. I have had positions as a psychiatric staff nurse, head nurse, supervisor, and liaison nurse. I have advanced through the ranks of academia as a faculty member at Case Western Reserve University's Frances Payne Bolton School of Nursing. All of these positions provided role models and mentors that helped me acquire additional leadership skills. I believe that I have benefited from every job I have ever had, as well as by every position I've held as an officer in several nursing organizations. It is essential to learn what your weaknesses are and how to accommodate for them by having good people around you. As an agent of change, one has to be flexible and know how to delegate tasks appropriately to others and evaluate the accomplishments. Leaders have to be open to exploring and listening, and they have to take criticism as a means of helping them grow personally and professionally. Through the years, I have learned to use different leadership styles for a variety of situations, for different people and at different times, while valuing the servant-leader role.

Hopefully, good leaders take care of their physical and mental health, stopping once in a while to "smell the roses." Achieving a balanced life requires consideration of family as part of the perspective of work to be done and is of equal importance in becoming a successful leader. A sense of spirituality provides leaders with a more rounded view of their work with others, and it underscores the development of interpersonal skills and the ability as leaders to juggle all of their tasks and responsibilities.

One of the important features of good leaders is their ability to build leadership in others and share their vision. In gerontological nursing, exceptional leaders who understand the concerns of an older population are vitally needed. It is critical that we play a part in helping others develop leadership skills. The following are ways we can promote gerontological nursing and support gerontological nurse leaders:

- Develop partnerships and mentorships to support each other, because honest feedback is essential for growth.
- Collaborate with other disciplines to build clinical research programs to improve the care for older adults.
- Participate with our nursing and geriatric organizations to disseminate information broadly.
- Strive for excellence in gerontological nursing education and translation of research findings into practice and policy.

Working together, we can build leaders in gerontological nursing for the twenty-first century, leaders who will address the special physical, developmental, and psychosocial needs of a growing older population and improve their quality of life through quality care.

May Wykle

May Wykle, PhD, RN, FAAN, FGSA
Dean and Florence Cellar Professor of Gerontological Nursing
Frances Payne Bolton School of Nursing
Case Western Reserve University
Cleveland, Ohio

Organizational Stewardship

Good **organizational stewardship** requires leaders to understand the mission, vision, and values of the organization and to act accordingly when representing that organization. The manner in which the mission and values of an organization are implemented may be undergoing rapid changes, so the leadership needs to continuously monitor the situation within their organization and communicate changes to others. In addition, the leader may need to help the organization understand when certain changes do not fit its mission by effectively communicating to management and administration these concerns.

Those model behaviors, attitudes, and actions should result from:

- Accepting accountability for the development of the organization
- Accomplishing the organizational business plan to improve health care
- Managing fiscal, social, physical, and human resources responsibly
- Empowering and trusting others to carry out their responsibilities
- Integrating the organization into the larger health care community
- Promoting opportunities for future change and development

An important component of leadership is assuming the responsibilities that go along with benefits of leadership, particularly leadership positions (McConnell, 2003). This means focusing on the needs of the organization and others, and not just the potential benefits of being a leader. A good leader serves as a mentor and works to develop others to be able to support the organization's development. A leader is also a role model in demonstrating the ethics and values of the organization.

Systems Thinking

Leaders who demonstrate **systems thinking** understand the roles ands value of all persons who provide health care, help others better understand their role in the big picture, are invaluable in explaining to others how change will affect them, and help create a climate of collaboration, rather than of competition. Characteristics of a person who is good at systems thinking include:

- Sees the big picture
- Never underestimates the value of anyone
- Helps others think in the broader context
- Encourages and rewards collaboration
- Remembers that the purpose of health care is to improve health
- Keeps an eye on the bottom line

The leader needs to continuously monitor developments in the field of health care, including legal issues, financial issues, organizational issues, and professional issues. For example, leaders today need to understand the changing relationships between employees and employers resulting from the mobility of workers, outsourcing of services, and shifting of loyalties (Porter-O'Grady, 2003a). These changes require leaders to have greater skills in communication, negotiation, and team building with an ever-changing workforce.

Customer Service

Good **customer service** entails the recognition of who the customer is. Depending upon the situation, it may be a patient, a family member, a student, a colleague, the media, a business, or an organization. The following attributes are necessary for a good leader to maintain and improve good customer service:

- Understands that customer service is critical to good care
- Sets up protocols to effectively address customer complaints promptly
- Uses customer feedback to improve services
- Identifies and rewards good customer service

Henry (2002, p. 1275) states that "nursing leadership entails ensuring high quality and cost effective services that are accessible to those most in need and provided by competent, satisfied workers." Nurses have always served as patient advocates, a role that can be extended to groups and communities (Davies & Hughes, 2002). As a result, nurses are in a good position to help ensure quality care is provided in a way that also provides good customer service.

Creative Thinking

Creative thinking requires that leaders demonstrate a willingness to generate new ideas and challenge assumptions, and encourage others to do the same. To do this, a leader must:

- Always be looking beyond the "status quo"
- Identify opportunities for providing better health care
- Reward both risk-taking and failure
- Learn as much from mistakes as from successes

Fasnacht (2003, p. 201) has defined creativity as "a process that occurs in response to a need or desire and generates a unique outcome" and states that it may be influenced by the environment. From another perspective, Myra Levine (1973) defined creativity as "the marriage of the art and science of nursing." With the future challenge of so many older patients, gerontological nurses will require creativity to identify ways to provide adequate and appropriate care to this growing population. The same old ways of doing things will not be possible, and we will need creative solutions for a new set of problems. Gerontological nurses will need to use their art and science to develop new models of care.

Flexibility and Adaptability

Flexibility and adaptability in leaders requires that they walk a fine line between appearing to be open to new ideas from others and appearing to be unable to think for themselves; being respectful and tolerant of differences in the workplace and being thought of as uncaring about traditions; being responsive to changes in priorities and being unable to hold any convictions. Because change requires embracing the new without disrespecting the old, a leader who is truly flexible must know how to:

- Respond appropriately to change
- Remain calm under pressure
- Be able to integrate the old and the new work objectives
- Seek out and incorporate input from others
- Understand change management

Good leaders are able to fulfill the traditional managerial roles of planning, organizing, directing, and controlling (Anderson & Robinson, 2001) when needed to accomplish organizational tasks. In addition, leaders need to be flexible enough to assume broader roles as clinical leaders, advocates, policy shapers, and many other positions as needed.

Technical Expertise

A leader who demonstrates **technical expertise** has maintained a level of knowledge and skills commensurate with maintaining a safe and up-to-date environment in which appropriate health care can be provided. In order to accomplish this, a leader must:

- Maintain skill levels appropriate to perform assigned duties
- Demonstrate functional and technical literacy
- Keep current with new developments in health care
- Participate in quality improvement and in performance measurement
- Know how to effectively use available technology

With the rapid advances in health care, gerontological nurses must commit to lifelong learning to stay current and up-to-date regarding practice, education, and/or research in health care in general and in their specialty in particular. In addition, leaders must learn to embrace the new technologies and obtain the skills to keep up. For example, advanced practice nurses now use personal digital assistants (PDAs) to help with scheduling and managing their practice. In addition, these devices can be used as a handy reference for drug information, clinical guidelines, and other important information. The good leader will also use judgement in adopting new approaches and technologies, using methods from evidence-based practice for evaluating new practices before adopting them, and evaluating changes once they are made to assure that they are useful.

Interpersonal Effectiveness

Interpersonal effectiveness is a necessary trait at all levels of patient care, whether it is eliciting an accurate patient history, working with a family to build consensus for treatment of a comatose patient, negotiating with office staff to change billing procedures, or lobbying the state legislature to pass legislation more favorable to Medicaid patients. Traits used at all of those levels include:

- Soliciting and incorporating other opinions
- Showing sensitivity and compassion for others
- Building consensus
- Earning trust
- Communicating well, orally and in writing

The ability to build relationships with a broad range of people and groups will serve the gerontological nursing leader well. For example, the nurse needs to work with patients, families, many levels of nursing personnel, physicians and other health care professionals, administrators, policymakers, third-party payers, the media, and the public at large. The National Association of Clinical Nurse Specialists (2004) has identified the three spheres of influence for the nurse: patient/client care, practice of other nurses and nursing personnel, and health care organizations (Figure 23-1). The nursing leader uses the skills and knowledge of their specialty practice in each sphere to affect patient care.

Developing and refining communication skills are critical to building successful relationships. Kerfoot (2004, p. 157) describes leaders who inspire others by creating "an environment that meets the needs of the people first, not the leader's needs." Strong interpersonal effectiveness will ensure that the leader understands the needs of others, including patients and other health care workers.

In summary, all of these leadership competencies are similar whether they apply to health care, business (Demming, 1993), or learning organizations (Senge, 1994). These attributes are not innate in many of us. However, they can be acquired through study and hard work. All of these competencies require continuous learning, constant development of skill sets, and consistent application of these skills to both work and personal scenarios.

Several nurses have also drawn our attention to the fact that nursing leadership is critical in dealing with changes in health care today (Anderson & Robinson, 2001; Antrobus & Kitson, 1999; Laurent, 2000; Perra, 2000; Porter-O'Grady, 1997, 1999; Sullivan & Decker, 2004). The rest of this chapter will serve to make the case that nurses must embrace leadership in their personal lives, within the profession, and across interprofessional lines, in order to be the agents of constructive change that will improve health care in this country.

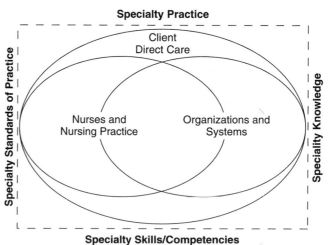

Figure 23-1 Spheres of influence of the clinical nurse specialist. (From National Association of Clinical Nurse Specialists. [2004]. *Statement on clinical nurse specialist practice and education.* Harrisburg, PA: National Association of Clinical Nurse Specialists.)

LEADING THROUGH CHANGE

The twenty-first century has arrived on the heels of many changes. One of the truer descriptions of modern health care is that change is constant. In health care, these changes have included the introduction of continuous quality improvement, the acknowledgment that the patient is a valued member of the health care team, an awareness of the ethical conundrums of health care, health care reform, the introduction of managed care, Medicare and Medicaid reforms, the new role of interdisciplinary care, and the rising numbers of uninsured to over 45 million people.

Change is also a normal part of the life cycle of organizations (Bruhn, 2004). Change is important in improving patient care and incorporating new practices (Buonocore, 2004). Unless a leader embraces change, they will be left behind. As Porter-O'Grady (2003a, 2003b) notes, nurses today need to incorporate changes quickly, even before they can adjust to the impact of these changes.

Components of Change

Concepts that need to be addressed concerning change leadership include the following: (1) What are the components of change? (2) How have strategies of leadership changed in the twenty-first century? (3) Which core competencies are most needed to effect change? The following discussion covers each of these issues.

A number of theories have been introduced that describe change as a process that individuals and groups pass though in adopting or making a change. Lewin (1951) was one of the early writers who described the change process as having three stages: unfreezing, moving, and refreezing. In the unfreezing stage, the individual or group considers making a change and then moves to do it. When the change is adopted, then refreezing has taken place. Many variations on this basic theory exist, and we will discuss further the components of change according to one set of authors: Cooperrider & Whitney (2000).

- **Recognition:** To effectively negotiate change, a leader must recognize that there is a need for change. Along with that recognition must be an understanding of who the stakeholders are that may be affected, and what the impact of change will be for each of them.
- **Forming a new vision:** Unless the stakeholders can grasp where change will take them, very few will be convinced to take the risks required to make that change. A vision must include a new image of the organization and a plan of how to achieve that new image. This is best accomplished by including all of the stakeholders in the development of the plans for change.
- **Letting go:** The old order must be laid to rest. Until a leader can identify and remove barriers to change (e.g., attitudes, people, habits, fear), the current state of affairs will interfere with acceptance of any change.
- **Accepting:** New ways of accomplishing the mission must become second nature. These ways include new attitudes, behaviors, policies, and communication channels between individuals and throughout the organization.
- **Celebration:** Success is always worth celebrating. Acknowledgment of individual and group achievements through change serves to validate the change and reinforces the new order of business. It also makes further change easier to navigate.

CHANGES IN STRATEGIES OF LEADERSHIP

Leaders of the twenty-first century have discovered that an educated workforce is both a bane and a boon. Health care is not possible without proper training, but an educated person is not a passive follower. As a result of this, leadership in health care has become more collaborative and less dictatorial. Leaders must now be more cooperative and less competitive because they can no longer advance an idea without the support of the entire workforce.

This symbiotic relationship between leader and follower has caused the development of heretofore foreign concepts, such as as partnerships, continuous quality improvement, continuing education, and constant change. Perhaps the most difficult concept, especially for more senior leaders and for students, is that it has become more important to know what new questions to ask rather than to know the answers to old questions. These changes in leadership style, plus the fact that health care providers are, more often than not, self-motivated and rewarded more by seeing improvement in others rather than by self-improvement, suggest that transformational leadership (Bass, 1985; Bennis & Nanus, 1985; Marriner-Tomey, 1993) styles are worth promoting for gerontological nurses.

Transformational leadership is more than the process of managing people or tasks. It includes the idea of being visionary, being able to express this vision, and extending this vision to others (Anderson & Robinson, 2001). The transformational leader can help effect change in organizations or groups in a positive way. Transformational leadership allows for the emergence of a new order of business from the old. There is a focus on the potential of the new vision, and all members of the organization are encouraged to participate in transforming the system. The logistics of change become a communal charge. Several core competencies are required to effect transformational leadership.

In order to effect change through transformational leadership, a leader must involve all of the stakeholders in all phases of change. This allows for the final product to be adopted more rapidly and be fully accepted by all. Kouzes & Posner (1995) identified five practices of exemplary leadership that characterize the transformational leader:

- Encouraging the heart
- Inspiring a shared vision
- Modeling the way
- Challenging the process
- Enabling others to act

These and additional constructs of the processes of transformational leadership are associated with the core competencies described earlier in this chapter, and this relationship is identified in Table 23-2. Working on core leadership competencies will assist the nurse in developing as both a leader and a transformational leader. These skills will also assist the nurse to serve as a change agent in any clinical setting. While the magnitude of the vision and change may vary, the skills and process of change are the same.

Effective leaders, no matter how public or private their actions may be, have several attributes in common. Many of these traits that are the hallmarks of a leader in nursing are listed below in the mnemonic **leadership in nursing**

- **L**—Learns from setbacks
- **E**—Effects change
- **A**—Adapts to change
- **D**—Demonstrates competence
- **E**—Exceeds expectations of others
- **R**—Relates well to people
- **S**—Shares the vision
- **H**—Honors commitments
- **I**—Is insightful when motivating others
- **P**—Projects a positive self-image
- **I**—Includes all stakeholders
- **N**—Negotiates with others
- **N**—Notices opportunities for change
- **U**—Understands consequences of actions
- **R**—Relies on others for input
- **S**—Strikes a balance
- **I**—Innovates
- **N**—Needs to continuously learn new things
- **G**—Graciously interacts with others

The application of these attributes can vary with any given situation. The relative importance of each of these traits depends upon the context within which leadership is needed, as well as the phase of the project. In Table 23-3 the relative importance (with 1 being the most important and 3 being less important) of each of these traits for success in leadership for various nursing sites of practice (education, research, clinical care, and interdisciplinary care) is shown. These numbers represent the relative importance of each of these traits under unstressed circumstances and are based on personal experiences of the authors. These numbers will differ during times of stress and change. The table is offered as a guideline to assist readers in understanding and assessing their own circumstances and priorities during times of change. A leader influences others to help in the successful completion of change by using varying combinations and amounts of the skills described previously to accomplish a specific goal.

DEVELOPING LEADERSHIP SKILLS

While much of the content in this chapter seems like a discussion of lofty ideals, the nurse can use a number of methods to develop as a leader. It is really no different than learning other nursing skills. Books and articles can increase awareness of leadership issues and trends. Continuing education opportunities include formal courses, workshops, and conferences. Many nursing organizations provide leadership development

Table 23-2 *Transformational Leadership Constructs and Associated Core Competencies*

Construct	Core Competency
Encouraging the heart	Interpersonal effectiveness
Having a vision for change	Creative thinking
Challenging the process	Organizational stewardship
Creating a context for change	Systems thinking
Inspiring a shared vision	Interpersonal effectiveness
Allowing work to continue through the change	Flexibility/adaptability
Build consensus for change by creating common goals and objectives	Interpersonal effectiveness
Incorporate new technology into changes	Technical expertise
Modeling the way	Personal mastery
Seek continuous feedback during change	Customer service
Bestow personal empowerment upon others to effect change	Organizational stewardship
Lead by personal example	Personal mastery

Table 23-3 *Mnemonic of Leadership Traits in Nursing and Their Relative Importance in Practice Settings*

Mnemonic	Education	Clinic	Research	Interdisciplinary Practice
Learns from setbacks	2	1	1	2
Effects change	1	1	2	2
Adapts to change	2	1	2	2
Demonstrates competence	1	1	1	1
Exceeds expectations of others	2	2	1	3
Relates well to people	2	1	3	1
Shares the vision	1	2	3	1
Honors commitments	1	1	1	1
Insightful when motivating others	1	1	3	1
Projects a positive self-image	1	1	2	2
Includes all stakeholders	1	1	2	1
Negotiates with others	1	1	3	1
Notices opportunities for change	1	1	1	1
Understands consequences of actions	1	1	1	1
Relies on others for input	2	1	3	1
Strikes a balance	1	1	1	2
Innovates	1	2	1	2
Needs to continuously learn new things	1	1	1	1
Graciously interacts with others	2	1	3	2

Key: 1 = important all of the time; 2 = important some of the time; 3 = important only occasionally.

opportunities, for example, Sigma Theta Tau. Getting involved in local organizations is a good place to start networking with other developing leaders and interacting with more advanced leaders. Organizations that specialize in gerontology, gerontological nursing, and geriatrics also provide opportunities for leadership development. These organizations include the Gerontological Society of America, the National Gerontological Nurses Association, and the American Geriatrics Society.

Mentoring is an excellent method that is fostered in gerontological nursing to develop leaders. Less experienced nurses are encouraged to connect with mentors who are willing to share time and experience for leadership development. A mentoring arrangement can be informal and just include casual conversations when the nurse and mentor are together. Other arrangements may be formal, where there is an agreement that mentoring will be fostered. In this case, the nurse may develop goals and objectives and specific activities to complete with the assistance or advice of the mentor. Gerontological nursing is lucky to have many exceptional senior leaders that want to develop the next generation of leaders in practice, education, and research.

SUMMARY

Gerontological nurses can learn and develop competencies that will help them assume leadership roles in practice or administrative positions. The core competencies include personal mastery, organizational stewardship, systems thinking, customer service, creative thinking, flexibility and adaptability, technical expertise, and interpersonal effectiveness. These competencies will help the nurse advocate for good patient care for older adults, impact health care organizations and systems, and even influence health policy. Nurses are encouraged to continue to seek out learning opportunities that will help them develop these leadership skills.

REFERENCES

American College of Hospital Administration. (1997). *Journal of Hospital and Health Services Administration, Special Issue on Veteran's Health Administration, 42*(3), 285-459.

Anderson, M. M., & Robinson, D. (2001). Leadership in the health care delivery system. In D. Robinson & C. P. Kish (Eds.), *Core concepts in advanced practice nursing.* St. Louis: Mosby.

Antrobus, S., & Kitson, A. (1999). Nursing leadership: Influencing and shaping health policy and nursing practice. *Journal of Advanced Nursing, 29,* 746-753.

Bass, B. (1985). *Leadership and performance beyond expectations.* New York: Free Press.

Bennis, W., & Nanus, B. (1985). *Leaders: The strategies of taking charge.* New York: Harper and Row.

Bruhn, J. G. (2004). Leaders who create change and those who manage it. *Health Care Manager, 24*(2), 132-140.

Buonocore, D. (2004). Leadership in action: Creating a change in practice. *AACN Clinical Issues, 15*(2), 170-181.

Cooperrider, D. L., & Whitney, D. (2000). *Appreciative inquiry: Collaborating for change.* San Francisco: Berrett-Koehler.

Covey, S. (1990). *The seven habits of highly effective people.* New York: Simon and Schuster.

Davies, B., & Hughes, A. M. (2002). Clarification of advanced nursing practice: Characteristics and competencies. *Clinical Nurse Specialist, 16*(3), 147-152.

Deming, W. E. (1993). *The new economics.* Boston: MIT Press.

Fasnacht, P. H. (2003). Creativity: A refinement of the concept for nursing practice. *Journal of Advanced Nursing, 41*(2), 195-202.

Flannery, T. P., Hofricher, D. S., & Platten, P. E. (1996). *People, performance and pay: Dynamic compensation in changing organizations.* New York: Free Press.

Goleman, D. (1998). *Working with emotional intelligence.* New York: Bantam Books.

Grossman, S., & Valiga, T. M. (2000). *The new leadership challenge: Creating the future of nursing.* Philadelphia: F.A. Davis.

Henry, B. (2002). Leadership is about quality, cost access, and morale. *Journal of Advanced Nursing, 31*(6), 1275-1276.

Huber, D. L., Maas, M., McCloskey, J., Scher, C. A., Goode, C. J., & Watson, C. (2000). Evaluating nursing administration instruments. *Journal of Nursing Administration, 30*, 251-272.

Kerfoot, K. (2004). The leader's challenge: Meetings, spiritual energy, and sneaker ratio. *Nursing Economics, 22*(3), 157-158.

Kouzes, J. M., & Posner, B. Z. (1995). *The leadership challenge.* San Fransico: Jossey- Bass.

Laurent, C. L. (2000). A nursing theory for nursing leadership. *Journal of Nursing Management, 8*, 83-87.

Levine, M. E. (1973). On creativity in nursing. *Image, 3*(3), 15-19.

Lewin, K. (1951). *Field theory in social science.* New York: Harper.

Marriner-Tomey, A. (1993). *Transformational leadership in nursing.* St. Louis: Mosby.

McConnell, C. R. (2003). Accepting leadership responsibility: Preparing yourself to lead honestly, humanely, and effectively. *The Health Care Manager, 22*(4), 361-374.

National Association of Clinical Nurse Specialists. (2004). *Statement on Clinical Nurse Specialist Practice and Education.* Harrisbug, PA: National Association of Clinical Nurse Specialists.

Perra, B. M. (2000). Leadership: The key to quality outcomes. *Nursing Administration Quarterly, 24*, 56-61.

Porter-O'Grady, T. (1997). Quantum mechanics and the future of healthcare leadership. *Journal of Nursing Administration, 27*, 15-20.

Porter-O'Grady, T. (1999). Quantum leadership: New roles for a new age. *Journal of Nursing Administration, 29*, 37-42.

Porter-O'Grady, T. (2003a). A different age for leadership, part 1: New context, new content. *Journal of Nursing Administration, 33*(2), 105-110.

Porter-O'Grady, T. (2003b). Of hubris and hope: Transforming nursing for a new age. *Dermatology Nursing, 15*(3), 255-256, 265-267.

Roberts, L. (1987). *Leadership secrets of Atilla the Hun.* London: Warner Books.

Senge, P. (1994). *The fifth discipline: The art and practice of the learning organization.* New York: Doubleday.

Sullivan, E. J., & Decker, P. J. (2004). *Effective leadership and management in nursing* (6th ed.). Menlo Park, CA: Addison Wesley.

Tourangeau, A. E. (2003). Building nurse leader capacity. *Journal of Nursing Administration, 33*(12), 624-626.

Wheatley, M. J. (1992). *Leadership and the new science.* San Francisco: Berrett-Koehler.

Chapter 24

Therapeutic Groups for Older Adults

James H. Cook, Jr. & Candace M. Ball

Objectives

Highlight a brief historical overview of therapeutic groups and provide a foundation for understanding why groups are effective.

Discuss groups commonly used with older adults and/or their caregivers.

Examine leader facilitation skills and explain how they are used in a group context.

Describe steps for planning groups for older adults and identify special considerations for this population.

Therapeutic groups have emerged as a distinct clinical discipline, with effective techniques resulting in proven outcomes (Hsieh & Wang, 2003; Ormont, 2000). Although group research is complex because of the many variables focusing on individual members or the group as a whole, recent publications (Burlingame, Fuhriman, & Johnson, 2002; Burlingame, Fuhriman, & Mosier, 2003) empirically demonstrated that group work is indeed effective. A meta-analysis of 20 years of published group research supports the notion that group work is overall as effective as individual therapy (Burlingame et al., 2003).

Group work with older adults has also provided favorable results for a variety of issues affecting this age-group, including dementia (Junn-Krebs, 2003), depression (Hsieh & Wang, 2003), intellectual disabilities (Kessel, Merrick, Kedem, Borovsky, & Carmeli, 2002), and chronic mental illness (Evans, Chisholm, & Walshe, 2001), and also for women in cognitive behaviorally focused activity counseling (Focht, Brawley, Rejeski, & Ambrosius, 2004). Additionally, group work has been used as a training method for nurses working with older adults (Murphy et al., 2000).

This chapter provides an introduction to using group interventions when working with older adults. It lays the groundwork for understanding the basic components of groups and discusses considerations needed when working with older adults in a group context. Included in the chapter is a brief history of the evolution of group work, types of groups used with older adults and their caregivers, and a practical overview of the application of leadership skills. The chapter concludes with pregroup planning and special considerations for older adults.

EVOLUTION OF GROUP WORK

It is helpful to look briefly at the historical evolution of groups to achieve a perspective on how the conceptual knowledge of groups has evolved. Groups are as old as civilization. Different types of therapeutic groups have existed and been developed throughout the twentieth century. Some of the earliest groups were developed by Joseph Pratt for patients who were suffering from tuberculosis (Gladding, 1999). The World Wars also created the need for groups to provide therapy for returning soldiers as well as to train the troops to become ready for war. There were many self-help groups developed in the 1930s to help people deal with issues such as alcohol abuse. While these early groups provided some therapeutic benefit, the focus was on the structure and organization of the group, rather than the skills and qualities of the leader.

The groups discussed in this chapter are based upon methods discovered primarily by Kurt Lewin, who in the 1940s established the field theory that focused on the individual in that person's surroundings. He recognized that the Gestalt notion of the whole (the group) being more than a sum of its parts (individual members) applied to the groups he was studying (Gladding, 1999; Yalom, 1995). Much of the present knowledge about group work is derived from the research conducted by Irvin Yalom (1995). He systematically studied groups and identified the factors that lead to group effectiveness. He named these powerful forces therapeutic factors. Whereas his groups were primarily psychotherapeutic in structure, these factors play an integral role in many types of groups.

For our purposes, group work is defined as a comprehensive professional practice involving the intentional application of theory and facilitation skills to build a therapeutic group alliance (ASGW, 2000; Ward, 2003). The leader's responsibility is to distribute communication within the group to build relationships that lead to group and individual progress. "The goals of the group may include the accomplishment of tasks related to work, education, personal development, personal and interpersonal problem solving, or remediation of mental and emotional disorders" (ASGW, 2000, p. 2). Whereas group work can be used across numerous populations, settings, and topics, here we address group work with older adults.

TYPES OF GROUPS USED WITH OLDER ADULTS

From nursing homes to community centers, group work is extensively used with older adults. Because of this popularity, nurses are likely to encounter a variety of group interventions that serve many different purposes. This section highlights common groups used with older adults (Table 24-1). It begins by introducing groups that require minimal leader training (reality orientation, remotivation therapy, and reminiscence therapy) and then progresses to those groups in which leaders need substantial education and supervised practice (counseling, psychotherapy, and psychoeducational groups).

Reality Orientation Groups

Reality orientation groups are designed to orient confused older adults as to time, place, and person. Developed by Taulbee and Folsom in the 1960s, these groups were initially used with patients at the Veterans Administration Hospital in Tuscaloosa, Alabama (Burnside, 1984). Although the method has changed since its original conception, the primary goal of reality orientation groups remains the same—to retard or decrease mental disorientation.

Reality orientation groups are generally used with older adults who are in the early stages of dementia or Alzheimer's disease (Junn-Krebs, 2003) or who have delerium. Educational in focus, these groups use various memory aids to assist in orienting members. For in-

stance, the group leader may use a large board containing information such as the date, year, weather, and current activities. Staff are asked to provide orienting cues throughout the days, such as, "It's nearly time for dinner." After reviewing the information, the group leader asks questions in a nonconfrontational manner and gently corrects any disorientation.

Reality orientation groups typically meet once a day for approximately 30 minutes. However, the time may be longer or shorter, depending on the tolerance of the members. These groups usually consist of three or four members when the problems are severe, and seven or eight members for those less confused. A component of the reality orientation program is that it must be extended, on an individual basis, outside of the group setting (e.g., in a nursing home) (Gladding, 1999).

Because these groups are loosely structured, there has been a lack of scientific rigor devoted to studying the groups. As a result, it is difficult to evaluate the true effectiveness of reality orientation groups. Most positive research evidence is anecdotal and cannot be validated (Donahue, 1984). Although leaders must have an understanding of how to facilitate reality orientation groups, there are no other special educational requirements. For this reason, these groups are often led by paraprofessionals such as nursing assistants and hospital technicians. Reality orientation groups are uncommon today.

Remotivation Groups

Developed in the 1950s, remotivation groups have been used in mental health centers and nursing homes to help older adults live in the present. These groups are designed to help members increase their involvement in activities of daily living (Erwin, 1996), improve socialization skills, and stimulate cognitive processes (Gladding, 1999). Remotivation groups use a structured curriculum that does not focus on personal problems. Topics of discussion might include current events, the arts, and hobbies.

Leaders use learning aids so that participants can experience session topics through one or more of the five senses. For instance, during a discussion on baking, the leader may pass around a small container of flour for participants to touch and then later hand out a small

Table 24-1 *Common Types of Groups Used with Older Adults*

Group	Purpose	Setting
Reality orientation	Improve orientation	Long-term care or geropsychiatric settings
Remotivation	Increase engagement	Long-term care or rehabilitation setting
Reminiscence	Provide therapeutic recollections	Community and long-term care settings
Counseling and psychotherapy	Manage problems and learn coping skills	Inpatient or outpatient older adults, caregivers
Psychoeducational	Education and psychological support	Older adults and/or caregivers

sample of baked goods to taste. By engaging participants in this manner, it is believed that this will lead to increased attention and interest in the topic.

Remotivation groups often have no more than 15 members and are held 3 times a week for a minimum of 4 weeks. These groups typically meet for 30 to 60 minutes (Capuzzi & Gross, 1990). Studies conducted in the 1960s and 1970s found that remotivation groups were moderately effective in raising self-concept, increasing self-esteem, and creating a higher degree of life satisfaction (Dennis, 1984).

Reminiscence Groups

Reminiscence groups use recollections of the past as a vehicle to therapeutically reach older adults. The theoretical beginnings of these groups date back to the classic work of Butler (1963) that rejected the notion that reminiscent storytelling is a maladaptive sign of old age. Instead, it was redefined as an important developmental process that helps older adults transition into late adulthood and accept the finality of life.

Reminiscences are natural, unorganized, and random recollections from the past (Brady, 1999). Reminiscence groups use these recollections to highlight member's successes, help them rethink critical life moments, and discover new ways of coping with the present (Soltys, Reda, & Letson, 2002). It is by revisiting important life events that members feel a sense of completeness and resolve with their past (King, 1984).

The literature divides reminiscence groups into simple reminiscence and life review. Reminiscence groups use recollections of the past as a vehicle for sharing, discussion, and communication among members. These groups do not have a defined structure, so conversation is spontaneous in nature (Erwin, 1996). Like reminiscence groups, life review groups also use recollections from the past. However, this group is structured to more systematically, comprehensively, and deeply explore the meaning of the member's life events (Brady, 1999; Minardi & Hayes, 2003).

Reminiscence groups are usually planned to last for 1 hour and often meet 1 or 2 times a week. There can be anywhere from 6 to 10 group members (Burnside, 1984; Capuzzi & Gross, 1990). Reminiscence groups provide promise as a viable therapeutic intervention to treat depression (Hsieh & Wang, 2003) and increase self-esteem (Lappe, 1987; Myers & Harper, 2004). However, more research on how to best deliver this type of intervention is needed (e.g., number of sessions, ideal number of participants per group) (Hsieh & Wang, 2003). Also, since paraprofessionals who are untrained in counseling sometimes lead these groups, there is some concern that issues might arise in the group that the leaders are not trained to therapeutically resolve (Myers & Harper, 2004).

Counseling and Psychotherapy Groups

Counseling and psychotherapy groups are usually led by mental health professionals whose training and authorized scope of practice includes one or both of these intervention strategies (e.g., licensed psychiatric/mental health registered or advanced practice nurses, licensed professional counselors, social workers, psychologists). Through an interactive process of feedback and sharing, members discover personal strengths, gain insight into problems, and develop new ways of coping. Counseling groups are different from psychotherapy groups because they are short-term, problem-solving interventions that focus on developmental and/or situational problems (e.g., relationship issues, adjusting to retirement) (Gladding, 1999). Members of these groups are generally normally functioning individuals who need emotional support. Psychotherapy groups, on the other hand, target psychologically distressed individuals who experience impaired functioning because of chronic mental health issues such as major depression or thought disorders. The primary purpose of these groups is to correct maladaptive behavior. This occurs through reexamining current behavior in the context of antecedent behavior (Corey & Corey, 2002).

Counseling groups are typically short-term interventions, usually requiring 12 or more sessions. Psychotherapy groups vary in session number from many months to possibly years. Overall, group work with older adults needing counseling has produced favorable research results. The literature provides support for both "topic-specific groups (e.g., as widowhood, specific health challenges, adjustment to retirement, and creation of leisure lifestyles) and participant-specific groups (e.g., groups designed for older men, older women, bereaved persons, and older adults dealing with substance abuse)" (Myers & Harper, 2004, p. 214).

Psychoeducational Groups

Older adults often experience problems in which both educational information and psychological support are needed (e.g., weight loss, smoking cessation, exercise maintenance, parenting grandchildren). Psychoeducational groups are recommended because members learn new skills and information that will help them overcome knowledge, affective, and/or behavioral deficits. Leaders of psychoeducational groups prepare a structured curriculum based on a general theme. For example, Schneider & Cook (2005) developed a psychoeducational group for older adults who wanted to maintain an exercise program. The psychoeduational group used cognitive behavioral therapy to help members identify and modify unrealistic thoughts related to exercise. The group addressed thoughts about exercise, personal barriers to exercise, myths, and exercise goals.

Psychoeducational groups use many different mediums to impart information to members. For example, leaders use experiential exercises that sometimes incorporate art, music, or role playing. While minilectures are sometimes used, leaders should keep in mind that activities are interactional in nature. The role of the leader is to encourage communication among members—not to dominate the group (Schneider & Cook, 2005). Leaders of these groups must also be knowledgeable of group theory and able to help members see the building process of knowledge from one session to the next (Conyne, Wilson, & Ward, 1997).

Whereas psychoeducational groups commonly have 8 to 10 sessions, 16 to 20 sessions maximize group development and enhance learning (Brown, 1997). Groups generally meet for 50 to 120 minutes (Gladding, 1999). For older adults, Schneider & Cook (2005) found that 1 hour was sufficient for both covering information and reducing the chance of participant fatigue. Likely benefits of psychoeducational groups are improved self-esteem and optimism (Burnside, 1984; Capuzzi, & Gross, 1990). A study of groups for grieving individuals, members displayed fewer symptoms of depression and had less physical complaints (Folken, 1991).

Caregiver Groups

Most of the care provided for older adults who need assistance is done by family members (Peacock & Forbes, 2003). This responsibility can leave the caregiver with stress, depression, anger, and guilt (Coon, Thompson, Steffen, Sorocco, & Gallagher-Thompson, 2003). Recently, substantial research was devoted to the use of group interventions for caregivers of older adults who primarily presented with Alzheimer's disease or dementia (Brodaty, Green, & Koschera, 2003; Coon et al., 2003; Perraud, Farran, Loukissa, & Paun, 2004; Sorensen, Pinquart, & Duberstien, 2002) and terminal illnesses (Witkowski & Carlsson, 2004). Most groups focused on providing support, education about the disability, and coping strategies designed to lessen the burden felt by the caregiver (Mittelman, Roth, Coon, & Haley, 2004; Sorenson et al., 2002). One meta-analysis provided support for involving both the older adult with early dementia and the caregiver in combined groups (Brodaty et al., 2003). These combined groups led to a delay in nursing home admission for the care receiver.

In planning groups for caregivers, the leader must consider several variables. Respite care may be necessary to allow the caregiver the opportunity to be involved in

---

BOX 24-1 *Reflections on Leading a Support Group for Persons with Dementia*

The experience of directing a support group for persons with dementia is humbling, insightful, rewarding, and positive. Many family members have asked me how we keep the attention of the person with dementia for 90 minutes, what the person actually contributes, and how we assist them with participation. My response is universal. The person with dementia makes consistently meaningful contributions without prompting, especially if the 'right' question is asked—one that either strikes at the heart of an issue for the person or reflects part of their personal experience. Poignant, heartfelt experiences, many of which are unpleasant or demeaning for the person with dementia, are shared. When advice is sought by the person with dementia, group members make meaningful contributions to help resolve the issue or dilemma, drawing on their own experiences. Even if a group member repeats a 'story' or experience within the same meeting, other members are incredibly respectful and will sit in rapt attention, even though the story may be one they just heard! I am always amazed by this ability to attend to and follow what another is saying, even in the face of cognitive impairment.

*One caregiver shared with me that her husband rarely knew what day of the week it was or the time of day, but would know every other week when it was his 'group' day and when it was time to leave to attend the group meet-*ings. *The group had grown to mean so much to him in his struggle with dementia. Group members talk consistently about the importance of having a 'shared' experience with others, the sense of feeling 'safe' in the group, the importance of being understood, and the respect they feel for one another. Group members will often ask about a missing member (remember, these members have marked memory loss) or ask someone about something that was shared 2 to 4 weeks previously. I believe this is due to the importance of the group to each member's personal experience with the disease and their need for this type of support. Each meeting is ended on a positive note—generally with an uplifting idea, suggestion, or song. Even though 90 minutes may seem like a long time for persons with dementia to sit, listen, and share verbally, I have universally ended each meeting over the past 7 years while the group members will continue talking and sharing. The group just means that much to each of them. I tell the group as often as is appropriate that they are truly the 'bravest people I know.' And they are.*

Sandy C. Burgener

Sandy C. Burgener, PhD, APRN-BC, FAAN
Associate Professor
University of Illinois College of Nursing
Chicago, Illinois

BOX 24-2 Guidelines for Development and Conduct of Support Groups for Persons with Dementia

Group Participant Characteristics
Able and Willing to Interact with Others
- Mental status scores not necessarily good indicators of participation quality.
- Ability to stay in the here-and-now helpful for meaningful interactions.

Acceptance of the Disease not Necessary
- Coping with the diagnosis is one outcome of the support group process.
- Acceptance of the diagnosis evolves within the group interactions and support.

Group Leader Characteristics
A Working Knowledge of Dementia
- Understands and is attuned to the limitations of participants.
- Has adequate understanding of the disease process to recognize participant limitations and methods to compensate for losses.

Open, Accepting Attitude
- Persons with dementia readily recognize insincerity or discomfort in others.
- Conducts the group with an attitude to preserving and protecting the participants' sense of self, self-control, and self-esteem.

Group Process Characteristics
Select Topics of General Interest to the Total Group That Are Nonthreatening
- Participants rarely, if ever, want to talk about 'future planning' of anticipated losses.

- NEVER force participants to contribute to a discussion or share feelings.
- Focus on the positive, instilling hope when possible in a realistic manner.

Facilitate Participation by all Attendees
- Compensate for a participant's deficits if at all possible (e.g., filling in gaps in the person's language).
- Allow time for everyone to respond: Remember, response time is delayed in dementia.
- Gently shift the attention back to the present if some participants dwell on past events of limited interest to the total group.

Ensure Confidentiality of all Interactions and Discussions
- Family members should attend the group for the first meeting only.
- Do not discuss what is said in the group with family members or outside the group unless a participant's safety is at risk.

Ensure Continuing Participation
- Participants should not be forced to 'graduate' or exit the group after a limited time period, such as 10 sessions.
- Participants generally self-select themselves out of the group (e.g., disease progression occurs and the person changes living situation).

---

a group. The focus of the group and the participants selected will determine the type of group that is most effective in meeting the objectives of its members. A psychoeducation group or a counseling group led by a knowledgeable professional and a leader trained in counseling could provide effective, comprehensive leadership to assist caregivers coping with a myriad of challenges.

More recently, support groups have been created specifically for those with dementia, usually for those in the early stages of memory loss. In Box 24-1, Dr. Sandy Burgener discusses her experiences in leading such a group. Additional information on developing and conducting this kind of group is provided in Box 24-2.

GROUP LEADERSHIP SKILLS

In 1955, Glover surveyed a group of psychoanalysts and discovered widespread disagreement regarding treatment practices and interventions. This discovery led him to believe that "without some reliable form of standardization of technique there can be no science of

psychoanalysis" (Glover, 1955, p. 383). Although these comments were made 5 decades ago about psychoanalysis, they parallel the state of treatment practices in group work today. In the past, the training of group leaders focused little attention on specific group skills (Dye, 1996; Harvill, West, Jacobs, & Masson, 1985; Robison, Jones, & Berglund, 1996), which resulted in an inability to describe effective leadership skills. Recently, scholars have recognized that because group work is a unique form of treatment, the skills for leading it are different from those used for individual-based interventions. Group training literature has subsequently emerged (e.g., Cook, 2004; Smaby, Maddux, Torres-Rivera, & Zimmick, 1999; Toth, 1995) that sheds light on the skills that are important to lead therapeutic groups.

Cook (2004) conducted a Delphi survey of group work experts to determine, among other things, the skills that were important to effective group leadership (Box 24-3). The following is a brief overview of a few important skills that were identified by the experts in his study.

BOX 24-3 Group Leadership Skills

- Attending to group participants
- Reflecting group/members feelings
- Linking members to each other
- Guiding group discussion:
  a. Using open-ended questions
  b. Shifting the focus as needed
  c. Holding the focus to complete a discussion
- Scanning the group to pick up nonverbal communication
- Assisting the group in processing the group experience

Attending Skills

Attending skills are a collection of behaviors that show group members that the leader is listening and following what is being said. These behaviors include maintaining eye contact, using verbal encouragers to prod members to continue their line of thinking, and asking questions that follow a who, what, when, where, and why format.

- **Reflections of feelings** are statements that show that the leader is accurately sensing the group's or individual member's emotional climate. The primary purpose of these skills is to assist the group or individual members to become aware of emotional themes that emerge in the group. For example, a group leader might say, "The group seems to be heading in different directions. I sense some feel quite comfortable with where we are heading while others may be a bit tense talking about this" (Ivey, Pederson, & Ivey, 2001, p. 96).
- **Linking** is a skill where leaders connect members based on their similarities to one another. Such similarities may include common traits, characteristics, or experiences (Corey & Corey, 2002). For instance, a group leader may notice that a male member is shaking his head while a female member shares her pain over the death of her mother. From noticing this nonverbal behavior, the leader may later ask the male member if something he heard about the situation or emotion relates to his own experience.
- **Open-ended questions** are those that cannot be answered with a simple "yes" or "no." Such questions encourage conversation and elaboration of thought. For example, a group leader may ask, "Where should we begin today?" or "Tell me about your sadness."
- **Scanning** is a skill where the leader continually looks around the room to observe nonverbal messages from members. By observing members' behaviors, group leaders may use these observations in formulating other interventions (e.g., linking for commonality).
- **Shifting the focus** is the purposeful attempt by the leader to change from an activity, topic, or person to another activity, topic, or person (Jacobs, Masson, Harvill, & Riley, 1998). For example, a leader may shift the focus from one member to another by stating that, "Much of our attention today has been on helping Louis understand his relationship with his son. Who else has had problems with family relationships?"
- **Holding the focus** is a skill where the leader attempts to keep group conversation on a specific topic, person, or activity (Jacobs et al., 1998). For example, after a particularly intense revelation a group member may change the topic of conversation. The group leader would hold the focus by saying, "Thelma, hold your thought for just a moment, I'd like to finish with Monroe before moving on."
- **Processing** is where leaders ask members questions as a way to encourage them to reflect on their group experience and attribute meaning to it. Such questions can encourage members to reflect on topics discussed in the group, an activity conducted during a group session, or interactions that occurred in the group. Leaders use processing at the end of structured activities, during a group session, and/or during the termination session (Jacobs et al., 1998). For example, at the end of an activity on goal setting, a group leader might ask, "How is it helpful to pinpoint long-term goals?"

Group skills are the basic and universal "mechanics" of leadership. While a good understanding of the various skills is necessary, leaders should also understand certain theoretical group concepts. These concepts will help the group leader recognize the skills appropriate to the given situation and suggest how to implement them. What follows is a discussion of four important group concepts termed here-and-now orientation, process and content, therapeutic factors, and stages of group development.

Here-and-Now Orientation

Working in the here-and-now orientation means the group is focusing on the present. While the here-and-now orientation is a technique used in many psychotherapies (such as Gestalt), here it is referred to as a distinct group concept. This concept relates to limiting discussion to events that have occurred within the group and which all group members share (Ivey et al., 2001). Use of the here-and-now technique enables the leader to identify patterns of behavior that serve as a basis for formulating appropriate interventions. For example, a group leader may notice that while Stephen is talking about the death of his father, group members consistently shift the conversation to neutral topics such as gardening and cooking. By maintaining a here-and-now orientation, the group leader is able to identify this pattern (that is, shifting the topic during emotional conversations) and then intervene by noticing out loud that the group shifts to benign topics.

Because group members learn about themselves through the feedback and interactions of others, the group leader must be mindful of the here-and-now to encourage member-to-member communication. Use of the here-and-now is generally more applicable to counseling, psychoeducation, and psychotherapy groups. "To the degree that the therapy group focuses on the here-and-now, it increases in power and effectiveness" (Yalom, 1995, p. 27). An understanding of this concept may make the difference between a productive group outcome and the digressions that so often bog down committee or social meetings.

Process and Content

Content consists of the actual words and ideas of a conversation. Quite simply, it is the topic of discussion (Yalom, 1995). For example, group members Minerva and Harley have a heated discussion about assisted suicide. During this conversation, both make substantive pro and con arguments. Process, on the other hand, is how members interact and relate to one another and the leader (Corey & Corey, 2002; Gladding, 1999; Yalom, 1995). In the previous example, while Minerva and Harley discuss issues related to assisted suicide, the group leader may notice, for example, that one member seems disengaged from the conversation, another group member is dominating the conversation, and other group members avoid meaningful discussion by trying to change the topic.

The leader's interventions and the movement of the group all rely on process. Process leads us to question the meaning behind behaviors. While we might think it is easy to interpret behaviors, the true meaning can only be known by the person exhibiting the behavior. Another way in which process moves the group is through reflection on critical incidents that occur in the session. Through understanding the dynamics of an incident, members gain insight into their own and other members' behavior, which leads to both individual and group development.

Therapeutic Factors

Eleven therapeutic factors were identified by Yalom (1995) to account for individual change that occurs through participation in groups. While these factors are applicable to counseling and psychotherapy groups, most are generalizable to other groups (e.g., psychoeducational groups) (Gladding, 1995). These factors are interwoven and are not viewed as separate entities, but rather they are dependent upon the stage of group development and the type of group. The following is a brief description of these factors:

- Instillation of hope—gaining confidence that problems can be resolved with the help of the leader and through work within the group
- Universality—realizing that many members are struggling with similar concerns
- Imparting information—providing information about mental health or wellness
- Altruism—doing something for the common good while not expecting anything in return
- Corrective recapitulation of the primary family group—correcting past family conflicts through present group introspection and resolution (for example, by examining Joe's conflictual behavior with Sally, it may shed insight into his turbulent relationship with his mother)
- Development of socializing techniques—learning socially appropriate behaviors (e.g., using "I" statements when giving feedback, looking at the person to whom the member is speaking)
- Imitative behavior—incorporating appropriate behaviors modeled by group leaders and other members
- Interpersonal learning—gaining insights through group interaction
- Group cohesiveness—feeling attraction toward the leader, its members, and the group
- Catharsis—expressing deeply held thoughts and emotions
- Existential factors—recognizing that while others can empathize with our problems, we are ultimately responsible for our own behavior

Stages of Group Development

Although every group is different, groups tend to evolve through similar developmental stages. During the initial stage (also known as the forming stage), members are anxious and unfamiliar with the group and its members. Conversation tends to be superficial, impersonal, and chatty, often accompanied by nervous laughter. Erwin (1996) noted that groups with older members usually spend more time in this stage. Establishing trust and rapport may be more difficult for some older adults, and because of their upbringing, they may view participation as a stigma or a sign of weakness. Negative feelings can be reduced through the leader's use of appropriate attending skills such as reflections of feelings and linking. By helping members gain a sense of universality and feelings of hope, the leader can help the group progress to the next stage of development.

The transition (or confronting) stage of development is characterized by overly critical statements about others' behavior. Conflict develops because members are attempting to find their role within the group. The leader is often the target of hostility and testing, but member trust can be gained through self-disclosure and nondefensive acceptance of criticism, while keeping the group safe for members. "The leader has more to gain by promoting safe, slow steps toward risk taking and acceptance than by challenging resistance or defenses" (Erwin, 1996, p. 8). While conflict may be uncomfortable for both leaders and members, well-managed conflict is an essential component for the group's progression into the next stage. Leaders can help the group resolve conflict through processing problematic interactions so that members can gain insight as a result of interpersonal learning.

During the working stage of development (norming and performing), the influence of therapeutic factors is increasingly apparent and effective (Yalom, 1995). Group members honestly share constructive feedback and readily self-disclose at a deeper level. Implicit norms become explicit and true norming materializes in this stage. Members become more able to self-regulate appropriate behavior, resulting in a decreased dependence on the leader. More time is spent working toward goal attainment and working through intrarelational conflict among members. Even though the group has demonstrated behaviors characteristic of the working stage, there is an ebb and flow in development. Some issues may cause the group to regress to an earlier stage. For example, a group in the working stage that experiences the loss of a member may return to earlier stages until the group develops sufficient cohesiveness.

Termination (or leaving) is the final stage of group development. This is a time for members to take stock of both individual and group accomplishments. There is an emphasis on generalizing information and skills gained from the group to future situations outside the group. Leaders must ensure that any unfinished business is resolved before the group ends. An important task of this stage is for members to acknowledge and express appreciation for how others contributed to their personal growth and attainment of goals. Although it may be helpful to prepare members in advance (e.g., two sessions before the group ends), discussing termination too early can lead to premature closure and an avoidance of effective closure activities. Termination may be a stressful and emotional parting for group members, which can cause resistance to saying goodbye. The leader must structure discussion and activities so that closure is achieved.

PREGROUP PLANNING AND SCREENING

Pregroup planning involves carefully selecting the type of group (e.g., counseling group, psychoeducational group) with a focus that is relevant to older adults. The leader must also consider the number and length of sessions appropriate for an older adult population. Physical facilities and other logistical elements must be resolved. Because some older adults have hearing and/or vision problems, group leaders need to be mindful of the physical environment. The group room should be large enough to comfortably seat every member, yet small enough for conversation. Outside noise can be reduced by shutting windows and doors. It is also advisable that the room is handicap-accessible and located near a restroom.

After deciding on a group format and securing the appropriate place to conduct a group, leaders are advised to conduct individual screening interviews with potential members to determine if they are appropriate for treatment (Brown, 1997; Gladding, 1999). Brown (1997) noted that screening interviews serve five important purposes. These purposes, discussed below, are the following: (1) determine if member's goals are consistent with the goals of the group, (2) inform members of their ethical rights relative to group treatment, (3) provide an assessment of member readiness, (4) prepare members for the group, and (5) assess member commitment to the group. Brown's (1997) list of screening purposes provides a useful organizing structure when applying these to working with older adults.

Determine If Member's Goals Are Consistent with the Goals of the Group

In the screening interview, potential members must identify issues that are affecting them. Common problems faced by older adults include grief, lack of social contact, fear, hopelessness, loss of independence and control over their lives, health problems, financial issues, and facing the inevitability of death (Corey & Corey, 2002; Gladding, 1999). Leaders must assess whether the member's problems are consistent with the goals and purpose of the group. Also, leaders must determine whether the potential member's problems can be met through the process of the group, or whether another form of treatment (such as individual work or case management) is more appropriate. This is the time to clarify misconceptions about group treatment. This might include attitude toward self-disclosure and willingness to work in a group format.

Older adults sometimes have the impression that groups are for persons identified as mentally ill. Their cultural and social norms may dictate that it is inappropriate to share personal information outside of the family, believing instead that their problems should be handled independently. In addition, by sharing personal limitations in a group, older adults may fear that others will think them incapable of independent living.

This being said, the leader's responsibility is to evaluate whether the member's goals are compatible with those of the group and are capable of being met in a group context. Potential members may have a fuzzy impression of potential problem areas, but have not operationalized these into attainable goals. Therefore the leader must help members identify specific areas of concern in order to determine how the group can help them achieve their goals. Because older adults might have less knowledge about groups intended for personal growth and education, it is incumbent upon the leader to impress on members that the overall purpose of the group is to empower its members.

Inform Members of Their Ethical Rights Relative to Group Treatment

It is standard ethical practice that leaders develop an informed consent document that outlines the purpose of the group, roles of leaders and members, structure of the group, limits of confidentiality, and possible benefits and limitations of group participation. To accommodate older adults, this document should be printed in large bold type in language that is clearly written, easily understood, and free of jargon. To fully ensure that the older adult understands the informed consent document, the leader should discuss the rights of group members, ethical obligations, and the qualifications of the leader.

Because confidentiality is an important ethical concern in treatment, it is vital to understand how it differs in a group context. Confidentiality can be guaranteed in some settings (e.g., individual counseling or medical treatment), but it cannot be guaranteed in a group setting. A group leader ensures that members commit to confidentiality by signing intake paperwork and including it in the group guidelines, but the leader cannot control members' release of other members' personal information shared outside the group.

Other ethical considerations involve participation, the right to reject advice received from other members, and the right to terminate if the member deems the group is no longer beneficial to them. Although participation is encouraged and essential for group development, members can elect not to participate in some discussions. It is important for members to know that unsolicited advice may be given by other members. Leaders should encourage members to evaluate these suggestions and to either accept or reject their relevance. In most cases, even though members commit to a minimum number of sessions, they retain the right to terminate membership.

Provide an Assessment of Member Readiness

To determine each member's suitability for group treatment, the leader must identify possible member strengths and limitations. Strengths might be a willingness to participate, ability to clearly conceptualize personal and group goals, and logistical considerations (such as transportation, time availability, and financial resources). Although it is important to recognize the strengths that older adults bring to groups, it is equally important to identify possible limitations. For example, older adults may not be able to physically negotiate stairs, may lack the stamina for long group sessions, or may have significant hearing or vision loss. Careful pregroup planning (e.g., site selection, length of sessions, number of breaks) can accommodate for many physical deficits; however, some of these limitations may preclude some member's ability to fully participate in the group. In this case, referral to other treatment options might be advisable. Brown (1997) suggests that leaders cautiously approach referrals to alternate forms of treatment so that the person will feel supported rather than rejected.

Potential members may lack the mental acuity required for group participation as a result of dementia or other health condition. If the leader perceives that a problem exists, there are instruments developed to assess cognitive function. For example, instruments such as the Folstein Mini-Mental State Examination (Folstein, Folstein, & McHugh, 1975) or the Delayed Word Recall test (Knopman & Ryberg, 1989; O'Carroll, Conway, Ryman, & Prentice, 1997) will detect cognitive processing deficits. The purpose and goals of the group will help the leader determine if individuals would be appropriate to participate in a specific group.

Similar to cognitive deficits, certain emotional difficulties may preclude members from participating in a group. Crisis situations (such as death of a spouse, terminal illnesses, abuse, or violent assault) may limit a member's ability to function as a group member and may require more intense individual attention than can be delivered in a group. Depending on the type and purpose of the group, depression or other diagnosed psychiatric illness can make group treatment less appropriate for those individuals. Shyness, lack of social skills, and other personality traits could indicate that these individuals are not appropriate for group. Although the identification of some of these traits is nebulous, the leader must decide if the severity of these deficits could interfere with group development.

Prepare Members for the Group

The screening procedure allows time for building rapport with potential members. Having established rapport with the leader, members are less likely to experience apprehension because they are fully informed about the group and are acquainted with the leader. During the screening procedure, leaders can emphasize how members can be helpful to one another. Members should understand that self-disclosure and feedback are essential to an effective group. Additional information about the format and types of activities as well as procedural information about the group can be shared.

When and where the group meets, session length, number of sessions, and cancellation notification are points to be covered.

Assess Member Commitment to the Group

As mentioned earlier, members must be willing to make a commitment to attend a predetermined number of sessions before deciding to terminate membership. Members must also make a verbal or written contract of attendance. By openly discussing the importance of regular attendance, leaders are setting the foundation for acceptable group behavior.

GROUP LEADER TRAINING

Bernard (2000) noted that group therapy often attracts unqualified leaders because of unregulated professional designations such as "psychotherapist." Subsequently, incompetent leaders often lead groups that should be reserved for trained professionals. While many of the groups discussed in this chapter do not require extensive education, working with people in a group context requires extensive knowledge about how people work together in groups. Because of the complexities of leading psychotherapeutic groups (e.g., counseling, psychotherapy, psychoeducation), it is imperative that nurses lead groups appropriate to their scope of practice and seek out additional experiences and education if needed. Box 24-4 contains contact information for several professional organizations that specialize in group work. These organizations provide professionals with information about current group research, new skills and methods for group leadership, training opportunities, and networking with others who have similar professional interests.

SUMMARY

Groups offer a therapeutic intervention that has the potential to help older adults resolve common problems. This chapter focused on practical aspects of working with older adults in groups. Exposing the reader to knowledge about the mechanics of group leadership, this chapter is intended to demonstrate that group work is an intentional intervention that requires specialized training. Combining this knowledge with information about universal group theory provides a comprehensive framework for understanding group work. The work involved in planning a group is described, underscoring the need for understanding the membership and the focus of the group. Resources for additional training and information are provided.

BOX 24-4 Professional Group Work Associations

American Society of Group Psychotherapy and Psychodrama
301 North Harrison Street, Suite 508
Princeton, NJ 08540
(609) 452-1339
www.ASGPP.org

American Psychological Association
Division 49, Group Psychology and Group Psychotherapy
750 First Street, NE
Washington, DC 20002-4242
(202) 336-6013
www.pitt.edu/~cslewis/GP2/Hello.html

The American Group Psychotherapy Association
25 East 21st Street, 6th Floor
New York, NY 10010
(877) 668-2472
www.groupsinc.org

The Association for Specialists in Group Work
(an affiliate organization of the American Counseling Association)
5999 Stevenson Avenue
Alexandria, VA 22304
(800) 347-6647
www.asgw.org

REFERENCES

Association for Specialists in Group Work. (2000). *Professional standards for the training of group workers.* Alexandria, VA: Author.

Bernard, H. S. (2000). The future of training and credentialing in group psychotherapy. *Group, 24*(2/3), 167-175.

Brady, E. M. (1999). Stories at the hour of our death. *Home healthcare nurse, 17*(3), 177-180.

Brodaty, H., Green, A., & Koschera, A. (2003). Meta-analysis of psychosocial interventions for caregivers of people with dementia. *Journal of the American Geriatrics Society, 51*(5), 657-664.

Brown, B. (1997). Psychoeducation group work. *Counseling and Human Development, 29*, 1-14.

Burlingame, G. M., Fuhriman, A., & Johnson, J. E. (2002). Cohesion in group psychotherapy. In J. C. Norcross (Ed.), *Psychotherapy relationships that work.* New York: Oxford University Press, pp. 71-87.

Burlingame, G. M., Fuhriman, A., & Mosier, J. (2003). The differential effectiveness of group psychotherapy: A meta-analytic perspective. *Group Dynamics: Theory, Research, and Practice, 7*, 3-12.

Burnside, I. (1984). *Working with the elderly: Group processes and techniques* (2nd ed.). Monterey, CA: Wadsworth.

Butler, R. N. (1963). The life review: An interpretation of reminiscence in the aged. *Psychiatry, 26*, 65-76.

Capuzzi, D., & Gross, D. (1990). Recent trends in group work with elders. *Generations, 14*(1), 43-48.

Conyne, R. K., Wilson, F. R., & Ward, D. E. (1997). *Comprehensive group work: What it means and how to teach it.* Alexandria, VA: American Counseling Association.

Cook, J. H., Jr. (2004). A description of core group leadership skills through a modified Delphi technique. *Dissertation Abstracts International, 65*(01), 75A (UMI No. 3120536).

Coon, D. W., Thompson, L., Steffen, A., Sorocco, K., & Gallagher-Thompson, D. (2003). Anger and depression management: Psychoeducational skill training interventions for women caregivers of a relative with dementia. *The Gerontologist, 43*(5), 678-689.

Corey, M. S., & Corey, G. (2002). *Groups: Process and practice* (6th ed.). Pacific Grove, CA: Brooks/Cole.

Dennis, H. (1984). Remotivation therapy. In I. Burnside (Ed.), *Working with the elderly: Group processes and techniques* (2nd ed.). Monterey, CA: Wadsworth, pp. 187-197.

Donahue, E. M. (1984). Reality orientation: A review of the literature. In I. Burnside (Ed.), *Working with the elderly: Group processes and techniques* (2nd ed.). Monterey, CA: Wadsworth, pp. 165-176.

Dye, A. (1996). Afterword: Confirmations, contrasts, and conjecture. *Journal for Specialists in Group Work, 21*, 178-180.

Erwin, K. T. (1996). *Group techniques for aging adults: Putting geriatric skills enhancement into practice.* Washington, DC: Taylor & Francis.

Evans, S., Chisholm, P., & Walshe, J. (2001). A dynamic psychotherapy group for the elderly. *Group Analysis, 34*(2), 287-298.

Focht, B. C., Brawley, L. R., Rejeski, W. J., & Ambrosius, W. T. (2004). Group-mediated activity counseling and traditional exercise therapy programs: Effects on health-related quality of life among older adults in cardiac rehabilitation. *Annals of Behavioral Medicine, 28*(1), 51-61.

Folken, M. H. (1991). The importance of group support for widowed persons. *Journal for Specialists in Group Work, 16*, 172-177.

Folstein, M. F., Folstein, S. E., & McHugh, P. R. (1975). "Mini-mental state." A practical method for grading the cognitive state of patients for the clinician. *Journal of Psychiatric Research, 12*(3), 189-198.

Gladding, S. T. (1999). *Group work: A counseling specialty* (3rd ed.). Upper Saddle River, NJ: Prentice Hall.

Glover, E. (1955). *The technique of psychoanalysis.* New York: International Universities Press.

Harvill, R., West, J., Jacobs, E. E., & Masson, R. L. (1985). Systematic group leader training: Evaluating the effectiveness of the approach. *Journal for Specialists in Group Work, 10*, 2-13.

Hsieh, H. F., & Wang, J. J. (2003). Effect of reminiscence therapy on depression in older adults: A systematic review. *International Journal of Nursing Studies, 40*, 335-345.

Ivey, A. E., Pederson, P. B., & Ivey, M. B. (2001). *Intentional group counseling: A microskills approach.* Belmont, CA: Brooks/Cole.

Jacobs, E. E., Masson, R. L., Harvill, R. L., & Riley, L. (1998). *Group counseling: Strategies and skills* (3rd ed.). Pacific Grove, CA: Brooks/Cole.

Junn-Krebs, U. (2003). Group work with seniors who have Alzheimer's or dementia in a social adult day program. *Social Work with Groups, 26*(2), 51-64.

Kessel, S., Merrick, J., Kedem, A., Borovsky, L., & Carmeli, E. (2002). Use of group counseling to support aging-related losses in older adults with intellectual disabilities. *Journal of Gerontological Social Work, 38*(1/2), 241-251.

King, K. S. (1984). Reminiscing, dying, and counseling: A contextual approach. In I. Burnside (Ed.), *Working with the elderly: Group processes and techniques* (2nd ed.). Monterey, CA: Wadsworth, pp. 272-286.

Knopman, D. S., & Ryberg, S. (1989). A verbal memory test with high predictive accuracy for dementia of the Alzheimer type. *Archives of Neurology, 46*, 141-145.

Lappe, J. M. (1987). Reminiscing: The life review therapy. *Journal of Gerontological Nursing, 13*(4), 12-16.

Minardi, H., & Hayes, N. (2003). Nursing older adults with mental health problems: Therapeutic interventions—part 2. *Nursing Older People, 15*(7), 20-27.

Mittelman, M. S., Roth, D. L., Coon, D. W., & Haley, W. E. (2004). Sustained benefit of supportive intervention for depressive symptoms in caregivers of patients with Alzheimer's disease. *The American Journal of Psychiatry, 161*(5), 850-856.

Murphy, P., Kreling, B., Kathryn, E., Stevens, M., Lynn, J., & Dulac, J. (2000). Description of the SUPPORT intervention. *Journal of the American Geriatrics Society, 48*(5), 154-161.

Myers, J. E., & Harper, M. C. (2004). Evidenced-based effective practices with older adults. *Journal of Counseling and Development, 82*, 207-218.

O'Carroll, R. E., Conway, S., Ryman, A., & Prentice, N. (1997). Performance on the delayed word recall test (DWR) fails to differentiate clearly between depression and Alzheimer's disease in the elderly. *Psychological Medicine, 27*, 967-971.

Ormont, L. R. (2000). Where is group treatment going in the 21st century? *Group, 24*(2/3), 185-192.

Peacock, S. C., & Forbes, D. A. (2003). Interventions for caregivers of persons with dementia: A systematic review. *The Canadian Journal of Nursing Research, 35*, 88-107.

Perraud, S., Farran, C. J., Loukissa, D., & Paun, P. (2004). Alzheimer's disease caregiving information and skills, part III: Group process issues and concerns. *Research in Nursing & Health, 2*(2), 110-120.

Robison, F., Jones, E., & Berglund, K. (1996). Research on the preparation of group counselors. *Journal for Specialists in Group Work, 21*, 172-177.

Schneider, J. K., & Cook, J. H. (2005). Planning psychoeducational groups to increase health behavior. *Journal of Gerontological Nursing, 31*(8), 33-38.

Smaby, M., Maddux, C., Torres-Rivera, E., & Zimmick, R. (1999). A study of the effects of a skills-based versus a conventional group counseling training program. *Journal for Specialists in Group Work, 24*, 152-163.

Soltys, F. G., Reda, S., & Letson, M. (2002). Use of the group process for reminiscence. *Journal of Geriatric Psychiatry, 35*(1), 51-61.

Sorensen, S., Pinquart, M., & Duberstein, P. (2002). How effective are interventions with caregivers? An updated meta-analysis. *The Gerontologist, 42*(3), 356-372.

Toth, P. (1995). Teaching the "here and now" intervention to master level group counseling students using a microcounseling skill based approach: The effect on skill acquisition and the level of self-efficacy (doctoral dissertation, Indiana University, 1995). *Dissertation Abstracts International, 55*, 2285.

Ward, D. E. (2003). Connections: Fundamental elements of a comprehensive approach to group work. *The Journal for Specialists in Group Work, 28*, 191-194.

Witkowski, A., & Carlsson, M. E. (2004). Support group programme for relatives of terminally ill cancer patients. *Supportive Care in Cancer: Official Journal of the Multinational Association of Supportive Care in Cancer, 12*(3), 168-175.

Yalom, I. (1995). *Theory and practice of group psychotherapy* (4th ed.). New York: Basic Books.

Chapter
25 Team Work: Interdisciplinary Geriatric Care

Helen W. Lach

Objectives

Discuss the importance of teams in meeting the complex needs of older adults.

Describe different team members and their preparation and approach to care.

Examine issues in training, development, and working together in interdisciplinary teams.

Discuss the nurse's contribution to the team process.

Many older patients presenting to the health care system have complex conditions with intertwined medical, psychological, and social problems. The common geriatric complaints such as falls, dementia, and incontinence are characterized by multiple risk factors, causes, and outcomes. These problems are optimally managed through complementary approaches provided by a variety of health professionals, each with their own expertise, working as a team. The importance of interdisciplinary care for older adults is described in Box 25-1. This chapter will discuss the structure and function of geriatric teams, as well as issues in teamwork that can help nurses clarify and strengthen their role in team processes.

INTRODUCTION TO TEAMS AND THEIR IMPORTANCE

Studies show that team management improves outcomes for older patients in a variety of settings (Rubenstein, 2004). Nurses are often integral parts of teams, and may be team leaders. The idea of interdisciplinary teams reminds one of the old parable of the blind men and the elephant. In this parable, three blind men approach an elephant; each touches the beast and based on his findings, describes it. The first blind man finds the elephant's leg and describes the elephant to be like a tree—round and strong. The second man reaches the elephant's side and thinks the elephant is wide and flat—resembling a wall. The third blind man comes upon the beast's squirming trunk. He proclaims the elephant is most like a snake! Each man argued for his point of view, and the blind men could not agree on a description of the elephant. Each of the blind men was partially correct in describing the elephant, but consider how much clearer and complete the description could have been if they had been able to combine their views of the elephant!

So it is with interdisciplinary teams. Each member sees the patient through his or her own particular lens of training, experience, and assessment. Each can provide important information necessary to understanding and caring for any particular patient, but a much more complete patient assessment can be provided when there is a team of professionals who see the patient from a variety of angles and lenses. Also, care can be much more comprehensive when the knowledge and skills of a variety of professionals can be considered.

The strength of the interdisciplinary team is also its weakness. When various disciplines endeavor to work together, the differences in training and skills can also result in misunderstandings and mistrust. Productive and effective geriatric teams do not develop without hard work and a combination of a shared mission, an appropriate structure, and good communication. Yet health professionals have inadequate educational experiences to prepare them for this type of work. Recommendation to increase interdisciplinary training was provided by the reports of the Health Professions' Commissions in the 1990s (Bellack & O'Neil, 2000). More recently, the 2003 report on health professions' education from the Institute of Medicine identified the ability to work in interdisciplinary teams as one of the core competencies needed by health professionals of

Box 25-1 *Reflections on Interdisciplinary Care for Older Adults*

Long before the current push for interdisciplinary care came into being (i.e., the National Institutes of Health Roadmap), I was a strong proponent of interdisciplinary geriatric care and research. As a practitioner, administrator, educator, and investigator, I have always believed that true collaboration (that is, the sharing of talent, resources, responsibilities, and expertise while putting aside traditional disciplinary boundaries) yields better outcomes. I also believe that geriatric nurses are essential members and leaders of interdisciplinary teams, in practice, research, and education.

From a clinical perspective, for example, an interdisciplinary team can tackle the challenging interplay of chronic and acute medical and psychosocial problems of persons with dementia, patients who are dying, or elders with unremitting pain, all of which may be too complex for any one provider to handle alone. Further, compelling evidence supports that comprehensive geriatric team care results in desired treatment outcomes such as reduced length of stay, improved functional status, lower mortality, and greater patient and family satisfaction to name but a few. A functional interdisciplinary care or research team is not without its challenges, however, and failure to be open, ethical, tolerant of review and critique, accepting of new ideas and perspectives, as well as personality clashes, "power plays" and oneupsmanship, can be a death knell for any collaborative effort.

As an administrator at an academic health center with five health sciences colleges, joint planning, decision-making, and goal-setting efforts across disciplines were essential to the success of virtually every new educational, policy, or clinical initiative we set forth. Regardless of how much information any one health profession has, interdisciplinary collaboration has the best chance of resulting in appropriate and effective services. Interdisciplinary approaches at an academic health center can facilitate efficiency of education, appreciation of other professions, and improved interpersonal relationships on campus, but the system must find a way to reward interdisciplinary ef-

forts, for example, during the promotion and tenure process.

As an educator, I often wondered how we can expect health care professionals to work together collaboratively in "the real world" if we do not educate them together. In recent years reports from the U.S. Department of Health and Human Services, the IOM, AACN, Healthy People 2000, the Pew Commission, and others have highlighted the need to inculcate interdisciplinary health care values while attending to the strengths of the individual professions. These organizations have also called for a restructuring of health profession education that supports a new model of health care delivery to which all disciplines contribute. However, the challenges associated with interdisciplinary education are immense and often logistical in nature. For example, I recently taught an interdisciplinary health policy and law course with students from three different colleges, two of which were on completely different semester schedules, with different grading expectations and writing requirements. We ended up offering the class from 6 to 9 PM on Sunday nights to accommodate the divergent schedules of students from various disciplines.

Finally, as a geriatric nurse researcher, the types of questions I and others address require multiple skills and access to diverse settings and populations that beg for an interdisciplinary research team approach that blends members with various types of expertise. In addition the enhanced resources that may result from pooled finances, equipment, and access to more settings, more subjects, and increased subject recruitment all serve to facilitate the research enterprise. Some of my best research experiences and outcomes have come from working with interdisciplinary research teams.

Kathleen C. Buckwalter
Kathleen C. Buckwalter, PhD, RN, FAAN
Sally Mathis Hartwig Distinguished Professor of Nursing
University of Iowa
Iowa City, Iowa

the future. Much work in the educational arena is now focused on increasing interdisciplinary experiences during basic training for students in the health professions (Skinner, 2001).

Drinka & Clark (2000, p. 6), who have studied and written about teamwork for more than 2 decades, provide the following definition of an Interdisciplinary Health Care Team (IHCT):

"An IHCT integrates a group of people with diverse training and backgrounds who work together as an identified unit or system. Team members consistently collaborate to solve patient problems that are too complex to be solved by one discipline or many disciplines in sequence. In order to provide care as efficiently as possible, a team creates formal and informal structures that encourage collaborative problem solving.

Team members determine the team's mission and common goals, work interdependently to define and treat patient problems; and learn to accept and capitalize on disciplinary differences, differential power, and overlapping roles. To accomplish these, they share leadership that is appropriate to the presenting problem and promote the use of differences for confrontation and collaboration. They also use differences of opinion and problems to evaluate the team's work and its development."

While teams consist of professionals from diverse backgrounds, the goal is for all members to identify more as a collective unit than as individuals and to value the team processes more than individual work. Yet studies of geriatric teams have revealed that team members often report the following obstacles to working effectively as a team: turf issues, conflict or communication difficulties, the team process, and organizational constraints (Clark, 2002). Team performance is influenced by a variety of structural and functional factors including the structure and design of the team, the members who make up the team, and even how long the team has been working together. Learning about these factors can help health professionals and teams understand and improve their group process in ways that will help improve performance and minimize these problems. These factors are described in the following paragraphs, with some examples from the work setting, starting with an exploration of the structure of health care teams.

STRUCTURES OF TEAMS: THEY ARE NOT ALL ALIKE

Four types of teams are common in geriatric health care: ad hoc, unidisciplinary, multidisciplinary, and interdisciplinary (Drinka & Clark, 2000). Ad hoc teams are generally short term, such as a task force. People come together to solve a problem or work on a specific project, and then disband. For example, a primary care nurse practitioner may have a geriatric patient in crisis and assemble a geriatric care manager, physical therapist, and hospice referral nurse to determine a course of action. Teams like this may meet physically, or connect completely by phone or e-mail. While a more consistent team may be ideal, the use of ad hoc teams may become increasingly common in situations where health care dollars are scarce. This model has been popular in the corporate world, where teams may collaborate on a project and then dissolve, with the members joining other teams.

Unidisciplinary teams are made up of members from only one profession. For example, an older patient may be under the care of an internist, cardiologist, ophthalmologist, and urologist. Each of these physicians provides care based on their specialty. There may or may not be any communication between the physicians. The multidisciplinary team involves professionals from different disciplines, but the assessment and patient care tasks are again carried out independently. There may be little communication between the professionals. For example, a home care nurse and physical therapist may make separate visits to an older woman at home but do not discuss the case together or see each other's paperwork. However, there is some doubt as to whether this constitutes a true team by definition: a group organized to work together (www.yourdictionary.com). If these caregivers do not share information, the patient does not have the benefit of a team in care coordination.

The type of team that has the potential to make the most contribution to care of the elderly is the geriatric interdisciplinary team. This team includes a variety of disciplines, or at least a minimum of two, but as noted in the prior definition, there is true collaboration in planning, implementing, and evaluating care. There may be sharing of information, leadership, and responsibilities, and the lines between disciplines become blurred. The overlap of roles requires communication and negotiation to work well as a team. Some people prefer the newer term for this collaborative care of "interprofessional" teams. However, for this book, the authors have chosen to use the term "interdisciplinary," which is more familiar to many readers.

Geriatric interdisciplinary teams ideally include a physician, advanced practice nurse, social worker, pharmacist, physical therapist, occupational therapist, and nutritionist. Depending on the resources of the program or health system, these professionals may all be core team members, but some may only be available as consultants. Geriatric interdisciplinary teams may offer specialized geriatric assessments through outpatient or inpatient programs in academic medical centers, clinics, or hospitals. In addition, geriatric teams are used in many settings, including rehabilitation, home health care, acute care, and long-term care, to promote comprehensive care for older adults.

The nurse's role on the team may be to perform nursing assessments, assist with history and physical examinations, administer screening tests, or collect information. In the acute care setting, teams may be part of specialized units or set up as consultation teams. Staff nurses often participate on acute care teams or at least provide input about the patients under their care. Advance practice nurses may serve as team members or coordinate teams for specialized units. In the rehabilitation and long-term care settings, nurses may serve on teams in a variety of formal roles, including care plan coordinator or case manager.

The structure of the team sets the stage for providing collaborative care by organizing who works together. While this is a key factor in providing care, another important component is how long the team has worked together. Learning to collaborate is a process that evolves over time (Gardner, 2005). How long the team has been together may determine whether it has worked through the tasks that groups commonly experience as they learn to collaborate. A discussion of these "stages" of team development follows with implications for team performance.

STAGES OF TEAM FORMATION

Teams typically pass through a series of stages as they form and develop:

- Team *forming*—team members are identified
- Team *norming*—the process of integration of members into the goals and values of the team, and the group process

- Team *confronting*—conflicts are identified and resolved
- Team *performing*—team members achieve a level of performance focused on the goal or patient, rather than the process or each other
- Team *leaving*—team may disband or lose members

This process of group development was originally described by Tuckman (1965), but has been used by many authors studying the formation of groups (Burbank et al., 2002). For interdisciplinary teams, different challenges can arise depending on the stage of a particular team. It is useful to understand the stages and common problems as well as interventions that can promote better team performance.

Forming

In this stage, members join a new or ongoing team. Members get to know each other and attempt to understand their roles and functions within the group. A newly formed team has the opportunity to develop its own goals, organizational structure, and process for the team's work; member roles, including leadership, as well as a plan for evaluating the team's progress can also be determined during this stage. This can be a good team exercise but also is very time-consuming; therefore it can take a significant amount of time for a new team to get started. However, even with a well-established team, new team members may cause a group to reorganize or reshape its structure. Useful activities in the forming stage will help group members get to know each other and feel that they can openly share and solve problems. Orienting new members to the team's structure and processes can help smooth the transition.

Norming

This stage involves the integration of new members into the team as they provide care to patients. The team begins working together, learning how to incorporate the goals and values of the team and use the group process. Members begin establishing roles and relationships. Informal leadership patterns emerge. Members learn more about working with each other and the expectations of various team members. Conflict may develop during this time as differences in members' expectations of each other or the team process become more obvious. Formalizing the team's structure and process and the roles of members, with team input, helps team members understand how they fit in and how to perform their work. Scheduling part of team meetings to discuss how the team is functioning can help the team recognize and deal with conflicts early. The focus of these discussions should be on patient successes and failures and improving team processes, rather than blaming team members for problems. One often effective approach is for team facilitators or leaders to ask team members during the team update part of meetings what would allow them to be more effective in their roles.

Confronting

The confronting stage is also called storming. As the team members become familiar with each other, conflict becomes more obvious and methods of dealing with conflict come into play. Conflict is an inevitable part of teamwork, and goal achievement suffers when teams are unable to deal effectively with conflicts. Members may use positive or negative coping methods to deal with conflicts. Examples are discussed later in the chapter.

Performing

When a team is well developed, members work together with a focus on team goals and patient problems, rather than process. Team members demonstrate trust in each other and collaborate and share responsibilities without undue interpersonal problems. Ongoing management of patient and process issues helps teams maintain a high level of functioning long term. In one study (Faulkner-Schofield & Amodeo, 1999), the support provided by well-functioning teams was shown to improve staff morale in situations where workers have large, complex caseloads.

Leaving

During this stage, the team may disband or individual team members may leave. Depending on the circumstances, anger or regret may impact team performance during this stage. Any changes may cause the team to reenter the forming stage. Unfortunately, organizational changes are common today, with resulting impact on health care teams. Teams may face system changes and reorganizations in addition to changing team members, and may even need to advocate for their own continuation (Clark, Leinhaas, & Filinson, 2002). As a result, teams may be in this stage as well as the forming stage more frequently than they would like.

The stage of team development is thus an important factor in team performance, as well as the way the team is designed. Awareness of developmental stage can assist a team in determining training or methods that may be helpful in the case of problems. In addition, the makeup of the team has an influence on team operations, and is discussed next.

VARIOUS TEAM MEMBERS AND THEIR PREPARATION

Health professionals may or may not learn about the preparation and expertise of those in other disciplines. Often this information is learned informally during training experiences or later in the work environment.

Because this learning is informal, it is usually incomplete. The perceptions of a profession may relate more to experience with particular team members and their knowledge and skills, rather than an understanding of their professional preparation and area of expertise. When team members change, the perception is generalized to new members of the same profession. These perceptions can be totally inaccurate and result in poor communication and resentment among team members. Think of the confusion caused by the many levels of nurses and the variations in their training! Other disciplines may not recognize the extent of the educational difference between a licensed practical nurse, professional nurse, and advanced practice nurse.

Team training programs encourage understanding and appreciation for the skills and knowledge of various team members (Drinka & Clark, 2000; Hyer et al., 2003). Table 25-1 provides a listing of the health professionals that nurses commonly encounter in teamwork, along with their preparation and key areas of expertise. Teams members may need education and information about all of their teammates in order to understand their style and approach to patient care.

While educational preparation provides a background for professionals, new team members may also have extensive experience or training that influences their skills and expertise. As a result, a new team should spend some time finding out about each other's disciplines, experiences, and expertise. If possible, team members should spend time observing the practice and activities of other team members to increase familiarity with them. When new members are introduced to an existing team, information should include the educational background and experiences they bring to the team, in order to enhance understanding and appreciation among team members.

Recent studies of geriatric interdisciplinary team training programs indicate that attitudes toward team participation vary among professionals. Studies showed that nurses and social workers were more positive toward teamwork than resident physicians (Leipzig et al., 2002) and also less likely to see the team's role as assisting the physician; nurses and social workers also tended to believe that the physician did not have the right to unilaterally alter team treatment plans. These preconceived ideas may in part be based on differences in the educational preparation of different professionals. Some professionals, such as dietitians, rarely see themselves as leaders on the team (Dahlke, Wolf, Wilson, & Brodnik, 2000).

The goal is to integrate team experiences into training for all health care professionals to foster positive attitudes toward interdisciplinary care. Specific education and training may be needed for team members who have not had this type of experience previously, and learning about each other is a key part of any team participation.

Role of the Patient and Family

The patient and family are considered part of the team, and should participate in providing information and shaping the plan of care. Ideally patients and their significant others provide input about the situation, and the patient and family preferences should carry the most weight in decision making. Challenges arise when patients are unable to speak for themselves because of severity of illness or cognitive impairment. Family members may be unavailable or out of town. The team must consider the possible sources of information, such as advance directives, and determine the ability of family members or others to speak on the patient's behalf. Methods to receive adequate input may include phone conferences, after-hours calls, and other adjustments to obtain adequate information from all needed sources. Once information is obtained, the patient and family should be part of ongoing implementation, evaluation, and future planning.

CONDUCTING EFFECTIVE TEAM MEETINGS

After consideration of the structure, membership, and stage of the health care team, we can proceed to the process of how teams usually conduct their work: through the team meeting. Team meetings can be efficient and effective; however, they can also be the source of a great deal of conflict. Everyone on the team needs to agree on the ground rules for team meetings in order to be respectful of members' time and expertise and still conduct a meeting as comprehensive as possible. The following are points that help create efficient and effective team meetings.

Regular Meeting Times

Plan a schedule for team meetings so members can arrange their calendars.

Agenda

Prepare an advance agenda for each meeting. In many cases the agenda will be a list of the patients that need to be discussed. Team members can then suggest modifications in advance, or when the team meeting is ready to begin.

Reporting Format

Determine an order for team members to give their reports on individual patients so that the information is assembled in a useful way. In the case study at the end of this chapter, the social worker sets the stage by describing the patient situation and the psychosocial assessment. The advanced practice nurse builds on this

Table 25-1 *Various Interdisciplinary Team Members and their Roles*

Members	Practice Roles/Skills	Education/Training	Licensure/Credentials
Nurse	Licensed vocational nurse (LVN)—basic nursing skills that are dictated by the facility; registered nurse (RN)—associate degree, BA, or higher; RN has increased scope of practice, including planning for optimal functioning, coordination of care, teaching, and direct and indirect patient care	LVN—1 year of traning; RN with associate degree—2 years of training, usually in a community college; BS, RN—4 years in college; MS, RN—2 years of postgraduate specialty study; PhD, RN—3 to 4 years of post graduate studies.	LVN—exam required for licensing; CE requirements. RN—can be RN; BS, RN; APN; MS, GNP, or other specialty RNs; PhD, RN: all must pass the national licensure exam and are required to have 20 hours of CEUs per year.
Nurse practitioner	Health assessment, health promotion, histories and physicals in outpatient settings; order, conduct, and interpret some lab and diagnostic tests; teaching and counseling	Master's degree with a defined specialty area such as gerontology (GNP).	In addition to RN licensure, NP must pass a National Certification Exam in the appropriate specialty area (e.g., gerontology, family practice).
Physician	Diagnose and treat diseases and injuries, provide preventive care, do routine checkups, prescribe drugs, and do some surgery	Physicians complete medical school (4 years) plus 3 to 7 years of graduate medical education.	State licensure required for doctor of medicine degree; exam required and possible exams required for specialty areas. CE requirements.
Geriatrician	Physician with special training in the diagnosis, treatment, and prevention of disorders in older people; recognizes aging as a normal process and not a disease state	Completion of medical school, residency training in family medicine and internal medicine, and 1-year fellowship program in geriatric medicine.	Completion of fellowship training program and/or passing examination for Certificate of Added Qualifications in Geriatric Medicine (CAQ). Recertification by examination is required every 10 years and begins in the eighth year because it is a 2-year process.
Physician assistant	Practice medicine with the supervision of licensed physicians, exercise autonomy in medical decision making, and provide a broad range of diagnostic and therapeutic services; practice is centered on patient care	Specially designed 2-year PA program at medical colleges and universities. Most have bachelor's degree and over 4 years of health care experience before entering a PA program.	State licensure or registration plus certification by NCCPA. Recertification every 6 years by examination. Requires 100 hours CME every 2 years.
Social worker	Assessment of individual and family psychosocial functioning and provision of care to help enhance or restore capacities; this can include locating services or providing counseling	There is a 4-year college degree (BSW); 2 years of graduate work (MSW); and a doctoral degree (PhD); 15 hours of continuing education is required every year.	State certification is required for clinical social workers. The LMSW (for master's level); LSW (BS level); SWA is a social work associate with a combination of education and experience. ACP signifies licensure for independent clinical practice.
Psychologist	Assessment, treatment, and management of mental disorders; psychotherapy with individuals, groups, and families	Graduate training consists of 5 years beyond undergraduate training; most course work includes gerontology and clinical experience.	PhD, or EdD or PsyD are degrees awarded. State licensure; the American Psychological Association has ethics codes, as do most states.

Table 25-1 *Various Interdisciplinary Team Members and their Roles—cont'd*

Members	Practice Roles/Skills	Education/Training	Licensure/Credentials
Psychiatrist	Medical doctors who treat patients' mental, emotional, and behavioral symptoms	Medical school and residency specializing in psychiatry. Residency includes both general residency training and 2 to 3 years in area of specialization (e.g., geriatrics, pediatrics).	State exam to practice medicine; Board of Psychiatry and Neurology offers exam for diplomat in psychiatry, though not required for psychiatric practice in Texas.
Pharmacist	Devise and revise a patient's medication therapy to achieve the optimal regime that suits the individual's medical and therapeutic needs; information resource for the patient and medical team	Pharmacists can receive a baccalaureate (BS)—5-year program; or doctorate degree (PharmD). Annual CEUs required range from 10 to 15 hours.	State exam required—Texas uses the national exam (NABPLEX); given every quarter; RPh is the title for a registered pharmacist in Texas; board certifications in specialties available (pharmacotherapy, nuclear pharmacy, nutrition, psychiatric, and oncology in near future).
Occupational therapist	One who utilizes therapeutic goal-directed activities to evaluate, prevent, or correct physical, mental, or emotional dysfunction or to maximize function in the life of the individual	BS or MS in OT with a minimum of 6 months of field work; for OT assistant, an associate degree or OT assistant certificate is required with a mimimum of 2 months' field work.	State exam required for the credential of OTR (occupational therapist registered). Exam also required for COTA (certified occupational therapy assistant). These exams are given at least twice per year.
Physical therapist	Evaluation, examination, and utilization of exercises, rehabilitative procedures, massage, manipulations, and physical agents including, but not limited to, mechanical devices, heat, cold, air, light, water, electricity, and sound in the aid of diagnosis or treatment	A 4-year college degree in physical therapy is required to be eligible for the state exam; master's degree in physical therapy is available; 3 CEUs every 2 years are required.	PT is the credential that is used by licensed physical therapists and PTA is the credential for licensed physical therapist assistant. To use either of these titles, one must pass a state exam. CEUs are required for both; titles and licenses must be renewed biennially.
Chaplain	Provide visits and ministry to patients and family	Master's degree in theology, plus a minimum of 1 year of clinical supervision if fully certified. Can work in some settings without being fully certified.	Certification is through the Chaplaincy Board of Certification; credentials for this are BCC; however, credentials are not normally used. Most, but not all, chaplains are ordained ministers. CEUs required are 50 hours per year.
Dietitian	Evaluate the nutritional status of patients; work with family members and medical team to determine appropriate nutrition goals for patient	BS degree in food and nutrition and experience are required to be eligible for exam; CEs are required for both the LD (6 clock hours per year) and RD (75 clock hours every 5 years); MS degree is available also.	RD is the credential for a registered dietitian in the state of Texas. For RD, must pass the national exam of the American Dietitian Association; LD is the credential for a licensed dietitian in the state of Texas; same exam is required but processing of paperwork/fees is different.

Reprinted from Long, D. M., & Wilson, N. L. (2001). *Geriatric interdisciplinary team training: A curriculum from the Huffington Center on Aging.* Houston, TX: Baylor College of Medicine's Huffington Center on Aging.

Note: Continuing education requirements vary by state, and licensing and certification titles vary (LVN or LPN; LISW or LMSW; CSW, CISW, or CICSW).

information with details of the functional and cognitive assessment. Finally, the physician describes the positive findings from the history and physical examination. A list is then developed with problems and recommendations. Different clinical situations may call for a different order for presentation of information. New groups may need to try various orders to determine the method that works best for their particular clinical situation and patient population. Box 25-2 notes techniques for effective team meeting communications.

Goal Setting Process

Determine a format for care planning. Once reports have been given, the team discusses their findings to identify goals for the patient, to obtain a consensus on the approaches and priorities, and to develop a care plan. The team identifies problems and interventions based on the patient and family goals as well as the resources and severity of problems. Criteria are determined so that success of the plan can be evaluated. This process should include all involved team members who discuss their ideas and opinions, and make joint decisions on how to proceed. Team members may easily agree on approaches for patients or may need to explore issues further to negotiate the best path to take. This negotiation is what often results in team conflict, as the values, approaches or communication techniques of different team members come into play through this process (see more on conflict later in the chapter). A plan of care should be developed for each patient discussed, including goals and strategies.

Time Frame

Allocate the amount of time for each patient, including, if helpful, how much time each professional has to present his or her information. Be sure to include time for

---

BOX 25-2 Communication Techniques for Effective Team Meetings

- Informative reports and questions
- Opinions are solicited and given
- Coordination to see that all are given the opportunity to participate
- Enumeration of problems
- Analysis of information and problems
- Development of solutions to problems
- Encouragement of team members
- Recognition and solution of conflict
- Distribution of specific tasks
- Recording of problems and team decisions
- Evaluation of team processes

---

discussion, planning recommendations, and actions. The team should discuss how to handle unusually complex cases that take longer than expected, so that everyone will know how to proceed. For example, the team may meet frequently enough that some patient cases can be held for discussion at the next meeting if time expires.

Assignment of Tasks

Make assignments so that every team member leaves the meeting knowing who will follow up with each task related to each patient by an agreed upon deadline.

Recording of Information

Devise a system for recording the results of the team discussion and assignments. The case study at the end of the chapter provides a sample problem list with goals and recommendations.

Managing Interruptions and Distractions

Determine ways to minimize interruptions. Interruptions and distractions disrupt team meetings, decreasing their efficiency. Interruptions are the result of busy team members with many responsibilities. Beepers have long intruded on the discussion and flow of meetings, and now cell phones seem to only increase the frequency of these interruptions. Ideally, team members can agree to turn off the phones and pagers during team meetings. In the clinical setting, this may not be possible. However, the team members can agree to attempt to eliminate those unnecessary interruptions so that the meeting can proceed as efficiently as possible.

The most common distraction during team meetings is the off-topic discussion, which often is about the weather, news, or personal issues. It is natural for team members to want to connect with other members. Positive relationships between team members help foster a positive work environment. However, the team leader needs to direct the conversation back on track when this occurs. Planning lunches or other time for members to get together and have more personal discussions is helpful.

Managing Team Meetings When Team Members Are Absent or Cannot Meet in Person

Vacations and other circumstances will result in team members missing meetings from time to time. The team should agree on how to handle these situations. Because there is overlap among professional roles, sometimes other team members can assume duties typically carried out by a different team member. The member who is missing may delegate the person taking over the actual patient care in his or her absence to provide the update to the team. Another option is to assign someone to contact the missing member and review patient cases they need to know. The ease of electronic communication today helps minimize these problems—team care plans or documents can be e-mailed and updated if needed when the missing team member returns.

It is now possible to consider virtual teams that communicate entirely by computer or other electronic methods—a model that has been used in education (Vroman & Kovacich, 2002) and the business world. The options of tele-health, conference calls, and video-conferencing all open possibilities for health professionals to work together both as ad hoc teams and as ongoing virtual teams. Integrated systems and devices are being developed to facilitate communication and data transfer to make the work of virtual teams easier, especially in the home care setting (Pitsillides et al., 2004). These exciting opportunities make it possible to enhance care for patients and to use scarce geriatric specialists in new ways. However, technology does not eliminate the need for teams to communicate and work together, so the issues of face-to-face teams can also arise in virtual teams. The principles described in this chapter also apply to digitized teams.

LEADERSHIP

Leadership is another major factor in health care teams. Perhaps this is because, as Drinka & Clark (2000) suggest, leadership is a system rather than a person when conducting interdisciplinary teamwork. They identify a set of tasks (Table 25-2) that facilitate interdisciplinary functions that could be performed by different team members at different times. Certain professionals may be more suited to perform some tasks than others, in part based on their training, but also based on their individual personalities and level of confidence. Because many tasks are not assigned to specific team members, there can be multiple members attempting to perform the same tasks and other necessary tasks that are not completed.

Some negotiation of these tasks develops as a team works together, and members learn each other's professional and individual skills and strengths. For example, different team members may have the role of "expert" in specific areas, so questions on those topics are targeted to them. For example, one may have expertise in falls and another in dementia or psychiatric problems. Someone who is acquainted with many people in the health system where the team functions may be assigned as "ambassador" to deal with issues that require outside help. Assignment of other tasks can be built

into the team's structure, such as a timekeeper or the role of "finisher."

Often in healthcare teams, physicians are the assumed, if not assigned, leaders because of various cultural and legal responsibility issues. In fact, physicians rarely have management training, and often have the least amount of time to deal with logistical problems that the assigned "leader" is expected to manage. However, hierarchies within and between professions and professionals are a reality that cannot be ignored (Drinka, 2002). Developing a general mechanism for decision making can avoid some leadership conflicts. This mechanism should identify who will be involved in decision making, how decisions are made, and who is responsible for following up decisions. In many cases, this will be shared work, with leadership roles determined by patient needs. Any member of the health care team with good consensus-building and leadership skills could potentially manage these tasks. Ideally, team members share responsibility for patient care and leadership, although overall leadership for the team may need to be a clearly designated responsibility (if everyone is in charge, no one is).

TEAM CONFLICT

At best, conflicts can lead to inefficiencies in team functioning; at worst, they can damage the team's ability to manage patients. Members may develop low morale and decrease their involvement. However, whenever people are working together to solve problems, there are bound to be disagreements about what to do or how to do it. Conflict helps the team consider a variety of options. A healthy discussion of differences can help the team solve similar problems more quickly in the future. Four kinds of team conflicts are described by Drinka & Clark (2000): intrapersonal, interpersonal, intrateam, and interteam.

Intrapersonal

Intrapersonal conflict occurs within an individual, resulting from personal issues or factors. For example, a new member may have difficulty adjusting to the way the team handles situations, or a new member may not feel prepared to carry out the work expected by the team. Individual team members may disagree with the team priorities, how resources are allocated, or how certain patient problems are managed. They may not understand the team's mission or goals. Team members can experience role conflicts because they do not have adequate time to meet all the demands of their various roles.

Another example of intrapersonal conflict could be a situation where a team member identifies a new method of assessing or managing problems, or a new resource,

---

Table 25-2 *Leadership Tasks That Facilitate Interdisciplinary Teamwork*

Organizer/Mover	Finisher	Expert
Initiate team development Identify team tasks Identify strengths/weaknesses Call meetings Provide structure Review team needs Identify appropriate patients	Impose time constraints Focus on outputs (patients treated, goals achieved) Seek progress Show high commitment to task Manage projects	Have special expertise Offer professional viewpoint Identify interdisciplinary patient problems Use expertise of other disciplines Understand patient needs Know team's expertise and limits
Ambassador	**Diplomat**	**Supporter**
Build external relationships Promote awareness of the team's work Build bridges Show concern for external team environment	Build understanding between members Negotiate Mediate Facilitate decision making	Build team morale Put team members at ease Ensure job satisfaction Help patient work with team
Judge/Evaluator	**Process Analyzer**	**Facilitator**
Listen critically Evaluate clinical process Evaluate clinical outcomes Help team reflect Promote appropriate treatment Act logically Seek truth	Identify team problems Analyze team problems Consult with team members Offer observations Offer potential solutions to team problems	Identify member conflicts Help team members find ways to resolve conflicts Help implement solutions
Creator	**Innovator**	**Challenger**
Generate new ideas Visualize new programs/projects Visualize new alliances	Discover resources Identify opportunities Transform ideas to strategy Propose new methods	Offer skepticism Look in new ways Question accepted order
Reviewer	**Quality Controller**	**Conformer/Follower**
Observe Review team performance Promote review of process Give feedback Mirror team's actions	Check output alignment Act as conscience regarding team goals Inspire higher standards Assure team reviews outcomes	Seek agreement Fill gaps in teamwork Cooperate Help relationships Avoid challenges Maintain continuity
Guard	**Teacher**	**Learner**
Protect team from too much output Protect team from too much input	Help new members learn the norms and values of the team Teach shared leadership skills to other members Recognize members' leadership potential Teach others when to seek specialty advice	Raise questions to enhance understanding across disciplines or areas Raise questions regarding need for interdisciplinary input

---

Reprinted from Drinka, T. J. K., & Clark, P. G. (2000). *Health care teamwork: Interdisciplinary practice and teaching.* Reproduced with permission of Greenwood Publishing Group, Inc., Westport, CT.

but the team is resistant to making changes. Individuals may also be resentful of the roles or leadership of other team members. In each of these conflict examples, individuals must solve their own problem or issue. However, these problems can escalate and begin to impact the entire team.

Interpersonal

Interpersonal conflicts exist between two team members. Sometimes these conflicts are a result of personality factors. Team members may not like each other, and this becomes an issue while working together.

Members' expectations of each other may be unclear or undefined.

People also have different styles of working or communicating, and the interplay during meetings can cause these differences to result in conflict. For example, team member Joan likes to discuss various options before reaching a decision about a patient problem. Team member Tom likes to give his recommendation and move to making the decision. Each time Tom discusses a case, Joan asks a lot of questions about management options, clearly irritating Tom, who has made his decision about what to do. Their exchanges show irritation on both sides as Joan pushes for more information and Tom tries to end the discussion.

Members may not agree about interventions or who should be providing certain care. They may also have different priorities for a patient's care. For example, an older patient, Mrs. M, is living alone and experiencing functional difficulties. One team member thinks, because Mrs. M used to be very social and is now lonely, that Mrs. M would be much happier in assisted living with people around her. The team could encourage such a move. However, another team member knows Mrs. M really does not want to leave her home and values her autonomy, so she thinks the team should help Mrs. M stay in her home and not discuss a move.

Two team members could be trying to assume the same roles on the team, either formally or informally. They may try to show each other up, get attention, or make the other team member look bad. This problem is common on teams where there is no structure for the team. Because there is no plan for accomplishing the work, individuals may eventually do things their own way. There is constant struggle because there is no decision about how to do things and people continually try to superimpose a structure.

In other situations, one team member may try to dominate another member because of disagreement about patient decisions. Team member Joe tends to overlook the input of social worker Saundra concerning adult day care. He does not think it works very well, while she has had good day care experiences with her patients. He ignores Saundra's suggestions about patients, or makes negative comments about her input (we all know what *Saundra* is going to say) in an attempt to discount her ideas or embarrass her. This may cause Saundra to stop contributing suggestions so that Joe can make the decision without any discussion.

Intrateam

Intrateam conflicts involve several team members at once, and may develop from the prior types of conflicts discussed, as additional team members get involved. If Saundra from the prior example begins to complain to other team members about her problems with Joe, they may get involved. In team meetings, other team members may try to encourage Saundra to speak up, introduce things for her, or address Joe's comments directly. If Joe has team members who take his side, then two groups of team members develop a conflict. Drinka & Clark (2000) suggest that intrateam conflicts often arise from disagreements about values, such as complicated problems of autonomy and patient competency.

Interteam

Interteam conflicts occur between the team and outside forces. For example, some primary care providers do not think specialized geriatric assessments are needed for their patients. If they treat a number of older patients, these providers may assume they have all the knowledge and skills necessary to provide good care. They may not appreciate geriatric specialists and may react negatively to the team or even patients and family members who seek this care. Conflict between the team and the primary care provider results, putting patients and families in a difficult position, perhaps not knowing whose advice to follow, and the team needs to help resolve the problem.

MANAGING TEAM CONFLICT

Team conflict is usually obvious to observers. Inappropriate exchanges among team members may be frequent. Team members may be spending time smoothing things over with one or more other members. The team may have frequent disagreements and difficulty making decisions. Some participants may feel like they cannot introduce certain issues, as it may cause arguments or disagreeable responses. The team may feel that it is walking on eggshells, and performance suffers.

Some team conflict is unavoidable, and may even be healthy and necessary for the effective functioning of the team. The real issue is how team members or the group as a whole deals with it. Ideally, the team can introduce problems, discuss them openly, and develop solutions. Identifying conflict is a good first step. Going back to our example of the conflict over adult day care, the nurse Joan states at a meeting that the team seems to have a problem discussing adult day care as people have such strong opinions on the topic. She asks each of the staff to talk about the experiences of their patients, so that they can think about what patients would be good candidates for day care to facilitate future discussions.

Good team leadership, as we have previously stated, is essential, and can prevent some types of conflict. The leader should monitor team functioning, identifying member's contributions and communication patterns that might indicate problems. The leader can discuss concerns with individual team members and help them rectify any difficulties. For example, the team leader may notice irritation expressed by a team member as in our prior example of Tom and Saundra. The leader may choose to meet with them separately or together, or both, to help them identify and resolve the conflict.

Group issues can be discussed with the team as a whole, and appropriate methods can be used to resolve issues. Clark (1995) suggests that diversity among team members should enhance creativity, and that the difference among team members should be recognized and appreciated. For some issues, it may be appropriate for the team to vote on a resolution. In other cases, making a decision may require more of a consensus or compromise among team members. The leader or a team member may be able to moderate such a discussion. If an issue is particularly difficult, an outside moderator who can be objective may be more helpful. Conflicts with those outside the team may need to be resolved through meetings or negotiations.

Orientation of new team members may help avoid potential conflicts. In addition to participating in team meetings, the new member may be given the opportunity to work with other experienced team members for a period of time. The preceptor can then discuss the team processes and rationale with the new member. Reviewing examples of prior paperwork or team care plans also may be helpful.

EVALUATING THE EFFECTIVENESS OF TEAMS

Given the potential problems in teamwork, it is helpful to think about how a team would appear when it is functioning effectively. The Geriatric Interdisciplinary Team Training Curriculum Guide (Hyer et al., 2003, p. 10) describes the following characteristics of effective teams:

- Purpose, goals, and objectives are known and agreed upon.
- Roles and responsibilities are clear.
- Communication is open, sharing, and honest. There is disagreement without tyranny and constructive criticism without personal attack.
- Team members listen to each other.
- Team members are competent, professional, and personally effective, and make appropriate contributions.
- Teams cooperate and coordinate activities. Decisions are reached by consensus.
- When decisions are made, assignments are made clearly, accepted, and carried out.
- Leadership shifts, depending on the circumstances.
- Team members support each other and act as different resources for the group.

- Team members trust one another, minimize struggles for power, and focus on how best to get the job done.
- The team evaluates its own operations.

ETHICAL ISSUES

Despite the potential benefits of interdisciplinary team care, a variety of ethical problems are possible (Kane, 2002):

- A team can overwhelm clients both by their numbers and by their expertise, particularly when the patient or family has goals that differ from the professional team.
- Individual team members may be squelched by other team members, as in the example discussed earlier, or may feel unwelcome to express their ideas.
- The team can get into a rut of always handling problems the same way, leading to "groupthink" or exclusion of new ideas.

The team process itself can cause difficulties for clients. For example:

- Group decision making can take longer than individual decision making, causing delays in action.
- Because many disciplines are frequently involved, there can be lack of accountability.

Teams should evaluate their effectiveness in terms of patient outcomes and satisfaction and discuss complaints and difficult issues as part of their team maintenance work to minimize ethical problems. In addition, teams may want to contact their health system ethics committee for consultation when complex ethical problems cannot be solved.

TRAINING

Training members can help the team to avoid some of the potential pitfalls discussed in this chapter. Historically the Veterans Administration Geriatric Research, Education, and Clinical Centers as well as Geriatric Education Centers funded by the Health Resources and Services Administration (HRSA) have promoted interdisciplinary training of health professionals. More recently the John A. Hartford Foundation funded a national program to promote geriatric interdisciplinary team training (GITT). As a result, curricula and training materials including videotapes of team meetings are available (Hyer et al., 2003; Long & Wilson, 2001). Box 25-3 describes the advanced practice nurse's role in geriatric interdisciplinary teams as developed by the Nursing Interest Group of the John A. Hartford GITT program (Hyer et al., 2003), and the additional competencies they can attain with specialized team training.

BOX 25-3 Advanced Practice Nurses Roles on Interdisciplinary Teams

Developed by the Nursing Interest Group of the John A. Hartford Foundation GITT program, including Dr. Joan Bezon, Sally Brooks, Kathy Echvarria, Dr. Vaunette Fay, Dr. Karen Feldt, Dr. Ellen Flaherty, Dr. Terry Fulmer, Mary Gleason, Sherry Greenberg, Dr. Lois Halstead, Dr. Kathryn Hyer, Dr. Mary Jirovec, Ernestine Kotthoff-Burrell, Dr. Valerie Matthieson, Dr. Mathy Mezey, Dr. Linda Moody, Dr. Maura Ryan, Dr. Ingrid Venhor, Dr. Maria Vezina, and Elisabeth Weingast.

In compiling these competencies, the Nursing Interest Group relied on the American Nurses Credentialing Center Guidelines for Graduating Nurse Practitioners, National Organization of Nurse Practitioner Faculty, and the American Nurses' Association Standards of Practice for the Primary Health Care Practitioner. Competencies have been modified to include an interdisciplinary focus reflecting the group's recognition of the importance of interdisciplinary care for elders.

Upon completion of a formal educational program, gerontological nurse practitioners are able to do the following:

■ Elicit a comprehensive health history from the client and/or caregivers, including an evaluation of developmental maturation, physiological/psychosocial/functional status, cultural orientation, perception of health, health-promoting behaviors, risk factors for illness, response to stressors, activities of daily living (instrumental and functional), service utilization, and support systems.
■ Complete a comprehensive functional assessment, mental status assessment, and psychoemotional assessment.
■ Perform a complete physical examination on the older adult, employing techniques of observation, inspection, palpation, auscultation, and percussion.
■ Discriminate among normal findings, normal changes of aging, pathological findings, and abnormal findings that require collaboration with a physician.
■ Use pertinent screening tools to determine health status.
■ Order and/or perform pertinent diagnostic tests.
■ Analyze the data collected in collaboration with the health care team to determine health status and need for consultation with or referral to other agencies or resources.
■ Formulate a problem list.
■ Develop and implement (with the client, caregivers and/or significant others, and health care team) a plan of care to promote, maintain, and rehabilitate health.
■ Evaluate the client's response to the health care provided and the effectiveness of the care with the client.
■ Collaborate with other health professionals and agencies involved in the client's care.
■ Modify the plan and intervention as needed.
■ Record all pertinent data about the client, including the health history, functional assessment, physical examination, problems identified, interventions planned and/or provided, results of care, and plans for consultation or referral.
■ Coordinate the services required to meet the client's need for primary health care and/or long-term care and monitor outcomes.
■ Act as an advocate for the older adult to improve his/her health status.
■ Provide for continuity of care over time and in a variety of settings.
■ Provide patient-centered and family-centered care.
■ Participate in life-long learning, peer review, and continuous quality improvement.

In addition to the above areas, gerontological nurse practitioners who have completed the GITT program will be able to:

■ Define the gerontological nurse practitioner's role in various health care settings.
■ Identify and implement assertiveness and leadership strategies to strengthen the gerontological nurse practitioner's role in various health care settings.
■ Identify complex geriatric cases that would most benefit from collaboration of other health care team members.
■ Demonstrate sensitivity to cultural and economic issues of clients in planning care as a team.
■ Identify team dynamics that promote collaboration among disciplines.
■ Develop skills in communicating and networking with health care team members.
■ Demonstrate knowledge of conflict management techniques for resolving conflict among health care team members.
■ Demonstrate skills in leading and coordinating health care team meetings.
■ Develop and implement strategies that have a positive effect on the advancement of knowledge, political and regulatory processes, and systems affecting the health and welfare of older adults, gerontological nurse practitioners, and the health care system.

Reprinted from the Nurses Special Interest Group of the John A. Hartford Foundation GITT program.

BENEFITS OF THE INTERDISCIPLINARY APPROACH: COMPREHENSIVE GERIATRIC ASSESSMENT

Interdisciplinary care for the elderly is often delivered through comprehensive geriatric assessment (CGA) programs. These programs provide evaluation of the older person in a variety of domains, typically physical, functional, psychological, and social. The purpose of the CGA is to uncover, describe, and explain the multiple problems of the older person and to identify the person's strengths and resources. The hallmark of the CGA is the role of the interdisciplinary team as described at the beginning of this chapter.

The goal of CGA is to systematically identify and tackle problems, and organize a coordinated plan of care for better outcomes. The team may provide a consultative service, where problems are identified and an initial plan developed. In this case, the patient returns to his or her primary provider, who implements the plan and provides ongoing care. In other situations, the CGA team provides ongoing care, monitors progress, and makes changes in the plan of care as needed. While these are usually outpatient programs, some providers offer inpatient options.

The rationale for the interdisciplinary approach is grounded in the understanding that older persons typically present with clinically complex, interrelated problems that require more complex evaluation and intervention than can realistically be provided by a single discipline. This is particularly true for the older, frailer patient, who may present with one or more geriatric syndromes. The comprehensive evaluation and care that can be provided by the team are geared toward improved outcomes. Rubenstein (2004) reports that the need for CGA arises from problems in care of the older patient, including undiscovered disease and disability, unnecessary nursing home admissions, neglect of rehabilitation needs, and iatrogenic problems.

CGA was developed in the 1970s. By the late 1980s, the National Institutes of Health held a consensus conference concluding that CGA was effective in improving health outcomes for older persons in various health settings. A meta-analysis of studies on inpatient geriatric care (Stuck et al., 1993) showed improved survival and function for CGA older patients, compared to those receiving usual care. Studies since then have looked at a variety of assessment models, with mixed outcomes. A new meta-analysis, again by Stuck and colleagues (2002), found that CGA is more effective when the team provides intensive follow-up care than when CGA is provided as a consultative process.

Comprehensive geriatric assessment is a time-consuming process, taking up to 3 hours to complete. In light of the cost as well as the amount of time and effort that various disciplines contribute, the use of CGA should be targeted to those who most need this intensive approach. While specific criteria are not available, older adults with complex medical problems who are frail, who have acute illness with complications, or who are being evaluated for placement in long-term settings are most appropriate for comprehensive assessment (Rubenstein, 2004).

On the other hand, healthy older adults can usually be adequately managed in the regular primary care setting. Those whose status falls in between, who may be developing functional decline or complicated geriatric problems, should have further assessment and intervention to prevent deterioration or improve management of chronic disease states. Common geriatric problems may be managed using clinical guidelines, protocols for care, or care pathways such as Clinical Glidepaths (Flaherty, Morley, Murphy, & Wasserman, 2002) before more intense services are recommended. Targeted appropriately, CGA provides a care technology that uses the interdisciplinary team to improve care for older adults with complex medical/social/psychological problems.

CASE STUDY OF A COMPREHENSIVE GERIATRIC ASSESSMENT

The following is a case study from a comprehensive geriatric assessment program at an academic medical center. In this case the core team includes a physician (MD), advanced practice nurse (APN), social worker (SW), and pharmacist (Pharm D). The following is a summary of their reports at a team meeting following an initial assessment of this patient, and a care plan developed for this patient.

The Case of Mrs. Jones

The social worker presented first, providing a summary of the psychosocial assessment including issues with family, and/or living arrangements, screening for depression, and other issues:

Mrs. Jones was brought to the CGA program by her daughter Joella, who is concerned about her mother's memory and ability to continue to live in her home. Mrs. Jones has become forgetful, is misplacing items, and is forgetting appointments and recent conversations. The daughter works full time and tries to help her out, but Mrs. Jones always tells her things are fine. Joella recently checked her mother's refrigerator and found that her mother had little food (with some of it spoiled) even though she claimed that a neighbor had taken her to the grocery store. One of her mother's heart medications had expired, and Mrs. Jones did not have it refilled. Joella reported that Mrs. Jones has lost weight and has had swollen ankles, but her health has been pretty good. Joella is the primary caregiver and a single mother with two children. Joella has a brother who lives out of town. Mrs. Jones has little income, and her medical insurance includes Medicaid and Medicare.

Mrs. Jones is very quiet with few complaints. She states that she does not want to be a burden to her daughter. She admits to being lonely and not getting to church or seeing friends as much as she would like, but states she is doing just fine. She is sad sometimes, and reminisces about her sisters who have recently died. A close neighbor of Mrs. Jones also died in the past year. Mrs. Jones denied being depressed, but her screening depression test is suggestive of mild to moderate depression. She wants to stay in her home for as long as she can.

The advanced practice nurse reported on the patient's functional status, management of health, and cognitive screen:

Mrs. Jones and her daughter felt that she was able to perform activities of daily living (ADLs) independently, including walking, bathing, dressing, feeding herself, and toileting. However, inspection of her current condition suggests she may not be changing clothes frequently, or taking care of her hair or nails. She has difficulty walking more than a short distance, because of pain in her knees and edema in her ankles. Although Mrs. Jones denies falling, her daughter believes that she has fallen at least once because she observed bruises on her mother's legs.

Mrs. Jones needs assistance with many instrumental ADLs such as cleaning and laundry, and does not appear to have adequate assistance. A neighbor takes Mrs. Jones to the store once a week for shopping, and she has the neighbor bring a "thing or two" if she does not have the energy to make the trip. She does not cook very much, but will make "a little soup" for supper. Mrs. Jones reports taking her medication every day, as directed. Mrs. Jones uses the phone and calls her daughter regularly, but relies on others to take her places. She has never driven a car. Cognitive testing is well within the impaired range, and her clock drawing was abnormal.

The geriatrician reported positive findings from the medical history and physical examination (in some cases the advanced practice nurse may perform part or all of the history and physical examination):

Mrs. Jones has hypertension that may not be managed by her medications, although it is unclear how regularly she is taking them. In addition, she has symptoms of hypothyroidism, a condition that can impair memory. She complains of knee pain when rising from a chair and during walking. Her gait is unsteady, with short steps and a wide stance, and her balance is impaired. She needs to use her arms to rise from a chair. The combination of lower extremity weakness, slow and widened gait, and balance impairment makes her a high fall risk. In reviewing her mood, she meets DSM-IV criteria for a major depression.

Finally the pharmacist reviewed the medications, noting those that might affect memory and mood.

The medications for this patient may be affecting her cognition, mood, and appetite, and changes should be considered to simplify her regimen and decrease the potential for side effects.

After discussing the case, the team developed a plan of care for Mrs. Jones that included management of her medical problems, educating the patient and family about her dementia, and working with the daughter to provide increased assistance. For this particular team, a nutritionist was included to provide additional input on patient problems. The team agreed that the goal was to attempt to increase the support and supervision for Mrs. Jones to help her stay at home for as long as possible, understanding that this may not be a permanent solution. Strategies that would increase her socialization and supervision, such as adult day care, were seen as the best approaches. The team identified a variety of options with little conflict (the plan of care including a problem list, goals, and interventions is provided in Table 25-3, adapted from a standardized care plan).

The next steps would be completed with input from the patient and daughter at a family conference to discuss the findings and recommendations, any additional information or tests that were recommended, and how the plan could be implemented. The recommendations would also be sent to Mrs. Jones' primary care provider. The appropriate team members would continue to work with Mrs. Jones and her primary care provider over the next few months to implement or adapt the plan to provide Mrs. Jones with increased support and supervision.

In this case, a frail patient with potential physical, psychological, and social problems was an appropriate candidate for comprehensive geriatric assessment. While there is potential overlap among the roles of team members, they each have designated roles that complement each other for the final assessment and treatment plan. They may have conflicts in determining the specific recommendations. For example, can they find adequate resources to keep her in her home? What other options might be acceptable to Mrs. Jones and her family? What will Mrs. Jones gain or lose by making different choices? The situation plays out over time as the team works with the patient and family.

SUMMARY

Interdisciplinary teams have the potential to improve care for many older adults, especially those with complex medical and psychosocial problems. Yet health professionals are often unprepared to work in these situations, and differences in the preparation and values of various professionals can develop into conflicts or poor care. This chapter discussed information about the structure of teams, common sources of conflict, and methods for operating team meetings that can help interdisciplinary teams function more effectively. Nurses educated in the team approach have the potential to impact the work of interdisciplinary teams and provide leadership to minimize the challenges of this work environment.

Table 25-3 *Interdisciplinary Team Care Plan for Mrs. Jones**

Problem/ Diagnosis	Goal	Overall Goal: Increase Services to Maintain Patient at Home in Safer Environment for as Long as Possible	
		Strategy	Team Member Responsible
Cognitive impairment: probable Alzheimer's disease	1. Establish diagnosis, rule out treatable and contributing factors	Review laboratory tests from primary doctor and obtain, if not available, CBC, CMP, folate, B_{12}, vitamin D, TSH Discuss possibility of head scan	MD
Lack of knowledge regarding health condition	2. Educate patient and family about findings	Discuss presence of memory problem, medical workup, and findings Explain disease process and prognosis Present goal of managing patient problems and symptoms rather than seeking cure	MD
	3. Identify medical options	Discuss medications that may help slow progression of disease Explain options to maintain health and provide activities and stimulation Identify drug studies or other options	MD, Pharm D
	4. Discuss need for assistance and supervision and options for providing care	Discuss need for supervision of medications, assistance with meals and personal care, concern about falling, and increased socialization Discuss options for providing care including family help and community resources Adult day care program would be a good choice and would provide transportation, supervision, meals, medication oversight, and socialization Consider PACE (Program of All-inclusive Care for the Elderly) for comprehensive supportive health services Consider move to more supportive environment if options are not viable	APN and SW
	5. Provide resources for learning about disease and coping	Give packet of information on managing memory problems Refer to Alzheimer's Association classes and support groups Encourage readings (i.e., The 36 Hour Day [Mace & Rabins, 2001])	APN
	6. Plan for legal and medical issues	Discuss financial and health care directives Discuss patient's ability to execute documents	APN
Impaired mobility/risk for injury: falls	Prevent injury	Physical therapy evaluation of gait and recommendations regarding assistive device Exercise prescription Home safety evaluation	MD and APN
Osteoarthritis	Reduce pain and promote mobility	Consider regimen of regularly scheduled acetaminophen Physical therapy/exercise as noted above	MD

Table 25-3 *Interdisciplinary Team Care Plan for Mrs. Jones*—cont'd

	Overall Goal: Increase Services to Maintain Patient at Home in Safer Environment for as Long as Possible		
Problem/ Diagnosis	Goal	Strategy	Team Member Responsible
Underweight	Encourage goal weight of 135 pounds	Assistance with meals as noted Consider meals-on-wheels for some days Liberalize diet so patient has more choices of foods that she likes Discuss foods that have high nutrients Discontinue digoxin	APN
Depression	Promote improved mood	Monitor mood with supportive services and consider medication if no improvement Increase socialization through adult day care or different home environment	SW
Hypertension	Maintain blood pressure <160/90 mm Hg	Recommend once daily regimen of medications with less potential for side effects than current drug Supervise blood pressure medication and monitor blood pressure to determine if regimen is working	MD, Pharm D
Hypothyroidism	Maintain T_3, TSH within appropriate range	Check blood level and adjust dose of Synthroid as needed, with supervised medication administration	MD, Pharm D

*Adapted from the Older Adult Health Center, Division of Geriatrics and Gerontology, Washington University School of Medicine.

REFERENCES

Bellack, J. P., & O'Neil, E. H. (2000). Recreating nursing practice for a new century: Recommendations and implications of the Pew Health Professions Commission's final report. *Nursing & Health Care Perspectives, 21*(1), 14-21.

Burbank, P. M., Owens, N. J., Stoukides, J., Evans, E. B., Leinhaas, M. M., & Evans, J. M. (2002). Developing an interdisciplinary geriatric curriculum: The perils and payoffs of collaboration. *Educational Gerontology, 28*, 451-472.

Clark, P. G. (1995). Quality of life, values and teamwork in geriatric care: Do we communicate what we mean? *Gerontologist, 35*(3), 402-411.

Clark, P. G. (2002). Evaluating an interdisciplinary team training institute in geriatrics: Implications for teaching and practice. *Educational Gerontology, 28*, 511-528.

Clark, P. G., Leinhaas, M. M., & Filinson, R. (2002). Developing and evaluating an interdisciplinary clinical team training program: Lessons taught and lessons learned. *Educational Gerontology, 28*, 401 410.

Dahlke, R., Wolf, K. N., Wilson, S. I., & Brodnik, M. (2000). Focus groups as predictors of dieticians' roles on interdisciplinary teams. *Journal of the American Dietetics Association, 100*, 455-457.

Drinka, T. J. K. (2002). From double jeopardy to double indemnity: Subtleties of teaching interdisciplinary geriatrics. *Educational Gerontology, 28*, 433-449.

Drinka, T. J. K., & Clark, P. G. (2000). *Health care teamwork: Interdisciplinary practice and teaching.* Westport, CT: Auburn House.

Faulkner-Schofield, R., & Amodeo, M. (1999). Interdisciplinary teams in health care and human services settings: Are they effective? *Health and Social Work, 24*(3), 210-219.

Flaherty, J. H., Morley, J. E., Murphy, D. J., & Wasserman, M. R. (2002). The development of outpatient Clinical Glidepaths. *Journal of the American Geriatrics Society, 50*, 1886-1901.

Gardner, D. B. (2005). Ten lessons in collaboration. *Online Journal of Issues in Nursing, 10*(1), 61.

Healy, J., Victor, C. R., & Sergeant, J. (2002). Professionals and post-hospital care for older people. *Journal of Interprofessional Care, 16*(1), 19-29.

Hyer, K., Flaherty, E., Fairchild, S., Botrell, M., Mezey, M., Fulmer, T., et al. (2003). *Geriatric interdisciplinary team training program (GITT): Curriculum guide.* New York: GITT Resource Center, New York University.

Institute of Medicine. (2003). *Health professions education: A bridge to quality.* Retrieved September 1, 2004, from www.iom.edu/report. asp?id=5914.

Kane, R. A. (2002). Avoiding the dark side of geriatric teamwork. In M. D. Mezey, C. K. Cassel, M. M. Bottrell, K. Hyer, J. L. Howe, & T. T. Fulmer (Eds.), *Ethical patient care: A casebook for geriatric health care teams.* Baltimore: Johns Hopkins University Press.

Leipzig, R. M., Hyer, K., Ek, K., Wallenstein, S., Vezina, M. L., Fairchild, S., et al. (2002). Attitudes toward working on interdisciplinary healthcare teams: A comparison by discipline. *Journal of the American Geriatrics Society, 50*, 1141-1148.

Long, D. M., & Wilson, N. L. (2001). *Geriatric interdisciplinary team training: A curriculum from the Huffington Center on Aging.* Houston,

TX: Baylor College of Medicine's Huffington Center on Aging.

Mace, N. L., & Rabins, P. V. (2001). The 36-Hour Day: Family guide to caring for persons with Alzheimer's disease, related dementing illnesses, and memory loss in later life. New York: Warner Books.

Mellow, M. J., & Lindeman, D. (1998). The role of the social worker in interdisciplinary geriatric teams. *Journal of Gerontological Social Work, 30*(3/4), 3-7.

Pitsillides, B., Pitsillides, A., Samaras, G., Andreou, P., Georgiadis, D., Christodoulou, E., & Panteli, N. (2004). User perspective of DITIS: Virtual collaborative teams for home care. *Studies in Health Technology & Informatics, 100,* 205-216.

Rubenstein, L. Z. (2004). Comprehensive geriatric assessment: From miracle to reality. *Journal of Gerontology, 50A,* 473-477.

Skinner, J. H. (2001). Transitioning from multidisciplinary to interdisciplinary education in gerontology and geriatrics. *Gerontology and Geriatrics Education, 21*(3), 73-85.

Sommers, L. S., Marton, K. I., Barbaccia, J. C., & Randolph, J. (2000). Physician, nurse, and social worker collaboration in primary care for chronically ill seniors. *Archives of Internal Medicine, 160,* 1825-1833.

Stuck, A. E., Siu, A. L., Wieland, G. D., & Rubenstein, L. Z. (1993). Comprehensive geriatric assessment. *Lancet, 342,* 1032-1036.

Stuck, A. E., Egger, M., Hammer, A., Minder, C. E., & Beck J. C. (2002). Home visits to prevent nursing home admission and functional decline in elderly people: Systematic review and meta-regression analysis. *Journal of the American Medical Association, 287*(8),1022-1028.

Tuckman, B. W. (1965). Developmental sequence in small groups. *Psychological Bulletin, 63*(6), 384-399.

Vroman, K., & Kovacich, J. (2002). Computer-mediated interdisciplinary teams: Theory and reality. *Journal of Interprofessional Care, 16*(2), 159-170.

Wells, J. L., Seabrook, J. A., Stolee, P., & Borrie, M. J. (2003). State of the art in geriatric rehabilitation. Part 1: Review of frailty and comprehensive geriatric assessment. *Archives of Physical and Medical Rehabilitation, 84,* 890-897.

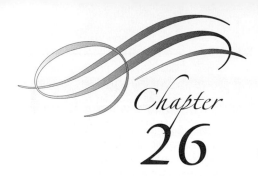

Chapter
26 Case Management

Todd M. Ruppar

Objectives

Identify the purpose and benefit of case management of older adults.

Identify case manager role functions.

List case-management principles to consider when working with older clients.

List patient and institutional outcomes of case-management programs.

Describe common components of case-management programs and explain how they can work together.

OVERVIEW OF CASE MANAGEMENT

Case management in health care in the modern era emerged in the early to mid-1980s as a way to improve both clinical and financial outcomes. Efforts were generally focused first in acute care settings, but as the number of successful programs grew, case-management approaches were applied to community, long-term care, and primary care settings.

Many definitions and approaches to case management exist in the literature, highlighting the fact that case management is a nursing role that has been adapted to multiple client populations and across varied care settings. A comprehensive definition from the Case Management Society of America is provided by Conger (1996) as "a process of assessment, planning, implementation, coordination, monitoring, and evaluation of health care services and outcomes in an attempt to meet client needs in a cost-effective manner" (p. 231). Several models of case management exist, though most involve a case manager who coordinates services for clients and matches them with appropriate resources. The case manager is typically a nurse, but may also be a social worker or even a physician.

Case management provides an important tool to improve health care for older adults because of the high prevalence of multiple chronic diseases and the complex nature of many of their health problems. This, coupled with the fragmentation of the health care system, places older adults at great risk of complications and poor outcomes, as well as duplication of services or the alternative of services not even being offered. Case management, particularly nursing case management, has the potential to increase quality of care and improve both patient and financial outcomes (Mahn-DiNicola & Zazworsky, 2005). This chapter provides an overview of case management as well as some specific information about case management with older adults. Box 26-1 describes the experiences of providing private case management for older adults from a nurse filling this role.

BASIC GOALS OF CASE MANAGEMENT

Case-management goals tend to vary in specifics among different patient populations and case-management models, but the basic goals have a tendency to remain constant. The general goals of case management include:

- Improving the quality of care
  1. Health promotion
  2. Early detection of disease
  3. Disease management/prevention of complications
- Controlling costs
  1. Decreasing length of stay
  2. Appropriate use of resources (Cohen & Cesta, 2005; Flarey & Blancett, 1996)

Quality of Care

Since its beginning, case management has been strongly linked with quality of care. Case managers are frequently charged with evaluating care interventions for therapeutic outcomes and often ensuring that clinical practice guidelines, protocols, or clinical pathways are followed. The impact of case management can be directed across the continuum from primary prevention in the form of health promotion to tertiary prevention

BOX 26-1 *Reflections on the Practice of Case Management in Two Settings*

Nurses serve as case managers in many types of settings. The following describes my experiences as a case manager as well as a member of a case management team caring for older adults in the community.

Experiences with a PACE Program Interdisciplinary Team

The PACE (Program of All-Inclusive Care of the Elderly) model utilizes an interdisciplinary approach to the care of older persons, incorporating all aspects of health care and support for the patient's social systems. These programs provide services to the frail older adult population in a community-based setting utilizing an adult day center, primary care clinics, and home care services. In doing this, the interdisciplinary team is charged with case management of the patient to maintain quality of care, efficiency, and overall quality of life. Essentially, everyone caring for and about the patient are case managers, including primary care providers, nurses, rehabilitation professionals, social workers, and recreational therapists, nursing assistants, van drivers, and dietary personnel.

A standard procedure at a PACE site is a daily meeting during which all team members meet with one another about issues and events concerning the patients. Problems and possible solutions are discussed until a consensus is reached. Solutions are always sought that are focused on maintaining the highest possible quality of life and quality of care while balancing financial costs and efficiency.

Considering the variety of roles and levels of staff involved, in conjunction with the frailty of the patient population served by the PACE program, the nurses on the team often assume the primary case manager role. Combining communication and collaboration skills with technical knowledge of pathophysiology, pharmacology, and aging, nursing professionals are well positioned to guide the team in decision making, short- and long-term planning, and realistic goal setting.

Private Geriatric Case Management

The challenges associated with caring for an older person can be trying and overwhelming. Because of this, the role of the private geriatric care manager is becoming more valuable, and nurses are increasingly serving in these

roles. Often called in to assist families in care decisions and coordination of health care services, the support and guidance offered by geriatric care managers is invaluable.

Many organizations now specialize in nursing-oriented geriatric care management, including consultation, assessment, recommendations, and ongoing care management services. Patients include older adults living in their own homes and those living in various types of long-term care facilities. The care manager is contacted by a family member overwhelmed with or needing advice about care, or by families living out of the area who are unable to provide close supervision of often tenuous situations. Services offered include the following:

- *Expert advice on geriatric care and services*
- *Assessment of in-home patients' needs in preparation for a move to another setting or to recommend changes and promote safety and independence*
- *Assistance with initiation of in-home services*
- *Long-term monitoring and coordination of in-home services to ensure effectiveness and quality*
- *Follow up for patients in long-term care facilities to evaluate the care being provided and to assist with changes as needed*
- *Guidance with the selection of and transfer to an appropriate long-term care setting*
- *Resources for individuals and family members on specific health care issues*
- *Referrals and information regarding medical, legal, and financial services*

The primary goal of the geriatric care manager is to promote each individual's optimal level of independence while maintaining well-being and dignity. Nurses in this role serve as unique and innovative resources for those facing the difficult task of providing care or planning care for themselves or their loved ones. This kind of care is challenging but rewarding, requiring a vast army of skills and knowledge and providing the practitioner with opportunity to interact with and improve the quality of life of patients in a variety of settings.

Mary M. Austin

Mary M. Austin, MSN, RN, NHA
President, Senior Pathways
Phoenixville, Pennsylvania

in preventing complications or negative sequelae of acute events or chronic disease.

Cost Control

In addition to minimizing health care costs by controlling length of stay, case management also works to control health care costs by overseeing factors that influence

the costs incurred by the patient, facility, and/or third-party payer.

Length of Stay

With the advent of Diagnosis-Related Groups (DRGs), case-management programs were frequently charged with working to minimize length of stay to control hospitalization costs. Longer length of stay can also be a risk factor for complications of hospitalization (for example, nosocomial infections).

Resource Utilization

Case management is designed to contribute to the appropriate use of health care resources. The supervision provided by case managers helps to link patients with helpful and appropriate resources, as well as minimize the inappropriate use of health care resources. Connection with appropriate resources may help older adults remain in the community and prevent premature nursing home placement.

CASE-MANAGEMENT MODELS

Nursing literature contains several different models of case management, each of which organizes services in different ways. The first factor considered in choosing a model, and thus a primary factor used in differentiating models, is the source from which case-management services are being provided (Box 26-2). From there, the case-management program can be tailored to meet the situation, population, and available resources.

Case Management by Third-Party Payers

A third-party payer may provide case-management services. The third-party payer is typically an insurance company or managed care organization such as a health maintenance organization (HMO) or preferred provider organization (PPO). These companies employ case managers, who oversee services to covered patients who fall into a certain population that is at high risk for hospitalization or for the development of sequelae leading to increased health care costs. Diabetes mellitus and asthma/COPD are two common conditions managed

---

BOX 26-2 Case-Management Service Providers

Third-Party Payers
1. Health maintenance organizations
2. Preferred provider organizations

Health Care Providers
1. Acute care providers
2. Ambulatory care providers
3. Home care providers
4. Long-term care providers
5. Rehabilitation providers

Outside Providers
1. Private case-management services

From Cesta, T. G., & Tahan, H. A. (2003). *The case manager's survival guide* (2nd ed.). St. Louis: Mosby.

---

by third-party payers. Generally, these case managers are able to follow their clients across health care settings, both inpatient and outpatient (Cesta & Tahan, 2003). Case managers for HMOs and PPOs may also work to guide high-risk clients into outpatient educational or symptom self-management programs. In some instances, managed care organizations contract with outside organizations to provide case-management services for older adults (Enguidanos et al., 2003).

In some managed care organizations, the primary care provider is considered the case manager. This is particularly true when patients have a primary care provider who serves as a 'gatekeeper' that must provide referrals for outside services or specialists. In this situation, the primary care provider ensures that health care resources are being appropriately used by only referring patients for specialty services when deemed necessary. A potential conflict of interest can occur when financial incentives are offered to case managers who reduce the amount of resources used by patients.

Case Management by Health Care Providers

Case managers who are health care providers (or work for health care providers) deliver case-management services at the point of care. This may be in an acute care setting (such as a hospital), in an outpatient setting (for example, a doctor's office or clinic), in a long-term care facility (such as a nursing home), or in the home, if the client is receiving home care. These models have typically been set up with the case manager working only within the facility or agency where they are employed. In recent years, however, more institutions are implementing case-management programs that collaborate with outside providers and reach beyond the organizational boundaries. One example of this is the trend of hospital case-management programs to add postdischarge follow-up as part of their standard services. In these cases, a hospital case manager will contact the patient or patient's family at home following discharge to ensure that discharge instructions are understood and being followed, that appropriate outpatient follow-up is completed, and that any postdischarge complications are addressed and managed in a timely manner (Ball & Peruzzi, 1997). This additional service is designed to decrease postdischarge complications and reduce hospital readmission rates.

Tucker and DiRico (2003) used a geriatric inpatient case manager in a pilot study to identify and follow the highest risk elderly patients on all units of the hospital. Patients were identified using an algorithm that predicted their likelihood for complications leading to increased hospital costs. These high-risk patients were then followed by the geriatric case manager during their hospital stay and referred to an affiliated service for community case management after discharge. While the study looked primarily at economic outcomes, this model showed reductions in both length of stay and readmission rates among case-managed patients.

In primary care (outpatient) settings, case managers typically focus on patients with chronic illnesses (Cesta & Tahan, 2003). The case manager will work with the patients to better manage their chronic conditions, with the goal of preventing hospitalizations and reducing the need for outpatient office visits. Strategies used in a primary care case-management model include patient self-management education and monitoring of routine measures of illness severity and management (for example, laboratory or radiologic testing). Primary care case managers may also serve as a first contact for their clients when a change in their health status occurs. The case manager can then assess the client's care needs and facilitate efficient access to the health care system.

The goal of case management in long-term care settings is generally to promote the greatest functional status possible for patients while at the same time working to prevent any new health problems. The long-term care (LTC) case manager may lead the interdisciplinary team in reviewing resident progress and care needs. The case manager may also work with staff to evaluate a resident's functional status, health status, social supports, and overall well-being so that realistic goals can be set for improving or maintaining health, function, and quality of life. Long-term care case management can also be instrumental in the implementation of programs to address issues such as falls, prevention of skin breakdown, and wound care (Theodos, 2003).

Rehabilitation, which for older adults often occurs in the subacute care setting, has a primary focus of restoring function, often so that the older individual can return home after illness or injury. Mosqueda and Brummel-Smith (2002) identify two phases of this process in which the case manager may be involved in coordinating services such as physical and occupational therapy. The first is promoting adaptation of the person to his or her environment, which may include adjusting to adaptive equipment or assistive devices. The second is adapting the environment to the person (e.g., making home modifications to improve safety).

Case Management by Outside Providers

There are situations where people may benefit from case-management services but not be in a situation where they are able to receive such services from a health care provider. In these cases, the patient or the patient's family may contract with a private case manager or care manager. The case manager works directly for the patient and the patient's family and serves as a source of assessment information and health care referrals as well as an advocate and guide through the health care system. The private case manager is sometimes considered to be the most impartial case manager, because he or she is accountable only to the client (Cesta & Tahan, 2003). Private case managers are most often paid directly by the client on some type of fee schedule, although in some cases reimbursement may be available through the client's health insurance.

Private case managers may specialize in providing services for older adults, including assessments, referrals, and monitoring of services. In some cases, families who live out of town may contract with case managers to assist an older adult in a variety of ways that they cannot provide themselves. The case manager may make home or nursing home visits, check on the older adult, or make any necessary arrangements for services.

In some areas, older adults have access to geriatric case-management programs run by nonprofit agencies. These programs are frequently managed by social-service agencies in the community and provide some degree of health and functional status assessment and monitoring, as well as referrals to other agencies to meet clients' unmet needs. These services are often funded through donations or grants, but may also charge a small fee, often on a sliding scale based on the client's income. One example of this model is the Seniors-at-Home program run by Jewish Family and Children's Services in San Francisco, California (Rassen, 2003). This program has collaborated with health care providers to refer frail older adults at risk for decline to their program. The Seniors-at-Home program care manager then meets with the client to assess the client's needs, makes referrals, and follows the client's progress to see that needs are met. If the client was referred from a health care provider, the care manager sends a report to the provider.

THE CASE MANAGER ROLE

It is important to keep in mind that case management is more than the case manager role. Case management is a process, involving multiple health care professionals spanning across disciplines. The case manager is the individual who coordinates the staff, disciplines, and agencies involved to focus on providing smooth, efficient care. To do this, the case manager role requires a myriad of both clinical and organizational skills. Case managers will function as assessors, planners, facilitators, and advocates (Conger, 1996). The case manager role is one that, in most settings, originated as a nurse-filled role. The role does require some additional skills that are not typically ascribed to nursing or are not unique to the nursing profession, such as communication skills, financial skills, and an understanding of sociological issues (Box 26-3).

BOX 26-3 contents:

BOX 26-3 Role Functions of Case Managers

- Patient identification and outreach
- Service planning
- Resource identification
- Linking clients with services and resources
- Communication between other disciplines
- Monitoring resource utilization
- Client advocacy
- Client education
- Outcome evaluation
- Program manager
- Staff resource

From Flarey, D. L., & Blancett, S. S. (1996). *Handbook of nursing case management.* Gaithersburg, MD: Aspen; Wells, N., Erickson, S., & Spinella, J. (1996). Role transition: From clinical nurse specialist to clinical nurse specialist/case manager. *Journal of Nursing Administration, 26*(11), 23-28; and Taylor, P. (1999). Comprehensive nursing case management: An advanced practice model. *Nursing Case Management, 4*(1), 2-13.

Clinical Skills

Case managers must be able to formulate assessments of clients' health care needs. In the often demanding work environments in today's health care setting, it is important that the case manager be able to make efficient, thorough assessments to ascertain clients' resource needs and assess for effectiveness of ongoing interventions. Knowledge of gerontology and care of older adults is critical for case management of older patients.

Current clinical skills also allow the case manager to have a realistic understanding of the capabilities of other staff working with the client. The case manager's clinical skills will prevent the arrangement of interventions or goals that are outside the abilities or scope of the health care providers involved in a client's care. The case manager will better recognize when to introduce additional providers or resources. A good working knowledge of community resources available to older adults is important.

Organizational Skills

Case managers must have effective organizational skills to coordinate client care, often from multiple providers. Case managers are frequently responsible for coordinating care from providers outside their institution (e.g., setting up and supervising home care services for hospital clients following discharge). Case managers may also be responsible for scheduling testing or medical imaging services from outside providers.

In some settings, case managers are an integral part of an interdisciplinary team, possibly even the team leader. In such cases, the case manager is responsible for coordinating between different providers and/or departments within her or his own institution. Content on interdisciplinary team work is provided in Chapter 25.

Communication Skills

Case managers spend a significant amount of time communicating with clients, outside providers, and insurance companies/third-party payers. These contacts may be face-to-face, by telephone, through electronic means such as e-mail, or through printed correspondence. All these forms of communication require the case manager to have strong communication skills to minimize confusion and ensure that client services are arranged efficiently, accurately, and promptly. The case manager must understand the language and culture of all the various players.

Financial Skills

Cost control has always been one of the driving forces behind case-management efforts. To more effectively evaluate progress toward this goal, case managers should have the ability to interpret and understand health care financial data (Conger, 1996). Such an understanding may enable case managers to show administrators the results of their efforts and, if necessary, to justify their positions.

ADVANCED PRACTICE NURSES AS CASE MANAGERS

Advanced practice nurses (APNs) are generally well suited to filling case manager roles. It is well within the scope of the advanced practice nurse to consult and collaborate with multiple care providers, often across different care settings (American Nurses Association [ANA], 2004). APNs generally have training and experience in working with systems and collaborating with other providers in an interdisciplinary environment. This, combined with clinical expertise, makes the APN well qualified to guide patients through the health care system (Foss & Koerner, 1997). It has been documented that when advanced practice nurses spend time with hospitalized older adults, patient outcomes improve and health care costs are reduced (Brooten, Youngblut, Deatrick, Naylor, & York, 2003). This also applies to older adults in long-term care facilities. Studies have shown that newly admitted long-term care residents who received case-management services from an APN implementing evidence-based protocols had less incontinence, fewer pressure ulcers, and less aggressive behavior (Naylor, 2002).

Both clinical nurse specialists and nurse practitioners have been successfully utilized in case manager roles

(Conger, 1996; Davidson, 1999; Wells, Erickson, & Spinella, 1996). The clinical nurse specialist role is historically considered to be one of clinician, consultant, change agent, educator, researcher, and leader (Mick & Ackerman, 2002). These attributes make the clinical nurse specialist ideal as a case manager. Clinical nurse specialist case managers are most often found in hospital settings, either linked to acute care for the elderly (ACE) units or specialty units (such as a stroke or CHF unit) or functioning as a geriatric inpatient case manager for the entire hospital (McCormick, 1999; Topp, Tucker, & Weber, 1998; Tucker & DiRico, 2003; Wells et al., 1996).

A nurse practitioner has additional skills in providing direct care as well as health promotion and disease management. While they also work in case manager roles in inpatient settings, nurse practitioners are particularly well suited to primary care settings (Mick & Ackerman, 2002). In the primary care setting, the NP can be used to manage all aspects of his or her clients' care. The NP serves as the primary care provider, and serves as a case manager to coordinate care from all other providers that may be involved.

CASE-MANAGEMENT OUTCOMES IN THE OLDER ADULT POPULATION

Recent research into case-management programs geared to older adult populations has shown success in a number of areas. This has led to the development of a number of outcome measures for evaluating case-management programs in older adult populations.

Length of Stay

Case management has been shown to be effective in contributing to decreasing length of stay in older acute care patients (Ball & Peruzzi, 1997; Dzyacky, 1997; George & Large, 1995; Peruzzi, Ringer, & Tassey, 1995; Topp et al., 1998). Decreasing length of stay contributes to lower costs of hospitalization, and has been shown to contribute to improved recovery in many cases. Reductions in length of stay through case management are frequently achieved through improvements in the efficiency of care delivery. In one example, Ball & Peruzzi (1997) discuss how their facility used a system where outcome-focused protocols were used to guide the plan of care for congestive heart failure patients. These protocols provided some standardization in the care provided and in assessments of patients' recovery and readiness for discharge. The case manager assisted and guided nursing staff in following the protocols and coordinating care with other disciplines. The case manager was also able to work across different nursing units, such as the inpatient floor and the emergency department, to keep the various departments working toward the same goals.

Readmission

Following initial efforts to decrease costs through decreasing length of stay, rates of readmission to acute care hospital units became an issue. Case management has been shown to reduce readmission rates while keeping length of stay down (Kim & Soeken, 2005), but results have not been consistent (Taylor et al., 2005). This is accomplished through case management's improved coordination of services, patient education, and discharge planning. Many case-management programs involve a postdischarge component, either as a simple follow-up or as a continued outpatient case-management program. Such postdischarge follow-up facilitates earlier, more efficient management of common issues that occur during recovery and often would otherwise lead to readmission.

Other Outcomes

Studies have also shown case management to have some significant clinical outcomes. These include reducing falls in nursing homes and reducing rates of urinary tract infection through the implementation of prevention programs or through improved monitoring of patients' status (Peruzzi et al., 1995; Theodos, 2003). Case management has also been shown to reduce costs for the patient, for the health care provider, and for insurance companies and Medicare (Tucker & DiRico, 2003).

IMPACT OF CASE MANAGEMENT ON OLDER ADULTS

Much of the research into the effectiveness of case management has been focused on improving outcomes for specific populations or diagnoses. These are generally high-cost and/or high-volume diagnoses. Two of the more prominent case-managed populations are acute stroke and congestive heart failure.

Despite efforts to screen and treat for risk factors, cerebrovascular disease remains the third leading cause of death in the United States (Anderson & Smith, 2003). Studies of case management for stroke patients in acute care settings show that various approaches have been used, often with differing results. Early studies of acute stroke management focused primarily on morbidity and mortality, and over time poststroke longevity and cost of care goals were added (Baker, Miller, Sitterding, & Hajewski, 1998). Researchers have modified methods to find ways to achieve additional goals including decreased length of stay, improved functional status at discharge, long-term survival, improved patient satisfaction, lower readmission rates, decreased costs, improved communication with rehabilitation providers, and more timely access to hospital services (Baker et al., 1998; Brown, 2000). Box 26-4 gives an example of a case-management program targeted toward stroke patients.

Heart disease remains the leading cause of death in the United States, both for the general population and for the elderly (Anderson & Smith, 2003). As with cerebrovascular disease, case management has been shown to improve outcomes for patients with heart disease. In the acute care setting, advanced practice nurse case managers have been shown to have a significant impact on reducing hospital charges and length of stay for congestive heart failure patients (Topp et al., 1998).

Postdischarge case management designed to coordinate and manage care following hospitalization for congestive heart failure has also shown to be effective (Box 26-5). Such transitional case management has been shown to improve health-related quality of life while reducing emergency department visits and readmission rates (Harrison et al., 2002; Laramee, Levinsky, Sargent, Ross, & Callas, 2003).

FUTURE TRENDS IN CASE MANAGEMENT

As case management continues to demonstrate positive outcomes for clients, providers, and payers, innovative case-management programs are investigating the use of new technologies. Programs have been developed that evaluate the use of telephone and Internet-based case-management programs for certain populations' disease processes (Riegel, Carlson, Glaser, Kopp, & Romero, 2002; Southard, Southard, & Nuckolls, 2003). Such programs allow clients easy access to case-management services from their home at times that are convenient to them, and in their own language. The program can be easily customizable for different clients based on their risk factors. Additionally, the new technologies allow for improved communication between case manager and clients, as wells as between health care providers.

Evidence is also showing the need for case-management services that follow patients from hospital to home and coordinate between multiple providers of care (Harrison et al., 2002; Naylor, 2002; Naylor et al., 1999). Outcomes are improved when case managers are able to collaborate with primary care providers (Laramee et al., 2003). Better outcomes are also noted when case managers are able to oversee clients' transitions between care settings (Naylor, 2002).

SUMMARY

The coordination of services provided by case managers can help improve outcomes for older adults as well as help control health care costs. A variety of methods and models can be employed to provide case management, and the setting and population will determine the exact methodology for a particular case manager.

BOX 26-4 Case Example: Acute Stroke Patients

While working to develop a case-management program for stroke patients, a team at Columbus Regional Hospital in Columbus, Indiana, discovered that the existing literature revealed that for stroke patients, clinical pathways appeared to provide the best improvement in outcomes by improving the efficiency by which hospital services are delivered. Critical pathways are diagnosis-specific guidelines outlining what key events must happen at certain time points of care to achieve certain goals (Flarey & Blancett, 1996). Critical pathways can also be used to identify deficiencies or 'weak spots' in the efficient delivery of health care services.

The team conducted a pilot study that showed that clinical pathways for stroke had been successful regardless of whether they were used in a dedicated stroke unit or in a decentralized fashion across standard medical/surgical units.

From Baker, C. M., Miller, I., Sitterding, M., & Hajewski, C. J. (1998). Acute stroke patients: Comparing outcomes with and without case management. *Nursing Case Management, 3*(5), 196-203.

BOX 26-5 Case Example: Congestive Heart Failure

One particular example of APN case management with congestive heart failure (CHF) patients used a four-component approach: (1) early discharge planning and care coordination, (2) comprehensive individualized patient and family education, (3) telephone follow-up and monitoring for 12 weeks, and (4) focus on optimal CHF medications and medication doses consistent with existing clinical practice guidelines.

The case manager also coordinated with other disciplines (physical and occupational therapy, dietary resources, social work, home care) as well as the hospital physician and, where possible, the patient's primary care physician and primary cardiologist.

This case-management program found significant difference in adherence to treatment, medication appropriateness, and patient satisfaction from those patients without APN case management, as well as lower readmission rates in cases where the case manager was able to collaborate with the patient's primary cardiologist.

From Laramee, A. S., Levinsky, S. K., Sargent, J., Ross, R., & Callas, P. (2003). Case management in a heterogeneous congestive heart failure population: A randomized controlled trial. *Archives of Internal Medicine, 163,* 809-817.

Gerontological nurses have the clinical expertise to serve as excellent case managers for older adults by promoting quality of care and evaluating outcomes to ultimately improve health care for this growing population.

REFERENCES

American Nurses Association. (2004). *Scope and standards of gerontological nursing practice*. Washington, DC: American Nurses Association.

Anderson, R. N., & Smith, B. L. (2003). Deaths: Leading causes for 2001 [Electronic version]. *National vital statistics reports, 52*(9), Hyattsville, MD: National Center for Health Statistics.

Baker, C. M., Miller, I., Sitterding, M., & Hajewski, C. J. (1998). Acute stroke patients: Comparing outcomes with and without case management. *Nursing Case Management, 3*(5), 196-203.

Ball, C., & Peruzzi, M. (1997). Case management improves congestive heart failure outcomes. *Nursing Case Management, 2*(2), 68-74.

Brooten, D., Youngblut, J. M., Deatrick, J., Naylor, M., & York, R. (2003). Patient problems, advanced practice nurse (APN) interventions, time and contacts among five patient groups. *Journal of Nursing Scholarship, 35*, 73-79.

Brown, M. J. (2000). Stroke management: Beginnings. *Outcomes Management for Nursing Practice, 4*(1), 34-38.

Cesta, T. G., & Tahan, H. A. (2003). *The case manager's survival guide* (2nd ed.). St. Louis: Mosby.

Cohen, E. L., & Cesta, T. G. (2005). *Nursing case management: From essentials to advanced practice applications* (4th ed.). St. Louis: Elsevier Mosby.

Conger, M. M. (1996). Integration of the clinical nurse specialist into the nurse case manager role. *Nursing Case Management, 1*(5), 230-234.

Davidson, J. U. (1999). Blending case management and quality outcomes management into the family nurse practitioner role. *Nursing Administration Quarterly, 24*(1), 66-74.

Dzyacky, S. C. (1997). Case management for the self-insured hospital. *Nursing Case Management, 2*(5), 219-225.

Enguidanos, S. M., Gibbs, N. E., Simmons, W. J., Savoni, K. J., Jamison, P. M., Hackstaff, L., et al. (2003). Kaiser Permanente Community Partners Project: Improving geriatric care management practices. *Journal of the American Geriatrics Society, 51*, 710-714.

Flarey, D. L., & Blancett, S. S. (1996). *Handbook of nursing case management*. Gaithersburg, MD: Aspen.

Forbes, M. A. (1999). The practice of professional nurse case management. *Nursing Case Management, 4*(1), 28-33.

Foss, N., & Koerner, J. (1997). The advanced practice nurse's role in differentiated practice: Martha's story. *AACN Clinical Issues, 8*(2), 262-270.

George, E., & Large, A. (1995). Reducing length of stay in patients undergoing open heart surgery: The University of Pittsburgh experience. *AACN Clinical Issues, 6*(3), 482-488.

Harrison, M. B., Browne, G. B., Roberts, J., Tugwell, P., Gafni, A., & Graham, I. D. (2002). Quality of life of individuals with heart failure: A randomized trial of the effectiveness of two models of hospital-to-home transition. *Medical Care, 40*(4), 271-282.

Kim, Y. J., & Soeken, K. L. (2005). A meta-analysis of the effect of hospital-based case management on hospital length-of-stay and readmission. *Nursing Research, 54*(4), 255-264.

Laramee, A. S., Levinsky, S. K., Sargent, J., Ross, R., & Callas, P. (2003). Case management in a heterogeneous congestive heart failure population: A randomized controlled trial. *Archives of Internal Medicine, 163*, 809-817.

Mahn-DiNicola, V. A., & Zazworsky, D. J. (2005). The advanced practice nurse as case manager. In A. B. Hamric, J. A. Spross, & C. M. Hanson (Eds.), *Advanced practice nursing: An integrative approach* (3rd ed.). St. Louis: Elsevier.

McCormick, S. A. (1999). Advanced practice nursing for congestive heart failure: Role of the advanced practice nurse in an ICU. *Critical Care Nursing Quarterly, 21*(4), 1-8.

Mick, D. J., & Ackerman, M. H. (2002). New perspectives on advanced practice nursing case management for aging patients. *Critical Care Nursing Clinics of North America, 14*, 281-291.

Mosqueda, L., & Brummel-Smith, K. (2002). Rehabilitation. In R. J. Ham, P. D. Sloane, & G. A. Warshaw (Eds.), *Primary care geriatrics: A case-based approach* (4th ed.). St. Louis: Mosby.

Naylor, M. (2002). Transitional care of older adults. In P. Archbold & B. Stewart (Eds.), *Annual review of nursing research*, Vol. 20, New York: Springer, pp. 127-147.

Naylor, M. D., Brooten, D., Campbell, R., Jacobsen, B. S., Mezey, M. D., Pauly, M. V., & Schwartz, J. S. (1999). Comprehensive discharge planning and home follow-up of hospitalized elders. *Journal of the American Medical Association, 281*(7), 613-620.

Peruzzi, P., Ringer, D., & Tassey, K. (1995). A community hospital redesigns care. *Nursing Administration Quarterly, 20*(1), 24-46.

Rassen, A. G. (2003). Seniors-at-Home: A case management program for frail elders. *Journal of Clinical Outcomes Management, 10*(11), 603-607.

Riegel, B., Carlson, B., Glaser, D., Kopp, Z., & Romero, T. E. (2002). Standardized telephonic case management in a Hispanic heart failure population: An effective intervention. *Disease Management and Health Outcomes, 10*(4), 241-249.

Southard, B. H., Southard, D. R., & Nuckolls, J. (2003). Clinical trial of an internet-based case management system for secondary prevention of heart disease. *Journal of Cardiopulmonary Rehabilitation, 23*, 341-348.

Taylor, P. (1999). Comprehensive nursing case management: An advanced practice model. *Nursing Case Management, 4*(1), 2-13.

Taylor, S. J., Candy, B., Bryar, R. M., Ramsay, J., Vrijhoef, H. J., Esmond, G., Wedzicha, J. A., & Griffiths, C. J. (2005). Effectiveness of innovations in nurse-led chronic disease management for patients with chronic obstructive pulmonary disease: Systematic review of evidence. *British Medical Jorunal, 331*(7515), 485-492.

Theodos, P. (2003). Fall prevention in frail elderly nursing home residents: A challenge to case management: Part I. *Lippincott's Case Management, 8*(6), 246-251.

Topp, R., Tucker, D., & Weber, C. (1998). Effect of a clinical case manager/clinical nurse specialist on patients hospitalized with congestive heart failure. *Nursing Case Management, 3*(4), 140-147.

Tucker, D., & DiRico, L. (2003). Managing costly Medicare patients in the hospital. *Geriatric Nursing, 24*(5), 294-297.

Wells, N., Erickson, S., & Spinella, J. (1996). Role transition: From clinical nurse specialist to clinical nurse specialist/case manager. *Journal of Nursing Administration, 26*(11), 23-28.

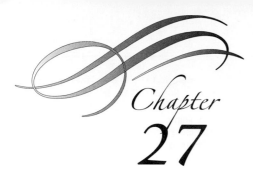

Chapter 27

Health Promotion and Health Education for Older Adults

Helen W. Lach

Objectives

Define the concept of health promotion.
Discuss the benefits and barriers of health promotion with older adults.
Describe common theories of health behavior change.
Discuss key components important for health in older adults.
Review techniques for targeting health promotion and health education to an older adult population.

As Americans live longer, the public's interest in health promotion activities is fueled by a desire to remain active and independent. Our youth-oriented society has an aging generation of baby boomers who also value looking and feeling good. From an individual perspective, many people are interested in developing healthier habits in later life. This may be the result of experiencing aging changes or health conditions that motivate them to improve health habits. From a national perspective, the ever-rising costs of health care should be motivation to support health promotion as a means of delaying the onset of costly chronic illness and disability for as many older people as possible.

Given the incentives, why do so few people engage in the health behaviors that would be so beneficial? What changes have the potential to make a difference in the lives of older adults? What are the barriers to adopting health habits? And what techniques can health professionals, particularly nurses, use to help older adults adopt healthier lifestyles? This chapter explores these issues in detail.

Nurses should be the key health professional delivering health education and health promotion programs for older adults. Nurses have advanced knowledge of health, disease, medicine, disease management, and the health care system that provides an excellent background for teaching health-related topics. In addition, nurses are trained to deliver health teaching to the lay learner, translating medical jargon into understandable terms. These skills and knowledge make nurses especially suited to develop and deliver health promotion and health education. Yet often physicians are the ones asked to give health talks and programs. Public health professionals often develop and provide health promotion programs. Nurses need to market their knowledge and skills to further develop this niche in the health care field that is so well suited to them.

Looking beyond what individuals can do to maintain and improve their health, gerontological nurses also can address the many other determinants of health that may be related to community and public policy initiatives, such as the stresses of poverty or crime. For example, older adults who live in communities with high crime and crumbling sidewalks have little opportunity for walking or getting out for physical activity. Poor urban communities may have few opportunities for residents to shop for affordable, healthy foods. Seeman and Crimmins (2001) have identified the relationship between health and personal social relationships, individual socioeconomic status, and community social characteristics. Gerontologists are just beginning to learn about the role the environment plays in supporting healthy aging (George, 2005). Many clinical, research, and educational approaches are needed to address the disparities in health that exist between white and minority groups.

This chapter is designed to provide an overview of health promotion issues for older adults at all levels of prevention. The first section looks at the concept of health and the benefits and barriers to providing effective health promotion to this population. The following section discusses key components of a healthy lifestyle. A review of secondary prevention, including screening and health maintenance for the older adult, is covered in the next section. The final sections address behavior change theories and strategies and techniques for use in delivering health promotion and health education, so that they are targeted and appropriate for an older audience.

WHAT IS HEALTH PROMOTION?

To explore health promotion, it helps to consider a definition of health. A widely held holistic view was originally put forth by the World Health Organization (1946) that defines *health* as "a state of complete physical, mental, and social well-being and not merely the absence of disease or infirmity." Illness can be thought of as a separate but related continuum that is parallel to health. Pender, Murdaugh, and Parsons (2005) describe this relationship by pointing out that "poor health can exist even if disease is not present, and good health can be present in spite of disease" (p. 25). Both of these states can be observed in the older adult. Many older adults have productive, healthy lives in spite of the presence of chronic disease, whereas others have multiple risk factors for disease that is not yet manifest.

So what constitutes health in later life? A popular expression is "successful aging," originally coined by Havighurst (1961). A major exploration of successful aging was conducted through the MacArthur Foundation Research Network on Successful Aging (Rowe & Kahn, 1998). Over more than a decade, researchers studied factors beyond genetic endowment to determine their impact on health and aging. A goal of these studies was to discover whether typical decline in physical and mental health with age is normal and to be expected with aging, or the result of disease processes. They hypothesized that because some people age well, the decline seen in many was really not normal aging. They found much support for their hypothesis.

The MacArthur Foundation studies identified factors important for maintaining health in later years in three major categories (Rowe & Kahn, 1987): (1) avoidance of disease (reducing risk factors for disease), (2) maintaining and improving physical and mental health, and (3) active engagement with life (Figure 27-1). As a result, it is important to reduce risk factors for disease, make healthy lifestyle choices, and maintain social connections and cognitive challenges to promote successful aging. These factors were found to be important, even when changes were made in later life. The results of these groundbreaking studies can be used to combat the myths about aging and educate older adults and the public about what they can do to improve their own aging.

Health promotion is any activity designed to improve health and well-being, and has been described as

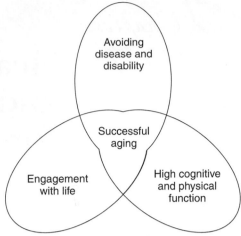

Figure 27-1 Successful aging model. (From Rowe, J. W., & Kahn, R. L. [1998]. Successful aging. *Gerontologist, 37*[4], 433-440. Copyright by The Gerontological Society of America. Adapted by permission of the publisher.)

"the central global strategy for improving health" (Pender, Murdaugh, & Parsons, 2005, p. 16). Health promotion is also sometimes seen as a broad approach to improving health, including social, political, and economic activities (Whitehead, 2004), whereas the narrower view of health programs and teaching are considered "health education." These terms are often used interchangeably. As a result, nurses pursue health promotion for populations through a variety of strategies, including providing education, services, and advocacy for older adults. Box 27-1 describes the experiences of a gerontological nurse who worked to improve dental health in her community through all three of these approaches. Through collaboration with other health professionals, the health system, and advocacy approaches, nurses are making a difference in the lives of underserved seniors.

Health promotion has been operationalized in the United States through the "Healthy People" program that establishes national health objectives that can be used for planning and program development. The current program, *Healthy People 2010*, was developed from scientific evidence and consultation with experts and has two overall goals: (1) increase quality and years of healthy life and (2) eliminate health disparities (U.S. Department of Health and Human Services [USDHHS], 2002). Under these major goals, there are 28 focus areas related to the following 10 leading health indicators:

- Physical activity
- Overweight and obesity
- Tobacco use
- Substance abuse
- Responsible sexual behavior
- Mental health
- Injury and violence
- Environmental quality

Box 27-1 *Reflections on Providing Dental Health Services for Underserved Older Adults*

Oral health is an often overlooked issue that is critical to the overall health of older adults. Research has provided evidence of a direct association between the bacteria involved in periodontal disease and cardiovascular disease, stroke, and heart attack (National Institutes of Health, 2005). Evidence has shown that untreated tooth decay in adults is linked to other adverse health conditions as well, including pneumonia, cancer, and poorly controlled blood sugar levels in diabetic patients. Quality of life is greatly affected when dental disease results in limited social interaction, interrupted sleep, and reduced nutritional intake.

Although water fluoridation and routine dental care have allowed more people than ever before to keep their teeth throughout their lives, as people age, they become more susceptible to poor oral health. This increased susceptibility is due to medications that reduce salivary flow, visual impairments, dementia, and reduced dexterity caused by arthritis or neurological diseases, such as Parkinson's disease and stroke. Therefore it is important, from a public health and economic perspective, to ensure that all older adults, particularly those who are vulnerable to disease, receive routine dental care. As a result, a local hospital set up a dental clinic to provide preventive and maintenance dental care for seniors in the local community. This describes the experiences of implementing this important community service in a midwestern state.

Providing routine dental care for all older adults is not an easy goal to reach. The United States is in the midst of a shortage of dentists, dental hygienists, and registered nurses that is expected to intensify as the number of older adults increases and the need for oral care grows. There are 2666 licensed dentists and 1777 dental hygienists in the state of Missouri (Centers for Disease Control and Prevention [CDC], 2003a). Since 1994, the number of dentists and dental hygienists has experienced a steady decline, and unfortunately this trend is projected to continue (CDC, 2003a). Additionally, the statewide vacancy rate for nurses in Missouri has been around the 10% mark since 2001 (Missouri Hospital Association, 2005). Only by working collaboratively can nursing and dental health care professionals provide quality oral health care in our current environment, in which the complex needs of a growing older population exceed the capabilities of either profession alone.

Working together, myself, a registered nurse, and a licensed dentist decided to find a way to address the dental health care needs of the approximately 1600 residents of 32 long-term care facilities and 3500 underserved, frail, community-dwelling older adults who desperately needed dental care. Approximately 95% of this population were over 65; 97% of them were below the federal poverty level, and nearly all were physically or mentally disabled (or both). We found volunteers to provide basic dental services; dental suppliers to donate necessary equipment;

and hospital administrators to provide space and monetary support. This strategy reflects our belief that the only way to solve the dental care access problem is through a multipronged, coordinated strategy, including provision of dental care at community health centers; implementation of educational programs; and influencing state Medicaid policies.

Our first objective was to provide dental care at a community health center. We approached the administration at our local hospital, St. Joseph Health Center (SJHC), a 328-bed facility located in St. Charles, Missouri. SJHC is a member of one of the largest Catholic health care systems in the country, and their mission is to bring comprehensive services to persons of all ages and social strata, with special concern for the poor. SJHC had an existing Senior Services Program that provided handicapped-accessible transportation, staff, and facilities for specialty physician examinations and coordination of outpatient services for long-term care residents. The existence of the Senior Health Clinic provided the space, staff, and transportation services for implementing the Dental Clinic. Our primary service population for the dental clinic consisted of the residents of the 32 extended care facilities located within three local counties. The services provided include treatment of infection, restorative care, prophylaxis, denture fabrication, and oral surgery. Recently, we expanded our services when we opened another Senior Dental Clinic at another SSM hospital. Both clinics are open Monday through Friday. Currently, the dental clinics are staffed by 11 volunteer dentists, 1 volunteer oral surgeon, and 2 dental hygienists. The volunteers donated nearly 6500 hours of professional dental health care in the first 4 years.

The clinic receives critically needed funds through multiple sources, including reimbursement from Medicaid; generous donations of funds and equipment from national, regional, and local organizations and individuals; and the financial support provided by the hospital. Our annual expenses average around $270,000. The only paid staff includes one full-time dental hygienist and a part-time dental director. The dental hygienists and our dental director are paid jointly by a grant from a local foundation and the hospital.

The Dental Health Clinic has provided care to more than 4000 older adults. Most have been diagnosed with periodontal disease, oral cancer, and tooth decay. In addition, at SJHC, approximately 30 people every month were entering our emergency department seeking dental care. Each dental case treated as an emergency costs $263.00 in uncompensated care; this equated to $94,680.00 annually. The number of patients seeking dental care in our emergency department has been reduced by approximately 60%.

To meet our second objective, implementing education programs, we developed a strategy to provide educational

Continued

Box 27-1 *Reflections on Providing Dental Health Services for Underserved Older Adults — cont'd*

services to encourage low-income adults to practice routine dental hygiene. We are implementing the educational strategy because, although common dental diseases are preventable, not everyone is informed about appropriate oral health-promoting measures (Joint Commission On Accreditation of Healthcare Organizations, 2000). We believe that educating caregivers about the importance of routine dental care and sharing tips for providing care to older adults is a means to reduce neglect in the long-term care setting.

We have two methods to affect our state's policymakers. First, our Dental Director is an active member of state and local dental societies. He works with state and local policymakers as they attempt to devise methods to reduce barriers to participation in Medicaid. Indeed, some barriers have been addressed, such as the use of different reporting codes and the high rate of claim rejections. Despite these efforts, our vulnerable populations have yet to experience access improvement. This situation is unlikely to improve because of continued state budget pressures. In fact, Missouri is 1 of the 16 states that have already begun to limit access to Medicaid by increasing insurance premiums charged to low-income families.

Second, we developed the Dental Advisory Board, whose members consist of dentists, community volunteers, and hospital professionals. Our goals are to provide community education, because we believe that raising awareness about the importance of oral health is an essential first step, and to build endowment funds to ensure the ongoing existence of our programs.

We are all proud of our successes; however, we still face many challenges. Barriers include competing for space within the hospital environment and recruitment of additional dental volunteers. All of our volunteers have

busy lives, and many volunteers provide services on their day off. Others are retired. And most have other volunteer obligations. Therefore we often struggle to provide dental services 5 days a week.

The bottom line is that lack of access to dental care for low-income older adults is an important and complex problem. National attention was brought to the issue of oral health disparities by multiple documents, including the Surgeon General's first report on oral health (National Institute of Dental and Craniofacial Research, 2000) and more recently by a report generated by the Senate Aging Committee (2003). However, additional effort and academic dialogue must generate continued interest in this often overlooked, critical issue. Nurses play an important role in helping patients access oral health services and providing care to hospitalized patients. As recommended by Coleman (2005, p. 35), "protocols developed and tested collaboratively between nursing and dentistry offer a best practices approach to improving oral health care" for older adults. Lack of good oral health care will not be solved by simply throwing more money into Medicaid reimbursement rates without addressing these other factors and developing new, creative methods of providing the necessary services. There is no doubt that good dental health is vital to maintaining the quality of life of older adults. In their words, "to smile, to bite into a crisp apple, and to laugh with my grandchildren" describes what it means to have a healthy mouth.

Rebecca A. Lorenz

Rebecca A. Lorenz, RN, MHS, PhD(c)
Saint Louis University
St. Louis, Missouri

- Immunization
- Access to health care

These health indicators and their corresponding categories (listed in Box 27-2) are tracked to determine how effective health promotion efforts are in improving the health and well-being of Americans. Some components are targeted specifically to older adults; for example, the section addressing unintentional injury has objectives that address reducing deaths from falls and reducing hip fractures among older adults.

Prevention

Health promotion also can be considered as prevention. Most nurses are familiar with the concept of prevention, which occurs at three levels:

- *Primary prevention* is designed to help prevent the development of disease, such as immunizations or other activities to help avoid the occurrence of disease.
- *Secondary prevention* takes place once disease is present and is designed to detect the presence of disease early so that action can be taken to treat it or prevent complications. Measures such as mammograms and screening for hypertension are considered secondary preventive measures.
- *Tertiary prevention* occurs to reduce complications or disability related to illness or injury, such as rehabilitation after a hip fracture.

Health promotion is important at all levels of prevention with older adults as with other age-groups. We often think of health promotion as occurring before the onset of disease, but in fact many older adults have

Box 27-2 Health Indicators for *Healthy People 2010*

1. Access to quality health services
   - Quality of care
   - Clinical preventive services
   - Health insurance
   - Primary care
   - Emergency medical services
   - Long-term care
2. Arthritis, osteoporosis, and chronic back conditions
   - Arthritis
   - Osteoporsis
   - Back care
3. Cancer
   - Cancer
4. Chronic kidney disease
   - End-stage renal disease
   - Kidney diseases
   - Organ transplant
5. Diabetes
   - Diabetes
6. Disability and secondary conditions
   - Disabilities
7. Educational and community-based programs
   - Community-based programs
8. Environmental health
   - Environmental health
9. Family planning
   - Family planning
10. Food safety
    - Food safety
11. Health communication
    - Patient education
    - Doctor and patient communication
    - Health communication
    - Consumer Internet
    - Literacy
12. Heart disease and stroke
    - Heart disease
    - Stroke
13. Human immunodeficiency virus (HIV)
    - HIV infection
14. Immunization and infectious diseases
    - Immunization
    - Infectious diseases
15. Injury and violence prevention
    - Abuse
    - Injuries
    - Violence
16. Maternal, infant, and child health
    - Infant health
    - Maternal health
17. Medical product safety
    - Drug safety
18. Mental health and mental disorders
    - Mental health
    - Mental disorders
19. Nutrition and overweight
    - Nutrition
    - Obesity
20. Occupational safety and health
    - Occupational health
    - Occupational safety
21. Oral health
    - Oral health
22. Physical activity and fitness
    - Physical activity
23. Public health infrastructure
    - Public health functions project
    - Public health professionals
    - Public health statistics
24. Respiratory diseases
    - Respiratory diseases
25. Sexually transmitted diseases
    - Sexually transmitted diseases
26. Substance abuse
    - Substance abuse
27. Tobacco use
    - Tobacco
28. Vision and hearing
    - Visual impairment
    - Hearing impairment

From U.S. Department of Health and Human Services. (2002). *Healthy people 2010: Improving health* (2nd ed.). Washington, DC: U.S. Government Printing Office.

chronic conditions. As a result, our goal is to help people strive for their own highest levels of wellness possible. Each person has the potential to maintain or improve health, from her or his own starting point. All of the concepts discussed, health, successful aging, and prevention, help identify the parameters of health promotion and health education for the older population. Suggestions for promoting physical, cognitive, and emotional health in later life have been identified by Hartman-Stein and Potkanowicz (2003):

- Physical health
  - Exercise, including aerobic, strength training, and flexibility components
  - Nutrition, including adequate calcium and vitamin D intake
- Cognitive health
  - Mental stimulation using puzzles or crosswords
  - Learn new information by reading, attending classes, or other
  - Visit new places or travel

- Emotional health
  - Stay involved with other people
  - Plan things you like to do regularly
  - Find meaning in your life
  - Seek treatment for any mental health issues

Barriers to Health Promotion for Older Adults

Two misconceptions get in the way of providing good health promotion and health education for the older population. The first is the misconception that older adults cannot or will not change, as in the saying, "You can't teach an old dog new tricks." This ageist attitude results in the belief that health promotion is not needed for older people, because they are unlikely to be successful anyway. Some perceive that because life expectancy is limited, the resources for health promotion for older adults are wasted. However, research is showing that changes even later in life can reduce costly premature disability, improve quality of life, and reduce health care costs (Rowe & Kahn, 1998).

The second misconception comes from lack of knowledge about the special needs of the older adult. As a result, the same approaches and materials that are used for any adults are used for older adults as well. The reality is that many of the principles that apply to teaching adults also apply to teaching the older learner. However, a number of adaptations must be made to accommodate the range of cognitive, physical, functional, and sensory changes that are common when teaching an older population, who may have different needs and interests as well.

The outcome of these misconceptions is limited opportunities for health promotion activities that are targeted to the older adult's problems and needs. For example, the typical exercise program at the local gym may be too intense for the out-of-shape older person to participate in safely. A lower-level introductory class would be more appropriate for the older adult who is debilitated. In addition, the instructors are often young, thin, and flexible, hardly role models for the older class participant. Even if older exercisers overcome these concerns and join a class, they may overdo activities and experience an injury. They may not attempt to exercise again, fearing more injuries and assuming that exercise is not right for them. Although some excellent senior exercise programs exist, they need to be made available to a wider population of older people.

Older adults have much to gain from health promotion and health education activities. Lack of motivation to make changes is not a natural part of aging. In fact, older adults face many changes, which require adaptation and coping. Examples include retirement; loss of spouse or other loved ones, including pets; relocation to new environments; and changes in physical health,

social status, and financial capacities. When we consider that the resources of older adults for coping with change may be shrinking both in terms of physical reserves to cope with stress and illness and in terms of social and role losses, it makes sense that older adults want a good reason to consider additional changes.

For example, an older diabetic may not understand the relationship between high blood sugar and complications or see the importance of maintaining good glucose control. As a result, he or she will probably not pay a lot of attention during a teaching session or class on nutrition or be motivated to change his or her diet. The health behavior models discussed next give us more information on motivating people to learn and change and are useful in approaching health promotion and health education. Making teaching relevant means finding out the individual's goals and showing how information ties into those goals. Assessing the needs of the individual or target population is an important step in designing relevant health promotion and health education (Lorig, 1996).

Older adults may make decisions to change their health behavior when they experience an illness or when they identify a change in their physical status that makes them aware of their health (Schneider, Eveker, Bronder, Meiner, & Binder, 2003). These may constitute "teachable moments" where health promotion interventions may be successful. Other important strategies can be used to help people make health changes and are discussed in a later section.

Health Disparities

Older adults as a group may have barriers to health promotion and greater levels of health problems than younger people, but older ethnic and cultural minorities have the highest levels of chronic disease and functional limitations and the lowest levels of health promotion activities (Johnson & Smith, 2002). These facts led to the *Healthy People* major objective of reducing health disparities mentioned earlier. Tailoring and targeting health promotion activities for various-age ethnic and cultural groups is discussed further later in the chapter as a mechanism to reduce health disparities.

Making Health Promotion in Aging a Priority

Health promotion for older adults is gradually becoming a priority. In addition to the interest of other government agencies, the Centers for Disease Control and Prevention (CDC) has developed a model describing its approach to promoting health (Figure 27-2) as part of an initiative started in 2000 (Lang, Moor, Harris, & Anderson, 2005). Lang and colleagues (2005, p. 25) define *healthy aging* as the "development and maintenance

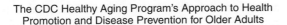

The CDC Healthy Aging Program's Approach to Health Promotion and Disease Prevention for Older Adults

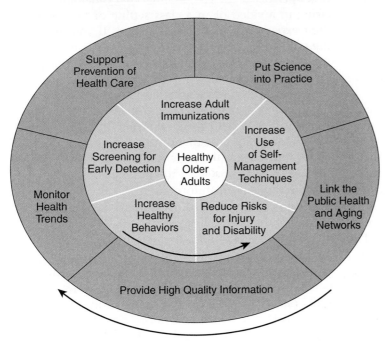

Figure 27-2 CDC model for health promotion. (Reprinted with permission from Lang, J. E., Moore, M. J., Harris, A. C., & Anderson, L. A. [2005]. Healthy aging: Priorities and programs of the Centers for Disease Control and Prevention. *Generations, 29*[2], 24-29. Copyright 2005 by American Society on Aging, San Francisco, California, www.asaging.org.)

of optimal physical, mental and social well-being and function in older adults." The CDC has several key strategies for healthy aging, similar to topics already discussed:

- Increasing healthy behaviors
- Reducing the prevalence of hazards and risk factors leading to injury and disability
- Increasing the use of immunizations and preventive screenings
- Assisting older adults in managing existing chronic conditions

Gerontological nurses should play a role in health promotion for older adults in all settings from health care systems to community-based organizations. Programs and interventions need to have a strong evidence base to promote the most effective approaches to improving health. Organizations need to share best practices to increase the level of programming. The following sections review several theoretical models that nurses can use to help in promoting health and health promotion changes for individuals and groups.

MODELS AND STRATEGIES FOR HEALTH BEHAVIOR CHANGE

Information is usually not enough to get people to change their health behaviors. Making health changes can be difficult, and even when people know what to do, they may not do it. Exercise is a good example of this problem. As a result, many models of health behavior change have been developed and tested to help

guide health promotion and health education to make it more effective. The following are major advantages of using health behavior models or theories as described by Doak, Doak, and Root (1996):

- Theories provide a predictable framework to plan interventions that are more likely to succeed.
- Theories offer a means to explain and justify interventions to colleagues.
- Theories give us a blueprint to replicate successful interventions.
- Theories offer a systematic process to analyze success or failure.

Health behavior models help us understand why individuals may or may not perform certain behaviors, or why they make health changes. Several important health behavior theories are described here that are helpful in working with older adults, including the Health Belief Model, Self-Efficacy Theory, and the Transtheoretical Model. Studies have demonstrated that interventions using these models can change people's knowledge, attitudes, and beliefs and ultimately health behaviors (Glanz, Rimer, & Lewis, 2002). Other strategies, including goal setting and motivational interviewing, are then discussed.

Health Belief Model

A nurse may want to understand how to increase the number of older women who get mammograms. The Health Belief Model (Becker, 1974) has been used to examine this behavior (Champion, 1999). Using this model, we can think of mammogram behavior as resulting from several beliefs a woman may have about the procedure:

- *Perceived threat*—belief that she is really at risk of getting breast cancer
- *Perceived benefits*—belief about the benefits of getting a mammogram, that mammograms will find any cancer and that catching cancer early is beneficial
- *Perceived barriers*—things a woman thinks would prevent her from getting a mammogram, such as cost or lack of transportation
- *Perceived self-efficacy*—belief that she can make the appointment and carry out getting the mammogram

By looking at women's beliefs in these areas, we can develop interventions to increase mammogram use. Education can include information about the increased risk of getting breast cancer with age and the benefits of early detection. In addition, interventions should help women learn to overcome any barriers that are preventing them from getting a mammogram. Showing women that many other older women like them have easily obtained a mammogram can help them feel that they can do it too. The Health Belief Model can be used by a nurse or health professional on an individual basis when talking to patients during a health care interaction. The model can also guide the development of programs for groups, written materials, or other new delivery methods such as interactive computer programs. Regardless of the method, the same issues are addressed to help increase mammogram use.

Self-Efficacy Theory

Self-Efficacy Theory is an important component of Social Cognitive Theory (Bandura, 1997). Self-Efficacy Theory states that people's confidence in their ability to perform certain behaviors predicts motivation and behavior. In addition, individuals' expectations of the outcome of behaviors is also important. As Bandura (1997) states, "People take action when they hold efficacy beliefs and outcome expectations that make the effort seem worthwhile" (p. 24). Four mechanisms help enhance self-efficacy and are integrated into programs designed to increase self-efficacy: skills mastery, modeling, reinterpretation of symptoms, and social persuasion (Lorig, 2001).

Skills mastery is a method to help people feel comfortable with tasks by learning and practicing them in small steps. As they become successful with practice, it builds their confidence to attempt larger steps and eventually make changes. *Modeling* occurs when individuals see that other people who are like them have accomplished the task that they are attempting. This can be integrated into health promotion programs by having participants meet or hear from other older adults who serve

as role models for the behavior. If the goal is to get an older person to exercise, seeing other older adults exercising in a video or in a class setting or talking about their experiences provides modeling. If you are working with older ethnic or minority women, it is helpful to include older role models from that participants' group.

It is important to identify individuals' beliefs regarding their health or health conditions. The health professional can then help them *reinterpret* these beliefs in a way that will support them in making health changes. By exploring what the patient knows and thinks about the health issue you want to address, you can uncover and address any misinformation. For example, people may think that resting joints is better for arthritis than exercising them.

Health professionals, family, friends, or support peers can help provide *persuasion* by encouraging behavior change or action. Information can sometimes be persuasive as well. Taken together, the techniques of skills mastery, modeling, reinterpretation, and persuasion can be used in interventions and counseling approaches to help older adults make behavior changes.

Transtheoretical Model

Another useful model for behavior change is the Transtheoretical Model (TTM) described by Prochaska and colleagues (Prochaska, DiClemente, Velicer, & Rossi, 1993; Prochaska, Norcross, & DiClemente, 1994), developed to help explain how people make changes. An important feature of the TTM is that it describes change as a process that occurs over time. Individuals go through a series of *stages of change* in adopting new behaviors and sustaining them over time. These stages are described in Table 27-1 and range from the individual not even thinking about a behavior change, to thinking about and preparing for change, to making the change, and finally to maintaining the change. Individuals use different cognitive and behavioral "processes of change" as they move through these stages. For example, individuals may become aware of an important health issue such as colon cancer screening at a health fair, a process of consciousness raising.

Exploring the individual's stage of readiness to make changes can help guide health promotion and health education because different interventions are more useful to individuals at different stages of making a behavior change. Early in the change process as people consider making a change, they look at the pros and cons or "decisional balance" of engaging in behaviors. Self-efficacy as discussed before is also considered important in the TTM, so the methods discussed earlier are also used in this model. Some strategies for helping people at each stage of change are noted in Table 27-1.

Table 27-1 *The Stages of Change Model: Examples and Strategies for Helping Older Adults Make Health Behavior Changes*

Stage	Examples	Strategies to Help
Precontemplation: Not even thinking about change	"It won't make any difference if I start exercising at my age."	Raise the awareness of individuals about why the behavior or change is important.
Contemplation: Considering the possibility of making a change	"Maybe exercise would help my joint pain and help me keep up my strength."	Point out all of the benefits of making a change and provide encouragement.
Preparation: Planning to make a change in the next month	"I signed up for a chair exercise program at the community center."	Give detailed information so that the individual can set up realistic plans for making the change.
Action: Have made the change within the past 6 months	"I've been going to class for 3 months and am feeling good."	Provide encouragement and support to keep up the change.
Maintenance: Have sustained the change for at least 6 months	"This month I am trying a Tai Chi class to work on my balance."	Help identify methods to stick with the change and prevent relapse, such as a variety of exercise classes and indoor/outdoor walking options.

Data from Prochaska, J. O., Norcross, J. C., & DiClemente, C. C. (1994). *Changing for good.* New York: Morrow.

Goal Setting

Goal setting, or making a health plan or contract, is a good strategy to assist people who want to make health behavior changes and is used in many practice and class settings (Stecher et al., 1995). Goal setting offers several benefits. First the individual uses this mechanism to make a specific plan, an important step to help increase the chances of making a successful change. Second, goal setting usually includes identifying some kind of positive reinforcement or reward when the individual meets her or his goal. Another benefit is that writing down the goal makes it a formal commitment (Haber, 2003). In many cases, the health care provider is involved in the goal-setting process, increasing communication about health issues. Another important feature of goal setting is to identify barriers to reaching the goal and planning ways to overcome these barriers before they occur. Although research is limited on the use of goal setting in health behavior change (Shilts, Horowitz, & Townsend, 2004), these steps equate to good planning.

Goals should be realistic, and individuals may set goals too low or too high. Lorig and Holman (2003) recommend that once individuals have developed a goal, they should determine their level of confidence in meeting that goal. A scale of 1 to 10 or 0% to 100% can be used. Their research indicates that if the person rates his or her confidence at 70% or greater, the person is likely to be successful. Those who rate their confidence lower should revise their goal to include a more realistic plan, or break up the goal into manageable steps. Goals should be high enough to motivate the individual, without being overwhelming (Stecher et al., 1995). If the person is not really interested in reaching the goal, these techniques may not help.

Motivational Interviewing

Motivational interviewing is a patient-centered counseling or health coaching method to enhance motivation to change by exploring and resolving ambivalence to making changes (Rollnick & Miller, 1995) and uses concepts from health models. Four main approaches are used according to Bennett and colleagues (2005, p. 188):

- Expressing empathy, including acceptance of the patient's feelings and skillful reflective listening
- Supporting self-efficacy, including giving responsibility to the patient for carrying out the change
- Rolling with resistance, including not arguing for change and recognizing that the patient is the primary resource for solutions
- Developing discrepancy, including recognizing that change is motivated by a patient's perceived discrepancy between present behavior and personal goals and values

Motivational interviewing can be provided in sessions lasting from a few minutes to an hour, and in person or by phone (Dupree-Jones, Burckhardt, & Bennett, 2004). Research on this technique has been positive, and it has been shown to help people increase physical activity (Burke, Arkowitz, & Dunn, 2003; Kirk, Mutrie, MacIntyre, & Fisher, 2003). Use of techniques from behavior change models probably enhances this process.

Implementing Health Models and Strategies in Practice

Nurses working with older adults should be aware of how they can use behavior change theory and strategies in working with older patients. This process is sometimes called *health coaching*. It can be applied to many situations where the older adult has to deal with health promotion issues, as well as health conditions. For example, a patient may need to exercise to lose weight, keep from losing bone mass, and maintain functional status. Other patients may need to learn how to manage conditions such as diabetes so that they can prevent complications that result from poor blood sugar control. Even caregivers of older adults may need to make changes to help manage their loved one's health, for example, when caring for someone with dementia or Alzheimer's disease. Although the person with dementia cannot make changes, the caregiver may need to make changes in the home, activities, and supervision of the person with dementia.

Using motivational interviewing and goal setting, the nurse can encourage positive changes. In addition, a simple method for addressing health changes in primary care practice, described in the section on smoking cessation, is the "five A's" (ask, advise, assess, assist, and arrange). This technique is helpful when there is little time to spend on these complex issues. When more in-depth assistance is needed, older adults should be referred to classes, personal trainers, health coaches, counselors, or others for more in-depth support and assistance.

Theoretical models can be used to develop health promotion programs or educational programs targeted to individuals or groups. For example, the author helped develop a health promotion program called HealthStages for a national education program for older adults, the Older Adult Service and Information System (OASIS) (Everard, Lach, & Heinrich, 2000; Lach, Everard, Highstein, & Brownson, 2004). The program used the concepts of the TTM model for program planning, curriculum development, and program evaluation. Different types of health promotion classes and activities were developed to reach people at all stages of readiness to make health changes for six major topic areas important for older adult health.

For example, an older woman may become aware of the need to exercise at a health fair where her fitness level is tested. As she considers what kind of exercise to do, she could attend an exercise sampler class where she could try water exercises, aerobics classes, Tai Chi, walking, and strength training. Finding an enjoyable form of exercise is important, because if she finds a class that is of interest she will be more likely to follow through with the exercise program. After taking a class and getting used to exercise, she may try different kinds of exercise so that she maintains exercise as a routine part of her life.

The HealthStages Programming Grid (Figure 27-3) describes a comprehensive health promotion program based on meeting all of the health topics at each of the stages of change. HealthStages incorporated techniques from the TTM in the curriculum to help people make health changes, such as activities to increase self-efficacy. Program evaluation focused on whether a local program was able to provide a comprehensive program by offering classes and activities in all areas of the grid. Evaluation of the HealthStages program showed that local sites were able to increase the numbers and variety of classes, and increase participation by the target audience (Lach

Class Level		Awareness	Knowledge	Skill Building/ Behavior Change	Maintenance
	Stage	Precontemplation Contemplation	Contemplation Preparation	Action	Maintenance
Topic					
General Health Promotion					
Physical Activity/Fitness					
Nutrition					
Mental Health/Wellness					
Disease Management					
Memory					
Sensory Health					

Figure 27-3 HealthStages Programming Grid. (From Lach, H. W., Everard, K. M., Highstein, G., & Brownson, C. A. [2004]. Application of the Transtheoretical Model to health education for older adults. *Health Promotion Practice, 5*[1], 88-93.)

et al., 2004). Use of theory in health promotion programs provides structure and direction. Next, health topics are explored.

COMPONENTS OF A HEALTHY LIFESTYLE

The following sections provide an overview of health promotion issues on topics related to the *Healthy People 2010* Health Indicators. The first eight are discussed in this section and are related to components of a healthy lifestyle and the environment. The last two topics are related to the provision of health care and preventive services for older adults for health promotion and prevention.

Physical Activity/Exercise

It is well accepted that regular physical activity is an important part of a healthy lifestyle. The following provide just a few examples of the evidence supporting this claim. Participation in regular physical activity can delay the onset of functional decline, giving support to the conventional wisdom that you must "use it or lose it." Women age 65 who participate in regular exercise can expect to have approximately 6 more years of active life expectancy than women who are sedentary (Ferucci et al., 2000). Physical activity aids both primary and secondary prevention related to many chronic diseases such as diabetes, heart disease, osteoporosis, arthritis, and hypertension.

Unfortunately, research indicates that only about 40% of older people get regular physical activity or exercise (Active Aging Partnership, 2001). In fact, 23.1% of adults age 65 to 74 and 39.5% of adults over age 75 are *inactive*, meaning that they do not participate in any leisure or other physical activity. Given the significant evidence that exercise and activity provide dramatic health benefits to older adults, and the low percentage of older people who engage in it, a national coalition of organizations developed a white paper to address this problem, "National Blueprint: Increasing Physical Activity among Adults Aged 50 and Older" (Active Aging Partnership, 2001). This white paper was developed with input from experts and senior organizations and provides a roadmap of strategies for addressing this issue. The recommendations address strategies from public policy to medical approaches, and form a call to action for practitioners, organizations, and government agencies to help increase physical activity among older adults. An "Active Aging Toolkit" and resources for providers and individuals are available (Active Aging Partnership, 2005).

The American College of Sports Medicine (ACSM) recommends that older adults regularly participate in four kinds of exercise (Pyron, 2003):

- *Aerobic or endurance exercise* to improve cardiac and respiratory fitness
- *Muscle strengthening or resistance exercises* to build muscles and strengthen bones
- *Balance exercises* to improve balance and prevent falls
- *Flexibility exercises* to stretch muscles and tissues to prevent injuries

As far as general health promotion, a pyramid for physical activity modeled on the Food Guide Pyramid is an easy way to convey general goals for physical activity (Figure 27-4). Older adults with injuries or problems may need individual evaluation and assistance from physical therapists or exercise specialists. In addition, classes and activities need to provide a wide range of options for those older adults, including those who are out of shape and are not ready for advanced physical activity usually provided by exercise programs.

Nurses in all settings can discuss and encourage exercise with all older patients. This process is enhanced when the nurse knows what resources are available to older adults in their local community, including classes for older adults at all fitness levels, personal trainers, physical therapy programs, walking groups, and so on. The motivation to exercise for older adults is often to maintain health and independence, but social reasons for exercising are also important (Dacey & Newcomer, 2005). As a result, group exercise is often the best format for older adults. Walking is also a very popular form of exercise for older adults, so provide options for group or individual walking. Nurses can encourage individuals to start increasing physical activity in any way they can, or just start moving, and then gradually work toward larger goals.

Overweight and Obesity

Healthy eating, as well as obesity and weight management, is discussed in Chapter 8. However, the methods and techniques for promoting healthy behaviors in this chapter also apply to nutrition, so we will briefly mention some key points about healthy eating here. A growing number of older adults meet criteria for obesity, which usually includes having a body mass index greater than 30. Researchers estimate that there will be just over 22 million adults over age 60 who are obese by 2010 (Arterburn, Crane, & Sullivan, 2004), and cases will only increase in the decades that follow. Weight management and healthy eating should regularly be included as an important part of health promotion programs, as well as clinical practice.

Tobacco Use

The current generation grew up in a time when smoking was considered glamorous and exciting. Still, smoking is considered the leading preventable cause of premature

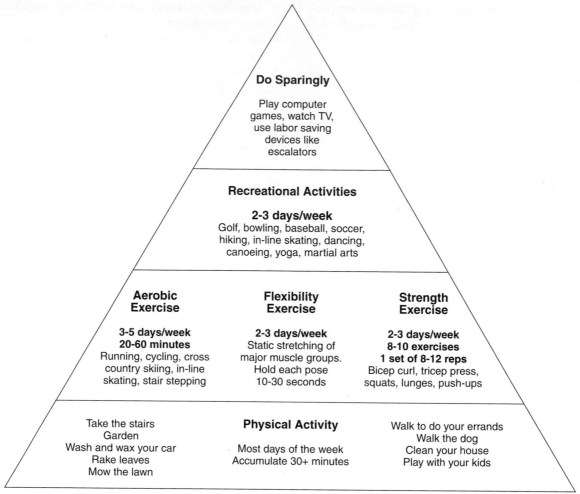

Figure 27-4 Physical activity pyramid. (From Georgia State University. [1999]. Physical activity pyramid. *Exercise and Physical Fitness Page.* Retrieved November 10, 2005, from www2.gsu.edu/~wwwfit/physicalactivity.html.)

death (CDC, 2005a). The prevalence of smoking in the United States continues to decline and the rate decreases with age, but studies suggest that 8.8% of current older adults report smoking. This includes older adults in long-term care settings (Guilmette & Shadel, 2002). A 2003 report from the Surgeon General connects smoking in older adults to decreased bone density, hip fractures, cataracts, and chronic obstructive pulmonary disease. Other negative effects of tobacco use include cardiovascular disease, cancer, disability, and death. However, little research has focused specifically on smoking or how to promote smoking cessation for this population (Cataldo, 2003).

As with other health promotion and disease prevention measures, primary care providers may not ask about smoking or discuss the need to stop with older patients. Older smokers need information about the relationship between smoking and health when health events occur, because they may be motivated to make health changes when illness occurs (O'Connell, 2001).

The U.S. Department of Health and Human Services provides a free reference for health care providers on how to help patients quit smoking (Fiore et al., 2000). Brief interventions can be offered during health care encounters, are effective, and should be part of routine practice (Rice & Stead, 2002). The individual who wants to quit smoking can be helped by following the five *As* (ask, advise, assess, assist, and arrange):

- *Ask* about tobacco use at every health care encounter
- *Advise* patients to quit smoking
- *Assess* if the individual is ready to quit
- *Assist* the individual to develop a plan and provide appropriate adjunct therapies such as medications, classes, support, counseling, or other
- *Arrange* for follow-up to provide support and accountability

For individuals who are not ready to stop smoking, additional methods discussed in this chapter on models and techniques to help with health behavior changes may be useful. Many times people take several attempts to stop smoking successfully, so continued attempts should be encouraged. The five *As* can be used in clinical practice with many health promoting behaviors.

Substance Abuse

Substance abuse in older adults is an often overlooked or ignored problem. Older drug abusers are often poor, frail, and hidden from health professionals and service providers. The stigma associated with these problems keeps them, as well as family members, from coming forward to report problems. Although substance abuse in older adults is lower than in younger people, it is a significant and growing problem with the increase in the older population. In 2002, 62 million adults age 55 and over were admitted to a substance abuse treatment program, and this figure is expected to increase to 5 million by 2020 according to the Substance Abuse and Mental Health Services Administrations (SAMHSA) (2005a). Alcohol abuse is a far greater problem than illicit drug use in this age-group.

SAMHSA reports the following prevalence of alcohol use in 2003: 45.1% of older adults had an alcoholic drink, 12.2% reported binge drinking (having five or more drinks on one occasion), and 3.25% reported heavy alcohol use (SAMHSA, 2005b). Screening for alcohol abuse needs to be part of routine screening for older patients (Knauer, 2003), and tools to help the practitioner are noted in Chapter 3. Other health problems such as falls or depression may increase suspicion that a problem exists, because increased alcohol use may be a response to pain or losses, and, as with younger alcoholics, it tends to run in families.

Some older adults may need to limit alcohol intake because of medications or health conditions that put them at risk (Masters, 2003). For those needing treatment, Alcoholics Anonymous continues to be a mainstay treatment approach, with free supportive groups. Inpatient and outpatient programs may also be available and may be the best choice for those with medical conditions that complicate withdrawal. Treatment needs to be individualized based on the psychological, physical, and functional abilities of the patient, as well as available resources.

It is important to note that alcohol has health benefits when used in moderation, which is usually defined as having two drinks or less per day. These benefits as summarized by Luggen (2006) include decreased risk of heart attack, stroke, some dementias and cancers, renal disorders, and cataracts. Some report improved sleep. However, the potential side effects for older adults must be considered because alcohol may alter the effects of medications or other health conditions. The nurse should explore alcohol use with patients and individualize recommendations.

Frequency of illicit drug use is reported in approximately 1.8% of adults over age 50 (marijuana 1.1%, prescription drug misuse 0.7%, and cocaine 0.2%). The problem is also reflected in the figures for substance abuse treatment of older adults. Because older adults are a small percentage of drug users, little is known about how to manage the problem in this age-group. Substance abuse in later life is often a continuation of a lifelong pattern (Benshoff & Harrawood, 2003). New substance abusers in later life tend to use alcohol rather than illicit drugs. The effects of aging create increasing difficulties for drug abusers, particularly those who inject drugs (e.g., hardening of the veins). Anderson and Levy (2003) describe the challenges of older abusers, who no longer fit in the drug culture of younger users and are fearful of being victimized. It is difficult to maintain drug habits with the physical and social changes of aging, which are often compounded by drug use.

Treatment for older drug users, as with alcoholics, needs to be individualized. Programs may not address the special needs of older patients. Tuchman (2003) explores how little is known about methadone treatment for older women in menopause; even less is known for the frail aging adult. With the increase in older people who have alcohol and substance abuse problems, gerontological nurses can play a role in identifying better ways to assess and treat these problems.

Responsible Sexual Behavior

There is little emphasis on sexually transmitted diseases (STDs) or human immunodeficiency virus/acquired immunodeficiency syndrome (HIV/AIDS) in the older population. However, even though the numbers of victims are smaller, older adults remain sexually active and at risk for STDs. Myths of later life as asexual contribute to the attitude that these issues are not important in the older population. Older adults themselves also may not perceive themselves as at risk and may engage in high-risk sexual behavior. As a result, older adults may not be asked about sexual behavior or diseases or be tested. Wilson (2003) reports that half of older adults are sexually active, including about 25% of those over 80, and these numbers may increase as younger cohorts age. Older adults make up a small percent of all STD cases (CDC, 2003b):

- Syphilis—2.3% of men, 0.2% of women
- Chlamydia—9.6% of men, 8.2% of women
- Gonorrhea—21.1% of men, 3.1% of women
- AIDS—10% to 12% (CDC, 2002), not including those who have HIV infection but have not yet been diagnosed with AIDS

Older adults often contract HIV through sexual contact, usually homosexual contact.

Nurses can provide counseling and education for older adults regarding protection against STDs, including abstinence and the use of condoms. In addition, elders should be encouraged to ask sexual partners about their sexual history, drug use, and history of blood transfusions in developing countries, or in the United States between 1978 and 1985 (National Institute on Aging, 2005). It is also helpful to dispel myths about how HIV is spread and provide information about current treatments to ensure that older adults have a good understanding of this and other STDs.

Mental Health

Mental health promotion often takes a back seat to physical issues in health education, but it is crucial to the well-being of the older adult (see Chapter 20 for an in-depth discussion). Older adults have to adapt to and cope with significant changes that are common in later life, including retirement, changes in health and function, and loss of friends and family, just to name a few. These changes and losses increase their vulnerability to mental health problems (Edwards & Chapman, 2004). The idea that the later years are stress free and older adults just sit on the porch and rock is a myth. In fact, older adults may be dealing with the most stressful events of their life, while addressing the developmental tasks of facing mortality and coming to grips with their life experiences. Many still think that depression is a normal part of aging and treatments are unacceptable, and therefore not worthy of mentioning to health care providers.

Older adults express an interest in learning more about topics that support personal development. Health promotion programs and professionals should address the following mental health topics:

- Managing stress and relaxation techniques
- Communication skills and active listening
- Relationships with family and friends
- Anger management
- Adapting to changes in activities and finding enjoyable replacements if needed
- Maintaining social engagement
- Managing negative stereotypes of aging
- Problem solving
- Using humor
- Developing positive attitudes and avoiding negative thoughts and feelings
- Improving self-esteem
- Assertiveness skills, especially for women
- Empowerment to express
- Bereavement
- Life review
- Spirituality

Nurses will want to explore these topics related to emotional health with older adults to promote mental health, prevent depression, and promote positive aging (Hartman-Stein & Potkanowicz, 2003; Rowe & Kahn, 1998). Older adults with problems should be referred to classes, counseling, psychotherapy, mental health professionals, support groups, and other resources. Discuss such topics without using terms such as *mental health, psychiatry,* and other words that have a negative stigma, particularly in this age-group, to avoid a negative reaction from the older adult. Using terms considered more positive such as *stress management, personal development,* or *coping* will often be more acceptable. Helping older adults address mental health problems and learn skills to promote good mental health can make aging a more positive experience.

Injury and Violence

Injury is the eighth leading cause of death among older adults, making it an important health promotion or prevention issue for clinicians and health educators. The top causes of injury-related death are falls (30%) and motor vehicle crashes (18%) (Dellinger & Stevens, 2005). Because many older adults remain active, we would be remiss in not mentioning such issues as bicycle and motorcycle accidents where helmet use is important. Violence-related injuries in the older population are most often due to elder abuse, discussed in Chapter 21.

Fires in the home are a less frequent cause of death for older adults, but this age-group is at increased risk of injury and death if a fire occurs (CDC, 2005b). Most fires occur in the home, with cooking and smoking the primary causes. Smoke detectors are an important warning system and should be explored with older patients during home assessments and discussed in health promotion programs.

Falls are a common accident among older adults and become more important with age because of the increasing rate of injuries that result from falls. About 30% to 40% of adults in the community fall each year (Stevens, 2002), and about 5% result in a serious accident, 3% being hip fractures. Hip fractures are a significant outcome of falls and can result in reduced functional ability, nursing home placement, and death. Falls are the sixth leading cause of death among older adults. Psychological outcomes of falls are also a problem, because many older adults may develop fear of falling that causes them to cut down excessively on their activities. This emerging public health problem may result in isolation and functional decline (Lach, 2005).

Guidelines for managing falls were developed by experts from the American Geriatrics Society, British

Geriatrics Society, and American Academy of Orthopedic Surgeons Panel on Falls Prevention (2001). A number of risk factors for falls have been identified:

- Muscle weakness
- History of falls
- Gait deficit
- Balance deficit
- Use of assistive device
- Visual deficit
- Arthritis
- Impaired activities of daily living
- Depression
- Cognitive impairment
- Age over 80 years

The guidelines recommend routine assessment of community-dwelling older adults to identify the presence of the risk factors listed and implementation of interventions as appropriate. Most important are gait training, education on the use of assistive devices, and referral for exercise. Medications should be reviewed for potential effects on balance and falls and regimens revised as needed. Medical conditions should be explored and treated, including postural hypotension, cardiac arrhythmias, and other cardiovascular disorders. A home safety assessment should be conducted and hazards modified. It is not known how often primary care providers actually provide assessment and referral regarding falls.

Older adults need education on the risk factors for falls and strategies to prevent them. Home safety checklists are widely available, but older adults may need encouragement to complete them. Low-cost resources for making home modifications are available in some communities. Nurses can address falls by asking about fall history and risk factors for falls, and referring older adults to education and exercise resources in the community.

Motor vehicle crashes are more common in older drivers than younger ones, and they have a higher fatality rate (Insurance Institute for Highway Safety, 2003). A number of age-related issues may put older drivers at disproportional risk, including medications, health conditions, and functional problems. The Older Driver's Project has been initiated by the American Medical Association together with the National Highway Traffic Safety Administration to develop approaches to improve safety (Wang & Carr, 2004). This program advocates maximizing the driver's health through management of health conditions, particularly those related to driving such as visual problems and cardiovascular problems, or functional problems. Drivers should be referred for rehabilitation, including evaluation of the patient and vehicle, adaptation as needed, or driver training.

The driving environment could be improved as roads are built or updated and signage changed to make it easier for older drivers to maneuver (Federal Highway Administration, 2001). Vehicle designs could also be improved to make them safer for older drivers. In some cases, the older adult should be encouraged to stop driving and families counseled on methods to help with this process. Nurses should be aware of driving issues and address them in care and education.

Environmental Quality

With the aging population, scientists and the U.S. Environmental Protection Agency (EPA) have increased concerns about the impact of the environment on the health of older adults. This interest is fueled in part by the possibility that older adults may be more susceptible to hazards in the environment than younger people, and by the fact that little research addresses this issue. Major health conditions such as heart and lung diseases can be aggravated by environmental factors (Adler, 2003), and pollutants may affect the aging process itself. The accumulated exposure to environmental hazards over a lifetime may also have an impact on aging and health. Important environmental hazards laid out by the EPA (2005) include the following:

- Indoor air pollutants—radon, secondhand smoke, carbon monoxide
- Outdoor air pollutants—ozone, lead, particulate matter
- Drinking water contaminants—microbes, disinfectants and by-products, volatile organic compounds (paint, glue, etc.)
- Pesticides
- Heavy metals—lead and mercury (primarily from coal-fired plants)

Older workers may also have special health needs related to environmental hazards (Chalupka, 2005). Gerontological nurses should consider these issues, as well as environmental effects on health and disease, in the care of older patients. For example, air pollution may contribute to pulmonary or cardiac conditions. Environmental issues vary by geographical locations, so nurses need to be aware of environmental issues in their own region.

The EPA launched an aging initiative in 2002 to develop a national agenda for protecting the health of older Americans and to guide future research and programs to address these issues (Sykes, 2005). The program included six national public forums around the country to explore issues, develop alliances among agencies and experts, and plan funding for training, outreach, and program development related to aging and the environment. Gerontological nurses can also participate in this initiative, as well as the environmental debate, and advocate for issues that affect older adults.

Health Maintenance and Clinical Preventive Services

The final health promotion topics are from *Healthy People 2010* indicators that are related to clinical services from health care professionals. They include both primary and secondary prevention that are often used in the primary care setting. The topics covered here are health maintenance activities, immunizations, and dental care.

Health Maintenance. For good health care, annual checkups are recommended for older adults to assess health status, including current health condition, medications, screening for new problems, and providing health promotion. Most older adults report having a place to go for routine medical care (96%) (Administration on Aging, 2004) and average nearly seven visits per year. Only 2.5% of older adults cannot afford medical care. This low number is in part due to

Table 27-2 *Health Screening Guidelines for Older Americans*

Screening	Men/Women	Age-Group	
		50 to 64	**65 and Older**
Height, weight, body mass index, and blood pressure; counseling for weight loss as appropriate[1]	M/W	Annually at each preventive examination	Annually at each preventive examination
Papanicolaou (Pap) smear/pelvic[2]	W	Yearly until three normal and then every 3 years	Yearly until three normal and then every 3 years
Mammogram[2]	W	Annually as long as patient is in good health	Annually as long as patient is in good health
Fasting cholesterol panel[4]	M/W	Every 5 years	Every 5 years
Colon and rectal cancer[2]	M/W	Starting age 50, should follow one of five schedules: ■ Yearly fecal occult blood test (FOBT) ■ Flexible sigmoidoscopy every 5 years ■ Yearly FOBT plus sigmoidoscopy every 5 years ■ Double-contrast barium enema every 5 years ■ Colonoscopy every 10 years	
Breast clinical examinaiton[2]	W	Annual	Annual
Bone density test[3]	W	At age 60 with risk factors	One at age 65 if normal
Digital rectal examination and prostate-specific antigen assay[2]	M	Annual	Annual
Dental examination[5]	M/W	Regularly	Regularly
Eye examination[6]	M/W	Every 2-4 years	Every 1-2 years
Hearing examination[7]	M/W	Every 3 years	Every 3 years

Sources of recommendations:

1. Regence Blue Cross Blue Shield of Oregon: www.or.regence.com/provider/clinicalcorner/index.html. Under *Guidelines,* select *Periodic Screening.*
2. American Cancer Society: www.cancer.org/docroot/PED/content/PED_2_3X_ACS_Cancer_Detection_Guidelines_36.asp?sitearea=PED.
3. U.S. Preventive Services Task Force: www.ahrq.gov/clinic/uspstf/uspsoste.htm.
4. American Heart Association: www.americanheart.org/presenter.jhtml?identifier=541.
5. American Dental Association (ADA): www.ada.org/public/index.asp. NOTE: According to the ADA Department of Public Information, the ADA does not have a recommendation concerning the frequency of dental visits. The time between recall visits is determined by the dentist, based on the patient's past and current oral health status.
6. American Academy of Ophthalmology: www.medem.com/MedLB/article_detaillb.cfm?article_ID=ZZZ08DZO3SC&sub_cat=2015.
7. American Speech-Language-Hearing Association: www.asha.org/public/hearing/testing/.

Medicare and Medicaid programs that provide coverage for older Americans. However, those without care are disproportionately ethnic and racial minorities.

General components of the history and physical examination are discussed in the assessment section in Chapter 2, but our emphasis here is on prevention and early detection of disease. Recommended health screenings for older adults are listed in Table 27-2, along with the frequency with which they should be provided. Older adults may need education and assistance to complete all of the recommended screenings. Some of the listed elements are completed in the course of an office visit with the health care provider (e.g., blood pressure and weight). Blood tests may also be obtained during regular office visits. However, additional tests must be scheduled and completed, usually at another site and time, such as mammograms and bone density tests. As a result, health behavior factors come into play, and the nurse should educate patients regarding the need for tests and use behavior change techniques if needed to increase the use of screenings.

If screening is not expected to change treatment, or if detected health problems would not be addressed, the utility of continued screening diminishes. With advanced age or the presence of major illness, such as advanced dementia, the clinician should use judgment about continuing screening (Takahashi, Okhravi, Lim, & Kasten, 2004). Patients and families should be included in these decisions.

Immunizations. Immunizations are an important preventive measure for older adults. Table 27-3 describes the recommended immunizations for all older adults.

The following provides a brief overview of each of the recommended immunizations.

Older adults have the highest mortality rate from influenza, so all adults over age 65 should get an annual flu vaccine (CDC, 2005c). The best time to get vaccinated is in the fall, usually October or November. The influenza vaccine is developed annually and is designed to protect the public against the worst influenza viruses expected for that year. Usually the vaccine provides protection against two type A viruses and one type B virus, which is typically a milder flu. The shot uses inactivated virus, and the nasal spray is an attenuated or weakened live virus.

Older adults may have many misconceptions about the flu vaccine, including the belief that they can get the flu from the vaccine and concerns about serious side effects, and need education regarding the vaccine. The CDC annually provides updated information for providers and the public that can be downloaded from their Web site.

The pneumococcal vaccine provides protection against 23 of the common bacteria that cause pneumonia (CDC, 2005c). Nurses should encourage adults to obtain the vaccination at age 65, again because the most serious disease and highest mortality rates are among older adults. Some individuals with chronic lung or health conditions may get vaccinated at a younger age and may take a second dose when they reach 65. For most people, the vaccination is only given once.

Tetanus is another important immunization that needs to be updated regularly, but much less frequently than the flu shot. Individuals should receive a primary set of three tetanus shots (given typically with diphtheria

Table 27-3 *Recommended Adult Immunization Schedule in United States, 2003-2004*

Vaccine	Dosage
Tetanus, diphtheria (TD)	One dose booster every 10 years
Influenza	One dose annually
Pneumococcal	One to two doses (50 to 64 years of age); one dose (65 years of age and older)
Hepatitis B	Three doses lifetime (0, 1-2, and 4-6 months)
Hepatitis A	Two doses (0 and 6-12 months or 0 and 6-18 months)
Varicella	Two doses (0 and 4-8 weeks)
Meningococcal	One or more doses

From the Centers for Disease Control and Prevention's National Immunization Program Web site: www.cdc.gov/nip. Schedule approved by Advisory Committee on Immunization Practices, and accepted by the American Academy of Family Physicians. For more information on indications or contraindications, check the Web site or call the National Immunization Hotline at 1-800-232-2522 (English) or 1-800-232-0233 (Spanish).

as a combined shot). After the initial series, booster shots should be given every 10 years. Men who served in the military received the primary tetanus series, but some older women never had the initial set of shots. If the immunization status of an adult is unknown, she or he should receive this initial set. Although tetanus is rare and there were only 20 cases in 2003 (CDC, 2005c), most cases occur in people over age 50 and are related to injuries or puncture wounds obtained in and around the home.

Several other vaccines are available for common communicable diseases and are recommended for older adults who are exposed to the disease or who are at risk for exposure. Immunizations include hepatitis A, hepatitis B, varicella, and meningococcal vaccines. As with influenza, information on communicable disease and recommendations for immunization are readily available from the CDC Web site.

Immunization status should be routinely checked with all older patients. Although immunization rates among older adults have been increasing, research indicates that older ethnic and racial minorities are much less likely to receive these important preventive measures (Bonito, Lenfestey, Eicheldinger, Ianacchione, & Campbell, 2004), in spite of the fact that Medicare covers these services. Nurses should work to help reduce this health disparity by identifying the immunization status of all older adults, providing education on the need for immunizations, and providing information on where and how they can be obtained. Another problem with vaccination occurs in older adults who are very frail and have severely impaired nutritional status who may not be able to develop antibodies in response to the vaccination. Their response to vaccination may need to be monitored.

Dental Health. Oral and dental health is increasingly an important component of a healthy lifestyle (Bailey, Gueldner, Ledikwe, & Smiciklas-Wright, 2005). General oral care should include daily brushing using a toothbrush and fluoride toothpaste and daily flossing. Dental checkups and care by a dentist should be conducted regularly. Although regular medical care may be available to most older adults, dental care may be less available, especially for underserved groups, and requires additional attention (Pyle & Stoller, 2003). See Box 27-1 for additional information on dental health issues. Maintaining oral health for those in long-term care or who cannot provide their own dental care is a major problem, with many barriers (Bailey et al., 2005). The Surgeon General has called for improved dental care and services for older people to try and sustain oral health throughout life, rather than continuous oral restorative care (USDHHS, 2000). Dental care and dental health services should be part of health maintenance and health promotion in every setting.

Advancing the Health Agenda

Key topics related to the health indicators set forth in *Healthy People 2010* have been reviewed in this section. They provide important information that health care providers and older adults need to understand and address. Gerontological nurses are in positions to educate both professionals and the lay public and should use their expertise to increase awareness and knowledge in these areas to advance the health agenda for this growing population. As we move into the next section, techniques for providing health education are discussed that can make this process more effective.

HEALTH EDUCATION FOR OLDER ADULTS: MATERIALS AND TECHNIQUES

Health education is an important method for delivering information to older adults about promoting or maintaining health, as well as managing chronic disease. The prior sections have addressed the content of health promotion and approaches to promote behavior change. This section of the chapter addresses practical issues and techniques in providing health education for older adults. The section begins by addressing adult education principles and the problem of health literacy. Later, the impact of aging changes on educational processes and specific techniques for targeting health education to older adults are described.

Teaching older adults has been described as "geragogy" (John, 1988), a methodology to address the special educational needs of this population that combines principles of adult education with knowledge of aging changes. Knowles (1984) has written much on the topic of adult learning and identified the following assumptions for addressing older adults as learners (Knowles, 1987, p. 5):

1. Older adult learners are self-directed.
2. Older adults bring a wealth of knowledge and experience that can be a resource for learning and teaching others.
3. Older adults become ready to learn when they want to function more effectively in life situations.
4. Older adults want to learn skills or gain information to solve problems.
5. Older adults are motivated by internal sources rather than external sources such as grades.

As a result, older adults want to be engaged in the learning process. If you are planning health education activities, include older adults in planning topics, identifying learning objectives, and developing the plan. Although learning can be easier and is best when related to past life experiences, sometimes habit or prior misinformation can inhibit learning (Bille, 1980). Therefore educational activities should address up-to-date information about health topics and include discussion so that each participant's individual needs are met (Box 27-3). Activities and exercises should assist older adults to integrate knowledge into their daily lives and provide for sharing of ideas and experiences.

Health Literacy

Health literacy has been defined as the "degree to which individuals have the capacity to obtain, process, and understand basic health information and services needed to make appropriate health decisions" (Ratzan & Parker, 2000). Health literacy includes the ability to read, the ability to perform basic math skills, comprehension, and the ability to make health care decisions

---

BOX 27-3 Health Promotion Topics of Interest to Older Adults

General
Managing your health
What tests are recommended and when
Talking to your doctor
Using medications safely
Women's health issues
Men's health issues
Legal and financial planning
Exercise*
Sexuality
Healthy eating
Fad diets
Sleeping well
Home safety
Fall prevention
Safe driving
Smoking cessation
Alcohol use
Mental wellness—positive aging
Stress management
Assertiveness
Relationships
Memory improvement

Disease Oriented
Living with chronic diseases
Arthritis
Memory problems
Heart disease
Diabetes
Osteoporosis
Managing chronic pain
The blues (depression)
Vision problems
Hearing

*NOTE: A wide variety of options are needed, such as aerobics, walking groups, Tai Chi, and others, including programs for those who have not been exercising and who are out of shape.

---

and function as a health care consumer (Speros, 2005). Beyond educational issues, cultural or ethnic differences can influence understanding of health issues (Cutilli, 2005). The Institute of Medicine has set forth recommendations for improving health literacy among all Americans (Nielsen-Bohlman, Panzer, & Kendig, 2004). The following discussions promote careful development of health education for older adults to make information accessible for as wide an audience of older adults as possible. To assess reading level of individuals, Davis and colleagues (1993) developed the Rapid Estimate of Adult Literacy in Medicine (REALM) literacy test.

Cultural Appropriateness

Beyond the issue of health literacy is cultural appropriateness. Growing awareness of health disparities and increased diversity in the older population has stimulated interest in delivering programs to minorities or underserved populations (Resnicow, Braithwaite, Dilorio, & Glanz, 2002). This includes two factors, the first of which is targeting or delivering programs or education to the population of interest. The other is tailoring, which involves designing the approach to the material or program to address the population's norms, values, and interests. Developing culturally appropriate programs and education involves the following strategies (Kreuter et al., 2003):

- *Peripheral strategies*—packaging programs and materials so that they have appeal to the target group
- *Evidential strategies*—providing information that helps the target audience see the importance of the issue
- *Linguistic strategies*—translating information if needed into other languages, using terms the group relates to
- *Constituent-involving strategies*—such as hiring people to deliver programs or materials who are from the targeted group
- *Sociocultural strategies*—addressing issues in a way that takes the culture of the group into account, such as their views of health, family, values, and beliefs
- *Cultural tailoring*—using information derived from assessment of the population and individuals within the population to design programs and materials that fit

All of these steps are important to reach diverse audiences of older adults, in addition to the special needs related to aging changes discussed next.

Adapting Teaching for Aging Changes

Aging changes are presented in detail (system by system) in Section 3 of this text system and need to be considered when developing health education programs or materials for older adults. The process of learning involves taking in information through the senses, storing or registering the information in the brain, and recalling information later. Aging changes affect these memory processes in various ways:

- Visual changes can impair ability to read (handouts, slides, reading lips)—decreased visual acuity; yellowing of the lens makes differentiation of colors more difficult, especially greens, blues, and purples; smaller pupil size so need more light to see well, sensitivity to glare
- Hearing changes can impair ability to hear—decreased hearing acuity; presbycusis results in difficulty hearing high-pitched voices or music; problems differentiating words or letters (s, z, t, f, and g are especially difficult); increased difficulty hearing with background noise, need to supplement hearing with lip reading
- Older adults may take longer to learn new information—repetition and concentration are important to ensure that information is stored in memory; time limitations will affect learning; distractions can interfere with learning (e.g., background noise, TV, conversations, etc.)
- Retrieving information stored in the brain takes longer—the experience of feeling that something is on the tip of the tongue is more frequent, information that is not linked to other information or reference cues is harder to recall
- Medical or functional problems—may pose additional challenges, including getting out to attend programs, fatigue, cognitive impairment

Assessment

Using the prior information about learning, conduct assessment of individuals, groups, or communities to inform the design of health promotion and education programs, materials, and approaches. The following should be assessed:

- Health goals and interests
- Prior knowledge or experiences with the topic
- Educational history/health literacy
- Cultural influences
- Choice of learning style
- Cognitive abilities
- Sensory abilities
- Psychomotor skills
- Medical conditions
- Readiness to learn or make changes

The information gained from the assessment can be used to develop materials that are tailored to the target individual or group. Additional techniques for developing materials for education and health promotion for older populations are discussed next.

Written Materials

Factors to be considered when developing written health materials for older adults include culture, health literacy, and adapting for visual changes. Use a font size of at least 14 points (Hayes, 2005). The size may need to be increased to 16 or 18 points if the materials are targeting older adults with vision difficulties. Provide adequate spacing between letters and lines, and white space on pages. The standard settings on most computers are usually set appropriately. The print color should provide high contrast with the paper or background, such as black on white. Select colors that are light, such as yellow or off-white. Paper should be low gloss to prevent glare (Lighthouse International, 2005).

If you are translating written materials, it may not be enough to use a computer-generated translation program. Materials should be translated into the other language, and then translated back into English to be sure the meaning has not been changed. A person from the target audience should also review the material to ensure that cultural differences do not change the meaning of the contents. In addition, people in different parts of the country may have different dialects in the language they use, so a booklet developed for Hispanic diabetics in New York may need to be adapted for a Hispanic population in New Mexico. Be specific for your target population.

Older adults today have a range of educational experiences and literacy levels, so materials should be written in a way to be accessible to a wide audience. A large number of older adults today did not complete high school or college, because the opportunities were much more limited when they were younger. As a result, you have to gear the educational level of materials to an appropriate grade level to be sure that they can be comprehended. A sixth-grade reading level is readable for about 75% of adult Americans (Doak, Doak, & Lorig, 1996) and is an appropriate level for most written materials.

There are a number of methods to determine reading level. Word processing software may do this automatically, calculating the grade level of a written document using the spelling or grammar check tool. Written formulas can also be used (e.g., the Simplified Measure of Gobbledygook [SMOG] reading test) (McLaughlin, 1969). Box 27-4 provides an assessment tool for evaluating written educational materials adapted from Doak, Doak, and Lorig (1996).

Group Presentations

Older adults enjoy learning in a group setting, especially when programs provide opportunities for sharing and learning from each other. Depending on the purpose of the presentation, the format, size of the group,

BOX 27-4 Assessment for Health Education Materials

Use the following items to evaluate educational materials for older adults.

1. Content
   a. Can patients easily understand the purpose of the material? If not, they may not pay attention to the rest of the material or they may miss the main point.
   b. Is there clear, behavior-specific content that helps patients solve their problems? Often materials address what health professionals think people ought to know, rather than what they want to know. Does the content provide information that will help the person deal with the health issue in his or her daily life?
   c. Is the scope limited to the objectives? Sometimes materials contain more information than patients want, need, or can reasonably learn.
   d. Is there a review or summary of the key points? This is important because readers often miss the key points on the first exposure.

2. Literacy demands
   a. Is the material written at a sixth-grade reading level or below?
   b. Is the material presented in a conversational style using active voice? Long or multiple phrases included in a sentence slow down the reading process and generally make comprehension more difficult.
   c. Does the material use common and explicit words? (For example, "doctor" rather than "physician," "pain lasting more than 5 minutes" rather than "excessive pain.") Whenever possible, use image words. These are things that people can see or feel (e.g., "vegetables" rather than "dietary fiber," "runny nose" rather than "mucus").
   d. Are there organizers such as headers or topic captions that tell what is coming? These advance organizers make material look less formidable and also prepare the reader for the next topic. They also help the busy reader pick and choose what she or he wants to read.

3. Graphics
   a. Is the cover graphic engaging? Does it convey an appropriate message? Some people do judge a booklet by its cover. Is the cover graphic interesting? Does it show what the material is all about?
   b. Are the illustrations simple and realistic without distracting details? Visuals are accepted and remembered better when they portray the familiar. Viewers may not recognize the meaning of medieval textbook drawings or abstract art or symbols. Photos should be limited in the amount of detail shown. Nonessential details such as room background, elaborate borders, or unnecessary color can be distracting.
   c. Do the illustrations tell the key points graphically?
   d. Are all graphics carefully and fully explained in text near the graphic? Explanation and directions are essential and do little good if they are not in close proximity to the graphic.
   e. Are captions used to explain graphics and illustrations? Captions can quickly tell the reader what the graphic or illustration is all about. A graphic without a caption is usually an inferior illustration and represents a missed learning opportunity.

4. Layout and typography
   a. Are illustrations near related text?
   b. Are there usual cueing devices such as boxes or arrows to point to key information?
   c. Is there adequate white space?
   d. Does the material look cluttered?
   e. Is there high contrast between the print and paper?
   f. Are more than six types of fonts or sizes used on one page? Too many makes the material appear confusing.
   g. Are ALL CAPS used? Type in ALL CAPS slows down reading comprehension.
   h. Are there more than five to seven subheadings? Few people can remember more than seven independent items. For adults with lower literacy skills, the limit may be three to five items. Longer lists need to be partitioned into smaller chunks.

5. Learning stimulation/motivation
   a. Is interaction included in the text and/or graphic? Readers should be asked to do something, such as solve a problem, make a choice, or demonstrate something.
   b. Are desired behaviors shown in specific terms and modeled? People learn more readily by observation and doing rather than by reading or being told.
   c. Are the behaviors presented as doable? People are more motivated when they believe that tasks are doable. Telling people with emphysema to "exercise" is not very motivating. Telling them that "everyone can walk for 10 minutes a day by walking 1 minute for each hour that he or she is awake" is much more motivating.

From Doak, C., Doak, L., & Lorig, K. (1996). Selecting, preparing, and using materials. In K. Lorig (Ed.), *Patient education: A practical approach* (ed 2). Thousand Oaks, CA: Sage.

Continued

BOX 27-4 Assessment for Health Education Materials—cont'd

6. Cultural appropriateness
   a. Do the language, logic, experience, and illustrations match the population?
   b. Are the images culturally appropriate, positive, and realistic? Using Grandma Moses as a positive image of aging may be meaningless to a Hispanic population.
   c. Does the material convey respect? There is a tendency to infantilize materials for people of other cultures or older people. People with low literacy or other languages have the same ability to learn if taught properly.

---

and audiovisual aids should be planned with the older learner in mind. A brief presentation on a health problem is effective for any size group, large or small, if you are trying to increase awareness of a topic. However, a common mistake is to try to include too much content and cover too many details. It is more effective to provide key information and schedule adequate time so that you can present your material and still allow time for questions and discussion. Build in ways for the participants to process information; do not just lecture.

Group presentations are an effective way to deliver information when you have a large group. A class size of 15 to 20 people is a good size that is conducive to discussion so that people have a chance to participate.

- Rooms should be arranged in a circle or U shape so that people can see and hear the presenter, as well as each other.
- Include group and individual exercises to increase engagement of participants with the material.
- Plan a break during the presentation so participants do not have to sit too long, getting stiff or sore.
- Allow time for a bathroom break and to stretch and move around.
- Provide refreshments; they are always a nice treat during programs, and often increase attendance.

Oral presentations should be carefully delivered. Even if you have a fairly loud voice, those with hearing difficulties may still not be able to hear. Using a microphone will allow you to lower your voice and annunciate more carefully so that the audience can discriminate between sounds and words. Speak slowly and face the audience or group so that your lips can be seen. Wearing lipstick can enhance the audience's ability to read your lips as you speak.

Audiovisual Aids

Overhead or computer slides may be used to enhance a presentation, but modifications need to be made for an older audience. As with written materials, use a large font for text and high contrast between the text and the background. Include even less content per slide than you would for a presentation to a younger audience. Avoid using a background template for computer slides that is busy or that decreases the contrast between the print and background on the slide.

When making a presentation, leave light in the room so that participants can take notes and see you to read your lips. If you can, copy the slides (in full page for those with visual impairment) and give them to participants so that they can follow along. This was a helpful addition to a class for older adults with visual impairment, who were expected to have difficulty reading overheads. It may work better to use a blackboard to write down key points as they are presented or just give out handouts. The room usually needs to be darker to use slides, which can affect viewing the speakers. Audiovisual presentations that include sound need to be clear, low in pitch, and loud enough for participants to hear.

Web Sites

The Internet offers an easy way for older adults to connect with other people and find information on a wide variety of topics (Kiel, 2005). However, many perceive a "digital divide," and adults over 50 who are not in the workforce have the lowest Internet use of groups over age 5 (U.S. Department of Commerce, 2004). In fact, finding health information is one of the top reasons older adults use the Internet (*Wall Street Journal Online,* 2005). Web sites, like other materials for older adults, need to be organized so that they are clear and legible, and developed in a way that will make their use easier for the older Web surfer.

Modifications for Web sites targeting older adults include using larger fonts with uppercase and lowercase letters, avoiding italics, and including more white space (Age Light Institute, 2000). Sans serif fonts are preferred, because letters remain clear if the writing is enlarged. A text-enlarging feature is very helpful to older adults and is available on some Web sites (SPRY Foundation, 1999). Studies have documented that navigation should be simple, with static links with large areas (Age Light Institute, 2000). Material should be presented in sections, using lists rather than paragraphs. Web pages should be evaluated by older adults as part of the Web development process, a technique used by the National Library of Medicine in developing its senior Web site for health information, MedlinePlus (Miller, LaCroix, & Backus, 2000).

In conclusion, a number of techniques are important to make health promotion and education accessible for older adults. Gerontological nurses can use this information in developing programs and materials, evaluating current resources to see if they are age friendly, and providing appropriate health education for older patients.

Program Evaluation

Evaluating health promotion and education programs is important so that effective strategies can be identified and shared. It is beyond the scope of this chapter to provide details on these methods; however, resources for program planning and evaluation are available to the gerontological nurse. The PRECEDE-PROCEED model offers a systematic method for assessment and planning for health promotion programs or interventions so that they can be evaluated (Gielen & McDonald, 2002). Another method is the RE-AIM framework (Glasgow, 2002). RE-AIM is an acronym for the elements of evaluation:

- *Reach*—how many people participate in a program?
- *Efficacy*—what impact did the program have?
- *Adoption*—how many are using the information from the intervention?
- *Implementation*—is the intervention delivered as designed?
- *Maintenance*—what are the long-term effects for individuals and groups?

Evaluating program outcomes is essential so that successful programs can be shared and replicated.

SUMMARY

This chapter explores the concept of health promotion and how gerontological nurses can provide effective health promotion and education for older adults. Despite the barriers to providing health promotion for older people, a growing recognition of the potential benefits is clear to address this burgeoning population. Gerontological nurses have many resources to help them provide effective health promotion. Evidence is increasing for behavior change theories and techniques, and this chapter describes three common theories: the Health Belief Model, Self-Efficacy Theory, and the Transtheoretical Model. Important topics are reviewed as set forth by *Healthy People 2010*, from physical activity to environmental issues. Additionally, clinical preventive services are discussed. Techniques for tailoring materials to address the physical and cognitive changes of older adults, as well as adult learning principles, are described. Gerontological nurses can provide leadership in promoting effective health promotion and health education to ultimately improve quality of life for our older patients.

REFERENCES

Active Aging Partnership. (2001). National blueprint: Increasing physical activity among adults aged 50 and older. Retrieved June 5, 2005, from www.agingblueprint.org.

Active Aging Partnership. (2005). First step to active health. Retrieved November 20, 2005, from www.firststeptoactivehealth.com/index.htm.

Adler, T. (2003). Aging research: The future face of environmental health. *Environmental Health Perspectives, 111*(14), A761-A765.

Administration on Aging. (2004). A profile of older Americans 2004. Retrieved November 20, 2005, from www.aoa.gov/prof/Statistics/profile/2004/14.asp.

Age Light Institute. (2000). *A guide for Web design usability for users of all ages.* Clyde Hill, WA: Author.

American Geriatrics Society, British Geriatrics Society, & American Academy of Orthopedic Surgeons Panel on Falls Prevention. (2001). Guidelines for the prevention of falls in older persons. *Journal of the American Geriatrics Society, 49*, 664-672.

Anderson, T. L, & Levy, J. A. (2003). Marginality among older injectors in today's illicit drug culture: Assessing the impact of aging. *Addiction, 98*, 761-770.

Arterburn, D. E., Crane, P. K., & Sullivan, S. D. (2004). The coming epidemic of obesity in elderly Americans. *Journal of the American Geriatrics Society, 52*, 1907-1912.

Bailey, R., Gueldner, S., Ledikwe, J., & Smiciklas-Wright, H. (2005). The oral health of older adults: An interdisciplinary mandate. *Journal of Gerontological Nursing, 31*(7), 11-17.

Bandura, A. (1997). *Self-efficacy: The exercise of control.* New York: W. H. Freeman.

Becker, M. (1974). The Health Belief Model and personal health behavior. *Health Education Monographs, 2*, 236.

Bennett, J. A., Perrin, N. A., Hanson, G., Bennett, D., Gaynor, W., Flaherty-Robb, M., et al. (2005). Health aging demonstration project: Nurse coaching for behavior change in older adults. *Research in Nursing and Health, 28*, 187-197.

Benshoff, J. J., & Harrawood, L. K. (2003). Substance abuse and the elderly: Unique issues and concerns. *Journal of Rehabilitation, 69*(2), 43-48.

Bille, D. A. (1980). Educational strategies for teaching the elderly patient. *Nursing and Health Care, 1*(5), 256-263.

Bonito, A. J., Lenfestey, N. F., Eicheldinger, C., Ianacchione, V. G., & Campbell, L. (2004). Disparities in immunizations among elderly Medicare beneficiaries. *American Journal of Preventive Medicine, 27*(2), 153-160.

Burke, B. L., Arkowitz, H., & Dunn, C. (2003). The efficacy of motivational interviewing and its adaptations. In W. R. Miller & S. Rollnick (Eds.), *Motivational interviewing: Preparing people for change.* New York: Guilford Press.

Cataldo, J. K. (2003). Smoking and aging. Clinical implications. Part I: Health and consequence. *Journal of Gerontological Nursing, 29*(9), 15-20.

Centers for Disease Control and Prevention. (2002). *HIV/AIDS Surveillance Report, 13*(2), 1-41.

Centers for Disease Control and Prevention. (2003a). Oral health resources. Retrieved September 29, 2004, from www2.cdc.gov/nccdphp/doh.

Centers for Disease Control and Prevention. (2003b). STD surveillance 2003: Trends in reportable sexually transmitted diseases in the United States, 2003—national data on chlamydia, gonorrhea and syphilis. Retrieved November 10, 2003, from www.cdc.gov/std/stats03/trends2003.htm.

Centers for Disease Control and Prevention. (2005a). Cigarette smoking among adults—United States, 2004. *Morbidity and Mortality Weekly Report, 54*(44), 1121-1124.

Centers for Disease Control and Prevention. (2005b). Fire deaths and injuries: Fact sheet. Retrieved November 10, 2005, from www.cdc.gov/ncipc/factsheets/fire.htm.

Centers for Disease Control and Prevention. (2005c). Adult immunization schedule. Retrieved November 20, 2005, from www.cdc.gov/nip/default.htm.

Chalupka, S. (2005). Environmental health: An opportunity for health promotion and disease prevention. *AAOHN Journal, 53*(1), 13-28.

Champion, V. L. (1999). Revised susceptibility, benefits and barriers scale for mammography screening. *Research in Nursing and Health, 22*(4), 341-348.

Coleman, P. (2005). Opportunities for nursing-dental collaboration: Addressing oral health needs among the elderly. *Nursing Outlook, 53*(1), 33-39.

Cutilli, C. C. (2005). Health literacy: What you need to know. *Orthopaedic Nursing, 24*(3), 227-231.

Dacey, M. L., & Newcomer, A. R. (2005). A client-centered counseling approach for motivating older adults towards physical activity. *Topics in Geriatric Rehabilitation, 21*(3), 194-205.

Davis, T., Long, S., Jackson, R., Mayeaus, E., George, R., Murphy, P., & Crouch, M. (1993). Rapid estimate of adult literacy in medicine: A shortened screening instrument. *Family Medicine, 25*(6), 391-395.

Dellinger, A. M., & Stevens, J. A. (2005). Identifying risk and providing protection are important public health goals. *Generations, 29*(2), 60-64.

Doak, C., Doak, L., & Lorig, K. (1996). Selecting, preparing, and using materials. In K. Lorig (Ed.), *Patient education: A practical approach.* Thousand Oaks, CA: Sage.

Doak, C. C., Doak, L. G., & Root, J. H. (1996). *Teaching patients with low literacy skills.* Philadelphia: Lippincott.

Dupree-Jones, K., Burckhardt, C. S., & Bennett, J. A. (2004). Motivational interviewing may encourage exercise in persons with fibromyalgia by enhancing self-efficacy. *Arthritis and Rheumatism, 51*(5), 864-867.

Edwards, H., & Chapman, H. (2004). Contemplating, caring, coping, conversing: A model for promoting mental wellness in later life. *Journal of Gerontological Nursing, 30*(5), 16-21.

Environmental Protection Agency. (2005). What is the EPA aging initiative? Retrieved November 10, 2005, from www.epa.gov/aging/pdfs/factsheet.pdf.

Everard, K. M., Lach, H. W., & Heinrich, B. (2000). The development of HealthStages: A unique university and not-for-profit collaboration to enhance successful aging. *Journal of Educational Gerontology, 26*, 715-724.

Federal Highway Administration. (2001). Guidelines and recommendations to accommodate older drivers and pedestrians. Retrieved November 20, 2005, from www.tfhrc.gov/humanfac/01105/cover.htm.

Ferucci, L., Penninx, B. W., Leveille, S. G., Corti, M. C., Pahor, M., & Wallace, R. (2000). Characteristics of nondisabled older persons who perform poorly in objective tests of lower extremity function. *Journal of the American Geriatrics Society, 48*(9), 1102-1110.

Fiore, M., Baily, W. C., Cohen, S. J., et al. (2000). *Treating tobacco use and dependence: Quick reference guide for clinicians.* Rockville, MD: U.S. Department of Health and Human Services, Public Health Service. Retrieved November 20, 2005, from www.surgeongeneral.gov/tobacco/tobaqrg.htm.

George, L. K. (2005). Socioeconomic status and health across the life course: Progress and prospects. *Journal of Gerontology, Special Issue II, 60b,* 135-139.

Georgia State University. (1999). Physical activity pyramid. *Exercise and Physical Fitness Page.* Retrieved November 10, 2005, from www2.gsu.edu/~wwwfit/physicalactivity.html.

Gielen, A. C., & McDonald, E. M. (2002). Using the PRECEDE-PROCEED planning model to apply health behavior theories. In K. Glanz, B. K. Rimer, & B. M. Lewis (Eds.), *Health behavior and health education: Theory, research and practice.* San Francisco: Jossey-Bass.

Glanz, K., Rimer, B. K., & Lewis, B. M. (2002). The scope of health behavior and health education. In K. Glanz, B. K. Rimer, & B. M. Lewis (Eds.), *Health behavior and health education: Theory, research and practice.* San Francisco: Jossey-Bass.

Glasgow, R. E. (2002). The RE-AIM model. In K. Glanz, B. K. Rimer, & B. M. Lewis (Eds.), *Health behavior and health education: Theory, research and practice.* San Francisco: Jossey-Bass.

Guilmette, T. J., & Shadel, W. G. (2002). Suggestions for a smoking-cessation program in the long-term care setting. *Annals of Long-Term Care, 10*(3), 43-48.

Haber, D. (2003). *Health promotion and aging: Practical applications for health professions.* New York: Springer.

Hartman-Stein, P. E., & Potkanowicz, M. A. (2003). Behavioral determinants of healthy aging: Good news for the baby boomer generation. *Online Journal of Issues in Nursing, 8*(2). Retrieved June 5, 2005, from www.nursingworld.org/ojin/topic21/tpc21_5.htm.

Havighurst, R. J. (1961). Successful aging. *Gerontologist, 1*(1), 8-13.

Hayes, K. (2005). Designing written medication instructions: Effective ways to help older adults self-medicate. *Journal of Gerontological Nursing, 31*(5), 5-10.

Insurance Institute for Highway Safety. (2003). Fatality facts 2004: Older people. Retrieved November 20, 2005, from www.iihs.org/research/fatality_facts/pdfs/olderpeople.pdf.

John, M. (1988). *Geragogy: A theory for teaching the elderly.* New York: Hearth Press.

Johnson, J. C., & Smith, N. H. (2002). Health and social issues associated with racial, ethnic and cultural disparities. *Generations, 26*(3), 25-32.

Joint Commission on Accreditation of Healthcare Organizations. (2000). Improving oral health assessment. Retrieved January 1, 2001, from www.va.gov.publ/innivatn/oral.htm.

Kiel, J. M. (2005). The digital divide: Internet and e-mail use by the elderly. *Medical Informatics and the Internet in Medicine, 30*(1), 19-23.

Kirk, A. F., Mutrie, N., MacIntyre, P. D., & Fisher, M. B. (2004). Promoting and maintaining physical activity in people with type 2 diabetes. *American Journal of Preventive Medicine, 27*(4), 289-296.

Knauer, C. (2003). Geriatric alcohol abuse: A national epidemic. *Geriatric Nursing, 24*(3), 152-154.

Knowles, M. (1984). *The adult learner: A neglected species* (3rd ed.). Houston, TX: Gulf Publishing.

Knowles, M. (1987). Older adults as learners. *Perspective on Aging, 16*(1), 4-5.

Kreuter, M. W., Lukwago, S. N., Bucholtz, D. C., Clark, E. M., & Sanders-Thompson, V. (2003). Achieving cultural appropriateness in health promotion programs: Targeted and tailored approaches. *Health Education and Behavior, 30*(2), 133-146.

Lach, H. (2005). Incidence and risk factors for developing fear of falling in older adults. *Public Health Nursing, 22*(1), 45-52.

Lach, H. W., Everard, K. M., Highstein, G., & Brownson, C. A. (2004). Application of the Transtheoretical Model to health education for older adults. *Health Promotion Practice, 5*(1), 88-93.

Lang, J. E., Moore, M. J., Harris, A. C., & Anderson, L. A. (2005). Healthy aging: Priorities and programs of the Centers for Disease Control and Prevention. *Generations, 29*(2), 24-29.

Lighthouse International. (2005). Making text legible: Designing for people with partial sight. Retrieved September 24, 2005, from www.lighthouse.org/print_leg.htm.

Lorig, K. (1996). How do I know what patients want and need? Needs assessment. In K. Lorig (Ed.), *Patient education: A practical approach.* Thousand Oaks, CA: Sage.

Lorig, K. (2001). Arthritis self-management. In E. A. Swanson, T. Tripp-Reimer, & K. Buckwalter (Eds), *Health promotion and disease prevention in the older adult.* New York: Springer.

Lorig, K. R., & Holman, H. R. (2003). Self-management education: History, definition and mechanisms. *Annals of Behavioral Medicine, 26*(1), 1-7.

Luggen, A. S. (2006). Alcohol and the older adult. *Advance for Nurse Practitioners, 14*(1), 47-53.

Masters, J. A. (2003). Moderate alcohol consumption and unappreciated risk for alcohol-related harm among ethnically divers, urban elders. *Geriatric Nursing, 24*(3), 155-161.

McLaughlin, G. (1969). SMOG grading: A new readability formula. *Journal of Reading, 12*(8), 639-646.

Miller, N., LaCroix, E. M., & Backus, J. E. B. (2000). MEDLINEplus: Building and maintaining the National Library of Medicine's consumer health Web service. *Bulletin of the Medical Library Association, 88*(1), 11-17.

Missouri Hospital Association. (2005). MHA's Missouri Hospital Workforce report 2005. Retrieved January 5, 2006, from http://web.mhanet.com/asp/Workforce/pdf/2005_workforce_report.pdf.

National Institute of Dental and Craniofacial Research, National Institutes of Health. (2000). Oral health in America: A report of the Surgeon General. Retrieved September 19, 2005, from www.nidcr.nih.gov/aboutnidcr/surgeongeneral/executivesummary.htm.

National Institute on Aging. (2005). HIV, AIDS, and older people. Retrieved November 10, 2005, from www.niapublications.org/agepages/aids.asp.

National Institutes of Health. (2005). Study finds direct association between cardiovascular disease and periodontal bacteria. *NIH News.* Retrieved February 11, 2005, from www.nih.gov/news/pr/feb2005/nidcr-07.htm.

Nielsen-Bohlman, Panzer, A. M., & Kendig, D. A. (2004). *Health literacy: A prescription to end confusion.* Washington, DC: Institute of Medicine.

O'Connell, K. A. (2001). Smoking cessation among older clients. In E. A. Swanson, T. Tripp-Reimer, K. & Buckwalter (Eds.), *Health promotion and disease prevention in the older adult.* New York: Springer.

Pender, N. J., Murdaugh, C. L., & Parsons, M. A. (2005). *Health promotion in nursing practice.* (5th ed.). Upper Saddle River, NJ: Pearson Prentice Hall.

Prochaska, J. O., DiClemente, C. C., Velicer, W. E., & Rossi, J. S. (1993). Standardized, individualized, interactive and personalized self-help programs for smoking cessation. *Health Psychology, 12*(5), 399-405.

Prochaska, J. O., Norcross, J. C., & DiClemente, C. C. (1994). *Changing for good.* New York: Morrow.

Pyle, M. A., & Stoller, E. P. (2003). Oral health disparities among the elderly: Interdisciplinary challenges for the future. *Journal of Dental Education, 67*(12), 1327-1336.

Pyron, M. (2003). Never too late to start when it comes to exercise. *ACSM Fit Society Page.* Retrieved November 10, 2005, from www.acsm.org/health+fitness/pdf/fitsociety/fitsc303_rev.pdf.

Ratzan, S. C., & Parker, R. M. (2000). Introduction. In C. R. Selden, M. Zorn, S. C. Ratzen, & R. M. Parkerm (Eds.), *National library of medicine current bibliographies in medicine: Health literacy.* Bethesda, MD: National Institutes of Health.

Rensicow, K., Braithwaite, R. L., Dilorio, C., & Glanz, K. (2002). Applying theory to culturally diverse and unique populations. In K. Glanz, B. K. Rimer, & B. M. Lewis (Eds.), *Health behavior and health education: Theory, research and practice.* San Francisco: Jossey-Bass.

Rice, V. H., & Stead, L. F. (2002). Nursing interventions for smoking cessation. Cochrane Review. *Cochrane Library, 3.*

Rollnick S., & Miller, W. R. (1995). What is motivational interviewing? *Behavioural and Cognitive Psychotherapy, 23,* 325-334.

Rowe, J. W., & Kahn, R. L. (1987). Human aging: Usual and successful. *Science, 237*(4811), 143-149.

Rowe, J. W., & Kahn, R. L. (1998). Successful aging. *Gerontologist, 37*(4), 433-440.

Schneider, J. K., Eveker, A., Bronder, D. R., Meiner, S., & Binder, E. F. (2003). Exercise training program: Incentives and disincentives for participation. *Journal of Gerontological Nursing, 29*(9), 21-31.

Seeman, T. E., & Crimmins, E. (2001). Social environment effects on health and aging: Integrating epidemiologic and demographic approaches and perspectives. *Annals of the New York Academy of Science, 954,* 88-117.

Senate Aging Committee Report. (2003). Nothing to smile about on older Americans oral health report card. Retrieved September 29, 2004, from www.oralhealthamerica.org/legislation.htm.

Shilts, M. K., Horowitz, M., & Townsend, M. S. (2004). Goal setting as a strategy for dietary and physical activity behavior change: A review of the literatures. *American Journal of Health Promotion, 19*(2), 81-93.

Speros, C. (2005). Health literacy: Concept analysis. *Journal of Advanced Nursing, 50*(6), 633-640.

SPRY Foundation. (1999). *Older adults and the World Wide Web: A guide for Web site creators.* Washington DC: Author.

SPRY Foundation. (2005). Evaluating health information on the World Wide Web. Retrieved November 10, 2005, from www.spry.org/sprys_work/education/evaluating_health_content.html.

Stecher, V. J., Seijts, G. H., Kok, G. H., Latham, G. P., Glasgow, R., DeVillis, B., et al. (1995). Goal setting as a strategy for health behavior change. *Health Education Quarterly, 22*(2), 190-200.

Stevens, J. (2002). Falls among older adults: Public health impact and prevention strategies. *Generations, 26*(4), 7-14.

Substance Abuse and Mental Health Services Administrations. (2005a). Older adults in substance abuse treatment: Update. *DASIS Report,* May 5, 2005. Retrieved November 10, 2005, from www.oas.samhsa.gov/2k5/olderAdultsTX/olderAdultsTX.cfm.

Substance Abuse and Mental Health Services Administrations. (2005b). Older adults in substance abuse treatment: Update. *DASIS Report,* May 5, 2005. Retrieved November 10, 2005, from www.oas.samhsa.gov/2k5/olderadults/olderadults.cfm.

Sykes, K. (2005). A healthy environment for older adults: The aging initiative of the Environmental Protection Agency. *Generations, 29*(2), 65-69.

Takahashi, P. Y., Okhravi, H. R., Lim, L. S., & Kasten, M. J. (2004). Preventive health care in the elderly population: A guide for practicing physicians. *Mayo Clinic Proceedings, 79*(3), 416-427.

Tuchman, E. (2003). Methadone and menopause: Midlife women in drug treatment. *Journal of Social Work Practice in the Addictions, 3*(2), 43-55.

U.S. Department of Commerce. (2004). A nation online: Entering the broadband age. National Telecommunication and Information Administration. Retrieved November 20, 2005, from www.ntia.doc.gov/reports/anol/index.html.

U.S. Department of Health and Human Services. (2000). Oral health in America: A report of the Surgeon General. Retrieved November 20, 2005, from www2.nidcr.nih.gov/sgr/sgrohweb/execsum.htm#chal.

U.S. Department of Health and Human Services. (2002). *Healthy people 2010: Improving health* (2nd ed.). Washington, DC: U.S. Government Printing Office.

Wall Street Journal Online. (2005, February 23). Web. What's that? *Wall Street Journal Online.* Retrieved June 5, 2005, from http://online.wsj.com/public/us.

Wang, C. C., & Carr, D. B. (2004). Older driver safety: A report from the Older Driver's Project. *Journal of the American Geriatrics Society, 52,* 143-149.

Whitehead, D. (2004). Health promotion and health education: Advancing the concepts. *Journal of Advanced Nursing, 47*(3), 311-320.

Wilson, M. M. (2003). Sexually transmitted diseases. *Clinics in Geriatric Medicine, 19,* 637-655.

World Health Organization. (1946). Preamble to the Constitution of the World Health Organization as adopted by the International Health Conference, New York, 19-22 June, 1946. *Official Records of the World Health Organization,* no. 2, p. 100. New York: World Health Organization.

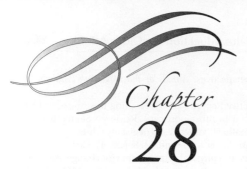

Chapter 28

Quality Improvement

Carolyn D. Philpot § Julie K. Gammack §
Susan J. Taylor § John E. Morley

Objectives

Discuss the importance of quality improvement in health care.

Explore trends in the quality improvement movement.

Describe methods for promoting quality of care.

Examine quality improvement in various settings, particularly long-term care.

Providing high-quality, cost-effective medical care is essential in meeting the health system demands of a rapidly expanding aging population. It is necessary to critically evaluate not only treatments and techniques but also the process by which health care is delivered to the consumer. As our society becomes more knowledgeable about health through information obtained from television, the Internet, and other educational opportunities, there is increasing awareness of quality in health care. Additionally, the increased access to information about quality indictors in health care is driving further demand for quality care. As a result, improving the quality of health services has become a routine part of all health care services.

The nursing profession is active in promoting quality care. National nursing organizations have developed educational programs and credentialing standards to promote safety and efficiency in many health care settings. Clinical practice guidelines and nursing protocols have been created to improve patient care and the nursing care environment. Many health care settings have interdisciplinary programs and projects designed to address quality of care. Gerontological nurses should be active participants in quality improvement (QI) initiatives to address quality of care, which can improve outcomes as well as patient satisfaction, while providing nurses with increased career satisfaction. This chapter will address the history of QI, describe the process of QI, and give examples, particularly from the long-term care setting, of how QI can be delivered.

QUALITY IMPROVEMENT IN GERONTOLOGICAL NURSING

Older adults are prone to abrupt health care events. When health care delivery is fragmented, adverse outcomes may occur. Research has confirmed that those persons over the age of 65 are at twice the risk for an adverse hospital event (Miller et al., 2001). As a result, monitoring for quality care is essential to prevent complications and adverse events as much as possible.

Gerontological nurses have been educated and trained to identify health care issues for older adults. They obtain a detailed nursing assessment for each patient. By identifying risk factors and geriatric syndromes, the nurse can help to prevent unfavorable outcomes by establishing a plan of care for that person. Once a patient's care plan has been developed, it should be readily available to the other members on the health care team. If there are any changes in the patient's status or condition, the care plan should be updated. Changes in condition may identify safety issues before a decline in health and function. Nurses can help ensure that processes are in place to ensure this quality of care is provided.

By effectively providing early intervention through a QI process, unfavorable outcomes can be minimized and patient satisfaction can be improved. Numerous studies have shown that interventions such as patient education and counseling and staff training can improve patient outcomes. Quality of care as well as patient satisfaction can be improved (Scott, Setter-Kline, & Britton, 2004; Wengstrom, Haggmark, Strander, & Forsberg, 1999). The history of the QI movement is described next.

HISTORY OF QUALITY IMPROVEMENT IN NURSING

Quality has been an issue in health care dating back to ancient Babylon (Spiegel, 1997). King Hammurabi (1700 BC) established a system that set payment rates for medical service, health care coverage for slaves, and strict responsibility for the outcomes of treatments. Physicians were well compensated, but operated under an "eye for an eye" model of punishment for poor outcomes. Nurses, which in those days were "wet nurses," were strictly monitored to be sure they did not take on extra children. If a wet nurse was convicted of nursing extra children, "her breasts shall be cut off" (Spiegel, 1997). The Egyptians also established punishments for poor treatment outcomes. If a patient receiving care unnecessarily lost an eye, for example, the physician would lose his right hand (Hartman & Moore, 1976).

In modern times, nursing has been involved in assessing quality of health care issues for over a century. Florence Nightingale (1820-1910), the founder of nursing as we know it today, was also a founder of QI (Hartman & Moore, 1976). While caring for British soldiers during the Crimean War, she observed that military hospitals were crowded and dirty. Adequate sanitation practices were lacking. She collected data and formulated a record-keeping practice that tracked sanitary conditions and patient outcomes within city and medical hospitals. Using these data, Nightingale was able to track death rates and show that deaths decreased with improved sanitary conditions (Miller et al., 2001).

During the nineteenth century, the care and treatments provided in hospitals and asylums for the mentally ill were frequently inadequate. Investigations into institutional care for those with mental illness captured public attention, and led to several radical reforms including the development of standards for nursing education (Hartman & Moore, 1976). These were first developed by The American Society of Superintendents of Training Schools for Nurses, established in 1893. This organization was renamed the National League for Nursing Education in 1912, and later merged with other nursing organizations in 1952 to become the National League for Nursing (NLN). The NLN has a mission to advance "excellence in nursing education that prepares the nursing workforce to meet the needs of diverse populations in an ever-changing health care environment" (NLN, 2005). After addressing the education of nurses, the movement shifted.

Throughout the twentieth century, as health care and technology advanced, nursing care has evolved to addressing the quality of health care provided to patients. The Nurses Associated Alumnae of the United States and Canada was renamed the American Nurses Association (ANA) in 1911; this association promoted proper training for nurses and developed a code for nursing education (ANA, 2005). The ANA also promoted admission requirements for nursing schools, regulation of workdays (down to 12 hours originally, and later 8-hour shifts), and state licensing for practicing nurses. An overabundance of nurses in the 1920s and 1930s resulted in economic hardships for nurses and nursing schools. The Works Progress Administration employed many nurses during this time, until World War II when nurses became in high demand.

After World War II, economics and advances in health care required a greater emphasis on training and better organization of health care services. The ANA and labor unions fought for a better working environment, increased salaries, and greater respect for nursing professionals. The number of nursing schools and nurses grew.

While nursing was making strides in addressing quality of care in nursing, Dr. W. Edwards Deming and others were developing processes for QI in business. The movement toward total quality management (TQM) gradually became popular in the health care field, as interest in both reducing costs and meeting consumer demands developed. This QI process, introduced by Dr. Deming in Japan, led to a revolution in the manufacturing industry. Nursing also gradually became involved in monitoring the quality of nursing care through the nursing audit, discussed in the next section. The Joint Commission on Accreditation of Healthcare Organizations (JCAHO) increasingly enforced ongoing QI among its members.

Nursing Audits

Florence Nightingale was an early pioneer of the nursing audit, as well as the QI process. Through careful observation, she identified a problem, collected statistical data, and then assessed the outcome. If the outcome was not satisfactory, she developed a plan for improvement, implemented the plan, and then reevaluated the outcome. Nightingale used what was later known as the nursing audit of patient care. Over time, the nursing audit has evolved to include three distinct forms: (1) the structure audit, (2) the process of care audit, and (3) the care outcome audit.

The structure audit entails the environment in which the care is given. This type of audit looks at the organizational structure, the individuals providing care, and the equipment that is used. Policies and standards for the organization are established and then evaluated. If the standards set by the organization have been met, then good medical care is likely to have been rendered. The first nursing audit appeared in the literature in 1955 (Hartman & Moore, 1976). This audit evaluated nurse's notes. At that time it was felt that if nurse's notes were accurate and complete, then good quality nursing care had been given.

In 1960 an administrative tool was developed for nursing service directors to evaluate the quality of patient care being provided in the hospital. This tool was a precursor to the development of an audit team that would make rounds in nursing divisions and conduct care audits. The members of the audit team set the standards by which care was measured, and the results were reported to the nursing divisions and to individual nurses.

The second type of nursing audit is the process audit. This type of audit evaluates the flow of patient care and the end result of health care events. The process audit is performed by the direct observation of care or by a chart review. Process audits evaluate whether an individual has adequately performed his or her duties. The process audit is not as scientifically sound as the structure audit because it lacks a uniformly accepted standard against a process of care that can be measured. Process audits may also be biased because of conflicting views held by different audit monitors or by standards set by an organization. Process audits are very time-consuming and may take several hours to conduct properly. Despite these limitations, there is some evidence that the process of care can be effectively changed through the use of guidelines and the audit process (Thomas et al., 1998).

Historically, several individuals and institutions have fostered the development of the process audit. Maria C. Phaneuf formulated an audit focused on seven functions in nursing that resulted in several books on the audit process (Phaneuf, 1972, 1976). Dr. Eleanor Lambertsen developed another standard process audit format (Lambertsen, 1995). Several years later, the Medical Center of Vermont developed a system using various resources, such as chart reviews; interviews with patients, families, and nursing staff; and direct observation of care and safety (Hartman & Moore, 1976).

The third type of audit is the outcome audit. This audit evaluates the end result of the care process for a patient and is usually conducted retrospectively. In 1973, JCAHO introduced an outcome audit process for hospitals. The audit was conducted at the time of patient discharge to determine if a successful clinical outcome was achieved. If the patient did not have the expected outcome, deficiencies in care were noted. A cause for deficiencies was then identified, and a plan of correction was established. Areas of deficiency were later reviewed to evaluate the effectiveness of the new plan. Health care organizations may use all three types of audits to monitor quality of care.

EVALUATING QUALITY

Before evaluating quality of care, one must first define quality. Quality has been defined as "services that are free from deficiencies and meet customer needs" (Gray, Anderson, & Robinson, 2001, p. 86) and is measured to a set standard of care. We have discussed the development of some standards of care for nursing. The standard may be set by an external governing or regulatory board or internally by the members within a health care organization. Patients and their families may also have an expectation of the quality of care. Consumers expect the health care delivery to meet or exceed the standard of care, but may not realize what constitutes a reasonable standard. Nurses may need to educate patients and families about accepted standards so that they have realistic expectations of care.

Maintaining high quality care can be a costly endeavor requiring constant observation, monitoring, and evaluation. Nurses in management positions are responsible for ensuring that their staff can perform at appropriate skill levels. To accomplish this, nursing managers must supervise and oversee nursing care, with the expectation that quality care is given. While setting high standards, managers must maintain a dialogue with nursing staff to discuss problems and identify areas needing improvement. Communication is key (Bolton & Goodenough, 2003).

Identifying Quality Problems

There are a number of means by which quality problems are identified. For example, problems may be presented to nurses from patients or families, or other staff. Problems could be identified by reports such as infection control data and safety or risk management reports. Institutions, nursing units, or staff may collect data on a particular issue, such as falls that occurred over a period of time.

Nursing needs to be aware that all areas of concern are important. If performance is substandard, it needs to be identified and corrected immediately. A good flow of communication is essential to recognize problems, facilitate resolutions, and attain positive outcomes. Interdisciplinary team meetings and patient care conferences offer an opportunity to identify problems where QI is needed. Once problems are identified, prompt evaluation, planning, and correction are vital components in upholding quality. Timeliness often affects outcome.

Impressions of quality affect patient and family attitudes. In one example, a patient from a hospital entered a long-term care (LTC) facility for rehabilitation. The patient arrived at the facility accompanied by family. They enter the patient's room in the nursing home, and it was not clean and the bed was not made. The patient and family may correlate the dirty room with poor nursing care. This bad first impression led the family to question the quality of care. In another example, a patient and family were greeted at the door of a long-term care facility and escorted to a room that was clean. On the bed was a personal written acknowledgment and welcome note from the administrator and staff. The patient and family would be more likely to have a good, positive perception of the nursing care in that facility as compared to the previous illustration where the facility was not prepared to receive them.

THE QUALITY MODEL

The quality assurance (QA) model was an early process used by nursing to evaluate quality of care. In this model there was a set standard or regulation that had to be met. Information was gathered by observation or chart review (chart audit) to determine if those standards were met. If proposed practices were correctly followed, the organization or process was considered to be in compliance. On the other hand, if proposed practices deviated from the regulation or set standard, those deviations needed to be identified, and corrected. Once corrected, reevaluation was necessary to assure compliance in meeting the standard.

QI processes in health care organizations have changed over the years. These processes evolved from the unidirectional regulation-compliance QA method to a multidirectional interactive total quality improvement (TQM) model. The TQM model focuses on a continuous process of monitoring and improving care. TQM addresses the multifactorial issues related to health care and looks beyond the individual practitioner to the health care system as a whole. The TQM model employs team members of an interdisciplinary nature. In this model, the members identify target areas of concern and review current performance and practices.

The goals of TQM must take into account current resources, environmental limitations, financial concerns, time, and staffing competence. In this model, outside resources may be used to implement an action plan to obtain the goals set by the committee. An individual or subcommittee may be appointed to carry out the new protocol or goals and be responsible for periodic reports at future committee meetings. If the goals are not met, factors obstructing attainment of the goal are explored by an appointed committee member or subcommittee. Once obstacles are identified, a proposal is presented to the committee to develop other strategies to reach the goal. Newly developed interventions are initiated, and performance is monitored until the goal is achieved.

QI is a structured process within an organization to improve organizational structure, standards of care, and patient outcomes. There are several models available to use when developing and maintaining a QI process within the organization. Advance practice nurses are often asked to be leaders in this effort, so it is important to understand and be able to implement a model for QI. One commonly used structured process of QI is the combination of the FOCUS model and the PDSA

model, or FOCUS-PDSA model (Walton, 1990). The FOCUS piece of the model is used to identify the processes in need of improvement. The PDSA part is the structure used to guide, identify, and implement the change in or replacement of the process. The FOCUS model is described in five steps from the mnemonic:

- *Finding* a process or quality problem to improve
- *Organizing* an interprofessional team or group and its resources to improve the process
- *Clarifying* the current knowledge about the process needing improvement
- *Understanding* the sources of process variation
- *Selecting* the improvement or intervention to initiate to improve the process

The FOCUS process is then followed by the PDSA or Plan-Do-Study-Act process. There is some overlap when the models are combined. During *planning*, the team determines interventions to improve care, which is similar to the *selecting* process of the FOCUS model. The *doing* part of the process involves implementing the changes on a small scale or a trial basis. *Studying* is the phase where the trial results are analyzed to see if the results meet the teams' original expectations. If the expectations of the team are met, then the team *acts* to implement the process system-wide. If the change is not positive, further refinements or change may need to be evaluated.

Another structured process model of QI is the Continuous Process Improvement 4 Step model (Figure 28-1). This model is described by a gerontological nurse practicing in an acute care setting in Box 28-1. QI practices in different settings of care are addressed next,

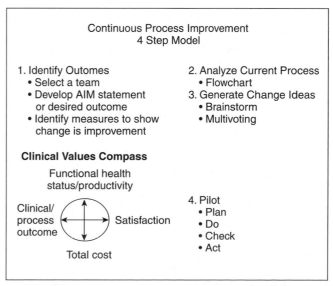

Figure 28-1 Continuous Process Improvement 4 Step Model. (Data from Nelson, E. C., Mohr, J. J., Batalden, P. B., & Plume, S. K. [1996]. Improving health care. Part 1: The clinical value compass. *Journal of Quality Improvement, 22*[4], 243-258.)

Box 28-1 *Reflections on Clinical Effectiveness and Quality Improvement*

Rapid and dynamic changes in health care delivery and policy environments have placed the issues of patient safety and quality care at the center of health care and the nursing profession. Nurses are caring for frail, complex elders with multiple acute and chronic comorbidities as well as functional and cognitive impairments. Consumers are able to access "score-cards" that identify how well individual facilities provide quality nursing care. No matter what role gerontological nurses play, it is their responsibility and within their scope of practice to improve resident outcomes guided by evidence-based nursing practice. This box describes a model that we used in an acute care setting that has helped improve outcomes for older patients.

Staff nurses play a substantial role in quality improvement, specifically those areas that are nursing sensitive. As defined by the American Nurses Association, nursing-sensitive quality indicators are those indicators that "capture care or its outcomes most affected by nursing care" (ANA, 2005). Nursing-sensitive indicators reflect the structure, process, and outcomes of nursing care. The structure of nursing care is indicated by the supply and skill level of nursing staff, and the education/certification of nursing staff. Process indicators measure facets of nursing care such as assessment and interventions. Outcomes that are determined to be nursing sensitive are those that improve if there is a greater quantity or quality of nursing care (for example, pain, pressure ulcers, falls, IV infiltrations).

To initiate a quality improvement program, leadership and interdisciplinary team members work collaboratively to identify a model to drive their process. One such version is the Continuous Process Improvement 4 Step model. This model is depicted in Figure 28-1, and the steps in the process are described below. Box 28-2 provides an overview of the process using an example from our skin committee designed to reduce pressure ulcers. Using this or other models, nurses can make a big difference in outcomes for patients.

Continuous Process Improvement 4 Step Model
Step 1
- What are the desired resident outcomes? Select a population or problem, for example:
  1. Mortality/morbidity
  2. Functional status
  3. Satisfaction
  4. Costs
- What is the scientific evidence for care?
- What is the aim? The Clinical Values Compass identifies issues to consider.

Step 2
- What is your current process of giving care to this type of resident?

1. Access
2. Assessment
3. Diagnosis
4. Treatment
5. Follow-up

Step 3
- What ideas do we have for changing the process?
- What is being done to get better results? Several major change concepts are listed below:
  1. Improve work flow
  2. Manage variation
  3. Design systems to avoid mistakes
  4. Eliminate waste
  5. Optimize inventory
  6. Change the work environment
  7. Enhance producer/customer relationships
  8. Manage time
  9. Focus on the product or service

Step 4
- Pilot
- Do
- Check
- Act

Pilot
- Plan
  1. Who does what? When? With what tools and training?
  2. Determine baseline data to be collected and displayed in run, control, and pie charts.

Do
- Implement the plan.

Check
- Collect and display data.
- Evaluate the results.
- Did improvement happen?

Act
- Implement the change or abandon the effort.
- Monitor, to hold the gain or continue to improve.

Deborah Marks Conley
Deborah Marks Conley, MSN, APRN, BC, CS, FNGNA
*Certified Gerontological Clinical Nurse Specialist
Nebraska Methodist Hospital
Assistant Professor of Nursing
Nebraska Methodist College, Department of Nursing
Omaha, Nebraska*

with a major focus on the long-term care setting (Box 28-2).

ACUTE CARE SETTING

The acute care setting addresses quality in a variety of ways. The ANA describes nursing quality indicators for the hospital setting (Box 28-3). Hospitals are required to have a QI committee that meets monthly. Members represent a variety of departments of the hospital. Committee members may be asked to make rounds in certain divisions or departments and record any discrepancies in care. Reports are generated and reviewed during committee meetings and then returned to the appropriate department or division. The committee may recommend changes, or departments may be charged with developing a plan for improvement. Safety issues are increasingly the focus of QI. The Agency for

---

BOX 28-2 Example of the Continuous Process Improvement 4 Step Model for Skin Care

Step 1
Desired Outcomes
- Nurses consistently demonstrate interrater reliability on the Braden Scale and implementation of the Skin Risk Assessment.
- Benchmark for incidence of pressure ulcers in our facility is at or <3% (national average is 7% or less).

Aim
- An opportunity exists to maintain and/or improve skin integrity of all inpatients at our facility. The process starts with admission to the facility and ends with discharge of the resident.
- Pressure ulcers are costly and painful to the resident, may cause greater lengths of stay in subacute care, increase the nurse's workload, increase facility liability, and decrease resident, family, and community satisfaction with nursing care.

Step 2
Present Practice
- Skin Risk Assessment includes three components of the integumentary system:
    1. Predisposing risk factors (all from the literature)
    2. Pressure points' assessment
    3. Braden Scale for Skin Risk Assessment
- Assessment is performed by nurse on admission, every 48 hours, and when there is any change in the patient's condition.

Step 3
Ideas for Changing the Process
- Brainstorm with the team about what needs to be done differently.
    1. Develop a Skin Risk Assessment competency for all nurses to complete on hire, and yearly thereafter.
- Use evidence-based practice to guide these decisions.

What Is Being Done to Get Better Results?
- Manage variation to validate competency of all nursing staff on the components of the Skin Risk Assessment and the interrater reliability of the Braden Scale.

Step 4
Pilot
- Who does what? When? With what tools and education/training?
    1. Clinical nurse specialists and wound care nurses develop modules.
    2. Modules placed on Internet for easy access and to manage registration and completion.
- Baseline data should be collected and displayed in run, control, and pie charts.
    1. Preintervention data are collected quarterly based on participation in the study on the prevalence and incidence of pressure ulcers and also during an additional yearly prevalence and incidence study—both with outside organizations.
    2. Nurses conduct monthly active audits (open computerized chart) on units and give immediate feedback to staff and mentor on best practices for skin care.

Do
- Implement the plan.
    1. Upon hire and annually thereafter, all nurses must complete the computer-based Skin Risk Competency.

Continued

BOX 28-2 Example of the Continuous Process Improvement 4 Step Model for Skin Care—cont'd

Check
- Collect and display data.
  1. Data should be displayed in a variety of ways to all nursing staff.
- Evaluate the results.
- Did improvement occur?
  2. Yes; improvements occurred.
  3. Incidence of pressure ulcers is 3% (for past 2 years), and improvement occurred in the interrater reliability and implementation of the Skin Risk Assessment based on data.

Act
- Implement the change or abandon the effort.
  1. Implemented the change (educational program) along with various nursing interventions that were not all discussed in this example.
- Monitor, to hold the gain or continue to improve.
  2. Postintervention data should be collected quarterly based on participation in a study on prevalence and incidence of pressure ulcers and also during an additional yearly prevalence and incidence study—both with outside organizations.
  3. Nurses conduct monthly active audits (open computerized chart) on units and give immediate feedback to staff and mentor on best practices for skin care.

Healthcare Research has developed quality patient safety indicators that describe hospital patient outcomes (Savitz, Jones, & Bernard, 2005) (provided in Box 28-3).

Model nursing-led units (NLUs) at hospitals can improve the quality of patient care. Two projects compared NLUs with usual care and demonstrated that NLU patients were better prepared for discharge and had a higher level of function (Griffiths et al., 2004; Griffiths et al., 2005). In geriatrics, acute care for the elderly (ACE) units were developed in the 1990s to reduce the functional impairments that so often occur in hospitalized older adults. The elements of ACE units are (1) environmental alterations, (2) patient-centered care, (3) interdisciplinary care planning, and (4) medical care review. Nurses play an integral role in ACE units (Siegler, Glick, & Lee, 2002).

The American Nurses Association has developed the Magnet recognition program to identify hospitals that demonstrate commitment to a high quality of care (Bolton & Goodenough, 2003). The Magnet program promotes a continuous QI model and provides a vehicle for disseminating successful practices and strategies.

HOME HEALTH CARE

Home health care provides another important service for older adults who are not able to leave their homes. Nurses are a primary provider of home health care, which has been shown to prevent nursing home admission and functional decline (Stuck et al., 2002). In this setting, quality of care can be assessed through chart reviews or retrospective audits, peer review, and patient case conferences. The patient conference involves all of the disciplines involved in a particular patient's care, who meet to review patient care and create a plan for future care. Standards are available for developing quality indicators for home care agencies (Box 28-4). The indicators are used to compare agencies with each other and ensure proper care (Zuber, 2005). Additional work is being done to develop quality indicators from the Minimum Data Set—Home Care (MDS-HC) similar to what are available for nursing homes (Hinder et al., 2005).

QUALITY IMPROVEMENT IN LONG-TERM CARE

In the United States, the federal government developed markers for quality in long-term care. These markers are termed "quality indicators"; they serve as triggers for possible unwanted outcomes in LTC settings and activate the need for further assessment and changes in care. Examples include accidents, infection control, and psychotropic drug use. The quality indicators are derived from the required resident evaluation form for long-term care called the minimum data set (MDS). MDS information is generally obtained upon admission to a nursing facility and then reviewed; it is updated quarterly or after any change in the patient's status or condition. For example, hospital admission, significant weight loss, or changes in health may trigger an update of the patient's MDS and plan of care.

Nursing plays a large role in gathering information entered into the MDS. Ideally, MDS data are obtained

---

BOX 28-3 Hospital Quality Indicators

American Nurses Association Nursing Quality Indicators
- Staff mix
- Total nursing care hours per patient day
- Pressure ulcer rates
- Patient injury, falls, and falls with psychiatric assault
- Pediatric pain and IV infiltration
- Nurse education and satisfaction

Agency for Healthcare Research and Quality Patient Safety Indicators
- Complications of anesthesia
- Death in low-mortality diagnosis-related groups (DRGs)
- Decubitus ulcer
- Failure to rescue
- Foreign body left during procedure
- Iatrogenic pneumothorax
- Selected infections because of medical care
- Postoperative hip fracture
- Postoperative hemorrhage or hematoma
- Postoperative respiratory failure
- Postoperative pulmonary embolism or deep vein thrombosis
- Postoperative sepsis
- Postoperative wound dehiscence
- Accidental puncture or laceration
- Transfusion reaction
- Birth trauma
- Obstetric trauma

Data from American Nurses Association (ANA). (2006). The National Center for Nursing Quality Indicators. The National Database of Nursing Quality Indicators (NDNQI). Retrieved March 6, 2006, from www.nursingworld.org/quality; and Savitz, L. A., Jones, C. B., & Bernard, S. (2005). Quality indicators sensitive to nurse staffing in acute care settings. From *Advances in patient safety* (vol 4). Retrieved November 10, 2005, from www.ahrq.gov.

BOX 28-4 Home Care Quality Indicators

The National Quality Forum (as of May, 2005) endorses these national voluntary consensus standards for home health care:
- Improvement in ambulation/locomotion
- Improvement in bathing
- Improvement in transferring
- Improvement in management of oral medications
- Improvement in pain interfering with activity
- Improvement in status of surgical wounds
- Improvement in dyspnea
- Improvement in urinary incontinence
- Increase in number of pressure ulcers
- Emergent care for wound infections and deteriorating wound status
- Emergent care for improper medication administration and medication side effects
- Emergent care for hypoglycemia and hyperglycemia
- Acute care hospitalization
- Discharge to community
- Emergent care

Data from National Quality Forum. (2005). National Quality Forum closes work on home health performance measures project. *Current News and Notes.* Retrieved July 10, 2005, from www.qualityforum.org.

The Center for Management Services then compares facilities with each other both locally and nationwide. The facilities that fall below others in particular domains or specific indicators are "flagged" and may be a target of further investigation by state and federal regulatory nursing home boards. Quality indicators may be a valuable resource to administrators or facility QI teams.

In one example, a long-term care facility had several residents with fractures during a review period. During a QI meeting at the facility, the medical director asked for more information about each fracture. All health care disciplines were represented at this meeting, and the pharmacy representative noted that some residents with a diagnosis of osteoporosis had not been treated. The medical director recommended that a list of residents falling into this category be identified and that their health care providers be notified. With notification, evidence-based educational materials would be submitted to the health care providers, supporting the need for treatment. The pharmacy or nursing personnel were assigned to follow-up on the recommendation. Updates on progress were then presented at future QI meetings. In addition, therapy and nursing staff were given additional education on the care and treatment of patients with osteoporosis. Quarterly reviews were monitored to see if fracture rates declined. This total quality management process has been shown to improve care

and entered by nurses that know and care for an individual. Inadequate data collection or documentation of the MDS can lead to misrepresentation of patient care and unnecessary inquiry. In some facilities, nurses must complete MDS data forms for unfamiliar patients that they are not treating.

There are 24 quality indicators for long-term care (Table 28-1). Domains of these quality indicators include accidents, behavior or emotional patterns, clinical management, cognitive patterns, elimination and incontinence, infection control, nutrition and eating, physical functioning, psychotropic drug use, quality of life, and skin care. Every long-term care resident is assessed in each of these domains by the long-term care facility, and that information is included in the MDS.

Table 28-1 *Nursing Home Quality Indicators*

Domain	Quality Indicator
Accidents	Fractures
	Falls
Behavior	Behaviors
	Depression without treatment
	Depression with treatment
Clinical management	Number of medications
Cognition	Cognitive impairment
Elimination	Bowel/bladder incontinence
	Incontinence without toileting plan
	Indwelling catheter
	Fecal impaction
Infection	Urinary tract infection
Nutrition	Weight loss
	Tube-feeding
	Dehydration
Physical function	Bedridden
	Loss of activities of daily living
	Range of motion
Psychotropic medication	Psychotropics without psychosis
	Use of anxiolytics
	Frequent hypnotics
Quality of life	Physical restraints
	Physical activity
Skin care	Pressure ulcers

and promote quality of life for long-term care residents (Caramania, Cousino, & Petersen, 2003).

Quality Improvement Meetings

Many long-term care facilities hold quarterly meetings to discuss quality of care, which is not frequent enough. Monthly meetings are ideal to maintain good communication and keep members focused on quality issues. Members of the QI team should include individuals from nursing, pharmacy, attending physicians, the medical director, administration, therapies, social service, medical records, dietary, laboratory, radiology, and maintenance.

During the QI meetings, various departments present areas that are of concern or that need improvement. Each department identifies an area to be reviewed and describes the importance of this area to resident care. Data are obtained and compared to the standard that has been set for that particular area. If the data show a problem, then a plan of correction is developed and discussed with the QI team. Periodic reviews are planned to monitor the issue until the standards are consistently met. Important issues may require continuous review, even when they meet acceptable standards; this ensures that these issues do not fall below the standard and remain unnoticed. For example, infection rates and falls are usually monitored on a regular basis.

Key Players in the Quality Improvement Process

To illustrate the process and key personnel that must be involved in the QI process, the roles of personnel in the long-term care setting follow. The process may be similar to that used in other settings, but the size of most facilities allows all of the departments to participate in the process. Meetings must be scheduled at regular intervals, and data must be tracked over time. Members of the team must feel free to share ideas, present both good and bad results without reprimand, and participate in the planning and evaluation process. The roles of various players are described.

The Administrator. The administrator is ultimately responsible for the overall care within the facility and should attend QI meetings. The administrator oversees all complaints and areas of concern. When a problem is identified, information is then broken down, categorized, and delegated to the appropriate person or department head for investigation and resolution, and often presented to the QI team. Administrators need to be active in the QI process and empower the employees to maintain high quality performance. The administrator should be visible and accessible to families, residents, and physicians, as well as staff. A caring attitude and high visibility may help prevent unwanted outcomes.

Overall, many complaints or areas of concern originate from family members or patients. If the number of complaints has decreased, then the facility is likely doing a good job meeting resident needs and expectations. When the number of complaints increases, then the administrator needs to investigate the situation and take steps to correct any problems. Common areas of complaint are nursing care, laundry/housekeeping, and food. The QI team and process are a valuable tool for the administrator (Caramania et al., 2003; Dyck, 2005).

Nursing Staff. There are numerous factors involved when studying quality nursing care. The nursing staff must be proficient in performance of certain tasks and skills. Nurse's assistants (aides) must be knowledgeable in assisting residents with personal care including eating, dressing, transferring, basic hygiene, and toileting. Key areas for aides are promoting good skin care and identifying when residents are not feeling well, and then notifying the nurse when the patient exhibits any changes. Licensed nurses are responsible for assessment, documentation, medication administration, and information distribution that is important for the resident's health care provider. Ongoing education of staff, especially given the frequent turnover, is an important quality issue.

Long-term care facilities are increasingly using geriatric advance practice nurses as educators and consultants. The geriatric advanced practice nurse can help the administration identify patient care skills that need to be developed and assist in educating the nursing staff. This education can include proper use and care of patient care equipment, which can prevent negative patient medical outcomes.

High-quality nursing care is delivered using a "systems" approach. Key elements of the system are how the nursing staff is structured and then how it functions.

Systems' issues include staffing patterns, delegation of work assignments, and designation of responsibilty for specific duties. For example, it is vital to develop a formalized procedure to see that ordered laboratory tests are drawn, and results are obtained in a timely manner and then reported to the health care provider. Nurses may use a tracking log for laboratory tests to ensure that each step is carried out. Good documentation helps the flow of good communication and is a crucial part of the needed nursing systems' process. The systems' process includes nursing staff on all shifts (Carboneau, 1999).

Another systems' process example is that of obtaining resident weights (Figure 28-2). In long-term care, weights are generally obtained on a monthly basis. Studies have documented that weights obtained by one person are more accurate than when weights are obtained by several different staff members. In the case where several people were responsible for weight measurements, no one person was responsible in overseeing that the weights were done properly. If a weight was questioned, there was no single person responsible to ask. Ownership of tasks is important.

Unit _____   Year _____

Room	Resident Name Admission Date	Current		Weight History						Other Issues			
				30 Days Ago			180 Days Ago						
		Date	Wt	Date	Wt	% Change	Date	Wt	% Change	BMI	Pressure Ulcers	Falls	Recent Hosp

Comments

_____

_____

Figure 28-2   Sample quality improvement weight loss report.

Care provided by nursing staff is often judged by families and patients by the visibility of the staff. A floor or unit may be perceived as understaffed if nursing personnel are not readily seen. Response time to residents' call lights is frequently considered a quality indicator by residents and family members.

The director of nursing (DON) is ultimately responsible for the nursing care provided at all times in that facility. The DON may use several resources to evaluate how nursing care in the facility is perceived. The DON may make random inspections to units or sections during any shift, or have staff or hired consultants conduct inspections. Concerns may be solicited from residents either individually or through resident councils. Nursing staff, families, and other facility staff should be comfortable expressing concerns to the DON. If deficiencies are found, further investigation may be needed, and the QI process initiated.

HIGH-RISK SITUATIONS. Nursing staff needs to identify high-risk situations for unfavorable outcomes, and monitor these issues consistently. In long-term care, some examples are skin breakdown, falls, aspiration, dehydration, depression, fecal impaction, and elopement. Nursing staff should track these issues and take actions if they occur to prevent complications. For example, staff should identify residents with pressure ulcers, including those developed within the facility and those

acquired elsewhere. Data on pressure sores that develop within the facility should be scrutinized to determine if there are patterns. Did they occur on a particular unit or shift? If so, then the QI process can be used to address the identified problem.

Other examples of high-risk situations are restraints and significant weight loss. Facilities should strive to be free of restraints. If physical restraints are used, then nursing staff should track the types of restraints, the safety measures used, the alternatives to restraints undertaken, and the timely removal of restraints. Deficiencies should be investigated further. Cases of significant weight loss (5% of body weight in 30 days, or 10% of body weight in 180 days) should be presented at QI meetings; probable causes for weight loss and a plan of correction can be discussed for each case. QI meetings can help promote awareness of problems and gain the support of all disciplines in determining solutions.

Laundry/Housekeeping. An important indicator of quality of care, especially in long-term care, is cleanliness. The administrator must convey to employees that everyone is expected to participate in keeping the facility clean. If anyone sees trash on the floor, they are expected to pick it up. Equipment that is not being used or is soiled or damaged should be quickly removed from hallways. Scheduled maintenance and protocols

Unit _____ Year _____

	Jan	Feb	Mar	April	May	June	July	Aug	Sept	Oct	Nov	Dec
Medication Usage												
Average number of routine medications												
Average number of PRN medications												
Psychotropic Usage												
Number of residents receiving antipsychotics												
Number of residents receiving hypnotics												
Number of residents receiving anxiolytics												
Number of residents receiving antidepressants												
Pain Management												
Number of residents receiving routine pain meds												
Number of residents receiving prn and NOT routine pain meds												
Total number of residents receiving pain meds												

Figure 28-3 Sample quality improvement medication report.

for cleaning of equipment should be reviewed. Strong or foul odors are another factor equated with poor quality care. If odors are noticed, they should be addressed quickly.

Residents and families frequently have complaints about laundry, including complaints that clothes are lost or not returned from the laundry in a timely manner. Lost clothing may be minimized by individually marking each item with a permanent marker or tape and/or placing that person's clothing in a special washing garment bag. Laundry problems may be curtailed by instructing the resident/family upon nursing home admission what the facility's laundry department can and cannot wash. Some clothing may not be able to withstand the rigor of industrial washing and should be replaced or cleaned by family members.

Food Service. Food is a common complaint in health care facilities. It is very hard to please everyone when serving food to a large group of people on a daily basis. Common complaints from residents are that the food is cold when it should be hot and that food is not presented in a timely manner. Food preferences should be reviewed with the dietitian upon admission and periodically if there are any complaints or changes in weight. Liberalizing diets increases satisfaction, improves quality of life, and aids in the prevention of weight loss, and is now recommended by the American Dietetics Association (Niedert, 2005). Allowing patients to participate in special meals or buffets may improve pleasure in dining.

Pharmacy. Pharmacy personnel need to attend the QI meeting each month and present data on current medication usage. Monthly data collection should include the average number of routine and PRN medications, as well as a list of high-cost or potentially problematic medications (Figure 28-3). Medication errors should be noted and discussed. Trends in medication errors may show the need for additional education for nursing staff. For those facilities that do not have an on-site pharmacy, it is also important to track how long it

Unit _____ Year _____

	Jan	Feb	Mar	April	May	June	July	Aug	Sept	Oct	Nov	Dec	Total
Number of new residents on antibiotics													
Number of cultures													
Number of negative cultures													
Number of URIs													
Number of LRIs													
Infiltration by CXR													
Wound/skin infections													
Eye infections													
GI infections													
Number of UTIs													
Number of catheters													
Number of catheters with UTIs													
Nosocomial infections													
Isolations													
Numer of pressure ulcers													
Number of ongoing pressure ulcers													
Number of new pressure ulcers													
Admissions with pressure ulcers													
Census													

Figure 28-4 Sample quality improvement infection control report. *CXR,* Chest x-ray; *GI,* gastrointestinal; *LRI,* lower respiratory infection; *URI,* upper respiratory infection; *UTI,* urinary tract infection.

takes for an ordered medication (both stat and routine) to be delivered to the facility. The pharmacy may be able to provide a list of high-cost medications as well as lower cost alternatives so that health care providers can make educated choices on residents' prescriptions.

Laboratory. The laboratory staff should report the number of microbial cultures performed during the last month and the number of positive cultures. Antibiotic sensitivity patterns and clustering of infections within the facility should be reviewed (Figure 28-4). Low numbers of negative cultures compared to the number of positive cultures may be an indicator that nursing is not identifying or reporting infections. The laboratory personnel should also track the frequency of laboratory ordering and the timeliness of reporting the results to the facility. The handling of routine and stat orders should be clear to the staff and health care providers. Timeliness of laboratory services should be monitored.

Medical Records. The medical records' department should report on the accuracy, completeness, and timeliness of medical record completion. The facility census should be reviewed at each QI meeting. Data can be presented on a flow chart with other information such as admissions, readmissions, discharges, transfers, and deaths.

When examining admissions, it is valuable to look at the source of admissions. Did the new resident come from home, or a nearby hospital (and which hospital)? A flow sheet should include data from previous months to observe for any trends in admissions (Figure 28-5). The day and time of admissions should also be examined. For example, if admissions are usually on a Thursday or Friday evening, then additional staff may need to be scheduled around that time so that new residents have a good transition into the facility.

Emergency transfers to the hospital or emergency department should be explored each month and compared to previous months on a flow sheet. Information should include the day and time of the transfer, floor/division, staff person arranging the transfer, adverse events associated with the transfer, reasons for the transfer, and outcomes of the transfer. This information may provide insight into the need for additional training, education, and/or staffing.

In summary, all of the departments in a long-term care facility have a part to play in QI. Working together through regular QI meetings, monitoring of key quality indicators, and following a QI process can lead to

Unit _____   Year _____

	Jan	Feb	Mar	April	May	June	July	Aug	Sept	Oct	Nov	Dec	Total
Admissions													
Readmissions													
Transfers to hospital													
Transfers to another facility													
Discharges to home													
Discharges to another facility													
Deaths													
Transfers due to:													
Hip fracture													
Other fractures													
Sutures													
Other injury													
Restorative program													
Bowel/bladder training													
Chemical restraints													
Physical restraints													
Contractures													
Hotline calls													

Figure 28-5   Sample long-term quality improvement report.

improved quality of care in long-term care. Gerontological nurses play a part in this process by participating on QI teams in these or other facilities.

SUMMARY

Monitoring and assuring quality care is an important function in health care today. The history of the QI movement and current methods are reviewed in this chapter. Gerontological nurses play a key role, particularly in the long-term care setting. In addition to nursing personnel, representatives from all departments in a facility need to participate in QI, including administration, food service, pharmacy, laundry, and laboratory. Working together to identify problems, create action plans, and monitor improvements, facilities can successfully participate in the continuous process of providing quality care.

REFERENCES

American Nurses Association. (2005). Nursing sensitive outcomes. Retrieved November 20, 2005, from www.nursingworld.org/readroom/nurssens.htm.

American Nurses Association (ANA). (2006). The National Center for Nursing Quality Indicators. The National Database of Nursing Quality Indicators (NDNQI). Retrieved March 6 2006, from www.nursingworld.org/quality.

Bolton, L. B., & Goodenough, A. (2003). A Magnet nursing service approach to nursing's role in quality improvement. *Nursing Administration Quarterly, 27*(4), 344-354.

Brown, S. A., & Grimes, D. E. (1993). *Nurse practitioners and certified nurse-midwives: A meta-analysis of studies on nurses in primary care roles.* Washington, DC: ANA Publications.

Caramania, L., Cousino, J. A., & Petersen, S. (2003). Four elements of a successful quality program: Alignment, collaboration, evidence-based practice, and excellence. *Nursing Administration Quarterly, 27*(4), 336-343.

Carboneau, C. E. (1999). Achieving faster quality improvement through the 24-hour team. *Journal for Healthcare Quality, 21*(4), 4-10 (quiz 10, 56).

Center for Health Systems Research and Analysis. (1999). Facility guide for the nursing home quality indicators national data system. Retrieved November 10, 2005, from www.cms.hhs.gov/medicaid/mds20/qifacman.pdf.

Cohen, I. B. (1984). Florence Nightingale. *Scientific American, 250*(3), 128-137.

Dyck, M. J. (2005). Evidence-based administrative guideline: Quality improvement in nursing homes. *Journal of Gerontological Nursing, 31*(2), 4-10.

Gray, P. M., Anderson, M. M., & Robinson, D. (2001). Quality management: Implications for nursing. In D. Robinson & C. P. Kish (Eds.), *Core concepts in advanced practice nursing.* St. Louis: Mosby.

Griffiths, P., Edwards, M., Forbes, A., & Harris, R. (2005). Post-acute intermediate care in nursing-led units: A systematic review of effectiveness. *International Journal of Nursing Studies, 42*(1), 107-116.

Griffiths, P. D., Edwards, M. H., Forbes, A., Harris, R., & Ritchie, G. (2004). Effectiveness of intermediate care in nursing-led in-patient units. *Cochrane Database Systematic Review, 18*(4), CD002214.

Hartman, M., & Moore, R. C. (1976). Pathways to quality care. *National League for Nursing,* 1-40.

Hirdes, P., Fries, B. E., Morris, J. N., Ikegami, N., Zimmerman, D., Dalby, D. M., et al. (2005). Home care quality indicators (HCQIs) based on the MDS-HC. *Gerontologist, 44,* 605-679.

Kleinpell, R., & Gawlinski, A. (2005). Assessing outcomes in advanced practice nursing: The use of quality indicators and evidence-based practice. *Clinical Issues, 16*(1), 43-57.

Lambertsen, E. C. (1995). A glance back in time, 1968: The emerging health occupation. *Nursing Forum, 30*(2), 22-26. Reprinted from *Nursing Forum, 7*(1), 87-97.

Leap, L. L., Brennan, T. A., & Laird, N. (1991). The nature of adverse events in hospitalized patients. Results of the Harvard Medical Practice Study II. *New England Journal of Medicine, 324,* 277-284.

Miller, M. R., Elixhauser, A., Zhan, C., & Meyer, G. S. (2001). Patient safety indicators: Using administrative data to identify potential patient safety concerns. *Health Services Research, 36,* 110-132.

National League for Nursing. (2005). The NLN mission—Our purpose. Accessed January 19, 2006, from www.nln.org/aboutnln/wourmission.htm.

National Quality Forum. (2005). National Quality Forum closes work on home health performance measures project. *Current News and Notes.* Retrieved July 10, 2005, from www.qualityforum.org.

Nelson, E. C., Mohnr, J. J., Batalden, P. B., & Plume, S. K. (1996). Improving health care, part 1: The clinical value compass. *Journal of Quality Improvement, 22*(4), 243-258.

Niedert, K. C. (2005). Position of the American Dietetic Association: Liberalization of the diet prescription improves quality of life for older adults in long-term care. *Journal of the American Dietetic Association, 105*(12), 1955-1965.

Phaneuf, M. C. (1972). *The nursing audit: Profile for excellence.* New York: Appleton-Century-Crofts.

Phaneuf, M. C. (1976). *The nursing audit: Self regulation in nursing practice.* New York: Appleton-Century-Crofts.

Rantz, M. J., Popejoy, L., Petroski, G. F., Madsen, R. W., Mehr, D. R., Zwygart-Stauffacher, M., et al. (2001). Randomized clinical trial of a quality improvement intervention in nursing homes. *Gerontologist, 41*(4), 525-538.

Savitz, L. A., Jones, C. B., & Bernard, S. (2005). Quality indicators sensitive to nurse staffing in acute settings. From *Advances in patient safety* (vol 4). Retrieved November 10, 2005, from www.ahrq.gov/qual/advances/vol4/Meurer/doc.

Scott, L. D., Setter-Kline, K., & Britton, A. S. (2004). The effects of nursing interventions to enhance mental health and quality of life among individuals with heart failure. *Applied Nursing Research, 17*(4), 248-256.

Siegler, E. L., Glick, D., & Lee, J. (2002). Optimal staffing for acute care of the elderly (ACE) units. *Geriatric Nursing, 23*(3), 152-155.

Spiegel, A. D. (1997). Hammurabi's managed health care—Circa 1700 B.C. managed care. Stezzi Communications. Retrieved January 18, 2006, from www.managedcaremag.com/archives/9705/9705.hammurabi.shtml.

Stuck, A. E., Egger, M., Hammer, A., Minder, C. E., & Beck, J. C. (2002). Home visits to prevent nursing home admission and functional decline in elderly people: Systematic review and meta-regression analysis. *Journal of the American Medical Association, 287*(8), 1022-1028.

Thomas, L. H., McColl, E., Cullum, N., Rosseau, N., Soutter, J., & Steen, N. (1998). Effect of clinical guidelines in nursing, midwifery, and the therapies: A systematic review of evaluations. *Quality Health Care, 7*(4), 183-191.

Walton, M. (1990). Deming management at work. New York: Perigee.

Wengstrom, Y., Haggmark, C., Strander, H., & Forsberg, C. (1999). Effects of a nursing intervention on subjective distress, side effects and quality of life of breast cancer patients receiving curative radiation therapy—A randomized study. *Acta Oncology, 38*(6), 763-770.

Zimmerman, D. R., Karon, S. L., & Arling, G. (1995). Development and testing of nursing home quality indicators. *Health Care Finance Review, 16*(4), 107-127.

Zuber, R. (2005). Home health quality measures: Inside the National Quality Forum Steering Committee. *Home Healthcare News, 23*(7), 402-408.

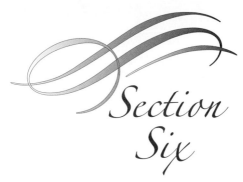

Section Six

Gerontological Nursing in the Context of Care

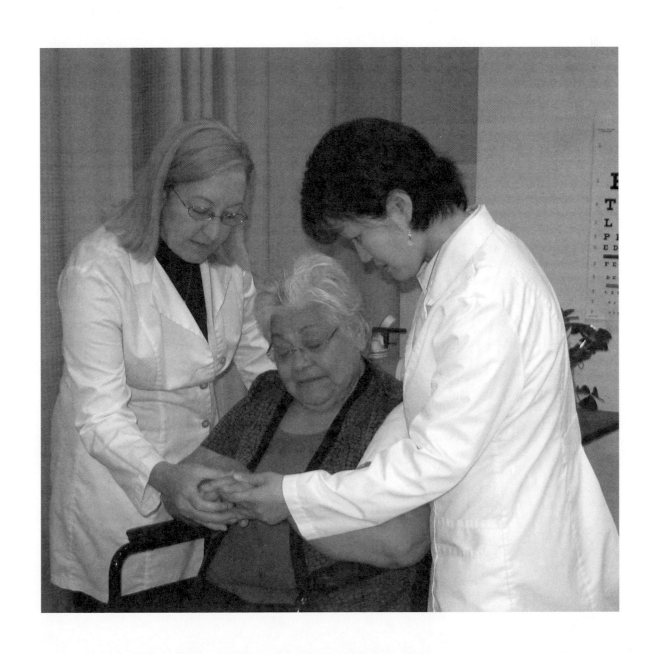

Chapter 29

The Geriatric Continuum of Care

Susan A. Ruzicka

Objectives

Identify the types of services available to older adults, including primary care services, community health services, hospital-based services, and residential care options.

Explore the variables that affect health care delivery.

Discuss the concept of aging in place.

Discuss care of older adults as a continuum.

Describe the benefits and limitations of Medicare and Medicaid in health care for older adults.

Analyze the implications of patterns of health care utilization by older adults.

Geriatric care, well-done, is a tapestry. It is a weaving of resources through an individual's life in a way that produces a seamless work of art. Poorly done, it is a tangled mass of knots and loose ends. The goal of gerontological health care is to provide the older adult with appropriate resources at the appropriate time within the context of the individual's value system. This chapter provides an overview of the range of resources and services available, the variables that affect the delivery of health care to older persons, and the concepts of aging in place and continuity of care. The remaining chapters in this section provide more detailed discussion of specific settings and the roles of the nurse in each.

PATTERNS OF HEALTH CARE UTILIZATION

Many individuals remain independent and relatively healthy until shortly before death; however, advancing age for others is marked by declining function and health status that requires increasing support and care over time. In the United States, where the life expectancy

is now 77.6 years, the implications for the health care system are enormous. Consider the following:

- Chronic disease accounts for 70% of health care expenditures in the United States (National Center for Health Statistics [NCHS], 2004).
- In 1999 82% of Medicare beneficiaries aged 65 and older had at least one chronic condition, and 65% had more than one condition (Wolff, Starfield, & Anderson, 2002).
- Of the 10 leading causes of disease in the United States, 7 are chronic diseases (NCHS, nd) (Box 29-1).
- The dependency ratio (ratio of dependent people to the working age population) is increasing on a global scale (Harwood, Sayer, & Hirschfeld, 2004).
- The hospital discharge rate for individuals ages 65 and older is 3 times higher than that of younger persons.
- The length of hospital stay is almost a day longer for older adults than younger adults.
- Older adults have almost twice as many doctors' office visits as younger persons.
- Per capita Medicare expenditures for Medicare beneficiaries in 1999 averaged $211 for individuals with no chronic conditions, and $13,973 for those with four or more chronic conditions (Wolff et al., 2002).

OVERVIEW OF RANGE OF SERVICES

When most of today's older adults were born, health care was provided in the home, the physician's office, or a general hospital. As health care became more sophisticated and specialized, the range of health care services available expanded dramatically. It now includes a vast array of options that can be classified as primary care, outpatient, multimodal outpatient, intermediate ambulatory, acute ambulatory, or inpatient residential (Kiser, Lefkovitz, & Kennedy, 2001). For the system to be used

827

effectively, individuals must be matched with the most appropriate service component at a given point in time. The selection of a service is guided by the characteristics of the older individual. Many algorithms exist to facilitate aligning clients with the proper services (Kiser et al., 2001).

Primary, Secondary, and Tertiary Care Services

Primary care services have great potential not only to reduce morbidity and mortality, but also to enhance the quality of life in older adults. Nursing professionals can significantly influence the older adult's health practices and health outcomes (Baileff, 2000; Beck, Daughtridge, & Sloane, 2002) through effective communication, client education, and role modeling. Primary care services can be classified in terms of primary, secondary, or tertiary prevention.

Primary Prevention. Primary preventive care services, which aim to prevent a disease or adverse event, most commonly are delivered in public health programs or physicians' offices. On average, three of every four people in the United States see a physician each year. The majority of those visits are to primary care practitioners (such as physicians and nurse practitioners), who are an important source of health care information (Chakravarthy, Joyner, & Booth, 2002; Davidson, MacIntosh, McCormack, & Morrison, 2002). Although less common, facilities operated by independent nurses are growing and gaining respect and public acceptance for the holistic care provided. Many

primary care services focus on the leading causes of death in the United States (Box 29-1). For example, smoking cessation reduces the risk of COPD, and proper nutrition may reduce the risk of heart disease and some types of cancer.

BARRIERS TO PRIMARY CARE. Barriers to primary care are listed in Box 29-2. The identified physician barriers could be applied to nurses as well because knowledge, experience, and attitude influence how all health care providers view preventive care for older adults. Providers must work to break down patient barriers that often are based on lack of knowledge and fears of cost or discomfort. Nurses also have a role in addressing barriers imposed by the health system itself. Within any system of care, nursing professionals have the opportunity to move health care systems in directions that better serve the older adult.

Secondary Prevention. Secondary prevention involves screening for early detection of a disease or condition that is asymptomatic. In many cases, early detection and appropriate treatment improve the chance of cure or slow the progression of a disease. For example, mammography, TB testing, colonoscopy, and blood pressure monitoring all are employed in secondary prevention. Also, early recognition of probable Alzheimer's disease and the prescription of cholinesterase inhibitors have been shown to slow the disease progression.

Tertiary Prevention. Tertiary prevention, which focuses on prevention of negative consequences of existing clinical disease, is especially applicable to the older population because of the prevalence of chronic disease. A good example of tertiary prevention is cardiac rehabilitation focused on preventing a second myocardial infarction (Hensrud, 2000; Longlett, Kruse, & Wesley, 2001).

Community Health Services

Services provided to older persons in the community can be viewed on two levels. Community/public health and community health nursing strive to meet the needs of aggregates whereas many other community-based services are directed toward individual needs.

Community-based services aim to promote the independence of older adults, and to provide an alternative to institutional care. Community services are provided in physician and nurse practitioner offices, clinics, HMOs, nurse-managed centers, nutrition sites and senior centers, mental health clinics, day hospitals and outpatient surgery clinics, board and care homes, and day care centers. Although these settings provide a vast array of services, they can pose a problem for the older adult who does not know which service to use or needs multiple services. Subsequent chapters in this unit will discuss various settings in greater detail.

Informal support groups provide the majority of community services to older adults who have disabling health problems but live outside institutions. Relatives represent 84% of all caregivers for males and 79% for females. More wives than husbands provide care to disabled spouses, reflecting the difference in the average life spans of males and females. Care of persons residing in the community is discussed in detail in Chapter 30.

Hospital-Based Services

The hospital setting provides the most intensive opportunity for health professionals to stabilize, monitor, and educate patients. For the older adult, however, it also may be the most foreign and stressful environment for health care. Because care is at risk for fragmentation during an acute illness, a strong interdisciplinary team is needed to facilitate smooth transitions to and from hospitals and to provide continuity of care.

At any given time, older adults typically comprise approximately 75% of the hospitalized population in the United States (http://www.aoa.gov/prof/Statistics/profile/2003/14.asp). The most common first-listed diagnoses for hospitalized older adults in 2001 were heart disease, injuries and poisoning, malignant neoplasms, pneumonia, and cerebrovascular diseases (CDC, 2003). A study of Medicare recipients showed that the use of acute medical care services increased significantly when older adults with at least one chronic condition also had a depressive syndrome (Himelhoch, Weller, Wu, Anderson, & Cooper, 2004). Older adults living with nonrelatives are three times as likely to be admitted for short hospital stays as those living with spouses. An Italian study identified the independent risk factors for prolonged hospitalization in older persons as the number of ADL functions lost, pressure sores, hip fractures, peripheral arterial disease with critical ischemia, and hyponatremia (Zanocchi et al., 2003).

Race, perceived health status, family relationships, and activities of daily living (ADLs) also are significant predictors of hospitalization among older individuals. Among older adults, whites are most likely to be admitted to the hospital. Those who rank their health status as fair or poor are 3 times as likely to be hospitalized as those who perceive their health status as excellent. Individuals with impairments in activities of daily living are twice as likely to be hospitalized as those who have no impairments (Aliyu, Adediran, & Obisesan, 2003). The profile of specific hospitalized patients may vary by race, as demonstrated in one study that examined a sample of individuals with CHF. In an insured population, older black patients with CHF had substantially more hospital use than older white patients. The increased use was not explained by differences in CHF outpatient management (Lafata, Pladevall, Divine, Ayoub, & Philbin, 2004). Care of the older adult in acute care is covered in Chapter 32.

Residential Care Options

Alternate housing arrangements exist to accommodate the older adult as changes occur that make living independently unsafe or undesirable. Many options exist, with the most prevalent being private homes, continuing care retirement communities, assisted living facilities, and skilled nursing facilities. These options are described briefly here, and are covered in detail in Chapters 30, 31, and 34.

Continuing Care Retirement Communities. Continuing care retirement communities offer a long-term contract to provide for the evolving needs of older persons within a single community. Both single and married older adults may enjoy a fully independent lifestyle. A progression of options range from independent living to assisted living to skilled nursing care, if and when it is needed. This arrangement allows the older adult to age in place, in familiar surroundings with familiar people.

Assisted Living Facilities (ALFs). The concept of assisted living is hardly a new one, but only in recent decades has it been formalized as a level of care for older adults. Assisted living facilities may be free-standing or one component of a residential community. They are designed for individuals who are able to live independently but need or desire some level of help with activities of daily living, meals, housekeeping, and/or transportation. The setting provides a sense of security for those who live alone because help is readily available and someone may check on the older person routinely. Residents in assisted living typically pay a base monthly rent with additional fees incurred for additional services (Medicare, 2005a). Many ALFs enable the individual to age in place by permitting the individual or family to bring in outside skilled care if the resident's needs for assistance increase. See Chapter 31 for a more complete discussion of assisted living facilities.

Long-Term Care Facilities. A long-term care facility offers skilled and custodial nursing care on an ongoing basis. A nursing home is a type of long-term care facility. A report prepared by the U.S. Senate Special Committee on Aging (in February of 2000) described long-term care as differing from other types of health care because the aim is to maintain an optimal level of functioning rather than to achieve a cure. To achieve this aim, long-term care provides medical, nursing, social, and personal services in addition to specialized housing for those with some functional impairment.

In 2001, nearly 1.5 million people lived in nursing homes in the United States, about 9 million of those ages 65 and older (CDC, 2003; Medicare, 2005b). The risk of nursing home placement increases with age. A study by the U.S. Department of Health and Human Services states that people who reach age 65 will likely have a 40% chance of entering a nursing home, with about 10% of those residing at the nursing home for 5 or more years (Medicare, 2005b). Among severely impaired individuals, 31% of those ages 65 to 70 receive care in a nursing home compared with 61% of those 85 years and older (Gabrel, 2000). For the most part, nursing home residents are not acutely ill although they may have significant physical and/or mental disabilities. According to the U.S. Department of Health and Human Services (September 2000), the proportion of the older population receiving long-term care has declined, but the level of disability and cognitive impairment among those in long-term care has risen sharply. By 2020 it is projected that 12 million older Americans will need long-term care. The majority of those will be cared for at

home by family and friends (Medicare, 2005b). For a more complete discussion of nursing home care, see Chapter 34.

Patient Classification and Health Policy in LTC. Long-term care encompasses a variety of levels of interventions. Patient classification generally is graded by use of skilled services such as physical therapy, respiratory care, kinesiology, speech therapy, psychological services, and occupational services. The goal for health in long-term care is to enable the individual as much as possible. However, this becomes difficult as the individual loses the capacity to regain these abilities and these services no longer facilitate a progressive trajectory toward health. At this point, the individual is said to require maintenance care. The focus is to maintain rather than rehabilitate, and health policy is geared to reimburse little for this stage of life. It can place the family and institution in a quandary for financial considerations.

VARIABLES AFFECTING HEALTH CARE DELIVERY

Variables affecting health care delivery are related to the delivery system, the health care professional, and the consumer (older adult). The present health care delivery system is burdened and fragmented. Whereas health care needs have changed dramatically over the past decades, the system still is operating under the original framework, resulting in gaps in care and disjointed and sometimes overlapping services.

Health Care Delivery System Issues

The health care system is facing an unprecedented volume of older adults and changes in delivery of care. This is a global issue. In North America and in Europe, the growth rate of the older population is exceeding that of the total population growth (Flesner, 2004). Health care system issues that impact care include access to services, increased outcome orientation, and implementation of evidence-based practice across settings.

Access to Services. The older adult facing personal health issues often is at a loss in terms of proper access. Linking individuals with services that best meet their needs is an important function of the gerontological nurse.

Figure 29-1 demonstrates the improvement in health care access between 1992 and 1996. The percentage of Medicare enrollees reporting difficulty in obtaining health care declined from 5% to 2% during that time. Also, delayed use of health care services because of cost declined from 10% to 6%. However, disparities remain among various sectors of the population. For example, in 1996 the percentage of older Americans who reported

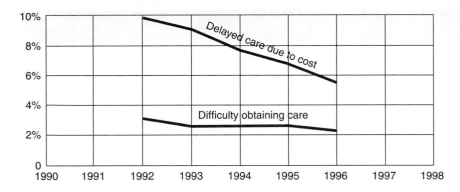

Figure 29-1 Percentage of Medicare beneficiaries age 65 and older who reported having had problems with access to health care 1992-1996. Reference population: These data refer to noninstitutional Medicare beneficiaries. (From Federal Interagency Forum on Aging-Related Statistics. [2000]. Older Americans 2000: Key indicators of well-being. Retrieved January 8, 2006, from www.agingstats.gov/chartbook2000.)

delays because of cost was highest among non-Hispanic black persons (10%), followed by Hispanic persons (7%), and non-Hispanic white persons (5%) (Federal Interagency Forum on Aging-Related Statistics, 2000).

One goal of *Healthy People 2010* is the elimination of disparities in health. Based on data obtained primarily from federal data collection sources, the Agency for Healthcare Research and Quality (AHRQ) published the National Healthcare Disparities Report. The seven key findings and specific examples from The National Healthcare Disparities Report are presented in Box 29-3.

Outcome Orientation. The focus of the health care system has shifted from place-oriented services to outcome-oriented services (Flesner, 2004). One example of health care initiatives focused on outcomes is *Healthy People 2010*. This initiative uses specific outcome-oriented measures to guide and evaluate public and private sector programs. It specifically focuses on health promotion and disease prevention. The two major goals of *Healthy People 2010* are to increase quality and years of healthy life and to eliminate health disparities. The objectives and outcomes provide directions for health care professionals and can be accessed at www.aoa.gov/prof/adddiv/healthy/addiv_healthy.asp.

Evidence-Based Practice. A general concern in health care, not just care of older adults, is the need to adopt health standards and to integrate evidence-based practice. At the national level, numerous initiatives are at work to accomplish these goals. The proposed National Quality Measurement and Reporting System (NQMRS) aims to integrate evidence-based practice to improve health care. To this end, the Strategic Framework Board has recommended that national goals:

- Be achievable by actions taken within health care delivery systems
- Represent areas in which patients experience a substantial burden of illness, injury, or disability or areas that substantially affect health and functioning
- Be based on evidence that progress on the goal is possible

- As a set, address the quality problems faced by diverse populations, covering a range of ages and including diverse racial and socioeconomic groups
- Be compelling to expert groups and relevant constituents (McGlynn, Cassel, Leatherman, DeCristofaro, & Smits, 2003)

Digital health care is another model of health care delivery being researched. It uses the Internet capability to empower consumers and providers, and to transition the health plan toward more of a knowledge facilitator/integrator. Basically, as a facilitator, it eliminates the role of the traditional health plan (Box 29-4). The goal is an electronic health plan infrastructure bridging the current structure to the envisioned digital structure (Table 29-1). More information on digital health care can be accessed at http://conferences.mc.duke.edu/2000dpsc.nsf/contentsnum/y.

Nurses have an incredible opportunity to influence health care policy as legislators seek solutions to health care challenges of older citizens in the United States (Fitzpatrick, 2004). Nurse scientists have contributed much to the knowledge of geriatrics and gerontology. The ability to translate research into policy is a powerful and necessary step in better addressing the needs of the older adult and better managing resources.

Health Care Professionals

Variables related to health care professionals that impact care delivery include limited knowledge of gerontology and geriatrics, the lack of uniform standards of care and protocols for care of older adults, and limited awareness of or access to evidence-based practice and research outcomes. The expanding older population, increased emphasis on chronic illness, and the trend toward fewer and shorter hospitalizations are of great significance to the nursing profession. The knowledge base needed by the gerontological nurse includes normal aging changes, atypical responses of older patients, common health problems of older adults, adaptations in care mandated by changing physiological and psychosocial factors, health care services and resources available, and laws and regulations relevant to care of

BOX 29-3 National Healthcare Disparities Report: Key Findings and Specific Examples

Inequality in Quality Persists

- Minorities are more likely to be diagnosed with late-stage breast cancer and colorectal cancer compared with whites.
- Patients of lower socioeconomic position are less likely to receive recommended diabetic services and more likely to be hospitalized for diabetes and its complications.
- When hospitalized for acute myocardial infarction, Hispanics are less likely to receive optimal care.
- Many racial and ethnic minorities and persons of lower socioeconomic position are more likely to die from HIV. Minorities also account for a disproportionate share of new AIDS cases.
- The use of physical restraints in nursing homes is higher among Hispanics and Asian/Pacific Islanders compared with non-Hispanic whites.
- Blacks and poorer patients have higher rates of avoidable hospital admissions (i.e., hospitalizations for health conditions that, in the presence of comprehensive primary care, rarely require hospitalization).

Disparities Come at a Personal and Societal Price

- Without screening, cancers may not be detected until they grow large or metastasize to distant sites and cause symptoms. Such late-stage cancers are usually associated with more limited treatment options and poorer survival. Minorities and persons of lower socioeconomic status are less likely to receive cancer screening services and more likely to have late-stage cancer when the disease is diagnosed.
- Persons with diabetes of lower socioeconomic position are less likely to receive recommended diabetic services and more likely to be hospitalized for diabetes and its complications.
- Many racial and ethnic minorities and persons of lower socioeconomic position are less likely to receive recommended immunizations for influenza and pneumococcal pneumonia, the most common type of pneumonia. Once hospitalized, some ethnic and racial minorities, as well as lower income patients, suffer worse quality of care for pneumonia. These differential rates of vaccination and hospitalization present opportunities for provider-based and community-based interventions to reduce disparities.

Differential Access May Lead to Disparities in Quality

- Many racial and ethnic minorities and individuals of lower socioeconomic status are less likely to have a usual source of care.
- Hispanics and people of lower socioeconomic status are more likely to report unmet health care needs.
- While most of the population has health insurance, racial and ethnic minorities are less likely to have health insurance compared with whites. Lower income persons are also less likely to have insurance compared with higher income persons.
- Higher rates of avoidable admissions by blacks and lower socioeconomic position persons may be explained, in part, by lower receipt of routine care by these populations.

Opportunities to Provide Preventive Care Are Frequently Missed

- Blacks and persons of lower socioeconomic status tend to have higher rates of death from cancer. While rates of cancer death may reflect a variety of factors not associated with health care, such as genetic disposition, diet, and lifestyle, screening and early treatment of cancers can lead to reductions in mortality.
- Many racial and ethnic minorities and persons of lower socioeconomic position are less likely to receive screening and treatment for cardiac risk factors. The combination of reduced screening and effective treatment of risk factors, such as smoking among the uninsured, lend themselves to quality improvement initiatives that can potentially reduce heart disease disparities among populations at risk.
- Many racial and ethnic minorities and persons of lower socioeconomic position are less likely to receive childhood immunizations.
- Many racial and ethnic minorities and individuals of lower socioeconomic status are less likely to receive recommended immunizations for influenza and pneumococcal disease.

Knowledge of Why Disparities Exist Is Limited

- Many racial and ethnic groups, as well as poor and less educated patients, are more likely to report poor communication with their physicians.
- Many racial and ethnic minorities and poor patients report more problems with some aspects of the patient-provider relationships.

From *National healthcare disparities report: Summary.* (2004). Rockville, MD: Agency for Healthcare Research and Quality. Retrieved at www.ahrq.gov/qual/nhdr03/nhdrsum03.htm.

BOX 29-3 National Healthcare Disparities Report: Key Findings and Specific Examples—cont'd

Knowledge of Why Disparities Exist Is Limited—cont'd

- Many racial and ethnic minorities and lower income patients report more difficult patient-provider relationships.
- Asians, Hispanics, and those of lower socioeconomic status have greater difficulty accessing health care information, including information on prescription drugs.

Improvement Is Possible

- While blacks and poor patients are more likely to present with later stage cancers with higher death rates, black women have higher screening rates for cervical cancer and no evidence of later stage cervical cancer presentation. While it would not be possible to demonstrate a causal link, the significant investment in community-based cancer screening and outreach programs for cervical cancer may be responsible for the lack of disparity.
- Quality improvement efforts have resulted in demonstrable reductions in black-white differences in hemodialysis. A targeted intervention within a quality improvement culture may offer important lessons in disparity reduction.
- Black patients are more likely to receive blood pressure monitoring without any disparity in blood pressure management. A greater perceived risk for significant cardiovascular disease among blacks may result in appropriately increased screening rates and treatment for risk factors. Directed public education campaigns about cardiac risk factors and the importance of being an active patient may play an important role in the lower observed rate of cardiac disparities among blacks.

Data Limitations Hinder Targeted Improvement Efforts

- Not all health care organizations routinely collect data on patient characteristics.
- Some individuals are reluctant to share personal demographic information.

BOX 29-4 The Practice of Medicine

Old	New
Reactive	Proactive
Find it; fix it	Predict it; prevent it; fix it
Sporadic intervention	Health care planning
Physician directed	Interactive
Fractionated delivery	Integrated delivery system
Experience based	Evidence based
Cost insensitive	Cost sensitive

From Synderman, R., & Duke Private Sector Conference. (2000). *Academic health systems in transition. Bringing it all together.* Duke Medical Center and Health Systems. Retrieved January 26, 2006, from http://conferences.mc.duke.edu/privatesector/dpsc2000/y.htm.

---

older adults. Basic nursing education often lacks depth in this component of the curriculum.

Some of the strategies to influence health care delivery and promote evidence-based practice for each older adult include clinical practice guidelines for a variety of disease processes and clinical problems with the intent of improved care and reduced medical costs (Doebbeling et al., 2002). Experts must continue to develop and disseminate research-based nursing practice guidelines for the management of care in specific situations.

The majority of nursing care for older adults takes place outside the acute care setting. Older adults leave hospitals "quicker and sicker" than in the past and have more procedures performed as outpatients. Appropriate referrals are vital to assure that clients have the support needed for the transition from one setting to another. The nurse often is the person who facilitates communication among members of the health care team, which helps to prevent gaps and duplication in services.

Outpatient management has its own set of challenges. Unlike the hospital setting where the patient is conveniently available at all times, outpatient care must be scheduled and coordinated with the patient and family. It is not unusual to have difficulty arranging a home visit or follow up with older adults because their schedule is so full! Health care conferences often must be coordinated to accommodate a family member's schedule to assure that they have the input, support, and information they need.

Consumers

At one time, older adults were not recognized as a discrete population in the health care system. When infectious disease was the leading cause of death, disability and chronic diseases received little attention. Much has changed as the life expectancy has increased from 47.3 years in 1900 to 77.6 years in 2003. In 2000 and 2001,

Table 29-1 *Infrastructure: Digital Health Plans*

Function	First Generation	Second Generation
Products	Health plan provides PPO, HMO, and POS options	Consumer creates individualized benefit plan by specifying key variables (e.g., copays, deductibles, ability to share risks, networks, quality improvement participation)
Market	Wired local markets move information in real-time	Leapfrog technology moves infrastructure functions to consumer
Health management	Plan removes restrictions to specific MD services and monitors periodically (e.g., 6 months)	Plan removes virtually all restrictions to MD services and monitors in real-time
Operations/customer service	Self-service enabled by Internet and IVR	Stakeholders have access to virtual service center online
Culture	Silos eliminated, corporate supports markets, physician-driven clinical decisions	Customer empowerment, health plan as knowledge integrator, and population health drives health plan

From Jacque, J., Sokolove, M. D., & Duke Private Sector Conference. (2000). *Academic health systems in transition. Bringing it all together.* Duke Medical Center and Health Systems. Retrieved January 26, 2006, from http://conferences.mc.duke.edu/privatesector/dpsc2000/y.htm.

chronic conditions such as hypertension, arthritic symptoms, all types of heart disease, cancer, sinusitis, and diabetes were among the most common health problems of older persons.

Older persons no longer are passive recipients of care. They are influential voters and paying customers who believe the system should be responsive to their unique health care needs. Older social activists have been one force in the expanded range of services over the past decade. They also are better educated than ever before and increasingly expect to be a partner in health care.

Health Care Expenditures

Although they comprise only about one eighth of the population, older Americans consume more than one fourth of trauma and critical care resources (Rosenthal & Kavic, 2004). A major percentage of health care expenditures, including those incurred by Medicare, occur during the last 3 months of life, with intensive hospital inpatient care accounting for most of this expense. Many changes have been made in the methods of Medicare reimbursement of hospitals, home health care, hospice, and long-term care in an effort to control health care expenditures.

Medicare and Medicaid. Established in 1965 as the Older Americans Act, Medicare and Medicaid were created as federal programs to assist in financing and regulating health care and social services for older adults. Medicare served 19 million older adults in 1966 and is projected to serve 77 million in 2050. Eligibility remains age 65 or over for Medicare, and less than 65 if one is disabled and on social security. Details of the history and critical milestones through the years are noted in Box 29-5.

Approval of The Medicare Adult Day Services Alternative Act of 2003, which acknowledges the significant role of adult day services, is pending at the time of this writing. If approved, it will provide specific funding for adult day services and would allow older adults to choose to receive Medicare home health services in an adult day location.

During the 1990s, Medicare HMOs and their enrollment accounted for approximately 16% of all Medicare beneficiaries. The Health Care Financing Administration (HCFA) paid these HMOs based on their enrolled beneficiaries' annual adjusted per capita cost, calculated by age, sex, Medicaid status, and type and county of residence—not by health status. Caring for healthy individuals is more cost-effective than caring for individuals with chronic disease, so there became a financial incentive to market and enroll healthy people and avoid enrolling sick people likely to require expensive health care. Plans inclusive of many ill individuals had to downsize or terminate their Medicare HMO contracts and return their members to the fee-for-service Medicare program. As a result, the HCFA was (over)paying for the care of the healthier-than-average subpopulation enrolled in HMOs at the same time that it was indemnifying the high costs of the sicker-than-average subpopulation in the fee-for-service Medicare program. The result was an increase in expenditures rather than the predicted decrease. Congress passed the Balanced Budget Act of 1997 (BBA 97), mandating that the HCFA develop a new "risk-adjusted" formula for computing

BOX 29-5 Medicare's Milestones

DATE	EVENT
July 30, 1965	Authorized under title XVIII of the Social Security Act, Medicare was enacted to cover the elderly. Seniors were the population group most likely to be living in poverty; about half had insurance coverage.
1966	Medicare was implemented and more than 19 million individuals enrolled on July 1.
1970	Over 20 million older Americans were enrolled in Medicare.
1972	Medicare coverage was extended to the disabled and those with permanent kidney failure. Two million new individuals subsequently enrolled in the program.
1977	The Health Care Financing Administration (HCFA) was established to administer the Medicare and Medicaid programs.
1982	While managed care plans could participate in the program since its inception, the Tax Equity and Fiscal Responsibility Act of 1982 (in provisions implemented in 1985) made it easier and more attractive for health maintenance organizations to contract with the Medicare program by introducing a risk-based option.
1983	A new prospective payment system (PPS) for hospitals was implemented to slow growth of hospital spending and preserve the life of the Hospital Insurance Trust Fund. The PPS, in which a predetermined rate is based on patients' diagnoses, was adopted to replace cost-based payments.
1988	The Medicare Catastrophic Coverage Act was repealed after higher income elderly protested new premiums. A new fee schedule for physician services was enacted.
1990	Additional federal standards for Medicare supplemental insurance policies were enacted.
1996	The Health Insurance Portability and Accountability Act of 1996 (HIPAA) was enacted to amend the Public Health Service Act, the Employee Retirement Income Security Act of 1974 (ERISA), and the Internal Revenue Code of 1986 to provide for improved continuity or "portability" of group health plan coverage and group health insurance provided through employment or through the individual insurance market (not connected with employment). HIPAA also allowed HCFA to regulate small and individual private health insurance markets. The act created the Medicare Integrity Program, which dedicated funding to program integrity activities and allowed HCFA to competitively contract for program integrity work. Furthermore, HIPAA enacted national administrative simplification standards for all electronic health care transactions.
1997	The Balanced Budget Act of 1997 included the most extensive legislative changes for Medicare since the program was enacted: Established as Part C of the Medicare program Medicare+Choice, creating an array of new managed care and other health plan choices for beneficiaries with a coordinated open enrollment process Developed and implemented several new payment systems for Medicare services to improve payment accuracy and to help further restrain the growth of health care spending Tested other innovative approaches to payment and service delivery through research and demonstrations; expanded preventive benefits
1998	The Internet site www.medicare.gov was launched to provide updated information about Medicare.
1999	The Balanced Budget Refinement Act (BBRA) made substantial investments to meet the needs of our nation's hospitals and their patients.
2000	Medicare served 39 million seniors and disabled Americans. Medicare trustees estimated that Medicare will be solvent through 2025. The Benefit Improvements and Protection Act of 2000 made additional investments to providers and expanded preventive benefits.
2030	Medicare will serve an estimated 77 million Americans.

From www.cms.hhs.gov/about/history/mcaremil.asp.

Medicare's capitation payments to HMOs, with higher capitation payments for HMO-enrolled beneficiaries at increased risk for requiring expensive care and lower payments for healthy individuals (Boulanger, 2002; Pacala, Boult, Urdangarin, & McCaffrey, 2003).

In transitional/extended care facilities, the Center for Medicare and Medicaid Services mandated a system of indicators using the Minimum Data Set (MDS). The MDS is a computerized database of comprehensive patient/resident assessment data. The data include cognitive patterns, communication, mood and behavior, psychosocial well-being, physical function, continence, disease diagnoses, health conditions, oral/nutritional status, oral/dental status, skin condition, activity patterns, medications, special treatments and procedures, and discharge potential. Upon admission to a facility, the MDS must be completed within 7 days, 14 days, 30 days, 60 days, quarterly, and annually. A new MDS also is completed any time there is a significant change in the patient's/resident's condition.

These MDSs are electronically transmitted to a national database that compiles the data into 11 domains of care, encompassing 24 quality indicators, and generates a facility quality indicator profile (FQIP). The areas of care include accidents, behaviors/emotional patterns, clinical management, cognitive patterns, elimination/incontinence, infection control, nutrition/eating, physical functioning, psychotropic drug use, quality of life, and skin care. The database also compiles information about each resident, in terms of the quality indicators. The FQIP provides data for quality improvement and allows individual facilities to observe how they compare to other regional facilities (Piette, Ellis, St. Denis, & Sarauer, 2002).

Regarding community health services, some of the challenges encountered included the 1997 Balanced Budget Act, welfare reform, and the transition to Medicaid managed care—all changes that hindered providers' ability to fund or cross-subsidize charity care. Fortunately, the economy during this time allowed states to expand public coverage options, benefitting uninsured people, who gained coverage through Medicaid expansions. Since 2000 to 2001, funding available through federal expansion grants for community health clinics (CHCs) and federal Community Access Program (CAP) grants has assisted communities in integrating care delivery for the uninsured. This economic burst began slowing in 2002, but with strong leadership and vision, facilities increased their capacities by enhancing and expanding facilities and services. They strengthened their finances to protect future viability, and the more vulnerable older adult had options in care. Generally, these changes have increased primary care and hospital services available to low-income people. Specialty services, mental health services, and dental services are less accessable to vulnerable populations of older adults (Shelley, 2000).

Legislation affecting the physician and nurse practitioner are The Ethics in Patient Referrals Act (also known as the Stark Act) and the anti-kickback statute—two examples of the legislation focus on protecting the individual from opportunistic priorities. "Stark I" became effective in 1995 and prevents physicians and their immediate family members who have an ownership or compensation relationship with a clinical laboratory services facility from making referrals to it. "Stark II" is broader, preventing physicians and immediate family members who have an ownership or compensation relationship with an entity providing "designated health services" from referring patients for these services where payment may be made under Medicare. The anti-kickback statute (Section 1128B of the Social Security Act/42 USC 1320a-7b) states individuals and entities are prohibited from "knowingly and willfully" making false statements or representations in applying for benefits or payments under all federal and state health care programs. This attempts to keep the focus on referral and use of resources that best meet the older adults needs, rather than serve the interests of the provider. The implication for nurses is reinforcement of awareness and responsibility in caring for older adults. Knowing the legislation, the guidelines, and the mechanisms to reinforce safe health care practice enables each nurse to provide the best care and resources to this vulnerable population.

PROGRAM OF ALL-INCLUSIVE CARE FOR THE ELDERLY (PACE). PACE is a capitated benefit that features integrated Medicare and Medicaid financing and a comprehensive service delivery system. Under this program, participants can receive services at home rather than be institutionalized. The Balanced Budget Act of 1997 allows states to provide PACE services to Medicaid beneficiaries as a state option. All services are delivered by an interdisciplinary team primarily in adult day health centers. In-home and referral services are available if needed by a client. To use PACE, a person must be at least 55 years old, live in the PACE service area, and be certified eligible for nursing home care. For participants, PACE becomes the sole source of services for Medicare- and Medicaid-eligible participants. Monthly Medicare and Medicaid capitation payments are paid to PACE providers for each eligible enrollee. Providers accept full financial responsibility for participant's care regardless of the amount, duration, or scope of services used. A person who is eligible for Medicare, but not Medicaid, can pay monthly premiums equal to the Medicaid capitation amount. No deductibles, coinsurance, or other cost-sharing apply (Center for Medicare and Medicaid Services, 2005).

Prospective Payment/DRGs. In the late 1960s, Yale University researchers developed a tool to assist clinicians and hospitals to monitor the use of services and quality of care. It was adopted by Medicare in 1983 as a method of reimbursing hospitals (Manitoba Centre for Health Policy, 2002). This was the origin of the Diagnosis-Related Groups, commonly referred to as DRGs. A fixed reimbursement amount was assigned to each of the 468 DRGs. Some adjustments were allowed for case severity, geographic labor costs, and teaching costs. Regardless of the length of stay or variety of services an individual receives, the hospital's reimbursement was limited to that assigned to the DRG. Following implementation of DRGs, hospital discharge planning increased and lengths of stay declined.

Long-term care hospitals, in general, are hospitals with an average Medicare inpatient length of stay greater than 25 days. Hospitals that provide extended medical and rehabilitative care for patients fall in this category. Services such as comprehensive rehabilitation, respiratory therapy, head trauma treatment, and pain management often are provided. The clients tend to be more clinically complex with multiple acute or chronic conditions. In mid-2004, Medicare & Medicaid Services made effective changes in reimbursement that increased the Medicare payment rates for long-term care hospitals (LTCHs) by 3.1%. More information can be found at the following Web sites as to specific changes made: www.cms.hhs.gov/providers/longterm/cms-1263-f.pdf; www.cms.hhs.gov/media/press/release.asp?Counter=1028; and www.medicare.gov.

Competitive Approaches to Control of Health Care Costs. In the United States, various facilities vie for customers. A competitive model is intended to encourage facilities that provide similar services to reduce costs in an effort to attract consumers of health care services. Health maintenance organizations (HMOs) and preferred provider organizations (PPOs) are examples of competitive approaches used to control costs. In HMOs, providers are paid a fixed amount for each enrolled client, thereby creating strong motivation to promote health and prevent disease. Access to specialists and costly interventions are controlled by the primary care provider who coordinates the client's care. The PPO model is different in that the third-party payer contracts with a list of providers who agree to provide specific services at specific reimbursement rates.

AGING IN PLACE

Aging in place refers to living in one residence throughout one's life. Few older adults choose to leave their home to live in a new and unfamiliar setting. The advantage to 'aging in place' is that the individual is comfortable in the surroundings and knows them intimately, which supports greater independence. The address, phone number, local grocer, pharmacy, neighbors, and streets are relatively unchanged. Moving is very stressful in all aspects: emotionally, physically, and psychologically. It often means downsizing and parting with treasures accumulated over the years; this can be overwhelming and depressing for the older individual already confronting physical losses, perhaps loss of independence, and loss of locus of control.

Disadvantages of aging in place may include the overwhelming repairs that often are needed in older homes, neighborhood changes that may create an unsafe environment, and the loss of familiar neighbors who have moved on. All of these factors can result in isolation of the older adult in a residence. The choice to age in place or not is difficult. Most older adults choose not to change routines.

Not all transitions are the result of crises, but careful planning can reduce the risk of crises being precipitated by a transition. Preventive health care strategies include discussions of the pros and cons of such a move while the older adult still is active and functional, prior to any major physical or emotional losses. If the individual is married, it is helpful to discuss this topic while both individuals are functioning at a high level. For example, one older couple chose to move from a home built in the inner city in 1904, for the World's Fair. They had discussed it with their children and between themselves for approximately 2 years before the move. They weighed the pros and cons; evaluated distance from family, health care centers, and grocery stores; and assessed the value of the neighborhood. The ultimate decision crystallized after observing friends lose their spouses, and then struggling with an older home alone. As the older couple transitioned to a duplex with fewer responsibilities, they stated they decided to move while they could do it together and age gracefully in new surroundings together. The important point in this couple's decision was that the decision was made while they both were in optimal health. It was not rushed and not done while they were in frail or vulnerable states of health. It was a decision they reached and made independently, and ultimately it was a gift to their children and a wonderful role model of graceful aging. It still was a difficult move, but made easier with the support of friends and family to encourage and offer insight when requested.

For a view of aging around the globe, see Box 29-6.

CARE AS A CONTINUUM

The following is an excerpt from a description of the health care system in New York City:

Thus we find a very confused picture—patients at home who should be in hospitals, patients in hospitals who should

Box 29-6 *Reflections on Global Aging*

Most of the content of this textbook relates to the health of older adults in the United States. As the world becomes smaller through ease of travel and communication, it is important to develop a more global perspective and consider the differences in aging and health across the globe. Most of the developed countries of the world are experiencing a demographic transition toward aging populations like that seen in the United States, including England, most European countries, and Japan (Grundy, 2003). Less developed countries have not experienced this trend to the same degree; however, with improved sanitation and medical care, even the less developed countries are expected to see an increase in the numbers of older people in the twenty-first century.

The world population of people over 60 is expected to increase from 600 million at the millennium to almost 2 billion in the year 2050 (United Nations, 2002). Older adults will reside in more urban areas in the developed countries, while less developed countries will have a larger aging population in rural areas. As in the United States, the oldest old will increase the most over this century, and women will outnumber men. As demography changes, countries will be challenged to provide resources.

Over the past few decades, the United Nations has considered the impact of global aging, which led to the International Year of Older Persons in 1999, and later to the International Plan of Action on Aging in 2002. This plan aims to ensure that persons everywhere are able to age with security and dignity and to continue to participate in their societies as citizens with full rights (United Nations, 2002). The plan provides a foundation for countries to use in developing their individual policies. The two priorities identified are (1) individual lifelong development or financial opportunity and (2) opportunities for health. The goal is equitable division of resources, even for vulnerable members of society.

Gerontological nurses need to consider the wide variation in care of older adults around the world, which is situated within the context and values of each country's culture (Swanson, 1999). In the following text, several nurses from around the world share their perspectives on aging and gerontological nursing within their respective countries of Taiwan, Zimbabwe, and the United Kingdom. The similarities and differences in the data presented above can be seen in these narrative descriptions. Gerontological nurses should partner with nurses and health professionals from around the world to ensure that research, education, and practice are available to promote the best opportunities for the health of older adults around the globe.

Taiwan

Taiwan is facing the challenge of a growing aging population. The Ministry of the Interior (2004) estimates that 9.5% of the population is over 65 years, and different kinds of long-term care facilities such as assistive care and skilled care facilities are rapidly increasing in order to help older

people and their caregivers. Dementia has become a common problem in Taiwan. The prevalence of dementia among the aging population is 5.44%, and the prevalence rates double approximately every 5 years, from rates of 1.2% in the category of 65 to 69 years to more than 30% in people ages 90 or above (Taiwan Alzheimer's Disease Association [TADA], 2004). About 79.6% of those with dementia live in the community (TADA, 2004), and the majority of caregivers are spouses, adult children, and daughters-in-law. The need for care for Taiwan's aging population is a challenge for caregivers and health care providers.

Most families prefer to take care of their elders at home as long as possible. An important factor in care decisions is traditional Chinese filial piety, which places a profound value and revered belief on children that it is their responsibility to care for their disabled parents. This traditional virtue highlights the fact that children need to reciprocate parents' love and care from childhood with gratitude. In this way, children gain social praise from their relatives and friends, and children who do not take care of their older parents are violators of traditional virtue.

When frail elders experience functional decline, family caregivers may not be able to provide care at home and have to make a decision about long-term care placement. Besides the traditional values, finances can influence this decision. Families may need to pay out of pocket for residency in a nursing home, ranging from $800 to $1000 (U.S. dollars) every month, which is a moderately high expense for a middle-class Taiwanese family. Paying for a caretaker to help at home is a solution used by some, although the quality of care may not be desirable. The conflict experienced by family caregivers in making decisions such as nursing home placement is a challenge, and nurses can assist families in making the best decision possible for their circumstances.

In Taiwan, there is no special certification for gerontological nursing, nor are there associations that focus on the specialty. Rather, gerontological nursing is a part of community health or psychiatric nursing. However, gerontological nursing has been recognized as a professional specialty for years, and some universities provide a master's level program.

Yu-Ping Chang
Yu-Ping Chang, PhD(c), MSN, RN
Nursing Instructor
Taiwan

Zimbabwe

There are many golden opportunities in living with an older adult. One of my favorite memories growing up was listening to endless stories and learning about my culture from my grandmother. Older adults are respected custodians of information and tradition in Zimbabwe. They are consulted about home remedies, and their skills are sought for a range of issues such as upbringing, dowry, marriage, and funeral rights. Select groups of elderly women function

Box 29-6 *Reflections on Global Aging*—cont'd

as traditional birth attendants or midwives and offer a valuable service in most of their communities.

A reciprocal exchange takes place with older adults and their families; the elderly provide child-care assistance, while their families offer socioeconomic support. Older adults often rely on members of their immediate and extended family for support. Care of older adults is embedded within norms of respect for older adults and responsibility and obligation for the younger generation to care for the older generation.

Few nurses in Zimbabwe have specialized in gerontological nursing because the population of older adults is less pronounced. Gerontology issues are emphasized within different types of nursing specialization, such as psychiatric, critical care, and public health nursing. Zimbabwe has a youthful population, with a median age of about 19 years. The percentage of Zimbabweans aged 65 and older was estimated to be 3.7% in 2005, which was only 474,254 out of a total population of over 12 million. There are two types of nursing homes in urban areas: private nursing homes and public social welfare-funded nursing homes. Because of the stigma associated with sending ones' parents to a nursing home, few Africans send their parents to expensive private nursing homes. Publicly funded nursing homes often have older adults of different nationalities and a few Zimbabwean.

There is a lot of diversity in living arrangements for older adults, with more extended families in rural communities than in urban communities. Coresidence or a separate living arrangement for older adults depends on an older adult's personal choice and the family's financial ability. Older adults often live with a married son, where the daughter-in-law is expected to provide care. In some cultures, the youngest son has the responsibility to live with parents. When an older adult has separate living arrangements, they are linked to formal and informal support resources provided by family, neighbors, and friends. In the past, fewer older adults lived alone; they frequently lived with an adult child. As mentioned, overall living arrangements are often complimentary; older adults receive socioeconomic support and in return assist in the care of children and other culturally acceptable family chores.

Unlike developed countries, Zimbabwe does not provide an extensive social security and pension system to support older adults' personal and family income. Zimbabwe has established a Social Dimension Fund (SDF) for low-income households to help mitigate the negative effects of food shortages in many areas, which is augmented by various nongovernmental organization programs. Older adults are included among special population groups, such as children and mothers, targeted for nutrition programs. Older adults are eligible to receive free health services within the public health system.

A special issue for nurses in Zimbabwe is to focus research in quality of life outcome measures for older adults—in particular, the psychosocial problems related to the HIV/AIDS epidemic. HIV/AIDS reversed earlier advances; the life expectancy has declined from about 60 years in the early 1990s to around 40 years. Zimbabwe is among the most severely affected countries, with over 20% of adults estimated to be HIV positive. Increasingly, more households with AIDS orphans are headed by a grandmother. As a result, the ratio of older adults to the working population continues to increase, also increasing the demand for health care and food security. Older adults who rely on their land for food face more challenges during droughts and are at increased risk of malnutrition.

In addition to HIV/AIDS challenges, current data indicates that noncommunicable conditions such as cancer, hypertension, heart diseases, diabetes, and malnutrition are the most common conditions affecting older adults in Zimbabwe. About 60% of the population lives in rural areas because such rural areas have a higher proportion of older adults, yet specialized health care services for chronic conditions are concentrated in urban areas. Because data were recently aggregated by age and gender in the early 2000s, a clear picture on health issues for older adults will emerge. There is also growing evidence of declining HIV prevalence in Zimbabwe, based on samplings of rural populations. The findings show a modest decrease in overall adult HIV prevalence and may imply an increase in the population of older adults. This shift can influence a change from the predominant infectious and parasitic diseases to a profile of chronic, degenerative noncommunicable diseases associated with older adults, such as cardiovascular conditions and the related health challenges of longevity. These changes will likely have a major effect on the demand for and provision of social and support services and related policy implications.

Social networks play an important role in the care of older adults. Social and economic trends have a significant outcome on the living patterns for older adults. Educational and economic aspirations of young families also impact the living arrangements of older adults who may seek employment opportunities in urban areas and in other countries. With several young Zimbabwean families in the diaspora, it is not surprising to find older adults living alone, because their children are away. However, informal support networks continue to be provided by extended family members, kin, and neighbors. The children remain responsible for the financial obligations to support their parents. Ingrained in the continuum of care for older adults is a principle that emphasizes care for those who are young so that they will take care of their elders when they age. Families tend to accept requests for care of young people within the extended family.

Gerontological nurses with an interest to practice in Zimbabwe should be aware of the diversity of living arrangements and family responsibilities. Although nurses need to be mindful of interwoven social networks, such assumptions tend to overlook negative challenges within the family milieu that may not enhance the care of

Continued

Box 29-6 *Reflections on Global Aging*—cont'd

older adults. Special attention needs to be paid to the discharge plan as decisions requiring inclusion of the family can override the views of the older adult. Implementing effective health promotion and disease prevention programs that reduce the degenerative risk factors will have a major impact on Zimbabwe's future burden of disease. This change will increase research interests in quality of life as an outcome measure for older adults. The focus needs to shift to providing care across the continuum of care for older adults and should not be limited to acute care in urban health care facilities, but expanded to rural areas that tend to have a higher population of older adults. Perhaps then a demand for nurses to specialize in gerontology will arise.

Sithokozile Maposa

Sithokozile Maposa, RN, BA, MSN
Community Health Nurse
Zimbabwe

United Kingdom

Consistent with countries across Europe, the average age of the population of the United Kingdom has been steadily increasing. Long-term trends of lower birth rates, improvements in health, and rising longevity have combined to produce constant growth in the proportion of the population who are ages 60 years and over, and in 2003, 18.5% of the total population were over pensionable age (60 for women and 65 for men). The most rapid increases are among those ages 80 and over, and this group generally has far higher levels of health needs secondary to multiple chronic diseases. Consequently, within the United Kingdom, older people are the main users of health and social care services (General Household Survey, 2004), and most nurses will come into regular contact with older people in their day-to-day practice.

Other demographic factors shaping older people's use of health and social care services include the decline in coresidence between generations and the increase in women's employment outside the home. The trend towards smaller family size is also reducing the number of potential caregivers. Changes in family structure, resulting from increased geographical mobility and the impact of divorce, are also affecting families' ability to provide informal networks of support for older people who need help to remain in the community (Victor, 2005). Despite this, it is important to recognize that even amongst very frail older people only a minority require residential care, with less than 5% of those ages 65 and over living in a care home.

In response to these changes, services for older people and their families within the United Kingdom have been continuously refigured over recent years. In particular, the goal of enabling older people to remain in their own homes in the community as long as possible has been an important driver and has resulted in the creation of new roles for nurses. The role of health visitors and practice nurses (attached to family doctors) has evolved to include health promotion work with older people. Simultaneously, community health development activities, which encourage consumer participation in the identification of health needs and the development of services to meet those needs, are increasingly involving older people as active participants. Programs such as intermediate care schemes intended to reduce hospital admission and length of stay are resulting in new roles for nurses. In a recent initiative, community matrons are being appointed to provide one-to-one support to the most vulnerable patients with long-term conditions (Department of Health, 2005). These nurses will work alongside other community-based nurses to provide intensive case management for older people with complex health needs. Increasingly, gerontological nurses are learning to work in partnership with older people and their families and to recognize that most older people and their caregivers are experts in the management of their own conditions.

During the past 20 years, long-term care for older people has been relocated within the independent sector, and there are now very few continuing care beds within the National Health Service. The nursing role within care homes for older people has become primarily a management and leadership role as day-to-day caregiving is increasingly undertaken by non-nursing personnel. Primary care trusts, which hold responsibility for the provision of community health services, are beginning to develop senior nursing posts to support staff working in care homes. Many of these outreach posts are aimed at reducing avoidable hospital admissions but are also providing staff in care homes with crucial links to networks of support.

Finally, in recognition of the fact that most users of acute care services will be older people, some acute units have established specialist nurse roles in gerontology, often known as consultant nurses, to act as advisors to nurses who may lack specialist training. An important goal for many of these nurses is to protect the privacy and dignity of older adults during an acute hospital stay.

In summary, key issues in the development of gerontological nursing in the United Kingdom are:

- Diversity in the provision of care services, resulting in greater choice for older people and their families
- Development of gerontological nurses as leaders in a range of care settings, with responsibility for managing and developing less qualified staff
- Recognition of the value of working in partnership, with older people, their families, and members of the multidisciplinary team

Susan M. Davies

Susan M. Davies, PhD, MSc, BSc, RGN, RHV
Senior Lecturer in Gerontological Nursing
School of Nursing and Midwifery
Sheffield, United Kingdom

be in less complex institutions, patients in homes for the aged that are not prepared to minister to their needs, patients in convalescent homes occupying beds needed for another purpose. A mad confusion of patients and institutions. It is really a scene of the greatest disorder that presents itself as the report unfolds the many types of agencies that contribute to the care of the chronic sick: public and private hospitals, homes for the aged, convalescent homes, nursing and visiting doctor services, aftercare agencies for sheltered work, medical social service departments, and family service agencies (Thomas, 1969, quoting Boas, 1933).

Although this document was written in 1933, many of the same issues remain today. A central concern is coordination of the components of the health care system to provide better services and reduce consumer frustration. This section addresses some of the issues related to continuity of care and efforts to bring about positive change.

The brief overview of the range of health care services presented at the beginning of this chapter illustrates the complexity of the health care system in the United States. The conglomerate of services sometimes is described as a continuum of care, which may be defined as including all aspects of health care: prevention, detection, management, rehabilitation and palliation. In the best sense, the term "continuum of care" suggests that a variety of services are available that provide progressive levels of care based on the amount of care a person needs. This simple concept might work well when a usually healthy person has a single acute health deviation. However, it is lacking if one considers individual health services as squares of a quilt that have not yet been sewn together. The pieces may be lovely, but they will not keep you warm. Only when the pieces are joined together in a systematic way do they create a functional product. A challenge for the health care system is to link the pieces so that the consumer can move readily from one service to another as their needs change. A well-designed continuum of care not only would serve the needs of the consumer but also would facilitate the work of the health care provider. The importance of a user-friendly system is particularly evident in the care of older adults who commonly receive care in multiple settings and from multiple providers.

Too often the older adult is overwhelmed or exasperated when trying to deal with health care services. Too often one listens to the lament of the older adult who has given the same information to multiple care providers and has been to a sundry of facilities, yet the initial problem still exists. Too often the health industry has just added to the individual's stress level instead of resolving the basic problem. That is not effective care nor is it the intention of any health profession.

A sadly typical scenario may begin when a community-dwelling older person is hospitalized for an acute event, followed by discharge to a skilled nursing facility for rehabilitation, and then moved to an assisted living facility. A subsequent hospitalization for another acute event can then start the cycle over. Movement between settings is neither linear nor predictable, but based on the older adult's abilities or losses at each stage, as depicted in Figure 29-2 (Kissam et al., 2003). This situation often results in fragmented care and crisis-driven care transitions that result in duplication of services, inappropriate or conflicting care recommendations, medication errors, patient/caregiver distress, and higher costs of care (Parry et al., 2003).

Barriers to a Continuum of Care

Because older adults often require complex, continuous care, the services they need commonly require multiple practitioners in multiple settings. The advantages of access to many specialists may be diminished when those practitioners operate without knowledge of the care provided by others. In the United States, a trend is for practitioners to restrict their practices to a single setting so that patients moving about the health care system must also move to new care providers. During transitions, complex patients particularly are at risk for medical errors, service duplication, inappropriate care, and critical omissions in care. The effects of poorly planned and executed transitions may include patient dissatisfaction, poor clinical outcomes, and inappropriate use of services such as emergency department visits that could have been handled in a clinic (Coleman & Boult, 2003).

Stakeholders in the Continuum of Care

One factor that contributes to the complexity of health care systems is the number of stakeholders who stand to gain or lose something. For example, the consumer

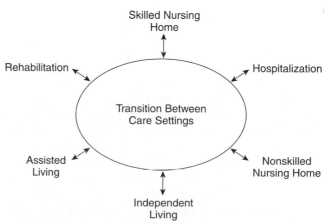

Figure 29-2 Continuum of care. (From Kissam, S., Gifford, D. R., Mor, V., & Patry, G. [2003]. Admission and continued-stay criteria for assisted living facilities. *Journal of the American Geriatrics Society, 51*[11], 1651-1654.)

wants convenient high-quality health and illness care at an affordable price. Health care professionals expect fulfillment and financial reward for the provision of high-quality care in a supportive environment. Vendors seek to obtain fair reimbursement for their products in a fair market atmosphere that stimulates product research. Agencies aim to meet their goals, provide a service that is appreciated by professionals and consumers, and employ sufficient personnel to provide the service. Some are entrusted with evaluating the care provided by others. The government has a stake in maintaining public health and assuring care for all citizens for both humane and economic reasons.

Though all stakeholders share some common goals, conflict necessarily arises at many points. To illustrate, unlicensed nursing personnel in a long-term care facility expect to be paid a living wage for providing direct care to residents. The administrator is looking to cover the budget, or in some cases make a profit. Regulating agencies need to determine whether minimum standards of care are being maintained regardless of the resources of the agency. Consumers and their families expect compassionate, skilled care in a clean, pleasant environment at a price that is within their means. The difficulties in balancing all these priorities are obvious.

Strategies to Improve Continuity of Care

For the patient trying to navigate this system, some questions that commonly arise are the following:
- What should I be doing to stay healthy?
- Which service do I need for a health problem I am having?
- How do I access the services I need?
- What services am I eligible to receive?
- Are there any resources to help me if I cannot pay for a service I need?
- Is there a single place I can go for all my health care needs?

To answer these questions and to make the access to care manageable, health services need to be coordinated as a continuum of care.

Careful management focused on the individual may minimize the fragmentation of care. Transitional care may involve moves between hospitals, assisted living facilities, skilled nursing facilities, the individual's home, the primary physician's office, and specialty physicians' offices. The seamless transition of care is based on a comprehensive plan of care and health care practitioners who are well trained in chronic care, communicate well, and are well informed of the patient's goals, preferences, and clinical status. Logistical arrangements, patient and family education, and coordination among the health professionals are essential aspects involved in the transition (Coleman & Boult, 2003).

AONE Strategic Plan. The American Organization of Nurse Executives (AONEs) identified some of the critical elements needed to accomplish an effective continuum of care and identified competencies for the professional nurse executive (AONE, 2003). AONE's strategic plan for 2004 involves "commitment to incorporating technology, diversity and patient safety in all of its educational and research programs." The three education and research priorities are as follows: (1) Stewards of Leadership, (2) Future Patient Care Delivery Models, and (3) Creating Positive and Healthy Work Environments (Box 29-7).

Achieving care coordination involves the following components (AONE, 2003):
- Coordinated planning and management
- Uniform information systems
- Quality management and measurement
- Integrated financing
- Interdisciplinary staffing

COORDINATED PLANNING AND MANAGEMENT. Collaborative arrangements and contractual agreements or ownership of all elements of the continuum could reduce or simplify transitions.

UNIFORM INFORMATION SYSTEMS. An understandable, easily accessed electronic medical record could greatly facilitate care coordination. This concept, which was in its infancy in 1998, is now the standard for many organizations and it continues to evolve. For example, International Business Machines (IBM) and the Mayo Clinic have agreed to a multiyear collaboration involving one of the world's largest medical databases, containing complete records on nearly 4.4 million patients. The intended outcome is to establish an information system that enables a physician examining a patient to ask an online computer system how the last 100 Mayo Clinic patients with the same gender, age, and medical history responded to particular treatments. The hope is that applying those same tools to medical records will help them find patterns that currently are discovered mostly by chance (Bulkeley, 2004).

To build a new health information infrastructure, a National Health Information Technology Coordinator has been appointed within the U.S. Department of Health and Human Services. The coordinator will head the development of a network that will link electronic health records and provide health professionals with access to a wealth of treatment information. The goals of this endeavor are to inform clinical practice, interconnect clinicians, personalize care, and improve population health. A new set of standards related to electronic health records is being developed that will be used in the development and implementation of new information technology systems. Examples are vocabulary standards

---

BOX 29-7 American Organization of Nurse Executives Education and Research Priorities

I. Stewards of Leadership

AONE is the national leader in strengthening America's future nursing leadership across the continuum of care in all types and sizes of health care settings. AONE's central role in education and research is to assist its members—from aspiring nurse leaders to senior executives—to develop and increase evidence-based leadership capacity. AONE members are leaders in the use of technology to complement patient care, act with a diverse workforce and a diverse patient population, and provide safe patient care and safe protocols for caregivers. AONE supports education and research that promotes the value of nursing leadership. Additionally, AONE senior nurse members are committed to mentoring aspiring nurse leaders and engaging in effective succession planning.

II. Future Patient Care Delivery Models

AONE is the leading provider of tools and resources for nurse leaders who seek to be knowledge leaders in the design, implementation, and evaluation of future patient care delivery models. The design and development of patient care delivery models that leverage new technologies, improve provider and patient safety, and honor a diverse workforce are key education and research priorities for AONE. AONE is committed to educating and supporting its members in these efforts to promote the use of technology and enhance patient safety, as well as acknowledge diversity in the work environment. In addition, AONE supports education and research for patient care delivery models that support quality care and satisfying work for nurses.

III. Creating Positive and Healthy Work Environments

AONE is a national leader in creating positive and healthy work environments in nursing and health care. Practice environments that attract and retain nurses are essential. Nurse leaders are accountable for guiding the development of the workforce and promoting professional growth and continuous learning, including mentoring of staff nurses. An adequate number of qualified nurses is essential for quality patient care, and positive practice environments are vital for attracting and retaining nurses. AONE supports education and research initiatives for healthy environments that encompass judicious use of technology, develop provider and patient safety guidelines, and promote diversity in the workforce.

Approved by AONE Board of Directors, December 7, 2003. From American Organization of Nurse Executives Education & Research Priorities. Accessed at www.aone.org/aone/index.jsp.

---

for demographics, units of measure, and immunizations; and SNOMED CT (Systematized Nomenclature of Medicine Clinical Terms) for laboratory results, anatomy, and other terms.

The Agency for Healthcare Research and Quality (AHRQ) has designed the Integrated Delivery System Research Network (IDSRN), which is a model of field-based research designed to connect researchers with large health care systems to facilitate research solutions on priority issues in health care.

The network creates, supports, and disseminates scientific evidence about what works and what does not in terms of data and measurement systems and organizational best practices related to care delivery and research. It also provides a number of delivery-affiliated researchers and sites to test ways to adapt and apply existing knowledge.

AHRQ also has established three new centers of excellence to research how market forces are affecting the quality of health care, access to care, and health care costs (Box 29-8).

QUALITY MANAGEMENT AND MEASUREMENT. Quality indicators and universal health standards, protocols, and goals based on clinical evidence across the various settings must be developed. For example, *Healthy People 2010*, which was discussed earlier, demonstrates established standards, goals, and quality indicators to measure progress.

INTEGRATED FINANCING. An example of a mechanism to establish congruent incentives to minimize costs and facilitate care would be a delivery system that offers multiple elements of health care (e.g., labs, offices, outpatient surgery centers, home care, hospital, hospice) organized in a single system to provide care to a defined population within the same financial network.

INTERDISCIPLINARY STAFFING. Patient care providers working together with the sole focus on planning care for the older adult across the continuum could minimize overlapping and duplication of services, thereby enabling smoother, more effective delivery of care services to the older adult.

Transitions between Health Care Settings

Almost 5 million older adults had over 15.1 million transitions between health care settings from 1992 to 1994. The majority of older adults had only one or two transitions into or out of institutional and community-based settings, but almost 10% of that population endured seven or more transitions. A significant percentage (22.4%) of those who endured multiple transitions subsequently needed health care services. Transitions from acute care hospitals to rehabilitation centers, long-term care facilities, or assisted living facilities represent a little more than 20% of all transitions and are associated with increased risk of subsequent health problems. The greatest number of problems occurred following transitions from hospital to nursing home, home to nursing home, nursing home to paid home care, and rehabilitation facility to paid home care. Problem indicators included ER visits, avoidable hospitalizations, all hospitalizations, and return to an institution from the community (Murtaugh & Litke, 2002). More than one third of all transitions (36.4%) were from a short-term general hospital to a postacute or long-term care setting. About 20% of the transitions were to residential homes. Transitions from hospitals to paid home care tended to be followed by the greatest number of potential problems, such as emergency department visits and subsequent readmissions to hospitals. An analysis of 12 months of posthospital data on 1055 older adults was conducted to determine transition patterns. During the first 3 months after hospital discharge, more than two thirds of the individuals had two or three transitions; another 14% had four to six transfers (Ma, Coleman, Fish, Lin, & Kramer, 2004).

Impact. Transition involves change for the individual, the family, and the institutions involved in coordinating the care. The cost to quality of life for the individual and family when thorough assessment is lacking is monumental. Needless suffering, complications, and costs in actual health status, as well as in time and money, can be averted with holistic evaluation of the individual's total quality of health before transition in care.

Management. Better care coordination has proven effective in reducing hospital and nursing home admissions. General strategies for improving the outcome of postacute and long-term care transitions are to:

■ Better integrate the clinical and supportive care provided to frail older adults
■ Develop interventions aimed at persons with a relatively high risk for transition problems
■ Develop interventions aimed at settings with relatively high rates of potential transition problems (Boockvar & Vladeck, 2004; Murtaugh & Litke, 2002)

The Position Statement of The American Geriatrics Society Health Care Systems Committee on Improving the Quality of Transitional Care for Persons with Complex Care Needs offers direction for professional practice (Box 29-9). Relevant data and the plan of care must be communicated among care providers, professional staff, older adults, and their families. All should be kept informed about care provided and changes in the care plan. Coordination of drug therapy during transitions is especially important because a dose may have been changed, or medications added or deleted. When changes in environment or medication regimens are necessary, vigilant assessment of physiological and emotional status is needed to facilitate adjustment of the older adult.

Follow up is essential to evaluate the outcomes of the care provided. Once again, the importance of communication cannot be overstressed. For example, after hip replacement surgery, 78-year-old Mrs. D is being discharged to her home on oral anticoagulant therapy. Mrs. D, her family, and her home health nurse and physical therapist all must be aware of this fact, know to

BOX 29-9 *American Geriatrics Society Position Statement: Improving the Quality of Transitional Care for Persons with Complex Care Needs*

Definition

For the purpose of this position statement, transitional care is defined as a set of actions designed to ensure the coordination and continuity of health care as patients transfer between different locations or different levels of care within the same location. Representative locations include (but are not limited to) hospitals, sub-acute and post-acute nursing facilities, the patient's home, primary and specialty care offices, and long-term care facilities. Transitional care is based on a comprehensive plan of care and the availability of health care practitioners who are well-trained in chronic care and have current information about the patient's goals, preferences, and clinical status. It includes logistical arrangements, education of the patient and family, and coordination among the health professionals involved in the transition. Transitional care, which encompasses both the sending and the receiving aspects of the transfer, is essential for persons with complex care needs.

Rationale

Persons whose conditions require complex continuous care frequently require services from different practitioners in multiple settings. Practitioners in each setting often operate independently, however, without knowledge of the problems addressed, services provided, information obtained, medications prescribed, knowledge of informal support, or preferences expressed in previous settings. This potential for fragmentation of care is heightened by the growing national trend for physicians and other clinicians to restrict their practices to single settings (e.g., hospitals, skilled nursing facilities, ambulatory clinics) and to not follow complex patients as they move between settings. During transitions, these patients are at risk for medical errors, service duplication, inappropriate care, and critical elements of the care plan "falling through the cracks." These risks are especially threatening for frail older patients with multiple co-morbid conditions. Ultimately, poorly executed care transitions lead to poor clinical outcomes, dissatisfaction among patients, and inappropriate use of hospital, emergency, post-acute, and ambulatory services.

The rationale for this position statement is consistent with the release of the timely and compelling Institute of Medicine Report, *Crossing the Quality Chasm: A New Health System for the 21st Century,* which states, "Care for the chronically ill needs to be a collaborative, multidisciplinary process. Effective methods of communication, both among caregivers and between caregivers and patients, are critical to providing high-quality care. Personal health information must accompany patients as they transition from home to clinical office setting to hospital to nursing home and back" (2001, p. 9).

Position 1: Clinical Care Needs

During a care transition, older patients require:
- Preparation for what to expect at the next care site.
- The opportunity to provide input about their values and preferences into the plan of care.
- Clear advice on how to manage their conditions, how to recognize warning symptoms that may indicate their condition has worsened, how to contact a health professional who is familiar with their plan of care, and how to seek immediate care in the setting to which they have transitioned.
- Arrangements for the next level of care (e.g., admission to a rehabilitation facility or a home health agency or an appointment and arrangements for transportation to a follow-up ambulatory visit).
- Stronger adherence to the practice standard that requires timely evaluation by the receiving clinician to identify or verify areas of concern and ensure implementation of the care plan.

During a care transition, the "sending" and "receiving" health care professionals require:
- A uniform plan of care to facilitate communication and continuity across settings.
- An accessible record that contains a current problem list, medication regimen, allergies, advance directives, baseline physical and cognitive function, and contact information for all professional care providers as well as informal care providers.
- Input from informal care providers who are involved in the execution of the plan of care.
- The opportunity to coordinate care with a "coordinating" health professional who oversees both the sending and receiving aspects of the transition. This professional should be skilled in identification of changes in health status, assessment and management of multiple chronic conditions, managing medications, and collaboration with members of the interdisciplinary care team and informal care providers.

Retrieved January 8, 2006, from http://www.americangeriatrics.org/products/positionpapers/complex_carePF.shtml. Used with permission from the American Geriatrics Society.

Continued

BOX 29-9 **American Geriatrics Society Position Statement: Improving the Quality of Transitional Care for Persons with Complex Care Needs—cont'd**

Position 2: Policy Needs

Policymakers need to recognize the critical role of transitional care in the quality and outcomes of care experienced by persons with complex care needs and commit to improving care by:

- Developing new performance indicators designed to measure the effectiveness of transitional care across different delivery settings.
- Launching new quality improvement efforts to address transitions between care settings. Both the "sending" and "receiving" providers of care would be accountable for the success or failure of the patient's transition. Whenever possible, transitional care performance in both fee-for-service and capitated practice environments should be monitored by quality improvement entities such as NCQA, HEDIS, QIOs, JCAHO or a new quality improvement entity.
- Removing barriers and creating incentives to develop electronic communication systems that facilitate the appropriate transfer of essential clinical data between providers with heterogeneous information systems.
- Creating financial incentives for providing transitional care. Essential elements of transitional care should become Medicare benefits (e.g., inter-institutional and inter-professional communication to coordinate their execution of each patient's care plan).
- Discussing the opportunity to link payment to the quality of care delivered, including transitional care, in the formulation of Medicare+Choice capitation.

Position 3: Education Needs

Professional educational institutions, specialty certification boards, licensing boards, and quality improvement programs should seek to improve, evaluate, and monitor health professionals' ability to collaborate across settings in order to execute a common plan of care. Core competencies include the incorporation of patients' and informal care providers' preferences into a plan of care, active communication (telephonic, electronic, or printed paper) with health care professionals across settings, attention to and coordination of individual elements of the plan of care, and ensuring timely transfer to the next level of care or follow-up in the ambulatory setting.

Position 4: Research Needs

In order to advance the understanding and practice of high-quality transitional care, research is needed to:

Develop and test systems of care designed to optimize transitional care. Such interventions need to be patient-centered and be designed to facilitate external adoption in different delivery systems and under different payment mechanisms.

Better understand how to empower persons with complex care needs and their informal care providers to express their preferences and manage their care needs across health care settings. This line of inquiry further necessitates attention to the needs of persons from various ethnic and racial groups.

Develop and test performance indicators and quality improvement technologies that focus on the quality of transitional care.

Determine the most effective incentive strategies for encouraging clinicians and institutions to improve transitional care.

Improve the effectiveness of training health care professionals in transitional care.

Advance and disseminate state-of-the-art information technology systems that facilitate inter-institutional and inter-practitioner communication and collaboration (with appropriate safeguards in place to ensure patient confidentiality).

---

monitor for bleeding, and understand what procedures to follow if bleeding occurs. Mrs. D should understand that she should not take other drugs such as aspirin that also affect coagulation. Plans should include periodic evaluations of prothrombin time/international normalized ratio (INR), and the drug should be discontinued at the appropriate time. If a visit to the dentist is required, Mrs. D should know to inform the dentist about the anticoagulant therapy. Knowledge of the assessment parameters to monitor and the appropriate action to take if a complication arises can have a dramatic influence on outcomes for the older adult.

Telephone follow-up of persons going to residential homes is one method to assess adjustment and to encourage appropriate self-care. It gives the older adult time to settle in, and clarify what questions he/she may have in the actual setting. A call also gives the individual a sense of security that there is someone knowledgeable available to answer questions should they arise. Questions or difficulties may surface in the new setting that had not been apparent in the previous setting. Follow-up calls to long-term or intermediate care facilities may be beneficial as well.

Ombudsman programs provide representation for older adults and their families. Table 29-2 clarifies the role and function of the ombudsman and protection of the older adult's rights.

Proper Placement in Levels of Care. Proper placement in the level of care is critical to the overall well-being and health of the individual. Placing an individual in an environment that requires more abilities to function than the individual possesses sets the individual up for failure physiologically and emotionally and creates further detriment. Placing individuals in an environment that does not allow them to use their skills and abilities enhances the risk of losing those abilities and creating unnecessary dependence. Enforced dependence may cause the individual to act out through difficult or aggressive behaviors, and may contribute to depression.

The best way to assure proper placement and healthy aging is comprehensive assessment. The assessments are best done using a multidimensional approach. Attention to all aspects of the individual's life is important as they overlap and affect the representation of the individual as a whole. One may jump to the conclusion that an individual has cognitive or functional loss, when the reality is that the individual is depressed. An assessment that includes the older adult's abilities, life events, and emotional and functional status provides a basis for appropriate expectations and the identification of needed resources and assistance.

SUMMARY

A helpful way to manage the situation of health care delivery and proper use of health system modalities is to view it from the perspective of the individual, and from the overall system of health care. Centering on the older adult as a multifaceted individual promotes the practice of continuity of care (Andrews, Manthorpe, & Watson, 2004). This is the best viewpoint to facilitate the individual's journey through graceful aging.

Understanding the patterns of health care utilization by older adults and identifying the types of services available to older adults are some of the basic essentials health care providers need to facilitate the older adult's experience. Each individual, while sharing in universal aspects of aging, has his or her own journey with specific variables that need to be considered in this continuum of care.

Organizations are not institutional machines with a staff that function as "parts" of the machine. Organizations are complex adaptive systems capable of change over time. The health care system is adaptable and will change in time based on the decisions and behaviors of the individuals guiding and creating the system. It will never be without flaws, nor will it ever meet all needs, but it can reflect the critical thinking, the vision, and the behaviors of the leaders and team within the system. It

Table 29-2 *Responsibilities of Long-Term Care Ombudsman and Resident's Rights*

Ombudsman Responsibilities	Resident's Rights
Identify, investigate, and resolve complaints made by or on behalf of residents	Be free from chemical and physical restraints
Provide information to residents about long-term care services	Manage own finances
Represent interests of residents before governmental agencies and seek administrative, legal, and other remedies to protect residents	Voice grievances without fear of retaliation
Analyze, comment on, and recommend changes in laws and regulations pertaining to health, safety, welfare, and rights of residents	Associate and communicate privately with any person
	Send and receive personal mail
	Have personal and medical records kept confidential
	Apply for state and federal assistance without discrimination
Educate and inform consumers and general public regarding issues and concerns related to long-term care and facilitate public comment on laws, regulations, policies, and actions	Be fully informed before admission of rights, services available, and all charges
Promote development of citizen organizations to participate in program	Be given advance notice of transfer or discharge
Provide technical support for development of resident and family councils to protect well-being and rights of residents	
Advocate for changes to improve residents' quality of life and care	

Source: Agency on Aging. Retrieved from www.aoa.gov/eldfam/Elder_Rights/LTC/LTC.asp.

is a daunting task that is both a challenge and a great opportunity for health professionals.

Helpful Web sites for additional information include the following:

- www.ahrq.gov
- www.cms.hhs.gov/researchers/
- www.cms.hhs.gov/healthplans/research/ PPOFactSheet.pdf
- www.aoa.gov
- www.cdc.gov/nchs/agingact.htm
- www.hschange.com/index.cgi?topic=topic02
- www.census.gov/population/www/socdemo/ age.html
- www.aone.org/aone/edandcareer/priorities.html

REFERENCES

Aliyu, M. H., Adediran, A. S., & Obisesan, T. O. (2003). Predictors of hospital admissions in the elderly: Analysis of data from the Longitudinal Study on Aging. *Journal of the National Medical Association, 95*(12), 1158-1167.

American Organization of Nurse Executives (AONE), (2003). American Organization of Nurse Executives education and research priorities. Retrieved June 2, 2006, from www.aone.org/aone/index.jsp.

Andrews, J., Manthorpe, J., & Watson, R. (2004). Involving older people in intermediate care. *Journal of Advanced Nursing, 46*(3), 303-310.

Baileff, A. (2000). Integrated nursing teams in primary care. *Nursing Standard, 14*(48), 41-44.

Beck, R. S., Daughtridge, R., & Sloane, P. D. (2002). Physician-patient communication in the primary care office: A systematic review. *Journal of the American Board of Family Practice, 15*(1), 25-38.

Boas, E. (1933). Foreword. In M. C. Jarrett (Ed.), *The problem of chronic illness. Volume 1: Chronic illness in New York City.* New York: Columbia University Press, p. xiii.

Boockvar, K., & Vladeck, B. C. (2004). Improving the quality of transitional care for persons with complex care needs. *Journal of the American Geriatrics Society, 52*(5), 855-856.

Boulanger, J. (2002). Letter with enclosures to Medicare + Choice organizations on risk adjustment. Retrieved August 8, 2004, from www.cms.hhs.gov/healthplans/rates/2003/cover-2003.pdf.

Bulkeley, W. M. (2004). Mayo, IBM join to mine medical data. *The Wall Street Journal,* August 4, p. B1.

Centers for Disease Control and Prevention National Center for Health Statistics. (2003). National Hospital Discharge Survey. Retrieved January 8, 2006 from www.cdc.gov.

Center for Medicare and Medicaid Services. (2005). Program of All-inclusive Care for the Elderly: Overview. Retrieved January 8, 2006, from http://new.cms.hhs.gov.

Chakravarthy, M. V., Joyner, M. J., & Booth, F. W. (2002). An obligation for primary care physicians to prescribe physical activity to sedentary patients to reduce the risk of chronic health conditions. *Mayo Clinic Proceedings, 77*(2), 165-173.

Coleman, E. A., & Boult, C. (2003). Improving the quality of transitional care for persons with complex care needs. *Journal of the American Geriatrics Society, 51,* 556-557.

Davidson, P., MacIntosh, J., McCormack, D., & Morrison, E. (2002). Primary health care: A framework for policy development. *Holistic Nursing Practice, 16*(4), 65-74.

Department of Health. (2005). *Supporting people with long term conditions: Liberating the talents of nurses who care for people with long term conditions.* London, England: Department of Health.

Doebbeling, B. N., Vaughn, T. E., Woolson, R. F., Peloso, P. M., Ward, M. M., Letuchy, E., et al. (2002). Benchmarking Veterans Affairs Medical Centers in the delivery of preventive health services: Comparison of methods. *Medical Care, 40*(6), 540-554.

Federal Interagency Forum on Aging-Related Statistics. (2000). Older Americans 2000: Key indicators of well-being. Retrieved January 8, 2006, from www.agingstats.gov/chartbook2000.

Fitzpatrick, J. J. (2004). Applied nursing research: Translating clinical research into health policy. *Applied Nursing Research, 17*(2), 71.

Flesner, M. K. (2004). Care of the elderly as a global issue. *Nursing Administration Quarterly, 28*(1), 67-72.

Foote, C., & Stanners, C (2002). *Integrating care for older people: New care for old, a systems approach.* Philadelphia: Jessica Kingsley Publishers.

Gabrel, C. S. (2000). *Characteristics of elderly nursing home current residents and discharges: Data from the 1997 National Nursing Home Survey. Advance data from vital and health statistic, No. 312.* Hyattsville, MD: National Center for Health Statistics.

General Household Survey. (2004). Living in Britain: Results from the 2004 General Household Survey, National Statistics. Tables 1.4, 7.27, and 7.30.

Grundy, E. D. (2003). The epidemiology of aging. In R. C. Tallis & H. M. Fillit (Eds.), *Brocklehurst's textbook of geriatric medicine and gerontology* (6th ed.). London: Churchill Livingstone.

Harwood, R. H., Sayer, A. A., & Hirschfeld, M. (2004). Current and future worldwide prevalence of dependency, its relationship to total population, and dependency ratios. *Bulletin of the World Health Organization, 82*(4), 251-258.

Hensrud, D. D. (2000). Clinical preventive medicine in primary care: Background and practice: 2. Delivering primary preventive services. *Mayo Clinic Proceedings, 75*(3), 255-264.

Himelhoch, S., Weller, W. E., Wu, A. W., Anderson, G. F., & Cooper, L. A. (2004). Chronic medical illness, depression, and use of acute medical services among Medicare beneficiaries. *Medical Care, 42*(6), 512-521.

Institute of Medicine Report. (2001). *Crossing the quality chasm: A new health system for the 21st century.* Washington DC: National Academy Press.

Jacque, J., Sokolove, M. D., & Duke Private Sector Conference. (2000). *Academic health systems in transition. Bringing it all together.* Duke Medical Center and Health Systems. Retrieved January 26, 2006, from http://conferences.mc.duke.edu/privatesector/dpsc2000/y.htm.

Kiser, L. J., Lefkovitz, P. M., & Kennedy, L. L. (2001). *The integrated behavioral health continuum: Theory and practice.* Washington, DC: American Psychiatric Publishing.

Kissam, S., Gifford, D. R., Mor, V., & Patry, G. (2003). Admission and continued-stay criteria for assisted living facilities. *Journal of the American Geriatrics Society, 51*(11), 1651-1654.

Lafata, J. E., Pladevall, M., Divine, G., Ayoub, M., & Philbin, E. F. (2004). Are there race/ethnicity differences in outpatient congestive heart failure management, hospital use, and mortality among an insured population? *Medical Care, 42*(7), 680-689.

Longlett, S. K., Kruse, J. E., & Wesley, R. M. (2001). Community-oriented primary care: Critical assessment and implications for resident education. *Journal of the American Board of Family Practice, 14*(2), 141-147.

Ma, E., Coleman, E. A., Fish, R., Lin, M., & Kramer, A. M. (2004). Quantifying posthospital care transitions in older persons. *Journal of the American Medical Directors Association, 5*(2), 71-74.

Manitoba Centre for Health Policy. (2002). Diagnostic Related Groupings (DRGs). Retrieved January 1, 2006, from www.umanitoba.ca/centres/mchp/concept/dict/DRG_overview.html.

McGlynn, E. A., Cassel, C. K., Leatherman, S. T., DeCristofaro, A., & Smits, H. L. (2003). Establishing national goals for quality improvement. *Medical Care, 41*(suppl; 1), 116-129.

Medicare. (2005a). Glossary. Retrieved January 7, 2006, from www.medicare.gov/Glossary.

Medicare. (2005b). Long term care. Retrieved January 7, 2006, from www.medicare.gov/LongTermCare.

Murtaugh, C. M., & Litke, A. (2002). Transitions through postacute and long-term care settings: Patterns of use and outcomes for a national cohort of elders. *Medical Care 2002, 40,* 227-236.

National Center for Health Statistics (NCHS). (2004). Data warehouse on trends in health and aging. Retrieved January 8, 2006, from www.cdc.nchs/agingact.htm [8/2004].

National Center for Health Statistics. (n.d). Deaths—Leading causes. Retrieved January 7, 2006, from www.cdc.gov/nchs/fastats/lcod.htm.

National healthcare disparities report: Summary. (2004). Rockville, MD: Agency for Healthcare Research and Quality. Retrieved from www.ahrq.gov/qual/nhdr03/nhdrsum03.htm.

Pacala, J. T., Boult, C., Urdangarin, C., & McCaffrey, D. (2003). Using self-reported data to predict expenditures for the health care of older people. *Journal of the American Geriatrics Society, 51*(5), 609-614.

Parry, C., Coleman, E. A., Smith, J. D., Frank, J., & Kramer, A. M. (2003). The care transitions intervention: A patient-centered approach to ensuring effective transfers between sites of geriatric care. *Home Health Care Services Quarterly, 22*(3), 1-17.

Piette, M., Ellis, J. L., St. Denis, P., & Sarauer, J. (2002). Integrating ethics and quality improvement: Practical implementation in the transitional/extended care setting. *Journal of Nursing Care Quality, 17*(1), 35-42.

Population Trends. (2004). PT 118, National Statistics, Table 1.4.

Rosenthal, R. A., & Kavic, S. M. (2004). Assessment and management of the geriatric patient. *Critical Care Medicine, 32*(suppl; 4), S92-S105.

Shelley, P. (2000). Evaluating Research. *International Journal of Psychiatric Nursing Research, 6*(1), 649.

Swanson, E., (1999). The world it is a-aging. *Journal of Gerontological Nursing, 25*(12), 35-37.

Synderman, R., & Duke Private Sector Conference. (2000). *Academic health systems in transition. Bringing it all together.* Duke Medical Center and Health Systems. Retrieved January 26, 2006, from http://conferences.mc.duke.edu/privatesector/dpsc2000/y.htm.

Taiwan Alzheimer's Disease Association (TADA). (2004). Retrieved March 30, 2006, from www.tada2002.org.tw/~tada/.

Taiwan Ministry of the Interior. (2004). Retrieved May 9, 2006 from www.ris.gov.tw/ch4/statis/st27-1-94.doc.

Thomas, W. C., Jr. (1969). *Nursing homes and public policy: Drift and decision in New York State.* Ithaca, NY: Cornell University Press.

United Nations. (2002). Madrid International Plan of Action on Aging: 2002. Retrieved January 13, 2006, from www.un.org/esa/socdev/ageing/waa/a-conf-197-9b.htm.

U.S. Department of Health and Human Services. (1999). *Mental health: A report of the Surgeon General.* Rockville, MD: U.S. Department of Health and Human Services, Substance Abuse and Mental Health Services Administration, Center for Mental Health Services, National Institute of Mental Health, National Institutes of Health.

U.S. Senate Special Committee on Aging. (2000). Patients in peril: Critical shortages in geriatric care. Retrieved July 1, 2006 from www.access.gpo.gov/congress/senate/senate22sh107.htm.

Victor, C. (2005). *The social context of ageing: A textbook of gerontology.* London, England: Routledge.

White-Means, S. I. (2000). Racial patterns in disabled elderly persons' use of medical services. *Journals of Gerontology B: Psychological Science, Sociological Science, 55,* S76-S89.

Wolff, J. L., Starfield, B., & Anderson, G. (2002). Prevalence, expenditures, and complications of multiple chronic conditions in the elderly. *Archives of Internal Medicine, 162*(20), 2269-2276.

Zanocchi, M., Maero, B., Francisetti, F., Giona, E., Nicola, E., Margolicci, A., et al. (2003). Multidimensional assessment and risk factors for prolonged hospitalization in the elderly. *Aging—Clinical and Experimental Research, 15*(4), 305-309.

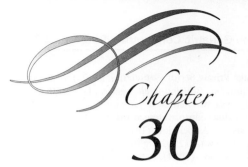

Chapter
30 Community Care

Mary Z. Dunn

Objectives

Define the concept of community and discuss the relationship of the community to health and older adults.

Describe the health services available to older individuals and their families in the community.

Discuss the history of community health nursing and the role of the community health nurse in caring for older adults.

Explain the components of the community assessment with a focus on aging and formulate a plan for nursing intervention with the community as the client.

Describe the characteristics of older adults who reside in the community.

Explain the components of the assessment of an older adult in the community.

Derive nursing diagnoses and design plans of care for the community and individual.

COMMUNITY

Communities are where people live and derive the social meaning in their lives. Gerontological nursing should therefore always be concerned with the communities of older clients.

Definition

The idea of community has many definitions. Anderson & Carter (1974, p. 47) view community as:

"a consciously identified population with common needs and interests, which may include occupation of common physical space, which is organized and engages in common activity including differentiation of functions and adaptation to its environment in order to meet the common needs. Its components include the individuals, groups, families, and organizations within its population and the institutions it forms to meet its needs. Its environment is the society within which it exists and to which it adapts, and other communities and organizations outside itself that impinge on its functioning."

Modern day community health nurses learn that the community is a place where health and illness occur. Communities may be perceived as the location of multiple individual, organizational, and social and cultural resources and assets. Visionaries of community change for health, Kretzman & McKnight (1993, pp. 1-11) describe the assets within communities as follows*:

"Each community boasts a unique combination of assets upon which to build its future. A thorough map of those assets would begin with an inventory of the gifts, skills and capacities of the community's residents. Household by household, building by building, block by block, the capacity mapmakers will discover a vast and often surprising array of individual talents and productive skills, few of which are being mobilized for community-building purposes. This basic truth about the "giftedness" of every individual is particularly important to apply to persons who often find themselves marginalized by communities. It is essential to recognize the capacities, for example, of those who have been labeled mentally handicapped or disabled, or of those who are marginalized because they are too old, or too young, or too poor. In a community whose assets are being fully recognized and mobilized, these people too will be part of the action, not as clients or recipients of aid, but as full contributors to the community-building process.

In addition to mapping the gifts and skills of individuals, and of households and families, the committed community builder will compile an inventory of citizens' associations. These associations, less formal and much less dependent upon paid staff than are formal institutions, are the vehicles through which citizens in the U.S. assemble to solve problems, or to share common interests and activities. It is usually the case that the depth and extent of associational life in any community is vastly underestimated. This is particularly true of lower income communities. In fact, however, though some parts of associational life may have dwindled in very low income neighborhoods, most communities continue to harbor significant numbers of associations with religious, cultural,

---

*Reprinted with permission of Kretzmann, J. P., & McKnight, J. L. (1993). *Building communities from the inside out: A path toward finding and mobilizing a community's assets.* Evanston, IL: Institute for Policy Research, pp. 1-11.

athletic, recreational and other purposes. Community builders soon recognize that these groups are indispensable tools for development, and that many of them can in fact be stretched beyond their original purposes and intentions to become full contributors to the development process.

Beyond the individuals and local associations that make up the asset base of communities are all of the more formal institutions which are located in the community. Private businesses; public institutions such as schools, libraries, parks, police and fire stations; nonprofit institutions such as hospitals and social service agencies—these organizations make up the most visible and formal part of a community's fabric. Accounting for them in full, and enlisting them in the process of community development, is essential to the success of the process. For community builders, the process of mapping the institutional assets of the community will often be much simpler than that of making an inventory involving individuals and associations. But establishing within each institution a sense of responsibility for the health of the local community, along with mechanisms that allow communities to influence and even control some aspects of the institution's relationships with its local neighborhood, can prove much more difficult. Nevertheless, a community that has located and mobilized its entire base of assets will clearly feature heavily involved and invested local institutions."

Etzioni (1993, p. 31) addressed another aspect of community: "When the term community is used, the first notion that typically comes to mind is a place in which people know and care for one another. . . . Communities speak to us in moral voices. They lay claims on their members. Indeed, they are the most important sustaining source of moral voices other than the inner self."

These definitions encompass many of the aspects of the community that contribute to the health and well-being of its citizenry.

Description

One method for describing the community is to examine the environment in which it is situated. Every community has a unique physical location with geographic boundaries as well as man-made and natural physical structures such as schools, waterways, factories, and parks. The physical environment can be very important to health if we consider environmental pollutants and occupational risks. A second way of describing the community is in terms of its social, cultural, and political components and their interactions. The model of community that is presented in the figure depicts determinants of health from an ecological perspective (Figure 30-1). The people are at the core of any community, and health is determined by multiple factors including the social and physical environment and heredity. People's health practices together with their biological inheritance and the environment shape experiences with health, illness, productivity, sense of well-being, and prosperity. Social capital—aspects of a community reflecting trust, security, neighborhood ties, and other benefits of strong social and economic relationships—improves health (Franzini, Caughy, Spears, & Esquer, 2005). Health care is limited by problems of discrimination, inadequate communication, and limited access to care. People need help to improve their "health literacy"

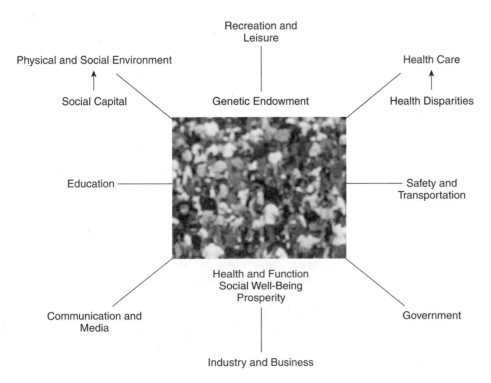

Figure 30-1 Model of community. (From Anderson, E. T., & McFarlane, J. M. [2003]. *Community as partner: Theory and practice in nursing* [4th ed]. Philadelphia: J. B. Lippincott.)

(i.e., their ability to negotiate health care and communicate with health care providers).

Finally, another way to think about communities is from larger to smaller. For example, neighborhoods are smaller communities where people share similar housing and incomes. Neighborhood families may share similar values as well and provide for each other in times of need. In some neighborhoods older adults are the primary population, especially in retirement communities.

Communities, Health, and Aging

Communities have informally and formally provided for the health of their members for all recorded history. Since the late nineteenth century, Western civilization has made formal efforts to provide health services to the community (Clemen-Stone et al., 1991). Nurses have been key professionals in recognizing and resolving community health problems. Problems associated with aging represent a community health challenge for a number of reasons:

- Many of the problems associated with aging are preventable through lifestyle modifications (McGinnis & Foege, 2003).
- Older people are the most frequent consumers of primary health care services of any age- group in the country (United States Senate Special Committee on Aging, 1991).
- Per 100 persons, individuals ages 65 and older have 2 to 3 times the number of visits as younger adults to physicians' offices, hospital outpatient services, and emergency departments (CDC, National Center for Health Statistics, 2004).
- Every year, each person 65 years and older makes approximately 10 health care visits (Federal Interagency Forum on Aging-Related Statistics, 2004).
- Older people are most likely to require long-term, supportive services to maintain independence in the community (Bremer, 1989; Johnson, 1990).

The changing composition of the United States population with escalating numbers of older persons is applying increasing pressure on the health care system. The ability of families to take care of older family members who have disabilities is changing as more women work, and the divorce rate remains high. Families may have to shift care of older members to public and social programs.

Because of these demographic trends, there is concern that health care costs for the older population will continue to grow dramatically. Per capita expenditures for older persons living in the community were more than 3 times those of the nonelderly in 1996—$5644 versus $1865 (Cohen et al., 2000)—and were projected to increase to $7674 (in 1996 dollars) by 2005 (Medical Expenditure Panel, 1996). Medicare and Medicaid long-term care expenditures were also projected to double by 2005 (Burner & Waldo, 1995). These projected increases in taxpayer-funded costs will place great pressure on these programs to reduce costs. Consequently, there is apprehension that continuing and rising pressures to contain costs will adversely affect health care quality and access.

Furthermore, the rapid changes in the health care system that have already occurred have significantly affected the care provided to older persons. For example, previous efforts to control costs have resulted in an increase in Medicare managed care, market instability, and shifting of care to ambulatory settings. There also have been significant changes in the provision and financing of long-term care, with growing use of community-based long-term care such as home care and assisted living communities. The role of institutions has also changed, with nursing homes being used more extensively for subacute care. Nursing homes are confronting many other changes, such as capitation and prospective payment for skilled nursing home care and quality measurement and reporting. There are many unanswered questions about the effect of these changes on quality and cost.

Caring for older people involves clinical complexities that are difficult to coordinate at the health system level and, because of fragmented financing, are also difficult to manage financially. Aging results in both pathophysiological and pharmacokinetic changes that must be addressed in clinical practice. Comorbidity is common, presenting a challenge to clinical management. End-of-life decision making grows in importance, focusing attention on quality of life. Family members often play an important role in providing and managing care, and require education, support, and assistance in these tasks (Eliopoulos, 2005).

Community care is influenced by family attitudes and behaviors in several ways. Family and cultural values shape and reinforce lifestyles, which in turn influence health status. Families provide most of the informal health care its members receive. To help people adopt healthier lifestyles, an attempt should be made to understand the family lifestyle and the individual purposes served by the current lifestyle (Hinds, Chaves, & Cypess, 1992). Provision of services from a health or social service agency is usually only an adjunct to ongoing family care. Therefore careful assessment of family strengths, limitations, and goals is essential in providing appropriate supportive services to meet the goals of both the individual and the family.

Area Agencies on Aging. To find solutions to problems associated with aging in the community care setting, goals should be formulated to guide problem solving. For the *community*, the goal is to recognize and prioritize health needs, and then to mobilize the resources necessary to bring about a healthy community. The community should recognize the problems associated with aging, prioritize the problems that are most urgent, and mobilize the community itself to solve the problems. For the *family,* the goal is to help older people meet their needs in a personally desirable way within the family context. The older person's values should predominate, but collaboration with family members should also take place, so that needs are met and the family network remains intact. For *older individuals,* the goal is to stay as functionally independent as long as possible according to their lifestyles and to maintain a personally satisfying quality of life. Therefore their wishes and preferences must be respected as they are assisted in maintaining their independence (Area Agencies on Aging [AAA], n.d.).

In response to the needs of Americans aged 60 and over, AAAs were established in every local community under the Older Americans Act (OAA) in 1973. The OAA also helps fund aging programs under Title VI to meet the unique needs of older American Indians, Aleuts, Eskimos, and Hawaiians. "The mission of AAAs is to make it easier for older persons to live independently in the comfort of their own surroundings" (AAA, n.d.).

For older adults who wish to remain in their own homes, AAAs in communities across the country plan, coordinate, and offer services that enable them to do just that. AAAs make a range of options available such as meals-on-wheels, homemaker assistance, and other services to make independent living possible (AAA, n.d.). The types of services available through AAA and Title VI agencies are classified as information and access services, community-based services, in-home services, and housing and elder rights. A range of programs is available within each category. These are listed in Box 30-1 (AAA, n.d.).

Among the roles of AAAs and Title VI agencies are to:
- Assess community needs and develop programs to meet those needs
- Advocate for improved services for older persons and their families
- Serve as portals to care, assessing multiple service needs, determining eligibility, authorizing or purchasing services, and monitoring service appropriateness and cost-effectiveness
- Provide direct services and contract with local providers to furnish other community services
- Support a range of home- and community-based services that are specific to the community being served

To find Area Agencies on Aging and Title VI programs across the country, call the nationwide, toll-free Eldercare Locator at (800) 677-1116 (AAA, n.d.).

Healthy Aging Initiative. The Health Services and Resources Administration of the U.S. Department of Health and Human Services has a Healthy Aging Initiative with a mission to increase access to comprehensive primary health care for underserved persons age 50 and older. The initiative focuses on reimbursement, outreach, quality, and modeling of effective approaches for adaptation in other communities.

DESCRIPTION OF COMMUNITY-DWELLING RESIDENTS

A review of the literature by Hays (2002) provided a description of older persons in the United States who live in the community. Almost 96% of older persons reside in the community. Of these, 75% live in single family homes, 20% in multiunit structures, and 6% in manufactured housing. Three fourths of older citizens own their homes with the proportion of homeowners decreasing with older age. About 8% reside in older adult housing such as retirement communities and assisted living facilities.

About half of older persons live with a spouse whereas 31% live alone, 13% live with a relative who is not a spouse, and 2% live with persons who are not relatives. Household composition varies greatly by cohort, gender, race, population density, and social class (Hays, 2002). Data from the *Asset and Health Dynamics Among the Oldest Old* study were used to examine the relationships among health, living arrangements, and marital status (Liang, Brown, Krause, Ofstedal, & Bennett, 2005). For those who were not married, functional status and cognitive function were significantly associated with living arrangements. Among married people, health conditions were not related to living arrangements. With the same functional status, unmarried persons were more likely than married persons to reside with their children or other people. The investigators concluded that a spouse is the greatest guarantee of support in old age (Liang, Brown, Krause, Ofstedal, & Bennett, 2005).

One topic of interest relates to community-dwelling older persons who live alone. Whereas earlier research found more depression in those who lived alone, a large study of Southern California residents found that those who lived with others had higher levels of depression and poorer functioning than those who lived alone (Gustavson & Lee, 2004).

A review of data on living arrangements among older people in Europe revealed an increase in the number of older persons living alone between 1970 and 1990. The trend stabilized or declined between 1990 and 2000. Variations among countries were attributed to different attitudes towards residential care and parent-child coresidence (Tomassini, Glaser, Wolf, Broese van Groenou, & Grundy, 2004).

COMMUNITY SETTINGS OF CARE

The goal of community-based services is to promote the independence of older persons and to provide an alternative to institutional care. Community-based services include public and private hospitals, community health

BOX 30-1 Services Available through AAA and Title VI Agencies

Information and Access Services

- **Information and Referral/Assistance**—a source for locating services available from a AAA or Title VI agency or from another service agency in the community
- **Health Insurance Counseling**—helps beneficiaries understand their options and rights under Medicare, Medicare1Choice, and Medicaid and obtain information on Medigap and other insurance alternatives
- **Client Assessment**—a determination of the client's needs and eligibility for services
- **Care Management**—a review of an individual's social, psychological, and physical health challenges, resulting in a "plan of care" for services or treatment, if appropriate
- **Transportation**—transportation to critical destinations such as a doctor's office or the grocery store
- **Caregiver Support**—education and resources that enable caregivers to provide care for an older family member while maintaining their own quality of life
- **Retirement Planning and Education**—help for older adults as they prepare for their retirement, with a focus on issues such as pensions, health concerns, legal issues, and work and leisure options

Community-Based Services

- **Employment Services**—a way to help the individual find meaningful work, including assessment, testing, job counseling, education, and placement
- **Senior Centers**—a gathering place where older adults can enjoy social, physical, and recreational activities; senior centers may serve as congregate meal sites
- **Congregate Meals**—group meals served at senior centers, schools, and other sites for the purpose of providing a nutritious meal in a social environment
- **Adult Day Care Services**—a community-based group program designed to meet the needs of functionally impaired adults and provide respite for their caregivers
- **Volunteer Opportunities**—a way for healthy older adults to continue to contribute to their community

In-Home Services

- **Meals-on-Wheels**—midday and evening meals delivered to individuals who cannot shop or prepare their own meals, often by a volunteer who also provides a sense of security and social contact to a homebound individual
- **Homemakers**—assistance with tasks essential to maintaining a household, such as food shopping and housekeeping
- **Chore Services**—a step beyond homemaking: includes minor home repairs, yard work, and general home maintenance
- **Telephone Reassurance**—regular, prescheduled calls to homebound older adults to reduce isolation and provide a routine safety check
- **Friendly Visiting**—periodic neighborly visits to homebound older adults to provide social contact and reassurance
- **Energy Assistance and Weatherization**—payment of fuel bills and home weatherization for low-income people
- **Emergency Response Systems**—electronic devices that allow individuals to contact a response center in the case of an emergency, such as a fall
- **Home Health Services**—a variety of services, including skilled nursing care, health monitoring, dispensing of medication, physical and other forms of therapy, and instructing individuals and family members about home care
- **Personal Care Services**—assistance with bathing, feeding, walking, and other daily activities
- **Respite Care**—a break for family members from caregiving responsibilities for a short period of time

Housing

- **Senior Housing**—housing designed to accommodate the needs and preferences of independent older adults
- **Alternative Community-Based Living Facilities**—a range of housing facilities that bridge the gap between independent living and nursing homes, such as assisted living and adult foster care

Elder Rights

- **Legal Assistance**—advice and counsel for older persons and their families faced with financial and legal concerns
- **Elder Abuse Prevention Programs**—designed to alleviate situations of abuse, neglect, or self-neglect; includes programs such as adult protection and guardianship/conservatorship
- **Ombudsmen Services for Complaint Resolution**—ombudsmen investigate and, when possible, resolve complaints made by or on behalf of older adults who are residents of long-term care facilities

centers (CHCs), local health departments, free and school-based clinics, and physician charity care. Providers, such as community health centers and public hospitals, that serve low-income people including the uninsured remain the anchor for community care. The nation's health care community safety net for low-income and uninsured people has become somewhat stronger over the past 8 years. Uniform access throughout the United States remains a goal as service gaps and financial planning and strategies still vary across communities (Felland, Kinner, & Hoadley, 2003; U.S. Department of Health and Human Services [USDHHS] Agency for Healthcare Research and Quality, 2004).

Physician Outpatient Services

Use of physician services increases with age. Physician visits and consultations increased from about 1.8 visits per person in 1990 to more than 13 visits per person in 1998 (Table 30-1). In the United States, physicians are gatekeepers to many other services within the continuum of care for older adults, including hospitals, nursing homes, laboratory services, rehabilitation services, nursing services, and pharmaceutical services. Some physicians practice a team approach to medical care, meaning that they routinely consult with members of other disciplines in assessing the needs of older patients and in planning their care. Some share office space with members of other disciplines such as nurses, psychologists, and nutritionists. More commonly, however, in private practice, physicians provide medical care in their offices and make referrals with minimal interaction with other care providers.

Historically, individuals looked to family physicians to address all their health needs. Those age 85 years and older may remember the days of the general practitioner who made house calls and was a community figure as well as a care provider. Currently few physicians are able to manage all of the older adults' needs because of time and financial constraints, the increased complexity of specialty care, and the lack of control over the services provided by the multidisciplinary helping network such as physical therapy, personal care attendants, and family members.

Older adults are more involved in guiding their care now than in the past (Andrews, Manthorpe, & Watson, 2004). The media and the Internet have greatly expanded access to health care information. Therefore, older adults may come armed with carefully researched current information that is relevant to their situation. Clients expect the health care provider to be well-informed and willing to consider what the client thinks. On the other hand, older adults sometimes hear or see information from unreliable sources, or take information that is based on a single study and apply it inappropriately to their situation.

The effective health care professional in the office setting must be informed, clarify information, and thoughtfully apply that information to the particular situation. Borders, Rohrer, Xu, & Smith (2004) surveyed 5000 community-dwelling older adults and found that those who never rated their medical care as satisfactory were those who were skeptical of prescription drugs, felt they knew more than their physician, and worried about their health consistently.

Outpatient Clinics

Outpatient clinics often are associated with community or teaching hospitals, or with community service agencies. Their focus generally is on patients with chronic disease problems, such as diabetes and hypertension, but patients with any medical or surgical problem, acute or chronic, might be seen. The goal is to diagnose and treat the presenting illness.

Outpatient clinics may offer physician services, nursing services, rehabilitative services, and laboratory and diagnostic services. In large hospitals, the clinics usually are organized along medical subspecialty lines. This can be problematic for older persons, who frequently have multiple chronic diseases and thus may be cared for in several clinics, rather than receiving coordinated medical and health care in one central location. This situation is improving with an increase in interdisciplinary clinics.

Nurses in community care strive to determine the least costly and most sustainable ways to respond to disablement while promoting the autonomy and well-being of chronically ill elders and their caregivers (Capitman, 2003). While effectively managing the older adult's chronic conditions, health promotion remains a priority. Nurse-led clinics are becoming more common and are greatly valued by older adults. An example from the literature is a nurse-led program in a diabetes clinic that was found to significantly improve the detection and management of diabetic nephropathy (Craig et al., 2004).

Mental disorders comprise 4 of the 10 leading causes of disability for persons age 55 and older, with major depression being the leading cause of disability in developed countries (U.S. Department of Health and Human Services, 1999). Twenty percent of individuals in this age-group experience a mental illness, with some evidence that the prevalence among Americans age 55 and older may be underreported (Administration on Aging, 2004). Older adults tend to underuse mental health services for a variety of reasons: social stigma, transportation problems, costs, and misconceptions about aging and mental health. Believing that mental health disorders and treatment are shameful or will lead to a loss of autonomy causes many older adults in need of treatment either to deny the mental health problem or to refuse treatment by a mental health provider.

Table 30-1 *Number of Mental Health Organizations by Type of Organization: United States, Selected Years 1970–1998**

Type of Organization	1970	1976	1980	1986	1990	1992	1994	1998
NUMBER OF MENTAL HEALTH ORGANIZATIONS								
All organizations	3005	3480	3727	4747	5284	5498	5392	5722
State and county mental hospitals	310	303	280	285	273	273	256	229
Private psychiatric hospitals	150	182	184	314	462	475	430	348
Nonfederal general hospitals with separate psychiatric services	797	870	923	1351	1674	1616	1612	1707
VA medical centers[†]	115	126	136	139	141	162	161	145
Federally funded community mental health centers	196	517	691	—	—	—	—	—
Residential treatment centers for emotionally disturbed children	261	331	368	437	501	497	459	461
All other mental health organizations[‡]	1176	1151	1145	2221	2233	2457	2474	2832
NUMBER WITH 24-HOUR HOSPITAL AND RESIDENTIAL TREATMENT SERVICE								
All organizations	1734	2273	2526	3039	3430	3415	3827	3729
State and county mental hospitals	310	303	280	285	273	273	256	229
Private psychiatric hospitals	150	182	184	314	462	475	430	348
Nonfederal general hospitals with separate psychiatric services	664	791	843	1287	1571	1517	1531	1593
VA medical centers[†]	110	112	121	124	130	133	135	123
Federally funded community mental health centers	196	517	691	—	—	—	—	—
Residential treatment centers for emotionally disturbed children	261	331	368	437	501	497	459	461
All other mental health organizations[‡]	43	37	39	592	493	520	1016	975
NUMBER WITH LESS THAN 24-HOUR CARE[§]								
All organizations[†]	2156	2318	2431	3146	3189	3390	4087	4387
State and county mental hospitals	195	147	100	83	84	75	70	60
Private psychiatric hospitals	100	60	54	114	176	198	347	263
Nonfederal general hospitals with separate psychiatric services	376	303	299	497	633	618	875	965
VA medical centers[†]	100	113	127	137	141	161	148	129
Federally funded community mental health centers	196	517	691	—	—	—	—	—
Residential treatment centers for emotionally disturbed children	48	57	68	99	163	167	227	210
All other mental health organizations[‡]	1141	1121	1092	2016	1992	2171	2420	2760

Sources: Published and unpublished inventory data from the Survey and Analysis Branch, Division of State and Community Systems Development, Center for Mental Health Services. In Manderscheid, R. W., Atay, J. E., Hernandez-Cartagena, M. D. R., Edmond, P. Y., Male, A., Parker, T. C. E., & Zhang, H. (2006). Mental health, United States 2000. Retrieved January 7, 2006, from http://mentalhealth.samhsa.gov/publications/allpubs/SMA01-3537/chap14.asp.

*Some organizations were reclassified as a result of changes in reporting procedures and definitions. For 1979 to 1980, comparable data were not available for certain organization types, and data for either an earlier or a later period were substituted. These factors influence the comparability of 1980, 1986, 1990, 1992, and 1994 data with those of earlier years.

[†]Includes Department of Veterans Affairs (formerly Veterans Administration) (VA) neuropsychiatric hospitals, VA general hospital psychiatric services, and VA psychiatric outpatient clinics.

[‡]Includes freestanding psychiatric outpatient clinics, partial care organizations, and multiservice mental health organizations. Multiservice mental health organizations were redefined in 1984.

[§]The 1994 survey format was changed, and partial care is now included with outpatient; together these are called "less than 24-hour care."

Legislation in the 1960s resulted in a movement to deinstitutionalize care of mental illness in the United States. From 1963 to 1980, the census in state and county mental hospitals declined by about two thirds. Federal funds supported the establishment of more than 500 community mental health centers (CMHCs)

(Rochefort, 1984). Centers were designed to prevent psychiatric hospitalization. In some communities, they have developed into sites for outpatient psychotherapy services. In other communities, they serve as screening points for people referred for psychiatric hospitalization and provide only limited aftercare services for those discharged from mental hospitals. Funding difficulties have reduced their potential for impact, primarily in the area of prevention (Bird & Parslow, 2002).

Information on specialty mental health organizations in the United States is compiled both by The Survey of Mental Health Organizations and General Hospital Mental Health Services and by Managed Behavioral Health Care Organizations (SMHO) (Sources and Qualifications of Data from the Survey of Mental Health Organization, 2005). Table 30-2 summarizes the types of organizations that offer mental health services. An outpatient mental health clinic provides only ambulatory

Table 30-2 *Major Age-Related Health Problems and Associated Risk Factors*

Major Age-Related Problems	Associated Risk Factors
Stroke	Smoking Sedentary lifestyle Cardiovascular disease Hypertension
Cancer	Environmental exposure to carcinogens Tobacco use (both smoking and smokeless tobacco) Family history of cancer Presence of "premalignant lesions" Diet
Cardiovascular disease (including congestive heart failure and peripheral vascular disease)	Smoking Sedentary lifestyle Diet high in cholesterol High serum triglycerides Family history of cardiovascular disease
Chronic lung disease	Smoking Exposure to environmental toxins, such as coal dust, cotton dust, asbestos
Dementing disorders	Hypertension, as in Binswanger's dementia or multi-infarct dementia Social isolation Sensory deprivation
Depression	Multiple losses Family history Social isolation Multiple drug use (as adverse side effect of drug therapy)
Adult-onset diabetes mellitus	Obesity Sedentary lifestyle Family history
Digestive disorders	Diet
Substance abuse	Family history Limited coping resources Social isolation
Hip fracture	Osteoporosis Frequent falls Depression Dementia Reduced physical agility

Continued

Table 30-2 *Major Age-Related Health Problems and Associated Risk Factors—cont'd*	
Major Age-Related Problems	**Associated Risk Factors**
Inappropriate institutionalization	Shortage of community-based supportive services Lack of geriatric multidimensional assessment services Lack of preinstitutionalization screening program
Elderly neglect or abuse	Inadequate family resources for long-term care Inadequate community-based services for long-term care
Poverty	Inadequate planning for postretirement income Catastrophic medical illness with inadequate insurance coverage
Family caregiver burnout	Insufficient knowledge of difference between normal aging process and results of disease Insufficient information about techniques of care Inadequate community support services Inadequate access to rehabilitatively oriented care Inadequate emotional support

mental health services. A psychiatrist generally assumes the medical responsibility for all patients/clients and/or for direction of the mental health program.

The importance of mental health care for older adults was voiced by Josefina G. Carbonell (2003), the Assistant Secretary for Aging, who said, "Too many of our elders struggle to cope with difficult life situations or mental health and substance abuse concerns that negatively affect their ability to participate fully in life."

Depression is a major mental health problem among older people. An estimated 20% of older adults in the community and up to 37% in primary care settings experience symptoms of depression (USDHHS, 1999). One factor that places the older adult at higher risk for depression is the comorbidity of chronic disease. Anxiety symptoms also are common in both depressed and nondepressed older people (AAA, 2004; Maynard, 2003; Mehta et al., 2003). Because of the underuse of community mental health clinics, the primary care provider must be especially alert to recognize and intervene when mental health care is needed by the older adult. Assessment and treatment often are handled by the primary physician, without a referral to a specialist in psychiatry. Without collaboration between the primary practitioner and the subspecialty areas of health care, mental conditions may not be properly diagnosed and treated.

A disturbing phenomenon that is being detected with increasing frequency is elder abuse. It most often occurs when an older person becomes more dependent and requires increased care (Turkoski, 2003). It may be undetected because it usually occurs at home, and is committed by spouses, children, or other family members.

This places the home health nurse in a key position to detect situations that foster abuse or the actual occurrence of abuse.

Home Health Care

The Boston Dispensary created the first home care program in the United States in 1796. The three founding principles were:

1. The sick, without being pained on a separation from their families, may be attended and relieved in their own houses.
2. The sick can, in this way, be assisted at less expense to the public than in any hospital.
3. Those who have seen better days may be comforted without being humiliated, and all the poor receive the benefits of a charity, the more refined as it is the more secret (Goodwin, 1871-1955).

More information concerning The Boston Dispensary can be accessed at www.simmons.edu/libraries/archives/char_coll/char_coll_027.htm.

During the late eighteenth and early nineteenth century, the poor and homeless received care in the hospital, whereas the wealthy patients were treated at home. In the late 1800s, lay persons organized and offered home nursing services. Voluntary agencies, such as the Henry Street Settlement founded by nurse Lillian Wald, began providing home nursing care around this time, and these later became visiting nurse associations. Around 1900, graduate nurses began to provide home nursing care. With advancing technology and improving sanitation and living conditions, health care needs shifted from communicable diseases to long-term illnesses. Hospitals became overcrowded and attempted to alleviate this problem by developing home care for discharged hospital patients. By the mid-1940s home health care providers included government agencies, voluntary health associates, private insurance companies, and hospital-based programs.

Although most of the home care received by older persons with disabilities is unpaid, the use of informal care as an exclusive means of assistance is declining. The percentage of older Americans with disabilities who received only informal care declined from 74% in 1982 to 64% in 1994, while the percentage of older persons who received both informal and formal care increased from 21% to 28% over the same period.

This excerpt from one of Florence Nightingale's letters reflects her crusade for home health:

"We will now deal with the PRESENT STATE OF RURAL HYGIENE, which is indeed a pitiful and disgusting story, dreadful to tell. For the sake of giving actual facts, it is no use lecturing upon drainage, water supply, wells, pigsties, storage of excrement, storage of refuse, etc., etc., in general; they are dreadfully concrete, I take leave to give the facts of one rural district, consisting of villages and one small market town, as described by a Local Government Board official this year; and I will ask the ladies here present whether they could not match these facts in every county in the kingdom. Perhaps, too, the lady lecturers on Rural Hygiene will favour us with some of their experiences" (quoted in Seymer, 1957).

She discussed the state of rural hygiene, proposed a strategy to educate the community one woman at a time, and successfully changed the health for the whole community. Home health nursing was one facet of nursing that she envisioned.

Fast forward to the present day when home health care is a well-established component of the health care system. In 2001, approximately 3.5 million older and disabled Americans received care from nearly 7000 Medicare-certified home health agencies (Fermazin, Canady, Milmine, Perron, & Cooper, 2004). Home health care is provided in the individual's own home, and involves skilled care, personal care, and/or education for self-care. According to the Centers for Medicare and Medicaid Services (2005), individuals who are eligible for nursing facility services under their state's Medicaid plan also are eligible for home health services. A physician must order these services as part of a plan of care, and must review that plan every 60 days. The plan must include nursing services, as defined in the state's Nurse Practice Act. Home health aide services and medical supplies, equipment, and appliances suitable for use in the home may be provided as well. "Physical therapy, occupational therapy, speech pathology, and audiology services are optional services that states may choose to provide." See http://new.cms.hhs.gov for more information about home health services.

The establishment of Medicare in 1965 had great impact on the expansion of home care during the next 2 decades, with federal regulations for home care agencies requiring them to provide nursing and one additional service. In recent years, cost-containment efforts, because of the rising cost of health care, have increased the focus on home health care.

Today the majority of older persons with disabilities live in the community with the assistance of family members. Although most of the care they receive is informal and voluntary, individuals with more severe disabilities are likely to use both informal and formal long-term care. The percentage of older Americans has gradually declined despite a slight rise in the total number of older Americans receiving assistance. The decreasing percentage of older adults needing assistance may be explained by the improving health status of the older population, the increasing number of residential options, such as assisted living, and the availability of environmental modifications and adaptive tools that enable disabled individuals to function more independently in the community.

The use of formal (paid) care has been increasing, possibly because of the growing frail population aged 85 and older, the improved financial status of many older adults, the increased numbers of individuals with supplemental health care coverage, the liberalization of home health coverage rules under Medicare, and the expansion of home and community-based services under Medicaid (National Alliance for Caregiving & American Association of Retired Persons [AARP], 1997).

Several sources of information are available to help in the selection of a home health care agency. Internet availability offers health care professionals and consumers a fast and easily accessible view of valid and reliable information related to the care practices of every Medicare-certified home health agency (HHA) in the country. Nationally reported quality measures for HHAs are posted on Medicare's Home Health Compare Web site (www.medicare.gov) for every Medicare-certified HHA in the United States (Box 30-2). Phase I of the Home Health Quality Initiative (HHQI) began in 2003 with the publication of home health quality measures for eight states. HHQI has two core goals: (1) to provide assistance to HHAs to help them continue to improve care; (2) to provide information about home health quality to help consumers make informed decisions. The HHQI rates home health agencies on the basis of 11 descriptive quality measures. Measures now are available for home health agencies nationwide at www.cms.hhs.gov/HomeHealthQualityInits/. The measures for the HHQI are a subset of a larger set of outcomes assessment and information set (OASIS) outcome measures that are well-known to the home health agencies (Box 30-3). Four measures are related to improvement

BOX 30-2 ANA Nurse Sensitive Quality Indicators

INDICATOR	RECOMMENDED DEFINITION
Pressure ulcers	(Number of patients with NPUAP-AHCPR stage I, II, III, or IV ulcers)/(number of patients in prevalence study) $\times$ 100
Patient falls	(Total number of patient falls $\times$ 1000)/(total number of patient days)
Patient satisfaction with pain management	Patient opinion of how well nursing staff managed their pain as determined by scaled responses to uniform series of questions designed to elicit resident views regarding specific aspects of pain management
Patient satisfaction with educational information	Patient opinion of nursing staff efforts to educate them regarding their conditions and care requirements as determined by scaled response to uniform series of questions designed to elicit patient views regarding specific aspects of patient education activities
Patient satisfaction with nursing care	Patient opinion of care received from nursing staff during hospital stay as determined by scaled responses to uniform series of questions designed to elicit patient views regarding satisfaction with key elements of nursing care services
Patient satisfaction with overall care	Patient opinion of care received during hospital stay as determined by scaled responses to uniform series of questions designed to elicit patient views regarding global aspects of care
Mix of RNs, LPNs, and unlicensed staff care for patients	Percent of registered nursing care hours as a total of all nursing care hours
Total nursing care hours provided per patient per day	Total number of productive hours worked by nursing staff with direct patient care responsibilities per patient day
Nurse staff satisfaction*	Job satisfaction expressed by nurses working in hospital settings as determined by scaled response to uniform series of questions designed to elicit nursing staff attitudes toward specific aspects of their employment situations

From Mueller, C., & Karon, S. L. (2004). ANA nurse sensitive quality indicators for long-term care facilities. *Journal of Nursing Care Quality, 19*(1), 39-47.
*Not included in this research study.

in mobility, four measures are related to meeting basic daily needs, two measures are related to patient medical emergencies, and one measure is related to improvement in mental health. Keepnews, Capitman, & Rosati (2004) examined the use of the OASIS data to analyze patient-level outcomes of home health care and noted the benefit of analysis of patient-level functional outcomes of short-term home health services.

The Centers for Medicare and Medicaid Services (CMS) Home Health Compare Web site gives consumers access to home health quality measures to help them choose a home health agency. The Home Health Compare Web site (www.medicare.gov) also offers case managers and discharge planners easily accessible data for helping clients select a HHA. The CMS (2004) cre-

ated the pamphlet *Medicare and Home Health Care,* which was designed to help people find and compare home health agencies. It includes information about eligibility for Medicare coverage of home health care, services that Medicare does and does not cover, quality of care, and resources for more information. It can be accessed on the Internet or a hard copy can be ordered. A list of questions to ask when selecting and comparing home health agencies is a helpful tool for older adults and their families (Figure 30-2) and can be accessed through the Internet at www.cms.hhs.gov/quality/hhqi/HHBenefits.pdf.

Research has explored various aspects of home health care. Validation of the value of home care is one area that has been a topic of scrutiny. Inglis et al.

BOX 30-3 Assessment Model for Home Health Care

I. Assessment of Need
  A. *Overview of health care system*
    1. Organization
    2. Payment systems
    3. Health care providers
  B. *Needs of health care consumers*
    1. Medical diagnoses
    2. Nursing diagnoses and nursing needs
    3. How needs best met

II. Assessment of Services
  A. *Federal and state regulations*
  B. *Home health services*
    1. Number
    2. Location
    3. Type
    4. Services provided
  C. *Interagency relationships*
    1. Hospital discharge planning
    2. Coordination of care
    3. Communication among health care professionals

III. Implications for Nursing
  A. *Education*
  B. *Service*
  C. *Research*

(2004) demonstrated fewer readmissions, fewer days of hospitalization, and fewer fatal events among persons with atrial fibrillation who were managed with a nurse-led multidisciplinary home-based intervention.

Improving the fit of those home services that people need with the services that are available is the ultimate goal of the nurse in guiding the best care for each client within the community. In the process of examining the fit between the needs of long-term patients and the actual use of home care, Algera, Francke, Kerkstra, & van der Zee (2004) were able to develop a profile of people with long-term conditions who used home care. In general, it was found that older, non-white women with multiple chronic diseases and impairments, and who had recently had inpatient care, tended to make more use of professional home care. The investigators recommended examination of the system- and patient-related characteristics to determine the reason for the common mismatch between care need and use (Algera et al., 2004).

When care is provided in the home, communication between all involved parties can become complicated. Larsson, Larsson, & Carlson (2004) studied communication among care providers, recipients of care, and the families of older adults receiving care. They found that patients' views of the quality of care were congruent with the opinions of family members if they lived together and shared the same daily experiences. This is significant because family members of older adults often are not in close proximity. The positive effect of home health care on family functioning also has been demonstrated by the finding that people living with their family demonstrated more independence in making decisions about their illness and life than those who were hospitalized (Kanervisto, Paavilainen, & Astedt-Kurki, 2003).

Types of Home Health Agencies. Home health care is provided by hospitals, private profit and nonprofit agencies, and public agencies. All home health care shares the characteristic of being tertiary (acute) care. Home health care is distinguished from home health visits, which are focused on health promotion (primary prevention).

HOSPITAL-BASED HOME HEALTH AGENCIES. Hospitals may provide posthospitalization services directly or arrange referral of patients to existing home health agencies. Hospitals establish their own home health agencies to maintain control of these services. The advantages of hospital-based home health agencies are threefold: financial, organizational, and community. Financial benefits include providing an additional source of revenue for the hospital and retaining patients within the hospital system. Smooth patient referrals to home health agencies or skilled nursing facilities help to reduce hospital length of stay and therefore costs of care. Organizational benefits include the use of available health staff, management, and support services and increased control of health care services. Services also can be provided where there is a gap in existing home health services. Advantages to the community include continuity of care between the hospital and the community, integration of health programs and services, and use of the community as a hospital referral source.

Robinson and Street (2004) studied the role of acute care nurses in discharge planning of older patients from hospital to home. They found that acute care nurses had limited knowledge and understanding of the care system of older persons and how to access appropriate services. The investigators concluded that acute care nurses need to learn more about services available to support older people following discharge. They recommended that nurses in acute care be offered interactive continuing education using a case study approach to enhance their knowledge and empower them to become more involved in discharge planning. Recent changes in Medicare limit the services available in homes so that discharge planning is not nearly as prevalent as it was when funding for these services was more readily available. Because changes in funding for health care occur frequently, continual updates are necessary for nurses to remain currently informed.

Is/Does the Agency:	Yes	No	Comment
1. Medicare-certified?			
2. Medicaid-certified?			
3. Offer the specific health care services I need (such as nursing or physical therapy)?			
4. Meet my special needs (such as language or cultural preference)?			
5. Offer the personal care services I need (such as bathing, dressing, and using the bathroom)?			
6. Offer the support services I need (such as help with laundry, cooking, shopping, or housekeeping), or help me arrange for additional services, such as meals-on-wheels, that I may need also?			
7. Have staff available to provide the type and hours of care my doctor ordered, and can start when I need them?			
8. Recommended by my hospital discharge planner, doctor, or social worker?			
9. Have staff available at night and on weekends for emergencies?			
10. Explain what my insurance will cover, and what I must pay out-of-pocket?			
11. Perform background checks on all staff?			
12. Have letters from satisfied patients, family members, and doctors that testify to the home health agency staff providing good care?			

Figure 30-2 Questions to ask about home health. (Taken from U.S. Department of Health and Human Services, Centers for Medicare and Medicaid Services, Publication No. CMS-0969, April, 2003.)

PROFIT/NONPROFIT/PUBLIC HOME HEALTH AGENCIES. Profit-making or proprietary home care companies are licensed by individual states for governmental reimbursement. Nonprofit agencies provide essentially the same services as for-profit agencies; however, each agency is autonomously run by members of local communities. They are governed by a board of directors made up of community members with various areas of expertise such as registered nurses, physicians, allied health care providers, business people, and community leaders. Agencies are funded by reimbursement from federal, state, and private insurance (Medicare, Medicaid, Blue Cross), direct payment from the patient, and contributions.

Hospice

Hospice is a concept of care for dying patients that emphasizes family-centered care, sophisticated pain and symptom management in terminal illness, and care of the bereaved. The focus of care is on terminally ill patients and their families, with the expressed goal of helping them to live as fully as possible until death occurs.

Services included in such a program of care vary according to the nature of the particular hospice. Approximately 80% of hospice care is provided in the home of the patient or family member or in nursing homes. Most provide round-the-clock professional nurse availability, chaplain service, medical services, and a strong volunteer service. Inpatient hospice facilities are sometimes available to assist with caregiving but are not the common modality of hospice (http://www.hospicefoundation.org).

Hospice offers a multidimensional team that facilitates not only the family but also the health care professionals involved in the care of the family member. The Institute of Medicine described a decent or good death as "free from avoidable distress and suffering for patients, families, and caregivers; in general accord with patients' and families' wishes; and reasonably consistent with clinical, cultural, and ethical standards" (Field & Cassell, 1997, p. 24).

Eligibility requirements for hospice care are:
- Eligible for Medicare Part A (hospital insurance)
- Physician's certification that the individual is terminally ill and probably has less than 6 months to live

- A statement choosing hospice care instead of routine Medicare-covered benefits for terminal illness (Medicare will still pay for covered benefits for any health problems that are not related to the terminal illness)
- Care provided by a Medicare-approved hospice program

A common question asked by a prospective hospice client is the following: "What if I don't die in six months?" Hospice care is authorized for two 90-day periods, followed by an unlimited number of 60-day periods (http://www.medicare.gov/Publications/Pubs/pdf/02154.pdf).

More than 3100 hospice programs exist in the United States, Puerto Rico, and Guam. Hospice programs cared for nearly 540,000 people in the United States in 1998. Although hospice is a vital care option, it is underused by older adults. One study showed that less than 10% of patients with end-stage heart failure actually enroll in hospice programs for which they may be eligible (Zambroski, 2004).

In assisting individuals and families to find the best hospice, the following questions are suggested by the National Hospice and Palliative Care Organization:

- What services are provided?
- What kind of support is available to the family/caregiver?
- What roles do the attending physician and hospice play?
- What does the hospice volunteer do?
- How does hospice work to keep the patient comfortable?
- How are services provided after hours?
- How and where does hospice provide short-term inpatient care?
- Can hospice be brought into a nursing home or long-term care facility?

The Centers for Medicare and Medicaid Services (2005) have allowed coverage for hospice care and have made recent changes to facilitate use of these services. They offer a valuable handbook titled *Medicare Hospice Benefits*, updated in July 2005 that is also available in large print through the Internet at www.medicare.gov/Publications/Pubs/pdf/02154.pdf. Medicare pays nearly all the following costs for hospice patients: physician services, nursing care, medical equipment (such as wheelchairs or walkers), medical supplies (such as bandages and catheters), medication for symptom control and pain relief, short-term care in the hospital (including respite care, home health aide, and homemaker services), physical and occupational therapy, speech therapy, social worker services, dietary counseling, and grief counseling.

Research has illuminated various aspects of hospice care. DeSilva, Dillon, & Teno (2001) found that one in five families felt that more could have been done to make their loved one comfortable. Families that are able to care for their dying family member are better able to participate in decision making, and receive spiritual support during this difficult period. Families using hospice services in the nursing home setting stated it provided, but did not duplicate, services for their family member (Casarett, Karlawish, Morales, Crowley, Mirsch, & Asch, 2005; Forbes, Bern-Klug, & Gessert, 2000; Hanson, Danis, & Garrett, 1997). Chapter 22 provides additional discussion of end of life care.

Assisted Living

Assisted living is a more recent development in living arrangements for older adults. Assisted living meets older adults' needs for food preparation, housework, and home maintenance, while allowing them to conduct other activities of daily living independently. Many assisted living facilities are part of elder residences with levels of care ranging from independent living apartments to nursing home care. This assures that older adults will be able to spend the rest of their lives in the same basic environment with the same neighbors. The term "boarding home" also may be used to describe this type of facility. Adult family homes are residential homes that provide room, board, laundry, necessary supervision, ADL assistance, personal care, and social services. These homes are licensed to care for a maximum of six residents (King County Long-Term Care Ombudsman, n.d.).

One reason for considering assisted living relates to the neurological changes of aging. As people age, they may have diminished executive function—that part of the working brain that is necessary for multiple step activities such as meal preparation. Individuals with poor executive function are more likely to leave the stove burners on, forget what they are doing in the middle of a chore, or find that they cannot complete a task. Managing food preparation and caring for a house are difficult for individuals who have lost this functional ability; thus assisted living is one arrangement families may consider.

Changing health and functional status may necessitate a change in living arrangements from assisted living to more direct or supervised care. Reasons for discharge from assisted living to other types of care have been identified as progression of dementia, need for more assistance with activities of daily living, incontinence, wandering, changes in physical condition, and aggressive behaviors (Aud, 2004). The most important consideration is to find a balance between safety, health, and the elder's desire to live independently. Decisions about changes in living arrangements, especially those that require separation from an environment that is known and comfortable, require the input of an interdisciplinary team of providers and family members. See Chapter 31 for further discussion of assisted living.

Nutrition Sites/Senior Centers

Older people who are in need of socialization and a good meal may participate in senior center programs. Supported by the Older Americans Act that was amended in 1972 to provide a national nutrition program, nutrition centers provide lunch to participants at no cost or for a small fee commonly based on a sliding-scale. These programs offer much more than food; often it is the highlight of the day for the homebound older adult. These programs offer interaction and a sense of caring. In addition to recreational activities such as singing, playing cards, and participating in arts and crafts, some centers serve a linkage function that facilitates access to other community services. Health-related assessments and learning experiences (such as blood pressure and oral cancer screening, nutrition counseling, and exercise programs) are also provided. Transportation to the centers usually is provided.

Home-delivered meals, provided through churches serving the communities or through programs such as meals-on-wheels, offer one hot meal per day to homebound individuals who are unable to prepare their own meals. Special diets often can be accommodated, and some programs deliver meals on weekends and holidays. The Meals On Wheels Association of America (MOWAA) is the oldest and largest organization in the United States that provides meal services to the elderly. They have approximately 900 meal programs in communities throughout the United States. More than 300,000 volunteers help prepare, serve, or deliver more than 1 million meals each day through the older adult nutrition programs (see www.suite101.com/welcome.cfm/meals_on_wheels).

Day Care Services

Day care programs for older adults are appropriate providers of community-based care for individuals with multiple and special needs such as Alzheimer's disease, developmental disabilities, traumatic brain injury, and vision and hearing impairments. This service helps to reduce family caregiver strain, enables family members to work while the older adult is living with them, and provides the older adult with appropriate stimulation and social interaction.

As defined by the National Adult Day Services Association (n.d.), "Adult day services are community-based group programs designed to meet the needs of functionally and/or cognitively impaired adults through an individual plan of care." These programs provide a variety of health, social, and other related support services

in a protective setting. Benefits of adult day services include increased socialization, individualized therapeutic activities, nutrition and health monitoring, and medication management. In addition, they enable family caregivers to continue working, and sustain the individual in the community, which allows for "aging in place." Adult day centers generally operate during normal business hours 5 days a week. Some programs offer services in the evenings and on weekends, but none provide 24-hour care (see www.nadsa.org for more information).

Many of these services are funded through the Older Americans Act. Roles for nurses and other health professionals in this service network vary. Usually the services operate on a social model rather than a medical or health model, so that social workers and paraprofessional workers predominate. Nurses and other health professionals provide their expertise in the role of teacher, consultant, assessor, researcher, and coordinator of care.

Naturally Occurring Retirement Communities

It is common for older adults to remain in the houses where they were married and reared children; thus there are neighborhoods with most housing occupied by older individuals or couples. Growing older without having to relocate in order to meet one's basic needs is referred to as "aging in place." Inherent in this concept is the assumption that one's own home is the place where a person can exercise the most autonomy and experience the best quality of life. For aging in place, health services conform to the needs of the patient rather than requiring the patient to conform to the service (Kunstler, 2002). Out of the aging in place phenomenon has come the identification of naturally occurring retirement communities (NORCs), which are residential buildings or communities that were not designed specifically for older adults, but have become populated mainly by persons 60 years of age and older. A NORC provides supportive and health services to eligible residents. Well-developed NORCs are found in New York City, where large numbers of people reside in cooperative apartment buildings. A successful NORC has programs that (Ormond, 2004, cited in Kunstler, 2002):

- Reflect residents' needs as expressed through surveys, focus groups, forums, and advisory committees
- Follow a social (not medical) model emphasizing community building and socialization
- Are provided by an experienced social service agency familiar with the residents' needs
- Are governed by a representative committee
- Have volunteer services provided by residents themselves

Disease Management Services

Disease management services are a relatively recent development. These services provide patient monitoring and education mostly over the telephone. Because it is assumed that education and monitoring will reduce costs of care, private insurance often pays for this service to eligible individuals. After being referred by a physician, patients are invited to participate in the services. Those who accept are enrolled during an in-depth telephone interview conducted by a nurse. Periodic communication then is scheduled and a teaching plan devised. During teaching sessions, nurses also gather data about the patient's health status, such as blood glucose level or blood pressure readings, collected by the patient or a caregiver. If the nurse has concerns about the patient's immediate well-being, a home health nurse is sent to evaluate the situation in person.

COMMUNITY AS CLIENT

Community health nursing standards in 1999 (American Nurses Association [ANA], 1999) recommended that the nurse treat the community as client. By caring for individuals, families, and groups, the nurse improves the health of the community as a whole. The community health nurse uses the guideline, "the greatest good for the greatest number" when making decisions about the use of resources. Thus it is common for community health nurses to focus on preventing health problems in older adults. However, chronic illness is more common in older adults, and therefore preventing the complications of chronic illness is an important nursing goal. In public health, community/public health nurses may be responsible for population health, or identifying and treating health problems common to certain population groups.

Nursing in the Community

Nurses working in community health settings, such as public health agencies, nurse-managed health centers, ambulatory care clinics, home health agencies, and other community-based agencies, have a tremendous opportunity to influence the health of aging people at both community and individual levels of care.

The concept of community/public health nursing originated with the activities of public health nurses who were social reformers as well as caregivers for the sick since the formation of district nursing associations (Buhler-Wilkerson, 2001). Many years ago, Wald identified the *community* as the focus of public health nursing and emphasized the nurse's responsibility in collaborating with others in the community to promote health:

Our basic idea was that the nurse's peculiar introduction to the patient and her organic relationship with the neighborhood should constitute the starting point for universal service to the region. Our purpose was in no sense to establish an isolated undertaking. We planned to utilize, as well as to be implemented by, all agencies and groups of whatever creed which were working for social betterment, private as well as municipal. Our scheme was to be motivated by a vital sense of the interrelation of all these forces. For this reason, we considered ourselves best described by the term "public health nurses" (Wald, in Anderson, 1983).

Harmer (Skrovan et al., 1974) saw nursing as "linked with every social agency which strives for . . . the preservation of health . . . and is . . . not only concerned with the care of the individual, but with the health of a people." In the 1960s, the American Nurses Association, Ad Hoc Committee, Public Health Nurses' Section (1964) recognized that public health nursing had responsibility in "diagnosis, planning and treatment of *community* ills—those of the body politic." In addition, "Public health nurses integrate community involvement and knowledge about the entire population with personal, clinical understandings of the health and illness experiences of individuals and families within the population."

A role for the community health nurse, who sees the *community* rather than the individual or family unit as the client, has evolved. The newest model for working in communities is an empowerment to action approach with the community leading the definition of problems and their solutions. Community nurses are taught skills of community development, needs' assessment, and evaluation. To establish trust and rapport with the community as well as to act as an effective facilitator, community nurses should be active participants in community groups, such as churches, schools, clinics, and community centers. Sources of assessment data may include census records, police reports, clinic records, and vital statistics (Anderson & McFarlane, 1988; Clark, 1992).

The community health nurse must first work with the community to define what it sees as its health problems and possible resources and solutions. The Minnesota Department of Health suggests using the following Community Health Planning Guidelines:

- A community-wide assessment of issues, needs, strengths, and resources: analysis of people's values, interests, customary practices, and needs as they relate to health, especially within the perspective of other perceived priorities
- Prioritization of public health problems
- A plan for addressing specific problems including establishing long-range goals and short-term objectives
- Identification of community resources and positive and negative factors that affect health practices

- Descriptions of existing collaborative activities, grants, and various ongoing activities that would influence the plan
- Interventions based on the above information
- Evaluation of the influence of the intervention(s) on health-related behavior, and modification of the intervention as necessary

Levels of Prevention. A prevention model to explain the natural history of any disease was first developed in the field of mental health, then adapted by public health officials. Later adaptations of this model were used to describe mental, social, and physical health interventions (Leavell & Clark,1965).

These levels were described well by George L. Carlo, PhD, JD, of The Science and Public Policy Institute in his testimony before the Energy and Environment Subcommittee of the Committee on Science of the U.S. House of Representatives in Washington, DC, on July 15, 1998:

Public health protection has a long and rich history spanning the past two hundred years, with fundamental tenets having been developed, tested, and verified that support the use of the Public Health Paradigm. These tenets include primary, secondary, and tertiary prevention.

Historically, public health protection has been achieved through the optimal use of these three tenets in combination. Primary prevention reduces or limits exposures. Risks are identified and characterized, and standards are established to provide primary intervention in most areas.

However, comprehensive public health protection is attained only through the incorporation of secondary and tertiary prevention in conjunction with reasonable standards regulating exposure. Secondary and tertiary preventions are disease-based approaches that involve screening, diagnosis, and treatment. Secondary prevention includes the identification and characterization of high risk groups at whom to target intervention, the identification and implementation of secondary interventions such as screening programs, and the identification of tertiary interventions such as research into the treatment of identified illnesses.

Tertiary prevention includes the implementation of interventions such as treatment and rehabilitation, which are typically implemented by the medical and public health communities. In reality, secondary and tertiary interventions must be coordinated with primary prevention to obtain the optimum public health benefit.

This model of prevention provides a useful framework for identifying areas of assessment and intervention.

Community Assessment: Focus on Aging

Numerous community assessment guides are available in the community health nursing literature; one focuses explicitly on the aging population as a community (Mezey et al., 1993). Assessment of the aging population in a community should provide a basis for the development of programs to achieve primary, secondary, and tertiary prevention of the common problems afflicting older people and their families. Defining aging as a life-long process allows the community health nurse to consider people of *all* ages as potential recipients of prevention services. The focus on prevention of problems associated with advanced age is an important focal point for the community health nurse.

The continued evolution of the community health nurse is evidenced in the emergence of positions titled case managers in managed care settings. The nurse is the professional who has the breadth of education and experience to be able to assist a client in the community to make use of the most appropriate services in the timeliest manner (Zander, 1988). Currently, professional organizations representing nursing are working on establishing these roles as nursing roles. In the end, the role of case manager may be extended to a variety of individuals including nurses and social workers.

An accurate and useful community assessment begins with observation and vital statistics information. The nurse interested in the older adult portion of the population can focus on that aggregate while also assessing the community as a whole for its assets and resources. For example, using an asset-focused assessment (recall the community definition by John McKnight) of the community chooses to focus on providing activities for youth to avoid the challenges faced by adolescents attracted to illegal or inappropriate activities. To this end, the community health nurse could explore developing a program where adolescents and elders were matched so that the needs of each for interaction and life purpose could be met. Thus older persons who might voluntarily become housebound out of fear would have the assistance of a capable young person for company or errands. The older person does not suffer from lack of activity and social contact. Consequently, mental and physical health could be enhanced. Hogue (1977) suggested that members of the community be involved in defining and addressing their health needs. Thus the following questions may be used as a guide for community assessment with elders:

1. How do elders define their health needs and problems?
2. Who seems to have this need or problem?
3. What causes this need or problem to occur?
4. How severe is the need or problem?
5. What do you think would be solutions for reducing or controlling this need or problem?
6. What is available in the community for each possible solution?

Specific community assessment efforts made by nurses concerned with prevention of age-associated disability and premature mortality should include evaluation of the:

- Prevalence of risk factors for age-related problems
- Existing programs for early identification of risk factors (screening) with lifestyle modification
- Functional status of elders in activities of daily living, independent activities of daily living, and especially related factors such as sensory loss and cognitive loss
- Existing programs for assisted living and long-term care

Each element of the community assessment is described more fully in the paragraphs that follow.

Risk Factors for Aging-Related Problems. It

is interesting that older adults generally take better care of their health than do younger persons (United States Senate Special Committee on Aging, 1991). Even so, most problems experienced by older persons have a behavioral component that can be altered (Fries, 1992). The list of age-related problems and associated risk factors contained in Table 30-3 is generated from national statistics on age-related disability and mortality, the gerontology and geriatrics literature, and the author's experience in common problems associated with aging.

Estimated prevalence rates of these disorders often can be obtained from regional or state planning offices,

universities, or direct care providers. When prevalence rates for a specific community or aggregate are not available on a disease or disability of interest, it is possible to design methods to evaluate the prevalence of the problem using community survey methods or key informant methods. For more detailed assistance with these methods, see Anderson and McFarlane (1988). Estimation of the prevalence of a problem is often necessary to justify allocating resources to a specific program. When the prevalence rate of a specific disorder in a given community greatly exceeds national or state averages, special programming may be indicated.

Lifestyle Modification Programs. Develop-

ment of healthy lifestyles in people of all ages is likely to reduce age-related disability and premature death (Topp, Fahlman, & Boardly, 2004). Many of the diseases that plague older people, including heart disease, cancer, diabetes, stroke, chronic lung disease, and substance abuse, are partially amenable to prevention through lifestyle modification. It is estimated 400,000 people die each year from tobacco-related illness. Unhealthy nutrition and physical activity patterns account for another 300,000 deaths. Application of the interventions offered through primary care services could change the current status of the health of older adults.

Table 30-3 *Examples of Community-Based Wellness Programs Designed to Promote Healthy Aging*

Target Aggregate	Program Description	Rationale
Young people, unselected for risk factors	1. Educational programs on: *Aging* as a normal, lifelong process, influenced by lifestyle choices *Exercise* as a key element of healthy aging and disease prevention	Increase understanding and coping skills for dealing with aging-related changes Sedentary lifestyle implicated in significant age-related pathology (e.g., hypertension, cardiovascular disease, diabetes, obesity, depression)
	Nutrition as a key element of healthy aging and disease prevention	Poor nutrition implicated in significant age-related pathology (e.g., hypertension, cardiovascular disease, obesity, cancer)
	Substance abuse: alcohol, drugs, and cigarettes as major problems in our society that adversely affect health	Significant morbidity and early mortality associated with substance abuse (e.g., organic brain disease, liver disease, chronic lung disease)
	Stress reduction and management	Increased coping skills may decrease reliance on drugs as escape
	2. Facilities for: *Access* to recreational pursuits	Reinforce educational programming Actions speak louder than words Build healthy lifestyle habits early
	Access to examples of high-quality nutrition (e.g., in school cafeteria) *Exposure* to role models who exemplify successful stress reduction techniques rather than turning to substance abuse	

Continued

Table 30-3 *Examples of Community-Based Wellness Programs Designed to Promote Healthy Aging—cont'd*

Target Aggregate	Program Description	Rationale
Employment-age adults, unselected for risk factors	1. Educational programs on: *Exercise* and health protection *Nutrition* and disease prevention *Stress management* techniques *Aging process* and its impact on emotional health, family relationships *Availability of community resources* to care for dependent older family members 2. Facilities to promote and reinforce healthy lifestyles: *Work safety program* to identify and control health hazards in workplace *Access to exercise places* and equipment (in workplace or community) *Cafeterias* and other eating places that promote and reinforce good nutrition *Access to support groups* for developmental and health-related life crises (e.g., unemployment and job-finding skills, new parenthood, caring for dependent adult relatives, and disease-specific conditions)	Same as for school-aged children Provide opportunity for adults to learn what they did not learn as children Lifestyle modification still possible and useful in adulthood
Older adults (postretirement age)	1. Educational programs in: *Difference* between normal aging process and disease Importance of *exercise* in maintaining health despite disease Importance of proper *nutrition* in maintaining normal body function Importance of maintaining and developing *social ties* as buffer against losses associated with aging *Availability of resources* for exercise, nutrition, and socialization *Availability of resources* to care for dependent older family members or friends *Availability of home maintenance* and repair programs 2. Programs that provide: *Age-appropriate exercise classes* *Educational opportunities* in retirement *Transportation* to exercise and social opportunities	Know when to seek professional help for disease symptoms Same as for younger age-groups; lifestyle modification is still possible and potentially effective in staving off end-stage disability
Not age specific	Air pollution controls Water pollution controls Hazardous waste disposal	Needed to prevent morbidity and premature mortality from lung disease and malignancies

Modifiable lifestyle factors implicated in these disorders include:

- Diets that are too high in calories, cholesterol, fat, or sodium
- Lack of regular moderate activity
- Tobacco use
- Inadequate coping resources and stress-reduction skills

Because the adverse effects of lifestyle commonly are not experienced until middle age or old age, it is important for younger people to become more knowledgeable about the aging process so that they understand the rationale for modifying their lifestyles in young adulthood. Wellness-type programs that help promote healthy lifestyles include both educational offerings and facilities and programs that promote or support the desired behavior. For example, educational programs in secondary schools about the hazards of smoking may be beneficial, but smoking cessation groups focus more on promoting and supporting a change in lifestyle. Similarly, health education about the benefits of regular exercise may help to persuade some people to begin a personal exercise program, but the development of high-quality facilities for exercise, such as those available at Young Men's Christian Associations (YMCAs) or provided by some employers, is also a useful element of a lifestyle modification effort.

INVENTORY. The community assessment should include an inventory of the existing wellness programs as well as programs that have been tried and found unsuccessful in the past. Because there are no generally accepted standards for minimum community efforts for promoting wellness, the community assessor must consider the priorities of the community and the prevalence of specific problems in the community to make decisions about the adequacy of the range of existing programs.

QUALITY AND ACCESSIBILITY. Once existing programs have been catalogued, the quality and accessibility of the programs should be determined. Quality is most difficult to assess because the field of health and wellness promotion is so young. However, standards for the establishment of fitness programs are emerging. Accessibility is somewhat easier to estimate. For example,

evaluation of the accessibility of a fitness program might include some of the following questions:

- Are most of the fitness programs developed by employers for current employees and thus not accessible to retirees or unemployed persons?
- Are the programs developed by the government underfunded so that they operate only Monday through Friday during usual working hours, thus excluding access by most employed persons?
- Are the waiting lists prohibitively long?
- Finally, is access to the fitness program restricted by finances? What is the enrollment fee for most programs?

The same types of questions can be applied to other health promotion activities, such as weight reduction support groups, classes on "You and Your Aging Parent," and preretirement planning groups. Table 30-4 summarizes some examples of community-based wellness programs that are likely to affect health positively in old age (Leigh & Fries, 1992-1993). Programs that are entirely missing from or inaccessible to large segments of the community suggest a need for further program development. Program development must always proceed according to the jointly derived priorities of the assessor and the community. Priorities in health promotion programming are particularly susceptible to influence from individuals in the community because there is a relative lack of evidence about the efficacy of strategies for lifestyle modification relative to cost, which might outweigh individual opinion.

FUNCTIONAL STATUS OF OLDER ADULTS. Knowledge of the proportion of older people in the community who suffer from disabilities should underlie the development of assessment and support services for elderly individuals, so that secondary and tertiary

Table 30-4 *Use of Health Care Services**

Utilization Measure	1992	1993	1994	1995	1996	1997	1998	1999	2000
RATE PER THOUSAND									
Hospital stays	306	300	331	336	341	351	354	365	361
Skilled nursing facility stays	28	33	43	50	59	67	69	67	69
Physician visits and consultations	11359	11600	12045	12372	12478	n/a[†]	13061	n/a[†]	13,346
Home health care visits	3822	4648	6352	7608	8376	8227	5058	3708	2295
DAYS									
Average length of hospital stay	8.4	8.0	7.5	7.0	6.6	6.3	6.1	6.0	5.9

From Centers for Medicare and Medicaid Services. (2000). Medicare claims and enrollment data. Retrieved from www.agingstats.gov/chartbook2000/healthcare.html.
*Note: Data for Medicare enrollees in fee-for-service only. Data on physician visits and consultations are not available for 1997 and 1999. Physician visits and consultations include all settings, such as physician offices, hospitals, emergency departments, and nursing homes. Beginning in 1994, managed care enrollees were excluded from the denominator of all utilization rates because utilization data are not available for them. Prior to 1994, managed care enrollees were included in the denominators; they comprised 7% or less of the Medicare population. Reference population: These data refer to Medicare enrollees.
[†]n/a, Data not available.

prevention services can be most effectively developed and targeted (CDC, 2004). As is the case with determining the prevalence of selected conditions that commonly affect older people, much of the necessary information can be derived from existing community surveys that are available from local, regional, or state agencies. When the information is not available, several approaches can be used to ascertain the extent of functional disability in the aged. Methods such as the Older Americans Resources and Services (OARS) instrument have been applied to large community samples using trained interviewers rather than professional assessments (Pfeiffer, 1975; see also Chapter 2). Other assessments include the Hebrew Rehabilitation and Care for the Aged (HRCA) Vulnerability Index (Morris et al., 1984). The HRCA combines self-report or proxy report of performance and capability on key instrumental and personal activities of daily living (ADLs), orientation, and activity level. In addition, screening assessment tools that allow estimation of the prevalence of specific age-associated disabilities, such as musculoskeletal impairment, and that are appropriate for large population studies are prevalent and available to the public via the Internet. For example, data from a series of Longitudinal Studies of Aging and in the Data Warehouse on Trends in Health and Aging are available through the National Center for Health Statistics (NCHS). These data sets are used in research studies by those with research questions about aging in the United States.

Screening and Assessment Programs.
Secondary prevention of disease (illness and disease management) is based on the ability to identify disease as early as possible, so that the disease can be more readily treated or managed and adverse sequelae prevented. Third-party payment for preventive health care has been improving. Medicare pays for many preventive services, as seen in the following list. Additional information on this topic can be accessed at www.cms.hhs.gov/PrevntionGenInfo/.

- One-time "Welcome to Medicare" physical examination
- Cardiovascular screening
- Cancer tests

Breast cancer screening (mammograms)
Cervical and vaginal cancer screening (Pap test and pelvic examination)
Colon cancer screening (colorectal)
Prostate cancer screening (PSA)

- Immunizations

Influenza
Pneumococcal pneumonia
Hepatitis B

- Bone mass measurements
- Diabetes screening, supplies, and self-management training

- Glaucoma screening
- Other health information
- Smoking cessation
- Medical nutrition therapy

Some public health agencies have provided multiphasic screening clinics to screen for common treatable diseases such as anemia, hypertension, tuberculosis, glaucoma, diabetes, and certain malignancies. Other communities accomplish the same goal through the use of community health and wellness fairs, in which professionals volunteer their time on a periodic basis to provide screening services. Where screening programs exist, it is important to evaluate the effectiveness of follow-up from the screening tests. If a potential disease is identified but appropriate evaluation and treatment are not carried out, then the screening has not accomplished the goal of secondary prevention.

Another issue in secondary prevention programs for older adults is identification of the full range of assessment and screening that should be applied to older people. For example, multiphasic screening approaches have traditionally focused on *diseases* that first manifest themselves in middle age rather than on *disabilities* that manifest themselves in late life. There is no question that screening maneuvers specific to the elderly, such as the detection of mobility problems, should be undertaken with the goal of preventing disability in advanced old age. In the elderly, secondary prevention should have a multidisciplinary focus that emphasizes prevention of disabilities (Stuifbergen, Seraphine, & Roberts, 2000). A growing number of studies are demonstrating the efficacy of comprehensive geriatric screening programs in the prevention of mortality and morbidity in the aged (Fleming, Evans, Weber, & Chutka, 1995).

Examples of useful screening maneuvers specific to older persons can be gleaned from clinical anecdotes. For example, one astute clinician has noticed that many older people, because of reduced joint mobility and lower extremity muscle weakness, tend to fall down into chairs rather than transferring gently, possibly predisposing to compression fractures and increased musculoskeletal pain. If screening programs included assessment of transfer abilities, specific exercises could be prescribed to remedy the incorrect transfer technique, perhaps preventing further musculoskeletal impairment. Another example pertains to drug screening. Adverse drug reactions increase with the number of medications taken. Many older people consult more than one primary care provider, who has little or no knowledge of what the other practitioner is prescribing. Periodic drug regimen review by a qualified professional is a screening maneuver that can prevent adverse drug reactions or interactions.

Yet another example of screening based on clinical observation is intended to detect factors related to falls. Falls are not just accidents and often can be prevented with appropriate interventions. Assessing the individual for relevant risk factors frequently associated with falling is critical. These factors can include medications that contribute to postural hypotension or vertigo, muscular and/or skeletal impairment, confusion, and decreased sensorial functioning. Environmental factors in the home should also be examined and include the presence of unanchored scatter rugs, crumbling flooring or sidewalks, slick floors, and inadequate handrails (Edwards et al., 1993; Kippenbrock & Soja, 1993). More recent screening programs seek to identify family history and personal health practices that could pose a risk for health conditions. Nurses then intervene with risks that are modifiable.

The community assessor has the responsibility to consider the availability of screening and assessment services to older persons in the community and whether the services are adequate to prevent common problems confronting the aged. This aspect of community assessment is particularly difficult because most screening and assessment services for the aged are not segregated and clearly identified but are included in other primary health care packages. Thus the assessor must become knowledgeable about the nature of the services provided to the older population in primary care settings as well as the services provided in senior centers, rest homes, adult day programs, public health departments, and pharmacies.

Programs for Care of Dependent Older People.
Tertiary prevention (rehabilitation) is concerned with rehabilitation and the return of optimal functioning, to the extent possible given the underlying cause of problems. The purpose of many community-based, long-term care services is to promote independence in the community without compromising the health of younger family members. The hazards of institutionalization are well described in the literature and include increased mortality, decreased social opportunity, and learned helplessness.

IDENTIFICATION OF GAPS IN THE SERVICE NETWORK. Communities differ greatly in the extent and depth of the community support services that are available. The community assessor should identify gaps in the network of services as well as the accessibility of the services. Barriers to obtaining services include financial, bureaucratic, cultural (including language and beliefs), and transportation or personal mobility barriers. Extensive waiting lists, limited service hours, and highly centralized locations of services are all signals that service delivery may not be matched to service need. Waiting lists generally indicate either that there is insufficient service for all who need it or that services are inappropriately targeted. One North Carolina survey showed that a high percentage of people receiving chore services (such as general home maintenance or minor repairs) had no documented functional impairment (Nelson, 1986), yet there were large numbers of functionally impaired people on the waiting list.

ASSESSMENT OF QUALITY OF SERVICES. Another element in the evaluation of existing programs for dependent older people includes an assessment of the quality of the service. Selective interviews with care recipients and their family members as well as with the personnel delivering the service are indicated. Anecdotal reports sometimes indicate that problems exist with caregivers. Notation of this in the community assessment and development of a strategy to address the problem are important tasks for the community health nurse interested in high-quality long-term care in the home. Monitoring the quality of care in highly decentralized care systems such as home care is recognized to be difficult. More and more agencies are employing a managed care approach.

DETERMINING HOME HEALTH CARE NEEDS. One model for determining home health care needs in a local community lists three components to be assessed: need for services, services already provided, and implications for nursing education, service, and research. Information acquired to determine need for service should include an overview of both the types of health care needs of the consumers and the health care system, especially its organization, payment systems, and health care providers. Services provided should be described in terms of the existing relationships among the various components of the long-term care continuum (primary care, hospital, long-term care institutions, home care), discharge planning, and availability of professional services. Implications for nursing education, service, and research are directly related to provision of care in the home health setting. Nurses must be educated to provide services to homebound clients, and they should be conducting research to enhance their assessment practices (Figure 30-3, Box 30-4, and Figure 30-4).

Nursing Diagnoses

Nursing diagnosis statements at the level of the community are consistent with nursing diagnoses for individuals. Each diagnosis has three parts: there is a problem or need, an etiology, and a list of characteristics. For example, the following diagnosis would be relevant to the community level: Elders at risk for depression related to social isolation as evidenced by lack of public transportation, loss of spouse and friends, comorbid illnesses, low vision and hearing, and reduced mobility.

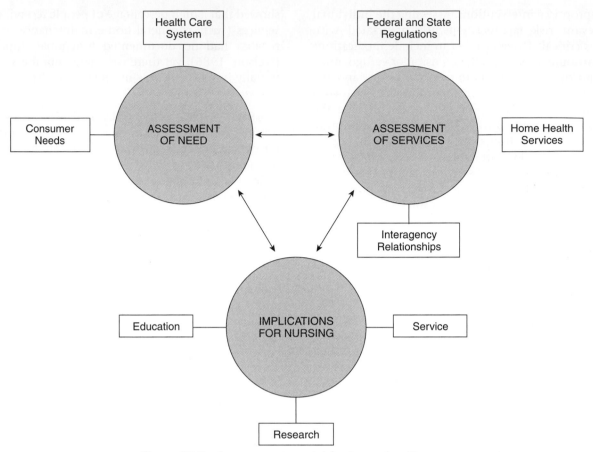

Figure 30-3 Assessment model for home health care.

Goals and Interventions

Planning at the community level is an extremely complex activity that requires knowledge of the community power structure as well as knowledge of the needs of the community. Factors other than simply the assessed needs of the community may dictate the types of community health programming in a specific community. In programming for older individuals, this situation is further complicated by the fact that problems of older persons typically transcend a number of service agency boundaries. For example, older people may simultaneously receive services from a home health agency, a community mental health center, a social services agency, voluntary organizations, and an ambulatory care clinic. Achieving consensus on the priorities for preventive services for older adults among the various community agencies may be difficult indeed, particularly when the needed services may have to compete for funding with more familiar and popular services, such as day care for children.

The specific techniques and subtleties of planning at the community level for older persons are beyond the scope of this book. Interested readers should consult

---

BOX 30-4 The Health Care Environment/ Digital Health Care

Concept
Digital Health Care—Application of Internet/ Web-based technology to health care practices and processes, thus:
- Empowering consumer/provider responsibility for health care
- Reducing administrative costs
- Introducing "real" (for the first time) mass customization to the industry

Definition
The "Digital" Health Plan—Consumer-focused, Internet-centered health information integrator that will enable patients, providers, and health care product/service suppliers to seamlessly facilitate health care solutions at all levels

From Sokolov, J. J. (2000). Bringing it all together. 2000 Duke Private Sector Conference: Academic health systems in transition. Retrieved January 26, 2006, from http://conferences.mc .duke.edu/privatesector/dpsc2000/y.htm.

Independent Living Assessment

1. RESIDENT'S WISHES
Desired living site _____
Ambivalence _____
Plans to manage at site successfully _____

2. FAMILY CONCERNS
Informant _____
Relationship _____
Ambivalence _____
Support needs seen _____
Plans to get support needs met _____

3. INDEPENDENCE OF RESIDENT IN ACTIVITIES OF DAILY LIVING

	INDEPENDENT	WITH HELP	SPECIFY KIND OF HELP AND BY WHOM
Mobility in apartment			
Walks to meals			
Gets own mail			
Feeds self			
Bathes			
Dresses			
Takes medications			
Maintains personal hygiene			

4. RESIDENT'S SAFETY

	ADEQUATE	DEFICIENT	SPECIFY HOW
Overall mental status			
Appropriate in relationships			
Hearing			
Mobility			
Vision			
Communication			
Ability to make decisions			

5. FINANCIAL/LEGAL CONSIDERATIONS
Financial constraints _____
Power of attorney _____
Helper with business affairs _____

Summary of recommendations:

Date _____   Signature _____

Figure 30-4   Independent living assessment.

the community health planning, community health nursing, and community organization literature for specific information on this topic (Spradley, 1985). The case examples in this chapter provide some insights into the complexity of planning for the needs of older people at the community level. The paragraphs that follow provide an overview of the kinds of programs that might be stimulated by a community nursing professional interested in prevention of aging-related problems.

A prevention model to explain the natural history of any disease was first adapted by public health officials. Later adaptations of this model were used to describe mental, social, and physical health interventions (Leavell & Clark, 1965).

These levels were described well by Carlo (1998) and are presented under Levels of Prevention. The levels of prevention provide one framework for interventions for communities and individuals.

Prevention Programming. The nurse's specific role in the community usually influences the opportunities chosen to develop various preventive programs. For example, public health nurses whose responsibilities include serving in an outpatient clinic as well as providing home health services have the opportunity to use their knowledge about preventable musculoskeletal disabilities seen in the home to enhance musculoskeletal screening and intervention in the outpatient clinic. Occupational health nurses may identify the need for middle-aged workers to have information about changes with aging and services for older family members and may then develop an educational series in collaboration with a local home health care provider. Nurses in an ambulatory care clinic, noting the high prevalence of obesity and hypertension, may stimulate the development of a weight-reduction support group in their community.

Development of Needed Services. At the tertiary level of prevention (rehabilitation), the case-management approach has been advocated both as a way to coordinate a complex array of services and as a means of systematizing needs' assessment for long-term care services. Case managers, who assess complex cases and design care plans with the comprehensive needs of the patients and their families in mind, have a special opportunity to document the lack of needed services because of the comprehensiveness of the service they provide (Eloniemi-Sulkava et al., 2001; Glickman, Stocker, & Caro, 1997; Lazarus, 2001). If the administration of the case-management service is attuned to presenting data about the gaps in services to community decision makers, then case management serves an important function in the community as well as for individual patients. Unfortunately, there is seldom a systematic means of assessing when the range of services is inadequate to serve the long-term needs of the elderly. Generally, new services are developed in response to some perceived crisis or as a response to a funding initiative.

Evaluation

Five criteria can be applied to the effectiveness of the nursing process at the community level:

- Effectiveness—How well did the resources meet the needs of the population?
- Efficiency—How do the benefits of the care compare to the costs?
- Adequacy—How much impact does the program have on the population?
- Appropriateness—Are the services acceptable to the population?
- Unintended consequences—What findings were not expected?

Starfield (1974) suggested a set of criteria to evaluate quality of care based on a continuum of levels of well-being with a focus on individual functional levels. The categories are listed according to complexity of measurement, beginning with the best-defined categories:

1. Longevity and prognosis: normal versus premature death
2. Activity: functional versus disabled
3. Comfort: comfortable versus distressed
4. Satisfaction: acceptance of one's health status or health care
5. Disease/morbidity: not detectable versus permanent
6. Achievement or level of accomplishment: achieving versus not achieving
7. Resilience (the ability to cope with adversity, including resisting a health threat and responding to stress): resilient versus vulnerable

Care is evaluated in terms of how well a provider helps a client move toward the positive end of the continuum. Evaluation of prevention-oriented programming is difficult but should be incorporated in planning to provide feedback to community planners about which programs increase well-being among older adults.

Few guidelines specify the definition of a "reasonable sum of money" to be expended on community health for older persons; a great deal depends on the community's values concerning the importance of caring for older persons and its beliefs about the efficacy of preventive services. Because various ethnic groups and communities differ in their willingness to institutionalize dependent older persons, the community health budget cannot be evaluated without considering the values and health care expenditures of the community as a whole. Communities differ in the degree to which they expect families to shoulder the burden of dependent care and the degree to which they expect support from government or industry.

Cost of community care must also be evaluated according to the outcomes obtained. Unfortunately, many cost studies on alternatives to long-term care have neglected to include adequate measures of effectiveness. For example, community-based alternatives to long-term care have been criticized as not being cost-effective compared with nursing home care because the average longevity of the client is greater in the community than in the nursing home (Weissert, 1985). If the goal is to care for dependent older people until they die, then the nursing home seems to be the more cost-effective alternative. If, however, the goal is to promote health and prevent premature mortality, the nursing home, although less costly, is not the most effective alternative.

Delivering care in the least restrictive environment means that institutionalization is forestalled whenever possible, and maximum autonomy is promoted. Access to the full range of community health and support services must be available for this goal to be achieved.

The prevalence of selected disorders in the community is an index of the effectiveness of certain prevention programs. Communities with accessible, well-developed fitness programs may over time demonstrate reductions in some diseases. Care must be taken in selecting target disabilities to allow an appropriate length of time to see the effects of the preventive effort. For example, in 1964 over one half of the adult American population smoked. After the initiation of broad-based prevention programming, the number dropped to 33% in 1981. Education and awareness efforts were continued, and by 1984 the number had decreased to 26%. This success is tempered by the fact that smoking remains one of the primary public health problems, causing 175,000 "excess" deaths (35% of all cancer deaths) per year (Weissert & Weissert, 1996).

Likewise, the impact of a hypertension screening program on the prevalence of stroke-related disabilities may take 20 years or more to assess. The impact of reinforcing healthy lifestyles in school-aged children and in the workplace may take even longer to evaluate. However, the impact of an educational program on body mechanics for family caregivers of older people may be evaluated by comparing the incidence of back strain complaints in the specific age range served in the clinic where the course was offered before and after the course was presented. Community health nurses should remember that significant decreases in such disorders may take a generation or more to achieve, and the time frame for evaluation of health promotion strategies should be modified to account for the long-range nature of the effects of these interventions.

DEVELOPMENT OF COMMUNITY HEALTH SERVICES

Suppose that a gerontological nurse specialist with expertise in psychiatric/mental health nursing was hired to direct the services of a community mental health center (CMHC) in a rural southeastern community. The goal was to see a caseload of older outpatient psychotherapy clients and to develop preventive, educational, and therapeutic programs according to the needs of the community. This example describes the steps of the nursing process used by the nurse specialist.

Assessment

A general systems model guided the community assessment. The goals of the assessment were to:
1. Identify factors in the community that contribute to or detract from the *emotional well-being* of older people and their families

2. Describe the *range of services* available to older persons and their families

The nurse specialist collected data over a 6-month period and organized it into the following categories: *contextual data, inputs, process,* and *products.*

Contextual Data. The major employers in this rural, conservative, southeastern community are two textile mills and one large defense contractor. The people have strong church affiliations, and the churches are active in community affairs and problems. There is a history of coordinated community action to address local problems. The CMHC has a reputation for implementing innovative prevention and treatment programs and fostering interagency working relationships. The goal of the CMHC is to increase the number of older persons served by the center.

Inputs. The community assessment revealed that funding sources for mental health programs came from several sources: federal and state grants, county funding, fee-for-service arrangements, insurance (including Medicare and Medicaid), United Way agencies, and other charitable contributions. A statewide Title XX needs' assessment discovered that loneliness and poverty were widespread for older people in the area, and there were only 250 nursing home beds.

Three important considerations would influence the development of a mental health program:
- National estimates suggest that *50% to 80%* of the older adults may require some type of mental health service.
- Family members' inability to cope with relatives suffering from *dementia* is a common outpatient problem.
- *Depression and adjustment reaction to late life* is a commonly diagnosed problem in outpatient therapy populations.

The nurse specialist grouped the inputs under three headings: governmental human services agencies, nongovernmental agencies, and informal groups.

INPUTS FROM GOVERNMENTAL HUMAN SERVICES AGENCIES. The public health department was the *only* provider of home health services. The department of social services operated a small-chore worker program and supervised rest home operators. The CMHC had a strong consultation and education component, a liaison with industry and area businesses through employee assistance programs, adult outpatient service clinicians involved with an adult day hospital program, a substance abuse program, and a long history of providing high-quality consultation and preventive services. A Community Action Agency sponsored five congregate nutrition sites throughout the county. The housing authority operated two congregate housing projects for senior citizens, with social workers based at each project. The recreation department runs the only senior center in the county and provides staff support for the council on aging, a senior volunteer program, and a senior transportation program; the department also convenes a forum of presidents of senior citizens' clubs throughout the county. The community college operates a licensed practical nurse program and has a broad array of adult education and noncurricular programs.

INPUTS FROM NONGOVERNMENTAL AGENCIES. Meals-on-wheels, a private nonprofit organization, does friendly visiting in addition to delivering meals; it is interested in writing a proposal for funding a homemaker/home health aide program. Several Protestant church ministers are concerned about the problems of and ministry to the aged; some senior citizens' clubs operate through the churches. There are two hospitals in the county—one with an inpatient psychiatric unit and a skilled nursing facility attached. Two intermediate care nursing homes besides the hospital facility are in the area. Several small domiciliary homes are operated throughout the county; the larger rest home, with about 60 beds, has a large census of chronic psychiatric patients.

INPUTS FROM INFORMAL GROUPS. A loose confederation of clergy is concerned about community problems. The community council is composed of members from key county and nonprofit agencies as well as charitable organizations; it discusses community problems and considers new programs for development. An interagency luncheon group of people from governmental human services meets monthly to facilitate communication between county agencies.

Process
INTRAAGENCY COMMUNICATIONS. The community assessment identified three sources of intraagency communications: regular staff meeting, biweekly grand rounds, and the lunchroom.

INTERAGENCY COMMUNICATIONS. On the individual client level, many workers believed that CMHC employees do not readily share client information, which impedes service delivery. Others believed that criteria for being screened at the mental health center were unduly restrictive. On the program level, openness was expressed about joint ventures, such as collaboration on training, patient evaluation, family conferences, and grant development. On the community service planning level, informal exchanges usually preceded a formal presentation at the community council or interagency groups.

DAY-TO-DAY INTERACTIONS. The CMHC had to improve certain aspects of its current programs for older adults and their families. Patients may be reluctant to come into the mental health center to be served, and the staff is not trained to recognize normal aging changes and their impact on the function of the aged. On the other hand, approximately one third of the staff in adult services are particularly interested in working with older persons.

The senior center and congregate meal sites provide accessible, pleasant environments that are conducive to socialization but cannot serve persons with severe functional or cognitive impairments.

The housing authority has people on its social work/outreach staff who are very concerned about maintaining the independence of marginally functional individuals as much as possible. The staff is attentive to subtle changes in clients' behavior. The agency is limited, though, because it can only provide direct services to clients who live independently.

Products. Specific mental health services for elders include family counseling, inpatient psychiatric services, sheltered workshop (old people have low priority because of their limited remaining worklife), a day hospital program (most clients are younger adults), and substance abuse counseling.

There are also three specialized geriatric services available: outpatient psychotherapy, preventive group work, and case-oriented and program-oriented consultation to rest homes and nursing homes regarding behavioral problems in older residents.

Gaps in the service delivery network for old people include no adult day care service, no respite services, and few home health aide providers. In addition, many family members have unresolved problems in caring for relatives suffering from dementia or depression.

Conducting the Assessment. The nurse specialist used a variety of means to collect the assessment data. Key members of the community, including workers in all relevant human service agencies, were interviewed to ascertain their view of the community's approach to the problems of older people and their families. Specific questions were asked about the adequacy of services, unmet needs, and barriers to increasing services to older people. Each element in the service delivery network was assessed in terms of how it approached services to older people and how its mission to older people was conceived.

Diagnostic Summary
Strengths of the community include the following:
- Good mental health center commitment to preventive as well as treatment services

- Many possible funding sources to support service expansion
- Good working relationships between formal and informal service providers
- Most elements of a continuum of long-term care services already in place
- Strong life span approach to preventive community mental health
- Orderly interagency communications processes and community problem-solving processes

Problems with providing mental health service to older persons and their families include:

- Gaps in services (no homemaker/home health aide service, no adult day care, no family-centered prevention, and limited department of social services interest in the aged)
- No ongoing consultation or direct service provision in rest homes or nursing homes
- Difficult access to outpatient mental health services by debilitated older people
- Space in mental health center too small to permit program expansion; not barrier-free for physically handicapped
- Mental health center staff not perceived as good team players by other agency staff
- Lack of training in aging by all community human service professionals
- Lack of awareness of special problems of the aged in obtaining human services from bureaucracies

Planning

The many strengths of the community in human services' delivery suggested that much could be accomplished to strengthen the network of services to older adults and their families. The nurse specialist elected to work toward several goals simultaneously for two reasons: (1) progress was likely to be slow on some fronts, and (2) success in achieving some goals would increase her credibility and in turn her ability to achieve more complex goals.

The highest priority for services in the community was lack of an *adult day care* program, but development of this would also be the most difficult to achieve because it required new space, start-up funding, and new staff. Other high priorities included:

- Development of preventive services for family members of dependent older people
- Development of ongoing consultation and direct services to nursing homes and rest homes
- Education of other human service professionals in the community about the aging process and addressing the special needs of older persons
- Increasing access to mental health services for dependent older persons

Areas in which special opportunities existed but were of less urgency included developing support groups for individuals with specific aging-related problems (such as widowhood, sensory loss, or chronic diseases) and fostering the development of preretirement counseling in the community through a liaison with industry or the community college's adult education program.

Interventions

To build on existing strengths in the mental health center, the nurse specialist first moved to affirm the efforts of the mental health center staff who had been working with older persons before her arrival. She negotiated with two other therapists from adult services to continue the weekly "sharing" group they had begun in a senior nutrition site as a preventive and outreach service while expanding the service to two other nutrition sites. She acquired new psychotherapy patients by referral only from the existing outpatient therapists and was available for consultation on problems of the aged for individual, family, and group psychotherapy sessions.

Next, the nurse specialist proceeded to know the other agency personnel in the community. No educational or speaking engagement was turned down during the first 6 months. Such invitations offered opportunities to foster trust with other community members while increasing the visibility of the mental health center's commitment to geriatric care. In addition, community consciousness was raised, and people became aware of the special needs of older persons and their families.

In the community at large, the nurse specialist affirmed some of the concerns voiced about access to the mental health center for dependent older people and pledged to work diligently to improve access. She scheduled joint home visits with some of the nurses at the public health department and social workers at other community agencies to provide mental health consultation and to foster enhanced interdisciplinary communication.

Finally, an advisory or "steering" committee for program development of geriatric services was formed consisting of the nurse specialist, the heads of consultation and education and adult services, the program evaluator for the mental health center, therapists from adult services with expressed interest in working with the aged, the head of the substance abuse prevention program, the director of nursing in the public health department, the chair of the senior citizens' club coalition, the head of the home-delivered meals' agency, and one of the active ministers in town. It is important to note that this steering committee was an informal group. The nurse specialist frequently consulted these key people for advice on program development but never convened the entire group for a meeting. The rationale behind not having the committee as a whole meet was to avoid the slowness of a highly bureaucratized group and to avoid the group process impeding the development of fresh ideas and programs. Subgroups met as needed to enhance efficiency, or when it was desirable to brain-storm in small groups, or when programmatic decisions would affect some segment of the larger group.

The community assessment outlined was shared with the advisory committee, along with a preliminary plan for addressing the prioritized needs. The advisory committee's ideas were particularly helpful in developing approaches for new services. For example, the advisors encouraged work on all goals simultaneously and facilitated introductions to key members of the community, such as the fiscal officer of the mental health center and members of the community council. The advisors also suggested that an attempt to revitalize the council on aging would be an excellent way to increase visibility and to provide a ready forum for receiving feedback about program development ideas.

The progress of program development then became opportunistic. As opportunities for collaborative work with other individuals or agencies were presented that were consistent with the overall plan of development, such projects were taken on. For example, the agency in charge of home-delivered meals prepared a proposal to develop a homemaker/home health aide service. The nurse specialist wrote letters of support for the proposal and, once it was funded, assisted in part of the curriculum development and training for the new workers that emphasized helping skills and teaching about the normal aging process. When the substance abuse division chief wanted to develop a grant proposal to enhance prevention services directed toward women, the nurse specialist successfully lobbied to focus the proposal on women in transition throughout the life cycle, thus beginning work on preventive mental health services for women in times of transition, such as retirement, widowhood, and assuming a caregiver role for dependent older family members.

A program of regular, case-oriented consultation was established with all three nursing homes and one rest home in the area. This increased the accessibility of both direct psychotherapy services to dependent older people and education to staff regarding techniques that foster positive adjustment to institutional life.

Education about the benefits of an adult day care program targeted toward the needs of dependent older people and their families was directed at diverse groups in the community, including the clergy, the mental health center staff, and other human service agencies.

A family education and support group was led with another mental health center clinician as cotherapist. It was a close-ended, weekly group of six sessions, designed to enhance the knowledge base of family members about the normal aging process and human responses to various chronic diseases. Selected other members of

the community were enlisted to assist with some of the teaching. At the first group of sessions, many of the participants were agency personnel (for example, public health nurses) who came both because they had to help older persons and their families professionally and because they wanted help with personal situations.

Evaluation

The nurse specialist left the mental health center before the full impact of the program development efforts could be assessed. The major accomplishments of the geriatric program development in the community 3 years later included:

- Two geriatric day care centers in the county: one managed by the mental health center and one privately operated, but both receiving extensive community support
- Increased willingness on the part of mental health center staff to consult with staffs of rest homes and nursing homes
- Continued support for a geriatric mental health specialist
- Increased numbers of older people receiving outpatient psychotherapy services
- Increased availability of prevention services to older people and their families
- Increased knowledge of the special problems of older people by human service workers in the county

MULTIDISCIPLINARY TEAM ASSESSMENT OF LONG-TERM CARE SERVICES

A nurse responsible for management of human services in a mixed urban/rural county in the southeast was able to identify difficulties in the long-term care services' delivery system for older persons in her county. Indications that the system was in trouble included:

- Long waiting lists for some in-home services
- Significant numbers of patients in the county hospital remaining longer than medically necessary because no nursing home beds were available
- A fragmented community service system
- Discontent in the professional community about the comprehensiveness of home care services offered

The nurse contracted with a university-based, multidisciplinary team to assess the long-term care service delivery system in the county. The team was also asked to develop and implement a case-management program for older persons in need of long-term care. The team was composed of a health care administrator with expertise in adult education and a pastoral care background, an occupational therapist with extensive experience working with severely handicapped individuals, a gerontological nurse specialist, a medical social worker with training in counseling psychology, and an internist interested in problems of the aged.

Assessment

A community assessment similar to the one in the previous example was conducted using a general systems' framework. The three assessment goals were to:

1. Identify the status of long-term care in the community
2. Identify barriers to optimal long-term care for older adults
3. Identify the components of the long-term care system

Contextual Data. There was increased concern about containing hospital costs both nationally and locally and a state limitation on construction of new nursing homes as well as heightened awareness of the problems of older persons in long-term care.

Inputs. Inputs were from old people with functional impairments, families trying to care for old people, governmental agencies (for example, the public health department, department of social services, and community mental health centers), and private sector agencies (proprietary home health care agencies, six proprietary nursing homes, several proprietary domiciliary homes, and one proprietary hospital). The voluntary sector was represented by two hospitals, the council on aging, a hospice, and meals-on-wheels. Reimbursors included Medicare, Medicaid, and private insurers. The new Medicaid waiver project reimbursed chore services, meals-on-wheels, case management, adult day care, increased professional nursing care, and rehabilitative therapies.

Process. Interagency communications were hindered by several factors. There was little joint program planning, except between the council on aging and the public health department. Multiple assessments were performed by different agencies, and little information was shared. There were multiple points of entry into the long-term care system and long waiting lists. Clinicians did not have specialized training in geriatrics, which resulted in decreased sensitivity to the special needs of older people, barriers to receiving care, and inadequate time frames for rehabilitation. The various agencies adopted narrow concepts of coordinated care within a highly bureaucratized system of care.

Products. Limited competition and minimal teamwork among agencies resulted in fewer service options for old people and their families. Patients were poorly served because of regulations, fiefdoms created by various funding sources, and restricted social work practice in the hospital.

Conducting the Assessment. The multidisciplinary team identified key agencies that provided long-term care services in the community. Heads of agencies as well as individual clinicians were interviewed to determine:

- Their ideas about how care for the aged was carried out
- The criteria for admission to and discharge from various service programs
- How eligibility for services was assessed
- How services were delivered
- How agencies interacted with each other
- What gaps in service were perceived

These data were combined with statistical information available from the county manager's office and the state department of human resources concerning the amount and sources of funding expended for long-term care in the county. Individual older people and their families as well as physicians in private practice in the community were interviewed regarding unmet but needed services and the availability of existing services.

Diagnoses

1. Older persons and their families have difficulty obtaining continuous, reliable care because of fragmented delivery of long-term care related to diverse funding sources and unduly restrictive sets of services being offered by single agencies.
2. Patient and family choices of care providers are limited because of unfair restraint of private agencies' growth by county agency dominance of referral patterns and caseloads.
3. Service options for older people and their families are limited.
4. Bias exists toward institutional care for dependent older people.

Planning and Intervention

Based on the community assessment data, the community nurse gave the multidisciplinary assessment team sanction to lead a series of interventions designed to improve the coordination and quality of community-based, long-term care services to older adults and their families. Two goals of the project were the following: (1) better coordination of care in order to provide comprehensive care options for patients and their families at the lowest possible cost; (2) lobbying to change existing barriers to better coordination of care.

First, a plan for implementation of a Medicaid Section 2176 community-based, long-term care waiver project was developed, using a centralized, hospital-based case-management approach. Plans were also developed for expanding the service to community-based sites pending evaluation of the effectiveness of the hospital-based program. The rationale for beginning with a hospital-based program was that patients in the hospital were most vulnerable to inappropriate institutionalization because of three factors: (1) the pressures to discharge patients from the hospital to the first available setting, regardless of its appropriateness; (2) the vulnerability of older adults to functional decline while in the hospital environment; and (3) the county's concern about wasting scarce hospital resources on patients who no longer required acute care, even though there was no long-term care facility available.

The team formed and staffed a community long-term care provider forum for the purpose of facilitating communications. The assessment team also recommended that a community long-term care advisory board be formed to begin to address some of the financial and administrative barriers to efficient, comprehensive, readily accessible, community-based long-term care. A policy board was formed that included members of the state legislature, advisory board members of each of the key human services' agencies in the county, and a consumer representative. The case-management project actively sought, assessed, and then presented to the board for their consideration cases that exemplified some of the systemic dilemmas in long-term care. Examples of cases presented to the board included the following:

- A case highlighting the need for less cumbersome guardianship procedures as well as the need for a public guardian other than the social services agency
- A case highlighting the bias toward institutionalization by Medicaid eligibility determinations because institutions have a higher nonmedical care cost of living allowance and have greatly streamlined eligibility recertification procedures
- Cases demonstrating how limited Medicare reimbursement adversely affects clinical decisions about need for rehabilitative services, despite the presence of alternative sources of funding
- Cases demonstrating the adverse effects of the virtual monopoly on services held by one of the home health agencies in the county

Evaluation

The project was operational for 18 months. During this time the following objectives were accomplished:

1. A total of 303 patients qualifying for institutional long-term care were served in the community at an average cost that was 40% of the current nursing home reimbursement rate.
2. Legislators and other community leaders gained increased understanding of the barriers to

expanded community-based long-term care services, including different Medicaid eligibility rules for institutional and community populations that favor institutionalized residents, and the fragmentation of services among various agencies.
3. A uniform assessment tool for long-term care services was developed and accepted for statewide use but was not adopted by all local agencies for intake assessment.

According to the criteria for evaluation of community care presented earlier, the nursing service to the community was successful at delivering care in a high-quality, cost-effective manner in the least restrictive environment possible to 303 elderly persons in need of long-term care. No data were collected that allow comparison of the incidence or prevalence rates of preventable disorders in this population with those in institutional settings or in those receiving traditional community long-term services.

The intervention was not successful in sustaining itself. The other community agencies lobbied successfully with the county commissioners to terminate the project on the grounds that it duplicated existing services in the community. Thus although an intervention or new service may be successful according to objective criteria, it may be politically unsupportable.

PROPER PLACEMENT OF RESIDENTS IN A RETIREMENT COMMUNITY

A private, nonprofit life care community has 320 older persons living independently in their own apartments. There is a 60-bed inpatient facility with 30 skilled nursing beds and 30 domiciliary home beds to accommodate residents with acute, chronic, rehabilitative, or terminal care needs. Primary care services are delivered on site by a geriatric nurse practitioner and a part-time clinic physician as well as by community physicians in their offices. There is a home health nurse/wellness coordinator who sees residents in their apartments for acute and chronic problems. Inpatient care is delivered by nursing staff led clinically by another nurse practitioner who specializes in care of older adults.

The level of care committee is an interdisciplinary group that meets every 2 weeks to discuss proper placement for residents who have borderline functional ability or those in transition from one level of care to another.

Community Health Problems

Although the health care system was designed to allow residents with functional dependencies to transfer to the inpatient facility, many residents prefer to stay in their apartments as long as possible despite chronic illness and functional disabilities.

General Needs of the Borderline Residents

Residents who have borderline function have the following general needs:

- Supervision of health care conditions, including multiple medical disorders
- Supervision of medication regimens
- Varying amounts of help with activities of daily living (ADLs)
- Varying amounts of help with instrumental ADLs
- Social support
- Coordination of caregiving activities
- Regular evaluation of functional status
- Regular evaluation of safety within own environment
- Respect for the wishes of clients to be as autonomous as possible
- Varying amounts of help from family members
- Freedom from caregiving of more frail residents by neighbors

System Constraints

The health care system in this particular community operates under a number of constraints. First, it is committed to maintaining an environment of independent living and wellness to attract other active, independent retirees as new residents; in addition, the socialized payment system must be fair so that the very dependent residents do not consume more than their share of health care resources. Limited home health services are available because Medicare does not fund home health services provided by the community staff, since the facility is not licensed as a home health agency. (A certificate of need would not be extended for this license, because home health services would be provided only to a very small number of persons, and there is already an operational home health agency in the area.) The facility is reluctant to use the local home health agency because of the need for close coordination of care, and many of the needs are not for reimbursable "skilled nursing."

There is a great need for custodial care among the residents, but there is a reluctance to use multiple privately hired nursing assistants who require supervision and coordination in the independent living units. On the other hand, 24-hour per day qualified nursing care is provided in the inpatient unit, where nursing needs can be met more efficiently by the staff than in the community at large.

Assessment

In view of the preceding needs and constraints, the need is for development of a plan to honor the residents' desire for independent living in the least restrictive environment while not taxing the socialized system of health care for the general community and destroying the norm of independent living for the retirement community.

Planning

1. Evaluate the needs of individual residents in terms of the general needs listed earlier. See the assessment form in Box 30-3.
2. Develop a specific care plan for each resident that the home health nurse will administer and coordinate.
3. Help residents and their families hire needed private aides for necessary help with activities of daily living and instrumental activities of daily living, and supervise these caregivers.
4. Discuss the care plan at the level of care meeting so that an interdisciplinary team, including an administrator, may have input about the appropriateness of the use of health care resources.
5. Incorporate the families and residents' physicians in planning and supporting the individualized care plans.
6. Allow residents to have short stays at the health center as necessary, to decrease resistance to possible institutionalization and to acclimate the resident to the supportive environment.
7. Schedule regular outpatient visits to the clinic as residents are able to obtain health care services independently.
8. Allow input from independent living residents about the proper solution to the appropriate level of care problem through the residents' association.
9. Hire a private aide to work with the home health nurse to increase services and decrease supervisory needs, but require that residents pay an additional charge for this service.
10. Require that residents wear street clothes in public areas.

Evaluation

The foregoing plan has worked well, with the decision making and evaluation taking place at the semimonthly level of care meeting. At that time, caregivers present individualized care plans and hear other relevant information from the administration, the residents, and the director of nursing regarding the availability of inpatient beds. When a resident's functional status is quite limited, the group acts as a forum for an objective critique of the care plan and the appropriateness of placement. The committee thus evaluates whether the care plan is adequate and the resident seems sufficiently functional to remain in the apartment without unduly taxing the community's health care resources. A system of checks and balances at level of care meetings works well to individualize patient care and preserve the autonomy of residents, in keeping with the facility's concern for overall fairness and emphasis on promoting functional independence.

THE INDIVIDUAL IN THE COMMUNITY AS CLIENT

Most older persons prefer to stay in their own homes in familiar communities for as long as possible. As people get older, they often fear that they may have to leave home for health reasons. Their fear is realistic because acute and chronic health problems associated with aging often dictate at least temporary changes in environment, leading older adults to reside in places they do not prefer. Their desire to stay at home challenges the health care system to study their special needs and devise solutions that will accommodate them in the most acceptable way. Nurses working in the community who focus on care for individual clients use different specific approaches in the nursing process. The goals of prevention of excess disability and promotion of health apply at both the community and the individual client levels.

Social Engagement

Social engagement is another factor that must be considered in planning care for an individual in the community. The importance of social engagement and activity in old age is a topic of debate that is reflected in numerous theories, including activity, disengagement, continuity, subculture, and age stratification.

Activity Theory. According to the activity theory, older persons who are more socially active are more likely to adjust well to aging (Lemon, Bengtson, & Peterson, 1972). This theory is based on the assumptions that social activity is necessary for continued role enactment, that role enactment is essential to maintain a positive self-concept, that people who have a wide range of roles have many opportunities to reaffirm this positive self-concept, and that people with increased social opportunity have more chances for role enactment, which is the substance of self-concept. Studies have shown that those with higher social involvement have higher morale and better life satisfaction, personal adjustment, and mental health than those who are less involved. Activities that involve close personal contact are of special value. Both the number and the quality of activities are believed to be important. If activities or roles are given up and not replaced, the older person no longer has a social function.

Critics of activity theory argue that the aging process is too complex to be characterized by such a simplistic formulation. It has also been noted that there is insufficient research data to support the theory in its current form. Some studies have produced little evidence to support a relationship between life satisfaction and social activity; in addition, a relationship has not been found between role losses, such as widowhood or retirement, and decreased life satisfaction. Critics conclude that other intervening variables are needed to explain responses to aging.

Disengagement Theory. Disengagement theory states that there is a mutual withdrawal or disengagement between the aging person and others in his or her social system—a withdrawal initiated by the individual or by others in the system (Cumming & Henry, 1961). Such a withdrawal keeps older persons from being frustrated in roles that they are no longer able to competently fulfill, while making a place in society for younger members to fulfill important roles. This is characterized as a normal, intrinsic, inevitable, and universal process.

Among the criticisms of disengagement theory are the following:
- It does not account for the many well-adjusted older persons who are active and highly engaged
- It is not a universal process because it varies among cultural groups
- It may have described older Americans in the late 1950s, but it might not predict what is normal for future cohorts
- Confirming research is limited.

Continuity Theory. Some theorists believe that personality and lifestyle are important factors to consider in adjustment to aging. According to Havighurst, Neugarten, Munichs, and Thomae (1969), the critical factor in adjustment to old age is previously acquired coping abilities and the ability to maintain continuity with previous roles and activities. Four patterns of personality and coping have been identified. *Integrated personalities* are those who are mature and happy but have varied activity levels from highly active to disengaged. *Defended personalities* are those who maintain middle-age values and norms and who are distressed by the losses that accompany old age. *Passive-dependent personalities* include those who have high dependency needs or who are apathetic. Last, *unintegrated personalities* are those who exhibit mental illness.

According to continuity theorists, individuals who were never highly involved with society adjust best to old age if they are able to maintain the same level of involvement. Their adjustment is *not* facilitated by encouraging them to become more socially active. Conversely, individuals who have been highly active socially should not endeavor to disengage from such pursuits but should maintain the same level of activity. Critics of continuity theory argue that it is too simplistic and does not take into account the myriad of variables that affect people's adjustment to aging.

Other Sociological Theories. Other theories of interest are the subculture theory and the age stratification theory. Subculture theory described the older population as a subculture with their own norms, habits, and beliefs. The age stratification theory describes age cohorts as having unique characteristics depending on their social history.

Assessment

Nurses in primary care settings have the most interaction with older individuals. As health promotion activities gain greater acceptance among older persons, it can be expected that the sophistication of this aspect of assessment will increase. If current health care reform reimbursement systems change to prepaid models, the emphasis on health promotion and disease prevention should become more pronounced.

Home health nurses have already experienced changes in the nature of their client population because of the advent of prospective payment for hospitals under Medicare. There is now an increased demand for technologically oriented care and an increased level of acute care for patients in the home, necessitating certain clinical skills in home health nurses previously required only in the hospital setting (Haddad, 1987). Although the focus of nursing care in home and clinic settings is changing to include more acutely ill patients, nurses must remain attentive to the preventive and rehabilitative aspects of care if older people are to be well served.

Primary Care Settings. In primary care, the purposes of assessment are to identify the risk factors for functional impairment, to assist in early detection of treatable disease, and to develop a database for providing continuous care. Primary care providers generally have the advantage of ample opportunity to gather assessment data over an extended period of time rather than being under pressure to perform a comprehensive assessment on the first visit. Although the older person's and family members' concerns should be conscientiously assessed on each visit, other parameters should also be routinely assessed, including:

1. Activities of daily living: walking, transfer, bathing, dressing, continence, eating
2. Instrumental ADLs: telephone use; household chores, including meal preparation; transportation and shopping; and administering one's own medication
3. Mental status

4. Lifestyle, including exercise, diet, use of social drugs
5. Nutrition
6. Social support network
7. Family support
8. Recent life changes
9. Review of desires in regard to a living will, aggressiveness of care
10. Sensory impairments: hearing, vision, peripheral sensation
11. Immunizations
12. Cancer detection protocol: breast, colorectal, prostate, cervical, oral
13. Fall-related injuries
14. Review of medications for possible adverse reactions

More in-depth assessment of these domains is required in selected cases, depending on the individual situation. For more detailed discussion of assessment maneuvers, see Chapter 2.

Individuals without functional impairment should receive an assessment that is focused on health maintenance and health promotion, with in-depth assessment of health problems guided by findings from the history, review of systems, and physical examination. Baseline measures of basic and instrumental ADLs, cognitive status, and social support should be obtained but in less detail than in the multiply impaired individual.

Home Care Settings. People seen in home care settings often have complex problems and suffer from multiple impairments. A comprehensive, multidimensional assessment therefore is indicated and should be obtained as soon as possible following admission to the home care service. Domains to be assessed include:

- Environment
- Activities of daily living
- Instrumental ADLs
- Mental status
- Lifestyle
- Social support network
- Family history
- Recent life change screening
- Review of desires in regard to living will, aggressiveness of care
- Sensory impairment
- Fall-related injury potential
- Review of medications for possible adverse reactions
- Physical assessment to document baseline pathological findings
- Pressure sore risk
- Need and adequacy of care given by others.

The conduct of the assessment is highly individualized according to the needs of the patient and the family and according to the style of the nurse. The end point of the assessment process should be a comprehensive database from which changes can be observed, along with a concise listing of nursing diagnoses.

Nursing Diagnoses

Nursing diagnoses that might apply to the older patient in the community include:

- Impaired home maintenance management related to physical limitations, financial status
- Risk for injury related to environmental obstacles, perceptual deficits, motor impairments, cognitive deficits
- Diversional activity deficit related to social isolation or withdrawal, lack of transportation, financial status, physical or cognitive impairment
- Noncompliance related to lack of knowledge, inadequate financial resources, lack of motivation
- Caregiver role strain related to physical and emotional demands of caregiving, competing demands

Goals and Intervention

Two goals in community-based care of older adults are:

- The older community-dwelling person with multiple impairments will reside in the most appropriate location.
- Families of community-dwelling individuals with multiple impairments will receive adequate support.

Disposition Determination. Determining the ultimate disposition or living situation for an older person can be particularly difficult. Often, elderly people want to remain independent at home, but there may be questions about the wisdom of such a decision. A person's mental or physical health may have a direct impact on where that person can safely live. Use of practical guidelines for making realistic determinations is possible.

Three fundamental questions must be addressed in determining the disposition of an older person who wants to live alone but is at risk for some untoward event: (1) What does the older person want? (2) Can the basic care needs of the person be met at home? (3) Is the older person basically safe at home alone? These three questions have been expanded into an assessment form that can guide the deliberations of an interdisciplinary team that decides with the client and the family where the older person will live (see the independent living assessment in Figure 30-4).

CLIENT DESIRES. Asking older adults what they want sounds rather obvious; however, health care providers often listen more attentively to the opinions of the older person's children than to the older person. The feelings and desires of the older person cannot be ignored, because to do so violates that person's basic human rights. Legally, older people cannot be forced to do something against their will unless they have been declared incompetent. The reasons for the individual's choice should be explored thoroughly. The nurse should determine why the person wants to live at home—specifically, what problems or advantages are foreseen, and what difficulties are anticipated in living in another place. Parnell (1982) noted that the costs of keeping a frail person at home come in two forms: (1) financial expense to pay for needed services in the home and (2) emotional expense of family concern over the risky situation.

FUNCTIONAL STATUS. Evaluation of a client's ability to get basic needs met at home involves assessment of the capacity in ADLs as well as ability to perform instrumental ADLs, such as food preparation, telephone use, medication administration, laundry, and housekeeping. These requirements may be met in many ways, such as through the use of home-delivered meals and in-home help for part of the day. Family, neighbors, or privately paid helpers may enable an older adult to stay at home longer (Wilson et al., 1989). Although assessments are imprecise, the primary provider can monitor whether needs are being met adequately by recording the client's weight at regular intervals, observing for evidence of falls, and observing the home for cleanliness and orderliness.

SAFETY CONSIDERATIONS. Assessing safety in the home is also important. Does the individual know how to summon emergency help? Are home adaptations made to compensate for decreased mobility and dexterity? Cognitive impairments often present a more serious threat to safety than do physical impairments. Judgment and insight should be assessed. For example, people who know they are having problems are likely to call for help and remain safely in the home until help arrives. Individuals with impaired judgment may present a hazard to themselves as well as to their neighbors, as when an older person forgets to turn off the stove. In isolated instances, a choice may be made to preserve the older person's autonomy at the risk of serious injury; however, few would agree that the impaired older person has a right to put others at risk of serious injury. In such cases, interventions such as disconnecting the stove and receiving meals from an outside source may be a reasonable compromise.

Medication use is another important factor to consider when evaluating whether or not an older person can safely remain at home alone. Sometimes the deciding factor in whether or not a cognitively impaired individual can remain at home alone is the nature of the medication regimen. Some individuals do not require medications or can do without drugs, such as calcium supplements, if necessary, whereas others must have medication regularly to maintain health. There are various systems to help forgetful persons take their medicines (see examples in Chapter 18). Preparing and labeling medications for each day is one strategy for simplifying medication administration. Medication calendars that show each type of pill with its time of administration and have a space for marking when the pill is taken are useful to individuals with early memory impairment.

Functionally impaired individuals who want to stay at home but require assistance or supervision with ADLs are often helped by paraprofessional personnel (see Chapter 20). Some controversy exists about the amount of training and supervision necessary for paraprofessionals to function effectively in a helping role with older adults, and requirements vary from state to state. A number of curricula and training guides have been developed, although none is universally accepted. The National Homecaring Council has made recommendations about the minimum training and supervison required of home care workers

Family Caregivers.

A discussion of community-based care is incomplete without acknowledging the importance of "informal supports" that provide the majority of community services to older adults with disabling conditions who live outside institutions. The contribution of family caregivers in the United States is substantial. The Administration on Aging (n.d.) reports that 22.4 million persons in the United States are informal caregivers for older people who live in the community and have at least one limitation in self-care.

Additional interesting findings related to caregiving that emerged from a Bureau of the Census survey (Arno, Levine, & Memmott, 1999) included:

- In the month before the survey, 9.3 million people reported providing regular, unpaid care to a family member or friend.
- The average length of time spent on caregiving was about 8 years.
- About one third of the respondents provided care for 10 or more years.
- The most common types of care/assistance provided by caregivers were helping with expenses, food, transportation, and medications.
- On average, caregivers helped with expenses for 2 to 6 years, spending a total of $19,525 in out-of-pocket expenses.
- The value of the labor contributed by informal caregivers was estimated at $196 billion (about 18% of total national health care spending) in 1997 (Arno et al., 1999).

POTENTIAL STRESSORS. Most family members are concerned and involved with their older relatives, and serve as a natural support network. However, the tasks and responsibilities related to care of an older person in the community must be clearly delineated, and family members must be willing and able to share in accomplishing these tasks. Needs that a family member cannot meet must be identified and then obtained through community agencies, volunteers, friends, or privately paid helpers. Caring for older family members presents many potential stressors on the family unit because of altered role relationships, value conflicts between younger and older adults, the need to confront one's own aging and mortality, financial burdens, and the difficulty of obtaining needed resources and services from the long-term care and health care systems. However, there is a potential for mutual benefit in a caregiving relationship that ranges from financial benefits to deepening of satisfying emotional relationships. Nurses should be skilled at assessing family support and signs of caregiver strain.

TECHNIQUES TO ENHANCE FAMILY FUNCTION. The community-based gerontological nurse's repertoire should include techniques to enhance family function and reduce caregiver burden. Factors associated with positive relationships between older adults and their family members include shared decision making and shared values (Stuart & Snope, 1981), a history of open communication and discussion of conflicts and feelings as they occur, physical proximity, a well-developed sense of self and one's priorities, an ability to have fun together, an ability to set limits without guilt, mutual expression of support and affection, and regular communication. When the older person is supported by a large extended family, it is worthwhile determining how equitably the workload is distributed. If only one or two family members are providing the bulk of support, consider in what ways the others might contribute, such as through financial assistance or provision of nonpersonal care services, such as occasional meal preparation, assistance with yard work, or shopping. When family stress is high, it is important to consider temporary care alternatives outside the family, such as respite care services.

SUPPORT GROUPS. Another useful method of supporting caregiving family members is the formation of support groups (Kernich & Robb, 1988; Pesznecker & Zahlis, 1986; Russell et al., 1989). Hartford & Parsons (1982) identified the following problems while working with caregivers of aged relatives and friends:

- Difficulty in deciding about relocation of an older person
- Acting on a decision to relocate an older person

Box 30-5 *Reflections on Disaster Preparedness: We Need Nurses Who Can "Zoom"*

At last! Some good ideas on handling future disasters have come out of our experiences with Hurricanes Katrina and Rita. Katrina and Rita were level five and four hurricanes, respectively, that devastated the Gulf Coast Region around New Orleans and Sabine Pass, located in the east coast of Texas, on those eventful days in September of 2005. As a volunteer responder in these two natural disasters (Pattillo, 2005), I gained a new understanding of what nurses can offer in these situations.

For months, all people talked about were the unnecessary deaths, unanswered calls for help, rooftop rescues, drained gas pumps, and 2.8 million people caught in snarled traffic. Finally, a task force in Texas recommended that the governor, not county judges or mayors, should have the authority to order mandatory evacuations in an emergency such as a hurricane, so a coordinated state response could be ensured.

- About 60 people, including 23 residents of a Houston suburb assisted living facility, died during the evacuation in advance of Hurricane Rita. Most of the deaths were caused by heat exhaustion while sitting in sweltering heat waiting for the traffic gridlock to open up. The 23 residents died when then their bus caught fire while they were trying to evacuate to Dallas.
- The task force incorporated public input from across the state. There are plans to locate fuel stations and aid stations along evacuation routes. The task force also suggested that nursing homes create and update evacuation plans and that local officials maintain a database of people who may require special assistance during an emergency.
- A single voice that has the clear command and control of the evacuation is needed for a large state like Texas. As the Governor expects the Department of Public Safety to assume control of evacuation routes, he is also expected to work closely with the local officials, especially on issues of shelter plans for pets and the use of bus drivers from school districts.

Why is all this important for gerontological nurses? Although many arguments could be raised for or against certain recommendations, I believe nurses working with older adults in the community should be able to have a macro view as well as micro view on the problem of disasters. I call it being able to "zoom in" and to "zoom out." in disaster response. Here is what I mean.

Zooming Out

Nurses practice in diverse settings, from hospitals to long-term care settings to the community itself. True disaster preparedness means "awareness" and competency in national response, state response, and local response. Nurses can either get caught up in the disaster and be a victim or be prepared so that they can help with response and recovery efforts. Nurses have to realize that all disasters are "local"; that is, the best people who know how to respond and recover are the people who live in the community themselves. The events of September 11, 2001, and the subsequent realignment of the Federal Emergency Management Administration (FEMA) with the Department of Homeland Security have changed the way we all need to look at disasters. Even "small" disasters may have an impact on the national security, economic health, and federal resources.

Nurses have to know the major players in times of a disaster because, like it or not, we have to play with them. And as patient advocates, we have to know how to get what we need in order to maintain a safe environment for ourselves, our families and our older patients. Katrina and Rita made it clear that, especially in times of chaos, we are all interconnected and interdependent on each other. A wise disaster nurse appreciates this and realizes that having relevant knowledge is power. So, get involved and find out about your local community and state disaster plans and provide input that will help your older patients.

Zooming In

Nurses who respond to disasters need skills of basic first aid, psychological first aid, and clinical assessment. Disasters have a way of removing the trappings of wealth and power to reveal the basic survival human needs for safe food, safe water, safe air, safe surroundings, and an intact body. We need to know that nursing in times of "peace" (when skill mix ratios and patient acuity scores are calculated and important) is very different from nursing in times of mass casualties (when nurses may be working along side an EMT, a fireman, a retired physician, or a dentist). Often, allied health professionals look to the nurse to provide the leadership in patient care. We need to be able to render care without electricity, with minimal running water, in the cold, in the heat, and in the dark. A wise disaster nurse realizes what we nurses have always known—that the bottom line in any situation is the human touch (the essence of caring) and some creative problem solving.

So, the experience learned from Katrina and Rita has not been for naught. We have learned much from our experiences in response to one major hurricane that devastated a wonderful vibrant city and another to follow soon after that caused much angst among Texas responders on how to evacuate over 2 million people from Houston and surrounding areas in 4 days. Nurses care very much how people are evacuated because we have to care for them at shelters, in full hospitals, and in their homes. They are from all age groups; they arrive cold, wet, dirty, hungry, worried, and with or without their medications, mobility aids, and caregivers. We have to answer questions from everyone! The public trusts nurses and thinks nurses know all the answers!

Box 30-5 *Reflections on Disaster Preparedness: We Need Nurses Who Can "Zoom"—cont'd*

Marilyn Pattillo

Marilyn Pattillo, PhD, RN, APRN
Gerontological Nurse Practitioner
University of Texas at Austin School of Nursing
Disaster Volunteer Nurse Responder to Approximately
  5000 Evacuees
Convention Center, Hurricanes Katrina and Rita
August-September 2005
Austin, Texas

There are many opportunities for nurses to learn more about preparing for and managing in times of disaster (Lach, Langan, & James, 2005). For example, see the Web sites for the Federal Emergency Management Association, Red Cross, and Center for Disease Control provide helpful information. We need to provide leadership, inside and outside of nursing, to assure good community disaster preparedness and response. Our older patients depend on it. The flexibility of our practice is an asset. What we need are good nurses who can zoom in and zoom out!

- Deciding when it is appropriate to make decisions for the older person
- Involvement with other caregivers who offer either too much or too little help
- Coping with feelings of entrapment, frustration, and guilt
- Dealing with the older person's fear of loss of control or fear of being a burden

Knowledge of strategies for managing these difficult issues facilitates coping with the stressors inherent in caring for an impaired relative. Nurses can foster the development of family support groups to meet this goal.

The Older Americans Act Amendments of 2000 established the National Family Caregiver Support Program (NFCSP) that appeals for all states to work in partnership with area agencies on aging and local community service providers to provide:

- Information to caregivers about services available
- Assistance to caregivers in accessing these services
- Individual counseling, organization of support groups, and caregiver training
- Respite care for caregivers
- Limited supplemental services

Coordination of Services. The role of the gerontological nurse in the primary health care setting depends on the nurse's job as negotiated with the employer. Increasingly, nurses in primary care settings are responsible for counseling in health promotion, coordination of needed in-home services and referrals to other providers, monitoring of response to chronic diseases, and teaching about self-care practices for disease-related conditions. Nurses with geriatric nurse practitioner preparation offer the additional services of diagnosis and management of acute and chronic problems, including prescribing medication, as allowed in some states. Nurses in home health settings have greater interaction with family members than do nurses in primary care settings. The nurse may be the primary support person and teacher of caregiving techniques, and the nurse is often the primary resource person when the patient's condition changes. The nurse has first-hand data about the home environment and its effects on patient and family coping and should take responsibility for communicating this information to other caregivers as indicated. Finally, home health nurses often are responsible for supervising home health aides and other paraprofessionals in the home.

Managed Care and the Older Person. Most older people receive funding for health care through the Medicare/Medicaid system. However, many are enrolled in health maintenance organizations (HMOs) or other prospective payment organizations, which are managed care-based systems. Even those in community agencies may find that they have a case manager whose job is to coordinate appropriate services relevant to their needs. This trend has been necessitated by the rising cost of health care and the disorganization surrounding provision of varying services.

The goal of HMO coverage is to provide access to medical care while containing costs. This goal is to be accomplished by using the most cost-efficient methods of treatment and eliminating unnecessary care. However, the cost incentive involved causes the HMO to increase volume of services. There is concern that older adults do not benefit from enrollment in a managed care system as opposed to remaining in a fee-for-service situation. Both health care providers and recipients are concerned about the impact of cost containment on the quality of care (Boland, 1993).

At the same time, organizations that employ a kind of community-based managed care that uses the services of a case manager show promising outcomes. This team approach is not necessarily new but is appropriate in the current health care environment, which has so

Text continued on p. 892.

Nursing Care Plan: The Ambulatory Care Patient

Assessment Data

A 67-year-old African American woman is seen in a general medical clinic for the following problems: type 2 diabetes mellitus, heart failure, and obesity. She lives with some of her children and works full-time as a housekeeper in the hospital.

The assessment was conducted during the course of several visits to the clinic and included one home visit. Orem's Self-Care Deficit Theory (1995) was used as a nursing "review of systems," and the framework outlined earlier in the section on primary care was used to collect the remainder of the assessment information. The data are as follows:

Universal Self-Care Demands:
1. Air: no difficulties
2. Fluid: takes diuretic to control fluid retention
3. Food: consumes more calories than needed for activity level
4. Elimination: no problems
5. Rest activity: experiences episodes of dizziness while working; often fatigued after work
6. Solitude/social interaction: feels that she has to help with babysitting family members, even when she would rather be alone
7. Injury prevention: engages in regular foot care regimen; has evidence of peripheral neuropathy
8. Normalcy: continues employment despite being older than retirement age and despite multiple chronic diseases; has leadership role in extended family network

Health-Deviation Self-Care Demands:
1. Diabetes mellitus: does not understand relationship between activity, diet, and insulin; has no regular system for monitoring blood glucose level, is frequently hyperglycemic when seen in clinic, and has symptoms attributable to poor blood glucose level control (dizziness, fatigue)
2. Heart failure: adheres to medication regimen but has poor understanding of heart failure and relationship between exercise, diet, and medication requirements

Developmental Self-Care Requisites:
1. Acceptance of chronic disease
2. Adjustment to role changes accompanying aging

Aging-Specific Assessment Parameters:
1. Activities of daily living status: independent in all basic ADLs and all instrumental ADLs except driving
2. Mental status: no evidence of cognitive impairment
3. Nutritional status: obese, 20% over ideal body weight; hematological indices normal, hyperglycemic
4. Social support: lives with three children (of six), who provide transportation and assist with grocery shopping; patient provides assistance with grocery shopping, contributes financially to the household; patient does not identify a confidante, is active in local church and neighborhood activities, has many friends in the workplace, and is referred to by many as "Mama"
5. Family assessment: family communications not completely open, although children do communicate with each other about patient's health status and needs
6. Recent life changes: none identified
7. Review of desires regarding living will, aggressiveness of care: deferred because of other priorities in assessment and care
8. Sensory impairment screening: no hearing impairment evident on "whispered word" test; able to read small print with glasses, distance visual acuity = 20/40 by Snellen chart; decreased sensitivity to light touch and pinprick in lower extremities to calf
9. Immunization status: tetanus, influenza, and Pneumovax up to date
10. Cancer detection status: does not perform breast self-examination, has had Papanicolaou smear within past year, stools negative for occult blood, mammogram 1 year ago negative
11. Fall-related injury assessment: risk factors include dizziness, cluttered home environment, four steps to enter home, uneven sidewalks in neighborhood
12. Medications: insulin glargine, metformin, captopril, hydrochlorothiazide

Nursing Diagnoses (Johnson, Bulechek, Dochterman, Maas, & Moorhead, 2001)

Noncompliance with therapeutic diet related to lack of understanding of dietary management of diabetes mellitus

Risk for Injury related to neuropathy and dizziness secondary to diabetes mellitus and environmental obstacles

Ineffective Coping related to unsatisfactory support systems

Goals/Outcomes

- The patient will verbalize the relationships among her symptoms of dizziness, blood glucose level, diet, and activity.
- The patient will express intent to modify lifestyle to achieve better control of diabetes.
- The patient will remain free of injury in her home and work environments.
- The family will provide increased support and decrease expectations of patient.

NOC Outcomes (Moorhead, Johnson, & Maas, 2004)

Adherence Behavior
Risk Control

Nursing Care Plan: The Ambulatory Care Patient—cont'd

Coping
Information Processing
Social Support

NIC Suggested Interventions (Dochterman & Bulechek, 2004)

Major interventions: Environmental management: Safety (6486), Fall Prevention (6490), Behavior Modification (4360), Health Education (5510), Learning Readiness Enhancement (5540), Family Involvement Promotion (7110), Coping Enhancement (5230)

- Identify safety hazards in the environment.
- Remove hazards from the environment when possible.
- Provide patient with emergency phone numbers.
- Provide assistive devices to steady gait.
- Teach patient how to fall so as to minimize injury.
- Avoid clutter on floor surface.
- Provide adequate lighting for increased visibility.
- Provide nightlight at bedside.
- Educate family members about risk factors that contribute to falls and how they can decrease these risks.
- Establish a personal relationship with the patient and family members who will be involved in care.
- Facilitate understanding of the medical aspects of the patient's condition for family members.
- Encourage focus on any positive aspects of the patient's situation.
- Inform family members of factors that may improve patient's condition.
- Determine patient's motivation to change.
- Give feedback in terms of feelings when patient is noted to be free of symptoms and looks relaxed.
- Avoid showing rejection or belittlement as patient struggles with changing behavior.
- Identify behaviors to be changed.
- Break behaviors to be changed into smaller, measurable units of behavior.
- Identify internal or external factors that may enhance or reduce motivation for healthy behavior.
- Determine current health knowledge and lifestyle behaviors.
- Help patient to identify the information she is most interested in obtaining.
- Encourage verbalization of feelings, perceptions, and fears.
- Prioritize identified learner needs based on client preference, skills of nurse, resources available, and likelihood of successful goal attainment.
- Provide factual information concerning diagnosis, treatment, and prognosis.
- Provide the patient with realistic choices about certain aspects of care.
- Avoid use of fear or scare techniques as strategy to motivate people to change health or lifestyle behaviors.
- Emphasize immediate or short-term positive health benefits to be obtained by positive lifestyle behaviors.
- Involve individuals, families, and groups in planning and implementing plans for lifestyle or health behavior modification.
- Encourage gradual mastery of the situation.
- Design and implement strategies to measure client outcomes at regular intervals during and after completion of program.
- Provide time for the patient to ask questions and discuss concerns.
- Assist the patient to develop confidence in ability.
- Assist the patient to realize the severity of the illness, the treatment options that exist, the susceptibility to complications, and the ability to control the progression of the illness.

Evaluation Parameters

Occurrence of falls or other injuries, blood glucose levels, peripheral edema, patient knowledge of diabetes and heart failure, adherence to prescribed medications, ability to measure blood glucose level, weight, patient activity tolerance, frequency of dizziness, family involvement in patient management of conditions, patient expressions of ability to manage conditions, patient intent to adhere with medical plan of care

Follow-up

In this case study, for 2 months the patient declined offers of instruction on blood glucose level monitoring at home. At this time, she was hospitalized in a hyperosmolar state. The primary care nurse visited her in the hospital to assess the nature of the diabetic teaching being provided and to determine whether the patient's readiness to learn had changed.

Both the patient and one daughter had become highly motivated to learn about home glucose level monitoring and how to improve dietary control over diabetes. Home health referral was made for teaching home blood glucose level monitoring during convalescence from the hospitalization. The clinic nurse and home health nurse were in close communication about the pacing of instruction and about the patient's recording her activity and diet information along with blood glucose levels. The patient was able to master the skill of blood glucose level monitoring and used the information to understand the effect of diet and exercise on glucose levels and symptoms.

Her activity level improved as a result of losing approximately 30 pounds and because she was no longer dizzy. Her comfort level increased because she no longer experienced daily episodes of dizziness and fatigue. Through mastery of a new skill, she was able to achieve better control over a chronic disease and make active choices about lifestyle modifications rather than blindly following a behavior pattern that contributed to poor control of her chronic diseases.

Nursing Care Plan: The Terminally Ill Patient

Assessment Data

Mr. H is a 70-year-old retired white male referred to home health for terminal care after discharge from the hospital. His diagnoses include metastatic brain cancer, seizure disorder, bilateral pleural effusions, and a history of alcoholism. He lives alone in a subsidized housing project.

Universal Self-Care Requisites:

1. Air: becomes short of breath with moderate activity
2. Fluid: drinks sufficient liquids without difficulty
3. Food: is unable to shop for groceries or prepare meals independently but can eat independently
4. Elimination: no problems
5. Activity/rest: lethargic at times; denies sleep disturbance
6. Solitude/social interaction: no longer meets friends at local convenience store because "They wouldn't want to see me like this."
7. Safety: at high risk for fall-related injury
8. Normalcy: in terminal stage of illness but is adamant about not going to a nursing home until "I can't make it on my own any more." Does not believe that time is now.

Health-Deviation Self-Care Requisites:

1. Requires twice-daily dexamethasone (Decadron) to control cerebral edema; has history of steroid psychosis in the past because of improper dosing
2. Requires twice-daily phenobarbital to control seizure disorder (not able to tolerate phenytoin)
3. Requires assistance with activities of daily living because of weakness related to cerebral edema, pleural effusions, cognitive impairment

Developmental Self-Care Requisites:

1. Acceptance of one's own mortality
2. Completion of unfinished business

Assessment Parameters for Home-Based Care:

1. Environmental assessment: lives alone in a two-story subsidized housing project apartment, where bedroom and toilet are upstairs. He sleeps on the sofa and has a bedside commode.
2. Activities of daily living status: requires assistance with meal preparation, grocery shopping, medication administration, dressing, and bathing. Can eat, transfer, ambulate, and toilet self independently using bedside commode but cannot empty bedside commode alone.
3. Mental status: has focal defects, including poor short-term memory, poor judgment, and limited reasoning ability. However, states a strong desire to remain at home as long as possible despite admittedly limited reserve. Can verbalize risks of staying at home alone.
4. Lifestyle assessment: lived a "drifter's life" for many years. Is used to making his own decisions, managing his own affairs. Has alienated most of his family, although his sister, who lives nearby, expresses sporadic interest in his care. Recreational activities before present illness included playing checkers at neighborhood store daily.
5. Social support status: one neighbor across terrace looks out for him in a friendly way—checks to see that he gets up each morning, fixes occasional meals. Sister willing to assist with finances, but patient resists this. Formal agencies involved include home health agency, council on aging, social services. Hospice not involved because patient has not identified a primary caregiver.
6. Family status: no children. Only relatives nearby are a sister who is inconsistently involved. She feels he should be in a nursing home or living with her, which he refuses to do. He would prefer to go to a nursing home first.
7. Recent life changes: no recent changes other than onset of cancer and its resultant functional limitations.
8. Desires regarding aggressiveness of care: does not want heroic measures taken. Has been through course of palliative radiation therapy. Says he will agree to go to nursing home when he can no longer care for self. Understands that he has cancer, and that it is not curable.
9. Sensory impairment: hemiparesis (left-sided), although he has only weakness, not true paralysis; decreased sensation to pinprick and light touch. Vision and hearing intact.
10. Fall-related injury risk: at high risk. Risk secondary to environmental problems (e.g., steep stairs) and intrinsic factors such as hemiparesis, weakness, poor judgment, lethargy from medications, and seizure disorder.
11. Medications include dexamethasone and phenobarbital.
12. Baseline pathological findings include left-sided hemiparesis, bilateral pleural effusions, dysarthria, and dependence in activities of daily living.
13. Risk of pressure sore development at present: mild, with a Norton score of 16. This is based on his relative functional independence (ability to ambulate, continence).

Nursing Diagnoses

Impaired Home Maintenance related to chronic debilitating disease (cancer) and impaired mental status

Self-Care Deficit: Bathing/Hygiene, Dressing/ Grooming, Instrumental (medication administration) related to cognitive and physical deficits

Ineffective Coping related to terminal illness

Spiritual Distress related to crisis of illness and lack of support network

Nursing Care Plan: The Terminally Ill Patient—cont'd

Risk for Injury related to altered cerebral function, environmental hazards, and alcoholism

Activity Intolerance related to pleural effusion

Goals/Outcomes

- The patient will remain free of injury in the home setting.
- The patient's basic needs will be met with assistance as needed.
- The patient will participate in decisions about the care setting.
- The patient will verbalize that his spiritual needs have been met.

NOC Outcomes

Safe Home Environment
Adaptation to Physical Disability
Acceptance: Health Status
Coping
Decision Making
Spiritual Health
Fall Prevention Behavior
Energy Conservation
Endurance

NIC Suggested Interventions

Major interventions: Home Maintenance Assistance (7180), Fall Prevention (6490), Self-Care Assistance: Bathing/Hygiene (1801), Self-Care Assistance: Dressing/Grooming (1802), Coping Enhancement (5230), Decision-Making Support (5250), Spiritual Growth Facilitation (5246), Energy Management (0180), and Self-Care Assistance: IADL (1805)

- Provide information on how to make home environment safe and clean.
- Monitor gait, balance, and fatigue level with ambulation.
- Provide assistive devices (e.g., cane, walker) as appropriate.
- Instruct patient about use of cane or walker, as appropriate.
- Teach patient how to fall so as to minimize injury.
- Provide elevated toilet seat for easy transfer.
- Provide a means of summoning help.
- Avoid clutter on floor surfaces.
- Provide nightlight at bedside.
- Ensure that the patient has shoes that fit properly, fasten securely, and have nonskid soles.
- Provide assistance until patient is fully able to assume self-care.
- Reinforce efforts to dress self.
- Facilitate assistance of a barber, as necessary.
- Determine whether there are differences between the patient's view of own condition and the view of health care providers.
- Inform patient of alternative views or solutions.

- Help patient identify the advantages and disadvantages of each alternative.
- Facilitate collaborative decision making.
- Serve as a liaison between patient and other health care providers.
- Provide factual information about diagnosis, prognosis, and treatment.
- Evaluate the patient's decision-making ability.
- Seek to understand the patient's perception of a stressful situation.
- Encourage the use of spiritual resources, if desired.
- Support the use of appropriate defense mechanisms.
- Encourage verbalization of feelings, perceptions, and fears.
- Appraise the patient's needs/desires for social support.
- Assist the patient to solve problems in a constructive manner.
- Assist the patient to grieve and work through the losses of disability.
- Demonstrate caring presence and comfort by spending time with patient.
- Encourage conversation that assists the patient in sorting out spiritual concerns.
- Assist patient with identifying barriers and attitudes that hinder growth or self-discovery.
- Offer prayer support, as appropriate.
- Refer for pastoral care as issues warrant.
- Encourage verbalization of feelings about limitations.
- Encourage alternate rest and activity periods.
- Assist the patient in assigning priority to activities to accommodate energy levels.
- Provide for methods of contacting support and assistance people.
- Provide cognitive enhancing techniques.
- Determine whether monthly income is sufficient to cover expenses.
- Refer to community services as needed.

Evaluation Parameters

The patient will experience no falls, burns, or other traumatic injuries. The patient will accomplish dressing, grooming, and hygiene with support as needed. The patient will maintain decision-making capacity, and will express acceptance of his condition and a sense of peace with his terminal state. Other specific indicators of outcome achievement are the following: identifies plan to meet ADLs, balances activity and rest, adapts lifestyle to energy level, recognizes reality of health situation, verbalizes acceptance of situation, chooses among alternatives, expresses feelings of peacefulness, uses personal alarm system, and stores assistive devices in an accessible location.

Continued

Nursing Care Plan: The Terminally Ill Patient—cont'd

Follow-up

The health care team, including the home health nurse, physician, and case manager, agreed to support the patient's goal of staying at home as long as possible. To assist with instrumental ADLs and to supervise one time slot of medication administration, homemaker services were obtained. This individual was assigned to perform light housekeeping, meal preparation, and grocery shopping and to empty the bedside commode, as well as to provide some social stimulation. The homemaker visited for 3 hours each day in the afternoon, 7 days per week. The presence of the homemaker, combined with daily home health aide visits, allowed for a twice-daily checking on the patient and the ability to call for help if the patient had fallen. A home health aide visited 7 days per week in the morning to assist with personal care, fix a hot breakfast, and supervise morning medication administration. She was supervised by the home health nurse, who also provided some limited counseling services to the patient. The home health nurse organized the medication administration schedule so that it was as simple as possible for the patient and helpers to understand. A medication calendar was used, with administration times set at breakfast and at bedtime. The home health agency was on call on a 24-hour per day basis to the patient and family, as well as to the paraprofessional helpers. The nurse/case manager was responsible for coordinating the overall plan of care, ensuring that accurate financial records were kept to continue Medicaid coverage for services, as well as communicating with the patient's sister. The case manager was also responsible for requesting adult protective services if the patient's situation became blatantly unsafe, so that nursing home placement could be arranged. The case manager provided assistance with life review and acceptance of dying, as well as counseling about obtaining more assistance if needed.

In less than 1 week, the patient became too weak to be able to care for himself adequately during the times when there was no help available. His increasing lethargy caused him to be admitted to the hospital emergency department pending identification of a nursing home bed. His total time in the hospital was less than 24 hours. He died within 1 week of admission to the nursing home.

---

many unrelated services that can be of benefit to older adults who wish to remain independent as long as possible. A demonstration project has been undertaken in Arkansas. The North Little Rock Community Seniors Health Services project has a goal to assist older adults to manage their own health care, maintain or improve their health, and continue living in their own homes (Leath & Thatcher, 1991). Each client who enrolls is given a comprehensive assessment of all health and social needs. Team members include a clinical nurse specialist as team coordinator, a gerontological nurse practitioner, a clinical pharmacist, a clinical nutritionist, a geriatrician who works with the client's private physician, and a social worker. After the initial evaluation, the agency then provides direct service delivery, health promotion services, and disease prevention services; coordinates resource referrals; and monitors clients' health status as long as they wish. The preliminary reports of the success of this project are very positive (Leath & Thatcher, 1991).

Evaluation

No matter who the primary provider of care for the older person is, the essentials of caring for older adults consist of competence, comprehensiveness, continuity, and coordination. *Competence* indicates that the care is based on scientific principles of gerontological care, drawing from research in the nursing, biomedical, pharmacological, nutritional, psychosocial, and rehabilitation literature. Satisfactory care is delivered only when care providers understand their limitations as well as their strengths and refer to other providers appropriately to maximize the functional potential of their clients.

Comprehensiveness specifies that the approach to the client is holistic. Every need the client perceives is related to health—be it physical, emotional, social, or spiritual. Distress is felt by the older adult in many ways, and one system may affect another. In other words, psychological or spiritual distress may manifest itself through the body in the form of a headache, abdominal cramping in an irritable colon, or an ulcer. Effective care must deal with the source of the problem as well as its physical manifestations. (For specific ideas about psychosocial care, see Chapters 20 and 21.) Comprehensiveness also means that the patient's environment is important and must be included in assessing and managing a patient's problem. Death of a spouse, a move to another house or community, or a lack of access to transportation all affect a person's health and must be dealt with in a comprehensive health program. Comprehensive care means that the nurse must view elderly clients from many perspectives, including health habits and lifestyle characteristics.

Continuity means that persons are cared for whatever their location. Because their care extends over time, their history and caretaking are relevant to any immediate problem. It is essential to gather baseline data on every older client. Only then can a provider know whether an dysrhythmia is an old or a new finding or whether a blood pressure reading is abnormal. Follow-up is also essential for both acute and chronic problems. Ideally, every time an older client leaves an encounter with a primary care clinician, a follow-up appointment should be made. Patients should know that if a problem is not improving, they should not hesitate to call their primary care clinician. Many older people need to know that some problems are not curable but can be controlled. Accurate, complete documentation is essential for continuity of care. Older clients often have long problem lists, the contents of which should be addressed individually over time and at regular intervals. Acute or chronic problems should be easily traced, and their status should be quite clear from review of the chart. For example, the presence of chronic bibasilar rales is important in assessing or monitoring a client with cardiopulmonary problems.

Coordination is another essential ingredient in geriatric care that involves many providers, disciplines, and agencies. The nurse can provide the link among all the professionals who are treating a patient and may not be aware of each others' actions. For example, one specialist physician may be prescribing a drug that is essentially the same as that prescribed by another physician or is contraindicated given the long list of other medications prescribed for various chronic illnesses. None of the providers may be aware of all the over-the-counter medications an older person is taking. As health care reform is implemented, the use of case managers may improve overall coordination.

A paramount goal of all primary care is to help clients be as functional and independent as possible within their preferred lifestyle. Nearly all older people dread becoming dependent. Achieving the aims cited above within a complex, fragmented health care delivery system requires scrupulous attention to the four hallmarks of high-quality elder care: competence, comprehensiveness, continuity, and coordination.

The nursing care plans describe some of the complexities of care for individuals in the community setting. The first plan focuses on an ambulatory care patient with multiple chronic problems. The second involves a terminally ill client, estranged from his family, who wants to remain at home as long as possible and requires sophisticated and well-coordinated care.

Also, for information on nursing care in disaster situations, see Box 30-5.

REFERENCES

Administration on Aging. (2004). Mental health and aging. Accessed December 15, 2005 at www.aoa.gov.

Administration on Aging. (n.d). Family caregiving. Retrieved January 4, 2006, from www.aoa.gov.

Algera, M., Francke, A. L., Kerkstra, A., & van der Zee, J. (2004). Home care needs of patients with long-term conditions: Literature review. *Journal of Advanced Nursing, 46*(4), 417-429.

American Nurses Association. (2005). Public health nursing: Scope and standards of practice. Retrieved December 24, 2005, from http://nursingworld.org.

American Nurses Association. (1999). *Scope and standards of public health nursing practice.* Washington, DC: ANA.

American Nurses Association, Ad Hoc Committee, Public Health Nurses' Section. (1964). *Nature of public health nursing.* New York: ANA.

Anderson, E. (1983). Community focus in public health nursing: Whose responsibility? *Nursing Outlook, 31,* 44-48.

Anderson, E. T., & McFarlane, J. M. (1988). *Community as partner: Theory and practice in nursing* (4th ed). Philadelphia: J. B. Lippincott.

Anderson, R. E., & Carter, I. E. (1974). *Human behavior in the social environment: A social systems approach.* Chicago: Aldine, p. 47.

Andrews, J., Manthorpe, J., & Watson, R. (2004). Involving older people in intermediate care. *Journal of Advanced Nursing, 46*(3), 303-310.

Area Agencies on Aging (AAA). (n.d.). A link to services for older adults and their caregivers. Retrieved January 3, 2006, from http://www.n4a.org/aboutaaas.cfm.

Arno, P. S., Levine, C., & Memmott, M. M. (1999). The economic value of informal caregiving. *Health Affairs, 18*(2), 182-188.

Aud, M. A. (2004). Residents with dementia in assisted living facilities: The role of behavior in discharge decisions. *Journal of Gerontological Nursing, 30*(6), 16-26.

Bird, M. J., & Parslow, R. A. (2002). Potential for community programs to prevent depression in older people. *Medical Journal of Australia, 177*(suppl), S107-S110.

Boland, P. (1993). *Making managed health care work: A practical guide to strategies and solutions.* Gaithersburg, MD: Aspen Publishing.

Borders, T. F., Rohrer, J. E., Xu, K. T., & Smith, D. R. (2004). Older persons' evaluations of health care: The effects of medical skepticism and worry about health. *Health Services Research, 39*(1), 35-52.

Bremer, A. (1989). A description of community health nursing practice with the community-based elderly. *Journal of Community Health Nursing, 6*(3), 173-184.

Buhler-Wilkerson, K. (2001). No place like home: A history of nursing and home care in the U.S. *Home Healthcare Nurse, 20*(10), 641-647.

Burner, S., & Waldo, D. (1995). Data view: National health expenditure projections 1994-2005. *Health Care Financing Review 1995, 16*(4), 221-242.

Capitman, J. (2003). Effective coordination of medical and supportive services. *Journal of Aging and Health, 15*(1), 124-164.

Carbonell, J. G. (2003). Press release: HHS and NCOA issue new resource to improve health of older adults. Retrieved January 28, 2005, from www.aoa.gov/press/pr/2003/06_jun/06_30_03.asp.

Carlo, G. L. (July 15, 1998). Testimony before Energy and Environment Subcommittee of the Committee on Science. U.S. House of Representatives, Washington, DC.

Casarett, D., Karlawish, J., Morales, K., Crowley, R., Mirsch, T., & Asch, D. A. (2005). Improving the use of hospice services in nursing homes: A randomized controlled trial. *Journal of the American Medical Association, 294*(2), 211-217.

Centers for Disease Control and Prevention, National Center for Health Statistics. (2004). Health care visits to doctor's offices and hospital outpatient and emergency departments by selected characteristics: United States, selected years 1995-2002. Bethesda, MD: National Institutes of Health.

Centers for Medicare and Medicaid Services. (2004). Medicare and home health care (publication no. CMS-10969). Retrieved May 9, 2006, from www.medicare.gov/Publications/Pubs/pdf/10969.pdf.

Centers for Medicare and Medicaid Services. (2000). Medicare claims and enrollment data. Retrieved May 9, 2006, from www.agingstats.gov/chartbook2000/healthcare.html.

Centers for Medicare and Medicaid Services. (2005). Medicare hospice benefits. Publication No. HCFA 02154-LE. Retrieved May 9, 2006, from www.medicare.gov/Publications/Pubs/pdf/02154.pdf.

Clark, M. J. (1992). *Nursing in the community*. Norwalk, CT: Appleton & Lange.

Clemen-Stone, S., Eigsti, D. G., & McGuire, S. L. (1991). *Comprehensive family and community health nursing* (3rd ed.). St. Louis: Mosby-Year Book.

Cohen, J., Machlin, S., Zuvekas, S., et al. (2000). Health care expenditures in the United States, 1996. *MEPS research findings 12*, AHRQ Publication No. 01-0009. Rockville, MD: Agency for Healthcare Research and Quality.

Craig, K. J., Donovan, K., Munnery, M., Owens, D. R., Williams, J. D., & Phillips, A. O. (2004). Identification and management of diabetic nephropathy in the diabetes clinic. *Diabetes Care, 26*(6), 1806-1811.

Cumming, E., & Henry, W. (1961). *Growing old: The process of disengagement*. New York: Basic Books.

DeSilva, D. L., Dillon, J. E., & Teno, J. M. (2001). The quality of care in the last month of life among Rhode Island nursing home residents. *Medicine & Health, Rhode Island, 84*(6), 195-198.

Dochterman, J. M., & Bulechek, G. M. (2004). *Nursing interventions classification* (4th ed.). St. Louis: Mosby.

Edwards, N., Cere, M., & Leblond, D. (1993). A community-based intervention to prevent falls among seniors. *Family Community Health, 15*(4), 57-65.

Eliopoulos, C. (2005). *Gerontological nurisng*. Philadelphia: Lippincott Williams & Wilkins.

Eloniemi-Sulkava, U., Notkola, I., Hentinen, M., Kivela Sivenius, J., & Sulkava, R. (2001). Effects of supporting community living demented patients and their caregivers: A randomized trial. *Journal of the American Geriatrics Society, 49*(10), 1282-1287.

Etzioni, A. (1993). *The spirit of community*. New York: Crown Publishers.

Federal Interagency Forum on Aging-Related Statistics. (2004). *Older Americans 2004: Key indicators of well-being* (chartbook). Washington, DC: Federal Interagency Forum on Aging-Related Statistics, U.S. Government Printing Office.

Felland, L. E., Kinner, J. K., & Hoadley, J. F. (2003). The health care safety net: Money matters but savvy leadership counts. *Issue Brief/Center for Studying Health System Change, 66*, 1-4.

Fermazin, M., Canady, M. O., Milmine, P., Perron, J., & Cooper, L. (2004). Home health compare: Web site offers critical information to consumers and professionals. *Home Healthcare Nurse, 22*(6), 408-416.

Field, M. J., & Cassell, C. K. (1997). *Approaching death: Improving care at the end of life* (report of the Institute of Medicine Task Force). Washington, DC: National Academies Press.

Fleming, K. C., Evans, J. M., Weber, D. C., & Chutka, D. S. (1995). Practical functional assessment of elderly persons: A primary-care approach. *Mayo Clinic Proceedings, 70*(9), 890-895.

Forbes, S., Bern-Klug, M., & Gessert, C. (2000). End of life decision making for nursing home residents with dementia. *Journal of Nursing Scholarship, 32*(3), 251-258.

Franzini, L., Caughy, M., Spears, W., & Esquer, M. E. F. (2005). Neighborhood economic conditions, social processes, and self-rated health in low-income neighborhoods in Texas: A multilevel latent variables model. *Social Science & Medicine, 61*(6), 1135-1150.

Fraser, K. D., & Strang, V. (2004). Decision making and nurse case management: A philosophical perspective. *Advances in Nursing Science, 27*(1), 32-43.

Fries, J. F. (1992). Strategies for reduction of morbidity. *American Journal of Clinical Nutrition, 55*(suppl; 6), 1257S-1262S.

Glickman, L. L., Stocker, K. B., & Caro, F. G. (1997). Self-direction in home care for older people: A consumer's perspective. *Home Health Care Services Quarterly, 16*(1/2), 41-54.

Goodwin, C. (1871-1955). *The Boston Dispensary records*. Boston: Simmons College Library.

Gustavson, K., & Lee, C. D. (2004). Alone and content: Frail seniors living in their own homes compared to those who live with others. *Journal of Women and Aging, 16*(3-4), 3-18.

Haddad, A. M. (1987). *High tech home care: A practical guide*. Rockville, MD: Aspen Publishing.

Hanson, L. C., Danis, M., & Garrett, J. (1997). What is wrong with end of life care? Opinions of bereaved family members. *Journal of the American Geriatrics Society, 45*(11), 1339-1344.

Hartford, M., & Parsons, R. (1982). Groups with relatives of dependent adults. *Gerontologist, 22*(3), 394-398.

Havighurst, R. J., Neugarten, B. L., Munichs, J. M. A., & Thomae, H. (Eds.). (1969). *Adjustment to retirement: A cross-national study*. Netherlands: Van Gorkum.

Hays, J. C. (2002). Living arrangements and health status in later life: A review of recent literature. *Public Health Nursing, 19*(2), 136-151.

Hinds, P. S., Chaves, D. E., & Cypess, S. M. (1992). Context as a source of meaning and understanding. *Qualitative Health Research, 2*(1), 61-74.

Hogue, C. C. (1977). Epidemiology for distributive nursing practice. In J. Hall & B. R. Weaver (Eds.), *Distributive nursing practice: A systems approach to community health nursing*. Philadelphia: Lippincott, pp. 193-210.

Hubert, H. B., Bloch, D. A., & Fries, J. F. (1993). Risk factors for physical disability in an aging cohort: The NHANES I Epidemiologic Followup Study. *Journal of Rheumatology, 20*(3), 480-488.

Inglis, S., McLennan, S., Dawson, A., Birchmore, L., Horowitz, J. D., Wilkinson, D., & Stewart, S. (2004). A new solution for an old problem? Effects of a nurse-led, multidisciplinary, home-based intervention on readmission and mortality in patients with chronic atrial fibrillation. *Journal of Cardiovascular Nursing, 19*(2), 118-127.

Johnson, M., Bulechek, G., Dochterman, J. M., Maas, M., & Moorhead, S. (2001). *Nursing diagnoses, outcomes, & interventions*. St. Louis: Mosby.

Johnson, M. A. (1990). Growing old in America: Health care for the elderly. In S. J. Wold (Ed.), *Community Health Nursing: Issues and Topics*. Norwalk, CT: Appleton & Lange.

Kanervisto, M., Paavilainen, E., & Astedt-Kurki, P. (2003). Impact of chronic obstructive pulmonary disease on family functioning. *Heart and Lung, 32*(6), 360-367.

Keepnews, D., Capitman, J. A., & Rosati, R. J. (2004). Measuring patient level clinical outcomes of home health care. *Journal of Nursing Scholarship, 36*(1), 79-85.

Kernich, C. A., & Robb, G. (1988). Development of a stroke family support and education program. *Journal of Neuroscience Nursing, 20*(3), 193-197.

King County Long-Term Care Ombudsman. (n.d.). Choosing a long-term care facility. Retrieved January 3, 2006, from http://www.ltcop.org/ChoosingFacilityMain.htm.

Kippenbrock, T., & Soja, M. D. (1993). Preventing falls in the elderly: Interviewing patients who have fallen. *Geriatric Nursing, 14*(4), 205-209.

Koop, C. E. (1991). *The memoirs of America's family doctor*. New York: Random House.

Kretzmann, J. P., & McKnight, J. L. (1993). *Building communities from the inside out: A path toward finding and mobilizing a community's assets*. Evanston, IL: Institute for Policy Research, pp. 1-11.

Kunstler, R. (2002). Therapeutic recreation in the naturally occurring retirement community (NORC): Benefiting "aging in place" (electronic version). *Therapeutic Recreation Journal, 36*(2), 186-202.

Lach, H. W., Langan, J. C., & James, D. C. (2005). Disaster planning: Are gerontological nurses prepared? *Journal of Gerontological Nursing, 31*(11), 21-27.

Larsson, B. W., Larsson, G., & Carlson, S. R. (2004). Advanced home care: Patients' opinions on quality compared with those of family members. *Journal of Clinical Nursing, 13*(2), 226-233.

Lazarus, A. (2001). Integrating end of life care with disease management programs: A new role for case managers. *Managed Care Interface, 14*(3), 76-79.

Leath, C., & Thatcher, R. M. (1991). Team-managed care for older adults: A clinical demonstration of a community model. *Journal of Gerontological Nursing, 17*(7), 25-28.

Leavell, H. R., & Clark, E. G. (1965). *Preventive medicine for the doctor in his community: An epidemiological approach.* New York: McGraw-Hill.

Leigh, J. P., & Fries, J. F. (1992-1993). Associations among healthy habits, age, gender, and education in a sample of retirees. *International Journal of Aging and Human Development, 36*(2), 139-155.

Lemon, B. W., Bengtson, V. L., & Peterson, J. A. (1972). An exploration of the activity theory of aging: Activity types and life satisfaction among in-movers to a retirement community. *Journal of Gerontology, 27*, 511-523.

Liang, J., Brown, J. W., Krause, N. M., Ofstedal, M. B., & Bennett, J. (2005). Health and living arrangements among older Americans: Does marriage matter? *Journal of Aging & Health, 17*(3), 305-335.

Manderscheid, R. W., Atay, J. E., Hernandez-Cartagena, M. D. R., Edmond, P. Y., Male, A., Parker, T. C. E., & Zhang, H. (2006). Mental health, United States 2000. Retrieved January 7, 2006, from http://mentalhealth.samhsa.gov/publications/allpubs/SMA01-3537/chap14.asp.

Maynard, C. K. (2003). Differentiate depression from dementia. *Nurse Practitioner, 28*(3), 18-19, 23-27, quiz 27-9.

McGinnis, J. M., & Foege, W. H. (2003). The immediate vs the important. *Journal of the American Medical Association, 291*(10), 1263-1264.

Medical Expenditure Panel. (1996). *Preliminary estimates from the 1996 Medical Expenditure Panel Survey, projections 1998-2008.* Rockville, MD: AHRQ.

Mehta, K. M., Simonsick, E. M., Penninx, B. W. J., Schulz, R., Rubin, R. M., Satterfield, S., & Yaffe, K. (2003). Prevalence and correlates of anxiety symptoms in well-functioning older adults: Findings from the health aging and body composition study. *Journal of the American Geriatrics Society, 51*(4), 499-504.

Mezey, M. D., Rauckhorst, L. H., & Stokes, S. A. (1993). *Health assessment of the older individual* (2nd ed.). New York: Springer, p. 246.

Moorhead, S., Johnson, M., & Maas, M. (2004). *Nursing outcomes classification (NOC)* (3rd ed.). St. Louis: Mosby.

Morris, J. N., Sherwood, S., & Mor, V. (1984). An assessment tool for use in identifying functionally vulnerable persons in the community. *Gerontologist, 24*, 373-379.

Mueller, C., & Karon, S. L. (2004). ANA nurse sensitive quality indicators for long-term care facilities. *Journal of Nursing Care Quality, 19*(1), 39-47.

National Adult Day Services Association. (n.d.). What are adult day services? Retrieved January 3, 2006, from http://www.nadsa.org/.

National Alliance for Caregiving and American Association of Retired Persons (AARP). Comparative analysis of caregiver data for caregivers to the elderly 1987 and 1997. Retrieved May 9, 2006, from www.caregiving.org.

Nelson, G. M. (1986). *Functional assessment of elderly subjects in four public welfare settings.* Working paper, Durham County Department of Social Services, Community Alternatives Program, Durham, NC.

Orem, D. (1995). *Nursing: Concepts and practice* (5th ed.). St. Louis: Mosby-Year Book.

Ormond, B. A., Black, K. J., Tilly, J., & Thomas, S. (2004). *Supportive services programs in naturally occurring retirement communities.* Washington, DC: USDHHS.

Parnell, J. (1982, September 22). Clinical comment. *Nursing Mirror, 46.*

Pattillo, M. (2005). City-wide efforts to provide shelter and care to elderly evacuees. *Journal of Gerontological Nursing, 31*(11), 21-27.

Pesznecker, B. L., & Zahlis, E. (1986). Establishing mutual-help groups for family-member care givers: A new role for community health nurses. *Public Health Nurse, 3*(1), 29-37.

Pfeiffer, E. (1975). *Multidimensional functional assessment: The OARS methodology.* Durham, NC: Duke University Center for the Study of Aging and Human Development.

Robinson, A., & Street, A. (2004). Improving networks between acute care nurses and an aged care assessment team. *Journal of Clinical Nursing, 13*(4), 486-496.

Rochefort, D. A. (1984). Origins of the "Third psychiatric revolution": The Community Mental Health Centers Act of 1963. *Journal of Health Politics, Policy and Law, 9*(1), 1-30.

Russell, V., Proctor, L., & Moniz, E. (1989). The influence of a relative support group on carers' emotional distress. *Journal of Advanced Nursing, 14*(10), 863-867.

Seymer, L. R. (1957). *Florence Nightingale.* London: Faber and Faber.

Skrovan, C., Anderson, E., & Gottchalk, J. (1974). Community nurse practitioner: An emerging role. *American Journal of Public Health, 64*, 847-853.

Sokolov, J. J. (2000). Bringing it all together. 2000 Duke Private Sector Conference: Academic health systems in transition. Retrieved January 26, 2006, from http://conferences.mc.duke.edu/privatesector/dpsc2000/y.htm.

Sources and qualifications of data from the survey of mental health organization. Retrieved January 25, 2005, from www.mentalhealth.org/publications/allpubs/SMA01-3537/appendixa.aspns.

Spradley, B. W. (1985). The community: Assessment and planning. In B. W. Spradley (Ed.), *Community health nursing: Concepts and practice* (2nd ed.). Boston: Little, Brown.

Starfield, B. (1974). Measurement of outcome. *Milbank Memorial Fund Q, Winter,* 39-50.

Stewart, R., & O'Rawe Amenta, M. (1993). Policy, politics, legislation, and public health nursing. In J. Swanson & M. Albrecht (Eds.), *Community health nursing: Promoting the health of aggregates.* Philadelphia: W. B. Saunders.

Stuart, M., & Snope, F. (1981). Family structure, family dynamics, and the elderly. In A. A. Somers (Ed.), *The geriatric imperative.* New York: Appleton-Century-Crofts.

Stuifbergen, A. K., Seraphine, A., & Roberts, G. (2000). An explanatory model of health promotion and quality of life in chronic disabling conditions. *Nursing Research, 49*(3), 122-129.

Tomassini, C., Glaser, K., Wolf, D. A., Broese van Groenou, M. I., & Grundy, E. (2004). Living arrangements among older people: An overview of trends in Europe and the USA. *Population Trends, 115,* 24-34.

Topp, R., Fahlman, M., & Boardly, D. (2004). Healthy aging: Health promotion and disease prevention. *Nursing Clinics of North America, 39*(2), 411-422.

Travis, S. S., Loving, G., McClanahan, L., & Bernard, M. (2001). Hospitalization patterns and palliation in the last year of life among residents in long-term care. *Gerontologist, 41*(2), 153-160.

Turkoski, B. B. (2003). Ethical dilemma: Is this elder abuse? *Home Healthcare Nurse, 21*(8), 518-521.

United States Senate Special Committee on Aging, American Association of Retired Persons, Federal Council on the Aging, and United States Administration on Aging. (1991). *Aging America: Trends and projections.* Washington, DC: U.S. Government Printing Office.

U.S. Department of Health and Human Services (USDHHS). (1999). *Mental health: A report of the Surgeon General.* Rockville, MD: USDHHS.

U.S. Department of Health and Human Services (USDHHS) Agency for Healthcare Research and Quality. (2004). *2004 National health-care quality report* (AHRQ publication no. 05-0013). Rockville, MD: USDHHS.

Vetter, N. J., Jones, D. A., & Victor, C. R. (1984). Effect of health visitors working with elderly patients in general practice: A randomized controlled trial. *BMJ, 289,* 369-372.

Weissert, C. S., & Weissert, W. G. (1996). *Governing health: The politics of health policy.* Baltimore: Johns Hopkins University Press.

Weissert, W. G. (1985). Seven reasons why it is so difficult to make community-based long-term care cost effective. *Health Services Research, 20*(4), 423-433.

Wilson, R. W., Patterson, M. A., & Alford, D. M. (1989). Services for maintaining independence. *Journal of Gerontological Nursing, 15*(6), 31-37.

World Health Organization, Regional Office for the Eastern Mediterranean. (1978, April/June). Health education with a special reference to the primary care approach. *International Journal of Health Education,* suppl.

Zambroski, C. H. (2004). Hospice as an alternative model of care for older patients with end stage heart failure. *Journal of Cardiovascular Nursing, 19*(1), 76-85.

Zander, K. (1988). Nursing case management: Resolving the DRG paradox. *Nursing Clinics of North America, 23*(3), 503-520.

Objectives

Describe the assisted living care setting and resident characteristics.

Describe the services available to older residents of assisted living facilities.

Discuss the role of the nurse caring for older adults in the assisted living setting.

Explore gerontological nursing issues in the assisted living setting.

Explain the components of the assessment of an older adult in the assisted living setting.

Develop nursing diagnoses and plans of care to address common needs of residents in assisted living.

As the nation's population ages, more adults must contend with the physical, cognitive, and psychosocial issues associated with chronic illnesses. Many affluent and middle-class Americans do not want to move into long-term care facilities when they can no longer safely maintain themselves at home. According to the National Center for Assisted Living (2001), assisted living facilities are an acceptable alternative for older adults who need more assistance than available in a retirement community or private home, but less assistance than skilled nursing facilities provide. Assisted living facilities provide residential housing and personalized supportive services including non-acute health care services. These services enable older adults to be essentially independent while living in a stable environment. Residents are able to maintain their quality of life with personal choice and privacy, and still receive assistance with activities of daily living (Johns Hopkins Medicine, 2004; Lassey & Lassey, 2001, p. 181; Senior Housing Net, nd).

POPULATION CHARACTERISTICS

According to the 2004 report of Bentley (Senior Policy Director for the National Center For Assisted Living), the age requirement to enter an assisted living facility varies among states. While some residents are as young as 60 years of age, the average age of residents is between 80 and 85. Most residents are female and need assistance with two activities of daily living, usually bathing and dressing (National Center for Assisted Living, 2001, p. 2).

SETTING DESCRIPTION

There are no federal regulations for assisted living facilities. State regulations set the basic guidelines for assisted living facilities, which include the following: (1) physical setting requirements; (2) administrator and staff qualifications; (3) continuing education requirements for staff; (4) scope of care to be provided; (5) type and frequency of health assessments; (6) medication management; (7) level of personal assistance and care; (8) Alzheimer's unit requirements; (9) training of staff for Alzheimer's units; (10) prohibited care; and (11) discharge of residents. Each state enacts laws and regulations deemed appropriate to the needs of older adults in their respective states. Therefore assisted living facilities vary greatly from state to state in available services, physical settings, and even in terminology prescribed by law (Bentley, 2004; California Code of Regulations, 2005).

There are seven federal statutes that impact employers and employees of assisted living facilities in every state. These are the following: (1) Americans With Disabilities Act (ADA), (2) Civil Rights Act of 1991, (3) Fair Housing Amendments Act (FHAA), (4) Fair Labor Standards Act (FLSA), (5) Occupational Safety and Health Act (OSHA), (6) Family and Medical Leave Act

(FMLA), and (7) Rehabilitation Act of 1973. The ADA, the FHAA, and the Rehabilitation Act of 1973 are three federal statutes that directly concern residents in assisted living facilities. If residents or guests meet the definition of 'disabled', the ADA mandates that they will be entitled to 'reasonable accommodations' in order to access the facility and its services on a nondiscriminatory basis (Assisted Living Federation of America, 2005, p. 1). The FHHA prohibits discrimination against any resident renting or being sold a place to live on the basis of disability (Assisted Living Federation of America, 2005, p. 3). The Rehabilitation Act of 1973 protects individuals on Medicaid (Medi-Cal in California) by allowing assisted living facilities to receive their Medicaid funds without discontinuing a person's eligibility to receive federal assistance should there be a change in living situation. In the event of a change in living situation, the funds would follow the person without the need to reapply for federal assistance (Assisted Living Federation of America, 2005, p. 2).

In a two-part report by Pettey (2003) of the American Medical Directors Association to the Senate Special Committee on Aging in July and September of 2003, the lack of uniformity of rules and regulations concerning health care services in assisted living facilities among different states caused much confusion to consumers regarding available services. However, in all states, assisted living facilities provide the following: (1) 24-hour 'awake staff' oversight; (2) assistance with activities of daily living; (3) health-related services such as medication management; (4) social services; (5) recreational activities; (6) transportation services; (7) personal services such as three meals a day, housekeeping, and laundry. In addition some facilities provide basic cable television and all utilities except telephone service.

Most assisted living homes are privately financed and house as few as six residents to as many as several hundred. Married residents live in individual apartments. Nonmarried residents have the choice to live alone or have a roommate. Each apartment is a secured living space with an emergency button that summons a health care worker when immediate attention is needed. Emphasis is placed on community living with common areas such as dining rooms and recreation areas, laundry services, and planned activities. The grounds around the facility are usually nicely landscaped with common outdoor sitting areas. Some facilities allow residents to have small pets. This relaxed, homelike environment encourages older adults to remain active.

Levels of Assisted Care

Table 31-1 describes two main types or levels of care in assisted living facilities (ALFs). Some assisted living facilities further subdivide the types of care into levels of service and base the service plan on functional and cognitive ability and capacity to manage own behavior.

Table 31-1 *Levels of Care in Assisted Living Facilities*

AFL Type I (or Level I)	AFL Type II (or Level II)
Safe, clean accommodations	Safe, clean accommodations permit 'aging in place' so that person can stay in same setting as assistance needs increase
Three meals/day	Three meals/day
Minimal assist with ADLs to significant assist with up to two ADLs	Semi-independent; may need assistance in more than two ADL categories
Mobility without assistance	Mobility with one person assistance
Assist with medications to medications administered by a nurse	Assist with medications to medications administered by a nurse
Receive home health services through individual contract with home health agency	Receive home health services through individual contract with home health agency
Receives 24/7 general monitoring	Receives 24/7 individualized personal and health-related services
Receive general nursing care according to facility policy	Receive general nursing care from facility staff
Have stable health and free from communicable diseases	Free from communicable diseases
Resident participation in developing service plan	Resident participation in developing service plan

Based on www.health.utah.gov/hflcra/facinfo/HFLevelsOfCare.pdf.

VARIATIONS IN COSTS FOR ASSISTED CARE

The cost of assisted living varies with the level of nursing care services needed and the extent of privacy desired. The level of privacy is related to the desire for a private room or the willingness to share a room with one or two other people. While some assisted living facilities (ALFs) have a single rate, many of the nation's ALFs (59%) have multiple rates, depending on whether the resident's need is for minimal nursing assistance/minimal privacy, maximum nursing service/minimal privacy, or maximum nursing service/maximum privacy. Monthly fees can range from $1373 to $1940, with some residents paying $26,000 per year for maximum nursing service/maximum privacy. As the baby boomer generation ages, it is anticipated that ALFs will become more in demand because of preferences for residential environments that provide dignity, autonomy, independence, and the opportunity to age in a home-like supportive environment as nursing care needs increase. This concept is referred to as 'aging in place' (Hawes, Rose, & Phillips, 1999, pp. 63-66, 69).

KEY ISSUES IN ASSISTED LIVING FACILITIES
Medication Errors

McCoy and Hansen (2004) reported in the cover story of *USA TODAY* that many residents in assisted living facilities face major problems daily concerning administration of medications. These problems include the following: (1) overmedication or undermedication, (2) improper labeling of residents' medications, or (3)

Table 31-2 *Examples of Educational Differences of Non–Nursing Care Providers in Different States*

State	Initial Hire	Continuing Education	Alzheimer's Disease Unit Initial Hire	Alzheimer's Disease Unit Continuing Education
Alabama	16-hour course in first year*	None specified	"Special training"*	None specified
California	Has ability to provide services requiring specialized skills; personnel qualified with recognized professional standards*	None specified	6 hours of dementia care orientation	8 hours of in-service/year*
District of Columbia	None specified	None specified	None specified	None specified
Florida	6 hours*	None specified	8 hours*	4 hours/year*
Indiana	In-service in advance of care	4 hours/year	6 hours within 6 months*	3 hours/year*
Kansas	Orientation with regular in-services on principles of assisted living including disaster and emergency preparedness training	None specified	Hours not specified, in-service education on treatment of behavioral symptoms	None specified
Maryland	Must be certified nursing assistant	None specified	None specified	None specified
New York	Complete personal care or home health aide training course	None specified	Special requirements for dementia units*	None specified
Wyoming	Must be certified nursing assistant	None specified	None specified	None specified

*Note: No specification of standards or required content of training.

untrained staff administering the medications. Sloane and colleagues (2004) reported that in a study of 328 subjects with congestive heart failure, over 50% were not receiving the appropriate medications for their medical condition. In July of 2005, *Consumer Reports* conducted an investigative examination of the 10 largest providers of assisted living facilities. Only 3 of the top 10 companies provided any information concerning who administers medications in their facilities (Consumers Union of United States, Inc., 2005). Carlson (2005) conducted a national study examining critical issues in assisted living facilities. He reported that of the 50 states, 21 states authorize nurses to delegate administration of medications to non-nurses. There are no nationwide educational standards for the non-nurses who administer medications. Table 31-2 illustrates variations among states for educational preparation of non-nursing care providers (Bentley, 2004).

Qualified Personnel

The shortage of registered nurses across the nation coupled with the increased number of older adults has the potential to decrease the quality of care offered in assisted living facilities. This may lead to increased use of less qualified non-nursing caregivers.

ROLE OF THE NURSE

Just as the definitions and settings for assisted living vary from state to state, educational requirements and roles of nurses in assisted living settings vary. Table 31-3 illustrates typical variability of nurse licensure and educational requirements among states (Bentley, 2004).

The role of nursing supervisor includes (1) working directly with residents to evaluate needs and services, (2) providing ongoing training of staff in all levels of nursing care provided by the facility, (3) analyzing and interpreting state and federal regulations, (4) conducting regular resident/family meetings to ensure needs are being met, (5) maintaining documentation of problems regarding nursing including functional status concerns, (6) ensuring availability of transportation to physician's office or other health-related services, (7) maintaining 24-hour accountability and availability by phone or pager, (8) collaborating with other health care providers, (9) providing management reports to consulting RNs and the administrator, (10) providing tools for assessments of residents, and (11) providing educational training necessary for staff.

NURSING CARE

As adults age and become frail with some degree of reduced functional ability, assisted living facilities can provide a positive living environment for older adults

Table 31-3 *Examples of Variations in Type of Nurse Licensure and Education Required by Different States*

State	Nursing Licensure Required
Alabama	RN for consultant role; staff training for residents in cognitive deficit units must receive 'special training' before resident contact; all other staff training nonspecified
District of Columbia	None specified
Florida	RN or pharmacist required to receive 4 hours of medication training; staff in special units for residents with cognitive deficits must have 8 hours of initial training and 4 hours of continuing education/year
Indiana	'Licensed nursing personnel' (licensure not specified)/staff in special units for residents with cognitive deficits must have 6 hours of specific training within 6 months and 3 hours of continuing education/year; all other nursing personnel must have 8 hours of continuing education/year
Kansas	'Licensed nurse' (not specified), licensed social worker, administrator, or operator must conduct admission functional assessment on resident; amount of staff training not specified
Maryland	None specified
New York	None specified
Wyoming	RN, LPN, or CNA in facility each shift; amount of staff training for continuing education not specified

Data from Assisted Living State Regulatory Review 2004. Prepared by the National Center for Assisted Living. Lynn Bentley, Senior Policy Director, March 2004.

who can no longer live independently but who do not need 24-hour skilled nursing care. Four common nursing problems evident in many residents in assisted living facilities are self-care deficit, mild cognitive impairment, interrupted family processes, and spiritual distress.

SUMMARY

With the increase in longevity for older adults, the role of nursing professionals in assisted living facilities will become increasingly complex because of the multifaceted issues that occur with the precarious physiological balance of the aging body (Box 31-1). Other concerns requiring well-educated nursing professionals include the following: diminished body reserves, chronic illnesses that impact multiple organ systems, decreased functional ability, decreased cognitive abilities, and altered ability to cope with change. The complex medical regimens and rapid advances in pharmacological therapies require nurses to have an extensive knowledge base related to the side effects and consequences of medications for older adults. Professionals need a high level of nursing knowledge and well-developed critical thinking ability to anticipate and prevent further cognitive and functional deficits. Nurses working in assisted living facilities also will need to have strong communication and collaboration skills to work effectively with medical teams and acute care hospital nurse discharge planners. As residents from assisted living have exacerbations of chronic illnesses that lead to hospitalizations, nurses' responsibility and accountability will increase. Nurses

Text continued on p. 906

Nursing Care Plan: The Caregiver for the Older Adult with Dementia

Assessment Data

Robert and Betty moved into an assisted living facility 1 year ago when Robert was diagnosed with probable early Alzheimer's disease. Betty wants to keep Robert with her as long as she can manage to provide good care. Betty notes that Robert requires increasing assistance with grooming and dressing. He sometimes becomes upset and frustrated when he is unable to complete these activities without assistance.

Betty has hypertension and osteoarthritis. She takes multiple medications that she has carefully organized. She claims to feel well "most days" but sometimes experiences fatigue. Betty's physical examination reveals that she has full range of motion in all joints except her hips and knees. Other findings are normal.

Nursing Diagnoses (Johnson, Bulechek, Dochterman, Maas, & Moorhead, 2001)

Self-Care Deficit related to inability to independently dress and groom self

Goals/Outcomes

- Robert will maintain ability to dress/groom self.
- Robert will accept assistance in dressing and grooming.

NOC Suggested Outcomes (Moorhead, Johnson, & Maas, 2004)

Self-Care: Activities of Daily Living (ADLs)
Self-Care: Dressing/Grooming
Self-Care: Hygiene

NIC Suggested Interventions (Dochterman & Bulechek, 2004)

Major interventions: Dressing (1630), Fall Prevention (6490), Foot Care (1660), Hair Care (1670), Nail Care (1680), Oral Health Promotion (1720)

- Obtain history of neurological, sensory, or psychological impairment.
- Encourage use of prescribed corrective lenses and other assistive devices while dressing/grooming.
- Assess self-care abilities, including knowledge of and use of adaptive equipment: front fasteners; zipper pull; buttonhook; long-handled shoehorn; shoe fasteners adapted with elastic laces; and Velcro closures of garments and shoes. Observe functional ability.
- Place matching clothes together on hangers.

If Robert's need for help increases, other interventions that may be helpful include:

- Give two choices of clothing to wear. Choose clothing that is loose fitting with wide sleeves and pant legs. Lay clothes face down on bed in the order in which they will be needed to dress.
- Provide nonverbal cues during dressing.
- Hand resident one item of clothing at a time.
- Place each shoe beside corresponding foot.
- Medicate PRN for pain 30 minutes before dressing/grooming activities if appropriate.
- Allow sufficient time for dressing and undressing, assessing for energy depletion, pain, and degree of difficulty.
- Assist with dressing and grooming: fasten clothes, comb hair, clean nails, and supervise brushing of teeth as needed.
- Encourage as much independence as possible for as long as possible.

Evaluation Parameters

Robert is appropriately dressed and groomed with the help of assistive devices and with assistance by caregiver as needed. More specific indicators of outcome achievement are: selects clothing, puts clothing on upper and lower body, buttons clothing, uses fasteners and zippers, puts on shoes and socks, ties shoes, maintains personal cleanliness and neat appearance (Moorhead et al., 2004).

Nursing Care Plan: The Older Adult with Memory Impairment

Assessment Data

Maria has been in an assisted living apartment since recovering from a stroke 2 years ago. She has some residual paralysis but manages well with a cane. She has been complaining about her poor memory. This was confirmed by her daughter, who reports that her mother has missed some appointments and failed to pay her utility bill. Maria has been charging numerous unnecessary items purchased from television sales channels and phone solicitations. When assessed by the nurse, Maria expressed difficulty remembering dates and days of the week. It was noted that Maria was unable to recall the nurse's name even though the two have had regular contact. A neurological assessment revealed no changes from previous evaluations.

Nursing Diagnoses (Johnson et al., 2001)

Disturbed Thought Processes related to uncertain etiology as manifested by memory deficit/problems

Impaired Memory related to neurological disturbances as manifested by reported experiences of forgetting, forgetting to perform a behavior at a scheduled time, inability to recall factual information

Goals/Outcomes

Maria will use memory resources effectively within 1 month as evidenced by the following indicators:

- Comes to all meals on time.
- Does not miss any appointments with caregivers.
- Is able to state which people have visited her each week.
- Reports no more than three episodes of lost belongings each week.
- Verbally reports feeling less stressed about memory problems.
- Verbally identifies the day of week and approximate time of day accurately.

NOC Suggested Outcomes (Moorhead et al., 2004)

Cognition
Cognitive Orientation
Decision Making
Information Processing

NIC Suggested Interventions (Dochterman & Bulechek, 2004)

Major interventions: Anxiety Reduction (5820), Cognitive Stimulation (4720), Decision-Making Support (5250), Reality Orientation (4820), Memory Training (4760)

- Ask Maria for history of CVA, degenerative brain disorder, head injury, psychiatric disorder, anxiety, depression, losses in past few years, stress, pain, sleeplessness, and use of alcohol and recreational or prescription mediations.
- Assess neurological status including cognition, memory, judgment, orientation, motor ability, and sensory ability.
- Assess self-care status including ability to perform activities of daily living and instrumental activities of daily living through observation of functional ability.
- Assess potential sources of memory problems, changes in memory function, and degree of impairment. Provide treatment as indicated.
- Involve in mentally stimulating activities such as games and crossword puzzles to conserve and/or improve memory.
- Use visual images and auditory and written cues.
- Ask family to provide family photos (labeled with name and relationship).
- Instruct staff and family to spend time with resident to encourage memories and discussion of current and past events.
- Keep schedule and activities as routine as possible.
- Post calendar with daily activities in room.
- Provide a clock that is easily read with an alarm to use as a reminder of appointments and meal times.
- Instruct older adult/family to write things down and put in appropriate places as reminders.
- Provide a visitors' book for visiting family and friends to use to help the older adult to remember who has been in to visit.

If Maria's cognitive status worsens over time, she may need a higher level of care or a caregiver residing in her apartment. Interventions that may be needed for more severe memory impairment include:

- Assess personal and family coping abilities.
- Identify resources to assist in awareness of time and date, including calendar, clock, other residents and staff, TV, and/or radio.
- Maintain safe, structured environment and protect from injury.
- Have familiar items in living environment and keep items in same place.
- Be sure all staff wear name identification badges that can be easily read. Have them identify themselves with each contact unless Maria addresses them by name.
- Have other residents and staff provide prompts and reminders of activities.
- Orient Maria to reality as necessary including use of name, place, time, and date. Use orientation

Nursing Care Plan: The Older Adult with Memory Impairment—cont'd

board, television, and radio to augment orientation. Orient to sight, sounds, and smells in environment. Call her by name.
- Ask family to provide Maria with family photos (labeled with name and relationship on back).
- Instruct staff/caregiver and family to spend time with Maria to encourage memories and discussion of past events.
- Have familiar items in living environment. Keep items in same place. Maintain safe environment and protect from injury.
- Carry out medical regimen to treat underlying cause of cognitive deficit.
- Provide structured environment for Maria. Post daily activities in room.
- Instruct Maria/family to write things down and put in appropriate places as reminders. Use visual images and auditory cues with written cues.
- Organize information into logical categories.

- Divide information into small 'chunks' that can be remembered.
- Encourage Maria/family members to voice feelings and concerns about loss of memory.
- Help family members identify a community support group.

Evaluation Parameters

Maria uses memory strategies to maintain orientation to date and time and to attend scheduled activities. She will be safe and protected from injury, verbalize need for assistance, and comply with medical regimen. Other specific indicators of outcome achievement might include the following: identifies correct day, month, and year; demonstrates recent and immediate memory; makes appropriate decisions; exhibits organized and logical thought processes (Moorhead et al., 2004).

Nursing Care Plan: The Newly Relocated Assisted Living Resident

Assessment Data

Amanda moved into an assisted living high-rise apartment 2 weeks ago. After her husband of 60 years died last year, Amanda sold her home and moved in with a daughter and her family because she was unable to maintain her large home. Amanda had several falls, one resulting in a hip fracture. The adult children agreed that assisted living would be a better option for their mother after she completed her rehabilitation. They informed her of their decision, and Amanda agreed because she felt that she had no choice. The only acceptable facility that had an apartment available was 30 miles from her daughter's home.

Since moving into the facility, Amanda rarely leaves her apartment. When visited by the nurse, she expressed anger at her children for 'making' the decision to place her in assisted living, and stated that she felt like her family did not want her. She also feels that her life has no meaning because she is useless and has nothing to do. She misses seeing her grandchildren and her former neighbors and friends. Her daughter visits once or twice weekly.

The health history and physical examination revealed mobility problems related to arthritis and stiffness following the hip fracture, which make traveling difficult for Amanda. Amanda also reports communication problems related to impaired hearing.

Nursing Diagnoses (Johnson et al., 2001)

Interrupted Family Processes related to admission to an assisted living setting manifested by feelings of isolation and role confusion

Goals/Outcomes

Amanda will express feelings of being connected with family and experiencing positive interactions with family within 1 month as evidenced by the following indicators:
- Verbally expresses feelings of satisfaction with daughter's visits and time with grandchildren.
- Verbally expresses enjoyment of regular phone conversations with family and friends.
- Expresses increased comfort and increased ability to move, enabling her to travel to visit sister and spend the weekend with daughter.
- Verbalizes recognition that she needs the care provided by assisted living in order to avoid further injury from falls.

NOC Suggested Outcomes (Moorhead et al., 2004)

Adaptation to Physical Disability
Family Coping

Continued

Nursing Care Plan: The Newly Relocated Assisted Living Resident—cont'd

Family Functioning
Psychosocial Adjustment: Life Change
Social Involvement

NIC Suggested Interventions (Dochterman & Bulechek, 2004)

Major interventions: Family Process Maintenance (7130), Family Integrity Promotion (7100), Normalization Promotion (7200)

- Assess hearing problems and provide appropriate equipment including hearing aids and telephone equipment for hearing impaired.
- Assess mobility problems, provide appropriate assistive devices, and involve resident in physical rehabilitation activities to maximize mobility.
- Assist Amanda in recognition of need for assisted living placement.
- Assess family communication patterns and use positive patterns to improve family cohesiveness.
- Assist Amanda in expressing negative feelings related to family and exploring appropriate ways of resolving these feelings.
- Assist Amanda to recognize family caring behaviors.

- Explore with Amanda ways to feel like a contributing family member.
- Assist family in exploring ways of helping Amanda feel included and useful in the family.
- Problem-solve with Amanda's children regarding ways to maintain family contacts with Maria on a regular basis.
- Assist family in exploring activities they can do with Amanda.

Evaluation Parameters

Amanda expresses acceptance of need for level of care provided in assisted living facility, and maintains close communication with family and friends. Other specific indicators of outcome achievement might include the following: adapts to functional limitations, identifies ways to cope with life changes, reports decrease in negative feelings, expresses feelings and emotions freely among (family) members, maintains stable core of traditions, adapts to developmental transitions, (family) members spend time with one another, reports feeling useful, verbalizes optimism about present and future, uses available social support, expresses satisfaction with living arrangements, reports feeling socially engaged (Moorhead et al., 2004).

Nursing Care Plan: The Resident in Spiritual Distress

Assessment Data

Joe, age 85, moved to assisted living 3 months after his wife died following a long illness. He has no close relatives and had lost contact with friends during his wife's illness. Joe attends group activities occasionally, but appears sad and withdrawn. When some neighbors invited him to attend church services with them, he replied that he had not attended church since his wife died. He expressed feelings of being abandoned by God because of the suffering endured by his wife. He said, "A loving God would not allow such a good person to endure such misery. Maybe it was His way of punishing me for mistakes in my life." He also questions why God would let him continue living when he is lonely and no longer has a purpose in life.

Nursing Diagnoses (Johnson et al., 2001)

Spiritual distress related to wife's suffering and death, lack of significant relationships, and loss of sense of purpose manifested by feelings of being punished

by God and questioning why God is allowing these things to happen

Goals/Outcomes

Joe will express feelings of spiritual well-being and feeling connected to God and will express feelings of hope and purpose in life within 2 months as evidenced by the following indicators:

- Verbalizes understanding that God cares about what is happening.
- Verbalizes increased feelings of connectedness with God and other people.
- Participates in religious activities and expresses feelings of satisfaction with help received from these activities.
- Discusses beliefs and values with others, indicating positive feelings about own relationship with God and hope for future.
- Verbalizes recognition that there is a continued purpose in life.
- Verbalizes sense of spiritual well-being and understanding that God accepts and values person as precious to Him.

NOC Suggested Outcomes (Moorhead et al., 2004)

Hope

Spiritual Health

NIC Suggested Interventions (Dochterman & Bulechek, 2004)

Major interventions: Spiritual Support (5420), Hope Instillation (5310)

■ Assess Joe's spiritual/religious background and practices to enable appropriate interventions.

■ Assess Joe for possible depression and provide appropriate medications if indicated.

■ Listen to Joe's spiritual concerns, questions, and beliefs about current situation.

■ Problem-solve with Joe to determine what he feels would help in resolving spiritual distress.

■ Facilitate visits from spiritual advisor of Joe's choice if he desires.

■ Facilitate contact by phone, letters, and visits to reestablish/maintain long-term relationships with friends.

■ Encourage Joe's participation in religious activities appropriate to beliefs.

■ Involve Joe in activities to promote development of new relationships with other residents.

■ Involve Joe in volunteer activities in which he helps others, to promote feelings of self-worth and usefulness.

■ Facilitate expectation of future enjoyable activities for Joe to anticipate.

Evaluation Parameters

Joe expresses feelings of hope, purpose, and a renewed connection to spiritual beliefs. Other specific indicators that might reflect outcome achievement are the following: expresses expectation of a positive future; expresses faith; expresses inner peace, meaning, and purpose in life; experiences spirituality; ability to pray and worship (Moorhead et al., 2004).

Box 31-1 *Reflections on Assisted Living and Nursing*

Older adults and their families are often faced with a puzzling array of living options when living independently is no longer feasible. Assisted living facilities offer a good option for the older adult who needs a supportive living situation. Decisions about where to move are often made in times of great stress: the recent loss of a spouse, a change in health status, or a growing awareness of cognitive changes noted by family members. Family members often struggle with the decision to move, hoping that their elderly parent will decide on his/her own, even when decisional capacity has become impaired. Family members can become so paralyzed by the decision to move the elder out of the home that the older adult stays in the community until complete skilled care is needed and assisted living is no longer an option. Family members often seek information from hospital nurses, home health care providers, or case managers in community settings during this time.

Nurses need to be aware of the emotional turmoil that older adults and families face when confronted with changes in care needs. Knowing care options for elders in the community and encouraging proactive decision making while an older adult is still able to participate are important for the well-being of older adults and their family members.

Older adults who move to assisted living before major changes occur may be able to stay in the assisted living facility for a much longer time than anticipated. The social setting of assisted living also can reduce depression and loneliness that an isolated person in the community may experience.

Assisted living settings vary widely in the types of services they offer, the kinds of residents that they serve, the amount and type of staffing available, and the costs of care. Families are often surprised that the focus of many assisted living settings is a social model, not a medical model. Nurses can best help older adults or their families by identifying whether the setting will meet the older adult's needs. For example, Mrs. J was discharged from the hospital after a hip fracture, and she had developed a lower extremity decubitus ulcer. Her family wanted care in an assisted living setting rather than a skilled nursing home during Mrs. J's rehabilitation after hospitalization. The assisted living facility was staffed only to provide for personal care needs, not 24-hour medical monitoring or skilled nurses for dressing changes. Once the family understood that only unskilled staff were available for personal care, not a registered nurse to monitor and assess medical status, they approved the decision to send Mrs. J to a skilled facility for the rehabilitation and monitoring she needed. However, after Mrs. J's wound healed and she was able to walk with a walker, her personal care needs were easily managed in the assisted living setting.

Older adults often make more than one move in the last years of their lives as their care needs change. Nurses who assess elders can provide a careful listing of needs to assist residents and/or their family members in making a decision that will best meet those needs. Supportive listening and empathy for the difficulty of these decisions are essential as the nurse assists older adults or their families in the decision-making process.

Karen S. Feldt

Karen S. Feldt, PhD, RN, GNP
Chief of Community Health
ERA Care Communities
Seattle, Washington

will be required to provide accurate assessments of clinical status to determine if the residents need a higher level of care than the assisted living facility can provide.

If older adults are to receive the care they need to maintain maximum independence, each assisted living organization should use advance practice nurses with a gerontological nursing specialty as consultants. This will ensure (1) that licensed staff are held accountable for critical thinking assessments and care plans for residents and (2) that nonlicensed nursing caregivers receive in-depth training to ensure the provision of quality care to older adults in assisted living environments.

REFERENCES

Assisted Living Federation of America. (2005). Federal statutes that impact assisted living. Retrieved October 20, 2005, from www.alfa.org/public/articles/details.cfm?id=43.

Bentley, L. (2004). *Assisted living state regulatory review 2004.* Washington, DC: National Center for Assisted Living.

California Code of Regulations. (2005). Title 22, Division 6, Chapter 8: Residential care facilities for the elderly. Manual letter no. CCL-05-11, effective June 15, 2005.

Carlson, E. (2005). *Critical issues in assisted living: Who's in, who's out, and who's providing care.* Washington, DC: National Senior Citizens Law Center.

Carpenito, L. (2000). *Nursing diagnosis: Application to clinical practice* (8th ed.). Philadelphia: Lippincott Williams & Wilkins.

Consumers Union of United States, Inc. (2005). Assisted living: How much assistance can you really count on? *Consumer Reports, 70*(7), 28-33.

Dochterman, J. M., & Bulechek, G. M. (2004). *Nursing interventions classification (NIC).* St. Louis: Mosby.

Doenges, M., Moorhouse, M., & Geissler-Murr, A. (2005). *Nursing diagnosis manual: Planning, individualizing, and documenting client care.* Philadelphia: FA Davis.

Hawes, C., Rose, M., & Phillips, C. (1999). National study of assisted living for the frail elderly: Results of a national survey of facilities. U.S. Department of Health and Human Services and Meyers Research Institute. Retrieved October 11, 2005, from http://aspe.hhs.gov/daltcp/reports/facres.htm.

Johns Hopkins Medicine. (2004). Elderly in assisted living facilities have rates of dementia and other psychiatric disorders. Retrieved October 11, 2005, from www.hopkinsmedicine.org/Press_releases/2004/10_04c_04.html.

Johnson, M., Bulechek, G., Dochterman, J., Maas, M., & Moorhead, S. (2001). *Nursing diagnoses, outcomes, interventions: NANDA, NOC, and NIC Linkages.* St. Louis: Mosby.

Lassey, W., & Lassey, M. (2001). *Quality of life for older people: An international perspective.* Upper Saddle River, NJ: Prentice Hall, p. 181.

McCoy, K., & Hansen, B. (2004, May 24). *USA TODAY.* Retrieved October 11, 2005, from www.usatoday.com/money/industries/health/2004-05-24-assisted-living-cover_x.htm.

Moorhead, S., Johnson, M., & Maas, M. (2004). *Nursing outcomes classification (NOC).* St. Louis: Mosby.

North American Nursing Diagnosis Association (NANDA). (2005). *Nursing diagnoses: Definitions and classification 2005-2006.* Philadelphia: NANDA International.

National Center for Assisted Living. (2001). 2001 Edition of facts and trends: The assisted living sourcebook. Retrieved October 4, 2005, from www.ncl.org/about/resident.htm.

Pettey, S. (2003). Assisted living report neglects medical coordination. *Caring for the ages.* Philadelphia: Lippincott Williams & Wilkins, vol. 4, pp. 12-13. Retrieved October 20, 2005, from www.amda.com/caring/september2003/al_report.htm.

Ralphs, S., & Taylor, C. (2005). *Sparks and Taylor's nursing diagnoses reference manual* (6th ed.). Philadelphia: Lippincott Williams & Wilkins.

Senior Housing Net. (nd). Assisted living. Retrieved October 20, 2005, from www.seniorhousingnet.com/seniors.kyo/assisted_living.html.

Sloane, P., Gruber-Baldini, A., Zimmerman, S., Roth, M., Watson, L., Boustani, M., et al. (2004). Medication undertreatment in assisted living settings. *Archives of Internal Medicine, 164*(18), 1957-1959.

32 Acute Care

Maria B. Carroll

A large percentage of personal health care dollars in the United States is spent on hospital care. Typically, hospitals serve as the setting for managing acute illnesses of rapid onset, short duration, and greater severity or complexity. Hospitalization usually occurs when diagnosing, monitoring, and treating a health condition requires 24-hour care by multiple health care disciplines. Providing nursing care for the older adult in the hospital presents a unique set of challenges. Although dealing with acute illness and hospitalization may be difficult for persons of any age, it is especially hard on older persons. The focus on cure or reversal of a specific, admitting diagnosis in a fast-paced, high-technology environment can obscure the goals of gerontological nursing and lead to a variety of adverse events. Nurses spend more time at the bedside than any other discipline, placing them in an ideal position to get to know older patients, individually and comprehensively, and to improve care for them globally.

This chapter provides an overview of the hospital setting and characteristics of hospitalized older adults, including their unique responses to acute illness and treatment. The role of nurses in preserving function and preventing complications in this special population is emphasized.

POPULATION CHARACTERISTICS

Hospitalization rates declined between 1979 and 2000 for all age-groups except older persons, whose hospitalization rates increased by 23% (Habel, 2004). Representing 12% of the U.S. population, older adults have a disproportionately higher hospital use than younger adults (Morrill & Elixhauser, 2005). In 2002, 35% of discharges from hospitals and 46% of days of care in hospitals were for patients age 65 years and older (Hall & DeFrances, 2003). In contrast, people age 18 to 44 represent 41% of the U.S. population but only 27% of hospitalizations, almost one half of which are for pregnancy and childbirth (Morrill & Elixhauser, 2005).

Approximately 80% of older Americans have at least one chronic illness or functional disability, and hospitalization is often required for exacerbation of those conditions (Habel, 2004). The most common diagnoses for older hospitalized patients are coronary atherosclerosis, congestive heart failure (CHF), pneumonia, acute myocardial infarction, chronic obstructive pulmonary disease (COPD), cerebrovascular accident (CVA), cardiac dysrhythmia, hip fracture, urinary tract infection, degenerative joint disease, fluid and electrolyte disorders, and rehabilitation care (Morrill & Elixhauser, 2005). The rate of hospitalizations for older adults with CHF was 62% higher in 2001 than in 1980 (Hall & DeFrances, 2003). Far exceeding the growth of the Medicare population, there was an unexplained rise by 108% and 310% in annual discharge rates for unspecified and pneumococcal septicemias, respectively (Baine, Yu, & Summa, 2001a). Over a similar period, hospitalizations for aspiration pneumonia nearly doubled in this population (Baine, Yu, & Summa, 2001b).

Over one half of all hospitalized patients have at least one comorbidity, and about one third have two or more comorbidities. Top comorbidities in hospitalized patients over age 65 include hypertension, COPD, diabetes mellitus, CHF, anemias, hypothyroidism, peripheral vascular disease, neurological disorders, heart valve disease, and fluid and electrolyte disorders. Major causes of death in the hospital for patients between the ages of 65 and 84 are pneumonia, myocardial infarction, CVA, septicemia, respiratory failure or arrest, CHF, metastatic cancer, and fluid and electrolyte disorders. For those over the age of 80, death in the hospital was most often related to pneumonia, myocardial infarction, septicemia, CHF, CVA, respiratory failure or arrest, fluid and electrolyte disorders, hip fracture, GI bleeding, and intestinal obstruction without hernia (Morrill & Elixhauser, 2005).

Older patients who require hospital admissions are among the sickest of patients anywhere. Owing to multiple factors, hospitals are used only as a last resort. Advances in technology and drug therapy have led to early diagnosis and treatment of acutely ill people as outpatients. Between 1980 and 2000, hospital admissions declined by 10% and outpatient visits increased by 150%. One half of all hospital-based surgeries take place on an outpatient basis as procedures have become safer and less invasive (Board on Health Care Services, Institute of Medicine [BHCS, IOM], 2004). Increased enrollment in managed care plans has also served to limit hospital use. A government-sponsored study of Pennsylvania hospitals found a 21% increase in hospital patient acuity between 1991 and 1996 (Stanton, 2004). Medicare's prospective payment system, growth in utilization review programs, and the development of more post–acute care alternatives have resulted in significant decreases in hospital lengths of stay. U.S. hospital stays for patients age 65 or older in 2001 averaged 5.8 days, less than half as long as they were in 1970 (Hall & DeFrances, 2003).

SETTING DESCRIPTION

Acute hospital care takes place in emergency departments (EDs), medical and surgical nursing care units, and intensive care units, where unfamiliar sights, sounds, odors, and tastes abound. Approximately 43% of all admissions are through the ED. More than 55% of admissions for people ages 65 to 79 begin in the ED; for persons ages 80 and older, 64% begin in the ED (Morrill & Elixhauser, 2005). Care is planned, managed, and delivered by multiple disciplines with the support of ancillary services and high-technology machinery. Diagnostic tests and procedures are often invasive and can be noxious.

Over the last 20 years, specialized inpatient geriatric nursing units have emerged. Guided by a gerontological philosophy focused on the whole, functioning

individual, these units, which have been referred to as geriatric evaluation and management (GEM) or acute care for elders (ACE) units, have demonstrated positive effects on mortality rates (Saltvedt, Opdahl, Fayers, Kaasa, & Sletvold, 2002), lower percentages of patients discharged to nursing homes (Asplund et al., 2000; Counsell et al., 2000; Landefeld, 2003), and greater recognition of geriatric syndromes such as dementia, depression, and delirium (Saltvedt et al., 2002). Perhaps the most striking outcome in clinical trials of these units is improvement in functional status or decreased functional decline (Cohen et al., 2002; Counsell et al., 2000; Landefeld, 2003). Other outcomes on specialized units as compared with usual care include more effective management of pain (Cohen et al., 2002), decreased length of stay (Asplund et al., 2002), and increased patient and staff satisfaction (Counsell et al., 2000). Most of these units report no increase in overall cost over time (Cohen et al., 2002; Counsell et al., 2000).

Basic components of most ACE units include the following: (1) a "prepared" environment specially designed to promote early mobility and reduce hazards, (2) patient-centered care with nurse-driven protocols, (3) frequent, if not daily, interdisciplinary rounds to review care and eliminate unnecessary medications and treatments, and (4) discharge planning that begins on admission. Physical features such as carpeting or nonskid flooring, handrails, nonglare lighting, and congregate rooms minimize injury, encourage mobility, and promote socialization. Nursing care plans aimed at function and all health domains include interventions for self-care, fall prevention, skin integrity, continence, delirium prevention, and restraint avoidance. Patients on such units usually have few, if any, days of bed rest and receive high-risk medications less frequently. Other disciplines such as social work and physical therapy are consulted more frequently and usually earlier in the course of the admission.

Despite demonstrated positive outcomes, these units have been criticized for reaching too few older patients. Jacelon (1999) asserts that it would be better to have younger patients isolated on separate units and improve the geriatric knowledge and competence of all caregivers, including staff nurses, physicians, and families, as well as older adults themselves. Prompted by similar concerns, Inouye, Bogardus, Baker, Leo-Summers, and Cooney (2000) propose the Hospitalized Elder Life Program (HELP) as a viable alternative. Designed for incorporation throughout hospitals, the program is not restricted to dedicated units. According to the authors, this model targets common, modifiable, evidence-based risk factors with feasible interventions requiring only a devoted staff with geriatric expertise. A team consisting of a geriatrician, a gerontological clinical nurse specialist, "elder life specialists," and volunteers implements protocols according to risk factors found on admission and discussed in twice-weekly interdisciplinary rounds. The elder life specialists hold bachelor's or master's degrees in a health or human services field and are experienced in geriatrics. They supervise volunteers who complete 16 hours of didactic training and 16 hours of one-on-one training with a mentor on the unit. The program has been successful in reducing rates of delirium and cognitive and functional decline. Surveys of patients and families demonstrate a 90% satisfaction rating. An estimated $1500 is saved in hospital costs per patient with the program (Inouye et al., 2000).

Some researchers suggest that broader dissemination of sound geriatric practice has occurred. Noting less dramatic reduction in mortality rates in randomized, multicenter trials of GEM units in the Veterans Administration system over an 18-year period, Cohen and colleagues (2002) conclude that this may be due to the growth of geriatrics, the spread of geriatric principles, and increased use of the team model in the system to the point that usual care has become progressively more like the specialized care of earlier studies. Likewise, Counsell and colleagues (2000) suggest that attenuated results in a 4-year interval between studies may be due to their successful establishment of a geriatric program with inpatient consultation. Further, because there currently is a shortage of specially trained care providers, they recommend triaging elderly patients so those most likely to benefit will receive care on the specialized geriatrics units. Saltvedt and colleagues (2002) used specific criteria to identify frail patients at greatest risk for nursing home placement and death. Reduction in patient mortality rate, which lasted up to 12 months after discharge, was attributed, in part, to this type of targeting. Still, although an estimated 30% of patients age 75 and older requiring hospital admission were assessed as needing specialized geriatrics care, only 18% were admitted to the GEM unit because of inadequate bed availability.

Working with what they already have, hospitals can more widely apply ACE and GEM concepts if they concentrate efforts on providing sound, intensive education for staff and stress early, interdisciplinary rehabilitation and discharge planning. Asplund and colleagues (2000) noted that when cared for by interdisciplinary teams emphasizing comprehensive assessment and early rehabilitation, acute stroke patients had improved functional outcomes whether they were treated on a medical, neurological, or geriatric unit. Most ACE units described in the literature have been established on general medicine divisions. Pilot studies suggest that adopting an ACE model of care may yield similar, positive results for older patients in specialty areas such as acute oncology and cardiac units, who share risk factors and have issues in common with general medicine geriatric patients (Flood, Carroll, Esker, & Carr, 2004; Flood, Emory, Le, Rich, & Carr, 2004).

ROLE OF THE NURSE
Background

Hospitals employ 59% of the nation's 2.2 million nurses (BHCS, IOM, 2004). Hospitalized elders are in great need of health care providers who understand their special needs. Older adults develop a myriad of concerns when hospitalized. They worry about the added responsibilities for their spouses, the potential for medical errors and complications, losing their independence, and inability to manage their care at discharge. They describe a "demeaning experience" with "nervous waiting," procedures that deplete their energy, and needless physical and mental suffering (Huckstadt, 2002, pp. 26, 27).

Nurses provide the majority of the 24-hour direct care in hospitals and are depended on to monitor clinical problems. Thus they are in a prime position to influence improved care for these vulnerable patients in keeping with gerontological nursing practice's emphasis on "maximizing functional ability in ADLs; promoting, maintaining, and restoring health, including mental health; preventing and minimizing the disabilities of acute and chronic illness; and maintaining life in dignity and comfort until death" (American Nurses Association [ANA], 2000, p. 7). Nursing interventions to prevent complications are based on knowledge of age-related changes discussed in the systems chapters of Section 3. Nursing process in the hospital setting is described next. Descriptions of the role of the nurse are interspersed in the discussion of gerontological issues in the hospital.

Nursing Process

Assessment. In the setting of decreased lengths of stay and rapid intervention, assessment begins immediately. Recognizing older adults as the most heterogeneous of persons of any age, the nurse thoroughly assesses them to identify individual strengths, weaknesses, and factors that increase their risk for incomplete recovery or further decline. Such assessment should include interview of the patient to learn more about his or her health and medication history, baseline functional status, history of falls, adaptive and medical equipment, and social supports/living arrangements, as well as the patient's perception of his or her health status. Verifying information with someone who knows the patient well and by using standardized screening tools adds strength to the assessment and may elucidate issues such as depression, cognitive impairment, or poor insight regarding abilities. Nursing's role is to coordinate thorough assessment by gathering information, administering screens, observing and physically examining the patient, and referring to other professionals for discipline-appropriate evaluations. Note and report any sign of abuse or neglect. Even in the ED, comprehensive geriatric assessment can be effective in reducing nursing home admissions (Mion, Palmer, & Meldon, 2003) (see also Chapter 2).

Nursing Diagnosis and Outcome Identification.
In the analysis of assessment findings leading to diagnosis, nurses must apply knowledge of normal age-related changes and be alert for common abnormalities with potentially unusual manifestations. The fast pace of acute care necessitates careful prioritization of nursing diagnoses. Problems considered more critical are those that may impede resolution of treatable acute illness, affect overall function, or result in unexpected institutionalization, as well as those that are most important to the patient.

Individualized care planning is guided by carefully selected expected outcomes and discharge criteria. Formulating realistic interventions involves the patient to determine the risks and burdens he or she is willing to bear. The nurse considers the cumulative effects of multiple chronic illnesses or degenerative processes as they will likely complicate treatment and recovery. Cognizant of the high risk for iatrogenesis in this setting, the nurse includes prevention strategies.

The complex nature of comprehensive care for older adults demands expertise from a number of different health care providers (ANA, 2000). Hospitals are fortunate to have greater availability of resources, services, and a wide variety of professional disciplines. The routine multidisciplinary approach does not use this advantage to its full potential, however, and may even lead, inadvertently, to fragmentation of care. Effective, integrated care begins with interdisciplinary planning where teams meet regularly for timely, pertinent communication. (A full discussion of interdisciplinary care is provided in Chapter 25.) Hospitalizations are short, and the complex geriatric patient is likely to have unresolved, though less acute, health issues at time of discharge. Interdisciplinary discharge planning helps predict discharge date and the degree to which self-care abilities will have recovered by that time. It has demonstrated a positive effect on reducing readmission rates and shortening readmission stays (Palmer & Meldon, 2003). Interdisciplinary plans enable the provision of appropriate discharge follow-up care and any necessary equipment.

Intervention.
Plans should be implemented swiftly because complications are often realized within a day or two of admission. Interventions should be based on current best practice and research (ANA, 2000). The older adult's spiritual, psychological, and developmental domains should not be overlooked while attending to his or her physical health. Nurses can help allay patients' fears by providing explanations and implementing care plans with confidence and compassion. Reminiscing and life review can be encouraged while starting an intravenous line or changing a dressing, serving to distract the patient and demonstrate personal interest.

"Hand-off of responsibility is a common cause of human error, and discontinuities in care probably adversely affect processes of care and patient experiences" (Landefeld, 2003, p. 424). Thus a primary nursing care model or consistency in assigning caregivers may reduce the risk for iatrogenesis while allowing for the stronger development of rapport and a greater chance that individualized care can be realized.

The majority of family caregivers want to help care for their hospitalized older relatives (Li, 2002). They may be accustomed to providing care for the patient or may be required to when the patient is discharged. Preferences regarding the degree and type of involvement in care will vary based on religion, culture, their own health and other obligations, the patient's health and complexity of care, and personal family dynamics (Li, 2002). Including them in the planning and delivery of care provides an educational opportunity, as well a chance to evaluate whether or not they will be capable of managing the care outside the hospital.

Nurses provide and coordinate patient education, an essential intervention in all care plans. Teaching is based on individual learning needs, preferred style, and ability of the patient. The nurse assesses the acutely ill patient for fatigue, anxiety, or pain that may diminish the patient's capacity to learn and attempts to alleviate these factors. The nurse must identify and teach an appropriate surrogate when necessary. Other health education considerations are discussed in full in Chapter 27.

Evaluation.
Evaluation of responses to and outcomes of interventions and continual reassessment are the responsibilities of the nurse in collaboration with the interdisciplinary team. Include assessment of energy and coping. Keep in mind that longer lengths of stay in hospitals are associated with increased complications (Jacelon, 1999). Assessment findings on day 10 are likely to be vastly different than findings on admission. Because of the nature of care and the frequency and intensity of contact, nurses are in the best position to notice small changes that potentially signal the beginning of iatrogenic cascade. Working with the interdisciplinary team, nurses encourage steady progress in assisting the patient in meeting discharge criteria. Signs that indicate a patient should remain in the hospital because they have been associated with death in the 30 days following discharge include the following: new finding of incontinence, chest pain, dyspnea, delirium, tachycardia, hypotension, fever above 38.3° C, and diastolic blood pressure above 105 mm Hg (Palmer & Meldon, 2003). As soon as the acute illness is stabilized, patients

should be discharged to a setting most appropriate for follow-up care and rehabilitation. The nurse ensures continuity by providing all relevant information to those assuming care at discharge. (Chapter 26 includes information regarding coordination of care between settings.)

Quality Improvement

Serving in quality improvement groups, nurses can evaluate the process of care for high-risk older persons, promote evidence-based practice to reduce iatrogenesis, and advocate for models of care better geared for the frail and vulnerable in the hospital setting. (For a full explanation of quality improvement, see Chapter 28.) Nurses are role models for improving other hospital caregivers' attitudes toward older persons, eradicating myths, and demonstrating a philosophy of respect for the older patient as a whole individual. When less than 5% of the U.S. population was over age 65, a few visionary nurses recognized nursing care for older adults as a specialty (ANA, 2000). Yet, today, there remains some lack of appreciation of the distinct body of knowledge and skills required and a persistent shortage of nurses adequately prepared to care for our aging population. Some believe that geriatric nursing is a specialty meant for practice only in nursing homes. Gerontological nurses must promote their field as the specialty that it is and demonstrate its applicability in the acute care setting. Specialized gerontological nurses can serve as mentors to those developing competence in delivering age-specific care. Lobbying for programs to reduce nurse turnover and educate larger numbers of nurses in gerontology can ultimately improve hospital care of older persons.

GERONTOLOGICAL NURSING ISSUES IN THE HOSPITAL

The following descriptions of key issues and related nursing suggestions are not meant to be exhaustive because many of the same issues are discussed in greater detail elsewhere in this book. Aspects unique to the hospital are highlighted.

Patient Self-Determination

Ethical issues frequently encountered in hospitals include informed consent, confidentiality, artificial nutrition and hydration, advanced life support, experimental care, and surrogate decision making. Patient self-determination is foremost. Since 1990, hospitals are required by law to give all patients information regarding their rights to refuse or accept treatment and to complete an advance directive (AD). Per research, patients who talk with their families or doctors about end-of-life

preferences have less fear and anxiety, feel more able to influence and direct their care, and believe their physicians have a better understanding of their wishes (Kass-Bartelmes & Hughes, 2004).

Unfortunately, studies have found that ADs do not guarantee that older patients' wishes will be followed. In one study, between 65% and 76% of physicians were not aware when their patients had ADs, and having one did not increase documentation of preferences in the medical chart. ADs helped make end-of-life decisions in less than one half of the cases where an AD existed (Kass-Bartelmes & Hughes, 2004). Nearly 50% of deaths occur in hospitals (Last Acts, 2002). The care of seriously ill patients is increasingly delegated to hospitalists who make more decisions about life-sustaining treatments but do not know the patients as well as the primary care physicians. Most ADs are very general, but ADs that include scenarios have been found to increase the accuracy of treatment decisions made by hospital-based physicians and reduce the likelihood of overtreatment (Coppola, Ditto, Danks, & Smucker, 2001). Families are not always reliable surrogate decision makers. In one study, even with scenarios and discussion of AD content with their loved ones, spouses and children of patients were two to three times more likely to make errors of overtreatment than undertreatment (Ditto et al., 2001). Complicating matters further is the tendency of older patients to change their judgment about quality of life over time (Lockhart, Ditto, & Danks, 2001) and to change their treatment preferences once they are hospitalized and confronted with actual situations (Kass-Bartelmes & Hughes, 2004).

Advance directives are sometimes invoked prematurely. Well-meaning family members may request that information not be shared with the patient for fear of unduly stressing him or her. The cognitively impaired may be presumed incompetent and excluded from decision making. There is a tendency in hospitals to document mental status only as it relates to orientation. Decision-making capacity involves short-term memory and the ability to concentrate, apply abstract reasoning, problem solve, use judgment, and express oneself. Pyschometric tools are designed to test these abilities. Usually, a person's ability to make decisions falls on a continuum between completely capable and completely incapable, rather than one or the other (Drickamer, 2003).

The gerontological nurse's role is to identify ethical dilemmas and seek available resources to help formulate ethical decisions (ANA, 2000). During the admission process, the nurse inquires about ADs and provides related education as needed. Copies of any existing AD documents are placed in the chart and called to the attention of the physician. Patients should be encouraged to review and update them frequently and to share with their durable power of attorney (DPOA) for health care and physicians any preference changes. Clearly explaining tests and treatments enables patients to better make informed choices.

While considering the needs of the patient and his or her family, the nurse places those of the patient first. Nurses protect the patient's right to privacy, discussing matters with the patient first and gaining his or her consent before sharing information with others. When DPOAs are called on to make treatment decisions, the nurse validates their feelings while reminding them that their role as surrogate is to base decisions on the patient's preferences. The nurse reassures them that a do-not-resuscitate order will not change the quality of care provided. In the absence of an AD, different family members may have conflicting ideas and agendas. Nurses facilitate family conferences. Referrals to spiritual care and social work professionals in these situations can be invaluable. Cognitively impaired individuals should be involved to the degree appropriate. The systematic evaluation by a specialist may be helpful. An ethics consultation is appropriate when the nurse, despite her or his advocacy, is concerned that a patient's rights or best interests may be violated.

Patients are often overwhelmed during acute illness when presented with information regarding advance directives. Nurses can lead efforts to educate the community about advance directives and encourage thoughtful consideration outside the hospital setting (see also Chapters 9 and 22).

Iatrogenesis

Older patients experience complications of hospital care three to five times more frequently than younger patients (Inouye et al., 2000). Because of diminished physiological reserves and tenuous homeostatic mechanisms, the older adult is less able to adapt to an unfamiliar environment and more prone to decline, especially during acute illness. Normal changes associated with aging as discussed in previous chapters place older patients at increased risk of postoperative complications such as delayed wound healing, pneumonia, deep vein thrombosis, paralytic ileus or bowel obstruction, and infection (Dixon, 2002). In fact, postoperative complications (including myocardial infarction, pulmonary embolism, respiratory failure, and renal failure) more than double in patients age 70 to 79 and nearly triple in those over 80 when compared with those younger than 60 (Polanczyk, Marcantonio, & Goldman, 2001).

Age, frailty, and comorbidities are not the only etiologies for complications in the acute care setting. Coupled with an inherent propensity of the older patient for adverse outcomes is the added risk posed by the hospital environment and treatment. Iatrogenesis refers to adverse events from diagnosis, intervention, or omission involving a reasonable clinical standard and

to poor outcomes worse than what would be expected as a natural consequence of the patient's underlying disease process. Iatrogenesis occurs disproportionately in older adults (Jacelon, 1999). Sometimes one adverse event is the beginning of a series of such events, or *cascade iatrogenesis* (Habel, 2004). Landefeld (2003, p. 423) lists the following "hospital-associated barriers to recovery and promoters of decline": negative expectations, depersonalization and isolation, immobility and starvation resulting in deconditioning, and unintended consequences of drugs and procedures.

The current nursing shortage creates additional risk for this vulnerable population. The average registered nurse (RN) vacancy rate in U.S. hospitals is 13% and is expected to reach as high as 29% by 2020. In a recent survey of over 13,000 nurses, 83% reported an increase in the number of patients assigned to them in the previous year and 44.8% reported a deterioration in the quality of care in their hospital during that same time frame. More nonlicensed staff members are providing care at the bedside. Lower nurse-to-patient ratios have been associated with adverse outcomes such as higher rates of nosocomial infections, pressure ulcers, and falls (Stanton, 2004). In 2000, 21% of all hospital nurses left their position. Inpatient units with less experienced staffs have higher rates of medication errors and patient falls (BHCS, IOM, 2004).

Functional Decline

Functional decline is the leading complication of hospitalization for older patients (Inouye et al., 2000). In a study of more than 2000 older patients hospitalized in the general medicine divisions of two hospitals, Covinsky and colleagues (2003) found that 35% of all patients age 70 and older and more than 50% of those 85 and older had worse activities of daily living (ADLs) function at discharge than they did 2 weeks before to admission. Those over age 89 were twice as likely to fail to recover function lost in the period between onset of illness and admission to the hospital and three times more likely to develop new functional losses while in the hospital than those patients age 70 to 74. Factors besides age that are independently associated with risk for decline in or failure to recover ADLs function include cognitive impairment, depression, malnutrition, and unsteadiness (Landefeld, 2003).

Recovery of functional status takes longer than resolution of the acute illness (Jacelon, 1999). The degree of functional dependence figures predominantly in issues of quality of life, caregiver burden, and costs. Eleven percent of all patients discharged from U.S. hospitals go to some type of long-term care facility. For those patients age 65 to 84, the percentage nearly doubles (21%), and for those 85 and older, the percentage nearly quadruples (41%) (Morrill & Elixhauser, 2005).

Nurses play a vital role in aiding older hospitalized patients to prevent and recover functional loss, beginning with assessment of functional status and risk factors. Bed rest must be avoided except in very rare circumstances. Nurses must place as much emphasis on increasing patients' activity levels as on other treatments and educate patients, families, and nurse aides about the hazards of immobility. If a patient can safely be assisted to the bathroom, a bedside commode should not be used. Chairs in the hallway or at a window strategically placed so as not to impede safety can break up a long corridor and encourage patients to get out of their room for a walk. Ambulating patients can be delegated to non-licensed caregivers and suggested to families and volunteers when appropriate. Patients should be encouraged to perform ADLs to the extent they are capable. Physical and occupational therapy consultations are helpful in further defining strengths and limitations, prescribing appropriate assistive devices and exercises, and teaching energy conservation. Collaboration is essential to ensure treatment carryover between therapy sessions. Nurses reinforce rehabilitation teaching, ensure that assistive devices are available and put to use, and communicate individualized strategies to maximize functional independence to other team members. To facilitate early discontinuation of equipment that restricts mobility (e.g., indwelling catheters, intravenous lines, and oxygen tubing), nurses can encourage oral fluid intake (when not contraindicated) and provide relevant information to physicians such as patients' intake and output measurements and oxygen saturation percentages.

Falls

Falls are the single largest category of incidents in acute care hospitals (Corrigan et al., 1999; Halfon, Eggli, Van Melle, & Vagnair, 2001; Perell et al., 2001), and, per some studies, more than half of all falls in hospitals are in patients over age 65 (Corrigan et al., 1999; Halfon et al., 2001; Hitcho et al., 2004). Fall incident rates are almost three times greater in hospitals than in the community for people in this age range (American Geriatrics Society, British Geriatrics Society, and American Academy of Orthopaedic Surgeons Panel on Falls Prevention, 2001). In a study of 634 falls during a 1-year period in one hospital, falls (defined as those observed by the nurse, those reported by the patient, or a patient found lying on the floor) occurred more frequently in medical than in surgical departments (Halfon et al., 2001). Medicine and neurology services had the highest fall rates in a study of 200 consecutive falls (defined as a sudden, unexpected descent from a standing, sitting, or horizontal position, including slipping from a chair to the floor, a patient found on the floor, and assisted falls) in another hospital during a 13-week period (Hitcho et al., 2004). In the studies by Halfon and colleagues (2001) and Hitcho and colleagues (2004), injuries resulted from 37% and 42% of first falls, respectively. Falls without injuries also can devastate older persons by diminishing their confidence, leading to decreased mobility, isolation, and increased dependence. Sometimes a fall in the hospital prompts restraint use.

Risk factors for falls, besides age, specifically identified by research in hospitals include the following: use of psychotropic medicine, including neuroleptics, benzodiazepines, and antidepressants (American Geriatrics Society et al., 2001; Hitcho et al., 2004); general muscle weakness (Hitcho et al., 2004); a previous fall (Corrigan et al., 1999; Halfon et al., 2001); gait disorders (Halfon et al., 2001); greater comorbidity (Halfon et al., 2001; Hitcho et al., 2004); depression (Halfon et al., 2001); and cognitive impairment (American Geriatrics Society et al., 2001; Halfon et al., 2001; Hitcho et al., 2004). About 50% of the 183 patients who fell in Hitcho and colleagues' study (2004) were engaged in elimination-related activities at the time of the fall, and older patients were more likely to have an elimination-related fall than younger patients. Additionally, these falls were nearly 2.5 times more likely to cause injury. A bedside commode was a risk factor for serious injury. Less than 6% of the 53 patients (29%) who reported using an assistive device routinely at home were using one at the time of their fall in the hospital. The call light was not used just before falls in 97% of the cases, often because the patients did not believe they needed assistance. In more than one third of the falls reviewed by Halfon and colleagues (2001), the staff person reporting the fall judged the incident to be preventable. Environmental factors have been implicated in 8% to 14% of hospital falls (Corrigan et al., 1999; Halfon et al., 2001).

Nursing assessment of risk factors for falls at admission and each shift using a consistent, systematic approach is paramount to preventing falls in hospitals. A standardized screening tool should be selected based on its demonstrated reliability, sensitivity, specificity, and applicability to nursing in the hospital setting. The Hendrich and Morse are two such appropriate instruments that are simple and quick to use (Corrigan et al., 1999; Perell et al., 2001). Identifying all risk factors is imperative. Multiple risk factors interact synergistically so that the risk of falling rises dramatically with the number of risk factors (American Geriatrics Society et al., 2001). Observing the patient walk is essential. Self-report of abilities is helpful in comparing the patient's perceived and actual abilities. Some patients underestimate the toll acute illness has taken on their strength and stability. Others underreport their limitations for fear of increased dependence and possible institutionalization. These patients are more likely to attempt to get up alone.

Some prevention strategies are universal whereas other must be guided by individual risk factors. Many are simple but are dependent on nursing implementation. Only multifactorial interventions targeting both intrinsic and environmental risk factors have resulted in significant reduction of falls in people who are high risk (Halfon et al., 2001). Necessary items such as facial tissue, telephones, water, urinals, glasses, hearing aids, and call lights must be within easy reach of patients. Urinals should be emptied frequently. At the beginning of each shift, ask patients to demonstrate their ability to use the call light, and reinforce instructions to wait for assistance before getting up. Older people are frequently unaware of their risk for falling (American Geriatrics Society et al., 2001). Educate them about the ways in which acute illness and the hospital environment may increase their risk for falling. Nearly 60% of drug-related injuries are the sequelae of falls (Walker, Foreman, & the NICHE Faculty, 1999). Warn patients when they have been given a medication that may increase their risk for falls. Answer call lights as promptly as possible. Institute scheduled toileting rounds. Consult physical and occupational therapists for gait and transfer training. Provide and reinforce the use of prescribed assistive devices. Use gait belts when appropriate. Instruct patients to rise slowly and teach them exercises such as ankle pumps to improve circulation while in bed. Provide proper footwear. Eliminate unnecessary medical equipment and reduce clutter. Ensure that bedside commodes are stable and beds are locked and in their lowest position. Patients should be alerted to rolling equipment (such as overbed tables) and instructed not to hold onto them to walk. Ensure adequate lighting. Night-lights should be used in bathrooms. Turning on full light after coming from relative darkness can be blinding. Extent of side rail use is case dependent. Raising two upper rails can aid patient mobility. Full use of side rails is no longer best practice in hospitals and is considered a restraint. Raising all bed rails does not guarantee protection from falls. Serious injuries have resulted when patients have climbed over bed rails. Entrapment and death is a risk of side rail use especially in patients with advanced age, altered mental status, or low body weight (Talerico & Capezuti, 2001).

Cognitively impaired patients require more frequent reminders and increased supervision. Pressure sensing alarms can signal when the patient is attempting to get up and needs assistance. Consider using a low bed to reduce the chance of injury in high-risk patients likely to get up alone. Provide sitters or ask family members if they can take shifts staying with the patient. Anticipate patients' needs and check on them frequently. Sufficient evidence does not exist to support using restraints to prevent falls (American Geriatrics Society et al., 2001). Restraint use is fraught with problems and may actually increase the risk for serious injury.

Following a fall, the patient should be promptly evaluated and the cause thoroughly investigated. Falls are often red flags of underlying problems that require attention. Discuss the fall in interdisciplinary rounds. Because multiple fallers tend to repeat the type and location of the fall on subsequent falls (Hitcho et al., 2004), communicate the incident and circumstances to essential personnel caring for the patient.

Track fall and injury rates and set goals for reduction. Not all findings from studies of falls are consistent or generalizable. Review postfall evaluations to determine any patterns on individual nursing units. Trends and details of any fall-related sentinel events should be shared at staff meetings. Hospital nurses do not always see the full effect of falls on individual patients and become desensitized to their seriousness. Quality improvement efforts should include activities to heighten nurses' awareness of the adverse effects of falls in older adults. There is paucity in the literature regarding falls in older persons in acute hospital settings (American Geriatrics Society et al., 2001; Halfon et al., 2001; Hitcho et al., 2004). Nurses can contribute to and publish research specific to this area and lead efforts to encourage universal adoption of a uniform definition for falls. (For a complete discussion of fall risk assessment and prevention, see Chapter 11.)

Polypharmacy

Older patients with acute illnesses are at increased risk for adverse events associated with polypharmacy. An average of nine different medications are administered to hospitalized older adults, increasing the odds of producing an adverse reaction to nearly 100% (Walker, Foreman, & the NICHE Faculty, 1999). Multiple new medications are often prescribed simultaneously in the hospital setting. Acute illness, superimposed on chronic illnesses and age-related changes, may compound alterations in drug absorption, distribution, metabolism, and excretion. Preventable adverse drug reactions have been linked to depression, constipation, confusion, falls, hip fracture, and immobility (Fick et al., 2003). They are associated with excess length of stay, higher costs, and increased mortality rates in hospital patients.

A complete list with dosages of prescription and over-the-counter medications used by the patient just before admission must be documented in the medical record. It is also helpful to know how long the patient has been on each medicine and if the patient has ever experienced an adverse drug reaction. Benzodiazepines should be titrated off to avoid withdrawal. Antidepressants should be continued unless contraindicated. An essential role of nursing is to monitor for and report adverse effects of medications. Nurses should be knowledgeable of drugs that commonly cause adverse events in older persons. In hospitals where nurses use computerized medication orders to administer medicines, systems can be maximized to provide "pop-up" reminders on those that are high risk. Changes in hospital formularies can reduce the use of high-risk medications. Lower initial doses and slow titration should govern prescribing. As members of the interdisciplinary team planning care, clinical pharmacists should be consulted to regularly review medications for drug-drug and drug-disease interactions. Unnecessary or inappropriate drugs based on up-to-date criteria such as the Beers (Fick et al., 2003) should be discontinued. Safer alternative drugs and nonpharmacological alternatives should be recommended.

Patient education regarding purpose, side effects, and administration accompanies all prescriptions. How patients will manage their medications outside the hospital must also be considered. Can they afford their medications? Do they have a safe system for taking a complicated medication regimen? Can medications dosed over multiple times a day be converted safely to an extended- or slow-release form? Will cognitive or functional abilities limit compliance? (Chapter 7 provides a full discussion of pharmacological considerations.)

Infection

Weakened conditions in acute illness, in combination with age-associated changes in immune, urinary, and respiratory systems, increase the hospitalized older adult's susceptibility to nosocomial infections. Virulent microorganisms such as *Clostridium difficile* and vancomycin-resistant enterococcus become commonplace in hospital nurses' minds, and their devastating effects in older patients are often realized too late. Opportunistic infections further weaken the older patient and complicate recovery and discharge planning. Isolation beds may be hard to come by in an extended care facility, and diarrhea can be difficult to manage at home.

Good handwashing, proper attention to infection control, and strict adherence to isolation guidelines are basic prevention strategies. Early mobility should be facilitated and use of incentive spirometers encouraged. Indwelling catheters should be avoided except in cases of urinary retention not manageable with intermittent catheterizing, acute renal failure or other conditions where strict measurement of output is required and the patient is incontinent, stage III or greater pressure sores in areas where incontinent urine will impede wound healing, or end-of-life care when an indwelling catheter might aid comfort (Evans, 1999; Ouslander & Johnson, 2003). To reduce risk for infection when indwelling catheters must be used, bags should be emptied at least three times each day and never allowed to become full. Daily and after each bowel movement, the perineum and catheter should be cleansed with soap and water or

a perineal cleanser from the urethral meatus outward (Evans, 1999). Ensure catheter care competence in non-licensed nursing staff. Catheters should be discontinued as soon as possible because the length of time the catheter is in place is a major factor influencing infection and other complications (Evans, 1999; Ouslander & Johnson, 2003). Diarrhea should be monitored and reported. Patients should be given an opportunity to wash their hands before eating or taking medications.

Pressure Ulcers

Frail hospitalized older persons must be protected from developing skin breakdown. A standardized tool such as the Norton Scale or Braden Scale should be used to assess risk for breakdown. Risk factors are reassessed routinely and systematically because the acutely ill older adult is prone to experience changes in mobility, continence, and nutrition during the course of the admission. Pressure relieving and prevention strategies such as frequent repositioning, barrier creams, and mattress overlays are used based on individual risk factors. On admission and every shift, the nurse inspects the patient's skin for integrity with careful attention to areas prone to pressure and friction such as the sacrum, coccyx, heels, shoulder blades, and trochanters. Location, size, and staging of ulcers are precisely documented with a description of the wound bed and periwound skin. Treatments are based on the type of the wound. Nurse-driven skin care protocols facilitate prevention and rapid intervention. Consulting enterostomal therapists or wound care experts is helpful in cases of severe or multiple surface ulcers. Rehabilitation therapists can suggest positioning strategies and prescribe splinting devices. Referral to a registered dietitian enables appropriate nutritional supplementation. Nurses provide education to patients, families, and unlicensed staff regarding skin care and participate in quality improvement measures to reduce incidence and prevalence of hospital-acquired pressure ulcers. (More information is provided in Chapter 10.)

For more on acute care, see Box 32-1.

Undernutrition

Early and detailed attention must be paid to nutrition for its role in the development of the condition requiring admission and in recovery. Older patients who are hospitalized for exacerbation of chronic illnesses are often undernourished. Protein-energy malnutrition (PEM) and other nutrient deficiencies are especially common and contribute to excess risk of death (Evans, 2001; Palmer & Meldon, 2003). Therapeutic diets and days of nothing by mouth when tests are tentatively scheduled, cancelled, and rescheduled are nutrition roadblocks in the hospital, as is staff inattention at

Box 32-1 *Reflections on Acute Care*

As we age, changes in the skin increase the potential for injury to the skin to occur. In the acute care setting, skin injuries can come from needle sticks for blood draws, IVs or other procedures, tape abrasions, friction and shearing, and pressure ulcers. The epidermis thins, dermal fibroblasts cease replicating, collagen and elastin shrink and degenerate, production from sweat and sebaceous glands decreases, and subcutaneous fat is lost; these are some of the age-related skin changes that occur in the geriatric population. The net effect of all these changes is thin, dry, inelastic skin that cannot insulate to provide warmth, protect from injury, or provide padding over bony prominences. In addition, pain perception is dulled as one ages and skin reactivity is reduced upon exposure to skin irritants, heat, hot water, heating pads, or hot burners; thus burns and other skin injuries can occur.

The thin, fragile skin of older patients needs to be handled by caregivers delicately and with special care. Gentle cleansing with a mild pH balanced emollient soap and warm water every couple of days is generally sufficient for skin hygiene. Acute care nurses want to bathe patients daily in their usual routine, which can be very drying and irritating to the geriatric skin. The liquid emollient body washes contain moisturizers and are less drying to the skin than bar soap. It is best to use a soft cloth to pat the skin dry rather than rubbing with a towel and creating friction. Forceful scrubbing and use of harsh cleansers and caustic agents can be harmful to the skin.

It is a challenge in the acute care setting to prevent skin injury. Nurses know the basics of assessing skin and bony prominences for redness, turning and repositioning patients frequently, and elevating heels off the bed, but these tasks can be a low priority for nurses when heavy patient care assignments and involvement in technical care supersede these basic components. However, nursing interventions to prevent skin injury far outweigh the cost of wound care, which includes dressings, nursing care time, and possible placement in a skilled nursing facility or long-term care facility. Wound healing in geriatric patients is slower due to disease processes that interfere with healing, inadequate nutrition and hydration, decreased or altered mobility, medications, and age-related changes that occur in the skin. Therefore prevention is a cost effective measure.

Our facility participated in a study to learn more about pressure ulcers in the acute care setting. We found a pressure ulcer prevalence rate of 11.4%, which tells us how many patients have pressure ulcers at one point; the national average ranges from 3.5% to 29.5%. The incidence rate for pressure ulcers was 6.64% for 2005, which tells us how many new cases of pressure ulcers occurred, compared to a national average of 2.7% to 29.5%. These rates both declined since we evaluated pressure ulcers in 2001, when we found a prevalence of 17.01% and an incidence of 6.85%. Since we are a tertiary care center, our patients are high risk, but our rates are not as high as many facilities, and we are proud of reducing our rates. Through these studies we identified high-risk nursing units, stages of pressure ulcers, and anatomical locations where the majority of pressure ulcers occur, and we implemented a plan of action for decreasing and treating pressure ulcers. Some key risk factors related to pressure ulcers include an albumin level less than 3, a prealbumin level less than 10, lengthy surgery, fragile skin, dehydration, obesity, diabetes, immobility, a Braden score less than 16, incontinence, poor circulation, sensory loss, being bedbound, being chairbound, and comorbidities.

As a gerontological clinical nurse specialist on an acute care for the elderly unit, I find nursing staff are diligent about keeping the skin clean and dry. During care, they avoid friction with bathing, avoid using incontinent briefs, use barrier creams to protect the skin, turn and reposition patients frequently, and elevate heels off the bed. We have a low incidence of pressure ulcers and skin tears. The nursing staff take great pride in caring for older patients, and they treat them like family. Providing diligent skin care is a part of the routine, yet special, care that our geriatric population deserves.

Marsha McGuire

Marsha McGuire, RN, BC, GCNS, CWOCN
Geriatric Clinical Nurse Specialist
Certified Wound, Ostomy, Continence Nurse
Saint Louis University Hospital
Saint Louis, Missouri

mealtimes. In a study of 497 patients 65 years of age and older who were admitted to a Veterans Administration hospital for 4 or more days, 21% had an average daily in-hospital intake of less than 50% of their caloric requirements (Evans, 2001).

At admission, nurses should record patient height and weight and ask about the patient's appetite and any unintended weight loss. Look for signs of dehydration and poor wound healing. Laboratory values should be reviewed. Unexplained anemia and low serum albumin, cholesterol, and protein levels should alert the nurse.

An interdisciplinary approach is helpful in modifying risk factors for PEM such as functional dependency, limited access to food, cognitive impairment, chronic medical illnesses (e.g., CHF and COPD), social isolation, and poor dentition (Palmer & Meldon, 2003). If assessment suggests that the patient is or is at risk for becoming undernourished, refer to a dietitian for in-depth evaluation and suggestions for appropriate, palatable supplements and strategies. Analyze diet orders to determine which are aiding disease management and which may be hindering recovery. To encourage intake, liberalize diets as much as possible and encourage families to bring in patients' favorite foods. Assist patients with meal selection and feeding to the degree necessary. Record intake percentages at each meal and report them to the interdisciplinary team during rounds. Promote oral care and ensure access to clean dentures. Get patients out of bed for meals. Administer oral medications with a cup of nutritional supplement instead of water. Ask families or volunteers to visit during mealtime. Suggest congregate meals when appropriate. Smaller, more frequent meals are often better tolerated in acutely ill elders. Alter food consistency only to the degree required to compensate for a chewing problem. Manage constipation. Seek a speech-language pathology consultation if swallowing problems are suspected and an occupational therapist to improve independence in eating. Ensure that the patient will have access to food at discharge. Consult a social worker to set up additional services, such as meals-on-wheels, as needed and agreeable to the patient.

Feeding by artificial means is indicated in select situations such as acute illness where the prognosis is good but adequate oral intake will not be possible for a prolonged period (Palmer & Meldon, 2003). Percutaneous esophagogastrectomy (PEG) tubes have not been shown to prevent aspiration or improve survival in end-stage dementia (Borum et al., 2000). (A full discussion of nutritional considerations is provided in Chapter 8.)

Constipation

Prone to constipation because of normal changes with aging, the older adult encounters additional risk during acute illness and hospitalization. Alterations in fluid balance and nutrition are likely during this time, as is decreased mobility. Many medications prescribed in the hospital, such as opiates and calcium channel blockers, are constipating. Nurses tend to minimize the older patient's complaint of constipation and underestimate the extent of complications constipation may cause. Even the cognitively intact older adult can lose track of time in the hospital and may not reliably report bowel movements. Bowel elimination should be monitored daily and documented in a consistent place. Constipation should be prevented with nurse-driven protocols and treated with a consistent bowel regimen based on severity and etiology. (More information is provided in Chapter 16.)

Sleep Disturbance

With aging, deep sleep and sleep efficiency decrease while night awakenings increase. Sleep problems in older adults, according to the National Sleep Foundation, are related to medical illnesses such as heart disease, lung disease, stroke, depression, cancer, arthritis,

Parkinson's disease, dementia, benign prostatic hypertrophy, and gastroesophageal reflux disease (Stimmel & Aiso, 2004). Acute illness and hospitalization compound sleep problems. Anxiety about illness, noise, interruptions, and alteration in routines all play a role in keeping the older person awake in the hospital. Medications that can aggravate sleep problems include aminophylline, phenytoin, levodopa, decongestants, caffeine, nicotine, and glucocorticoids (Coll, 2001). Sleep is restorative and vital for survival. Poor sleep slows reaction time and causes daytime sleepiness, fatigue, inattention, and memory problems, increasing the risk for falls and accidents (Coll, 2001; Stimmel & Aiso, 2004). Sleep deprivation in the hospital setting is a significant risk factor for delirium (Inouye, 2000). Inadequate sleep in an acutely ill older adult can delay recovery.

Nonpharmacological strategies are the most appropriate approach to aid the older patient who is trying to get adequate sleep in the hospital. Hypnotics leave patients feeling less rested. Benzodiazepines can worsen sleep apnea and sleep problems caused by depression (Coll, 2001; Stimmel & Aiso, 2004). Both carry dangerous side effects for older persons, increasing their risk for falls and delirium in an unfamiliar hospital environment. Sedatives or benzodiazepines the patient was taking regularly at home must be continued or tapered to prevent withdrawal. Chronic sleep problems are best managed in the outpatient setting. Assess for and treat aggravating conditions such as uncontrolled pain and unresolved depression.

A three-part nonpharmacological sleep protocol consisting of a back rub, a warm drink of milk or herbal tea, and relaxation tapes with nature sounds or music was tested in a group of 111 patients age 70 and older hospitalized on a general medicine service. The program was successful in reducing the use of sedative-hypnotics from a baseline preintervention rate of 54% to 31%. Quality of sleep increased with the number of protocol parts implemented. Program feasibility is suggested by the overall adherence rate of 74% during the study period (Inouye, 2000). Learn what helps the individual patient sleep at home and reproduce the conditions as much as possible. Increase the time the patient is out of bed and his or her exposure to light during the day. Take the patient for a walk in the late afternoon. Offer reassurance and opportunities for the patient to verbalize anxiety. Limit nighttime disruptions. Do not give stimulating medications or caffeine within 4 to 6 hours of bedtime. Lead a quality improvement effort to reduce noise on the unit at night.

Some patients may require a medication on a time-limited basis to get sleep adequate for healing and recovery. Zolpidem (Ambien) and zaleplon (Sonata) preserve normal sleep structure and have a much better safety profile, with minimal rebound and no development of tolerance (Stimmel & Aiso, 2004). Zaleplon is best for those who need help falling asleep, whereas zolpidem helps patients who need help falling asleep and staying asleep. Anticipate the need for such medications and administer them 30 to 60 minutes before the patient's usual hour of sleep. Do not administer sedatives after midnight to avoid perpetuating a sleep-wake cycle disturbance.

Depression

In older adults, mood disorders can accompany physical illness, functional dependence, pain, and losses. The risk for depression in older persons rises with the severity of their medical illnesses and functional disabilities (Kurlowicz & the NICHE Faculty, 1999). An estimated 20% to 30% of hospitalized older adults have depression, but physicians frequently fail to recognize or treat it (Kurlowicz & the NICHE Faculty, 1999; Palmer & Meldon, 2003). Untreated depression can impede recovery and amplify pain and disability.

Nurses can be instrumental in identifying signs of depression. The challenge comes in distinguishing symptoms of the acute illness from those depression may be causing or aggravating. Ask patients about their mood and how it affects their day-to-day function. History of depression is pertinent because recurrence with acute illness and hospitalization is common (Kurlowicz & the NICHE Faculty, 1999). The patient may endorse feeling "blue" or "down in the dumps" rather than being depressed. Some older patients accept low mood as a normal or expected aspect of aging or illness. The depressed patient may lack insight. Families often detect changes in mood and can provide pertinent information. Manifestation may be different in the older patient. Anxiety out of proportion for the illness and hospital experience; excessive negativity or pessimism; obsession with vague, somatic complaints; neediness greater than functional assessment suggests is appropriate; apathy; and lack of interest in recovery are suspect.

Minor depression is two to four times more common in older adults than major depression (Kurlowicz & the NICHE Faculty, 1999). Even minor depression can hinder function and quality of life. Such depression often responds as well as major depression to antidepressants and nonpharmacological approaches. Antidepressants should be selected based on low side-effect profile and targeted to specific symptoms such as insomnia, anxiety, or decreased appetite.

Nurses can alleviate depression aggravators in the hospital such as isolation, depersonalization, and boredom. Maximize personal control and autonomy. Provide therapeutic activities. If the hospital does not have recreational therapists, hospital auxiliaries can be solicited for donations and volunteers. Social workers and chaplains complement nursing by making therapeutic visits that allow patients additional opportunities to vent their feelings, find meaning in their experiences of illness and hospitalization, review their lives, and identify remaining strengths. Depressed patients need follow-up of their mood and monitoring for compliance with health care protocols after discharge (see also Chapters 7 and 20).

Delirium

Delirium is most common in hospitalized older adults. Reportedly, between 14% and 24% of older adults are admitted with delirium, and new cases arise in 6% to 56% of older patients in the hospital (Inouye, 1999). In a study of 111 mechanically ventilated patients in a hospital intensive care unit (ICU), 83.3% were delirious sometime during their short stay (Reuters Health Information, 2001). Delirium is a serious condition with associated increases in mortality rates, hospital lengths of stay, institutionalization, and health care costs (Inouye, 2000).

Delirium is usually the combined effect of patient vulnerability and noxious insults (Inouye, 2000). Although more than 30 predisposing and 25 precipitating factors for delirium can be identified, research suggests focusing on the ones with the greatest relative risk and most clinical relevance to the hospital setting. Reporting on a delirium prevention program, Inouye (2000) refers to two foundation studies identifying risks in hospitalized general medicine patients age 70 and older. Visual acuity worse than 20/70, severe illness, cognitive impairment with Mini-Mental State Examination (MMSE) score less than 24, and dehydration with blood urea nitrogen (BUN)–to–creatinine ratio greater than 18 were found to be significant factors on admission that increased the risk for delirium. Patients with three or four risk factors were nine times more likely to develop delirium than those with no risk factors. Physical restraints, malnutrition, the addition of more than three medications on the previous day, an indwelling bladder catheter, and any iatrogenic event were key precipitating factors. The relative risk for delirium rose from 1.0 in patients who had experienced none of those factors to 22.7 in those experiencing three or more. Analysis of the effect of precipitating factors superimposed on predisposing risk factors suggests a multiplicative rather than an additive effect.

Six risk factors amenable to intervention strategies that can feasibly be implemented in hospitals were targets selected by Inouye and colleagues (2000) for a multicomponent prevention program designed to reduce the incidence of delirium in older patients at intermediate to high risk for developing it. Which interventions a patient received depended on the presence of cognitive impairment, sleep deprivation, immobility, visual impairment, hearing impairment, and dehydration. Cognitively impaired patients received reality orientation and therapeutic activities. Sleep was protected with noise-reducing strategies and rescheduling of treatments and procedures to allow uninterrupted sleep periods. The nonpharmacological sleep protocol described previously in the sleep disturbance section of this chapter was used to limit the use of psychoactive medications. Mobility-impaired patients were assisted to ambulate or exercise three times per day, and equipment interfering with activity was minimized. Sensory-impaired patients were provided with visual aids, working hearing aids, and wax disimpaction when necessary. Dehydration was recognized early and fluids repleted. Effectiveness of this program, the Hospital Elder Life Program (HELP), was studied in a controlled clinical trial of 852 patients age 70 and older; 426 patients received the intervention and 426 patients served as controls. Overall, the risk of delirium was reduced by 40% in the intervention group. The incidence and total number of days of delirium were significantly lower among those who were enrolled in the prevention program versus those who received usual care (Inouye et al., 2000).

Delirium is a medical emergency in older patients (Henry, 2002), but before it can be treated, it must be recognized. Studies suggest that delirium is underrecognized by physicians and nurses in hospitals (Milisen et al., 2002). Poor recognition of delirium has been connected with inaccurately or incompletely evaluating mental status changes and misattributing them to dementia, normal aging, or acute illness (Milisen et al., 2002). Hypoactivity is common in older patients with delirium but complicates recognition of the syndrome in hospitals because the patients are easier to care for than those with agitation (Milisen et al., 2002) and decreased activity is often considered normal during acute illness.

Routine, systematic, and comprehensive assessment facilitates recognition of delirium. The Confusion Assessment Method (CAM) has reliably demonstrated specificity and sensitivity and is the most widely used tool to detect delirium (Henry, 2002; Inouye, 2000; Milisen et al., 2002). The CAM-ICU is a valid tool with high sensitivity and specificity for identifying delirium in mechanically ventilated patients and takes only 2 minutes to administer (Reuters Health Information, 2001). In hospitals, documentation of mental status is frequently limited to orientation, and nurses often form a gestalt about the patient's orientation rather than actually questioning him or her. Standard tools such as the MMSE aid assessment of overall cognitive function, but accuracy depends on the education and ethnicity of the individual (Berg, 2003). The best indicator of cognitive impairment is a change in cognition from the patient's baseline. Consider the case of a patient who gets up alone despite frequent instruction to call for help and asks the nurse when he will get his medicines—20 minutes after the nurse administered them. Is his behavior caused by anxiety, dementia, depression, delirium, or a combination of problems? Information regarding the onset and course of any cognitive impairment is critical to making the differential diagnosis.

Assess for predisposing risk factors on admission. Be alert for signs of the development of delirium in the first 2 to 3 days after admission (Foreman et al., 1999), the first 5 days after surgery (Milisen et al., 2002), and in patients transferred from the ICU. Signs of delirium may be more noticeable in the late afternoon or evening because of fatigue and the cumulative effect of a full day of stimulation or lack of appropriate stimulation. Family members' reports of abnormal changes in patient behavior must be taken seriously. Short interactions with patients may preclude delirium recognition by physicians in the hospital setting. Consistent assignment of nursing staff and daily discussion of the patient's mental status and usual behavior in shift-to-shift reports and interdisciplinary rounds increase the chance that signs of delirium will be noticed.

For patients admitted with delirium and for those in whom prevention strategies fail, identifying and eliminating or minimizing causative factors and providing a therapeutic environment become the cornerstones of treatment. Medication toxicity, infections, fluid and electrolyte imbalances, metabolic disturbances, and hypoxia are frequent culprits. Etiology is usually multifactorial. Continual assessment to uncover causes is essential even after one or more sources have been identified. All of the prevention strategies should be continued. Patients with delirium are at increased risk for injury and require more frequent observation. A commonly recommended strategy is to place the patient nearer to the nurses' station (Henry, 2002) or in a chair in the hallway. Be mindful of the increased exposure to noise and commotion in these areas. Even when patients are delirious, they should be included in their care; however, complex information, instructions, and choices can be overwhelming. Use simple language, a low voice, and a gentle approach, but do not patronize. Do not argue with them. Seeing a relative in the throes of delirium can be frightening. Families need education from nurses to understand delirium and how they can help. Medications with lower anticholinergic and extrapyramidal side effects (e.g., risperidone, seroquel) may be appropriate temporarily to promote comfort and safety in a delirious patient with agitation. Many patients who develop delirium have a previously unrecognized, underlying dementia. Older patients who have experienced delirium in the hospital should be referred for a full dementia workup after resolution of acute illness.

Acute Urinary Incontinence

Approximately 90% of community-dwelling older adults are continent most of the time (Ouslander & Johnson, 2003). Many who ordinarily are continent experience incontinence within a few days of hospitalization. In a study of over 6500 women age 60 and older admitted for hip fracture to hospitals in four states, 21% developed new incontinence while in the hospital and were incontinent at discharge (Palmer, Baumgarten, Langenberg, & Carson, 2002). Urinary continence depends not only on intact structural and neurological functions but also on the ability to recognize the need to void and get to a toilet, motivation to remain continent, and an environment that facilitates the process (Bradway, Henley, & the NICHE Faculty, 1999). Functional incontinence is caused by impairments in these nongenitourinary factors. Insertion of indwelling catheters as routine treatment in hospital EDs impedes assessment and maintenance of continence. Functional and cognitive impairments may be exacerbated by acute illness. Mobility may be limited by equipment and tubing. Research suggests that nursing home residency, confusion, and mobility impairments before hospital admission increase the risk for hospital-acquired incontinence (Palmer et al., 2002).

Urinary incontinence in acute care can lead to infection, skin breakdown, and decreased activity (Bradway et al., 1999). Incontinence can affect self-esteem and promote self-isolation. It is hard to manage at home and is a primary factor in deciding on nursing home placement (Mason, Newman, & Palmer, 2003).

Patients should be asked about usual voiding patterns and history of incontinence. Symptoms such as frequency, nocturia, dribbling, leakage with sneezing or coughing, and rushing to the bathroom help diagnose the type of incontinence and direct the plan of care. A voiding diary can be helpful if kept for even 1 day and is considered the gold standard in obtaining information about a patient's voiding pattern and incontinence severity. When urinary incontinence is of recent onset, look for causes. Transient or acute incontinence can be precipitated by restricted mobility; diuretic, anticholinergic, narcotic, calcium channel blocking, and beta-adrenergic medications; excessive urine production with hyperglycemia and hypercalcemia; urinary tract infection; stool impaction; depression; and delirium (Bradway et al., 1999; Ouslander & Johnson, 2003). Older adults with CHF and lower extremity venous insufficiency may have nocturnal polyuria (Ouslander & Johnson, 2003).

Treatment of functional incontinence is based on eliminating or reducing the causative factors. Functional incontinence is reversible, and its management rests primarily with the nursing staff. Reduce obstacles and the distance to the bathroom. Keep urinals within reach for male patients. Offer assistance with toileting on a schedule appropriate to the individual patient. Assist the patient to void before leaving the unit for tests, at bedtime, and when administering a diuretic or sedating medication. Indwelling catheters are not indicated for

this type of incontinence and should be avoided to reduce the risk of associated complications. Consult occupational and physical therapists when indicated for toilet transfer training and to improve ambulation. Reassure the patient that he or she can expect return of normal bladder function. Discourage the patient from self-restricting fluids as a solution to incontinence. Avoiding caffeine and limiting fluids after dinner if adequate fluid has been consumed during the day is appropriate. Incontinence that persists several weeks after hospitalization requires further evaluation (Ouslander & Johnson, 2003). Provide emotional support. Assist with hygiene and skin care. (Incontinence is discussed in greater detail in Chapter 16.)

Acute Pain

Acute illness is often accompanied by pain. The incidence of pain-causing conditions increases with age. Many geriatric patients in the hospital experience both acute and chronic pain. If not controlled, pain can disrupt sleep, impair function and mobility, lead to depression, and delay recovery (Otis & McGeeney, 2000).

Older hospitalized adults are at risk for inadequate treatment of pain because of misconceptions of staff and patients alike. Aging does not alter the neurophysiological processes necessary for pain perception (Sheehan & Schirm, 2003). The gold standard in pain assessment is patient report. However, patients must be asked. "The most common reason for unrelieved pain in U.S. hospitals is the failure of staff to routinely assess pain and pain relief" (American Pain Society [APS], 1999, p. 3). If not specifically asked about pain, some patients will tolerate it. Standardized pain scales help patients rate their pain intensity. Most adults can score their pain intensity on numerical, category, or visual analog scales (APS, 1999). The nurse should have multiple tools close at hand so that the patient may choose the one with which he or she is most comfortable. Explore why a patient might be underreporting pain. The patient may not want to alarm loved ones or admit that his or her disease may have worsened. The nurse should inquire about the location, quality, and duration of the pain, as well as any precipitating or alleviating factors. Ask how pain has affected the patient's function. Help the patient define acceptable pain levels and the degree of sedation or side effects he or she is willing to tolerate.

Give special attention to pain assessment and management in older adults who are at greatest risk for inadequate pain relief: those who abuse alcohol or drugs, the frail and debilitated, the cognitively impaired, and those who are reluctant to report pain (Sheehan & Schirm, 2003). Culture and ethnicity influence the experience of pain and, along with language barriers, should be considered in the assessment of pain. Tachycardia, hypertension, and diaphoresis often, but do not always, accompany acute pain (APS, 1999). In studies of moderately cognitively impaired patients, 60% to 83% of them could reliably and validly complete at least one pain tool (Feldt, 2000). The 0-to-10 pain intensity number scale requires abstraction from a verbal description into a number and ranking, a task that may be too complex for some. Try uncomplicated pain intensity scales that use simple language. Observe for withdrawal, decreased activity, increased irritability, aggressive behaviors, or resistance to personal care that requires movement. Family members who know the patient better may notice changes in the patient's personality. In a study by Feldt (2000) of cognitively intact and impaired older post–hip surgery patients, the Checklist of Nonverbal Pain Indicators (CNPI) guided observations of pain behaviors such as grimacing, wincing, restlessness, guarding, rubbing, sighing, grunting, moaning, profanity, and verbalizations such as "don't" and "stop." It was considered simple and reliable. Noting significantly fewer pain behaviors at rest, Feldt cautions the nurse to include use of the assessment tool during patient activity. The faces pain scale may be an appropriate alternative for the cognitively impaired (Herr, 2002), hospitalized older adults, and the less educated (Taylor & Herr, 2002).

Acute pain should be treated immediately. Analgesics need not and should not be withheld in order to diagnose. Per the APS (1999, p. 4), drug therapy, including opioids and nonopioids, is the "mainstay" for the management of acute pain and cancer pain in all age-groups. Alterations in drug absorption, distribution, and metabolism and susceptibility to side effects create challenges in treating acute pain in older adults. Analgesics should be selected based on their ability to provide the greatest relief with the fewest side effects (Otis & McGeeney, 2000). Propoxyphene and meperidine should not be used in older patients (Fick et al., 2003; Fine, 2000). All pain treatment regimens should include a nonopioid even if pain is severe enough to require the addition of an opioid. Nonsteroidal antiinflammatory drugs are helpful in treating most types of pain and should be used unless contraindicated (APS, 1999). Scheduled acetaminophen is usually tolerated by older adults and may reduce amounts of opioids needed. For patients over age 70, starting doses of opioids should be 25% to 50% lower and slowly titrated up to achieve pain relief (APS, 1999). Placebos are never indicated. For patients with difficulty communicating pain, provide analgesics for conditions or procedures known to be painful.

Use the oral route when possible. Administration of medications intramuscularly results in more rapid falloff of action. Injections are painful and absorption is inconsistent, especially in older adults with muscle atrophy. Intravenous administration is useful for rapid onset but has the shortest duration of action (APS, 1999). Administer medications routinely rather than as required for acute pain that is present most of the day. Sustained-release analgesics can be put on a schedule and immediate-release analgesics ordered as required for breakthrough pain. The transdermal route offers continuous release, but uptake and distribution are inconsistent in people with altered subcutaneous fat and water (Fine, 2000). In the best circumstances, substantial therapeutic effect with transdermal fentanyl takes 12 to 16 hours and steady-state blood concentrations may take 48 hours to achieve (APS, 1999). Thus titration is also delayed. For these reasons, transdermal fentanyl is not the first choice for older adults with acute pain. Patient-controlled analgesia may be warranted for the treatment of severe, acute pain. Enhancing patient control can help alleviate patients' feelings of frustration, despair, and loss of confidence in care (Fulmer, Mion, Bottrell, & the NICHE Faculty, 1999).

Expect the patient to experience some sedation or other cognitive change, respiratory depression, nausea, and constipation with opioid use. Prevent, monitor, and treat side effects. Tolerance to side effects usually develops within 48 to 72 hours. Maintaining relatively constant blood levels and avoiding high peak levels by using sustained-release preparations or by decreasing the dose and the time interval between doses can reduce side effects. If intolerable side effects persist and are not amenable to treatment, switching to another analgesic in the same class may help because there is incomplete cross tolerance. Because of its lower side effect profile, an equianalgesic dose of transdermal fentanyl may be appropriate after shorter-acting opioids have been titrated to relief (APS, 1999).

Studies of the efficacy of nonpharmacological treatments for pain have not been of sufficient quantity or quality to draw any generalizable conclusions (Agency for Healthcare Research and Quality [AHRQ], 2001). Alternative therapies may be explored once the crisis of acute pain has subsided (Fulmer et al., 1999). Positioning and reassurance may aid relief. Application of heat or cold, massage, physical and occupational therapy, relaxation, distraction, and guided imagery may help. Promote sleep. A cyclical relationship exists between sleep and pain. Pain disrupts sleep and sleep deprivation can lead to lowered pain thresholds, resulting in increased pain during the first week of hospitalization (Bursch, 2004). Before discharge, ensure that pain is adequately controlled and can be managed in the setting to which the patient will be discharged. Usually, this means that a nonintravenous route of administration with dosing less frequent than four times a day has been adequate to control pain in the 24 hours preceding discharge.

Older patients worried about addiction or how they might act may be reluctant to take pain medications

Nursing Care Plan: The Older Adult in Acute Care

Assessment Data (on Admission)

78-year-old white man admitted from the ED where he sought treatment for severe pain in the right hip. History of prostate CA status post radiation therapy 3 years ago, osteoarthritis, mild coronary artery disease, hypercholesterolemia, and mild hypertension. Medications at home include HCTZ, atorvastatin (Lipitor), and baby aspirin. NKDA.

Current pain rating is 7/10 severity on a 0-to-10 numerical rating scale (0 being no pain and 10 being the worst pain imaginable). The pain is a deep and constant ache, sometimes throbbing. He is rubbing his hip and grimacing, but states that he does not want to take anything for it. "I just had something downstairs. I better not take anything more yet." 2 mg morphine was administered intravenously 3 hours ago in the ED for pain rated 9/10 severity, and the pain initially subsided to 4/10. He admits that he would like his pain level to be 3/10 or less severe. He cannot identify any precipitating factors. He notes that he usually takes a 1-mile walk each day. When the pain first started about 10 days ago, he continued his walks, hoping that would help. The pain has progressively worsened to where, for the past 3 days, he could only walk short distances in the house. He tried one of his wife's Darvocet N100s this morning. "That didn't really help. It made me feel a little weird. I've never really needed anything for my arthritis. I usually turn on the ballgame or go do something else to get my mind off of it."

Vital signs are as follows: temperature, 37.6° C; pulse, 88 beats per minute; respirations, 22 breaths per minute; blood pressure, 150/90 mm Hg; pulse oximetry, 97% on room air. Lungs clear to auscultation. Complete blood count and comprehensive metabolic blood panel (CMP) are within normal limits, but hemoglobin (Hgb) and hematocrit (Hct) are borderline low. Urine assay (UA) is negative. Prostate-specific antigen is elevated. X-ray results are not available. Fully oriented, MMSE = 25. Wife states that he is "sharp as a tack." Height, 5 ft 11 in; weight, 170 lb.

His appetite began declining about 3 days before admission, but he has not lost weight. He reports feeling a little nauseated now. Last bowel movement was yesterday. He usually has a bowel movement every morning. Abdomen is soft, nontender, and nondistended. Bowel sounds are hypoactive in all four quadrants. Skin is intact. Braden Score = 19.

He remained independent in all ADLs. Normally capable of independence in all instrumental activities of daily living (IADLs) but limited in heavier chores in the last 3 days because of pain. He has had no falls or near falls. He uses no adaptive equipment at home.

Slow limping gait from bed to bathroom, reaching for support. Vision is adequately corrected with bifocals. Able to hear normal tones of voice without hearing aid.

Increased risk for falling secondary to age, altered gait, new environment, and opioid use. Mood: denies depressive symptoms.

Retired professor of literature. Married for 51 years, wife considered to be in good health. Three children, one living nearby, two out of state. Rare alcohol use. Hobbies: reading, attending symphony concerts, gardening, and following baseball.

Code status: full. Wife is DPOA.

Nursing Diagnosis 1 (Johnson, Bulechek, Dochterman, Maas, & Moorhead, 2001)

Pain, acute, related to tissue injury of unknown etiology at this time

Goals/Outcomes

- Patient will report pain to nurse and pain level will be maintained at 3/10 or less.

NOC Suggested Outcomes (Moorhead, Johnson, & Maas, 2004)

Pain control
Pain level
Pain: disruptive effects
Comfort level

NIC Suggested Interventions (Dochterman & Bulechek, 2004)

Major interventions: Analgesic Administration (2210), Pain Management (1400)

- Ask the patient to rate his pain severity each shift and 1 hour after administering as-required pain medication.
- Document pain ratings in a consistent place.
- Educate the patient about the myths associated with opioid use (e.g., addiction, inability to achieve pain relief if pain gets worse over time).
- Instruct the patient to report pain before it becomes severe.
- Instruct the patient to inform the nurse if pain is not relieved.
- Ask the patient to discuss his level of satisfaction with pain management.
- Report patient pain ratings and discuss pain management strategies in interdisciplinary rounds.
- Adjust frequency and dosage of analgesics as indicated by pain assessments.
- With each dose adjustment, monitor pain relief, side effects, and physical and psychosocial function.

Nursing Care Plan: The Older Adult in Acute Care—cont'd

- Maximize use of nonopioid pain medications.
- Help the patient find a comfortable position.
- Administer immediate-release analgesic before painful events such as transferring to a stretcher or wheelchair for a diagnostic test.
- Help him address lower extremity hygiene and dressing.
- Plan physical therapy and occupational therapy evaluations when pain is less severe.
- Ask his wife to bring in his headset and favorite music.
- Adjust temperature in the room to the patient's preference.
- Promote adequate rest and sleep.
- Start a bowel regimen.
- Administer an antiemetic with a lower side effect profile (e.g., Zofran) as needed.
- Monitor respiratory status.
- Monitor for cognitive changes.

Evaluation Parameters

The patient expresses satisfaction with pain management and experiences minimal side effects. Pain scores are documented at least each shift and 1 hour after each dose of as-required analgesia. Specific indicators of outcome achievement might include the following: usual pain rating of 3/10 or lower, the patient reports pain before it becomes severe and without being asked, and the patient returns to usual independence in performing ADLs.

Assessment Data (on Day 3)

The patient appears excessively sleepy. He rouses for vital signs in the morning (temperature, 37.2° C; pulse, 78 beats per minute; respirations, 18 beats per minute; blood pressure, 130/70 mm Hg; pulse oximetry, 95% on room air) and asks, "What are we having for supper?" His breakfast tray is set up in front of him on his overbed table, but he dozes back off. His bed and gown are wet with urine. When asked to rate his pain with the 0-to-10 scale he had been using, he responds, "It's not too bad." His face and body appear relaxed, but when assisted to transfer he grunts a little. He is fully awake and with appropriate conversation at 10:30 AM, but at 4:00 PM his wife comes to the nurses' station and says, "He's talking out of his head in there. He looked like he was trying to get out of bed. I asked him what he was trying to do and told him to wait a second, and the next thing he was urinating."
- Oriented to person and place. CAM positive.
- Braden Score = 17, skin remains intact.
- He has not been eating or drinking well since admission. He had a bowel movement yesterday.

- Physical therapist evaluated patient yesterday during a period of pain relief. Recommended walking short distances with quad cane and assist, twice each day in addition to physical therapy sessions.
- Hgb and Hct have been stable. Hct up slightly today compared with Hct drawn in ED. $Na^+ = 148$, BUN 32, serum creatinine 1.6. Laboratory values are otherwise within normal limits.
- Preliminary results of a bone scan yesterday are suggestive of boney metastasis in the right hip.
- Assessment is otherwise unchanged.
  Medications include the same medications he was on at home at the same dosages, plus MS Contin 30 mg twice a day, Celebrex twice a day, senna S twice a day, acetaminophen 650 mg q4-6hr as required, Percocet 5/325 q4-6hr as required, and Zofran 4 mg intravenously as required.

Nursing Diagnosis 2 (North American Nursing Diagnosis Association [NANDA], 2005)

Acute confusion related to delirium secondary to dehydration, opioid use

Goals/Outcomes

Patient will return to baseline mental status.

NOC Suggested Outcomes (Moorhead, Johnson, & Maas, 2004)

Cognitive orientation
Information processing
Safety behavior: personal
Sleep

NIC Suggested Interventions (Dochterman & Bulechek, 2004)

Major interventions: Delirium Management (6440), Cognitive Stimulation (4720), Environmental Management: Safety (6480), Fall Prevention (6490), Reality Orientation (4820), Sleep Enhancement (1850)
- Encourage oral intake of fluids; with each interaction, offer noncaffeinated fluids the patient likes and educate family to do the same.
- Administer Zofran before breakfast and evening meals and monitor for effect on intake.
- Monitor intake and output, BUN, and serum creatinine; avoid placing indwelling catheter (see Nursing Diagnosis 3 for plan of care for functional incontinence).
- Prepare to run intravenous fluid bolus; convert to saline lock as soon as possible.

Nursing Care Plan: The Older Adult in Acute Care—cont'd

- Confer with clinical pharmacist and physician for medication changes. Medication changes might include the following: Hold HCTZ and continue to monitor blood pressure each shift. Hold Celebrex until resolution of dehydration. Attempt lowering MS Contin dose and monitor for response, including subsequent pain ratings, nonverbal pain behaviors, and frequency of requiring breakthrough pain medication. Administer Tylenol 650 mg four times daily. Change breakthrough medication to one that is not combined with acetaminophen to avoid exceeding 4 g daily limit.
- Assign consistent caregivers.
- Clean and give the patient his glasses.
- Point out the clock and orientation board to the patient and orient him as needed.
- Slip orienting cues into conversation (e.g., "What a beautiful fall afternoon out there! A good day to plant bulbs if we weren't at the hospital").
- Keep the room lit during the day.
- Minimize daytime sleeping but allow for adequate rest periods.
- Take the patient for short walks with quad cane as recommended by the physical therapist.
- Use television judiciously (e.g., so patient can watch a baseball game, a gardening show, or a concert) but not left on continuously.
- Reduce noise and interruptions at night.
- If patient awakens during the night, offer a back rub, a warm noncaffeinated drink, and his headset with music he finds relaxing.
- Encourage wife to visit and ask if adult child can visit at alternate times to increase patient supervision. Suggest mealtime visits to promote nutrition intake.
- Educate family on the cause of acute confusion and provide emotional support.
- Teach family communication techniques therapeutic for their delirious relative (e.g., calm, supportive tone; avoiding arguments; orienting omments).
- Suggest therapeutic activities to the family or request a volunteer visit (e.g., read the baseball results to him from the newspaper).
- Keep call light in reach and ask the patient to show you how to use it. Provide frequent instructions to wait for help before getting up and explain why.
- Use a bed alarm when visitors are not with the patient.
- Check on the patient more frequently and continue to monitor mental status.

Evaluation Parameters

Patient is fully oriented, with CAM negative, and maintains admission baseline MMSE score of 25 or greater. Other outcome indicators in this situation might include the following: patient reports pain using the 0-to-10 pain severity tool, patient is awake most of the day and asleep most of the night, and patient does not fall and remains free of injury.

Nursing Diagnosis 3 (NANDA, 2005)

Urinary incontinence, functional related to mobility and cognitive impairments

Goals/Outcomes

- Patient will be continent of urine.

NOC Suggested Outcomes (Moorhead, Johnson, & Maas, 2004)

Urinary continence
Urinary elimination
Tissue integrity: skin and mucous membranes

NIC Suggested Interventions (Dochterman & Bulechek, 2004)

Major interventions: Urinary Habit Training (0600), Urinary Incontinence Care (0610).

- Place urinal within the patient's reach, explain its use, and remind him that it is there.
- Empty urinal promptly each time the patient voids in it.
- Every 2 hours during waking hours, just before bedtime, before administering opioids, and before sending the patient off the unit for a test, encourage him to walk to the bathroom or stand at the bedside to void into the urinal with the staff's assistance.
- Document incontinent and continent episodes and adjust voiding schedule accordingly (e.g., increase toileting interval by 1 hour if patient is unable to void at two or more scheduled toileting times or has had no incontinent episodes for 3 consecutive days; decrease interval by 30 minutes if more than three incontinent episodes in 24 hours).
- Keep call light within patient's reach; demonstrate call light use and ask for return demonstration. Answer call light as promptly as possible.
- Offer fluids frequently during the day.
- Apply moisture barrier cream to genital skin.
- Check routinely for wetness, and promptly wash and dry genital skin after any incontinence episode.
- Promptly clean up any wet areas on the floor.
- Explain etiology of the problem to the patient and his wife, and explain how it can be helped; assure them that it is a temporary problem.
- Consult occupational therapy.
- If incontinence persists, repeat UA and assess for other types/causes of incontinence.

Evaluation Parameters

Patient is dry during the day and urinating in either the urinal or toilet. Other specific indicators of outcome achievement might include the following: genital skin is intact and without redness or irritation, recognizes urge to void, responds to urge in timely manner, and voids in appropriate receptacle.

(Fulmer et al., 1999). Dispelling myths and educating patients about pain and pain management is crucial. "Analgesics benefit the patient only if the clinician monitors pain relief and side effects frequently and adjusts the regimen accordingly" (APA, 1999). Nurses are the physician's eyes and ears and must be aware when doses have been adjusted. Documentation of pain assessment and response to treatment, including physical and psychosocial functioning, is crucial. A study of 709 hip fracture patients over age 65 in 12 midwestern hospitals illuminated poor pain management practice despite nurses' knowledge of current recommendations. The greatest barrier to proper pain management, according to the nurses, was trouble in contacting physicians to discuss the best regimen for individual patients (Ferri & Safer, 2004). Nurse participation in interdisciplinary planning meetings can facilitate nurse-physician communication for improved pain management. Research suggests that the greater the exposure to others' expressions of pain, the less often observers acknowledged it (Tsao, 2004). Hospital nurses see pain every day. They must be aware of their beliefs and values regarding pain management and guard against becoming desensitized to their patients' pain experiences.

SUMMARY

The goal of admission to a hospital is to enable accurate, timely diagnosis and treatment of acute illness in a 24-hour continuum with the availability of multiple disciplines and high technology all in one setting. Unfortunately, hospital care historically has not been in tune with the special needs of vulnerable older patients and has often led to preventable, functional decline despite resolution of the acute illness. Though hospitalization has long been recognized as hazardous for frail, older adults, the development and dissemination of validated, effective interventions have been slow. The traditional goals focusing on treatment or cure of a specific disease entity must be meshed with those of gerontological nursing to preserve function and dignity and to promote comfort and quality of life. Care for older adults in hospitals is complex and requires careful oversight by professionals competent in gerontology. Nurses are in the best position to protect patients from iatrogenesis; promote functional independence while providing dignified, appropriate acute care; and advocate for the adoption of proven models of care as standard for all frail patients in the hospital.

REFERENCES

Agency for Healthcare Research and Quality. (2001). Management of cancer pain. Summary. *Evidence report/technology assessment: Number 35.* AHRQ pub. no. 01-E033. Rockville, MD: Author. Retrieved July 5, 2004, from www.ahrq.gov/clinic/epcsums/canpainsum.htm.

American Geriatrics Society, British Geriatrics Society, & American Academy of Orthopaedic Surgeons Panel on Falls Prevention. (2001). Guideline for prevention of falls in older persons. *Journal of the American Geriatrics Society, 49*(5), 664-672.

American Nurses Association. (2000). *Scope and standards of gerontological nursing practice.* Washington, DC: Author.

American Pain Society. (1999). *Principles of analgesic use in the treatment of acute pain and cancer pain* (4th ed.). Glenview, IL: Author.

Asplund, K., Gustafson, Y., Jacobsson, C., Bucht, G., Wahlin, A., Peterson, J., et al. (2000). Geriatric-based versus general wards for older acute medicine patients: A randomized comparison of outcomes and use of resources. *Journal of the American Geriatrics Society, 48*(11), 1381-1388.

Baine, W. B., Yu, W., & Summa, J. P. (2001a). The epidemiology of hospitalization of elderly Americans for septicemia or bacteremia in 1991-1998: Application of Medicare claims data. *Annals of Epidemiology, 11*(2), 118-126.

Baine, W. B., Yu, W., and Summa, J. P. (2001b). Epidemiologic trends in the hospitalization of elderly Medicare patients for pneumonia, 1991-1998. *American Journal of Public Health, 91*(7), 1121-1123.

Berg, A. O. (2003). Screening for dementia: Recommendations and rationale. *American Journal of Nursing, 103*(9), 87, 89, 91, 93, 95.

Board on Health Care Services, Institute of Medicine. (2004). *Crossing the quality chasm summit: Redesigning care and improving health in priority areas.* Retrieved May 20, 2006, from www.iom.edu/CMS/3809/9868.aspx?printfriendly=true.

Borum, M. L., Lynn, J., Zhong, A., Roth, K., Connors, A. F., Jr., Desbiens, N. A., et al. (2000). The effect of nutritional supplementation on survival in seriously ill hospitalized adults: An evaluation of the SUPPORT data. *Journal of the American Geriatrics Society, 48*(5), S33-S38.

Bradway, C., Henley, S., & the NICHE Faculty. (1999). Urinary incontinence in older adults. In I. Abraham, M. M. Bottrell, T. Fulmer, & M. D. Mezey (Eds.), *Geriatric nursing protocols for best practice.* New York: Springer.

Bursch, B. (2004). Physiologic correlates of pain during sleep. Highlights of the 2nd joint scientific meeting of the American Pain Society, May 6-9, 2004. Retrieved August 2, 2004, from www.medscape.com/viewprogram/3174_pnt.

Cohen, H. J., Feussner, J. R., Weinberger, M., Carnes, M., Handy, R. C., Hsieh, F., et al. (2002). A controlled trial of inpatient and outpatient geriatric evaluation and management. *New England Journal of Medicine, 346*(12), 905-912.

Coll, P. P. (2001). Sleep disorders. In A. M. Adelman & M. P. Daly (Eds.), *20 common problems in geriatrics.* New York: McGraw-Hill.

Coppola, K. M., Ditto, P. H., Danks, J. H., & Smucker, J. D. (2001). Accuracy of primary care and hospital-based physician's prediction of elderly outpatients' treatment preferences with and without advance directives. *Archives of Internal Medicine, 161*(2), 431-440.

Corrigan, B., Allen, K., Moore, J., Samra, P., Stetler, C., Thielen, J., et al. (1999). Preventing falls in acute care. In I. Abraham, M. M. Bottrell, T. Fulmer, & M. D. Mezey (Eds.), *Geriatric nursing protocols for best practice.* New York: Springer.

Counsell, S. R., Holder, C. M., Liebenauer, L. L., Palmer, R. M., Fortinsky, R. H., Kresevic, D. M., et al. (2000). Effects of a multicomponent intervention on functional outcomes and process of care in hospitalized older patients, a randomized controlled trial of acute care for elders (ACE) in a community hospital. *Journal of the American Geriatrics Society, 48*(12), 1572-1581.

Covinsky, K. E., Palmer, R. M., Fortinsky, R. H., Counsell, S. R., Stewart, A. L., Kresevic, D., et al. (2003). Loss of independence in activities of daily living in older adults hospitalized with medical illnesses: Increased vulnerability with age. *Journal of the American Geriatrics Society, 51*(4), 451-458.

Ditto, P. H., Danks, J. H., Smucker, W. D., Bookwala, J., Coppola, K. M., Dresser, R., et al. (2001). Advance directives as acts of communication. *Archives of Internal Medicine, 161*(2), 421-430.

Dixon, L. (2002). Postoperative complications and the older adult. *Geriatric Nursing, 23*(4), 203.

Dochterman, J. M., & Bulechek, G. M. (2004). *Nursing interventions classification (NIC)*. St. Louis: Mosby.

Drickamer, M. A. (2003). Assessment of decisional capacity and competency. In W. R. Hazzard, J. P. Blass, J. B. Halter, J. B. Ouslander, & M. E. Tinetti (Eds.), *Principles of geriatric medicine and gerontology* (5th ed.). New York: McGraw-Hill.

Evans, E. (1999). Indwelling catheter care: Dispelling the misconceptions. *Geriatric Nursing, 20*(2), 85-89.

Evans, W. J. (2001). Aging and malnutrition: Treatment guidelines. *Medscape Nursing Clinical Management, 3*. Retrieved September 24, 2001, from www.medscape.com/Medscape/Nurses/ClinicalMgmt/CM.v03/pnt-CM.v03.html.

Feldt, K. S. (2000). The Checklist of Nonverbal Pain Indicators (CNPI). *Pain Management Nursing, 1*(1), 13-21.

Ferri, R. S., & Safer, D. (2004). Pain management in older adults: When will research evidence become practice? *American Journal of Nursing, 104*(2), 19.

Fick, D. M., Cooper, J. W., Wade, W. E., Waller, J. L., Maclean, J. R., & Beers, M. H. (2003). Updating the Beers criteria for potentially inappropriate medication use in older adults. *Archives of Internal Medicine, 163*, 2716-2724.

Fine, P. G. (2000). Pain and aging: Overcoming barriers to treatment and the role of transdermal opioid therapy. *Clinical Geriatrics, 8*(12), 28-36.

Flood, K. L., Carroll, M., Esker, D. A., & Carr, D. B. (2004, May). A descriptive pilot study on an oncology-acute care of the elderly (OACE) unit. Poster session presented at the annual scientific meeting of the American Geriatrics Society.

Flood, K. L., Emory, V., Le, C. V., Rich, M. W., & Carr, D. B. (2004, May). Prevalence of geriatric syndromes on an inpatient cardiology unit. Poster session presented at the annual scientific meeting of the American Geriatrics Society.

Foreman, M. D., Mion, L. C., Trygstad, L. J., Fletcher, K., & the NICHE Faculty. (1999). Acute confusion/delirium: Strategies for assessing and treating. In I. Abraham, M. M. Bottrell, T. Fulmer, & M. D. Mezey (Eds.), *Geriatric nursing protocols for best practice*. New York: Springer.

Fulmer, T. T., Mion, L. C., Bottrell, M. M., & the NICHE Faculty. (1999). Pain management. In I. Abraham, M. M. Bottrell, T. Fulmer, & M. D. Mezey (Eds.), *Geriatric nursing protocols for best practice*. New York: Springer.

Habel, M. (2004). The hospitalized older adult. Entering a danger zone. *Nurse Week, 5*(2) 26-27.

Halfon, P., Eggli, Y., Van Melle, G., & Vagnair, A. (2001). Risk of falls for hospitalized patients: A predictive model based on routinely available data. *Journal of Clinical Epidemiology, 54*, 1258-1266.

Hall, M. J., & DeFrances, C. J. (2003). *2001 National Hospital Discharge Survey. Advance data from vital and health statistics; no. 332*. Hyatsville, MD: National Center for Health Statistics.

Henry, M. (2002). Descending into delirium. *American Journal of Nursing, 102*(3), 49-56.

Herr, K. (2002). Pain assessment in cognitively impaired older adults. *American Journal of Nursing, 102*(12), 65-67.

Hitcho, E. B., Krauss, M. J., Birge, S., Dunagan, W. C., Fischer, I., Johnson, S., et al. (2004). Characteristics and circumstances of falls in a hospital setting. A prospective analysis. *Journal of General Internal Medicine, 19*, 732-739.

Huckstadt, A. A. (2002). The experience of hospitalized elderly patients. *Journal of Gerontological Nursing, 28*(9), 24-29.

Inouye, S. K. (1999). Delirium in hospitalized older patients. *Clinical Geriatric Medicine, 14*, 745-763.

Inouye, S. K. (2000). Prevention of delirium in hospitalized older patients: Risk factors and targeted intervention strategies. *Annals of Medicine, 32*(4), 257-263.

Inouye, S. K., Bogardus, S. T., Baker, D. I., Leo-Summers, L., & Cooney, L. M., Jr. (2000). The Hospital Elder Life Program: A model of care to prevent cognitive and functional decline in older hospitalized patients. *Journal of the American Geriatrics Society, 48*(12), 1697-1706.

Institute of Medicine (IOM). (2004). *Keeping patients Safe: Transforming the work environment of nursing*. Washington, DC: National Academy Press. Available online at www.nap.edu/catalog/1085l.html.

Jacelon, C. S. (1999). Preventing cascade iatrogenesis in hospitalized elders: An important role for nurses. *Journal of Gerontological Nursing, 25*(1), 27-33.

Johnson, M., Bulechek, G., Dochterman, J. M., Maas, M., & Moorhead, S. (2001). *Nursing diagnoses, outcomes, and interventions: NANDA, NOC, and NIC linkages*. St. Louis: Mosby.

Kass-Bartelmes, B. L., & Hughes, R. (2004). Advance care planning. Preferences for care at the end of life. Retrieved July 6, 2004, from www.ahrq.gov/research/edliferia/endria.htm.

Kurlowicz, L., & the NICHE Faculty. (1999). Depression in elderly patients. In I. Abraham, M. M. Bottrell, T. Fulmer, & M. D. Mezey (Eds.), *Geriatric nursing protocols for best practice*. New York: Springer.

Landefeld, C. S. (2003). Improving health care for older persons. *Annals of Internal Medicine, 139*(5), 421-424.

Last Acts. (2002). *Means to a better end: A report on dying in America today*. Retrieved August 11, 2004, from www.lastacts.org/files/misc/meansfull.pdf.

Li, H. (2002). Family caregivers' preferences in caring for their elderly relatives. *Geriatric Nursing, 23*(4), 204-207.

Lockhart, L. K., Ditto, P. H., & Danks, J. H. (2001). The stability of older adults' judgments of fates better and worse than death. Retrieved July 5, 2004, from www.ahrq.gov/research/may02/v502RA13.htm.

Mason, D. J., Newman, D. K., & Palmer, M. H. (2003). Changing UI practice. *American Journal of Nursing, 3*(suppl), 2-3.

Milisen, K., Foreman, M. D., Wouters, B., Driesen, R., Godderis, J., Abraham, I., et al. (2002). Documentation of delirium in elderly patients with hip fracture. *Journal of Gerontological Nursing, 28*(11), 23-29.

Mion, L. C., Palmer, R. M., & Meldon, S. W. (2003). Case finding and referral modes for emergency department elders: A randomized clinical trial. *Annals of Emergency Medicine, 41*(1), 57-68.

Moorhead, S., Johnson, M., & Maas, M. (2004). *Nursing outcomes classification (NOC)*. St. Louis: Mosby.

Morrill, C. T., & Elixhauser, A. (2005, June). Hospitalization in the U. S., 2002 (HCUP fact book #6). Rockville, MD: AHRQ pub. no. 05-0056. Retrieved May 9, 2006, from www.ahrq.gov/data/hcup/factbk6.

North American Nursing Diagnosis Association. (2005). *Nursing diagnoses: Definitions and classification*. Philadelphia: NANDA International.

Otis, J. A., & McGeeney, B. (2000). Managing pain in the elderly. *Clinical Geriatrics, 8*(1), 48-62.

Ouslander, J. G., & Johnson, T. M., II. (2003). Incontinence. In W. R. Hazzard, J. P. Blass, J. B. Halter, J. B. Ouslander, & M. E. Tinetti (Eds.), *Principles of geriatric medicine and gerontology* (5th ed.). New York: McGraw-Hill.

Palmer, M. H., Baumgarten, M., Langenberg, P., & Carson, J. L. (2002). Risk factors for hospital-acquired incontinence in elderly female hip fracture patients. *Journal of Gerontology: Medical Sciences, 57*(10), M672-M677.

Palmer, R. M., & Meldon, S. W. (2003). Acute care. In W. R. Hazzard, J. P. Blass, J. B. Halter, J. B. Ouslander, & M. E. Tinetti (Eds.), *Principles of geriatric medicine and gerontology* (5th ed.). New York: McGraw-Hill.

Perell, K. L., Nelson, A., Goldman, R. L., Luther, S. L., Prieto-Lewis, N., & Rubenstein, L. Z. (2001). Fall risk assessment measures: An analytic review. *Journal of Gerontology, 56A*(12), M761-M766.

Polanczyk, C. A., Marcantonio, E., & Goldman, L. (2001). Impact of age on perioperative complications and lengths of stay in patients undergoing noncardiac surgery. *Annals of Internal Medicine, 134*(8), 637-643.

Reuters Health Information. (2001). Delirium common in ventilated patients, reliably detected with nonverbal tool. Retrieved December 17, 2001, from http://nurses.medscape.com/reuters/prof/2001/12/12.11/2001121-clin017.html.

Saltvedt, I., Opdahl, E., Fayers, P., Kaasa, S., & Sletvold, O. (2002). Reduced mortality in treating acutely sick, frail older patients in a geriatric evaluation and management unit. A prospective randomized trial. *Journal of the American Geriatrics Society, 50*(5), 792-798.

Sheehan, D., & Schirm, V. (2003). End-of-life care of older adults. Debunking some common myths about dying in old age. *American Journal of Nursing, 103*(11), 48-58.

Stanton, M. W. (2004). Hospital nurse staffing and quality of care. *Research in Action,* issue 14. Retrieved July 5, 2004, from www.ahrq.gov/research/nursestaffing/nursestaff.htm.

Stimmel, G., & Aiso, J. (2004). Managing insomnia in the elderly. *Geriatric Times, 5*(2), 21-24.

Talerico, K. A., & Capezuti, E. (2001). Myths and facts about side rails. *American Journal of Nursing, 101*(7), 43-48.

Taylor, L. J., & Herr, K. (2002, April). Evaluation of the faces pain scale with minority older adults. *Journal of Gerontological Nursing,* pp 15-23.

Tsao, J. C. (2004). Judging pain in others. Highlights of the 2nd joint scientific meeting of the American Pain Society, May 6-9, 2004. Retrieved August 2, 2004, from www.medscape.com/viewprogram/3174_pnt.

Walker, M. K., Foreman, M. D., & the NICHE Faculty. (1999). Ensuring medication safety for older adults. In I. Abraham, M. M. Bottrell, T. Fulmer, & M. D. Mezey (Eds.), *Geriatric nursing protocols for best practice.* New York: Springer.

Chapter

33 Subacute Care

Elizabeth A. Capezuti

Objectives

Explain the nature of subacute care.

Discuss the role of the nurse in caring for older adults in subacute care.

Explore gerontological nursing issues in the subacute care setting.

Identify important assessment data to be obtained for older adults in subacute care.

Develop nursing diagnoses and plans of care to address common needs of older adults in acute care settings.

Subacute care is "a hybrid between the hospital and the nursing facility" (Willging, 1993) addressing the medical and rehabilitative needs of those who are "sufficiently stabilized to no longer require acute (hospital) care services but are too complex for treatment in a conventional nursing center" (Hyatt, 1993). Subacute care is provided in freestanding facilities or units within a hospital or nursing home (USDHHS, 1994). More than three fourths of subacute care is offered in nursing homes (Levenson, 1994). Older adults are the primary users of subacute care (Carr, 2000).

Although the number of providers of subacute care has risen sharply in the last decade, subacute care for older adults is a permutation of "post-acute care" that has been available since the inception of the Medicare program in 1965 (Levenson, 1999). This level of care was established as the skilled nursing facility category following hospitalization, such as for postsurgical rehabilitation. Advances in technological and other medical interventions have resulted in an increase in survivors of serious illnesses and injury as well as new options for those with complex chronic illnesses (Levenson, 1999). Thus subacute care has expanded its target population to include all age-groups with medical conditions resulting in recovery periods that do not require intensive hospital-based intervention. The major impetus underlying the development of this "new" level of care is the reduction of health care costs and the diminution of acute care hospital bed use (Kelly, 2000).

This chapter will address this rapidly expanding sector of health care by defining this level of care and describing the types of units, populations served, and interventions provided. Clinical problems that have been studied in the subacute care settings and risk management issues specific to the complex recovery needs of the patients will be described. Because the persons receiving this level of care do not reside in the facility for long periods of time, they are referred to as "patients" instead of "residents" in this chapter.

SETTING AND POPULATION CHARACTERISTICS
Definition of Subacute Care

Subacute care is also referred to as "post-acute," "transitional," "near-acute," or "super-skilled" (USDHHS, 1994). Nursing home providers use the term "subacute" to distinguish it from traditional nursing home care (Knapp, 2001).

The American Health Care Association (AHCA), the Joint Commission on Accreditation of Healthcare Organizations (JCAHO, 1994), and the Association of Hospital-Based Skilled Nursing Facilities have developed a definition of subacute care:

Subacute care is comprehensive inpatient care designed for someone who has an acute illness, injury, or exacerbation of a disease process. It is goal oriented treatment rendered immediately after, or instead of, acute hospitalization to treat one or more specific active complex medical conditions or to administer one or more technically complex treatments, in the context of a person's underlying long-term conditions and overall situation (Hyatt, 1993).

Similarly, the International Subacute Healthcare Association defines subacute care as:

A comprehensive, cost-effective and outcome oriented approach to care for patients requiring short-term, complex medical and/or rehabilitation interventions provided by a physician directed interdisciplinary, professional team. Subacute services should be administered through defined programs without regard to setting. Subacute programs typically are utilized as an inpatient alternative to an acute hospital admission or an alternative to an acute hospital admission or an alternative to continued hospitalization, and may be a component of a vertically integrated health care system. (Hyatt, 1993)

In other words, the patient's condition does not require high-technology monitoring or complex diagnostic procedures characteristic of hospital/acute care. However, the patients do need a higher level of health care supervision and often more complex technological nursing or rehabilitative interventions than provided in the traditional nursing home setting. Examples of technologies monitored or administered in this setting include ventilators, intravenous infusion, tracheotomies, and feeding tubes (Levenson, 1996). Subacute care can be delivered in a separate unit or dispersed throughout the nursing home (Knapp, 2001).

Subacute Care Categories

As the field has developed, subacute care is categorized in a variety of ways: type of patient problem, length of stay, or scope of services (USDHHS, 1994).

Patient Problem Type. Patient care needs in subacute care settings can be divided into those requiring mostly rehabilitation (such as walking or swallowing retraining) versus medical/nursing interventions (for example, ventilators, dialysis, or intravenous infusion).

Rehabilitation subacute care refers to conditions requiring intense rehabilitative therapies (such as physical, occupational, and/or speech) for specific conditions (for example, stroke, hip fracture, or amputation surgery) or general deconditioning (for example, muscle weakness and decreased aerobic capacity) following lack of mobilization (such as walking, transferring in/out of bed/chair, self-care) associated with hospitalization or a medical condition (for example, muscle strain). Such care can be provided in rehabilitation hospitals; however, most Medicare recipients receive rehabilitation in subacute units if they can only tolerate 90 minutes of therapy per day.

Stroke patients are equally distributed between nursing homes and rehabilitation hospitals (Kramer et al., 1997). Positive patient outcomes (ability to walk, discharge to community) following stroke are generally improved when post-acute care is provided in a rehabilitation hospital compared to subacute care nursing home units (Kramer et al., 1997). Subacute care nursing home units have demonstrated better outcomes following stroke than traditional nursing home units (Kramer

et al., 1997). There are no differences in outcomes for patients following rehabilitation in the subacute care setting versus rehabilitation in a hospital setting following hip fracture surgery (Kramer et al., 1997). Most subacute care patients are discharged to community-based settings, although this varies by condition: 67% for stroke patients and 94% for those with joint replacement (Deutsch, Fiedler, Iwanenko, Granger, & Russell, 2003).

A large survey of more than 39,000 patients from 180 subacute units/facilities reported that, in general, patients cared for in subacute rehabilitation programs demonstrated significant functional improvements (Deutsch et al., 2003). One study of 20 facilities reported that subacute units within nursing homes provided more intensive therapy than subacute units in hospitals (Chen, Heinemann, Granger, & Linn, 2002). Therapy intensity was found to be weakly associated with functional gains (Chen et al., 2002). A high number of patients with medical comorbidities and depression resulted in poorer functional outcomes (Allen, Agha, Duthie, & Layde, 2004; Deutsch et al., 2003; Likourezos et al., 2002).

More than three fourths of all subacute care patients receive some physical or occupational therapy service during their stay (Johnson, Kramer, Lin, Kowalsky, & Steiner, 2000). In the last decade, however, there are a growing number of patients receiving subacute care for unstable or chronic medical conditions.

Medical subacute care refers to skilled nursing services for medical conditions that require frequent medical monitoring. The most common medical diagnoses that receive this care include congestive heart failure, infection (lung, urinary tract, blood, heart lining, or bone), and chronic obstructive lung disease; patients recovering from heart bypass surgery may also be recipients of medical subacute care services (Johnson et al., 2000). One study of 290 medical subacute care recipients reported a wide assortment of medical hospital discharge diagnoses (Johnson et al., 2000). Conditions affecting the heart and lungs represented about one half of the sample (Johnson et al., 2000). No single diagnosis accounted for greater than 10% of patients except coronary artery disease (13.8%) (Johnson et al., 2000).

Medical subacute care patients spend significantly more days in the acute care hospital but significantly fewer days in subacute care when compared to rehabilitation subacute care patients (Johnson et al., 2000). Nursing care includes frequent evaluation of symptoms (for example, glucose levels of diabetic patients), management of ventilators and associated technologies (for example, suctioning, respiratory treatments, and tracheostomy care), administration of intravenous medications (such as antibiotics and chemotherapy), treatment of complex wounds, feeding via tubes inserted in the nose or directly into the abdomen, and management of ostomies (Knapp, 2001). Also, many of these patients suffered significant functional decline in the ability to walk and transfer independently during their acute care hospitalization. Thus they receive both medical and rehabilitation services during their subacute care stay. Significant improvements in functional abilities have been demonstrated among medical subacute care patients (Johnson et al., 2000).

Length of Stay. The number of days the patient resides in the subacute unit or facility—the length of stay—can be defined as short, medium, or long. Short stays of 3 to 30 days are usually for either medical or rehabilitative care while medium stays of 31 to 90 days are provided to patients requiring both medical and rehabilitative services. Long stays of over 90 days are for those patients necessitating a slow recovery because of a catastrophic injury or illness (such as advanced pressure ulcer treatment) (Banta & Richter, 1993). The average length of stay is between 1 and 3 weeks (Marcantonio & Yurkofsky, in press). Longer stays are associated with increasing numbers of comorbidities (ongoing chronic medical conditions) (Likourezos et al., 2002).

Scope of Services. Combining patient problems and length of stay, this categorization divides care services into three groups—short-term, intermediate-term, and long-term services. Short-term subacute care delivers care to those patients requiring short-term intravenous therapy to receive hydration, antibiotics for infections such as pneumonia, and chemotherapy (Weinberg, 2000). Patients recovering from stroke, orthopedic surgery (for example, fracture or joint replacement surgery), uncomplicated head trauma, and other routine postoperative rehabilitation (Weinberg, 2000) can also be included in the short-term service category. Short-term respiratory services are limited to only those patients requiring oxygen or respiratory treatments (Weinberg, 2000). Blood transfusions, hospice/postoperative pain management, and hospice care are also considered short-term subacute services, but the length of stay can be longer for certain individuals (Weinberg, 2000).

Intermediate-term services include long-term intravenous antibiotic treatment for serious infections such as endocarditis (inflammation of the lining of the heart and its valves) and osteomyelitis (infection of the bone), hospice care, chemotherapy, and complicated pressure ulcer ("bed" sore) management (Weinberg, 2000).

Finally, chronic or long-term subacute units manage cancer patients or those requiring hemodialysis or peritoneal dialysis. Also included in this category are patients receiving ventilator support and total parenteral nutrition (Weinberg, 2000).

Specialized Subacute Programs

To increase cost efficiency, some subacute units or facilities specialize in focused areas of care. These may include ventilator support, brain injury care, extensive wound care, pain management, dialysis, or chemotherapy (AHCA, 1998). According to an American Health Care Association 1998 survey of 98 nursing home subacute care programs, most provide several specialty services within their facility or unit (AHCA, 1998). Subacute care hospital units compared to subacute care nursing home units are similar in the proportion of some program specialties such as postsurgical care (52% versus 51%), respiratory therapy (52% versus 54%), and complex medical management (57% versus 59%). Subacute care hospital units are more likely to provide dialysis (26% versus 16%) and chemotherapy/oncology (13% versus 8%) (AHCA, 1998) while subacute care nursing home units are more likely to provide ventilator support, brain injury care, extensive wound treatment, pain management, cardiac care, and especially intensive rehabilitation (AHCA, 1998).

Subacute Care Reimbursement

Subacute care is reimbursed by Medicare, Medicaid, private insurers, and managed care companies (Press, 2000). Medicare's hospital prospective payment system, which initiated Diagnosis-Related Groups (DRGs) in 1983, resulted in patients being discharged from hospitals "quicker and sicker" (Manton, Woodbury, Vertrees, & Stallard, 1993). The DRG reimbursement formula encourages hospitals to discharge Medicare beneficiaries into alternative care settings including comprehensive outpatient rehabilitation facilities, home care, hospital-based skilled nursing facilities, and nursing homes (Knapp, 1995). Thus subacute nursing home units were developed to provide health care to these patients in a less expensive setting (Knapp, 1995). Managed care providers are primarily responsible for the growth of this level of care because of the high costs of hospital care for older patients as well as children and young/middle-aged adults with certain illnesses requiring long recovery (e.g., head trauma) (Knapp, 1995). Subacute units are less expensive sites for recovery and/or rehabilitation compared to a general medical-surgical, intensive care, or rehabilitation unit within a hospital (Marcantonio & Yurkofsky, in press). Savings are estimated to be between 40% and 60% compared to hospital-based costs (Carr, 2000).

Subacute Care Regulations

There are no specific "subacute" regulations for nursing homes; rather, the Medicare regulations associated with Medicare Part A skilled care coverage determine eligibility and reimbursement (Knapp, 2001). Further, OBRA (Omnibus Budget Reconciliation Act of 1987) and accompanying regulations for nursing homes apply to subacute care. Thus subacute care is considered an industry category rather than a regulatory category (Berezny & Howells, 2000).

The quality of subacute care services is evaluated by the Centers for Medicare and Medicaid Services via 24 indicators of care that are generated from the electronic submission of minimum data set information. Data, such as percentage of patients with weight loss and dehydration, are compared among nursing home facilities. State surveyors use these indicators to focus their annual Medicare recertification surveys of facilities (Knapp, 2001).

Since 1995, both the Joint Commission on Accreditation of Healthcare Organizations (JCAHO) and the Commission on Accreditation of Rehabilitation Facilities (CARF) have designated standards specific to subacute accreditation (Berezny & Howells, 2000). Accreditation is voluntary and does not substitute for state survey requirements. Approximately 42% of subacute care nursing home units are accredited by JCAHO, 3% by CARF, and an additional 3% by both (AHCA, 1998).

SUBACUTE CARE ADMINISTRATORS AND CLINICIANS

Since subacute care is governed by the same state and federal regulations as any other nursing home, then the administrative and clinical standards of nursing homes apply. The complexity of the environment has led professional organizations and facilities to address the unique characteristics of this setting. For example, the American Health Care Association certifies subacute care administrators via a national examination. Eligibility requires individuals to hold a license as a nursing home or hospital administrator or clinician (registered nurse, respiratory therapist, occupational therapist, physical therapist, speech therapist, home health services manager/executive, social worker, physician, or psychologist), to have relevant experience, and to have received 40 clock hours of continuing education relevant to subacute care administration and/or management (Hyatt, 1993).

Physicians and Advanced Practice Clinicians

A major physician role in the subacute units, especially those providing rehabilitative care, is the identification of realistic functional goals for the patients, based on knowledge of the impact of concurrent medical illnesses (Marcantonio & Yurkofsky, in press). This includes the ability to provide medical expertise on the

prognosis, establish obtainable functional goals, decide if the medical condition necessitates hospitalization or if improvement in function is unlikely , assist with ethical treatment decisions such as insertion of a feeding tube), communicate with the patient and family about the medical limits to recovery, determine the medically indicated length of stay, and select an appropriate discharge setting.

Advanced practice clinicians who may be nurse practitioners or physician assistants provide routine care such as taking an admission history and performing a physical examination. They also provide acute episodic care such as evaluation of symptoms/signs, diagnostic workup, and treatment of noncomplicated acute illnesses and technical interventions including insertion of intravenous line and management of feeding tubes in a collaborative arrangement with an attending physician (Levenson, 1999; Marcantonio & Yurkofsky, in press). These clinicians can work as employees of the physician, multiphysician practice, medical school, or nursing home; as partners in a multidisciplinary practice; or as independent clinicians, depending on their state's State Practice Acts (Marcantonio & Yurkofsky, in press).

Medical Director

For most subacute units, the medical director is the same as the director for the entire facility. Because both physician expertise and physician accessibility differ from typical nursing home units, some nursing homes designate a separate medical director for the subacute care unit. Either unit-specific medical directors or overall medical directors are ultimately responsible for the provision of appropriate medical care for the patients in their unit/facility (Weinberg, 2000).

Case Managers/Admission Directors

The 1997 Balanced Budget Act capitates Medicare reimbursement for rehabilitative services, nursing homes, long-term care hospitals, and home health care services via a prospective payment system (Carr, 2000). The reimbursement rate is based on the facility's MDS (minimum data set) report and the patients' resource utilization group classification (Carr, 2000). Errors in documentation can lead to reduced payments; therefore facilities employ case managers to coordinate care and optimize reimbursement (Carr, 2000). Case managers or admission directors working closely with the medical or nursing director ensure that the patients admitted meet the facility's established criteria and capabilities (Weinberg, 2000). Furthermore, the marketing director's efforts should be consistent with these policies (Megan, 2000; Weinberg, 2000).

ISSUES SPECIFIC TO SUBACUTE NURSING HOME CARE
Integrated Team Approach

Typical nursing home care is provided mostly by certified nursing assistants under the supervision of licensed professionals including physicians, registered/vocational nurses, nursing home administrators, and social workers. Other specialists and therapists are involved on an "as needed" basis. In contrast, the type of licensed health care providers working in subacute units is more varied (e.g., orthopedics, pulmonary medicine, cardiology, nephrology, physiatry, speech and respiratory therapy), and there is a higher ratio of licensed provider to nursing assistant care provision (Levenson, 1996). The patients' problems require more than one discipline, and thus successful subacute units rely on organizing their "package" of services efficiently (Levenson, 1999).

Because the lower costs of subacute care are partially derived from time restrictions, the coordination of the multidisciplinary team in meeting the discharge goals in a timely manner is crucial. A systematic approach to how providers interact and communicate their findings to each other and to the patient/family is essential, but individual providers must be "team players"—they should be comfortable with this interdisciplinary approach to care (Weinberg, 2000). Inadequate team functioning and poor communication may result in poor patient outcomes. For example, if a patient frequently interrupts the physical therapy sessions because of urinary urgency but the therapist does not inform the nursing staff of this development, then the patient's urinary tract infection or other urological problem may not be treated in a timely fashion. Similarly, a patient refusing to atttend therapy may have an untreated depression. Communication among the various disciplines is essential. The patient care plan should reflect how the team communicates using electronic/voice messages, facsimile, patient record, patient rounds, or team meetings, as well as the outcomes of this team interaction. A case manager, who is either a nurse or a social worker, usually coordinates the various disciplines to "optimize patient outcomes at the lowest possible cost" (Carr, 2000).

Physician Expertise

Many physicians trained in internal medicine or family/general practice lack formal training in rehabilitation (Marcantonio & Yurkofsky, in press). Thus the inclusion of on-site physicians specializing in physical medicine and rehabilitation (also know as physiatrists) or unit-specific areas (e.g., a pulmonologist for a ventilator unit) as consultants is often needed to promote realistic and obtainable goals. Alternatively, geriatricians with their focus on functional status are also well equipped to provide this needed expertise. Although rare, physicians who work exclusively in subacute units are referred to as "SNFist" or "Subacutist," just as "Intensivist" is the new term for those physicians specializing in intensive care medicine (Marcantonio & Yurkofsky, in press).

Nurse Education and Staffing

Similar to physicians, nurse education rarely includes rehabilitation content or experience in a rehabilitation setting. In rehabilitation subacute care units, the patients may receive between 1 and 3 hours of therapy a day. Nurses and their assistants need to incorporate the principles learned in therapy sessions to the patient's "non-therapy" activities, such as transferring out of bed independently or teaching a patient how to use a cane while walking in the unit hallway.

In the hospital setting, subacute care is viewed as a "step-down" or lower level of care provision while in the nursing home it is a "higher" or more intense level of care. Thus nurses with mostly nursing home experience may not be qualified to administer relatively "high" technology interventions. Likewise, nurses with mostly hospital "medical-surgical" or "critical care" backgrounds may not be familiar with regulations specific to nursing homes such as resident rights (e.g., privacy issues) and documentation requirements (e.g., MDS, RAPS).

CLINICAL ISSUES IN THE SUBACUTE SETTING

Because subacute care is a relatively new setting in health care, there are few research-based outcomes reported in the literature. Most research is concerned with functional outcomes following subacute care. Negative outcomes or complications that may develop in the subacute care setting mirror the problems seen both in acute care of older adults and in nursing home residents. For some of these complications, it is unclear if the problem first developed in the hospital setting, if it reflects the patient's overall poor health status, or if it is the result of care practices in the subacute setting. For example, a study evaluating the nutritional status of 837 patients newly admitted to a subacute facility found that approximately one third were malnourished and another two thirds were at risk for malnutrition (Thomas et al., 2002). Malnutrition at the time of admission predicted a longer length of stay, and rehospitalization was more likely among malnourished patients as compared to well-nourished patients. Although it was unclear if the poor nutritional status reflected poor nutritional care in the hospital or the severity of illness of the subjects, nutritional status is clearly a priority issue in subacute care.

Similarly, in a study of 2158 patients, a high (16%) incidence of delirium was found within 72 hours of admission to a subacute facility from an acute care hospital (Kiely et al., 2003). Again, it was unclear if the delirium began during hospitalization or was the result of the transfer or the patient's medical problems. Nevertheless, the implication to practice is clear—subacute nurses need to effectively assess mental status.

Another mental health problem to carefully assess on admission to subacute care is depression. Depression is associated with increased risk of negative consequences during hospitalization and decreased likelihood of improvement following hospitalization (Covinsky, Fortinsky, Palmer, Kresevic, & Landefeld, 1997). Patients in acute rehabilitation settings with major depression demonstrate significantly lower functional status on discharge compared to those without depression (Diamond, Holroyd, Macciocchi, & Felshenthal, 1995). One study conducted in a subacute care setting found that even minor depression was associated with poor functional recovery (Allen et al., 2004). Thus both cognitive status and affect need to be carefully assessed in subacute patients.

Falls are a common problem in hospital and institutional settings, especially during rehabilitation (Mahoney et al., 2000). One intervention study found that a targeted fall prevention program that included fall risk assessment and awareness, exercise, and use of hip protectors was associated with significantly fewer falls and fall-related injuries when compared to a control group (Haines, Bennell, Osborne, & Hill, 2004). Given the high propensity for falling during patient transfers between settings and also in the convalescent phase of an illness, fall prevention is another important subacute care issue.

Hospital-acquired infection is a significant complication of hospital care and is considered the major pathway for serious infections, such as methicillin-resistant *Staphylococcus aureus* (MRSA), to enter long-term care facilities. A study of one large nursing home facility found that 6.2% of patients were MRSA carriers and that the majority of these patients came from the subacute units (Mendelson et al., 2003). It was assumed that these patients brought the infection from the hospital to the subacute units and eventually to the long-term care unit. Thus nursing homes with subacute units need to be especially vigilant in their infection control practices in order to prevent widespread influx of serious infections.

Since many patients are admitted to a subacute unit following surgery or a stroke, the prevention of deep vein thrombosis is a concern. A multisite study of 36 facilities found that deep vein thrombosis was detected in almost 16% of subacute patients, representing a rela-

tively high incidence of this potentially fatal problem (Bosson et al., 2003). Prophylaxis use varied widely among the facilities, from 20% to 87%, regardless of several risk factors for deep vein thrombosis. Both increased evaluation of patients for deep vein thrombosis and greater use of thromboembolism prophylaxis are important implications for care of high-risk subacute patients.

Risk Management

Although all the clinical problems seen in the nursing home are applicable to the subacute care setting, subacute care differs significantly from traditional nursing home care and thus presents unique risk management considerations. Most of these concerns focus on the facility's ability to provide this unique level of care, including appropriate admission criteria, physician supervision, and staff expertise (Fromhart, 1995).

Admission Criteria. Patients are admitted to subacute care based on their ability to regain their prehospitalization functional abilities such as independent walking, transferring out of a chair, and self-feeding. Effective admission screening of rehabilitation potential is one of the major reasons why the large majority of subacute patients are discharged to the community (Iwanenko, Feidler, & Granger, 1999; Iwanenko, Fiedler, Granger, & Lee, 2001; Levenson, 1999; Likourezos et al., 2002). Because poor cognitive function is strongly associated with potentially poor rehabilitation outcomes, most patients that are admitted to subacute care have higher cognitive function compared to those in a general nursing home unit (Likourezos et al., 2002).

Subacute units should have clear admission criteria, which include obtaining specific hospital discharge or transfer information that is required before admission to the unit (Weinberg, 2000). Information such as "any history of falling, wandering, or abusive, violent, or sexually inappropriate behavior" is necessary for the facility to activate preventive strategies (Weinberg, 2000). One way to ensure that the patient meets the facility's admission criteria is for the admissions coordinator, director of nursing, case manger, or medical director to evaluate the patient in the hospital before discharge to the nursing home (Carr, 2000). Considering the medical acuity of the prospective patients, the medical director should play an active role in evaluating the patient's clinical status and recovery potential (Weinberg, 2000). A meeting with the potential patient and/or family before admission also encourages realistic expectations of the subacute care setting and the patient's prognosis (Carr, 2000; Weinberg, 2000). A tour of the facility should be offered to all prospective patients and their families.

Nursing Care Plan: The Older Patient in Subacute Care

Assessment Data

A 70-year-old male is transferred to a subacute unit following 22 days of hospitalization. He had been found unconscious on a sidewalk, the apparent victim of a hit-and-run accident. Police records indicated he is a day laborer who rents a small room in a boarding house. The patient had numerous abrasions and a deep scalp wound. A femoral fracture required total hip replacement surgery. Physical therapy progressed slowly because of generalized weakness and episodes of delirium that were attributed to alcohol withdrawal. Enteral feedings were required initially to provide adequate nutrition; however, he has now resumed a regular oral diet. Recovery was slowed by pneumonia.

Data on admission to subacute care are as follows: 5 feet, 9 inches; 123 pounds; vital signs within normal limits; oriented times 3; walks slowly with a walker, pauses about every 6 to 8 steps. Surgical wound margins are closed. Scalp wound remains open and requires daily care and dressing changes. Wound bed is pink and free of exudate. The patient says for many years he has been drinking beer every night if he has the money to buy it. He has been alienated from his family for "a long time" because of his alcohol use.

Nursing Diagnosis 1

Delayed surgical recovery related to preexisting malnutrition

Goals/Outcomes

- The patient's wounds will heal completely as evidenced by closed margins and absence of swelling or tenderness.
- The patient's endurance will continue to improve as evidenced by the ability to walk progressively greater distances and to perform hygiene and dressing without tiring.

NOC Suggested Outcomes

Wound Healing: Primary Intention
Wound Healing: Secondary Intention
Endurance

NIC Suggested Interventions (Dochterman & Bulechek, 2004)

Major interventions: Incision Site Care (3440), Wound Care (3660), Nutrition Management (1100), Self-Care Assistance (1800)

- Monitor incision for signs and symptoms of infection.
- Note characteristics of any drainage.
- Monitor the healing process in the incision site.
- Cleanse the area around the incision with an appropriate cleansing solution.
- Change the dressing at appropriate intervals.
- Teach the patient how to care for the incision and the open wound.
- Assist patient to obtain supplies (at discharge).
- Ascertain patient's food preferences.
- Determine, in collaboration with dietitian as appropriate, number of calories and type of nutrition needed to meet nutrition requirements.
- Encourage increased intake of protein, iron, and vitamin C, as appropriate.
- Monitor recorded intake for nutritional content and calories.
- Weigh patient at appropriate intervals.
- Provide appropriate information about nutritional needs and how to meet them.
- Determine patient's ability to meet nutritional needs.
- Assist patient in receiving help from appropriate community nutritional programs, as needed.
- Monitor patient's ability for independent self-care.
- Provide assistance until patient is fully able to assume self-care.
- Encourage patient to perform normal activities of daily living to level of ability.
- Encourage independence, but intervene when patient is unable to perform.

Evaluation Parameters

The patient's incision and scalp wound will be well healed. The patient will be performing daily self-care activities without assistance. The patient will consume required caloric intake and maintain or gain weight. Other specific indicators of outcome achievement include rested appearance, muscle endurance, and energy restored after rest.

Nursing Diagnosis 2

Activity intolerance related to deconditioning secondary to impaired mobility and pneumonia

Goals/Outcomes

- The patient will resume self-care activities without assistance.
- The patient will engage in progressive ambulation without tiring.

NOC Suggested Outcomes

Activity Tolerance
Endurance
Energy Conservation
Self-Care Status
Self-Care: Activities of Daily Living
Self-Care: Instrumental Activities of Daily Living

Nursing Care Plan: The Older Patient in Subacute Care—cont'd

NIC Suggested Interventions (Dochterman & Bulechek, 2004)

Major interventions: Energy Management (0180), Self-Care Assistance: IADLs (1805)

- Determine patient's physical limitations.
- Determine what and how much activity is required to build endurance.
- Monitor patient for evidence of excess physical and emotional fatigue.
- Monitor cardiorespiratory response to activity.
- Monitor/record patient's sleep pattern and number of sleep hours.
- Encourage alternate rest and activity periods.
- Plan activities for periods when the patient has the most energy.
- Assist the patient to establish realistic activity goals.
- Encourage patient to choose activities that gradually build endurance.

Evaluation Parameters

The patient will resume full self-care in ADLs with ease. Patient will tolerate progressive increases in physical activity. Specific indicators that may reflect outcome achievement include the following: pulse rate, respiratory rate, blood pressure, and ease of breathing with activity; walking pace; walking distance; stair climbing tolerance; upper and lower body strength; energy restored after rest; balances activity and rest; adapts activity to energy level; reports adequate endurance for activity. Upon discharge, it will be important that the patient be able to perform household tasks and obtain needed household items, recognize safety needs in the home, and prepare food and fluid for eating.

Nursing Diagnosis 3

Knowledge deficit of self-care, rehabilitation, and substance abuse control

Goals/Outcomes

- Before discharge, the patient will obtain resources to assist with nutrition and rehabilitation.
- The patient will verbalize understanding of the consequences of continued substance abuse.
- The patient will have information about resources to assist with control of substance abuse.

NOC Suggested Outcomes

Knowledge: Health Behavior
Knowledge: Substance Abuse Control
Knowledge: Health Resources

NIC Suggested Interventions (Dochterman & Bulechek, 2004)

Major interventions: Teaching: Individual (5606), Counseling (5240), Mutual Goal Setting (4410), Substance Use Treatment (4510)

- Determine learning needs.
- Appraise the patient's current level of knowledge and understanding of content, educational level, ability to learn specific information.
- Determine the patient's motivation to learn specific information.
- Enhance the patient's readiness to learn as appropriate.
- Set mutual, realistic learning goals with the patient; identify learning objectives to meet those goals.
- Appraise the patient's learning style; select appropriate teaching methods/strategies.
- Instruct the patient when appropriate.
- Evaluate the patient's achievement of learning objectives.
- Select new teaching methods/strategies, if previous ones were ineffective.
- Refer the patient to other specialists/agencies to meet the learning objectives, as appropriate.
- Establish a therapeutic relationship based on trust and respect.
- Demonstrate empathy, warmth, and genuineness.
- Provide factual information as necessary and appropriate.
- Assist patient to identify the problem or situation that is causing the distress.
- Ask patient to identify what he can and cannot do about his situation.
- Identify any differences between patient's view of the situation and the view of the health care team.
- Assist patient to identify strengths, and reinforce these.
- Encourage substitution of undesirable habits with desirable habits.
- Determine patient's need for assistance with IADLs.
- Provide for methods of contacting support and assistance people.
- Determine whether patient's monthly income is sufficient to cover ongoing expenses.
- Refer to community services as needed.
- Determine needs for safety-related changes in the home.
- Identify with patient the goals of care.
- Recognize the patient's value and belief system when establishing goals.
- Avoid imposing personal values on patient during goal setting.
- Assist the patient in examining available resources to meet goals.

Continued

Nursing Care Plan: Older Patient in Subacute Care—cont'd

- Develop a scale of upper and lower levels related to expected outcomes for each goal.
- Identify with patient those factors that contribute to chemical dependency.
- Encourage patient to take control over own behavior.
- Discuss with patient the impact of substance abuse on general health, daily functioning, and relationships.
- Discuss with patient the effect of associations with other users during leisure or work time.
- Assist patient to learn alternate methods of coping with stress or emotional distress.
- Assist patient to select an alternative activity that is incompatible with the substance abused.

- Identify support groups in the community for long-term substance abuse treatment.

Evaluation Parameters

The patient describes how basic self-care can be accomplished. The patient identifies resources to assist with health maintenance and promotion needs and substance abuse control. Other specific indicators of outcome achievement might include the following: descriptions of adverse health effects of substance abuse, benefits of eliminating substance abuse, personal responsibility in managing substance abuse, threats to substance abuse control, actions to prevent substance abuse, actions to prevent and manage relapses in substance abuse.

Box 33-1 Reflections on the Subacute Setting from a Family Perspective

Families often find that when a loved one is the nursing home, it is a turning point in that person's life, which impacts the family as well. The individual is usually placed in this setting after being in the hospital to regain the strength and ability for self-care, so that he or she can hopefully return home. After living through this issue with my own mother and my husband's parents, there are several problems that families have to grapple with. The following questions had to be answered each time we were in this situation, and each time different family members had different ideas about what to do:

- "What does mom or dad really want?"
- "How much time can be devoted to mom or dad?"
- "How much will the solution cost?"

The following is an example of one of my family's experiences:

Linus had cared for his wife Gert at home for 14 years after she suffered a stroke, until she died. He had several years at home by himself until he was diagnosed with lung cancer at the age of 90. He ended up in the subacute setting after one hospitalization. It became apparent that he could not stay by himself, so we had to consider our options. Linus was adamant about staying in the house he'd lived in for over 50 years, where he raised his children and cared for his wife.

Linus needed 24-hour care. For this to work, the family all had to pitch in and help. Deciding how to split up the work and care was a huge challenge, even though everyone wanted to keep him at home. However, reality set in. One daughter lived in Florida, and had a job, so she was limited to short trips home. One brother lived in a small town an hour away, and his wife had recently died of lung cancer. The two sons here worked and there was no on who could devote full time to providing care.

After much discussion, Linus agreed to hire an in-home helper during the day if he could have family members

spend the night. But who would do it? Realizing that this would be a temporary situation, his two sons agreed they could help stay with Linus at night. One of the older grandchildren was able to help out as well. In this way, Linus was able to stay in his home for several months until he became very ill just a week before he died.

Each family has to answer the above questions and decide how they can help older family members. Children want to set up situations that follow their parents' wishes; at the same time, they need to be realistic about what they can do and for how long. The older adult may have the financial ability to hire help or pay for resources, but he or she may not want to spend the money. Families need help identifying what their older relative needs, determining what options are available for providing care, and coming up with a plan for what to do. They also need to know how to monitor the situation and what signs to look for to see if more help is needed.

Gerontological nurses and other health professionals can help by giving families information about who can help and what kind of services are available. Most people don't even understand what is covered by Medicare and what must be paid for by individuals. They may want a referral to a private care manager to help make arrangements, or they may not even know that this service exists. Families appreciate hearing examples of how other people have handled similar situations because they may not have any experiences with these decisions. Supporting families through this process can help ease family tensions and help people avoid guilt and second-guessing regarding these difficult decisions.

Sheila Hoffmeister
Sheila Hoffmeister
Journalist and family member
St. Louis, Missouri

Physician/Other Primary Care Supervision.

Subacute patients require more intensive medical supervision than most nursing home residents; therefore the facility must have adequate physician or other primary care provider (nurse practitioners or physician assistants) coverage of the unit. This means more frequent on-site visits and quick accessibility of staff to physicians by phone, electronic mail, or facsimile. JCAHO accreditation standards require physicians to closely and frequently monitor patients in subacute care settings (JCAHO, 1994). Thus risk of liability can occur if a patient's medical condition worsens and there is documentation that the nursing staff was unable to access a physician or other primary care provider in a timely manner. The medical director is responsible for monitoring the performance of all physicians in responding to any patient's medical needs. Although there are no governmental standards for on-site physician visits, Dr. Andrew Weinberg, Director of Geriatrics and Extended Care Service at the WJB Dorn Veteran's Administration Medical Center, asserts that "weekly visits to each patient would be the lowest acceptable frequency . . . with very stable patients" (Weinberg, 2000, p. 6).

Staffing and Staff Expertise.

Because of the complexity of care provided in the subacute care setting, this part of a nursing home will usually require higher staff to patient ratios compared to other units of a nursing home. A study conducted between 1992 and 1996 of 1471 nursing homes found that nursing homes with a higher percentage of subacute care beds were associated with greater numbers of all types of staff, especially ancillary staff (Yeh, Wan, & Neff-Smith, 2002). Thus nursing homes with staffing problems may increase their liability risk. Furthermore, nursing staff expertise to manage technological interventions is essential. For example, staff in a ventilator unit require substantial orientation and continuing education regarding how to handle emergencies such as accidental dislodgement of a patient's tracheostomy tube (Birdsall & Gutekunst, 1995). Unlike a hospital where a physician, anesthetist, or respiratory therapist is available on-site to reinsert a tube, nurses in a subacute ventilator unit must stabilize the patient until an ambulance arrives (Birdsall & Gutekunst, 1995).

Nursing homes willing to admit patients with highly complex care needs are more likely to have a higher ratio of registered professional nurses to licensed practical/vocational nurses (Yeh et al., 2002). Mary T. Knapp, MSN, RN, Senior Director in the Post Acute Consulting Group at ZA Consulting (www.hipaapros.com/mary.html) and author of *The Definitive Guide to Hospital Based Nursing Facilities*, reports that daily nursing care to patients averages 4.5 to 5.5 direct care hours in subacute units (Knapp, 2001).

SUMMARY

Subacute nursing home care represents a growing trend in health care (Marcantonio & Yurkofsky, in press). The complexity of care provided in these units, compared to typical nursing home care, results in unique clinical care and administrative and risk management issues.

For more on subacute care from a family perspective, see Box 33-1.

REFERENCES

Allen, B. P., Agha, Z., Duthie, E. H., Jr., & Layde, P. M. (2004). Minor depression and rehabilitation outcome for older adults in subacute care. *Journal of Behavioral Health, 31*(2), 189-198.

American Health Care Association. (1998). *Facts and trends: The subacute care sourcebook 1998.* Washington, DC: AHCA. Retrieved from www.ahcabookstore.com. Available online at www.ahca.org/research/subdata.htm.

Banta, M. G., & Richter, T. B. (1993). The future of the nursing home field. *Dean Witter—Facility-Based Long Term Care Industry, 23.*

Berezny, L., & Howells, J. (2000). Rehabilitation service delivery issues in a managed care environment. In M. W. Kelly (Ed.), *Subacute care services: The evolving opportunities and challenges.* Chicago: Irwin Professional Publishing, pp. 149-177.

Birdsall, C., & Gutekunst, M. (1995). Preparing staff for opening of a new ventilator unit in long-term care. *Journal of Gerontological Nursing, 21*(5), 39-43.

Bosson, J. L., Labarere, J., Sevestre, M. A., Belmin, J., Beyssier, L., Elias, A., et al. (2003). Deep vein thrombosis in elderly patients hospitalized in subacute care facilities: A multicenter cross-sectional study of risk factors, prophylaxis, and prevalence. *Archives of Internal Medicine, 163*(21), 2613-2618.

Carr, D. D. (2000). Case management for the subacute patient in a skilled nursing facility. *Nursing Case Management, 5*(2), 83-92.

Chen, C. C., Heinemann, A. W., Granger, C. V., & Linn, R. T. (2002). Functional gains and therapy intensity during subacute rehabilitation: A study of 20 facilities. *Archives of Physical Medicine and Rehabilitation, 83*(11), 1514-1523.

Covinsky, K. E., Fortinsky, R. H., Palmer, R. M., Kresevic, D. M., & Landefeld, C. S. (1997). Relation between symptoms of depression and health status outcomes in acutely ill hospitalized older persons. *Annals of Internal Medicine, 126*(6), 417-425.

Deutsch, A., Fiedler, R. C., Iwanenko, W., Granger, C. V., & Russell, C. F. (2003). The uniform data system for medical rehabilitation report: Patients discharged from subacute rehabilitation programs in 1999. *American Journal of Physical Medicine & Rehabilitation, 82*(9), 703-711.

Diamond, P. T., Holroyd, S., Macciocchi, S. N., & Felshenthal, G. . (1995). Prevalence of depression and outcome on the geriatric rehabilitation unit. *American Journal of Physical Medicine & Rehabilitation, 74*, 214-217.

Dochterman, J. M., & Bulechek, G. M. (2004). *Nursing interventions classification* (4th ed.). St. Louis: Mosby

Fromhart, S. (1995). How have higher-acuity residents affected your operations? *Contemporary Long Term Care, 18*(9), 34.

Haines, T. P., Bennell, K. L., Osborne, R. H., & Hill, K. D. (2004). Effectiveness of targeted falls prevention programme in subacute hospital setting: Randomised controlled trial. *BMJ, 328*(7441), 676.

Hyatt, L. (1993). Subacute care: An important new trend. *Nursing Homes, 7/8*, 9.

Iwanenko, W., Fiedler, R., & Granger, C. (1999). The uniform data system for medical rehabilitation: Report of first admissions to subacute rehabilitation for 1995, 1996 and 1997. *American Journal of Physical Medicine & Rehabilitation, 78*(4), 384-388.

Iwanenko, W., Fiedler, R., Granger, C., & Lee, M. K. (2001). The uniform data system for medical rehabilitation: Report of first admissions to subacute rehabilitation for 1998. *American Journal of Physical Medicine & Rehabilitation, 80*(10), 56-61.

Johnson, M. F., Kramer, A. M., Lin, M. K., Kowalsky, J. C., & Steiner, J. F. (2000). Outcomes of older persons receiving rehabilitation for medical and surgical conditions compared with hip fracture and stroke. *Journal of the American Geriatrics Society, 48*(11), 1389-1397.

Joint Commission on Accreditation of Healthcare Organizations (JCAHO). (1994). *Digest: Subacute care protocol*. Oakbrook Terrace, IL: Author.

Kelly, M. W. (2000). *Subacute care services: The evolving opportunities and challenges*. Chicago: Irwin Professional Publishing.

Kiely, D. K., Bergmann, M. A., Murphy, K. M., Jones, R. N., Orav, E. J., & Marcantonio, E. R. (2003). Delirium among newly admitted postacute facility patients: Prevalence, symptoms, and severity. *Journal of Gerontology: Medical Sciences, 58A*, 441-445.

Knapp, M. T. (1995). *Subacute care: The definitive guide to hospital-based nursing facilities*. Gaithersburg, MD: Aspen.

Knapp, M. T. (2001). Subacute care. In M. D. Mezey (Ed.), *The encyclopedia of elder care*. New York: Springer Publishing, pp. 620-622.

Kramer, A. M., Steiner, J. F., Schlenker, R. E., Eilertsen, T. B., Hrincevich, C. A., Tropea, D. A., et al. (1997). Outcomes and costs after hip fracture and stroke: A comparison of rehabilitation settings. *Journal of the American Medical Association, 277*(1), 396-404.

Levenson, S. A. (1994). Subacute care: Why nursing home practitioners should take notice. *Nursing Home Medicine, 2*(3), 23-24.

Levenson, S. A. (1996). *Subacute and transitional care handbook*. St. Louis: Beverly-Cracin.

Levenson, S. A. (1999). Subacute care: Role and implications for a modernized health care system. In P. Katz, R. Kane, & M. Mezey (Eds.), *Emerging systems in long-term care* (4th ed.). New York: Springer Publishers.

Likourezos, A., Si, M., Kim, W. O., Simmons, S., Frank, J., & Neufeld, R. (2002). Health status and functional status in relationship to nursing home subacute rehabilitation program outcomes. *American Journal of Physical Medicine & Rehabilitation, 81*(5), 373-379.

Mahoney, J. E., Palta, M., Johnson, J., Jalaluddin, M., Gray, S., Park, S., et al. (2000). Temporal association between hospitalization and rate of falls after discharge. *Archives of Internal Medicine, 160*(18), 2788-2795.

Manton, K. G., Woodbury, M. A., Vertrees, J. C., & Stallard, E. (1993). Use of Medicare services before and after introduction of the prospective payment system. *Health Services Research, 28*(3), 269-292.

Marcantonio, E. R., & Yurkofsky, M. Subacute care. In W. Hazzard, J. Blass, , J. Halter, J. G. Ouslander, & M. Tinetti (Eds.), *Principles of geriatric medicine and gerontology* (6th ed.). New York: McGraw-Hill (in press).

Megan, L. A. (2000). Marketing subacute care: Issues in developing a successful marketing program. In M. W. Kelly (Ed.), *Subacute care services: The evolving opportunities and challenges*. Chicago: Irwin Professional, pp. 15-47.

Mendelson, G., Yearmack, Y., Granot, E., Ben-Israel, J., Colodner, R., & Raz, R. (2003). *Staphylococcus aureus* carrier state among elderly residents of a long-term care facility. *Journal of the American Medical Directors Association, 4*(3), 125-127.

Press, S. H. (2000). Financing for subacute facilities. In M. W. Kelly (Ed.), *Subacute care services: The evolving opportunities and challenges*. Chicago: Irwin Professional, pp. 84-92.

Thomas, D. R., Zdrowski, C. D., Wilson, M., Conright, K. C., Lewis, C., Tariq, S., & Morley, J. E. (2002). Malnutrition in subacute care. *American Journal of Clinical Nutrition, 75*, 308-312.

U.S. Department of Health and Human Services, Office of Disability, Aging and Long-Term Care Policy and Lewin-VHI, Inc. (1994, December). Subacute care: Review of literature. Available online at www.aspe.hss.gov/daltcp/reports/scltrves.htm.

Weinberg, A. D. (2000). The medical director's role in screening high-acuity admissions to subacute units. *Annals of Long-Term Care, 8*(2), 1-7.

Willging, P. (1993). New directions in long term care. *Provider, 18*(8), 22-28.

Yeh, S. J., Wan, T., & Neff-Smith, M. (2002). Subacute care in nursing homes. *Journal of Nursing Administration, 32*(7/8), 369-370.

Chapter 34 Long-Term Care

Adrianne Dill Linton § Helen W. Lach

Objectives

Describe the long-term care setting and population characteristics.

Discuss personnel and staffing issues in the long-term care setting.

Explore approaches to care to promote function and quality of care.

Analyze the issue of relocation for nursing home residents.

Describe the processes of care and implications for quality improvement in long-term care settings.

Admission to a long-term care nursing facility is a significant event in the lives of older persons and their families. Although only about 4.5% of the older population resides in a long-term care nursing facility at any one time, it is estimated that more than half of all older persons will be admitted to such a facility at some point in their life (Administration on Aging [AOA], 2004). The individual and family member may anticipate the transition to a nursing facility with both optimism and reluctance. Older persons often prefer to "age in place," that is, to remain in their own familiar and secure environment, even as their ability to safely do so may be questioned. A transition of this magnitude may be feared because of the disruption and uncertainty that this change may bring.

For many, continuing care in a long-term care nursing facility offers security, stability, needed care and services, and safety. In this most challenging setting, nurses have an enormous opportunity to provide creative, innovative care in working with residents, their families, and other health professionals. However, the setting has trouble attracting and retaining qualified staff at all levels. The complexity of the service delivery within the nursing facility organization and the unique needs of the residents demand gerontological nursing leadership and management expertise, as well as clinical expertise. This chapter explores gerontological nursing in the long-term care setting and addresses key issues in promoting quality care and quality of life for the long-term care population.

LONG-TERM CARE SETTING

A nursing home is a type of long-term care facility that offers skilled and basic nursing care on an ongoing basis. A report prepared by the U.S. Senate Special Committee on Aging (2000) described long-term care as differing from other types of health care because the aim is to maintain an optimal level of functioning rather than to achieve a cure. To achieve this aim, long-term care facilities may provide medical, nursing, social, restorative, and personal services in addition to specialized housing for those with some functional impairment or skilled nursing needs. Gerontological nurses have a large role to play in this setting. The following describes the history of the setting before exploring the current state of long-term care.

History of Long-Term Care

The long-term care nursing facility is a health care institution with a rich history of social, demographic, and legislative change. During the nineteenth century, religious orders and benevolent citizens established almshouses and poor farms to care for dependent, chronically ill patients. At the turn of the century, as the number of hospitals grew and hospital stays grew shorter, almshouses and poor farms were gradually replaced by private charitable homes, board and care homes, and rest homes. As medical and technological advances led to prevention of communicable diseases, quicker recovery from illness, and increased survival, the population of older and disabled persons increased, as did the need for institutional long-term care (Elderweb, 2005).

Social changes occurring after World War II introduced trends toward the dissolution of family caregiving networks. Many adult children left their home communities to seek career opportunities in distant locations. As parents aged, fewer family members were available to provide assistance. Friends and community-based services became increasingly important in meeting instrumental and caregiving needs.

A number of legislative initiatives helped establish the nursing home industry as a dominant provider of long-term care. The Social Security Act passed in 1935 created a source of funds that individuals could use to pay for their own health services. Because payment with these funds to public facilities was restricted, the growth of for-profit facilities began. The Medicare and Medicaid amendments to the Social Security Act, which passed in 1965, created payment systems for the elderly and the poor while fostering the growth of long-term care in the private sector. Hospitals concentrated on acute care because they had little incentive to develop long-term services (Tellis-Nayak, 1988). The need for long-term care beds was also affected in the 1960s by the discharge of many older adults with mental illness from institutions, and few community-based alternatives were available. Social changes since the 1960s raised society's awareness of the nontherapeutic conditions under which many residents received care in nursing homes, creating growing consensus about patients' rights and quality of care (Institute of Medicine, 1986). Nursing homes developed during this time were based on a hospital or acute care model.

In the 1980s, additional demand for long-term care resulted from change in Medicare. The prospective payment system was imposed on hospitals, resulting in a higher rate of discharge from the hospital of older persons who were still acutely ill. Reform also continued. The Omnibus Budget Reconciliation Act (OBRA), passed by Congress in 1987, introduced substantial reform in residents' rights, the facility survey process, nurse staffing and training standards, and quality monitoring in the nursing facility. As standards for excellence and quality in long-term care have evolved, innovative long-term care nursing facilities have increasingly developed and implemented models that enrich the quality of life of residents and have the potential to provide a challenging and stimulating practice environment for nurses. The nursing home setting could provide monitoring to prevent acute exacerbations of illness and improve management of chronic diseases, and nurses in long-term care are challenged to provide quality care.

The Contemporary Long-Term Care Nursing Facility

Long-term care nursing facilities today offer continuing care for chronically ill, disabled, and medically frail persons, with a goal of promoting the highest quality of life possible for all residents. Ouslander and Weinberg (2003) formulated medical goals for care in the long-term care setting. Many of these goals are common to all members of the health care team; others that represent the unique contributions of nursing have been added:

- Provide a safe and pleasing environment that supports engagement and independence.
- Ensure that basic physiological, psychological, social, and spiritual needs are met.
- Maintain or improve function.
- Maximize the quality of life.
- Manage symptoms of acute and chronic conditions to prevent complications and promote health.
- Prevent suffering and treat discomfort.
- Prevent excess disability.
- Preserve dignity.
- Encourage autonomy.
- Support the family unit.
- Provide compassionate end-of-life care.

The population characteristics and the service delivery in the long-term care nursing facility create a paradoxical view. For example, the long-term care nursing facility is both a home to many residents and a health care institution offering a number of health services. Many long-term care nursing facilities offer a full range of rehabilitation and specialized services that facilitate discharge to the home, particularly in their subacute care units, described in Chapter 33.

Although the nursing facility is commonly associated with the care of older persons, a small percentage of residents are chronically or terminally ill infants, children, or young adults; patients with acquired immunodeficiency syndrome; and those with spinal cord injuries. The intensity of care is often perceived as long term or nonemergent; however, this setting in fact often resembles acute care with high acuity levels and frequent acute episodic illnesses requiring a variety of nursing and medical resources and various laboratory and diagnostic technologies. Although advanced technologies and health professional resources may not predominate in most nursing facilities, these resources are increasingly available to improve resident care outcomes. Facilities struggle with decisions about when to transfer individuals to acute care facilities and when to treat acute illness themselves. They also struggle with terminal care and when to treat illness or transfer patients to a higher level of care and when to provide comfort care.

The name "nursing facility" or "nursing home" is another paradox in long-term care. Although the primary service in this setting relates to nursing care, few positions are actually filled by professional nurses, and most direct care is provided by certified nursing assistants. This is unfortunate because professional nurses have assessment and care skills that can improve quality of care and quality of life for older long-term care residents. These skills are the focus of this chapter.

Reimbursement for Long-Term Care

Long-term care is expensive, costing $64,000 per year for a semiprivate room, depending on the geographical area where people live (MetLife, 2005). About one third of nursing home care is paid by individuals or their families, with the rest covered by government programs. Many people mistakenly think that Medicare, the government health insurance program for older adults, pays for much nursing home care. In fact, Medicare covers short-term skilled nursing care or rehabilitation; it does not pay for help with basic activities of daily living such as eating, bathing, and dressing. As a result, most nursing home care is paid by individuals or the joint federal-state Medicaid program.

Medicaid provides health insurance and nursing home coverage for the indigent and is means-tested, so it is based on the individual's income and personal assets. In addition, there are usually requirements to ensure that nursing home care is needed. Documentation of the need for nursing home care may require assessment data. Older adults who do not qualify for Medicaid must pay for nursing home care until they "spend down" their personal assets to qualify for coverage. Medicaid pays for about half of all nursing home care and therefore has a large interest in the care provided in this setting.

Medicaid requirements vary from state to state; therefore it is beneficial to clarify details with a social worker or the Medicaid office of the state where the individual resides. Planning how to pay for nursing home care must be handled carefully, and some attorneys specialize in this area. Assets must be used to pay for care if available, and some states penalize individuals for gifting personal assets away instead of spending them down on the needed nursing home care.

Long-term care insurance is a growing method to help cover the high cost of nursing home care. In 2001, somewhere between 3.4 and 4 million people had policies to cover long-term care (Cohen, 2003). These policies are particularly appealing to individuals who want to protect their assets and avoid the need to depend on family for help. In some states, long-term care insurance is tax deductible to encourage participation. Although nursing home care is covered, many policies also provide home care services that may ultimately serve to decrease the time spent in nursing homes. Individuals with insurance may also have more options in choosing a nursing home or in choosing what kind of room they have, such as a private room. Surveys show that people are generally satisfied with their long-term care insurance policies (Cohen, 2003).

Characteristics of Long-Term Care Residents

In 2001, over 1.5 million people lived in nursing homes in the United States (Centers for Disease Control and Prevention [CDC], 2003). By 2020, it is projected that 12 million nursing home beds will be needed. A study by the U.S. Department of Health and Human Services predicts that people who reach age 65 will have a 40% chance of entering a nursing home with about 10% of those residing there for 5 or more years (Medicare, 2005, 2006).

Long-term nursing home residents are primarily women over age 80 who have dementia and functional deficits (AOA, 2004). In addition, the majority are white (90%), with only a small percentage of African Americans, Hispanics, and other ethnic groups. Ouslander and Weinberg (2003) categorize nursing home residents into three groups based on their types of impairments:

- Residents with cognitive impairment
- Residents with impaired physical functioning
- Residents with both physical and cognitive impairments

Nursing homes may choose to provide care for these three groups in different geographical locations because they may require different kinds of care.

Physical impairments are typically the result of several comorbid chronic medical conditions that complicate the care of the older adult in long-term care. Stroke, severe chronic heart disease, osteoarthritis, diabetes, and chronic obstructive pulmonary disease are just some of the most common conditions in this population. Other common problems are falls, pain, urinary incontinence, pressure sores, constipation, immobility, nutrition, and dehydration. Infections are the leading cause of death and hospitalization for nursing home residents (Sloane & Boustani, 2002). Common sites of serious infections are the respiratory and urinary tracts. Because of the high number of chronic conditions, residents are often on complex medication regimens. Each year, approximately 10% of nursing home residents have to be transferred to a hospital for acute care (Sloane et al., 2005).

Dementia, a common diagnosis in residents of long-term care, often precipitates nursing home placement. Studies suggest that over half of nursing home residents have dementia (Zimmerman, et al., 2003). Many residents with physical problems also have dementia. The changes in memory and thinking associated with dementia are usually moderate to severe by the time the older adult moves to the long-term care setting. Therefore such individuals often require assistance with activities of daily living. In addition, behavioral problems may occur when the disease is at the point where the residents cannot understand situations and explanations, or make appropriate decisions even about simple tasks. As a result, most long-term residents with dementia require skillful and patient care.

Mental health problems are also prevalent in the long-term care setting. Frequently concomitant to dementia, depression has been reported in as many as 30% of older residents, with some depressive symptoms being reported by additional older individuals (Gruber-Baldini et al., 2005). Often, depression is not diagnosed and may not be adequately treated (Brown, Lapane, & Luisi, 2002).

Residents often spend their last days in the nursing home, so end-of-life care is an important component of the setting (Forbes-Thompson & Gessert, 2005). Families and staff struggle with issues such as weight loss, dehydration, pain management, and treatment decisions. Optimal end-of-life care is not the norm. Staffing issues, lack of education, and other problems contribute to a lack of adequate care (Kayser-Jones et al., 2003).

According to the AOA (2004), the proportion of the older population receiving long-term care has declined, but the level of disability and cognitive impairment among those in long-term care has risen sharply. Among U.S. nursing home residents who are age 65 and older, 80.3% are dependent for mobility; 65.7% are incontinent; 47.3% are dependent for eating; and 36.9% are dependent for mobility and eating, in addition to being incontinent (CDC, 2003). Several risk factors are consistently associated with nursing home placement: age, cognitive impairment, functional dependence, and medical burden (Bharucha, Pandav, Shen, Dodge, & Ganguli, 2004). Studies show that 31% of those age 65 to 70 receive care in a nursing home compared with 61% of those 85 years and older (Gabriel, 2000). Dementia has been documented as the most potent predictor of placement, increasing the risk of nursing home placement by nearly 6 times (Bharucha et al., 2004). Medical problems tend to be more significant for people without cognitive impairment.

The characteristics of nursing home residents make them an interesting and challenging group that requires a high degree of gerontological nursing skill to manage appropriately. However, financial and regulatory issues may prevent adequate staffing to ensure quality care. We next explore the nursing and other personnel in the long-term care setting and their roles.

STAFF IN NURSING HOMES

A variety of professionals play an important role in the lives of long-term care residents. Health problems of nursing facility residents require complex systems of care that involve numerous services and therapies that cut across professional domains. Health professionals can include nurses, physicians, physical and occupational therapists, speech therapists, dietitians, activity direc-

tors, pharmacists, and many more. Of paramount importance is that all the disciplines work together and see themselves as part of a unified team that provides care to the residents; no single member's approach should be considered in isolation from that of other disciplines. Box 34-1 describes the experiences of a gerontological nurse practitioner in working with all of the staff in nursing facilities to address a common health issue: dehydration. The following section describes the roles of various professionals in the nursing facility.

Nursing Staff

Nurse staffing in the long-term care facility can be viewed as a pyramid structure, with licensed nursing staff such as registered nurses (RNs) and licensed practical nurses (LPNs) at the top of the pyramid, denoting their lesser number, and certified nursing assistants (CNAs) forming the base of the pyramid, denoting their greater number. The adequacy of nursing staff directly affects quality of care for residents and is the subject of much current debate.

Labor costs account for approximately 60% of costs in the nursing facility. The current federal standards for nurse staffing require the following (Harrington, 2005):

- A licensed nurse must be on duty for 8 consecutive hours each day, 7 days a week, and at least 8 hours must be provided by an RN.
- The director of nursing must be an RN.
- The director of nursing may also serve as charge nurse in facilities with no more than 60 residents.
- Staff levels must be sufficient to provide adequate care to residents (there are no federal standards for nursing assistants).

RN requirements may be waived if recruiting is a problem, as often occurs as a result of low salaries offered in long-term care. Beyond federal regulations, minimum staffing standards are defined by each state, and are in part driven by the cost of long-term care borne by each state through the Medicaid program. Staffing levels are evaluated as part of each state's survey process.

CNAs have the most frequent contact with residents and provide the majority of care. According to the most recent National Nursing Home Survey (CDC/National Center for Health Statistics, 1999), for every 100 nursing home beds, there were 32.9 CNAs, 7.6 RNs, and 10.6 LPNs. These figures varied among regions of the United States. The highest numbers of RNs and CNAs per 100 beds was in the Northeast. The South had the lowest number of RNs, but the highest number of LPNs. The Midwest had the lowest numbers of LPNs and CNAs. Differences also were noted in terms of affiliation; independent nursing homes had higher rates of all levels of nurses than chain nursing homes. Increasing patient

Box 34-1 *Reflections on Collaborating in the Long-Term Care Setting to Prevent Dehydration*

"He's been restless all night, calling out for help," the nurse told me. "I gave him a pain pill and something for anxiety, but he just won't settle down." She was referring to a 92-year-old nursing home resident who had recently been admitted to a hospice program because of end-stage cardiomyopathy and congestive heart failure.

His feeble cries for help grew louder as I approached. His legs were edematous, his abdomen swollen with ascites, and his respirations—despite the oxygen—appeared labored. "Howard, what can I do to help you?" I asked. "Help me. Please help me," he responded. His lips were cracked and his tongue parched. I got a glass of water and, putting his recliner upright, I offered him the straw. He drank quickly and steadily until the glass was empty. I refilled it and offered him another drink. Again he consumed the full glass. After the third glass of water, he looked at me and said, "Thank you." Shortly thereafter, he fell asleep.

Ensuring adequate fluid intake in the long-term care setting is a challenging undertaking. Dehydration is the most common fluid and electrolyte disturbance in older adults. A decrease in thirst perception and reduced response to serum osmolality (hypodipsia), as well as decreased ability to concentrate urine following fluid deprivation, occurs even in healthy aging.

Many disease processes affecting the mental or physical capabilities of older adults reduce access to fluids and reduce the ability to recognize or express thirst, as in this resident's situation. With such a large concentration of physically and mentally disabled people, long-term care residents are by far the most vulnerable to experience fluid deprivation.

Vigilance on the part of nursing home staff is necessary to recognize and respond to situations that can contribute to dehydration. A history of decreased food or fluid intake, febrile illness, vomiting, diarrhea, use of diuretic agents, or the presence of chronic renal disease or a known infection should alert the nurse to the possibility of dehydration. When these variables are present, closer monitoring and attention to fluid administration are necessary.

Volume depletion and dehydration manifest in a variety of ways, including altered mental status, lethargy, light-headedness, and syncope. On physical examination, decreased skin turgor, dry mucous membranes, tachycardia, and orthostatic hypotension provide further support for the clinical diagnosis, but these findings may be present in elderly individuals whose hydration status is normal.

Dehydration can be prevented if a comprehensive hydration program is in place. An effective hydration program in the long-term care setting requires the efforts of all staff, including administrators, ancillary staff, and caregivers. This is one area where a team approach is truly mandatory for goals to be realized. Successful hydration programs in facilities where I have practiced have all involved collaborative strategies.

In one facility, the administration completely eliminated water pitchers, because few of the residents are able to pour themselves a drink. Instead, disposable cups of water with lids and straws are handed to the residents on a four-times-daily schedule between meals. Wheelchairs and walkers have cup holders attached to keep fluids portable as they traverse to therapies and other activities.

The activity therapy department can play a vital role in the hydration program by incorporating drinks into all activity sessions. We have found that unit-based activity programs are the most conducive to supporting a hydration program. This approach allows nursing staff on the unit to assist the activity therapist with fluid administration and make modifications for those who require fluid consistency adjustments.

The cocktail hour is a popular time to focus attention on drinking, whether or not alcohol is served. Sparkling beverages in clear glass stemware, with fruit garnishes, can be served in place of alcohol for residents who enjoy the social ritual. An attractive presentation tends to induce more fluid consumption, as it does with food.

Part of the bedtime routine in our facility centers around fluid consumption. The certified nursing assistants are responsible for dispensing the evening "nightcap" of hot cocoa, cider, or our popular nonalcoholic apricot "cognac." This activity generally takes place in the lounge where a movie can be shown or music played to establish a relaxing atmosphere before bedtime.

Because fluid consumption during exercise is important, another hydration program includes fluid distribution whenever a resident participates in an exercise activity. Physical therapists, occupational therapists, and restorative therapists are required to administer fluids during their one-on-one sessions with residents and must document the volume of fluid consumed in the progress note. A refrigerator with beverages and a cold water dispenser made available in the rehabilitation or workout rooms facilitates hydration for more functional residents who choose to "work out."

Timing the introduction of fluids at mealtime is also an effective strategy. Fluids are the first items served at mealtime, including water, juices, soups, teas, palate-cleansing sorbets, and Jell-O. Once these are consumed, the dietary staff proceed with serving salads and the main entrée.

The housekeeping department supports our hydration program by making certain that each nursing division has an ample supply of disposable cups, lids, and straws. Even the maintenance department is involved in supporting the hydration program because it is responsible for installing and maintaining the cup holders on all walkers and wheelchairs. The medical director and nurse practitioner round out the hydration team, by taking the "pop cart" along when making rounds and offering drinks to residents after they have been examined.

Each department's involvement in the hydration program is crucial to ensuring an effective outcome. Defining the role that each staff member plays in providing for the fluid needs of the residents is the key ingredient to preventing dehydration in the long-term care setting.

Kathryn A. Houston

Katherine A. Houston, GNP
Private Practice
St. Louis, Missouri

care acuity levels of residents, combined with a therapeutic focus in care mandated by OBRA regulations, has fostered renewed attention on the role of the RN. The following describes the roles of each type of nursing personnel.

Licensed Professional Nurses

Professional nurses in nursing homes consist of three groups: administrative nurses (nurse administrators and directors of nursing), staff nurses (RNs and LPNs), and nurses with advanced clinical preparation in the care of older adults, including nurse practitioners and clinical nurse specialists. The RN has increased authority and autonomy in the coordination of resident care from assessment, intervention, and evaluation to ongoing quality monitoring of resident outcomes.

Registered nurses have responsibility for resident assessment and care planning, supervising and evaluating the implementation of resident care plans, supervising and directing the care given by nursing assistants, and administering direct care, treatments, medications, and other procedures. Both RNs and LPNs can serve in charge nurse roles. Nurses in the nursing facility not only assume major responsibility for the residents' health care but also function as unit managers with day-to-day responsibility for management of staff issues. LPNs fulfill a wider range of resident care and managerial responsibilities in the nursing facility than in other settings of care. Therefore, management and leadership skills are as critical as clinical expertise to ensuring quality care.

Staffing levels have been related to quality of care in nursing homes. Among the factors associated with insufficient nursing staff and inadequately trained staff are poor resident feeding, inadequate nutritional intake, hospitalization, malnutrition, and dehydration (Harrington, 2005). A study of California nursing homes found that the minimum threshold at which quality of care improved was 4.1 total nursing staff hours for each resident per day. However, the average number of minutes of care provided by nursing staff to each resident was 42 minutes per day in 2001 (Rosenfeld & Harrington, 2003). Another California study reported that the nursing homes with the greatest number of nursing staff had resident care loads of 7.6 residents per nursing assistant. Other homes reported resident care loads of 9 to 10. Homes with lower resident care loads performed significantly better on 13 of 16 measures of quality of care (Schnelle et al., 2004).

Hours per resident day (HPRD) is a figure used to quantify the availability of staff to provide care for each resident. See Table 34-1 for recommended staffing levels from various agencies and experts. Research shows that staffing varies widely among nursing facilities and among different states, despite regulations (Mueller et

al., 2006). Although states with higher staffing standards are associated with higher staffing levels, low standards have little effect, and may result in lower staffing. The low number of budgeted RN positions in the long-term care nursing facility continues to be a concern, particularly in light of increasing resident care acuity levels and complexity of care and treatment.

The commonly cited barrier to increasing nursing staff is economic. However, the cost of increased staff must be weighed against the cost of negative outcomes related to inadequate staffing. A national study of staffing ratios and frail residents at risk for urinary tract infection, decubitus ulcer, and hospitalization demonstrated an annual net savings of $3191 per resident in facilities with sufficient staff to provide 30 to 40 minutes of RN direct care time per resident per day (compared with facilities in which staffing allowed less than 10 minutes of RN direct care per resident per day) (Dorr, Horn, & Smout, 2005).

A challenge for nursing homes is recruitment and retention of good nursing staff. Nursing staff turnover in

Table 34-1 *Recommended Nursing Home Staffing Standards*

Source	Recommendations
U.S. Centers for Medicare and Medicaid Services (CMS)	Did not recommend a specific federal minimum staffing standard, but reported that facilities with less than 0.75 RN HPRD, 0.55 LVN/LPN HPRD, and 2.8 NA HPRD placed residents in jeopardy.
Institute of Medicine Reports	24 hour/day RN care and increased levels of total nurse staffing to be adjusted based on resident case mix. CMS should institute minimum standards.
Hartford Institute for Geriatric Nursing Expert Panel	RN as director of nursing, assistant director of nursing for facilities with more than 100 beds, RN supervisor on duty at all times, full-time RN director of in-service education. Ratio of direct caregivers to residents—1:5 on day shift; 1:10 on evening shift; 1:15 on night shift. Increased staffing for residents with higher needs. Minimum of 4.44 HPRD total nursing time.

HPRD, Hours per resident day; *LVN/LPN,* licensed vocational nurse/licensed practical nurse; *NA,* nursing assistant; *RN,* registered nurse.

nursing homes is a significant problem. The nursing home industry has one of the highest turnover rates in the health care field. In addition to adverse effects on residents, turnover has a negative impact on staff morale, task efficiency, and satisfaction. Studies of turnover have measured numerous variables, including staff characteristics (age, education, sex, ethnicity, attitudes, knowledge about older people), facility characteristics (ownership, physical environment, staff patterns, turnover and absenteeism, salary and benefits, management patterns), and resident characteristics (age, acuity, functional impairments).

Nursing facilities with low turnover rates demonstrate attributes of a moral and cultural environment that is committed to service and caring. Caring for and about employees is as important as caring for residents. In outstanding nursing facilities, a pervasive philosophy based on mutual respect, trust, expectations, pride, and recognition for the employees' work is communicated to the employees. There is open two-way communication and commitment to solving problems as a team. In addition to a positive organizational culture, specific rewards to motivate staff, including job mobility, educational advancement, and good salary and benefits, can be effective in increasing staff retention (Cocco, Gatti, deMendonca Lima, & Camus, 2003). The work environment can be designed to reduce excess stress by means such as staff support, promoting teamwork, offering stress reduction activities, and workload management (Kennedy, 2005).

Certified Nursing Assistants

Certified nursing assistants (CNAs) provide 80% to 90% of care delivered to nursing home residents (Pennington, Scott, & Magilvy, 2003). The primary focus of CNAs is direct care related to bathing, toileting, feeding, and other activities of daily living, although they may also help maintain the patient care environment. A minimal level of training is required for certification (only about 75 hours), which was mandated by the Nursing Home Reform Act of 1987. CNAs must pass a written and performance-based examination, and participate in continuing education to maintain certification. Some states train CNAs to administer routine oral medications; these personnel are called certified medication aides. Little is known about the safety of using medication aides, but preliminary reports suggest that their use does not compromise patient safety (Nelson, 2005).

CNAs provide care under the supervision of professional nurses. Wages are typically low, but above minimum wage, and CNAs may not have health insurance benefits, or they may be too expensive for CNAs to afford. CNAs are vital members of the nursing care team, but turnover for them is also high, with some facility turnover rates as high as 400% per year. Many factors

are related to the high levels of CNA turnover (Mitty, 1997, 2000), including the following:

- Poor wages and benefits
- Inadequate preparation for the role
- Poor management (i.e., frequently changing assignments, inadequate supplies, inadequate input into care, poor policies and rules, supervisors who do not listen)
- Racial bias
- Difficult or heavy care patients
- Inadequate staffing

Injuries may also be a factor in CNA retention, and the Occupational Safety and Health Administration has developed voluntary ergonomic guidelines to reduce injuries in this high-risk group (Clinical Rounds, 2003). Responding to a survey (Metcalf, 2002), CNAs in North Carolina reported a need for more training for the skills they needed. The two most important factors related to job satisfaction were "ability to work as a team" and the "number of residents I care for each day." Strategies to improve CNA training and retention could significantly affect the quality of care provided. Barry (2002) described nurse aide empowerment strategies that had a positive effect on CNA turnover. Nursing homes with supportive charge nurses who delegated to CNAs had lower CNA turnover rates, whereas homes that offered more rewards had higher turnover rates.

Interviews of CNAs in another study found the following issues to be important to them: job enrichment opportunities, personal growth opportunities, recognition, responsibility, and sense of achievement (Pennington et al., 2003). Mather and Bakas (2002) found that perceptions of CNAs provided important information for developing continence care programs. When rewards were given to CNAs in another study, homes experienced a lower incidence of pressure ulcers, and when CNAs were involved in care decisions, homes had better social environments (Barry, Brannon, & Mor, 2005). Nursing homes that address these needs may not only improve retention of CNAs, but improve resident outcomes as well.

Nursing Administrators

Nurse administrators and directors of nursing form the core of administrative personnel in the nursing facility, retaining 24-hour accountability for residents and staff, in contrast to acute care, in which managerial and clinical responsibilities are shared by a bureaucracy of nursing, medical, and administrative staff. Larger nursing facilities may have additional nursing positions for an assistant director of nursing, staff development, and quality improvement personnel. In many facilities, these responsibilities are carried out by the same person, but in smaller facilities, the director of nursing may also be responsible for these duties. Roles and responsibilities of the nurse administrator and director of nursing have been described to broadly encompass the following (Lodge, 1987; Mueller, 1998):

- Organizational management: establish goals, policies, procedures, budget, and quality assurance
- Human resources management: recruiting and retaining staff, scheduling, and creating work climate
- Management of nursing and health services: developing philosophy, goals, and objectives for nursing; implementing and evaluating nursing; and ensuring residents' rights
- Addressing regulations
- Professional nursing and long-term care leadership: creating linkages with community resources, affecting public policy, and continuing professional growth

Nursing administrators and directors influence the quality of life of institutionalized older persons, and directors with more experience tend to show better resident outcomes (Anderson, Issel, & McDaniel, 2003). In spite of this, administrative positions experience as much turnover as other staff positions. The scope of influence and authority of this position significantly affects the quality and the effectiveness of the work environment and organizational climate, which is dependent on knowledgeable, effective nursing leaders.

Box 34-2 lists the roles, responsibilities, and qualifications of nurse administrators/directors of nursing in long-term care.

Advanced Practice Nurses

Gerontological nurse practitioners (GNPs) are increasingly practicing in long-term care facilities, often in collaborative practices with medical providers. Their preparation makes them especially qualified to work closely with patients and their families to educate them across the long-term care experience and to promote successful health maintenance, chronic care management, and end-of-life care. A chronic care management model encompasses preparation of the patient to participate actively in setting health goals and patient education on self-reliance and self-management of the chronic illness. At end of life, GNPs can provide important resident and family services, including symptom management, advanced care planning, counseling, and coordination of care (Henderson, 2004). Among the key factors that GNPs identify that keep them in long-term care are appreciation from patients and families, and primary care responsibility (Karlin, Schneider, & Pepper, 2002). The following were identified as deterrents to attracting clinically competent nurses to long-term care: lack of appropriate staffing, peers holding negative image, public image of long-term care, and lack of money.

Early studies suggested that nurse practitioners are cost-effective providers and have a positive impact on quality indicators, such as reducing hospitalization and improving functional status in residents (Kane et al., 1989, 1991). Evidence of the value of nurse practitioners

(NPs) in long-term care facilities is growing. Out of 870 respondents to a survey of members of the American Medical Directors Association, 63% reported NP involvement in care of residents in their facilities (Rosenfeld, Kobayashi, Barber, & Mezey, 2004). These NPs were reported to evaluate residents for acute problems, make required regulatory visits, and provide preventive care, hospice care, and wound care. The medical directors specifically noted the effectiveness of NPs in maintaining physician, resident, and family satisfaction.

Krichbaum, Pearson, Savik, and Mueller (2005) demonstrated improvements in resident incontinence, pressure ulcers, and aggression when gerontological advanced practice nurses provided direct care and taught staff protocols to manage specific resident problems. In a subsequent study, these investigators demonstrated significant improvement in resident depression after the GNPs implemented organization-level interventions, including staff collaboration and membership on the facility quality assurance committee.

Medical Director

The medical director is a licensed physician who helps coordinate care and provide clinical guidance and oversight of resident care (CMS, 2005). The director is ideally board certified in geriatrics. The position of medical director was created in the 1970s as a means of improving physician participation and improving the medical care in the nursing facility. Since then, federal regulations have required all nursing facilities to have a medical director (Elon, 1993). Medical directors have both administrative and clinical responsibilities. In general, the medical director assists the nursing home administration to conduct the following activities:

- Develop and revise policies and standards
- Address medical and clinical concerns
- Communicate with attending physicians about policies, standards, and patient problems
- Assist with in-service training
- Arrange for medical coverage when necessary
- Help ensure that emergency care is available
- Help identify and correct problems in quality of care by serving on committees (utilization review, quality assurance, infection control)
- Carry a caseload of residents for whom they are the primary physicians

Employee health activities, such as preemployment screening and annual physical examinations, may also be responsibilities of the medical director. Participation in nursing home processes by the medical director may be limited by the level of reimbursement currently available for such activities, but surveyors are increasingly directed to determine whether medical directors are actively involved in facility oversight (Elon, 2005). In some cases, physicians serve as medical directors for several nursing homes and spend little time at each, or else

BOX 34-2 Statement of Roles, Responsibilities, and Qualifications of Nurse Administrators/Directors of Nursing in Long-Term Care

Assumptions
- Long-term care is where professional nursing will have a major impact.
- The health care delivery system of the future will be different from the present system.
- The aging population is increasing and requires additional and different kinds of health care services.
- The national movement toward self-care and personal responsibility for health has direct implications for nursing services.
- Better educated, more articulate consumers have higher expectations of the quality of nursing services they will receive.
- Changing family structures and relationships influence nursing services for the elderly.
- The frail elderly population increasingly makes up a greater percentage of institutionalized persons and requires more complex nursing care.
- The nurse administrators/directors of nursing are responsible for the management and improvement of nursing care delivery.
- The compensations of nurse administrators/directors of nursing will be commensurate with their role, responsibilities, and qualifications.
- The complexity of the role requires that the nurse administrators/directors of nursing place increased emphasis on administrative responsibilities.
- There is a common core of knowledge for nurse administrators/directors of nursing.
- Knowledge about aging is also essential for the nurse administrator/director of nursing in long-term care.
- The standards developed by nursing organizations as they relate to nursing administration are criteria for quality nursing services and education.
- Increasing competition in the health care industry requires a marketing orientation by nurse administrators/directors of nursing.
- Cost containment is and will continue to be a major issue in health care.
- Quality long-term care requires collaboration among individuals and professional organizations.

Roles and Responsibilities
The nurse administrator in long-term care has four major roles with related responsibilities: organizational management (member of management team), human resources management, nursing/health services management, and professional nursing and long-term care leadership.

Organizational Management
As a member of the management team, the nurse administrator/director of nursing in long-term care
- Serves as a member of the executive staff of the organization and develops effective working relationships with the chief executive officer and the medical director
- Participates in development of institutional policies
- Shares in development of long-range plans for the institution
- Participates in development and administration of an evaluation plan for the institution based on institutional goals and objectives and on nursing standards
- Works in establishing and facilitating effective employer-employee relations
- Minimizes legal risks
- Participates in establishing and maintaining management information systems to facilitate administration of the institution's nursing department
- Designs and implements organizational structure for the nursing department
- Formulates and administers policies and procedures for the nursing department
- Implements federal, state, and local regulations pertaining to nursing service
- Develops long-range plans for the nursing department
- Formulates and administers the departmental budget based on nursing department goals and projected revenue
- Participates in establishing a competitive wage, salary, and benefit plan for nursing services staff
- Operates the department in a cost-effective manner
- Designs and implements a quality assurance program for nursing care
- Formulates and administers an evaluation plan for nursing services in relation to the department's established goals, objectives, and standards
- Raises consciousness, educates, and participates in formulating policy relative to bioethical issues
- Initiates research projects that address problems and issues specific to the nursing department

From Lodge, M. P. (1987). *Professional education and practice of nurse administrators/directors of nursing in long-term care. Executive summary.* Kansas City, MO: American Nurses' Foundation.

Continued

BOX 34-2 Statement of Roles, Responsibilities, and Qualifications of Nurse Administrators/Directors of Nursing in Long-Term Care—cont'd

Human Resources Management in Nursing
As the person responsible for nursing personnel, the nurse administrator/director of nursing in long-term care
■ Recruits, selects, and retains qualified nursing staff
■ Develops and implements a master staffing plan based on patient needs and nursing service goals and standards
■ Initiates and approves position descriptions for nursing personnel
■ Promotes a scheduling system that balances employee and patient needs
■ Formulates, implements, and evaluates a departmental plan for orientation and staff development
■ Assists individual staff members in development of career plans
■ Designs and implements a performance appraisal system for nursing
■ Promotes resolution of conflicts
■ Promotes and implements personnel policies
■ Creates a work climate that promotes a high-quality work life

Nursing/Health Service Management
As the person ultimately responsible for the quality of nursing care, the nurse administrator/director of nursing in long-term care
■ Develops philosophy, goals, and objectives for the department of nursing
■ Assesses the implementation of effective strategies and methods for delivery of nursing services
■ Implements actions to meet and maintain nursing care standards
■ Cooperates in developing and implementing a process for an interdisciplinary approach to health care services
■ Facilitates creative use of community resources
■ Ensures that patients' rights are protected
■ Encourages independence of patients through use of self-care and rehabilitation concepts
■ Initiates formal or informal testing of nursing interventions
■ Evaluates the organization of nursing care
■ Evaluates plans of nursing care

Professional Nursing and Long-Term Care Leadership
As the professional nurse and leader in long-term care, the nurse administrator/director of nursing in long-term care
■ Plans for future health and nursing care actions based on social, economic, political, and technological changes
■ Promotes changes in community health care systems based on social, economic, political, and technological changes
■ Encourages innovative methods for delivery of long-term care
■ Encourages entrepreneurial activities associated with development of nursing models for health care delivery focusing on health promotion, health education, and direct services
■ Establishes linkages with existing community resources
■ Influences public policy affecting long-term care and nursing
■ Establishes relationships with colleges and universities to promote formal educational opportunities for nursing staff, faculty practice, student learning experiences, and research
■ Promotes a positive image of long-term care and long-term care institutions
■ Seeks opportunities for personal and professional growth
  In addition, curriculum implications for each role and responsibility were suggested for graduate programs in nursing.
  The following qualifications were recommended for the nurse administrator in long-term care:
■ 1982: baccalaureate in nursing
■ 1992: master's degree in nursing with specialized preparation in administration; experience in nursing practice required, with middle-management and long-term care nursing experience desirable
■ Certification in nursing administration for long-term care highly desirable

---

they serve in name only, having little impact on care. The American Medical Directors Association (AMDA) offers certification, training, clinical practice guidelines, and resources for medical directors, as well as others interested in long-term care.

Social Worker

A full-time social worker is required in Medicare-approved nursing facilities with more than 120 beds. The social worker is often involved in the admission process to ascertain admission status and financial arrangements and to help families resolve considerations associated with the resident's transition to the nursing facility. The social worker is also involved in obtaining the social history and in participating in the comprehensive care plan. Social workers interact with residents and families to facilitate admission to the nursing facility, as well as to help plan discharge activities and coordinate the use of community resources. Social workers may also conduct group activities as part of the activities program in addition to conducting one-on-one counseling sessions. Smaller homes may not have a social worked or may have only part-time social work involvement.

Dietitian

The registered dietitian assesses, supervises, and evaluates the diets provided to residents. Residents receiving special diets should be provided with tasteful food choices that are consistent with specified dietary guidelines. On a regular basis, residents are assessed, using nutritional indicators to determine the adequacy of nutritional intake and to ascertain any changing needs that may warrant a change in diet. Monthly weight, food intake patterns, and other nutritional data, such as laboratory values for glucose, albumin, and protein levels, are evaluated.

Abnormal changes in weight and intake patterns trigger in-depth assessment and follow-up. Registered dietitians must be very creative in providing tasteful food choices to large numbers of residents with widely varying food preferences. The dietary department can be extremely helpful in the implementation of programs that address fluids for residents prone to dehydration, fiber supplementation for residents with chronic constipation, and restorative feeding programs in residents advancing from tube feeding to a pureed or semisolid diet.

Pharmacist

Pharmacy services are typically outsourced by nursing homes today, and a number of national companies provide much of the distribution of medications for the nursing home industry. Pharmacists, often provided by the pharmacy companies, have an active role in monitoring medication regimens to assist in reducing polypharmacy, drug-drug interactions, adverse side effects, suboptimal dosage, and long-term complications. Regulations provide for at least a quarterly review of each resident's medications to evaluate efficacy and document any problems the resident may be experiencing as a result of the medication regimen. For some medications, such as psychotropic drugs, adverse signs and symptoms related to the drug are documented on a flow sheet and reviewed by the pharmacist. Based on periodic medication review, recommendations for changes

in the drug, dosage, and schedule may be made, as may suggestions for a drug holiday or discontinuation of drug therapy.

Speech Therapist

Speech therapists are increasingly involved in long-term care to assist in evaluation and treatment of speech, language, and swallowing problems. These problems are common given the neurological, respiratory, and other chronic problems experienced by this population. Speech therapists can provide assistance in evaluating eating and swallowing problems and oversight of restorative dining programs for residents. They may also complete swallowing studies and make recommendations regarding the thickness of liquids needed to promote oral hydration and feeding.

Recreational Therapy

Most nursing homes have an activities director or a recreational therapist who oversees therapeutic and recreational activities for nursing home residents. While boredom is a major issue in the nursing home setting, many facilities provide recreational services and activities to improve health and well-being. Therapeutic recreation is provided by professionals who are trained and certified, registered, or licensed to provide therapeutic recreation (American Therapeutic Recreation Association, 2005). Long-term care facilities are responsible for providing a schedule of daily activities that foster an environment that is interesting, stimulating, and meaningful. An active volunteer force is helpful in providing for programs that occur in groups as well as singly. General group activities may include current events discussions, organized singing, cards and games, book clubs or book readings, ice cream socials, and religious services. Pet therapy, music therapy, art therapy, exercise, and horticulture therapy are among the more specialized activity programs. In addition to social activities, the activities director may facilitate meetings of the residents' councils or resident clubs.

Family

Family members continue to experience stress after placing a loved one in a nursing facility (Hagen, 2001), and sometimes concerns over care cause increased stress. Placement results in new roles that families have to negotiate with the nursing staff. Many times family members want to continue to be involved in care and have helpful information, but may not be included in the patient care team, resulting in conflicts with staff (Maas et al., 2001). Family members should be considered an important part of the team. Use of a structured intervention using a written agreement between family and staff members has been shown to improve family perceptions of care and staff perceptions of families (Maas et al., 2004).

Nursing Home Administrators

Administrators in nursing homes are required to have a license and complete continuing education. Although they do not provide direct care, they have influence over the budget and therefore the resources of the facility. They are responsible for hiring other administrative staff, who also report to them, so their influence is felt through others. As the manager, they can also influence the facility culture. Like other nursing home staff, administrators have a high turnover rate of 43% (Castle, 2001a), and turnover of administrators is associated with quality of care (Box 34-3).

GENERAL APPROACHES TO LONG-TERM CARE

For decades the nursing home industry has battled the image of their facilities as warehouses that provide marginal care. Modern, well-run nursing homes strive to provide social and physical environments that are therapeutic and homelike. The dynamic interaction between the individual and the environment (physical and social) is a powerful influence that can foster independence and competence, as well as create and perpetuate unnecessary dependency.

Functional decline of residents in nursing homes has been considered the norm, with the typical resident declining as much as 32% in 6 months (Rosen et al., 1999). Resnick and Simpson (2003) identify several factors associated with functional decline, including environmental factors, lack of motivation, social issues and cultural expectations, fear of falling, and comorbid diseases. Learned helplessness is another cause of functional decline and occurs when the care provided serves to increase dependency. Often staff find it easier to assist residents with self-care activities or perform care for the residents, rather than encourage and support self-care. Long-term care institutions foster dependency with inflexible daily routines, rigid policies and procedures, and lack of choice in all but a few matters. Certain features of the physical and social environment reinforce dependent behavior or fail to reward and reinforce independent behavior. Promoting resident autonomy in making choices, even if the choices seem insignificant, can help increase a sense of independence, personal decision making, and control. We will address the nursing home environment from two perspectives: the psychosocial environment and the physical environment.

BOX 34-3 Quality Indicators for Nursing Homes

Accidents
- Incidence of new fractures
- Prevalence of falls

Behavioral/emotional patterns
- Prevalence of behavioral symptoms affecting others
- Prevalence of symptoms of depression
- Prevalence of depression without antidepressant therapy

Clinical management
- Use of nine or more medications

Cognitive patterns
- Incidence of cognitive impairment (new since prior assessment)

Elimination
- Prevalence of bladder or bowel incontinence
- Prevalence of occasional or frequent bladder or bowel incontinence without a toileting plan
- Prevalence of indwelling catheters
- Prevalence of fecal impaction

Infection control
- Prevalence of urinary tract infections

Nutrition/eating
- Prevalence of weight loss
- Prevalence of tube feeding
- Prevalence of dehydration

Physical functioning
- Prevalence of bedfast residents
- Incidence of decline in late-loss ADLs (bed mobility, transferring, eating, toileting)
- Incidence of decline in range of motion

Psychotropic drug use
- Prevalence of antipsychotic use in the absence of psychotic or related conditions
- Prevalence of antianxiety/hypnotic drug use
- Prevalence of hypnotic use more than two times in last week

Quality of life
- Prevalence of physical restraints
- Prevalence of little or no activity

Skin care
- Prevalence of stage 1 to 4 pressure ulcers

From Center for Health Systems Research and Analysis. (2005). Quality indicators: Nursing homes. Retrieved January 13, 2006, from www.chsra.wisc.edu/chsra/qi/domaindesc.htm; and Center for Health Systems Research and Analysis. (2005). QI domains and descriptions. Retrieved November 20, 2005, from www.chsra.wisc.edu/chsra/qi/domaindesc.htm#accidents.

Psychosocial Environment

Physical frailty is noticed more often in the long-term care setting than psychological frailty. The losses, changes, and health problems experienced by most nursing home residents put them at risk for depression and mental health problems. A supportive psychosocial environment can buffer the impact of institutional living. A study of older adults' perceptions of their satisfaction with their living situation identified seven priority areas (Paulas & Jans, 2005), most related to the psychosocial environment:

- Human contact with management, staff, and other residents
- Relationships with others outside the institution
- Accommodations (i.e., meals, rooms, etc.)
- Quality of care experienced
- Activities
- Respect for the individual
- Financial issues

Social interaction is a basic human need that does not end when individuals enter a long-term care facility. Therefore the social environment plays a major role in quality of life for nursing home residents. The therapeutic social environment should provide a humane and caring milieu in which older persons receive confirmation of who they were and who they are now. A positive, supportive environment should foster communication, self-confidence, and hopefulness and enhance expectations. The essential features of the milieu include an atmosphere of acceptance, trust, and positive expectations. Positive expectations are conveyed through touch, words of encouragement, and articulation of choices to be made by the resident. Involving the residents in decision making improves activity levels and psychological outlook.

For the institutionalized older adult, the natural support system of the family and other social groups dwindles, and many social ties may no longer be available. Nursing personnel become significant participants in the resident's social network, but interactions with staff may not fully meet residents' needs for communication and affiliation. Too commonly, a negative communication style is used that portrays a patronizing or childlike "baby talk" approach to older residents; some authors have called this communication style *elderspeak*. This type of talk includes short and simple speech, exaggerated tones, using terms such as "honey," calling people by first names or nicknames without asking, or using the collective pronoun "we" instead of talking to the person directly. Williams, Kemper, and Hummert (2003) tested an intervention to enhance communication between CNAs and residents that decreased negative communication styles and resulted in more respectful styles.

Visits from family and friends can buffer the overwhelming effects of being in an institutional environment, and residents who have more visitors tend to do better than those with fewer visitors. Unfortunately, studies show that about one third of nursing home residents have no visitors from the outside. Gueldner and colleagues (2001) explored telephone conversations of nursing home residents and concluded that the telephone can provide an important means of maintaining social ties with the world outside the home. Staff may need to help residents in maintaining telephone contact with friends and family as part of a positive psychosocial environment.

For individuals without family or friends, a few selected staff members and residents can be designated to assist and support the resident. Ascertaining the residents' previous socialization patterns is crucial to avoid imposing unrealistic demands and expectations. For some older persons who lived alone for a long time, group living situations may be very stressful. For many older persons, one confiding and trusting relationship can have a greater positive effect than multiple, superficial contacts. Overall, the psychosocial environment may be more important than the physical environment, which is explored next.

Physical Environment

Functional impairment and sensory deficits are prevalent among nursing home residents. The design and structure of the nursing home must take these characteristics into consideration in order to promote function and safety of the residents. The physical environment should encourage the resident to move about and pursue activities independently without fear of overexertion or of getting lost or injured. Structural and design measures to simplify the environment promote resident function and mobility.

Visual impairments are common in nursing home residents. This problem is made worse by the fact that some residents cannot be tested for visual acuity and therefore cannot be effectively treated (West et al., 2003). Therefore caregivers must assume some degree of visual impairment. Furniture, carpet, drapes, and other fixtures can blend together if in like colors, making it difficult for residents to distinguish the boundaries of chairs, pathways, and other objects. This may inhibit residents from moving about freely without feeling cautious. Bright colors and different textures should be used in the design of the environment. Walls and doors painted in contrasting colors to identify bathrooms, social spaces, and exits provide visual markers for room recognition. Lettering on doorways and signs should be large and clearly marked. A study of various aspects of visual impairment as risk factors for falls found that contrast sensitivity, but not reported sensitivity to glare, was a factor in recurrent falling (de Boer et al., 2004).

No specific studies were found that attributed falls to glare. However, any factor that negatively impacts vision has the potential to affect function and safety. An unshaded window at the end of a hall could impair vision for a person walking toward the window. Tiled floors and light-colored walls reflect light, which may blur the resident's field of vision. Glare can be painful for the person with cataracts. Lighting decisions should take into consideration the increased illumination needed by older persons and the hazards posed by both glare and shadows. Lighting should be indirect and should come from natural sources if possible. Louvered window shades can divert the bright rays of the sun and still allow natural light to enter.

Hallways should be wide to allow for easy passage of wheelchairs and other carts and equipment. Recessed spaces should be designed to accommodate food, linen, and medication and housekeeping carts. Recessed spaces could also accommodate several chairs for residents who need a rest when walking or who just like to "people watch."

Furniture should be selected with consideration of the physical characteristics of the residents. It can be difficult for older people to get in and out of chairs with low seats and without arms. Chair selection should take into account the height, width, and depth of the chair and the elevation of the arms; the chairs also should be stable. Upholstery should be firm, to provide support and to prevent the person from sinking too deeply into the seat. Furniture should be arranged in a way that promotes socialization and activity. Units should provide interesting places to go and interesting things to do.

Advantages of carpeted floors are that they buffer noise, reduce the abrasive impact of falls, and create a homelike atmosphere. Analysis of 6641 falls revealed that the risk of fracture was significantly reduced when the fall occurred on a carpeted surface with wooden sub-flooring; the other types of flooring were non-carpeted with wooden sub-flooring, concrete subfloor with carpet, and concrete subfloor without carpet (Simpson, Lamb, Roberts, Gardner, & Grimley-Evans, 2004). In another smaller study, the risk of fracture decreased fourfold when a fall occurred on a 7-mm thick carpet as opposed to a vinyl floor (Gardner et al., 1998).

Wheelchair-bound residents should be able to reach light switches, sinks, mirrors, shelves, desks, windows, and other utilities. Wall pictures and news items posted on bulletin boards should be at eye level. Residents should be encouraged to personalize their rooms by having familiar objects in view to promote a sense of familiarity and comfort. Personal mementos serve as a reminder of important events from the resident's life history. They also stimulate interest and conversation in staff, other residents, and visitors. All residents need some territory or space to call their own, a place to be physically separated from others. Nurses should always be sensitive about personal boundaries and private space.

One of the most important outcomes of the OBRA regulation has been the limitation in the use of physical restraints. The restraint reform of OBRA mandates that the rights of nursing home residents to humane care and alternatives to restraints must be upheld. The use of physical restraints once was commonplace in nursing homes to prevent falls or tampering with medical devices such as catheters. Rows of residents could be seen parked in their wheelchairs and secured with vest or waist restraints. That scenario began to change with the passage of OBRA. Today the goal is restraint-free care, with attention to the environmental issues described earlier, restorative efforts to maintain muscle strength and walking abilities, and appropriate use of technologies for safe patient handling. Research has shown that care can safely be provided without the use of restraints, and this may actually decrease the number of falls, or at least reduce the number of falls resulting in injury. (Dimant, 2003).

A Cochrane Review concluded that the most effective fall prevention approaches are multidisciplinary, multifactorial interventions that address both resident and environmental factors. Muscle strengthening and balance training when implemented by a trained health professional has been found to be effective in home settings. Other patient interventions that have been effective are withdrawal of psychotropic medications and cardiac pacing for selected individuals (Gillespie et al., 2006).

Having described details about creating a functional and pleasing environment in nursing homes, we encourage you to access an essay by Karen Bermann entitled "Love and Space in the Nursing Home" that was published in *Theoretical Medicine* in 2003. This thoughtful essay captures a dimension of architecture that is missing from this discussion.

New Trends and Approaches to Care

A variety of new approaches to long-term care are discussed in the literature, and some of these are briefly described here. First is the idea of restorative care. This nursing approach is used primarily by direct care staff and is designed to help assist nursing facility residents in maintaining or improving functional abilities (Resnick & Simpson, 2003). Residents are encouraged to increase exercise and activity and assist with self-care in activities of daily living. Pilot studies are exploring the outcomes of using this model (Resnick et al., 2004).

The Eden Alternative is a model of care developed in the 1990s to improve conditions in nursing homes. With a goal of decreasing loneliness, boredom, and helplessness, the model encourages nursing homes to create a "Human Habitat" by including pets, plants, and children in the daily environment (Eden Alternative, 2002). The program reports members across the United States, as well as other countries. Little research has examined the Eden model, but one study comparing two facilities did not show a change in cognition, function, or other parameters (Coleman et al., 2002). However, another study compared residents from a facility implementing the Eden model with a control facility, and found a decrease in boredom and helplessness after 1 year (Bergman-Evans, 2004).

An additional movement in long-term care is what has been called "person-centered care." This approach started as a grassroots effort and is now organized into a group called the "Pioneer Network" (Pioneer Network, 2005). The Pioneer Network includes a board of directors, local contacts, and resources for people interested in improving long-term care. The Pioneer Network Web site promotes individualized care for older adults, based on knowing the person, building relationships and community, supporting self-determination, and working for positive change. Ideas to make nursing homes more homelike are shared through meetings and resources.

Special Care Units. Special care units evolved in response to the identified needs of residents with cognitive impairment in an effort to group residents and provide targeted therapeutic services to promote adaptive behavior and social interaction. The designation is usually reserved for units that have the following five characteristics (Maas & Specht, 2000):

1. Admission of residents with dementia
2. Special staff specifications, selection, and training
3. Activity programming tailored to residents with dementia
4. Family programming and involvement
5. A segregated and modified physical and social environment

The goals of care are to maintain function and dignity while allowing individuals to live a meaningful life (Gerdner, Shue, & Beck, 2000). Special care units offer a controlled environment and a staff that is skilled in the principles of creating and implementing a therapeutic milieu. The use of psychotropic drugs is typically limited, and the use of restraints is avoided. Environmental awareness is increased through the use of enriched environmental cues (calendars, clocks, and reality orientation boards). Residents are prompted and gently guided through activities of daily living to help them maintain the maximum functional level possible, including dressing, eating, and toileting. The therapeutic environment of the special care unit should provide a setting in which the resident may become more socially adjusted and less agitated, be free to move around, be free of restraints, receive fewer drugs, and achieve a balance of physical activity and rest.

Although the benefits of special care units are difficult to document, studies have shown that the cost is not increased and that family members prefer this type

of care (Maas & Specht, 2000). However, the use of the term *special care unit* is not regulated, so that any facility can say that it has such a unit without providing any actual specialized care. Therefore family members should be aware of the difference so they can determine whether facilities indeed provide special care for residents with dementia within such units.

The physical environment of Alzheimer's units has been the topic of numerous studies, possibly because these units have controlled access and exit. The setting is, in a sense, the resident's whole world much of the time. Also, environmental features have been noted to contribute to or reduce some behavioral symptoms in persons with dementia. One study of 15 special care units found that factors related to less aggressive and agitated behavior included privacy, personalization in bedrooms, residential character, and an ambient environment that residents understand. Common areas and camouflaged exit doors were associated with decreased depression, social withdrawal, misidentification, and hallucinations. To evaluate each setting, investigators used the Environment Rating Checklist Indicators tool (Zeisel et al., 2003). See Table 34-2 for a list of the concepts included and indicators assessed.

Quality of Care in Nursing Homes

Because the nursing facility is home to many aging adults, not just a temporary place, the quality of care takes on an even greater importance than in other settings. As a result, increasing efforts to monitor and address quality issues have been mandated. The following gives some background on the history of the quality movement in nursing homes followed by the current regulatory process for managing quality in long-term care.

History of Quality of Care in Nursing Homes. During the 1960s and 1970s, concern about the quality of care in long-term care facilities prompted the development of complex regulatory standards. However, the effectiveness of those regulations in terms of quality of care was questionable. In the 1980s, several important events propelled the emphasis away from structure and process and toward outcomes. In 1985, the National Citizens' Coalition for Nursing Home Reform reported on a project titled *A Consumer Perspective on Quality Care: The Resident's Point of View*. This project developed recommendations for nursing home reform based on interviews with over 450 residents across the country who identified important staff characteristics and services, particularly staff with good attitudes toward residents, who promptly attended to their needs, and who provided good care. Findings from this report strongly influenced the development of legislation by articulating resident/consumer expectations for care.

Table 34-2 *Sample Concepts from the Environment Rating Checklist Indicators: Indicators Assessed*

Concept	Indicators Assessed
Exit control	Camouflaging techniques Immediacy of controls
Walking paths	Continuous with destination Way finding
Individual space	Individual privacy Personalization opportunities
Common space	Uniqueness of common spaces Appropriate number of common spaces
Outdoor freedom	Accessibility of outdoor space Appropriate plan and design of outdoor space
Residential character	Residential size Homelike character
Autonomy support	Safety Support for independence
Sensory comprehension	Staff control Understandable sensory input

Data from Zeisel, J., Silverstein, N. M., Hyde, J., Levkoff, S., Lawton, M. P., & Holmes, W. (2003). Environmental correlates to behavioral health outcomes in Alzheimer's special care units. *Gerontologist*, 43(5), 697-711.

In 1986 the Institute of Medicine released a report on a 2.5-year study titled *Improving the Quality of Care in Nursing Homes*. This report contained more than 400 pages of analysis and recommendations that focused on regulatory changes addressing a number of issues, including quality of care, residents' rights, staffing and training, and survey and certification processes. The outstanding panel of experts who participated in the development of this document strongly supported major change in the long-term care nursing facility.

The implementation of the Nursing Home Reform Act (PL 100-203) of the Omnibus Budget Reconciliation Act (OBRA) in 1987 heralded a new era in the quest for quality of care and residents' rights in the long-term care nursing facility. The achievement of nursing home reform came after years of consumer activism, health professional advocacy, and legislative initiatives on behalf of nursing facility residents. At the core of the OBRA legislation is the recognition of the need to define and articulate quality in long-term care and to hold the long-term care nursing facility accountable for meeting high-quality standards. OBRA states that the purpose of the long-term care nursing facility is to bring each resident to the highest practicable level of mental, physical, and psychosocial well-being in an environment that emphasizes residents' rights. This is achieved by focusing on quality of life, as well as on quality of care.

OBRA included new regulatory requirements that must be met by nursing facilities as conditions of participation in the Medicare and Medicaid programs and thus be eligible for reimbursement. The methodology for evaluating the quality of care in the nursing facility changed from an emphasis on documentation of policies and procedures and structural characteristics (termed *paper compliance*) to an emphasis on outcomes of care and services as evidenced by direct observation of, and interaction with, residents. The outcome-oriented survey process shifted the focus to measuring the effectiveness of resident care.

Processes to review and promote quality care have been described in Chapter 28, and the mandated individualized assessment and care planning processes are described later in this chapter. However, providing good fundamental nursing care is the key to quality nursing homes. Recent research found the following key elements among nursing facilities that provided good care as measured by resident outcomes (Rantz & Zwygart-Stauffacher, 2004):

- Residents were assessed for high-risk problems.
- Staff helped residents walk or restore walking if possible.
- Alternatives to restraints were used.
- Good food and appropriate feeding techniques were used.
- Toileting plans were carried out.
- Pain management techniques were routinely used.

The authors encourage renewed attention on these fundamental nursing actions as an important part of quality improvement.

Monitoring of Quality. Nursing home care is monitored through audits or surveys coordinated by each state. These surveys are required for all facilities receiving Medicare or Medicaid funds. Surveys are conducted at least annually, and additional surveys are conducted if there are serious complaints or incidents. The surveys are not announced and are conducted by trained health care professionals. Reports are compiled and sent to the nursing homes, and if standards are not met, the homes must develop a plan to correct deficiencies and follow-up surveys may be conducted. Information is also entered into a national database, the Online Survey Certification and Reporting (OSCAR) database, for use by CMS and to provide information that can be used to compare nursing homes.

Quality Indicators. Processes are the activities carried out by staff, such as bathing, feeding, and ambulating, and the activities that facilitate resident care, such as staff education. Outcomes are the products of one or more processes and may include pressure ulcers, weight loss, and falls (Joint Commission on Accreditation of Healthcare Organizations [JCAHO], 1992). Many aspects of care may be seen as both processes and outcomes; however, the indicator must be measurable in objective terms.

A number of quality indicators are evaluated as evidence of substandard care. Monitoring specific quality-of-care indicators should be part of an ongoing quality improvement plan in the nursing facility. A high prevalence of problems associated with quality indicators suggests systemic problems with care. Table 34-2 lists a number of important quality indicators. State surveyors evaluate these quality indicators during their review of care to determine whether the nursing facility would be charged with deficiency penalties.

Recent statistics indicate that 18% of nursing homes were cited with a deficiency for actual harm or jeopardy of the residents (Gibson, Gregory, Houser, & Fox-Grage, 2004). Survey deficiencies vary by state (Castle, Degenholtz, & Engberg, 2005) and class of ownership. Not-for-profit facilities continue to average fewer deficiencies than government and for-profit facilities.

JCAHO Accreditation of Long-Term Care Facilities.
JCAHO accreditation of long-term care facilities has been available since 1966. It became an option for assisted living facilities in 2002, but is being discontinued in 2006 because of the lack of market demand (JCAHO, 2005a). The stated purpose of the accreditation process is to support the delivery of safe, quality resident care. Standards assessed for accreditation of long-term care facilities are noted in Box 34-4. In addition to the standards, facilities must meet additional criteria that demonstrate compliance with National Patient Safety Goals and Recommendations (NPSGs). NPSGs focus on specific actions intended to prevent medical errors. The goals that apply to a particular facility depend on the services that facility provides.

JCAHO's 2006 NPSGs included some new requirements under existing goals, as well as some new goals and requirements for long-term care facilities. These are summarized in Box 34-5. In addition, a new quality measure for long-term care was added to the priority focus process. The new measure is concerned with residents who lose too much weight (JCAHO, 2005c).

Facilities seeking JCAHO accreditation first submit a written application, which is then followed by an onsite survey (Box 34-6). In long-term care, the survey is

---

BOX 34-5 2006 JCAHO New National Patient Safety Goals and Requirements

New Requirements under Existing Goals

2E. Implement a standardized approach to "hand off" communications, including the opportunity to ask and respond to questions

9B. Implement a fall reduction program and evaluate the effectiveness of the new program

New Goals and Requirements

14. Prevent health care-associated pressure ulcers (decubitus ulcers)

14A. Assess and periodically reassess each resident's risk for developing a pressure ulcer or decubitus ulcer, and take action to address any identified risks

Data from Joint Commission on Accreditation of Healthcare Organizations (JCAHO). (2005). LTC update. Retrieved January 20, 2006, from www.jcaho.org.

BOX 34-6 JCAHO: The Onsite Survey Agenda

- Opening conference
- Leadership interview
- Validation of organization's implementation and monitoring of the plan(s) of action emanating from the periodic performance review (PPR)
- Visits to care and service areas guided by the priority focus process using the tracer methodology
- Environment of care review
- Human resources review
- Credentials review
- System tracers, that is, specific time slots devoted to in-depth discussion and education regarding the use of data in performance improvement (as in core measure performance and the analysis of staffing), medication management, infection control, and other current topics of interest to the organization
- Closing conference

Source: Shared visions—New pathways Q&A. *New Pathway: The Onsite Survey Process.* Retrieved from www.jcaho.org.

BOX 34-4 JCAHO Standards for Long-Term Care

Resident-Focused Functions

Ethics, rights, and responsibilities
Provision of care, treatment, and services
Medication management
Surveillance, prevention, and control of infection

Organization Functions

Improving organization performance
Management of the environment of care
Management of human resources
Management of information

conducted by a masters-prepared nurse, physician, or administrator. All surveyors are experienced long-term care professionals, most of whom are currently practicing in long-term care. As of 2006, all reaccreditation surveys are unannounced. Organizations undergoing initial surveys are informed of the date of the visit. The process has been modified for Medicare/Medicaid-certified facilities to eliminate duplications in the evaluation process. JCAHO provides a variety of services including publications, seminars, and educational programs to assist facilities to prepare for the accreditation process (JCAHO, 2005b).

An independent information services company specializing in long-term care conducted a study of nursing facilities in 2002. Agencies that were JCAHO accredited were compared with those that were not. Among the findings were that JCAHO-accredited facilities had the following characteristics (JCAHO, 2002):

- Significantly fewer severe quality-of-care deficiencies
- Higher compliance with the Life Safety Code
- Significantly fewer medication errors
- Fewer complaints and fewer substantiated complaint allegations
- Lower rates of facility-acquired pressure ulcers
- Higher occupancy

The JCAHO ORYX initiative integrates performance measurement data into the accreditation process. The intent of the measurement requirements is to support accredited organizations in quality improvement. Sets of standardized performance measures are being developed for each accreditation program. An organization's use of core measure sets to improve performance is assessed during on-site surveys. At this time, ORYX long-term care measures have not been identified (JCAHO, 2005d).

Evaluating and Choosing a Long-Term Care Nursing Facility.

Selecting a long-term care facility is a daunting task for the older adult and his or her family. First, available nursing facilities should be identified. Names of nursing facilities may be obtained from local councils on aging, the department of social services, the state department of human resources, and the nursing facility association. Evaluating and choosing a long-term care nursing facility are affected by subjective opinions and first impressions that may or may not reflect usual practices. A systematic evaluation of structure, process, and outcome variables can be accomplished by using various sources of information. State surveys of the nursing facility are mandated by law to be accessible to the public. Information about deficiencies and citations may be obtained from state agencies responsible for surveying nursing facilities. Nursing Home Compare (CMS, 2005) is a federal database on the Internet that provides information on nursing home deficiencies and quality of care from recent residents'

assessment data that can help you evaluate the quality of care of specific nursing homes.

When visiting a facility, it is important to carefully interview the administrators of the nursing facility with regard to the philosophy of care; the resources available to meet the prospective resident's needs; the availability of RNs, advanced practice nurses, and physicians to meet ongoing and episodic needs of residents; nurse staffing patterns; and conditions under which residents may be transferred out of the facility. Clarify financial details concerning what is and is not covered in the daily rate or by insurance carriers. It is also important to observe care being delivered to residents at different times of the day and to observe staff communication patterns. Guides to evaluating and selecting a nursing home are available from Medicare, the American Association of Retired Persons, the Alzheimer's Association, and other sources (Rantz, Popejoy, & Zwygart-Stauffacher, 2001).

RELOCATION AND TRANSITIONS

Relocation is always an issue in long-term care, and even when residents want to make this change, the process can be difficult. Burnette (1986, p. 8, cited in Castle, 2001b) defined *relocation* as "moving from one environment to another for various reasons." Risk factors for relocation in the 6-month period after hip fracture included absence of dementia, in-hospital delirium, one or more new impairments at hospital discharge, hospital discharge other than to home, and not living at home alone before the fracture (Boockvar et al., 2004). Relocations are common among older adults, and may be classified as interinstitutional, intrainstitutional, residential, or residential or institutional, and may have negative or positive benefits. Examples of *interinstitutional* relocations are moves to and from home, hospital, and rehabilitation facilities. Moves within a single facility are termed *intrainstitutional*. A move from one home to another is a *residential* relocation. When the move occurs between home and an institution, it is a *residential* or *institutional* relocation (Castle, 2001b).

Numerous factors necessitate relocation of older persons. Smallegan (1985) noted that a decision to enter a nursing home is always a result of inadequacy—finances, health, social supports, emotional strength, or other ability to cope. Interviews with decision makers for newly admitted nursing home residents about problems preceding admission revealed that the residents were receiving substantial care from family members and friends before admission. Multiple functional impairments and complex medical and social circumstances interact to produce excessive caregiving burdens. The study findings substantiated that families do make significant contributions in caring for their older members and usually do not inappropriately or prematurely admit them to institutions. When the burden of managing care exceeds the family's ability to provide such care, nursing home placement becomes an important option.

Organizational reorganizations, which are common in the nursing industry, often require relocation as facilities are merged, closed, or relocated. One estimate is that some 75,000 nursing home residents are relocated each year for these reasons (Castle, 2001b). Within an institution, relocations may be associated with remodeling, extension, or consolidation of facilities. Changes in level of care needed, financial resources, and roommate problems also can trigger moves. Various databases suggest that 6.8% to 8% of nursing home residents are moved each year within a facility. Using these figures, Castle (2001b) concluded that approximately 120,000 nursing home residents per year are relocated within their facilities of residence.

Stages of Relocation

The process of relocation can be divided into three stages: preinstitutionalization, immediately after institutionalization, and postinstitutionalization. Preinstitutionalization is characterized by a search for an appropriate facility, medical and legal consults, and decisions about the patient's personal property. This stage commonly is stressful for both the older adult and the family involved in the care decisions. Feelings of helplessness, vulnerability, and abandonment are most common in the period immediately after institutionalization. A state of physical, social, and mental disorganization may persist for up to 3 months (Jackson et al. in Hsueh-Fen, Travis, & Acton, 2004). During postinstitutionalization, residents' perceptions of the amount of control they retain affect their psychological response to relocation. Assimilation into the long-term care routine may require many months (Hsueh-Fen, Travis, & Acton, 2004).

Brooke (1989) described adaptation to the nursing facility environment as a socialization continuum with four phases: disorganization, reorganization, relationship building, and stabilization (Figure 34-1). In the disorganization phase, the resident may feel a pervasive sense of loss and grieving about his or her health status and new environment. The resident may also feel overwhelmed by the challenge of learning about a new living situation. In the reorganization phase, the resident attempts to understand the environment and to find meaning and autonomy in daily experiences. The resident may attempt to justify and resolve being in a nursing facility and may see personal benefit. During the relationship-building phase, the resident forms emotional links with other residents and staff and may experience conflict or frustration in these attachments.

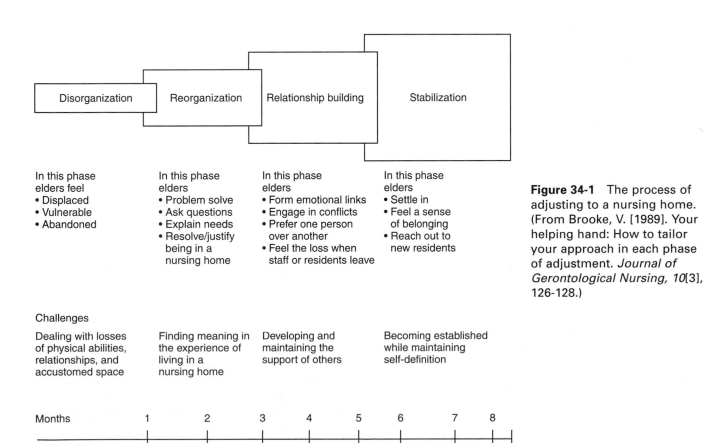

Figure 34-1 The process of adjusting to a nursing home. (From Brooke, V. [1989]. Your helping hand: How to tailor your approach in each phase of adjustment. *Journal of Gerontological Nursing, 10*[3], 126-128.)

When the stabilization phase is reached, the resident's roles and routines are established, but he or she may still have fears and anxieties about the future.

Outcomes of Relocation

Abrupt change in the living situation challenges the older person's coping abilities, putting the individual at high risk for loss of physical or psychological function. Unfamiliar environments are particularly stressful because there is a loss of personal control and routines. Transition from the home or hospital to the nursing facility, whether temporary or permanent, is a stressful event for the older person. The degree to which the person exercises control over the environment and participates in the decision-making process can positively influence the transition. Preadmission visits should be encouraged, and prospective residents should be given opportunities to express concerns and realistically appraise the options. Rosswurm (1983) noted that the predictability of the move, the reason for the move, and the degree of control the older person has in the decision-making process and in other events surrounding the move all affect the relocation. Planned preparation for transition to the nursing facility is widely acknowledged to be essential to successful transition.

Castle (2001b) reviewed the literature on relocation from 1970 to 1999. A concern with many of these studies was the small sample sizes. Other sources of possible bias were the diversity of procedures used to analyze effects, common lack of comparative control groups, and no standard periods of observation for effects of relocation. The potential negative outcomes of relocation were classified as mortality, morbidity, and psychological and social changes. The outcome studied most often was mortality.

Mortality

Early studies on the negative consequences of relocation to new environments, including mental hospitals and nursing facilities, concluded that mortality rate was high during the first month and during the first year (Camargo & Preston, 1945; Whittier & Williams, 1956). These studies helped generalize the opinion that relocation itself was hazardous, even life threatening, apart from conditions associated with the move (Coffman, 1981). Terms such as *transplantation shock, transfer trauma, relocation trauma,* and *relocation effect* described the perceived dangers of relocation. Subsequent reviews of these studies have determined that methodological flaws in the studies made those conclusions questionable and probably overrated (Borup, 1981, 1983; Coffman, 1981). Although the effect of relocation on mortality rate in later studies was shown to be insignificant, it is believed that certain factors mediate relocation,

including the degree of environmental change, the type or quality of environmental change, the degree of preparation for the change, and whether the relocation was voluntary or involuntary (Mirotznik & Ruskin, 1984).

Castle (2001b) found few commonalities among the 35 studies published between 1970 and 1999 that addressed mortality rate following relocation. Postrelocation mortality rates ranged from 0% to 43%. Notably, some individuals benefited from relocation, especially those most in need of care. For example, the health status of a frail, malnourished person living alone might improve after moving into assisted living. Mortality rates related to intrainstitutional moves ranged from 4% to 36%. In relation to both interinstitutional and intrainstitutional relocation, disparate results could be attributed to study design, period of observation, study setting, and statistical power. Insufficient studies of residential relocation were available on which to base conclusions (Castle, 2001b).

A 2004 study followed older persons with mental illness after discharge from a psychiatric hospital to community-based extended care units over an 18-month period. During the study period, 21.7% of these individuals died and 11.6% had been transferred to nursing homes. The investigators determined that those who died had significantly higher levels of physical ill health than their counterparts, and that the mortality rate in the study period was more likely related to initial health status rather than to relocation trauma (Meehan, Robertson, Stedman, & Byrne, 2004).

Morbidity

It is commonly assumed that physical health may be affected by relocation, but this has not been validated by the research literature. Most morbidity studies in Castle's (2001b) review were in relation to interinstitutional relocation. Outcomes addressed included a variety of variables such as measures of general health (e.g., activities of daily living [ADLs]), vision, hearing, locomotion, and daily functioning. Most studies found either improvement in general health or no change following relocation. Findings were similar in the small number of studies (five) that focused on intrainstitutional relocation. Only two studies of residential relocation were examined; however, one of these (Lawton & Cohen, 1974, cited in Castle, 2001b) had the largest sample size of any of those reviewed. In this large study ($n = 574$), functional health declined significantly following residential relocation. Engle and Graney (1993) reported on a large prospective study of residents during the first and second week after nursing home admission. These findings documented improvement in hygiene, grooming, dressing, and transferring, whereas feeding, ambulation, urination, and defecation were stable.

Psychological or Social Changes

Societal norms for transition to, and living in, the nursing facility are lacking. Aside from the personal distress that may be caused by other losses encountered in nursing home admission—perhaps one's home, belongings, social network, health status, and finances—the resident may feel a lack of social context within which health-directed and goal-directed behavior can occur. As a result, passive, dependent behavior may prevail, along with feelings of loss of control and helplessness. New environments can be overwhelming, disorienting, and exhausting to the new resident. Individuals with cognitive and sensory deficits who are physically frail are the most vulnerable and have the most serious adverse relocation effects. Changes in appetite, physical activity, mood, and cognitive function leading to acute confusion or delirium may represent signs of distress.

About half of the studies of psychological or social changes in the period reviewed by Castle (2001b) focused on interinstitutional relocation. Among the many outcomes studied were IQ, personality, morale, and psychosocial health. Overall, there appeared to be few psychological or social changes. Once again, generalization was difficult because of small sample sizes. However, the study in this group with the largest sample ($n = 389$) showed significant positive effects for some outcomes and negative effects for others in geriatric psychiatric patients (Castle, 2001b). In general, studies of psychological and social changes following intrainstitutional relocation did not find significant change.

One frequently cited study (Borup, 1982) introduced the concept of degree of change resulting from relocation. In this work, residents undergoing a moderate relocation change demonstrated significant decreases in hypochondria and violent behavior, and significant increases in compliance, reality perception, and social adjustment. A radical relocation was associated with significant decreases in hypochondria and a significant increase in aggression. Measures of life satisfaction, environmental responsiveness, alienation, and self-concept showed no change in either group (Castle, 2001b).

A study by Washburn (2005) compared residents moving to a new nursing home with those remaining in a nursing home. Based on measures of salivary cortisol, pulse, blood pressure, anxiety, and affect, the investigators concluded that older nursing home residents may experience stress before relocation; however, the increase in stress is short-lived. One week before the move, persons to be relocated had a significantly greater rise in late-afternoon cortisol than those who would remain in the original facility.

Waldron, Gitelson, and Kelley (2005) studied gender differences in social adaptation to a retirement community over a 4-year period. In relation to the number of persons providing personal support, practical assistance,

advice, and help with illness, men reported gains whereas women reported losses or no change. The use of e-mail was positively correlated with perceived social support by both sexes.

Depressive symptoms related to relocation have been a focus of numerous studies. A longitudinal (18 months) study of depressive symptomatology compared older persons discharged from medical rehabilitation to live alone in their own homes, to live with others, and to live in nursing homes (Loeher, Bank, MacNeill, & Lichtenberg, 2004). Before their medical rehabilitation, all participants had lived alone. Individuals who lived in nursing homes for the duration of the study had the highest levels of depression, whereas those discharged home alone had the lowest levels of depressive symptoms. The investigators concluded that the move to live with others or to nursing homes represented a loss of independence that was linked to depressive symptomatology (Loeher et al., 2004). The loss of independence also was a theme in a study of Swedish elders' reflections on relocation to sheltered housing (Sviden, Wikstrom, & Hjortsjo-Norberg, 2002). Keister (2004) studied the predictive value of variables at the time of admission on relocation outcomes. Depressive symptoms were found to be associated with lower challenge appraisal and greater harm/loss appraisal. Lower depressive symptoms were associated with greater mastery and increased emotional social support. Variables that were associated with lower levels of anxiety were greater mastery and greater benign appraisal.

Variables in addition to depression have been explored. When residents of a long-term care facility were moved to a new facility, investigators collected data on antipsychotic drug use in persons relocated to the new facility and persons in a facility not undergoing relocation. The use of antipsychotics remained stable (around 30%) in the nonrelocating site. In the facility that was being relocated, antipsychotic use rose from a baseline of 21.5% to 32.6% immediately after the move, to 36.9% 6 months after the move. Most prescriptions did not document the indication for the drugs (Hagen et al., 2005).

The timing of data collection relevant to a transition may significantly alter findings. Patnaik and colleagues (1974) studied resident and staff behavior patterns before and after involuntary relocation and found that the relocated residents were observed to restrict themselves to their bedrooms, fewer were observed in the lounge, and more passive behavior was exhibited (more staff were noted to be performing tasks for the resident). This behavior was interpreted as an appropriate way for residents with diminished competence to orient themselves to a new environment; however, longitudinal measurements of these behaviors that would note permanent declines in behavior patterns were not taken (Patnaik et al., 1974). Brody, Kleban, and Moss (1974) reported that personality variables, including depression, aggression, resistance, anger, demandingness, neurosis, and anxiety, all increased after relocation, especially anxiety and depression, but returned to baseline status after 2 weeks. Engle and Graney (1993) reported similar findings during the first and second weeks after nursing home admission. Tired and depressed moods improved, and other affective states, such as anger, loneliness, fear, and cheerfulness, remained stable. This study provided data suggesting that negative aspects of nursing home admission may be less than anticipated.

Resident characteristics thought to be associated with the outcomes of relocation include physical status, cognitive and emotional status, gender, age, life satisfaction, previous health care experience, timing, duration of the relocation, preparation, quality of the new environment, and the community setting of the new residence (Castle, 2001b). Clearly, additional studies of factors that enhance positive outcomes are needed.

Benefits of Relocation

Despite the focus on adverse responses to relocation, residence in a nursing facility offers numerous benefits. Factors that can make this setting attractive include access to professional nursing services and other health professionals; health monitoring; timely evaluation and treatment of illness; the convenience of having available basic services, such as meals, laundry, housekeeping, and personal assistance; and the stability of being in a safe setting of care. Many individuals can function at a higher level when the appropriate services are available. Special environmental design features in the nursing home can enhance physical mobility and social interaction. For the person needing round-the-clock personal assistance and care, the nursing home may be the most economical and practical solution (Sloane & Gwyther, 1980). Smith and Bengtson (1979) reported on the positive effect of nursing facility placement on family relationships. More than two thirds of family members of nursing home residents interviewed indicated that they experienced a renewed closeness and strengthening of family ties, a discovery of new love and affection, or a continuation of closeness. In only 10% were there negative patterns, and there was no evidence that the resident had been abandoned. Family relationships may actually be renewed or strengthened, at least in part because of the release of the family from the strain of caregiving.

The Impact of Resident Relocation on Others

Relocation affects not only the older adult who moves, but also the individuals who were their caregivers before relocation. Often a family caregiver had been caring for the older adult until circumstances made that no longer feasible. Entrusting their loved one to strangers can be a difficult transition for the family. The majority of family caregivers are female spouses, followed by daughters, and then daughters-in-law. Although it would seem that institutionalization would relieve caregiver burden, new issues arise that continue to cause stress. Feelings of guilt and uncertainty may overshadow the relief of physical labor. A study of Taiwanese family caregivers found that a higher caregiver burden at the time of placement was associated with the level of the care recipient's dependence or the caregiver's poor health. Four months after nursing home placement, perceived global burden decreased, particularly in relation to lack of family support, impact of schedule, and impact of health. Burden scores on caregiver esteem and impact of finances were not altered by placement. The only demographic factor predicting change in global burden was duration of caregiving (Yeh, Johnson, & Wang, 2002).

Following admission of the older adult to a nursing home, some family members maintain close relationships with the older adult and others do not. The nature of family involvement varies and might include participation in direct care, collaboration with staff, and participation in decision making. Family members who are concerned about the quality of care provided may visit often to oversee care. Those who disengage from the older resident may do so because of distress over the resident's deterioration, uncertainty over their role in the setting, or feeling unwelcome in the facility. Among the benefits of family involvement are

- Reduced distress of institutionalization
- Enhanced sense of identity for the resident
- A sense of order in a foreign environment
- Maintenance of a basic link for the resident to the outside world
- Break in the monotony of nursing home life
- Reduced sense of abandonment

CARE OF OLDER ADULTS IN NURSING HOME SETTINGS

The care of older adults in the nursing home setting today is organized through interdisciplinary team meetings that are held regularly to review each resident's care and to communicate each discipline's plan for the resident and evaluate the plan's effectiveness. These team meetings typically are structured around the care planning process required by Medicare/Medicaid (Health Care Financing Administration, 1995). This process includes a document for assessment, care planning, and intervention and evaluation of outcomes, similar to the nursing process.

Resident assessment in the long-term care setting revolves around the Minimum Data Set (MDS), the standardized screening and assessment tool to measure physical, medical, psychological, and social functioning of residents. The general categories of data and health status items in the MDS include the following: demographics and patient history, cognition, communication/hearing, vision, mood/behavior patterns, psychosocial well-being, physical functioning, continence, diagnoses, health conditions, medications, nutritional and dental status, skin condition, activity patterns, special treatments and procedures, and discharge potential. Assessment to provide MDS data is required by the Center for Medicare and Medicaid Services (CMS, 2002) for all nursing homes receiving federal money, and reports are regularly submitted electronically to CMS.

The MDS is administered on admission, quarterly, annually, or whenever the resident experiences a significant change in status, whenever the resident experiences readmission from a hospital, or whenever the facility identifies a significant error in a prior assessment. The MDS is the core source of assessment information for an individualized care planning process, which is documented on the Resident Assessment Instrument (RAI), which is required each time the MDS is administered. Many facilities have a single MDS coordinator who manages the process of routine assessment and care planning for residents (Taunton, Swagerty, Smith, Lasseter, & Lee, 2004), who ideally knows the residents well and solicits input from all staff to complete MDS data. If the MDS coordinator is able to develop positive relationships with staff, he or she has the potential to influence quality of care (Piven et al., 2006). Nurses usually fill this important role in the nursing home setting.

When scored, the RAI data identify nursing care problems that should be addressed in the residents' care plans, for example, weight loss or falls. Resident Assessment Protocols (RAPs) are given to address these problem areas that can be further individualized to address the residents' particular issues. Depending on the resident's condition, special attention must be directed toward common problems such as confusion, urinary retention or incontinence, urinary tract infection, instability, constipation, weight loss, breaks in the skin, weakness, muscle contractures, and pain. Risk factors for problems such as falls and pressure sores must also be documented. Prescribed medications should be assessed for appropriate dosage, potential interactions, and both therapeutic and adverse effects. The team can contribute to the MDS assessment data and participate in formulating the plan of care to address identified problems.

Once developed, resident care plans are communicated to all nursing care staff and information is transferred to other documents used by staff to plan and document daily care. The gerontological nurse is essential in providing a leadership role on interdisciplinary care planning teams, because nursing represents the vital link in development and implementation of the plan of care 24 hours a day. The gerontological nurse integrates treatment recommendations into a coherent plan of care and is in frequent contact with the resident and family to evaluate its effects.

The involvement and role of the CNA are also key in the implementation of the care plan. Even though CNAs provide the majority of direct physical care to residents, they are typically underused as key participants during interdisciplinary team meetings. They may have daily interchanges with other team members, but not as a member of the formal organizational structure. Systematic mechanisms for involving nursing assistants in patient care planning meetings affirm their important role in implementation of the care plan and ongoing observation of the resident's status and response to care. This also ensures that the caregiver responsible for most of the direct care fully understands the goals of the care plan and individual role responsibilities.

Nursing Diagnoses

The list of nursing diagnoses that might apply to nursing home residents is unlimited. Many of these have been addressed in Section 3, including activity intolerance, chronic confusion, constipation, risk for falls, risk for injury, impaired physical mobility, self-care deficits, disturbed sensory perception, impaired skin integrity, social isolation, impaired swallowing, ineffective tissue perfusion, impaired walking, wandering, imbalanced nutrition: less than body requirements, impaired oral mucous membrane, chronic pain, urinary incontinence, and risk for imbalanced fluid volume. This section focuses on the most common diagnoses related to adaptation to the nursing home setting.

- Impaired adjustment related to low state of optimism, intense emotional state, multiple stressors, disability, or health status changes requiring change in lifestyle
- Anxiety related to unmet needs, situational crisis, threat to self-concept, stress, change in role status, health status, environment
- Ineffective coping related to inadequate level of perception of control, situational crisis
- Compromised family coping related to prolonged disease or progression of disability that exhausts supportive capacity of significant people
- Deficient diversional activity related to environmental lack of diversional activity
- Interrupted family processes related to shift in health status of a family member, situation transition, or crises
- Hopelessness related to (perceived) abandonment, failing or deteriorating physiological condition
- Powerlessness related to health care environment, lifestyle of helplessness
- Relocation stress syndrome related to isolation from family/friends, recent losses, lack of adequate support system

Nursing Goals/Outcomes

In relation to the listed nursing diagnoses, appropriate goals for the resident include (1) healthy adaptation to new environment; (2) reduced feelings of anxiety, hopelessness, and helplessness; (3) enhanced sense of control; (4) participation in diversional activities of choice; and (5) diminished stress related to relocation. Goals for the family might include (1) improved coping with resident status and relocation, and (2) restoration of family processes.

Interventions

Interventions to meet the goals can be clustered as those designed to facilitate successful resident adaptation and those that promote family adjustment.

Interventions to Facilitate Successful Adaptation.

A variety of premove and postmove strategies to promote successful adaptation have been proposed. Ideally, older adults who are moving from home to a long-term care facility should have the opportunity to visit prospective sites and to participate in decision making. Family meetings that include the older adult can address concerns and establish the older adult's routines and preferences. As much as possible, the environment should be adapted to accommodate the new resident. Assimilation of the older adult into the new setting marks the end of the postinstitutionalization stage.

The importance of nursing home staff in facilitating adjustment of the new resident cannot be overstated. Care must be individualized. The move must be coordinated between the discharging and the receiving facilities to avoid redundant procedures and incomplete records and nursing care plans. Nurse-to-nurse communication of timely information facilitates the prompt development of an effective plan of care for the newly admitted nursing home resident (Cortes, Wexler, & Fitzpatrick, 2004). A transition team to minimize anxiety and reduce stress and trauma associated with transfers is suggested (Smith, 2004).

Specific nursing approaches proposed by Brooke (1989) focus on learning the resident's perceptions, goals, and feelings regarding the new living situation. Frequent one-on-one contacts should be used to orient the resident to new routines; determine the resident's preferences and habits so they may be incorporated into the care plan; and understand and acknowledge the emotional state of the resident. Reminiscence therapy may help residents examine and accept losses and separate past from present events. Obtaining a list of important dates such as anniversaries and birthdays can stimulate discussion about fond memories. Problem solving in difficult situations should involve the resident and

ask that he or she take initiative in identifying needs, previous coping mechanisms, and choices possible for that situation.

Wolanin (1978), a pioneer in gerontological nursing, advised orienting the new residents to the facility, staff, and routines gradually to avoid overwhelming them. Paying extra attention to rest and comfort needs and maintaining previous routines (meals, therapy, elimination, ADLs, and recreational activities) can help the resident adjust. The resident should be encouraged to personalize his or her living space with special belongings.

Amenta, Weiner, and Amenta (1984) recommended the following steps for successful relocation:

- Use a film strip to describe the new facility to persons who will be moved there.
- Take ambulatory residents to visit the new facility.
- Inventory personal possessions before the move.
- Provide individual counseling regarding the move as needed.
- Whenever possible, permit residents to select their own roommates.

Other strategies that have been suggested for successful relocation include assessing resident preferences for a new home, transferring friends together, and using trusted staff members in the process (Castle, 2001b). Based on the relocation experience of a 90-year-old man, Renzenbrink (2004) stressed the importance of challenging ageist attitudes and derogatory labels, validating the older person's response to loss and change, and adopting an empowerment approach. Self-expression through art therapy might be used to negotiate the differing needs of identity and self (Emberley, 2005).

Research has moved from simply identifying the outcomes of relocation to attempting to identify the conditions most likely to have positive outcomes. A qualitative retrospective study of the adaptation of older adults to new living arrangements after hospitalization identified sense of plan and sense of self as the two major themes that were indicative of effective adaptation (Hersch, Spencer, & Kapoor, 2003).

A study designed to determine the effectiveness of planning and preparing to move a group of elderly veterans to a new facility showed that the group that received preparation interventions experienced fewer illnesses, such as fever, pneumonia, and urinary and respiratory infection, and fewer transfers to the hospital, than did a control group who did not receive the interventions (Petrou & Obenchain, 1987). In the intervention group, several months were devoted to preparation, which included frequently discussing key aspects of the move, selecting one's roommate, seeing photos of the new location, and conducting site visits to the new location. The time spent building familiarity with the new facility and presenting opportunities for individual decision making facilitated the residents' acceptance of the move and eased the transition.

Using the Schumacher and Meleis nursing model of transitions, Rossen and Knafl (2003) identified three distinct relocation transition styles among older women relocating to congregate living facilities. The styles used and the percent of participants who employed each were as follows: full integration (45%), partial integration (42%), and minimal integration (13%).

Some studies have used specific strategies to prevent or manage negative effects of relocation. Mitmansgruber and colleagues (2002) reported that depressive symptoms declined markedly when a psychological intervention was implemented during the first few weeks of relocation. The older persons who seemed to benefit most from this pilot study were those who were distressed because of existing psychological problems and those who experienced overload with relocation.

After reviewing the literature related to older people's experiences with residential care placement, Lee, Woo, and MacKenzie (2002) concluded that the actual experiences of older individuals as they adapt to relocation has not been adequately described. This lack of knowledge has impeded the development of strategies to help elders adjust to residential care placement with dignity and success. Likewise, Sandberg, Lundh, and Nolan (2002) identified the need for more research exploring the dynamics of the placement process, including the role of adult children in the process. The decision-making process related to relocation, particularly among ethnic elders, is another area recommended for additional study (Johnson & Tripp-Reimer, 2001).

Interventions to Promote Family Adjustment. Good family-staff relationships are desirable, but sometimes difficult to maintain. If family members are viewed as visitors, servants, patients, team members, or workers, this will affect the way staff interacts with them. Staff members need to be educated about the need of most family members to maintain some level of involvement in the resident's life. They need to consider the grief and guilt that families often experience when an older adult moves into a nursing home. Good communication helps to clarify the roles of family and staff and create a negotiated relationship that benefits all (Bauer & Nay, 2003) (Box 34-7).

Evaluation

Evidence of goal achievement for the resident might be (1) healthy adaptation to new environment; (2) reduced feelings of anxiety, hopelessness, and helplessness; (3) enhanced sense of control; (4) participation in diversional activities of choice; and (5) diminished stress related to relocation. Goals for the family might include (1) improved coping with resident status and relocation, and (2) restoration of family processes.

BOX 34-7 Interventions to Promote Good Staff-Family Relationships

- Offer a facility orientation for new residents, family members, and significant others
- Explain the roles of various types of nursing home staff
- Suggest how the family members can make a visit meaningful for the resident or be involved in care
- Clarify staff and family responsibilities
- Negotiate an agreement between staff and family members regarding family involvement in care
- Stress the role of the family in personalizing and individualizing resident care
- Involve families in problem solving and decision making as much as possible

Data from Bauer, M., & Nay, R. (2003). Family and staff partnerships in long-term care: A review of the literature. *Journal of Gerontological Nursing, 29*(10), 46-53; and Maas, M. L., Reed, D., Park, M., Specht, J. P., Schutte, D., Kelley, L. S., Swanson, E. A., Tripp-Reimer, T., & Buckwalter, K. C., (2004). Outcomes of the family involvement in care intervention for caregivers of individuals with dementia. *Nursing Research, 53*(2), 76-86.

OTHER ISSUES IN LONG-TERM CARE
Clinical Teaching in the Nursing Facility

The use of the long-term care nursing facility as a clinical teaching site for nursing students has been a long-debated academic topic in schools of nursing. Disadvantages in the use of this setting are often cited. However, literature documenting the unique advantages of this setting strongly supports the inclusion of long-term care nursing facility experience for all nursing students (Burke & Sherman, 1993; Heine, 1993). When nursing homes are used for clinical experiences, it usually is seen as a place to perform simple skills such as bathing, feeding, and transferring, and to practice doing assessments. Chen, Melcher, Witucki, and McKibben (2002) listed advantages and disadvantages of clinical experiences in nursing homes. These are summarized in Box 34-8.

The clinical teaching experience in the long-term care nursing facility should be recognized as an environment that is quite different from acute care, where most clinical teaching in many schools of nursing occurs. The long-term care nursing facility is a setting that requires a shift in thinking about what would constitute a rich learning experience for the student. In many ways, the long-term care nursing facility is an ideal context for the student to assimilate the full scope of the nursing process in a resident-centered environment. The long-term care nursing facility clinical experience offers numerous opportunities:

1. To focus on the resident as a unique individual, working with well older persons as well as with those who are acutely and chronically ill

---

Box 34-8 Advantages and Disadvantages of Clinical Experience in Nursing Homes

Advantages

- Provides experience with chronic illness and health promotion
- Acuity of hospital patients makes them too complex for beginning students
- Opportunity to work with residents over a period of weeks or months
- Prepares student for care of older persons with various functional abilities
- Opportunities for comprehensive assessments
- Greater opportunities to practice age-appropriate, individualized, holistic nursing care
- Opportunity to experience nursing in long-term care
- Can promote increased comfort in working with older persons
- Students can inspire nurses to reevaluate their care
- Increased interest in nursing home care when acuity is increasing and more registered nurses will be needed

Disadvantages

- Lack of adequate role models
- Possibility of creating negative stereotypes of older people
- Students may feel unprepared because many programs do not include gerontological content
- Few faculty are educated for gerontological nursing

Data from Chen, S., Melcher, P., Witucki, J., & McKibben, M. A. (2002). Nursing home use for clinical rotations: Taking a second look. *Nursing and Health Sciences, 3,* 131-137.

---

2. To focus on health promotion, health maintenance, chronic disease management, and acute, episodic illness management under conditions that emphasize resident-centered continuity of care

3. To develop an appreciation for the aging experience by interacting with the nursing facility resident over an extended period of time

4. To learn and master advanced assessment skills and comprehensive functional assessment techniques and strategies

5. To experience the implementation of a nursing model that emphasizes function, individual choice, self-care, and teaching and learning

6. To experience the full richness of interdisciplinary team function and collaboration in the implementation of resident-focused care

7. To develop and participate in organized activities and groups for special needs or interests among residents

8. To articulate and come to value the purpose and significance of the role of the gerontological nurse in contributing to quality of care in the nursing facility

9. To implement managerial leadership skills with nursing staff and interdisciplinary team members

10. To understand the impact of public policy on the quality of care for residents and on nursing practice, particularly OBRA regulations and the role of quality improvement in long-term care

11. To cultivate sensitivity in working with older adults and to consider future opportunities for working in long-term care nursing facilities

12. To differentiate the organizational culture and management practices of the long-term care nursing facility from those of other settings of care

Development of a clinical partnership between academic institutions and long-term care nursing facilities signifies an investment in the quality care of the resident. The reciprocal relationship between long-term care practice settings and academic institutions offers innovative solutions to challenges faced in both domains. For long-term care nursing facilities, keeping abreast of state-of-the-art innovations in care is stimulated by nursing faculty and students who have expertise, opportunity, and technical resources to explore special resident care problems in depth. For nursing students, developing and mastering skills that will prepare them to be competent nurses in the care of well, acutely ill, and frail older persons occur in a well-planned long-term care clinical experience. The teaching nursing home innovations have laid the groundwork for the design of successful clinical partnerships and clinical teaching experiences. Widespread adoption of the lessons learned in the teaching nursing home projects about designing long-term care nursing, facility-based experiences with older individuals is crucial to nursing's future in the care of older persons.

Professional Associations for Gerontological Nurses in Long-Term Care

The National Gerontological Nursing Association (NGNA) offers its members continuing education through regional and national conferences, and a network for communication. The focus of NGNA is on clinical care of older adults in diverse settings. Membership is open to clinicians, educators, and researchers with varied educational preparation, positions, and interests.

Professional certification through the American Nurses' Credentialing Center is available for several positions. Diploma, ADN, and BSN nurses are eligible for Gerontological Nurse certification; however, they take different examinations. Certification as a clinical specialist in gerontological nursing and gerontological nurse practitioner requires master's level preparation (American Nurses' Credentialing Center [ANCC], 2006).

Many nurses belong to national organizations such as the Gerontological Society of America (GSA), whose members represent researchers, educators, practitioners, and policymakers from various disciplines. GSA publishes two journals: *The Gerontologist* and *The Journals of Gerontology*. The American Geriatrics Society (AGS) is open to anyone with an interest in geriatric health care. The membership comprises mostly health care professionals. AGS promotes professional and public education, high-quality research, and quality care of older adults.

The National Association of Directors of Nursing Administration/Long Term Care (NADONA/LTC) is a nursing association established in 1986 to provide education, communication, and services to nursing professionals in long-term care. The services available include a mentor system for members, a reference research library, educational materials, a quarterly journal *(The Director)*, scholarships for all educational stages, a director of nursing certification program, and educational conferences. The association has adopted a code of ethics that delineate guidelines for the profession. Mentors provide assistance by telephone, by mail, or on site. With a membership of over 5000 and growing, this organization provides a professional network for directors of nursing administration in long-term care.

The National Association of Geriatric Nursing Assistants (NAGNA) was established in 1995 by two former CNAs who both had moved up to positions of leadership in long-term care. This organization works to ensure the highest quality of care to older adults by raising the standing and performance of CNAs. NAGNA recognizes outstanding achievements, provides development training for CNAs and mentoring programs intended to reduce CNA turnover, and advocates for issues relevant to long-term care and CNAs.

SUMMARY

Gerontological nursing in the long-term care nursing facility offers opportunities for professional growth in clinical practice, managerial leadership, research, and public policy. Nurses practice in this setting for the rewarding caregiving experiences and the opportunity to lend their professional nursing expertise to make a significant difference in the lives of residents. The expertise, power, and influence of nurses are critical to facilitating change to meet new challenges, foster innovation, and sustain high standards of nursing practice.

REFERENCES

Administration on Aging. (2004). Older Americans 2004: Key indicators of well-being. Retrieved January 13, 2006, from http://agingstats.gov.

Administration on Aging (AOA). (2005). A profile of older Americans, 2005. Retrieved August 15, 2006, from www.aoa.gov/prof/statistics/profile/2005/6asp?pf=true.

Amenta, M., Weiner, A., & Amenta, D. (1984, Nov.-Dec.). Successful relocation. *Geriatric Nursing*, pp. 356-360.

American Nurses Credentialing Center. (ANCC). (2006). Certification and certification renewal. Retrieved August 4, 2006, from www.nursecredentialing.org.

American Therapeutic Recreation Association. (2005). About ATRA. Retrieved November 20, 2005, from www.atra-tr.org/about.htm.

Anderson, R. A., Issel, L. M., & McDaniel, R. R., Jr. (2003). Nursing homes as complex adaptive systems: Relationship between management practice and resident outcomes. *Nursing Research, 52*(1), 12-21.

Barry, T. (2002). The impact of nurse aide empowerment strategies on nursing home resident outcomes. Dissertation abstract, Pennsylvania State University.

Barry, T., Brannon, D., & Mor, V. (2005). Nurse aide empowerment strategies and staff stability: Effects on nursing home resident outcomes. *Gerontologist, 45*(3), 309-317.

Bauer, M., & Nay, R. (2003). Family and staff partnerships in long-term care: A review of the literature. *Journal of Gerontological Nursing, 29*(10), 46-53.

Bergman-Evans, B. (2004). Beyond the basics: Effects of the Eden Alternative model on quality of life issues. *Journal of Gerontological Nursing, 30*(6), 27-34.

Bermann, K. (2003). Love and space in the nursing home. *Theoretical Medicine, 24*, 511-523.

Bharucha, A. J., Pandav, R., Shen, C., Dodge, H. H., & Ganguli, M. (2004). Predictors of nursing facility admission: A 12-year epidemiological study in the United States. *Journal of the American Geriatrics Society, 52*, 434-439.

Boockvar, K. S., Litke, A., Penrod, J. D., Halm, E. A., Morrison, R. S., Silberzweig, S. B., et al. (2004). Patient relocation in the 6 months after hip fracture: Risk factors for fragmented care. *Journal of the American Geriatrics Society, 52*(11), 1826-1831.

Borup, J. H. (1981). Relocation: Attitudes, information network and problems encountered. *Gerontologist, 21*(5), 501-511.

Borup, J. H. (1982). The effects of varying degrees of interinstitutional environmental change on long-term care patients. *Gerontologist, 22*(4), 409-417.

Borup, J. H. (1983). Relocation mortality research: Assessment, reply, and the need to refocus on the issues. *Gerontologist, 23*, 234-242.

Brody, E., Kleban, M., & Moss, M. (1974). Measuring the impact of change. *Gerontologist, 14*, 299-305.

Brooke, V. (1989). Your helping hand: How to tailor your approach in each phase of adjustment. *Journal of Gerontological Nursing, 10*(3), 126-128.

Brown, M. N., Lapane, K. L., & Luisi, A. F. (2002). The management of depression in older nursing home residents. *Journal of the American Geriatrics Society, 50*, 69-76.

Burke, M., & Sherman, S. (1993). *Gerontological nursing: Issues and opportunities for the twenty-first century*. National League for Nursing, Pamphlet #14-2510, p. 97.

Camargo, O., & Presston, G. H. (1945). What happens to patients who are hospitalized for the first time when over 65? *American Journal of Psychiatry, 102*, 168-173.

Castle, N. G. (2001a). Administrator turnover and quality of care in nursing homes. *Gerontologist, 41*(6), 757-767.

Castle, N. G. (2001b). Relocation of the elderly. *Medical Care Research and Review, 58*(3), 291-333.

Castle, N. G., Degenholtz, H., & Engberg, J. (2005). State variability in indicators of quality of care in nursing facilities. *Journal of Gerontology: Medical Sciences, 60A*(9), 1173-1179.

Center for Health Systems Research and Analysis. (2005a). Quality indicators: Nursing homes. Retrieved January 13, 2006, from www.chsra.wisc.edu/chsra/qi/domaindesc.htm.

Center for Health Systems Research and Analysis. (2005b). QI domains and descriptions. Retrieved November 20, 2005, from www.chsra.wisc.edu/chsra/qi/domaindesc.htm#accidents.

Center for Medicare and Medicaid Services. (2002). Resident assessment instrument. Retrieved November 20, 2005, from http://new.cms.hhs.gov/NursingHomeQualityInits/downloads/MDS20rai1202ch1.pdf.

Center for Medicare and Medicaid Services. (2005). Nursing homes—Advance issuance of revised interpretive guidelines for TAG F501, medical director. Retrieved December 20, 2005, from www.cms.hhs.gov/medicaid/survey-cert/sc0529.pdf.

Centers for Disease Control and Prevention (CDC). (2003). *Health: United States 2003. Trend tables and chartbook.* Hyattsville, MD: Department of Health and Human Services.

Centers for Disease Control and Prevention/National Center for Health Statistics. (1999). Number and rate per 100 beds of full-time equivalent employees by occupational categories, according to selected nursing home characteristics, United States. Retrieved January 14, 2006, from www.cdc.gov.

Chen, S., Melcher, P., Witucki, J., & McKibben, M. A. (2002). Nursing home use for clinical rotations: Taking a second look. *Nursing and Health Sciences, 3,* 131-137.

Clinical Rounds. (2003). New guidelines watch your back. *Nursing2003, 33*(6), 34.

Cocco, E., Gatti, M., deMendonca Lima, C. A., & Camus, V. (2003). A comparative study of stress and burnout among caregiers in nursing homes and acute geriatric wards. *International Journal of Geriatric Psychiatry, 18*(1), 78-85.

Coffman, T. L. (1981). Relocation and survival of institutionalized aged: A re-examination of the evidence. *Gerontologist, 21,* 483-500.

Cohen, M. A. (2003). Private long-term care insurance: A look ahead. *Journal of Aging and Health, 15*(1), 74-89.

Coleman, M. T., Looney, S., O'Brien, J., Ziegler, C., Pastorino, C. A., & Turner, C. (2002). The Eden Alternative: Findings after 1 year of implementation. *Journals of Gerontology, 57*(7), M422-M427.

Cortes, T. A., Wexler, S., & Fitzpatrick, J. J. (2004). The transition of elderly patients between hospitals and nursing homes. Improving nurse-to-nurse communication. *Journal of Gerontological Nursing, 30*(6), 10-15.

DeBoer, M. R., Pluijm, S. M., Lips, P., et al. (2004). Different aspects of visual impairment as risk factors for falls and fractures in older men and women. *Journal of Bone and Mineral Research, 19*(9), 1539-1547.

Dimant, J. (2003). Avoiding physical restraints in long-term care facilities. *Journal of the American Medical Directors Association, 4*(4), 207-215.

Dobbs, D. (2004). The adjustment to a new home. *Journal of Housing for the Elderly, 18*(1), 51-71.

Dorr, D. A., Horn, S. D., & Smout, R. J. (2005). Cost analysis of nursing home registered nurse staffing times. *Journal of the American Geriatrics Society, 53*(5), 840-845.

Drozkick, L. W. (2003). Adjustment to relocation to an assisted living facility. *Dissertation Abstracts International Section B: The Sciences and Engineering, 64*(6-B), 2913.

Eden Alternative. (2002). The Eden Alternative principles. Retrieved January 13, 2006, from www.edenalt.com/10.htm.

Elderweb. (2005). LTC backwards and forwards. Retrieved January 13, 2006, from www.elderweb.com.

Elon, R. (1993). The nursing home medical director role in transition. *Journal of the American Geriatrics Society, 41,* 131-135.

Elon, R. (2005). Medical direction in nursing facilities: New federal guidelines. *Annals of Long-Term Care, 13*(10), 43-46.

Emberley, A. (2005). Responding to the crisis of relocation: Cultural difference, self psychology and art therapy. *Canadian Art Therapy Association Journal, 18*(1), 9-19.

Engle, V. F., & Graney, M. J. (1993). Stability and improvement of health after nursing home admission. *Journal of Gerontology, 48*(1), S17-S23.

Evans, D., Wood, J., & Lambert, L. (2002). Patient injury and physical restraint devices: A systematic review. *Journal of Advanced Nursing, 41*(3), 274-282.

Forbes, S. (2001). This is Heaven's waiting room: End of life in one nursing home. *Journal of Gerontological Nursing, 27*(11), 37-45.

Forbes-Thompson, S., & Gessert, C. (2005). End of life in nursing homes: Connections between structure, process and outcomes. *Journal of Palliative Medicine, 8*(3), 545-555.

Futrell, M., & Melillo, K. D. (2005). Gerontological nurse practitioners: Implications for the future. *Journal of Gerontological Nursing, 31*(4), 19-24.

Gabriel, C. S. (2000). An overview of nursing home facilities: Data from the 1997 National Nursing Home Survey. *Advance Data, 311,* 1-12.

Gardner, T. N., Simpson, A. H. R., Booth, C., Sprukkelhorst, P., Evans, M., Kenwright, J., & J. Grimley-Evans. (1998). Measurement of impact force, simulation of fall and hip fracture. *Medical Engineering and Physics, 20,* 57-65.

Gerdner, L. A., Shue, V. M., & Beck, C. K. (2000). Dementia: Long-term care. In J. J. Fitzpatrick, T. Fulmer, M. Wallace, & E. Flaherty (Eds.), *Geriatric nursing research digest.* New York: Springer.

Gibson, J. J. Gregory, S. R., Houser, A. N., & Fox-Grage, W. (2004). Across the states; profiles of long-term care. Retrieved December 20, 2005, from www.aarp.org/research/reference/statistics/across_the_states_profiles_of_longterm_care_2004.html.

Gillespie, L. D., Gillespie, W. J., Robertson, M. C., Lamb, S. E., Cumming, R. G., & Rowe, B. H. (2006). Interventions for preventing falls in elderly people. *Cochrane Database for Systematic Reviews, 2.*

Gruber-Baldini, A. L, Zimmerman, S., Boutani, M., Watson, L. C., Williams, C. S., & Reed, P. S. (2005). Characteristics associated with depression in long-term care residents with dementia. *Gerontologist, 45*(special issue 1), 50-55.

Gueldner, S. H., Smith, C. A., Neal, M., Penrod, J., Ryder, J., Dye, M., Bramlett, M. H., & Hertzog, L. (2001). Patterns of telephone use among nursing home residents. *Journal of Gerontological Nursing, 27*(5), 35-41.

Gurvich, T., & Cunningham, J. A. (2000). Appropriate use of psychotropic drugs in nusing homes. *American Family Physician, 61*(5), 1437-1446.

Hagen, B. (2001). Nursing home placement: Factors affecting caregivers' decisions to place family members with dementia. *Journal of Gerontological Nursing, 27*(2), 44-53.

Hagen, B., Esther, C. A., Ikuta, R., Williams, R., Navenec, C. C., & Aho, M. (2005). Antipsychotic drug use in Canadian long-term care facilities: Prevalence, and patterns following resident relocation. *International Psychogeriatrics, 17*(2), 179-193.

Harrington, C. (2005). Nurse staffing in nursing homes in the United States: Part II. *Journal of Gerontological Nursing, 31*(3), 9-15.

Health Care Financing Administration. (1995). *Long-term care facility resident assessment instrument (RAI) users manual for use with version 2.0 of the Health Care Financing Administration's Minimum Data Set, resident assessment protocols, and utilization guidelines.* Baltimore, MD: Health Care Financing Administration.

Heine, C. (1993). *Determining the future of gerontological nursing: Partnerships between nursing education and practice.* New York: National League for Nursing Press.

Heisler, E., Evans, G. W., & Moen, P. (2004). Health and social outcomes of moving to a continuing care retirement community. *Journal of Housing for the Elderly, 18*(1), 5-23.

Hendel, T., Fradkin, M., & Kidron, D. (2004). Multicultural aging: Physical restraint use in health care settings: Public attitudes in Israel. *Journal of Gerontological Nursing, 30*(2), 12-19.

Henderson, M. L. (2004). Gerontological advanced practice nurses as end-of-life care facilitators. *Geriatric Nursing, 25*(4), 233-237.

Hendrix, C. C., & Wojciechowski, C. W. (2005). Chronic care management for the elderly: An opportunity for gerontological nurse practitioners. *Journal of the American Academy of Nurse Practitioners, 17*(7), 263-267.

Hersch, G., Spencer, J., & Kapoor, T. (2003). Adaptation by elders to new living arrangements following hospitalization: A qualititative, retrospective analysis. *Journal of Applied Gerontology, 22*(3), 315-339.

Hodgson, N., Freedman, V. A., Granger, D. A., & Erno, A. (2004). Biobehavioral correlates of relocation in the frail elderly: Salivary cortisol, affect, and cognitive function. *Journal of the American Geriatrics Society, 52*(11), 1856-1866.

Hsueh-Fen, K., Travis, S. S., & Acton, G. J. (2004). Relocation to a long-term care facility. *Journal of Psychosocial Nursing, 42*(3), 10-16.

Hughes, C. M., & Lapane, K. L. (2005). Administrative initiatives for reducing inappropriate prescribing of psychotropic drugs in nursing homes. *Drugs and Aging, 22*(4), 339-351.

Institute of Medicine. (1986). *Improving the quality of care in nursing homes.* Washington, DC: National Academies Press.

Johnson, R. A., & Tripp-Reimer, T. (2001). Relocation among ethnic elders: A review—Part 2. *Journal of Gerontological Nursing, 27*(6), 22-27.

Joint Commission on Accreditation of Healthcare Organizations. (1992). *Quality improvement in long term care: How quality improvement can help fulfill OBRA '87 requirements.* Oakbrook Terrace, IL: Joint Commission on Accreditation of Healthcare Organizations.

Joint Commission on Accreditation of Healthcare Organizations. (2002). JCAHO accreditation helps nursing facilities achieve better outcomes. Retrieved January 21, 2006, from www.jcaho.org.

Joint Commission on Accreditation of Healthcare Organizations. (2005a). Long term care update: Issue 3. Retrieved January 21, 2006, from www.jcaho.org.

Joint Commission on Accreditation of Healthcare Organizations. (2005b). Long term care update: Issue 2. Retrieved January 21, 2006, from www.jcaho.org.

Joint Commission on Accreditation of Healthcare Organizations. (2005c). Long term care accreditation overview guide. Retrieved January 21, 2006, from www.jcaho.org.

Joint Commission on Accreditation of Healthcare Organizations. (2005d). Facts about ORYX: The next evolution in accreditation. Retrieved January 21, 2006, from www.jcaho.org.

Kane, R. L., Garrard, J., Buchanan, J. L., et al. (1991). Improving primary care in nursing homes. *Journal of the American Geriatrics Society, 89,* 359-367.

Kane, R. L., Garrard, J., Skay, C. L., et al. (1989). Effects of a geriatric nurse practitioner on process and outcome of nursing home care. *American Journal of Public Health, 79*(9), 1271-1277.

Karlin, N. J., Schneider, K., & Pepper, S. (2002). Issues of attraction, retention, and affective states for geriatric nurse practitioners in long-term care. *Geriatric Nursing, 23*(6), 324-329.

Kayser-Jones, J., Schell, E., Lyons, W., Dris, A. E., Chan, J., & Beard, R. L. (2003). Factors that influence end-of-life care in nursing homes: The physical environment, inadequate staffing and lack of supervision. *Gerontologist, 43*(special issue 2), 76-84.

Keister, K. J. (2004). Relocation appraisal of nursing home residents (abstract). Case Western Reserve University Health Sciences.

Kennedy, B. R. (2005). Stress and burnout of nursing staff working with geriatric clients in long-term care. *Journal of Nursing Scholarship, 37*(4), 381-382.

Krichbaum, K., Pearson, V., Savik, K., & Mueller, C. (2005). Improving resident outcomes with GAPN organization level interventions. *Western Journal of Nursing Research, 27*(3), 322-337.

Lee, D. T. F., Woo, J., & MacKenzie, A. E. (2002). A review of older people's experiences with residential care placement. *Journal of Advanced Nursing, 37*(1), 19-27.

Lodge, M. P. (1987). *Professional education and practice of nurse administrators/directors of nursing in long-term care. Executive summary.* Kansas City, MO: American Nurses' Foundation.

Loeher, K. E., Bank, A. L., MacNeill, S. E., & Lichtenberg, P. A. (2004). Nursing home transition and depressive symptoms in older medical rehabilitation patients. *Clinical Gerontologist, 27*(1/2), 59-70.

Looney, M. T., O'Brien, J., Ziegler, C., Pastorino, C. A., & Turner, C. (2002). The Eden Alternative: Findings after 1 year of implementation. *Journals of Gerontology, 57*(7), M422-M427.

Maas, M., Reed, D., Specht, J., Swanson, S., Tripp-Reimer, T., & Buckwalter, K., et al. (2001). The caring partnership: Staff and families of persons institutionalized with Alzheimer's disease. *Journal of Alzheimer's Disease and Related Disorders, 9,* 21-30.

Maas, M. L., Reed, D., Park, M., Specht, J. P., Schutte, D., Kelley, L. S., et al. (2004). Outcomes of the family involvement in care intervention for caregivers of individuals with dementia. *Nursing Research, 53*(2), 76-86.

Maas, M. L., & Specht, J. P. (2000). Alzheimer's disease: Special care units in long-term care. In J. J. Fitzpatrick, & T. Fulmer (Eds.), *Geriatric nursing research digest.* New York: Springer.

Mather, K. F., & Bakas, T. (2002). Nursing assistants' perceptions of their ability to provide continence care. *Geriatric Nursing, 23*(2), 76-81.

Medicare. (2005). Long-term care. Retrieved January 25, 2005, from www.medicare.gov/LongTermCare/Static/Home.asp.

Medicare. (2006). Nursing home compare. Retrieved January 13, 2006, from www.medicare.gov/NHCompare/Static/Related/ImportantInformation.asp?dest=NAV|Home|About|NursingHomeCompare#TabTop.

Meehan, T., Robertson, S., Stedman, T., & Byrne, G. (2004). Outcomes for elderly patients with mental illness following relocation from a stand-alone psychiatric hospital to community-based extended care units. *Australian and New Zealand Journal of Psychiatry, 38*(11/12), 948-952.

Metcalf, R. C. (2002). Certified nursing assistants in long-term care facilities: Perceptions of their initial training and competency evaluation program. North Carolina State University.

Metlife. (2005). Market survey of nursing home and home care costs, September, 2005. Retrieved January 13, 2006, from www.metlife.com/wpsassets/4383861060113829355 6V1F2005NHHCsurvey.pdf.

Mirotznik, J., & Ruskin, A. P. (1984). Inter-institutional relocation and its effects on health. *Gerontologist, 24,* 286-291.

Mitmansgruber, H., Baumann, U., Feichtinger, L., & Thiele, C. (2002). Psychological intervention supporting the relocation into residential care: Concept and pilot study [abstract]. *Zietschritf fur Gerontopsychologie and Psychiatrie, 15*(4), 185-204.

Mitty, E. (2000). Certified nursing assistants. In J. J. Fitzpatrick, T. Fulmer, M. Wallace, & E. Flaherty (Eds.). *Geriatric nursing research digest.* New York: Springer.

Mitty, E. L. (1997). Role of nursing in long-term care. *Health Care Management, 3*(1), 55-75.

Mueller, C. (1998). Education for long-term care directors of nursing: A need or a demand? *Nursing Management, 29*(11), 39-42.

Mueller, C., Arling, G., Kane, R., Bershadsky, J., Holland, D., & Joy, A. (2006). Nursing home staffing standards: Their relationships to nurse staffing levels. *Gerontologist, 46*(1), 74-80.

National Center for Health Statistics. (1999). *Health, United States, 1999: Health and aging chartbook.* Hyattsville, MD: National Center for Health Statistics.

National Citizens' Coalition for Nursing Home Reform. (1985). Executive summary. In *A consumer perspective on quality care: The resident's point of view.* Retrieved September 24, 2005, from www.nccnhr.org/public/50_155_495.cfm.

Nelson, R. (2005). Certified medication aides: Do they free up nurses' time? Or do they water down care? *American Journal of Nursing, 105*(9), 28-29.

Ouslander, J. G., & Weinberg, A. D. (2003). Institutional long-term care services in the USA. In R. C. Tallis & H. M. Fillit (Eds.), *Brocklehurst's textbook of geriatric medicine and gerontology* (6th ed.). London: Churchill Livingstone.

Patnaik, B., Lawton, M. P., Kieban, M. H., et al. (1974). Behavioral adaptation to the change in institutional residence. *Gerontologist, 14,* 305-307.

Paulas, D., & Jans, B. (2005). Assessing resident satisfaction with institutional living: Developing a tool. *Journal of Gerontological Nursing, 31*(8), 6-11.

Pennington, K., Scott, J., & Magilvy, K. (2003). The role of certified nursing assistants in nursing homes. *Journal of Nursing Administration, 33*(11), 578-584.

Petrou, M. F., & Obenchain, J. V. (1987). Reducing incidence of illness post-transfer. *Geriatric Nursing, 8*(5), 264-266.

Pioneer Network. (2005). Toward a new culture of aging. Retrieved November 10, 2005, from www.pioneernetwork.net/.

Piven, M. L., Ammarell, N., Bailey, D., Corazzini, K., Colon-Emeric, C. S., Lekan-Rutledge, D., et al. (2006). MDS coordinator relationships and nursing home care processes. *Western Journal of Nursing Research, 28*(3), 294-309.

Rantz, M., Popejoy, L., & Zwygart-Stauffacher, M. (2001). *The new nursing homes: A 20-minute way to find great long-term care.* Minneapolis, MN: Fairview.

Rantz, M. J., & Zwygart-Stauffacher, M. (2004). Back to the fundamentals of care: A roadmap to improve nursing home quality. *Journal of Nursing Care Quality, 19*(2), 92-94.

Rapp, M. P. (2003). Opportunities for advance practice nurses in the nursing facility. *Journal of the American Medical Directors Association, 4*(6), 337-343.

Renzenbrink, I. (2004). Home is where the heart is: Relocation in later years. *Illness, Crisis and Loss, 12*(1), 63-74.

Resnick, B., & Simpson, M. (2003). Restorative care nursing activities: Pilot testing self-efficacy and outcomes expectation measures. *Geriatric Nursing, 24*(2), 82-89.

Resnick, B., Simpson, M., Bercovitz, A., Galik, E., Gruber-Baldini, A., Zimmerman, S., & Magaziner, J. (2004). Testing of the Res-Care Pilot Intervention: Impact on nursing assistants. *Geriatric Nursing, 25*(5), 292-297.

Rosen, A. K., Berkowitz, D. R., Anderson, J. J., Ash, A. S., Kazis, L. E., & Moskowitz, M. A. (1999). Functional status outcomes for assessment of quality in long-term care. *International Journal for Quality in Health Care, 11*(1), 37-46.

Rosenfeld, P., & Harrington, C. (2003). Nursing home care for the elderly. *American Journal of Nursing, 103*(9), 97.

Rosenfeld, P., Kobayashi, M., Barber, P., & Mezey, M. (2004). Utilization of nurse practitioners in long-term care: Findings and implications of a national survey. *Journal of the American Medical Directors Association, 5*, 9-15.

Rossen, E. K., & Knafl, K. A. (2003). Older women's response to residential relocation: Description of transition styles. *Qualitative Health Research, 13*(1), 20-36.

Rosswurm, M. A. (1983). Relocation and the elderly. *Journal of Gerontological Nursing, 9*, 632-637.

Sacco-Petersen, M., & Borrell, L. (2004). Struggles for autonomy in self-care: The impact of the physical and socio-cultural environment in a long-term care setting. *Scandinavian Journal of Caring Sciences, 18*(4), 376-386.

Sandberg, J., Lundh, U., & Nolan, M. (2002). Moving into a care home: The role of adult children in the placement process. *International Journal of Nursing Studies, 39*(3), 353-362.

Sanders, S., Bowie, S. L., & Bowie, Y. D. (2003). Lessons learned on forced relocation of older adults: The impact of Hurricane Andrew on health, mental status, and social support of public housing residents. *Journal of Gerontological Social Work, 40*(4), 23-35.

Schnelle, J. F., Simmons, S. F., Harrington, C., Cadogan, M., Garcia, E., & Bates-Jensen, B. M. (2004). Relationship of nursing home staffing to quality of care. *Health Services Research, 39*(2), 225-250.

Seligman, M. (1975). *On depression, development and death.* San Francisco: W. H. Freeman.

Simpson, A. H. R., Lamb, S., Roberts, P. J., Gardner, T. N., & Grimley-Evans, J. (2004). Does the type of flooring affect the risk of hip fracture? *Age and Aging, 33*, 242-246.

Sloane, P., & Boustani, M. (2002). Institutional care. In R. J. Ham, P. Sloane, & G. Warshaw. *Primary care geriatrics: A case-based approach.* St. Louis, Mosby.

Sloane, P., & Gwyther, L. (1980). Nursing homes. *Journal of the American Medical Association, 244*, 1840-1841.

Sloane, P. D., Zimmerman, S., Gruber-Baldini, A. L., Hebel, J. R., Magaziner, J., & Konrad, T. R. (2005). Health and functional outcomes and health care utilization of persons with dementia in residential care and assisted living facilities: Comparison with nursing homes. *Gerontologist, 45*(special issue 1), 124-132.

Smallegan, M. (1985). There was nothing else to do: Need for care before nursing home admission. *Gerontologist, 25*(4), 364-369.

Smith, K., & Bengston, V. L. (1979). Positive consequences of institutionalization: Solidarity between elderly parents and their middle-aged children. *Gerontologist, 19*, 438-447.

Smith, L. (2004). Relocation trauma: Residents are particularly vulnerable and often die within days of being transferred. *Canadian Nursing Home, 15*(3), 5-12.

Sviden, G., Wikstrom, G., & Hjortsjo-Norberg, M. (2002). Elderly persons' reflections on relocating to living at sheltered housing. *Scandinavian Journal of Occupational Therapy, 9*(1), 10-16.

Taunton, R. L., Swagerty, D. L., Smith, B., Lasseter, J. A., & Lee, R. H. (2004). Care planning for nursing home residents: Incorporating the minimum data set requirements into practice. *Journal of Gerontological Nursing, 30*(12), 40-49.

Tellis-Nayak, V. (1988). *Nursing home exemplars of quality: Their paths to excellence.* Springfield, IL: Charles C. Thomas.

U.S. Senate Special Committee on Aging. (2000, February). *Developments in aging: 1997 and 1998* (vol. 1.). Report 106-229. Washington, DC.

Waldron, V. R., Gitelson, R., & Kelley, D. L. (2005). Gender differences in social adaptation to a retirement community: Longitudinal changes and the role of mediated communication. *Journal of Applied Gerontology, 24*(4), 283-298.

Washburn, A. M. (2005). Relocation puts elder nursing home residents at risk of stress, although the stress is short-lived. *Evidence-Based Mental Health, 8*(2), 49.

West, S. K., Friedman, D., Munoz, B., Roche, K. B., Park, W., Deremeik, J., et al. (2003). A randomized trial of visual impairment interventions for nursing home residents: Study design, baseline characteristics, and visual loss. *Ophthalmic Epidemiology, 10*(3), 193-209.

Whittier, J. R., & Williams, D. (1956). The coincidence in constancy of mortality figures for aged psychotic patients admitted to state hospitals. *Nervous and Mental Disorders, 124*, 618-620.

Williams, K., Kemper, S., & Hummert, M. L. (2003). Improving nursing home communication: An intervention to reduce elderspeak. *Gerontologist, 43*(2), 242-247.

Wolanin, M. O. (1978). Relocation of the elderly. *Journal of Gerontological Nursing, 44*(3), 47-50.

Yeh, S., Johnson, M. A., & Wang, S. (2002). The changes in caregiver burden following nursing home placement. *International Journal of Nursing Studies, 39*(6), 591-600.

Zeisel, J., Silverstein, N. M., Hyde, J., Levkoff, S., Lawton, M. P., & Holmes, W. (2003). Environmental correlates to behavioral health outcomes in Alzheimer's special care units. *Gerontologist, 43*(5), 697-711.

Zimmerman, S., Gruber-Baldini, A. L., Sloane, P. D., Eckert, J. K., Hebel, J. R., Morgan, L. A. (2003). Assisted living and nursing homes: Apples and oranges? *Gerontologist, 43*, 107-117.

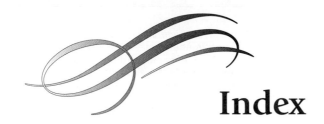

Index

A

AARP, 696
Abandonment, 703
Abdominal assessment
  bowel function and, 40
  in gastrointestinal disorder, 470
Absorption, drug, 141
Absorptive gel for pressure ulcers, 248
Abuse
  alcohol, 663
  assessment for, 46
  elder, 699-705, 701*b*, 701*t*, 705*t*
    as legal issue, 212-213
Academic detailing in evidence-based
      practice, 98*b*
Access
  to community program, 869
  to health care, 830-831, 831*f*
Accommodation, visual, 602
Accreditation of long-term care facility,
      955-956, 955*b*
Acetaminophen, 276
Acetinobacter, 372
Acetohexamide, 545
Acetophenazine, 425
Acetylcholine
  in Alzheimer's disease, 423
  overactive bladder and, 507
Achalasia, 449
Acinus
  in emphysema, 367-368
  secretion of, 528
Acquired immunity, 576-577
Acquired immunodeficiency disease,
      587-590
  clinical manifestations of, 588
  prevalence of, 587-588
  special concerns about, 588-589
  treatment of, 589-590, 589*t*, 590*b*
Acral lentiginous melanoma, 239
Acrochordon, 232, 233*f*
Action statement in evidence-based practice,
      113
Activities of daily living
  in Alzheimer's disease, 423
  assessment of, 40, 42
    in musculoskeletal disorder, 292
  in dementia, 418-419
  Katz Index of, 57, 58*f*, 59*f*, 60
  Lawton instrumental, 60-62, 61*f*
  in Multidimensional Functional
      Assessment Questionnaire, 62

Activities of daily living (*Continued*)
  respiratory disease and, 389
  self-care deficit and, 286-288
    of bathing/grooming, 304
    of dressing/grooming, 305
    of feeding, 303-304
    of toileting, 305-306
Activity. *See also* Activities of daily living;
      Exercise
  motor, 409-410
  in respiratory disease, 395*t*
Activity checklist, 62-63
Activity-exercise pattern
  assessment of, 40-42
  diagnoses concerning, 31*b*
Activity intolerance
  in heart failure, 336
  in musculoskeletal disorder,
      293
  in respiratory disease, 394
  self-care and, 287
  in stroke, 340
Activity theory, 882
Acuity, visual, 602
Acupuncture, 282
Acute bowel, 455*t*
Acute care, 907-927
  focus of, 7
  in hospital, 911-925. *See also* Hospitalized
      patient
  population of, 907-908
  quality improvement in, 815-816
  reflection on, 916*b*
  role of nurse in, 909-911
  setting for, 908-909
Acute disease, patterns of, 5
Acute renal failure, 491-492
Acyclovir, 240
Adalat, 149*t*
Adalimumab, 281*f*
Adaptability, 742
Adaptation
  to chronic pain, 91
  to long-term care facility, 962-
      963
  visual, 602
Adaptation model, 87
Adaptive immunity
  age-related changes in, 582
  characteristics of, 576-577
Addiction to pain medication, 921,
      925

Adenocarcinoma
  esophageal, 451-452
  gastric, 454
Adipocyte, 528*t*
Administration, drug, 163
Administrator
  nursing home, 950
  quality improvement and, 818
  of subacute care facility, 931
Admission criteria for subacute care, 933
Admission director for subacute care, 931
Adrenal cortex
  age-related changes in, 531
  function of, 526-527
  hormones of, 527*t*
Adrenal gland, 531-532, 542*t*
Adrenal medulla, 527*t*
Adrenocorticotropic hormone
  function of, 527*t*, 529*f*
  for gouty arthritis, 284
  pituitary gland and, 525
Advair, 366*t*
Advance directive, 209-210, 714, 716-717,
      716*b*, 716*f*
  instruments for, 75*t*
  technology and, 203
Advanced activities of daily living, 62-63
Advanced care planning, 36-37
Advanced glycation end product, 133
Advanced practice nurse, 7, 84
  as case manager, 781-782
  in evidence-based practice, 114*b*, 115
  function and education of, 22*t*
  on interdisciplinary team, 771*b*
  in long-term care facility, 946
  medical diagnosis used by, 32
  role of, 21
  for subacute care, 931
Adverse drug reaction
  to antihypertensive drug, 322-323
  to antitubercular drug, 380-381
  epidemiology of, 143-144
  nursing process and, 158
  risk factors for, 144-153
    drug interactions as, 145, 150-151
    inappropriate prescribing as, 145, 146*t*-
        151*t*
  skin disorder as, 236
Advertising, drug, 139
Advocate
  against ageism, 698*t*
  nurse as, 708-709, 709*b*

Page numbers followed by *b*, *t*, or *f* indicate boxes, tables, or figures, respectively.

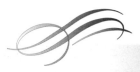